W9-BPL-087

Physical Therapy
for Children

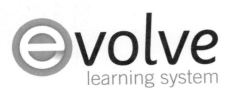

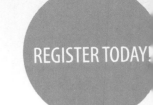

To access your Student Resources, visit:

http://evolve.elsevier.com/Campbell/PTchildren/

Evolve Student Learning Resources for Campbell: Physical Therapy for Children, 4e, offers the following features:

- Critical Thinking Questions—Helps reinforce what's covered in the chapters
- Pediatric Clinical Specialist Examination Questions and Answers—Sample test questions and answers modeled after the Pediatric Specialty Exam
- References—End-of-chapter references linked to the MEDLINE abstract
- Five UNIQUE: E only chapters—Chapters covering gait, genomics, hemophilia, assistive technology, and screening for referral
- Video—Over 40 video clips that correspond to case studies found throughout the text
- Weblinks—An exciting resource that lets you link to hundreds of websites carefully chosen to supplement the content of the textbook.

ELSEVIER

Physical Therapy for Children

Fourth Edition

Suzann K. Campbell, PT, PhD, FAPTA

Professor Emerita
Department of Physical Therapy
Director of Mentoring Services
Center for Clinical and Translational Science
University of Illinois at Chicago
Chicago, Illinois

Robert J. Palisano, PT, ScD

Professor
Physical Therapy and Rehabilitation Sciences
Drexel University
Philadelphia, Pennsylvania

Margo N. Orlin, PT, PhD

Associate Professor
Physical Therapy and Rehabilitation Sciences
Drexel University
Philadelphia, Pennsylvania

ELSEVIER
SAUNDERS

3251 Riverport Lane
St. Louis, Missouri 63043

PHYSICAL THERAPY FOR CHILDREN   ISBN: 978-1-4160-6626-2

Notices

Knowledge and best practice in this field are constantly changing. As new research and experience broaden our understanding, changes in research methods, professional practices, or medical treatment may become necessary.

Practitioners and researchers must always rely on their own experience and knowledge in evaluating and using any information, methods, compounds, or experiments described herein. In using such information or methods they should be mindful of their own safety and the safety of others, including parties for whom they have a professional responsibility.

With respect to any drug or pharmaceutical products identified, readers are advised to check the most current information provided (i) on procedures featured or (ii) by the manufacturer of each product to be administered, to verify the recommended dose or formula, the method and duration of administration, and contraindications. It is the responsibility of practitioners, relying on their own experience and knowledge of their patients, to make diagnoses, to determine dosages and the best treatment for each individual patient, and to take all appropriate safety precautions.

To the fullest extent of the law, neither the Publisher nor the authors, contributors, or editors, assume any liability for any injury and/or damage to persons or property as a matter of products liability, negligence or otherwise, or from any use or operation of any methods, products, instructions, or ideas contained in the material herein.

Vice President and Publisher: Linda Duncan
Executive Editor: Kathy Falk
Senior Developmental Editor: Christie M. Hart
Publishing Services Manager: Julie Eddy
Senior Project Manager: Richard Barber
Book Designer: Amy Buxton

Last digit is the print number: 9 8 7 6 5 4 3 2 1

Contributors

Jennifer L. Agnew, BScPT, BHK
Physiotherapist
Respiratory Medicine Division
Hospital for Sick Children
Lecturer,
Department of Physical Therapy
University of Toronto
Toronto, Ontario
Canada

Amanda Arevalo, PT, MS, PCS
Owner
Amanda Arevalo, P.C.
Pediatric Private Practitioner
Berwyn, Illinois

Donna Bernhardt Bainbridge, PT, EdD, ATC
Special Olympics Global Advisor for FUNfitness & Fitness
    Programming
Adjunct Faculty
University of Indianapolis
Project Consultant
The University of Montana Rural Institute on Disability in
    Rural Communities

Yvette Blanchard, PT, ScD
Professor of Physical Therapy
Department of Physical Therapy
Sacred Heart University
Fairfield, Connecticut

Brenda Sposato Bonfiglio, MEBME, ATP
Clinical Assistant Professor
Department of Disability and Human Development
Project Coordinator for Seating and Wheeled Mobility
    Services
Assistive Technology Unit
University of Illinois at Chicago
Chicago, Illinois

Suzann K. Campbell, PT, PhD, FAPTA
Professor Emerita
Department of Physical Therapy
Director of Mentoring Services
Center for Clinical and Translational Science
University of Illinois at Chicago
Chicago, Illinois

Tricia Ann Catalino, PT, MS, PCS
Physical Therapist
Pediatric Clinical Specialist
Chicago, Illinois

Lisa A. Chiarello, PT, PhD, PCS
Associate Professor
Drexel University
Physical Therapy and Rehabilitation Sciences
Philadelphia, Pennsylvania

Nancy A. Cicirello, PT, MPH, EdD
Professor
School of Physical Therapy
College of Health Professions
Pacific University, Oregon
Hillsboro, Oregon

Colleen Coulter-O'Berry, PT, DPT, PhD, PCS
Physical Therapist IV, Team Leader Limb Deficiency Program
Clinical Coordinator Residency Program
Children's Healthcare of Atlanta
Atlanta, Georgia

Maureen Donohoe, PT, DPT, PCS
Clinical Specialist
Nemours/ Alfred I.duPont Hospital for Children
Department of Therapeutic Services
Wilmington, Delaware

Antonette K. Doty, PT, MPH
Portage County Educational Service Center
Kent, Ohio

Helene M. Dumas, PT, MS
Research Center for Children with Special Health Care Needs
Franciscan Hospital for Children
Boston, Massachusetts

Stacey Dusing, PT, PhD
Assistant Professor
Department of Physical Therapy
Virginia Commonwealth University
Richmond Virginia

Susan K. Effgen, PT, PhD, FAPTA
Professor
University of Kentucky
Department of Rehabilitation Sciences
College of Health Sciences
Lexington, Kentucky

Heidi A. Frere, PT, DPT
Senior Physical Therapist
Children's Memorial Hospital
Chicago, Illinois

Carrie G. Gajdosik, PT, MS
Missoula, Montana

Richard L. Gajdosik, PT, PhD
Missoula, Montana

Brian Giavedoni, MBA, CP, LP
Senior Prosthetist
Limb Deficiency Program
Children's Healthcare of Atlanta
Atlanta, Georgia

Andrew M. Gordon, PhD
Professor of Movement Science
Teachers College, Columbia University
Department of Biobehavioral Sciences
New York, New York

Suzanne M. Green, PT
Senior Physical Therapist
Childrens Memorial Hospital
Chicago, Illinois

Laura H. Hansen, PT, MS
Research Associate
Family, Infant, and Preschool Program
J. Iverson Riddle Developmental Center
Morganton, North Carolina

Susan R. Harris, PhD, PT, FAPTA, FCAHS
Professor Emerita
University of British Columbia
Department of Physical Therapy, Faculty of Medicine
Vancouver, British Columbia
Canada

Paul J.M. Helders, PhD, MSc, PT, PCS
Professor and Chair in Clinical Health Sciences
Faculty of Medicine
Utrecht University
Director Child Development and Exercise Center
University Children's Hospital and Medical Center
Utrecht, the Netherlands

Kathleen A. Hinderer, PT, PhD
Executive Director
Michigan Abilities Center Equine Assisted Therapy
Ann Arbor, Michigan

Steven R. Hinderer, PT, MD
Associate Professor, Department of Physical Medicine and Rehabilitation
Director, PM&R Oakwood Residency Program
Wayne State University School of Medicine
Dearborn, Michigan

Betsy A. Howell, PT, MS
Physical Therapist II
Department of Physical Medicine and Rehabilitation
C.S. Mott Children's Hospital
University of Michigan Medical Center
Ann Arbor, Michigan

Mary Wills Jesse, PT, DHS, OCS
Staff Physical Therapist
Decatur Memorial Hospital
Decatur, Illinois

Therese E. Johnston, PT, PhD, MBA
Assistant Professor
University of the Sciences
Department of Physical Therapy
Philadelphia, Pennsylvania

Linda Kahn-D'Angelo, PT, ScD
Professor
University of Massachusetts Lowell
Department of Physical Therapy
Lowell, Massachusetts

Marcia K. Kaminker, PT, DPT, MS, PCS
Department of Student Services
South Brunswick Township Public Schools
South Brunswick, New Jersey

Karen Karmel-Ross, PT, PCS, LMT
Clinical Specialist
Department of Rehabilitation Services
University Hospitals Case Medical Center
Rainbow Babies and Children's Hospital
Cleveland, Ohio

Michal Katz-Leurer, LPT, MPH, PhD
Lecturer, Department of Physical Therapy
University of Tel Aviv Ramat Aviv
Campus ISRAEL
Research Counselor
Alyn Hospital, Pediatric and Adolescent Rehabilitation Center
Jerusalem, Israel

M. Kathleen Kelly, PT, PhD
Assistant Professor and Vice-Chair
Department of Physical Therapy
University of Pittsburgh
Pittsburgh, Pennsylvania

Susan E. Klepper, PhD, PT
Assistant Professor of Clinical Physical Therapy
Columbia University
New York, New York

Thubi H.A. Kolobe, PT, PhD, FAPTA
Professor
Department of Rehabilitation Science
University of Oklahoma Health Sciences Center
Oklahoma City, Oklahoma

Christin H. Krey, PT, MPT, ATP
Physical Therapist
Shriners Hospital for Children-Philadelphia
Philadelphia, Pennsylvania

Carrie J. Yenne-Laker, PT, DPT, CWS
Physical Therapist
University of Washington Burn Center
Harborview Medical Center
Seattle, WA

Judy Leach, PT
Physical Therapy Consultant
Pahoa, Hawaii

Venita Lovelace-Chandler, PT, PhD, PCS
Associate Director and Professor
School of Physical Therapy
Texas Woman's University
Dallas, Texas

Linda Pax Lowes, PT, PhD
Clinical Therapies Research Coordinator
Nationwide Children's Hospital
Columbus Ohio

Richard A. Magill, PhD
Professor and Chair
Department of Teaching and Learning
New York University
New York, NY

Teresa L. Massagli, MD
Associate Professor of Rehabilitation Medicine and Pediatrics
University of Washington and Children's Hospital and
    Regional Medical Center
Seattle, Washington

Mary Massery, PT, DPT
Owner, Massery Physical Therapy
Glenview, IL
DSc Candidate
Rocky Mountain University of Health Professions
Provo, Utah

Sarah Westcott McCoy, PT, PhD
Associate Professor
University of Washington
Department of Rehabilitation Medicine
Seattle, Washington

Irene R. McEwen, PT, DPT, PhD, FAPTA
Professor
University of Oklahoma Health Sciences Center
Department of Rehabilitation Sciences
Oklahoma City, Oklahoma

Margaret C. McGee, PT, PhD, BSN, PCS
Assistant Professor
Department of Physical Therapy
University of Central Arkansas
Conway, Arkansas

Sandra M. McGee, PT, PCS
Department of Physical Therapy
Children's Hospital of Philadelphia
Philadelphia, Pennsylvania

Beth McManus, PT, ScD, MPH
Robert Wood Johnson Health & Society Scholar
Department of Population Health Sciences
School of Medicine and Public Health
University of Wisconsin—Madison
Madison, Wisconsin

Mary J. Meiser, PT, MS
Physical Therapist
Easton, Maryland

Cheryl Missiuna, PhD, OTReg(Ont)
Professor, School of Rehabilitation Science
Director, *CanChild* Centre for Childhood Disability Research
McMaster University
Hamilton, Ontario, Canada

Merilyn L. Moore, PT
Rehabilitation Therapies Manager
University of Washington Burn Center
Harborview Medical Center,
Seattle, Washington

Janjaap van der Net, PhD, BSc(PT), PCS
Associate Professor in Clinical Health Sciences
Assistant Professor in Pediatrics
Faculty of Medicine
Utrecht University
Senior Researcher and Pediatric Physical Therapist Child
Development & Exercise Center
University Children's Hospital and Medical Center.
Utrecht, the Netherlands

Joan A. O'Keefe, PT, PhD
Assistant Professor
Department of Anatomy and Cell Biology
Rush University Medical Center
Chicago, Illinois

Margo N. Orlin, PT, PhD
Associate Professor
Physical Therapy and Rehabilitation Sciences
Drexel University
Philadelphia, Pennsylvania

Roberta Kuchler O'Shea, PT, PhD
Associate Professor
Physical Therapy Department
Governors State University
University Park, Illinois

Blythe Owen, MScPT, HBSc
Physiotherapist
Respiratory Medicine Division
Hospital for Sick Children
Lecturer
Department of Physical Therapy
University of Toronto
Toronto, Ontario
Canada

Robert J. Palisano, PT, ScD
Professor
Physical Therapy and Rehabilitation Sciences
Drexel University
Philadelphia, Pennsylvania

Lesley A. Palmgren, PT, MPT
Physical Therapist
University of Washington Burn Center
Harborview Medical Center
Seattle, Washington

Mark V. Paterno, PT, MS, MBA, SCS, ATC
Coordinator of Orthopaedic and Sports Physical Therapy
Sports Medicine Biodynamics Center
Division of Occupational and Physical Therapy
Cincinnati Children's Hospital Medical Center
Assistant Professor
Division of Sports Medicine, Department of Pediatrics
Cincinnati Children's Hospital Medical Center
University of Cincinnati School of Medicine
Cincinnati, Ohio

Cheryl R. Patrick, PT, MBA
Senior Physical Therapist
Children's Memorial Hospital
Chicago, Illinois

Nancy Pollock, MSc, OTReg(Ont)
Associate Clinical Professor
School of Rehabilitation Science
McMaster University
Hamilton, Ontario
Canada

Lisa Rivard, PT, BSc(PT), MSc
Doctoral Student
School of Rehabilitation Science and *CanChild* Centre for
    Childhood Disability Research
McMaster University
Hamilton, Ontario
Canada

Hemda Rotem, PT, BPT, MSc(PT)
Senior Physical Therapist
Alyn Hospital, Pediatric and Adolescent Rehabilitation Center
Jerusalem, Israel

Laura C. Schmitt, PT, PhD (PT)
Cincinnati Children's Hospital Medical Center
Cincinnati, Ohio

Kristine A. Shakhazizian, PT
Physical Therapist
West Grove, Pennsylvania

David B. Shurtleff, MD
Professor Emeritus
Seattle Children's Hospital, Research and Foundation
Seattle, Washington

Meg Stanger, PT, MS, PCS
Director of Physical Therapy and Occupational Therapy
Children's Hospital of Pittsburgh of UPMC
Pittsburgh, Pennsylvania

Jean L. Stout, PT, MS
Research Physical Therapist
James R. Gage Center for Gait and Motion Analysis
Gillette Children's Specialty Healthcare
St. Paul, Minnesota

Wayne A. Stuberg, PT, PhD, PCS
Professor and Associate Director for Education
Director, Physical Therapy & Motion Analysis Lab
Munroe-Meyer Institute, UNMC
Omaha, Nebraska

Michelle Sveda, PT
PT Clinical Lead
Nationwide Children's Hospital
Columbus, Ohio

Tim Takken, PhD, MSc
Associate Professor in Clinical Health Sciences
Faculty of Medicine
Utrecht University
Senior Researcher and Medical Physiologist
Child Development & Exercise Center
Wilhelmina Children's Hospital
University Medical Center Utrecht
Utrecht, the Netherlands

Chris Tapley, PT, MS
Physical Therapy Clinical Specialist
Department of Physical Medicine and Rehabilitation
C.S. Mott Children's Hospital
University of Michigan
Ann Arbor, Michigan

Darl W. Vander Linden, PT, PhD
Professor
Department of Physical Therapy
Eastern Washington University
Spokane, Washington

Linda Wallman, BScPT
Physiotherapist
Niagara Peninsula Childrens Centre
St. Catharines, Ontario
Canada

Marilyn Wright, BScPT, MEd, MSc
McMaster Children's Hospital
Assistant Clinical Professor
Department of Pediatrics & School of Rehabilitation Sciences
McMaster University
Hamilton, Ontario, Canada

Preface

As Cherry[1] said in a description of philosophy and science in pediatric physical therapy, specialty practice in pediatrics derives from the general philosophy of physical therapy but must address additional concerns that are different from those of physical therapy for adults. For example, clinical decision making must be guided by the knowledge that the natural development of children interacts with disability. As a result, physical therapists must anticipate and provide for childrens' changing needs. In addition, interventions must address the issues and problems identified by children and their caregivers. To the extent possible, children and caregivers must be intimately involved in both developing the plan of care and in its implementation in natural settings for children—the home, school, and community. The philosophy of family-focused care continues to guide the editors and authors of this book. In keeping with the challenges that face youth with disabilities as they approach adulthood, the fourth edition of *Physical Therapy for Children* includes an exciting new chapter, "Transition to Adulthood for Youth with Disabilities."

In this edition of *Physical Therapy for Children*, the editors continue to use two conceptual models to guide the updating of existing chapters and the development of both new chapters. These models also guided the development of new technological information resources such as videos of typically developing children and those with disabilities, as well as a dedicated website organized by the contents of each chapter. The conceptual models that guide our work include the International Classification of Functioning, Disability and Health (ICF)[2] of the World Health Organization and the *Guide to Physical Therapist Practice*[3] of the American Physical Therapy Association. Descriptions of these conceptual models can be found in the opening chapter on the evidence-based practice of pediatric physical therapy. We recommend that readers commence using this book with Chapter 1 as a guide to our philosophy, terminology, and conceptual framework for *Physical Therapy for Children*.

The *Guide to Physical Therapist Practice* should, of course, be used by all pediatric physical therapists in developing plans of care. We have, however, chosen to use the ICF as our model of the disabling process, rather than the model used in the *Guide*, because the ICF presents the dimensions of disability in a positive light, emphasizing activity rather than functional limitations, and participation rather than disability. The editors believe that all interventions provided by physical therapists should have as their goal the promotion of activity and participation as defined in the ICF model. Use of this model is helpful in directing attention to the ultimate purpose of providing intervention for children and education for their parents; therefore, this book focuses on prevention of disability throughout childhood and during the transition to living successfully as an adult.

The goal of our book continues to be the provision of a comprehensive reference for pediatric practice. To accomplish this goal, the remaining chapters in Section I of *Physical Therapy for Children* provide foundational knowledge in development, motor control, and motor learning. The chapters in this section should lead to understanding motor performance in children. These chapters provide information on the development of functional motor skills and the musculoskeletal structures, motor control and learning, evidence-based clinical decision making, and health-related physical fitness. Chapters on gait and on genomics complete this section and have been moved to the EVOLVE website to take advantage of the ability to show illustrations in color and include videos as an integral part of the content.

Sections II through IV of the book describe the impairments of body function and structure and the physical therapy management of activity and participation limitations common in pediatric musculoskeletal, neurologic, and cardiopulmonary conditions, respectively. Each chapter has been updated for the new edition, and application of the content is illustrated with evidence-based case studies and videos from the authors' practice. Select case studies and other topics are accompanied by video clips and include a movie icon in the margin of the text, as shown on the thumb margin of this page.

Finally, Section V addresses special settings and special considerations, including the burn unit, the special care nursery, early intervention, the educational environment, and public laws addressing disabilities in childhood. An addition to this section is the new chapter on the transition to adulthood. A chapter on assistive technology is again included but moved to the EVOLVE website including video material. New to the fourth edition is the chapter on the EVOLVE website entitled "Screening for Referral and Differential Diagnosis." This chapter addresses competencies that are now included in physical therapy education programs and important for direct access.

With this edition we continue to develop material on the dedicated EVOLVE website. Here instructors, students, researchers, and clinicians will find a host of useful resources, including links to websites for research laboratories, organizations serving families of children with disabilities, and many other Internet sites. Instructors, students, and clinicians preparing for pediatric specialist certification will find questions and educational exercises on the website to reinforce their learning.

The editors are grateful to the authors of this new edition, including several distinguished new international authors, and to the editorial and media consultants at Elsevier for creating the features that bring this book alive and connect pediatric physical therapists to the world at large through the resources of the Internet. I would also like to thank my co-editors, Robert J. Palisano and Margo N. Orlin, for their valuable contributions to all aspects of the work.

Suzann K. Campbell
Senior Editor
Chicago, Illinois

1. Cherry, D. B. (1991). Pediatric physical therapy: Philosophy, science, and techniques. *Pediatric Physical Therapy*, 3, 70–75.
2. World Health Organization (2001). *International Classification of Functioning, Disability and Health*. Geneva: World Health Organization.
3. American Physical Therapy Association (2001). *Guide to physical therapist practice*, 2nd ed. *Physical Therapy*, 81(1).

Contents

1

Evidenced-Based Decision Making in Pediatric Physical Therapy

ROBERT J. PALISANO, PT, ScD • SUZANN K. CAMPBELL, PT, PhD, FAPTA • SUSAN R. HARRIS, PT, PhD, FAPTA, FCAHS

Every day, pediatric physical therapists make several types of decisions that affect the lives of children, youth, and their families. These decisions include (1) who needs services and why; (2) what are the desired outcomes of intervention and how should they be documented; (3) the plan of care including communication and coordination of services and providing information, education, and instruction, and procedural interventions; (4) the number of visits required to achieve desired outcomes; and (5) how the overall clinical program should be evaluated for effectiveness and efficiency. On what basis do we make these important decisions? Physical therapy has long used the empirical base of collective experience or practice knowledge that is passed down from clinicians and educators to successive generations of new practitioners. Practice knowledge,[78] also called professional craft knowledge,[138] involves the integration of propositional knowledge (largely acquired through professional education) and procedural knowledge (acquired through actual practice). Practice knowledge is often implicit and embedded in the decisions of therapists.[167] Although practice knowledge has served therapists and their clients well, today's health care and education systems require more. Increasingly, physicians and other health professionals, third-party payers, administrators implementing policies for serving children in educational settings, and the public expect that physical therapists will use research evidence and valid and reliable decision-making methods as the basis for their practice.

The overall objectives of this chapter are to optimize the ability of pediatric physical therapists to (1) apply processes and strategies associated with evidence-based practice, (2) identify barriers to and solutions that facilitate translation of scientific findings into everyday practice, and (3) reflect on the assumptions and rationale for their clinical decisions. The chapter is written for the pediatric physical therapist attempting to provide "best practices" and serves as a resource for other chapters in this textbook. A primary tenet is that decisions on physical therapy services for children and their families are often complex and multifaceted.

EVIDENCE-BASED PRACTICE

Evidence-based practice refers to the use of current knowledge and research to guide clinical decision making within the context of the individual client.[149] This is accomplished through "integration of best research evidence with clinical expertise and patient values."[150] In 1992, the Evidence-Based Medicine Working Group described evidence-based practice as an emerging paradigm.[48] In this paradigm, evidence from clinical research is emphasized in decision making, whereas intuition, unsystematic clinical experience, and pathophysiologic rationale are de-emphasized. Evidence-based practitioners must critically appraise research and translate evidence to practice. These competencies reflect the perspective that health care providers have the responsibility to document the effectiveness of interventions, including the ability to provide quality care and a desirable cost/benefit ratio.[100]

The model of evidence-based decision making by Haynes, Devereaux, and Guyatt[75] has utility for pediatric physical therapy practice. Decision making is a process by which options are identified, compared, and a choice is made. In the model, research evidence is applied within the context of the values and preferences of individual patients, clinical expertise of the practitioner, and health care resources.[63] A model of evidence-informed decision making adapted from Haynes et al.[75] is presented in Figure 1-1. The wording has been modified for pediatric physical therapy. The process begins with identification of the child and family strengths and needs. This involves consideration of the home and community environment, including family resources and availability and accessibility of services. Second, research on the effectiveness and efficiency of each intervention option is appraised. Third, child and family preferences are considered. What options are the child and family ready and able to engage in? A fourth consideration is the physical therapist's practice knowledge including expertise in providing the interventions under consideration. The statement "Evidence alone does not make decisions, people do" by Haynes

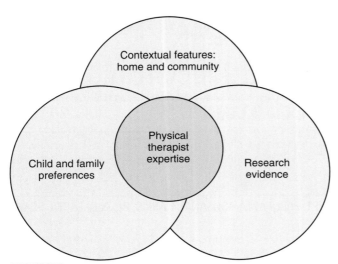

Figure 1-1 Model of evidence informed decision making. (Adapted from Haynes, R. B., Deveaux, P. J., & Guyatt, G. H. [2002]. Physician's and patients' choices in evidenced based practice. *British Medical Journal, 324,* 1350.)

et al.[75] reflects the integral role of the physical therapist in translation of research evidence to practice. Therapists must apply evidence in ways that address the needs of children and families. Interventions must not only be evidence informed but also acceptable to children and families and meaningful to their daily life. Clearly, evidence-based practice is a process that involves more than knowledge of current research; this may explain why in health care, transfer of evidence to practice is slow and sometimes does not occur.[25]

To what extent do pediatric physical therapists base their clinical decisions on the best available knowledge and research evidence? Therapists make decisions related to examination, selection of tests and measures, prognosis, outcomes, the plan of care, and coordination of care on a daily basis. Yet the evidence on which decisions are based is of variable quality. High-quality, peer-reviewed research provides the strongest evidence. Often, however, research is limited or lacking. Other sources of evidence that inform decision making include expert consensus, information from textbooks and continuing education courses (propositional knowledge), advice from a colleague, and personal experience (procedural knowledge).[164] School-based pediatric physical therapists reported that they continue to depend on these types of resources to inform their practice despite an expressed belief in the value of using evidence to guide their decision making.[151] Therapists who have been involved in research, however, are more likely to use evidence to guide practice.

RESPONSIBILITY TO PROVIDE EVIDENCE-BASED INTERVENTIONS

Traditionally, physical therapists have assumed that practice knowledge is sufficient and that it is the responsibility of researchers to determine the effectiveness of interventions.

We disagree with this perspective and support the viewpoint that all members of a profession have the responsibility to provide evidence-based interventions.[73] Objective documentation of goals and outcomes[137] and reflection on determinants of outcomes are important for deciding on the most appropriate interventions and evaluating outcomes. Such an approach was modeled successfully in a study by Ketelaar and colleagues.[94] Children with cerebral palsy who received physical therapy that emphasized functional motor abilities had greater achievement of individualized goals compared with a reference group of children with cerebral palsy whose intervention focused on improving quality of movement. Collaboration among children, families, practitioners, and researchers is important to identify critical research questions. Readers are strongly encouraged to consider the evidence that informs their clinical decisions. The impact of decisions based on expert opinion and practice knowledge should be carefully monitored and alternatives considered, should the child's progress be less than desirable.

FINDING EVIDENCE

Physical therapists are interested in evidence for tests and measures, prognosis, methods of service delivery, intensity of services, the effectiveness of procedural interventions, and outcomes of physical therapy for children with specific health conditions. Parents frequently ask questions such as "When will my child walk?" "Should my child receive more therapy?" "Will practice on a treadmill improve my child's walking?" This section provides an overview of how to find high-quality evidence through searching electronic databases for published research. Lou and Durando[105] recommend a five step process: (1) formulate a clinical question, (2) select appropriate information sources, (3) select the best databases or printed sources, (4) apply the search strategy, and (5) modify the search strategy.

FORMULATE A CLINICAL QUESTION

A clear and concise clinical question is an important first step in finding evidence. Herbert et al.[76] group clinical questions into four categories: (1) effects of intervention, (2) patients' experiences, (3) prognosis, and (4) accuracy of diagnostic tests. Category 3 can be expanded to include physical therapist diagnosis, whereas category 4 can include evidence of responsiveness of outcome measures. The mnemonic PICO is useful for remembering the parts of a well-written clinical question related to intervention:

P—Patient or problem
I—Intervention or management strategy
C—Comparative intervention
O—Outcome

For questions where two interventions are not being compared, the (C) is omitted. Examples of clinical questions written using the PICO format are provided in Box 1-1.

Box 1-1   EXAMPLES OF CLINICAL QUESTIONS WRITTEN USING THE PICO FORMAT

For (P) children with developmental coordination disorder, is (I) cognitive motor learning more effective than (C) sensory integration in improving (O) motor function?

For children (P) with hemiplegia, is (I) bimanual coordination therapy more effective than (C) constraint induced movement therapy in improving (O) arm and hand motor function?

For (P) infants with torticollis, what (I) physical therapy interventions improve (O) head and neck alignment and range of motion?

For (P) children with Duchenne muscular dystrophy, is (I) resistive exercise effective in (O) maintaining the ability to walk?

For (P) parents of infants born preterm, does (I) support, education, and instruction in the neonatal intensive care nursery improve (O) confidence and skill in handling and caring for their infants upon discharge to home?

IDENTIFY APPROPRIATE INFORMATION SOURCES

The second step is to identify appropriate information sources. Peer-reviewed journals are the primary source for original research. Peer-reviewed journals also publish systematic reviews that synthesize the results of several original research studies in an effort to summarize the overall evidence for an intervention. Peer review involves appraisal of articles submitted for publication by reviewers selected for their content expertise. The decision on whether to publish a manuscript is based on the recommendations of the reviewers and the editor. To minimize the potential for reviewer bias, many journals do not disclose the names or affiliations of authors to reviewers. This type of peer review is referred to as a masked or blinded review. Similarly, names of the reviewers are not disclosed to authors. Information on editorial policy is included in a journal and the journal's website. Contemporary editorial standards also typically require that authors reveal any conflicts of interest, such as research funding from commercial sources. Textbooks provide a secondary source of research. Book chapters generally are not peer-reviewed. Authors of textbooks cite published research and thus textbooks are a secondary source, but the authors may interpret findings based on personal perspectives. Another factor that limits the usefulness of information from textbooks is the time lag between preparation of text and publication. As a result, evidence cited in textbooks is at least 1 to 2 years out of date. Newsletters, magazines, and reports published by health care, professional, and consumer organizations also typically are secondary sources and information and not peer-reviewed.

SELECT THE BEST DATABASES AND PRINTED SOURCES

Electronic databases are the most efficient method for finding evidence. Electronic databases provide bibliographic references to thousands of peer-reviewed journals and can be searched from a personal computer via the Internet. In addition to the complete reference, databases provide links to the abstract and increasingly the full text of published articles. Many journals provide online access to articles before publication in print. Some electronic databases are within the public domain; others require a paid subscription or access to a university library or health care system that subscribes to the database. The Open Door: APTA's Portal to Evidence-Based Practice is a service available to members of the American Physical Therapy Association (APTA). The website is designed to facilitate evidence-based physical therapy services including the databases Cumulative Index to Nursing and Allied Health Literature (CINAHL), the Cochrane Library, and ProQuest Nursing and Allied Health Source that otherwise requires a paid subscription. Other strategies for finding evidence include the reference lists of recently published journal articles, the websites of professional organizations, and contacting authors for more detailed information about a study and the implications for practice (the e-mail of the author to whom to direct correspondence is included in the journal article).

MEDLINE, published by the National Library of Medicine with bibliographic references to more than 4600 biomedical journals and more than 12 million citations, is the largest health science database. MEDLINE is available on the Internet at no cost through the National Library of Medicine Gateway and PubMed. The National Library of Medicine Gateway is a web-based system that allows users to search simultaneously in multiple retrieval systems. In addition to journal citations, users can search monographs, serials, audiovisual materials, and several other databases maintained by the National Library of Medicine. PubMed was developed by the National Center for Biotechnology at the National Library of Medicine in conjunction with publishers of medical literature. Citations may include links to full-text articles from PubMed Central or publisher websites. Of particular interest to practitioners is the Clinical Queries option that allows users to frame their search as a clinical question. The web address for PubMed is ncbi.nlm.nih.gov/pubmed. The home page includes links to tutorials.

The Cumulative Index to Nursing and Allied Health Literature (CINAHL) is an electronic bibliographic database that indexes more than 2800 journals, books, and dissertations in nursing and 17 allied health disciplines, including physical therapy. Articles published in smaller or newer journals of interest to physical therapists are more likely to be located through CINAHL than MEDLINE. Herbert et al.[76] recommend CINAHL for clinical questions that are best addressed using qualitative research, such as child and family lived experiences and preferences.

The Cochrane Library is a product of the Cochrane Collaboration, an international, independent, not-for-profit organization dedicated to making up-to-date, accurate information about the effects of health care readily available worldwide. *The Cochrane Library* is a collection of six databases that contain different types of high-quality, independent evidence to inform health care decision making, and a seventh database that provides information about groups in the Cochrane Collaboration. The Cochrane Database of Systematic Reviews is of particular interest to practitioners. Updated and expanded regularly, the reviews focus on controlled trials and are highly structured. As of 2010, the Cochrane Database of Systematic Reviews contained 4186 reviews.

The Educational Resources Information Center (ERIC) is an online digital library of education research and information sponsored by the Institute of Education Sciences and the U.S. Department of Education. ERIC is available at no cost at eric.ed.gov. Users have access to educational research and information to improve practice in learning, teaching, and educational decision making. Physical therapists working in educational settings may find ERIC a useful resource.

PEDro is a free database of more than 16,000 randomized trials, systematic reviews and clinical practice guidelines in physical therapy (pedro.org.au). PEDro was established in 1999 by a small group of clinical and academic physical therapists in Australia. PEDro is currently produced by the Centre for Evidence-Based Physiotherapy (CEBP) at the George Institute for International Health. Its mission is to maximize the effectiveness of physiotherapy services by facilitating the clinical application of the best available evidence. All trials indexed in PEDro are independently assessed for quality. These quality ratings are used to quickly guide users to trials that are more likely to be valid and to contain sufficient information to guide clinical practice. Physiotherapy Choices is a companion website (physiotherapychoices.org.au) of the CEBP that was designed for use by consumers of physiotherapy services, including patients, their friends and families, health service managers, and insurers. The database provides a catalog of research evidence on the effectiveness of physical therapy interventions.

Hooked on Evidence, sponsored by the American Physical Therapy Association, is a database of extractions of published research articles relevant to physical therapy practice that is available to members. Therapists who contribute to the database follow a standardized format to review current clinical trials, cohort studies, case-control studies, case reports, single-subject experimental designs and cross-sectional studies. As of 2010, more than 5700 extractions of research articles were included in the database.

Turning Research into Practice (TRIP) is a meta-search engine that was developed in 1997 to address clinical questions using the principles of evidence-based medicine. Based in South Wales, United Kingdom, the database is available

through the Internet at no cost (tripdatabase.com/index.html). TRIP allows users to search across a variety of health-related websites using simple keywords.

APPLY AND MODIFY THE SEARCH STRATEGY

Selection of the keywords and phrases that will identify research articles relevant to your clinical question is the most important step in conducting a literature search. Knowledge of the topic and titles, abstracts, and keywords from relevant articles previously read provides a starting point. In MEDLINE, terms to describe the content of an article come from a standardized list of vocabulary and definitions called MeSH, or Medical Subject Headings. In CINAHL, articles are indexed by subject terms, which are similar to MeSH. The advantage of MeSH headings and subject terms is that articles that use any of the terms listed for a MeSH heading or subject term are identified. In contrast, when keywords or phrases are entered as text words, only articles in which the exact word or phrase appears in the title or abstract are identified. A text word search, also referred to as free text search, is most useful for keywords or phrases that are new or not common.

A common strategy is to combine two or more searches using "AND" or "OR" (referred to as Boolean operators or Boolean logic). The Boolean operator "AND" narrows a search, retrieving only articles containing at least one term from each concept. The AND operator is very good for narrowing a search to retrieve those guidelines most relevant to your topic. The Boolean operator "OR" broadens a search, retrieving all articles containing at least one of the search words entered, but not necessarily both. The use of double quotation marks around a search phrase (e.g., "developmental screening") is used to narrow a search to find articles that contain the specific phrase. Additional strategies for combining keywords, limiting and expanding the scope of the search, are used depending on the topic and purpose of the search. Following the initial search, the titles and abstracts of relevant articles are useful in modifying and refining searches.

Regular literature searches by a clinical program or therapy staff is an excellent strategy for quality assurance and to stay abreast of current best evidence. Always remember to save your searches. Saved searches are easy to update at regular intervals. Tutorials for performing searches and instructions on how to create an account to save searches are provided in PubMed and CINAHL.

APPRAISING RESEARCH EVIDENCE

Evidence-based decision making is predicated on the physical therapist's ability to analyze and apply research knowledge. This process involves access to current research, appraisal of research, and determination of how findings apply to individual children and their families. Harris[73] and Golden[57] posed several thought-provoking questions for professionals to ask themselves when analyzing the scientific merit of an intervention:

1. Is the theory on which the intervention is based consistent with current knowledge?
2. Is the population for whom the intervention is intended identified?
3. Are the goals and outcomes of intervention consistent with the needs of the intended population?
4. Are potential adverse effects of the intervention identified?
5. Is the overall evidence critiqued?
6. Are advocates of the intervention open to discussing its limitations?

A negative response to one or more of these questions is a warning sign that an intervention is not evidence based.

TYPES OF RESEARCH

Awareness of the distinction between *efficacy* and *effectiveness* is important for therapists attempting to translate research to practice. Efficacy refers to outcomes of interventions provided in a controlled setting under experimental conditions. Effectiveness refers to outcomes of interventions provided within the scope of clinical practice. The *randomized controlled trial* (RCT) is an experimental design that provides evidence of efficacy. Subjects are randomly assigned to an experimental or control group, and the researchers specify the intervention, permitting the strongest inferences about cause and effect. (Did the experimental intervention cause the documented outcomes?) Although the RCT provides the strongest evidence of a cause-effect relationship between the intervention and outcomes, trials are costly and challenging to implement with children with developmental disabilities. To adhere to the rigor of an experimental design, the intervention is often provided under conditions that are not representative of many practice settings. Consequently, when attempting to apply the results of an efficacy study, therapists must consider whether subject characteristics generalize to children on their caseloads and whether the intervention is feasible within their practice settings.

Effectiveness research typically involves quasi-experimental (subjects are not randomly assigned to an experimental or control group), observational designs (no control group or the intervention is not specified by the researchers or both) that describe current practice and predictive designs for identifying child, family, and environmental factors that are determinants of outcomes. *Cohort, case control,* and *case series* are designs used in clinical epidemiology that provide evidence of effectiveness. *Clinical practice improvement* (CPI) methodology is a type of effectiveness research with the purpose of identifying specific strategies and procedures that are associated with outcomes and determinants of outcomes.[80] Horn contends that the RCT is designed to investigate a single intervention as opposed to the combination of strategies and procedures that constitute a typical physical therapy intervention. In CPI, standardized forms are created to document intervention strategies and procedures and time spent on each activity. Data are also collected on variables that potentially influence outcomes. Variables might include child characteristics (age, severity of condition, interests, cognition, and communication), family characteristics (family dynamics, interests, resources, supports), and features of the physical, social, and attitudinal environment. Multivariate statistical analyses are used to discriminate among all of the interventions documented those that are associated with favorable outcomes and determinants of outcomes. This type of information is appealing to physical therapists because it informs the decision-making process. Although clinical practice improvement is feasible to implement in practice settings, multivariate analyses require large numbers of subjects.

Because reviewers of research frequently lament the fact that the existing evidence lacks clinical relevance, an argument has been made that research designs that meld the best characteristics of efficacy and effectiveness studies should be more widely utilized and supported by major funding agencies.[168] *Pragmatic or practical clinical trials* (PCTs) are specifically designed to answer a clinically important question. The PCT is characterized by comparison of clinically relevant interventions, inclusion of subjects from diverse populations and practice settings, and measurement of a wide range of outcomes.[168] Comparison of two interventions is similar to the RCT, whereas the other characteristics are similar to CPI methodology. PCTs are needed to address knowledge gaps, such as long-term outcomes and effects on function in daily life, but are expensive because of the requirements for large numbers of subjects and use of multiple research sites. Nevertheless, influential organizations such as the Veterans Administration in the United States and health systems in England and Canada have successfully used this approach to improving care and reducing costs.

Qualitative methods of inquiry have been used in nursing and occupational therapy and increasingly more often in physical therapy.[67,139] *Qualitative research* is well suited for understanding processes associated with effective communication, coordination, and documentation, and child and family related instruction, two of the three components of all physical therapist interventions. Qualitative methods were used by Palisano et al.[128] to better understand the mobility experiences of youth with cerebral palsy and Hutzel et al.[83] to learn about the experience of fitness instructors in leading an exercise program for children with juvenile arthritis. The experiences and values of consumers (e.g., children and families), practitioners, and administrators are integral components of health services research that are too often missing in clinical research.

In qualitative studies, data collection typically involves interviews and focus groups that are recorded and transcribed verbatim. Interviews include neutrally worded, open-ended questions followed by prompts to encourage participant reflection. Other methods of data collection include observation and examination of artifacts such as medical records and clinical documentation. In qualitative research, theory emerges from analysis of data that are *grounded* in the social world of the people being studied. This is in contrast to experimental and quantitative research that is based on the researcher's preconceived hypothesis. *Phenomenology* and *grounded theory* are the two qualitative approaches that are used most frequently in health care research. Both are concerned with understanding the lived experiences of the population of interest. In both approaches, themes or theory emerge from analysis of data that are *grounded* in the social world of the people being studied. Qualitative methods are distinct from those used in experimental research, especially with respect to sample size. Greenhalgh's[61] overview of qualitative research is recommended as a foundation for reading journal articles, whereas the textbook by Creswell[31] provides a more extensive understanding of qualitative research.

Participatory action research involves collaboration of consumers, practitioners, and researchers to address specific questions or issues. Children and their families and practitioners are participants or co-researchers who provide input about the questions or issues to address, feasibility of proposed practices, and dissemination of information in usable formats. The preferences and values of consumers and practitioners, therefore, are incorporated into the design and implementation of research. Schreiber et al.[152] used participatory-action research to collaborate with pediatric physical therapists to identify strategies for implementation of evidence-based practice.

Recently published *systematic reviews* provide an efficient way for therapists to inform themselves of current evidence. A systematic review is a "study of studies"! All relevant research is analyzed in an effort to determine the overall evidence for an intervention. In a well-conducted systematic review, the author(s) (1) define a focused clinical question, (2) identify criteria for inclusion of a study in the review, (3) perform a comprehensive literature search, (4) appraise the internal validity of each relevant study, (5) indicate how results were analyzed, and (6) interpret findings in a manner that enhances application to clinical practice.[30] Just like a research report, therapists must critique a systematic review. A systematic review is only as good as the quality of each study included.

Meta-analysis is a mathematical synthesis of the results of two or more research reports. A meta-analysis can be performed on studies that used reliable and valid measures and report some type of inferential statistic (e.g., t-test, analysis of variance.) Effect size, odds ratio, and the weighted mean difference are examples of statistics used for meta-analysis.

Effect size is the mean difference on the outcomes of interest between subjects in experimental and control groups. The most basic measure of effect size is the d-index. The d-index is the mean difference between groups in terms of the common standard deviation. Cohen[28] provided the following guidelines for interpretation of the d-index: d = 0.2

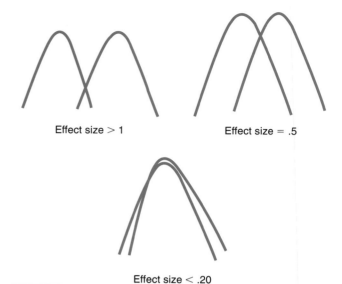

Effect size > 1   Effect size = .5

Effect size < .20

Figure 1-2 Distribution of scores of subjects in the experimental and control groups for small, medium, and large effect sizes (illustrations not drawn to scale).

TABLE 1-1   **Interpretation of Effect Size Based on Cohen's Criteria[28]**

Effect Size	Interpretation	Overlap of Scores*
0.00	No effect	100%
0.20	Small	85%
0.50	Medium	67%
0.80	Large	53%
1.70		25%

*Overlap in individual scores of subjects in the experimental and control groups.

represents a small effect, d = 0.5 represents a medium effect, and d = 0.8 represents a large effect. Figure 1-2 and Table 1-1 present the overlap of scores between subjects in the experimental and control group for selected effect sizes. The overlap in distribution of scores has important implications for clinical decision making. A finding that the mean score on the outcome measure was significantly higher for subjects in the experimental group *does not* indicate whether all subjects or even most subjects in the experimental group scored higher than subjects in the control group. As illustrated in Table 1-1, even for a large effect size (.80) there is 53% overlap in scores of subjects in the experimental and control groups. Consequently, when applying the evidence to clinical decisions for an individual child, the therapist would not be certain of that child's outcome.

The Forest Plot Diagram is used to graphically present the results of a systematic review. Figure 1-3 illustrates a Forest Plot Diagram for a meta-analysis of four randomized

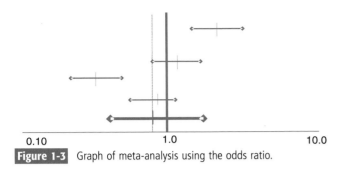

Figure 1-3   Graph of meta-analysis using the odds ratio.

controlled trials. The odds ratio is used to present the results of each study and the meta-analysis. The odds ratio is presented on a scale of 0.10 to 10.0; 1.00 is the line of no effect. Each study is represented on the graph by a horizontal line. The vertical mark in the middle of the line is the odds ratio and the diamonds at the far left and right indicate the boundaries of the 95% confidence interval. If a horizontal line crosses the line of no effect, the odds ratio is *not* significantly greater than 1 ($p > 0.05$). When the horizontal line is to the right of the line of no effect, the odds ratio is significantly greater than 1 ($p < 0.05$). In Figure 1-3, the odds ratio for only one study is significantly greater than 1 (top study). The horizontal lines for the remaining three studies cross the line of no effect, indicating the odds ratio is not significantly greater than 1. The thicker horizontal line at the bottom is the overall odds ratio for the four studies. The overall odds ratio is 0.90 ($p > 0.05$) indicating that subjects who received the experimental intervention were not more likely to improve compared to subjects who did not receive the experimental intervention (control group). Miser[111] suggested an odds ratio of 2.0 or greater represents a strong intervention effect. An odds ratio of 2.0 indicates that subjects who received the intervention are two times more likely to have improved on the outcomes measured compared with subjects who did not receive the intervention.

Examples of systematic reviews of interest to pediatric physical therapists include strength training programs for children with cerebral palsy,[112] management of the upper limb of children with hemiplegia,[147] treadmill training and body weight support in pediatric rehabilitation,[32] treadmill training programs for high-risk infants and children with cerebral palsy,[106] exercise therapy for children with juvenile idiopathic arthritis,[162] and physical activity for youth with disabilities.[88] In most databases, searches can be limited to systematic reviews. This is a good strategy for determining whether a systematic review has been published on the clinical question of interest.

LEVELS OF EVIDENCE AND GRADE OF RECOMMENDATION

Systems have been developed to classify strength of evidence of a single research study and grades of recommendation

from multiple studies based on the type of design and the quality of the methods (also referred to as internal validity). Sackett[148] proposed a five-level system that relates the research design to levels of evidence and grades of recommendation. This system has subsequently been expanded and refined by the Centre for Evidence Based Medicine at the University of Oxford (2010) to include sublevels and categories of research: (1) therapy/prevention, etiology/harm, (2) prognosis, (3) diagnosis, (4) differential diagnosis/symptom prevalence, and (5) economic and decision analyses. For research on therapy interventions, a systematic review of randomized controlled trials (RCT) provides the strongest evidence (level 1A), whereas a single RCT of high quality provides 1B evidence. A systematic review of cohort studies is classified as level 2A evidence and an individual cohort study or RCT of low quality is classified as 2B evidence. Inferences on cause and effect are more limited for quasi-experimental designs in which group assignment is not randomized (levels 3 and 4) or when there is no control group (level 5). The Centre for Evidence Based Medicine also provides criteria for Grades of Recommendation. Grade A indicates that outcomes are supported by consistent level 1 studies. Grade B indicates outcomes are supported by consistent level 2 or 3 studies. Grade C indicates that outcomes are supported by level 4 studies. Grade D indicates outcomes are supported by level 5 evidence or inconsistent or inconclusive studies of any level.

The American Academy for Cerebral Palsy and Developmental Medicine (aacpdm.org) uses a five-level system for assigning levels of evidence for group research designs that is simplified compared with the system developed by the Centre for Evidence Based Medicine. The academy has also created a five-level system for single subject design studies. Both systems, guidelines for preparing evidence reports, and evidence reports that have been prepared for the academy are available on the website. Daly et al.[35] have developed a hierarchy of evidence for assessing qualitative health research.

The *critically appraised topic* (CAT) provides a format for therapists to summarize the research evidence from a literature search conducted as part of clinical practice.[51] A critically appraised topic is a one- to two-page summary of research related to a focused clinical question that includes implications for practice. The format is intended to facilitate transfer of evidence to practice.

PRACTICE GUIDELINES AND PATHWAYS

Practice guidelines are systematically developed statements to assist patient and practitioner decisions about management of a health condition. The emergence of practice guidelines within the U.S. health care system was precipitated by large variation among health care providers in the type and amount of services for patients with similar conditions. Practice guidelines are intended to provide current standards for quality practice in order to improve effectiveness and efficiency of health care. The focus is generally on people with a particular condition or disorder (e.g., preterm infants at risk for developmental disabilities), and many guidelines are discipline specific (e.g., guide for physical therapist intervention in the neonatal intensive care unit). In general, practice guidelines include recommendations for the following:

- Who should receive intervention
- Expected outcomes
- Documentation including selection of reliable and valid tests and measures
- Utilization of services (frequency and duration, number of visits)
- Procedural interventions
- Coordination of care
- Discharge planning

Recommendations in practice guidelines should be derived from systematic review of peer-reviewed research and, when research is limited or lacking, consensus statements based on expert opinion. In 1990, the Section on Pediatrics of the American Physical Therapy Association sponsored a consensus conference on the effectiveness of physical therapy in the management of children with cerebral palsy.[18] The summary statements described interventions supported by some research evidence, interventions that lacked supporting research, and interventions that lacked supporting research but, based on the clinical opinion of conference participants, were judged to warrant investigation.

The following are competencies and guidelines for pediatric physical therapy:

Competencies for Physical Therapists in Early Intervention,[26] working in the schools[40], Providing Physical Therapy Services Under Parts B and C of the Individuals with Disabilities Education Act (IDEA),[109] and Neonatal Physical Therapy Practice Guidelines and Training Models.[160,161]

These competencies and guidelines are based primarily on expert opinion and informal consensus (as opposed to formal consensus development by a large group or organization). Kaplan[92] provides a list of Internet sites for access to practice guidelines, including the U.S. Agency for Healthcare Research and Quality (ahrq.gov/clinic/cpgonline), the Canadian Medical Association INFOBASE (mdm.ca/cpgsnew/cpgs/index.asp), and the Centre for Evidence Based Physiotherapy in the Netherlands (cebp.nl).

A *clinical pathway* is a type of practice guideline that is developed by a provider organization to standardize patient episodes of care for specific conditions. A clinical pathway is a multidisciplinary tool that indicates the usual interventions and expected outcomes in a definitive length of time for management of a patient population in a specific setting. Clinical pathways are most common for high incidence conditions and the acute and subacute settings. The impetus for clinical pathways is to increase the efficiency of health care (favorable outcomes that are cost efficient) by reducing unexplained variation in type and intensity of intervention and improving coordination of care. Typically, a pathway

specifies the sequence and components of care for each day, the discipline responsible for each component of care, and the expected goals and outcomes. Critical pathway and care paths are other terms used to describe a standard care plan.

The evidence to support published clinical pathways varies considerably and, for many pathways, the effectiveness has not been evaluated. Methods of evaluation include the impact of the clinical pathway on the following:

- Intensity of service
- Quality assurance
- Patient satisfaction with how care is provided
- Patient outcomes

Campbell[21] suggested a clinical pathway for follow-up examination of infants at risk for developmental disabilities during the first year of life based on the psychometric qualities of various assessment tools. Byrne developed a clinical path to guide physical therapy management of infants in the neonatal intensive care unit (NICU) based on evidence in the literature, and Goldstein designed a parallel care path specifically to educate parents of infants born preterm as they manage their infant's needs and progress toward discharge.[16]

APPRAISAL OF PRACTICE GUIDELINES AND PATHWAYS

In 1998, an international group of researchers and policy makers formed the AGREE collaboration to improve the quality and effectiveness of clinical practice guidelines. AGREE stands for Appraisal of Guidelines for Research and Evaluation. The collaboration includes members from Denmark, Finland, France, Germany, Italy, the Netherlands, Spain, Switzerland, the United Kingdom, Canada, New Zealand, and the United States. An instrument was designed to assess clinical practice guidelines developed by local, regional, national, or international groups and government organizations. The AGREE instrument is a useful resource for physical therapists deciding whether to implement recommendations in a practice guideline or pathway. The instrument provides guiding questions and a response scale to assess the scope and purpose of a guideline, the people involved in development, rigor of development, clarity and presentation of recommendations, applicability, and editorial independence. The instrument and training manual are available on the AGREE website (agreecollaboration.org).

Researchers studying the application of guidelines in everyday practice find that failure to incorporate recommendations is often related to the large number of guidelines produced by a formal consensus process and the fact that reorganization of the practice structure is often needed in order to comply with the recommended guidelines.[34,130] Because it is frequently the case that following one or more of the many guidelines provided results in 80% to 90% of the expected improvement in outcomes, they recommend that clinicians begin with implementing one or two of the primary recommendations rather than give up because of the perceived enormity of the task.

CHILD AND FAMILY PERSPECTIVES

Evidence-based decision making encompasses the perspectives of the child and family. Presentation of information to families in useful and acceptable formats encourages their active participation in decision making. By presenting evidence in family-friendly format, pediatric therapists can enhance informed shared decision making on the part of their young clients.[172] In fact, research has shown that patients who are more informed and more involved in their own decision making are more likely to adhere to their treatment regimens and experience better health outcomes.[156,158]

Parents of children with disabilities have also become active providers of information by using the power of the Internet. It is not uncommon for a parent to ask a question about information from the Internet that is unfamiliar to the therapist. Because the quality and accuracy of information available on websites vary greatly, the physical therapist can assist a family to critique information and determine its relevance to the child and family. Examples of websites for families of children with disabilities are as follows:

1. *Family Voices* (familyvoices.org) is a national grassroots network of families and professionals who are advocates for health care services for all children and youth with special health care needs; the services are family centered, community based, comprehensive, coordinated, and culturally competent.
2. *Beach Center on Disability's* (beachcenter.org) mission is to make a difference in the quality of life of families and individuals affected by disability and of those who are closely involved with them. Located at the University of Kansas and an affiliate of the Department of Special Education, the website includes a section for families, knowledge-to-action guides, and a Community of Practice on Facebook to share evidence, values, and wisdom among families, practitioners, researchers, and policy makers about early childhood family supports.
3. *Pathways Awareness Foundation* (pathwaysawareness.org) is a national nonprofit organization dedicated to raising awareness about the benefit of early detection and early therapy for children with physical movement differences.
4. *Bright Foundation* (BRain Injury Group–Hope through Treatment) (brightfoundation.tripod.com/main) is a nonprofit parent group with involvement of clinical and research professionals whose focus is infants and children with acquired brain injury. The website includes current research reviews, therapy effectiveness reviews, advocacy information, and a practical advice and support forum.

A consumer's guide to therapeutic services for families of children with disabilities was developed through the combined efforts of several professional and parent organizations.[82] Included in the guide is a consumer checklist that consists of the following six questions:

1. Will achievement of goals make a real difference in the lives of the child and family?
2. Is there a formal process to discontinue or change the course of intervention if there is no progress?
3. Are interventions as much a part of the child's day-to-day life as possible?
4. Are parents, teachers, and other individuals present in the child's daily life as involved in the planning and provision of intervention as they could be?
5. Are the professionals involved in assessing the child and planning intervention experienced in serving children with similar disabilities?
6. Are sources of financial support sufficient for the cost of the planned intervention?

From the perspective of the child and family, the answer to all six questions should be yes.

PRACTICE KNOWLEDGE AND CLINICAL REASONING

Physical therapists must have a strong knowledge base and the abilities to problem solve and make sound clinical judgments to effectively transfer research knowledge to practice. Research on problem solving has repeatedly confirmed that skill in problem solving is problem specific, indicating that one can solve problems better with a comprehensive base of knowledge about the problem. Clinical reasoning refers to the many ways a practitioner thinks about and interprets an idea or phenomenon and incorporates knowledge, experience, problem solving, judgment, and decision making.[52] Higgs, Titchen, and Neville[78] proposed that health care practitioners use three types of knowledge: propositional (derived from theory and research), professional or craft (derived from professional experience), and personal (derived from self). Mattingly[107] suggested that pediatric therapists incorporate a minimum of five domains of knowledge into their thought processes: (1) understanding of the child's motivation, commitments, and tolerances; (2) assessment of the environment in which the task is taking place; (3) knowledge of the child's physical and cognitive deficits and capacities; (4) perception of the therapeutic relationship; and (5) immediate and long-term goals.

Mattingly[107] proposed an interpretive or meaning-centered model of clinical reasoning in occupational therapy that emphasizes implicit and embodied knowledge. She conceptualized clinical reasoning as the process of deciding on the appropriate action for an individual patient at a particular time. Knowledge is viewed as a starting point but not as a strict plan for action. As part of the process of individualizing intervention, the therapist makes judgments and improvises in moving from general practice guidelines to the requirements of a specific situation. Mattingly suggested that judgment and improvisation are often guided by knowledge that is embodied in the therapist's hands or eyes. Part of the therapist's expertise, therefore, is reflected in implicit thought processes that are translated into habitual ways of observing and interacting with patients. The perspective that clinical reasoning involves more than the ability to apply theory and learned technical skill may explain the frustration of physical therapy students when they first attempt to apply classroom material to the clinical setting.

Embrey and associates[41,42,43,45] used qualitative research methodology to describe the thought processes of three experienced (greater than 10 years of pediatric experience) and three novice (less than 2 years of pediatric experience) pediatric physical therapists while providing direct intervention to children with cerebral palsy. The experienced therapists appeared to make procedural changes and respond to the emotional and social needs of children with fewer interruptions of the therapeutic process, whereas the novice therapists appeared to be limited in their clinical options when they perceived that therapy goals were not being achieved. The investigators suggested that within a treatment session, therapists make rapid, on-the-spot, clinical decisions based on improvisation and intuition.

In their framework for reflective practice within physical therapy, Donaghy and Morss[38] contend that knowledge must be explicit for evidence-based practice. Higher-order cognitive processes, including critical inquiry, problem solving, and clinical reasoning, are encouraged. Through reflection and self-appraisal, knowledge becomes more explicit and subject to further appraisal. In their study of expert practice in physical therapy, Jensen et al.[86] concluded that "Reflection was a critical element for our experts and the means for their continued learning and development of knowledge from their experience (p. 40)."

What are characteristics of expert physical therapists? The model of expert practice in physical therapy developed by Jensen et al.[86] using grounded theory includes four dimensions: (1) multidimensional knowledge that is patient centered and evolves through reflection, (2) clinical reasoning processes that are embedded in collaborative problem-solving with the patient, (3) focus on movement that is centered on function, and (4) virtues of caring and commitment. A great deal remains to be learned about expert practice including how to optimize clinical reasoning and knowledge gained from professional experience. Pediatric physical therapists are encouraged to strive for better understanding of their thought processes, not only to enhance their own professional development but also to serve their clients and educate physical therapy students more effectively. A better understanding of how to integrate research, consumer preferences, and practice knowledge is essential for the development of decision models that reflect the broad scope and complexity of pediatric physical therapy. A description of the thought process related to decision making for a child with Down syndrome complicated by significant health issues is presented in Box 1-2.

INTERNATIONAL CLASSIFICATION OF FUNCTIONING, DISABILITY AND HEALTH

The International Classification of Functioning, Disability and Health (ICF) was developed by the World Health Organization[175] to provide a scientific basis for understanding and studying health and health-related states, outcomes, and determinants. The ICF also is intended to provide a common language in order to improve communication among people with disabilities, health care providers, researchers, and policy makers. The ICF emphasizes "components of health" rather than "consequences of disease" (i.e., participation rather than disability) and environmental and personal factors as important determinants of health. The ICF model is available on the World Health Organization website (www.who.int/classifications/icf/en). A children and youth version (ICF-CY) was published by the World Health Organization in 2007.[176] The model is the same as the ICF, but codes for components of health, personal, and environmental factors were modified and new codes added to reflect development and environments of children and youth from birth to 18 years.

The diagram of the ICF model is presented in Figure 1-4. The ICF has two parts. Part 1: Functioning and Disability includes three components of health: body functions and structures, activities, and participation. Part 2: Contextual Factors include environmental and personal factors that influence components of health. For example, the impact of activity (ability to walk) and participation (ability to travel with classmates at school when going to lunch) may be influenced by the environment (distance from classroom to cafeteria and time to travel this distance) and personal factors (the child's fitness and motivation to walk). The bidirectional arrows are inclusive of all possible relationships. The challenge when applying the ICF is to identify the relationships that are most relevant for an individual child and family.

Body functions are the physiologic and psychologic functions of body systems. Physiologic functions include respiration, vision, sensation, muscle performance, and movement. Psychologic functions include attention, memory, emotion, thought, and language. *Body structures* are the anatomic parts of the body such as the brain, organs, bones, ligaments, muscles, and tendons. *Impairments* are problems in body functions and structures. Examples of impairments are limited ability to plan and execute movement, poor processing of sensory information, reduced cardio-respiratory endurance, lack of sensation, muscle weakness, balance difficulties, skeletal deformity, and joint contracture. *Activity* is the performance of a task or action by an individual. Activities represent the integrated use of body functions and vary in complexity. Examples of activities are maintaining and changing body positions, walking and moving around, lifting and carrying objects, fine hand use, and self-care. *Activity limitations* are difficulties in performing age-appropriate

Box **1-2** EXAMPLE OF COMBINING EVIDENCE FROM THE RESEARCH LITERATURE WITH FAMILY VALUES AND INDIVIDUAL CLIENT CHARACTERISTICS IN CLINICAL DECISION MAKING

RESEARCH EVIDENCE

Research on treadmill training for children with Down syndrome suggests that independent walking can be achieved on average 4 months earlier after about 10 months of five times per week treadmill training.[169] How does this research apply to my client with Down syndrome who has complicated health issues?

Child's Status

Caleb is a 2½-year-old child with Down syndrome complicated by infantile spasms, visual impairment, and Hirschsprung's disease, necessitating three surgeries to correct. The last surgery was successful and he is now gaining weight and shows more endurance for physical activity. He sits alone and rolls but does not crawl, pull to stand, or take weight on his feet in standing.

FAMILY CONSIDERATIONS

Parents are professionals with college educations, have heard about the treadmill training research, and have specified their early intervention goals for Caleb to include learning to walk. They are interested in trying treadmill training if it can be done at home.

DECISIONS TAKEN

Because the treadmill training study started children on the training regimen when they could sit alone for at least 30

seconds and take weight on their feet on the treadmill, Caleb's home program for early intervention was revised to place more emphasis on improving his sitting balance and trunk strength and on working standing into his daily routines. This included placing him against the couch in his living room while providing manual stability for extension of the legs. Within a couple weeks, he was pulling up into kneel-standing in his crib and also at the couch.

INTRODUCTION OF TREADMILL TRAINING

At this point, a treadmill was brought into the home and Caleb was placed on it for a trial of stepping. On the first day, he took no steps but did support his weight briefly in standing and seemed interested in the treadmill. His parents tried placing him on the treadmill daily and, at the therapist's next visit, he was able to take six to eight steps per trial. It was decided that his parents wanted to incorporate this training into Caleb's home program; the therapist made sure that they understood that the length of training required in the study of children with Down syndrome was an average of 10 months and that Caleb might require more time because of his more fragile health situation. Because he was not able to support his trunk in the upright position, a harness to provide partial weight support will also be needed.

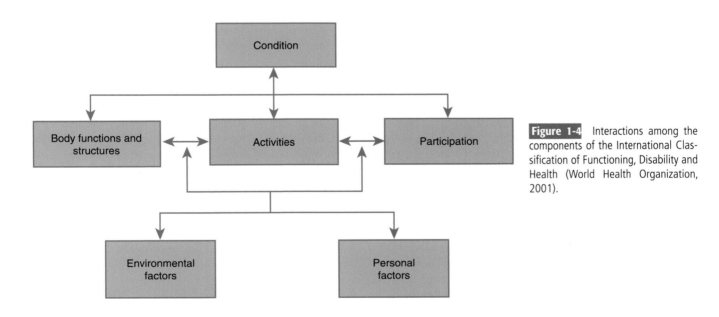

Figure 1-4 Interactions among the components of the International Classification of Functioning, Disability and Health (World Health Organization, 2001).

tasks or actions. *Participation* is involvement in a life situation. Most children participate in home life, school, community activities and organizations, and social relationships with friends. Participation is highly individualized. What is important to one child may be of little consequence to

another child. *Participation restrictions* are problems in involvement in life situations. *Environmental factors* make up the physical, social, and attitudinal environments in which people live and conduct their lives. *Personal factors* are the particular background of the individual's life and living that

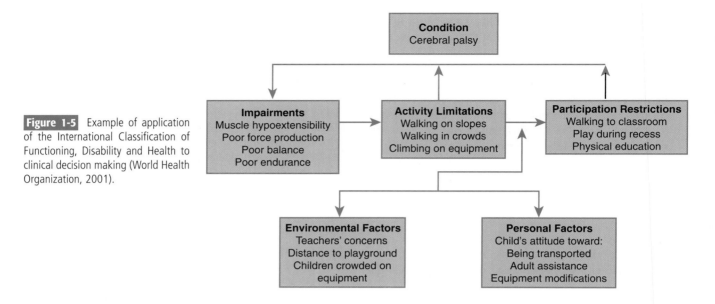

Figure 1-5 Example of application of the International Classification of Functioning, Disability and Health to clinical decision making (World Health Organization, 2001).

are not part of a health condition or disorder. These factors may include gender, race/ethnicity, age, fitness, lifestyle, habits, coping styles, and past and current experiences.

The decision to adopt the ICF model for the third, and now fourth, edition of *Physical Therapy for Children* was made because of the emphasis on components of health and on environmental and personal factors as important determinants of health. The *Guide to Physical Therapist Practice*[2] is based on a disablement framework. The model Person with a Disability and the Rehabilitation Process[114] is referenced in the guide and provided a conceptual framework for the first two editions of *Physical Therapy for Children*. A case report illustrates using the ICF to inform clinical decision making and how child and family priorities change over time.[120]

An example of a child with spastic diplegia will be used to illustrate application of the ICF for clinical decision making (Figure 1-5). The child's impairments in the neuromuscular and musculoskeletal systems include hamstring and gastrocnemius muscle hypoextensibility, reduced muscle force production, poor balance, and limited muscular endurance. The child's activity limitations include difficulties in walking on a sloping surface, walking amid people, and climbing playground equipment. At school, the child occasionally falls when walking from the bus to the classroom. Although the child has several friends and enjoys physical activity, participation in recess and physical education is restricted. Social and physical environmental factors that may contribute to restricted participation include the following: teachers are concerned that the child will get injured; the child's classroom is located at the end of the school most distant from the playground; the terrain of the school yard is uneven; and students are crowded on the playground equipment. In applying the ICF framework, the therapist is encouraged to identify what the child does do (strengths) in

addition to impairments, activity limitations, and participation restrictions that limit or restrict what the child wants to or needs to do. The challenge is to hypothesize cause-effect relationships. For example, what are the causes of a student's restricted participation during recess and physical education? There is evidence that an exercise program to improve muscle strength and endurance will improve gait characteristics.[112] Is there evidence that instruction and practice in climbing on playground equipment (motor learning) will improve participation? Collaboration with the teachers to discuss their safety concerns and the feasibility of modifications to playground equipment are environmental considerations. The child's feelings about energy conservation (e.g., being transported to the playground), modifications of playground equipment, and support from adults are examples of personal factors to consider in formulating an intervention plan. Note that in Figure 1-5, only the hypothesized interactions are depicted. The arrow from the participation restrictions and activity limitation to impairments represents a secondary impairment.

The ICF framework will be considered further when problems and processes for making diagnostic, prognostic, outcomes evaluation, and program evaluation decisions are discussed. The ICF will also be applied throughout the text. Box 1-3 lists considerations for applying the ICF to clinical decision making.

PHYSICAL THERAPY DIAGNOSIS AND PROGNOSIS

Historically, answers to the question "Who needs treatment by a physical therapist and what for?" were simple to obtain. Physicians identified the problem (the medical diagnosis) and referred children to physical therapists, sometimes with a specific prescription, or at other times for "evaluation and

BOX 1-3	CONSIDERATIONS FOR USING THE INTERNATIONAL CLASSIFICATION OF FUNCTIONING, DISABILITY, AND HEALTH AS A FRAMEWORK FOR CLINICAL DECISION MAKING

IMPAIRMENTS

- Not all impairments are modified by physical therapy
- Not all impairments cause activity limitations and participation restrictions
- Relate impairments to activity limitations and participation restrictions
- Impairments are identified from examination and evaluation of body functions and structures

ACTIVITIES

- Relate activity limitations to participation restrictions
- Activity limitations can cause secondary impairments
- Activities are often measured by norm-referenced and criterion-referenced assessments

PARTICIPATION

- Reflects child and family perspectives
- Is context-dependent (environmental and personal factors)
- Is one aspect of health-related quality of life
- Is measured by child and parent self-report
- Is measured by observations in natural environments as well as parent and child self-report

treatment" at the therapist's discretion. For many of the disorders managed by pediatric physical therapists, physicians remain the primary diagnosticians for identification of the health condition. Unfortunately, standardized practice guidelines are not available to guide physicians in deciding who would benefit from therapy (and when) so physicians' practices vary widely. For example, research on physicians' decisions regarding referral for physical therapy of children with suspected cerebral motor dysfunction indicates that the decision to refer is related to the physician's diagnostic certainty, perceived severity of the child's involvement, and belief in the value of physical therapy.[22] The diagnostic certainty expressed by physicians in this study, who reviewed a series of standardized videotaped cases, varied widely. Furthermore, the probability of referral varied with physician specialty. Orthopedists were less likely and physiatrists more likely to refer a child younger than 2 years of age for physical therapy than were pediatricians or neurologists.

Research also demonstrates that disclosure practices can be improved. Despite recommended guidelines for sharing diagnostic information, which leave about 75% of families satisfied with the manner and structure of disclosure of diagnostic information, about half of parents remain dissatisfied with the information content delivered.[8] It is recommended that information about the diagnosis should present a

balanced viewpoint rather than just a list of problems and that a follow-up appointment be scheduled not too far after the original disclosure to enable parents to continue to discuss the diagnosis. Parents should be sent written material soon after the initial disclosure as a back-up to the verbal information, and it is important that accurate information be provided at all stages of service delivery. Parents often have questions years after the initial diagnosis. An example from clinical practice is provided in Box 1-4.

Under the current health care system and evolving state licensure laws, physical therapists increasingly serve as the point of entry into physical therapy services, either as independent practitioners, as part of a comprehensive diagnostic and intervention team, as related service providers in educational settings, or as practitioners in other venues. To be worthy of such a powerful role, physical therapists need valid and reliable decision-making procedures that result in the provision of truly necessary services in the most cost-effective manner. They also need skill in information sharing with families, especially during periods of uncertainty regarding the diagnosis and prognosis, because families often believe that their concerns are not heard.[99] Most important, therapists must identify when referral to another practitioner is warranted. This topic is addressed in the chapter, Screening for Referral and Differential Diagnosis on the Evolve website.

The diagnostic and prognostic decisions that physical therapists make fall within the realm of impairments, activity limitations, and participation restrictions. In the *Guide to Physical Therapist Practice*,[2] a diagnosis is defined as a cluster of signs, symptoms, syndromes, or categories, the purpose of which is to guide the physical therapist in determining the most appropriate intervention for a child and family. Prognosis refers to the predicted level of improvement in function and the duration and frequency of intervention needed to achieve the expected outcomes. For example, therapists are best qualified to make decisions regarding whether a client has impairments of body functions, such as in strength or passive range of motion, the presence of and degree to which a client has activity limitations because of mobility issues, and the presence of developmental gross motor delay and the types of impairments contributing to that delay.

Clinical prediction rules have been developed for physical therapy and other disciplines to help clinicians to incorporate multiple types of data into decisions such as making a diagnosis, establishing a prognosis, or matching patients to optimal procedural interventions.[27] Developing a clinical prediction rule involves (1) reviewing the scientific literature to identify predictors of the outcome of interest and developing a statistical analysis incorporating these factors to test its predictive power, (2) trying out the prediction equation with a new sample of clients or in a different setting to further test its validity, and (3) conducting an impact analysis study to test the hypothesis that applying the clinical prediction rule will improve outcomes, increase

---

| Box **1-4**   EXAMPLE OF INFORMATION NEEDS OF A FAMILY |

CHILD

Ali was diagnosed with encephalitis that ensued after a childhood vaccination when he was 18 months old. Previously, he was typically developing. Following in-patient rehabilitation, he was referred for early intervention services. At the time of referral, he was able to sit alone precariously and walk 10 feet with maximum support at the trunk, but he could not crawl or pull to stand. His condition was characterized by severe ataxia and better use of the right hand than the left. He had no expressive language. Over time, he gained weight at an alarming rate and nutritional concerns became a major issue.

FAMILY

Ali's parents were immigrants. His mother spoke no English, so management of Ali's care was done by his father who had been in the United States for 10 years before bringing his wife and children, including a newborn, to live with him. His command of English was good for everyday purposes, but understanding complicated medical communications and completing forms for insurance and the transition from early intervention to the educational system were challenging. Numerous providers perceived the family to be "difficult," and several providers either stopped delivering services or were dismissed by the family during Ali's time in early intervention.

FAMILY GOALS

The goals of Ali's family were for him to regain normal function. Their expectations of a physical therapist were that she would manipulate Ali's arms and legs and perform hands-on care. Family expectations were different from the expectations of the early intervention service providers. The focus of the early intervention program was teaching families to incorporate activities pertaining to the child's goals into daily routines.

INTERVENTION

Gradually the family came to understand and accept their role in working toward Ali's goals, but the therapist's probes regarding their understanding of Ali's condition revealed major misconceptions and knowledge gaps. The parents did not understand that Ali had sustained permanent brain damage and that regaining his previous level of function would be problematic. They began to feel that Ali was lazy and not motivated to regain function. They also believed that the large size of his legs meant that they were strong, leading to a lack of concern about his increasing obesity. They were concerned, however, about the fact that Ali seemed to have frequent respiratory infections but did not connect this with the fact that the father smoked in the small studio apartment the family occupied. All of these issues were addressed gradually with the family, resulting in the assistance of a nutritional consultation, a referral for state-provided services for smoking cessation, and more realistic expectations of Ali's progress on the part of the family. The therapist also gained an understanding of the respective roles of parents within this family's culture, their expectations regarding children's play and general development, and their view of the role of health professionals in managing health and disability. A significant challenge was presented by the lack of English language skills on the part of the mother because the early intervention program did not have a translator available in the family's native language.

---

patient satisfaction, and decrease costs once implemented in everyday clinical practice. In physical therapy, this method has been applied primarily to orthopedic problems like management of back pain and no examples for pediatric practice have yet been published.

THE PROBLEM OF PREDICTABILITY

Most often, the decision regarding who needs physical therapy revolves around the diagnosis of developmental delay or the presence of signs of aberrant development, such as those seen in the motor control dysfunction associated with cerebral palsy. Only a few diagnostic tests, however, have adequate sensitivity and specificity to identify and define the impairments and functional limitations we hope to diagnose. The most useful means for assessing delayed development are standardized developmental scales that have been normed on large populations. The positive predictive validity of the tests that currently exist, however, is often low because a proportion of children with delayed development in early infancy demonstrate recovery at older ages. Aylward (1997) described the need to evaluate tests further for both diagnostic classification accuracy and also relative risk—that is, the probability of a child later displaying a developmental problem if results of an earlier screening test were abnormal or suspect.[3]

What do we know about prediction of outcomes from early developmental assessment? The bulk of the older literature on assessment in infancy suggests that little regarding outcome in later years can be successfully predicted for individual children.[70,97,131,142] For example, poor motor performance scores early in life have some capacity for identifying children at risk for developmental problems, but sometimes in a nonspecific way. Poor motor scores may later be associated with cerebral palsy, cognitive impairment, or even blindness and behavioral problems.[23,49,115] The process of recovery from early medical complications and the environment that a family provides for optimal recovery and facilitation of development also contribute to the difficulty in predicting developmental outcomes.

Unfortunately, test scores at any single point in time may be inadequate for making a decision regarding whether a child's development is permanently impaired until the time for maximally effecting important long-term outcomes has already passed. A conceptual framework that encompasses the complexity involved in early brain lesions or atypical development is needed. Aylward and Kenny[4] and Gordon and Jens[59] have suggested models for early identification of developmental disabilities,[19] and Campbell[21] suggested a clinical pathway for follow-up examination of infants at risk for developmental disabilities in the first year of life.

A test that showed promise in the prediction of poor motor outcome, the Alberta Infant Motor Scale,[33] was included in the clinical pathway for follow-up examination of infants under 10 months of age.[21] Recently, Campbell and colleagues[24] demonstrated that the Test of Infant Motor Performance (TIMP) has a sensitivity of 92% and specificity of 76% at 3 months for predicting 12-month AIMS performance. Furthermore, the TIMP performed better than the AIMS at 3 months for identifying the delay associated with a later diagnosis of cerebral palsy[9] and with motor outcomes at 5 to 6 years of age.[98] Thus, the TIMP may be a more useful test in the period prior to 4 months of age, although this test, like others, has the problem of over identification of at-risk infants.[24]

Use of the TIMP in conjunction with the General Movement Assessment[46] might reduce the number of misidentifications. Decision making for diagnostic purposes could be improved by the development of clinical prediction rules based on published research on prediction of developmental outcomes.[27] For example, Lekskulchai and Cole[104] showed in a controlled clinical trial that the TIMP at hospital discharge could be used to identify a group of children born prematurely who would benefit from a physical therapy home program. TIMP test scores in conjunction with other factors such as health status, infant behavioral organization,[117] and home environment conditions could be used to develop a clinical prediction rule for high risk infants to guide NICU discharge planning and early intervention.

Despite imperfect predictability from early assessment, general agreement exists that use of standardized testing instruments represents best practice for the purposes of diagnosis. Yet Jette and colleagues[87] reported that only about half of the physical therapists surveyed in their research used such instruments on a regular basis. More that 90% of those who used standardized tests believed that use of such measures improved communication with patients and helped to direct care planning. Barriers to use of tests included lack of access to testing materials, insufficient time for clients to complete and therapists to analyze results, and perceived difficulties of clients in completing tests. Jette and colleagues[87] suggested that further efforts to educate physical therapists about the value of standardized testing is needed and that development of electronic software to assist in interpretation of scores, comparison with norms, and classification of patients by severity or improvement after intervention would facilitate more widespread use of formal tests. Fortunately, a number of tests used in pediatric practice are available in electronic formats, including the Gross Motor Function Measure,[145] the Pediatric Evaluation of Disability Inventory,[65,66] and the Test of Infant Motor Performance.[24]

CLASSIFICATION SYSTEMS

Use of taxonomic classification systems for describing impairments, activity limitations, and participation restrictions is a means to improve clinical decision making. All therapists know that no two children with the same disorder are exactly alike. Establishing taxonomies for the description of constellations of impairments or functional limitations occurring in children with particular conditions can lead to improved diagnosis and prognosis on which to base clinical decisions. Taxonomic classification is also useful in generating studies of differential intervention effects for subcategories of disability and studies of whether different types of interventions are most appropriate for children classified by severity of impairment or activity limitations. But are there ways to identify the underlying impairments at the systems level, and are there clinically practical means for classification of children based on either impairment or activity limitation? This section presents classification systems that have been developed for infants, children, and youth with cerebral palsy. Classification systems for other developmental disabilities are not as well developed. Given the diversity of abilities of children with autistic spectrum disorders and the number of different interventions applied to this population, there is a great need for classification systems based on activity and participation.

Research on the General Movement Assessment suggests that the pathologic movement qualities characteristic of cerebral palsy can be reliably identified in the first few months of life with a sensitivity of 95% and specificity of 96%.[50,135] All pediatric clinicians know that children with cerebral palsy are characterized by stereotypic movement patterns and lack of selective control. Prechtl and colleagues have developed an assessment of general movement that characterizes the movement pattern in cerebral palsy as being one of "cramped synchrony," with a paucity of selective joint movements, especially in the rotational components.[49] Their work has also demonstrated that clinical examination of children with known signs of brain pathophysiologic impairment can identify the effects of such lesions on movement. These effects can then be qualitatively and quantitatively described longitudinally and used to predict recovery or nonrecovery from early nonoptimal medical conditions and events. The test is totally noninvasive because it involves observation of spontaneous movement from 15-minute to 1-hour videotapes (depending on age). Use of this general movement examination to diagnose high risk for cerebral palsy has the potential to eliminate the problem of late referral because of diagnostic uncertainty identified by Campbell et al.[22] Westcott and Bradley (Chapter 3) reviewed the research demonstrating the exceptionally strong predictive validity of this test.

Three five-level classification systems have been developed for describing gross motor function, manual ability, and communication function of children and youth with cerebral palsy. Descriptions for each level represent functional abilities that are meaningful in everyday life. The Gross Motor Function Classification System (GMFCS) for children with cerebral palsy[121,126] has become the standard for classification of gross motor function of children and youth with cerebral palsy. The GMFCS is translated into over 15 languages and has been cited in more than 800 peer-reviewed journal articles. The GMFCS was developed for children with cerebral palsy who are 12 years of age and younger and subsequently expanded to include a 12- to 18-year age band and revised to include environmental and personal considerations for the 6- to 12-year and 12- to 18-year bands. This five-level system is based on the perspective that classification based on functional abilities and limitations should enhance communication among professionals and families with respect to (1) efficient utilization of medical and rehabilitation services, (2) the creation of databases describing the development of children with cerebral palsy, and (3) comparing and generalizing the results of program evaluations and outcomes research. The terms *functional related groups, severity of disability, case-mix complexity,* and *risk adjustment* have been used to describe methods of grouping patients for evaluating internal quality standards or for comparative analysis of intervention outcomes across sites (benchmarking).

A classification is made by determining which of the five levels best represents the child's current abilities and limitations in gross motor function in home, school, and community settings. Classification is based on the child's self-initiated movement with emphasis on sitting and walking. The description for each level is broad and not intended to describe all aspects of the motor function of individual children. For each level, separate descriptions are provided for children in the following age bands: less than 2 years, 2 to 4 years, 4 to 6 years, and 6 to 12 years. A summary of the 6- to 12-year age band is included in Table 1-2. Distinctions among levels of gross motor function are based on functional limitations, the need for handheld assistive mobility devices (walkers, crutches, canes), wheeled mobility, and, to a lesser extent, quality of movement. The scale is ordinal with no intent that the distances between levels be considered equal or that children with cerebral palsy are equally distributed among the five levels. Parents can apply the GMFCS reliably to their own children's functional status[113] and value being able to understand their child's level of function and what that means in terms of understanding future needs. Evidence of inter-rater reliability, stability, content,

TABLE 1-2 **Summary of Level of Mobility That a Child Is Expected to Achieve between 6 and 12 Years of Age for Each of the Five Levels of the Gross Motor Function Classification System**

Level	Abilities and Limitations
I	Walks without restrictions; limitations in more advanced gross motor skills
II	Walks without assistive devices; limitations in walking outdoors and in the community
III	Walks with assistive mobility devices; limitations in walking outdoors and in the community
IV	Self-mobility with limitations; children are transported or use powered mobility outdoors and in the community
V	Self-mobility is severely limited, even with the use of assistive technology

construct, and predictive validity has been reported[121,122,125,174] Gorter et al.[60] found that that classification of infants less than 2 years of age is less precise than classification of older children and recommended reclassification at age 2 or older as more clinical information becomes available.

The Manual Ability Classification System (MACS)[47] is a five-level system to classify hand use of children with cerebral palsy, 4 to 18 years of age. Classification is based on the child's typical performance in handling objects during daily activities. Distinctions among the levels are based on the child's ability to handle objects and the amount of assistance or adaptation the child needs to complete tasks of daily living. Reliability and validity of the MACS have been demonstrated.[47,132]

The Communication Function Classification System (CFCS)[77] is a five- level system to classify usual communication function of individuals with cerebral palsy. A classification is based on everyday performance for all methods of communicating, including speech, gestures, eye gaze, facial expressions, and augmentative and alternative communication. Distinctions among the levels are based on the performance of sender and receiver roles, the pace of communication, and the type of conversational partner. Examination of reliability and validity is in progress.

GROSS MOTOR DEVELOPMENT CURVES

Pediatric physical therapists use standardized measures normed on children with typical development to identify infants and children with delays in motor development and to qualify children for services in early intervention and educational settings. For children with identified health conditions characterized by motor impairments and activity limitations, the value of such measures to plan interventions and document change is controversial. An alternative approach for measuring change over time or in response to an intervention in children with physical disabilities is to compare performance with expectations for children of the same age with a similar disability. This approach is dependent on disability-specific data.

The 66-item version of the Gross Motor Function Measure (GMFM-66)[145] and the GMFCS enabled researchers at the CanChild Centre for Developmental Disability Research to create gross motor development curves for children with cerebral palsy. This research was guided by the perspective that, for children with cerebral palsy, knowledge of prognosis for gross motor function would assist in determining (1) goals and management plans that are consistent with a child's potential and (2) the extent to which interventions improve gross motor function beyond expectations based on age and severity of impairment. Rosenbaum et al.[141] and Hanna et al.[68] conducted prospective longitudinal studies on a cohort of children with cerebral palsy randomly selected from an accessible population of 2108 children in the province of Ontario (Canada). Children were stratified by age and GMFCS level. Each child's classification level at the start of the study was used to create five motor development curves. The first study[141] included 657 children who were administered the GMFM-66 an average of 4.3 times. The model that provided the best "fit" of GMFM-66 scores was nonlinear and included two parameters: the *rate parameter*, an estimate of how fast children approach their limit of gross motor function, and the *limit parameter*, an estimate of maximum potential for gross motor function.

A subsequent study was completed that followed 229 of the 343 older children in the original cohort for an additional five years during adolescence and early adulthood.[69] A consideration in deciding how to model the curves was the possibility that some youth might demonstrate a decline in gross motor function. To account for this possibility, a model was examined that included a third parameter to allow for a peak and decline in GMFM-66 scores, prior to a long-term limit. The data were modeled using both two and three parameters. The two-parameter model provided the best fit for children and youth in levels I and II, whereas the three-parameter model provided the best fit for children and youth in levels III, IV, and V. The gross motor development growth curves are presented in Figure 1-6.

The gross motor development curves represent the average pattern of development for children and youth in each of the five classification levels. For all five curves, children progress faster to their maximum GMFM-66 score at younger ages and then demonstrate a leveling of scores (levels I and II) or a decline followed by a leveling (levels III-V). The predicted average maximum GMFM-66 score differs significantly for each level. On average, children in level I achieve a maximum score of 90, whereas children in level V achieve a score of 24 at age 6, which then declines to 17 age 21. Children and youth in levels III, IV, and V are predicted, on average, to demonstrate a decline in GMFM-66 score of 4.7 to 7.8 points.

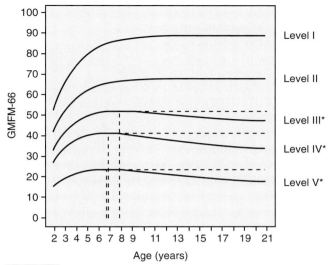

Figure 1-6 Predicted average Gross Motor Function Measure (GMFM-66) scores of children and youth with cerebral palsy as a function of age by Gross Motor Function Classification System level. *GMFCS levels with significant average peak and decline. (Reprinted with permission from Hanna, S. E., Rosenbaum, P. L., Bartlett, D. J., et al. [2009]. Stability and decline in gross motor function among children and youth with cerebral palsy aged 2 to 21 years. *Developmental Medicine and Child Neurology, 51,* 295–302.)

How should the gross motor development curves be used in decision making? Rosenbaum and associates[141] anticipated that the curves will help children and families understand the outlook for gross motor function. The curves should prove useful for planning interventions, enabling families and professionals to collaborate and make informed decisions about the most appropriate therapy goals for a child. The curves also provide an effective way to assess whether a child's motor progress is consistent with patterns of children of similar age and disability severity. Rosenbaum and associates[141] believe that the gross motor development curves will have important implications for evaluation of interventions by providing evidence of the extent to which a particular intervention improves a child's gross motor function beyond what is predicted by the curves.

When sharing the gross motor curves with children, families, and other health care providers, therapists must clearly explain w*hat the curves do* and *do not measure.* The GMFM-66 measures activities, specifically what a child "can do" in a standard condition. The activities measured are usually achieved by age 5 in children without motor impairments. The number of children below age 2 and the number above age 18 were low; therefore, the ends of the curves may not reflect actual development. The gross motor development curves do not measure many components of health that are important for children with cerebral palsy. These components include the following:

• Movement efficiency and endurance
• Adapted function (achieved with mobility aids)
• Wheeled mobility

- Performance of mobility during daily activities and routines (child-environment interaction)
- Wellness and physical fitness
- Prevention of secondary impairments (e.g., skeletal alignment, range of motion, pain)

Prognosis for goals and outcomes that are not measured by the GMFM-66 *should not* be inferred from the motor development curves!

An example of application of GMFCS, GMFM-66, and gross motor development curves to physical therapist examination, evaluation, and prognosis is provided in Box 1-5. The example is described in more detail in Palisano.[120] The *CanChild* research team also has constructed gross motor development curves for children with Down syndrome, using a model similar to the one used for children with cerebral palsy.[123]

PROBABILITY ESTIMATES FOR METHODS OF MOBILITY

Another type of data that is useful for decision making is performance of mobility in daily life. Performance of mobility or how children actually move at home, school, and in the community involves the interaction of the child and environment. Performance, therefore, is potentially influenced by several factors, including the child's physical capacity, the physical, social, and attitudinal features of the environment, and the child's (or family's) personal preference and choice. As part of the two longitudinal studies that led to creation of the motor development curves, parents of a population-based sample of 642 children reported their children's mobility at home, school, and outdoors at 6- or 12-month intervals for a mean of 5.2 times.[129] The data were analyzed to model the probabilities that children and youth with cerebral palsy walk (with or without mobility devices), use wheeled mobility (self-propelled or self-powered mobility), or use methods of mobility that require physical assistance (e.g., carried, takes steps with assistance, transported) as a function of age and environmental setting.

By age 3, almost all children in level I walked in all environmental settings, whereas only a small number of children and youth in level V moved without physical assistance of a person (powered mobility). Among children and youth in levels II, III, and IV, however, usual method of mobility varied by age and environmental setting. Figure 1-7 presents the estimated probabilities for children and youth in level III. At younger ages, there is a high probability that children are transported or carried outdoors. The probability of walking increases from age 4 and peaks at age 9 in the school setting (68%), age 11 in the outdoors setting (54%), and age 14 in

---

Box **1-5** APPLICATION OF THE GROSS MOTOR FUNCTION CLASSIFICATION SYSTEM (GMFCS), GROSS MOTOR FUNCTION MEASURE (GMFM-66), AND THE GROSS MOTOR DEVELOPMENT CURVES TO PHYSICAL THERAPIST EXAMINATION, EVALUATION, AND PROGNOSIS

Teresa Spataro is a 17-month-old twin born at 31 weeks gestational age with a birth weight of 1570 g. She was recently diagnosed as having cerebral palsy and referred for physical therapy. During the initial interview, Mrs. Spataro identified the following needs and priorities: (1) information on when Teresa will walk, (2) concerns about leg stiffness, and (3) recommendations for what to do. Teresa crawls on hands and knees with leg reciprocation and is beginning to pull to stand and cruise. Using the GMFCS, the therapist classified Teresa's gross motor function at level II. The therapist uses the algorithm developed by Russell et al.[146] to identify the item set to administer (set B that includes 29 items). Teresa achieved a GMFM-66 score of 44. As illustrated, her score is slightly above the average score predicted at 17 months of age for children in level II. Children with a GMFM-66 score of 56 have a 50% chance of walking 10 steps unsupported. On average, children at level II achieve a score of 56 at age 3 years. The therapist shared this evidence with Mr. and Mrs. Spataro when addressing their question, "When will Teresa walk?"

At age 4, Teresa continues to be classified at level II. She walks indoors and short distances outdoors. She has difficulty with initiation of walking, changing directions, and stopping. GMFM-66 item set C (39 items) was administered and Teresa achieved a score of 60 on the GMFM-66. Hanna et al.[68] created percentiles for the GMFM-66 for children with cerebral palsy ages 2 to 12 years (not pictured). Teresa's score is at the 80th percentile. The therapist shares this information with Teresa and her parents. Teresa is proud saying she only has "a little cerebral palsy" and her parents express their delight at Teresa's progress in gross motor function.

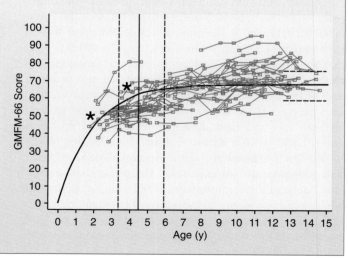

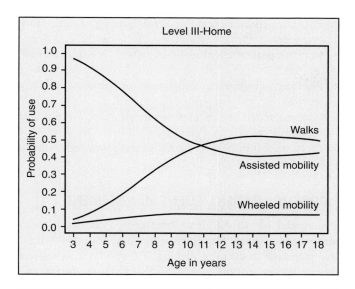

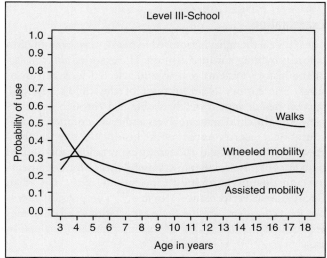

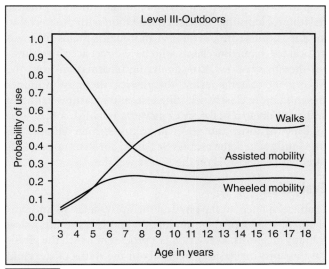

Figure 1-7 Estimated probabilities of walking, wheeled mobility, and mobility with physical assistance as a function of age and environment for children and youth in GMFCS level III. (Reprinted from Palisano, R. J., Hanna, S. E., Rosenbaum, P. L., & Tieman B. [2010]. Probability of walking, wheeled mobility, and assisted mobility for children and youth with cerebral palsy. *Developmental Medicine and Child Neurology, 52,* 66–71.)

the home setting (52%). The probability of walking at age 18 is about 50% in all three settings. At home, youth who do not walk as their usual method of mobility are more likely to move with physical assistance than use wheeled mobility. At school and outdoors, youth who do not walk as their usual method of mobility are almost as likely to use wheeled mobility as assisted mobility.

The probability estimates provide evidence that usual methods of mobility of children and youth with cerebral palsy are influenced by age and environmental setting. The probabilities are modeled from a population-based sample and, therefore, are likely to generalize to populations elsewhere whose resources and services are comparable to those in Ontario, Canada. The results have implications for long-term planning, clinical decision making, and family-centered services. Discussion of mobility options with children and families and involving children in decision making is recommended, with the understanding that the method of mobility that optimizes participation in one setting may not be the preferred method in another setting. Efficiency, safety, self-sufficiency, and environmental features such as distance and time requirements are important considerations when making decisions regarding goals and interventions for mobility. Therapists are encouraged to evaluate features of everyday environments when planning interventions to improve mobility.

HYPOTHESIS-ORIENTED ALGORITHM FOR CLINICIANS II

The Hypothesis-Oriented Algorithm for Clinicians (HOAC) was developed by Rothstein and Echternach[39,143] to provide physical therapists with a systematic method for clinical decision making and patient care that is independent of methods of examination and intervention philosophy. An algorithm uses a branching approach to decision making, involving several steps that are intended to narrow the focus of the problem and direct the practitioner to the appropriate plan of action. The Hypothesis-Oriented Algorithm for Clinicians II (HOAC II)[144] was designed to be more compatible with contemporary practice and to include the concept of prevention. HOAC II is not supported by a database, is not computer generated, and is not intended to provide specific guidelines for examination and intervention decisions. Rather, the HOAC II provides a format to guide the physical therapist through the decision-making process.

The focus of the HOAC II is on patient-centered outcomes. The patient or therapist identifies existing and anticipated problems. For each identified problem, the therapist generates hypotheses as to the cause(s), formulates an intervention plan that addresses the hypothesized cause(s), and documents outcomes. Children who receive physical therapy often have several primary and secondary impairments that can cause activity limitations and participation restrictions. When using the HOAC II, therapists are encouraged to consider all possible hypotheses, how each hypothesis relates to the others, and to prioritize the changes most likely to occur through physical therapy. Management of anticipated problems is a unique aspect of the HOAC II. For children with neuromuscular and musculoskeletal impairments who experience excessive or asymmetrical weight-bearing forces while walking, anticipated problems might include skeletal deformity and joint contracture. For anticipated problems, intervention is aimed at eliminating risk factors. In this example, depending on the rationale for why the child is likely to have skeletal deformity and joint contracture, interventions might involve muscle strengthening, stretching, an orthosis, and reducing weight-bearing forces through use of wheeled mobility when traveling long distances. The HOAC II model is compatible with the elements of patient/client management in the *Guide to Physical Therapist Practice*[2] described in the next section.

GUIDE TO PHYSICAL THERAPIST PRACTICE

The *Guide to Physical Therapist Practice*[2] is a consensus document based on the opinions of more than 800 physical therapist clinicians. A third edition of the guide is in production. The purpose of the guide is to (1) describe generally accepted physical therapist practice, (2) standardize terminology, and (3) identify preferred practice patterns that describe common sets of management strategies used by physical therapists for selected patient/client diagnostic groups. The guide represents a first step in the development of practice guidelines (which are usually based on a comprehensive search of peer-reviewed literature) in that it classifies patients/clients and identifies the range of current options for care. A patient is an individual who receives physical therapy and procedural intervention. A client is someone who is not necessarily sick or injured but could benefit from physical therapy. Clients are also businesses, school systems, and others to whom physical therapists offer services. The guide is not based on clinical research but is intended to promote outcomes research. In addition to physical therapists, the guide was developed for use by health care policy makers, third-party payers, managed care providers, and other health care professionals.

The guide incorporates the concepts of disablement, prevention, and wellness. Part One describes the elements of patient/client management and explains the tests, measures, and interventions performed by physical therapists. Part Two includes the preferred practice patterns grouped into four areas: musculoskeletal, neuromuscular, cardiovascular/ pulmonary, and integumentary. As the guide is presently constituted, the term "preferred practice pattern" is misleading. Practice patterns are broad in scope and inclusive of all procedural interventions that are justifiable. Interventions that are supported by research evidence are not distinguished. The guide is intended to do the following:
1. Enhance the quality of physical therapy

2. Enhance coordination of care among health care providers
3. Improve patient/client satisfaction with physical therapy services
4. Promote appropriate utilization of physical therapy services
5. Increase efficiency of and reimbursement for physical therapy services
6. Promote cost reduction through prevention and wellness initiatives

MODEL OF PATIENT/CLIENT MANAGEMENT

The model of patient/client management is designed to maximize outcomes through a systematic and comprehensive approach to decision making. The model includes five elements: examination, evaluation, diagnosis, prognosis, and intervention leading to optimal outcomes (Figure 1-8).

Examination

The physical therapist is required to perform an examination before providing any intervention. The examination consists of the history, systems review, and selected tests and measures. The history is an account of the child's past and current health status, which is obtained through an interview with the child and caregivers and review of medical and educational records. As part of the history, the physical therapist identifies the child and family expectations and desired outcomes of physical therapy. A useful means for documenting and quantifying family expectations is the Canadian Occupational Performance Measure.[102] The physical therapist then considers whether these expectations and outcomes are realistic in the context of examination and evaluation data.

The systems review is a brief screening that is intended to help focus the subsequent examination and identify possible health problems that require consultation with or referral to another health care provider. A thorough systems review is critical for managing clients who have direct access to physical therapy services. After analyzing information from the history and systems review, the physical therapist examines the child more closely, selecting tests and measures to obtain sufficient data to make an evaluation, establish a diagnosis and a prognosis, and select appropriate interventions. As previously stated, the chapter Screening for Referral and Differential Diagnosis is on the Evolve website.

Evaluation

Evaluation refers to the physical therapist's analysis and synthesis of results of the examination and leads to a physical therapy diagnosis. Evaluation is a process in which the physical therapist makes judgments about the status of the child based on the information gathered from the examination. This step includes judgment of the relationships among impairments in body functions and structures, activity

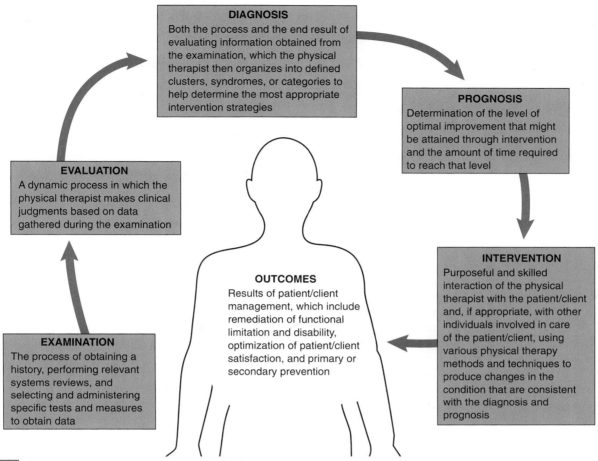

DIAGNOSIS
Both the process and the end result of evaluating information obtained from the examination, which the physical therapist then organizes into defined clusters, syndromes, or categories to help determine the most appropriate intervention strategies

PROGNOSIS
Determination of the level of optimal improvement that might be attained through intervention and the amount of time required to reach that level

EVALUATION
A dynamic process in which the physical therapist makes clinical judgments based on data gathered during the examination

OUTCOMES
Results of patient/client management, which include remediation of functional limitation and disability, optimization of patient/client satisfaction, and primary or secondary prevention

INTERVENTION
Purposeful and skilled interaction of the physical therapist with the patient/client and, if appropriate, with other individuals involved in care of the patient/client, using various physical therapy methods and techniques to produce changes in the condition that are consistent with the diagnosis and prognosis

EXAMINATION
The process of obtaining a history, performing relevant systems reviews, and selecting and administering specific tests and measures to obtain data

Figure 1-8 The elements of patient/client management leading to optimal outcomes. (Reprinted from *Guide to Physical Therapist Practice* with the permission of the American Physical Therapy Association.)

limitations, participation restrictions, and the influence of environmental and personal factors. We encourage therapists to consider child, family, and community strengths as part of the evaluation process. Strength-based and ability-focused interventions build on the strengths and resources of the youth, family, and community.[140]

Diagnosis

The physical therapy diagnosis is a label encompassing a cluster of signs, syndromes, or categories. The diagnosis is reached through the evaluation process and is intended to guide the physical therapist in determining the most appropriate interventions for each child and family. Diagnosis as an element of physical therapy management does not refer to the medical diagnosis (disease or pathophysiology). Rather, the diagnosis involves patients/clients who are grouped by impairments of the musculoskeletal, neuromuscular, cardiopulmonary, or integumentary system. Diagnosis is associated with a preferred pattern of patient/client management that identifies the range of current options for care. A more

in-depth discussion of diagnosis is provided in the Evolve chapter Screening for Referral and Differential Diagnosis.

Prognosis

Perhaps the greatest challenge to patient/client management is determination of the likely outcomes of intervention. Prognosis refers to the predicted optimal level of improvement in function and the amount or intensity of service needed to reach that level (frequency and duration of intervention). A trend in managed health care is to use periodic and episodic intervals of therapy services based on specific functional problems. This approach is a marked departure for children with developmental disabilities for whom ongoing services have traditionally been reimbursed based on medical diagnosis. Presently, therapists have limited evidence to guide decisions on level of service. At this point in the process of patient/client management, the physical therapist establishes a plan of care that includes the following:
1. Long-term and short-term goals and expected outcomes
2. Intervention procedures and techniques

3. Recommendations for duration and frequency of intervention
4. Discharge criteria

In the guide, expected outcomes are the changes that are anticipated as a result of implementing the plan of care. Expected outcomes should be measurable and time limited. Outcomes of therapy include changes in health, wellness, and fitness, an emerging area of pediatric practice.

Having identified the need for intervention, the therapist's next important decision is the plan of care. What are the goals and expected outcomes, what interventions should be implemented, how often, and for how long? Such decisions are frequently sources of professional conflict because members of each discipline view the child's needs from their unique perspectives and may identify entirely different outcomes and potential solutions for the same constellation of impairments, activity limitations, and participation restrictions. Even when clinicians agree on overall outcomes, priorities may differ.[15] The resolution of such conflicts through the use of effective team consensus-building processes, however, can lead to elegant program plans that truly meet clients' needs. Both preventive and ameliorative approaches may be necessary; however, both stages of life and stages of the disease or condition affect the decision regarding which outcomes are the most important to attain in the limited time that is likely to be available.[20]

For example, if primary impairments can be limited by early therapy, some activity limitations that would otherwise result as a part of the natural history of a condition may be avoided. Thus, prevention involves attempts to limit impairment resulting from the lesion or disorder and to promote developmentally appropriate, functional abilities. For example, most therapists believe that early intervention for children with spastic diplegia produces a more efficient later gait. Little research exists to document such effects, however. One of the few studies that suggests such a relationship is a comparison of early (before 9 months) versus late Vojta therapy that reported that children whose treatment began before 9 months of age walked earlier, on average, and with better postural alignment than did those treated later.[91] Theoretically, early intervention should also result in prevention or reduction of secondary impairments, such as contractures and skeletal deformities that are not generally present as primary impairments in early infancy. Rather, they develop later as a result of habitual movement using compensatory patterns or overactive muscles with paretic antagonists or as a result of overall poverty of movement and disuse. Barbosa and colleagues[9] have also shown that infants who are later diagnosed as having cerebral palsy may show regression in lower extremity skills at 3 to 4 months of age. Research is needed to evaluate whether this loss of skills could be prevented. Until we develop tests that clearly separate elements of underlying impairment from activity limitations that may be primary or may result from use of compensatory strategies to enhance function, we will be unable to document the value of early or preventive intervention for cerebral palsy and other conditions present in early childhood. With appropriate measurement tools available, studies of the efficacy and effectiveness of early intervention at the impairment level will be possible. Until such time as this information is available, however, therapists will continue to come into conflict with physicians and other professionals (including other therapists) who believe that intervention does not need to begin early or can be carried out solely by parents, does not need to include procedural interventions by therapists, and should be aimed at provision of compensatory strategies to increase function rather than address underlying impairment.

When activity limitations persist for long periods and are not remediable or cannot be compensated for, children may fail to succeed in normal life roles, such as participation in school, play, or family activities. Therapy planning should start with interdisciplinary assessment of activity and participation in natural environments when a condition that impairs developmental progress and functional capabilities is already well established. This involves asking which roles and skills are needed and appropriate for a child at his or her particular stage of life and must involve the family and teachers as full participants in the examination process. In the case of our example of the child with spastic diplegia, walking in the community is a long-term goal but an important decision is whether the child should be transported at the moment to allow him or her greater participation in family outings. Other members of the rehabilitation team will have their own unique contributions to make to the solution of the problems of lack of mobility and other functional limitations. Giangreco[56] emphasized that *all* professionals should have the same goals rather than separate disciplinary goals when intervention takes place in a school setting.

Environmental setting is an important consideration for deciding on mobility methods and interventions. Research suggests that children with cerebral palsy are more dependent on adult assistance and use wheeled mobility most often when outdoors or in the community.[124,165] Therapy services for children in educational settings in the United States is, by law, aimed at improving participation in the education program in the least restrictive environment. Therapists, teachers, families, and other professionals must all be clear regarding these priorities and realize that decision making for school therapy may not address all the therapy needs of children with disabilities.

Research on intensity of therapy services is limited and perspectives often vary considerably among families, therapists, administrators, policy makers, and health insurers. Palisano and Murr[127] presented five considerations for decision making: (1) episodes of therapy with identified goals versus continuous services, (2) the child's readiness to achieve goals for activity and participation, (3) method of service delivery, (4) the distinction between intensity of therapy and amount of time spent practicing a motor skill, and (5) the relationship between skill level and method of service delivery. Research has primarily addressed intensity of direct individual therapy services. Other methods of service delivery that have received less attention include small group, large group, consultation, and monitoring. These methods are discussed in Chapter 30: The Educational Environment. A child who receives 1 hour/week of physical therapy for 3 months spends 12 hours practicing under the supervision of a therapist. If the child spends 15 minutes/day for 3 months practicing the activity in natural settings, the total amount of practice outside of scheduled therapy is 22.5 hours. The authors concluded that method of service delivery and intensity of therapy may differ for each episode of therapy based on contextual factors, including child and family priorities and goals. In most situations, more than one method of service delivery can and should occur simultaneously.

Intervention

Intervention is the purposeful and skilled interaction of the physical therapist with the patient/client and, when appropriate, with other individuals involved in patient/client care. Various physical therapy procedures and techniques are used during intervention to enable the child and family to achieve goals and outcomes that are consistent with the child's diagnosis and prognosis. Physical therapy intervention has three components: (1) coordination, communication, and documentation; (2) patient/client instruction; and (3) procedural interventions.

Coordination, Communication, and Documentation

These services are provided for all children and their families to ensure appropriate, coordinated, comprehensive, and cost-effective care and efficient integration or reintegration into home, community, and work (job/school/play). Services may include (1) case management, (2) coordination of care with family and other professionals, (3) discharge planning, (4) education plans, (5) case conferences, and (6) documentation of all elements of patient/client management. Based on our experience in tailoring continuing education experiences for the needs of physical therapists, this is an area of particular challenge. Children with disabilities are managed in a variety of settings, from public schools to private offices or rehabilitation facilities to specialty clinics for orthotics, surgery, and assistive technology. Therapists in each of these settings complain of the lack of coordination of services among settings and the paucity of effective and timely information sharing among health professionals, teachers, and families.

Patient/Client-Related Instruction

These services are provided for all families to provide information about the child's current condition, the plan of care, and future transition to home, work, or community roles. Methods of instruction include demonstration; modeling;

verbal, written, or pictorial instruction; and periodic reexamination and reassessment of the home program. The educational backgrounds, needs, and learning styles of family members must be considered during this process. As part of family-centered services, therapists collaborate with children and families to identify how to incorporate exercise and practice of functional movements in daily activities and routines.

Procedural Interventions

Procedural interventions provided by physical therapists include (1) therapeutic exercise; (2) functional training in self-care and home management; (3) functional training in the community and at work (job/school/play); (4) manual therapy techniques; (5) prescription, application, and fabrication of devices and equipment; (6) airway clearance techniques; and (7) physical agents and mechanical modalities. The first three interventions listed are included most often in the plan of care.

Outcomes

At each step of patient/client management, the physical therapist considers the possible outcomes. The therapist also engages in outcome data collection and analysis. Outcomes include optimization of health status, activity and participation, prevention of disability, and optimization of patient/client satisfaction through achievement of goals deemed important by the child or family.[92] Horn and colleagues[81] have introduced and tested an innovation in documenting outcomes of intervention, which therapists can use to show that treatment of impairments results in functional improvements that generalize to settings outside the immediate treatment environment. Three domains that appear repeatedly in the research on interpersonal aspects of care are information exchange, respectful and supportive care, and partnership and enabling.[96] In a review of research on family-centered care, Rosenbaum and associates[140] concluded that parents of children with physical disabilities have positive perceptions of how services are provided to their children but are not as satisfied with information exchange.

PREFERRED PRACTICE PATTERNS

The preferred practice patterns in the *Guide to Physical Therapist Practice* are organized by the five elements of patient/client management. Most preferred practice patterns are applicable to both children and adults. The three patterns specific to children are Neuromuscular Pattern B: Impaired Neuromotor Development, Neuromuscular Pattern C: Impaired Motor Function and Sensory Integrity Associated with Congenital or Acquired Disorders of the Central Nervous System in Infancy, Childhood, and Adolescence, and Cardiovascular/Pulmonary Pattern G: Impaired Ventilation, Respiration/Gas Exchange, and Aerobic Capacity/Endurance associated with Respiratory Failure in the

Neonate. The *Guide to Physical Therapist Practice* does not specifically address physical therapist practice in early intervention and in the public schools. Public laws and guidelines for physical therapist practice in these settings are presented in Chapters 29, 30, and 32.

EVALUATING INTERVENTION OUTCOMES

Physical therapists typically evaluate the effectiveness of an intervention by comparing the child's performance on preset short- and long-term goals and outcomes developed in collaboration with the child and family. How can we be certain that the outcomes we identify are really the result of our intervention and not the effect of other interventions, of natural development, or of recovery? And how can we be sure that our interventions do not result in unintended negative consequences?

CASE REPORTS

A first step in assessing intervention outcomes (in a nonexperimental fashion) is to develop, conduct, and write a case report or series of case reports on one or more children in one's caseload. Although case reports do not employ the controls needed to establish cause-and-effect relationships, they *are* helpful in deriving clinical hypotheses or "hunches" about why a specific intervention may or may not be effective for a particular child.[7] In her excellent manual for clinicians on how to write case reports, McEwen[108] stated that a case report is intended to describe practice and does not involve research methodology. McEwen went on to point out that case reports provide an excellent mechanism to enable practicing therapists to integrate best research evidence with their own clinical expertise and patient values and choices. Case reports require that therapists review the relevant research literature, develop measurable therapy objectives for the children they plan to include, assess the reliability of those outcome measures, and describe the children's histories, previous treatments, examination results, and medical characteristics in rich detail. In the case reports manual, McEwen has outlined each of these steps, relating them to the *Guide to Physical Therapist Practice*. There are many diverse examples of case reports in the pediatric rehabilitation literature[1,11,90,93,110] as well as recent examples of case series.[37,53,89] However, there is a need for many more case reports and case series if we are to truly call ourselves evidence-based practitioners.

SINGLE-SUBJECT RESEARCH

One clinical decision tool that has been used increasingly by pediatric physical therapists to assess the effectiveness of their interventions is the single-subject research design. The single-subject design is an experimental paradigm that is particularly useful for practicing clinicians who wish to study intensively the effects of intervention on individual patients within their caseload.[58,72]

Nearly all pediatric physical therapists must develop individualized, measurable objectives for the children with whom they work as part of "best-practice" procedure, and the single-subject design represents a logical extension of this procedure. In developing individual behavioral objectives, therapists are required to specify patient outcomes that are expected to change as a result of introducing intervention. These behavioral objectives are analogous to outcome measures that are a form of *dependent variable,* a term that is universal to all types of experimental research designs.

A second major component of experimental research is selection of the independent variable or, in the case of physical therapy, the specific treatment technique that is being applied in an effort to effect positive change in the outcome variable. Obviously, careful treatment planning for the pediatric patient involves not only the selection of the outcome or target behavior, as represented in the individualized therapy objective, but also selection of a specific treatment technique that is designed to enhance change or facilitate improvement in the outcome behavior. In comparing the single-subject research design to physical therapy as it is typically provided in a clinical setting, Gonnella[58] stated that the first few steps are similar: the problem behavior is identified, baseline data are collected on the problem behavior, a treatment plan is developed and implemented, and changes in the problem behavior are assessed. However, several important differences exist between the single-subject design and the therapeutic model.

Whereas typically only one baseline assessment is taken in the therapeutic model, single-subject design mandates that a minimum of three data points be collected on the outcome behavior before treatment is introduced.[10] A second criterion of single-subject research is that a specific design should be implemented that involves sequential application and withdrawal of the intervention. Finally, performance must be measured repeatedly (and frequently) throughout each phase of the design. For a visual comparison of these two models as described and depicted by Gonnella[58] (Figure 1-9). Other important criteria of single-subject research designs are that the data collection procedures are both replicable and reliable.[118] Percentage agreement is typically used to assess consistency of scoring the behavioral objectives or outcome measures between two or more independent raters.

In his excellent text on single-subject designs for occupational and physical therapists, Ottenbacher[118] outlined six important steps for setting up such designs: (1) determining the setting in which the behavior or performance will be observed and recorded, (2) deciding on the method to collect data, (3) determining the length of time that the behavior will be observed and measured, (4) observing and recording client behavior, (5) recording and plotting the data collected, and (6) continuing the measurement and recording procedures until requirements of the design have been satisfied.

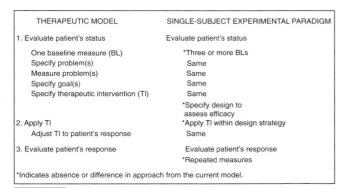

THERAPEUTIC MODEL	SINGLE-SUBJECT EXPERIMENTAL PARADIGM
1. Evaluate patient's status	Evaluate patient's status
One baseline measure (BL)	*Three or more BLs
Specify problem(s)	Same
Measure problem(s)	Same
Specify goal(s)	Same
Specify therapeutic intervention (TI)	Same
	*Specify design to assess efficacy
2. Apply TI	*Apply TI within design strategy
Adjust TI to patient's response	Same
3. Evaluate patient's response	Evaluate patient's response
	*Repeated measures

*Indicates absence or difference in approach from the current model.

Figure 1-9 Comparison of therapeutic process with single-subject paradigm. (From Gonnella, C. [1989]. Single-subject experimental paradigm as a clinical decision tool. *Physical Therapy, 69,* 603. Reprinted from *Physical Therapy* with the permission of the American Physical Therapy Association.)

Because the Ottenbacher text is no longer in print, pediatric physical therapists who wish to set up single-subject designs in their own clinical settings are advised to consult recent single-subject design texts by Gast[55] or Janosky and colleagues,[84] as well as other references in the physical therapy literature that describe this important clinical decision tool.[58,72]

Since the early 1980s, pediatric physical and occupational therapists have used single-subject designs to examine the effects of "tone-reducing" (inhibitive) casts and orthoses in improving gait and standing balance in children with cerebral palsy;[74,79] to evaluate the influence of some specific, well-defined, neurodevelopmental treatment techniques on increasing heel contact[101] and decreasing knee flexion during gait[44] in children with cerebral palsy; to assess the effects of two different treatment approaches (behavior modification and a neurophysiologic approach) in reducing tongue protrusion in young children with Down syndrome;[136] and to examine the effects of different modes of mobility on school performance of children with myelodysplasia.[54] These are but a sampling of the published reports that have used single-subject designs to examine treatment effectiveness in children with developmental disabilities. Single-subject designs have been used also to examine the effect of passive range-of-motion (ROM) exercises on lower-extremity goniometric measurements of six adults with cerebral palsy, ranging in age from 20 to 44 years,[17] and to determine the effectiveness of a modified version of constraint-induced movement therapy on a child under the age of 1 year with hemiplegic cerebral palsy.[29]

In the following paragraphs, two published single-subject studies will be described—one involving two children with spastic diplegia and the other involving three children with myelodysplasia. Reference will be made to the ICF model in discussing the goals and outcomes of each of these studies.

In a single-subject study published in 1988, Hinderer and colleagues set out to evaluate the relative effects of tone-reducing casts and standard plaster casts on gait

characteristics and functional locomotor activities in two young children with cerebral palsy.[79] The first child (case 1) was a 3.5-year-old boy with mild spastic diplegia and mild mental retardation; spasticity was greater on the right. Some of the impairments noted in this child included gait deviations such as moderate in-toeing on the right, decreased stride length on the left, toe-dragging, forefoot weight bearing, limited trunk rotation, and high-guard posture of the upper extremities. Activity limitations included the inability to walk up and down stairs without support and the inability to squat or rise to standing without support.

The second child (case 2) was a girl, age 5 years 9 months, with asymmetrical spastic diplegia (greater involvement on the left), moderate ataxia, and normal intelligence quotient (IQ). Impairments included poor static and dynamic balance and unsteady gait with frequent falling. Specific gait deviations consisted of mild in-toeing on the left and difficulty with left toe clearance, limited trunk rotation, and a wide base of support. Activity limitations that resulted from these impairments included the inability to walk backward and balance on one leg and the need for upper extremity support to climb stairs and to move from squatting to standing.

An A-B-A-C crossover single-subject design was used in this study to evaluate the effects of the two different types of casts (the independent variables or specific intervention techniques). Tone-reducing casts were defined as those that "maintain the ankle at zero degrees and stabilize the toes and foot in neutral alignment by incorporating a footplate which supports the toes and the metatarsal, peroneal and longitudinal arches of the foot."[79] Standard plaster casts held the ankle in neutral alignment but did not include a footplate.

The study began with both children in a baseline (A1) phase (no casts). In the second phase of the study, case 1 wore tone-reducing casts (B) and case 2 wore standard casts (C). Then the baseline condition (A2) was reinstituted for both subjects, after which the crossover of treatments occurred so that the design for case 1 was A1-B-A2-C and the design for case 2 was A1-C-A2-B.

Outcome measures (target behaviors) included footprint data used to analyze various gait parameters, specific developmentally appropriate fine motor tasks, and videotaped ratings by an interdisciplinary panel of experts on gait and functional motor activities. Data were collected two or three times per week for 19 weeks. The number of data points per phase ranged from 5 to 12. Inter-rater percentage agreement for the gait measures was 96.1% and for the fine motor measures was 97.4%. Anecdotal impressions were obtained also from parents of the two children and their treating therapists.

One of the benefits of sequential application and withdrawal of interventions, as occurs in single-subject designs, is the ability to control for natural history, developmental maturation, and practice effects. Analysis of the fine motor data for the children in this study revealed that their performance continued to improve even during the baseline (no-cast) phases, thus suggesting that practice of these tasks was contributing more to their improvement than were the specific interventions. In a typical therapeutic model as described by Gonnella[58] (see Figure 1-9), such control is not possible and the treating therapist might assume that the improvements are due to the intervention itself, whereas such improvements may, in fact, be due to practicing the task or to other intervening variables such as developmental maturation.

Another benefit of this particular crossover design is the opportunity to compare two different interventions. Greater increases in stride length were noted for both children during the tone-reducing cast phases as compared with the standard cast condition. Blinded videotape analysis by the panel of experts revealed mild gait improvements for case 2 during the tone-reducing cast phase and improvements in standing balance, ability to walk backward, and ability to squat and return to upright. Owing to poor adherence by case 1, a standardized sequence of gait and functional motor activities was not obtained.

Although this study provided some limited support for the relative benefits of tone-reducing casts as compared with standard casts, the authors concluded by making a plea for practitioners to document their own outcomes of tone-reducing casts and orthoses: "Single-subject research designs offer a clinically appropriate means for reliably studying their effectiveness, and are particularly indicated when studying a heterogeneous population, such as individuals with cerebral palsy, whose clinical presentation varies from day to day."[79]

Another single-subject study compared the relative effects of assistive device ambulation (walker or crutches) and wheelchair mobility on three school performance measures for children with myelodysplasia.[54] Subjects were three students aged 9, 10, and 15 years with L4 or L5 level myelomeningocele, all of whom had a physiologic cost index (an indicator of energy efficiency) of greater than 1.00 beat per meter when ambulating with assistive devices. The independent variables or specific interventions in this study were the assistive ambulation devices and the wheelchair. Outcomes assessed were reading fluency, visuomotor accuracy, and manual dexterity. A convincing rationale for this study was the frequent encouragement of ambulation for children with lumbar-level lesions in spite of the high energy costs.[171]

In the case of these children with lumbar-level lesions, the pathophysiologic condition (myelodysplasia) led to impairments, including lower extremity paralysis, which had then resulted in activity limitations in gait and upright mobility. Basically, this study sought to examine whether ambulation, when energy cost is high, had a negative effect on school performance (participation). To examine these questions, an alternating condition single-subject design was used in which phase 1 was wheelchair propulsion, phase 2 was ambulation with crutches or walker, and phase 3 was again wheelchair propulsion. Each phase was 1 week in length (5 school days), with data collected daily on the three outcome measures: correct words per minute of a 100- to 200-word reading passage (reading fluency); visuomotor accuracy as assessed by the Motor Accuracy Test, Revised;[5] and manual dexterity as assessed on the Purdue Pegboard Assembly subtest.[166] Although reading fluency was unaffected by the method of mobility and manual dexterity varied across the three subjects and the two treatment conditions, visuomotor accuracy scores were significantly lower for all three subjects during the assistive ambulation phase.

In an accompanying commentary on this article, Haley concluded the following:

> [I]mplications of this study may cause us to step back from our often aggressive posture toward functional ambulation at all costs. If assisted ambulation is not energy efficient, time efficient, or safe or leads to an interruption in social, emotional, or cognitive growth, then alternate means of mobility must be considered. Is not the aim of the physical therapist to promote overall development rather than to promote ambulation at a significant cost? Is not efficient, independent mobility the real functional goal for children and their families?[64]

It is exactly these types of questions that we face daily in our clinical decision making as pediatric physical therapists. Using single-subject studies to systematically examine effects of specific interventions and replicating these studies across other subjects in other clinical settings will assist in allowing us to answer such questions. Therapists are encouraged to consult three references[6,7,134] that provide more information and examples of different types of single-subject designs commonly used in rehabilitation settings. Levels of evidence and quality or rigor questions have been developed recently to enable critical review of published studies using single-subject research designs.[133]

It is the responsibility of all practicing therapists, be they clinicians, researchers, or educators, to provide ethically responsible and effective interventions for their clients. Systematic examination of intervention outcomes, through such strategies as the single-subject design, can assist us in attaining this goal. Despite the value of single-subject studies and case reports for generating evidence in support of practice, pediatric physical therapists can increase the generalizability of findings by going beyond an n-of-1 to study of the results of management of a group of clients with similar conditions from their own practice. Kaplan[92] provided instruction in using retrospective chart review to both study outcomes and improve documentation to increase the value of record review. She reminded us that if it is not in the record, it did not happen, and encouraged physical therapists to reflect on their practice by studying whether they are achieving the outcomes intended and whether these outcomes are systematically documented.

MONITORING SERVICES WITH A DATABASE

Developments in the area of monitoring services and tracking outcomes include computerized approaches to creating a database on patients served that may also provide systematic, structured individual patient reports to guarantee uniform reporting of significant information across both therapists and types of patients.[85,155,157] A database is a generalized set of computer programs that allows (1) entry of a variety of data by different authorized users; (2) organization of the data for storage; and (3) retrieval, updating, reorganization, and printing of output in the form of summary reports.[103] Yearly statistics can be rapidly collated, care trends can be monitored across time, and data can be used for prospective or retrospective research.[157] Use of a database approach can guard against errors of both omission and commission by structuring therapists' reports and by automatically providing checks of entered data against a range of appropriate responses. Development of national databases on specific client populations can form the basis for improving practice through comparison of institutional or regional differences in management strategies, identifying infrequent negative outcomes, and studying low-incidence conditions.

Slagle and Gould[157] emphasized that only 27% of tertiary care neonatal units, responding to a national survey of database use, monitored the accuracy of their data, an essential element of a high-quality plan. Users liked their system best if it generated patient records, such as discharge summaries. In addition to these critical issues, Jenkins[85] suggested that database developers should consider what aspects of care are likely to change over time in order to develop a system that is flexible in meeting long-term needs. Developers should consider how to collect enough data to be maximally useful for meeting such diverse needs as preparing annual reports and answering important research questions, while eliminating large amounts of data that are easy to collect but unlikely to be used.[157] In addition, a specific plan for maintaining overall quality of the database should be developed.[157]

In response to the growing trend for health care accountability, the Joint Commission on Accreditation of Healthcare Organizations (JCAHO) has incorporated the use of outcomes and other performance measures into the accreditation process.[153] JCAHO requirements focus on clinical performance measures designed to evaluate both the processes and outcomes of care. Processes of care include measures of patient satisfaction. The Measure of Processes of Caregiving[96] is a parent report measure for use in programs serving children with developmental disabilities. Two pediatric outcome measures for which there is an external data system are the Functional Independence Measure for Children[13] through the Uniform Data System for Medical Rehabilitation, Buffalo, New York, and the Pediatric Evaluation of Disability Inventory[65,66] through the Center for Rehabilitation Effectiveness, Boston, Massachusetts. Hashimoto and

McCoy[71] provided evidence of content validity of an activity-based data form developed for pediatric physical therapy practice. The form was designed to quickly document type of activity, time spent on each type of activity, and specific intervention strategies and procedures that are coded numerically. The form could be adapted for electronic data entry using a handheld computer.

PROGRAM EVALUATION

Although physical therapists frequently believe that they have done their professional jobs thoroughly when they have appropriately documented outcomes for individual children, professional practice requires additional evaluation of the overall impact and costs of physical therapy programs. Here, the tools include formal program evaluations and quality assurance strategies involving evaluation of record keeping; monitoring of therapist adherence to program policies; assessment of interactions with clients, other providers, and third-party payers; and evaluation of client satisfaction and long-term outcomes.

Formal program evaluation is a comprehensive approach to assessing program effectiveness.[154] The explicit purpose of formal program evaluation is to assess the effects of programs in meeting their stated goals for the purpose of improving subsequent decision making about the program and, in a broader sense, for improving future program planning. Evaluation theory, although initially idealistic, has been expanded and revised based on the experience of program evaluators operating in the real world. These experiences have led to the recognition that (1) the achievement of stated goals may not be the only useful product of a social program; (2) there are many stakeholders involved in the typical program, some of whom are more concerned that the interests of their particular group are addressed than that program goals have been achieved; and (3) politics always act on programs in ways that may be difficult to identify but may mean that program evaluation results are not likely to change programs effectively in major ways.

Program evaluation results are usually considered to be of two major types: formative (evaluation for the purpose of improving the program and understanding the processes by which the program operates) and summative (outcomes or products). The latter makes the supposition that an outcome of the evaluation itself might be abolition of the program; the former generally assumes that the program will continue to exist and that better ways of improving the product or the provision of services are sought. Because studies of the uses to which evaluation results are put have generally shown that effects trickle down into new-generation programs, producing slow, incremental change rather than resulting in revolutions in thinking and implementation, recent theorists have emphasized that evaluation results may be most usefully thought of as being "enlightening"—that is, having future use for program planners in thinking about issues, defining problems, and developing new perspectives and ideas.

Those who formulate policy and implement programs seldom actively search for evidence, or if they do, they tend to use whatever fits with their current understanding of the problem under study. Information such as this has led to important studies of the uses of program evaluation and theoretic formulations regarding how information can be most usefully disseminated. Whatever the purpose, program evaluation must be conducted based on the identified needs for the program and how well it satisfies the needs identified, as well as meets the needs that might not have been previously identified but happen to be satisfied by the program. The best program evaluation designs also search for potential negative effects, such as those identified by the study of Franks and colleagues[54] on mobility in children with myelodysplasia.

Arguments have arisen among program evaluation theorists regarding the value of quantitative versus qualitative evaluation methods. The randomized, controlled clinical trial remains, at least in medical arenas, the most highly valued summative assessment of intervention outcomes, and is especially valuable in studies of intervention with children because of the control needed to rule out the effects of maturation and other threats to internal validity[116,154] Combined with causal modeling of the theoretically and empirically derived processes and factors influencing outcomes, clinical trials are most powerful in studies with large numbers of subjects or in studies seeking to identify low-incidence but potentially highly dangerous unintended negative effects. Designing pragmatic or practical clinical trials to specifically address questions stemming from practice increases the value of such experimental designs.[168]

Qualitative methods offer flexibility, a dynamic quality, and a unique ability to reflect the world from the perspective of multiple program stakeholders and participants. They are especially well suited for gathering answers to formative questions about the quality of program implementation and its meaning to participants. Qualitative methods may also be used to study the processes by which programs achieve useful outcomes in meeting needs of patients and society. Of most importance, however, are methods appropriate to the level of development of the program (e.g., early development stage program, innovative demonstration project, established ongoing program), the problematic issues of concern to program stakeholders of various types, decisions under the control of the program to be made at a time when evaluation results will be available, and the level of uncertainty regarding critical program features. Methods tailored to these factors are most likely to result in effective use of program evaluation results.

The combination of formative and summative evaluation is recommended for examining methods of service delivery and the overall effectiveness of therapy programs. Wang and Ellett[170] used the term *program validation* to describe a form of evaluative research useful in the development and refinement of innovative educational programs. The major purposes of program validation are to (1) obtain empirical evidence of the effectiveness of an innovative program, (2) identify aspects of the program that require improvement in order to achieve the intended outcomes, and (3) evaluate the feasibility of implementing the innovative program. Wolery and Bailey[173] have proposed that a comprehensive evaluation of early intervention programs addresses the following questions:

1. Does the method of service delivery represent the best educational practice?
2. Is the intervention being implemented accurately and consistently?
3. Is an attempt being made to verify the effectiveness of the intervention objectively?
4. Does the program carefully monitor patient progress and demonstrate sensitivity to points at which changes in service need to be made?
5. Does a system exist for determining the adequacy of patient progress and service delivery?
6. Is the program accomplishing its goals and objectives?
7. Does the service delivery system meet the needs and values of the community and clients it serves?

The questions proposed by Wolery and Bailey offer a framework for program evaluation of physical therapy services provided in a variety of settings, including the school system, acute care and rehabilitation hospitals for children, and private practices.

Two studies serve to illustrate the scope of program evaluation and how questions are developed specific to particular programs. Both occurred in educational settings where research on physical therapy services is limited. Palisano[119] evaluated two methods of therapy service delivery provided to students with learning disabilities who attended public school. To adequately serve approximately 500 students receiving occupational therapy and physical therapy, the therapy staff of the intermediate unit had instituted group and consultation methods for providing services to students with learning disabilities who met eligibility criteria for therapy as a related service. The therapists and teachers of students who participated in the study had worked together during the previous school year using the two methods of service delivery. Students in classrooms that received a combination of large-group and small-group therapy were compared with students in classrooms that received large-group therapy and consultation. Methods of evaluation included student progress in motor, visuomotor, and visuoperceptual skills; the therapy needs of each group; teacher satisfaction; and use of available therapy resources. Both methods appeared to represent sound practice. Interaction between the therapist and the teacher in establishing goals and planning group sessions was identified as integral to the success of both methods of service delivery. Recommendations for the following year included placing greater emphasis on achievement of functional goals, establishing group behavioral objectives, and examining similarities and differences between the services provided by occupational therapy and physical therapy.

Stuberg and DeJong[159] performed a program evaluation of physical therapy as an Early Intervention and Related Service in a public school district that employed 18 physical therapists. The district's philosophy of service delivery was to initially provide consultation and then, as needed, direct services. Therapists were also instructed to make sure that goals for impairments had a clear relationship to the child's participation in either the home or school environment. Over two school years, data were collected on a non-random sample of 690 students using the Individualized Education Plan (IEP) and the Individualized Family Service Plan (IFSP) as the primary sources of data. Most children were classified as having other health impairments (diagnoses such as developmental coordination disorder, congenital heart defects, or mild juvenile rheumatoid arthritis) or orthopedic impairments (diagnoses such as spastic diplegic cerebral palsy, spina bifida, or amputee). Ninety-one percent of the 2228 IFSP and IEP objectives analyzed were scored as having been met or progress made. Seventy-three percent of the goals addressed functional limitations. The majority of objectives were addressed through integration of services into the education program (43%), followed by direct (35%) and consultative (22%) methods of service delivery. Of interest was the finding that children who received a total of 12 hours or less of physical therapy during the school year demonstrated higher scores for goal attainment than children who received greater than 12 hours of service. Factors that may have mediated this finding, such as severity of health condition, were not analyzed. The authors concluded that the high attainment of IEP and IFSP objectives suggests a positive effect of physical therapy on the educational programs of the children. They emphasized that a causal relationship between the therapy and the outcomes cannot be implied.

KNOWLEDGE TRANSLATION

Knowledge translation (KT) is the process by which relevant research information is applied to practice, planning, and policy making. Knowledge transfer, translation, utilization, and uptake are also used to describe the process by which research is applied to decision making in health care. Knowledge translation is based on the assumptions that "quality services" and "best practices" are evidence-based and that an intervention is modified or discarded when there is no evidence of effectiveness or it is not acceptable to patients. Technology such as the Internet has led to an explosion in availability and access to information. Despite technologic advances, research in health care is slow to be applied. Publications, presentations, and other means of dissemination

do not ensure that research will be applied to practice. As a consequence, federal agencies such as the Agency for Healthcare Research and Quality and the National Institutes of Health have advocated that research proposals include a plan for knowledge translation.

Given the plethora of evidence available in the literature, should we not expect that all pediatric physical therapists would practice evidence-based care? What motivates physical therapists to try a new intervention? To what extent are these decisions guided by evidence? Why do therapists persist with interventions despite evidence to the contrary? These questions illustrate that attitudes and beliefs may shape therapists' practice behaviors.

New studies are constantly emerging that examine the barriers to evidence-based practice. Rappolt and Tassone[163] identified the following themes regarding how physical therapists and occupational therapists gather, evaluate, and implement new knowledge: (1) unsystematic approach, (2) formal continuing education is highly valued, (3) informal consultation with peers, and (4) resigned to organizational barriers. Research has revealed the following types of barriers: time, lack of critical appraisal skills, the inertia of previous practice, contradictory and highly complex guidelines, and lack of incentives.[130,151,152] Data collected from across the health professions suggest that the time between publication of information that could be used to change practice and application of that knowledge in the everyday world is extremely lengthy.[34,130]

Grimshaw et al.[62] recommended the simultaneous use of multiple knowledge transfer strategies, especially active, interpersonal approaches. Strategies should be geared to the target group such as practitioners, administrators, or policy makers. Ketelaar et al.[95] described strategies used to increase knowledge translation and use of the Gross Motor Function Measure (GMFM) and the Gross Motor Function Classification System (GMFCS) in clinical practice in the Netherlands. Knowledge translation strategies included peer-reviewed publications, workshops, and posting information on websites. Peer-reviewed publications did not appear to impact clinical practice. Interactive workshops were more successful at increasing use, but a gap remained between knowledge and use; the transfer into clinical practice was not optimal.

The terms *change agents, knowledge transfer agents,* and *knowledge brokers* are used to describe service providers or program managers who take on a role within their settings to be the translators of new ideas and to support others to become aware of, and comfortable in using, new research findings. A *community of practice* refers to a group of people who share a concern or a passion for something they do and learn how to do it better as they interact regularly. Quality assurance activities, such as case reviews and journal clubs, facilitate communities of practice, as do local, regional, and national pediatric special interest groups. Physical therapy managers are encouraged to facilitate knowledge translation and consider providing release time to a staff member who is a champion of evidence-based practice. The website for Knowledge Translation Canada (http://ktclearinghouse.ca/ktcanada) is recommended as a resource.

SUMMARY

Evidence-based decision making is integral to determining who needs physical therapy and why, how cases should be managed, how outcomes should be documented, and what methods should be used for evaluating the effectiveness of interventions. Pediatric physical therapists are becoming increasingly aware of the need to base their clinical decisions on the best available knowledge and research evidence. This involves finding and appraising research reports, systematic reviews, clinical practice guidelines and pathways, and applying evidence to practice. Translation of evidence to practice occurs within the context of child and family identified needs. Sharing information with children and families in useful and acceptable formats encourages their active participation in decision making. The statement by Guyatt and colleagues[63] that "research is never enough" acknowledges the need for therapists to have a strong knowledge base, problem solve, and make sound judgments based on expert consensus and personal practice knowledge. Conceptual frameworks like the International Classification of Functioning, Disability and Health, the Hypothesis-Oriented Algorithm for Clinicians II, and the Elements of Patient/Client Management can improve clinical reasoning and the decision-making process. Practitioners can also become part of knowledge networks, reflect on their documentation practices as a basis for examining the outcomes of their work, and collaborate with researchers in academic institutions as strategies for rapidly transferring knowledge into everyday practice.

Although physical therapists typically evaluate outcomes on the basis of whether children achieve short- and long-term goals or demonstrate improvement on standardized assessments of motor development and function, these methods do not indicate whether the outcomes were the result of intervention, because children are also expected to change as a result of maturational processes. Single-subject research designs provide one clinical decision tool that enables pediatric physical therapists to evaluate the effectiveness of their interventions for individual patients and to discover information of use in future research. In addition to evaluations of individual patient outcomes, professional practice requires evaluation of the overall effectiveness and costs of physical therapy programs. Monitoring of program inputs, implementation, and outputs is enhanced by computerized programs that allow the creation of databases and are capable of generating systematic, structured, individual reports. Formal methods of program evaluation provide information for assessing whether programs meet important consumer and societal needs, are properly implemented for maximal impact, and actually serve targeted populations. Given the changing and complex nature of health care, pediatric physical therapists are challenged to enhance their use of more scientific evidence and more valid and reliable decision methods as the basis for their practice.

ACKNOWLEDGMENTS

The work reported in this chapter was partially supported by grants to S. K. Campbell from the Agency for Healthcare Policy and Research and the National Institute for Child Health and Human Development. S. K. Campbell is the managing member of Infant Motor Performance Scales, LLC, the publisher of the Test of Infant Motor Performance.

REFERENCES

1. Almeida, G. L., Campbell, S. K., Girolami, G. L., Penn, R. D., & Corcos, D. M. (1997). Multi-dimensional assessment of motor function in a child with cerebral palsy following intrathecal administration of baclofen. *Physical Therapy, 77*, 751–764.
2. American Physical Therapy Association. (2001). Guide to physical therapist practice (2nd ed.). *Physical Therapy, 81*, 9–744.
3. Aylward, G. P. (1997). Conceptual issues in developmental screening and assessment. *Developmental and Behavioral Pediatrics, 18*, 340–349.
4. Aylward, G. P., & Kenny, T. J. (1979). Developmental follow-up: Inherent problems and a conceptual model. *Journal of Pediatric Psychology, 4*, 331–343.
5. Ayres, A. J. (1972). *Southern California sensory integration tests.* Los Angeles: Western Psychological Services.
6. Backman, C. L., Harris, S. R., Chisholm, J. M., & Monette, A. D. (1997). Single-subject research in rehabilitation: A review of studies using AB, withdrawal, multiple baseline, and alternating treatment designs. *Archives of Physical Medicine and Rehabilitation, 78*, 1145–1153.
7. Backman, C. L., & Harris, S. R. (1999). Case studies, single subject research, and N of 1 randomized trials: Comparisons and contrasts. *American Journal of Physical Medicine and Rehabilitation, 78*, 170–176.
8. Baird, G., McConachie, H., & Scrutton, D. (2000). Parents' perceptions of disclosure of the diagnosis of cerebral palsy. *Archives of Diseases in Childhood, 83*, 475–480.
9. Barbosa, V. M., Campbell, S. K., Sheftel, D., Singh, J., & Beligere, N. (2003). Longitudinal performance of infants with cerebral palsy on the Test of Infant Motor Performance and on the Alberta Infant Motor Scale. *Physical & Occupational Therapy in Pediatrics, 23*(3), 7–29.
10. Barlow, D. H., Hayes, S. C., & Nelson, R. O. (1984). *The scientist practitioner: Research and accountability in clinical and educational settings.* Elmsford, NY: Pergamon Press.
11. Behrman, A. L., Nair, P. M., Bowden, M. G., Dauser, R. C., et al. (2008). Locomotor training restores walking in a non-ambulatory child with chronic, severe, incomplete spinal cord injury. *Physical Therapy, 88*, 580–590.
12. Reference deleted in page proofs.
13. Braun, S. (1998). Featured instrument. The Functional Independence Measure for Children (WeeFIM instrument):

Gateway to the WeeFIM System. *Journal of Rehabilitation Outcomes Measurement, 2,* 63–68.

14. Reference deleted in page proofs.

15. Butler, C. (1991). Augmentative mobility: Why do it? *Physical Medicine and Rehabilitation Clinics of North America, 2,* 801–815.

16. Byrne, E. M., & Campbell, S. K. (Eds). (forthcoming). A care path for physical therapy in the neonatal intensive care nursery. *Physical and Occupational Therapy in Pediatrics.*

17. Cadenhead, S. L., McEwen, I. R., & Thompson, D. M. (2002). Effect of passive range of motion on lower-extremity goniometric measurements of adults with cerebral palsy: A single-subject design. *Physical Therapy, 82,* 658–669.

18. Campbell, S. K. (Ed.). (1990). Proceedings of the consensus conference on the efficacy of physical therapy in the management of cerebral palsy. *Pediatric Physical Therapy, 2*(3), 121–176.

19. Campbell, S. K. (1993). Future directions for physical therapy assessment in early infancy. In I. J. Wilhelm (Ed.), *Physical therapy assessment in early infancy* (pp. 293–308). New York: Churchill Livingstone.

20. Campbell, S. K. (1997). Therapy programs for children that last a lifetime. *Physical and Occupational Therapy in Pediatrics, 17*(1), 1–15.

21. Campbell, S. K. (1999). Models for decision making. In S. K. Campbell (Ed.). *Decision making in pediatric neurologic physical therapy* (pp. 1–22). Philadelphia: Churchill Livingstone.

22. Campbell, S. K., Gardner, H. G., & Ramakrishnan, V. (1995). Correlates of physicians' decisions to refer children with cerebral palsy for physical therapy. *Developmental Medicine & Child Neurology, 37,* 1062–1074.

23. Campbell, S. K., & Wilhelm, I. J. (1985). Development from birth to three years of fifteen children at high risk for central nervous system dysfunction. *Physical Therapy, 65,* 463–469.

24. Campbell, S. K., Kolobe, T. H. A., Wright, B. D., & Linacre, J. M. (2002). Validity of the Test of Infant Motor Performance for prediction of 6-, 9-, and 12-month scores on the Alberta Infant Motor Scale. *Developmental Medicine and Child Neurology, 44,* 263–272.

25. Chassin, M. R., & Galvin, R. W. (1998). The urgent need to improve health care quality: Institute of Medicine National Roundtable on Health Care Quality. *Journal of the American Medical Association, 280,* 1000–1005.

26. Chiarello, L. A., Effgen, S. (2006). Update on competencies for physical therapists in early intervention. *Pediatric Physical Therapy, 18,* 148–158.

27. Childs, J. D., & Cleland, J. A. (2006). Development and application of clinical prediction rules to improve decision making in physical therapist practice. *Physical Therapy, 86,* 122–131.

28. Cohen, J. (1988). *Statistical power analysis for the behavioral sciences,* 2nd ed. Hillsdale, NY: Lawrence Erlbaum Associates.

29. Coker, P. M., Lebkicher, C. M., Harris, L. M., & Snape, J. (2009). The effects of constraint-induced movement therapy for a child less than one year of age. *NeuroRehabilitation, 24,* 199–208.

30. Cook, D. J., Mulrow, C. D., & Haynes, R. B. (1997). Systematic reviews: Synthesis of best evidence for clinical decisions. *Annals of Internal Medicine, 126,* 376–380.

31. Creswell, J. W. (2007). *Qualitative inquiry and research design* (2nd ed.). Thousand Oaks, CA: Sage.

32. Damiano, D. L., & DeJong, S. L. (2009). A systematic review of the effectiveness of treadmill training and body weight support in pediatric rehabilitation. *Journal of Neurological Physical Therapy, 33,* 27–44.

33. Darrah, J., Piper, M., & Watt, M. J. (1998). Assessment of gross motor skills of at-risk infants: Predictive validity of the Alberta Infant Motor Scale. *Developmental Medicine and Child Neurology, 40,* 485–491.

34. Davis, D., Evans, M., Jadad, A., et al. (2003). The case for knowledge translation: Shortening the journey from evidence to effect. *British Medical Journal, 327,* 33–35.

35. Daly, J., Willis, K., Small, R., et al. (2007). A hierarchy of evidence for assessing qualitative health research. *Journal of Clinical Epidemiology, 60,* 43–49.

36. Reference deleted in page proofs.

37. de Bode, S., Fritz, S. L., Weir-Haynes, K., & Mathern, G. W. (2009). Constraint-induced movement therapy after cerebral hemispherectomy: a case series. *Physical Therapy, 89,* 361–369.

38. Donaghy, M. E., & Morss, K. (2000). Guided reflection: A framework to facilitate and assess reflective practice within the discipline of physiotherapy. *Physiotherapy Theory and Practice, 16,* 3–14.

39. Echternach, J. L., & Rothstein, J. M. (1989). Hypothesis-oriented algorithms. *Physical Therapy, 69,* 559–564.

40. Effgen, S.K., Chiarello, L., & Milbourne, S.A. (2007). Updated competencies for physical therapists working in schools. *Pediatric Physical Therapy, 19,* 266–274.

41. Embrey, D. G., & Adams, L. S. (1996). Clinical applications of procedural changes by experienced and novice pediatric physical therapists. *Pediatric Physical Therapy, 8,* 122–132.

42. Embrey, D. G., & Hylton, N. (1996). Clinical applications of movement scripts by experienced and novice pediatric physical therapists. *Pediatric Physical Therapy, 8,* 3–14.

43. Embrey, D. G., & Nirider, B. (1996). Clinical applications of psychosocial sensitivity by experienced and novice pediatric physical therapists. *Pediatric Physical Therapy, 8,* 70–79.

44. Embrey, D. G., Yates, L., & Mott, D. H. (1990). Effects of neuro-developmental treatment and orthoses on knee flexion during gait: A single subject design. *Physical Therapy, 70,* 626–637.

45. Embrey, D. G., Yates, L., Nirider, B., Hylton, N., & Adams, L. S. (1996). Recommendations for pediatric physical therapists: Making clinical decisions for children with cerebral palsy. *Pediatric Physical Therapy, 8,* 165–170.

46. Einspieler, C., Prechtl, H. F. R., Bos, A. F., Ferrari, F., & Cioni, G. (2004). *Prechtl's method on the qualitative assessment of*

general movements in preterm, term and young infants. Clinics in Developmental Medicine No. 167. London: Mac Keith Press.

47. Eliasson, A. C., Krumlinde Sundholm, L., et al. (2006). The Manual Ability Classification System (MACS) for children with cerebral palsy: Scale development and evidence of validity and reliability. *Developmental Medicine & Child Neurology, 48,* 549–554.

48. Evidence-Based Medicine Working Group. (1992). Evidence-based medicine: A new approach to teaching the practice of medicine. *Journal of the American Medical Association, 268*(17), 2420–2425.

49. Ferrari, F., Cioni, G., & Prechtl, H. F. R. (1990). Qualitative changes of general movements in preterm infants with brain lesions. *Early Human Development, 23,* 193–231.

50. Ferrari, F., Cioni, G., Einspieler, C., et al. (2002). Cramped synchronized General Movements in preterm infants as an early marker for cerebral palsy. *Archives of Pediatric Adolescent Medicine, 156,* 460–467.

51. Fetters, L., Figueiredo, E. M., Keane-Miller, D., McSweeney, D. J., & Tsao C. C. (2004). Critically appraised topics. *Pediatric Physical Therapy, 16,* 19–21.

52. Fleming, M. H. (1991). Clinical reasoning in medicine compared to clinical reasoning in occupational therapy. *American Journal of Occupational Therapy, 45,* 988–996.

53. Fragala-Pinkham, M. A., Dumas, H. M., Barlow, C. A., & Pasternak, A. (2009). An aquatic physical therapy program at a pediatric rehabilitation hospital: a case series. *Pediatric Physical Therapy, 21,* 68–78.

54. Franks, C. A., Palisano, R. J., & Darbee, J. C. (1991). The effect of walking with an assistive device and using a wheelchair on school performance in students with myelomeningocele. *Physical Therapy, 71,* 570–577.

55. Gast, D. L. (2009). *Single subject research methodology in behavioral sciences.* London: Routledge.

56. Giangreco, M. F. (1995). Related services decision-making: A foundational component of effective education for students with disabilities. *Physical and Occupational Therapy in Pediatrics, 15*(2), 47–67.

57. Golden, G. S. (1980). Nonstandard therapies in the developmental disabilities. *American Journal of Diseases in Childhood, 134,* 487–491.

58. Gonnella, C. (1989). Single-subject experimental paradigm as a clinical decision tool. *Physical Therapy, 69,* 601–609.

59. Gordon, B. N., & Jens, K. G. (1988). A conceptual model for tracking high-risk infants and making early service decisions. *Journal of Developmental and Behavioral Pediatrics, 9*(5), 279–286.

60. Gorter, J. W., Ketelaar, M., Rosenbaum, R., Helders, J. M., Palisano, R. (2009). Use of the gross motor function classification system in infants with cerebral palsy: The need for reclassification at age 2 or older. *Developmental Medicine and Child Neurology, 51,* 46–52.

61. Greenhalgh, T. (2002). Integrating qualitative research into evidence based practice. *Endocrinology and Metabolism Clinics of North America, 31,* 583–601.

62. Grimshaw, J. M., Shirran, L., Thomas, R., et al. (2001). Changing provider behaviour: An overview of systematic reviews of interventions. *Medical Care, 39*(8) (Suppl 2)2–45.

63. Guyatt, G. H., Haynes, R. B., Jaeschke R. Z., et al. (2000). Users' guides to the medical literature: XXV. Evidenced-based medicine: Principles for applying the users' guide to patient care. *Journal of the American Medical Association, 284,* 1290–1296.

64. Haley, S. M. (1991). Commentary on "The effect of walking with an assistive device and using a wheelchair on school performance in students with myelomeningocele." *Physical Therapy, 71,* 577–578.

65. Haley, S. M., Coster, W. J., Kao, Y.-C., et al. (2010). Lessons from use of the Pediatric Evaluation of Disability Inventory: Where do we do from here? *Pediatric Physical Therapy, 22,* 69–75.

66. Haley, S. M., Coster, W. J., Ludlow, I. H., Haltiwanger, J. T., & Andrellos, P. (1992). *Pediatric evaluation of disability inventory.* Boston: PEDI Research Group.

67. Hammell, KW, & Carpenter, C. (2004). *Evidence-based practice in rehabilitation: informing practice through qualitative research.* Edinburgh: Elsevier.

68. Hanna, S. E., Bartlett, D. J., Rivard, L. M., & Russell, D. J. (2008). Reference curves for the Gross Motor Function Measure: Percentiles for clinical description and tracking over time among children with cerebral palsy. *Physical Therapy, 88,* 596–607.

69. Hanna, S. E., Rosenbaum, P. L., Bartlett, D. J., et al. (2009). Stability and decline in gross motor function among children and youth with cerebral palsy aged 2 to 21 years. *Developmental Medicine and Child Neurology, 51,* 295–302.

70. Harbst, K. B. (1990). Indicators of cerebral palsy 1985–1988. *Physical and Occupational Therapy in Pediatrics, 10*(3), 85–107.

71. Hashimoto, M., & McCoy, S. W. (2009). Validation of an activity-based data form developed to reflect interventions used by pediatric physical therapists. *Pediatric Physical Therapy, 21,* 53–61.

72. Harris, S. R. (2004). Single case designs for the clinician. In B. H. Connolly & P. C. Montgomery (Eds.). *Therapeutic exercise in developmental disabilities* (3rd ed., pp. 491–504). Thorofare, NJ: Slack.

73. Harris, S. R. (1996). How should treatments be critiqued for scientific merit? *Physical Therapy, 76,* 175–181.

74. Harris, S. R., & Riffle, K. (1986). Effects of inhibitive ankle-foot orthoses on standing balance in a child with cerebral palsy. *Physical Therapy, 66,* 663–667.

75. Haynes, R. B., Deveaux, P. J., & Guyatt, G. H. (2002). Physician's and patients' choices in evidenced based practice. *British Medical Journal, 324,* 1350.

76. Herbert, R., Jamtvedt, G., Mead, J., Hagen, K. B. (2005). *Practical evidence-based physiotherapy* (pp. 12–14). Philadelphia: Elsevier.

77. Hidecker, M. J. C., Paneth, N., Rosenbaum, P., et al. (2008). *Communication Function Classification System (CFCS) for individuals with cerebral palsy.* Unpublished manuscript.

78. Higgs, J., Titchen A., & Neville, V. (2001). In J. Higgs & A. Titchen, *Practice knowledge and expertise in the health professions* (pp. 3–10). Oxford, UK: Butterworth-Heinemann.

79. Hinderer, K. A., Harris, S. R., Purdy, A. H., et al. (1998). Effects of "tone-reducing" vs. standard plaster casts on gait improvement of children with cerebral palsy. *Developmental Medicine and Child Neurology, 30*, 370–377.

80. Horn, S. D. (1997). *Clinical practice improvement methodology: Implementation and evaluation.* New York: Faulkner & Gray.

81. Horn, E. M., Warren, S. F., & Jones, H. A. (1997). An experimental analysis of neurobehavioral motor intervention. *Developmental Medicine and Child Neurology, 37*, 697–714.

82. Human Services Research Unit. (1995). *Consumer's guide: Therapeutic services for children with disabilities.* Cambridge, MA: Human Services Research Institute.

83. Hutzel, C. E., Wright, F. W., Stephens S., Schneiderman-Walker, J., Feldman B. (2009). A qualitative study of fitness instructors' experiences leading an exercise program for children with juvenile idiopathic arthritis. *Physical & Occupational Therapy in Pediatrics, 29*, 409–425.

84. Janosky, J. E., Leininger, S. L., Hoerger, M. P., & Libkuman, T. M. (2009). *Single subject designs in biomedicine.* New York: Springer.

85. Jenkins, D. A (1989). Practical introduction to databases: Part 2. *Biomedical Instrumentation and Technology, 23*, 109–112.

86. Jensen, G. M., Gwyer, J., Shepard, K. F., & Hack, L. (2000). Expert practice in physical therapy. *Physical Therapy, 80*, 28–43.

87. Jette, D. U., Halbert, J., Iverson, C., Micelei, E., & Shah, P. (2009). Use of standardized outcome measures in physical therapist practice: Perceptions and applications. *Physical Therapy, 89*, 125–135.

88. Johnson, C. C. (2009). The benefits of physical activity for youth with developmental disabilities: a systematic review. *American Journal of Health Promotion, 23*(3), 157–167.

89. Johnston, T. E., Smith, B. T., Oladeji, O., Betz, R. R., & Lauer, R. T. (2008). Outcomes of a home cycling program using functional electrical stimulation or passive motion for a children with spinal cord injury: A case series. *Journal of Spinal Cord Medicine, 31*, 215–221.

90. Jones, M. A., McEwen, I. R., & Hansen, L. (2003). Use of power mobility for a young child with spinal muscular atrophy. *Physical Therapy, 83*, 253–262.

91. Kanda, T., Yuge, M., & Yamori, Y. (1984). Early physiotherapy in the treatment of spastic diplegia. *Developmental Medicine and Child Neurology, 26*, 438–444.

92. Kaplan, S. L. (2007). *Outcome measurement & management: First steps for the practicing clinician.* Philadelphia: FA Davis.

93. Karman, N., Maryles, J., Baker, R. W., Simpser, E., & Berger-Gross, P. (2003). Constraint-induced movement therapy for hemiplegic children with acquired brain injuries. *Journal of Head Trauma & Rehabilitation, 18*, 259–267.

94. Ketelaar, M., Vermeer, A., t'Hart, H., van Petegem-van Beek, E., & Helders, P. J. M. (2001). Effects of a functional therapy program on motor abilities of children with cerebral palsy. *Physical Therapy, 81*, 1534–1545.

95. Ketelaar, M., Russell, D., & Gorter J. W. (2008). The challenge of moving evidence-based measures into clinical practice: Lessons in knowledge translation. *Physical and Occupational therapy in Pediatrics, 28*(2), 191–206.

96. King, G. A., King, S. M., & Rosenbaum, P. L. (1996). Interpersonal aspects of care-giving and client outcomes: A review of the literature. *Ambulatory and Child Health, 2*, 151–160.

97. Kopp, C. B. (1987). Developmental risk: Historical reflections. In J. D. Osofsky (Ed.), *Handbook of infant development* (pp. 881–912). New York: Wiley.

98. Kolobe, T. H A, Bulanda, M., & Susman, L. (2004). Predicting motor outcome at preschool age for infants tested at 7, 30, 60, and 90 days after term age using the Test of Infant Motor Performance. *Physical Therapy, 84*, 1144–1156.

99. Knafl, K. A., Ayres, L., Gallo, A. M., Zoeller, L. H., & Breitmayer, B. J. (1995). Learning from stories: Parents' accounts of the pathway to diagnosis. *Pediatric Nursing, 21*, 411–415.

100. Lansky, D., Butler, J. B. V., & Waller, F. T. (1992). Using health status measures in the hospital setting: From acute care to outcome management. *Medical Care, 30*(5 Suppl), MS57–MS73.

101. Laskas, S. A., Mullen, S. L., Nelson, D. L., & Willson-Broyles, M. (1985). Enhancement of two motor functions of the lower extremity in a child with spastic quadriplegia. *Physical Therapy, 65*, 11–16.

102. Law, M., Baptiste, S., Carswell-Opzoomer, A., McColl, M. A., Polatajko, H., & Pollack, N. (1991). *Canadian Occupational Performance Measure manual.* Toronto, CA: CAOT Publications.

103. Lehmann, J. F., Warren, C. G., Smith, W., & Larson, J. (1984). Computerized data management as an aid to clinical decision making in rehabilitation medicine. *Archives of Physical Medicine and Rehabilitation, 65*, 260–262.

104. Lekskulchai, R., & Cole, J. (2001). Effect of a developmental program on motor performance in infants born preterm. *Australian Journal of Physiotherapy, 47*, 169–176.

105. Lou, J. Q., & Durando, P. (2008). Asking clinical questions and searching for the evidence. In M. Law & J. MacDermid (Eds.). *Evidence-based rehabilitation: A guide to practice* (pp. 95–117). Thorofare, NJ: Slack.

106. Luo, H.-J., Chen, P.-S., Hsief, W.-S., et al. (2009). Associations of supported treadmill stepping with walking attainment in preterm and full-term infants. *Physical Therapy, 89*, 1215–1225.

107. Mattingly, C. (1991). What is clinical reasoning? *American Journal of Occupational Therapy, 45*, 979–986.

108. McEwen, I. (Ed.). (2009). *Writing case reports: A how-to manual for clinicians* (3rd ed.). Alexandria, VA: American Physical Therapy Association.

109. McEwen, I. (Ed). (2009). *Providing physical therapy services under parts B & C of the individuals with disabilities education act (IDEA)* (2nd ed.). Alexandria, VA: Section on Pediatrics, American Physical Therapy Association.

110. Messersmith, N. V., Slifer, K. J., Pulbrook-Vetter, V., & Bellipanni, K. (2008). Interdisciplinary behavioral intervention for life-threatening obesity in an adolescent with Prader-Willi syndrome: A case report. *Journal of Developmental and Behavioral Pediatrics, 29,* 129–134.

111. Miser, W. F. (2000). Applying a meta-analysis to daily clinical practice. In J. P. Geyman, R. A. JP, Deyo & S. D. Ramsey (Eds.), *Evidence-based clinical practice: Concepts and procedures* (pp. 57–64). Woburn, MA: Butterworth-Heinemann.

112. Mockford, M., & Caulton, J. (2008). Systematic review of progressive strength training in children and adolescents with cerebral palsy who are ambulatory. *Pediatric Physical Therapy, 20,* 318–333.

113. Morris, C., Galuppi, B. E., Rosenbaum, P. L. (2004). Reliability of family report for the Gross Motor Function Classification System. *Developmental Medicine and Child Neurology, 46,* 455–460.

114. National Institutes of Health. (1993). *Research plan for the National Center for Medical Rehabilitation Research.* NIH Publication No. 93–3509. Bethesda, MD: National Institutes of Health.

115. Nelson, K. B., & Ellenberg, J. H. (1982). Children who "outgrew" cerebral palsy. *Pediatrics, 69,* 529–536.

116. Norton, B. J., & Strube, M. J. (1989). Making decisions based on group designs and meta-analysis. *Physical Therapy, 69,* 594–600.

117. Nugent, J. K., Keefer, C. H., Minear, S., Johnson, L. C., & Blanchard, Y. (2007). *Understanding newborn behavior & early relationships: The Newborn Behavioral Observations (NBO) System handbook.* Baltimore: Paul H. Brookes.

118. Ottenbacher, K. J. (1986). *Evaluating clinical change: Strategies for occupational and physical therapists.* Baltimore: Williams & Wilkins.

119. Palisano, R. J. (1989). Comparison of two methods of service delivery for students with learning disabilities. *Physical and Occupational Therapy in Pediatrics, 9*(3), 79–100.

120. Palisano, R. J. (2006). A collaborative model of service delivery for children with movement disorders: A framework for evidence-based decision-making. *Physical Therapy, 86,* 1295–1305.

121. Palisano, R., Rosenbaum, P., Walter, S., Russell, D., Wood, E., & Galuppi, B. (1997). Development and reliability of a system to classify gross motor function of children with cerebral palsy. *Developmental Medicine and Child Neurology, 39,* 214–223.

122. Palisano, R. J., Hanna, S., Rosenbaum, P., et al. (2000). Validation of a model of motor development for children with cerebral palsy. *Physical Therapy, 80,* 974–985.

123. Palisano, R. J., Walters, S., Russell, D., et al. (2001). Gross motor function of children with Down syndrome: Creation of motor growth curves. *Archives of Physical Medicine and Rehabilitation, 82,* 494–500.

124. Palisano, R. J., Tieman, B. L., Walter, S. D., et al. (2003). Effect of environmental setting on mobility methods of children with cerebral palsy. *Developmental Medicine and Child Neurology, 45,* 113–120.

125. Palisano, R. J., Cameron, D., Rosenbaum, P. L., Walter, S. D., & Russell, D. (2006). Stability of the gross motor function classification system. *Developmental Medicine and Child Neurology, 48,* 424–428.

126. Palisano, R. J., Rosenbaum, P., Bartlett, D., & Livingston, M. H. (2008). Content validity of the expanded and revised gross motor function classification system. *Developmental Medicine and Child Neurology, 50,* 744–750.

127. Palisano, R. J., & Murr, S. (2009). Intensity of therapy services: What are the considerations? *Physical and Occupational Therapy in Pediatrics, 29,* 107–112.

128. Palisano, R. J., Shimmell, L. J., Stewart, D., Lawless, J. J., Rosenbaum, P. L., & Russell, D. J. (2009). Mobility experiences of youth with cerebral palsy. *Physical and Occupational Therapy in Pediatrics, 29,* 133–153.

129. Palisano, R. J., Hanna, S. E., Rosenbaum, P. L., Tieman B. (2010). Probability of walking, wheeled mobility, and assisted mobility for children and youth with cerebral palsy. *Developmental Medicine and Child Neurology, 52,* 66–71.

130. Pierson, D. J. (2009). Translating evidence into practice. *Respiratory Care, 54,* 1386–1401.

131. Piper, M. C., Darrah, J., Pinnell, L., Watt, M. J., & Byrne, P. (1991). The consistency of sequential examinations in the early detection of neurological dysfunction. *Physical and Occupational Therapy in Pediatrics, 11*(3), 27–44.

132. Plasschaert, V. F., Ketelaar, M., Nijnuis, M. G., Enkelaar, L., & Gorter, J. W. (2009). Classification of manual abilities in children with cerebral palsy under 5 years of age: How reliable is the manual ability classification system? *Clinical Rehabilitation, 23*(2), 164–170.

133. Romeiser, L. R., Hickman R. R., Harris S. R., & Heriza C. B. (2008). Single-subject research design: Recommendations for levels of evidence and quality rating. *Developmental Medicine and Child Neurology, 50,* 99–103.

134. Portney, L. G., & Watkins, M. P. (2009). Single subject designs. In *Foundations of clinical research: Applications to practice* (3rd ed., pp. 235–272). Upper Saddle River, NJ: Pearson/Prentice Hall.

135. Prechtl, H. F. R., Einspieler, C., Cioni, G., Bos, A. F., Ferrari, F., & Sontheimer, D. (1997). An early marker for neurological deficits after perinatal brain lesions. *Lancet, 349,* 1361–1363.

136. Purdy, A. H., Deitz, J. C., & Harris, S. R. (1987). Efficacy of two treatment approaches to reduce tongue protrusion of children with Down syndrome. *Developmental Medicine and Child Neurology, 29,* 469–476.

137. Randall, K. E., & McEwen, I. R. (2000). Writing patient-centered functional goals. *Physical Therapy, 80,* 1197–1203.

138. Richardson, B. (2001). In J. Higgs & A. Titchen, *Practice knowledge and expertise in the health professions* (pp. 42–47). Oxford, UK: Butterworth-Heinemann.

139. Ritchie, J. E. (1999). Using qualitative research to enhance the evidenced-based practice of health care providers. *Australian Journal of Physiotherapy, 45,* 251–256.

140. Rosenbaum, P. L., King, S., Law, M., King, G., & Evans, J. (1998). Family-centered service: A conceptual framework and

research review. *Physical and Occupational Therapy in Pediatrics*, *18*(1), 1–20].

141. Rosenbaum, P. L., Walter, S. D., Hanna, S. E., Palisano, R. J., Russell, D. J., & Raina, P. (2002). Prognosis for gross motor function in cerebral palsy: Creation of motor development curves. *Journal of the American Medical Association*, *288*, 1357–1363.

142. Rosenblith, J. F. (1992). A singular career: Nancy Bayley. *Developmental Psychology*, *28*, 747–75892.

143. Rothstein, J. M., & Echternach, J. L. (1986). Hypothesis-oriented algorithm for clinicians: A method for evaluation and treatment planning. *Physical Therapy*, *66*, 1388–1394.

144. Rothstein, J. M., Echternach, J. L., & Riddle D. L. (2003). Hypothesis-oriented algorithm for clinicians II (HOAC II): A guide for patient management. *Physical Therapy*, *83*, 455–470.

145. Russell, D. J., Rosenbaum, P. L., Avery, L. & Lane, M. (2002). *Gross motor function measure (GMFM-66 & GMFM-88) user's manual: Clinics in developmental medicine no. 159*. London, England: Mac Keith Press.

146. Russell, D. J., Avery, L. M., Walter, S. D., et al. (2010). Development and validation of item sets to improve efficiency of administration of the 66-item Gross Motor Function Measure in children with cerebral palsy. *Developmental Medicine and Child Neurology*, *52*(2), e48–e54.

147. Sakzewski, L., Ziviani, J., & Boyd R. (2009). Systematic review and meta-analysis of therapeutic management of upper-limb dysfunction in children with congenital hemiplegia. *Pediatrics*, *123*, e1111–e1122.

148. Sackett, D. L. (1986). Rules of evidence and clinical recommendations on use of antithrombotic agents. *Chest*, *89*(2 Suppl), 2S–3S.

149. Sackett, D. L., Rosenberg, W. M. C., Gray, J. A. M., Haynes, R. B., & Richardson, W. S. (1996). Evidence based medicine: What it is and what it isn't. *British Medical Journal*, *312*, 71–72.

150. Sackett, D. L., Strauss, S. E., Richardson, W. S., et al. (2000). *Evidence-based medicine: how to practice and teach EBM* (2nd ed., p. 1). New York: Churchill Livingstone.

151. Schreiber, J., Stern, P., Marchetti, G., Provident, I., & Turocy, P. S. (2008). School-based pediatric physical therapists' perspectives on evidence-based practice. *Pediatric Physical Therapy*, *20*, 292–302.

152. Schreiber, J., Stern, P., Marchetti, G., & Provident, I. (2009). Strategies to promote evidence-based practice in pediatric physical therapy: A formative evaluation pilot project. *Physical Therapy*, *89*, 918–933.

153. Schyve, P. M. (1996). The evolving role of the Joint Commission for the Accreditation of Health Care Organizations. *Joint Commission Journal on Quality Improvement*, *11*, S54–S57.

154. Shadish, W. R., Jr., Cook, T. D., & Leviton, L. C. (1991). *Foundations of program evaluation: Theories of practice*. Newbury Park, CA: Sage.

155. Shurtleff, D. B. (1991). Computer databases for pediatric disability: Clinical and research applications. *Physical Medicine and Rehabilitation Clinics of North America*, *2*, 665–687.

156. Simpson, M., Buckman, R., Stewart, M., et al. (1991). Doctor-patient communication: The Toronto consensus statement. *British Medical Journal*, *303*, 1385–1387.

157. Slagle, T. A., & Gould, J. B. (1992). Database use in neonatal intensive care units: Success or failure. *Pediatrics*, *90*, 959–965.

158. Stewart, M., Brown, J. B., Boon, H., Galajda, J., Meredith, L., & Sangster, M. (1999). Evidence on doctor-patient communication. *Cancer Prevention & Control*, *3*, 25–30.

159. Stuberg, W., & DeJong, S. L. (2007). Program evaluation of physical therapy as an early intervention and related service in special education, *Pediatric Physical Therapy*, *19*, 121–127.

160. Sweeney, J. K., Heriza, C. B., Blanchard, Y., & Dusing, S. C. (2010). Neonatal physical therapy. Part II: Practice frameworks and evidence-based practice guidelines. *Pediatric Physical Therapy*, *22*, 2–16.

161. Sweeney, J. K., Heriza, C. B., & Blanchard, Y. (2009). Neonatal physical therapy. Part I: Clinical competencies and neonatal intensive care unit clinical training models. *Pediatric Physical Therapy*, *21*, 296–307.

162. Takken, T., Van Brussel, M., Engelbert, R. H. H., van der Net, J. J., Kuis, W., Helders, P. P. J. M. Exercise therapy in juvenile idiopathic arthritis. *Cochrane Database of Systematic Reviews* 2008, Issue 2. Art. No.: CD005954. DOI: 10.1002/14651858. CD005954.pub2

163. Rappolt, S., & Tassone, M. (2002). How rehabilitation therapists gather, evaluate, and implement new knowledge. *Journal of Continuing Education in the Health Professions*, *22*(3), 170–180.

164. Thomson-O'Brien, M. A., & Moreland, J. (1998). Evidence-based information circle. *Physiotherapy Canada*, Summer, 184–189.

165. Tieman, B. L., Palisano, R. J., Gracely, E. J., & Rosenbaum, P. L. (2004). Gross motor capability and performance of mobility in children with cerebral palsy: A comparison across home, school, and outdoors/community settings. *Physical Therapy*, *84*, 419–429.

166. Tiffin, J. (1968). *Purdue pegboard examiner manual*. Chicago: Scientific Research Associates.

167. Titchen, A., & Ersser, S. J. In Higgs, J., & Titchen, A. (2001). *Practice knowledge and expertise in the health professions* (pp. 35–42). Oxford, UK: Butterworth-Heinemann.

168. Tunis, S. R., Stryer, D. B., & Clancy, C. M. (2003). Practical clinical trials: Increasing the value of clinical research for decision making in clinical and health policy. *Journal of the American Medical Association*, *290*, 1624–1632.

169. Ulrich, D. A., Ulrich, B. D., Angulo-Kinzler, R. M., & Yun, J. (2001). Treadmill training of infants with Down syndrome: Evidence-based developmental outcomes. *Pediatrics*, *108*, E84, www.pediatrics.org/cgi/content/full/108/5/e84.

170. Wang, M. C., & Ellet, C. D. (1982). Program validation: The state of the art. *Topics in Early Childhood Special Education, 1*(4), 35–49.

171. Waters, R. L., & Lunsford, B. R. (1985). Energy cost of paraplegic locomotion. *Journal of Bone and Joint Surgery (American), 67*, 1245–1250.

172. Weston, W. W. (2001). Informed and shared decision-making: The crux of patient-centrad care. *Canadian Medical Association Journal, 165*, 438–439.

173. Wolery, M., & Bailey, D. D. (1984). Alternatives to impact evaluation: Suggestions for program evaluation in early intervention. *Journal of the Division for Early Childhood, 4*, 27–37.

174. Wood, E., & Rosenbaum, P. (2000). The gross motor function classification system for cerebral palsy: A study of reliability and stability over time. *Developmental Medicine and Child Neurology, 42*, 292–296.

175. World Health Organization. (2001). *International classification of function, disability, and health*. Geneva: World Health Organization.

176. World Health Organization. (2007). *International classification of function, disability, and health: children and youth version. Geneva: World Health Organization.*

2

The Child's Development of Functional Movement

SUZANN K. CAMPBELL, PT, PhD, FAPTA

Working knowledge of motor development is the basis of the practice of pediatric physical therapy. It provides the age standards (norms) for functioning of children at various ages that guide diagnosis and treatment planning through emphasis on selection of age-appropriate skills as functional outcomes. Development of effective plans of care for children also requires knowledge of the cognitive milestones that must be recognized in order to promote activities that are stimulating and motivating and to take advantage of interactions among cognitive, perceptual, and motor development.[200] Developing such an environment for the provision of intervention typically involves use of adapted play activities at a cognitive level appropriate for an individual child, regardless of the child's level of motor development. The challenge is perhaps greatest when motor and cognitive levels in a particular child are exceedingly different.

Movement, on the other hand, also promotes cognitive and perceptual development.[10,27,221,286] The two go hand in hand to foster functional performance. Therapists must consider in their intervention planning how to structure therapy and parent coaching to facilitate best all aspects of their clients' development and community participation and to take advantage of the interactive nature of developmental subsystems, especially when activity limitations are present and likely to be lifelong. The *Guide to Physical Therapist Practice*[8] suggests that goals of therapy should focus on treatment of impairments (e.g., strength, endurance, or range of motion), but anticipated outcomes of intervention should include minimization of functional and activity limitations, optimization of health status, prevention of disability in daily life (participation), and consumer satisfaction, including cost effectiveness (see Chapter 1). Nevertheless, when to emphasize treatment of physical impairments and activity limitations through exercise and other therapeutic modalities, when to concentrate on finding compensatory means to promote participation in a variety of social and developmental areas, and when to combine the two are important considerations in designing a plan of care that addresses family concerns.

This chapter describes important milestones in the development of functional movement in children and introduces a discussion of the processes by which development occurs, which is elaborated on in Chapter 3 on motor control. It seems appropriate first to define what is meant by functional movement and activity. Fisher[106] has reviewed the various meanings of the term "function" that rehabilitation professionals have used in the design and evaluation of tests and measures. Function is variously described as having a definite end or purpose and as being goal directed and meaningful. A functional limitation represents a failure of the individual's performance to meet a standard expectation. In the language of the International Classification of Function, Disability and Health (ICF),[297] functional limitations impair activity. When permanent, functional or activity limitations result in a reduction in behavioral skills, task accomplishment, or fulfillment of appropriate social roles. The alleviation of effects of activity limitations on behavior or social roles is defined in this volume as the promotion of participation (see Chapter 1 on clinical decision making for further elaboration of ICF definitions). In rehabilitation, impaired functional performance resulting in disabilities is frequently assessed by examining the degree of assistance the client needs to perform activities of daily living (ADL). The use of technology to compensate for functional limitations and promote activity, however, means that participation in age-appropriate social roles can be achieved through alternative means to promote quality of life[47] (see also the chapter on assistive technology on Evolve).

Certainly all therapists would agree that ADL should be considered under the rubric of "functional activity." But children engage in many meaningful movement activities that appear to lack a well-defined goal. Spinning, bouncing, and endless repetition of spontaneous or newly learned movements—such as arm waving, going up and down steps, and putting things into containers and taking them out—are just a few examples.[248] We would probably call this "play" or "practice," but regardless of terminology, therapists surely see these activities as important aspects of motor development, motor learning, and environmental mastery. In other words, they represent functional activities for the child's stage of development despite lacking apparent goals. Repetition of motor behaviors might serve a variety of useful functions, such as muscle strengthening, trial of a variety of approaches to assembling effective task-related movements, testing the limits of balance, and learning to deal with the reactive forces produced elsewhere in the body by muscle contraction of prime movers for a particular activity. Practice of tasks under constant conditions is believed to form the basis of scaleable response structures (general motor programs) in motor learning theory.[247] Certainly, children demonstrate a remarkable intensity of purpose when practicing emerging skills. Vander Linden (personal communication, 1993) provided several examples of his daughter Abby's development. Abby played almost compulsively with nesting cups for about 2 weeks, and when she could nest all 10, she was no longer interested in them. Similarly, she repeatedly went up and down a 4-inch step onto a screened porch in her home, insisting that her parents open the porch door for her to access the porch for stepping practice and resisting enticements to play with toys instead.

Based on many observations such as these, the definition provided by Fisher[106] that I prefer is that functional activity, or occupation in the framework of occupational therapy theory and practice, is "what people do" (p. 184). These words imply that movements are self-chosen, self-directed, and, therefore, meaningful in the life of the individual at his or her particular place in the life cycle.[106,208] Given this definition, our descriptive presentation will review information regarding what children do and the general order in which they do it, beginning with infants' spontaneously generated, that is, self-directed, movements, and gradually incorporating information on tasks that are easier for adults to identify as purposeful and goal directed.

In keeping with the importance to pediatric physical therapists of knowledge of functional motor development, the main objectives of this chapter are to (1) briefly review the history of theories of motor development, (2) describe current information and hypotheses regarding general processes and principles of motor development, and (3) provide an overview of the developmental course of acquisition of

upright posture and mobility and of object manipulation—the two most basic functions that underlie meaningful movement activities. Brief attention will be paid to issues in cognitive development, play, and the interaction of motor skill acquisition and perceptual-cognitive development, including memory for activities. The chapter concludes with an abbreviated review of tests of motor development and functional motor behavior of use to physical therapists from the point of view of the theoretic perspectives provided in earlier parts of the chapter.

MOTOR DEVELOPMENT THEORIES

Throughout the history of physical therapy, theories of child development have changed dramatically, eliciting successive revisions of intervention approaches to maximizing motor development and activity in children. Underlying the changes in developmental theory are differing conceptualizations of the respective roles of changing structure and function within the individual and of the influence of the environment on the developmental course. Thelen and colleagues[270] summarized the major theoretic approaches as encompassing three theories: (1) neural-maturationist, (2) cognitive, and (3) dynamical systems. Each has an interesting history that in itself makes fascinating reading because of the strong role that changing biases and accumulation of new knowledge play in how research efforts are designed and how their results are interpreted and judged.[24,80,266,267] These theories are reviewed briefly in this chapter, and their major distinguishing features are summarized in Table 2-1. Further elaboration can be found in Chapter 3 on motor control.

TABLE 2-1   **Comparison Of Developmental Theories**

	Neural-Maturationist	Cognitive: Behavioral	Cognitive: Piagetian	Dynamical Systems
View on "stages"	Stages of motor development occur as a result of CNS maturation	Stages are merely empirical descriptions of behavior	Stages represent alternating periods of equilibrium and disequilibrium	Apparent stages of development are actually states of relative stability arising from the self-organizing, emergent properties of a multitude of systems, each developing at its own continuous rate
Driving forces for development	Development spirals with alternating periods of flexor vs. extensor dominance and symmetry vs. asymmetry based on maturation of the CNS	Development occurs through interaction of the individual with the environment	Development occurs through interaction between cognitive-neural structures and environmental opportunities for action	The individual develops as the organism recognizes the affordances of the environment and selects (self-organizes) the most appropriate available responses to tasks
Building blocks of development	Reflexes	Pavlovian and operant responses to environmental stimuli	First actions using reflexes and later from voluntary actions	Multiple cooperating systems with individual rates of development and self-motivated exploration of the environment

NEURAL-MATURATIONIST THEORIES

The neural-maturationist point of view was pioneered by Arnold Gesell,[115,116,117,118,119,120] Shirley,[248] and others. This view proposed that the ontogeny of behavior is "an intrinsic property of the organism, with maturation leading to an unfolding of predetermined patterns, supported, but not fundamentally altered by the environment (p. 40)."[270] According to this approach, functional behaviors appear as the nervous system matures, with more complex behaviors being based on the activity of progressively higher levels of the nervous system. This theory, therefore, depends on the assumption of hierarchic maturation of neural control structures.

Gesell's point of view and research findings resulted in the development of important tests of motor milestones and other adaptive behaviors that have had, and continue to have, a monumental influence on practice in the area of diagnosis of developmental delay or deviance.[80,267] Virtually all subsequent tests of development contained items derived from Gesell's work. Gesell emphatically believed in stages of development as biologic imperatives. He did recognize that there are individual differences among children, was a strong believer in freedom of human action, and toward the end of his career came to recognize the role of environmental factors in development, particularly for their influence on cognitive development. Nevertheless, he never completely resolved the paradox between these beliefs and his insistence on maturation as the predominant force driving development. Gesell was a major force promoting the right to special education for children with both cognitive and physical disabilities.[80]

It is helpful to recognize that Gesell's views were strongly shaped by opposition to the behaviorist approach developed in the 1930s (described in the next section) that posited the environment as the critical force driving development.[80] Thelen and Adolph[267] also pointed out that among Gesell's less remembered contributions is the idea that the nature of development forms a spiraling function, with alternations between extremes in a variety of behavioral realms, including alternating dominance between flexor and extensor muscle activity. He believed in a principle of functional asymmetry in which the child must break free of symmetrical movement patterns to achieve functional goals such as manipulation.

Pediatric physical therapy developed according to this neural-maturationist theoretic model. As a result, emphasis was placed on examination of stages of reflex development and motor milestones as reflections of increasingly higher levels of neural maturation.[149] Treatment of the child with central nervous system (CNS) dysfunction was organized around inhibition of primary reflexes that were believed to persist and produce activity limitations, along with facilitation of righting and equilibrium reactions that were supposedly the underlying coordinative structures for

development of skilled voluntary motor behavior. It was generally assumed that functional outcomes would naturally follow. Research conducted according to neural-maturationist theory seeks to identify the timing of appearance of developmental milestones and the establishment of age standards for developmental advances. Work by Adolph and colleagues[6] demonstrated the inadequacy of most protocols used in longitudinal developmental research, a problem that must be addressed in future work. After assessing changes in behavior on a daily basis, they found that sampling at greater than 7-day intervals resulted in a large loss of information and was inadequate for work on theory development.

COGNITIVE THEORIES

Cognitive theories of motor skill development are of two types. One is based on the approach of B. F. Skinner and the other on the work of Jean Piaget.

Behavioral Theory

Skinner[252] developed a behavioral approach to development that emphasized the importance of contingent learning with reinforcement from the environment being the motivator and shaper of both motor and cognitive development.[30,66] In this theoretic approach, the environment is the site of developmental control.

In more contemporary developmental psychology, behavioral analysis theory was based on Skinner's later radical behaviorism and on the interbehaviorism of Kantor, in which the developing individual is conceived of as a pattern of psychologic responses in interaction with the environment.[30] Progressions in development depend on opportunities and circumstances inherent in the individual's make-up and in his or her past and present physical and social environments. Developmental progress occurs through Pavlovian responses to previous stimulation and by operant processes in which responses are controlled by consequences. Operant responses are acquired and maintained by contingent stimuli with acquired or primary reinforcing functions, and the strength of these interactions is affected by conditions such as timing and frequency of reinforcements. Although sometimes misused, behavior modification approaches have greatly aided the training of specific skills for children with cognitive delay,[30] and the knowledge base of the behavioral approach helped therapists to break down skills into component parts for easier learning by children with impaired neural control mechanisms. Angulo-Kinzler[11] used a behavioral approach to demonstrate the ability of 3-month-old infants to discover and adopt specific solutions to a movement problem—kicking within an experimenter-specified range of motion. Clinical problems are approached based on the beliefs that each problem has its unique history and that the intervention program should be individually tailored to the specific problem behavior.

A frequently misunderstood aspect of behavioral analysis theory is the role of individuals in their own development. The individual is not perceived of as passive and responding only when stimulated. Rather, the individual is considered to be adjusting in continual interaction with the environment. The critical feature of this theory is that it is a psychology of the individual in interaction with the environment. Unlike Gesell's concept of development,[117] stages of development are considered to be merely empirical descriptions and not in any sense causal explanations of behavior. The research methodology of behavioral analysis is, therefore, one of single-subject designs or within-subject comparisons designed to demonstrate functional relationships rather than to test theories. The elaboration of such designs has been a significant contribution to clinical research science in physical therapy.

Piagetian Theory

A second cognitive theory based primarily on the work of Piaget[219] emphasizes an interaction between maturation of cognitive-neural structures and environmental opportunities to promote action.[23,107] Control functions are found in the development of higher-level plans based on biologic structures, termed schemata in Piagetian theory or motor programs or subroutines in motor control theory.[44,73] (See also Chapter 3.) Cognitive mechanisms of all types are believed to derive from knowledge gained through action based at first on innate hereditary reflexes and instinctual capacities and later on experience forming concrete intelligent operations. Cognitive development culminates in abstract intelligence based on coordination of fundamental cognitive operations.

Piagetian theory had little effect on pediatric physical therapy from the perspective of planning the motor aspects of therapeutic programming because it was primarily a cognitive theory and because it continued to emphasize the evolution of functional behaviors from reflexive movements. These movements were believed to be practiced and coordinated with developing mental structures. Adaptive responses were thought to develop through psychologic processes interacting with maturation of neural structures. In this view, the most important processes are successive equilibration, disequilibrium, and re-equilibration, resulting from the interaction of maturation and experience. An important aspect of Piagetian theory is the view of the individual as possessing a self-regulating system of psychologic processes that provides balance between assimilation of environmental experiences and accommodation of existing cognitive structures to that experience. The individual is a homeorrhetic system that, by virtue of its self-regulating characteristics, constantly adjusts itself to maintain equilibrium despite disturbances from the environment, thus driving developmental progress. Viewing the operation of these psychologic processes in children who were observed while solving interesting problems led to theories of the mental structures

constructed by children as a result of their activity. Neo-Piagetian work has emphasized research on the functioning of these psychologic processes.[23]

The concept of stages played a major role in early Piagetian theory, although in his later conceptions of development, when faced with evidence contradicting some of his hypotheses, he realized that stage theory tended to lead one to think in terms of periods of rest or equilibrium, whereas development was, in fact, never static.[23] In later years, Piaget, like Gesell, tended to see development as a spiraling process, an important principle that we will return to later. Description of stages nonetheless forms the framework for discussions of development of cognitive systems in Piagetian theory.

Four main stages were posited, each with multiple substages. The first is the stage of sensorimotor intelligence from birth to about 18 to 24 months.[23] Repetition in action is a major factor in this stage, culminating in the major achievement of symbolic functioning. The second period of representational thought, from 1.5 to 2 through 6 years of age, involves the development of language and of one-way mappings of logical thought that allow classifications to be developed. Experiments detailing the errors of logical thought in this period were influential in revealing the lack of sophistication in children's mental constructions that was not previously obvious. More current work on classifications suggests that they can be performed perceptually much earlier than Piaget projected, probably as early as 3 months of age in a primitive form.[144] An example of recent work on the sensorimotor basis of children's thought processes is a study by Perry and colleagues revealing the ability of 2- to 3-year-olds to discriminate between the occluded paths of faster versus slower moving objects, a concept termed representational momentum.[218] In the third period of concrete operations, thought processes become reversible, allowing conservation of number, weight, and volume under transformation conditions. In the final period of cognitive development, formal operations beginning at about age 11 permit logical thinking in a hypothetico-deductive mode.

The impact of Piagetian theory on pediatric physical therapy was primarily on the inclusion of interesting spectacles and problem-solving activities in therapeutic programs to assist in the cognitive-motivational aspects of facilitating motor development. Therapists used problems such as the search for hidden objects (object permanence) and problems involving means-ends relationships and container-contained ideas as therapeutic media to motivate children to move and to examine and promote the perceptual-cognitive aspects of development and motor learning.[62,98]

DYNAMICAL SYSTEMS THEORY

Esther Thelen and colleagues[266,268,269,270,271,278] proposed a dynamical functional perspective on motor development that currently drives most research on motor development. Dynamical systems theory emphasizes process rather than product or hierarchically structured plans and places neural maturation on an equal plane with other structures and processes that interact to promote motor development. These "structures become progressively integrated with the self-organized properties of the system (p. 41)." to gradually optimize skilled function. Cooperating systems include musculoskeletal components, sensory systems, central sensorimotor integrative mechanisms, and arousal and motivation (see Chapter 3).[146,149,250,251,270] In this theoretic approach, both these internal components of the organism and the external context of the task are equivalent in determining the outcome of behavior because behavior is task-specific. In this model of infant motor development, therefore, the environment is as important as the organism. Because, however, the infant's cooperating systems, such as those involving strength and postural control, do not develop at the same rate, certain components are seen as rate limiting or constraining to the performance of any specific behavior.

In a seminal paper in the physical therapy literature, Heriza[146] described the basic concepts of dynamical systems theory and suggested various approaches to testing its utility in planning and assessing the outcomes of therapeutic interventions. For example, eight subsystems are postulated to be involved in the development of infant locomotion:

1. Pattern generation of the coordinative structure leading to reciprocal lower extremity activity, consisting primarily of alternating flexor muscle activation
2. Development of reciprocal muscle activity of flexor and extensor muscles
3. Strength of extensor muscles needed for opposing the force of gravity
4. Changes in body size and composition
5. Antigravity control of upright posture of the head and trunk
6. Appropriate decoupling of the tight synchronization characteristic of early reciprocal lower extremity movements, such that the knee moves out of phase with the hip and ankle
7. Visual flow sensitivity required to maintain posture while moving through the environment
8. Ability to recognize the requirements of the task and be motivated to move toward a goal

This listing makes it clear that the development of a particular motor pattern, in this case upright locomotion, depends on a combination of mechanical, neurologic, cognitive, and perceptual factors in addition to environmental contributions specific to both the task and the context of the infant's action. Each of the subsystems develops at its own rate but is constrained or supported by physical and environmental factors, such as a nutritional diet, especially one that is adequate in iron[186,196] and experiences providing the opportunity to practice antigravity trunk extension while prone, standing upright, and stepping. For example, since the implementation of advice to encourage parents to have infants sleep on their back,[7,264] investigators have shown that back-sleeping infants are less likely to roll over at 4 months of age than infants who sleep in the prone position[154] and have lower developmental scores at 6 months of age,[87] a difference that was no longer apparent at 18 months. Sleep position in a group of premature infants also affected ability to maintain the head elevated and lower it with control at 56 weeks' postconceptional age, although global developmental was not affected.[227] Fetters and colleagues demonstrated that prone sleep position was correlated with motor development in preterm as well as term infants at 1, 5, and 9 months of age,[103] and Salls and colleagues[242] reported that 2-month-old infants who spent 15 minutes or less awake time in the prone position differed significantly in gross motor milestone attainment from the normative population for the Denver II test. In keeping with dynamical systems theory, changing the environment available to the infant for practicing movements as a result of medical recommendations to prevent sudden infant death syndrome (SIDS) appears to have altered the timing of motor development. Spending a majority of one's time in supine also appears to be a reason for an increase in referral of infants to physical therapy for management of plagiocephaly;[29] these infants can also be expected to show delayed development.[161] As a result of accumulating evidence of the effects of limited prone experience on motor development, the American Academy of Pediatrics revised their guidelines to emphasize the slogan "Back for sleep; tummy for play," and many online sources are now available as handouts for parents to encourage "tummy time" play (Box 2-1, example 2).

In the dynamical systems view of development, the movements of locomotion are conceived not as derived from a set of instructions from the nervous system nor as built from chains of reflexes but as self-organizing and emergent as a result of the interaction of the subsystems described. The locus of control for function shifts over time, depending on the dominance or constraints of various subsystems. Spontaneous exploration of movement possibilities and flexible selection of the most appropriate movement synergy for accomplishing goal-directed actions are key processes in development in the view of the proponents of dynamical systems theory.[268] Transitional periods, when movement patterns appear more variable, are thought to be sensitive periods in development when intervention might be particularly effective. Research is needed to identify these sensitive periods in the development of specific functional behaviors, thereby providing new knowledge to guide intervention by therapists.

Based on dynamical systems theory, developmental change is seen not as a series of discrete stages but as a series of states of stability, instability, and phase shifts in which new states become stable aspects of behavior.[266] Research involves the search for collective variables or patterns of behavior that reflect the action of the component parts involved in a particular environment or task context.[203] An example of research designed to identify the collective

---

Box **2-1**   EXAMPLES OF HEALTH PROMOTION CONCERNS AND RESOURCES

1. Injury prevention education, including use of car seats and helmets and safe (or no) use of baby walkers,[45] swings, and other play equipment, cribs and youth beds, and toys. The American Academy of Pediatrics injury prevention program website can be accessed at www.aap.org/family/ tippmain.htm. A useful reference on typical injuries in children is Agran, P. H., Anderson, C., Winn, D., Trent, R., Walton-Haynes, L., & Thayer, S. (2003). Rates of pediatric injuries by 3-month intervals for children 0 to 3 years of age. *Pediatrics, 111*, e683–e692, 2003, accessed at www.pediatrics.org/cgi/content/full/111/6/e683. Falls are the leading cause of injury in this age group. Motor vehicle accidents are the most common cause of mortality in children 4 to 14 in the United States, yet use of restraint systems was seen in only 25% of vehicles bringing children to school in a study by Emery, K. D., & Faries, S. G. (2008). The lack of motor vehicle occupant restraint use in children arriving at school. *Journal of School Health, 78*, 274–279.

2. "Back-to-sleep" to prevent SIDS (sudden infant death syndrome; see Task Force on Sudden Infant Death Syndrome). The changing concept of sudden infant death syndrome: diagnostic coding shifts, controversies regarding the sleeping environment, and new variables to consider in reducing risk. *Pediatrics, 116*, 1245–1255, 2005, and www.healthychildcare.org/pdf/SIDStummytime.pdf on back to sleep and awake play in the prone position to promote motor development (Tummy Time). Children's Healthcare of Atlanta has Tummy Time tools available in six languages at www.choa.org/default.aspx?id=4892. A Tummy Time teaching session is shown in the videos accompanying this chapter.

3. Effects of second-hand smoke. A fact sheet from the National Cancer Institute at the National Institutes of Health in the United States is available at www.cancer.gov/cancertopics/ factsheet/Tobacco/ETS.

4. Nutrition and obesity prevention, including the value of breast-feeding through at least 6 months of age and need for a diet adequate in essential nutrients. A useful reference is de Onis, M., Garza, D., Victora, C. G., Onyango, A. W., Frongillo, E. A., & Martines, J. (2004). The WHO multicentre growth reference study: Planning, study design, and methodology. *Food and Nutrition Bulletin, 25*(1), S15–S26. Iron deficiency which impedes myelination plays a major role in delayed development in infants, especially in

developing countries, and effects are long-lasting despite treatment; see Lozoff, B. (2007). Iron deficiency and child development. *Food and Nutrition Bulletin, 28*(4 Suppl), S560–S571; Shafir, T, Angulo-Barroso, A, Calatroni, A, Jimenez, E, & Lozoff, B. (2006). Effects of iron deficiency in infancy on patterns of motor development over time. *Human Movement Science, 25*, 821–838. The role of folic acid use in improving gross motor development is discussed in Wehby, G. L., & Murray, J. C. (2008). The effects of prenatal use of folic acid and other dietary supplements on early child development. *Maternal and Child Health Journal, 12*, 180–187. Obesity prevention is addressed at www.aap.org/ pressroom/play-public.htm.

5. Encouraging an active lifestyle to prevent obesity. A useful review of environmental correlates of youth physical activity is Ferrerira, I., van der Horst, K., Wendel-Vos, W., Kremers, S., van Lethe, F. J., & Brug, J. (2007). Environmental correlates of physical activity in youth: A review and update. *Obesity Review, 8*, 129–154; Dyment, J. E., & Bell, A. C. (2008). Grounds for movement: green school grounds as sites for promoting physical activity. *Health Education Research, 23*, 952–962, describes the effect of greening school grounds on children's play and activity levels. The American Academy of Pediatrics has a website on the importance of unstructured play that can be accessed at www.aap.org/obesity/ index.html. See Chapters 6 on physical fitness and Chapter 32 on Transition to Adulthood for more information on this topic.

6. Clarifying myths regarding ill effects of immunizations. A useful reference is Wolfe, R. M., Sharp, L. K., & Lipsky, M. S. (2002). Content and design attributes of antivaccination web sites. *Journa of the American Medical Association, 287*, 3245–3248. Websites that discuss immunizations and this issue can be accessed at www.cdc.gov/vaccines and www.aap.org/immunization.

7. Promote mental health. Two useful references are Thomasgard, M., & Metz, W. P. (2004). Promoting child social-emotional growth in primary care settings: Using a developmental approach. *Clinical Pediatrics, 43*, 119–127; Petterson, S. M., & Albers, A. B. (2001). Effects of poverty and maternal depression in early child development. *Child Development, 72*, 1794–1813. A website based on the work of Kathryn Barnard can be accessed at http://cimhd.org.

---

variables that might show qualitative change as new movement patterns appear, as well as the control variables that limit or facilitate the transition between patterns, is the work on the developmental transition between walking and running of Whitall and Getchell.[289]

Although running has generally been described as differing from walking in having a flight phase, Whitall and

Getchell[289] did not find this to be the case in the early development of running. Nor could they find another variable that differed significantly between the two patterns of movement, suggesting that the transition was really one between two similar movements and not two qualitatively different patterns at all. These researchers recommended that the search for a collective variable for describing the qualitative difference between walking and running should be continued by assessing the possible role of arm movements. Young runners had difficulty generating both horizontal forces (reflected in a small increase in stride length over that used in walking) and vertical forces (reflected in little flight and little hip extension in running). Whitall and Getchell[289] surmised that the ability to produce or regulate force by the ankle extensors was a key control parameter for emergence of running. They suggested that another control parameter might be ability to organize posture during high-velocity movement.

A dynamical systems approach to studying the transition from reaching without grasping to reaching with grasping was more successful in showing a sharp transition from predominant use of one pattern to predominant use of the other over a period of approximately 1 to 2 weeks.[292,293] In keeping with the prediction of dynamical systems theory, in the weeks just before the shift from predominance of one mode of reaching to the other, infants showed instability of mode choice; that is, they frequently switched between types of reaching during a single session of reaching opportunities.[292] Individual infants demonstrated the phase shift at different ages (usually between 13 and 20 weeks of age), and a search for control parameters driving the change showed that arm weight and arm circumference (which increased with age in a continuous, linear fashion) were significantly related to the change in preferred mode of reaching.[293] Computer modeling of infant grasp learning is also revealing how the infant grasp reflex can be shaped to achieve a variety of arm movements leading to successful grasping without the need for visual guidance,[209] bringing back the old question of whether voluntary movements are derived from reflexes. The model proposes that two assumptions are sufficient for an infant to learn effective grasping: that infants can sense the effects of their motor activity and can use feedback to adjust movement planning parameters.

Other researchers have taken the investigation of learning to reach further back in developmental time to the period before reaching occurs successfully at 4 to 5 months of age.[175] This research demonstrated that the presence of a toy during the period just prior to appearance of spontaneous successful reaching changed the dynamics of elbow movements to a more adult-like coordination but did not affect shoulder movements in a similar way. The researchers surmised that the control of elbow spatial coordination may be more task specific than that of the shoulder. They believe that the role of the shoulder is to propel the arm forward to an approximate position near the object, whereas the role of the elbow is to fine tune arm and hand position. The transition from prereaching to successful reaching to contact an object thus involves discovering the properties afforded by the various arm segments during the many spontaneous movements generated by infants every day.

Although use of dynamical systems theory to drive therapeutic theory and practice in physical therapy is still in its infancy with no large efficacy studies reported to date,[42,180,275] it is already clear that this model focuses the attention of the therapist on a number of important aspects of the therapeutic process of facilitating functional activity and participation. These aspects include (1) search for the constraints in subsystems that limit motor behavior, such as contractures or weakness, leading to treatment goals related to reduction of impairments; (2) creation of an environment that supports or compensates for weaker or less mature (rate-limiting) components of the systems that contribute to development of motor control so as to promote activity and participation; (3) attention to setting up a therapeutic environment that affords opportunities to practice tasks in a meaningful and functional context, especially in the child's home and community with a high value placed on parent coaching rather than direct treatment by therapists; (4) use of activities that promote exploration of a variety of movement patterns that might be appropriate for a task; and (5) search for control parameters, such as speed of movement or force production, that can be manipulated by intervention to facilitate the attainment of therapeutic goals, especially during sensitive periods of development during which behavior is less stable.[99,100,146,175] Chapter 3 on motor control and Chapter 4 on motor learning explore these concepts as therapeutic guides in more detail.

Myrtle McGraw, although generally considered a member of the maturationist school, developed a theory of motor development in the 1930s that contained the rudiments of many of the components of the modern dynamical systems approach to understanding the development of motor skills.[24,80,192] McGraw was a psychologist who studied the effects of intensive intervention, beginning at 20 days of age, with Johnny, the weaker of twin boys named Johnny and Jimmy. Her research was conducted at the height of the nature-nurture controversy between maturationists (represented by Gesell) and behaviorists (represented by Skinner). In summary, her work showed that providing up to 7 hours a day of exercise of newly emerging developmental skills in the first year of life did not increase the rate of motor development. Her anecdotal comments, however, indicated that the exercised twin had more relaxed muscle tone and better coordination of movement than the twin whose movements and exploration had been restricted to a crib for much of the day, with no interaction with people other than for needed care.

McGraw's work was interpreted at the time as supporting the neural-maturationist theory that the environment had little effect on child development. In the second year of his life, however, McGraw provided Johnny with a stimulating environment and extensive practice opportunities (3 hours per day) for developing motor skills that were not otherwise likely to develop in a child younger than 2 years, such as roller skating, climbing inclines of 70°, and jumping off high pedestals. Under these conditions, Johnny excelled in physical growth, problem solving of difficult motor control situations, and attainment of skills that Jimmy refused even to try during the periodic testing sessions that occurred. McGraw also noted the remarkable persistence in tasks demonstrated by Johnny, as well as his extensive visual review of the situation before embarking on a task. Films of the twins at age 40 years, moreover, demonstrated that the twin who exercised intensively during the first 2 years had an impressive physique and elegantly coordinated movement compared with those of his twin. In recounting her life's work and its interpretation by herself and others, McGraw illustrated how the biases of the times are reflected in how research results are interpreted and received. Clearly, experience practicing novel skills enhanced the physical development of the trained twin.

Although the results of an analysis of two individual cases cannot be accepted as leading to fundamental laws of motor development, McGraw's study makes it clear that we have little idea of the possibilities inherent in the very young child who is seldom stimulated to achieve the full potential of early motor skill development. By analogy, we can assume that we have barely scratched the surface in our understanding of how therapeutic intervention might be used to mitigate the effects of conditions causing motor dysfunction. Research on treadmill training of infants,[36,279] behavioral shaping of movement exploration efforts,[11] mathematical modeling of developmental processes,[209] and robotic models of development[173,201,202] show promise for dramatically altering our approaches to research and intervention for children with disabilities in the future.

DEVELOPMENTAL PROCESSES AND PRINCIPLES

Based on her study of Johnny and Jimmy, as well as 68 other babies studied longitudinally without special intervention, McGraw constructed a set of developmental principles, many of which remain current (or are once again current) today. She conceived of movements as behaviors within an action system in which objects in the environment are as important a part of the action system as the movements themselves. "Any activity is composed of many ingredients, some of which may for convenience be considered as external and others as internal with respect to the organism, but none of these factors can be considered as external to the behavior."[192] McGraw also recognized that multiple components are interwoven in the development of behavior patterns:[192]

> The growing of a behavior pattern is likened to a design in the process of being woven, composed as it is of various colored threads. All of the threads do not move forward at the same time or at the same rate. The weaver picks up the gold thread and weaves it back and forth, though at the same time steadily forward. Then he drops it in order to bring the blue thread forward a distance, until finally the two become united to make the pattern complete. The design is

contingent upon the interrelation of the various threads. It is not the summation of the blue and gold threads but their position with respect to each other and to the piece as a whole that determines the design (pp. 302–303).

McGraw also described the uneven nature of development, in which a given behavior pattern has a period of "inception, incubation, consummation, and decline (p. 305)."[192] The results of her longitudinal studies on the intratask course of development of important motor patterns were published in 1945[193] and remain highly informative today (although her description of brain development itself has long been out of date). Because of her daily observations, she often saw a movement pattern appear only once or twice (examples of beginner's luck) and then disappear before becoming a stable part of the infant's repertoire. When first becoming stable, the activity seems overworked and exaggerated. Furthermore, she noted that "as the child begins to get control over a pattern or an aspect of a pattern, the activity itself becomes the incentive for repetition (p. 307)."[192] Thus, early in life, movement for the sake of movement is a functional activity. The daily observations of infant development conducted by Adolph and colleagues[6] confirmed that multiple daily transitions in performance skills are present before a stable new pattern emerges.

Therapists who perceive these evanescent periods of self-driven motivation to practice emerging movements and who follow the lead of children in the flow of therapy or parent coaching are likely to be among those whose clients are both happy and productive in intervention sessions. Because children with disabilities may have fewer options for exploration of movement opportunities, it is important to note that research supports the importance of caregiver guidance in assisting children with self-discovery efforts. For example, young children with developmental disabilities do have mastery motivation (i.e., persistent task-directed behavior in moderately challenging problem-solving situations) that is similar to that of other children, but their level of motivation is related to their mental, rather than chronologic, age and is improved in those who experience high levels of adaptive interaction with their mothers.[33,142] However, most research efforts aimed at exploring the relationship between maternal education or family socioeconomic status (SES) do not find these variables important in motor development,[229] the exception being in the presence of severe disadvantage.[194] Cognitive development, however, is negatively affected as a function of the total number of environmental risk factors present, even when controlling for SES.[243] For example, the presence of multiple-factor risk scores explained up to 50% of the variance in IQ in children at 4 and 13 years of age in Sameroff and colleagues' longitudinal study. As a result, parent education efforts should include exploring the family's understanding of infant development and fostering growth-promoting interactions with their children.

McGraw suggested that a stable movement pattern may seem to disappear as a part of the child's repertoire, becoming superseded by some rapidly developing new behavior, but ultimately the movement is restricted to its most specific and economic form. She was among the first to note the presence of normal regressions in motor behavior and has been credited as one of the first developmental psychologists to recognize the bidirectionality of neural and behavioral development.[24,28,208,224] A behavior may also become integrated with other behaviors to form a complex activity; thus, McGraw noted that the developmental course of a behavior may look quite different during different stages of its maturation. A "second wind" for a behavioral pattern in decline as a part of the movement repertoire was also noted.

Because McGraw noted these various characteristics across many developing movement patterns, she believed that fits and starts, spurts and regressions, and overlapping of patterns undergoing emergence, development, and decline were firm developmental principles and that snapshots of development, such as motor milestone tests, could not adequately reflect the underlying processes of development.[24] The work of Adolph and colleagues[6] confirms this belief. McGraw firmly believed that there were sensitive periods (she actually used the term "critical period" but later regretted it because of its "use it or lose it permanently" interpretation in biology) in which interventions could produce the most influence on developing behavioral patterns.[14] During a sensitive period, certain experiences have particularly influential effects on development, although these effects are not necessarily irreversible or nonmodifiable with subsequent experience.[40] A recent example is research demonstrating that in musicians matched for years of experience, those who began training before the age of 7 years performed better on a rhythmic tapping task than musicians who began training after 7 years.[217]

McGraw believed that the period of greatest susceptibility to exercise was one in which a behavior pattern was entering its most rapid phase of development. Delay did not mean that intervention could no longer affect the behavior pattern (the concept of critical period), but rather that the interference of other ongoing developmental programs, including changes in anthropometric configuration of the body with growth, can decrease effectiveness. Unfortunately, we still have little idea of how these developmental principles might be systematically applied in a therapeutic milieu, but dynamical systems theory has brought them back to the forefront of scientific thinking about the processes of motor development. When research provides prescriptions for most effectively structuring therapy based on a child's current repertoire and presence of instability in selection of behavioral response modes, readiness level for learning new skills, constraints that limit the possibility of change, and task or environmental characteristics that will be influential in evoking developmental progress, we are likely to make great strides in the

efficient packaging of therapeutic programs.[37] Even more important will be knowledge that helps therapists to coach parents in effectively assisting children in their own self-initiated attempts to drive developmental progress.

McGraw ended her monumental study of human development by foreseeing the development and potential of dynamical systems–based motion analysis. "Perhaps the time will come when the movements of growth can be expressed in mathematical formulas as precisely as the movements of celestial bodies, but until that time arrives we shall have to be content with cumbersome descriptive analyses (p. 312)."[192] The work by Wimmers and colleagues[293] on the developmental transition between two modes of reaching and Oztop and colleagues'[209] computational modeling of learning to grasp are just two examples of elegant quantitative descriptions of the processes of change during motor development that McGraw predicted. She would be amazed by current work in which developmental processes and principles are being explored with robots.[173,201]

CONTEMPORARY ISSUES IN UNDERSTANDING PRINCIPLES OF MOTOR DEVELOPMENT

Despite a current theoretic perspective that models development as encompassing multiple organismic components in the creation of coordinative structures for posture and movement and emphasizes the crucial role of the environment and task characteristics in organizing emergent movements, certain principles of motor development have consistently appeared in the conceptual framework of various students of motor development. These principles include the notions that development of motor skills generally proceeds in a cephalocaudal and proximodistal direction, that neural maturation is an important component of unfolding skill development, and that motor development appears, at least on the surface, to be more stagelike than continuous, having a spiraling nature in which regressions, consolidations, and reappearances of underlying fundamental processes occur.[28]

What is becoming clear is that these long-standing theoretic concepts must be revised and expanded to incorporate a new understanding of the underlying developmental processes. For example, new research on developmental processes discussed in Chapter 3 on motor control has revealed that certain factors are rate limiting to motor development, with strength, postural control, and perceptual analysis capabilities being among the most important. When compensations are provided experimentally to eliminate the effects of these rate-limiting factors, the developing motor system may display previously unrecognized potential. Patterns of movement appear that seem precocious because they were previously denied expression owing to immaturity of certain of the cooperating systems. Recent work has demonstrated constraints on motor development and learning that include planning for tool use in toddlers being constrained by hand preference, an internal organismic constraint,[78] and the ability of an infant to mimic adult actions being constrained by whether the infants' response was cued by sound or was visible to them or not, each external factors related to the task or environmental characteristics.[156]

Dynamical systems theory research has also demonstrated that stagelike external behavior, such as the switch from reaching without grasping to reaching with grasping[292,293] can emerge from continuously changing underlying processes. Here a new stage seems to appear de novo only because the continuous developments of a number of cooperating systems finally merge in a way that allows the new behavior to appear. The behavior appears to reflect an entirely novel stage of development when in fact the underlying processes in multiple systems were developing continuously in a gradually accretive fashion. We will use more information about the development of eye-hand coordination to illustrate these points.

CEPHALOCAUDAL AND PROXIMODISTAL DEVELOPMENTAL DIRECTION

The processes involved in the advanced stages of development of functional reaching include (1) visual fixation to localize the object and choose a hand transport program, (2) foveal analysis for perceptual identification of the object needed for anticipatory adaptation of the action to fit the characteristics of the object, (3) manual capture, and (4) object manipulation.[143] By the time of birth, a primitive body scheme has already developed that provides the infant with a hand transport program. Infants have been observed in utero during real-time ultrasound imaging to perform hand-to-mouth activities, touch other parts of their own bodies, and explore the uterine walls—all, of course, without visual guidance.[255] Shortly after birth, they are able to launch the hand toward an object, preferring one that is moving.[285,286] (This competence fits well with the known characteristics of early development of the retina, which is more mature in the movement-sensitive periphery than in the foveal area.[1]) The hand, although open, does not engage in actual grasping in most cases, and the coordination of the movement does not include corrections of direction or hand-shaping for the object's properties during the course of the reach.[284] In fact, the entire arm is launched as a single unit in a pattern that can best be described as a swipe, a coordinative strategy that is quite unlike the lift-project strategy typical of more mature reaching. Nevertheless, such reaches can sometimes result in use of precision-type grips very early in infancy. Oztop and colleagues[209] used information in the literature to guide the development of a computer model of the early stages of learning to grasp which demonstrates that arm movements along with the infant grasp reflex and tactile search can be used to guide the development of a variety of grasping strategies without the need for visual guidance in the early months of life.

Because we know that further development will include gradual refinement of hand use as part of reaching and grasping, this sequence of development would appear to follow the proximodistal developmental rule. The course of development, however, is much more complicated. First, reaching at 1 to 2 months is typically done with a fisted hand, rather than the open hand of the newborn, and reaching under visual control with an open hand begins at 4 to 5 months.[284] Furthermore, successful reach-and-grasp can often occur in the period from 1 to 2 months if the head is supported to eliminate a major problem in developing a successful coordinative strategy. Thus, when external controls are provided for the posturally incompetent head, the infant may be able to coordinate a reach-and-grasp successfully, even though, as we have seen, consistent use of reaching with grasping is not present until 13 to 20 weeks of age.[292]

These and other observations have led to the suggestions that postural control is a rate-limiting factor in early motor development[251] and that distal competence may be masked by deficiencies in postural control of the head and neck. In support of the importance of postural control in development, Viholanen and colleagues[283] reported that an early body control factor measured in infancy explained 38% of the variance in gross motor skills at age 3.5 years. Although it seems readily apparent that the ability to control the head to maintain stability of visual perception is an important competence in a general sequence of cephalocaudal progression of development, many aspects of proximal and distal control of the extremities are undergoing contemporaneous development that may not be overtly observable under normal conditions.[102,146,183] Many exceptions to a proximodistal progression of development have been found.[146]

An important consequence of understanding these research findings is that therapists should not conceive of individual body parts as developing independently, sequentially, or purely as a result of nervous system maturation when planning therapeutic intervention. Although various segments of the body may develop their patterns of control for any given task at different rates, any movement pattern is a composite, involving coordination of all the body subsystems. Furthermore, the apparent directionality of development does not appear to be inherent only in the genetic direction of nervous system development, but rather it is a result of the interactive functioning of the multiple systems children bring to exploration of the problems and possibilities inherent in a particular task at a particular point in their physical and cognitive development.[265] The characteristics and demands of the task are critical in organizing the response of the subsystems,[209] but each child's response is unique in its kinematics and time of appearance.[269,292] In early infancy, for example, the enormous mass of the child's head relative to the size of the rest of the body places constraints on the functions that are possible. Lifting the head and sustaining its upright position while the body is prone therefore entails coordinating the trunk and extremities to create a stable base for head movement. Until the head can be adequately stabilized in space, other movement functions of the body in the prone position cannot be fully expressed.

What seems to play a major role, then, in the general observation of cephalocaudal progression of development are the infant's strength of key muscle groups and anthropometric characteristics—that is, the ability to control the large mass of the head relative to the rest of the body and cope with the high center of mass. Although cephalocaudal progression is a notion that seems to hold as an overall generalization regarding the postural control of the whole body, most movements used by infants entail the coordination of multiple body parts if they are to be effective. The coordination of a prone-on-elbows-with-head-turn strategy for responding to an interesting sound with visual fixation is a good example.

In developing items for the Test of Infant Motor Performance,[57] an interesting sequence of development was discovered in the organization of a response to a sound made behind an infant's head as the infant lay in the prone position (Liao & Campbell, 2004, unpublished data). An immature response involved dragging the face across the surface to turn the head toward the sound and visualize it. By 4 months of age, typically developing infants were able to support themselves on their elbows with head lifted and turn toward the sound. Over the course of weekly examinations, however, we noticed that some infants tended to alternate for several weeks between the mature response described and one in which they lifted the head and extended the upper trunk, but they seemed unable to turn the head toward the sound source despite obvious interest in the stimulus. After several weeks in which the two modes of response alternated, the individual infant's response stabilized in its most mature form. What intrigued us was why an infant who could lift his head, but apparently could not organize his posture so as to turn it toward an interesting sound, would not choose to go back to an earlier, successful response—that is, putting his head down on the surface to turn it. It appears that once the infant has the ability to extend the neck and trunk in prone position, he would forgo successful task accomplishment (i.e., seeing the interesting sound source) in favor of an unsuccessful head lifting strategy that was used repeatedly over a period of a couple of weeks until he could consistently put together all the components of the most mature response strategy using prone-on-elbows as a base of support. Green and colleagues'[128] description of the changes in load bearing with development showed that body weight must be shifted caudally such that load-bearing surfaces include the lateral thighs and lower abdomen before successful head turning with the head erect occurs. Based on our data, this development appears to occur over a short period of a couple of weeks and represents an ability to dissociate movement of the upper part of the body from the pelvis and lower extremities.

The examples given earlier illustrate the power of the dynamical systems perspective by pointing out that multiple systems and processes are developing at any given time, each at its own rate and instantaneous level of competence. What then appears to be a newly appearing "stage" may merely be the time at which one or more rate-limiting factors finally achieve a level of development in a continuous trajectory that supports the appearance of a new, stable form of behavior. The new behavior appears discontinuous with what went before only because the underlying continuous processes were not visible. In the example from research on the Test of Infant Motor Performance, it can be recommended that a treatment plan for helping a child with motor dysfunction to achieve the ability to freely use head and later hands in a prone position might profitably include learning to organize the load-bearing parts of the lower body or use of a roll under the chest to passively position the load more posteriorly. Further research to identify the critical processes and subsystems that contribute to qualitative changes in infant behavior should be productive in refining intervention strategies to promote motor development in children with disabilities.

NERVOUS SYSTEM MATURATION AS ONE DRIVING FORCE FOR DEVELOPMENT

Although McGraw,[193] Gesell,[115,116] and Shirley[248] emphasized brain maturation as being the major force driving development (despite their own contrary evidence for the important role of external factors), dynamical systems theory has sometimes seemed to view neural maturation with less credence than I believe it deserves. The nervous system in dynamical systems theory is described as merely another system in its developmental contribution, no more important than any other system. In children with mental retardation or cerebral motor dysfunction, however, therapists are well aware of the serious limitations in adapting movement to functional purposes imposed by a compromised CNS. This chapter describes development and functions of the nervous system in movement; Chapter 5 provides information on another important cooperating component, the musculoskeletal system.

Research suggests that about 30% of the entire genome is expressed only in the brain,[206] but the effects of genetics differ even within the regions of the brain. For example, studies using twins to analyze the heritability versus environmental effects on cerebral cortical development suggest that early-developing regions such as the primary sensorimotor cortical areas show especially strong genetic effects early in childhood, whereas later developing regions, such as the prefrontal cortex and temporal lobes, show more prominent heritability effects later in childhood consistent with previous findings that IQ becomes more heritable later in the course of maturation.[178] Although it is true that we now know that experience drives brain development in just as important a way as do genetics,[129] the notion that no hierarchy of important functions or no unique function of structures exists is simply not true, especially in the human brain with its highly encephalized processes. What is true is that lower levels of the nervous system, such as the midbrain and the spinal cord, have been recognized to be capable of controlling many finely coordinated movements, not only simple reflexes, and that vast amounts of the CNS are involved in the production and control of even the most basic movements. For example, animal research described in Chapter 3 has revealed that well-coordinated stepping movements can be evoked from activation of spinal cord circuits. Involvement of higher levels of the nervous system, however, is necessary to control the body's overall equilibrium during gait and to express the intentionality of functional movements. Similarly, the modeling research of Oztop and colleagues[209] suggests that spinal circuits involved in the primitive grasp reflex can be used to organize more sophisticated grasping strategies through use of feedback derived from reaching activity. The locus of control for a given movement varies, however, depending on task requirements and previous experience with similar tasks. Thus, environmental demands become a part of the neural ensemble for producing movement, and the infant's practice of exploratory movements creates inputs that drive brain development.

To return to the example of development of eye-hand coordination, humans display a major shift from subcortically organized movement in the first 3 to 4 months to increasing involvement of cortical circuits at 4 to 5 months.[210] Infants with later evidence of cortical blindness, for example, may be able to track an object visually in the newborn period, using brain stem processing mechanisms. Although the organism's own activity is influential in directing the early course of neural plasticity,[129] this example of deviant development reinforces the concept that the higher levels of the CNS are necessary (but not sufficient) for normal human development to occur. Visual functions involving binocularity seem particularly dependent on development of cortical visual circuits. For example, most infants can align their eyes appropriately in the first month of life, but only when visual cortex dominance columns have been refined do they gain control of both the sensory (optical fusion) and the motor (eye convergence) aspects of binocularity.[274]

Reaching, too, differs fundamentally in the newborn and the 6-month-old.[210] Reaching is a unitary action in the young infant; a differentiation among reach, grasp, manipulation, and release will later result from maturation of cortical systems in conjunction with anthropometric changes[292,293] and learning gained from experiences in the world of objects.[96]

As seen in patients with a stroke that affects fine hand function, cortical activity is necessary for the more delicate aspects of motor control of the hand, and it cannot develop adequately unless the encephalic structures are intact. No examples have been reported in the literature of a capability of higher primates to develop or regain fine finger control in the absence of the primary motor cortex. Establishment of monosynaptic connections between the motor cortex and spinal cord motoneurons is associated with the appearance of selective control of digital movements in primates;[245] these connections are not present in neonatal monkeys and develop gradually during the first 8 months after birth. Improvement in monkeys' abilities to retrieve small pieces of food from indentations is seen when a wide range of rapid, small movements involving the forearm or shoulder joint appear to assist more efficient distal performance of the digits. This description is remarkably similar to descriptions of the development of fidgety movements in human infants at 2 to 3 months of age.[130] These movements herald the development of goal-directed movements, including the emergence of consistently effective reaching and grasping. These small synergistic movements in monkeys do not survive pyramidotomy, nor do selective digital movements.

At about the same time that fidgety movements develop, the appearance in infants of ballistic movements (swipes and swats) heralds the switch from coactivation of muscle groups to the reciprocal coordination of muscle activity that characterizes more mature motor patterns.[131] Wimmers and colleagues[293] suggested that use of coactivation patterns may also be correlated with reaching with a fisted hand and that the ability to reciprocally activate muscles may be related to both changes in arm circumference and the switch to reaching with an open hand. Although we do not know what leads to the appearance of reciprocal patterns of muscle activity, it is notable that this development does not seem to appear in children with cerebral palsy (CP).[179]

According to Paillard,[210] four features characterize the evolution of the primate nervous system, culminating in the human brain, and promote use of the hand as an elaborate tool for manipulating the environment. These features are (1) extension of the precentral cortex developed principally for fine sensory-guided steering and control of the hand and digits, which is included in the computer model of Oztop and colleagues;[209] (2) enlargement of the lateral cerebellum, again relating to control of forelimb segments and to timing and smoothing of movements; (3) specialization of the parietal association cortex for precise visual guidance of goal-directed arm and hand movements; and (4) prominent development of the frontal association areas that funnel information to motor control regions, mainly through basal ganglia loops. Here we see an example of multiple subsystems in the brain cooperating with the musculoskeletal structures characteristic of the human organism to produce functional movement.

Further evidence of the complex relationships among brain subsystems and environmental inputs and exploration by infants comes from research documenting the existence of mirror neurons that fire when an individual watches another person manipulate an object as well as during active manipulation by the individual himself.[26] A second class of neurons discharges when the same action is performed by either the hand or the mouth. Bernardis and colleagues[26] conjecture that these neurons are a source of the connection between gesture and speech during early language learning. As infants learn to gesture to indicate their wants during the period from 8 to 13 months, they usually vocalize at the same time. The researchers demonstrated that the vocalizations differ depending on whether an object is large or small in support of their hypothesis that manual interactions with objects contribute to language development before the use of first words.

The frontal areas of the cerebral cortex process information related to goal-directed behavior and anticipated consequences of intended acts involving the basic capacity to guide response choice by stored information.[124,210] Major developments in this area in the human infant begin at about 8 months and reach a maximum at 2 years of age. The ventrolateral prefrontal cortex is associated with rule representation and develops later than the supplementary motor area (SMA), which is involved in suppressing responses that are no longer successful.[79] The SMA is mature by adolescence, whereas the ventrolateral prefrontal cortex shows differences between adolescents and adults in functional magnetic resonance imaging studies. Activity in frontal areas cooperates in motor functions through basal ganglia circuits.[148] The basal ganglia are involved in the internal generation of automatic movements, the predictive monitoring of head and arm activities,[96] and the acquisition and learning of motor skills through their five parallel pallidal-thalamocortical loops, including projections to primary motor cortex, where the dynamics of movement patterns are selected.[113]

Eye-head-body orientation activities and target-reaching activities have been shown in lower vertebrates to be coordinated primarily by brain stem centers, prominently involving the superior colliculus.[210] In keeping with identification of these behaviors in very young infants, arm projection at that age is possible without cerebral cortical control. Functional manipulation, such as the fine digital control involved in food taking in experimental primates, however, depends on the additional coordinated action of cortical pathways from higher centers.[96] Elegant hand-grasping and manipulation movements of the primate are dependent on inputs from cerebral cortical levels that are coordinated with lower-level eye-hand-head activity. Overall, however, the primary role of higher-level CNS structures is to tune, guide, learn, and select, adapt, or inhibit execution of basic movements by lower levels of the nervous system. The therapist views this as increasing ability to control movements selectively and adapt them to functional purposes.

Motor control functions are not assumed at successively higher hierarchic levels, leaving behind previously used primitive behaviors and control centers; rather, many levels of the nervous system cooperate in the production of movement behaviors. Typically, no single active site for any

particular behavior can be identified; behavior is, rather, an emergent property of the cooperation of various subsystems, with task characteristics organizing the response.[26,269] That is, the characteristics of the task lead the nervous system with its distributed functions to select from a variety of currently available options for assembling a task-related action. The next section of this chapter elaborates on a theory of nervous system development and function that provides an appropriate explanatory model for how the developing organism actively constructs its own operating system for functional behavior.

THE THEORY OF NEURONAL GROUP SELECTION

According to a popular summary by Edelman[90] of current theories of nervous system functioning, previous psychologic theories have failed spectacularly in shedding light on how the human mind originates in the functioning of the physical brain because they have neglected the biology of the system. Popular models describing the brain as analogous to a computer with hardware (neurons) and software (motor programs) bear only superficial resemblance to the actual operation of the brain. Edelman's theory is based instead on facts that are garnered from biologic research but are also consistent with behavioral observations. Called the neuronal group selection theory, it has three basic tenets. These tenets describe how the anatomy of the brain is produced during development, how experience selects for strengthening certain patterns of responses from the anatomic structures, and how the resulting maps of the brain give rise to uniquely individual behavioral functions through a process called reentry. Sporns and Edelman[258] further described how such a system solves the problem of managing movement in an organism with multiple degrees of freedom, and Newell and Vaillancourt[203] described their new conceptualization of how changes in reorganization of the biomechanical degrees of freedom occur during motor learning.

The first tenet of Edelman's theory[90] is concerned with developmental selection by which the characteristic neuroanatomy of a species is formed. The genetic code of the species does not specify the wiring diagram but instead inscribes the constraints of the process of formation of neural networks, resulting in a primary repertoire of species-specific behavior. In humans, for example, these behaviors appear to include rhythmic movements of the lower extremities, expressed in kicking and neonatal stepping,[265] mouth-to-hand behaviors, visual following of moving objects, and projection of the arm toward objects.[285] An overproduction of early synaptic connections formed by activity and cell death or retraction of unexercised connections may explain why individual wiring diagrams vary somewhat yet still maintain the same general form across members of the species.

The second tenet of Edelman's[90] neuronal group selection theory involves the development of a secondary repertoire of functional circuits from the basic neuroanatomic network through a process of selective activation that strengthens or weakens synaptic connections based on individual experience. The secondary repertoire includes mechanisms underlying skilled motor behavior, memory, and other important functions and is unique to the individual. In a movement system with multiple degrees of freedom, a variety of ways to accomplish the movements involved in functional tasks can arise,[258] but to become incorporated into the secondary repertoire, the functional synergy selected must (1) accomplish the task and (2) allow for postural stability of the body during the task. Adolph[2] showed that the first movement strategy selected for a risky task such as descending a steep slope is goal directed and may be highly inefficient, even foolhardy. During development, however, infants try out a variety of movement strategies that happen to occur to them, often accidentally, before readily selecting the most safe and economical one for the task at hand. Similarly, Oztop and colleagues'[209] model of learning to grasp suggests that a variety of arm movements with differing coordinative structures among the joints of the arm are explored by the infant with feedback from tactile inputs shaping the selection of effective strategies.

Edelman's third tenet describes how the first two selectional processes interact to connect biology with psychology. The primary and secondary repertoires of species-typical and uniquely individual functional neural circuits must form maps connected by massively parallel and reciprocal connections. Edelman presented the example that the visual system of the monkey consists of more than 30 different maps, each with a unique degree of functional segregation for orientation, color, movement, and other functions and each linked to the others by parallel and reciprocal connections that can be accessed by the reentry process. By this process, a nervous system with distributed functions is formed.

Selection occurs over neuronal groups from various maps throughout the region and the nervous system as a whole to produce a particular behavior. The behavior is unique to the individual in whom it occurs because of variations in maps caused by the effects of individual experience on their development. The combination of neuronal groups from selected multiple maps of an area's function (for example, the hand motor area of primary cerebral motor cortex combined with selections from maps that are concerned with receipt of visual and tactile information and ones concerned with postural function of the neck and shoulder) allows the production of a movement that is precisely tuned to the environmental demands for functional performance yet unique to the individual's capacity for processing sensory inputs and for combining selections of neuronal groups from his or her individual regional maps. A selectionist system with distributed functions requires a repertoire of variable actions in order to provide adaptability; that is, a variety of means for responding to environmental demands and internal changes such as growth must be available.

A selectionist model of the nervous system is consistent with the research of Keshner and colleagues[163] demonstrating that when overtly similar movements are studied in a group of individuals, each person performs the movement with his or her own unique combination of synergistic muscle activation patterns. Thelen and colleagues[269] have demonstrated similar findings in infants learning to reach. Although a group of infants tended to use a similar strategy of coactivating muscular antagonists when first learning to reach, each infant came at the task in a unique way based on preferred posture, movement, and energy level. Two quiet infants, for example, organized their reaches by lifting their arms and extending them slowly forward. Two other infants, who were highly active and frequently engaged in bilateral arm flapping, needed to damp down their oscillations to reach successfully. These infants used high-velocity swipes to orient their arms toward the toy. In testing infants on the Test of Infant Motor Performance, we also observed variations in how infants approached the orientation-to-sound task in the prone position. For example, one infant extended his neck and trunk when he heard the sound, but being unable to shift his load bearing caudally and support himself on his elbows in order to turn his head, he instead flapped his arms and legs, causing his trunk to rock forward and backward, and eventually negotiated a partial turn of his trunk toward the sound source by pivoting on his abdomen (Campbell, 1998, unpublished data).

In keeping with each individual's march to a personal internal drum, each phenotypic neuronal group has a combination of excitatory and inhibitory connections, allowing the final motor output to be assembled selectively based on current demands and past experience with the task that has strengthened or weakened the tendencies to select particular groups from particular maps.[90,265] Essential to this development is exposure of the nervous system to a sufficient sample of coactivated sensory signals to permit the neuronal groups to respond differentially to various objects and events in the environment.[257] Obtaining such a sampling of experience occurs during development when an infant spontaneously explores the environment through movement. To have adaptive value, the responding neuronal groups must also contribute to functional activity in the organism. Resulting from these selections, higher-order dynamic structures called global maps are formed that link sensory and motor maps. Such correlated activity is essential to operation of a system based on variability in response units, which become strengthened through use and adaptive value. Such resulting global maps are able to interact with memory processes and other unmapped functions such as those of the basal ganglia and cerebellum. Global maps allow the connection between local maps and motor behavior, new sensory inputs, and further neural processing as important aspects of development and learning.

Neuronal group selection theory does not hold that programs are executed by the nervous system; rather, dynamic loops are created that continually match movements and postures to task-related sensory signals of multiple kinds. Functioning is based on statistical probabilities of signals, not coded signals or preformed programs. Georgopoulos and colleagues,[114] for example, have demonstrated that the precise directionality of a reaching movement can be specified by vectors calculated from the neural activity of large populations of cells in the motor cortex, each of which individually has a preferred directionality but also fires in relation to movements in multiple directions. Edelman[90] further theorized that the system has biologic "values" that are species-specific and drive the selective strengthening of synaptic activities based on experience. These values influence adaptive processes by linkage between the global mappings and activity in hedonic centers and the limbic system of the brain in a way that fulfills homeostatic needs of the organism that have been set through evolution. For example, the computer model of Oztop and colleagues[209] includes a variable labeled by the authors "joy of grasping," which models the sensory feedback received by the infant from achieving a successful stable grasp and that, in turn, strengthens the future selection of grasping strategies.

In a computer model of a visual system with a set "value" that prefers light to no-light conditions in the center of a "visual" field (similar to that produced in humans by evolution), initially nondirected movements of an "arm" have been shaped to target an object.[90,266] If one appreciates that newborn infants possess a primary repertoire that includes moving the mouth to the hand, seeking light, and producing head turns or arm projections in response to moving objects in the visual field, it is not difficult to perceive of the theory of neuronal group selection as an explanation for the gradual process of learning to reach successfully to grasp an object and put it into the mouth. The research of Oztop and colleagues[209] produced the first successful computational model of the process of learning to grasp.

With repeated experience in reaching and grasping as an "individual problem solver working each day,"[269] infants modulate their intrinsic dynamics, discovering the most stable trajectory, joint coordination, and patterns of muscle activation,[269] thereby creating their own personal maps. For example, Strick and Preston[261,262] have suggested that separate representations of hand motor patterns at cerebral cortical levels may reflect the modular organization of sensorimotor units underlying the distinctive uses of the hand for power gripping or as a palpatory sensory surface. Dynamical systems theory, however, emphasizes that the nervous system is only one subsystem infants use to self-organize exploration of the environment.

Map creation through an individual's use of movement to drive brain plasticity can go awry. Byl and colleagues,[48] for example, reported that when a monkey was trained and reinforced for performing a stereotyped movement thousands of times, the simultaneous activation of muscles and tactile-kinesthetic receptors resulted in degradation of the primary sensory cortex maps. Neurons in the cortical area related to hand function become responsive to stimulation almost anywhere on the hand (even the back of the hand), a condition Byl and colleagues describe as a dedifferentiation of the normally exquisitely organized response patterns of the sensory cortex. They believe that this animal model may reflect the process of repetitive strain injury with focal dystonia in humans and that the findings support use of a sensorimotor retraining approach to treating this disorder in order to redifferentiate sensory maps in the cerebral cortex. If we think of the constrained and repetitive movements used by infants with CNS dysfunction, it is not hard to conceive of the possibility that they also have a poorly differentiated sensory cortex. The key to understanding and treating this type of problem is recognition that maps are formed connecting various areas of the brain based on the simultaneous activity of sensory and motor systems. We learn (and train the brain to select) what we do. Stereotyped simultaneous activity leads to poorly differentiated brain maps, whereas learning to use a variety of flexible patterns to accomplish common tasks leads to rich, complex brain organization compatible with adaptability to environmental demands and the internal changes accompanying growth.

New developments in understanding how the early movements of infants drive the development of more mature sensorimotor strategies come from robotic studies. A humanoid robot developed by Natale and colleagues[201] explores its own body before turning its attention to the environment; the interaction of the robot's body during reaching and contacting objects in its external environment leads to acquisition of a visual model of the objects encountered. These developments then are used to guide an attentional system for later learning. Kuniyoshi and colleagues[173] simulated fetal/neonatal motor development with spontaneous exploration of a variety of motor patterns and showed that visual-motor self-directed learning can lead to imitation behaviors on the part of a neonate. The knowledge acquired from experiments such as these are rapidly being translated into the design of robots that can be controlled by human infants,[185] and that will soon evolve into useful designs for fostering activity and participation in children with disabilities.

EXPERIENCE-EXPECTANT AND EXPERIENCE-DEPENDENT NEURAL MATURATION

Greenough and colleagues[129] have also discussed the importance of environmental experience in driving development of the brain, and their work provides further elaboration on Edelman's theory of neuronal group selection in a maturational context. Although no scientific evidence exists to suggest that training or an enriched environment leads to development of new neurons, extensive evidence documents the effect of training and environment on numbers and properties of synaptic connections among neural cells. Greenough and colleagues[129] suggested that genetically specified directions lead to initial synaptic connectivities through a process of overproduction of populations of cells that are pruned by exposure to experiences common to all members of a species, such as the array of visual inputs to which infants are typically exposed. The result is species-typical behaviors akin to the primary repertoire described by Edelman.[90]

Greenough and colleagues[129] called this process experience-expectant development and suggested that it occurs through the death of cells that do not establish productive connections. It has been discovered, however, that the genetic code may actually program cell death.[17] If neurons have access to particular nerve growth factors, they may be able to escape their programmed fate. By such genetic-environmental interactions, development occurs by a size-matching process whereby the appropriate number of neurons survives to serve peripheral needs. By one's own developmental processes, therefore, each individual obtains a personal, unique structure and functional movement.

A second process, akin to Edelman's secondary repertoire and called experience-dependent neural maturation, is proposed to be the process by which each individual achieves further uniqueness in structure and function through exposure to an individualized set of experiences that establishes strong connectivities among cells based on strengthening of neural synapses that are "exercised" through both sensory and motor experiences.[129] The specific structure and function of a person therefore depend on both species-typical connectivities and the amount and strength of other connections resulting from personal experiences specific to each individual and his or her life history. Of most importance, in both aspects of neural plasticity, synaptic connectivity is linked to the individual's own activity in conjunction with genetic programs and environmental opportunities. Thus, the individual in a very real sense is the creator of his or her own unique brain and, by extension, functional motor behaviour.[265] Furthermore, Anderson and colleagues[10] argue that the acquisition of motor skills through self-produced motor activity orchestrates psychologic changes that expose infants to patterns of information that can be used in the acquisition and control of skills in a variety of other domains. The work by Bernardis and colleagues[26] suggests that hand use in object manipulation and during gestures along with hand-mouth coordination at the neural level and their relationship to language development is just one example.

SENSITIVE PERIODS IN DEVELOPMENT

Bertenthal and Campos,[27] in a commentary on Greenough and colleagues' theory, summarized research that may support the theory that experience-expectant and experience-dependent maturation of neural systems could be the basis of sensitive periods in development. They stressed that experience-dependent plasticity of the nervous system can initiate the generation of new synaptic connections and is available throughout the life span. The effects of experiences during a sensitive period, however, are expected to be qualitatively different from those at other points in the life span.[273] The theory also predicts that sensitive periods in experience-expectant development can be extended by various means, including deprivation of sensory inputs that allow synaptic competition for connections to persist longer than is usual.

Most of the animal research on the influence of environmental stimuli on neural plasticity has been on cerebral cortical areas, especially those devoted to visual function. Research has documented the existence of sensitive and in some cases critical periods for development of visual perceptual skills,[49,150,151,152,274] once again suggesting the superior benefits of intervention earlier, rather than later, in life. Some evidence also exists to suggest effects of interventions on the sensory cortex, the motor cortex, and the cerebellum.[129,207] For example, extensive practice of specific finger activities by monkeys led to enlarged areas of the motor cortex devoted to activation of the exercised fingers.[207]

Several sensitive periods in cognitive development have been demonstrated to occur during infancy.[105] At 2 to 4 months, infants demonstrate the ability to vary activity within a single action sequence to reach a simple goal, such as grasping a toy within reach. At 7 to 8 months, several actions can be related in a single functional unit, such as a delayed-response task, using vision to guide a manual manipulation or compare multiple objects, and using a string to activate a toy. By 12 to 13 months, a number of actions can be coordinated to perform a function such as putting a ball into a small hole in a toy box. At 18 to 21 months, symbolic representation is achieved in which a memory of an object can activate an action without the object's being present. Various types of evidence, such as changes in rates of synaptogenesis and electroencephalographic changes, show discontinuities at related time periods.

Unfortunately, only few data are available on the subject of sensitive periods as they affect motor skill development, particularly in children with acquired or congenital disabilities, and much of the evidence is correlational in nature. Zelazo and colleagues[298,299] demonstrated the effect of early stepping experience in human infants on maintenance of stepping behavior and earlier age of walking. Viholanen and colleagues[283] related an early body control factor in infancy to gross motor skills at toddler age with 38% of the variance explained. A large study of standing balance and chair rising ability showed that attainment of motor milestones at modal ages and higher scores on motor coordination in childhood were related to better physical performance in midlife.[172] Heriza[146] has proposed that sensitive periods exist in the development of locomotor behavior that can be identified through kinematic analysis of rhythmic alternating movements of the legs based on dynamical systems theory and hypothesized that these transitional periods are important points for intervention in children at risk for developmental disabilities. Piek and colleagues[222] extended the analysis of development of limb coordination patterns to the upper extremities. Dynamical systems theory suggests that when children vary in their selection of a movement strategy in response to a particular task, this period of instability represents a special opportunity for directing development.[175] Kanda and colleagues[158,159] have also reported superior benefits on quality of movement and walking in children with CP of early, as opposed to later or less intense, exposure to Vojta therapy, and Scherzer and colleagues[244] suggested that children with CP who were treated at an earlier age than others also demonstrated greater benefits. These preliminary suggestions that intervention to promote motor development may vary in effectiveness based on timing of therapy are tantalizing, and further research on this topic is direly needed for improving the scheduling of intervention for maximizing outcomes. To be successful, however, research designs must be tailored specifically to the search for answers to the sensitive period question.[40,273] Specifically, research to demonstrate a sensitive period requires that the same type, intensity, and duration of intervention be delivered at different stages of development.

PERIODIC EQUILIBRATION IN A SPIRALING PATTERN OF DEVELOPMENT

Piaget[219] suggested that the experience of acting on the world (assimilation) with whatever sensorimotor schema is currently dominant was frequently met with resistance because the objects of interest were not easily adapted to the current schema (e.g., handling a soft cookie when the motor activity of crumpling or shaking was currently popular). This misfit between the child's current sensorimotor functioning and the response of handled objects leads to disequilibrium, which drives developmental progress through the child's persistence in gradually accommodating to the properties of objects eliciting interest. In so doing, the child eventually develops a different approach to handling the cookie and thereby alters the cognitive structure as well. I would suggest that our infants' alternation over several weeks between symmetrical head and trunk extension versus supporting themselves on their elbows in response to a sound stimulus is an example of children learning to accommodate to new physical capabilities (head and trunk extension) while attempting to accomplish a task, in other words, flexible problem solving. Similarly, Lee and colleagues[176] demonstrated how the longitudinal development of grasping is influenced by the shape of objects. With age, infants continually differentiated their adaptive grip configuration to the properties of the prehension task.

Ames and colleagues,[9] following from Gesell's earlier observations, posited a similar process of alternating equilibrium and disequilibrium in behavioral characteristics that

they believed cycled periodically. For example, toddlers at 18 months are likely to be trying to their parents because they have definite wants but few words with which to express them; they may communicate with crying and tantrums instead. (The reader should note that in this and other sections of the chapter, ages given are normative or average times of appearance of described behaviors; individual developmental rates, of course, differ on the basis of experience, task, and other characteristics.) At 2 years, the child has developed more language and coordination and is emotionally on an even keel. Disequilibrium returns again at about 2.5 years, when this little person becomes more difficult to live with—bossy, rigid, and oppositional. Cooperation and sharing in play have not yet appeared, and the 2.5-year-old wants to hold onto any toy "he is playing with, has played with, or might in the future want to play with (p. 28)."[9] The age of 3 years is again an easy time emotionally, whereas at 3.5 years children are insecure and anxious, yet determined and self-willed. At 3, children need their security blankets and thumbs a great deal. The 4-year-old is described as wild and wonderful. This child loves humor and is secure and self-confident, although going overboard in either enthusiasm or anger, even threatening to run away when upset. Five-year-olds are more inwardly directed, prefer to stay within known boundaries, and have less interest in novel experiences. These children are careful to attempt only what can most definitely be achieved but are, nonetheless, expansive intellectually, loving to talk and learn about things. "Why?" is the word of choice. By 5.5 years, however, another period of disequilibrium seems to occur, but it is one characterized by extremes—shy at one moment, extremely bold the next. The child may seem to be in a constant state of tension, chewing on pencils and fidgeting. By 6.5 years, however, a calmer, more even-tempered child again emerges, moving toward the inner-directed 7-year-old.

Gesell,[146] Rood,[259] Bly,[34] and others have suggested that motor development also consists of an alternation and recombination of patterns of flexion, extension, and symmetry versus asymmetry, leading ever onward toward improved mobility and stability in posture and movement in opposition to the force of gravity. At different times, various patterns predominate, but an alternation between stability and instability of functioning characterized also by switches between symmetry and asymmetry is thought to be characteristic of normal developmental progression. Heriza has summarized these principles based on Gesell's early work as viewing growth "not as a linear process but a spiral one where structure and function jointly mature leading to regression, asymmetries, and reorganization.[146] Although Gesell is best known for his principles of direction of development and individuating maturation, his principle of reciprocal interweaving "foreshadows [a] contemporary systems view of motor development (p. 102)."[146] As we have seen, McGraw[192] held a similar view, but she and other early developmental researchers lacked the contemporary ability to reveal the underlying systems changes that produce these overtly observed patterns of development and tended to stress nervous system maturation as the driving force.

To summarize, studies have suggested that development proceeds in a continuous spiral characterized by "paired-but-opposed types of responses that occur in repeated alternation"[9] and with relative periods of stability and instability[146] that may reflect underlying developmental continuity within multiple subsystems involved in maturation. Regressions are also normal aspects of developmental processes[28,74,208,224] Ages 2, 5, 10, and 16 years are considered to be periods of emotional equilibrium; ages 3.5, 7, and 13 as periods of relative inwardness and withdrawal; and ages 4, 8, and 14 as periods of expansive behavior.[9] Research has suggested that periods of rapid behavioral changes of many kinds occur at approximately 4, 6 to 7, 10 to 12, and 14 to 16 years.[105] Similarly, Shumway-Cook and Woollacott[250] suggested that motor patterns in the development of postural stability undergo a period of disequilibrium between 4 and 6 years, when a physical growth spurt occurs. Changes in perceptual functions during this period offer an alternative, or possibly an additional, explanation.[164]

Whether these findings can be correlated with specific periods of brain growth is an interesting question. Overall brain growth stages have been correlated with mind growth, a process called "phrenoblysis."[92] Although Greenough and colleagues[129] cautioned that spurts in growth of the whole brain or in head circumference may not be reflective of relative differences in timing of growth rates in the various regions of the brain, Goldman-Rakic[124] has shown that concurrent spurts of synaptogenesis take place in many regions of the cerebral cortex of rhesus monkeys during the period of rapid behavioral growth in ability to perform delayed-response tasks. In humans, this stage occurs beginning at about 8 months, with rapid developments in understanding of object permanence, and can be correlated with rapid synaptogenesis in the visual cortex.[124,105] In humans, however, the prefrontal cortex, the area of the brain that has been related to delayed-response tasks, has an extensive period of synaptogenic development, peaking at 1 to 2 years and remaining high until about 7 years.

During the second postnatal brain growth stage (2 to 4 years), there are striking developments in sensory function, including binocularity, hearing, and language. Evidence suggests that earlier-occurring defects in these functions can be remedied only during the growth stage. For example, the fact that children with strabismus leading to amblyopia will never have normal three-dimensional (3-D) depth perception if the strabismus is not corrected before 60 days of constant misalignment during the first 9 months of life is important evidence of a critical period in development.[277] Surgical correction of esotropia is also correlated with improvement in rate of motor milestone development.[88]

In summary, significant principles of motor development include (1) the concept that an apparent cephalocaudal progression results not from genetically directed brain development but rather from a process of coordination of a variety of subsystems in response to the affordances of the environment for action, (2) spiraling development characterized by periods of relative stability and instability and sensitive periods in which development is especially responsive to environmental influences and therapeutic intervention, and (3) self-regulating active construction of developmental progress on the part of the child. Most developmentalists would now agree that the individual is formed through interaction among genetically determined processes, individual history, and environmental opportunities at least partially created by the organism itself. Seen in this light, the infant's actions structure the organization and complexity of her or his brain and psychologic development, not the other way around.[10] The paucity and limited patterns of movement available to children with disabilities presents a challenge to the physical therapist. Research is needed to identify means to increase the variety and flexibility of movement in these children to enable them to use self-directed exploration to foster increased complexity of their neural and other systems.

"STAGES" OF MOTOR DEVELOPMENT

Because a large number of researchers have documented that the behavior of children varies based on characteristics of tasks and environments,[18,25,176,233,234] it has become abundantly clear that the apparently invariant sequence of development of motor skills is an artificial creation of the particular tasks chosen by early investigators such as Gesell. Nevertheless, information on when children achieve various skills is of continuing importance in physical therapy and other fields because information about ages and stages of appearance of motor milestones is used in developmental diagnosis of delayed motor performance. Thus, this section elaborates on the observable "stages" of gross and fine motor development that represent milestones of developmental progress toward achieving the goals of upright posture, mobility, and manipulation—essential elements of environmental mastery and control. As infants attain and perfect these major developmental motor skills, they are incorporated into functional activities such as self-care, feeding, and play. Important milestones of motor development in later years of childhood will also be briefly addressed.

The major gross motor milestones of the first 12 to 18 months include achieving an indefinitely maintained upright head posture, attaining prone-on-elbows position, rolling from supine to prone, independent sitting, belly crawling, attaining hands-and-knees position, moving from sitting to four-point position and prone, creeping on hands and knees, pulling to a stand, cruising along furniture, crawling up and down stairs, standing independently, and walking

TABLE 2-2 Average Ages and Ranges of Attainment of Gross Motor Milestones from Two Studies

	Berger et al., 2007 (n = 732)		WHO Growth Study, 2006 (n = 816)	
	Mean Age (mo.)	Range (mo.)	Mean Age (mo.)	1st, 99th Percentile (mo.)
Sitting without support			6.0	3.8, 9.2
Belly crawl	6.8	2.7–11.7		
Stand with assistance			7.6	4.8, 11.4
Hands/knees crawl	8.1	4.6–12.7	8.5	5.2, 13.5
Cruise	9.3	4.3–14.1		
Walk with assistance			9.2	5.9, 13.7
Ascend stairs	11.0	6.1–19.1		
Stand alone			11.0	6.9–16.9
Walk alone	11.9	8.2–16.8	12.1	8.2, 17.6
Descend stairs	12.5	7.0–20.0		

independently.[25,281] As each position or skill is attained, further development will entail the perfecting of postural control in these positions and the ability to make rapid, effortless transitions from one position to another. These developments are discussed further in Chapter 3.

Results of large longitudinal studies of average ages of attainment for some of these major gross motor milestones have recently been reported. Table 2-2 compares results for a U.S. sample from Indiana, Pennsylvania, and New York City[25] with those for children from five countries, including Ghana, India, Norway, Oman, and the United States.[296] Ranges for accomplishment of early milestones are narrower than for later milestones and neither study noted gender differences. Of note, however, is that the order of attainment of mobility skills can vary a great deal. Berger and colleagues[25] found that 64% of their sample used one of 8 variations in the order of attainment of skill from belly crawling to stair descent, but in the sample as a whole 57 different orders of attainment were recorded.

Despite the greater complexity of our more recent view of the development of motor behavior, it is possible to summarize the perfection of use of various parts of the body in an overall schema of cephalocaudal direction. During the first quarter of the first year of life, infants develop the ability to control their heads in virtually all positions in space, although control will continue to be fine-tuned during successive months. The second quarter reveals major advances in control of the arms and upper trunk, although once again continued refinements occur later. Arm movements are aided by increasing ability to control the destabilizing effects of arm movements on other parts of the body. During the third quarter, initial stages involving mastery of control of the lower trunk and pelvis in the upright position occur, and the final quarter of the first year reveals the development of milestones in mobility and control of the lower parts of the legs in conjunction with upright stance and overall postural control.

INFANCY

Functional Head Control

At birth, infants already have the capacity to right the head from either full flexion or full extension when they are supported in an upright position. A stable vertical head position, however, cannot usually be sustained for more than a second or two, if at all. In supine, or with the head supported in a reclining position, head turning to either side of midline can usually be elicited by attracting the infant's visual orientation to a moving object. Shifts of gaze are typically preceded by rapid bursts of body movement.[232] Smooth visual pursuit is present by 6 weeks of age and is adult-like by 14 weeks.[286] At about 2 months, the infant can sustain the head in midline in the frontal plane during supported sitting but often appears to be looking down at his or her feet, so that the eyes are oriented about 30° below the horizontal plane as in Figure 2-1 (Campbell, S. K., Kolobe, T. H., Osten, E., Girolami, G., & Lenke, M., unpublished research, 1992). Turning of the unsupported head in the upright position is not usually possible. If the child can be enticed to lift the head to the vertical position, oscillations are typically seen with inability to maintain a stable upright posture. Finer synergistic control of neck flexor and extensor muscles typically appears in the third month, when the head is indefinitely stable in a vertical position and can be freely turned to follow visual stimulation, although sometimes with brief oscillations and loss of control.

When stabilizing control of the head in the upright position has been attained, the infant can typically organize head and trunk activity so that when placed prone with the arms extended along the sides of the body, the prone-on-elbows position is rapidly assumed by lifting the head and extending the thoracic spine while simultaneously bringing both arms up to rest on the elbows (Figure 2-2). Given the large weight of the head relative to the rest of the body at this age, a stabilizing postural function of the legs and pelvis must provide

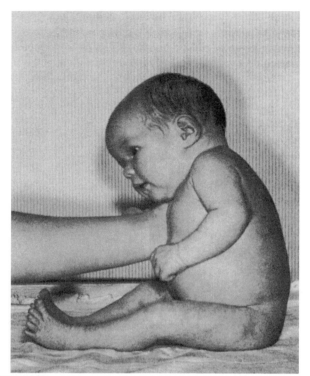

Figure 2-1 Early head control in space is characterized by ability to stabilize the head in midline but with eyes angled downward from the vertical. (From van Blankenstein, M., Welbergen, U. R., & de Haas, J. H. [1962]. Le développement du nourrisson: Sa première année en 130 photographies. Paris: Presses Universitaires de France, p. 26.)

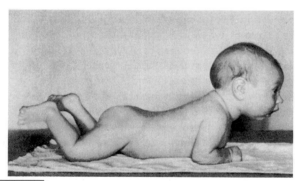

Figure 2-2 Early stage of prone-on-elbows posture with stable neck extension, elbows close to trunk, and flexed hips and knees. (From van Blankenstein, M., Welbergen, U. R., & de Haas, J. H. [1962]. Le développement du nourrisson: Sa première année en 130 photographies. Paris: Presses Universitaires de France, p. 25.)

a stable base of support for simultaneous neck and trunk extension with arm movement. Green and colleagues[128] demonstrated that the developmental progression in both supine and prone positions involves a gradual shifting of the load-bearing surfaces in a caudal direction.

Turning the head to either side while prone on the elbows may still be difficult to coordinate at this stage, and lateral head righting also remains imperfect. Nevertheless, by the

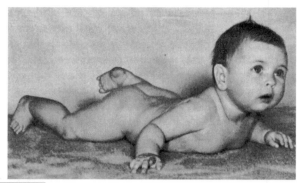

Figure 2-3 Advanced stage of prone-on-elbows posture, with free movement of head and arms and extended lower extremities. (From van Blankenstein, M., Welbergen, U. R., & de Haas, J. H. [1962]. Le développement du nourrisson: Sa première année en 130 photographies. Paris: Presses Universitaires de France, p. 34.)

end of the third or fourth postnatal month, the head, in conjunction with organized trunk and lower extremity extension, has largely perfected the maintenance of stable positioning in space appropriate for the further development of eye-head-hand control and of independent sitting to come (Figure 2-3). Bushnell and Boudreau[46] believe that a stable head is a prerequisite for initial ability to perceive depth cues from kinetic information (movement of an object relative to its surroundings or to self), which is present by 3 months of age. Once established by 4 or 5 months of age, binocular vision is used to identify depth cues.

Commensurate with acquisition of functional control of head positioning are important developments in control of the arms that are also related to positioning. For example, the prone position was effective in eliciting hand-to-mouth behavior in 0- to 2-month-old infants, whereas this behavior was elicited more often in sidelying when infants were 3 to 4 months old.[234] During the second and third months, generalized movements of the arms and body have altered their earlier writhing quality.[70] Small fidgety movements appear throughout the body, the arms and legs may show oscillations during movement, and ballistic swipes and swats with legs or arms appear for the first time.[130] For example, if the legs are flexed up to the chest and then released while the infant is supine, the legs may extend so that the heels pound the supporting surface, or when excited, the infant may make large arm-swiping movements in the air. As noted earlier, the first evidence of reciprocal activity of muscular antagonists about the shoulder underlies the ability to perform these ballistic movements.[131] Ferrari and colleagues[97] suggested the importance of these developing qualitative changes in spontaneous movement by demonstrating that they herald the appearance of goal-directed reaching and by indicating that they do not appear in children destined to be diagnosed as having CP. Children with spastic CNS dysfunction also tend to move in tight ranges characterized by simultaneity of activity in multiple limbs, referred to as cramped synchrony,

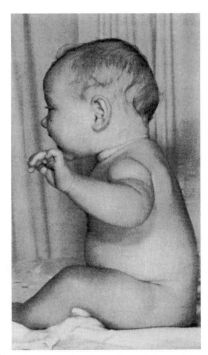

Figure 2-4 Early stage of independent sitting, with arms used for balance. (From van Blankenstein, M., Welbergen, U. R., & de Haas, J. H. [1962]. Le développement du nourrisson: Sa première année en 130 photographies. Paris: Presses Universitaires de France, p. 39.)

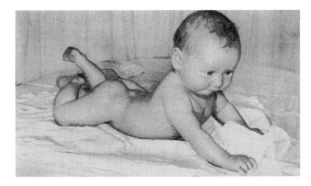

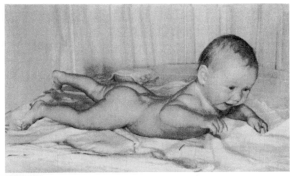

Figure 2-5 In the most advanced stage of the prone posture, arms and legs move freely from a stable trunk. (From van Blankenstein, M., Welbergen, U. R., & de Haas, J. H. [1962]. Le développement du nourrisson: Sa première année en 130 photographies. Paris: Presses Universitaires de France, p. 37.)

and general movements that tend to repeat monotonously. The characteristics of children with dyskinetic CP are different.[91] Until the second post-term month, these infants displayed a poor repertoire of general movements, circling arm movements, and finger spreading. These movements remained until 5 months when they became associated with lack of arm and leg movements toward the midline.

Upright Trunk Control

The initial ability to maintain sitting independently on propped arms when placed is achieved after the infant is able to (1) extend the head and trunk in prone position so as to use the legs and pelvis as the load-bearing surfaces and (2) control the pelvis and lower extremities while using the arms or moving the head in supine position, that is, has developed anticipatory stabilizing responses to counteract internally generated forces caused by movement.[128] Midway through the first year, the average child has achieved the ability to sit alone (Figure 2-4) and can successfully manipulate an object with one hand while the other hand holds it, although sitting and manipulating at once may still be a challenge. Poking fingers explore crevices and crumbs and herald the fine selective digital control that characterizes the human organism. Strong extension throughout the body in the prone position and caudal shift of the load bearing surfaces allows significant freedom of action for the arms and head (Figure 2-5). Bushnell and Boudreau[46] believe that ability to perceive

the characteristics of objects through their manipulation now allows the child to use configural cues from objects in depth perception. Despite these developments in arm control, the child in sitting lacks the fine pelvic and lower extremity control needed for moving into and out of the position or for turning the trunk freely on a stable base. Pelvic control functions begin to be developed at this time, however, in rolling from supine to prone position (Figure 2-6), pivoting while prone, and playing with the legs and feet while supine.

Lower Trunk Control in the Upright Position

During the third quarter of the first year, functional movements free the child from a spot on which others place him. Control of lower trunk and pelvis, combined with previously achieved upper body skills, provides new mobility when prone (Figure 2-7), crawling and creeping (Figure 2-8), pulling to a stand, moving from supine to four-point and sitting positions, and moving down to hands and knees or prone position from sitting (Figure 2-9). Inherent in each activity are freedom from a strong midline symmetry that previously characterized postural control and the continued refinement of rotational abilities within the axis of the trunk.

The presence of oscillations also continues to herald new developments. Rocking on four limbs before launching into creeping[4] and bouncing while standing before beginning to

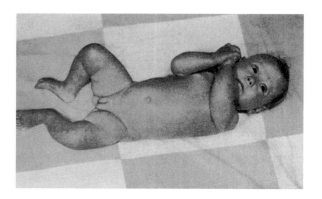

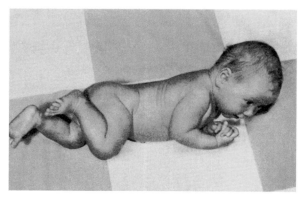

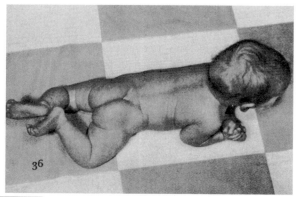

Figure 2-6   Rolling from supine to prone with head righting. (From van Blankenstein, M., Welbergen, U. R., & de Haas, J. H. [1962]. Le développement du nourrisson: Sa première année en 130 photographies. Paris: Presses Universitaires de France, p. 36.)

cruise along furniture are examples of self-induced actions that appear to be important precursors of functional skills.

Fine Lower Extremity Control in the Upright Position

Once the child has attained competence at standing and cruising along furniture, the legs and feet move toward perfection of selective control because the trunk and pelvis are increasingly reliable supports that permit freedom of lower extremity activities. In creeping, pelvic swiveling motions give way to reciprocal hip flexion and extension activity, and creeping velocity increases because an arm and a leg on the

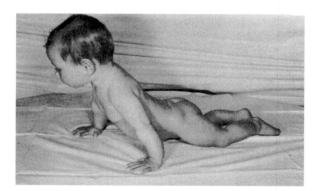

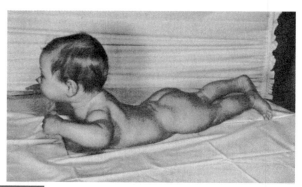

Figure 2-7   Dynamic play in prone position includes push-ups on extended arms and "flying" with strong trunk extension and scapular retraction. (From van Blankenstein, M., Welbergen, U. R., & de Haas, J. H. [1962]. Le développement du nourrisson: Sa première année en 130 photographies. Paris: Presses Universitaires de France, p. 47.)

same side of the body can be placed in simultaneous flight. The child can lower himself or herself from standing (Figure 2-10); bear-walk with dorsiflexed ankles, flexed hips, and partially extended knees (Figure 2-11); ascend stairs by crawling up at an average age of 11 months with descent several weeks later, usually by backing down,[25] and stand and walk independently at 9 to 15 months of age (Figure 2-12).[171] As an example of typical regressions in the course of development, the early stage of walking is accompanied by a return to two-handed reaching which declines again in frequency as balance control improves.[74] Chen and colleagues have also shown that learning to walk affects infants' sitting posture as the internal model for sensorimotor control of posture accommodates to the newly emerging bipedal behaviour.[67] Increased postural sway in sitting just prior to or at the onset of walking is commensurate with the idea that new motor behaviors arise during periods of high instability.

The gradual refinement of gait is described by Stout in the chapter on the Evolve website. In summary, during the first several months of walking experience, creeping is gradually abandoned and heel-strike in gait develops, allowing faster walking with longer strides. As children become bigger, older, and more experienced, steps become longer, narrower (reflecting a narrowing of the base of support), straighter

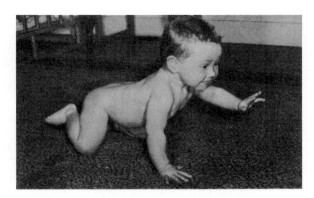

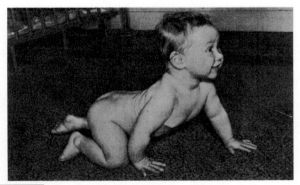

Figure 2-8 Creeping on hands and knees. (From van Blankenstein, M., Welbergen, U. R., & de Haas, J. H. [1962]. Le développement du nourrisson: Sa première année en 130 photographies. Paris: Presses Universitaires de France, p. 53.)

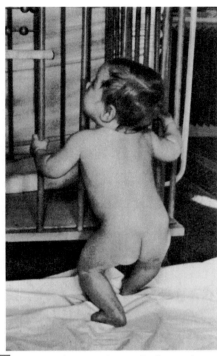

Figure 2-10 Lowering from standing to the floor with control. (From van Blankenstein, M., Welbergen, U. R., & de Haas, J. H. [1962]. Le développement du nourrisson: Sa première année en 130 photographies. Paris: Presses Universitaires de France, p. 57.)

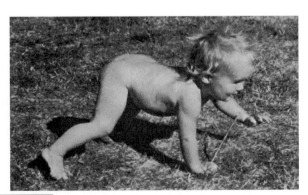

Figure 2-11 "Bear-walking" on hands and feet. (From van Blankenstein, M., Welbergen, U. R., & de Haas, J. H. [1962]. Le développement du nourrisson: Sa première année en 130 photographies. Paris: Presses Universitaires de France, p. 54.)

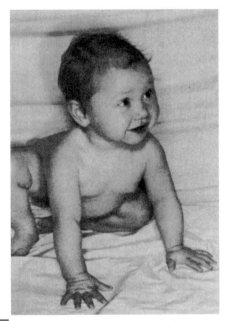

Figure 2-9 The infant moves from sitting to the four-point position over one leg. (From van Blankenstein, M., Welbergen, U. R., & de Haas, J. H. [1962]. Le développement du nourrisson: Sa première année en 130 photographies. Paris: Presses Universitaires de France, p. 57.)

(reflecting increasing control over the path of progression), and more consistent.[5] Walking practice is a stronger predictor of improvement in walking skill than age and duration of walking experience.

Roberton and Halverson[231] hypothesized the following temporal sequence of further development of foot locomotion patterns: walking; running; single leap, jumping down or bounce-jumping, and galloping (in uncertain order, but generally at about 2 to 2.5 years); hopping on dominant foot (seldom before age 3) and then nondominant foot; and skipping and sideways galloping or sliding. Although some

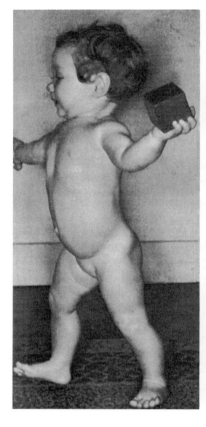
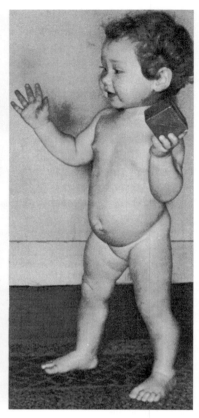

Figure 2-12   The infant walks and carries a toy, with wide-based gait and hands in "guard" position. (From van Blanken-stein, M., Welbergen, U. R., & de Haas, J. H. [1962]. Le développement du nourrisson: Sa première année en 130 photographies. Paris: Presses Universitaires de France, pp. 64–65.)

children may manage a skip by age 4, many reach an early level of proficiency only by age 7. A rhythmic step-and-hop movement is even more difficult and does not appear until well into the primary school years, when it may be used in many dance forms. Before describing the further development of gross motor skills in preschoolers, however, the sequence of development of functional hand use in infancy will be described.

Object Manipulation

Development of fine motor function entails two major features: control of the hand as a terminal device for reaching and grasping and object manipulation and release. Postural control for reaching and grasping has been briefly described earlier in this chapter and is further discussed in Chapter 3; Bard and colleagues edited an excellent volume devoted to development of all aspects of the capacity to reach, grasp, and release, as well as the functional use of the hands.[16] Oztop and colleagues[209] described the development of a computational model of the early phases of learning to grasp, and an important issue of Progress in Brain Research (Vol. 164) discusses hand function from an action-perception theoretic perspective, including computer models of infant development.[173,201] This chapter, on the other hand, emphasizes development of the manipulative functions of the hand that allow the child to engage in productive activity.

Wallace and Whishaw[287] showed that infants use four grasping patterns in the first 5 months, including fisted grasps, preprecision grips (thumb to side of index or middle finger), precision grips of objects, and self-directed grasps of their own body or clothing. Furthermore, Karniol[160] has documented the stages of object manipulation in the first year of life. These stages of spontaneous behaviors observed in daily life occur in a hierarchic form that progresses from rotation (angular displacement) to translation (movement parallel to the object itself) to vibration (rapid periodic movements of either translation or rotation). Later stages involve combinations of these actions and bimanual activities.[39] The invariant sequence of spontaneous behaviors documented by Karniol[160] is as follows:

Stage 1, rotation of held objects—by 2 months. With improvements in head stability and visual perception, holding objects becomes an intentional act. Objects are first held when they come directly into the infant's reach and are later (by 3 to 4 months) twisted while being held. Karniol[160] indicated that through this action infants learn that objects can be held and their appearance transformed by rotation.

Stage 2, translation of grasped objects—by 3 months. Typical of this stage is reaching for an object while in the prone position and bringing it to the mouth. The object may also be rotated. What the infant learns through these

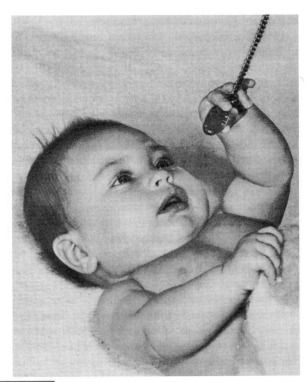

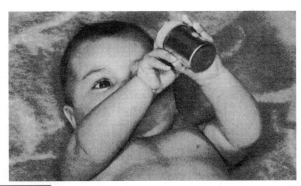

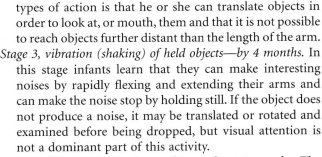

Figure 2-13 Bilateral hold of two objects. One hand holds the blanket, the other reaches for a keychain (stage 4 of Karniol).[160] (From van Blankenstein, M., Welbergen, U. R., & de Haas, J. H. [1962]. Le développement du nourrisson: Sa première année en 130 photographies. Paris: Presses Universitaires de France, p. 91.)

Figure 2-14 Coordinated action with a single object: holding a toy with one hand while poking at it with another (stage 7 of Karniol).[160] (From van Blankenstein, M., Welbergen, U. R., & de Haas, J. H. [1962]. Le développement du nourrisson: Sa première année en 130 photographies. Paris: Presses Universitaires de France, p. 93.)

types of action is that he or she can translate objects in order to look at, or mouth, them and that it is not possible to reach objects further distant than the length of the arm.

Stage 3, vibration (shaking) of held objects—by 4 months. In this stage infants learn that they can make interesting noises by rapidly flexing and extending their arms and can make the noise stop by holding still. If the object does not produce a noise, it may be translated or rotated and examined before being dropped, but visual attention is not a dominant part of this activity.

Stage 4, bilateral hold of two objects—by 4.5 months. The infant may hold an object in one hand and shake an object held in the other; infants thereby learn that it is possible to do more than one thing at a time (Figure 2-13).

Stage 5, two-handed hold of a single object—by 4.5 months. First use of bimanual holding is to hold an object, such as a bottle, steady, but it rapidly advances to holding (and often rotating) large objects that require the use of two hands. These actions allow the child to learn that two hands can steady and rotate objects better than can one hand, as well as permit the holding of large objects.

Stage 6, hand-to-hand transfer of an object—at 4.5 to 6 months. Transfer is usually followed by repeated actions on the object with the second hand; infants thereby learn

that whatever can be done with the right hand can also be done with the left.

Stage 7, coordinated action with a single object in which one hand holds the object while the other manipulates or bangs it—at 5 to 6.5 months. A quintessential example of this type of activity is holding a toy in one hand while picking at it with the other (Figure 2-14). Displacements of the object caused by handling are followed by rotational readjustments of the hand that holds it. These activities teach the infant that two hands can do more than can one hand alone and that noise can be produced from striking objects that do not respond to vibrating. Infants at this age tend to be unimanual reachers with reaching being space dependent rather than object dependent,[188] and it is not until 6 to 8 months of age that infants can take possession of two objects at the same time.[170]

Stage 8, coordinated action with two objects, such as striking two blocks together—at 6 to 8.5 months. Through these actions, the infant learns to produce interesting effects by moving one object toward another.[160]

Stage 9, deformation of objects—at 7 to 8.5 months. At this stage, the infant learns that it is possible to alter the way things look or sound by ripping, bending, squeezing, or pulling them apart.

Stage 10, instrumental sequential actions—at 7.5 to 9.5 months. These activities involve the sequential use of two hands for goal-oriented functions, so that the infant learns that coordinated use of the hands leads to desired outcomes. The infant may, for example, open a box with one hand and take out its contents with the other.

The achievement of these stages completes the development of the essentials of manual manipulation. More complex actions follow that are related to the functional characteristics of objects or to imaginary play in which an object can be whatever one pretends it to be.[160] Manual manipulations become automatized, leaving attention to be directed more toward the functional use of objects. At around 7 to 9 months of age, infants also develop the ability to predict the action goals of others if they have mastered the intended movements themselves.[94]

Based on the previously discussed research of Edelman,[90] Thelen,[265] Thelen and colleagues,[269] Oztop and colleagues,[209] and Keshner and colleagues,[163] we can hypothesize that, although functional hand use develops in a regular, invariant sequence when tested with a standardized series of tasks, it is likely that each infant uses unique coordinative patterns and kinetics to achieve manipulative goals that are circumscribed by individual variations in body structure, experiences, and rate of neural and physical maturation. One factor that has been shown to affect skill in managing multiple objects during the age range from 7 to 13 months is hand preference.[170] Infants with stable hand-use preference used more sophisticated sequences of activity when presented with multiple objects. Because the task characteristics structure the infant's unique response, parents play an important role in providing opportunities that support development.

Karniol[160] suggested that parents and others who choose toys for infants have two important functions: (1) helping infants to master the abilities of each stage by providing objects that are appropriate for emerging skills and (2) facilitating infants' developing sense of capability to control their world by providing objects that are responsive to current manipulative abilities.

Thus, Karniol and others believed that mastery of controlling objects in the environment is influential in development of the infant's general sense of competence and in providing initial sensorimotor knowledge of the permanence of objects and of cause-effect relationships. Karniol reviewed research demonstrating the influence on persistence at tasks and IQ at age 3 of play with objects that provide contingent feedback and are appropriate for the infant's manual manipulative competencies. Similarly, in a search for the correlates of performance of infants in descending slopes that varied in riskiness, Adolph[2] found that experience in dealing with steps and backing off furniture at home was related to superior ability to negotiate risky slopes. Furthermore, use of teaching strategies by Mexican American mothers was found to be correlated with their infants' motor development.[166]

As each stage is attained, the presentation of any object results in action appropriate to the motor stage, whether or not the object lends itself well to that action. Thus, in stage 3, all objects are considered shakable whether or not they make noise when shaken. When infants have a stable hand preference at 2 years of age, they persist in using the preferred hand for tool use, even when that might not be the most efficient approach for the task.[78] Infants who could crawl plunged recklessly down slopes too steep to negotiate safely in order to get to their mothers at the landing.[2] With more experience in crawling and walking, failures on risky slopes frequently led to accidental use of a different pattern (one that an infant already knew from previous activities) that was successful, such as sliding down the slope backward or in sitting. The alternative mode then became one that children purposely selected for descending slopes they perceived to be risky. These facts are not well explained by developmental theories that suggest that children perceive the affordances of the environment and act on them,[99,100,220,265] but Piaget recognized this type of function[107] and included it in his principle of assimilation. This principle states that when cognitive structures develop a particular schema, it is applied indiscriminately to objects in the environment, assimilating them to the existing cognitive structure. Piaget also posited that repeated experiences with attempted assimilations of inappropriate objects results in gradual accommodation to their properties and the appearance of both new behaviors and new cognitive structures.

On the other hand, a selectionist theory of motor development suggests that children must use online decision making to choose the appropriate motor synergy for use in a given situation.[2] Case-Smith and colleagues[65] have shown that the characteristics of objects, such as differences in size and presence of moveable parts, lead to immediate use of distinct actions when grasping that are appropriate to the object's characteristics. For example, a given infant might display more mature patterns of grasp when handling a toy with movable parts than when handling a pellet, so even infants do seem to have some capability to recognize the affordances for manipulation offered by different objects despite having preferred modes of operating on items in the environment. Recently Barrett and Needham[18] showed that 11- and 13-month-old infants used visual information from the shape of an object to grasp an asymmetrical object further from its center of mass than a symmetrical object. A surprising finding of Adolph's research on slope descent was that infants who had, week after week, practiced crawling down slopes that ranged from easy to hard, nevertheless did not transfer their experience with deciding which slopes were too risky to attempt to making the decision whether or not to traverse a risky slope once they learned to walk. Experienced crawlers, when faced as new walkers with slopes they had done over and over again for weeks on hands and knees, heedlessly plunged down slopes that were too risky for their immature walking skills. These infants did no better than control group subjects with no previous experience with slope descent. Only with more experience walking did infants become more cautious and choose to use an alternative mode of locomotion for difficult slopes. Because infants did make judgments indicating that they found some slopes too risky to attempt, Adolph surmised that children (1) used vision first to decide whether a slope was negotiable with just a quick glance, (2) then decided either to go or to take a longer look, and (3) then decided either to go or to use haptic exploration of the surface with actions such as a hand or foot pat, followed by (4) going using preferred current mode of locomotion (crawling or walking). With more experience, they became able to select an alternative, safer mode, such as sliding down backward. In a later study in which Adolph and Avolio[3] added lead weights to infants' bodies during slope traversal, infants recognized that slopes that were safe without weights were risky with added loads and those infants who engaged in exploratory activity on the starting platform displayed greater ability to produce adaptive responses to risky slopes rather than failed attempts to descend.

Because Adolph[2] did not find that previous extensive experience with slopes of varying riskiness was useful when the means of preferred locomotion changed from crawling to walking, she believes that a selectionist view of what infants learn from experience with everyday problem-solving challenges is appropriate to describe what children have learned from the slope experiments. Each new presentation of a slope presented a choice: to go with the currently preferred mode of locomotion, to choose an alternative (presumably safer) mode of locomotion, or to avoid the situation, using a detour attempt or simply sitting down and waiting for the caretaker to come to the rescue. Notably, the latter was seldom selected with slopes that were moderately risky; it seemed that infants were goal oriented rather than safety oriented. Their choice was made based on, first, visual information, and then if still uncertain, tactile and proprioceptive information. The choice was usually their preferred mode of locomotion until they had many weeks of experience and had, usually accidentally, discovered an already familiar motor strategy that appeared to be safer or more successful. As they gained experience crawling or walking, their choice was made more and more quickly; after many weeks of practice, a short glance was enough for making a decision. Near their ability boundary (slopes that generated less than predictable success in descending without falling), they appeared to have less than adequate knowledge of their own motor capabilities and instead made the decision based on desire to achieve the goal of returning to their caregiver and a quick judgment of whether or not to go based on visual or haptic information. Failure (i.e., falling) did not predict whether infants would choose to go on a subsequent trial, so they appeared to learn little between trials based on successful or unsuccessful outcomes. Adolph concluded that infants have extensive capability to use sensory inputs to make decisions about choice of motor actions, although they are not always right about their motor capabilities for solving the problem at hand. They choose to act rather than avoid a challenging situation, do not engage in trial-and-error learning, but rather continue to rely on their visual-haptic analysis of whether or not to engage in risky behavior. When useful motor synergies happened serendipitously, however, they seemed to recognize the adaptability of such patterns and used them on subsequent trials as alternatives to generally preferred modes of locomotion that were riskier to use in a given situation. Goldfield[123] summarized Adolph's[2] findings by indicating that "inexperienced infants tend to be drawn inexorably toward the goal, rather than stopping at a choice point, and apparently do not notice the available affordances.... Conversely, the experienced infant who has explored the available affordances may be overly conservative because the affordance information about slopes is inherently inhibitory; that is, it specifies ways for slowing, stopping, and changing direction" (p. 157). Thus, it seems that infants generate information visually, use their preferred mode of locomotion if the choice is to go, and then over time learn, accidentally or through a general wealth of experience with variable-level surfaces, to select from a variety of possible choices the most efficacious method of traversing risky terrain. One must conclude that adaptive locomotion (i.e., selecting the most appropriate method for the task at hand) requires exploratory movements to obtain information and a repertoire of available movement synergies from which to select.[2] This research once again emphasizes that advances in motor behavior depend on having a variety of movement patterns from which to choose when faced with challenging new opportunities for action. As a result, children with disabilities, who generally have a limited vocabulary of movement synergies, are constrained in their motor development by a lack of experience with a variety of movement patterns and may also have limited perceptual capabilities for making online judgments about the likelihood of successfully accomplishing a motor task even when they have an intense interest in the goal.

THE PRESCHOOL AND EARLY SCHOOL YEARS

Functional Motor Skills and Activity Levels in Preschoolers

We turn now to a description of the functional skills of preschool children, combining information on both gross and fine motor function in practical use. Toddlers operate with different anthropometric characteristics than infants. Toddlers gain about 5 pounds in weight and 2.5 inches in height each year, the latter resulting mostly from growth of the lower extremities.[71] Fifty percent of adult height is reached between the ages of 2 and 2.5 years. Children now walk well (although steps are still short and constrained) and enjoy the sheer pleasure of movement through running, climbing up and down stairs independently, and jumping off the bottom step.[9] The 2-year-old child can kick a ball and steer a push-toy, and by 2.5 years the child can walk on tiptoes, jump with both feet, stand on one foot, and throw and catch a ball using arms and body together. Galloping may appear, but only leading with the preferred foot.[231] The more practical pleasures of dressing independently (pulling on a simple garment at 2 years and pulling off pants and socks by 2.5 years) and eating with a spoon with little spilling also develop.[9] Food preferences can become a touchy subject by around 2.5 years; nevertheless, the toddler is gradually developing impulse control.[71]

The 3-year-old child can alternate feet easily when ascending stairs, can control speed of movement well, and takes pleasure in riding a tricycle.[9] Hopping may emerge, although it is often a momentary, single hop on the preferred foot.[231] Surprisingly, however, by 3.5 years, the child may seem less secure and physically coordinated, stumbling frequently and showing a fear of falling.[9] Hands may show excessive dysmetria during block stacking. Nevertheless, typical 3-year-olds feed themselves well and can hold a glass with only one hand. At 3.5 years, mealtime may again become trying because the food must be put on the plate in a certain way and the sandwich has to be cut just so. The same may be true of the dressing process, with special objection being expressed against clothing that goes over the head. The typical 3-year-old can put on pants, socks, and shoes, but buttoning may be difficult. Nearly all 3-year-olds are consistently dry during the daytime, and bowel training is well established as the physical skills and the emotional willingness to participate in toilet training come together.[71] The ability to delay gratification is developing, and toddlers strive for autonomy while continuing to intermittently seek reassurance from caregivers to whom they are securely attached.

Despite these generalizations, preschoolers exhibit a variety of individual behavioral styles.[71] About 10% of children are considered "difficult" because of increased levels of activity, emotional negativity, and low adaptability. Another 15% of children are described as "slow to warm up" because they take a long time to adapt to new situations.

Ames and colleagues[9] have described typical 4-year-olds as characteristically out-of-bounds in their exuberance. Behavior in all spheres is frequently wild, and self-confidence and bragging seem endless. The 4-year-old can walk downstairs with one foot per step, catch with hands only, and learn to use roller skates or a small bicycle. (But remember McGraw's experiments demonstrating that learning these skills is possible much earlier.) Athletic activities are particularly enjoyed, especially running, jumping, and climbing. Four-year-olds can button large buttons and lace shoelaces, feed themselves independently except for cutting, and talk and eat at the same time. The average Chinese child can use chopsticks to finish more than half the meal at 4.6 years.[295] Most children can take responsibility for washing hands and face and brushing teeth as well as dressing and undressing without help except for tying their shoes or differentiating front from back of some garments.[9]

Five-year-olds tend to be more conforming than the exuberant 4-year-old.[9] Children begin to learn to dodge well at 5 years[231] and can skip, long jump about 2 feet, climb with sureness, jump rope, and do acrobatic tricks. Handedness is well established, and overhand throwing is accomplished.[9] Current research suggests that hand preference is already stable by 12 to 13 months in most children.[93] The 5-year-old likes to help with household tasks, play with blocks, and build houses. Eating is independent, including using a knife except for cutting meat, although dawdling and wriggling in the chair may be trying to parents. The challenge of dressing oneself is past, so children age 5 may ask for more help than they need (usually only for tying shoes or buttoning difficult buttons), and overall, undressing is generally easier than dressing.

At age 6, children are constantly on the go, "lugging, tugging, digging, dancing, climbing, pushing, pulling (p. 49)."[9] Six-year-olds seem to be consciously practicing body balance in climbing, crawling over and under things, and dancing about the room. They swing too high, build too tall, and try activities exceeding their ability. Indoors, awkwardness may cause accidents, and the child seems less coordinated than during the previous year. Despite excellent eating skills, falling out of the chair or knocking over full glasses is not uncommon.

Because of the epidemic levels of obesity in the U.S. population (see Box 2-1, examples 4 and 5), concern about children's activity levels as an aspect of health has been heightened. In a study of the activity levels of 493 3- to 5-year-old children in 24 preschools, children were found to engage in moderate-to-vigorous physical activity during less than 3% of observations conducted with the Observational System for Recording Physical Activity in Children-Preschool Version.[214] Children were sedentary in more than 80% of the observation intervals. Boys were more active than girls, and younger boys were more active than older boys. An important observation was that activity levels varied by preschool, highlighting the importance of environmental variables in children's opportunities to engage in vigorous activity. An approach to describing middle school children's physical activity is under development by Pearce and colleagues.[215] This self-report questionnaire is computerized and is being developed in collaboration with children. See Chapter 6 on physical fitness for more information.

STEPS IN MOTOR SKILL DEVELOPMENT

In the various motor skills developed in the preschool and elementary school years, each body segment has its own developmental trajectory within the overall coordinative structure; one part can be at a different level of skill than another, although all parts tend to be at a primitive level early or at an advanced level when skills are well learned.[231] Furthermore, when demands of the task change (increased height, distance, or accuracy requirements) or when fatigue sets in, one body component may regress in its action while another continues to perform at an advanced level of skill. Thus, task requirements are once again seen to be influential in determining the characteristics of motor responses. For hopping and other skills, such as catching, throwing, and jumping, Roberton and Halverson[231] provided detailed analyses and photographs of the intratask developmental steps for each critical body component, instruction in how to make detailed observations to categorize the level of skill of body segments, and advice for guiding the learning of these childhood skills.

Physical therapists would find this information useful in planning intervention for children with mild physical disabilities or clumsiness. For example, as children learn to throw, the trunk goes through similar stages of development as those found in early developmental motor activities. The trunk is initially passive, then increasingly a stabilizer for the function of the extremities, and finally a participant in actively imparting force to the flight of the ball. Jumping changes from a functional activity characterized best as falling and catching to one of projection, flight, and landing, each with components that add force and speed or shock absorption to lend elegance and style to the activity.

Although many tests of motor development include assessment of hopping skills, most therapists probably would not view this as a particularly functional activity because children seldom hop spontaneously.[231] Physical educators, however, believe that hopping is an important developmental skill because a hop is often required in situations such as controlling momentum during sudden stops and in handling unexpected perturbations to balance, as well as for pleasurable play activities such as skipping. Hopping is also an excellent activity for describing the development of various strategies leading, finally, to skillful action.

Skillful hopping requires projected flight off the supporting leg and a pumping action of the swinging leg that assists in force production. Initial prehop attempts involve extension of the supporting leg as the child tries to lift off with the nonsupporting leg raised high. The first successful strategy, however, is usually a quick hip-and-knee flexion that pulls the supporting leg off the floor and into momentary flight (actually falling off balance and flexing the leg) while the swing leg remains inactive. At the next level of skill, the supporting leg again extends but with limited range and early timing relative to the point of takeoff. In skillful hopping, the swinging leg leads the takeoff, and extension of the supporting leg occurs late; thus, the action becomes one of "land, ride, and extend."[231] Just as with infants learning to descend risky slopes,[2] children learn through practice how to control their intrinsic dynamics to produce efficient movements that accomplish intended goals.

Sports and playground games become increasingly important parts of children's motor activities when they enter school and when complex feats of coordination become possible. Children have, however, individual rates of development of the components of motor skill, some undoubtedly innate, some based on cultural characteristics and family interest in development of physical skills. McGraw's[192] work demonstrates, for example, that toddlers can develop motor skills that are usually considered inappropriate, primarily because of safety issues. Furthermore, research has generally supported the belief that African American children have superior motor skills, especially those involving speed and agility, relative to white children.[69,174,223] Most authors have explained these differences on the basis of SES and differences in permissiveness of child rearing.[291]

INTERACTIONS BETWEEN PERCEPTUAL-COGNITIVE DEVELOPMENT AND MOTOR DEVELOPMENT

The work of Bertenthal and Campos[27] is significant in demonstrating that experience, not maturation alone, drives perceptual-cognitive development and that self-induced movement is critical in evoking advancements in a number of important cognitive processes. Through ingenious studies that varied locomotor experience levels by studying natural differences, such as length of time infants had been creeping and unusual childhood events (such as being confined to a cast for a long period or being given a walker to induce locomotion before it occurred independently), Bertenthal and Campos have shown that self-induced locomotion is a critical ingredient in the development of depth perception that mediates avoidance of heights when a child is placed on a visual cliff. This behavior normally develops between 7 and 9 months of age but is related more to degree of locomotor experience than to age at locomotion. Bertenthal and Campos also reviewed other evidence that self-produced locomotion promotes developmental progress in functions such as memory for locations and ability to localize objects objectively with reference to external landmarks rather than egocentrically. Children who did not creep have also been demonstrated to be cognitively delayed when compared with children with creeping experience.[191] Adolph[2] found that only 2 of 24 infants in her study of slope descent were able to transfer what they had learned from crawling on slopes to the choice of whether to traverse risky slopes as new walkers. Those infants were younger and smaller at crawling onset but older and more maturely proportioned at walking onset than infants who did not show transfer of learning from crawling on slopes to the decision regarding traversal by walking. These infants therefore had more experience with crawling than other infants. Infants who spent a long time as belly-crawlers also were able to descend steeper slopes than other infants. Two infants in the study who were consistently reckless (i.e., traversed hopelessly risky slopes despite repeated experiences of falling) were infants who spent little time as crawlers and walked very early. Adolph and colleagues[4] have also demonstrated that, although not all children go through a belly crawling stage, duration of experience with belly crawling is correlated with speed and efficiency at onset of creeping on hands and knees. These findings call into question the previous assumption that varying patterns of development of locomotion are merely that, variations without developmental significance for learning and future motor performance.

In general, therapists must take into account in treatment planning not only the precocity of an infant's abilities to perceive the basic affordances of the environment in terms of action possibilities but also the long period of development of motor skills and spatial-cognitive and other perceptual functions for fine-tuning choices regarding how to act on objects. For example, infants can adapt their reaching to the actual distance of an object at 3.5 to 5.5 months.[284] Depth perception is based on kinetic information at 3 months, binocular information at 5 months, and pictorial information at 7 to 9 months. Children preform the hand for the anticipated shape of an object at about 9 to 10 months and can adapt for anticipated weight by 14 to 16 months.[75] At 18 to 30 months, children sometimes fail to take into account object size, attempting impossible actions on miniature objects such as sitting in a dollhouse chair.[86] Children under the approximate age of 6 are not able to conserve the amount of a substance when the shape of its container is altered.[23] By 7 or 8 years of age, however, they recognize that pouring water from a wide container to one that is narrower has not increased the amount of water.[231] Weight, however, is not conserved until 9 or 10 years, and volume not until 11 or 12. As mentioned earlier, Bushnell and Boudreau[46] proposed that motor development is a rate-limiting factor in many of these perceptual-cognitive skills because movements make available information needed for the acquisition of related perceptual abilities. Although they believe that self-generated movements are the typical means for acquiring these abilities, they think that assistance with the necessary movements may also help infants to learn, an obvious area for research on intervention with children with disabilities.

Gibson used the term *differentiation* to describe the improvements that occur in perception over the course of development.[220] According to Pick, Gibson stated that "progressive differentiation occurs with respect to information specifying the meaningful properties of the world (p. 789)."[220] Gibson believed that perception involves an active effort to make sense of the world, but the action is exploratory, not executive in the sense of using physical manipulation. Perception improves because we detect more of the aspects, features, and nuances that convey the meaning of objects and events, such as how risky it might be to descend a steep slope. It seems likely that the alternations in apparent self-confidence, coordination, and other characteristics of children reported by Ames and colleagues[9] and Adolph[2] are related to their best attempts to make sense of the world as physical characteristics and control over intrinsic dynamics of the body, neural maturation, perceptual abilities, and other developmental subsystems change with growth and experience.

Although the importance of motor experience in the longitudinal development of many of the perceptual functions described earlier has not, to my knowledge, been explored by researchers aside from Adolph's[2] inquiry

regarding decisions about traversible slopes, the finding that self-directed activity is influential in some spatial-cognitive functions suggests the need to pay attention to providing compensations for functional limitations that may hinder children's development when physical disabilities are present. Bertenthal and Campos,[27] for example, have shown that use of a walker before endogenously produced locomotion was present positively affected performance on the visual cliff problem. Thus, maneuvering under self-control appears to be more important than does locomotor movement per se. Although a review of the literature on the influence of baby walker use on age of walking suggests that walking onset may be delayed by 11 to 26 days when a walker is used,[45] perhaps therapists should reconsider prohibitions regarding the use of walkers for children with developmental disabilities if safety during usage can be assured.

Bushnell and Boudreau[46] proposed that if infants are unable to engage in motor activities necessary to the acquisition or practice of specific perceptual or cognitive skills, the motor problem may block mental development. An example is that lack of self-generated mobility may lead to failure to begin to code spatial location based on environmental landmarks rather than in relation to self. In their review of the development of haptic perception (ability to acquire information about objects with the hands and to discriminate and recognize objects from handling them as opposed to looking at them), Bushnell and Boudreau[46] noticed a developmental timetable suggesting that infants under 7 months of age can already distinguish objects by characteristics such as temperature and hardness, that from 6 months on they can distinguish textures, and that ability to perceive weight emerges at about 9 months of age.

Finally, distinguishing objects by configurational shape emerges sometime after 12 to 15 months. These authors believe that this timetable is explained by constraints placed on infants by their motor development, specifically the exploratory procedures or hand movements they are capable of making at various ages. Rubbing with the fingers, for example, is typically used to assess the texture of an object, and repeatedly lifting and lowering an object is used to gauge weight. Until an infant can use the property most appropriate for gaining knowledge about an object's multiple characteristics, such perceptual knowledge cannot be gained or used. Temperature and hardness can be appraised by static contact or pressure; thus, these properties of objects would logically be among the first to be recognized by an infant. In Adolph's[2] study of slope behavior, it may be that infants used their vision and patting abilities only to decide that a risky slope provided a stable continuous path toward a landing below but were unable to consider whether their physical capabilities included sufficient balance to control gravitational and inertial forces that would result from their attempts to descend until they had sufficient experience with a variety of other movement patterns to help them learn about controlling intrinsic dynamics.

GROSS MOTOR ACTIVITY IN A FUNCTIONAL CONTEXT: PLAY

Research on children's activity memory, or ability to explicitly recall activities they observe or create, is helpful in considering how to structure therapeutic exercise to promote memory regarding what has been experienced. Ratner and Foley[228] reviewed the literature on activity memory and suggested that children remember activities better if (1) there was a clear outcome of the activity, (2) actions within the activity were logically sequenced such that cause and effect were obvious throughout the activity, and (3) the child engaged in planning of the actions involved in the activity in advance of carrying it out (not just mental imaging of it) or were asked to plan to remember what happened. Young children do not always profit from external memory cues, at least not until 3 years of age or older, depending on the type of cue. Nevertheless, children's behaviors show that they both consciously and verbally anticipate the unfolding and outcomes of activities by at least 2 years of age, even telling themselves "no, no" when about to perform some forbidden action.[228] At this point, imaginary play with objects that are not present appears, and children express surprise when outcomes of actions are not what they expected. Play then provides the opportunity for children to voluntarily act out intentions and to learn the difference between plans and outcomes. By 20 months of age, children are able to work toward a concrete goal, such as building a house from blocks, exhibit checking behaviors, correct mistakes, and acknowledge successful achievement of the goal. Repetition of an activity typically enhances memory of it when recall support is provided, and even infants 4 to 6 months of age can be shown to have some retrospective processing of events in that experiments demonstrate that they actively notice properties of an activity that were previously not noticed. Preschoolers allowed to demonstrate what happened will recall far more of an activity than if only verbal recall is elicited. Therapists should consider the mental ages of the children they treat with a mind toward creating therapeutic activities that provide children with disabilities the opportunity to develop cognitive skills such as planning and activity memory as they engage in exercise to reduce impairments.

When seen in its functional context as a learning device, motor activity can also be seen to have a stagelike character. Physical activity play (i.e., play with a vigorous physical component) has three developmental stages.[216] In infancy, babies engage in what Thelen[266] has called rhythmic stereotypies or repetitive gross motor activities without any obvious purpose, including body rocking, foot kicking, and leg waving. Whole-body, self-motion play is also called peragration, and Adolph[2] suggested that such activities are the most direct route to knowledge—infants plunge in and obtain important information as a result. These behaviors peak around the midpoint of the first year of life with as much as 40% of a 1-hour observation at 6 months being composed of such play.[216]

A second stage called exercise play begins at the end of the first year.[216] Such play can be solitary or with others, increases from the toddler to the preschool periods, and then declines during the primary school years. It accounts for about 7% of behavior observed in childcare settings. Activities included in exercise play include running, chasing, and climbing. Children with physical disabilities may need alternatives for participating in such play, particularly with other children.

The third phase of physical activity play is rough-and-tumble play such as wrestling, kicking, and tumbling in a social context. Often this type of play appears first in interaction with a parent, typically a father. Rough-and-tumble play increases through the preschool and primary school years and peaks just before early adolescence. No gender differences are noted in peragration activities, but males engage in more exercise play and rough-and-tumble play than females.

The functional benefits of physical activity play may be deferred or immediate. Pellegrini and Smith[216] suggested that the benefits of rhythmic play in infants is immediate in improving control of specific motor patterns, that is, the primary repertoire in Edelman's terms. Through active self-generated body movement, infants create perturbations to balance for which they gradually learn to accommodate or plan; such play also provides interesting visual and perhaps auditory spectacles for development of perceptual systems. Strength and endurance are also developed through such activities. Pellegrini and Smith[216] posited that the function of exercise play is specifically to promote muscle differentiation, strength, and endurance. Chapter 6 provides further information on health-related physical fitness, which may have its roots in early play behavior. Pellegrini and Smith[216] described animal research on the juvenile period, suggesting that it is a sensitive period for such development (recall McGraw's experiment with Johnny and Jimmy and their respective adult physiques). Play may also have cognitive benefits in terms of providing a break from attention-demanding activities, thus leading to distributed practice and creating an enhanced arousal level of benefit to subsequent engagement in mental activities. Seen in this light, recess becomes something more than a meaningless break in the routine.

Pellegrini and Smith[216] hypothesized that rough-and-tumble play serves a social function, especially for boys, related to establishing and maintaining dominance in social groups (girls are believed to use verbal skills more than boys in establishing dominance hierarchies). As a by-product, children also may use rough-and-tumble play as a way to code and decode social signals. For example, in early rough-and-tumble play with parents, children learn that this is "play" and not aggression. Rosenbaum[235] suggested that this view of motor activity raises the question of what goals we should pursue in therapeutic interventions. Is it more important to provide opportunities to "travel" than to concentrate on improving gait? Do children with disabilities benefit from adapted recreational activities such as horseback riding in terms of social skills and cognitive function, as well as in motor skills per se? What is lost in terms of self-esteem or ability to decode social signals in children with disabilities if they are "protected" from rough-and-tumble play? Such "differentness" begins even in infancy as babies born prematurely are less likely to be included in play date activities in community centers or the homes of other families as much as other babies, in part because of concern for exposure to illness. For children in early intervention services, such isolation may be reinforced by the current emphasis on home-based therapy for the 0-to-3 population.

USING DEVELOPMENTAL SEQUENCES AS A THERAPEUTIC FRAMEWORK

Most of our contemporary clinical approaches to developing intervention plans for children with disabilities were originally based on use of the developmental sequence as the primary framework for planning intervention. New theoretic models for understanding the achievement of functional motor skills suggest that this framework, as a rigid structure for approaching intervention, is inadequate. Atwater,[12] for example, suggested that a number of issues must be considered when deciding whether to follow a normal developmental sequence in planning treatment. These issues include the knowledge that (1) multiple underlying processes involving both distal and proximal function develop contemporaneously; (2) motor milestones and their components develop in overlapping sequences, with spurts and regressions being common; (3) many variations in the development of motor milestones occur in typically developing children, and thus motor milestones cannot be considered to be an invariant sequence leading to skill; (4) development in multiple domains must be considered; (5) the age of the child and the extent and type of disability are important considerations in determining which skills will be most functional for a child at any given time; and (6) child and family involvement in decisions regarding the goals of therapy must be considered. The discussion earlier in the chapter regarding contemporary theories of development and neural plasticity provides additional information in support of Atwater's suggestion.[12] She aptly quoted Bobath and Bobath[35] in stating that treatment should not attempt to follow the sequence of development regardless of the age and physical condition of the individual child. Rather, it should be decided what each child needs most urgently at any one stage or age, and what is absolutely necessary for him to participate for future functional skills, or for improving the skills he has but performs abnormally.[12]

I would add the suggestion that an emphasis on processes underlying developmental progress, such as the role of self-induced exploratory movement in both motor learning and in perceptual and cognitive development, and the motivation on the part of children to engage in repetitive, apparently goal-less, practice of activities during sensitive periods of development, should be considered in treatment planning conducted in conjunction with family input on goals they would like to have their child attain. Further information on sensitive periods of development for basic motor functions will be needed to target times appropriately for most effective intervention, especially for children with disabilities. Information such as this must be incorporated with knowledge of daily routines at home and in school and the community in order to individualize intervention goals. Bartlett and colleagues[19] are developing a Daily Activities of Infants Scale to document how infants spend their days and tests such as the School Function Assessment allows the child's educational team to describe performance in school-related activities.[77]

Also of great importance is identification of the most effective strategies for promoting the attainment of functional goals involving motor activity. Based on research on facilitation of cognitive development in disadvantaged children, early learning environments, and basic learning strategies, Ramey and Ramey[226] have identified the following essential daily ingredients to promote intellectual development in children: (1) encouragement of exploration; (2) mentoring in basic skills such as labeling, sequencing, and noting means-ends relations; (3) celebration of developmental advances; (4) guided rehearsal and extension of new skills; (5) protection from inappropriate disapproval, teasing, or punishment; and (6) provision of a rich and responsive language environment. Many of these ingredients are likely to be equally important in promoting motor development in children with physically challenging conditions; research on the design of specific teaching and learning strategies for such children is direly needed. Chapter 4 reviews what is known.

Atwater[12] recommended that treatment planning should focus on encouragement of functional independence to prevent cognitive retardation and learned helplessness that will be highly disabling in adolescence and adulthood, even when this means giving up goals for improving movement quality. Fetters[101] and Harris[136] agreed, suggesting that ecologically valid treatment programs have as their goals the movements that are necessary and useful to humans as they move about in their environment. Fetters,[101] however, emphasized that there may be trade-offs inherent in working for function of which therapists should be cognizant. Independence in ambulation may be accomplished only with high physiologic cost; the achievement of faster reaching may result in poorer trunk control.

Although I agree wholeheartedly with the recommendations and observations of these three thoughtful scientific practitioners, I have also argued that therapists must choose wisely when making decisions regarding use of compensatory patterns or assistive devices to facilitate functioning of children with CNS dysfunction. Wise decision making involves giving due consideration to whether use of compensatory patterns may lead to later secondary impairments of a musculoskeletal nature that could also be severely disabling in the future.[51] It is not acceptable to include in a treatment plan a goal for functional movement that does not also meet a requirement that working toward such an objective will not be likely to contribute to potential future deformity, skin breakdown, osteoporosis,[145] or other preventable secondary impairment.[53] A focus on health promotion and disease prevention, in addition to a focus on functional improvement to promote current and future activity and participation, is important, indeed, required as physical therapists assume responsibility for direct access care. Box 2-1 provides a sampling of health promotion concerns and resources that should be considered to be a part of the armamentarium of every pediatric physical therapist.

Research presented here on the processes of motor development also suggests that children (1) should have the opportunity to make decisions about choosing how to act (rather than being assisted or guided) when a task is presented so that they can exercise their perceptual capabilities, (2) need to engage in exploration through movement in order to develop their appreciation for the affordances of objects and the environment and for whether they possess the motor skill for successful action, and (3) benefit from having a variety of movement synergies available from which to select the most appropriate adaptive strategy in an online process of making decisions about how to achieve immediate task goals.

To promote these goals, Blauw-Hospers and colleagues[42] developed a theoretic approach to care of infants 3 to 6 months old that uses parent coaching to facilitate variation in motor behaviors and trial-and-error experiences for accomplishing motor tasks. When applied in a small clinical trial involving infants with abnormal general movements at 3 months corrected age, subjects in the experimental group had better sitting at 6 months than infants managed with traditional physical therapy. Although group differences were apparently not statistically significant, children in the experimental group deteriorated less in cognitive performance on the Bayley II mental scale[21] than infants managed traditionally. Larger studies are needed before superiority of the parent coaching approach is accepted as demonstrated.

To best accomplish these objectives and provide children with a variety of movement strategies with which they can approach the world of infinite possibilities for meaningful activity, we need both our extensive knowledge of biomechanics and more information on the natural history of conditions we treat. Indeed, I believe that the combination of attention to assisting persons with disabilities to improve their functional capabilities through promoting achievement of useful, meaningful activities performed as efficiently as possible, along with prevention of musculoskeletal and

other complications, constitutes the unique features of physical therapy. In Chapter 1 and throughout this book, we recommend that therapists use as frameworks for decision making the Guide to Physical Therapist Practice[8] and the International Classification of Function, Disability and Health of the World Health Organization[297] because of its positive outlook on disability and global acceptability.

Such a comprehensive approach to clinical decision making requires the use of appropriate assessments on which to base treatment planning and outcome evaluation. Tests of motor development and functional skills that meet appropriate psychometric standards and are useful in clinical settings are discussed in the next section. Other tests are described in Chapters 3 and 6 as well as in chapters throughout the book on examination and treatment of children with specific disabilities.

TESTS OF MOTOR DEVELOPMENT AND FUNCTIONAL PERFORMANCE

Physical therapists use motor milestone and functional performance tests to document children's developmental level in relation to age-related standards and to observe the activity strengths and limitations that may be present. Tests of specific functional skills, such as dressing and feeding, are also used to assess current levels of functioning and to document developmental progress and achievement of expected intervention and family education outcomes. Constraints causing functional limitations can be assessed with various tests of impairment. Those related to postural control and musculoskeletal impairment, such as the Alberta Infant Motor Scale, are described in Chapters 3 and 5. In conjunction with family interviews and home or school observations, therapists can examine competencies in fulfilling age-appropriate roles and identify areas of disability that should be addressed with a therapeutic program in consultation with other professionals and the family. In early intervention programs addressing family goals is paramount.

Although all tests to be described in this chapter are standardized scales with acceptable psychometric properties according to the American Physical Therapy Association's Standards for Tests and Measurements in Physical Therapy,[263] some tests remain under development, so complete information is not available. Those selected for brief discussion include the Test of Infant Motor Performance, Harris Infant Neuromotor Test, Miller First Step, Bayley III, Peabody Developmental Motor Scales, Bruininks-Oseretsky Test of Motor Proficiency, Gross Motor Function Measure, Pediatric Evaluation of Disability Inventory, Functional Independence Measure for Children, and the School Function Assessment. Tests selected for discussion were limited by space, and commonly used tests such as the Denver II[110,111] and the Gesell Revised Developmental Schedules[165] are not included because of poor specificity (43%) with high overreferral rates[122] and out-of-date norms. The reader may consult

Palisano[211] or Spittle and colleagues[256] for more information on these and other tests. Finally, the Pediatric Clinical Test of Sensory Interaction for Balance is briefly described as an example of a test of children's capability to use perception to control movement responses. The description of tests omits information on reliability, as one can assume that tests with demonstrated validity for the purposes for which they are intended will have also demonstrated appropriate reliability; information on this aspect of psychometric quality can be found in the references provided on each test.

Although the tests described are at various stages of development, none is a test of participation in daily life in which observations take place in an ecologically valid setting. Those that purport to assess disability do so through report of a knowledgeable informant, such as the parent, guardian, or teacher. Some tests are more useful for individual treatment planning, others for comparing global performance to age standards for diagnostic and classification purposes or for programmatic assessment of overall rehabilitation outcomes. Use of a combination of the tests would provide comprehensive assessment of functional skills in children with physical disabilities, although improved tests and well-thought-out, comprehensive protocols are still needed.[50,52,101,132,182] In a survey of standardized test use among physical therapists, fewer than half of therapists report regular use of such assessments.[155] Barriers to use of standardized tests include the time required to complete them and interpret results, but therapists who use them regularly report that use of such measures enhances communication with clients and helps to direct the planning of care.

SCREENING TESTS

The Harris Infant Neuromotor Test (HINT; www.thetimp.com)[138,140] is a 21-item screening test to identify developmental delay in infants from 3 to 12 months of age. The test includes items to assess neuromotor milestones, active and passive muscle tone, head circumference, stereotypic movement patterns, and behavioral interactions, plus the caregiver's assessment of the infant's development. Rather than reflecting a specific developmental theme, items were selected specifically because of research evidence suggesting sensitivity to delayed development. Age standards for the HINT were developed from testing a sample of 412 full-term infants in five Canadian provinces with at least 40 infants at each of 10 monthly age levels between 3 and 12 months.[140,141]

In a study of 54 high-risk infants,[139] concurrent validity with the Bayley II motor scale in the first year of life was −0.89 (high scores on the HINT indicate poorer performance, accounting for the negative correlation). The predictive validity of the HINT in the first year to Bayley II motor scale scores at 17 to 22 months was −0.49, accounting for 24% of the variance in Bayley II scores. Correlations with the Bayley II mental scale were lower. A later study compared the predictive validity of the HINT at two points in time (4 to 6 months and 10 to 12 months) with that of the AIMS to the Bayley II Motor Scale at 2 years of age and the gross and fine motor subscales of the Bayley III at 3 years of age in a sample of 144 high and low risk infants.[137] At time 1 the correlations with Bayley outcomes was higher for the HINT than the AIMS; at time 2 the HINT correlation with the 2-year Bayley was higher than that for the AIMS but the correlation with 3-year Bayley III scores were the same for the AIMS and the HINT (r = −0.55 for gross motor and r = −0.35 for the fine motor subtests). More important than predictive correlations for clinical purposes is an analysis of how well the HINT identifies children who are screened correctly as typically or atypically developing (i.e., sensitivity and specificity) when compared with a gold standard. Harris and colleagues[137] also completed a classification analysis for diagnostic purposes comparing HINT scores at the same two timepoints against 2-year and 3-year Bayley scores. Caregiver impressions concurred with motor development measured concurrently with the Bayley scales at a 60% level for sensitivity but the sensitivity for identifying delayed development on a concurrent Bayley examination was higher at 80%. When used to predict Bayley II performance at 2 years of age, a HINT score 1 SD below the mean at 4 to 6 months of age produced a sensitivity of 21%; the sensitivity for prediction at 10 to 12 months of age was 19%. The respective specificities of 99% were better using a 2 SD cutoff on the HINT at both time points. Thus the HINT is strongest at ruling out developmental deviance but misses a number of children with atypical development at both time points. Positive predictive validity, however, was excellent–that is, children who fail the HINT are unlikely to show later recovery so a positive finding of poor performance on the HINT should definitely be followed up with an appropriate intervention plan. The test takes less than 30 minutes to administer and score, is primarily observational, and can be used by a variety of health care professionals.

The Miller First Step Screening Test for Evaluating Preschoolers[195] is a screening test to identify children at risk for developmental delays. The test is appropriate for assessing cognitive, communicative, physical, social-emotional, and adaptive function in children from 2 years 9 months to 6 years 2 months of age. Function is defined as performance on games using toys that are entertaining and exciting for children in this age group. The test was normed on a U.S. sample of 100 boys and 100 girls in each 6-month age grouping. It takes 17 minutes to administer and score performance on the 18 games.

The TIMPSI or Test of Infant Motor Performance Screening Inventory[54,61] is a screening test for gross motor function in infants from 34 weeks postmenstrual age through 4 months post-term. It is described in more detail following discussion of the Test of Infant Motor Performance (TIMP) in the next section because it is a derivative of this comprehensive motor assessment.

COMPREHENSIVE DEVELOPMENTAL ASSESSMENTS

The Bayley Scales of Infant and Toddler Development,[22] better known as the Bayley III, is a revised and renormed version of the Bayley Scales of Infant Development (BSID)[20] Five subscales are available for assessing cognition, language (receptive and expressive), motor skills, social-emotional function, and adaptive behavior in children from 1 to 42 months. Functions assessed on the mental scale include object permanence, memory, and problem solving. The motor scale assesses fine manipulatory skills, coordination of large muscle groups, dynamic movement, postural imitation, and stereognosis. For the first time, the Bayley motor subscale was formatted so that it is possible to obtain separate gross motor and fine motor quotients, a significant improvement over past versions of the scale. The cognitive, language and motor scales were normed on 1700 U.S. children stratified according to gender, parental education, ethnicity, and geographic area. In a study of the effects of power mobility training in an infant with lumbar-level myelodysplasia from the age of 7 months to 12 months,[185] Bayley III scores for cognition and language increased at a rate faster than the child's chronologic age, suggesting that this new version of the test may be sensitive to intervention effects (for a driving demonstration, see online videos at http://links.lww.com/PPT/A3 and http://links.lww.com/PPT/A4). The Bayley III takes about 45 to 60 minutes to administer.

Because it was published so recently, little research is available on the new version of the scale. As a result the remainder of this section discusses research available for the previous 1993 version, the Bayley II.[21] The Bayley II was itself a revised and renormed version of the BSID necessitated by changes in infants' developmental rate since 1969.[60] The Bayley II was normed on a sample of 1700 U.S. children resulting in age standards for motor and mental performance for ages birth to 42 months of age as well as a criterion-referenced behavioral scale for examining such areas as affect, attention, exploration, and fearfulness. Use of the behavioral scale revealed the problems with self-regulation of very low birth weight preterm infants, supporting the need for neurobehavioral intervention in the first 6 months of life.[294] A strength of this version of the Bayley Scales was that items were carefully evaluated for bias based on cultural factors.

Scores of infants tested longitudinally in the first year with the 1969 motor scale have not been demonstrated to be stable,[76] and Bayley herself recommended that three consecutive tests be used to estimate performance during the first 15 months of life.[238] Research on various aspects of the validity of the Bayley II is reviewed by Koseck,[169] including potential scoring problems of which users should be aware. Harris and Daniels[139] reported the correlation between Bayley II motor scale scores in the first year of life with

scores at 17 to 22 months of age to be only 0.34. As a result, therapists are advised to be conservative in assuming predictive capabilities of the newest version of the test until further research on the Bayley III is available. In terms of diagnostic capabilities of the test when compared with other assessments, Campos and colleagues reported that scores on the Bayley II were highly correlated with Alberta Infant Motor Scale Scores (see Chapter 3) in infants born full term and tested at 6 months of age.[64] Concurrent validity for agreement on the identification of delay using the 5th percentile on the AIMS and 1 standard deviation below the mean on the Bayley had sensitivity 100%, specificity 78%, and overall agreement on child classification of 81%. Agreement was only 56% when the 10th percentile on the AIMS was used as the cutoff for comparison with the Bayley II. Use of the Bayley II as an outcome measure in intervention research is limited; a study of the effects of individualized developmental care (NIDCAP) in a prospective cohort experiment in a neonatal intensive care unit (NICU) in the Netherlands; however, reported no differences in performance at 24 months of age on the Bayley II and lower performance at term age in infants cared for in a NIDCAP nursery.[290]

MOTOR ASSESSMENTS

The TIMP[54,57] is a test for infants below 5 months of age, including prematurely born infants as young as 32 weeks of postmenstrual age. Function on this scale is defined as the postural and selective control needed for functional movements in early infancy, including head and trunk control in prone, supine, and upright positions. The TIMP was normed in 2004 on 990 U.S. infants stratified by age, ethnicity, and risk for poor developmental outcome based on medical complications in the perinatal period.[59] Version 5.1 of the TIMP has 13 items scored pass-fail on the basis of observations of spontaneous activity and 29 scaled items administered by the examiner according to a standardized format. Elicited items present the infant with problems to solve that require organization of head and trunk posture in space to orient to interesting spectacles, interact with the tester, or regain a preferred postural configuration. The TIMP takes approximately 25 to 35 minutes to complete. Scores are correlated with age (0.83), are sensitive to degree of medical complications experienced in the newborn period ($R^2 = 0.72$, $p < 0.00001$, when age and risk are used to predict test performance,[57] and discriminate among infants with varying risk for poor developmental outcome.[55] Rasch psychometric assessment of test results indicates that the test forms an interval-level scale.[63] At 3 months of age scores above and below 0.50 standard deviation below the mean on the TIMP identified 80% of the same children identified as above or below the 10th percentile on the AIMS at the same age.[56] The predictive validity of TIMP scores at 3 months to 12-month Alberta

Infant Motor Scale percentile ranks was sensitivity 0.92 and specificity 0.76.[58] TIMP scores at 3 months have a sensitivity of 0.72 and specificity of 0.91 for predicting Peabody Developmental Gross Motor Scale scores at preschool age.[167] TIMP scores in infancy are correlated with Bruininks-Oseretsky scores at school age (partial correlation = 0.36[108]). Tests done at earlier ages have limited predictability,[167,254,58] but they can be compared with age standards for peers for assessing the presence of delay.[59]

Ecologic validity of the TIMP has been demonstrated by research indicating that 98% of TIMP item-handling procedures are similar to demands for movement placed on infants by their caregivers in dressing, bathing, and play interactions.[199] The test is sensitive to changes in motor performance of preterm infants in the weeks prior to term age,[280] to developmental differences in infants who will later be diagnosed as having CP,[15] and to developmental change, including regression, of infants with spinal muscular atrophy type I.[104] Two studies have demonstrated that the test is sensitive to the effects of physical therapy in the form of neurodevelopmental treatment in the special care nursery[121] and in the form of a home program following nursery discharge.[177] Goldstein and Campbell[125] demonstrated that the TIMP is an effective parent education tool in the developmental follow-up clinic, and Dusing and colleagues[89] showed that a videotaped TIMP test was one of the preferred methods for parents to learn about infant motor development. A self-instructional CD (V.4.1) is available for use in learning to score the test.[181] A shorter screening version of the TIMP, the Test of Infant Motor Performance Screening Items (TIMPSI) was published in 2008 based on the performance of the 990 infants in the age standards study.[61] Concurrent validity with the TIMP is high but users need to be aware that TIMPSI scores in the 34- to 35-week age group tend to underestimate performance on a TIMP administered at the same age. The TIMPSI takes approximately 15 to 20 minutes to complete and its use can greatly reduce the time devoted to testing of infants in the NICU because performance above the cutoff for delay on the TIMPSI is highly reliable in ruling out the need for a full TIMP test.[61,54].

The Peabody Developmental Motor Scales (PDMS; www.pearsonassessments.com)[109,147] contain separate scales for gross and fine motor assessment for children from birth to 71 months of age. Functions examined by the gross motor scale include reflexes, balance, nonlocomotor and locomotor activities, and receipt and propulsion of objects. The fine motor scale examines grasp, hand functions, eye-hand coordination, and manual dexterity. The PDMS was renormed in 1997–1998 on 2003 children[109] and is generally now called the PDMS-2. Fine motor ratings were reported to be more reliable for children with delays (0.96) than for those without delays (0.76), but these results were related more to the statistical effect created by the greater variability of the delayed group than to actual disagreements between raters.[260] van Hartingsveldt and colleagues,[282] however, reported that the fine motor scale of the PDMS-2 appeared to lack sensitivity to mild problems with hand function. Further problems with the fine motor scale were identified in a Rasch psychometric analysis of item performance in 419 children, 77 of whom had fine motor problems.[68] A ceiling effect was found in typically developing children and a small subset of the items was found to provide maximum differentiation across levels of fine motor status. The authors suggested that the number of items could be reduced and scoring simplified to improve the psychometric quality of the fine motor scale.

Goyen and Lui[126] used the PDMS to demonstrate differences in gross and fine motor performance over time in "apparently normal" high-risk infants and reported that the presence of gross motor deficiencies increased over the period from 18 months to 5 years, but Darrah and colleagues[81] showed that serial assessments of motor function did not show stability over time, which could be a result of nonlinear development in children or because of the psychometric properties of test items themselves. Darrah and colleagues[82] also studied longitudinal performance of children on the PDMS-2 and again reported that scores across time were not highly correlated, ranging from .13 to .45. Furthermore, scores on the PDMS-2 were correlated at only .7 with concurrently obtained PDMS scores; mean scores for age and age-equivalents were not the same; thus the two versions of the test are not interchangeable. The finding of noncomparability of test scores from assessments intended for the same populations has been found repeatedly and is very important for therapists to realize. For example, Connolly and colleagues[72] compared scores on the PDMS-2 and the Bayley II Motor Scale in children at 12 months of age and reported that only the locomotion subtest of the PDMS-2 was highly correlated with age equivalent scores on the Bayley. Provost and colleagues[225] made the same comparisons in a large sample of 110 children aged three to 41 months who were referred to an early childhood program because of developmental concerns. They, too, found that the age equivalent scores on the locomotion subscale of the PDMS-2 agreed best with the Bayley II motor scale age equivalents, but when applying typical cutoffs to determine delay, the same decisions would not be obtained. More than 75% of the children whose Bayley scores supported eligibility for services would not have qualified for services if the PDMS-2 standard scores were used. Maring and Elbaum[187] compared PDMS-2 age equivalents and standard scores with scores on the Early Intervention Developmental Profile (EIDP) and found a high correlation (.91), indicating that children tended to be ranked the same, but age equivalent scores were very different with EIDP ages averaging 26% higher than PDMS-2 ages. Although the comparison of the PDMS-2 with the newer Bayley III might give different results for these two tests, for the present it must be noted that the various tests studied to date cannot be expected to give comparable results for decision making in clinical practice.

Kolobe and colleagues[168] examined the sensitivity to change in children with motor delay or CP of the gross motor scale of the PDMS and found it to be as sensitive to change over a 6-month period as the Gross Motor Function Measure[241] described in the next section. An interesting recent study of the meaning of a diagnosis of global developmental delay (GDD) in young children asked the question of whether this diagnosis (defined as performance more than 2 SDs below the mean in at least two developmental areas) was uniformly related to poor intellectual performance on an IQ test at 4 to 5 years of age.[230] The authors found that 73% of those with GDD displayed a global IQ score of 70 or more, and only the fine motor score on the PDMS-2 and expressive language scores were significantly correlated with later cognitive performance, thus calling into question the assumption that an early diagnosis of GDD predicts cognitive delay at a later age. The PDMS-2 takes 45 to 60 minutes to administer.

The Bruininks-Oseretsky Test of Motor Proficiency (BOT) is a test of gross and fine motor function originally developed for children from 4.5 to 14.5 years of age[41] which was renormed as the BOT-2 and extended to cover ages 4 to 21.[43] The test was normed on 1502 U.S. subjects stratified by sex, race/ethnicity, SES, and disability status (11.4% of the sample had special education status). Both a Short Form and a Complete Form are available.

The revision of the test was intended to increase its functional relevance as well as extend the age range. The test has four motor area composites, including Fine Manual Control, Manual Coordination, Body Coordination, and Strength and Agility. Other aspects of reliability and validity have been reviewed by Deitz and colleagues.[84] Several subtests have items that are clearly related to functional demands for school-age children, such as cutting within lines and ball activities and physical education skills such as sit-ups, shuttle-runs, and long jumping.

Limited research on the validity of the BOT-2 is available at this point, but the test has been demonstrated to distinguish between groups with and without disabilities. At the time of the normative study an additional clinical sample including children with autism, developmental coordination disorder, and mild to moderate cognitive delay was tested, and tables describing their performance are provided along with the normative results.[43] Each of the groups demonstrated lower performance than typically developing children matched by age, race/ethnicity and parent education. Scores on the BOT-2 are moderately to strongly correlated with related sections of the PDMS-2.[43] The earlier edition of the Bruininks-Oseretsky was sensitive to the differences in motor development of 8-year-old children with a history of bronchopulmonary dysplasia when compared with other preterm infants or full-term infants; furthermore, test scores were even poorer in those who had been treated with

steroids than in those who had not.[249] Shafir and colleagues[246] demonstrated the sensitivity of the Short Form to long-term effects of iron deficiency in infancy. Motor delay relative to a group without iron deficiency was still evident in early adolescence despite supplementation in infancy that corrected the deficiency. The test takes about 10 minutes to setup, 40 to 60 minutes to administer (15- to 20-minutes for the Short Form), and a minimum of 20 minutes to score. Deitz and colleagues[84] commented on the complexity of the scoring system and normative evaluation; software is available to assist in scoring and a training video is also available (www.Pearsonassessments.com). It also must be noted that the inclusion in the normative sample of children with disabilities means that cutoff scores used with the earlier version of the test may need to be revised to higher levels in order to avoid missing children who are delayed in motor skills.

ASSESSMENTS DESIGNED FOR CHILDREN WITH DISABILITIES

The Gross Motor Function Measure (GMFM)[236,240,241] is a test specifically designed and validated for measuring change over time in gross motor function in children with CP. The test has also been validated as useful in children with Down syndrome.[112] Function in this test is defined as the child's degree of achievement of a motor behavior (regardless of quality) when instructed to perform or when placed in a particular position. Spontaneously chosen movements are not assessed. The test's items are distributed over five dimensions to measure how much children can do, not the quality with which they do it. These dimensions include lying and rolling; sitting; crawling and kneeling; standing; and walking, running, and jumping. The test was validated for sensitivity to change over a 6-month period in children with CP from 5 months to 16 years of age. Change judged from blind evaluation of videotapes was correlated with GMFM test scores at 0.82. Kolobe and colleagues[168] found that, as would be expected, children with motor delay changed more on the GMFM over a 6-month period than did children with CP. Responsivity to change with development or intervention has also been demonstrated in research by Wang and Yang[288] and Josenby and colleagues.[157] The test has not been normed on a sample of able-bodied children, but generally all items are achievable by 5-year-olds with normal motor function. Rasch analysis of test items to create an interval-level test resulted in the formation of a new 66-item version called the GMFM-66.[13] Josenby and colleagues[157] followed 41 children post-rhizotomy to compare the responsiveness to change of the GMFM-88 and GMFM-66 over a 5-year follow-up period and found the GMFM-88 to show a larger effect size earlier than the GMFM-66 in both children who could walk prior to rhizotomy and those with more severe involvement. Neither assessment showed significant change after only 6 months; both showed significant change in motor development after 3 years. A computer program is available for scoring the GMFM-66. The full 88-item version of the test requires 45 to 60 minutes to administer.

The GMFM has been extensively used in research on interventions such as intensive physical therapy and selective dorsal rhizotomy, documenting its value for use in clinical practice and decision making.[31,157,205] Because children with CP are generally considered to be highly variable in performance from day to day, Bjornson and colleagues[32] studied test-retest reliability over a 1-week period and found intraclass correlations for all subsections to be at least 0.80. Russell and colleagues[239] assessed the responsivity of the GMFM to change in children with Down syndrome below age 6. They found that, although children showed significant changes in scores over a 6-month period that were also greater for the youngest children than those demonstrated by the Bayley II, the correlation between GMFM scores and parents' or therapists' judgments of change was poor and lower than that obtained in studies of change responsivity in children with CP. Correlations were improved if raters accepted parents' reports of item achievement when the child did not demonstrate the behavior during testing. GMFM-66 scores have also been found to explain over 80% of the variance in Pediatric Evaluation of Disability Inventory scores.[253] Finally, scores on the total GMFM and on the subsections using predominantly the legs are correlated with independently obtained assessments of leg strength, accounting for 55 to 65% of the common variance, but are not correlated with aerobic power or with arm strength.[213] The Gross Motor Performance Measure, a companion test of postural control in items from the GMFM,[38] is described in Chapter 3. A Gross Motor Function Classification System (GMFCS) for grouping children by level of disability, similar in nature to a disease staging system[212] is described in Chapter 1 on clinical decision making. The validity of the classification system for predicting developmental growth curves in children with CP has been demonstrated,[237] and the GMFCS is now the standard measure used in research to classify the severity of CP.

The Pediatric Evaluation of Disability Inventory (PEDI) is a discriminative device for detecting functional limitations and participation in terms of age-appropriate independence and is also a tool for program evaluation in tracking progress in individual children with disabilities.[95,133,134] Function in this scale is defined as ability to perform ADL with or without modifications or assistance as reported by a knowledgeable informant. On the PEDI, 197 items measure functional skills in self-care, mobility, and social function, and 20 items assess the extent of caregiver assistance and modifications needed to reduce or eliminate disabilities in each domain. The test was normed on 412 U.S. children without disabilities, and initial validity for discriminating function and assistance needed was derived from a clinical sample of 102 children

with various disabilities.[95] Both normative standard scores and scaled scores are provided for each of its three domains. The PEDI items are clustered at the lower end of the continuum of functional skills so that it is most useful for detecting small differences in young or slowly developing children.[190] In studies of sensitivity to change, a scaled score increase of about 11 points is proposed to represent an important clinical improvement.[153] The test takes 20 to 30 minutes to complete by therapists or teachers and 45 to 60 minutes by structured parent interview. Hey and colleagues at Boston Children's Hospital have developed a parent self-administered version of the PEDI that took an average of 35 minutes to complete in a sample of 110 parents (Hey, L.A., Kasser, J., Rosenthal, R., Ramsing, N., & Katz, J., unpublished data, 1992). Scoring software to obtain Rasch logit measures is available. Direct testing of children's performance in an ecologically valid setting is not specified but could be done.

Haley and colleagues[135] reviewed the history of development and use of the PEDI and described the forthcoming new version of the test called the PEDI-CAT, a test format using computer adaptive testing that allows administration of the minimal number of items necessary to estimate a child's level of performance. Development of the new version of the test also involved expanding the bank of items available to cover a wider range of age, changing rating scales to four levels to increase precision of measurement, and to be sensitive to cultural differences identified by users around the world. A new domain called Responsibility has been added to assess the extent to which a young person with a disability is managing tasks to enable independent living. When available dissemination will occur via the website at www.crecare.com under outcome assessments.

The Functional Independence Measure for Children (WeeFIM) is a discipline-free test of disability for assessing functions in self-care, sphincter control, mobility, locomotion, and communication and social cognition.[127,197] Function in this scale is defined as caregiver assistance needed to accomplish daily tasks. The WeeFIM is descriptive of caretaker and special resources required because of functional limitations and is useful in tracking outcomes over time across health, developmental, and community settings. Although insufficient detail is provided to be useful in making treatment decisions, it is an excellent tool for description of overall rehabilitation outcomes, for use in program evaluation, and for cross-disciplinary communication. The test has 18 items measured on a 7-point ordinal scale for use with children with developmental disabilities from 6 months to 12 years of age. Pilot normative work on a sample of 222 U.S. children demonstrated significant correlations between total WeeFIM scores and age (r = 0.80).[198] The test has been used with children with extreme prematurity, CP, Down syndrome, congenital limb disorders, myelodysplasia, and traumatic brain injury (Msall, ME, personal communication, 1992). The test requires 20 to 30 minutes to complete.

Because the WeeFIM was noted to be relatively insensitive to change in children between birth and 2 years of age who are not yet expected to have a large repertoire of ADL skills, a new downward extension of the test with 36 items called the WeeFIM 0-3 instrument was developed.[204] The WeeFIM 0-3 was administered as a parent report questionnaire. It measures precursors to functional independence including early skills in motor (16 items), cognitive (13 items) and behavioral perceptions (7 items) using Rasch psychometric methods to form interval-level scales for the 3 domains. In a series of validity studies of 527 children of whom 173 had impairments, subscale scores were found to be significantly correlated with age at r = .70 or higher, and as expected children with impairments scored less well than typically developing children. Total items on the WeeFIM 0-3 correctly predicted impairment status in 89% of the children. Because the purpose of the WeeFIM 0-3 is to measure the overall effects of interventions, more research is needed on the responsivity of the scales.[276]

The School Function Assessment[77] is a structured method for assessing and monitoring the performance of children in functional tasks and activities in elementary school social and academic settings. The assessment has three parts that assess participation in six major school settings, task supports including assistance and adaptations provided to the student, and activity performance in the task areas assessed globally in the previous sections. The SFA is a criterion-referenced test that can be used with children in grades kindergarten through 6. Although a variety of types of school personnel can use the test it is best performed by the whole team in order to adequately cover all activities in which children participate.[83] The School Function Assessment Technical Report available at www.pearsonassessments.com/NR/rdonlyres/D50E4125-86EE-43BE-8001-2A4001B603DF/0/SFA_TR_Web.pdf describes the standardization sample of 676 students, including 363 students with special needs from 112 sites in 40 U.S. states and Puerto Rico. Davies and colleagues[83] studied the discrimination validity of the SFA using known groups of children with learning disabilities, autism, and traumatic brain injury. Children with autism and learning disabilities were correctly classified into their known diagnostic groups, but those with traumatic brain injury did not fall into a systematic pattern of performance and were not as reliably distinguished from the other children. The individual scales can be completed in 5 to 10 minutes each.

Finally, given the evidence from studies such as Adolph's,[2] which illustrates how children use their perception of the affordances of the environment, one test that assesses children's ability to use their multiple senses to solve problems involving conflicting information for control of upright posture will be briefly mentioned; information on test findings in children with different disabilities is dis-

cussed in Chapter 3. Deitz and colleagues[85] developed the Pediatric Clinical Test of Sensory Interaction for Balance in order to assess children's standing stability under varying sensory conditions, including standing on stable versus foam surfaces, with and without vision, and with information from body sway relative to the surround occluded. Children must "select" the right sensory inputs to interpret their stability situation correctly, and these researchers have shown that children with learning disabilities and motor delays perform more poorly on the test than typically developing children. Lowes and colleagues[184] used the test to demonstrate the relationship of range of motion and strength to balance abilities in children with CP. Tests of impairment such as this should be useful clinically to differentiate movement problems caused by sensory processing difficulties from problems with coordination of the motor ensemble.

In summary, a number of well-designed tests are available for screening and examining functional motor performance in children, and several tests assess specific motor constructs, activity, and functional limitations of children with disabilities. Some of these tests require further validation in clinical practice, but early results are promising. No standardized tests have yet emerged from the new interest in contemporary theories of motor development and motor control, perhaps because dynamical systems theory emphasizes the process rather than products of development. Measures derived from dynamical systems theory should (1) include examination of a variety of subsystems related to the motor ensemble, such as the musculoskeletal system, perception, and movement patterns; and (2) use age-appropriate tasks and variation in the environment.[146] Measurement of periods of instability in patterns of movement selected by the child in response to tasks in varying contexts is deemed to be important. Long and Tieman[182] recently reviewed tests for conformity to the challenges of a dynamical systems perspective as outlined by Heriza.[146] They found that some tests examine age-appropriate tasks and subsystems performance but do not specifically address contextual variations or search for instability of selection of movement patterns just before systematic appearance of a qualitatively new motor behavior. The latter is a key issue in assessment of motor development from a dynamical systems perspective because such periods of instability are believed to be sensitive periods for effective intervention.

Evaluation of the results of tests of function and disability gives the therapist knowledge of what the child can do, with or without assistance from technology or caregivers. These results are important in diagnosis of developmental delay or deviance and for providing basic information regarding the child's motor competencies for accomplishing the important tasks of childhood play and for experiencing the joy of activity used for pleasure and for purposeful exploration of the world. More information, however, is needed for planning intervention when functional limitations are identified.

Roberton and Halverson[231] have described, in a beautifully succinct way, the process of developing a plan for helping a child to learn movement. Once having observed in what way and how the child responds to a movement task believed to be developmentally appropriate, the prospective coach must consider what the environment demands for the child to succeed at the task and also must interpret the child's response. "What is the meaning of a child's solution to a particular movement problem? Does it indicate a more advanced form of movement? Does it suggest improved perceptual functioning? Is the solution a cognitive attempt to avoid a balance-threatening position? Does the child's response suggest that the task is too stressful, too complex at that particular moment—that the child is not "ready" for it?"[231] According to dynamical systems theory, we would also ask what constraints in a variety of cooperating subsystems might be limiting performance and whether the child's selected movement strategy is stable or in transition. Based on task analysis and an interpretation of the child's solution, the teacher must decide whether to intervene or to leave the child and the environment alone. If the decision is to intervene, the teacher must decide whether to redesign the physical environment, verbally or physically coach the child, or show the child a possible solution. After implementing the decision, reexamination is used to evaluate the effectiveness of the intervention.

SUMMARY

Theories of motor development have evolved over time, but current thinking suggests that development is a complex outcome of the maturation of multiple physiologic systems in combination with demands placed on children by the environment and task-related experiences. In keeping with this idea, pediatric physical therapists use examination and interview processes to identify activity and participation needs of children along with impairments and environmental conditions that may present barriers to satisfying and efficient performance. Planning of intervention based on these results incorporates goals of parents and children. The other chapters in this foundational section provide further information to aid the physical therapist with these basic processes of examination, clinical instruction, and decision making. The information provided in these chapters will enable pediatric physical therapists to apply current concepts and research for the benefit of our clients—children with disabilities and their families.

ACKNOWLEDGMENTS

Partial support for work described in this chapter was provided by the Foundation for Physical Therapy and the National Center for Medical Rehabilitation Research of the U.S. National Institutes of Health. SK Campbell is the managing member of Infant Motor Performance Scales, LLC, the publisher of the TIMP, TIMPSI, and HINT.

REFERENCES

1. Abramov, I., Gordon, J., Hendrickson, A., Hainline, L., Dobson, V., & LaBossiere, E. (1982). The retina of the human infant. *Science, 217,* 265–267.
2. Adolph, K. E. (1997). Learning in the development of infant locomotion. *Monographs of the Society for Research in Child Development, 62*(3), 1–140.
3. Adolph, K. E., & Avolio, A. M. (2000). Walking infants adapt locomotion to changing body dimensions. *Journal of Experimental Psychology, 26,* 1148–1166.
4. Adolph, K. E., Vereijken, B., & Denny, M. A. (1998). Learning to crawl. *Child Development, 69,* 1299–1312.
5. Adolph, K. E., Vereijken, B., & Shrout, P. E. (2003). What changes in infant walking and why. *Child Development, 74,* 475–497.
6. Adolph, K. E., Robinson, S. R., Young, J. W., & Gill-Alvarez, F. (2008). What is the shape of developmental change? *Psychological Review, 115,* 527–543.
7. American Academy of Pediatrics Task Force on Infant Positioning and SIDS. (1992). Positioning and SIDS. *Pediatrics, 89,* 1120–1126.
8. American Physical Therapy Association. (2001). Guide to physical therapist practice, 2nd ed. *Physical Therapy, 81,* 9–746.
9. Ames, L. B., Gillespie, C., Haines, J., & Ilg, F. L. (1979). *The Gesell Institute's child from one to six: Evaluating the behavior of the preschool child.* New York: Harper & Row.
10. Anderson, D. I., Campos, J. J., Anderson, D. E., et al. (2001). The flip side of perception-action coupling: Locomotor experience and the ontogeny of visual-postural coupling. *Human Movement Science, 20,* 461–487.
11. Angulo-Kinzler, R. M. (2001). Exploration and selection of intralimb coordination patterns in 3-month-old infants. *Journal of Motor Behavior, 33,* 363–376.
12. Atwater, S. W. (1991). Should the normal motor developmental sequence be used as a theoretical model in pediatric physical therapy? In M. J. Lister (Ed.). *Contemporary management of motor control problems: Proceedings of the II STEP Conference* (pp. 89–93). Alexandria, VA: Foundation for Physical Therapy.
13. Avery, L. M., Russell, D. J., Raina, P. S., Walter, S. D., & Rosenbaum, P. L. (2003). Rasch analysis of the Gross Motor Function Measure: Validating the assumptions of the Rasch model to create an interval-level measure. *Archives of Physical Medicine & Rehabilitation, 84,* 697–705.
14. Bailey, D. B., Jr., Bruer, J. T., Symons, F. J., & Lichtman, J. W. (2001). *Critical thinking about critical periods.* Baltimore: Paul H. Brookes.
15. Barbosa, V. M., Campbell, S. K., Sheftel, D., Singh, J., & Beligere, N. (2003). Longitudinal performance of infants with cerebral palsy on the Test of Infant Motor Performance and on the Alberta Infant Motor Scale. *Physical & Occupational Therapy in Pediatrics, 23*(3), 7–29.

16. Bard, C., Fleury, M., & Hay, L. (Eds.). (1990). *Development of eye-hand coordination across the life span*. Columbia, SC: University of South Carolina Press.

17. Barinaga, M. (1993). Death gives birth to the nervous system. But how? *Science, 259*, 762–763.

18. Barrett, T. M., & Needham, A. (2008). Developmental differences in infants' use of an object's shape to grasp it securely. *Developmental Psychobiology, 50*, 97–106.

19. Bartlett, D. J., Fanning, J. K., Miller, L., Conti-Becker, A., & Doralp, S. (2008). Development of the Daily Activities of Infants Scale: A measure supporting early motor development. *Developmental Medicine and Child Neurology, 50*, 613–617.

20. Bayley, N. (1969). *Manual for the Bayley scales of infant development*. New York: Psychological Corporation.

21. Bayley, N. (1993). *Bayley II*. San Antonio, TX: Psychological Corporation.

22. Bayley, N. (2006). *Bayley scales of infant and toddler development*. San Antonio, TX: Psychological Corporation.

23. Beilin, H. (1989). Piagetian theory. In R. Vasta, (Ed.), Annals of child development, *Vol. 6* (pp. 85–131). Greenwich, CT: JAI Press.

24. Bergenn, V. W., Dalton, T. C., & Lipsitt, L. P. (1992). Myrtle B. McGraw: A growth scientist. *Developmental Psychology, 28*, 381–395.

25. Berger, S. E., Theuring, C., & Adolph, K. E. (2007). How and when infants learn to climb stairs. *Infant Behavior & Development, 30*, 36–49.

26. Bernardis, P., Bello, A., Pettenati, P., Stefanini, S., & Gentilucci, M. (2008). Manual actions affect vocalizations of infants. *Experimental Brain Research*, Epub 10.1007/s00221-007-1256-x, January 9.

27. Bertenthal, B. I., & Campos, J. J. (1987). New directions in the study of early experience. *Child Development, 58*, 560–567.

28. Bevor, T. G. (1982). *Regressions in mental development: basic phenomena and theories*. Hillsdale, NJ: Lawrence Erlbaum Associates.

29. Biggs, W. S. (2003). Diagnosis and management of positional head deformity. *American Academy of Family Physicians, 67*, 1953–1956.

30. Bijou, S. W. (1989). Behavior analysis. In R. Vasta (Ed.), Annals of child development, *Vol. 6* (pp. 61–83). Greenwich, CT: JAI Press.

31. Bjornson, K. F., Graubert, C. S., Buford, V. L., & McLaughlin, J. (1998a). Validity of the Gross Motor Function Measure. *Pediatric Physical Therapy, 10*, 43–47.

32. Bjornson, K. F., Graubert, C. S., McLaughlin, J. F., Kerfeld, C. I., & Clark, E. M. (1998b). Test-retest reliability of the Gross Motor Function Measure in children with cerebral palsy. *Physical and Occupational Therapy in Pediatrics, 18*(2), 51–61.

33. Blasco, P. M., Hrncir, E. J., & Blasco, P. A. (1990). The contribution of maternal involvement to mastery performance in infants with cerebral palsy. *Journal of Early Intervention, 14*, 161–174.

34. Bly, L. (1983). *The components of normal movement during the first year of life and abnormal motor development*. Oak Park, IL: Neuro-Developmental Treatment Association.

35. Bobath, B., & Bobath, K. (1984). The neuro-developmental treatment. In D. Scrutton, (Ed.), *Management of the motor disorders of children with cerebral palsy* (pp. 6–18). London: Spastics International Medical Publications.

36. Bodkin, A. W., Baxter, R. S., & Heriza, C. B. (2003). Treadmill training for an infant born preterm with a grade III intraventricular hemorrhage. *Physical Therapy, 12*, 1107–1118.

37. Bower, E., & McLellan, D. L. (1992). Effect of increased exposure to physiotherapy on skill acquisition of children with cerebral palsy. *Developmental Medicine and Child Neurology, 34*, 25–39.

38. Boyce, W., Gowland, C., Hardy, S., et al. (1991). Development of a quality of movement measure for children with cerebral palsy. *Physical Therapy, 71*, 820–832.

39. Brakke, K., Fragaszy, D. M., Simpson, K., Hoy, E., & Cummins-Sebree, S. (2007). The production of bimanual percussion in 12- to 24-month-old children. *Infant Behavior & Development, 30*, 2–15.

40. Bruer, J. T. (2001). A critical and sensitive period primer. In D. B. Bailey, Jr., J. T. Bruer, F. J. Symons, & J. W. Lichtman (Eds.), *Critical thinking about critical periods* (pp. 3–26). Baltimore: Paul H. Brookes.

41. Bruininks, R. H. (1978). *Bruininks-Oseretsky test of motor proficiency: Examiner's manual*. Circle Pines, MN: American Guidance Service.

42. Blauw-Hospers, C. H., de Graaf-Peters, V. B., Dirks, T., Bos, A. F., & Hadders-Algra M. (2007). Does early intervention in infants at high risk for a developmental motor disorder improve motor and cognitive development? *Neuroscience and Biobehavioral Reviews, 31*, 1201–1212.

43. Bruininks, R., & Bruininks, B. (2005). *Bruininks-Oseretsky test of motor proficiency* (2nd ed.). Minneapolis, MN: NCS Pearson.

44. Bruner, J. S. (1970). The growth and structure of skill. In K. Connolly, *Mechanisms of motor skill development* (pp. 63–94). New York: Academic Press.

45. Burrows, P., & Griffiths, P. (2002). Do baby walkers delay onset of walking in young children? *British Journal of Community Nursing, 7*, 581–586.

46. Bushnell, E. W., & Boudreau, J. P. (1993). Motor development and the mind: The potential role of motor abilities as a determinant of aspects of perceptual development. *Child Development, 64*, 1005–1021.

47. Butler, C. (1991). Augmentative mobility: Why do it? *Physical Medicine and Rehabilitation Clinics of North America, 2*(4), 801–815.

48. Byl, N. N., Merzenich, M. M., Cheung, S., Bedenbaugh, P., Nagarajan, S. S., & Jenkins, W. M. (1997). A primate model for studying focal dystonia and repetitive strain injury: Effects on the primary somatosensory cortex. *Physical Therapy, 77*, 269–284.

49. Braddick, O., & Atkinson, J. (2007). Development of brain mechanisms for visual global processing and object segmentation. *Progress in Brain Research 164*, 151–168.

50. Campbell, S. K. (1989). Measurement in developmental therapy: Past, present, and future. In L. J. Miller (Ed.), *Developing norm referenced standardized tests* (pp. 1–13). Binghamton, NY: Haworth Press.

51. Campbell, S. K. (1991). Framework for the measurement of neurologic impairment and disability. In M. J. Lister, (Ed.), *Contemporary management of motor control problems: Proceedings of the II STEP Conference* (pp. 143–153). Alexandria, VA: Foundation for Physical Therapy.

52. Campbell, S. K. (1996). Quantifying the effects of interventions for movement disorders resulting from cerebral palsy. *Journal of Child Neurology, 11*(Suppl 1), S61–S70.

53. Campbell, S. K. (1997). Therapy programs for children that last a lifetime. *Physical and Occupational Therapy in Pediatrics 17*(1), 1–15.

54. Campbell, S. K. (2005). *The Test of Infant Motor Performance Test user's manual version 2.0.* Chicago: Infant Motor Performance Scales, LLC.

55. Campbell, S. K., & Hedeker, D. (2001). Validity of the Test of Infant Motor Performance for discriminating among infants with varying risk for poor motor outcome. *Journal of Pediatrics, 139*, 546–551.

56. Campbell, S. K., & Kolobe, T. H. A. (2000). Concurrent validity of the Test of Infant Motor Performance with the Alberta Infant Motor Scale. *Pediatric Physical Therapy, 12*, 1–8.

57. Campbell, S. K., Kolobe, T. H. A., Osten, E., Lenke, M., & Girolami, G. L. (1995). Construct validity of the Test of Infant Motor Performance. *Physical Therapy, 75*, 585–596.

58. Campbell, S. K., Kolobe, T. H. A., Wright, B., & Linacre, J. M. (2002a). Validity of the Test of Infant Motor Performance for prediction of 6-, 9-, and 12-month scores on the Alberta Infant Motor Scale. *Developmental Medicine & Child Neurology, 44*, 263–272.

59. Campbell, S. K., Levy, P., Zawacki, L., & Liao, P.-J. (2006). Population-based age standards for interpreting results on the Test of Infant Motor Performance. *Pediatric Physical Therapy, 18*, 119–125.

60. Campbell, S. K., Siegel, E., Parr, C. A., & Ramey, C. T. (1986). Evidence for the need to renorm the Bayley Scales of Infant Development based on the performance of a population-based sample of twelve-month-old infants. *Topics in Early Childhood Special Education, 6*(2), 83–96.

61. Campbell, S. K., Swanlund, A., Smith, E., Liao, P.-J., & Zawacki, L. (2008). Validity of the TIMPSI for estimating concurrent performance on the Test of Infant Motor Performance. *Pediatric Physical Therapy, 20*, 3–10.

62. Campbell, S. K., & Wilson, J. M. (1976). Planning infant learning programs. *Physical Therapy, 56*, 1347–1357.

63. Campbell, S. K., Wright, B. D., & Linacre, J. M. (2002b). Development of a functional movement scale for infants. *Journal of Applied Measurement, 3*(2), 191–204.

64. Campos, D., Santos, D. C., Gonçalves, V. M., et al. (2006). Agreement between scales for screening and diagnosis of motor development at 6 months. *Journal of Pediatrics (Rio J), 82*, 470–474.

65. Case-Smith, J., Bigsby, R., & Clutter, J. (1998). Perceptual-motor coupling in the development of grasp. *American Journal of Occupational Therapy, 52*, 102–110.

66. Catania, A., & Harnad, S. (Eds.). (1988). *The selection of behavior—The operant behaviorism of B. F. Skinner: Comments and consequences.* New York: Cambridge University Press.

67. Chen, L.-C., Metcalfe, J. S., Jeka, J. J., & Clark, J. E. (2007). Two steps forward and one back: Learning to walk affects infants' sitting posture. *Infant Behavior & Development, 30*, 16–25.

68. Chien, C. W., & Bond, T. G. (2009). Measurement properties of fine motor scale of Peabody Developmental Motor Scales-Second Edition. *American Journal of Physical Medicine and Rehabilitation, 88*, 376–386. DOI: 10.1097/PHM.0b013e318198a7c9

69. Cintas, H. M. (1988). Cross-cultural variation in infant motor development. *Physical and Occupational Therapy in Pediatrics, 8*(4), 1–20.

70. Cioni, G., & Prechtl, H. F. R. (1990). Preterm and early post-term behaviour in low-risk premature infants. *Early Human Development, 23*, 159–191.

71. Colson, E. R., & Dworkin, P. H. (1997). Toddler development. *Pediatrics in Review, 18*, 255–259.

72. Connolly, B. H., Dalton, L., Smith, J. B., Lamberth, N. G., McCay, B., & Murphy, W. (2006). Concurrent validity of the Bayley Scales of Infant Development II (BSID-II). Motor Scale and the Peabody Developmental Motor Scale II (PDMS-2) in 12-month-old infants. *Pediatric Physical Therapy, 18*, 190–196.

73. Connolly, K. (1970). Skill development: Problems and plans. In K. Connolly (Ed.), *Mechanisms of motor skill development* (pp. 3–21). New York: Academic Press.

74. Corbetta, D., & Bojczyk, K. E. (2002). Infants return to two-handed reaching when they are learning to walk. *Journal of Motor Behavior, 34*, 83–95.

75. Corbetta, D., & Mounoud, P. (1990). Early development of grasping and manipulation. In C. Bard, M. Fleury, & L. Hay (Eds.), *Development of eye-hand coordination across the life span* (pp. 188–213). Columbia, SC: University of South Carolina Press.

76. Coryell, J., Provost, B. M., Wilhelm, I. J., & Campbell, S. K. (1989). Stability of Bayley Motor Scale scores in the first two years. *Physical Therapy, 69*, 834–841.

77. Coster, W., Deeney, T. A., Haltiwanger, J. T., & Haley, S. M. (1998). *School Function Assessment.* Boston: Boston University.

78. Cox, R. F. A., & Smitsman, A. W. (2006). Action planning in young children's tool use. *Developmental Science, 9*, 628–641.

79. Crone, E. A., Donohue, S. E., Honomichir, R., Wendelken, C., & Brunge, S. A. (2006). Brain regions mediating flexible

rule use during development. *Journal of Neuroscience, 26,* 11239–11247.

80. Dalton TC. Arnold Gesell and the maturation controversy. (2005). *Integrative Physiological & Behavioral Science, 40,* 182–204.

81. Darrah, J., Hodge, M., Magill-Evans, J., & Kembhavi, G. (2003). Stability of serial assessments of motor and communication abilities in typically developing infants—Implications for screening. *Early Human Development, 72,* 97–110.

82. Darrah, J., Magill-Evans, J., Volden, J., Hodge, M., & Kembhavi, G. (2007). Scores of typically developing children on the Peabody Developmental Motor Scales: infancy to preschool. *Physical & Occupational Therapy in Pediatrics, 27*(3), 5–19.

83. Davies, P. L., Soon, P. L., Young, M., & Clausen-Yamaki, A. (2004). Validity and reliability of the School Function Assessment in elementary school students with disabilities. *Physical & Occupational Therapy in Pediatrics, 24*(3), 23–43.

84. Deitz, J. C., Kartin, D., & Kopp, K. (2007). Review of the Bruininks-Oseretsky Test of Motor Proficiency, Second Edition (BOT-2). *Physical and Occupational Therapy in Pediatrics, 27*(4), 87–102.

85. Deitz, J. C., Richardson, P., Crowe, T. K., & Westcott, S. L. (1996). Performance of children with learning disabilities and motor delays on the Pediatric Clinical Test of Sensory Interaction for Balance (P-CTSIB). *Physical and Occupational Therapy in Pediatrics, 16*(3), 1–21.

86. DeLoache, J. S., Uttal, D. H., & Rosengren, K. S. (2004). Scale errors offer evidence for a perception-action dissociation early in life. *Science, 304,* 1027–1029.

87. Dewey, C., Fleming, P., & Golding, J. (1998). Does the supine sleeping position have any adverse effects on the child? II. Development in the first 18 months. *Pediatrics (CZE), 101,* E5.

88. Drover, J. R., Stager, D. R., Sr, Morale, S. E., Leffler, J. N., & Birch, E. E. (2008). Improvement in motor development following surgery for infantile esotropia. *Journal of the AAPOS, 12,* 136–140.

89. Dusing, S. C., Murray, T., & Stern, M. (2008). Parent preferences for motor development education in the neonatal intensive care unit. *Pediatric Physical Therapy, 20,* 363–368.

90. Edelman, G. M. (1992). *Bright air, brilliant fire: On the matter of the mind.* New York: Basic Books.

91. Einspieler, C., Cioni, G., Paolicelli, P. B., et al. (2002). The early markers for later dyskinetic cerebral palsy are different from those for spastic cerebral palsy. *Neuropediatrics, 33,* 73–78.

92. Epstein, H. T. (1979). Correlated brain and intelligence development in humans. In M. E. Hahn, C. Jensen, & B. C. Dudek (Eds.), *Development and evolution of brain size: Behavioral implications* (pp. 111–131). New York: Academic Press.

93. Fagard, J. (1990). The development of bimanual coordination. In C. Bard, M. Fleury, & L. Hay (Eds.), *Development of eye-hand coordination across the life span* (pp. 262–282). Columbia, SC: University of South Carolina Press.

94. Falck-Ytter, T., Gredebäck, G., & von Hofsten, C. (2006). Infants predict other people's action goals. *Nature Neuroscience, 9,* 878–879.

95. Feldman, A. B., Haley, S. M., & Coryell, J. (1990). Concurrent and construct validity of the Pediatric Evaluation of Disability Inventory. *Physical Therapy, 70,* 602–610.

96. Fentress, J. C. (1990). Animal and human models of coordination development. In C. Bard, M. Fleury, & L. Hay (Eds.), *Development of eye-hand coordination across the life span* (pp. 3–25). Columbia, SC: University of South Carolina Press.

97. Ferrari, F., Cioni, G., & Prechtl, H. R. F. (1990). Qualitative changes of general movements in preterm infants with brain lesions. *Early Human Development, 23,* 193–231.

98. Fetters, L. (1981). Object permanence development in infants with motor handicaps. *Physical Therapy, 61,* 327–333.

99. Fetters, L. (1991a). Foundations for therapeutic intervention. In S. K. Campbell (Ed.), *Pediatric neurologic physical therapy* (pp. 19–32). New York: Churchill Livingstone.

100. Fetters, L. (1991b). Cerebral palsy: Contemporary treatment concepts. In M. J. Lister (Ed.). *Contemporary management of motor control problems: Proceedings of the II STEP Conference* (pp. 219–224). Alexandria, VA: Foundation for Physical Therapy.

101. Fetters, L. (1991c). Measurement and treatment in cerebral palsy: An argument for a new approach. *Physical Therapy, 71,* 244–247.

102. Fetters, L., Fernandez, B., & Cermak, S. (1989). The relationship of proximal and distal components in the development of reaching. *Journal of Human Movement Studies, 17,* 283–297.

103. Fetters, L., & Huang, H. H. (2007). Motor development and sleep, play, and feeding positions in very-low-birthweight infants with and without white matter disease. *Developmental Medicine and Child Neurology, 49,* 807–813.

104. Finkel, R. S., Hynan, L. S., Glanzman, A. M., et al. (2008). The Test of Infant Motor Performance: Reliability in spinal muscular atrophy type I. *Pediatric Physical Therapy, 20,* 242–246.

105. Fischer, K. W. (1987). Relations between brain and cognitive development. *Child Development, 58,* 623–632.

106. Fisher, A. G. (1992). Functional measures, Part 1, What is function, what should we measure, and how should we measure it? *American Journal of Occupational Therapy, 46,* 183–185.

107. Flavell, J. H. (1963). *The Developmental Psychology of Jean Piaget.* Princeton, NJ: Van Nostrand.

108. Flegel, J., & Kolobe, T. H. A. (2002). Predictive validity of the Test of Infant Motor Performance as measured by the Bruininks-Oseretsky Test of Motor Proficiency at school age. *Physical Therapy, 82,* 762–771.

109. Folio, M. R., & Fewell, R. R. (2000). *Peabody Developmental Motor Scales* 2nd ed. Austin, TX: Pro-Ed, Inc.

110. Frankenburg, W. K., Dodds, J., Archer, P., Bresnick, B., Maschka, P., Edelman, N., & Shapiro, H. (1990). *Denver II.* Denver: Denver Developmental Materials.

111. Frankenburg, W. K., Dodds, J., Archer, P., Shapiro, H., & Bresnick, B. (1992). The Denver II. A major revision and restandardization of the DDST. *Pediatrics, 89,* 91–97.

112. Gemus, M., Palisano, R., Russell, D., Rosenbaum, P., Walter, S. D., Galuppi, B., & Lane, M. (2001). Using the Gross Motor Function Measure to evaluate motor development in children with Down syndrome. *Physical & Occupational Therapy in Pediatrics, 21*(2–3), 69–79.

113. Georgopoulos, A. P., Ashe, J., Smyrnis, M., & Taira, M. (1992). The motor cortex and the coding of force. *Science, 256,* 1692–1695.

114. Georgopoulos, A. P., Taira, M., & Lukashin, A. (1993). Cognitive neurophysiology of the motor cortex. *Science, 260,* 47–52.

115. Gesell, A. (1928a). *Infancy and Human Growth.* New York: Macmillan.

116. Gesell, A. (1928b). *The Mental Growth of the Pre-school Child: A Psychological Outline of Normal Development from Birth to the Sixth Year, Including a System of Developmental Diagnosis.* New York: Macmillan.

117. Gesell, A. (1945). *The Embryology of Behavior.* New York: Harper & Row.

118. Gesell, A., Amatruda, C. S., Castner, B. M., & Thompson, H. (1975). *Biographies of Child Development: The Mental Growth Careers of Eighty-four Infants and Children.* New York: Arno Press.

119. Gesell, A., Halverson, H. M., Thompson, H., Ilg, F. L., Castner, B. M., Ames, L. B., & Amatruda, C. S. (1940). *The First Five Years of Life.* New York: Harper & Row.

120. Gesell, A., Thompson, H., & Amatruda, C. S. (1934). *Infant Behavior: Its Genesis and Growth.* New York: McGraw-Hill.

121. Girolami, G., & Campbell, S. K. (1994). Efficacy of a neurodevelopmental treatment program to improve motor control of preterm infants. *Pediatric Physical Therapy, 6,* 175–184.

122. Glascoe, F. P., Byrne, K. E., Ashford, L. G., Johnson, K. L., Chang, B., & Strickland, B. (1992). Accuracy of the Denver-II in developmental screening. *Pediatrics, 89,* 1221–1225.

123. Goldfield, E. C. (1997). Toward a developmental ecological psychology. *Monographs of the Society for Research in Child Development, 62*(3), 152–158.

124. Goldman-Rakic, P. S. (1987). Development of cortical circuitry and cognitive function. *Child Development, 58,* 601–622.

125. Goldstein, L. A., & Campbell, S. K. (2008). Effectiveness of the Test of Infant Motor Performance as an educational tool for mothers. *Pediatric Physical Therapy, 20,* 152–159.

126. Goyen, T.-A., & Lui, K. (2002). Longitudinal motor development of "apparently normal" high-risk infants at 18 months, 3 and 5 years. *Early Human Development, 70,* 103–115.

127. Granger, C. V., Hamilton, B. B., & Kayton, R. (1989). *Guide for the Use of the Functional Independence Measure (WeeFIM) of the Uniform Data Set for Medical Rehabilitation.* Buffalo, NY: Research Foundation, State University of New York.

128. Green, E. M., Mulcahy, C. M., & Pountney, T. E. (1995). An investigation into the development of early postural control. *Developmental Medicine and Child Neurology, 37,* 437–448.

129. Greenough, W. T., Black, J. E., & Wallace, C. S. (1987). Experience and brain development. *Child Development, 58,* 539–559.

130. Hadders-Algra, M., & Prechtl, H. F. R. (1992). Developmental course of general movements in early infancy. I. Descriptive analysis of change in form. *Early Human Development, 28,* 201–213.

131. Hadders-Algra, M., Van Eykern, L. A., Klip-van den Nieuwendijk, A. W. J., & Prechtl, H. F. R. (1992). Developmental course of general movements in early infancy. II. EMG correlates. *Early Human Development, 28,* 231–253.

132. Haley, S. M., Baryza, M. J., & Blanchard, Y. (1993). Functional and naturalistic frameworks in assessing physical and motor disablement. In I. J. Wilhelm (Ed.), *Physical therapy assessment in early infancy* (pp. 225–256). New York: Churchill Livingstone.

133. Haley, S. M., Coster, W. J., & Faas, R. M. (1991). A content validity study of the Pediatric Evaluation of Disability Inventory. *Pediatric Physical Therapy, 3,* 177–184.

134. Haley, S. M., Coster, W. J., Ludlow, L. H., Haltiwanger, J. T., & Andrellos, P. J. (1992). *The Pediatric Evaluation of Disability Inventory: Development standardization and administration manual.* Boston: New England Medical Center Publications.

135. Haley, S. M., Coster, W. I., Kao, Y.-C., et al. (2010). Lessons from use of the Pediatric Evaluation of Disability Inventory: Where do we go from here? *Pediatric Physical Therapy, 22,* 69–75, DOI: 10.1097/PEP.0b013e3181cbfbf6.

136. Harris, S. R. (1990). Efficacy of physical therapy in promoting family functioning and functional independence for children with cerebral palsy. *Pediatric Physical Therapy, 2,* 160–164.

137. Harris, S. R., Backman, C. L., & Mayson, T. A. (2009). Comparative predictive validity of the Harris Infant Neuromotor Test and the Alberta Infant Motor Scale. *Developmental Medicine and Child Neurology,* Oct 26 epub. DOI: 10.1111/j.1469-8749.2009.03518.x.

138. Harris, S. R., & Daniels, L. E. (1996). Content validity of the Harris Infant Neuromotor Test. *Physical Therapy, 76,* 727–737.

139. Harris, S. R., & Daniels, L. E. (2001). Reliability and validity of the Harris Infant Neuromotor Test. *Journal of Pediatrics, 139,* 249–253. DOI: 10.1067/mpd.2001.115896.

140. Harris, S. R., Megans, A. M., & Daniels, L. E. (2010). *The Harris Infant Neuromotor Test (HINT) Test User's Manual Version 1.0 Clinical Edition.* Chicago: Infant Motor Performance Scales, LLC.

141. Harris, S. R., Megens, A. M., Backman, C. L., & Hayes, V. (2003). Development and standardization of the Harris Infant Neuromotor Test. *Infants and Young Children, 16,* 143–151.

142. Hauser-Cram, P. (1996). Mastery motivation in toddlers with developmental disabilities. *Child Development, 67,* 236–248.

143. Hay, L. (1990). Developmental changes in eye-hand coordination behaviors: Preprogramming versus feedback control. In

C. Bard, M. Fleury, & L. Hay (Eds.), *Development of eye-hand coordination across the life span* (pp. 217–244). Columbia, SC: University of South Carolina Press.

144. Hayne, H., Rovee-Collier, C., & Perris, E. E. (1987). Categorization and memory retrieval by three-month-olds. *Child Development, 58*, 750–767.

145. Henderson, R. C., Lark, R. K., Gurka, M. J., et al. (2002). Bone density and metabolism in children and adolescents with moderate to severe cerebral palsy. *Pediatrics, 110*, e5.

146. Heriza, C. (1991). Motor development: Traditional and contemporary theories. In M. J. Lister (Ed.), *Contemporary management of motor control problems: Proceedings of the II STEP Conference* (pp. 99–106). Alexandria, VA: Foundation for Physical Therapy.

147. Hinderer, K. A., Richardson, P. K., & Atwater, S. W. (1989). Clinical implications of the Peabody Developmental Motor Scales: A constructive review. *Physical and Occupational Therapy in Pediatrics, 9*(2), 81–106.

148. Hoover, J. E., & Strick, P. L. (1993). Multiple output channels in the basal ganglia. *Science, 259*, 819–821.

149. Horak, F. B. (1991). Assumptions underlying motor control for neurologic rehabilitation. In M. J. Lister (Ed.). *Contemporary management of motor control problems: Proceedings of the II STEP Conference* (pp. 11–27). Alexandria, VA: Foundation for Physical Therapy.

150. Horton, J. C. (2001). Critical periods in the development of the visual system. In D. B. Bailey, Jr., J. T. Bruer, F. J. Symons, & J. W. Lichtman (Eds.). *Critical thinking about critical periods* (pp. 45–65). Baltimore: Paul H. Brookes.

151. Hunnius, S. (2007). The early development of visual attention and its implications for social and cognitive development. *Progress in Brain Research, 164*, 187–209.

152. Hunnius, S., Geuze, R. H., Zweens, M. J., & Bos A. F. (2008). Effects of preterm experience on the developing visual system: A longitudinal study of shifts of attention and gaze in early infancy. *Developmental Neuropsychology, 33*, 521–535.

153. Iyer, L. V., Haley, S. M., Watkins, M. P., et al. (2003). Establishing minimal clinically important differences for scores on the Pediatric Evaluation of Disability Inventory for inpatient rehabilitation. *Physical Therapy, 83*, 888–898.

154. Jantz, J. W., Blosser, C. D., & Fruechting, L. A. (1997). A motor milestone change noted with a change in sleep position. *Archives of Pediatrics and Adolescent Medicine, 151*, 565–568.

155. Jette, D., Halbert, J., Iverson, C., Miceli, E., & Shah, P. (2009). Use of standardized outcome measures in physical therapist practice: Perceptions and applications. *Physical Therapy, 89*, 125–135. DOI: 10.2522/ptj.20080234.

156. Jones, S. S. (2007). Imitation in infancy. *Psychological Science, 18*, 593–599.

157. Josenby, A. L., Gun-Britt, J., Gummesson, C., & Nordmark, E. (2009). Longitudinal construct validity of the GMFM-88 total score and goal total score and the GMFM-66 score in a 5-year follow-up study. *Physical Therapy, 89*, 342–350.

158. Kanda, T., Pidcock, F. S., Hayakawa, K., Yamori, Y., & Shikata, Y. (2004). Motor outcome differences between two groups of children with spastic diplegia who received different intensities of early onset physiotherapy followed for 5 years. *Brain Development, 26*, 118–126.

159. Kanda, T., Yuge, M., Yamori, Y., Suzuki, J., & Fukase, H. (1984). Early physiotherapy in the treatment of spastic diplegia. *Developmental Medicine and Child Neurology, 26*, 438–444.

160. Karniol, R. (1989). The role of manual manipulative stages in the infant's acquisition of perceived control over objects. *Developmental Review, 9*, 205–233.

161. Kelly, Y., Sacker, A., Schoon, I., & Nazroo, J. (2006). Ethnic differences in achievement of developmental milestones by 9 months of age: The Millennium Cohort Study. *Developmental Medicine & Child Neurology 48*, 825–830.

162. Kennedy, E., Majnemer, A., Farmer, J. P., Barr, R. G., & Platt, R. W. (2009). Motor development of infants with positional plagiocephaly. *Physical & Occupational Therapy in Pediatrics, 29*(3), 236–238.

163. Keshner, E. A., Campbell, D., Katz, R., & Peterson, B. W. (1989). Neck muscle activation patterns in humans during isometric head stabilization. *Experimental Brain Research, 75*, 335–364.

164. Kirshenbaum, N., Riach, C. L., & Starkes, J. L. (2001). Nonlinear development of postural control and strategy use in young children: A longitudinal study. *Experimental Brain Research, 140*, 420–431.

165. Knobloch, H., Stevens, F., & Malone, A. F. (1980). *Manual of developmental diagnosis (rev. ed.)*. New York: Harper & Row.

166. Kolobe, T. H. (2004). Childrearing practices and developmental expectations for Mexican-American mothers and the developmental status of their infants. *Physical Therapy, 84*, 439–453.

167. Kolobe, T. H. A., Bulanda, M., & Susman, L. (2004). Predicting motor outcome at preschool age for infants tested at 7, 30, 60, and 90 days after term age using the Test of Infant Motor Performance. *Physical Therapy, 84*, 1144–1156.

168. Kolobe, T. H. A., Palisano, R. J., & Stratford, P. W. (1998). Comparison of two outcome measures for infants with cerebral palsy and infants with motor delays. *Physical Therapy, 78*, 1062–1072.

169. Koseck, K. (1999). Review and valuation of psychometric properties of the Revised Bayley Scales of Infant Development. *Pediatric Physical Therapy, 11*, 198–204.

170. Kotwica, K. A., Ferre, C. L., & Michel, G. F. (2008). Relation of stable hand-use preferences to the development of skill for managing multiple objects from 7 to 13 months of age. *Developmental Psychobiology, 50*, 519–529.

171. Kubo, M., & Ulrich, B. (2006). A biomechanical analysis of the 'high guard' position of arms during walking in toddlers. *Infant Behavior & Development, 29*, 509–517.

172. Kuh, D., Hardy, R., Butterworth, S., et al. (2006). Developmental origins of midlife physical performance: Evidence from a British birth cohort. *American Journal of Epidemiology, 164*, 110–121.

173. Kuniyoshi, Y., Yorozu, Y., Susuzki, S., Sangawa, S., Ohmura, Y., Terada, K., & Nagakubo, A. (2007). Emergence and

development of embodied cognition: A constructivist approach using robots. *Progress in Brain Research, 164,* 425–445.

174. Lee, A. M. (1980). Child-rearing practices and motor performance of black and white children. *Research Quarterly for Exercise and Sport, 51,* 494–500.

175. Lee, H. M., Bhat, A., Scholz, J. P., & Galloway, J. C. (2008). Toy-oriented changes during early arm movements. IV: Shoulder-elbow coordination. *Infant Behavior & Development, 31,* 447–469.

176. Lee, M.-H., Liu, Y.-T., & Newell, K. M. (2006). Longitudinal expressions of infant's prehension as a function of object properties. *Infant Behavior & Development, 29,* 481–493.

177. Lekskulchai, R., & Cole, J. (2001). Effect of a developmental program on motor performance in infants born preterm. *Australian Journal of Physiotherapy, 47,* 169–176.

178. Lenroot, R. K., Schmitt, J. E., Ordaz, S. J., Wallace, G. L., Neale, M. C., Lerch, J. P., Kendler, K. S., Evans, A. C., & Giedd, J. N. (2009). Differences in genetic and environmental influences on the human cerebral cortex associated with development during childhood and adolescence. *Human Brain Mapping, 30,* 163–174.

179. Leonard, C. T., Moritani, T., Hirschfeld, H., & Forssberg, H. (1990). Deficits in reciprocal inhibition of children with cerebral palsy as revealed by H reflex testing. *Developmental Medicine and Child Neurology, 32,* 974–984.

180. Levac, D., Wishart, L., Missiuna, C., & Wright, V. (2009). The application of motor learning strategies within functionally based interventions for children with neuromotor conditions. *Pediatric Physical Therapy, 21,* 345–355. DOI: 10.1097/ PEP.0b013e3181beb09d

181. Liao, P.-J. M., & Campbell, S. K. (2002). Comparison of two methods for teaching therapists to score the Test of Infant Motor Performance. *Pediatric Physical Therapy, 14,* 191–198.

182. Long, T. M., & Tieman, B. (1998). Review of two recently published measurement tools: The AIMS and the TIME. *Pediatric Physical Therapy, 10,* 62–66.

183. Loria, C. (1980). Relationship of proximal and distal function in motor development. *Physical Therapy, 60,* 167–172.

184. Lowes, L. P., Westcott, S. L., Palisano, R. J., Effgen, S. K., & Orlin, M. N. (2004). Muscle force and range of motion as predictors of standing balance in children with cerebral palsy. *Physical & Occupational Therapy in Pediatrics, 24*(1–2), 57–77.

185. Lynch, A., Ryu, J.-C., Agrawal, S., & Galloway, J. C. (2009). Power mobility training for a 7-month-old infant with spina bifida. *Pediatric Physical Therapy, 21,* 362–368. DOI: 10.1097/ PEP.0b013e3181bfae4c.

186. Lynch, S. R., & Stoltzfus, R. J. (2003). Iron and ascorbic acid: Proposed fortification levels and recommended iron compounds. *Journal of Nutrition, 133*(9), 2978S–2984S.

187. Maring, J. R., & Elbaum, L. (2007). Concurrent validity of the Early Intervention Devleopmental Profile and the Peabody Developmental Motor Scale-2. *Pediatric Physical Therapy, 19,* 116–120.

188. Marschik, P. B., Einspieler, C. S., Trohmeier, A., Plienegger, J., Garzarolli, B., & Prechtl, H. F. (2008). From the reaching behaviour at 5 months of age to hand preference at preschool age. *Developmental Psychobiology, 50,* 511–518.

189. Mazyn, L. I., Lenoir, M., Montagne, G., Delaey, C., & Savelsbergh, G. J. (2007). Stereo vision enhances the learning of a catching skill. *Experimental Brain Research, 179,* 723–726.

190. McCarthy, M. I., Silberstein, E. I., Atkins, E. A., et al. (2002). Comparing reliability and validity of pediatric instruments for measuring health and well-being of children with spastic cerebral palsy. *Developmental Medicine & Child Neurology, 44,* 468–476.

191. McEwan, M. H., Dihoff, R. E., & Brosvic, G. M. (1991). Early infant crawling experience is reflected in later motor skill development. *Perceptual and Motor Skills, 72,* 75–79.

192. McGraw, M. B. (1935). *Growth: A study of Johnny and Jimmy.* New York: Appleton-Century.

193. McGraw, M. B. (1963). *The neuromuscular maturation of the human infant.* New York: Hafner. (Original work published by Columbia University Press, 1945.)

194. McPhillips, M., & Jordan-Black, J.-A. (2007). The effect of social disadvantage on motor development in young children: A comparative study. *Journal of Child Psychology and Psychiatry, 48,* 1214–1222.

195. Miller, L. J. (1992). *The Miller First Step (screening test for evaluating preschoolers).* New York: Psychological Corporation.

196. Morbidity & Mortality Weekly Report. (2002). Iron deficiency: United States, 1999–2000. *Morbidity & Mortality Weekly Report, 51*(40), 897–899.

197. Msall, M. E., Braun, S., Duffy, L., DiGaudio, K., LaForest, S., & Granger, C. (1992a). Normative sample of the Pediatric Functional Independence Measure: A uniform data set for tracking disability (Abstract). *Developmental Medicine and Child Neurology, 34*(Suppl 66), 19.

198. Msall, M. E., Braun, S., Granger, C., DiGaudio, K., & Duffy, L. (1992b). *The Functional Independence Measure for Children (WeeFIM), developmental edition (version 1.5).* Buffalo, NY: Uniform Data Set for Medical Rehabilitation.

199. Murney, M. E., & Campbell, S. K. (1998). The ecological relevance of the Test of Infant Motor Performance Elicited Scale items. *Physical Therapy, 78,* 479–489.

200. Murray, G. K., Jones, P. B., Kuh, D., & Richards, M. (2007). Infant developmental milestones and subsequent cognitive function. *Annals of Neurology 62,* 128–136.

201. Natale, L., Orabona, F., Metta, G., & Sandini, G. (2007). Sensorimotor doordination in a "baby" robot: Learning about objects through grasping. *Progress in Brain Research, 164,* 403–424.

202. National Advisory Board on Medical Rehabilitation Research. (1993). *Research plan for the National Center for Medical Rehabilitation Research.* NIH Publication No. 93-3509. Bethesda, MD: National Institutes of Health.

203. Newell, K. M., & Vaillancourt, D. E. (2001). Dimensional change in motor learning. *Human Movement Science, 20,* 695–715.

204. Niewczyk, P. M., & Granger, C. V. (2010). Measuring function in young children with impairments. *Pediatric Physical Therapy, 22,* 42–51. DOI: 10.1097/PEP.0b013e3181cd17e8.

205. Nordmark, E., Jarnlo, G.-B., & Hagglund, G. (2000). Comparison of the Gross Motor Function Measure and Pediatric Evaluation of Disability Inventory in assessing motor function in children undergoing selective dorsal rhizotomy. *Developmental Medicine and Child Neurology, 42,* 245–252.

206. Nowakowski, R. S. (1987). Basic concepts of CNS development. *Child Development, 58,* 568–595.

207. Nudo, R. J., Milliken, G. W., Jenkins, W. M., & Merzenich, M. M. (1996). Use-dependent alterations of movement representations in primary motor cortex of adult squirrel monkeys. *Journal of Neuroscience, 16,* 785–807.

208. Oppenheim, R. W. (1981). Ontogenetic adaptations and retrogressive processes in the development of the nervous system and behavior: A neuroembryological perspective. In K. Connolly & H. F. R. Prechtl (Eds.), *Maturation and development: Biological and psychological perspectives* (pp. 73–109). Philadelphia: JB Lippincott.

209. Oztop, E., Bradley, N. S., & Arbib, M. A. (2004). Infant grasp learning: A computational model. *Experimental Brain Research, 180,* 480–503.

210. Paillard, J. (1990). Basic neurophysiological structures of eye-hand coordination. In C. Bard, M. Fleury, & L. Hay (Eds.), *Development of eye-hand coordination across the life span* (pp. 26–74). Columbia, SC: University of South Carolina Press.

211. Palisano, R. J. (1993). Neuromotor and developmental assessment. In I. J. Wilhelm (Ed.), *Physical therapy assessment in early infancy.* New York: Churchill Livingstone.

212. Palisano, R., Rosenbaum, P., Walter, S., Russell, D., Wood, E., & Galuppi, B. (1997). Development and reliability of a system to classify gross motor function in children with cerebral palsy. *Developmental Medicine and Child Neurology, 39,* 214–223.

213. Parker, D. F., Carriere, L., Hebestreit, H., Salsberg, A., & Bar-Or, O. (1993). Muscle performance and gross motor function of children with spastic cerebral palsy. *Developmental Medicine and Child Neurology, 35,* 17–23.

214. Pate, R. R., McIver, K., Dowda, M., Brown, W. H., & Addy, C. (2008). Directly observed physical activity levels in preschool children. *Journal of School Health, 78,* 438–444.

215. Pearce PF, Williamson, J., Harrell, J. S., Wildemuth, B. M., & Solomon, P. (2007). The Children's Computerized Physical Activity Reporter. *CIN: Computers, Informatics. Nursing, 25,* 93–105.

216. Pellegrini, A. D., & Smith, P. K. (1998). Physical activity play: The nature and function of a neglected aspect of play. *Child Development, 69,* 577–598.

217. Penhune, V., Watanabe, D., & Savion-Lemieux, T. (2005). The effect of early musical training on adult motor performance: Evidence of a sensitive period in motor learning. *Annals of the New York Academy of Science, 1060,* 265–268.

218. Perry, L. K., Smith, L. B., Hockema, S. A. (2008). Representational momentum and children's sensori-motor representations of objects. *Developmental Science, 11,* F17-F23.

219. Piaget, J. (1952). *The origins of intelligence in children.* New York: International Universities Press.

220. Pick, H. L., Jr. (1992). Eleanor J. Gibson: Learning to perceive and perceiving to learn. *Developmental Psychology, 28,* 787–794.

221. Piek, J. P., Dawson, L., Smith, L. M., & Gasson, N. (2008). The role of early fine and gross motor development on later motor and cognitive ability. *Human Movement Science, 27,* 668–681.

222. Piek, J. P., Gasson, N., Barrett, N., & Case, I. (2002). Limb and gender differences in the development of coordination in early infancy. *Human Movement Science, 21,* 621–639.

223. Plimpton, C. E., & Regimbal, C. (1992). Differences in motor proficiency according to gender and race. *Perceptual and Motor Skills, 74,* 399–402.

224. Provost, B. (1981). Normal development from birth to 4 months: Extended use of the NBAS-K. Part II. *Physical and Occupational Therapy in Pediatrics, 1*(3), 19–34.

225. Provost, B., Heimerl, S., McClain, C., Kim, N.-H., Lopez, B. R., & Kodituwakku, P. (2004). Concurrent validity of the Bayley Scales of Infant Development II Motor Scale and the Peabody Developmental Motor Scales-2 in children with developmental delays. *Pediatric Physical Therapy, 16,* 149–156. DOI: 10.1097/01.PEP.0000136005.41585.FE

226. Ramey, C. T., & Ramey, S. L. (1992). Effective early intervention. *Mental Retardation, 30*(6), 337–345.

227. Ratliff-Schaub, K., Hunt, C. E., Crowell, D., et al. (2001). Relationship between infant sleep position and motor development in preterm infants. *Developmental and Behavioral Pediatrics, 22,* 293–299.

228. Ratner, H. H., & Foley, M. A. (1994). A unifying framework for the development of children's activity memory. *Advances in Child Development and Behavior, 25,* 33–105.

229. Ravenscroft, E. F., & Harris, S. R. (2007). Is maternal education related to infant motor development? Pediatric *Physical Therapy, 19,* 56–61.

230. Riou, E. M., Ghosh, S., Francoeur, E., & Shevell M. (2009). Global developmental delay and its relationship to cognitive skills. *Developmental Medicine & Child Neurology, 51,* 600–606. DOI: 10.1111/j.1469-8749.2008.03197.x.

231. Roberton, M. A., & Halverson, L. E. (1984). *Developing children: Their changing movement. A guide for teachers.* Philadelphia: Lea & Febiger.

232. Robertson, S. S., Johnson, S. L., Masnick, A. M., & Weiss, S. L. (2007). Robust coupling of body movement and gaze in young infants. *Developmental Psychobiology, 49,* 2080215.

233. Rocha, N. A., Silva, F. P., & Tudella, E. (2006). The impact of object size and rigidity on infant reaching. *Infant Behavior & Development, 29,* 251–261.

234. Rocha, N. A., & Tudella, E. (2008). The influence of lying positions and postural control on hand-mouth and hand-hand behaviours in 0–4-month-old infants. *Infant Behavior & Development, 31,* 107–114.

235. Rosenbaum, P. (1998). Physical activity play in children with disabilities: A neglected opportunity for research? *Child Development, 69,* 607–608.

236. Rosenbaum, P., Russell, D., Cadman, D., Gowland, C., Jarvis, S., & Hardy, S. (1990). Issues in measuring change in motor function in children with cerebral palsy: A special communication. *Physical Therapy, 70,* 125–131.

237. Rosenbaum, P. L., Walter, S. D., Hanna, S. E., Palisano, R. J., Russell, D. J., & Raina, P. (2002). Prognosis for gross motor function in cerebral palsy: Creation of motor development curves. *Journal of the American Medical Association, 288,* 1357–1363.

238. Rosenblith, J. F. (1992). A singular career: Nancy Bayley. *Developmental Psychology, 28,* 747–758.

239. Russell, D., Palisano, R., Walter, S., Rosenbaum, P., Gemus, M., Gowland, C., Galuppi, B., & Lane, M. (1998). Evaluating motor function in children with Down syndrome: Validity of the GMFM. *Developmental Medicine and Child Neurology, 40,* 693–701.

240. Russell, D., Rosenbaum, P., Avery, L., & Lane, M. (2002). *Gross Motor Function Measure (GMFM-66 and GMFM-88), user's manual.* London: MacKeith Press.

241. Russell, D., Rosenbaum, P., Cadman, D., Gowland, C., Hardy, S., & Jarvis, S. (1989). The Gross Motor Function Measure: A means to evaluate the effects of physical therapy. *Developmental Medicine and Child Neurology, 31,* 341–352.

242. Salls, J. S., Silverman, L. N., & Gatty, C. M. (2002). The relationship of infant sleep and play positioning to motor milestone achievement. *American Journal of Occupational Therapy, 56,* 577–580.

243. Sameroff, A J, Seifer, R., Baldwin, A., & Baldwin, C. (1993). Stability of intelligence from preschool to adolescence: The influence of social and family risk factors. *Child Development, 64,* 80–97.

244. Scherzer, A. L., Mike, V., & Ilson, J. (1976). Physical therapy as a determinant of change in the cerebral palsied infant. *Pediatrics, 58,* 47–52.

245. Schoen, J. H. R. (1969). The corticofugal projection to the brain stem and spinal cord in man. *Psychiatry, Neurology and Neurosurgery, 72,* 121–128.

246. Shafir, T., Angulo-Barroso, A., Calatroni, A., Jimenez, E., & Lozoff, B. (2006). Effects of iron deficiency in infancy on patterns of motor development over time. *Human Movement Science, 25,* 821–838.

247. Shea, C. H., & Wulf, G. (2005). Schema theory: A critical appraisal and reevaluation. *Journal of Motor Behavior, 37*(2), 85–101.

248. Shirley, M. M. (1931). *The first two years: A study of twenty-five babies. Vol. I. Postural and locomotor development.* Minneapolis, MN: University of Minnesota Press.

249. Short, E. J., Klein, N. K., Lewis, B. A., et al. (2003). Cognitive and academic consequences of bronchopulmonary dysplasia and very low birth weight: 8-year-old outcomes. *Pediatrics, 112,* e359.

250. Shumway-Cook, A., & Woollacott, M. (1985). The growth of stability: Postural control from a developmental perspective. *Journal of Motor Behavior, 17,* 131–147.

251. Shumway-Cook, A., & Woollacott, M. (1993). Theoretical issues in assessing postural control. In I. J. Wilhelm (Ed.), *Physical therapy assessment in early infancy* (pp. 161–171). New York: Churchill Livingstone.

252. Skinner, B. F. (1972). *Cumulative record: A selection of papers* (3rd ed.). New York: Meredith.

253. Smits, D.-W., Gorter, J. W., Ketelaar, M., et al. (2009). Relationship between gross motor capacity and daily-life mobility in children with cerebral palsy. *Developmental Medicine and Child Neurology, 52,* e60-e66. DOI: 10.1111/j.1469-8749.2009.03525.x.

254. Snider, L., Majnemer, A., Mazer, B., Campbell, S., & Bos, A. F. (2009). Prediction of motor and functional outcomes in infants born preterm assessed at term. *Pediatric Physical Therapy, 21,* 2–11.

255. Sparling, J. W. (Ed.). (1993). *Concepts in fetal movement research.* New York: Haworth Press.

256. Spittle, A. J., Doyle, L. W., & Boyd, R. N. (2008). A systematic review of the clinimetric properties of neuromotor assessments for preterm infants during the first year of life. *Developmental Medicine & Child Neurology, 50,* 254–266. DOI: 10.1111/j.1469-8749.2008.02025.x.

257. Sporns, O. (1994). Selectionist and instructionist ideas in neuroscience. *International Review of Neurobiology, 37,* 3–26.

258. Sporns, O., & Edelman, G. M. (1993). Solving Bernstein's problem: A proposal for the development of coordinated movement by selection. *Child Development, 64,* 960–981.

259. Stengel, T. J., Attermeier, S. M., Bly, L., & Heriza, C. B. (1984). Evaluation of sensorimotor dysfunction. In S. K. Campbell (Ed.), *Pediatric neurologic physical therapy* (pp. 13–87). New York: Churchill Livingstone.

260. Stokes, N. A., Deitz, J. L., & Crowe, T. K. (1990). The Peabody Developmental Fine Motor Scale: An interrater reliability study. *American Journal of Occupational Therapy, 44,* 334–340.

261. Strick, P. L., & Preston, J. B. (1982a). Two representations of the hand in area 4 of a primate. I. Motor output organization. *Journal of Neurophysiology, 48,* 139–149.

262. Strick, P. L., & Preston, J. B. (1982b). Two representations of the hand in area 4 of a primate. II. Somatosensory input organization. *Journal of Neurophysiology, 48,* 150–159.

263. Task Force on Standards for Measurement in Physical Therapy. (1991). Standards for tests and measurements in physical therapy practice. *Physical Therapy, 71,* 589–622.

264. Task Force on Sudden Infant Death Syndrome. (2005). The changing concept of sudden infant death syndrome: diagnostic coding shifts, controversies regarding the sleeping

environment, and new variables to consider in reducing risk. *Pediatrics, 116,* 1245–1255.

265. Thelen, E. (1990). Coupling perception and action in the development of skill: A dynamic approach. In H. Bloch & B. I. Bertenthal (Eds.), *Sensory-motor organization and development in infancy and early childhood* (pp. 39–56). Dordrecht, Netherlands: Kluwer Academic.

266. Thelen, E. (1995). Motor development. A new synthesis. *American Psychologist, 50,* 79–95.

267. Thelen, E., & Adolph, K. E. (1992). Arnold L. Gesell: The paradox of nature and nurture. *Developmental Psychology, 28,* 368–380.

268. Thelen, E., & Corbetta, D. (1994). Exploration and selection in the early acquisition of skill. *International Review of Neurobiology, 37,* 75–102.

269. Thelen, E., Corbetta, D., Kamm, K., Spencer, J. P., Schneider, K., & Zernicke, R. (1993). The transition to reaching: Mapping intention and intrinsic dynamics. *Child Development, 64,* 1058–1098.

270. Thelen, E., Kelso, J. A. S., & Fogel, A. (1987). Self-organizing systems and infant motor development. *Developmental Review, 7,* 39–65.

271. Thelen, E., & Ulrich, B. D. (1991). *Hidden skills: A dynamic systems analysis of treadmill stepping during the first year. Monographs of the Society for Research in Child Development. Serial No. 223, Vol. 56, No. 1.* Chicago: University of Chicago Press.

272. Thelen, E., Ulrich, B. D., & Jensen, J. L. (1989). The developmental origins of locomotion. In M. H. Woollacott & A. Shumway-Cook (Eds.), *Development of posture and gait across the life span* (pp. 23–47). Columbia, SC: University of South Carolina Press.

273. Thompson, R. A. (2001). Sensitive periods in attachment? In D. B. Bailey, Jr., J. T. Bruer, F. J. Symons, & J. W. Lichtman (Eds.). *Critical thinking about critical periods* (pp. 83–106). Baltimore: Paul H. Brookes.

274. Thorn, F., Gwiazda, J., Cruz, A. A., Bauer, J. A., & Held, R. (1994). The development of eye alignment, convergence, and sensory binocularity in young infants. *Investigative Ophthalmology and Visual Science, 35,* 544–553.

275. Tscharnuter, I. (1993). A new therapy approach to movement organization. *Physical and Occupational Therapy in Pediatrics, 13*(2), 19–40.

276. Tucker, C. A., & Watson, K. E. (2010). Clinical bottom line: Measuring function in young children with impairments. *Pediatric Physical Therapy, 22,* 51.

277. Tychsen, L. (2001). Critical periods for development of visual acuity, depth perception, and eye tracking. In D. B. Bailey, Jr., J. T. Bruer, F. J. Symons, & J. W. Lichtman (Eds.). *Critical thinking about critical periods* (pp. 67–80). Baltimore: Paul H. Brookes.

278. Ulrich, B. D. (1989). Development of stepping patterns in human infants: A dynamical systems perspective. *Journal of Motor Behavior, 21,* 329–408.

279. Ulrich, D. A., Ulrich, B. D., Angulo-Kinzler, R. M., & Yun, J. (2001). Treadmill training of infants with Down syndrome: Evidence-based developmental outcomes. *Pediatrics, 108,* E84. Accessed at www.pediatrics.org/cgi/content/full/108/5/384.

280. Unanue, R. A., & Westcott, S. L. (2003). The responsiveness of the Test of Infant Motor Performance (TIMP) in preterm infants (abstract). *Pediatric Physical Therapy, 15,* 64.

281. van Blankenstein, M., Welbergen, U. R., & de Haas, J. H. (1962). *Le développement du nourrisson: Sa première anné en 130 photographies.* Paris: Presses Universitaires de France.

282. van Hartingsveldt, M. J., Cup, E. H., & Oostendorp, R. A. (2005). Reliability and validity of the fine motor scale of the Peabody Developmental Motor Scales-2. *Occupational Therapy International, 12*(1), 1–13.

283. Viholanen, H., Ahonen, T., Cantell, M., Tolvanen, A., & Lyytinen, H. (2006). The early motor milestones in infancy and later motor skills in toddlers: A structural equation model of motor development. *Physical & Occupational Therapy in Pediatrics, 26*(1–2), 91–113.

284. Vinter, A. (1990). Manual imitations and reaching behaviors: An illustration of action control in infancy. In C. Bard, M. Fleury, & L. Hay (Eds.), *Development of eye-hand coordination across the life span* (pp. 157–187). Columbia, SC: University of South Carolina Press.

285. von Hofsten, C. (1982). Eye-hand coordination in the newborn. *Developmental Psychology, 18,* 450–461.

286. Von Hofsten, C. (2006). Action in development. *Developmental Science, 10,* 54–60, Epub 20, Dec.

287. Wallace, P. S., & Whishaw, I. Q. (2003). Independent digit movements and precision grip patterns in 1–5-month-old human infants: Hand babbling, including vacuous then self-directed hand and digit movements, precedes targeted reaching. *Neuropsychologia, 41,* 1912–1918.

288. Wang, H. Y., & Yang, Y. H. (2006). Evaluating the responsiveness of 2 versions of the Gross Motor Function Measure for children with cerebral palsy. *Archives of Physical Medicine and Rehabilitation 87,* 51–56.

289. Whitall, J., & Getchell, N. (1995). From walking to running: Applying a dynamical systems approach to the development of locomotor skills. *Child Development, 66,* 1541–1553.

290. Wielenga, J.M., Smit, B.J., Merkus, M.P., Wolf, M.J., van Sonderen, L., Kok, J.H (2009). Development and growth in very preterm infants in relation to NIDCAP in a Dutch NICU: two years of follow-up. *Acta Paediatr, 98,* 291–297.

291. Williams, J. R., & Scott, R. B. (1953). Growth and development of Negro infants: Motor development and its relationship to child-rearing practices in two groups of Negro infants. *Child Development, 24,* 103–121.

292. Wimmers, R. H., Savelsbergh, G. J. P., Beek, P. J., & Hopkins, B. (1998a). Evidence for a phase transition in the early development of prehension. *Developmental Psychobiology, 32,* 235–248.

293. Wimmers, R. H., Savelsbergh, G. J. P., van der Kamp, J., & Hartelman, P. (1998b). A developmental transition in prehension modeled as a cusp catastrophe. *Developmental Psychobiology*, *32*, 23–35.

294. Wolf, M. J., Koldewijn, K., Beelen, A., Smit, B., Hedlund, R., & de Groot, I. J. (2002). Neurobehavioral and developmental profile of very low birthweight preterm infants in early infancy. *Acta Paediatrica*, *91*, 930–938.

295. Wong, S., Chan, K., Wong, V., & Wong, W. (2002). Use of chopsticks in Chinese children. *Child Care, Health & Development*, *28*, 157–161.

296. WHO Multicentre Growth Reference Study Group. (2006). WHO motor development study: Windows of achievement for six gross motor development milestones. *Acta Paediatrica* (Suppl. 450), 86–95.

297. World Health Organization. (2001). *International Classification of Function, Disability and Health*. Geneva: World Health Organization.

298. Zelazo, P. R. (1983). The development of walking: New findings and old assumptions. *Journal of Motor Behavior*, *15*, 99–137.

299. Zelazo, P. R., Zelazo, N. A., & Kolb, S. (1972). "Walking" in the newborn. *Science*, *176*, 314–315.

3

Motor Control: Developmental Aspects of Motor Control in Skill Acquisition

SARAH WESTCOTT MCCOY, PT, PhD • STACEY DUSING, PT, PhD

The term "motor control" is commonly used in both research and clinical arenas of physical therapy, perhaps so commonly as to erode a clear understanding of its meaning. This chapter seeks to familiarize the clinician with the research field of motor control and, more specifically, how motor control applies to issues of motor development by addressing four objectives. The first objective of this chapter is to briefly discuss some theories, hypotheses, and models that have shaped the direction of research and current views on motor control. Research conducted to test theories, hypotheses, and models of motor control, in turn, have led scientists to propose that physiologic, psychologic, and mechanical mechanisms or processes play select roles in the control of movement and can be studied under conditions of controlled observation. Thus, the second objective of this chapter is to describe some of the processes that may control movement initiation or execution. The third objective and emphasis of this chapter is to present the work of researchers that both describes motor skill acquisition and attempts to reveal the processes that drive or permit acquisition of skills such as posture, gait, reaching, and grasping. The fourth objective is to explore how a physical therapist might examine and address a child's movement problems employing current knowledge of motor control. If the four objectives are adequately addressed, the reader should ultimately understand how evidence about motor control can assist and guide physical therapy examination, evaluation, and intervention.

CLINICAL EXAMPLE

As you begin reading this chapter, consider a 20-month-old boy with mild spastic diplegic cerebral palsy (CP) who is an emerging walker eagerly attempting to reach for a bright shiny toy with one hand while standing and holding on to a table with the other hand. As you observe the child trying to capture the toy, you see that he is standing on his toes and leaning into the table. As he attempts to reach, he seems to have difficulty rotating his trunk, balancing on his legs, moving his shoulder forward to reach, and opening his hand to grasp. His movements appear jerky and stiff. Why is he having difficulty moving the way he wants to? What should the physical therapist assess and recommend that would help him learn to move more efficiently and effectively? As the picture of this child forms in the therapist's mind, she or he

will start to make assumptions about what the problems are, which should then lead to potential assessments to confirm the therapist's hypotheses and ultimately to the selection of the best interventions that will improve the child's movement ability. Dependent on the frame of reference of the therapist, different possible problems could be hypothesized to be the constraining factors; as a result, the issues that need to be assessed and the type of procedural interventions to employ will vary. Given this case scenario, we will start the process of learning about motor control with a discussion of theories, hypotheses, and models, which will help frame our problem solving for this child.

THEORIES, HYPOTHESES, AND MODELS

Defining the term "motor control" and describing many of the theoretic constructs common to the field are not easy tasks, in part because motor control is a multidisciplinary field of study drawing from a broad range of disciplines including, but not limited to, anatomy, physiology, psychology, kinesiology, engineering, and physical therapy. Historically, theories of motor control typically emerged from within a field such as anatomy or psychology, whereas hypotheses and models often emerged from the integration of ideas across fields. One consequence of this cross-pollination is that theoretic constructs and terminology have taken on slightly different definitions from one disciplinary view to the next, often leaving resolution of the discrepancy in definitions to the persevering student. In this section we will briefly review some of the more well-known theories, hypotheses, and models of motor control to gain an understanding of the ideas commonly embraced or challenged.

Theories of motor control attempt to unite various observations and laws that emerge from scientific study to explain why the observations/laws exist or how they relate to one another. Theories also provide the foundation for development of hypotheses, models, and new theories. Three distinctly different theoretic perspectives are currently encountered in motor control development literature: maturational, learning, and dynamic-based views. In the discussion to follow, we will briefly consider each view. Hypotheses, in contrast, attempt to predict the relationship between observations and defined (or experimental) conditions. For example, the maturational-based theory of motor control proposes that emergence of behavior is primarily attributable to maturational changes in the nervous system.[361] A hypothesis based on this theory is that independent finger movements emerge at 7 months of age because of specific physiologic changes occurring in the primary motor cortex, the corticospinal tract, or both just before 7 months. When experiments by a large number of scientists testing a hypothesis produce consistent findings, the hypothesis becomes a law. Thus, laws define highly predictable relationships between variables, and in some instances these relationships can be mathematically specified. Fitts's law, for example, states that accuracy requirements and the distance over which a movement occurs can be used to predict movement time.[162] Models, in contrast to laws, are idealized constructs that incorporate a few select variables believed to be most powerful in explaining relationships between events and are used by scientists to both visualize and test theories. A basic understanding of hypotheses and models is useful because they provide the rationale for most research designs and views currently found in motor control literature, as well as guidance for examination and intervention in physical therapy (Figure 3-1). For further elaboration on these topics, the reader is referred to discussions by Schmidt and Lee[434] and Shumway-Cook and Woollacot.[458]

MATURATIONAL-BASED THEORIES

In the late 1800s, the neurologist Ramón y Cajal discovered that Golgi silver stain could selectively label individual nerve cells. This advance led to the neuron doctrine and set the course for neurobiologic research and thinking in the twentieth century.[451] The notion of "structure-function" and the maturational-based theory of motor control are two theoretic products of the neuron doctrine. Using silver stain, anatomists found that structural features distinguish subpopulations of neurons within and between regions of the nervous system and that morphologic changes occur during development. The array of morphologic findings led to the view that structural organization of the nervous system determines behavioral function (structure-function).

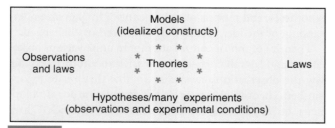

Figure 3-1 The development of theories stems from observations and known laws and is a fluid and regenerative process. Experiments are designed to test hypotheses developed from the theories, and models are created to depict relationships within theories. Both are examined and used to either support or modify theories. If a theory is supported many times, it can become a law, which can then support the development of further theories.

Physiologists provided evidence for structure-function control of behavior by isolating portions of the nervous system (reduced preparations) that produced stereotypic movements such as the stretch reflex, the brisk contraction of a muscle in response to a quick stretch of the muscle stimulating its proprioceptors. Based on his many studies of reflex function in the spinal cord of cats, dogs, and monkeys, Sherrington[452] espoused the view that behavior is hierarchically organized and the simple reflex (composed of a receptor, conductor, and effector organ) is the fundamental unit of neural integration. Furthermore, he proposed that motor behavior is the composite coordination of simple reflexes (e.g., reflex chaining) as excitatory and inhibitory actions are summated at the synapse.

Sherrington's notion of reflex chaining so dominated the study of physiology in the first half of the 20th century that physiologists gave little attention to other views of motor control in explanations of behavior.[177] Structure-function organization and reflex chaining were commonly employed rationales in studies of motor development as evidenced by the temporal correlations commonly drawn between emerging stimulus-evoked behavior and anatomic changes in neural pathways.[272] Thus, early studies identified the neuroanatomic changes occurring around the time a new behavior emerged without considering whether other variables contributed to the behavioral change. Consequently, scientists proposed that certain predictable changes during neural maturation are the causal determinants of behavioral development,[256,361] establishing the foundation for maturational theories. Concurrent with these developments, hierarchic reflex chaining evolved to include the notion that reflex behaviors are expressions of an animal's phylogenetic origins.[273] Such views merged into the notions that the earliest movements are primitive behaviors controlled by phylogenetically older neural structures and these movements eventually disappear as older neural structures are inhibited by later differentiating neural structures that are phylogenetically more recent.[501] These notions suggest that the development of control of movement is primarily a reflection of internal neural development. It appears there was little or no scientific challenge of these neuromaturational views into the latter half of the 20th century, perhaps because students of development took little notice of other directions in neurobiologic research that were emerging at the time.[177]

LEARNING-BASED THEORIES

During this same time period (20th century), psychologists were also attempting to form theories of development. Behaviorism looked to the role of factors external to the individual, such as the environment, and sought to determine what attributes of the environment trigger or shape behavior. Response chaining, for example, proposed that feedback becomes more strongly associated with action over practice, automating the sequences of action executed by the nervous system.[417] According to response chaining, the environment is the controller of the automating process. Response chaining, like reflex chaining, explains the ordering of movements as the consequence of feedback from one movement that in turn activates the next movement. Thorndike extended the notion of response chaining to address how motor skills are learned, and in the law of effect he proposed that skills emerge as we repeat actions that are rewarded.[434a]

The law of effect and emphasis on feedback can also be identified in theories and models of motor learning such as Adams's closed-loop theory.[2] Adams proposed that we develop a perceptual memory trace for what a correct movement should feel like (expected sensory consequences) based on intrinsic feedback generated during movement implementation. The perceptual trace evaluates the actual sensory consequences (feedback) of a movement each time it is executed and selects the movement attributes that are compatible with the perceptual memory trace to establish a memory trace for movement execution parameters. According to Adams's learning-based theory, feedback during movement is required to learn a movement, but subsequent research indicated that we do not need to monitor ongoing movements in order to reinforce desirable movement parameters.[489] This inconsistency between experimental results and theoretic prediction was subsequently addressed by Schmidt's schema theory.[435]

Schema theory, one of the most widely embraced of the learning theories, proposed that motor development is a function of learning rules to evaluate, correct, and update memory traces for a given class of movements.[435] Schema theory assumes the presence of three constructs: general motor programs and two types of memory traces, recall schema, and recognition schema. General motor programs are loosely defined as sets of instructions that are responsible for organizing the invariant or fundamental components of a movement. Recall schemas are defined as memories of relationships between past movement parameters, past initial conditions, and the *movement outcomes* they produced. Recognition schemas are defined as memories of relationships between past movement parameters, past initial conditions, and the *sensory consequences* they produced. It is theorized that recall schemas function to establish rules regarding the relationship between movement parameters of a general motor program, such as force or velocity, and movement outcome for a given set of initial conditions that can be used to plan similar movements under anticipated conditions. Recognition schema, in turn, are proposed to compare sensory consequences with movement outcome in light of initial conditions to form a second set of rules that can be used to predict the expected sensory consequences for similar movement outcomes during anticipated initial conditions. The expected sensory consequences are proposed to serve as a perceptual memory trace for evaluating new movements. When movements are generated too

quickly (ballistically) to be corrected by feedback as they are executed (i.e., open loop), it is theorized that a feedforward motor command can be compared with the expected sensory consequences to evaluate the movements after the movements are completed. In this manner the schema are established and refined as a function of practice. Research suggests that there may be an interdependence between parameters such as time and force during schema development. Motor learning related to manipulation of one parameter may have a negative effect on learning the other parameter.[450,538] See Chapter 4 for further discussion of motor learning theories.

Schema theory does not attempt to explain the establishment of general motor programs, nor does it attempt to ascribe them to specific neural structures. The term "motor program" is employed in a variety of ways by researchers from a variety of disciplinary backgrounds, which may help explain why there is no consensus as to what constitutes a motor program.[417,450] In motor learning literature, motor programs are commonly invoked to explain the stereotypic attributes of a complex movement pattern that persist as movement parameters or context is altered. For example, it has been suggested that we have a general motor program for writing our name and its instructions are recognized in the features common to signing our name under different conditions with different tools, different parameters of movement, even different sets of muscles.[405] Motor learning literature also ascribes to motor programs the ability to generate complex movements without benefit of concurrent feedback, such as reaching for a target after administration of a local anesthetic or tourniquet, as well as ballistic movements that may be completed before feedback can contribute to the movement (Schmidt & Lee, 1998). In each of these instances, motor programs are viewed as learned sets of instructions. Based on more recent motor learning research, this definition of and the presence of general motor programs has been suggested to be outdated.[450] Rather a "scalable response structure" that is not necessarily invariant has been suggested as the more appropriate construct.[450] The notion is that rather than a "memory state" (motor program), we have a "processing mechanism" (scalable response structure). Research involving the observation of infant development of walking when presented with various obstacles such as inclines, cliffs, and bridges has supported this notion, suggesting a process of "learning to learn" or a continual process of online problem-solving.[5,7]

While programs for higher-level behaviors are being challenged, it may be that these more basic networks exist. In neurobiology, "motor programs" are called "pattern generators" and are viewed as genetically inherited sets of instructions that control the stereotypic features of innate behaviors such as mating, defense, and locomotion.[311] Some of the strongest arguments in neurobiology for the existence of general motor programs refer to the many examples of an animal's ability to execute functional movements in the absence of feedback.[315,394,476,489] Where the movement instructions are stored is yet to be determined, but some investigators implicate the sensorimotor cortex,[14] primary motor cortex,[252] and cerebellum,[313,429] for motor learning, and the prefrontal association cortex,[176,311,448] basal ganglia,[446] and subcortical areas[476] for motor memory and planning.

As theories are tested, the outcomes reveal their shortcomings, clarify the boundaries of our understanding, and raise a new generation of questions. In contrast to maturationist theories, learning-based theories suggest that development of motor skill is the consequence of learning by trial and error to master and sequence units of action that in their rudimentary form are genetically determined. Connolly[96] proposed, for example, that genetics endow the infant with the equivalent of computer hardware (neurologic and biomechanical features) and the infant's cognitive activities, equivalent to computer software, function to modify and adapt rudimentary units of movement into skilled action.

DYNAMIC-BASED THEORIES

The most recent theory receiving broad interest that was established to explain the development of motor control is the dynamic systems theory proposed by Thelen and her colleagues.[460,491,492] The theory seeks to address what drives skill acquisition and a particular problem poorly handled by previous theories: How does a child move from one developmental stage of skill to another? A fundamental hypothesis of the theory is that there are multiple identifiable variables, such as muscle power, body mass, arousal, neural networks, motivation, and environmental forces (e.g., gravity and friction), that establish a context for movement initiation and execution. A second fundamental hypothesis is that the relationship (interaction) among these variables is in constant flux and therefore shapes the features of a movement as it unfolds. Thus, dynamic systems theory proposes that developmental changes in motor behavior and skill performance can be explained in terms of dynamics common to physical, biologic, and computational systems. Developmental stages are viewed as attractor states that are governed by a set of variables, and transitions in behavior are viewed as flips between attractor states powered by change in one or more of the variables. For example, an animal may be capable of producing coordinated limb movements for stepping but incapable of locomoting until related postural skills are sufficient.[53] Or the pattern of limb movements may abruptly vary with changes in movement parameters such as velocity.[491] Behavioral solutions are thus the composite solution of neural, biomechanical, and environmental forces acting in concert.[25,484] Variability in motor behavior, as opposed to deterministic movement, is thus a part of the development or learning process.[6,111] In fact it has been suggested that variability is a crucial feature of learning optimal motor behavior[409,431] and can be argued to be part of the generalized motor program for rhythmic interlimb coordination.[9]

Recent studies on the development of postural control have also documented changes in variability of postural control during the development of sitting balance using nonlinear analysis procedures.[122]

Theoretic work by Sporns and Edelman[466] has modified dynamic theory by developing the notion of dynamic selection. Rather than assuming the existence of genetically predetermined motor programs, they hypothesize that motor skills emerge from an interaction between development-related changes in movement dynamics and brain structure-function. Given that musculoskeletal anatomy and related biomechanics change dramatically over the course of development, the theory is primarily concerned with how the brain's circuitry can readily change to match or accommodate these changes. The theory incorporates three key hypotheses: a developing organism is genetically endowed with spontaneously generated behaviors that make up the basic movement repertoire; it is also endowed with a sensory system capable of detecting and recognizing movements having adaptive value; and the developing organism can select movements having adaptive value by varying synaptic strengths within and between brain circuits such that successive event selections will progressively modify the movement repertoire. In essence, the theory proposes that there is a "handshaking" relationship between evolving movement mechanics and ongoing maturation of brain circuits, all of which is edited or biased by the adaptive value of a movement experienced. Recognizing the value of a movement experience will increase the probability of repetition, strengthening a behavior; failure to recognize its value will reduce the probability of repetition, thereby weakening the behavior. Thus, this latter theory embraces attributes of maturational, learning, and dynamic theories to explain motor control development. This theoretic perspective has been supported by Hadders-Algra[212,214] based on the typical development of postural control and abnormalities that occur with this development in infants and children with CP and developmental coordination disorder (DCD).

In summary, theories of motor control and development attempt to explain complex and changing motor behavior and, as theories go, are also not static notions. Theory terminology, which stems from different fields of study, is often obtuse and difficult to understand without intense study. There is no one unifying theory of motor control related to motor development, and there are some overlapping tenets among the broad theoretic positions presented. This likely is influenced by the fact that we may control our movement in different manners dependent on the type of movement we are doing, for instance movements that repeat periodically (e.g., walking) versus movements for skills of the sort that are typically learned (e.g., playing a piano) and are not developed potentially from a special evolutionary base.[294] Theories, however, guide research and should guide our problem solving when assessing and determining interventions for children with motor dysfunction. Returning to our

TABLE 3-1 Example Considerations for Examination and Intervention Based on Different Developmental Motor Control Theories

Theories	Basis	Tenets	Developmental Prediction	Child's Major Problem	Broad Application: PT Examination	Broad Application: PT Intervention
Maturational	Neural maturation	Neural structure to functional movement dependence	Linear development of motor skills following neural maturation	Initial brain damage and altered neural maturation	Infrequent assessments to determine developmental delay; tests focused on assessment of neural maturation	Facilitation of motor development following neural maturation trajectory
Learning	Trial and error	Existence of motor program with development of force and timing parameters	Task dependent development of motor skills	Lack of exposure and practice of tasks	Task-specific assessment; tests focused on ability to do certain tasks	Practice of task specific skills with feedback controlled for best motor learning
Dynamic systems	Interaction of brain-body-environment	Emergence of behaviors dependent on task and environment	Nonlinear development	Difficulty using affordances of the environment	Frequent assessment to determine developmental delay; tests focused on observation of problem solving in typical environments	Movement exploration in multiple environmental circumstances

20-month-old child with CP, from the broad theoretic positions described earlier, we would assume certain notions based on each theory, which then leads us to assess and intervene in specific manners. Table 3-1 outlines just several of many potential possibilities for how physical therapy might vary based on the theory one is assuming to be most valid. The reader is encouraged to consider other possibilities. We next examine hypotheses and models related to motor control that perhaps simplifies the link between theories to the supporting evidence and may provide more specific guidance for physical therapy practice.

CURRENT HYPOTHESES OF MOTOR CONTROL

Rather than proposing some unifying theory, many current hypotheses of motor control attempt to identify controlling variables for specific types of movement. Central pattern generators (CPGs) are proposed to account for the basic neural organization and function required to execute coordinated, rhythmic movements, such as locomotion, chewing, grooming (e.g., scratching), and respiration. CPGs are commonly defined as interneuronal networks, located in either the spinal cord or brain stem that can order the selection and sequencing of motoneurons independent of descending or peripheral afferent neural input. Under normal conditions, however, neural input from select supraspinal regions, such as the brain stem reticular nuclei, activate CPGs, and peripheral afferents, propriospinal regions, and other supraspinal regions modulate the output of CPGs and adapt the

behavior to the movement context. Work in invertebrate species suggests that pattern generators can even alter their own configurations (i.e., intrinsic modulation) to produce more than one pattern associated with the same or different behaviors.[293] CPGs can also modulate the inputs they receive, gating potentially disruptive reflex actions such as nociceptive activation of the flexor withdrawal reflex when a limb is fully loaded during the stance phase of locomotion (further reviews of pattern generators are available[200,202,563]). Cellular studies appear to indicate that embryonic behaviors are the product of transient neural networks (discussed later in this chapter) that may have little or no participation in mature pattern-generating networks.[380] Work in this area is hindered, however, by the lack of full understanding of adult CPGs.[202,353,563] Nonetheless, a growing body of literature examining the continuum of stepping behaviors in fetuses, premature infants, term infants, and young infants is beginning to make a strong case for the view that human locomotion is also governed by CPGs.[52] Promising research in humans to substantiate the presence of CPGs for locomotion has centered around locomotor recovery studies in adults with spinal cord lesions and hemiplegia.[129,347] Research on infants and children with CP,[104,541] Down syndrome,[507,555] and spinal cord injury[26] who train on treadmills with partial body weight support has also shown positive improvements in these individuals' ability to ambulate faster and without assistive devices, to start walking at a younger age, and to demonstrate some facility in upright ambulation, respectively. Newer studies are documenting changes in cortical activity via functional magnetic resonance imaging[115,389] and changes in short latency reflexes in the peripheral nervous system.[243]

A recent motor control hypothesis suggests that we do not constrain or reduce the degrees of freedom (multiple muscle forces, joint angles, etc.) for production of coordinated movement synergies.[320] Rather we learn to use and adjust all the degrees of freedom for the most efficient (stable and flexible) movement according to a principle of abundance. (The idea of stable and flexible movement versus fixed synergies is consistent with Shea and Wulf's[450] suggestions about modernizing the term "general motor program" to be "scalable response structures.") Latash and colleagues have used this principle of abundance to develop their hypothesis about motor control, the so-called uncontrolled manifold (UCM) hypothesis.[318] Based on this hypothesis, the controller rather than reduce the degrees of freedom for movements via so called synergy production organizes all the elements into a manifold so that there can be ongoing compensation for internal and external errors. Thus, synergies of movement can be defined as co-varying changes in individual elemental variables of a multielement system that is stabilizing a performance variable in order to complete a particular motor action. For example, if one were examining the coordination of movements of two digits to produce a total force output, several key elements of coordination of this activity would be the individual force under each digit. Plotting these two forces (F_1 and F_2) across many trials would produce a constant line if perfectly coordinated, as depicted in the conceptual model in Figure 3-2, A. The "good" variability allows for flexibility of motor actions based on varied environmental conditions, and the "bad" variability hinders the coordination and makes the action "clumsy." These two types of variability are represented in the figure as the ellipse (cloud of data points from multiple trials) around the perfect coordination line, with "good" variability as the variation along the line of perfect coordination and "bad" variability as the variability perpendicular to the line of best coordination. If this represents a depiction of coordination, then after practice of an action that is known to improve coordination, one should see a change in the picture to represent for instance a decrease in bad variability and either an increase or no change in good variability. This is represented in Figure 3-2, B. This hypothesis has been supported based on studies of postural control movements[13,307,319,410] and multifinger force production in people with and without Down syndrome.[317,319,442] A surprising finding, however, from study using the UCM hypothesis on 8- to 10-year-old children with Down syndrome during walking[39] was that the children actually employ more "good" variability than children with typical development in controlling the center of mass at heel contact during treadmill walking. It was hypothesized that the children with Down syndrome need more solutions for maintenance of balance control during walking because of the presence of joint laxity, hypotonia, and potentially other

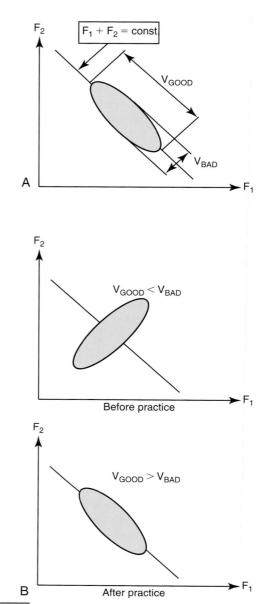

Figure 3-2 **A,** The diagram illustrates the relationship of the force under two fingers (F_1 and F_2) as they press simultaneously to produce one overall force. If the forces produced by each finger were perfectly coordinated, the person would produce a perfect and consistent overall force, which could be represented by a straight line. However, there is variability in how a person can produce the individual finger forces across time. This can be represented by "good" variability along the line of perfect force and "bad" variability perpendicular to the line representing perfect force. **B,** Using this relationship of "good" and "bad" variability as a measure of coordination, one can compare before and after interventions to demonstrate effectiveness of the intervention. The diagram represents in a cartoon manner changes in "good" and "bad" variability (V_{GOOD} and V_{BAD}) in persons with Down syndrome before and after 2 days of practice doing the finger-pressing task. (Adapted from Latash, M. L. [2007]. Learning motor synergies by persons with Down syndrome. *Journal of Intellectual Disability research, 51*[12], 962–971, Fig. 1 and Fig. 4.)

variables such as cognitive capacity. The children with Down syndrome were not seen as having greater coordination during walking on the treadmill as compared to the children without Down syndrome; rather they were thought to have learned an adaptive strategy based on their circumstances. This research was completed on children who were competent walkers. To date, no studies demonstrating changes in coordination with development of movement skills have been completed. Developmental studies using the UCM hypothesis could potentially assist in understanding coordination and help to guide intervention for children with developmental disabilities.

A number of hypotheses of motor control specifically attempt to explain how we control discrete arm movements. According to the equilibrium-point hypothesis, also called the mass-spring hypothesis, the nervous system strives to control joint position in space, and every position can be defined by a unique combination of agonist and antagonist muscle forces that result in a net stiffness.[154] It is argued that muscles function like springs, and once a motor program is sufficiently established, it activates the appropriate muscles to contract and move a limb segment until the segment reaches the point in space where all active and passive muscle forces are in equilibrium. The equilibrium points composing a trajectory or end point of movement are achieved as a function of neural commands that regulate coactivation of alpha and gamma motoneurons.[154] Experimental evidence for the latter point is found in studies of spinal-transected frogs, indicating that spinal neurons code for spatial equilibrium points of the leg during grooming;[37] however, other experimental studies using human subjects suggest that endpoint knowledge is insufficient and that the brain must also have some knowledge of the movement dynamic.[185,186,349] Proponents of the equilibrium-point hypothesis, however, argue that alternative interpretations of the data demonstrate support for the hypothesis[153] and that the hypothesis is so well supported that it now is more appropriate to call the fundamentals outlined as the threshold control theory.[152] The threshold control theory suggests that motor control is a combination of control of muscle activation thresholds with the steady state emerging from an interaction between the person and the environment.[152]

Other hypotheses attempt to distinguish whether we learn to control movement with respect to intrinsic body coordinates of joint position, referred to as joint space, or with respect to extrinsic coordinates, referred to as hand space in the case of reaching.[292,445] Finally, some hypotheses attempt to determine which parameters—such as time, distance, or force—are controlled during movement initiation before correction. Most notable among these, the impulse-variability model proposes that the nervous system controls movement by planning the phasing and duration of muscle contractions (for a review, see reference 363). For further discussions on hypotheses of motor control, the reader is referred to additional sources.[456,503,504]

Researchers are also investigating the use of models for motor control based on developments in the fields of robotics and neural networks. Both approaches seek to incorporate perception and action to explain control of movement. Robotic models are based on the physics of perception and movement, assigning mathematic values to known neural and biomechanical relationships to explain movement outcome. Currently, in the area of autonomous robotics there is interest in simulating principles of dynamic systems using a new method called computational neuroethology. The method attempts to account not only for the neural and biomechanical elements of a robot but also for environmental context and the new phenomena that may emerge during action within that environment.[93,352,474,525,564] Neural network models are based on the assumption that no simplistic, predictable relationship exists among nerve cells to explain movement, but rather it is the phenomenon of their complex interactions that is believed to explain the movement outcome. Thus, neural networks focus primarily on specifying the array of cellular and network properties that may govern how a population of neurons will self-assemble under a given set of conditions. For example, CPGs are typically modeled as discrete populations of neurons, but studies examining rhythmic behaviors in invertebrates[337] and chick embryos[380] suggest that at least in some systems, the behavior emerges from the populational dynamics of neural interactions. In a neural network model, rhythmicity is attributed to reiterative functions as a consequence of recurrent connectivity within the neuron population, and populational behavior is chiefly attributed to various inhibitory relays (i.e., reciprocal inhibition) and select intracellular mechanisms (i.e., inhibitory rebound). During development populational behavior may vary as a function of changing cellular properties; for example, some immature neurons have excessively negative resting membrane potentials such that inhibitory transmitters induce transient depolarizations and potentiate immature excitatory connections within a neural network, thereby producing spontaneous activity. Furthermore, the populational behavior of neural networks may flip between two or more stable states as a consequence of either intrinsic or extrinsic transmitter regulation.[293] Bernabucci and colleagues[30] developed a neural controller that learns to manage movements on the basis of kinematic information and arm characteristics. Other researchers through use of computer simulations have shown how neural dynamics lead to simulated grasping movements with human-like kinematic features.[529] Models of motor control are in a sense an end point, the assimilation of data from experiments testing hypotheses derived from theories. Models can then, in turn, be used to test the extent to which we can generalize the findings of studies testing hypotheses and theories. As ideas are put through these tests, we can become more confident in estimating how they may be effectively applied in addressing practical and clinical problems of motor control.

Revisiting our case, the child with CP, dependent on which of the various models or hypotheses for motor control you as the therapist favor, your assumptions about key components of movement would vary. This in turn would lead you to focus your assessments and interventions as related to the control components you believe in. Each therapist should give some time to this consideration, as in the end the intervention used is usually based on whatever is assessed. We will continue our overview of the motor control field with a discussion of motor control variables, as a basic understanding of this information will enhance our current understanding of the development of motor behaviors.

MOTOR CONTROL VARIABLES

Characteristic of contemporary motor control research is the notion that multiple variables contribute to the initiation and execution of a movement. Thus, it is generally assumed that to understand how movements are controlled, one must be able to identify which variables are important and determine how they interact during movement. Knowledge of this information could be very important for focusing assessment and intervention for children with motor dysfunction. This section identifies possible variables and considers how investigators currently think these variables contribute to motor control. Borrowing from the ideas of Bernstein,[31] some investigators speak of motor control variables as systems or subsystems of control composed of many intrapersonal and extrapersonal variables.[492] In more eclectic terms, variables may be anything, be it physical, physiologic, or psychologic, that has an impact on movement planning or execution. Thus, to identify the underlying processes that determine skill acquisition during development, one must know not only which variables are important at a given age, but also how each variable changes during development and the impact of that change on all the other variables involved. To successfully accomplish such a task requires an experimentalist's approach that controls as many variables as possible while methodically manipulating the one in question, a task that is rarely feasible in human studies. Furthermore, if a variable is dynamically context specific, even the experimental approach may be too artificial to truly understand its impact on motor control. Nonetheless, researchers are attempting to identify variables that are critical to motor skill acquisition. By nature, these variables are interactive, but for convenience we will refer to them here as being sensorimotor variables, mechanical variables, cognitive variables, and task requirements.

SENSORIMOTOR VARIABLES

Sensorimotor variables are those physiologic mechanisms or processes that reside within the nervous system. CPGs are an example of a sensorimotor variable. By selecting and timing the activity of motoneurons, they play a key role in determining the pattern of muscle activity during movement.[200,271,420] For example, in the case of locomotion, CPGs determine which muscles are active in the stance phase of gait and which are active in swing. CPGs can produce motor patterns or synergies similar to those produced during normal behavior even when deprived of afferent (sensory) information, but pattern generators are not the only determinants of the synergies that characterize rhythmic movements. When a cat rapidly shakes a paw to dislodge an irritant, for example, a novel combination of flexor and extensor activity is produced, referred to as a mixed synergy. The mixed synergy is partially determined by a spinal CPG and partially determined by motion-dependent feedback from the leg.[305] Many studies in animal models and humans have substantiated the effect of sensory feedback on the CPG activation.[271]

Movement synergies and neural mechanisms that alter or regulate them can also be viewed as sensorimotor variables controlling movement. A common view is that the formation of synergies for movement is the nervous system's solution to controlling the multiple degrees of freedom inherent in coordinating a multisegmented body.[31] Research has supported this hypothesis as relatively few (one to three) synergies have been identified in frogs' unrestrained kicking[103] and in human movements such as squats, walking, and going up and down a step.[473] Although synergies, such as flexor and extensor synergies, have long been viewed as the stereotypic motoneuron patterns inherent in spinal neural circuitry, current views suggest that movement synergies can be context specific and highly individualistic[296] and can change during the acquisition of coordination.[73a] Supporting this view, anatomic and physiologic data in cats suggest that motoneuron pools for biarticular muscles of the leg are actually a collection of smaller pools that can be separately recruited in a task-specific manner.[397] For example, portions or all of these pools may be recruited depending on movement parameters such as velocity or acceleration.[565] Other studies suggest that synergies characterizing voluntary movement, particularly of the upper extremity, may be controlled by premotor cortical areas because specific patterns of corticoneuronal activity in these areas can be recorded before the onset of practiced movements.[180,181,448] Sensorimotor variables that may contribute to regulation of muscle synergies to enhance performance include mechanisms controlling joint stiffness,[227,349] joint net torque,[260,560] visuomotor and visuospatial processes,[1,333,336,434] and, in essence, all other perceptuomotor processes tuned to participate in planning or executing a movement.[343,447,500] Developmental aspects of sensorimotor variables also include processes of change such as differentiation and refinement of neural networks, and changes in sensory perception, neural conduction characteristics, motor unit properties, and force-producing capabilities. The latter two topics are considered more fully with respect to musculoskeletal development in Chapter 5.

MECHANICAL VARIABLES

Mechanical contributions to motor control are of particular interest in many disciplinary areas of research. Changes in total body mass and relative distribution of mass during development are accompanied by changes in length and center of mass per body segment. These changes, in turn, alter inertial forces resulting from gravity and friction during movement.[565] In some instances these inertial forces may assist movement. In other instances they may oppose movement.[287] Together with other variables, they help shape movement.[93,565] Studies in animals and humans have demonstrated that motor skills are greatly affected by inertial forces[270,440] and that part of learning to perfect a skill is learning to anticipate and use these forces to execute a movement more efficiently.[300,440] The viscoelastic properties of musculoskeletal tissues are also an important mechanical variable in the control of movement.[486] The passive elastic attributes of these tissues contribute to action by absorbing and releasing energy and have been suggested to reduce neural programming requirements for movement execution.[349,565,440] Aberrations of the musculoskeletal system—for example, contractures or external bracing—can also change motor coordination patterns.[67,117]

COGNITIVE VARIABLES

Cognitive variables may include variables that are dependent on conscious and subconscious processes such as reasoning, memory, or judgment to optimize performance. Such variables might include arousal, motivation, anticipatory or feedforward strategies, the selective use of feedback, practice, and memory. Variations in arousal can probably modify any other control variable, such as pattern generation,[494] or even whether a behavior is demonstrated.[53] Motivation may make multiple contributions to the control of movement. In some instances it may serve primarily to trigger activity, and in other instances motivation may determine the form of the consequent movement.[196] For example, it has been suggested that hand path is straighter during reaches for a moving target than for a stationary one because the infant or child is more motivated to reach and make contact with a moving target.[251,339] Cognitive-related variables likely emerge with and assist in skill mastery; toddlers as young as 13 to 14 months of age having only a few weeks of standing experience can selectively determine when to use manual assistance for maintaining postural control while standing on an array of support surfaces[472] or when challenged with various obstacles.[6] Cognitive processes associated with action are also important for acquiring spatial maps (memories) of the movement environment,[359] are apparent in the earliest anticipatory behaviors during infancy (such as the anticipatory head and eye turning during games of peekaboo), and may be delayed or differently configured in children with Down syndrome.[11]

Cognitive processes for predicting the postural requirements and selecting timely anticipatory strategies, also called feedforward strategies, are a select form of anticipatory behavior characterized by movement adjustments time locked to voluntary movements.[355] Typically, as we become expert in a movement task, we learn to recognize those sensory cues most reliable for predicting how the environment may change during movement execution, and we learn to ignore less useful cues. Simultaneously, we learn to predict how our movements will change our relationship with respect to a more or less predictable environment and therefore determine the postural requirements for the task. In the control of posture, anticipatory strategies work to minimize equilibrium disturbance and may also assist in completing the desired movement. In other acts, anticipatory strategies minimize the amount of attention dedicated to monitoring feedback and making corrections after initial movement execution. In the adult, for example, when asked to rise onto tiptoes (from a plantigrade to digitigrade posture), ankle dorsiflexor muscles are activated nearly 200 ms before ankle plantar flexors, apparently to shift the center of pressure (COP) at the foot-floor interface a sufficient amount forward before onset of postural elevation.[204] Although anticipatory strategies are not usually conscious cognitive processes, they involve subconscious forecasting processes[355] that are essential for minimizing movement errors during perceptuomotor tasks[530] and sometimes require considerable training such as the anticipatory postural adjustments (APAs) observed in dancers.[372] Indeed, it is argued that anticipatory strategies are learned, that they are relatively fixed under stable conditions, and that they are adapted in less fixed situations only by learning from past movement experiences.[355] Anticipatory strategies are observed in postural adjustments before the onset of whole body movements,[374] postural adjustments prior to onset of arm movements,[265] shaping and orientation of the hand before contact with an object to be grasped,[280] and strategies to time body movements with timing demands of the environment.[530] Anticipatory strategies during preparation to grasp can also be observed as early as 9 months of age[165,245] and appear to be present by 4 postnatal months, as evidenced by postural adjustments in neck and trunk musculature when infants are about to be pulled to sit or picked up from supine[24] and adjustments in gaze as they anticipate an object's trajectory.[519]

Whether all of these anticipatory strategies share some fundamental means of regulation has not been addressed experimentally, to our knowledge, but it is speculated that similarities may exist between feedforward strategies in postural and arm trajectory control.[355] Nor is there any clear locus of control for any of the identified anticipatory strategies. It is generally thought that APAs are controlled by local spinal cord and brain stem networks, as well as by transcortical loops, including the motor and premotor cortices.[355] Models of feedforward control hypothesize that the controller is likely to be a network that receives and compares afferent feedback and information about the desired movement (efferent copy) to set gain adjustments for modifying movement commands as they are executed.[355] They may also function to reprogram postural responses[65,261] or delay initiation of the voluntary command[355] when the command is destabilizing.

The amount of attention dedicated to monitoring a movement is also viewed as a variable that can be modified to perfect a motor skill. It has been suggested that during development, children initially execute new movements in a ballistic manner, ignoring feedback, then swing to the opposite extreme attempting to process excessive amounts of feedback, before finally learning to selectively attend to feedback. An example of this transition proposed by Hay[231] is described under "Reaching" later in this chapter and shown in the videotape of the development of reaching attached to this chapter. It is generally thought that once the child (or adult) learns to selectively attend to feedback, more attention (or mental processing) can be assigned to reading the environment and predicting the environmental changes and movement outcome as the movement is executed.[295] Other cognitive variables related to learning, such as form and quantity of practice and the role of memory, are addressed within the context of motor learning in Chapter 4.

TASK REQUIREMENTS

Task requirements can also be considered to be distinct motor control variables. Task requirements may include any variable that can contribute to or in some way alter movement, including biomechanical requirements, meaningfulness, predictability, or any other variable associated with a given movement context. Physiologic recordings from several sensorimotor centers of the brain indicate that their participation in a task is context specific.[102,181,335] Task requirements shape motor strategies such as the response selection to postural perturbations; for example, after perturbation one could recover a posture, step into a new posture, or execute protective extension[65,261] or one can select from a variety of possibilities for how to move from sit to stand.[443] Task requirements can also result in the gating of reflexes; for example, a noxious stimulus applied to the foot may produce a flexor withdrawal response if the leg is in the swing phase of gait, but an extensor "contact" response if the leg is in the stance phase.[419] Similarly, task requirements may alter the strategy a child uses to reach for an object,[251] and evidence suggests that the meaningfulness of the task may enhance or mask performance.[523] The role of meaningfulness is demonstrated by comparing performance when a child is asked to complete a relatively abstract task (e.g., to repetitively pronate and supinate as far as possible) versus a concrete task (e.g., to strike a tambourine, a task requiring repetitive pronation and supination). Children with CP generate larger movement excursions following the concrete instructions than after the abstract instructions.[523] In summary, task requirements, like all other variables we

have considered, appear to play a crucial role in the control of movement. Control variables may add to or subtract from movement such that there may be multiple possible behavioral outcomes for a given set of centrally generated movement instructions.

For therapists interested in learning- or dynamic-based theories, thoughtful analyses of task requirements can generate both a deeper understanding of the minimal requirements for completing a task and an array of hypotheses as to why a client cannot complete the task. Analysis can also assist in determining how to modify and reduce task requirements so that a child can successfully complete the modified version of the task. For example, thinking again of our 20-month-old child with CP, if biomechanical variables are rate limiting (i.e., the task requires more muscle force or rate of change in force than the child can currently generate), the therapist may look for ways of scaling the amount of force required. If leg extensor muscles are too weak for the child to maintain standing balance without holding onto the furniture, treatment may consist of repeated movements that require leg extensor muscle activity such as standing from chairs of varying height, or from an array of surfaces under varying degrees of buoyancy (in a pool). If cognitive variables are rate limiting and the task requires analysis of the environment or anticipatory planning, the therapist may try to simplify the environment by reducing the number of distracting stimuli or range of possible choices that can be made and identify ways to enhance the interest in and focus on an essential cue for motor planning. For example, while initially working on eye-hand coordination with the child, distracting stimuli may be removed from the room, the amount of effort (i.e., strength, coordination, or postural context) required to reach may be reduced, and the amount of spatiotemporal uncertainty may be minimal to none (e.g., the toy located closer to the child). The task would include elements known to be of significant interest to the child (e.g., favorite toys, cartoon characters, colors, textures, sounds) so the child is motivated to reach for the toy. As success is achieved, the competing stimuli may be gradually returned, the amount of spatiotemporal uncertainty may be increased, the amount of effort required may be increased (strength, coordination, postural context), and an attempt to expand the child's interests or attention to the task may be made. Applying learning-based theories, the objective would be to provide an array of movement conditions associated with an array of possible movement consequences from which the child can formulate rules of association. Applying dynamic-based theories, the objective would be to provide an array of movement contexts that would allow the child to discover his or her own movement solutions.[11,323,377,509]

MOTOR SKILL ACQUISITION IN CHILDREN

This section examines specific areas of motor development in children and the variables currently viewed as critical to the process of skill acquisition. As will be demonstrated, many of the apparently key sensorimotor variables for control of a skill are already present in the earliest phases of postnatal development, suggesting that the basic neural substrate for orderly generation of skilled movement may be in place months to years before maturation of the nervous system is complete and adult-like behaviors are observed. Although neural maturation of sensorimotor variables for motor control is necessary to attain adult levels of skill, it is not sufficient to fully account for how or when skilled movement is achieved. Here we will consider some of the variables identified by researchers and how these variables may contribute to the control of four specific skill areas—postural control, locomotion, reaching, and grasping—during development.

POSTURAL CONTROL

Postural control is achieved via the cooperative interaction of neural sensory (e.g., visual, vestibular, and somatosensory systems) and motor systems and cooperating musculoskeletal systems so as to meet the behavioral goals of postural orientation and stability.[259,260] Although each of the three systems is considered essential to optimal control of both static and dynamic posture, each system can compensate to some extent for the other two,[259] and the relative importance of each system appears to vary with contextual or task demands.[260,263] As we will see, acquiring skill to process and use the ensemble of sensory information in selecting a motor strategy may more fully account for the postnatal development of postural control than indices of physiologic maturation of any given system. Achievement of postural control is often described in terms that emphasize the closed-loop or sensory feedback aspects of balance correction or reactive postural adjustments (RPAs). Adaptive postural control, however, also employs open loop or APAs. These anticipatory strategies function to minimize potential postural perturbations arising with movement initiation and to assist in achieving the desired movement. Thus, the process of establishing effective anticipatory strategies may more fully account for the development of postural control than indices of postnatal change or impairment in sensory feedback systems during development.[259,267] In this section, we will consider the contribution of sensory, motor, and musculoskeletal system variables contributing to the acquisition of postural control. Tables are presented with details related to developmental accomplishments based on the components of each of these variables.

SENSORY SYSTEM VARIABLES

Vision

Vison is perhaps the most powerful sensory system functioning to regulate posture, both for feedback correction and for selection of anticipatory postural strategies.[69,228,331,477] The

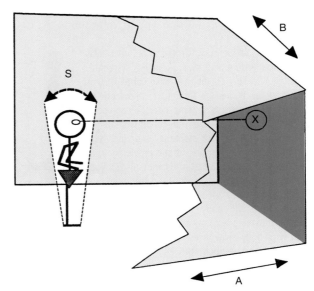

Figure 3-3 The subject is placed in the center of a partial room formed by three walls and a ceiling that can be slid along in direction A or B. When the subject is facing wall X, room motion in direction A creates a looming visual stimulus and triggers an increase in the magnitude of sway (S) in the anterior-posterior plane. Younger children are likely to sway closer to their limits of stability (noted by the dashed lines forming an inverted cone) when presented with a looming visual stimulus, but not when the visual stimulus moves side to side (direction B). (Adapted from Lee, D. N., & Aronson, E. [1974]. Visual proprioceptive control of standing in human infants. *Perception & Psychophysics, 15,* 529–532.)

first to ascribe a proprioceptive function to vision, Gibson[182] suggested that as light from the visual field strikes the retina, changes in light associated with movement create "optical flow patterns" interpreted by the brain to determine the position of the head and body with respect to the surrounding environment. It is argued that the large-amplitude postural sway observed in blind individuals is due to the absence of this optical flow information.[334] Optical flow patterns can evoke dramatic postural responses in both children and adults. In a now classic set of studies, Lee and Lishman[332] demonstrated that when an adult stands inside a closed space formed by three walls and a ceiling, a forward or backward movement of the wall facing the person (center wall, Figure 3-3) will trigger a larger sway amplitude (S) than under static visual conditions: a so-called "moving room" paradigm. The effect is greater if the postural task is made more difficult (e.g., standing on one leg) and if the visual stimulus moves along the anterior-posterior (AP) axis of vision (referred to as a looming visual stimulus, A), and it is least effective if it moves tangential (side to side, B) to the visual axis. In general, if the subject faces the center wall as it is slowly moved toward the subject, the subject will sway backward; if the wall is moved away from the subject, the subject will lean forward. If the entire enclosure is moved sideways from the subject's left to right (or vice versa); however, little or no change in posture is detected.

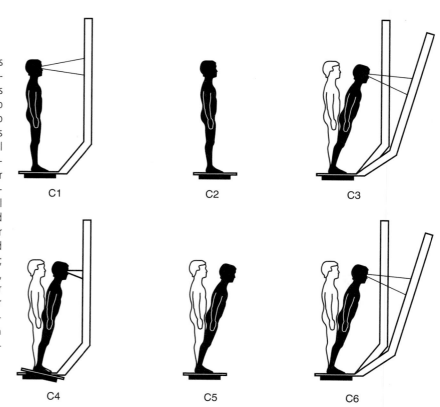

Figure 3-4 The Sensory Organization Test was designed to measure body sway during six systematically altered sensory conditions. These conditions, as depicted in the figure, are thought to allow one to determine which sensory systems a person can use to maintain standing balance. The conditions are as follows: condition 1: floor stable, eyes open, visual surround stable so all sensory systems providing accurate cues on body orientation; condition 2: floor stable, eyes closed, somatosensory and vestibular providing accurate cues; condition 3: floor stable, visual surround moves with body sway, somatosensory and vestibular providing accurate cues; condition 4: floor moves with body sway, eyes open, visual surround stable, vision and vestibular providing accurate cues; condition 5: floor moves with body sway, eyes closed, vestibular providing accurate cues; condition 6: floor and visual surround move with body sway, vestibular providing accurate cues. (From Steindl, R., Kunz, K., Schrott-Fischer, A., & Scholtz, A. W. [2006]. Effect of age and sex on maturation of sensory systems and balance control. *Developmental Medicine and Child Neurology, 48,* 477–482, Fig. 1.)

A second experimental paradigm employing computerized posturography tests has been used to determine how visual and other sensory system variables contribute to postural control development. The Sensory Organization Test (SOT) was first suggested by Nashner and colleagues.[164] This test consists of systematically varying the sensory conditions as a person is maintaining standing balance. The following six conditions are tested: (1) eyes open (EO), surface stationary (SS), visual surround stationary (VS); (2) eyes closed (EC), SS, VS; (3) EO, visual surround moving in synchrony with the person's body sway (VM); (4) EO, VS, surface moving in synchrony with the person's body sway (SM); (5) EC, SM; and (6) EO, VM, SM (Figure 3-4). By measuring the ability with which the person can control their standing balance (i.e., amount of body sway) in these conditions, one can make assumptions about how well the person can use each of the three sensory system variables. For example if a person has great difficulty maintaining standing in the fifth and sixth condition, where it is assumed that one must rely on the vestibular system for body orientation information, one can infer that there is a deficit in use of vestibular system cueing for postural control. If a person does very well in the first and third condition where visual information is "normal" but has difficulty in the EC or the conditions where the visual information provides inaccurate information regarding body position in relation to the environment, that person may be thought to rely too heavily on visual information and not be able to shift to somatosensory or vestibular information for postural stability. Using the moving room, the SOT, or simple eyes open versus eyes closed to vary visual input, researchers have examined the development of use of the visual system to assist in maintenance of postural control in sitting and standing.

Children begin to demonstrate distinct postural responses to optical flow patterns early in development.[69,331,477] Then they go through several visual dependence periods as they first develop sitting and standing control. Table 3-2 outlines this developmental process. It appears that if children lack visual information during development, they do not learn to minimize their postural sway to the same degree with increasing age as sighted children.[395,400] Prechtl and colleagues[400] suggested that the visual system exerts a calibrating effect on the proprioceptive and vestibular systems, which, when missing in children who are blind from birth, causes prolonged ataxia-like movements during postural control. Researchers studying adults have categorized individuals into those who appear to be visual field dependent and those who demonstrate visual field independence.[275] Based on the visual categorization, adults demonstrate different choices in motor responses to perturbations. When visual information is eliminated, individuals with visual field dependence utilize whole trunk stabilization responses (muscular co-contractions), whereas those who are visual field independent show more variable, flexible balancing ability.

TABLE 3-2   Typical Development of Postural Control: Sensory System

Components	Age	Skills/Behaviors
Vision	4 to 6 days old to 2 months	Activation of neck muscles following visual stimuli from looming visual stimulation in supported sitting[559]
	5 to 13 months	Scaling of postural responses to visual stimulation from moving room[32]
	5 months	Postural response to looming visual stimulation in stance[171]
	13 to 17 months and <7 months walking experience	Apt to fall in looming moving room[69]
	2 to 10 years	Decreased falls and reaction to eyes closed conditions in moving room, moveable platform, SOT[164,477,553]
Somatosensory		
	>6 months	Can control head and sitting balance using somatosensory input[331,457]
	4 to 6 years	Beginning ability to use somatosensory input for sensory conflict in standing during SOT[457]
	4 to 10 years	Ability to reweight within visual and somatosensory stimuli of various amplitudes by 4 years age; ability to reweight between visual and somatosensory input by 10 years[19]
	7 to 10 years	Adult-like ability to use somatoseonsory input to balance during sensory conflicts during SOT[172,457]
Vestibular		
	7 to 10 years	Adult-like ability to use vestibular input to balance during sensory conflict during SOT[91,550]
	12 to 16 years	Adult-like ability to balance during sensory conflict SOT[464,470]

VESTIBULAR AND SOMATOSENSORY SYSTEM VARIABLES

The vestibular system is activated and drives postural activity to regulate head control and to reference gravitational forces to prevent slow drift of the trunk during complicated postural control tasks.[76,258,262] The somatosensory system primarily triggers postural activity related to body positioning and righting. Evidence from study of adults suggests that the somatosensory and vestibular systems interact at premotoneuronal levels via common circuitry to influence the overall outcome of motoneuron activation.[266] When both head and body movement occur, as is common in many functional movements, the two sensory systems appropriately influence the motor outcome based on the various head/body configurations. The location of somatosensory input (i.e., the weight-supporting structure and the use or not of hands to support or balance the body) also greatly influences the postural muscle activity in reaction to or in anticipation of perturbations.[282] Changes in postural control based on fingertip support has been shown to vary dependent on the position of the arm (i.e., proprioceptive input).[402] Changes in the amplitude of the tilt of the support surface also seems to cause adults to shift from reliance on somatosensory input to reliance on vestibular input for standing balance maintenance.[388]

The vestibular and somatosensory systems are capable of generating directionally appropriate responses in the trunk and legs following AP displacements in infants and toddlers in sitting[225,239] and in stance.[481] Commonly used testing methods and leg responses are illustrated in Figure 3-5. It is likely that vestibular and somatosensory systems participate in these postural tests during infancy because directionally appropriate muscle responses are generated even when infants are blindfolded.[553] Variable responses also may be attributed to the availability of vision, for when vision is occluded infants produce more reliable vestibular and somatosensory-evoked neck responses following AP displacements in sitting than when vision is available.[553] Complete developmental information related to use of these systems is outlined in Table 3-2.

SELECTION AND INTEGRATION OF SENSORY INFORMATION

A new research paradigm to evaluate how a person relies on or weights visual information during standing and the ability to shift from visual weighting to use of somatosensory information has been developed[8,19,281] (Figure 3-6). The person first is asked to view a screen with oscillating shapes that move at barely perceptible amplitudes. After observing the screen for a few seconds, the person will begin to sway back and forth in tune with the visual stimuli, suggesting that he is using or entraining to the visual information as he balances in standing. If, however, the amplitude of the oscillating visual stimuli is increased enough to potentially destabilize the person, he will disengage or unweight his sway from the visual stimuli. When a touch pole is available to provide somatosensory information, again oscillating at very small amplitudes, the person can be observed to entrain to this sensory information, and again as the amplitude of the stimuli increases, the person will stop entraining to it. Children 4 to

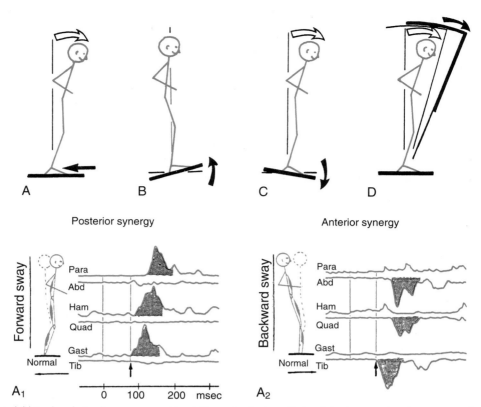

Figure 3-5   When a child is placed standing on a movable platform that is then displaced in the posterior direction at a fixed rate and duration (computer driven), the child sways forward and the posterior synergy is activated in a distal to proximal sequence over time to realign the head and trunk over the base of support **(A₁)**. Conversely, displacement of the platform in the anterior direction produces a posterior sway that is corrected by activation of the anterior muscle synergy, also in a distal to proximal sequence **(A₂)**. In both conditions illustrated, normal visual, vestibular, and somatosensory inputs are available. If the platform is rapidly rotated to produce ankle dorsiflexion **(B)** or plantarflexion (not shown), visual and vestibular inputs remain relatively stable throughout the perturbation, whereas somatosensory receptors register displacement. If, however, the platform is rapidly rotated in the same direction and synchronous with normal sway **(C)**, somatosensory input remains relatively stable because the ankle angle changes little during the perturbation, whereas vestibular and visual receptors register the postural sway. Visual information regarding sway can be altered during testing by closing the eyes or by placing a dome around the head to provide a stable visual field **(D)**. If vision is stabilized during platform translations, as in **A**, visual inputs will be in conflict with normal vestibular and somatosensory information. If vision is stabilized during platform rotations, as in **(B)**, both visual and vestibular inputs will be in conflict with somatosensory information. Finally, if vision is stabilized during platform rotations synchronized to normal sway **(C)**, visual and somatosensory inputs will be in conflict with normal vestibular information. (Adapted from Nashner, L. M., Shumway-Cook, A., & Marin, O. [1983]. Stance posture control in select groups of children with cerebral palsy: Deficits in sensory organization and muscular coordination. *Experimental Brain Research, 49,* 393–409, Fig. 1; and Horak, F. B., & Nashner, L. M. [1986]. Central programming of postural movements: adaptation to altered support-surface configurations. *Journal of Neurophysiology, 55,* 1369–1381, Fig. 2.)

8 years old have been shown to be able to entrain to the somatosensory information in a manner similar to adults, but the 4-year-olds did show a weaker coupling to the stimuli.[20] If both visual and somatosensory information are provided, each with its own frequency so the person's sway frequency can be matched to the sensory information that he is entraining to, one can demonstrate how people weight and unweight sensory information during typical standing. Bair and colleagues[19] have used this paradigm testing the sensory fusion process with children 4 to 10 years of age. See Table 3-2 for details on the developmental progression.

Initial limitations in postural control and progressive sensory integration can also be set forth in studies that test a child's ability to manage more blatant intersensory

conflict situations. The looming stimulus of the moving room presents a sensory conflict for the child; visual proprioception indicates that the relationship between posture and the environment has changed, whereas vestibular information regarding the relationship between posture and gravity and somatosensory information regarding the relationship between posture and support surface have not changed. Initially, infants will fall in reaction to the AP perturbation. Further study using the moving room test suggests that infants may start learning to reduce dependence on unreliable visual information shortly after they begin walking, but this relationship has been shown to be task dependent in that the children respond more strongly to an oscillating stimulus versus a nonoscillating one.[184] Using the

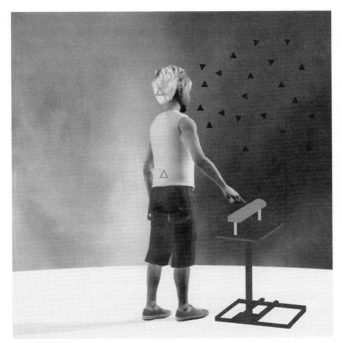

Figure 3-6 Standing balance is examined via subtle oscillation of geometric shapes in the visual scene and in a touch pole, which also oscillates at a different frequency from the geometric shapes. The amplitude of the oscillations of the visual scene and the touch pole are systematically varied and in this manner, one can determine changes in use of visual and somatosensory input for maintenance of standing balance. This test is unique from the SOT as the perturbations of sensory input are barely perceptible and the person is never taken near their limits of stability. (From Bair, W. N., Kiemel, T., Jeka, J. J., & Clark, J. E. [2007]. Development of multisensory reweighting for posture control in children. *Experimental Brain Research, 183*, 435–446, Fig. 1.)

SOT paradigm, both visual and somatosensory information can be attenuated so that the information the child receives from these systems is inaccurate for knowledge of body orientation. Examination of children developing typically suggests that the ability to resolve sensory conflicts continues to mature gradually to an adult-like state at 15 to 16 years of age.[470,528] Details on the developmental sequence can be found in Table 3-2. This continued maturation may be linked with practice and activity in the upright posture within varied environmental conditions.

Research on the SOT and a clinical version of this test, the Pediatric Clinical Test of Sensory Interaction for Balance,[125] and eyes open and closed paradigms on movable platforms has demonstrated that there are differences between children with disabilities in the development, use, and the ability to coordinate sensory information to trigger appropriate postural motor activity. Children with Down syndrome and general cognitive delays seem to continue to overrely on the visual system beyond when children developing typically shift to using somatosensory or vestibular input.[455,533] Children with ataxic CP demonstrate difficulty triggering motor responses when sensory information is conflicting.[375,424]

Children with DCD tend to have problems with utilizing vestibular information and reacting to sensory conflicts.[125,201] Children with fetal alcohol spectrum disorders are thought to overrely on somatosensory input for postural control.[413,414] Readers are directed to other reviews[119,534] and chapters in this volume on specific conditions for more detailed findings related to children with different disabilities.

MOTOR SYSTEM VARIABLES

Unperturbed Sitting and Standing Balance

Most research on development of postural control has been done using research paradigms that either externally perturb the infant or child in sitting or standing and examine the RPAs or ask the child to do an activity that internally perturbs the child's balance, and examine APAs. Some research is now unfolding that examines unperturbed sitting and standing balance control. Sitting development in five infants was examined from the time the infants could prop in sitting using arms on the support surface until they could sit freely using their arms to play.[224] Analyses indicated that as sitting balance improved the infants first moved from instability to a period of constraint of the degrees of freedom (i.e., more stability using very consistent unchanging motor coordination patterns). Then the infants moved to a period of releasing the degrees of freedom or using more variable motor coordination patterns, indicating a complex chain of control development. Harbourne and Stergiou[224] hypothesized that the increased variability in selection of motor coordination patterns reflects specific individual solutions to solve specific individual problems. This research could be construed to be supportive of Latash and colleagues' UCM hypothesis of development of coordination.

Chen and colleagues[89] examined nine infants' development of standing balance longitudinally from age 6 months until they had been walking for 9 months, while standing with and without support on a forceplate. They found rate-related changes in the children's postural sway. Sway developed toward a lower frequency and a slower, less variable velocity, but the infants did not show overall less amplitude of sway as they developed. This was hypothesized to be due to the child not just controlling sway to remain upright but also using sway to explore the limits of stability and learn about postural control. During the time the infants were tested, they also experienced both growth and development of sensorimotor control mechanisms.[89]

REACTIVE POSTURAL ADJUSTMENTS

During the earliest phases of skill acquisition in sit and stance, reactive muscle responses tend to be slower and more variable than at subsequent phases of skill acquisition.[209,234,236,457,481] As expected, latencies and consistency of response to tests of postural skill gradually approach adult levels of performance over childhood. It has been suggested that postural responses in infants and adults during sit and stance are produced by a CPG.[241] Argument for this view is that directionally appropriate responses to perturbations in sitting are generated as early as 1 to 5 months of age and before acquisition of independent sitting,[225,235] suggesting that the response patterns are not acquired by learning.[205] Furthermore, according to this view, correct response selections are available in established central networks, but retrieval or activation of possible responses is variable because afferent and efferent neural components are immature. It is also possible that early responses are variable because young infants have not yet experienced and stored associations between the nuances of intertrial mechanical variability and best response. It is equally possible, borrowing from Sporns and Edelman's[466] theoretic framework discussed earlier, that infants are inherently biased to produce a great array of responses so as to acquire sufficient memories for solving more challenging tasks at later ages.

In support of this view, studies have been done using sit and stance perturbation paradigms. Infants have been shown to generate appropriate muscle responses even before they can sit or stand independently. Muscle onset latencies under these conditions are greater and more variable than during independent stance at later ages.[209,241,481] Children 4 to 6 years of age often have muscle response latencies that are greater and more variable than children under 4 years of age. For example, when displaced in an anterior direction, children as young as 15 months of age sequentially activate the gastrocnemius and hamstring muscles, also referred to as the posterior synergy, at latencies within the ranges for children 7 to 10 years of age; however, the average and range in temporal values for these parameters are considerably greater in 4- to 6-year-olds.[457] It has been suggested that the greater variability observed in children 4 to 6 years of age may reflect a period of transition as vision becomes less important and somatosensory information becomes more important in the control of posture.[457,458] During this transition, children may be trying to process excessive amounts of information rather than selectively attending to the most pertinent sensory information, as has been suggested for other types of motor skill acquisition.[231] Children may also attempt to process excessive amounts of information as a strategy for coping with limited ability to anticipate change in the environment.[295] Yet another possible explanation for the variations in children's muscle response patterns may be found in variations in the biomechanics during testing.[225,241] Finally, several studies have noted that reactive postural responses are task dependent,[88,236] supporting the idea of a second phase of development. See Table 3-3 for detailed developmental information.

Some mention should be made regarding the failure of researchers to find distinct sequences of development in postural motor responses.[387] This probably reflects the fact that complex neuromuscular responses are available early in development, and a child's ability to select the most favorable

strategy is still developing. As well, the task requirements and the immediate context in question are critical determinants. Further, our methods of measurement may be limiting our ability to analyze movement across development. If an infant's sitting balance is examined starting from the infant's ability to prop sit to the ability to sit while freely moving arms, coordination is visually thought to improve, but examination across these abilities using linear measurements of COP paths does not discriminate between these developmental levels because of the variability in the data.[122] To document and potentially better understand these coordinative changes, methods to measure nonlinear behavior across time, which embrace variability as a component of development of coordination, are now being employed. These analyses methods (Figure 3-7) are showing discriminative differences among various levels of sitting balance ability in infants and between infants and children with and without motor delay.[222]

It is noteworthy that children with Down syndrome can produce correct neuromuscular patterns (i.e., the posterior synergy with a distal to proximal activation of leg and thigh muscles) in response to postural perturbations in stance, but the patterns are initiated at a greater latency than in other children of similar chronologic age.[455] Thus, in children with Down syndrome, motor patterns for postural control appear to be available and similar to those in children who are typically developing, but may not be adequately timed to effectively regain upright posture before reaching the boundaries of stability in stance. Perhaps to accommodate for this, protective responses appear to emerge before righting and equilibrium responses in children with Down syndrome,[217] providing a highly effective strategy for limiting injury and a reasonably adaptive strategy if one cannot rely on other postural strategies. Later in development, children and young adults with Down syndrome learn to use co-contraction motor patterns to maintain postural control, another effective adaptive strategy for delayed triggering of the motor adjustments.[11,455]

In children with CP, results of sitting perturbation studies[59,118] suggest the presence of disordered muscle activations (RPA cephalo-caudal muscle activation, simultaneous activation of ventral muscles, excessive co-contractions) for sitting postural control. In standing studies, children with spastic hemiplegia have poor timing and delayed muscle onset latencies as well as reversals in muscle activation (proximal to distal sequencing rather than the expected distal to proximal pattern of muscle activation) in the legs with spasticity.[375] Children with spastic diplegia showed nonselective activation of agonist and antagonist muscles with increased frequency of reversals (proximal to distal recruitment of leg and thigh muscles), increased recruitment of antagonist muscles, and decreased activation of trunk musculature in response to standing platform perturbations.[66,88,375,549,551,554] Some children with CP also showed an increase in COP displacement during standing, especially in a radial direction,

TABLE 3-3   Typical Development of Postural Control: Motor System

Components	Age	Skills/Behaviors
REACTIVE POSTURAL ADJUSTMENTS (RPA)		
Sitting		
	3 to 5 months	Single postural muscle groups activated or antagonist activated rather than an identifiable RPA sequence[206]
	5 to 6 months	Activation of directionally specific motor coordination patterns (agonists opposite to the side the child is falling)
		Slow and variable timing (co-contractions and reversals of proximal to distal patterns)
		Poor adaptation to task specific conditions[59,188,241]
	7 to 10 months	Decreased timing variability of directionally specific motor coordination patterns (activations of leg, trunk, neck muscles)[207]
	9 months to 3 years	Invariant use of directionally specific motor coordination patterns, some use of co-contractions
		Good modulation of pelvic muscles at base of support for adaptations to task specific conditions[206]
	> 3 years	Variability in directionally specific motor coordination patterns
		Less co-contraction and use of neck muscles to improve variability of postural control[206]
Standing		
	7 to 8 months	Infants who pull-to-stand show beginnings of ankle strategies[207,481]
	10 to 12 months	Adult-like RPA with grossly directionally specific (distal to proximal) motor coordination patterns[236,481]
	12 to 16 months	More consistent directionally specific motor coordination patterns although onset latencies longer[207]
	3 months walking experience	Compensatory stepping balance responses emerge[415]
	4 to 6 years	Increased variability of motor coordination patterns occurs (perhaps resulting from growth spurts or sensory integration changes)[164,458]
	7 to 10 years	Adult-like use of directionally specific motor coordination patterns[164,458]
ANTICIPATORY POSTURAL ADJUSTMENTS (APA)		
Movement in Sitting		
	6 to 8 months	APA in trunk muscles before lifting the arm in sitting[513,516]
		Can adapt to different sitting positions and velocities of reaching movement
	12 to 15 months	Consistent APA, particularly in neck muscles[512]
	2 to 11 years	APA variable and incomplete by age 11 years when compared to adults[517]
Movement in standing		
	10 to 17 months	APA activity in gastrocnemius muscles (to counteract the reach and pull movements with arms) in 10- to 13-month-old infants
		More consistent and temporally specific APAs in 16- to 17-month-olds[547]
	3 to 5 years	APA response variable, with immature as well as adult-like activity[438]
		Anterior shifts in COP are present before raising an arm while standing, but these are less well coordinated[229,407]
	4 to 6 years	APAs recorded in the following tasks: lever pull[164]
		Voluntary drop weight;[436] raise arm[229,238,239]
		APA may shift from a supporting function to movement to a compensatory function of postural stability

Continued

TABLE 3-3 **Typical Development of Postural Control: Motor System—cont'd**

Components	Age	Skills/Behaviors
	6 to 8 years	More continuous, systematic, and harmonious APA during a reaching movement
		APA show greater variability of muscle coordination patterns than in 9- to 12-year-olds[535]
	9 to 10 years	Some children exhibit insufficient APA before movement into digitigrade stance[204]
		APA shown only when postural control disturbances reached "perilous" limits[229]
		APA less variable during stand and reach[535]
		Modulation of APA in weighted and unweighted wrist reach task
	12 years	APA with forward leg raising similar to adults and both affected by segmental acceleration (slow versus fast movement) and sensory context (eyes open versus closed)[384]
Movement during Gait Initiation		
	1 to 17 months walking experience	Inexperienced walkers use gait initiation APAs involving lateral rather than posterior COP shifts and use both the upper and lower body to make the shifts[16]
	1 to 2.5 years	Variable APA in reaction to a perturbation (holding the limb back) during gait initiation[552]
		APA (posterior COP shift) present, but not coordinated with the velocity of the step forward[328]
	4 to 6 years	Adult-like APA patterns of anterior tibialis activity and posterior COP shifts during gait initiation[350]
		APA (decrease in latency and increase in amplitude of muscles for push-off) in reaction to a perturbation (holding the limb back) during gait initiation[552]
		With *4 to 5 years walking experience*, postural control motor coordination patterns move distally with ability to control gravitational forces with leg muscles during gait[56]
	6 to 8 years	APA (posterior COP shift) present and coordinated with the velocity of the step forward[328]

and slowed frequencies of sway. This rotational control contribution may be critical for postural stability in children with CP owing to their overall relatively poor ankle control as compared to children without CP.[155] Finally researchers are just starting to apply nonlinear analyses of variability to examine differences between children with and without CP.[122,124,123,130] Using these techniques applied to measurement of sitting in children with and without CP, researchers found that children with typical development have more complexity and variability, but at an optimal level for achieving sitting balance. This suggests that therapists should encourage exploration of balance in sitting. In standing, children 5 to 11 years old with CP were found to have more regular (i.e., less variable and potentially adaptable) sway than children with typical development.[130] Further, when children with CP were given an external visual cue, they were able to reduce the regularity of their sway. This suggests that therapists should consider use of external cues to practice movement versus asking children to concentrate on internal cues.

Collectively, these findings and previous points of discussion suggest at least one possible hypothesis regarding the emergence of postural skills. Namely, children may possess the potential to produce a particular postural response despite the inability to evoke it under given testing conditions. The more mature postural response may be masked or overridden by more simple but reliable strategies for a given context. The context specificity of a response is further underscored by the gradual changes in strategy observed over repeated trials when the postural perturbation is modified.[164] When children 4 to 6 years of age are subjected to repeated mechanical rotations of the ankle (into dorsiflexion) in stance, the posterior synergy is gradually suppressed because, under this context, activation of the synergy is potentially destabilizing.[457] Furthermore, it appears that children begin to either consciously or subconsciously select a postural strategy from an array of possibilities (e.g., step, squat, reach for support pole) based on context as early as 13 to 14 months of age.[472] Exploration of variability of responses may be very important in terms of development of optimal postural control. Both too little variability and too much variability may be detrimental to flexible and adaptive control.[471]

ANTICIPATORY POSTURAL ADJUSTMENTS

Anticipatory activity can be observed in infants when reaching from various lying and sitting positions.[512] Interestingly, these APAs appear primarily during goal-directed arm movements, as compared to spontaneous movements. As

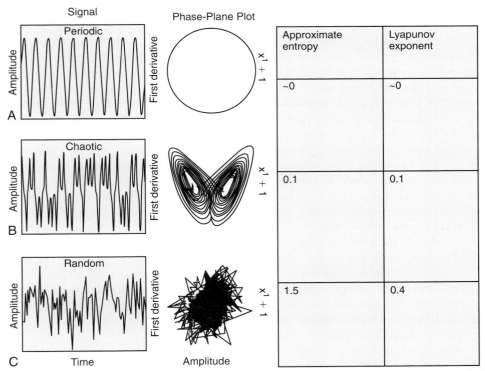

Figure 3-7 Subtle differences in coordination of complex movement, such as center of pressure (COP) changes during sitting balance, can be revealed using time series analysis methods for complex behavior. The figure shows the following phase-plane plots: **A,** Periodic signal with no variation across time. **B,** Chaotic behavior, which has a repeatable pattern embedded within a complex signal. **C,** Random signal, which has no periodic repeatable pattern. Approximate entropy and Lyapunov exponent are two examples of measurements from time series analysis that reflect changes across the three depicted categories of behavior. Movement reflecting good coordination would be expected to have a "just right" chaos to allow for modulations to adapt to changing environmental conditions, but not to be so chaotic, as this would not allow for optimization of motor control. (From Harbourne R. T., & Stergiou N. [2009]. Movement variability and the use of nonlinear tools: Principles to guide physical therapists practice. *Physical Therapy, 89,* 267–282, Fig. 2.)

early as 1 year of age, children have been shown to activate postural muscles in anticipation of destabilizing upper extremity movements.[164] In the standing position, the presence of APAs appears to depend on the time the child has practiced in standing and walking, becoming more consistently observed after practice.[16] Overall, developmental studies suggest that there is a progression and refinement or modulation of APAs that improves with experience in movement. See Table 3-3 for details on development of the APA. The overlap in refinements of feedback (perturbation-triggered corrections) and feedforward postural control in children between 1 and 10 years of age suggests that they are two distinct processes that emerge in parallel during development. Furthermore, it is suggested that children begin to learn anticipatory postural strategies to coordinate posture and locomotion with the onset of voluntary movements to sit, crawl, and walk.[204,547]

Evidence to date suggests that development of feedforward strategies is disrupted in some children with motor disabilities. Hadders-Algra and colleagues[216] suggested that infants and children with CP demonstrate variable APAs. Seemingly, these children cannot choose appropriate APA to use. As a result, they keep trying different strategies or using

immature strategies such as co-contractions.[210,339,375,537,562] A study of rapid arm raising in stance suggests that anticipatory activation of trunk muscles is appropriate but very delayed in individuals with Down syndrome when compared with age-matched control subjects,[11] underscoring the potential importance of cognitive-related processes in postural control. To cope with the large COP shifts of the feet, these individuals also appear to adopt more immature co-contraction strategies to maintain postural control. With enough practice however, children with Down syndrome have been shown to develop APA during gait for walking over obstacles after both low- and high-intensity treadmill training.[555] Children with dyslexia were shown to have difficulty with fast walking over uneven ground, also suggesting problems with APA development and use.[371]

MUSCULOSKELETAL SYSTEM VARIABLES

In children younger than 4 years of age, some key rate-limiting variables are biomechanical in nature. Most notably, in the first postnatal year, the center of mass is proportionately higher than at any other age because of the combination of a large head and short limbs, requiring large force generation and regulation by neck and upper trunk musculature to counter the inertial forces created by displacements of the head. Second, in young walkers, the actual distance between floor contact and the center of mass is small and results in much higher frequencies of postural sway with relatively larger arcs of motion than at later ages.[406,508] Consequently, younger children sway faster and closer to their limits of stability than older children and adults. Also, COP along the AP axis of the foot is more posterior at younger ages.[508] Although younger children can produce adult-like muscle synergies for postural correction at latencies similar to adult values, given the aforementioned biomechanical constraints, adult-like responses may be too slow for regaining upright posture. Some developmental studies have also reported that the biomechanics associated with head position and pelvic rotation during perturbation trials can be notably variable.[225,241]

It is likely that some trends in available postural data, such as the greater variability observed at younger ages, may be the consequence of small variations in postural alignment at onset of data collection trials rather than solely the consequence of an immature neural control system.[324] As well, variable postural responses may be associated with behavioral variables such as restlessness, fatigue, apprehension, and novelty during laboratory testing. For example, Aruin[12] demonstrated that when adults made fast bilateral shoulder extension movements from several different trunk alignment positions (erect and with forward upper body bend of 15° to 60°), the APA activity of individual muscles within muscle pairs varied to accommodate both the change in the postural muscle lengths and the altered stability of the person because of the forward bend.

Biomechanical alignment changes have also been examined in some children with disabilities. When children with mild to moderate CP (children who were able to ambulate independently either with or without adaptive equipment) were perturbed in erect (crossed legs position or tailor-sit position, mean pelvic angle 89°) and crouched (legs positioned forward, mean pelvic angle 135°) sitting postures, the mechanical configuration of the crouched posture provided a solution to instability in sitting. These children were shown to be able to modulate their RPA electromyographic (EMG) activity in the crouch position, whereas they could not do this in the erect position. Thus, the atypical musculoskeletal positioning used by these children improved their RPA postural responses.[58] The question remains, however, whether the children performed better in the crouch position because the position offered some specific biomechanical alignment advantage relative to the children's disability or if this is just the most practiced sitting position of children with mild to moderate CP. If the latter, the child may have learned the most adaptability in the crouch position.

In standing, when children with spastic diplegia or with typical development adopt a crouched position (hips and knees flexed and ankles dorsiflexed),[67,554] or when solid ankle-foot orthoses (AFOs) are worn,[67] the musculoskeletal constraints (different starting position, as well as the presence of spasticity) affect RPA muscle recruitment during balance perturbation in both groups. The motor coordination patterns used by the typically developing children became more like those of age- and gender-matched children with CP who were in a crouched position or wore the solid AFOs. A similar effect is found in APAs of children with typical development when asked to reach forward from a crouched standing position.[498] Most recently, during a stand and reach paradigm experiment, children with CP who were wearing dynamic AFOs were compared to children with typical development.[376] APAs were different and some of the differences appeared related to the orthoses; for example, when reaching, the children with CP did not show the typical pattern of integration between a pushing force under the leg on the reaching side and braking force under the leg on the nonreaching side. These studies support the hypothesis that musculoskeletal differences that lead to altered biomechanical resting postures contribute to postural control dysfunction.

LOCOMOTION

The locomotor capabilities of the neonate and young infant have been vigorously explored. The theoretic bases and experimental designs for these studies were drawn from approximately four decades of study into the control of locomotion in animals. Studies of locomotion and other rhythmic behaviors in animals have been important because they enabled investigations of motor control to move from a focus on classic reflex paradigms to the broader domain of natural, spontaneous motor behavior and the development of new research methods to study both naturally occurring behavior and corresponding physiologic systems under behaviorally restricted conditions. In particular, because locomotion is a rhythmic behavior with many kinematic and EMG features that are repeated across cycles in predictable patterns under stable conditions, studies typically focus on the production of these features to test specific hypotheses of locomotor control and theories of motor control more generally. Because animal studies have contributed significantly to both the knowledge of and methods used to study locomotion in humans, and because they continue to influence clinical studies, such as the assisted weight support paradigms for treadmill locomotion training, some animal studies on the control of locomotion will be considered briefly.[46,271,420] Note that this chapter section is relatively brief regarding the development of walking given that a detailed discussion on the refinement of locomotion during childhood is presented in the chapter on gait on the Evolve website by Stout.

Development of Locomotion in Animals

Animal studies demonstrate the potential to produce either locomotion or potentially related forms of rhythmic limb movements during embryonic or neonatal development.[50] Newborn kittens, when separated from their mothers during feeding, take a few very hypermetric and awkward steps to return to their mother's teats, often falling in the process.[51] During these efforts, steps are occasionally characterized by the stereotypic features of reciprocal flexor-extensor EMG patterns similar to those occurring during adult locomotion. Adult-like muscle activity patterns are most readily apparent, however, when kittens are posturally supported while stepping on the moving belt of a treadmill or making stepping motions midair (airstepping). Typically, steps over ground are accompanied by extensive coactivation of antagonists at the ankle, suggesting that coactivation may be a functional strategy for increasing joint stiffness to compensate for limitations in postural control or muscle force production.[51] The appearance of adult features for locomotion in muscle activity of newborn kittens, alternating flexor-extensor muscle synergies,[49] limb kinematics in chick embryos,[80] and cellular studies of spinal cord activity in neonatal mice[46,55] and rats[297] suggests that the neural networks for locomotion are established during embryogenesis. For more detailed review of animal research, the reader is referred to reviews by Hultborn and Nielsen[271] and Rossignol et al.[421]

Parallels between Developing Animals and Humans

The presence of stepping movements in the human fetus, early onset of infant stepping in premature infants, and rhythmic leg movements of infant kicking provide argument for development of basic stepping circuitry for locomotion in humans during embryogenesis as in other animals.[52] The presence of some potential for locomotion at birth raises the question of whether that potential is established early in fetal development. Here again a parallel may be drawn with animal studies. Ultrasound studies of human fetal movement indicate that isolated kicks are initiated during the ninth embryonic week and alternating leg movements, reported to resemble neonatal stepping, are initiated with postural changes ("backward somersaults") in utero during the fourteenth embryonic week.[121] Thus, human fetuses appear to exhibit stepping during the first half of the gestational period, about the same portion of the embryonic period when chicks exhibit organized EMG and kinematic features during spontaneous motility.[49,80] Given that low-risk preterm infants born at 34 weeks of gestational age demonstrate orderly kinematic patterns similar to those of full-term newborns, and that those features differing from full-term infants appear to be attributable to dynamic interactions emerging during movement,[179,237,283,284,346] the parallel between human fetuses and chick embryos appears reasonable (Figure 3-8). In other words, the neural foundations for locomotion in humans may be assembled during neurogenesis, as they appear to be in other animals.[50,68]

Several parallels can also be drawn between studies of neonatal animals and rhythmic, locomotor-like leg movements in human infants. When supported on the treadmill,

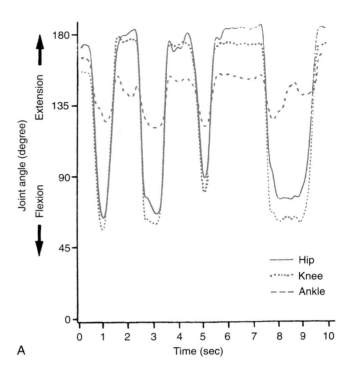

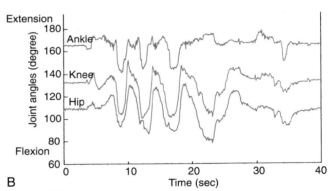

Figure 3-8 Kinematic analyses indicate that lower extremity movements are organized very early in development. When preterm infants initiate a sequence of several kicks at 40 weeks of gestational age, the alternation of flexion and extension at the hip is synchronous with motions of the knee and ankle in the same direction **(A)** and is similar to kicking movements during spontaneous motility in chick embryos in ovo at 9 embryonic days of age **(B).** (Adapted from Heriza, C. B. [1988]. Comparison of leg movements in preterm infants at term with healthy full-term infants. *Physical Therapy, 68,* 1687–1693, Fig. 2.)

infants perform repetitive leg movements characterized by several kinematic features similar to adult locomotor behavior.[492,506,557] Although infants 6 to 12 months of age become more reliable in producing a sustained pattern of alternating steps that is timed to the treadmill belt speed, even infants as young as 10 days of age occasionally demonstrate these features.[557] Neonatal infant stepping shares many features with early treadmill stepping. Most notably, hip, knee, and ankle joints are synchronously flexed during the swing phase and synchronously extended during the extensor phase; the excursions are accompanied by nonspecific EMG patterns; and there is an absence of both heel strike and push-off at the transitions between swing and stance.[169] These features are also characteristic of infant kicking within the first 1 to 3 postnatal months,[285,286] further suggesting that some of the mechanisms controlling treadmill stepping, and therefore locomotion, are already functional at birth.

Development of Locomotor Muscle Patterns in Humans

Until recently, it was believed that infant locomotion lacked adult-like features typically observed in EMG recordings. Failure to observe adult-like EMG patterns was often attributed to late myelinization of descending paths at caudal spinal levels,[479] late maturation of cortical structures,[167] or late myelination of peripheral nerves.[480] In a study of treadmill locomotion, however, infants as young as 10 days of age occasionally produced steps characterized by alternating activation of antagonist muscles, and the extent of coactivation decreased with practice.[557] The relative duration of flexor and extensor burst durations also varied with treadmill speed in a manner similar to that in adults. Furthermore, it has been demonstrated that prewalking infants, age 4 to 12 months, can respond with adult-like interlimb coordinated responses when given unilateral leg perturbations while supported to walk on a treadmill.[385,386] The failure to observe adult-like EMG patterns for locomotion in previous studies of prewalkers and early walkers may have been the result of adaptive strategies that masked this potential. For example, infants may have coactivated antagonist muscles to increase joint stiffness and stabilize limb posture as a compensation for insufficient postural control or control of force generation for supporting and transporting body mass.[51,381] Also, testing conditions may have masked the potential to generate adult-like locomotor EMG patterns—that is, support in stance or movement against gravity in supine likely altered the task requirements,[506] necessitating a different EMG pattern. Conversely, the testing conditions may have lacked key features for expressing locomotor EMG patterns. For instance, in cats, the velocity of limb movements contributes to the generation of certain EMG patterns.[565]

Although there is wide support for the view that basic features of locomotion are spinally mediated,[68,271] some argue that uniquely human features of gait emerge as spinal neural networks are transformed with maturation of higher neural centers.[167] Specifically, it is argued that the basic patterns of alternating flexion and extension observed during neonatal stepping persist with development of locomotion, but that maturing sensorimotor input suppresses activation of ankle extensor motoneurons to permit heel contact at the onset of stance. Also, the absence of heel strike in children with CP is thought to occur because cerebral injury impairs development of higher-center control over spinal neural networks for locomotion.[169] As further support for this view,

Luo and colleagues[346] studied infants who were born prematurely as compared to a similar group born at full term in their ability to walk while supported on a treadmill. The factors that contributed across the whole group to earlier attainment of independent walking were a higher percentage of alternating stepping pattern, a decreased association in hip/knee coupling and an increased association in hip/ankle coupling during swing phase as well as increased interlimb symmetry during stance. A small number of preterm infants were classified as "late walkers," and authors hypothesize that the presence of periventricular leukomalacia—i.e., a neural control deficit and/or chronic lung disease (either linked to muscle weakness and/or to a neural deficit related to poor oxygenation of the brain)—affected the infant's coordination and delayed the development of locomotion.

Conversely, many researchers now speculate that attributes of gait, such as heel strike, need not be specifically dictated by higher neural centers because they may emerge from the inertial interactions and associated feedback among body segments during different types of movement exploration from many practice sessions.[40,82,92,219,254,276,310,492,565] For example, when cats walk at relatively fast speeds, the sartorius muscle produces a two-burst pattern, one during late stance and one during late swing, but the second burst does not consistently occur at slower walking speeds. Kinematic and kinetic analyses suggest that the burst in late swing functions to counteract extensor forces at the knee during faster walking speeds, but it is not required and therefore not recruited at slower speeds because viscoelastic properties of knee flexors are sufficient to counter these forces. In adult humans, examination of muscle actions during the walk-to-run transition demonstrates lower swing-related ankle, knee, and hip flexor muscle activation and higher stance-related activation of the ankle and knee extensors during running than walking.[401] It is suggested that the exaggerated sense of effort in lower extremity flexors during swing of a fast walk may trigger the locomotor pattern to change from the walk to run pattern.

Whether the muscle activity associated with heel strike or other attributes of gait is due to centrally organized neural commands or is an emergent property of movement exploration and motion-dependent feedback has recently received more focused study related to the development of walking in infants. A study of treadmill training in a premature infant who sustained a left grade III/IV intraventricular hemorrhage demonstrated that the infant changed the right and left initial foot contact from a toe touch to either a flat foot or heel strike after 4 months of practice.[44] This improved motor pattern continued for a time after the treadmill training ended, then it reverted to the previous pattern. This finding might suggest that the absolute velocities or rate of change in velocity typically achieved during early overground locomotion are insufficient to force the infant to express adult-like ankle control in the step cycle. However, when given the higher velocities of the treadmill to stimulate the walking pattern, the appropriate heel-strike pattern emerges even though the infant had early brain damage. From study of early walking development in infants, researchers have demonstrated that the infant's walking pattern related to EMG control,[82] net joint moment control,[219] and coupling of AP and medial-lateral oscillations[308] seem to emerge in a nonlinear manner requiring cycles of perception and action to self-organize and stabilize. Other researchers have also examined the emergence of walking in children with typical development and with Down syndrome from the perspective of an escapement-driven inverted pendulum and spring model of gait shown in Figure 3-9.[40,255,505] In this model, the gait pattern is thought to emerge as a result of the dynamic resources available to the walker, including the force producing capability of the muscles (so-called impulse), the elastic energy of the muscles and tendons (passive stiffness), and energetics of the body with the gravitational field (use of centrifugal force resulting from the inverted pendulum). The model "assumes that during the stance/push-off phase a walker's system can be described as an inverted pendulum that conforms to natural mechanical and physical principles, with a small escapement function. This force (escapement function) initiates the forward and upward arc of motion of the center of mass which is sustained by gravity until the opposite limb touches down."[40] Examination of the early months of independent walking in children with and without Down syndrome has suggested that the pendular

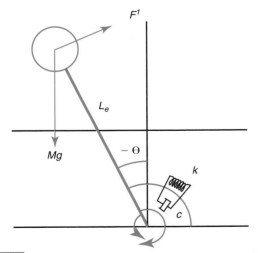

Figure 3-9 The escapement-driven inverted pendulum and spring model of gait is depicted in the figure as the swing leg at initial contact in the gait cycle. The model is composed of the person's body mass minus the mass of the stance foot (M) and the gravity constant (g), the equivalent length of the body (L_e), the escapement force (F^1), which is the active muscle force of the opposite leg push off across the angle θ, the coefficient of stiffness (k) because of tissue elasticity and active muscle contraction, and the damping coefficient (c) at the ankle. (From Ulrich, B. D., Haehl, V., Buzzi, U. H., Kubo, M., & Holt, K. G. [2004]. Modeling dynamic resource utilization in populations with unique constraints: Preadolescents with and without Down syndrome. *Human Movement Science, 23*, 133–156, Fig. 1.)

dynamics develop in a two-stage process.[40,253,254] In the first few months of walking, the infant learns through practice to insert the force impulse at the correct time to begin to achieve effective forward progression. Then a longer fine-tuning process to take advantage of the resonance characteristics of the body tissue and the use of gravity takes place to make the gait optimal in terms of energy conservation. Infants with Down syndrome appear to follow a similar, albeit more variable, development to the infants with typical developmental trajectories for the first 6 months of walking.[40]

BIOMECHANICAL VARIABLES

The emergence of locomotion during development is determined by the interactive aspects of anatomy and environment during movement. Typically, infant stepping is not readily elicited beyond the first to second postnatal month under standard testing conditions, and it was long argued that the behavior disappears as a consequence of encephalization processes (the taking over of control) by maturing higher motor centers.[360] However, the postnatal decreases in rate of stepping temporally correlate with rapid weight gain, suggesting that morphologic changes in body mass may contribute to the "disappearance" of infant stepping. Two lines of evidence support this hypothesis. One, when infants are submerged in water up to chest level, both stepping rate and amplitude increase in comparison with stepping out of water.[493] Two, if weights equivalent to the weight gains at 5 and 6 postnatal weeks are added to the ankles of infants at 4 postnatal weeks, both stepping rate and amplitude decrease in comparison with stepping without ankle weights.[493] Thus, buoyancy appears to diminish the dampening effect of body mass and gravitational interactions, whereas added weight appears to augment the effect of these interactions. Results of animal studies underscore the notion that morphologic features of the organism interact with the environment to either express or mask potential abilities. Fetal rat pups, for example, exhibit interlimb coordination during spontaneous movements under buoyant conditions several days before testing under nonbuoyant conditions.[27] Frog tadpoles exhibit coordinated leg movements several stages earlier in development if they can push off a mesh surface placed in an aquatic tank.[469] The latter point invites reconsideration of the discussion regarding heel contact in gait: heel strike may not be observed until independent walking is established because of immature morphologic characteristics of the infant foot interacting with a support surface. Given the considerable structural change the foot undergoes during the first postnatal year or more, it is conceivable that initial biomechanical features of the foot do not readily afford initiation of heel strike or push-off in the young infant. Recent study would also suggest that strength of the foot/ankle muscles plays a role. Vereijken et al.[527] have examined manipulation of body weight during the first 6 months of independent walking. They placed ankle, waist, or shoulder weights on the infant and observed changes in the infants' gait patterns. Ankle weights affected the gait most over these months of development, causing continued slower and shorter stepping patterns. This was hypothesized to occur due to immature strength and control at the ankle.

VARIABLES UNDER INVESTIGATION

The relative contributions of mechanical and neural variables underlying control of leg movements in infants are revealed as methods for study of kinematic and kinetic methods have become more affordable and less labor intensive. A collection of studies, for example, suggests that intersegmental dynamics are the critical determinants of leg coordination during kicking,[285,286,441] treadmill locomotion,[346,506] and the development of walking.[92,354] During both kicking and supported treadmill locomotion, active muscle forces are used to initiate hip flexion against gravity, but it appears that gravity and passive (inertial) forces largely determine the spatiotemporal patterns of corresponding knee and ankle excursions. Furthermore, the extent of synchrony between leg joint rotations during kicking varies with the infant's posture and appears to be greater when the infant is supported upright than when supine. The greater synchrony between leg joints in an upright posture may be due to the greater gravitation-related forces and therefore muscle force (and recruitment effort) required to overcome gravitational forces.[286] Conversely, the lesser synchrony between leg joints during supine kicking may be due to the more variable effects of gravity on the hip and ankle during the supine kick cycle. When the hip and ankle are positioned between 0° and 90°, gravity assists extension, whereas gravity assists flexion as joint position exceeds 90°.[441] During both kicking and treadmill locomotion, the swing phase appears attributable to active flexor (muscle) forces at the hip, whereas the extensor phase is primarily attributable to gravity and passive (inertial) forces and, to a lesser extent, active flexor (muscle) forces as hip flexor muscles lengthen (Figure 3-10). During the first 8 months of walking, phase shifts have been recorded with lower extremity range of motion (ROM) showing decreases, hip-knee-ankle relationships beginning to resemble mature gait patterns, time to peak angular velocity shortening, and stability of ankle angular velocity phasing improving.[354] Examining the intersegmental dynamics differently, the extent to which the covariation of thigh, shank, and foot angles were constrained on a plane in three-dimensional space was shown to improve rapidly (within <6 months from the onset of unsupported walking).[92] This was followed by slower changes that were hypothesized to be related to maturation of anthropometric parameters. These findings match with the previous discussion of the escapement-driven inverted pendulum results described earlier.

Paradigms developed to study spinal control of interlimb coordination have also been adapted to determine whether

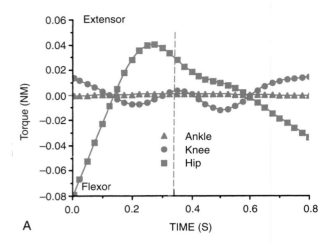

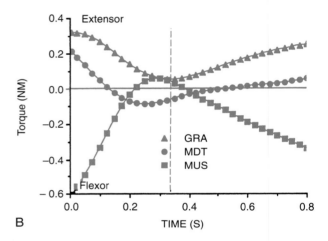

Figure 3-10 Motions of adjacent limb segments during kicking may arise from active forces resulting from muscle activity and passive forces resulting from gravity and inertia of the limb segments. For example, in the data presented here, an infant initiates a kick cycle starting from a semiextended position of 125° and achieves a peak flexion of 80° at 0.32 second *(vertical dashed line)* before the hip returns to the extended position. The motion into flexion is attributable primarily to an initial hip flexor force or torque that is maximal at the outset (0.0 s) and begins to drop off as the hip moves into flexion **(A)**. The hip flexor force is due to active muscle force (MUS) during the first 0.2 second **(B)**. An extensor force develops between 0.2 and 0.3 second **(A)** as active hip flexor force decreases to 0 newton-meter **(B)** and serves to slow and reverse the hip motion into extension (0.32 s). Throughout the extension of the hip, there are small passive extensor forces resulting from gravity (GRA) and inertia (MDT) and a growing active hip flexor force (MUS) to lower the leg **(B)**. (Adapted from Schneider, K., Zernicke, R. F., Ulrich, B. D., Jensen, J. L., & Thelen, E. [1990]. Understanding movement control in infants through the analysis of limb intersegmental dynamics. *Journal of Motor Behavior, 22,* 493–520, Fig. 3. Reprinted with permission of the Helen Dwight Reid Educational Foundation. Published by Heldref Publications, 1319 Eighteenth St., NW, Washington, DC 20036-1802. Copyright © 1990.)

similar neural mechanisms control stepping in human infants. For example, when infants are supported on a treadmill and one leg is blocked during swing phase, the stance phase of the contralateral leg is lengthened, as in adult cats and humans.[558] Responses vary with extent of loading in the stance limb (e.g., increases in load result in lengthening of extensor burst duration and delay in onset of swing), which indicates that human infants as young as 3 months of age possess mechanisms for adaptive stepping observed in cats and kittens and attributed to spinal circuitry.[385,558] Nonetheless, studies in cats show that cerebral cortical centers normally play an important role in these adjustments, indicating that perception and planning are important neural contributions to control of locomotion.[131] Animal studies also indicate that experience-based learning is important for refining rudimentary locomotor skills. For example, findings from a kinetic study of locomotion in neonatal chicks suggest that practice is required to acquire efficient energy absorption strategies for yield in stance.[373] Experience-based learning for refinement of locomotor skills appears to be under way before the onset of independent locomotion. In a recent study of infants 9 months of age or older, perturbation of two or more consecutive steps resulted in aftereffects characterized by increased vertical clearance of the toe for one to two steps after the perturbation was removed.[386] Experiments utilizing the UCM hypothesis to study changes in variability in coordination associated with practice of walking are under way. Black and colleagues[39] demonstrated in preadolescents with established walking patterns that the variability observed in the children with Down syndrome as compared to children with typical development was apportioned differently when walking on treadmills. Children with Down syndrome actually used more "good" variability than children with typical development. This was hypothesized to occur in order to stabilize gait resulting from the decreased dynamic resources of lax joints, low muscle tone, and potentially other internal differences related to having Down syndrome. Further studies utilizing the UCM model to examine how children initially learn to control variability during development of the gait pattern are warranted.

REACHING

Reaching is one of the first motor skills infants perform and provides an early window into the motor control of young infants. (See the video for Chapter 3 on the development of reaching from 2 weeks to 6 months.) The development of reaching is constrained by both internal and external factors. Internal factors include the infant's age, experience reaching, and postural control with each influencing the quality and accuracy of reaching. External constraints include body position, degree of support, seating configuration, and object properties. This section describes features that characterize the development of reaching skills. For additional discussion on the control of reaching, the reader may wish to refer to

TABLE 3-4 Age-Related Reaching Development

Age	Skills/Behavior
Newborn period	Arm movements appear to be purposeful[520] and spatiotemporally structured[246] Reaching is visually triggered[250] Hand is typically open during forward extension of the arm
7 weeks	Rate of reaching briefly decreases Infants seem more interested in looking at the object Hand posture is more likely to be fisted[249]
12 weeks	Frequency of reaching increases Hand prepared for reaching[34,249] Infants acquire ability to visually determine realistic reaching distances[157]
12 to 18 weeks	Acquire skill in aiming reaches[245] Infants can contact a moving object in as much as 90% of trials Between 15 and 18 weeks, contact shifts from just touching to catching the moving object[248]
19 weeks	Reaches include most movement units that are seen in adults Reaching path is not straight[251]
31 weeks	First movement unit is longer, and functions as the transport unit similar to adults Reaching path is straighter[251]
5 to 9 months	Variability in reaching path and movement units while reaching for a stationary object[156]

more comprehensive texts.[33,491,496,495] Table 3-4 is provided to summarize the development of reaching.

Intrinsic Factors Influencing Reaching in Infancy

A growing body of work suggests that arm movements of the neonate, like kicking movements, are rudimentary expressions of skilled reaching that emerge during the first postnatal year. Supported in a semireclined posture newborns demonstrate rudimentary eye-hand coordination in response to a moving target.[246,520]

When infants from 1 to 19 weeks of age are presented with a slowly moving object, they continue to display interest in the object, but during the weeks in which neonatal reaching transitions into functional reaching, the role of vision appears to change somewhat and there are periods when reaching is less readily observed. Age-dependent declines in reaching responses are reported to occur between 8 and 16 postnatal days[403] and in the seventh postnatal week.[244] As infants become more interested in looking at objects, visual attention may inadvertently extinguish neonatal reaching efforts.[29] Vision functions to elicit reaching throughout the transition from neonatal to functional reaching, but it is not used to guide hand trajectory[316,545] or to orient the hand toward the object before initial contact during this transitional period in skill level.[344] In fact, infants do not appear to require vision of their hands for initiating reaching or contact and grasp of an object.[94] These findings seem to suggest that younger infants initiate reaching using a ballistic strategy to aim the hand toward the target and then switch to a feedback strategy (vision, proprioception, or both) to make corrective movements for grasping once the object is contacted.[94] At 4 to 5 months of age, reaches are as good with vision as when vision is removed after onset of the reach,[94,545] and infants begin to adjust their gaze, anticipating the future trajectory of an object.[519]

During the period from 12 to 36 postnatal weeks, several major changes occur in the form of reaching that suggest the development of a new control strategy.[251] To determine how reaching is perfected and to investigate strategies used to control reaching during development, the velocity and distance paths of hand transport are measured from video records of infant performances. Based on standard research methods used in studies of adult behavior, trajectories are dissected into movement units, each containing one acceleration phase and one deceleration phase. Adult reaches are characterized by 1 to 2 movement units; the first unit functions to transport the hand 70% to 80% of the distance to the target and is relatively long in duration, and the second unit functions to home in on the object and is relatively short

in duration.[279] Between 19 and 31 postnatal weeks, infants progressively restructure reaches for a moving object from an average of four movement units per reach to two movement units;[251] yet even at 19 weeks, only 22% of reaches contain only one or two movement units. The sequencing of movement units is also modified. In the younger infant when there are greater than two movement units per reach, the transport unit can occur as one of the middle movement units rather than the first. In 19-week-old infants, the transport unit is the first movement unit in only half of the reaches, extending an average distance of 80 cm, whereas at 31 weeks, it is the first unit in 84% of reaches and extends 137 cm. Finally, the hand path trajectory straightens with age (Figure 3-11), suggesting that, by 31 weeks, improved spatial planning contributes to advances in aiming skill as the hand is now transported closer to the target in a more efficient manner during the first movement unit, requiring fewer subsequent units to correct for errors.[251]

Experience in reaching is frequently found to be related to an infant's age, but in a series of studies investigating changes in arm movements with and without a toy present, Bhat and colleagues demonstrated the importance of spontaneous movement and reaching experience on joint kinematics.[34,35,36,178,329] Similarly, the coordination of shoulder and elbow movements during the development of reaching provides evidence for the importance of spontaneous

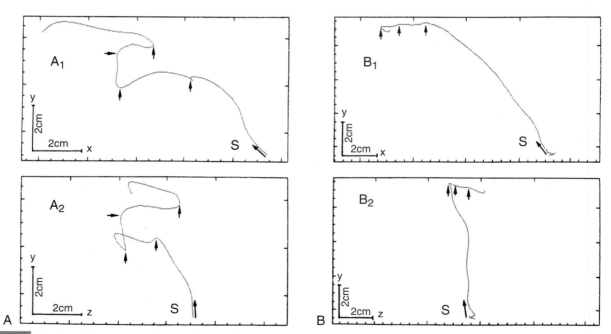

Figure 3-11   Hand paths become straighter and contain fewer movement units during the first postnatal year when reaching for a moving target. During a reach at 19 weeks of age (**A**), four movement units are identified (by arrows) in views from the front (**A₁**) and the side (**A₂**). Note that these movement units are similar in length. During a reach at 31 weeks of age in the same infant (**B**), only three movement units are identified from the front (**B₁**) and side (**B₂**). Note that most of the reaching distance is covered in the first movement unit. (Adapted from von Hofsten, C. [1991]. Structuring of early reaching movements: A longitudinal study. *Journal of Motor Behavior, 23,* 280–292, Figs. 3 and 4. Reprinted with permission of the Helen Dwight Reid Educational Foundation. Published by Heldref Publications, 1319 Eighteenth St., NW, Washington, DC 20036-1802. Copyright © 1991.)

movements for the development of reaching.[34,178] Infants alter the joint kinematics of their spontaneous arm movements in the presence of a toy months before the onset of reaching.[34] Clear stages of prereaching movements can be identified in the coordinated movement patterns of these healthy infants based on their reaching experience, not just their age. Carvalho[75] found that infants with less ability in reaching demonstrated fewer reaching attempts resulting in less practice reaching compared with more skilled reachers of the same age. Thus, age alone is not a good indicator of reaching ability; experience must be considered as well.

Another intrinsic factor influencing the improvements in typical infants' reaching is postural control.[119,514] As postural control improves in supine between 12 and 24 weeks of age, a decreased number of reaching movement units, a decreased length of the displacement path of the hand, and an increase in the length and duration of the first movement unit have been shown to be correlated.[147] Given that there is this pattern of control in young infants, the kinematic quality of reaching movements in preterm infants has been suggested as a possible construct to be examined to predict later motor coordination problems. Fallang and colleagues[148] have shown in a group of preterm and full-term infants without diagnosed motor disorders that the high-risk preterm group of infants performs nonoptimal reaching behavior at age 6 months, which differs from the low-risk preterm and full-term group. Preterm infants who used a "still trunk" posture at 6 months of age were more likely to have minor neurologic dysfunction and fine motor delays at 6 years of age.[150] Research on the postural muscle activation patterns, or APAs, in preparation for reaching has demonstrated the presence of organized muscle activation patterns before infants are able to successfully reach and during the onset of reaching.[119,513,514] Muscle activation patterns were less variable by 6 months of age, and infants with a "top-down" or cephalic-caudal temporally ordered recruitment pattern demonstrated a larger percentage of successful reaches that those using a less organized pattern of muscle activation.[119]

Developmental disability and risk for motor delays are intrinsic factors, which may contribute to the development of reaching in some groups of infants. Although the development of reaching is well described in typically developing infants, less research has been completed on the role of developmental disabilities in the development of reaching.[116] Preterm infants have been shown to have atypical postural adjustment and postural control strategies during reaching at 4 to 6 months of age.[149,150,515] Infants who were later diagnosed with CP have been shown to have atypical postural adjustment amplitude or organization depending on the type of CP.[211] Infants with Down syndrome have delayed reaching abilities, slower velocity, and less straight movement paths than typically developing infants.[71] These few examples demonstrate the impact of developmental disabilities on the motor control required for the development of reaching.

Extrinsic Factors Influencing Reaching in Infancy

Although age, reaching experience, posture, and developmental delay influence reaching abilities, task demands or extrinsic factors of the task may result in changes in reaching strategies as well. This section describes changes in reaching abilities under different task demands including a stationary versus a moving object, the removal of vision from a task, and changes in body position.

Infants 5 to 9 months of age who are typically developing appear to use the adult pattern of control when seated and reaching to grasp a stationary object placed on a horizontal (table) surface.[156] Under these conditions, movement units tend to be similar in duration (200 ms) for all ages, reaching distances, and positions (or order) within a reach (Figure 3-12). Furthermore, there may not be a decrease in the number of movement units within the path or a change in the straightness of hand path under these conditions between 5 and 9 months of age. Both hand path distance (equivalent to twice the shortest possible distance) and mean reaching duration (800 ms) also appear to be stable across ages and within adult limits, only more variable. These findings suggest that the movement speed and curvature of early functional reaching observed under stationary reaching conditions may be fundamental properties of both skilled and unskilled reaching controlled by biologic or physical constraints emerging from body-environment interactions.[156] These findings also point to the effect of task context on measurements used to explore control variables and the likelihood that control strategies vary with context.[251] It has been suggested, for example, that hand path is straighter when reaching for a moving object than when reaching for a stationary one.[248]

During the period from 5 to 9 months, infants begin to use visual information at the end of the reach as the hand approaches the target to correct for errors in hand path trajectory.[248] Before 5 months of age, they take little notice of the hand during flight, but thereafter, if vision of the hand is blocked, as when infants reach for a virtual (mirror image) object, performance is frequently disrupted.[316] Although infants continue to use a ballistic reaching strategy well into childhood, withdrawal of visual feedback begins to impair reaching skill at 6 to 7 months of age.[316,545] To determine how reaching movements are controlled, investigators have explored parameters that characterize the straightness of the hand trajectory. In adults, the curved hand path during reaching is composed of straight-line segments linked sequentially. The end of one segment and beginning of the next corresponds to a speed valley (deceleration and reacceleration) and a change in direction of the hand.[279] It is thought that each movement segment is ballistically generated and that corrections are made at these junctions between movement segments. To test whether path corrections are necessarily restricted to these speed valleys, Mathew and Cook[356] examined the curved hand path in reaching trials of

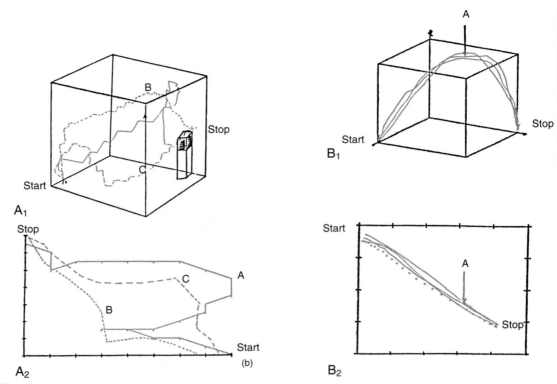

Figure 3-12 When reaching for a stationary object, infants exhibit reaches containing multiple movement units similar in duration. Three reaches are shown for a 9-month-old infant from a side view (**A₁**) and an overhead view (**A₂**). Note the irregularities both within and between reaches as compared with adult performance from the side view (**B₁**) and overhead view (**B₂**). (Adapted from Fetters, L., & Todd, J. [1987]. Quantitative assessment of infant reaching movements. *Journal of Motor Behavior, 19,* 147–166, Figs. 4 and 5. Reprinted with permission of the Helen Dwight Reid Educational Foundation. Published by Heldref Publications, 1319 Eighteenth St., NW, Washington, DC 20036-1802. Copyright © 1987.)

infants between 4 and 8 months of age who were presented with a suspended object having some motion. Three-dimensional analyses of hand trajectories indicated that the initial movement segment is directed toward the object at all ages tested and that changes in the path after reach onset tend to curve the hand toward the target to correct for error. Also, measures of hand speed within a movement segment correlate with veering of the hand toward the target within the movement segment, suggesting that error correction occurs continuously rather than only at discrete intervals in hand transport. The relationship between veering within a movement unit and target location may indicate that when vision is available, reaching is not executed using a ballistic strategy. On the other hand, continuous veering within a movement unit may be the biomechanical consequence of projecting the arm through space, a notion that is consistent with the equilibrium point hypothesis for joint position in the mass-spring model of arm control.[251,394]

During the first postnatal year, interlimb coordination of the arms and hands during reaching is characteristically variable. It has long been argued that early unilateral reaching is a consequence of asymmetrical tonic neck reflexes, and bilateral reaching emerges as these reflex influences lessen.[146] Other possible explanations for variability in reaching

strategies may be postural context during the reach and the characteristics of the target object.[128,146] In a longitudinal case study of one infant from 3 to 52 weeks of age, instances of bimanual reaching appeared to correlate with more variable kinetics, greater limb stiffness, and greater reaching velocities in the following arm as compared with the leading arm. These findings led the investigators to conclude that bimanual reaching predominates until infants learn to differentially control the following arm at approximately 6 to 7 months of age.[97] The degree of coupling between arms during reaching also appears to depend on the complexity of bimanual cooperation required, that is, whether one hand can remain relatively passive or must produce complementary movement patterns such as when holding a box lid up with one hand while extracting a toy with the other. Complementary bilateral reaching skill emerges at 9 to 10 months of age.[145]

A recent study comparing adults with Down syndrome to typical adults and children found that the individuals with Down syndrome were able to demonstrate stable bimanual coordination during a circle-drawing task that appeared adult-like.[411] In contrast, their unimanual ability was less coordinated and similar to the children examined in the study. This suggests that the individuals with Down syndrome have more mature bilateral reach and fine motor skill and less mature unilateral ability. This may be due to improved postural control via using both sides of the body during the bimanual activity, but this is yet to be examined experimentally.

The influences of object properties on grasping has been well documented (see the next section.), but the properties of objects also influence infants' reaching strategies.[98] Infants between 6 and 9 months of age frequently have a preferred reaching strategy, but they may be able to alter that movement strategy based on the task demands. In a study comparing the reaching and grasping strategies of 6- to 9-month-old infants for small balls, large balls, and large pompoms, Corbetta and Snapp-Childs[98] described the infants' ability to use sensorimotor information to alter their preferred reaching strategy. Older infants were better at altering their reaching strategy between unimanual and bimanual based on the task demands than were the younger infants. In addition, handling the object provided more cues to the infant than vision alone, leading to more appropriate changes in reaching strategy.[98]

Reaching in infants is routinely studied in a semireclined seated posture, but several groups have compared the development of reaching among infants in supine, upright, and semireclined postures. An early comparison of reaching in supine and upright sitting at 12 to 19 weeks of age and 20 to 27 weeks of age found that position had little impact on reaching abilities or quality between 20 to 27 weeks of age. Infants in the younger age group, however, demonstrated fewer reaches and grasps, and they had poorer quality of movement in supine.[430] Consistent in the research literature is the finding that younger, less experienced reachers are more influenced by changes in body position that those who have more experience and are older.[74,75,430] Carvalho and colleagues[75] suggested that the similarity of reaching performance of the more experienced reacher in either body position is an indication of the adaptability of the system to new constraints, which is not observed in the less adaptable, less experienced infant.

Reaching Strategies in School-Age Children

Studies in older children suggest that reaching strategies change very little from 9 months until approximately 7 years of age, at which time there appears to be a transitional period leading to an adult reaching strategy. When the visual field is displaced by a prism, children 5 years of age reach out to the apparent target location in one or two movement units before making corrective movements to move the hand to the actual target location.[231] In contrast, 7-year-olds execute multiple small movement units (referred to as early braking), producing hand paths that begin to veer toward the actual target location early in the path, and 9- to 11-year-olds execute an initial movement unit that approaches the virtual target location but is then followed by a second, corrective unit (referred to as smooth braking) that alters the path

before the hand reaches the virtual target location (Figure 3-13). These findings suggest that 5-year-olds continue to use ballistic strategies much like those of older infants, whereas 7-year-olds constantly monitor their movements in a closed-loop strategy to control their reaches. Between 9 and 11 years of age, children begin to combine these strategies to increase the efficiency of their movements and to reduce the amount of attention required.[231,295]

These changes in reach strategy appear to coincide with developmental changes in how children utilize sensory information for guiding and adjusting arm position during reach. Hay and colleagues[230] examined perceptual skill during an arm positioning task and found that, in the absence of vision, 8-year-olds produced greater errors in movement amplitude than both 6- and 10-year-olds, yet at the end of a trial, using kinesthetic information, they were able to detect and reduce the magnitude of their end-point error. A specific study of typical children's ability to correct forearm position when perturbed found that 4- to 9-year-old children gradually learn to master fine timing adjustments to perturbations.[436] In a study of accuracy and reaction time development, 6- to 9-year-olds demonstrated the development of adult-like motor planning.[151] Reaction time decreased initially followed by an improvement in accuracy. By 9 years of age the children had reaction times, movement times, and accuracy similar to adults when asked to reach quickly for an object. Furthermore, in a study of 4- to 11-year-old children with typical development in a goal-directed reaching protocol in which forearm movements reacted to externally applied forces, it was shown that as age increased, the children showed less variability in their movements to the target, and they adapted to external perturbations more quickly.[303] But even the 11-year-old children were not showing precision similar to the adults. Based on these studies, the child's ability to understand and utilize sensory information for reach correction continues to develop through at least the first 11 years.

Recent research on the coordination of head and trunk control in typically developing children provides evidence for a nonchronologic and protracted course of development.[15] Changes in head and trunk stabilization do not occur at the same rate in all planes, but children between 2 and 11 years old tend to use a head-stabilized-in-space pattern, whereas adults tend to use a head-stabilized-on-trunk pattern.[482] This evidence supports the relationship between postural control and reaching, as discussed in infants, and demonstrates a potential influence on the protracted development of reaching in children.[303,482]

In a related vein, one current view of the clumsiness seen in children with mild to moderate movement dysfunction is that a sensory or attention problem hinders the ability of these children to identify or selectively attend to the most pertinent information during a reach.[141,351,432,566] For example, study of hand paths during movement between two buttons in a repetitive tapping task in 8- to 10-year-olds with minimal

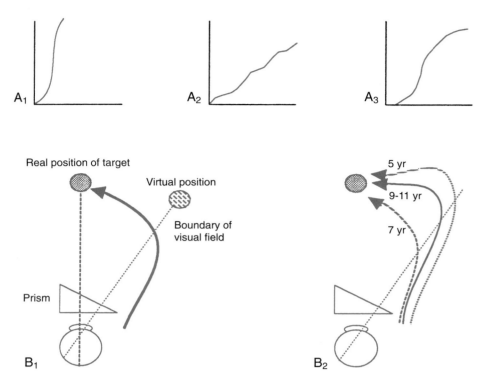

Figure 3-13 Hand paths during reaching to a stationary target correspond to the use of visual information to plan and control reaching. Ballistic reaches exhibit smooth trajectories with no distinct points of path correction, suggesting that they are preplanned and executed open loop **(A₁),** whereas early braking reaches are executed closed loop, using vision to continuously monitor and correct error **(A₂).** Late-braking reaches, in contrast, combine open loop and closed-loop strategies to maximize reaching efficiency by preplanning 70% to 80% of the trajectory and then correcting trajectory error in the final approach to the target **(A₃).** The use of these three strategies can be demonstrated by using a prism to displace the visual field **(B₁).** Under these conditions, it is apparent that children 5 years of age use a ballistic reaching strategy, because they correct their hand path only after they have reached or surpassed the target's virtual position **(B₂).** In contrast, 7-year-olds, using an early braking strategy, identify the discrepancy between real and virtual target position as soon as the hand enters the visual field, and 9- and 11-year-olds, using a late-braking strategy, almost reach the virtual target position before detecting the discrepancy. (Adapted from Hay, L. [1979]. Spatial-temporal analysis of movements in children: Motor programs versus feedback in the development of reaching. *Journal of Motor Behavior, 11,* 188–200, Figs. 1 and 4. Reprinted with permission of the Helen Dwight Reid Educational Foundation. Published by Heldref Publications, 1319 Eighteenth St., NW, Washington, DC 20036-1802. Copyright © 1979.)

neurologic dysfunction (DCD) suggests that these children must constantly monitor and correct their actions. It is believed that using this closed-loop strategy leaves little opportunity to attend to information for executing anticipatory adjustments and minimizing the amount of error correction required. In comparison with age-matched controls, children with minimal neurologic dysfunction also appear to execute more movement units per reach. The first movement unit is less likely to be the longest unit or to achieve the greatest acceleration, and each unit tends to contain more acceleration irregularities.[432] Not surprisingly, these children tend to have more difficulty maintaining task orientation. When asked to reach from a starting point to a stationary target, 8- to 10-year-old children with DCD were less accurate than typical peers as a result of spending less time in the deceleration phase of the reach.[461] When the visual conditions were manipulated (vision removed after reach began, or only target or target and hand visible), the group with DCD did

not seem to take advantage of the visual information available.[521] Similarly when children with DCD were asked to reach for a target with and without a visual perturbation (prism goggles), they used longer and more curved movement paths than a control group demonstrating that their response to altered vision was different than typically developing children.[566] In a different task, manual tracking of a continuously moving stimulus (a coincident-timing task) with a predictable path, children with motor coordination dysfunction (ages 6 and 11 years) were slower than age-matched controls.[521] Their movement distance during an acceleration phase was more variable than that of control children, their tracking motions were more delayed, and they performed more trials with apparently suboptimal attention. As an adaptive strategy, 7-year-olds with minimal brain dysfunction gave themselves more time to cope with less efficient reaching skills by planning a hand trajectory that would intercept a moving target further along its trajectory.[170] When these children were presented with an unpredictable tracking task, they had greater difficulty attending to the task than age-matched controls, perhaps because they could not identify a compensatory strategy.[141,522]

As was suggested for the infant during development, postural control may also affect the reaching behavior of children with DCD. Johnston and colleagues[290] documented differences in the APAs of shoulder and trunk muscles in 8- to 10-year-old children with and without DCD during a goal-directed reaching movement. The children with DCD demonstrated longer reaction times and movement times of their reach as compared to children who were typically developing. From a postural muscle perspective, the DCD group used earlier onsets of shoulder and posterior trunk muscle activity and later than typical activations of the anterior trunk muscles. Johnston and colleagues[290] hypothesize that the altered timing of postural muscle activation influences the speed and quality of the reach movement. Children with myelomeningocele, who frequently have atypical postural control and sensory deficits, used a different strategy for a similar task. The children with myelomeningocele did not alter their movement time while demonstrating a significant decrease in accuracy.[379] Whether the altered postural movements are part of the primary problem or a compensation for difficulty with necessary sensory integration to complete the task is yet to be determined.

In summary, the variables and processes that contribute to an emerging control of reaching skills during infancy and childhood are similar to variables contributing to those for posture and locomotion. In each instance, rudimentary aspects of control can be observed in very young infants if optimal conditions are provided, suggesting that precursors to functional skills may be established at very young ages. Each of these early skills, however, undergoes important transformations as children learn to perceive the task demands, monitor their movements, predict the potential consequences of their actions for a given context, and develop anticipatory strategies for efficient movement execution. As shown in the following section, these variables also contribute to the development of grasp control.

GRASPING

Hand function has long been viewed as one of the key control responsibilities of the motor cortex. Study of monkeys suggests that there are two cerebral cortical areas of importance to the grasping movement, the ventral premotor cortex containing the visuomotor neurons that respond to the location and components of the object, and the hand field of the primary motor cortex containing the neurons for finger muscle activation.[163] Classical studies linked onset of fine motor milestones with myelination of the lateral precentral gyrus.[326] Based originally on pyramidal lesion studies in monkeys,[327] it is generally accepted that reaching and grasping are also controlled by separate subcortical neural

systems. Following lesion of the lateral brain stem, monkeys cannot control hand movements independently of arm movements, yet they can use the limbs for walking and climbing. After lesion of the ventrolateral path, in contrast, monkeys can no longer control the posture of the limb, but they can pick up food with their hands. Studies suggest that the potential for coordinated hand movements may be present earlier than previously appreciated and that anatomic changes in descending neural paths, although necessary, may not be sufficient to account for development of hand control. For example, ultrasound recordings of human fetuses and observations of preterm infants indicate that extension of fingers during isolated arm movements begins by 12 weeks of gestation,[120,121,312] long before myelination of the corticospinal tract can account for these rudimentary actions. Furthermore, observation of spontaneous hand movements in neonates indicates that the hand is not always in a stereotypic posture of flexion (closed fist) or extension (open). The hands continuously move between these extremes and, in so doing, they exhibit considerable variability, suggesting that the potential for independent finger control is present at birth. This potential is underscored by recent neuroanatomic and neurophysiologic studies in infants, indicating that monosynaptic corticospinal connections are present at birth.[142,143] By 3 months, index finger forces can be clearly differentiated from those of other fingers during grasping.[314] If there is sufficient neural substrate to produce motor commands for independent finger actions at birth, why do fine motor milestones typically emerge several months later? This section reviews the acquisition of grasp control and studies identifying variables that may account for this finding.

Rudimentary Perceptual Control of Grasping

Although reaching and grasping skills are intimately related in a functional sense, control of grasping is distinguished from control of reaching by the different roles ascribed to the anatomic structures discussed previously and by apparent differences in perceptuomotor control of these two skills.[247] Early grasping behaviors can be observed in infants during spontaneous movements between 1 and 5 months of age.[531] Infants are observed to open and close their hands and to grasp their clothing and other objects that are near their hands during spontaneous movements. Fisting decreases while preprecision and precision grasp emerge around 2 to 4 months of age. Self-directed grasping and self-exploration increase around 4 months of age in typically developing children.[531] These early grasping behaviors may provide experience and help infants learn to anticipate grasping following reaching at older ages. The initial trajectory of reaching (phase 1 reaching) is based on visual definition of the object's location in space and executed using a ballistic or open-loop strategy, processes that do not appear to be linked with control of grasping. During execution of the reach (phase 2 reaching), visual feedback[278,279] or proprioceptive feedback[396] may be used to define arm position as part of a closed-loop strategy to correct for initial errors in trajectory. The hand is typically open during neonatal reaching; however, hand posture is independent of the reach trajectory and does not vary with or without visual fixation of the target.[244] By 3 months of age, the hand begins to open during reaching, but only when the infant visually fixates on the target.[244] Between 5 and 7 months infants show a transition from a tactile feedback-guided grasp to a visually based prospectively planned grasp.[546] Infants 5 to 6 months of age use visual information for adjusting grip configuration relative to object size.[378] Around 6 postnatal months, infants can occasionally execute an adult-like (phase 1 and 2) reach-to-grasp movement pattern, and by 9 months of age, they can execute the pattern reliably.[248]

Emergence of Anticipatory Control

With the onset of functional reaching, infants begin to develop perceptual abilities for reading the environment in such a way as to shape reaching and grasping skills. At the onset of functional reaching, they are not inclined to reach for objects that are placed at the perimeter of their reach.[156] At 5 months of age, they begin to orient their hand toward the object, either just before or at the beginning of the reach,[244,358] as well as shape the hand in anticipation of object size constraints during manipulation.[378] At this age, infants primarily rely on contact with the object to orient and successfully grasp the object, but over the next 3 months, infants begin to use visual information to both anticipate contact and orient their hand with respect to the object.[21,344] When adults reach to grasp an object, the distance between index finger and thumb is set with respect to object size at the onset of reaching.[277,279] Anticipation of object size is similarly observed in the hand posture of 9- to 13-month-old infants during reaching,[245] suggesting that young infants quickly learn to preprogram reaches for object size, location, and distance on the basis of visual information. The grasp of infants older than 9 months continues to exhibit some immature features, one being the relatively constrained range in hand opening when infants are presented with an assortment of objects varying in size.[329] The hand may open in exaggerated postures. Infants may open the hand widely as a strategy to compensate for limited ability to estimate the task requirements for grasping an object;[247] adults exhibit similar exaggerated hand postures when visual feedback is withdrawn, unpredictable,[277] or intermittent.[28] Finally this exaggerated hand opening in the infant could be due to the small size of the hand in relation to the object. A body-scaled relation of the grip configuration, based on an equation including the size and mass of the object to be grasped and the length and mass of the grasping hand, has been demonstrated to be invariant across young children (6 to 12 years of age) and adults.[78,79] The force applied during grasp, the duration of the grasp, and displacement phases of prehension have also been shown to adhere to the same body-scaled relationship.[77] These findings support the idea that mature grasp and displacement are ultimately controlled within a single action that relates to body size and object perception. Anticipatory strategies apparent in control of precision grip and load forces are discussed next.

Maturation of Precision Grip and Load Force Control

Once contact is initiated, the infant must coordinate normal (grip) and frictional (load) forces to grasp and lift an object.[288] Adults coordinate these forces synchronously, whereas infants and young children coordinate them sequentially.[165] To quantitatively examine grip control, infants are encouraged to pick up a toy that is equipped with force transducers to measure the grip forces of the opposing thumb and index finger and the load force necessary to lift the object off the table (Figure 3-14). During the preload phase (initial contact with the object), infants as young as 8 months contact the object with one finger before the other, creating a latency to onset of grip force that is significantly greater than in infants 18 months of age or older. Infants and young children also tend to press down on the object, creating a negative load force before reversing the direction of force to successfully lift the object off the table. Infants and young children generate a significant portion of the total grip force (often twice the magnitude of adult grasps) for grasping before initiating the load force, and during the load phase they typically exhibit multiple peaks in records for both of these forces. Adults, in contrast, scale the increases in grip and load forces in an economic, synchronous, and nearly linear manner with only a single peak near the middle of the load phase.[165] These findings suggest that the smooth execution of an adult grasp is the consequence of anticipating the object's weight so as to select an appropriate target force magnitude and scaling over time.[288] This anticipation of necessary grip-force adjustments for precision grip to lift, hold, and replace an object has been shown in adults to be related to experience with a predictable stimulus.[544] This collective experience, called central set, appears to affect the response gain of both voluntary and triggered rapid grip force adjustments to be set to a certain extent before perturbation onset in a similar manner as the effects of central set on lower extremity RPAs to platform perturbations. This suggests that in motor control there may be a general rule governing anticipatory processes.

The studies on control of grasp[165,166,167] are consistent with a reoccurring theme of this chapter: infants appear to possess the neural substrate to execute skilled motor patterns early in development, but demonstration of this potential is unreliable. First, these studies indicate that by 6 to 8 months of age infants can produce each of the actions required for a precision grip, and by 12 months of age infants can occasionally assemble all the components to produce adult-like force patterns, but there is considerable variability in performance across trials.[69] These studies also indicate that infants and young children use far more force than required, a common

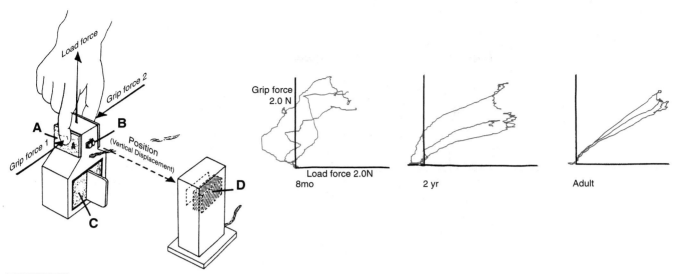

Figure 3-14   One method for quantitatively describing grasping skills and examining aspects of motor control is to measure the combination of grip and load forces over time. Precision grip force is the net normal force exerted by the index finger (Grip Force 1) and thumb (Grip Force 2), and load force is the tangential or friction force exerted when lifting the object against gravity (positive values) or pushing the object down into the table (negative force). The mass of the object can be varied by exchanging weights **(C)**, and displacement of the object can be detected by infrared diodes **(B)** and a sensor **(D)**. By 8 months of age, infants first press down on the object (negative X values), then they increase grip force (positive Y values) before initiating a load (positive X values) to lift the object. By 2 years of age, positive load and grip forces are scaled in a synchronous, more linear fashion similar to that in adults, and negative loading force is less apparent. (Adapted from Forssberg, H., Eliasson, A. C., Kinoshita, H., Johansson, R. S., & Westling, G. [1991]. Development of human precision grip. I. Basic coordination of force. *Experimental Brain Research, 85,* 451–457, Figs. 1 and 4.)

finding in studies of motor development.[295] Children as young as 2 years of age are able to adjust grip and load forces with respect to the degree of friction or potential slip during repeated lifts of the same object, but when the coefficient of friction is randomized over trials, they cannot adapt grip and load forces effectively. Thus, with sufficient practice they can formulate rules for more adult-like performance, but if confronted with uncertainty, they do not know how to draw from limited previous experience.

When typical children 6 to 8 years of age are asked to grasp and lift a 200-g object repeatedly, they initiate nearly synchronous, linear increases in grip and load forces with a single peak in magnitude, as do adults. Children with CP (diplegia or hemiplegia) and autism, in contrast, tend to initiate the forces sequentially, as do younger children with typical development.[113,138] Specifically, it appears that at least some children with CP and autism can produce the requisite forces, but they have difficulty selecting or executing efficient grasp strategies. Available data indicate that these children have difficulty regulating the timing and magnitude of force during both dynamic and static phases, and they tend to bear down on the object before lifting it (Figure 3-15). When these children are asked to grasp and lift objects of two different weights, presented in blocked and randomized trials, they also have difficulty scaling forces with respect to object weight during both nonrandom and random presentation of the two weights,[139] but if they are given a sufficient number of practice trials, they can anticipate and scale grasp force

parameters[140,468] and learn better precision isometric grip force, but not to the same extent as children of the same age who are typically developing.[510] Children with CP may also have difficulty stabilizing their gaze so that they can effectively use the available visual information.[333] Given that the normal acquisition of grasp control has a protracted period of development,[165,166,168] it is also probable that these children do not experience sufficient amounts and variety of practice to use available information for developing efficient strategies, an issue previously raised by Goodgold-Edwards.[187]

Refinements in the control of grasping continue to occur well into late childhood. Examination of the fine details of grip force amplitude and timing control has suggested that children age 7 to 8 years still do not exhibit finger force components typical of adult skill.[274] By 12 years of age, children approximate adult patterns of control and accuracy of bimanual isometric finger force production for both inphase (both hands pinching a load cell device at the same time) and antiphase (one hand pinching, then the other) activation.[221] When coordinating grasp and lift of objects, young children execute grasps characterized by multipeaked variations in grip and load forces and do not execute the smooth, coincident increases and decreases in these forces characteristic of adult grasping until approximately 8 years of age.[165] Transitions to smooth, single-peak force patterns may in part be due to gradual improvements in anticipatory strategies.[166] It appears that the scaling of grip and load force rates continues to change until approximately 8 to 15 years of age,

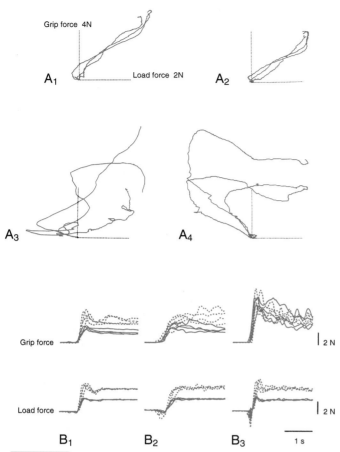

Figure 3-15 Children with cerebral palsy demonstrate some of the same force patterns during grasping to lift as those observed in younger typically developing children. Although age-matched (6- to 8-year-olds) normal children (**A₁**) exhibit synchronous scaling of grip and load forces, some children with diplegia (**A₃**) or hemiplegia (**A₄**) exhibit marked negative load force at the onset of a grasp, serial ordering of grip and positive loading forces, and grip force magnitudes twice that of normal children. However, children with less severely disabling cerebral palsy, such as one child with mild diplegia (**A₂**), may exhibit more normal, age-appropriate grasp patterns. In addition to difficulty coordinating grip and load forces, children with hemiplegia (**B₂**) and diplegia (**B₃**) have greater difficulty scaling grip force with respect to object weight than normal children (**B₁**). During lifts of a 400-g weight *(dashed lines)*, typically developing children apply larger grip forces than for a 200-g weight *(solid lines)*, and grip force quickly peaks and then drops to a stable level. Grip forces in children with cerebral palsy, in contrast, are slow to reach peak magnitude, are unstable during the static phase of the lift, and are not scaled reliably with respect to object weight. (**A,** Adapted from Eliasson, A. C., Gordon, A. M., & Forssberg, H. [1991]. Basic coordination of manipulative forces of children with cerebral palsy. *Developmental Medicine and Child Neurology, 33,* 661–670, Fig. 4. **B,** Adapted from Eliasson, A. C., Gordon, A. M., & Forssberg, H. [1992]. Impaired anticipatory control of isometric forces during grasping by children with cerebral palsy. *Developmental Medicine and Child Neurology, 34,* 216–225, Fig. 3.)

depending on the order of presentation of the weights, suggesting that anticipatory skills do not achieve adult levels until some point in this age range.[193]

Collectively, the studies described in this section demonstrate that grasping is a complex skill involving many different aspects of sensorimotor control. Rudimentary skills, biomechanics, experience, and other context-dependent variables probably contribute to the rapid changes in motor control observed in the first year of life. Even during earliest exercise of skill, infants are probably building a database of information for transforming their skills as they become increasingly more intent on shaping their experiences. Probably one of the views enjoying the greatest consensus among researchers in the field of motor control today is the view that all aspects of movement execution, including the basic physiology, biomechanics, perceptual processing, and development of strategies, must be closely examined under varying movement conditions to better understand the acquisition of motor control during typical development and when it goes awry.

MOTOR CONTROL RESEARCH: CLINICAL IMPLICATIONS

The implied assumption of motor control research is that it will advance clinical interventions to improve or restore motor function limited as a consequence of disease or injury. Collaboration between movement science researchers, rehabilitation clinician scientists, and clinicians is timely and important to improve examination and treatment of movement problems. New ideas and approaches are continually emerging as scientists and clinicians test the generality of theory-driven findings applied to various patient populations. It will take well-designed studies addressing specific links between science and practice, however, to know precisely the implications of motor control studies for specific problems encountered in rehabilitation practice. In this section, several likely implications of movement science for clinical practice are briefly discussed with respect to examination and intervention for motor control problems. Readers, however, are encouraged to apply their clinical and scientific knowledge to consider many more potential applications for translation of the research to practice.

CLINICAL EXAMINATION TOOLS

The majority of tools currently available for examination of motor control are based on neural maturation or learning theories, but some newer tools appear to reflect changing views of development, such as that espoused by the dynamic systems theory.[542] Maturational-based tools can be readily identified by an emphasis on reflex testing[383] or evoked behaviors because it is assumed that expression of these behaviors indicates the level of neural integration and function achieved.[501] In many of these tests, little or no consideration is given to other variables that may enhance, depress, or otherwise alter expression of the evoked behaviors. Even some maturational-based tools are beginning to consider broader views of motor development, however, as variables such as state behavior (e.g., level of arousal) are included in testing protocols or grading of responses. In many cases, the theoretic underpinnings of a given tool are not so clear. For instance, some motor assessment tools are composed of tests to determine milestone achievements and may be viewed as indicators of the extent of neural maturation and corticospinal control, as posed by McGraw,[360,361] or as behavioral indicators of cognitive maturation, as originally posed by Piaget.[295] In other instances, examinations are composed of milestones solely because they appear to display statistical or diagnostic significance.[257] Tools incorporating a dynamic-based view of development attempt to examine spontaneous, self-produced movements under more naturalistic conditions, recognizing that multiple variables contribute to movement.[208] All motor examinations provide some indication of ability or extent of control, but we have yet to realize tests that tell us precisely how and why control is limited or has broken down, and this is one of the greatest barriers in our efforts to bridge the gap between the highly controlled and constrained tests used in the research laboratory and those available for use in the clinical setting. This section reviews several tools that incorporate examination of self-produced movements that have been developed for use in identifying infants at risk for developmental disabilities, including the General Movement Assessment, Movement Assessment of Infants, and Alberta Infant Motor Scale. (See Chapter 2 for information on another current measure embodying these principles, the Test of Infant Motor Performance.) Following this discussion, two comprehensive tests that attempt to tease out the multiple variables that contribute to movement and the quality of movement of preschool and older children are highlighted, the Toddler and Infant Motor Evaluation and the Assessment of Motor and Process Skills. Then two more specific ways to measure components of motor coordination are highlighted, the Gross Motor Performance Measure and the Selective Control Assessment of the Lower Extremity.

Infant Examination

General Movement Assessment

The General Movement Assessment (GMA) is used to examine the spontaneous movements of preterm and term newborns and young infants, typically from a videotaped observation.[135] The GMA has been broadly applied to term and preterm infants with an array of clinical diagnoses and results suggest that it is an effective tool for predicting neurologic outcome at 2 years of age, for CP in particular.[135,399,465] The examination consists of observation and classification of spontaneous movements while the infant lies in the supine position. Only movements generated while the infant is in

an awake, noncrying state are analyzed and classified by movement quality. Classifications include writhing, fidgety, wiggling-oscillating, saccadic, and ballistic, and classification definitions distinguish frequency, amplitude, power, speed, flow, irregularity, and abruptness of the movements. Based on ethnologic methods, the design of the GMA reflects a theoretic view that maturation is not a fixed sequence of differentiation but rather a continuous transformation of behavior.[257] The theoretic framework of the GMA also incorporates the views that general spontaneous movement is a distinct, coordinated pattern of activity in the healthy newborn and that self-organizing neural networks, extrinsic factors, and endogenous maturational processes are likely contributors to the emergence of the different movement qualities.[208]

Recent applications of the GMA tool suggest that it has strong predictive potential for examining the neurologic status of a preterm, term, or young infant.[3,61,302,398] Intertester agreement appears to be good to excellent, sensitivity is high across age groups from preterm to 3 months corrected age, and specificity is high by 3 months of age.[135] Low specificity at earlier ages is attributed to spontaneous resolution of early dysfunction. A recent review suggests that prediction to developmental outcome is best at 2 to 4 months, which is the age of "fidgety GM."[213] Definitely abnormal fidgety movement, meaning an absence of this type movement, is reported to predict CP accurately 85% to 100% of the time. More specific analysis of GM also has suggested that particular types of CP (e.g., dyskinetic and hemiplegia CP) or impairments such as spasticity can be detected early on the basis of certain qualities of the movement observed.[3,134,203] If the infant with definitely abnormal GM does not go on to have CP, there is some suggestion that other developmental problems such as DCD will occur. Mildly abnormal GMs are also related to later development of DCD, attention deficit and hyperactivity disorders, and delayed development.[210,215,302] The GMA appears to be an effective and clinically useful tool for identifying infants who have early motor control deficits.

Movement Assessment of Infants

The Movement Assessment of Infants (MAI) is a tool designed for the purposes of identifying motor dysfunction, changes in the status of motor dysfunction, and establishment of an intervention program for infants from birth to 1 year of age.[81] The MAI is a criterion-referenced examination composed of 65 items selected to evaluate four areas: muscle tone, reflexes, automatic reactions, and volitional movement. Each item is scored on a scale of 0 to 4 or 0 to 6 points and checked for asymmetrical or rostrocaudal variations to obtain an "at-risk score" for motor dysfunction. Like other maturational-based assessment tools, the current version of the MAI contains many examiner-evoked test procedures, and it does not attempt to control for contextual variables such as state of arousal. It does include, however, items to examine spontaneous motor features such as self-initiated postures and behaviors commonly identified in milestone schedules of development that are scored for quality or level of proficiency. Theoretic justification for items of the MAI has not been specified, but it would appear that each is included for its statistical potential to discriminate abnormal deviations in motor development.

Several investigators have studied the psychometric properties of the MAI and the findings have been reviewed.[383] In general, studies indicate that rater reliability is weakest for items requiring handling of the infant by the examiner and greatest for those not requiring handling.[218] Studies also appear to indicate that the MAI is sensitive, readily identifying deviations in motor development that may predict motor dysfunction at later ages, but that it exhibits poor specificity because it also identifies some normal infants[439] and infants with transient medical problems as being at risk for later motor dysfunction.[226,483] It appears that the most consistently reliable and predictive portion of the MAI is the section on volitional movement, because it is the only section to exhibit a strong relationship with outcome (at 18 months of age) at both the 4-month and 8-month examinations.[483] Most recently, the predictability of the MAI has been examined in infants with extremely low birth weight[428] and infants at increased social risk.[416] Adequate sensitivity and high specificity for predicting CP at 1 and 2 years age were documented. Lower sensitivity and specificity were noted for prediction of more minor motor disorders such as DCD.[428] MAI scores were correlated with cognitive but not motor outcomes at 2 years of age for a group of 134 infants at risk of developmental delay because of their social environment.

Alberta Infant Motor Scale

The Alberta Infant Motor Scale (AIMS) was developed as a screening tool to identify infants at risk for motor dysfunction.[391,392] It is purely an observational scale, in which movement ability is documented in infants from birth to 18 months of age, with the infant in prone, supine, sitting, and standing positions. Item scoring criteria specify aspects of quality of movement that must be met in order to pass each item (e.g., postural alignment or weight distribution). High reliability (intraclass correlation coefficient [ICC] > 0.90) has been demonstrated in trained and untrained raters[41,392] and with different cultural backgrounds.[283] Normative information, based on 2022 infants from the Canadian province of Alberta, is also available for use of the test to document motor development delay.[391] This test is quick and easy to give and seems to estimate developmental levels most accurately between 4 and 10 months of age.[338] Discriminative validity for identifying infants with atypical movement as atypical was 89%.[112] Predictive validity of assessments at 4 and 8 months of age for identifying delayed motor development at 18 months of age revealed sensitivity and specificity of 77% and 82%, respectively, using cutoff scores below the

10th percentile at 4 months, and 86% and 93%, respectively, using cutoff scores below the 5th percentile at 8 months. A study of 800 preterm infants in the Netherlands found the normative AIMS data did not reflect the average motor ability of the included preterm infants.[524] Further, AIMS scores on infants in Taiwan at 6 months age[283] were only moderately predictive of motor function at 12 months. Both studies may indicate cultural differences or a need for new normative values for preterm infants. The test is not designed to document why an infant may have difficulty with movement, but by stepping back and observing the infant carefully across the different postures, the therapist can potentially focus on what the limiting factors may be. Then further testing of specific systems—such as force production capability, postural control, sensory acuity, cognitive capability, motivation—can ensue.

Childhood Examination

Toddler and Infant Motor Evaluation

The Toddler and Infant Motor Evaluation (TIME) was developed to quantify the theoretic construct of quality of movement in infants and children 4 months to 3.5 years of age for discriminative purposes and potentially to monitor change across time or because of therapeutic intervention.[367] Based on specific observation and quantification of quality of movement in children with motor delays, the authors developed the items for the test.[366] The test consists of five subtests—Mobility, Motor Organization, Stability, Social/Emotional Abilities, and an optional Functional Performance subtest. Also, there are three clinical subtests—Quality Rating, Atypical Positions, and Component Analysis. The majority of the assessment is completed via observation of the child with the parent or caregiver assisting to place the child in different positions or to provoke various movements. The test can be scored in real time or videotaped for later scoring. The parent or caregiver is also interviewed to determine the Functional Performance score. The test is child- and family-friendly in terms of stress during testing, and the subtests potentially can direct the therapist to specific systems that may be affecting movement success. The reliability and validity of the test are reported to be high, but the responsiveness (ability to show clinically meaningful change across time or with intervention) has yet to be fully evaluated.[366] A review of use of the test to monitor change across time in two children suggests that some changes in the test construction may improve the responsivity.[404] Recent reviews of the TIME suggest that although it is lengthy to administer the test, results may yield valuable information for determining potential causes of motor control dysfunction, but more research is needed to confirm this notion.[465,499]

Assessment of Motor and Process Skills

The Assessment of Motor and Process Skills (AMPS) was developed to evaluate motor skills and series of actions (called process skills) leading to completion of a task.[161] Design of the AMPS is based on sensory integration theory for the purpose of examining the behavioral manifestation of sensory integrative dysfunction in children[64] and adults.[161] Selection of specific items in the AMPS is based on the assumption that the items collectively represent the abilities underlying performance of common tasks and therefore can be used to estimate overall function and to identify specific deficits limiting function for use in planning therapeutic intervention. The AMPS contains 15 motor skills items to examine strength, posture, mobility, fine motor capabilities, and subtle postural adjustment capabilities, plus 20 process skills to measure attentional, conceptual, organizational, and adaptive capabilities. To evaluate these skills, the subject selects a common activity, such as fixing a sandwich, from a range of 30 possible activities listed in the AMPS manual. Each of the skills is then scored on a 4-point scale describing levels of competence displayed while the subject completes the activity. Scores for each of the motor skills are then adjusted for the level of task difficulty so that performance can be related to a continuum of performance capacity to compare and predict performance for tasks of lesser or greater difficulty. Studies published thus far on adult populations suggest that the AMPS is a valid tool across cultures[195] and gender.[132] The authors have developed a version specifically for children in the school setting, the School AMPS scale.[160] Support for the rater reliability, scale validity, and person response validity has been demonstrated,[160] as well as concurrent validity with the Peabody Developmental Fine Motor Scale.[158] Correlations with the Peabody Developmental Fine Motor Scale were higher with the School AMPS motor score than with the process score, which was expected and highlights the differences and potential advantage of the School AMPS.[158] The School AMPS has also been shown to be able to differentiate among children with and without congenital heart disease[199] and children at risk for delays.[159] Studies to document the responsivity of the test after physical or occupational therapy intervention in children need to be done. This test does incorporate the dynamic systems perspective through evaluation of components of movement for functional skill activities and should receive more use in the future.

Examples of Measures of Components of Motor Control

Pediatric Clinical Test of Sensory Interaction for Balance

The Pediatric Clinical Test of Sensory Interaction for Balance (P-CTSIB) was created based on a suggestion from the field by Shumway-Cook and Horak to assist in the identification of specific sensory components of balance dysfunction.[101a,454a] Measurements are made of a child's ability to balance in a standing position when sensory conditions are systematically altered. The P-CTSIB mimics the SOT (see Figure 3-4) in that standing balance is examined

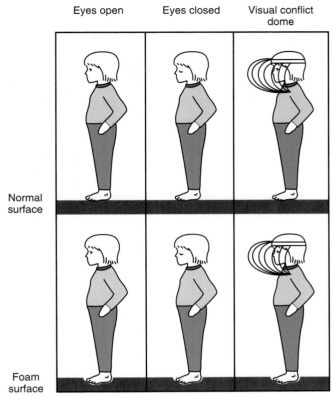

Figure 3-16   The Pediatric Clinical Test of Sensory Interaction for Balance (P-CTSIB) is a systematic way to examine a child's reaction to altered sensory conditions. It was designed as a clinical test to be similar to the SOT (Figure 3-4). The domelike hat simulates the moving visual surround and a piece of high-density foam simulates the moving surface of the SOT. (Adapted from Crowe, T. K., Deitz, J. C., Richardson, P. K., & Atwater, S. W. [1990]. Interrater reliability of the Clinical Test for Sensory Interaction for Balance. *Physical and Occupational Therapy in Pediatrics, 10*[4], 1–27.)

within combinations of three visual and two support surfaces conditions. Visual variables include eyes open, eyes closed, and eyes open while wearing a dome-like hat. Support surface variables are a flat hard surface and a foam surface that is firm but compliant. The six conditions, illustrated in Figure 3-16 are standing on a (1) hard surface with eyes open, (2) hard surface with eyes closed, (3) hard surface while wearing a visual conflict dome, (4) foam surface with eyes open, (5) foam surface with eyes closed, and (6) foam surface while wearing the visual conflict dome. Visual conflict is created by use of a hatlike apparatus made of a lightweight dome. The dome allows some diffuse light to come through, but impedes the peripheral vision. As the child sways, the dome moves in synchrony with the head to simulate the moving visual surround of the SOT.[101a] Somatosensory conflict is provided by having the child stand on a piece of medium-density closed-cell foam, which alters somatosensory input. Both the time the child can stand in a feet-together position as well as a rating of AP sway is recorded. Time and sway scores are combined into an ordinal scale and then into a sensory system scale (Westcott et al. 1994). Reliability, validity (with other general tests of balance) and pilot norms have been developed (Crowe et al., 1990; Deitz et al., 1991; Garner et al., 2005; Inder & Sullivan, 2005; Richardson et al., 1992; Vessey et al., 2005; Westcott et al., 1994, 1997). Using the sensory system scale, the clinician can classify the child as being able to balance appropriately, or not, when (1) vision provides accurate body orientation information (conditions 1 and 4); (2) vision is absent (conditions 2 and 5); (3) vision provides inaccurate body orientation information (conditions 3 and 6); (4) somatosensory provides accurate body orientation information (conditions 1, 2, 3); (5) somatosensory provides inaccurate body orientation information (conditions 4, 5, 6); and (6) vestibular provides accurate body orientation information (conditions 5 and 6). With this classification information, hypotheses can be made regarding the presence or absence of sensory components of a child's balancing dysfunction and appropriate targeted procedural interventions may be recommended. Researchers recently compared the P-CTSIB to the SOT in 6- to 12-year-old children without motor disability and found no correlation between the two tests on conditions with altered support surfaces.[176a] This raises concerns about the validity of the P-CTSIB given that it was developed to mimic the SOT; however, the researchers argue that the information derived from the P-CTSIB is different but complementary to the SOT and several previous studies on children with balance dysfunction demonstrated similar results for each test. More research needs to be undertaken to understand the differences between the two tests.

Gross Motor Performance Measure

The Gross Motor Function Measure (GMFM) (see Chapter 2) and its companion, the Gross Motor Performance Measure (GMPM), were specifically designed to examine the status and change in status of motor proficiency because of therapeutic interventions in children with CP.[47,198,423] The theoretic basis for design of the GMFM was the measurement property of responsiveness, or ability to show change in motor function, in a population of children from 5 months to 12 years of age who have CP. Studies suggest that the GMFM is both a responsive[423] and valid[38] measurement tool. The currently published GMPM consists of 20 motor skills commonly performed by children who are typically developing and younger than 5 years of age derived from the GMFM that measure proficiency in eight areas of motor function: activities in supine, prone, four-point, sitting, kneeling, and standing positions and during walking and climbing. Each item is scored for three attributes using a criterion-referenced scale to indicate the postural alignment, selective control and coordination, and stabilization of weight during the task. Most items involve either movements requiring a change in posture, such as during overground progression (crawling or walking) or action while maintaining a posture (extending

an arm while in sitting or four-point position). The GMPM was designed to examine qualities of movement believed by therapists to be problematic but amenable to intervention in children with CP. The use of physical aids or orthoses is noted on the score sheet, but use of these is not reflected in scoring and no other possible variables affecting motor control are considered. The GMPM does not examine qualities of performance such as speed, effort, or efficiency, nor can it specify the underlying cause of dysfunction in control. Studies of GMPM measurement properties by the authors suggest that overall interrater, intrarater, and test-retest reliability are good to excellent.[197,497] A recent study, however, that examined inter- and intrarater reliability from videotape recordings, while concurring that overall reliability was good, identified the determination of disassociated movements as the least reliable and in need of further modification in terms of test criteria to improve reliability.[463] Construct validity was demonstrated via differences in scores among children with varied diagnoses, severities of motor disorder, and ages. There appears to be moderate agreement between GMPM and GMFM scores for children with CP and age-matched controls but lower agreement between GMPM scores and therapists' ratings of performance. Nevertheless, there appears to be good agreement between changes in GMPM scores and therapists' indications of improvement in children with CP, suggesting that the GMPM is a responsive motor performance examination.[48] The reader is encouraged to follow the literature on the development of this test, as based on personal communication with the authors (e-mail correspondence with Virginia Wright, November 12, 2009), a new version focused on the examination of quality of movement in standing, walking, and climbing, entitled the Quality FM, became available for use in 2010.

Selective Control Assessment of the Lower Extremity

The Selective Control Assessment of the Lower Extremity (SCALE) was recently developed to quantify selective voluntary motor control, hypothesized to be mediated through corticospinal tracts, in children with CP.[174] The test is recommended for children age 4 years or older who do not have severe cognitive and motor deficits. During the test, the child is asked to perform individual movements at the hip, knee, ankle, subtalar, and toe joints from either a sitting or sidelying position. To judge selective voluntary motor control, one representative movement at each of these joints are observed to rate selective joint movement, involuntary movement at other joints, reciprocal movement, speed of movement, and generation of force through the child's available range. Movement at each joint is then scored to be either normal, impaired, or the child is unable to move.[174] Interrater reliability and content and construct validity of the test are purported to be acceptable for clinical use.[174] The authors suggest that the results of the test can be used as a prognostic indicator for treatment planning. For example, scores on the test might be used to help determine if various orthopedic surgeries might be beneficial or not for specific children. For instance, hamstring muscle lengthenings are commonly used in children with CP to improve the swing phase of gait by increasing knee extension ROM and decreasing spasticity, both of which are hypothesized as limiting the gait pattern. The outcome of such procedures, however, is not always beneficial. To determine if selective voluntary motor control could be a limiting factor in the gait pattern, researchers[173] examined the correlation between SCALE scores and the movements of the hip and knee during the swing phase of gait in a group of ambulatory children with CP. During swing phase, extension of the knee should occur while the hip is flexing. The ability to do this requires selective voluntary motor control at the hip and knee. Results of the study demonstrated that SCALE scores were significantly correlated to selective control of the hip and knee during the swing phase of gait and may be helpful for future determinations of effectiveness of various orthopedic procedures.[173] Other researchers considering the idea of predictive clinical reasoning have suggested that classification of children with CP based on measures of age, ROM, selective motor control, and spasticity may assist with the recommendation for intervention and the analysis of outcomes after interventions.[422] It is suggested that future study of the SCALE be focused on other forms of reliability and validity, the predictive value of the measurement of selective voluntary motor control for recommendations for intervention, and perhaps as an outcome measure for motor learning interventions.[173,174]

Shriners Hospital Upper Extremity Examination

The Shriners Hospital Upper Extremity Examination (SHUEE) was designed for children 3 years and older with hemiplegia for three main purposes: to determine the potential for improved function, to direct interventions, and to evaluate the effects of intervention to impairment elements that disrupt function.[453] During 16 functional activities, such as taking money from a wallet or unscrewing a bottle lid, an assessment of the child's spontaneous functional use of the affected arm/hand is used to assess the potential for improved use as presumably the more spontaneous use, the greater the child's potential. The child's movements during the activities are also scored for dynamic segmental alignment of the elbow, wrist or fingers, dependent on the activity. Lastly, the child's ability to grasp and release are observed with the wrist flexed, in neutral and extended. The child's performance during the test is videotaped and the scoring occurs later, therefore the examination can be completed in about 15 minutes. This test reflects some of the newer ideas about motor control given that judgments about motor control are made from the child's active movements during functional tasks rather than from passive movement tests. The authors of the test have documented excellent intrarater and interrater reliability of all three sections rated on the test and moderate concurrent and construct validity through comparison of children's performance on the SHUEE with two other tests of hand use and self-care skills.[114] A review of upper limb activity measures described the SHUEE as one of the five best measures available for children with hemiplegia and recommended its use especially if therapists wanted to measure change in unimanual function as a result of spasticity management, surgery, or specific training to reduce impairments.[183]

Other selective motor assessments with the aim of evaluating components or systems affecting movement are an array of upper extremity motor tests,[183] postural control assessments, some of which were reviewed in the postural development section of this chapter,[536] and prehensile movements.[467,468] Measurement of specific key behaviors may also move from the laboratory to the clinic such as measurement of rhythmic timing in upper extremity movement,[526] relative kicking frequency in infants,[232] and use of video coding for measurement of head control[72] and reaching behaviors.[233] With the advent of more user-friendly technology, more sensitive testing of motor control may be able to move from research laboratory protocols to clinical measurement systems utilizing EMG[175] and kinematics.[425] As efforts continue to extend research in motor control to issues of assessment, development of specific measures consistent with current knowledge of the processes and mechanisms of motor control will continue. These new tools, which borrow directly from current research methods in motor control, will represent a new generation of standardized tests.

IMPLICATIONS FOR TREATMENT

Conceptualization regarding application of contemporary research in motor control to intervention begins with understanding the theoretic basis for why a certain action is taken and specifying the expected consequences predicted by the theory enlisted. Excellent reviews of the theoretic bases and expected consequences from motor intervention during much of the 20th century[194,268,269] and the beginning of the 21st century are available,[4,240,259,298,458] and readers are encouraged to explore this literature in detail. Next we will only highlight some examples of possible implications for intervention drawn from motor control research. Much more research is needed to competently apply research in motor control[105,259,317] and motor learning to practice,[299] especially in the areas of development of motor control in infants and children.[6,548]

Evolving Bases for Treatment

The earliest neurotherapeutic approaches used in pediatric physical therapy were originally based on maturational-developmental theory, which typically ascribed to a hierarchic model of motor skill acquisition and enlisted a facilitation model of treatment. In practical terms, it was assumed that motor development in the child progressed in a specific sequence of reflexes, movement patterns, and milestones, and that a child had to experience each facet of this sequence to acquire normal, age-appropriate motor control. Such logic can be found in various forms of treatment adapted from theoretic neurorehabilitation models developed by (but not limited to) the Bobaths,[43] Brunnstrom,[62] Knott,[301] Ayres,[18] and Vojta.[17] Documented dissatisfactions with these approaches include poor carryover to functional activities, insufficient active movement by the patient, lack of attention to movement-related variables that are extrinsic to the nervous system, and failure to produce the expected normal movement patterns once abnormal muscle tone or primitive reflexes were inhibited.[104,259,268,475] Although some of these intervention approaches have been modified across time to reflect newer ideas of motor control and learning,[10] the evidence to support this type of intervention as a whole continues to be weak.[104,475]

Newer approaches, such as those developed by Carr and Shepherd,[73] Horak,[259] and Law and colleagues[325] are organized around goal-directed, functional behaviors and consider the importance of both peripheral and central neural function as well as the environment in learning to accomplish specific functional goals. The goal-oriented approach is based on the systems model of motor control.[31] According to this model, function of each contributing system and interaction among systems are dictated by the demands of task goals during a given movement (Figure 3-17, *A*). Thus, unlike other approaches, the goal-directed approach assumes that movement patterns will vary according to the goal and systems contributing to a given movement. Similarly, the goal-directed approach assumes that there may be multiple satisfactory movement pattern solutions for achieving a goal; therefore, a patient is encouraged to find multiple strategies for accomplishing a goal. Active, self-initiated movement is encouraged and principles of motor learning are used to enhance practice and learning of new movement strategies. Some aspects of this approach are yet undeveloped, such as methods for more precisely specifying the quality of movement and how to specifically enhance the motor learning processes, especially in children.[240,259,511] Nevertheless, this goal-directed treatment approach is the closest approximation to a dynamic theory-based (or systems) and learning-based model of rehabilitation currently found in clinical practice.

Shumway-Cook and Woollacott[458] have offered specific ideas regarding intervention for using a goal- or task-oriented approach with reference to physical therapy for children as well as adults. They suggest that the examination procedures focus on three areas: (1) functional skill ability in the area of interest (such as postural stability, gait, reach and grasp movements, etc.), (2) strategies (organization of sensory and perceptual information and movement patterns) used to complete these functional skills, and (3) impairments constraining the strategies used to complete the functional skills. The impairments constraining the strategies available to the client could come from any system, cognitive, sensory, or motor, involved in the control

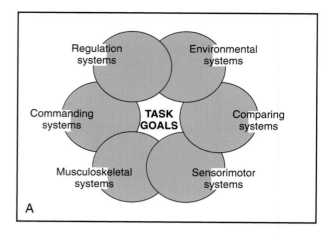

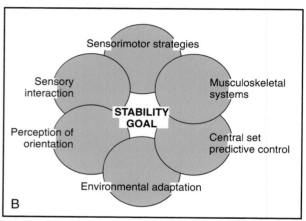

Figure 3-17 The Systems Model of Motor Control (**A**) and Systems Model of Rehabilitation (**B**) specify a collection of systems as contributing to the control of movement. The organization of these systems is heterarchic rather than hierarchic, suggesting that control shifts among the contributing systems as a function of the goal for a given task. (**A**, Adapted from Horak, F. B. [1991]. Assumptions underlying motor control for neurologic rehabilitation. In Lister, M. J. [Ed.], *Contemporary management of motor control problems, Proceedings of the II Step Conference* [pp. 11–28, Fig. 4-7]. Alexandria, VA: Foundation for Physical Therapy. **B**, Adapted from Horak, F. B. [1992]. Motor control models underlying neurologic rehabilitation. In Forssberg, H. & H. Hirschfeld [Eds.]. *Movement disorders in children, medicine and sport science* [Vol. 36, pp. 21–30, Fig. 2]. Basel: Karger.)

of the movements as depicted in Figure 3-17, *A*. To illustrate this for a specific class of goals, Horak[269] hypothesized that the systems involved in a postural stability goal would include those depicted in Figure 3-17, *B*. Starting from the upper right corner of the model, the musculoskeletal system contributes the net biomechanical forces for postural control resulting from active contractile forces, passive elastic forces, and displacements of multilinked body segments. The central set provides anticipatory strategies based on past experience to minimize the potential for postural instability as it emerges during movement. Environmental adaptation provides a means for using both feedforward and feedback control to adapt postural strategies to a

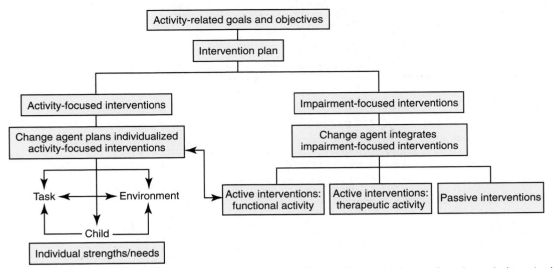

Figure 3-18   A model for organizing intervention in children with movement dysfunction is depicted. Starting from the goals determined by the child/family and therapist, the intervention plan has two components, the activity-focused interventions driven by both learning-based and dynamic systems theories, and the impairment-focused interventions related to changing constraints on the child's movement via both active and passive means. (From Valvano, J. [2004]. Activity-focused motor interventions for children with neurological conditions. *Physical and Occupational Therapy in Pediatrics, 24*, 79–107, Fig. 1.)

particular task or environment. Based on somatosensory, vestibular, and visual information, perception of orientation determines the postural orientation goal for the task at hand. Sensory interaction provides a means for adjusting the relative dominance of all sensory inputs based on current postural context and environment, previous postural experience, and postural expectations. Finally, sensorimotor strategies provide a collection of innate and learned movement strategies (that can be adapted by the actions of all other systems) to simplify planning of an action and effectively meet the postural goal. Intervention would then focus on three areas: (1) the resolution, reduction, or prevention of impairments affecting functional ability; (2) the development of effective (efficient) strategies to perform task-specific activities; and (3) the development of ability to utilize these strategies across changing task and environmental conditions.[458] Intervention strategies would be directed at changing the individual's constraining impairments and manipulating the task and environment to promote motor learning.[509] Valvano[509] has developed a model for this type of intervention in children (Figure 3-18). The figure depicts both the dynamic and learning based intervention to teach the child movement skill and the passive or active body function/structure interventions to decrease the constraints that might be affecting the ability to move in a more coordinated manner. Manipulation of the task and environment would occur through alterations of feedback and patterns or locations of motor skill practice based on motor learning principles that are explained in detail in Chapter 4. Use of strategies such as these in programs to increase children's participation and reduce disability in daily life are described in Chapter 27.

Applications of Motor Control Research to New Interventions

Several specific applications of the theoretic positions and research findings presented in this chapter follow to demonstrate how research in motor control has influenced pediatric physical therapy intervention. Most of the interventions described have a preliminary evidence base for use in clinical practice, but more research is necessary to truly define the appropriate populations, applications, doses, and benefits of the interventions. Treadmill and strength training for gait and functional mobility, constraint-induced movement therapy for upper extremity use, use of robotics and other external devices, cognitive interventions for improved coordination, and a discussion of the potential effects of the timing and intensity of intervention are briefly reviewed.

Improving gait and functional mobility are primary goals of many pediatric physical therapy interventions. Based on the motor control research suggesting the hypothesis that our locomotor gait pattern is controlled via a CPG, partial-weight-bearing treadmill training as a way of triggering the gait CPG has emerged as a possible effective intervention. As was noted earlier in the chapter, the use of this intervention has been evaluated in children with CP,[243,408,433,462] children born prematurely,[346] and children with Down syndrome.[507,556] Positive effects in terms of improvements in gait speed, cadence, stride length, and functional skills such as standing and transferring were attained in the children with CP who ranged from 1.7 to 18 years of age with Gross Motor Function Classification System levels of II to IV. Most recently, it has been demonstrated that treadmill training in children with CP can modulate the short latency reflexes during the swing phase of gait.[243] Infants with Down syndrome who used treadmill practice learned to walk on average approximately 3 to 4 months before a control group that did not have the practice.[507] This earlier walking behavior could potentially impact the rate of development in cognitive and behavioral skills through earlier ability to explore the environment, but this has not been examined experimentally at this time. Examination of dosing in children with Down syndrome demonstrated that a higher intensity of treadmill training that also included more complex walking via practice stepping over obstacles provided more long-term retention and earlier adaptive strategies for negotiating over obstacles than a less intense protocol that did not include obstacle walking practice.[556] Overall this type of task-specific training and extensive practice of the walking behavior appears to have efficacy in children with Down syndrome, but more controlled trials are needed to understand outcomes in children with other disabilities.[104]

On a somewhat different avenue to improve gait, researchers using a systems approach to examination have suggested that children with CP may have increased difficulty with gait owing in part to impaired force production capability of their lower extremity muscles. A series of studies by Damiano and colleagues documented that children with CP do have weakness in the majority of lower extremity muscles as compared to peers who are typically developing.[108] Children with CP were then shown to be able to improve their activation and strength in specific lower extremity muscles after a standard weight lifting protocol in a similar manner to children without disabilities and without any increase in spasticity.[110,348] Several studies have shown that the increase in muscle strength resulted in an improved gait pattern with less crouch, faster speed,[106,109,133] and improved gross motor ability (standing, sit-to-stand, walking, running, jumping activities).[42,107,306,348,370] Although this evidence is compelling, a recent meta-analysis of published studies on strengthening in children with CP raises questions as to the effect size of the intervention.[444] As always more research is needed to help direct clinical practice. Using the escapement-driven inverted pendulum and spring model, specific strength training to improve the impulse at push-off might be hypothesized as an effective intervention, but to date this analysis has not been done.

Constraint-induced movement therapy was designed based on research with nonhuman primates and adults after stroke who demonstrated a learned nonuse phenomenon specifically of the involved upper extremity with a measurable reduction of cerebral cortical representation of the involved limb.[127,487] Although this intervention does not easily stem from a motor control theoretic perspective or address issues of how we control movements, it has been examined experimentally and is receiving support in clinical practice.[475] It can be anchored well based on motor learning theory[434] and our understanding of neural plasticity.[289,298,548] This therapy has been applied to children with CP who have

one upper extremity more involved than the other in single subject or case study research[87,101,127,365,390] and experimental studies.[86,126,136,488,540] A multisite randomized clinical trial is currently under way.[144] Descriptions of the intervention can be found in multiple reviews on the topic.[54,83,242,426] The therapy essentially employs a restraint of the less involved upper extremity via use of slings or casts, and then it actively engages the child to practice movement using the more involved upper extremity. The length of time for the restraint and practice has ranged from 2 to 3 weeks, 4 to 6 hours a day in the original protocols, and it also has been completed in modified protocols with modified restraint (mitts) and practice times as low as 2 hours per day for several months.[137,188,190] Studies have documented changes in upper extremity use, and maintenance of benefits 3 to 6 months after the intervention ended. Repeated application of the intervention has been shown to be beneficial.[85] The age of the child thus far does not seem to degrade the effect,[45,95,189] but the specific diagnosis of the child may alter the outcome.[309] Several researchers have documented evidence for modulation in the cerebral cortex after the intervention.[291,478] Comparisons of the constraint with movement practice to movement practice (both unimanual and bimanual) alone have shown support of the practice aspect of the intervention separate from the constraint.[84,191,192] Further research would be helpful to determine more specifically when, how long, and under what specific situations this intervention is most beneficial as well as to identify any possible negative effects of using restraints.[459] See Chapter 4 for a video.

Changing coordination in children with less severe motor dysfunction such as DCD has been challenging. Motor control research has suggested that these children may have difficulty with utilizing and prioritizing sensory input to control motor output.[290,351] Several types of intervention are currently being studied to determine effectiveness of improving coordination. Metronome training,[304] based on capitalizing on the entrainment possibilities of the auditory system, has been examined in a randomized pretest, posttest control group study in children with attention deficit disorder.[23,449] The researchers documented significant positive outcomes in favor of the metronome group in attention, motor control, language, reading, and regulation of aggressive behaviors. More recently, beneficial effects on visual motor control and speed were shown but no changes in attention and motor inhibition.[99] A cognitive intervention, consisting of teaching problem-solving strategies and guided discovery of child- and task-specific strategies,[369] is based on several of the theoretic positions on motor control presented earlier in this chapter. Teaching these strategies has been shown to be as effective and more long lasting than the standard contemporary intervention in improving achievement of motor goals.[368,393,412] Another cognitive training technique, based on findings that children with DCD have difficulty with representation of visual-spatial coordinates of intended movement, focuses on imagery intervention designed to train the forward modeling of purposive actions and is delivered by an interactive CD-ROM.[543] Imagery plus active movement has been shown to cause greater transfer of learning in children with typical development than active movement alone.[485] The imagery protocol used with children with DCD was found to be as effective as a standard perceptual-motor training protocol in improving the development of motor skill. All these techniques for changing coordination need a larger evidence base to support widespread use in clinical practice.

Other new intervention techniques based on motor control theory and collaborations between engineering and neuroscientists are just beginning to receive experimental study. The reader should keep current with the literature on topics such as the use of robotic devices to assist with movement practice[364] and to manipulate the feedback the person receives with the aim of provoking greater motivation to move,[57] the use of virtual reality devices to manipulate sensory input during motor control,[63,88,539] and functional electrical stimulation or EMG biofeedback used during cycling or other types of movements.[330,362]

Research concerning the timing and intensity of therapeutic interventions is a final example of applications of motor control research to physical therapy. These issues of intervention are at a beginning level of theoretic research at this time. From a motor control perspective, Palisano and Murr[382] suggested that therapists should consider the child's readiness for activity and participation, perhaps related to a critical period for development of a particular motor behavior, if known, and practice of activity in natural environments versus the need for more time with the therapist. Researchers have demonstrated that parents can be trained to provide practice of movements leading to positive outcomes in motor behaviors.[233,341] Based on the Neuronal Group Selection Theory, Hadders-Algra[212] has suggested that infants with periventricular leukomalacia or white matter deficits need to be assisted at an early age to enlarge the primary neuronal networks. At a later age, these infants begin to demonstrate a problem in selection of the most efficient neuronal activity, perhaps because of problems with sensory processing. Intervention focus should then change to provision of ample opportunities for active practice to improve sensory processing and motor coordination.[471] In relation to older children, Bartlett and Palisano[22] have suggested we examine the multivariate determinants of motor change for children with CP in order to anticipate what areas we should focus on. Use of motor development curves drawn for different severity levels as designated by the Gross Motor Function Classification System, based on follow-up of children with CP age 1 to 21 years, potentially could assist with determination of specific intervention issues that should be the focus of treatment.[220,418] It has been our experience that intensity of intervention varies dependent on the setting the child is seen in (Early Intervention Program, School, Private Clinic, Hospital) from monitoring monthly to more intensive intervention recommended for short periods of time such as after surgery or within special programs such as constraint-induced movement therapy. Reasons for the selection of intervention intensity seem unclear and may reflect reimbursement agencies rules and regulations. Based on the motor control and motor learning literature, it can be hypothesized that a greater intensity of intervention from a therapist might be more beneficial during the early learning of a motor skill than while the skill is routinely practiced to consolidate the skill and refine coordination. From this perspective, Trahan and Malouin[502] examined the effects of an intensive intervention (four times a week for 4 weeks) alternating with 8-week periods without physical therapy over a total 6-month period. In their small sample of young (mean age 22.6 months) children with CP at Gross Motor Function Classification System levels IV and V, gains made during the intensive therapy were maintained over the longer periods without intervention. They hypothesized that this regimen may optimize motor training.

Application of Motor Control Theory to a Clinical Example

With the close of this chapter, we will again consider the 20-month-old child with spastic diplegic CP, Gross Motor Function Classification System level III, who is an emerging walker eagerly attempting to reach for a bright shiny toy with one hand while standing and holding on to a small piece of furniture with the other hand. Employing the model in Figure 3-17, *B*, and Figure 3-18, the goal is to remain standing while reaching for the toy. The systems can be reviewed first from a developmental perspective, based on the infant's age, size, and maturation of motor ability. The musculoskeletal system will contribute biomechanical variables such as a relatively high center of gravity resulting in a greater sway frequency (see the section on Musculoskeletal System Variables under Postural Control) and produce responses limited by a small and relatively undeveloped lever system at the leg-ankle-foot for generating force against the floor.[345] Because the infant is a new walker and has little experience, the central set will have limited predictive capacity and few anticipatory strategies from which to generate a plan for minimizing a shift in center of mass as the reach is initiated. Thus, the central set may be viewed as a limiting system in this task. Given limited predictive skills, environmental adaptations may only generate feedback strategies for correcting postural perturbations creating demands on attention that reduce the infant's attention to other tasks or interests. Because the infant has several months of experience in a gravitational environment, perception of orientation is not likely to be a limiting system in this task. The infant will likely rely almost exclusively on vision to control his or her posture because sensory interaction, also a limiting system, will not yet have determined how to adjust the relative dominance of each contributing sensory system. Because of biomechanical variables (faster sway and shorter distance to the limits of stability) and a dependence on feedback rather than feedforward correction strategies, the timing or sequencing of ankle (sensorimotor) strategies may not be sufficiently effective or reliable to correct posture before the infant sways to the limits of stability. The presence of spasticity may also hamper the emergence of more coordinated patterns. In this case, sensorimotor strategies may select to stabilize posture by increasing stiffness about the ankle (e.g., co-contracting antagonist ankle muscles) or to prepare to break a fall by selecting a directionally appropriate protective extension response. All of this will affect the child's ability to use the arm and hand to reach for and grasp the toy.

In contrast to hypothetical interpretations, immature motor skills or actions have typically been viewed as indicative of a nervous system not yet able to execute adaptive, coordinated motor commands. If one embraces multifactorial assumptions of motor control, however, immature motor actions may also be viewed as adaptive strategies to cope with inherent immaturity in one or more contributing systems. The failure to see a motor pattern associated with more mature responses need not mean that it cannot be produced by sensorimotor strategies; rather, the pattern may be potentially available but not emitted because other contributing systems cannot support it. Immature motor actions may also be the emergent consequences of biomechanical or other environmental constraints and affordances that contribute forces or cues and shape the movement differently as it is executed through a physical space or movement context. Studies by Thelen and colleagues provide a wide range of examples describing how infant kicking is altered with changes in biomechanics and environmental characteristics.[491]

When the presence of the infant's neural lesion (spastic diplegia) is added to the systems model analysis, consideration must also be given to the various direct and indirect effects of the lesion, including disuse, on each contributing system. Attempting to reach for the toy, the infant rises up on his toes, the heels seldom in contact with the ground, reducing the effectiveness of an ankle strategy and increasing the likelihood of a hip strategy for correcting postural sway. In this instance, in addition to the contributions of normal rate-limiting systems, weakness and changes in compliance of leg muscles further diminish the effectiveness of the postural lever system. Given the state of other systems, sensorimotor strategies may select to activate extensor muscles excessively in an effort to control posture for a number of possible reasons. For example, the extensor posture may keep the center of mass forward within a new cone of stability that is biomechanically more advantageous than if the center of mass shifts posteriorly; if the center of mass shifts posteriorly, strength or timing of the anterior postural synergy may not be sufficient to make a correcting anterior adjustment in posture. Another possible reason for selection of the extensor synergy may be to reduce the number of degrees of freedom and enhance stiffness where phasing or

force generation of muscle is insufficient. Because each system's participation is viewed as being organized around a specific task, even atypical motor behaviors can be interpreted as being the patient's current solution for attempting to achieve a goal.[317,323]

If we focus on the child's attempts to reach and grasp the toy, we would need to consider the internal and external factors that might be affecting the movements. Internally, the child's potential difficulty with postural control may not be allowing the child to reach out far away from his body. Also, he may not have had extensive practice with reaching, which is thought to relate to reach development, therefore he may show immature movement patterns as a result. The fact that he is visually regarding the toy and expressing interest in acquiring the toy facilitates the use of extensive practice with reaching when the child's body is supported as well as challenging his reaching when greater postural control is required.[233] Externally, the size and placement of the toy in relation to the child may not be facilitating success with the reach/grasp pattern that the child can produce. This can be varied to create a need for unimanual or bimanual reach/grasp. For grasping the child may have difficulty opening the hands sufficiently to grasp the toy and therefore may become frustrated with his attempts and lose interest in obtaining the toy. Use of easily grasped toys can be of assistance or "sticky" mitts can be used to encourage success with practice.[342]

According to the systems model, each contributing system is also influenced by the function of all other systems. Thus, another implication of the model is that if function of one or more systems is altered by a pathologic process, other systems will be altered as well. Similarly, if these systems have not fully matured at the time a pathologic process occurs, maturational processes of any or all systems may be seriously altered. Another implication for intervention is the need to anticipate both the direct and indirect effects of a pathologic process on each contributing system. For example, a lesion affecting the musculoskeletal system may result in a significantly reduced level of activity, practice, and variety of experiences necessary for maturation of the central set or any other contributing systems.

Given the outcome of the analysis of this child's difficulty with postural stability and reaching, specific interventions could be applied to improve impairments in force production capability (strengthening exercises, movement practice, etc.),[427] postural control (practice of recovery of postural control after perturbations[454,532] or active movement under a variety of sensory conditions), hypertonicity (handling techniques, AFOs, drug therapies), potential development of contractures (positioning, stretching, AFOs, etc.), and to improve functional ability through movement practice (treadmill training, active practice of skills in varied environments and tasks with varied feedback, etc.).

As one becomes discontented with the current state of knowledge, experience, or practice, it is difficult to not be somewhat frustrated and critical. Criticism of accepted practices may create the impression that the current state of affairs, in this case clinical practice, is not advancing fast enough. Such is not necessarily the case or necessarily the view of those generating the criticism. As discussed previously in this chapter, maturational-based views and approaches to practice have experienced considerable criticism. As research in motor control continues to advance, however, maturational-based approaches to treatment have also undergone modification by their creators,[43] a point not always appreciated by either the practitioners or critics of maturational-based views.[357] Yet for the profession to grow, it seems that study of specifically described interventions rather than using umbrella terms would provide the best direction for ultimate improvement in effectiveness studies. Future motor control research and efforts to link it with practice may even lead to preservation of some treatment approaches currently under scrutiny, but advances in knowledge may also suggest different reasons or different expected outcomes from those previously proposed.[458] A uniquely specified "motor control theory" does not exist; thus, it is illogical to say there is a motor control approach to examination or treatment. There is, however, a dynamic disciplinary field of motor control research that offers opportunities to develop, test, and thoughtfully critique assumptions underlying physical therapy practice and potentially lead to the development of new assessments and interventions.

SUMMARY

In this chapter, we described motor control theoretic information and processes as related to development of motor behaviors in children with and without motor disabilities. Using current research findings, several specific motor behaviors—locomotion, postural control, reaching, and grasping—were highlighted. Applications of motor control principles to the physical therapy management of children with motor disabilities were suggested in terms of examination options and intervention strategies.

REFERENCES

1. Abbruzzese, G., & Berardelli, A. (2003). Sensorimotor integration in movement disorders. *Movement Disorders, 18,* 231–240.
2. Adams, J. A. (1971). A closed-loop theory of motor learning. *Journal of Motor Behavior, 3,* 111–149.
3. Adde, L., Rygg, M., Lossius, K., et al. (2007). General movement assessment: predicting cerebral palsy in clinical practise. *Early Human Development, 83*(1), 13–18.
4. Adkins, D. L., Boychuk, J., Remple, M. S., & Kleim, J. A. (2006). Motor training induces experience-specific patterns of plasticity across motor cortex and spinal cord. *Journal of Applied Physiology, 101,* 1776–1782.
5. Adolph, K. E., & Berger, S. E. (2007). Learning and development in infant locomotion. *Progress in Brain Research, 164,* 237–255.
6. Adolph, K. E., Robinson, S. R., Young, J. W., & Gill-Alvarez F. (2008). What is the shape of developmental change? *Psychological Review, 115,* 527–543.
7. Adolph, K. E. (2008). Learning to move. *Current Directions in Psychological Science: A Journal of the American Psychological Society, 17*(3), 213–218.
8. Allison, L. K., Kiemel, T., & Jeka, J. J. (2006). Multisensory reweighting of vision and touch is intact in healthy and fall-prone older adults. *Experimental Brain Research, 175,* 342–352.
9. Amazeen, P. G. (2002). Is dynamics the content of a generalized motor program for rhythmic interlimb coordination? *Journal of Motor Behavior, 34,* 233–251.
10. Arndt, S. W., Chandler, L. S., Sweeney, J. K., Sharkey, M. A., & McElroy, J. J. (2008). Effects of a neurodevelopmental treatment-based trunk protocol for infants with posture and movement dysfunction. *Pediatric Physical Therapy, 20,* 11–22.
11. Aruin, A. S., & Almeida, G. L. (1997). A coactivation strategy in anticipatory postural adjustments in persons with Down syndrome. *Motor Control, 1,* 178–191.
12. Aruin, A. S. (2003). The effect of changes in the body configuration on anticipatory postural adjustments. *Motor Control, 7,* 264–277.
13. Asaka, T., Wang, Y., Fukushima, J., & Latash, M. L. (2008). Learning effects on muscle modes and multi-mode postural synergies. *Experimental Brain Research, 184,* 323–338.
14. Asanuma, H., & Keller, A. (1991). Neuronal mechanisms of motor learning in mammals. *Neuroreport, 2,* 217–224.
15. Assaiante, C., Mallau, S., Viel, S., Jover, M., & Schmitz, C. (2005). Development of postural control in healthy children: A functional approach. *Neural Plasticity, 12*(2–3), 109–118; discussion 263–272.
16. Assaiante, C., Woollacott, M., & Amblard, B. (2000). Development of postural adjustment during gait initiation: Kinematic and EMG analysis. *Journal of Motor Behavior, 32,* 211–226.
17. von Aufschnaiter, D. (1992). Vojta: A neurophysiological treatment. In H. Forssberg & H. Hirschfeld (Eds.). *Movement disorders in children, medicine and sport science* (Vol. 36, pp. 7–15). Basel: Karger.
18. Ayres, A. J. (1989). *Sensory integration and praxis tests.* Los Angeles: Western Psychological Services.
19. Bair, W. N., Kiemel, T., Jeka, J. J., & Clark, J. E. (2007). Development of multisensory reweighting for posture control in children. *Experimental Brain Research, 183,* 435–446.
20. Barela, J. A., Jeka, J. J., & Clark, J. E. (2003). Postural control in children: Coupling to dynamic somatosensory information. *Experimental Brain Research, 150,* 434–442.
21. Barrett, T. M., Traupman, E., & Needham, A. (2008). Infants' visual anticipation of object structure in grasp planning. *Infant Behavior & Development 31*(1), 1–9.

22. Bartlett, D. J., & Palisano, R. J. (2000). A multivariate model of determinants of motor change for children with cerebral palsy. *Physical Therapy, 80,* 598–614.

23. Bartscherer, M. L., & Dole, R. L. (2005). Interactive Metronome1 training for a 9-year-old boy with attention and motor coordination difficulties. *Physiotherapy Theory and Practice, 21*(4), 257–269.

24. Bayley, N. (1969). *Bayley scales of infant development.* New York: Psychological Corporation.

25. Beer, R. D. (2009). Beyond control: The dynamics of brain-body-environment interaction in motor systems. *Advances in Experimental Medicine and Biology, 629,* 7–24.

26. Behrman, A. L., Nair, P. M., Bowden, M. G., et al. (2008). Locomotor training restores walking in a nonambulatory child with chronic, severe, incomplete cervical spinal cord injury. *Physical Therapy, 88*(5), 580–590, Epub Mar 6.

27. Bekoff, A., & Lau, B. (1980). Interlimb coordination in 20-day rat fetuses. *Journal of Experimental Zoology, 214,* 173–175.

28. Bennett, S. J., Elliot, D., Weeks, D. J., & Keil, D. (2003). The effects of intermittent vision on prehension under binocular and monocular viewing. *Motor Control, 7,* 46–56.

29. Bergmeier, S. A. (1992). An investigation of reaching in the neonate. *Pediatric Physical Therapy, 4,* 3–11.

30. Bernabucci, I., Conforto, S., Capozza, M., Accornero, N., Schmid, M., & D'Alessio T. (2007). A biologically inspired neural network controller for ballistic arm movements. *Journal of Neuroengineering and Rehabilitation, 3,* 4, 33.

31. Bernstein, N. (1967). *The coordination and regulation of movements.* London: Pergamon.

32. Bertenthal, B. I., Rose, J. L., & Bai, D. L. (1997). Perception-action coupling in the development of visual control of posture. *Journal of Experimental Psychology: Human Perception and Performance, 23*(6), 1631–1643.

33. Berthier, N. E. & R. Keen, R. (2006). Development of reaching in infancy. *Experimental Brain Research, 169*(4), 507–518.

34. Bhat, A. N., & Galloway, J. C. (2006). Toy-oriented changes during early arm movements: Hand kinematics. *Infant Behavior & Development, 29*(3), 358–372.

35. Bhat, A. N., & Galloway, J. C. (2007). Toy-oriented changes in early arm movements III: Constraints on joint kinematics. *Infant Behavior & Development, 30*(3), 515–522.

36. Bhat, A. N., Lee, H. M., & Galloway, J. C. (2007). Toy-oriented changes in early arm movements II–joint kinematics. *Infant Behavior & Development, 30*(2), 307–324.

37. Bizzi, E., Mussa-Ivaldi, F. A., & Gisler, S. (1991). Computations underlying the execution of movement: A biological perspective. *Science, 253,* 287–291.

38. Bjornson, K. F., Graubert, C. S., Buford, V. L., & McLaughlin, J. (1997). Validity of the gross motor function measure. *Pediatric Physical Therapy, 10,* 43–47.

39. Black, D. P., Smith, B. A., Wu, J., & Ulrich, B. D. (2007). Uncontrolled manifold analysis of segmental angle variability during walking: Preadolescents with and without Down syndrome. *Experimental Brain Research, 183*(4), 511–521.

40. Black, D., Chang, C. L., Kubo, M., Holt, K., & Ulrich, B. (2009). Developmental trajectory of dynamic resource utilization during walking: toddlers with and without Down syndrome. *Human Movement Science, 28*(1), 141–154.

41. Blanchard, Y., Neilan, E., Busanich, J., Garavuso, L., & Klimas, D. (2004). Interrater reliability of early intervention providers scoring the Alberta Infant Motor Scale. *Pediatric Physical Therapy, 16,* 13–18.

42. Blundell, S. W., Shepherd, R. B., Dean, C. M., Adams, R. D., & Cahill, B. M. (2003). Functional strength training in cerebral palsy: A pilot study of a group circuit training class for children aged 4–8 years. *Clinical Rehabilitation, 17,* 48–57.

43. Bobath, K., & Bobath, B. (1984). The neuro-developmental treatment. *Clinics in Developmental Medicine, 90,* 6–18.

44. Bodkin, A. W., Baxter, R. S., & Heriza, C. B. (2003). Treadmill training for an infant born preterm with a grade III intraventricular hemorrhage. *Physical Therapy, 83,* 1107–1118.

45. Bollea, L., Rosa, G. D., Gisondi, A., et al. (2007). Recovery from hemiparesis and unilateral spatial neglect after neonatal stroke: Case report and rehabilitation of an infant. *Brain Injury, 21*(1), 81–91.

46. Bonnot, A., Whelan, P. J., Mentis, G. Z., & O'Donovan, M. J. (2002). Locomotor-like activity generated by the neonatal mouse spinal cord. *Brain Research Review, 40,* 141–151.

47. Boyce, W., Gowland, C., Hardy, S., et al. (1991). Development of a quality of movement measure for children with cerebral palsy. *Physical Therapy, 71,* 820–832.

48. Boyce, W., Gowland, C., Rosenbaum, P. L., et al. (1995). The Gross Motor Performance Measure: Validity and responsiveness of a measure of quality of movement. *Physical Therapy, 75,* 603–613.

49. Bradley, N. S., & Bekoff, A. (1990). Development of coordinated movement in chicks: I. Temporal analysis of hindlimb muscle synergies at embryonic days 9 and 10. *Developmental Psychobiology, 23,* 763–782.

50. Bradley, N. S., & Bekoff, A. (1989). Development of locomotion: animal models. In M. Woollacott & A. Shumway-Cook (Eds.), *The development of posture and gait across the lifespan* (pp. 48–73). Columbia: University of South Carolina Press.

51. Bradley, N. S., & Smith, J. L. (1988). Neuromuscular patterns of stereotypic hindlimb behaviors in the first two postnatal months. I. Stepping in normal kittens. *Developmental Brain Research, 38,* 37–52.

52. Bradley, N. S. (2003). Connecting the dots between animal and human studies of locomotion. Focus on "Infants adapt their stepping to repeated trip-inducing stimuli." *Journal of Neurophysiology, 90,* 2088–2089.

53. Bradley, N. S. (1992). What are the principles of motor development? In H. Forssberg & H. Hirschfeld (Eds.), *Movement disorders in children, medicine and sport science* (Vol. 36, pp. 41–49). Basel: Karger.

54. Brady, K., & Garcia, T. (2009). Constraint-induced movement therapy (CIMT), Pediatric applications. *Developmental Disabilities Research Reviews, 15*(2), 102–111.

55. Branchereau, P., Morin, D., Bonnot, A., Ballion, B., Chapron, J., & Viala, D. (2000). Development of lumbar rhythmic networks: from embryonic to neonate locomotor-like patterns in the mouse. *Brain Research Bulletin, 53,* 711–718.

56. Breniere, Y., & Bril, B. (1998). Development of postural control of gravity forces in children during the first 5 years of walking. *Experimental Brain Research, 121,* 3, 255–262.

57. Brewer, B. R., Klatzky, R., Markham, H., & Matsuoka, Y. (2009). Investigation of goal change to optimize upper-extremity motor performance in a robotic environment. *Developmental Medicine and Child Neurology, 51*(Suppl 4), 146–153.

58. Brogen, E., Forssberg, H., & Hadders-Algra, M. (2001). Influence of two different sitting positions on postural adjustments in children with spastic diplegia. *Developmental Medicine and Child Neurology, 43,* 534–546.

59. Brogen, E., Hadders-Algra, M. & Forssberg, H. (1998). Postural control in sitting children with cerebral palsy. *Neuroscience and Biobehavioral Reviews, 22,* 591–596.

60. Reference deleted in page proofs.

61. Bruggink, J. L., Cioni, G., Einspieler, C., Maathuis, C. G., Pascale, R., & Bos, A. F. (2009). Early motor repertoire is related to level of self-mobility in children with cerebral palsy at school age. *Developmental Medicine and Child Neurology, 51*(11), 878–885.

62. Brunnstrom, S. (1970). *Movement therapy in hemiplegia.* New York: Harper & Row.

63. Bryanton, C., Boss, J., Brien, M., McLean, J., McCormick, A., & Sveistrup, H. (2006). Feasibility, motivation, and selective motor control: Virtual reality compared to conventional home exercise in children with cerebral palsy. *Cyberpsychology & Behavior, 9*(2), 123–128.

64. Bundy, A. C., & Fisher, A. G. (1992). Evaluation of sensory integration dysfunction. In H. Forssberg & H. Hirschfeld (Eds.), *Movement disorders in children, medicine and sport science,* (Vol. 36, pp. 272–277). Basel: Karger.

65. Burleigh, A., & Horak, F. (1996). Influence of instruction, prediction, and afferent sensory information on the postural organization of step initiation. *Journal of Neurophysiology, 75,* 1619–1627.

66. Burtner, P. A., Qualls, C., & Woollacott, M. H. (1998). Muscle activation characteristics of stance balance control in children with spastic cerebral palsy. *Gait and Posture, 8,* 163–174.

67. Burtner, P. A., Woollacott, M. H., & Qualls, C. (1999). Stance balance control with orthoses in a group of children with spastic cerebral palsy. *Developmental Medicine and Child Neurology, 41,* 748–757.

68. Butt, S. J., Lebret, J. M., & Kiehn, O. (2002). Organization of left-right coordination in the mammalian locomotor network. *Brain Research and Brain Research Review, 40,* 107–117.

69. Butterworth, G., & Hicks, L. (1977). Visual proprioception and postural stability in infancy. A developmental study. *Perception, 6*(3), 255–262.

70. Butterworth, G., & Hicks, L. (1977). Visual proprioception and postural stability in infancy. A developmental study. *Perception, 6,* 255–262.

71. Cadoret, G., & Beuter, A. (1994). Early development of reaching in Down syndrome infants. *Early Human Development 36*(3), 157–173.

72. Cameron, E. C., Maehle, V. (2006). Comparison of active motor items in infants born preterm and infants born full term. *Pediatric Physical Therapy, 18*(3), 197–203.

73. Carr, J. H., & Shepherd, R. B. (1998). *Neurologic rehabilitation: Optimizing motor performance.* Oxford: Butterworth and Heinemann.

73a. Carson, R. G., & Riek, S. (2001). Changes in muscle recruitment patterns during skill acquisition. *Experimental Brain Research, 138,* 71–87.

74. Carvalho, R. P., E. Tudella, & Savelsbergh, G. J. (2007). Spatio-temporal parameters in infant's reaching movements are influenced by body orientation. *Infant Behavior & Development, 30*(1), 26–35.

75. Carvalho, R. P., Tudella, E., Caljouw, S. R., et al. (2008). Early control of reaching: effects of experience and body orientation. *Infant Behavior & Development, 31*(1), 23–33.

76. Cenciarini, M., & Peterka, R. J. (2006). Stimulus-dependent changes in the vestibular contribution to human postural control. *Journal of Neurophysiology, 95*(5), 2733–2750, Epub, Feb 8.

77. Cesari, P., & Newell, K. M. (2002). Scaling the components of prehension. *Motor Control, 6,* 347–365.

78. Cesari, P., & Newell, K. M. (2000). The body scaling of grip configurations in children aged 6–12 years. *Developmental Psychobiology, 36,* 301–310.

79. Cesari, P., & Newell, K. M. (1999). The scaling of human grip configurations. *Journal of Experimental Psychology: Human Perception and Performance, 25,* 927–935.

80. Chambers, S. H., Bradley, N. S., & Orosz, M. D. (1995). Kinematic analysis of wing and leg movements for type I motility in E9 chick embryos. *Experimental Brain Research, 103,* 218–226.

81. Chandler, L. S., Andrews, M. S., & Swanson, M. W. (1980). *Movement assessment of infants.* Rolling Bay, WA: Chandler, Andrews, & Swanson.

82. Chang, C. L., Kubo, M., & Ulrich, B. D. (2009). Emergence of neuromuscular patterns during walking in toddlers with typical development and with Down syndrome. *Human Movement Science, 28*(2), 283–296.

83. Charles, J., & Gordon, A. M. (2005). A critical review of constraint-induced movement therapy and forced use in children with hemiplegia. *Neural Plasticity, 12*(2–3), 245–261; discussion, 263–272.

84. Charles, J., & Gordon, A. M. (2006). Development of hand-arm bimanual intensive training (HABIT) for improving bimanual coordination in children with hemiplegic cerebral palsy. *Developmental Medicine and Child Neurology, 48*(11), 931–936.

85. Charles, J. R., & Gordon, A. M. (2007). A repeated course of constraint-induced movement therapy results in further improvement. *Developmental Medicine and Child Neurology, 49*(10), 770–773.

86. Charles, J. R., Wolf, S. L., Schneider, J. A., & Gordon, A. M. (2006). Efficacy of a child-friendly form of constraint-induced movement therapy in hemiplegic cerebral palsy: A randomized control trial. *Developmental Medicine and Child Neurology, 48*(8), 635–642.

87. Charles, J., Lavinder, G., & Gordan, A. (2001). Effects of constraint-induced therapy on hand function in children with hemiplegic cerebral palsy. *Pediatric Physical Therapy, 13*, 68–76.

88. Chen, J., & Woollacott, M. H. (2007). Lower extremity kinetics for balance control in children with cerebral palsy. *Journal of Motor Behavior, 39*(4), 306–316.

89. Chen, L. C., Metcalfe, J. S., Chang, T. Y., Jeka, J. J., & Clark, J. E. (2008). The development of infant upright posture: sway less or sway differently? *Experimental Brain Research, 186*, 293–303.

90. Chen, L. C., Metcalfe, J. S., Jeka, J. J., & Clark, J. E. (2007). Two steps forward and one back: Learning to walk affects infants' sitting posture. *Infant Behavior & Development, 30*, 16–25.

91. Cherng, R. J., Chen, J. J., & Su, F. C. (2001). Vestibular system in performance of standing balance of children and young adults under altered sensory conditions. *Perceptual and Motor Skills, 92*(3 Pt 2), 1167–1179.

92. Cheron, G., Bengoetxea, A., Bouillot, E., Lacquaniti, F., & Dan, B. (2001). Early emergence of temporal co-ordination of lower limb segments elevation angles in human locomotion. *Neuroscience Letters, 308*, 123–127.

93. Chiel, H., & Beer, A. R. (1997). The brain has a body: Adaptive behavior emerges from interactions of nervous system, body and environment. *Trends in Neuroscience, 20*, 553–557.

94. Clifton, R. K., Muir, D. W., Ashmead, D. H., & Clarkson, M. G. (1993). Is visually guided reaching in early infancy a myth? *Child Development, 64*, 1099–1110.

95. Coker, P., Lebkicher, C., Harris, L., & Snape, J. (2009). The effects of constraint-induced movement therapy for a child less than one year of age. *NeuroRehabilitation, 24*(3), 199–208.

96. Connolly, K. (1977). The nature of motor skill development. *Journal of Human Movement Studies, 3*, 128–143.

97. Corbetta, D., & Thelen, E. (1994). Shifting patterns of inter-limb coordination in infants' reaching: A case study. In S. P. Swinnen, H. Heuer, J. Massion, & P. Casaer (Eds.), *Interlimb coordination: Neural, dynamical, and cognitive constraints* (pp. 413–438). San Diego, CA: Academic Press.

98. Corbetta, D., & W. Snapp-Childs (2009). Seeing and touching: The role of sensory-motor experience on the development of infant reaching. *Infant Behavior & Development 32*(1), 44–58.

99. Cosper, S. M., Lee, G. P., Peters, S. B., & Bishop E. (2009). Interactive Metronome training in children with attention deficit and developmental coordination disorders. *International Journal of Rehabilitation Research, 32*(4), 331–336.

100. Crocker, M. D., MacKay-Lyons, M., & McDonnell, E. (1997). Forced use of the upper extremity in cerebral palsy: A single-case design. *American Journal of Occupational Therapy, 51*(10), 824–833.

101. Crocker, M. D., Mackay-Lyons, M., & McDonnell, E. (1997). Forced use of upper extremity in cerebral palsy: A single case design. *American Journal of Occupational Therapy, 51*, 824–833.

101a. Crowe, T., Deitz, J. C., Richardson, P. K., & Atwater, S. W. (1990). Interrater reliability of the Pediatric Clinical Test of Sensory Interaction for Balance. *Physical & Occupational Therapy in Pediatrics, 10*, 31–27.

102. Crutcher, M. D., & Alexander, G. E. (1990). Movement-related neuronal activity selectively coding either direction or muscle pattern in 3 motor areas of the monkey. *Journal of Neurophysiology, 64*, 151–163.

103. d' Avella, A., Saltiel, P., & Bizzi, E. (2003). Combinations of muscle synergies in the construction of a natural motor behavior. *Nature Neuroscience, 6*, 300–308.

104. Damiano, D. L., & DeJong, S. L. (2009). A systematic review of the effectiveness of treadmill training and body weight support in pediatric rehabilitation. *Journal of Neurologic Physical Therapy, 33*(1), 27–44.

105. Damiano, D. L. (2009). Rehabilitative therapies in cerebral palsy: The good, the not so good, and the possible. *Journal of Child Neurology, 24*, 1200–1204.

106. Damiano, D. L., & Abel, M. F. (1998). Functional outcomes of strength training in spastic cerebral palsy. *Archives of Physical Medicine and Rehabilitation, 79*, 119–125.

107. Damiano, D. L., & Abel, M. F. (1996). Relation of gait analysis to gross motor function in cerebral palsy. *Developmental Medicine and Child Neurology, 38*, 389–396.

108. Damiano, D. L., Dodd, K., & Taylor, N. F. (2002). Should we be testing and training muscle strength in cerebral palsy? *Developmental Medicine and Child Neurology, 44*, 68–72.

109. Damiano, D. L., Kelly, L. E., & Vaughan, C. L. (1995a). Effects of a quadriceps femoris strengthening program on crouch gait in children with cerebral palsy. *Physical Therapy, 75*, 658–667.

110. Damiano, D. L., Vaughan, C. L., & Abel, M. F. (1995b). Muscle response to heavy resistance exercise in children with spastic cerebral palsy. *Developmental Medicine and Child Neurology, 37*, 731–739.

111. Darrah, J., Hodge, M., Magill-Evans, J., & Kembhavi, G. (2003). Stability of serial assessments of motor and communication abilities in typically developing infants: Implications for screening. *Early Human Development, 72*(2), 97–110.

112. Darrah, J., Piper, M., & Watt, M. J. (1998). Assessment of gross motor skills of at-risk infants: Predictive validity of the Alberta Infant Motor Scale. *Developmental Medicine and Child Neurology, 40*, 485–491.

113. David, F. J., Baranek, G. T., Giuliani, C. A., et al. (2009). A pilot study: Coordination of precision grip in children and adolescents with high functioning autism. *Pediatric Physical Therapy, 21*(2), 205–211.

114. Davids, J. R., Peace, L. C., Wagner, L. V., Gidewall, M. A., Blackhurst, D. W., & Roberson, W. M. (2006). Validation of

the Shriners Hospital for Children Upper Extremity Evaluation (SHUEE) for children with hemiplegic cerebral palsy. *Journal of Bone and Joint Surgery, 88A*, 326–333.

115. de Bode, S., Mathern, G. W., Bookheimer, S., & Dobkin, B. (2007). Locomotor training remodels fMRI sensorimotor cortical activations in children after cerebral hemispherectomy. *Neurorehabilitation and Neural Repair, 21*(6), 497–508, Epub Mar 16.

116. de Campos, A. C., Rocha, N. A., Savelsbergh, G. J. (2010). Reaching and grasping movements in infants at risk: A review. *Research in Developmental Disabilities, 31*(1),70–80.

117. de Freitas, P. B., Freitas, S. M., Duarte, M., Latash, M. L., & Zatsiorsky, V. M. (2009). Effects of joint immobilization on standing balance. *Human Movement Science, 28*(4), 515–528.

118. de Graaf-Peters, V. B., Blauw-Hospers, C. H., Dirks, T., Baker, H., Bos, A. F., & Hadders-ALgra, M. (2007). Development of postural control in typically developing children and children with cerebral palsy: Possibilities for intervention? *Neuroscience and Biobehavioral Reviews, 31*, 1191–1200.

119. de Graaf-Peters, V. B., Bakker, H., van Eykern, L. A. et al. (2007). Postural adjustments and reaching in 4- and 6-month-old infants: An EMG and kinematical study. *Experimental Brain Research, 181*(4), 647–656.

120. de Vries, J. I., Wimmers, R. H., Ververs, I. A., Hopkins, B., Savelsbergh, G. J., & van Geijn, H. P. (2001). Fetal handedness and head position preference: A developmental study. *Developmental Psychobiology, 39*, 171–178.

121. de Vries, J. I. P., Visser, G. H. A., & Prechtl, H. F. R. (1982). The emergence of fetal behavior: I. Qualitative aspects. *Early Human Development, 7*, 301–322.

122. Deffeyes, J. E., Harbourne, R. T., DeJong, S. L., Kyvelidou, A., Stuberg, W. A., & Stergiou N. (2009). Use of information entropy measures of sitting postural sway to quantify developmental delay in infants. *Journal of Neuroengineering and Rehabilitation, 6*, 34.

123. Deffeyes, J. E., Harbourne, R. T., Kyvelidou A., Stuberg, W. A., & Stergiou N. (2009). Nonlinear analysis of sitting postural sway indicates developmental delay in infants. *Clinical Biomechanics* (Bristol, Avon), *24*(7), 564–570, Epub Jun 2.

124. Deffeyes, J. E., Kochi N., Harbourne, R. T., Kyvelidou A., Stuberg, W. A., & Stergiou, N. (2009). Nonlinear detrended fluctuation analysis of sitting center-of-pressure data as an early measure of motor development pathology in infants. *Nonlinear Dynamics, Psychology, and Life Sciences, 13*(4), 351–368.

125. Deitz, J., Richardson, P. K., Westcott, S. L., & Crowe, T. K. (1996). Performance of children with learning disabilities on the Pediatric Clinical Test of Sensory Interaction for Balance. *Physical & Occupational Therapy in Pediatrics, 16*, 1–21.

126. Deluca, S. C., Echols, K., Law, C. R., & Ramey, S. L. (2006). Intensive pediatric constraint-induced therapy for children with cerebral palsy: randomized, controlled, crossover trial. *Journal of Child Neurology, 21*(11), 931–938.

127. DeLuca, S. C., Echols, K., Ramey, S. L., & Taub, E. (2003). Pediatric constraint-induced movement therapy for a young child with cerebral palsy: Two episodes of care. *Physical Therapy, 83*, 1003–1013.

128. Diedrich, F. J., Highlands, T. M., Spahr, K. A., Thelen, E., & Smith, L. B. (2001). The role of target distinctiveness in infant perseverative reaching. *Journal of Experimental Child Psychology, 78*, 263–290.

129. Dobkin, B. H. (2009). Motor rehabilitation after stroke, traumatic brain, and spinal cord injury: common denominators within recent clinical trials. *Current Opinion in Neurology*, Aug 29 [Epub ahead of print].

130. Donker, S. F., Ledebt, A., Roerdink, M., Savelsbergh, G. J. P., & Beek, P. J. (2008). Children with cerebral palsy exhibit greater and more regular postural sway than typically developing children. *Experimental Brain Research, 184*, 363–370.

131. Drew, T. (1993). Motor cortical activity during voluntary gait modifications in the cat. I. Cells related to the forelimbs. *Journal of Neurophysiology, 70*(1), 179–199.

132. Duran, L. J., & Fisher, A. G. (1996). Male and female performance on the Assessment of Motor Process Skills. *Archives of Physical Medicine and Rehabilitation, 77*, 1019–1024.

133. Eagleton, M., Iams, A., McDowell, J., Morrison, R., & Evans, C. L. (2004). The effects of strength training on gait in adolescents with cerebral palsy. *Pediatric Physical Therapy, 16*, 22–30.

134. Einspieler, C., Cioni, G., Paolicelli, P. B., et al. (2002). The early markers for later dyskinetic cerebral palsy are different from those for spastic cerebral palsy. *Neuropediatrics, 33*, 73–78.

135. Einspieler, C., Prechtl, H. F., Ferrari, F., Cioni, G., & Bos, A. F. (1997). The qualitative assessment of general movements in preterm, term and young infants: Review of the methodology. *Early Human Development, 50*, 47–60.

136. Eliasson, A. C., Krumlinde-Sundholm, L., Shaw, K., & Wang, C. (2005). Effects of constraint-induced movement therapy in young children with hemiplegic cerebral palsy: An adapted model. *Developmental Medicine and Child Neurology, 47*(4), 266–275.

137. Eliasson, A. C., Shaw, K., Ponten, E., Boyd, R., & Krumlinde-Sundholm, L. (2009). Feasibility of a day-camp model of modified constraint-induced movement therapy with and without botulinum toxin A injection for children with hemiplegia. *Physical & Occupational Therapy in Pediatrics, 29*(3), 311–333.

138. Eliasson, A. C., Gordon, A. M., & Forssberg, H. (1991). Basic co-ordination of manipulative forces of children with cerebral palsy. *Developmental Medicine and Child Neurology, 33*, 661–670.

139. Eliasson, A. C., Gordon, A. M., & Forssberg, H. (1992). Impaired anticipatory control of isometric forces during grasping by children with cerebral palsy. *Developmental Medicine and Child Neurology, 34*, 216–225.

140. Eliasson, A. C., Gordon, A. M., & Forssberg, H. (1995). Tactile control of isometric fingertip forces during grasping in children with cerebral palsy. *Developmental Medicine and Child Neurology, 37*, 72–84.

141. Estil, L. B., Ingvaldsen, R. P., & Whiting, H. T. (2002). Spatial and temporal constraints on performance in children with movement co-ordination problems. *Experimental Brain Research, 147,* 153–161.

142. Eyre, J. A., Miller, S., Clowry, G. J., Conway, E. A., & Watts, C. (2000). Functional corticospinal projections are established prenatally in the human foetus permitting involvement in the development of spinal motor centres. *Brain, 123,* 51–64.

143. Eyre, J. A., Taylor, J. P., Villagra, F., Smith, M., & Miller, S. (2001). Evidence of activity dependent withdrawal of cortico-spinal projections during human development. *Neurology, 57,* 1543–1554.

144. Facchin, P., Rosa-Rizzotto, M., Turconi, A. C., et al. (2009). Multisite trial on efficacy of constraint-induced movement therapy in children with hemiplegia: study design and methodology. *American Journal of Physical Medicine & Rehabilitation, 88*(3), 216–230.

145. Fagard, J., & Pezé, A. (1997). Age changes in interlimb coupling and the development of bimanual coordination. *Journal of Motor Behavior, 29,* 199–208.

146. Fagard, J. (1994). Manual strategies and interlimb coordination during reaching, grasping, and manipulating throughout the first year of life. In S. P. Swinnen, H. Heuer, J. Massion, & P. Casaer (Eds.), *Interlimb coordination: Neural, dynamical, and cognitive constraints* (pp. 439–460). San Diego, CA: Academic Press.

147. Fallang, B., Saugstad, O. D., & Hadders-Algra, M. (2000). Goal directed reaching and postural control in supine position in healthy infants. *Behavioral Brain Research, 115,* 9–18.

148. Fallang, B., Saugstad, O. D., Grogaard, J., & Hadders-Algra, M. (2003). Kinematic quality of reaching movements in preterm infants. *Pediatric Research, 53,* 836–842.

149. Fallang, B., & Hadders-Algra, M. (2005). Postural behavior in children born preterm. *Neural Plasticity, 12*(2–3), 175–182; discussion 263–172.

150. Fallang, B., Oien, I., Hellem, E., et al. (2005). Quality of reaching and postural control in young preterm infants is related to neuromotor outcome at 6 years. *Pediatric Research, 58*(2), 347–353.

151. Favilla, M. (2006). Reaching movements in children: Accuracy and reaction time development. *Experimental Brain Research, 169*(1), 122–125.

152. Feldman, A. G., & Levin, M. F. (2009). The equilibrium-point hypothesis—Past, present and future. *Advances in Experimental Medicine and Biology, 629,* 699–726.

153. Feldman, A. G., Ostry, D. J., Levin, M. F., Gribble, P. L., & Mitnitski, A. B. (1998). Recent tests of the equilibrium-point hypothesis (lambda model). *Motor Control, 2,* 189–205.

154. Feldman, A. G. (1986). Once more on the Equilibrium-Point Hypothesis (l model) for motor control. *Journal of Motor Behavior, 18,* 17–54.

155. Ferdjallah, M., Harris, G. F., Smith, P., & Wertsch, J. J. (2002). Analysis of postural control synergies during quiet standing in healthy children and children with cerebral palsy. *Clinical Biomechanics, 17,* 203–210.

156. Fetters, L., & Todd, J. (1987). Quantitative assessment of infant reaching movements. *Journal of Motor Behavior, 19,* 147–166.

157. Field, J. (1977). Coordination of vision and prehension in young infants. *Child Development, 48,* 97–103.

158. Fingerhut, P., Madill, H., Darrah, J., Hodge, M., & Warren, S. (2002). Classroom-based assessment: Validation for the school AMPS. *American Journal of Occupational Therapy, 56*(2), 210–213.

159. Fisher, A. G., & Duran, G. A. (2004). Schoolwork task performance of students at risk of delays. *Scandinavian Journal of Occupational Therapy, 11,* 1–8.

160. Fisher, A. G., Bryze, K., & Atchison, B. T. (2000). Naturalistic assessment of functional performance in school settings: Reliability and validity of the school AMPS scales. *Journal of Outcome Measurements, 4,* 491–512.

161. Fisher, A. G. (1994). Development of a functional assessment that adjusts ability measures for task simplicity and rater leniency. In M. Wilson (Ed.), *Objective measurement: Theory into practice* (Vol. 2., pp. 145–175). Norwood: Ablex.

162. Fitts, P. M. (1954). The information capacity of the human motor system in controlling the amplitude of movement. *Journal of Experimental Psychology, 47,* 381–391.

163. Fogassi, L., Gallese, V., Buccino, G., Craighero, L., Fadiga, L., & Rizzolatti, G. (2001). Cortical mechanism for the visual guidance of hand grasping movements in the monkey: A reversible inactivation study. *Brain, 124,* 571–586.

164. Forssberg, H., & Nashner, L. M. (1982). Ontogenetic development of postural control in man: Adaptation to altered support and visual conditions during stance. *Journal of Neuroscience, 2*(5), 545–552.

165. Forssberg, H., Eliasson, A. C., Kinoshita, H., Johansson, R. S., & Westling, G. (1991). Development of human precision grip. I. Basic coordination of force. *Experimental Brain Research, 85,* 451–457.

166. Forssberg, H., Eliasson, A. C., Kinoshita, H., Westling, G., & Johansson, R. S. (1995). Development of human precision grip. IV. Tactile adaptation of isometric finger forces to the frictional condition. *Experimental Brain Research, 104,* 323–330.

167. Forssberg, H., Kinoshita, H., Eliasson, A. C., Johansson, R. S., Westling, G., & Gordon, A. M. (1992). Development of human precision grip. II. Anticipatory control of isometric forces targeted for object's weight. *Experimental Brain Research, 90,* 393–398.

168. Forssberg, H. (1992). Evolution of plantigrade gait: Is there a neuronal correlate? *Developmental Medicine and Child Neurology, 34,* 920–925.

169. Forssberg, H. (1985). Ontogeny of human locomotor control. I. Infant stepping, supported locomotion and transition to independent locomotion. *Experimental Brain Research, 57,* 480–493.

170. Forsström, A., & von Hofsten, C. (1982). Visually directed reaching of children with motor impairments. *Developmental Medicine and Child Neurology, 24,* 653–661.

171. Foster, E. C., Sveistrup, H., & Woollacott, M. H. (1996). Transitions in visual proprioception: A cross-sectional developmental study of the effect of visual flow on postural control. *Journal of Motor Behavior, 28*, 101–112.

172. Foudriat, B. A., Di Fabio, R. P., & Anderson, J. H. (1993). Sensory organization of balance responses in children 3–6 years of age: A normative study with diagnostic implications. *International Journal of Pediatric Otorhinolaryngology, 27*(3), 255–271.

173. Fowler, E. G., Goldberg, E. J. (2009). The effect of lower extremity selective voluntary motor control on interjoint coordination during gait in children with spastic diplegic cerebral palsy. *Gait Posture, 29*(1), 102–107, Epub 2008 Sep 10.

174. Fowler, E. G., Staudt, L. A., Greenberg, M. B., & Oppenheim, W. L. (2009). Selective Control Assessment of the Lower Extremity (SCALE), development, validation, and interrater reliability of a clinical tool for patients with cerebral palsy. *Developmental Medicine and Child Neurology, 51*(8), 607–614, Epub 2009 Feb 12.

175. Frigo, C., & Crenna, P. (2009). Multichannel SEMG in clinical gait analysis: A review and state-of-the-art. *Clinical Biomechanics* (Bristol, Avon), *24*(3), 236–245.

176. Fuster, J. M. (2000). Executive frontal functions. *Experimental Brain Research, 133*, 66–70.

176a. Gagnon, I., Swaine, B., & Forget, R. (2006). Exploring the comparability of the Sensory Organization Test and the Pediatric Clinical Test of Sensory Interaction for Balance in children. *Phys Occup Ther Pediatr, 26*(1–2), 23–41.

177. Gallistel, C. R. (1980). *The organization of action: A new synthesis.* Hillsdale, NJ: Lawrence Erlbaum Associates.

178. Galloway, J. C., Bhat, A., Heathcock, J. C., et al. (2004). Shoulder and elbow joint power differ as a general feature of vertical arm movements. *Experimental Brain Research, 157*(3), 391–396.

178a. Garner, J., Haas, A., Antone, A., Fenlason, C., Vessey, S., & Westcott, S. L. (2005). Reliability of a new single-rater version of the Pediatr Clinical Test of Sensory Interaction for Balance. *Pediatr Phys Ther, 17*, 68.

179. Geerdink, J. J., Hopkins, B., Beek, W. J., & Heriza, C. B. (1996). The organization of leg movements in preterm and full-term infants after term age. *Developmental Psychobiology, 29*, 335–351.

180. Georgopolous, A. P. (1990). Neurophysiology of reaching. In M. Jeannerod (Ed.), *Attention and performance XIII* (pp. 227–263). Hillsdale, NJ: Lawrence Erlbaum Associates.

181. Ghez, C. (1991). Voluntary movements. In E. R. Kandel, J. H. Schwartz, & T. M. Jessell, (Eds.). *Principles of neuroscience* (3rd ed., pp. 609–625). New York: Elsevier.

182. Gibson, J. J. (1966). *The senses considered as perceptual systems.* Boston: Houghton Mifflin.

183. Gilmore, R., Sakzewski, L., & Boyd, R. (2009). Upper limb activity measures for 5- to 16-year-old children with congenital hemiplegia: A systematic review. *Developmental Medicine and Child Neurology*, Oct 7. [Epub ahead of print].

184. Godoi, D., & Barela, J. A. (2008). Body sway and sensory motor coupling adaptation in children: Effects of distance manipulation. *Developmental Psychobiology, 50*, 77–87.

185. Gomi, H., & Kawato, M. (1996). Equilibrium-point control hypothesis examined by measured arm stiffness during multijoint movement. *Science, 272*, 117–120.

186. Gomi, H., & Kawato, M. (1997). Human arm stiffness and equilibrium-point trajectory during multi-joint movement. *Biological Cybernetics, 76*, 163–171.

187. Goodgold-Edwards, S. A. (1991). Cognitive strategies during coincident timing tasks. *Physical Therapy, 71*, 236–243.

188. Gordon, A., Connelly, A., Neville, B., et al. (2007). Modified constraint-induced movement therapy after childhood stroke. *Developmental Medicine and Child Neurology, 49*(1), 23–27.

189. Gordon, A. M., Charles, J., & Wolf, S. L. (2006). Efficacy of constraint-induced movement therapy on involved upper-extremity use in children with hemiplegic cerebral palsy is not age-dependent. *Pediatrics, 117*(3), e363–e373.

190. Gordon, A. M., Charles, J., & Wolf, S. L. (2005). Methods of constraint-induced movement therapy for children with hemiplegic cerebral palsy: Development of a child-friendly intervention for improving upper-extremity function. *Archives of Physical Medicine and Rehabilitation, 86*(4), 837–844.

191. Gordon, A. M., Chinnan, A., Gill, S., Petra, E., Hung, Y. C., & Charles, J. (2008). Both constraint-induced movement therapy and bimanual training lead to improved performance of upper extremity function in children with hemiplegia. *Developmental Medicine and Child Neurology, 50*(12), 957–958.

192. Gordon, A. M., Schneider, J. A., Chinnan, A., & Charles, J. R. (2007). Efficacy of a hand-arm bimanual intensive therapy (HABIT) in children with hemiplegic cerebral palsy: A randomized control trial. *Developmental Medicine and Child Neurology, 49*(11), 830–838.

193. Gordon, A. M., Forssberg, H., & Iwasaki, N. (1994). Formation and lateralization of internal representations underlying motor commands during precision grip. *Neuropsychologia, 32*, 555–568.

194. Gordon, J. (1987). Assumptions underlying physical therapy intervention: theoretical and historical perspectives. In J. H. Carr, & R. B. Shepherd (Eds.), *Movement science foundations for physical therapy in rehabilitation.* Rockville, MD: Aspen, 1987, pp. 1–30.

195. Goto, S., Fisher, A. G., & Mayberry, W. L. (1996). The assessment of motor and process skills applied cross-culturally to the Japanese. *American Journal of Occupational Therapy, 50*, 798–806.

196. Gottlieb, J., Balan, P., Oristaglio, J., & Suzuki, M. (2009). Parietal control of attentional guidance: The significance of sensory, motivational and motor factors. *Neurobiology of Learning and Memory, 91*(2), 121–128, Epub 2008 Nov 8. Review.

197. Gowland, C., Boyce, W., Wright, V., Russell, D., Goldsmith, C., & Rosenbaum, P. (1995). Reliability of the Gross Motor Performance Measure. *Physical Therapy, 75*, 597–602.

198. Gowland, C., Rosenbaum, P., Hardy, S., et al. (1998). *Gross Motor Performance Measure manual.* Kingston: Queen's University.

199. Granberg, M., Rydberg, A., & Fisher, A. G. (2008). Activities in daily living and schoolwork task performance in children with complex congenital heart disease. *Acta Paediatrica, 97*(9), 1270–1274.

200. Grillner, S. (1996). Neural networks for vertebrate locomotion. *Scientific American, 274,* 64–69.

201. Grove, C. R., & Lazarus, J. A. (2007). Impaired re-weighting of sensory feedback for maintenance of postural control in children with developmental coordination disorder. *Human Movement Science, 26,* 457–476.

202. Guertin, P. A., & Steuer I. (2009). Key central pattern generators of the spinal cord. A review. *Journal of Neuroscience Research, 87*(11), 2399–2405.

203. Guzzetta, A., Mercuri, E., Rapisardi, G., et al. (2003). General movements detect early signs of hemiplegia in term infants with neonatal cerebral infarction. *Neuropediatrics, 34,* 61–66.

204. Haas, G., Diener, H. C., Rapp, H., & Dichgans, J. (1989). Development of feedback and feedforward control of upright stance. *Developmental Medicine and Child Neurology, 31,* 481–488.

205. Hadders-Algra, M., Brogren, E., & Forssberg, H. (1998). Development of postural control: Differences between ventral and dorsal muscles? *Neuroscience and Biobehavioral Reviews, 22*(4), 501–506.

206. Hadders-Algra, M., Brogren, E., & Forssberg, H. (1998). Postural adjustments during sitting at preschool age: Presence of a transient toddling phase. *Developmental Medicine and Child Neurology, 40*(7), 436–447.

207. Hadders-Algra, M. (2005). Development of postural control during the first 18 months of life. *Neural Plasticity, 12,* 99–108.

208. Hadders-Algra, M., & Prechtl, H. F. R. Developmental course of general movements in early infancy. I. (1992). Descriptive analysis of change in form. *Early Human Development, 28,* 201–213.

209. Hadders-Algra, M., Brogren, E., & Forssberg, H. (1996). Ontogeny of postural adjustments during sitting in infancy: variation, selection and modulation. *Journal of Physiology, 493,* 273–288.

210. Hadders-Algra, M., & Groothuis, A. M. C. (1999). Quality of general movements in infancy is related to the development of neurological dysfunction, attention deficit hyperactivity disorder and aggressive behavior. *Developmental Medicine and Child Neurology, 41,* 381–391.

211. Hadders-Algra, M., & van der Fits, I. B. M., Stremmelaar, E. F., & Touwen, B. C. L. (1999). Development of postural adjustments during reaching in infants with CP. *Developmental Medicine and Child Neurology, 41,* 766–776.

212. Hadders-Algra, M. (2001a). Early brain damage and the development of motor behavior in children: Clues for therapeutic intervention? *Neural Plasticity, 8,* 31–49.

213. Hadders-Algra, M. (2001b). Evaluation of motor function in young infants by means of assessment of general movements: A review. *Pediatric Physical Therapy, 13,* 27–36.

214. Hadders-Algra, M. (2000). The Neuronal Group Selection Theory: A framework to explain variation in normal motor development. *Developmental Medicine and Child Neurology, 42,* 566–572.

215. Hadders-Algra, M. (2002). Two distinct forms of minor neurological dysfunction: Perspectives emerging from a review of data of the Groningen Perinatal Project. *Developmental Medicine and Child Neurology, 44,* 561–571.

216. Hadders-Algra, M., van der Fits, I. B., Stremmelaar, E. F., et al. (1999). Development of postural adjustments during reaching in infants with CP. *Developmental Medicine and Child Neurology, 41*(11), 766–776.

217. Haley, S. (1987). Sequence of development of postural reactions by infants with Down syndrome. *Developmental Medicine and Child Neurology, 29,* 674–679.

218. Haley, S. M., Harris, S. R., Tada, W. L., & Swanson, M. W. (1986). Item reliability of the Movement Assessment of Infants. *Physical & Occupational Therapy in Pediatrics, 6*(1), 21–39.

219. Hallemans, A., Dhanis, L., De Clercq, D., & Aerts, P. (2007). Changes in mechanical control of movement during the first 5 months of independent walking: A longitudinal study. *Journal of Motor Behavior, 39*(3), 227–238.

220. Hanna, S. E., Rosenbaum, P. L., Bartlett, D. J., et al. (2009). Stability and decline in gross motor function among children and youth with cerebral palsy aged 2 to 21 years. *Developmental Medicine and Child Neurology, 51*(4), 295–302.

221. Harabst, K. B., Lazarus, J. A., & Whitall, J. (2000). Accuracy of dynamic isometric force production: The influence of age and bimanual activation patterns. *Motor Control, 4,* 232–256.

222. Harbourne, R. T., Deffeyes, J. E., Kyvelidou, A., & Stergiou, N. (2009). Complexity of postural control in infants: Linear and nonlinear features revealed by principal component analysis. *Nonlinear Dynamics, Psychology, and Life Sciences, 13*(1), 123–144.

223. Harbourne, R. T., & Stergiou, N. (2009). Movement variability and the use of nonlinear tools: principles to guide physical therapist practice. *Physical Therapy, 89,* 267–282.

224. Harbourne, R. T., & Stergiou, N. (2003). Nonlinear analysis of the development of sitting postural control. *Developmental Psychobiology, 42,* 368–377.

225. Harbourne, R. T., Giuliani, C., & Mac Neela, J. (1993). A kinematic and electromyographic analysis of the development of sitting posture in infants. *Developmental Psychobiology, 26,* 51–64.

226. Harris, S. R. (1987). Early detection of cerebral palsy: Sensitivity and specificity of two motor assessment tools. *Journal of Perinatology, 7,* 11–15.

227. Hasan, Z. (1986). Optimized movement trajectories and joint stiffness in unperturbed, inertially loaded movements. *Biological Cybernetics, 53,* 373–382.

228. Hatzitaki, V., Zisi, V., Kollias, I., & Kioumourtzoglou, E. (2002). Perceptual-motor contributions to static and dynamic balance control in children. *Journal of Motor Behavior, 34,* 161–170.

229. Hay, L., & Redon, C. (2001). Development of postural adaptation to arm raising. *Experimental Brain Research, 139,* 224–232.

230. Hay, L., Fleury, M., Bard, C., & Teasdale, N. (1994). Resolving power of the perceptual and sensorimotor systems in 6- to 10-year-old children. *Journal of Motor Behavior, 26,* 36–42.

231. Hay, L. (1979). Spatial-temporal analysis of movements in children: Motor programs versus feedback in the development of reaching. *Journal of Motor Behavior, 11,* 188–200.

232. Heathcock, J. C., Bhat, A. N., Lobo, M. A., & Galloway J. (2005). The relative kicking frequency of infants born full-term and preterm during learning and short-term and long-term memory periods of the mobile paradigm. *Physical Therapy, 85,* 8–18.

233. Heathcock, J. C., Lobo, M., & Galloway, J. C. (2008). Movement training advances the emergence of reaching in infants born at less than 33 weeks of gestational age: A randomized clinical trial. *Physical Therapy, 88*(3), 310–322.

234. Hedberg, A., Carlberg, E. B., Forssberg, H., & Hadders-Algra, M. (2005). Development of postural adjustments in sitting position during the first half year of life. *Developmental Medicine and Child Neurology, 47,* 312–320.

235. Hedberg, A., Forssberg, H., & Hadders-Algra, M. (2004). Postural adjustments due to external perturbations during sitting in 1-month-old infants: Evidence for the innate origin of direction specificity. *Experimental Brain Research, 157,* 10–17.

236. Hedberg, A., Schmitz, C., Forssberg, H., & Hadders-Algra, M. (2007). Early development of postural adjustments in standing with and without support. *Experimental Brain Research, 178,* 439–449.

237. Heriza, C. B. (1988). Comparison of leg movements in preterm infants at term with healthy full-term infants. *Physical Therapy, 68,* 1687–1693.

238. Hirschfeld, H., & Forssberg, H. (1991). Phase-dependent modulations of anticipatory postural activity during human locomotion. *Journal of Neurophysiology, 66*(1), 12–19.

239. Hirschfeld, H., & Forssberg, H. (1992). Phase-dependent modulations of anticipatory postural adjustments during locomotion in children. *Journal of Neurophysiology, 68,* 542–550.

240. Hirschfeld, H. (2007). Motor control of every day motor tasks: Guidance for neurological rehabilitation. *Physiology & Behavior, 92*(1–2), 161–166.

241. Hirschfeld, H., & Forssberg, H. (1994). Epigenetic development of postural responses for sitting during infancy. *Experimental Brain Research, 97,* 528–540.

242. Hoare, B., Imms, C., Carey, L., & Wasiak, J. (2007). Constraint-induced movement therapy in the treatment of the upper limb in children with hemiplegic cerebral palsy: A Cochrane systematic review. *Clinical Rehabilitation, 21*(8), 675–685.

243. Hodapp, M., Vry, J., Mall, V., & Faist, M. (2009). Changes in soleus H-reflex modulation after treadmill training in children with cerebral palsy. *Brain, 132*(Pt 1), 37–44.

244. von Hofsten, C., & Fazel-Zandy, S. (1984). Development of visually guided hand orientation in reaching. *Journal of Experimental Child Psychology, 38,* 208–219.

245. von Hofsten, C., & Rönnqvist, L. (1988). Preparation for grasping an object: A developmental study. *Journal of Experimental Psychology: Human Perception and Performance, 14,* 610–621.

246. von Hofsten, C., & Rönnqvist, L. (1993). The structuring of neonatal arm movements. *Child Development, 64,* 1046–1057.

247. von Hofsten, C. (1990). A perception-action perspective on the development of manual movements. In M. Jeannerod (Ed.), *Attention and performance XIII* (pp. 739–762). Hillsdale, NJ: Lawrence Erlbaum Associates.

248. von Hofsten, C. (1979). Development of visually guided reaching: The approach phase. *Journal of Human Movement Studies, 5,* 160–178.

249. von Hofsten, C. (1984). Developmental changes in the organization of prereaching movements. *Developmental Psychology, 20,* 378–388.

250. von Hofsten, C. (1982). Eye-hand coordination in the newborn. *Developmental Psychology, 18,* 450–461.

251. von Hofsten, C. (1991). Structuring of early reaching movements: A longitudinal study. *Journal of Motor Behavior, 23,* 280–292.

252. Holdefer, R. N., & Miller, L. E. (2002). Primary motor cortical neurons encode functional muscle synergies. *Experimental Brain Research, 146,* 233–243.

253. Holt, K. G., Saltzman, E., Ho, C. L., Kubo, M., & Ulrich, B. D. (2006). Discovery of the pendulum and spring dynamics in the early stages of walking. *Journal of Motor Behavior, 38*(3), 206–218.

254. Holt, K. G., Saltzman, E., Ho, C. L., & Ulrich, B. D. (2007). Scaling of dynamics in the earliest stages of walking. *Physical Therapy, 87*(11), 1458–1467.

255. Holt, K. G., Fonseca, S. T., & LaFiandra, M. E. (2000). The dynamics of gait in children with spastic hemiplegic cerebral palsy: Theoretical and clinical implications. *Human Movement Science, 19,* 375–405.

256. Hooker, D. (1958). *Evidence of prenatal function of the central nervous system in man.* New York: American Museum of Natural History.

257. Hopkins, B., & Prechtl, H. F. R. (1984). A quantitative approach to the development of movements during early infancy. *Clinics in Developmental Medicine, 94,* 179–197.

258. Horak, F. B. (2009). Postural compensation for vestibular loss. Review. *Annals of the New York Academy of Sciences, 1164,* 76–81.

259. Horak, F. B. (2006). Postural orientation and equilibrium: What do we need to know about neural control of balance to prevent falls? Review. *Age Ageing, 35*(Suppl 2), ii7–ii11.

260. Horak, F. B., & MacPherson, J. M. (1996). Postural orientation and equilibrium. In L. B. Rowell & J. T. Sheperd (Eds.), *Handbook of physiology, Section 12, Exercise: Regulation and integration of multiple systems* (pp. 255–292). New York: Oxford University Press.

261. Horak, F. B., & Nashner, L. M. (1986). Central programming of postural movements: Adaptation to altered support-surface configurations. *Journal of Neurophysiology, 55,* 1369–1381.

262. Horak, F. B., Buchanan, J., Creath, R., & Jeka, J. (2002). Vestibulospinal control of posture. *Advances in Experimental Medicine and Biology, 508,* 139–145.

263. Horak, F. B., Diener, H. C., & Nashner, L. M. (1989). Influence of central set on human postural responses. *Journal of Neurophysiology, 62,* 841–853.

264. Horak, F. B., Earhart, G. M., & Dietz, V. (2001). Postural responses to combinations of head and body displacements: Vestibular-somatosensory interactions. *Experimental Brain Research, 141,* 410–414.

265. Horak, F. B., Esselman, P., Anderson, M. E., & Lynch, M. K. (1984). The effects of movement velocity, mass displaced, and task certainty on associated postural adjustments made by normal and hemiplegic individuals. *Journal of Neurology, Neurosurgery and Psychiatry, 47,* 1020–1028.

266. Horak, F. B., Nashner, L. M., & Diener, H. C. (1990). Postural strategies associated with somatosensory and vestibular loss. *Experimental Brain Research, 82,* 167–177.

267. Horak, F. B., Shumway-Cook, A., Crowe, T. K., & Black, F. O. (1988). Vestibular function and motor proficiency of children with impaired hearing, or with learning disability and motor impairments. *Developmental Medicine and Child Neurology, 30,* 64–79.

268. Horak, F. B. (1991). Assumptions underlying motor control for neurologic rehabilitation. In M. J. Lister (Ed.), *Contemporary management of motor control problems: Proceedings of the II Step Conference* (pp. 11–28). Alexandria, VA: Foundation for Physical Therapy.

269. Horak, F. B. (1992). Motor control models underlying neurologic rehabilitation. In H. Forssberg & H. Hirschfeld (Eds.), *Movement disorders in children, medicine and sport science* (Vol. 36, pp. 21–30). Basel: Karger.

270. Hoy, M. G., Zernicke, R. F., & Smith, J. L. (1985). Contrasting roles of inertial and muscle moments at the knee and ankle during paw-shake response. *Journal of Neurophysiology, 54,* 1282–1294.

271. Hultborn, H., & Nielsen, J. B. (2007). Spinal control of locomotion—from cat to man. *Acta Physiologica (Oxford), 189*(2), 111–121.

272. Humphrey, T. (1964). Some correlations between the appearance of human reflexes and the development of the nervous system. *Progress in Brain Research, 4,* 93–135.

273. Humphrey, T. (1970). The development of human fetal activity and its relation to postnatal behavior. *Advances in Child Development and Behavior, 5,* 1–57.

273a. Inder, J. M., & Sullivan, S. J. (2005). Motor and postural response profiles of four children with developmental coordination disorder. *Pediatr Phys Ther, 17*(1), 18–29, Spring.

274. Inui, N., & Katsura, Y. (2002). Development of force control and timing in a finger-tapping sequence with an attenuated-force tap. *Motor Control, 6,* 333–346.

275. Isableu, B., Ohlmann, T., Cremieux, J., & Amblard, B. (2003). Differential approach to strategies of segmental stabilisation in postural control. *Experimental Brain Research, 150,* 208–221.

276. Ivanenko, Y. P., Dominici, N., & Lacquaniti, F. (2007). Development of independent walking in toddlers. *Exercise and Sport Sciences Reviews, 35*(2), 67–73.

277. Jakobson, L. S., & Goodale, M. A. (1991). Factors affecting higher-order movement planning: A kinematic analysis of human prehension. *Experimental Brain Research, 86,* 199–208.

278. Jeannerod, M. (Ed.). (1990). *Attention and performance XIII: Motor representation and control.* Hillsdale, NJ: Lawrence Erlbaum Associates.

279. Jeannerod, M. (1981). Intersegmental coordination during reaching at natural visual objects in infancy. In J. Long & A. Baddeley (Eds.), *Attention and performance IX* (pp. 153–168). Hillsdale, NJ: Lawrence Erlbaum Associates.

280. Jeannerod, M. (1984). The timing of natural prehension movement. *Journal of Motor Behavior, 26,* 235–254.

281. Jeka, J., Oie, K. S., & Kiemel, T. (2000). Multisensory information for human postural control: Integrating touch and vision. *Experimental Brain Research, 134,* 107–125.

282. Jeka, J. J., & Lackner, J. R. (1994). Fingertip contact influences human postural control. *Experimental Brain Research, 100,* 495–502.

283. Jeng, S. F., Yau, K. I., Chen, L. C., et al. (2000). Alberta infant motor scale: Reliability and validity when used on preterm infants in Taiwan. *Physical Therapy, 80*(2), 168–178.

284. Jeng, S. F., Chen, L. C., & Yau, K. I. (2002). Kinematic analysis of kicking movements in preterm infants with very low birth weight and full-term infants. *Physical Therapy, 82,* 148–159.

285. Jensen, J. L., Thelen, E., Ulrich, B. D., Schneider, K., & Zernicke, R. F. (1995). Adaptive dynamics of the leg movement patterns of human infants: III. Age-related differences in limb control. *Journal of Motor Behavior, 27,* 366–374.

286. Jensen, J. L., Ulrich, B. D., Thelen, E., Schneider, K., & Zernicke, R. F. (1994). Adaptive dynamics of the leg movement patterns of human infants: I. The effects of posture on spontaneous kicking. *Journal of Motor Behavior, 26,* 303–312.

287. Jensen, R. K., Sun, H., Treitz, T., & Parker, H. E. (1997). Gravity constraints in infant motor development. *Journal of Motor Behavior, 29,* 64–71.

288. Johansson, R. S., & Westling, G. (1988). Coordinated isometric muscle commands adequately and erroneously programmed for the weight during lifting task with precision grip. *Experimental Brain Research, 71,* 59–71.

289. Johnston, M. V. (2009). Plasticity in the developing brain: Implications for rehabilitation. *Developmental Disabilities Research Reviews, 15*(2), 94–101.

290. Johnston, L. M., Burns, Y. R., Brauer, S. G., & Richardson, C. A. (2002). Differences in postural control and movement

performance during goal directed reaching in children with developmental coordination disorder. *Human Movement Science, 21,* 583–601.

291. Juenger, H., Linder-Lucht, M., Walther, M., Berweck, S., Mall, V., & Staudt, M. (2007). Cortical neuromodulation by constraint-induced movement therapy in congenital hemiparesis: An FMRI study. *Neuropediatrics, 38*(3), 130–136.

292. Kalaska, J. F., & Crammond, D. J. (1992). Cerebral cortical mechanisms of reaching movements. *Science, 255,* 1517–1523.

293. Katz, P. S., & Frost, W. N. (1996). Intrinsic neuromodulation: Altering neuronal circuits from within. *Trends in Neuroscience, 19,* 54–61.

294. Keele, S. W. (1998). Replies to J. J. Summers: Has ecological psychology delivered what it promised? Commentary 1, Programming or planning conceptions of motor control speak to different phenomena than dynamical systems conceptions. In J. P. Piek (Ed.), *Motor behavior and human skill* (pp. 403–408). Champaign, IL: Human Kinetics.

295. Keogh, J., & Sugden, D. (1985). *Movement skill development.* New York: Macmillan.

296. Keshner, E. A. (1990). Equilibrium and automatic postural reactions as indicators and facilitators in the treatment of balance disorders. In *Touch: Topics in pediatrics* (Lesson 4) (pp. 1–17). Alexandria, VA: American Physical Therapy Association.

297. Kjaerulff, O., & Kiehn, O. (1996). Distribution of networks generating and coordinating locomotor activity in the neonatal rat spinal cord in vitro: A lesion study. *Journal of Neuroscience, 16,* 5777–5794.

298. Kleim, J. A., & Jones, T. A. (2008). Principles of experience-dependent neural plasticity: Implications for rehabilitation after brain damage. *Journal of Speech, Language, and Hearing Research, 51*(1), S225–S239.

299. Kleim, J. A. (2006). III STEP: A basic scientist's perspective. *Physical Therapy, 86*(5), 614–617.

300. Klimstra, M. D., Thomas, E., Stoloff, R. H., Ferris, D. P., & Zehr, E. P. (2009). Neuromechanical considerations for incorporating rhythmic arm movement in the rehabilitation of walking. *Chaos, 19*(2), 026102.

301. Knott, M. (1966). Neuromuscular facilitation in the child with central nervous system deficit. *Journal of the American Physical Therapy Association, 7,* 721–724.

302. Kodric, J., Sustersic, B., & Paro-Panjan, D. (2009). Assessment of general movements and 2.5 year developmental outcomes: Pilot results in a diverse preterm group. *European Journal of Paediatric Neurology, 14*(2):131–137.

303. Konczak, J., Jansen-Osmann, P., & Kalveram, K. T. (2003). Development of force adaptation during childhood. *Journal of Motor Behavior, 35,* 41–52.

304. Koomar, J., Burpee, J. D., DeJean, V., Frick, S., Kawar, M. J., & Fischer, D. M. (2001). Theoretical and clinical perspectives on the Interactive Metronome: A view from occupational therapy practice. *American Journal of Occupational Therapy, 55*(2), 163–166.

305. Koshland, G. F., & Smith, J. L. (1989). Paw-shake responses with joint immobilization: EMG changes with atypical feedback. *Experimental Brain Research, 77,* 361–373.

306. Kramer, J. F., & MacPhail, H. E. A. (1994). Relationships among measures of walking efficiency, gross motor ability, and isokinetic strength in adolescents with cerebral palsy. *Pediatric Physical Therapy, 6,* 3–8.

307. Krishnamoorthy, V., Latash, M. L., Scholz, J. P., & Zatsiorsky, V. M. (2003). Muscle synergies during shifts of the center of pressure by standing persons. *Experimental Brain Research, 152,* 281–292.

308. Kubo, M., & Ulrich, B. D. (2006). Early stage of walking: Development of control in mediolateral and anteroposterior directions. *Journal of Motor Behavior, 38*(3), 229–237.

309. Kuhnke, N., Juenger, H., Walther, M., Berweck, S., Mall, V., & Staudt, M. (2008). Do patients with congenital hemiparesis and ipsilateral corticospinal projections respond differently to constraint-induced movement therapy? *Developmental Medicine and Child Neurology, 50*(12), 898–903.

310. Kuo, A. D. (2007). The six determinants of gait and the inverted pendulum analogy: A dynamic walking perspective. *Human Movement Science, 26*(4), 617–656.

311. Kupfermann, I. (1991). Localization of higher cognitive and affective functions: The association cortices. In E. R. Kandel, J. H. Schwartz, & T. M. Jessell (Eds.), *Principles of neuroscience* (3rd ed., pp. 823–838). New York: Elsevier.

312. Kurjak, A., Stanojevic, M., Andonotopo, W., et al. (2004). Behavioral pattern continuity from prenatal to postnatal life—a study by four-dimensional (4D) ultrasonography. *Journal of Perinatal Medicine, 32*(4), 346–353.

313. Lang, C. E., & Bastian, A. J. (1999). Cerebellar subjects show impaired adaptation of anticipatory EMG during catching. *Journal of Neurophysiology, 82*(5), 2108–2119.

314. Lantz, C., Melén, K., & Forssberg, H. (1996). Early infant grasping involves radial fingers. *Developmental Medicine and Child Neurology, 38,* 668–674.

315. Lashley, K. S. (1917). The accuracy of movement in the absence of excitation from the moving organ. *American Journal of Physiology, 43,* 169–194.

316. Lasky, R. E. (1977). The effect of visual feedback of the hand on the reaching and retrieval behavior of young infants. *Child Development, 48,* 112–117.

317. Latash, M. L. (2007). Learning motor synergies by persons with Down syndrome. *Journal of Applied Research in Intellectual Disabilities, 51,* 962–971.

318. Latash, M. L., Kang, N., & Patterson, D. (2002). Finger coordination in person s with Down syndrome: Atypical patterns of coordination and the effects of practice. *Experimental Brain Research, 146,* 345–355.

319. Latash, M. L., Krishnamoorthy, V., Scholz, J. P., & Zatsiorsky, V. M. (2005). Postural synergies and their development. *Neural Plasticity, 12,* 119–130.

320. Latash, M. L., Scholz, J. P., & Schoner G. (2007). Toward a new theory of motor synergies. *Motor Control, 11*(3), 276–308.

321. Reference deleted in page proofs.

322. Reference deleted in page proofs.

323. Latash, M. L., & Anson, J. G. (1996). What are normal movements in atypical populations? *Behavioral and Brain Sciences*, *19*, 55–106.

324. Latash, M. L., Ferreira, S. S., Wieczorek, S. A., & Duarte, M. (2003). Movement sway: Changes in postural sway during voluntary shifts of the center of pressure. *Experimental Brain Research*, *150*, 314–324.

325. Law, M., Darrah, J., Pollock, N., et al. (2007). Focus on function: A randomized controlled trial comparing two rehabilitation interventions for young children with cerebral palsy. *BMC Pediatrics*, *7*, 31.

326. Lawrence, D. G., & Hopkins, D. A. (1976). The development of the motor control in the rhesus monkey: Evidence concerning the role of corticomotorneuronal connections. *Brain*, *99*, 235–254.

327. Lawrence, D. G., & Kuypers, H. G. J. (1968). The functional organization of the motor system in the monkey: I. The effects of bilateral pyramidal lesions. *Brain*, *91*, 1–14.

328. Ledebt, A., Blandine, B., & Breniere, Y. (1998). The build-up of anticipatory behavior. *Experimental Brain Research*, *120*, 9–17.

329. Lee, H. M., Bhat, A., Scholz, J. P., & Galloway, J. C. (2008). Toy-oriented changes during early arm movements IV: Shoulder-elbow coordination. *Infant Behavior & Development*, *31*(3), 447–469.

330. Lee, S. C., Ding, J., Prosser, L. A., Wexler, A. S., & Binder-Macleod, S. A. (2009). A predictive mathematical model of muscle forces for children with cerebral palsy. *Developmental Medicine and Child Neurology*, *51*(12), 949–958.

331. Lee, D. N., & Aronson, E. (1974). Visual proprioceptive control of standing in human infants. *Perception & Psychophysics*, *15*, 529–532.

332. Lee, D. N., & Lishman, J. R. (1975). Visual proprioceptive control of stance. *Journal of Human Movement Studies*, *1*, 87–95.

333. Lee, D. N., Daniel, B. M., Turnbull, J., & Cook, M. L. (1990). Basic perceptuo-motor dysfunctions in cerebral palsy. In M. Jeannerod (Ed.), *Attention and performance XIII* (pp. 583–603). Hillsdale, NJ: Lawrence Erlbaum Associates.

334. Lee, D. N. (1980). The optic flow-field: The foundation of vision. *Philosophical Transactions of the Royal Society of London B*, *290*, 169–179.

335. Lemon, R. (1988). The output map of the primate motor cortex. *Trends in Neuroscience*, *11*, 501–506.

336. Levin, M. F., Lamarre, Y., & Feldman, A. G. (1995). Control variables and proprioceptive feedback in fast single-joint movement. *Canadian Journal of Physiology and Pharmacology*, *73*(2), 316–330.

337. Levitan, I. B., & Kaczmarek, L. K. (1997). *Neural networks and behavior. In the neuron. Cell and molecular biology* (pp. 451–474). New York: Oxford.

338. Liao, P. M., & Campbell, S. K. (2004). Examination of the item structure of the Alberta Infant Motor Scale. *Pediatric Physical Therapy*, *16*, 31–38.

339. Reference deleted in page proofs.

340. Liu, W. Y. (2001). *Anticipatory postural adjustments in children with cerebral palsy and children with typical development during forward reach tasks in standing*. Philadelphia: MCP Hahnemann University (pp. 111–173), dissertation.

341. Lobo, M. A., Galloway, J. C., & Savelsbergh, G. J. (2004). General and task-related experiences affect early object interaction. *Child Development*, *75*(4), 1268–1281.

342. Lobo, M. A., & Galloway, J. C. (2008). Postural and object-oriented experiences advance early reaching, object exploration, and means-end behavior. *Child Development*, *79*(6), 1869–1890.

343. Lockhart, D. B., & Ting, L. H. (2007). Optimal sensorimotor transformations for balance. *Nature Neuroscience*, *10*(10), 1329–1336, Epub Sep 16.

344. Lockman, J. J., Ashmead, D. H., & Bushnell, E. W. (1984). The development of anticipatory hand orientation during infancy. *Journal of Experimental Child Psychology*, *37*, 176–186.

345. Lowes, L. P., Westcott, S. L., Palisano, R. J., Effgen, S. K., & Orlin, M. N. (2004). Muscle force and range of motion as predictors of standing balance in children with cerebral palsy. *Physical & Occupational Therapy in Pediatrics*, *24*, 57–77.

346. Luo, H. J., Chen, P. S., Hsieh, W. S., et al. (2009). Associations of supported treadmill stepping with walking attainment in preterm and full-term infants. *Physical Therapy*, *89*(11), 1215–1225.

347. MacKay-Lyons, M. (2002). Central pattern generation of locomotion: A review of the evidence. *Physical Therapy*, *82*, 69–83.

348. MacPhail, H. E., & Kramer, J. F. (1995). Effect of isokinetic strength training on functional ability and walking efficiency in adolescents with cerebral palsy. *Developmental Medicine and Child Neurology*, *37*, 763–775.

349. Mah, C. D. (2001). Spatial and temporal modulation of joint stiffness during multijoint movement. *Experimental Brain Research*, *136*, 492–506.

350. Malouin, F., & Richards, C. L. (2000). Preparatory adjustments during gait initiation in 4–6-year-old children. *Gait and Posture*, *11*, 239–253.

351. Mandich, A., Buckolz, E., & Polatajko, H. (2003). Children with developmental coordination disorder (DCD) and their ability to disengage ongoing attentional focus: More on inhibitory function. *Brain and Cognition*, *51*(3), 346–356.

352. Marchal-Crespo, L., & Reinkensmeyer, D. J. (2009). Review of control strategies for robotic movement training after neurologic injury. *Journal of Neuroengineering and Rehabilitation*, *6*, 20 DOI:10.1186/1743-0003-6-20.

353. Marder, E., & Rehm, K. J. (2005). Development of central pattern generating circuits. *Current Opinion in Neurobiology*, *15*(1), 86–93.

354. Marques-Bruna, P., & Grimshaw, P. (2000). Changes in coordination during the first 8 months of independent walking. *Perceptual Motor Skills*, *91*, 855–869.

355. Massion, J. (1992). Movement, posture and equilibrium: Interaction and coordination. *Progress in Neurobiology, 38,* 35–56.

356. Mathew, A., & Cook, M. (1990). The control of reaching movements by young infants. *Child Development, 61,* 1238–1258.

357. Mayston, M. J. (1992). The Bobath concept: Evolution and application. In H. Forssberg & H. Hirschfeld (Eds.). *Movement disorders in children, medicine and sport science* (Vol. 36, pp. 1–6). Basel: Karger.

358. McCarty, M. E., Clifton, R. K., Ashmead, D. H., Lee, P., & Goubet, N. (2001). How infants use vision for grasping objects. *Child Development, 72,* 973–987.

359. McComas, J., Dulberg, C., & Latter, J. (1997). Children's memory for locations visited: Importance of movement and choice. *Journal of Motor Behavior, 29,* 223–229.

360. McGraw, M. B. (1940). Neuromuscular development of the human infant as exemplified in the achievement of erect locomotion. *Journal of Pediatrics, 17,* 747–771.

361. McGraw, M. B. (1945). *The neuromuscular maturation of the human infant.* New York: Hafner Press.

362. McRae, C. G., Johnston, T. E., Lauer, R. T., Tokay, A. M., Lee, S. C., & Hunt, K. J. (2009). Cycling for children with neuromuscular impairments using electrical stimulation: Development of tricycle-based systems. *Medical Engineering & Physics, 31*(6), 650–659, Epub Feb 4.

363. Meyer, D. E., Smith, J. E. K., Kornblum, S., Abrams, R. A., & Wright, C. E. (1990). Speed-accuracy tradeoffs in aimed movements: Toward a theory of rapid voluntary action. In M. Jeannerod (Ed.), *Attention and performance XIII* (pp. 173–226). Hillsdale, NJ: Lawrence Erlbaum Associates.

364. Meyer-Heim, A., Borggraefe, I., Ammann-Reiffer, C., et al. (2007). Feasibility of robotic-assisted locomotor training in children with central gait impairment. *Developmental Medicine and Child Neurology, 49*(12), 900–906.

365. Michaud, L. J., Klein, A., Hudson, P., Gehrke, K., & Custis-Allen, L. (2003). Constraint-induced movement therapy in pediatric hemiplegia: A case series. *Archives of Physical Medicine and Rehabilitation, 84,* E2.

366. Miller, L. J., & Roid, G. H. (1993). Sequence comparison methodology for the analysis of movement patterns in infants and toddlers with and without motor delays. *American Journal of Occupational Therapy, 47,* 339–347.

367. Miller, L. J., & Roid, G. H. (1994). *The T.I.M.E. Toddler and Infant Motor Evaluation, a standardized assessment.* San Antonio, TX: Therapy Skill Builders.

368. Miller, L. T., Polatajko, H. J., Missiuna, C., Mandich, A. D., & McNab, J. J. (2001). A pilot trial of a cognitive treatment for children with developmental coordination disorder. *Human Movement Science, 20,* 183–210.

369. Missiuna, C., Mandich, A. D., Polatajko, H. J., & Molloy-Miller, T. (2001). Cognitive orientation to daily occupational performance (CO-OP), Part 1— Theoretical foundations. *Physical & Occupational Therapy in Pediatrics, 20*(2/3), 69–81.

370. Mockford, M., & Caulton, J. M. (2008). Systematic review of progressive strength training in children and adolescents with

cerebral palsy who are ambulatory. *Pediatric Physical Therapy, 20,* 318–333.

371. Moe-Nilssen, R., Helbostad, J. L., Talcott, J. B., & Toennessen, F. G. (2003). Balance and gait in children with dyslexia. *Experimental Brain Research, 150,* 237–244.

372. Mouchnino, L., Aurenty, R., Massion, J., & Pedotti, A. (1990). Coordinated control of posture and equilibrium during leg movement. In T. Brandt, W. Paulus, W. Bles, et al. (Eds.), *Disorders of posture and gait* (pp. 68–71). Stuttgart: Georg Thieme.

373. Muir, G. D., Gosline, J. M., & Steeves, J. D. (1996). Ontogeny of bipedal locomotion: Walking and running in the chick. *Journal of Physiology, 493,* 589–601.

374. Nashner, L. M., & Forssberg, H. (1986). Phase-dependent organization of postural adjustments associated with arm movements while walking. *Journal of Neurophysiology, 55,* 1382–1394.

375. Nashner, L. M., Shumway-Cook, A., & Marin, O. (1983). Stance posture control in select groups of children with cerebral palsy: Deficits in sensory organization and muscular coordination. *Experimental Brain Research, 49,* 393–409.

376. Näslund, A., Sundelin, G., & Hirschfeld, H. (2007). Reach performance and postural adjustments during standing in children with severe spastic diplegia using dynamic ankle-foot orthoses. *Journal of Rehabilitative Medicine, 39*(9), 715–723.

377. Newell, K. M., & Valvano, J. (1998). Therapeutic intervention as a constraint in learning and relearning movement skills. *Scandinavian Journal of Occupational Therapy, 5,* 51–57.

378. Newell, K. M., McDonald, P. V., & Baillargeon, R. (1993). Body scale and infant grip configurations. *Developmental Psychobiology, 26,* 195–205.

379. Norrlin, S., Dahl, M., & Rösblad, B. (2004). Control of reaching movements in children and young adults with myelomeningocele. *Developmental Medicine & Child Neurology, 46*(1), 28–33.

380. O'Donovan, M. J., & Chub, N. (1997). Population behavior and self-organization in the genesis of spontaneous rhythmic activity by developing spinal networks. *Seminars in Cell and Developmental Biology, 8,* 21–28.

381. Okamoto, T., & Okamoto, K. (2001). Electromyographic characteristics at the onset of independent walking in infancy. *Electromyography and Clinical Neurophysiology, 41,* 33–41.

382. Palisano, R. J., & Murr S. (2009). Intensity of therapy services: What are the considerations? *Physical & Occupational Therapy in Pediatrics, 29*(2), 109–114.

383. Palisano, R. J. (1993). Neuromotor and developmental assessment. In I. J. Wilhelm (Ed.), *Physical therapy assessment in early infancy* (pp. 173–224). New York: Churchill Livingstone.

384. Palluel, E., Ceyte, H., Olivier, I., & Nougier, V. (2008). Anticipatory postural adjustments associated with a forward leg raising in children: Effects of age, segmental acceleration and sensory context. *Clinical Neurophysiology, 119*(11), 2546–2554, Epub Sep 12.

385. Pang, M. Y., & Yang, J. F. (2002). Sensory gating for the initiation of the swing phase in different directions of human infant stepping. *Journal of Neuroscience, 22,* 5734–5740.

386. Pang, M. Y., Lam, T., & Yang, J. F. (2003). Infants adapt their stepping to repeated trip-inducing stimuli. *Journal of Neurophysiology, 90,* 2731–2740.

387. Perham, H., Smick, J. E., Hallum, A., & Nordstrom, T. (1987). Development of the lateral equilibrium reaction in stance. *Developmental Medicine and Child Neurology, 29,* 758–765.

388. Peterka, R. J. (2002). Sensorimotor integration in human postural control. *Journal of Neurophysiology, 88,* 1097–1118.

389. Phillips, J. P., Sullivan, K. J., Burtner, P. A., Caprihan, A., Provost, B., & Bernitsky-Beddingfield, A. (2007). Ankle dorsiflexion fMRI in children with cerebral palsy undergoing intensive body-weight-supported treadmill training: A pilot study. *Developmental Medicine and Child Neurology, 49*(1), 39–44.

390. Pierce, S., Daly, K., Gallagher, K. G., Gershkoff, A. M., & Schaumburg, S. W. (2002). Constraint-induced therapy for a child with hemiplegic cerebral palsy: A case report. *Archives of Physical Medicine and Rehabilitation, 83,* 1462–1463.

391. Piper, M. C., & Darrah, J. (1994). *Motor assessment of the developing infant.* Philadelphia: W.B. Saunders.

392. Piper, M. C., Pinnell, L. E., Darrah, J., Maguire, T., & Byrne, P. J. (1992). Construction and validation of the Alberta Infant Motor Scale (AIMS). *Canadian Journal of Public Health, 83*(Suppl 2), S46–S50.

393. Polatajko, H. J., Mandich, A. D., Miller, L. T., & Macnab, J. J. (2001). Cognitive orientation to daily occupational performance (CO-OP), Part 2: The evidence. *Physical & Occupational Therapy in Pediatrics, 20*(2/3), 83–106.

394. Polit, A., & Bizzi, E. (1979). Characteristics of motor programs underlying arm movements in monkeys. *Journal of Neurophysiology, 42,* 183–194.

395. Portfors-Yeomans, C. V., & Riach, C. L. (1995). Frequency characteristics of postural control of children with and without visual impairment. *Developmental Medicine and Child Neurology, 37,* 456–463.

396. Prablanc, C., & Pélisson, D. (1990). Gaze saccade orienting and hand pointing are locked to their goal by quick internal loops. In M. Jeannerod (Ed.). *Attention and performance XIII* (pp. 653–676). Hillsdale, NJ: Lawrence Erlbaum Associates.

397. Pratt, C. A., & Loeb, G. E. (1991). Functionally complex muscles of the cat hindlimb. 1. Patterns of activation across sartorius. *Experimental Brain Research, 85,* 243–256.

398. Prechtl, H. F. (2001). General movement assessment as a method of developmental neurology: New paradigms and their consequences. *Developmental Medicine and Child Neurology, 43,* 836–842.

399. Prechtl, H. F. (1997). State of the art of a new functional assessment of the young nervous system: An early predictor of cerebral palsy. *Early Human Development, 50,* 1–11.

400. Prechtl, H. F. R., Cioni, G., Einspieler, C., Bos, A. F., & Ferrari, F. (2001). Role of vision on early motor development: Lessons from the blind. *Developmental Medicine and Child Neurology, 43,* 198–201.

401. Prilutsky, B. I., & Gregor, R. J. (2001). Swing- and support-related muscle actions differentially trigger human walk-run and run-walk transitions. *Journal of Experimental Biology, 204,* 2277–2287.

402. Rabin, E., DiZio, P., Ventura, J., & Lackner, J. R. (2008). Influences of arm proprioception and degrees of freedom on postural control with light touch feedback. *Journal of Neurophysiology, 99,* 595–604.

403. Rader, N., & Stern, J. D. (1982). Visually elicited reaching in neonates. *Child Development, 53,* 1004–1007.

404. Rahlin, M., Rheault, W., & Cech, D. (2003). Evaluation of the primary subtest of Toddler and Infant Motor Evaluation: Implications for clinical practice in pediatric physical therapy. *Pediatric Physical Therapy, 15,* 176–183.

405. Raibert, M. H. (1977). *Motor control and learning by the state-space. Tech. Rep. AI-TR-439.* Cambridge, MA: Massachusetts Institute of Technology, Artificial Intelligence Laboratory.

406. Riach, C. L., & Hayes, K. C. (1987). Maturation of postural sway in young children. *Developmental Medicine and Child Neurology, 29*(5), 650–658.

407. Riach, C. L., & Hayes, K. C. (1990). Anticipatory postural control in children. *Journal of Motor Behavior, 22,* 250–266.

408. Richards, C., Malouin, F., Dumas, F., Marcoux, S., LePage, C., & Menier, C. (1997). Early and intensive treadmill locomotor training for young children with cerebral palsy: A feasibility study. *Pediatric Physical Therapy, 9,* 158–165.

408a. Richardson, P. R., Atwater, S. W., Crowe, T. K., & Deitz, J. C. (1992). Performance of preschoolers on the Pediatric Clinical Test of Sensory Interaction for Balance. *American Journal of Occupational Therapy, 46,* 793–800.

409. Riley, M. A., & Turvey, M. T. (2002). Variability and determinism in motor behavior. *Journal of Motor Behavior, 34,* 99–125.

410. Robert, T., Zatsiorsky, V. M., & Latash, M. L. (2008). Multi-muscle synergies in an unusual postural task: Quick shear force production. *Experimental Brain Research,* DOI 10.1007/s00221-008-1299-7.

411. Robertson Ringenbach, S. D., Chua, R., Maraj, B. K., Kao, J. C., & Weeks, D. J. (2002). Bimanual coordination dynamics in adults with Down syndrome. *Motor Control, 6,* 388–407.

412. Rodger, S., Springfield, E., & Polatajko, H. J. (2007). Cognitive Orientation for daily occupational Performance approach for children with Asperger's syndrome: A case report. *Physical & Occupational Therapy in Pediatrics, 27*(4), 7–22.

413. Roebuck, T. M., Simmons, R. W., Mattson, S. N., & Riley, E. P. (1998). Neuromuscular responses to balance. *Alcoholism, Clinical and Experimental Research, 22,* 1192–1997.

414. Roebuck, T. M., Simmons, R. W., Mattson, S. N., & Riley, E. P. (1998). Prenatal exposure to alcohol affects the ability to maintain postural balance. *Alcoholism, Clinical and Experimental Research, 22,* 252–258.

415. Roncesvalles, N. C., Woollacott, M. H., & Jensen, J. L. (2000). Development of compensatory stepping skills in children. *Journal of Motor Behavior, 32*, 100–111.

416. Rose-Jacobs, R., Cabral, H., Beeghly, M., et al. (2004). The Movement Assessment of Infants (MAI) as a predictor of two-year neurodevelopmental outcome for infants born at term who are at social risk. *Pediatric Physical Therapy, 16*(4), 212–221.

417. Rosenbaum, D. A. (1991). *Human motor control.* San Diego, CA: Academic Press.

418. Rosenbaum, P. L., Walter, S. D., Hanna, S. E., et al. (2002). Prognosis for gross motor function in cerebral palsy: Creation of motor development curves. *Journal of the American Medical Association, 288*, 1357–1363.

419. Rossignol, S., & Drew, T. (1986). Phasic modulation of reflexes during rhythmic activity. In S. Grillner, P. S. G. Stein, D. G. Stuart, H. Forssberg, & R. M. Herman, (Eds.), *Neurobiology of vertebrate locomotion* (pp. 517–534). London: Macmillan.

420. Rossignol, S. (1996). Neural control of stereotypic limb movements. In L. B. Rowell, & J. T. Sheperd (Eds.). *Handbook of physiology, Section 12, Exercise: Regulation and integration of multiple systems* (pp. 173–216). New York: Oxford University Press.

421. Rossignol, S., Dubuc, R., & Gossard, J. P. (2006). Dynamic sensorimotor interactions in locomotion. *Physiological Reviews, 86*, 89–154.

422. Rozamalski, A., & Schwartz, M. H. (2009). Crouch gait patterns defined using k-cluster analysis are related to underlying clinical pathology. *Gait Posture, 30*, 155–160.

423. Russell, D. J., Rosenbaum, P. L., Cadman, D. T., Gowland, C., Hardy S., & Jarvis, S. (1989). The Gross Motor Function Measure: A means to evaluate the effects of physical therapy. *Developmental Medicine and Child Neurology, 31*, 341–353.

424. Saavedra, S., Woollacott, M., & van Donkelaar, P. (2010). Head stability during quiet sitting in children with cerebral palsy: Effect of vision and trunk support. *Experimental Brain Research, 201*(1), 13–23.

425. Sagnol, C., Debillon, T., & Debû, B. (2007). Assessment of motor control using kinematics analysis in preschool children born very preterm. *Developmental Psychobiology, 49*(4), 421–432.

426. Sakzewski, L., Ziviani, J., & Boyd, R. (2009). Systematic review and meta-analysis of therapeutic management of upper-limb dysfunction in children with congenital hemiplegia. *Pediatrics, 123*(6), e1111–e1122.

427. Salem Y., Godwin, E. M. (2009). Effects of task-oriented training on mobility function in children with cerebral palsy. *NeuroRehabilitation, 24*(4), 307–313.

428. Salokorpi, T., Rajantie, I., Kivikko, I., Haajanen, R., & Rajantie, J. (2001). Predicting neurological disorders in infants with extremely low birth weight using the Movement Assessment of Infants *13*, 106–109.

429. Sanes, J. N., Dimitrov, B., & Hallett, M. (1990). Motor learning in patients with cerebellar dysfunction. *Brain, 113*, 103–120.

430. Savelsbergh, G. J., & J. van der Kamp (1994). The effect of body orientation to gravity on early infant reaching. *Journal of Experimental Child Psychology, 58*(3), 510–528.

431. Schaal, S., Mohajerian, P., & Ijspeert, A. (2007). Dynamics systems vs. optimal control: A unifying view. Review. *Progress in Brain Research, 165*, 425–445.

432. Schellekens, J. M. H., Scholten, C. A., & Kalverboer, A. F. (1983). Visually guided hand movements in children with minor neurological dysfunction: Response time and movement organization. *Journal of Child Psychology and Psychiatry, 24*, 89–102.

433. Schindl, M. R., Forstner C., Kern, H., & Hesse, S. (2000). Treadmill training with partial body weight support in non-ambulatory patients with cerebral palsy. *Archives of Physical Medicine and Rehabilitation, 81*, 301–306.

434a. Schmidt, R. A., & Lee, T. D. (2005). *Motor control and learning: A behavioral emphasis.* Champaign, IL: Human Kinetics.

434b. Schmidt, R. A., & Lee, T. D. (1998). *Motor control and learning: A behavioral emphasis*, 3rd ed. Champaign, IL: Human Kinetics.

435. Schmidt, R. A. (1975). A schema theory of discrete motor skill learning. *Psychological Review, 82*, 225–260.

436. Schmitz, C., & Assaiante, C. (2002). Developmental sequence in the acquisition of anticipation during a new co-ordination in a bimanual load-lifting task in children. *Neuroscience Letters, 330*(3), 215–218.

437. Reference deleted in page proofs.

438. Schmitz, C., Martin, N., & Assaiante, C. (2002). Building anticipatory postural adjustment during childhood: A kinematic and electromyographic analysis of unloading in children from 4 to 8 years of age. *Experimental Brain Research, 142*, 354–364.

439. Schneider, J. W., Lee, W., & Chasnoff, I. J. (1988). Field testing of the Movement Assessment of Infants. *Physical Therapy, 68*, 321–327.

440. Schneider, K., Zernicke, R. F., Schmidt, R. A., & Hart, T. J. (1989). Changes in limb dynamics during the practice of rapid arm movements. *Journal of Biomechanics, 22*, 805–817.

441. Schneider, K., Zernicke, R. F., Ulrich, B. D., Jensen, J. L., & Thelen, E. (1990). Understanding movement control in infants through the analysis of limb intersegmental dynamics. *Journal of Motor Behavior, 22*, 493–520.

442. Scholz, J. P., Kang, N., Patterson, D., & Latash, M. L. (2003). Uncontrolled manifold analysis of single trials during multifinger force production by persons with and without Down syndrome. *Experimental Brain Research, 153*, 45–58.

443. Scholz, J. P., Reisman, D., & Schöner, G. (2001). Effects of varying task constraints on solutions to joint coordination in a sit-to-stand task. *Experimental Brain Research, 141*(4), 485–500, Epub Oct 20.

444. Scianni A., Butler, J. M., Ada L., Teixeira-Salmela, L. F. (2009). Muscle strengthening is not effective in children and adolescents with cerebral palsy: A systematic review. *Australian Journal of Physiotherapy, 55*(2), 81–87.

445. Scott, S. H., & Kalaska, J. F. (1995). Changes in motor cortex activity during reaching movements with similar hand paths but different arm postures. *Journal of Neurophysiology, 73,* 2563–2567.

446. Seidler, R. D., Bernard, J. A., Burutolu, T. B., et al. (2009). Motor control and aging: Links to age-related brain structural, functional, and biochemical effects. *Neuroscience and Biobehavioral Reviews,* Oct 19 [Epub ahead of print].

447. Seidler, R. D., Noll, D. C., & Thiers, G. (2004). Feedforward and feedback processes in motor control. *Neuroimage, 22*(4), 1775–1783.

448. Seitz, R. J., Stephan, K. M., & Binkofski, F. (2000). Control of action as mediated by the human frontal lobe. *Experimental Brain Research, 133,* 71–80.

449. Shaffer, R. J., Jacokes, L. E., Cassily, J. F., Greenspan, S. I., Tuchman, R. F., & Stemmer, P. J. Jr. (2001). Effect of interactive metronome training on children with ADHD. *American Journal of Occupational Therapy, 55,* 155–162.

450. Shea, C. H., & Wulf, G. (2005). Schema theory: A critical appraisal and reevaluation. *Journal of Motor Behavior, 37*(2), 85–101.

451. Shepherd, G. M. (1991). *Foundations of the neuron doctrine.* New York: Oxford University Press.

452. Sherrington, C. S. (1947). *The integrative action of the nervous system.* New Haven: Yale University Press. (Original work published 1906.)

453. Shriner's Hospital Upper Extremity Evaluation. (2005). Shriner's Hospital for Children, Greenville, SC, www.ejbjs.org/cgi/content/full/88/2/326/DC1.

454. Shumway-Cook, A., Hutchinson, S., Kartin, D., Price, R., & Woollacott, M. (2003). Effect of balance training on recovery of stability in children with cerebral palsy. *Developmental Medicine and Child Neurology, 45*(9), 591–602.

454a. Shumway-Cook, A., & Horak, F. B. (1986). Assessing the influence of sensory interaction of balance. Suggestion from the field. *Phys Ther, 66*(10), 1548–50, Oct.

455. Shumway-Cook, A., & Woollacott, M. (1985b). Dynamics of postural control in the child with Down syndrome. *Physical Therapy, 9,* 1315–1322.

456. Shumway-Cook, A., & Woollacott, M. (2001). *Motor control theory and practical applications.* Baltimore: Lippincott Williams & Wilkins.

457. Shumway-Cook, A., & Woollacott, M. (1985a). The growth of stability: Postural control from a development perspective. *Journal of Motor Behavior, 17,* 131–147.

458. Shumway-Cook, A., & Woollacot, M. H. (2007). *Motor control: Translating research into clinical practice* (3rd ed.). Philadelphia: Lippincott, Williams, & Watkins.

459. Siegert, R. J., Lord, S., & Porter, K. (2004). Constraint-induced movement therapy: Time for a little restraint? *Clinical Rehabilitation, 18,* 110–114.

460. Smith, L. B., & Thelen, E. (2003). Development as a dynamic system. *Trends in Cognitive Science, 7,* 343–348.

461. Smyth, M. M., Anderson, H. I., & Churchill, A. (2001). Visual information and the control of reaching in children: A comparison between children with and without developmental coordination disorder. *Journal of Motor Behavior, 33,* 306–320.

462. Song, W. H., Sung, I. Y., Kim, Y. J., & Yoo, J. Y. (2003). Treadmill training with partial body weight support in children with cerebral palsy. *Archives of Physical Medicine and Rehabilitation, 84,* E2.

463. Sorsdahl, A. B., Moe-Nilssen, R., & Strand, L. I. (2008). Observer reliability of Gross Motor Performance Measure and Quality of Upper Extremity Skills Test, based on video recordings. *Developmental Medicine and Child Neurology, 50,* 146–151.

464. Sparto, P. J., Furman, J. M., & Redfern, M. S. (2006). Head sway response to optic flow: effect of age is more important than the presence of unilateral vestibular hypofunction. *Journal of Vestibular Research, 16*(3), 137–145.

465. Spittle, A. J., Doyle, L. W., & Boyd, R. N. (2008). A systematic review of the clinimetric properties of neuromotor assessments for preterm infants during the first year of life. *Developmental Medicine and Child Neurology, 50*(4), 254–266.

466. Sporns, O., & Edelman, G. M. (1993). Solving Bernstein's problem: A proposal for the development of coordinated movement by selection. *Child Development, 64,* 960–981.

467. Steenbergen, B., Van Thiel, E., Hulstijn, W., & Meuelenbroek, R. G. J. (2000). The coordination of reaching and grasping in spastic hemiparesis. *Human Movement Science, 19,* 75–105.

468. Steenbergen, B., Hulstijn, W., Lemmens, I. H. L., & Meulenbroek, R. G. J. (1998). The timing of prehensile movements in subjects with cerebral palsy. *Developmental Medicine and Child Neurology, 40,* 108–114.

469. Stehouwer, D. J., & Farel, P. B. (1984). Development of hindlimb locomotor behavior in the frog. *Developmental Psychobiology, 17,* 217–232.

470. Stendl, R., Kunz, K., Schrott-Fischer A., & Scholtz, A. W. (2006). Effect of age and sex on maturation of sensory systems and balance control. *Developmental Medicine and Child Neurology, 48,* 477–482.

471. Stergiou, N., Harbourne, R., & Cavanaugh, J. (2006). Optimal movement variability: A new theoretical perspective for neurologic physical therapy. *Journal of Neurologic Physical Therapy, 30*(3), 120–129.

472. Stoffregen, T. A., Adolph, K., Thelen, E., Gorday, K. M., & Sheng, Y. Y. (1997). Toddlers' postural adaptations to different support surfaces. *Motor Control, 1,* 119–137.

473. St-Onge, N., & Feldman, A. G. (2003). Interjoint coordination in lower limbs during different movements in humans. *Experimental Brain Research, 148,* 139–149.

474. Stringer, S. M., Rolls, E. T., Trappenberg, T. P., & de Araujo, L. E. T. (2003). Self-organizing continuous attractor networks and motor function. *Neural Networks, 16,* 161–182.

475. Sugden, D., & Dunford, C. (2007). Intervention and the role of theory, empiricism and experience in children with motor impairment. *Dis Rehab, 29*(1), 3–11.

476. Summers, J. J., & Anson, J. G. (2009). Current status of the motor program: revisited. *Human Movement Science, 28*(5), 566–577, Epub Feb 23.

477. Sundermier, L., & Woollacott, M. H. (1998). The influence of vision on the automatic postural muscle responses of newly standing and newly walking infants. *Experimental Brain Research, 120*, 537–540.

478. Sutcliffe, T. L., Gaetz, W. C., Logan, W. J., Cheyne, D. O., & Fehlings, D. L. (2007). Cortical reorganization after modified constraint-induced movement therapy in pediatric hemiplegic cerebral palsy. *Journal of Child Neurology, 22*(11), 1281–1287.

479. Sutherland, D. H., Olshen, R., Cooper, L., & Woo, S. L. (1980). The development of mature gait. *Journal of Bone and Joint Surgery, 62*, 336–353.

480. Sutherland, D. H., Olshen, R. A., Biden, E. N., & Wyatt, M. P. (1988). The development of mature walking. *Clinics in Developmental Medicine, 104/105*, 1–227.

481. Sveistrup, H., & Woollacott, M. H. (1996). Longitudinal development of the automatic postural response in infants. *Journal of Motor Behavior, 28*, 58–70.

482. Sveistrup, H., Schneiberg, S., McKinley, P. A., et al. (2008). Head, arm and trunk coordination during reaching in children. *Experimental Brain Research, 188*(2), 237–247.

483. Swanson, M. W., Bennet, F. C., Shy, K. K., & Whitfield, M. F. (1992). Identification of neurodevelopmental abnormality at four and eight months by the Movement Assessment of Infants. *Developmental Medicine and Child Neurology, 34*, 321–337.

484. Swinnen, S. P., Heuer, H., Massion, J., & Casaer, P. (Eds.). (1994). *Interlimb coordination: Neural, dynamical, and cognitive constraints*. San Diego: Academic Press.

485. Taktek, K., Zinsser, N., & St-John, B. (2008). Visual versus kinesthetic mental imagery: efficacy for the retention and transfer of a closed motor skill in young children. *Canadian Journal of Experimental Psychology, 62*(3), 174–187.

486. Tardieu, C., Laspargot, A., Tabary, C., & Bret, M. (1989). Toe-walking in children with cerebral palsy: contributions of contracture and excessive contraction of triceps surae muscle. *Physical Therapy, 69*, 656–662.

487. Taub, E., Griffin, A., Nick, J., Gammons, K., Uswatte, G., & Law, C. R. (2007). Pediatric CI therapy for stroke-induced hemiparesis in young children. *Developmental Neurorehabilitation, 10*(1), 3–18.

488. Taub, E., Ramey, S. L., DeLuca, S., & Echols, K. (2004). Efficacy of constraint-induced movement therapy for children with cerebral palsy with asymmetric motor impairment. *Pediatrics, 113*(2), 305–312.

489. Taub, E., & Berman, A. J. (1968). Movement and learning in the absence of sensory feedback. In S. J. Freedman, (Ed.), *The neuropsychology of spatially oriented behavior*. Homewood, IL: Dorsey Press.

490. Reference deleted in page proofs.

491. Thelen, E., & Smith, L. B. (1994). *A dynamic systems approach to the development of cognition and action*. Cambridge, MA: MIT Press.

492. Thelen, E., & Ulrich, B. D. (1991). Hidden skills: A dynamic systems analysis of treadmill stepping during the first year. *Monographs of the Society for Research in Child Development, 56*, 1–98.

493. Thelen, E., Fisher, D. M., & Ridley-Johnson, R. (1984). The relationship between physical growth and a newborn reflex. *Infant Behavior & Development, 7*, 479–493.

494. Thelen, E., Fisher, D. M., Ridley-Johnson, R., & Griffin, N. J. (1982). Effects of body build and arousal on newborn infant stepping. *Developmental Psychobiology, 15*, 447–453.

495. Thelen, E., & Spencer, J. P. (1998). Postural control during reaching in young infants: a dynamic systems approach. *Neuroscience and Biobehavioral Reviews, 22*(4), 507–514.

496. Thelen, E., Corbetta, D., & Spencer, J. P.(1996). Development of reaching during the first year: role of movement speed. *Journal of Experimental Psychology: Human Perception and Performance, 22*(5), 1059–1076.

497. Thomas, S. S., Buckon, C. E., Philips, D. S., Aiona, M. D., & Sussman, M. D. (2001). Interobserver reliability of the Gross Motor Performance Measure: Preliminary results. *Developmental Medicine and Child Neurology, 43*, 97–102.

498. Thorpe, D., Zaino, C., Westcott, S., & Valvano, J. (1998). Comparison of postural muscle coordination patterns during a functional reaching task in typically developing children and children with cerebral palsy. *Physical Therapy, 78*, S80–S81.

499. Tieman, B. L., Palisano, R. J., & Sutlive, A. C. (2005). Assessment of motor development and function in preschool children. *Mental Retardation and Developmental Disabilities Research Reviews, 11*(3), 189–196.

500. Todorov, E., & Jordan, M. I. (2002). Optimal feedback control as a theory of motor coordination. *Nature Neuroscience, 11*, 1226–1235.

501. Touwen, B. C. L. (1984). Primitive reflexes—Conceptual or semantic problem? *Clinics in Developmental Medicine, 94*, 115–125.

502. Trahan, J., & Malouin, F. (2002). Intermittent intensive physiotherapy in children with cerebral palsy: A pilot study. *Developmental Medicine and Child Neurology, 44*, 233–239.

503. Turvey, M. T., & Fonseca, S. (2009). Nature of motor control: Perspectives and issues. *Advances in Experimental Medicine and Biology, 629*, 93–123.

504. Turvey, M. T. (2009). Nature of motor control: Not strictly "motor," not quite "control." *Advances in Experimental Medicine and Biology, 629*, 3–6.

505. Ulrich, B. D., Haehl, V., Buzzi, U., Kubo, M., & Holt, K. G. (2004). Modeling dynamic resource utilization in populations with unique constraints: Preadolescents with and without Down syndrome. *Human Movement Science, 23*, 133–156.

506. Ulrich, B. D., Jensen, J. L., Thelen, E., Schneider, K., & Zernicke, R. F. (1994). Adaptive dynamics of the leg movement patterns of human infants: II. Treadmill stepping in infants and adults. *Journal of Motor Behavior, 26*, 313–324.

507. Ulrich, D. A., Ulrich, B. D., Angulo-Kinzler, R. M., & Yun, J. (2001). Treadmill training of infants with Down syndrome: Evidence-based developmental outcomes. *Pediatrics, 108*, E84.

508. Usui, N., Maekawa, K., & Hirasawa, Y. (1995). Development of the upright postural sway of children. *Developmental Medicine and Child Neurology, 37,* 985–996.

509. Valvano, J. (2004). Activity-focused motor interventions for children with neurological conditions. *Physical & Occupational Therapy in Pediatrics, 24,* 79–107.

510. Valvano, J., & Newell, K. M. (1998). Practice of a precision isometric grip-force task by children with spastic cerebral palsy. *Developmental Medicine and Child Neurology, 40,* 464–473.

511. Valvano, J. (2004). Activity-focused motor interventions for children with neurological conditions. *Physical & Occupational Therapy in Pediatrics, 24,* 79–107.

512. Van der Fits, I. B., Otten, E., Klip, A. W., Van Eykern, L. A., & Hadders-Algra, M. (1999). The development of postural adjustments during reaching in 6- to 18-month-old infants. Evidence for two transitions. *Experimental Brain Research, 126*(4), 517–528.

513. Van Der Fits, I. B., & Hadders-Algra, M. (1998). The development of postural response patterns during reaching in healthy infants. *Neuroscience and Biobehavioral Reviews, 22*(4), 521–526.

514. Reference deleted in page proofs.

515. van der Fits, I. B., Flikweert, E. R., Stremmelaar, E. F., et al. (1999). Development of postural adjustments during reaching in preterm infants. *Pediatric Research, 46*(1), 1–7.

516. van der Fits, I. B., Klip, A. W., van Eykern, L. A., & Hadders-Algra, M. (1999). Postural adjustments during spontaneous and goal-directed arm movements in the first half year of life. *Behavioral Brain Research, 106,* 75–90.

517. van der Heide, J. C., Otten, B., van Eykern, L. A., & Hadders-Algra, M. (2003). Development of postural adjustments during reaching in sitting children. *Experimental Brain Research, 151*(1), 32–45.

518. Reference deleted in page proofs.

519. van der Meer, A. L. H., van der Weel, F. R., & Lee, D. N. (1994). Prospective control in catching by infants. *Perception, 23,* 287–302.

520. van der Meer, A. L. H., van der Weel, F. R., & Lee, D. N. (1995). The functional significance of arm movements in neonates. *Science, 267,* 693–695.

521. van der Meulen, J. H. P., Vandergon, J. J. D., Gielen, C. C. A., Gooskens, R. H. J., & Willemse, J. (1991a). Visuomotor performance of normal and clumsy children. 1. Fast goal-directed arm-movements with and without visual feedback. *Developmental Medicine and Child Neurology, 33,* 40–54.

522. van der Meulen, J. H. P., Vandergon, J. J. D., Gielen, C. C. A., Gooskens, R. H. J., & Willemse, J. (1991b). Visuomotor performance of normal and clumsy children. 2. Arm-tracking with and without visual feedback. *Developmental Medicine and Child Neurology, 33,* 118–129.

523. van der Weel, F. R., van der Meer, A. L. H., & Lee, D. H. (1991). Effect of task on movement control in cerebral palsy: Implications for assessment and therapy. *Developmental Medicine and Child Neurology, 33,* 419–426.

524. van Haastert, I. C., de Vries, L. S., Helders, P. J., et al. (2006). Early gross motor development of preterm infants according to the Alberta Infant Motor Scale. *Journal of Pediatrics, 149*(5), 617–622.

525. van Heijst, J. J., Vos, J. E., & Bullock, D. (1998). Development in a biologically inspired spinal neural network for movement control. *Neural Networks, 11,* 1305–1316.

526. Van Waelvelde, H., De Weerdt, W., De Cock, P., et al. (2006). Parameterization of movement execution in children with developmental coordination disorder. *Brain Cognition, 60*(1), 20–31.

527. Vereijken, B., Pedersen, A. V., & Storksen, J. H. (2009). Early independent walking: A longitudinal study of load perturbation effects. *Developmental Psychobiology, 51*(4), 374–383.

527a. Vessey, S. K., Antone, A., Fenlason, C., Garner, J., Haas, A., & Westcott, S. L. (2005). Validity Of A New Single-Rater Version Of The Pediatric Clinical Test Of Sensory Interaction For Balance. *Pediatr Phys Ther, 17,* 88–89.

528. Viel, S., Vaugoyeau, M., & Assaiante, C. (2009). Adolescence: A transient period of proprioceptive neglect in sensory integration of postural control. *Motor Control, 13*(1), 25–42.

529. Vilaplana, J. M., & Coronado, J. L. (2006). A neural network model for coordination of hand gesture during reach to grasp. *Neural Networks, 19*(1), 12–30, Epub 2005 Nov 21.

530. Viviani, P., & Mounoud, P. (1990). Perceptuomotor compatibility in pursuit tracking of two-dimensional movements. *Journal of Motor Behavior, 22,* 407–443.

531. Wallace, P. S., & Whishaw, I. Q. (2003). Independent digit movements and precision grip patterns in 1–5-month-old human infants: Hand-babbling, including vacuous then self-directed hand and digit movements, precedes targeted reaching. *Neuropsychologia 41*(14), 1912–1918.

531a. Westcott, S. L., Crowe, T. K., Deitz, J. C., & Richardson, P. (1994). Test-retest reliability of the Pediatric Clinical Test of the Sensory Interaction for Balance (P-CTSIB). *Phys Occup Ther Pediatr, 14,* 1–21.

531b. Westcott, S. L., Richardson, P. K., & Lowes, L. P. (1997). Evaluation of postural stability in children: Current theories and assessment tools. *Phys Ther, 77,* 629–645.

532. Washington, K., Shumway-Cook, A., Price, R., Ciol, M., & Kartin, D. (2004). Muscle responses to seated perturbations for typically developing infants and those at risk for motor delays. *Developmental Medicine and Child Neurology, 46*(10), 681–688.

533. Westcott, S. L., Lowes, L. P., Richardson, P. K., Crowe, T. K., & Deitz, J. (1997b). Difference in the use of sensory information for maintenance of standing balance in children with different motor disabilities. *Developmental Medicine and Child Neurology, 39* (Suppl 75), 32–33.

534. Westcott, S. L., & Burtner, P. (2004). Postural Control in Children: Implications for Pediatric Practice. *Physical & Occupational Therapy in Pediatrics, 24,* 5–55.

535. Westcott, S. L., & Zaino, C. A. (1997). Comparison and development of postural muscle activity in children during stand

and reach from firm and compliant surfaces. *Society for Neuroscience Abstract*, 23, 1565.

536. Westcott, S. L., Lowes, L. P., & Richardson, P. K. (1997a). Evaluation of postural stability in children: Current theories and assessment tools. *Physical Therapy, 77*, 629–645.

536a. Westcott, S. L., Zaino, C. A., Miller, F., & Thorpe, D. E. (1997). Comparison of Postural Muscle Activity in Children of Different Ages During Stand and Reach From Firm. Compliant, and Narrow Surfaces: 9. Pediatric *Physical Therapy, 9*(4), 207, Winter.

536b. Deitz, J. C., Richardson, P., Atwater, S. W., Crowe, T. K., & Odiorne, M. (1991). Performance of normal children on the pediatric clinical test of sensory interaction for balance. *Occup Ther J Res, 11*, 336–357.

537. Westcott, S. L., Zaino, C. A., Miller, F., Thorpe, D., & Unanue, R. (1998). Anticipatory postural coordination and functional movement skills by degree of cerebral palsy in children age 6–12 years. *Society for Neuroscience Abstracts, 24*, 149.

538. Whitacre, C. A., & Shea, C. H. (2000). Performance and learning of generalized motor programs: Relative (GMP) and absolute (parameter) errors. *Journal of Motor Behavior, 32*, 163–175.

539. Wille, D., Eng, K., Holper, L., et al. (2009). Virtual reality-based paediatric interactive therapy system (PITS) for improvement of arm and hand function in children with motor impairment: A pilot study. *Developmental Neurorehabilitation, 12*(1), 44–52.

540. Willis, J. K., Morello, A., Davie, A., Rice, J. C., & Bennett, J. T. (2002). Forced use treatment of childhood hemiparesis. *Pediatrics, 110*, 94–97.

541. Willoughby, K. L., Dodd, K. J., & Shields N. (2009). A systematic review of the effectiveness of treadmill training for children with cerebral palsy. *Disability and Rehabilitation, 31*(24), 1971–1979.

542. Wilson, P. H. (2005). Practitioner review: Approaches to assessment and treatment of children with DCD: an evaluative review. *Journal of Child Psychology and Psychiatry, 46*, 806–823.

543. Wilson, P. H., Thomas, P. R., & Maruff, P. (2002). Motor imagery training ameliorates motor clumsiness in children. *Journal of Child Neurology, 17*, 491–498.

544. Winstein, C. J., Horak, F. B., & Fisher, B. E. (2000). Influence of central set on anticipatory and triggered grip-force adjustments. *Experimental Brain Research, 130*, 298–308.

545. Wishart, J. G., Bower, T. G. R., & Dunked, J. (1978). Reaching in the dark. *Perception, 7*, 507–512.

546. Witherington, D. C. (2005). The development of prospective grasping control between 5 and 7 months: A longitudinal study. *Infancy 7*(2), 143–161.

547. Witherington, D. C., von Hofsten, C., Rosander, K., Robinette, A., Woollacott, M. H., & Bertenthal, B. I. (2002). The development of anticipatory postural adjustments in infancy. *Infancy, 3*, 495–517.

548. Wittenberg, G. F. (2009). Neural plasticity and treatment across the lifespan for motor deficits in cerebral palsy. *Developmental Medicine and Child Neurology, 51* (Suppl 4), 130–133.

549. Woollacott, M., Shumway-Cook, A., Hutchinson, S., Ciol, M., Price, R., & Kartin, D. (2005). Effect of balance training on muscle activity used in recovery of stability in children with cerebral palsy: A pilot study. *Developmental Medicine and Child Neurology, 47*(7), 455–461.

550. Woollacott, M. H., & Shumway-Cook, A. (1990). Changes in posture control across the life span: A systems approach. *Physical Therapy, 70*(12), 799–807.

551. Woollacott, M. H., & Shumway-Cook, A. (2005). Postural dysfunction during standing and walking in children with cerebral palsy: What are the underlying problems and what new therapies might improve balance? *Neural Plasticity, 12*, 211–219.

552. Woollacott, M., & Assaiante, C. (2002). Developmental changes in compensatory responses to unexpected resistance of leg lift during gait initiation. *Experimental Brain Research, 144*, 385–396.

553. Woollacott, M., Debu, B., & Mowatt, M. (1987). Neuromuscular control of posture in the infant and child. *Journal of Motor Behavior, 19*, 167–186.

554. Woollacott, M. H., Burtner, P., Jensen, J., Jasiewicz, J., Roncesvalles, N., & Sveistrup, H. (1998). Development of postural responses during standing in healthy children and children with spastic diplegia. *Neuroscience & Biobehavioral Reviews, 22*, 583–589.

555. Wu, J., Looper, J., Ulrich, B. D., Ulrich, D. A., & Angulo-Barroso, R. M. (2007). Exploring effects of different treadmill interventions on walking onset and gait patterns in infants with Down syndrome. *Developmental Medicine and Child Neurology, 49*(11), 839–845.

556. Wu, J., Ulrich, D. A., Looper, J., Tiernan, C. W., & Angulo-Barroso, R. M. (2008). Strategy adoption and locomotor adjustment in obstacle clearance of newly walking toddlers with Down syndrome after different treadmill interventions. *Experimental Brain Research, 186*(2), 261–272, Epub 2007 Dec 7.

557. Yang, J. F., Stephens, M. J., & Vishram, R. (1998b). Infant stepping: A method to study the sensory control of human walking. *Journal of Physiology, 507*, 927–937.

558. Yang, J. F., Stephens, M. J., & Vishram, R. (1998a). Transient disturbances to one limb produce coordinated, bilateral responses during infant stepping. *Journal of Neurophysiology, 79*, 2329–2337.

559. Yonas, A., Bechtold, A. G., Frankel, D., Gordon, F. R., McRoberts, G., Norcia, A., & Sternfels, S. (1977). Development of sensitivity to information for impending collision. *Perception and Psychophysics, 21*, 97–104.

560. Young, R. P., & Marteniuk, R. G. (1998). Stereotypic muscle-torque patterns are systematically adopted during acquisition of a multi-articular kicking task. *Journal of Biomechanics, 31*, 809–816.

561. Reference deleted in page proofs.

562. Zaino, C. A., & Westcott McCoy, S. (2008). Reliability and comparison of electromyographic and kinetic measurements during a standing reach task in children with and without cerebral palsy. *Gait and Posture, 27,* 128–137.

563. Zehr, E. P. (2005). Neural control of rhythmic human movement: the common core hypothesis. Review. *Exercise and Sport Sciences Reviews, 33*(1), 54–60.

564. Zentgraf, K., Green, N., Munzert J., et al. (2009). How are actions physically implemented? *Progress in Brain Research, 174,* 303–318.

565. Zernicke, R. F., & Smith, J. S. (1996). Biomechanical insights into neural control of movement. In L. B. Rowell & J. T. Sheperd, (Eds.), *Handbook of physiology, Section 12, Exercise: Regulation and integration of multiple systems* (pp. 293–330). New York: Oxford University Press.

566. Zoia, S., Castiello, U., Blason, L., et al. (2005). Reaching in children with and without developmental coordination disorder under normal and perturbed vision. *Developmental Neuropsychology 27*(2), 257–273.

4

Motor Learning: Application of Principles to Pediatric Rehabilitation

ANDREW M. GORDON, PhD • RICHARD A. MAGILL, PhD

Increasingly, physical therapists are recognizing that effective training of motor function in children requires motor learning. The child needs to be an active learner to problem-solve how to accomplish a specific task, given his or her constraints. Such task-oriented approaches[11] are becoming the predominant type of treatment in adult therapy. An important difference among children with disabilities, however, is that unlike adults, children are rarely trying to regain function, and thus they do not have a motor image of how the task should be performed. Rather, their learning must occur in the context of development, whereby age-appropriate skills must be learned for the very first time. Such learning can be considered as part of a triad consisting of the person, the task (i.e., skill or activity), and the environmental context in which the child performs the task.

In this chapter, we first discuss this triad and how it applies to adult motor learning, as well as the relevant learning principles derived from studies of adults without disabilities. Specifically, we discuss taxonomies of motor skills in relation to skill progression, types of knowledge gained during motor learning, different types and stages of learning, methods of instructions, feedback types and frequency, types of practice schedules, variability and specificity of training with whole and part practice, and benefits of mental practice. This information provides important theory and context for the training of motor skills in children. Oddly, there is a dearth of good studies on motor learning in typically developing children. We review what is known about motor learning in children and how learning in children may differ from that in adults. We discuss the implications of reduced information-processing capabilities and processing/memory in children and the implications for feedback, along with the type and amount of practice, and will show that skill emerges over enormous amounts of practice and extensive time periods. We continue by discussing the limited research on motor learning in pediatric rehabilitation, with emphasis on cerebral palsy (CP), the most common type of pediatric physical disability. We show that contrary to older notions, CP is not static, but rather motor function improves with development and practice. We provide examples of how intensity matters, models for providing intensive, task-oriented approaches (e.g., constraint-induced movement therapy, bimanual training), and information on how tasks and the environment can be used to optimize learning. We describe the importance of training specificity and provide important clues from the neuroscience literature on how to take advantage of and maximize neuroplasticity. Among these is the fact that neuroplasticity is enhanced when the tasks are meaningful to the performer. Increasingly, this means use of video gaming to maintain salience and motivation and to target specific motor impairments. It is suggested that motor learning in the context of gaming can be an important complement to, but not a replacement for, salient task-oriented activities in the real world. Finally, we discuss gaps in the existing knowledge and project where pediatric rehabilitation research needs to be directed to fully incorporate motor learning into practice.

MOTOR LEARNING PRINCIPLES

One way to address the many complexities of the therapist–patient interaction is to consider principles on which to base decisions that must be made during this interaction. One set of principles relevant to this situation relates to learning processes that underlie physical rehabilitation. Patients present not only specific motor skill capabilities and limitations when they initially engage the services of a physical therapist, but also future movement goals. The therapist is confronted with the need to determine a plan of action to enable the patient to attain achievable goals given the individual's capabilities and limitations. Implicit in the development of such a plan is an understanding of learning processes as they relate to the learning or relearning of motor skills. Accordingly, the goal of this section of the chapter is to provide a foundation on which the therapist can establish knowledge of these processes and apply that knowledge to developing and implementing effective intervention strategies.

BASIC ASSUMPTIONS

General Influences on the Learning of Motor Skills

When a person attempts to learn or relearn a motor skill, at least three different sets of characteristics influence that process: the person, the task (i.e., skill or activity), and the environmental context in which the person performs the task (Figure 4-1). These characteristics interact in ways that

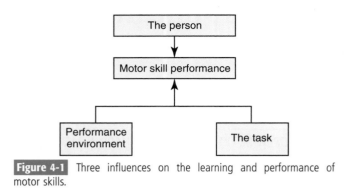

Figure 4-1 Three influences on the learning and performance of motor skills.

influence not only motor skill learning and performance but also the effectiveness of therapeutic intervention strategies. For the physical therapist, this interactive model should provide support for the view that there can be no "one size fits all" approach to creating interventions. As therapists are keenly aware, patients (the "person" part of the model) differ in their capabilities and limitations. However, the intervention planning process for a child must also incorporate specific characteristics of the skills or activities developed and the environmental contexts in which those skills will be performed.

Categories and Taxonomies of Motor Skills

Because the motor skill itself plays an important role in the learning and relearning process, it is important to understand key characteristics of motor skills that influence this process. Several different categorization and taxonomy schemes have been developed to identify characteristics of motor skills that make them distinct or similar.[72] The taxonomy that is most relevant to physical therapy is one developed in the United States by A.M. Gentile at Teachers College, Columbia University, which was based on the view that certain characteristics of motor skills place different types and quantities of attention and motor control demands on the person.[39] The full taxonomy consists of the interrelationship of four general characteristics of skills. Rather than discuss all of the categories of skills created by this interrelationship, we consider only three of the four general characteristics of skills that are especially relevant to the purposes of this chapter.

The first two characteristics concern the environmental context (i.e., all the components of the location and situation in which the skill is performed, such as the supporting surface, objects, and other people). The first of these relates to *whether the skill's regulatory conditions are stationary or in motion*. Gentile defined *regulatory conditions* as those features of the environmental context that specify the specific movement characteristics needed to achieve the skill's performance goal (note that Gentile used the term *action* goal).[39] Because a person could achieve a specific performance goal with different movement characteristics, the regulatory con-

ditions specify the movement characteristics required to achieve the performance goal in a specific situation. For example, the regulatory conditions associated with the performance goal of walking from one location to another would include the surface on which the child walks and the objects or other people in the pathway. These environmental context features influence the person's walking behavior by requiring him or her to alter certain movements to walk from one location to another. Consider, for example, how your walking movements would differ when you walk on a concrete sidewalk, a sandy beach, a moving bus, or a treadmill. Also consider how your walking movements would differ when you walk on a sidewalk with no other people on the sidewalk, or when you walk on one that is filled with people walking in various directions and at different speeds. In these examples of different situations involving the motor skill of walking, the regulatory conditions of the performance environment influence walking behavior in considerably different ways, depending on the specific characteristic of the regulatory condition and whether or not the regulatory condition is stationary or in motion. Skills for which the regulatory conditions are stationary are commonly referred to as *closed skills*, and skills for which the regulatory conditions are in motion are commonly referred to as *open skills*.

The second general characteristic of a motor skill concerns whether the regulatory conditions are the same or different on successive repetitions of performing the skill. Gentile referred to this characteristic as *intertrial variability*.[39] If the regulatory conditions are the same on successive repetitions, the skill has no intertrial variability. For example, stepping up a series of stair steps when each step is the same height requires repetitions of stepping with each repetition occurring in a performance context in which the regulatory conditions are the same for each repetition. In contrast, if the regulatory conditions are different on successive repetitions, the skill is classified as having intertrial variability. For example, when we drink a glass of water, each successive drink (i.e., repetition) removes some water from the glass, which means that the amount of water in the glass changes on each trial. The important point here is that although both stair-stepping skills and drinking skills are similar because each is a closed skill, they differ in the demands placed on the performer on succeeding repetitions of the skill. The skill with no intertrial variability (stair-stepping) requires the person to simply repeat each trial's movement characteristics, but the skill with intertrial variability (drinking from a glass) requires the person to adjust specific movement characteristics on each repetition.

The third general characteristic is whether or not an object must be manipulated when performing the skill. The same motor skill can place distinctly different attention and motor control demands on the child simply by adding or taking away an object as part of the performance requirement. Consider, for example, the different attention and motor control demands of walking on a sidewalk while carrying or not carrying a book bag.

Gentile organized the taxonomy on the basis of the complexity of each skill.[39] She defined complexity in terms of the amount of attention and motor control demands the skill places on the person performing the skill. The simplest skill, which is the closed skill with no intertrial variability and no object to manipulate, involves the lowest number of these demands. Skill complexity is increased by the addition of intertrial variability or an object to manipulate. Because of its systematic basis for identifying the complexity level of a skill, the taxonomy has practical value to the physical therapist. One use of the taxonomy is as a guide for evaluating a patient's movement capabilities and limitations. Another use is as a guide for systematically selecting a progression of activities to improve a child's functional capabilities.

Types of Knowledge Acquired During Learning

Learning of motor skills involves the acquisition of two types of knowledge: *explicit* (sometimes referred to as *declarative*) and *implicit* (sometimes referred to as *procedural*).[38,39] These types of knowledge are commonly distinguished on the basis of how accurately a person can verbally describe the knowledge. For example, if you were asked to provide evidence that you know how to tie your shoes, you could verbally describe how you do it, or you could physically tie them. The verbal description would indicate an explicit knowledge of the skill of shoe tying. But, if you were to have difficulty giving this verbal description, it could not be concluded that you don't have the knowledge of how to tie your shoes. Your knowledge may be in an implicit form and therefore difficult, if not impossible, to verbally describe. Evidence of this implicit knowledge of shoe tying could be revealed by a physical demonstration of performing the skill. Although some learning theorists typically view knowledge of how to perform a motor skill as implicit, or procedural, this view is too narrow to present a complete understanding of the knowledge structure underlying motor skill learning. In fact, motor skills involve the acquisition of both explicit and implicit knowledge.[119] Some researchers argue that the acquisition of explicit knowledge precedes that of implicit knowledge; others contend that the two types of knowledge are acquired simultaneously, but that certain skill characteristics are acquired explicitly or implicitly.[38,119] Clear evidence that they are separate comes from object rotation experiments. Subjects learn to grasp and lift an object with a symmetrical appearance but whose mass distribution is actually asymmetrical within one or two consecutive lifts by partitioning fingertip load forces asymmetrically before lift-off.[4,94,95] This involves learning to generate a compensatory moment in the opposite direction of the external moment, thus preventing object roll. However, despite subjects' explicit knowledge of the new center of mass (CM) location following object rotation, as determined by verbal cuing, they fail to generate a compensatory moment, resulting in object roll.[4,94,95,129] It is interesting to note that over repeated object rotations and lifts, subjects do reduce object roll through modulation of digit placement along the vertical axis (e.g., thumb lower than index finger when the center of mass is on the left side) but not tangential forces.[129] Thus the explicit knowledge influences the modulation of grasping kinematics but not kinetics. There is much that remains to be understood about these types of knowledge and their relationship to the skill learning process, but as you will see in later discussions in this chapter, the type of knowledge acquired has implications for several aspects of the therapist–patient interaction.

Stages of Learning

An important characteristic of the motor skill learning process is that people go through distinct stages, or phases, as they learn. Although several models have been proposed to identify and describe these stages,[72] we consider here one that is especially relevant to the physical therapy context. Gentile proposed a model of skill learning involving two stages.[36,37,39] The first stage, which Gentile called the *initial stage*, involves the learner attempting to attain some degree of success at achieving the performance goal of the skill. To do this, the person develops movement characteristics that match the regulatory conditions of the skill. In addition, the person acquires a movement coordination pattern that results in successful achievement of the skill's performance goal, although this achievement will be inconsistent from trial to trial. In the initial stage, the learner produces movement characteristics that often match, but sometimes do not match, requirements of the regulatory conditions. The result is that this stage is characterized by both successful and unsuccessful attempts. Eventually, the learner develops a movement coordination pattern that allows a reasonable amount of performance goal achievement, although the pattern is rather crude and inefficient. As Gentile described it, "Although the learner now has a general concept of an effective approach, he or she is not skilled. The action-goal is not achieved consistently and the movement lacks efficiency" (p. 149).[39]

In the second stage, which Gentile called the *later stages*, the learner needs to acquire three general characteristics: (1) the capability of adapting the movement pattern acquired in the initial stage to specific demands of any performance situation involving that skill; (2) consistency in achieving the performance goal of the skill on each attempt at performing the skill; and (3) efficiency of performance in terms of reducing the energy cost of performing the skill to a level that allows an "economy of effort."[39]

A distinct feature of the second stage is that the learning goals depend on whether the skill being learned is closed or open. Closed skills require what Gentile called *fixation* of the basic movement coordination pattern acquired in the first stage. This means that the learner must refine this pattern so that he or she can consistently achieve the action goal with little, if any, conscious effort and a minimum of physical energy. In contrast, open skills require what Gentile called *diversification* of the basic movement coordination pattern acquired in the first stage. This means that the movement pattern needs to be adaptable to the ever-changing spatial and temporal characteristics of the open-skill performance context.

Another characteristic of Gentile's learning stages model is the involvement of explicit and implicit learning processes in the two stages.[38] Although both types of learning processes occur in both stages, one type predominates over the other in each stage. In the initial stage, explicit learning processes predominate, whereas implicit processes predominate in the later stages. The basis for which type of learning process predominates is the characteristic of the skill being acquired at each stage. For example, Gentile proposed that during the initial stage the learner acquires knowledge about the regulatory conditions that influence the movements required to achieve the skill's performance goal. These conditions and the performer's own movements that must be learned are acquired through explicit learning processes. In contrast, the dynamics of force generation involved in performing a skill are acquired by implicit learning processes and become predominant in terms of what is learned in the later stages of learning.

PRACTICE CONDITIONS CONSIDERATIONS

Generalization: From the Clinic to the Everyday Experience

Physical therapists engage children in specific types of interventions because they want the interventions to ultimately allow patients to function in their everyday world. In the study of motor learning, this clinic-to-everyday-world relationship is known as *generalization*, or *transfer of learning*.[72] Because this type of generalization is such an essential goal of physical therapy practice, it is important to consider the factors that influence it.

The long-standing view of why generalization occurs is that it is due to the *similarity between the components of the skills or performance contexts* involved. More generalization occurs with increased amounts of skill or context similarity. Consider first the similarity of skills. If you analyze the movement components of skills or assess the movement goals of skills, you will find similarities as well as differences. For example, the skill of reaching for and grasping an object can involve a variety of skills that are distinct according to the characteristics of the object to be grasped and the intended use of the object, but are similar in terms of many of the movements required. The context in which a skill or activity is performed also must be considered as a factor influencing generalization, especially if the generalization involves performing a skill or activity in the clinic and then in the daily living environment. Again, more generalization

occurs as the degree of similarity increases between these two contexts. Taken to its logical conclusion, the greatest amount of generalization of skill performance from a clinical environment to the child's everyday living environment would occur when all the characteristics of the patient's everyday living environment are included in the intervention strategies, wherever they take place. Two implications for physical therapy practice of this view of generalization are the use of simulations in the clinic of a patient's daily living environment, and of children performing functional daily living skills in their own home or workplace.

Presenting Instructions About How to Perform a Skill: Demonstration and Verbal Instructions

If you want to give instructions to a child about how to perform a skill or activity, how would you do it? In any motor skill learning situation, the learner needs to know something about what he or she needs to do to perform the activity to be learned. The instructions can be as simple as a verbal description of the goal of the activity, such as "I want you to walk from this line on the floor to that table," or "I want you to pick up this coin and place it in the jar." This type of instruction works well for motor skills the child can already perform. But, if the person is not familiar with a skill or activity or does not know how to perform it, then some other type of instructions must be provided. The two most common ways therapists provide instructions are by demonstrating the skill or activity and by verbally describing what to do to perform the skill or activity. What do we know about these two forms of presenting instructions?

Demonstration

Sometimes referred to as modeling, demonstration is an effective way to communicate how to perform a skill or activity. It is especially effective when the skill or activity involves many movements that must be coordinated or sequenced in a way that the child has not experienced before, or if he or she would have difficulty following a long verbal description of the sequence of movements. After a demonstration of a complex activity, it is common to observe the person perform a reasonable approximation of the activity on the first attempt. Why does this happen? Most researchers agree that the observation of another person performing an activity engages a part of the brain that involves "mirror neurons."[60] These neurons are activated by vision as the person watches the activity being performed. In addition, when engaged in observing an activity, the visual system detects specific movement-related features of the activity that do not change from one performance of the activity to another. These features specify the coordinated movement patterns underlying performance of the activity. For example, if you observe another person walking and running, it is easy to distinguish each skill because each has a unique coordinated movement pattern. The combination of the mirror neurons registering the activity and vision detecting the specific movement pattern associated with the activity allows the observer to form a type of blueprint on which to base his or her own attempt to perform the activity.

Researchers also have shown that learning benefits occur when novice learners observe other novice learners.[72] The beneficial learning effect appears to be due to the cognitive problem-solving activity in which the observer engages while watching the novice practice the activity. This means that the observer sees what not to do as well as what to do to achieve the goal of the activity. One strategy that implements this use of demonstration is the pairing or grouping of children where one of the pair or group practices the activity while the others observe him. After a certain number of practice attempts or a specific amount of time, one of the observers practices the activity and the previous performer becomes an observer. This is consistent with the philosophy of conducting intensive therapies such as constraint-induced movement therapy in group or day camp settings,[16,24,42] as described later in the chapter.

Verbal Instructions

An alternative to demonstrating how to perform an activity is providing verbal instructions. Although evidence supports the value of verbal instructions, two factors are important to consider. One is that the *amount of instruction* given must be within the limits of the person's capacity to remember and think about them when he or she attempts to perform the activity. In general, this means that instructions should be few in number and concise in presentation, particularly when working with children or individuals with limited comprehension.

Another influential factor is where the instructions *focus the person's attention* while performing the activity. Researchers have compared the effects of focusing attention on the movements themselves (i.e., an *internal focus*), such as "be sure that your thigh is parallel to the floor before you place your foot on the step," versus focusing attention on the intended movement outcome (i.e., an *external focus*), such as "be sure to place your foot on the step." Typically better learning occurs with an external focus, that is, when the person's attention is directed to the intended movement outcome. (See Wulf et al.[126] for a review of this research and an experiment involving patients with Parkinson's disease learning to improve postural stability.)

We commonly think of verbal instructions as words that describe how to perform a skill or activity. But another way to use verbal instructions about how to perform a skill or activity is to describe a *visual metaphoric image* to help the person determine how to perform the skill. This type of image involves picturing in the mind what the skill or activity is like, rather than the skill itself. For example, the fundamental locomotion movement of hopping with two legs involves a complex array of movements that must be spatially and temporally coordinated. A verbal description of this array of movements to inform a child what to do to hop

may overwhelm the child. Although a demonstration of hopping would be an alternative way to provide information of what to do, telling the child to move from one place to another "like a bunny would move" describes a metaphoric image the child can use to determine how to hop.

Presenting Feedback During Practice

When a person practices a skill or activity, he or she typically performs some parts correctly and some incorrectly. The therapist provides essential information about these aspects of the person's performance by providing feedback. Although the term *feedback* is used in various ways, we use it here to denote the information the therapist provides to the child during or after the performance of an activity (this type of feedback is sometimes referred to as *augmented, external,* or *extrinsic* feedback to distinguish it from the feedback naturally available through the various sensory systems, such as visual, auditory, or tactile feedback).[72]

Feedback provided by the therapist can refer to the outcome of performing a skill (e.g., "you were 2 inches short of grasping the cup") or the movement characteristics that led to the performance outcome (e.g., "your elbow was not extended enough to allow you to reach the cup"). Motor learning researchers often refer to these two types of feedback as knowledge of results (KR) and knowledge of performance (KP), respectively.[72]

Feedback can play two roles in the motor skill learning process. One is to facilitate achievement of the skill's performance goal. Because feedback provides information about the degree of success achieved while performing a skill (e.g., the errors made or what was done correctly), the learner can determine whether what he or she is doing is appropriate, and what he or she should do differently to successfully perform the skill. In this way, feedback can help the person achieve successful performance of the skill more quickly or easily than could occur without the feedback. The second role of feedback is motivational. Feedback can motivate the child to continue striving toward a specific performance goal. In this role, the child uses feedback to compare his or her own performance to a specified performance goal. The person must then decide to continue to pursue that goal, to change the goal, or to stop performing the activity.

Feedback About Errors Versus Correct Aspects of Performance

An often debated issue is whether the performance information conveyed by feedback should refer to the mistakes the person made or those aspects of the skill or activity that were correctly performed. The resolution to this debate appears to be that both types of information are valuable, especially because each is related to a different role of feedback. Research evidence consistently has shown that error information is more effective for facilitating skill learning, and information about correctly performed aspects of an activity serves to inform the person that he or she is on track in learning the skill or activity, which should encourage the person to keep trying.[72]

Selecting the Skill or Activity Component for Feedback

When a child performs a skill or activity during a therapy session, he or she will undoubtedly make many errors. The challenge the therapist faces in this situation is determining which error, or errors, to give feedback about. The first step in addressing this challenge is to acknowledge that the feedback will relate to only one aspect or component of the person's performance. The rationale for this point relates to a similar point made in our earlier discussion about the amount of instruction to present, which emphasized the need to keep the amount of information given within memory and attention limits. To simplify the process of determining how much feedback to give, we recommend that the therapist focus on only one aspect or component of the child's performance.

The decision to give feedback about one of the many errors characterizing a person's performance of a skill or activity leads to another challenge. Of the many errors observed, which one should feedback be given about? The therapist should base this decision on the part of the skill that is most critical for achieving the performance goal of the skill. For example, if a child were attempting to step over an object, the most critical part of the skill would be looking at the object. If the child is not looking at the object, the therapist would provide feedback to correct this error. Additional errors to be corrected would be based on a priority list of errors that are most critical for successfully performing the skill.

Frequency of Giving Feedback

It is not uncommon for therapists to want to give error correction feedback after every attempt a patient makes at performing a skill, or even during the performance itself. However, sufficient research evidence shows that giving error correction feedback during or after every practice trial (referred to as 100% frequency) is not optimal for learning motor skills. Rather, a less than 100% frequency optimizes skill learning, at least in healthy adults.[71] The primary problem with 100% frequency is that it engages the patient in a fundamentally different, and less effective, learning process than when he or she receives error correction feedback less frequently. According to the *guidance hypothesis*,[96,120] the learner uses the feedback to guide his or her performance to achieve success, which occurs rather quickly. But there is a negative aspect to this guidance. The positive guidance benefit experienced during practice creates a dependency on the availability of feedback, which results in performance without the feedback that is poorer than if the feedback were available. In effect, the feedback becomes a crutch that is essential for performing the skill. In contrast, when feedback is available less frequently than on every practice attempt, the learner engages in more active learning strategies on

trials when no feedback is available. A concern here for pediatric physical therapists is the extent to which the guidance hypothesis as it relates to feedback frequency applies to children. As is discussed later in this chapter, some research evidence suggests that the frequency conclusion may not apply to children in the same way as it applies to adults.

Although motor learning scholars have not identified an optimal frequency for giving error correction feedback, they have reported various techniques that reduce the frequency to less than 100%.[72] One is the *fading technique*, which systematically reduces the frequency from high to low as the person progresses in learning the skill. Another technique (referred to as the *self-selection technique*) involves the patient receiving feedback only when he or she requests it. It is interesting to note that research has shown that when novice learners are allowed to request error correction feedback when they want it, they request it at a frequency that is less than 100%. Another technique involves the *interspersing of motivational and error correction feedback* during practice trials. Research has not established an optimal ratio for the interspersing of these two types of feedback.

Practice Structure

In addition to selecting specific activities for each child, an essential part of the physical therapist's decision making involves scheduling the sequence of those activities. This scheduling involves not only the within therapy session activities but also the activities to be completed from the first to the last session. Specific motor learning principles can guide the therapist in making these scheduling decisions.

Practice Variability

A practice structure characteristic that increases the chances for future performance success is the variability of the learner's experiences while he or she practices. This includes variations in the skill or activity itself, as well as variations in the context in which an activity is practiced. In the motor learning literature, inclusion of these variations is referred to as *practice variability*.[72] A common characteristic of theories of motor skill learning is their emphasis on the learning and performance benefits derived from practice variability. The primary benefit a learner derives from practice experiences that promote movement and context variability is an increased capability to perform a skill or activity in some future situation. This means that the person has acquired an increased capability not only to perform a practiced skill or activity, but also to adapt to performance context conditions that he or she may not have actually experienced before.

Practice variability can be included in practice sessions in various ways. One is by directly requiring the child to perform multiple variations of a skill that require different movement patterns or sequences to achieve the same action goal. For example, consider how in a child's daily activities he or she moves to achieve the goal of reaching, grasping, and drinking from a cup. The person may need to use various movement strategies to achieve this goal simply because of the location or shape of the cup, or various movement strategies will be required when the cup is completely full or almost empty. Another way to include practice variability in practice sessions is to vary the characteristics of the context in which the skill or activity is performed. Using the same reaching-grasping-drinking from a cup example, context characteristics can be varied by using different types and sizes of cups (e.g., cup with sippy cover, one or two handles, with a straw) or different types of contents in the cup.

Organizing Practice Variability

When variations of a skill or activity, or performance context, are included in therapy sessions, the therapist needs to determine how to organize or schedule those variations. Should each variation be practiced separately with a sufficient amount of time or number of practice trials for the person to demonstrate a desired amount of improvement? Or should each variation be practiced in a way that all variations are experienced within each session? Research comparing these two different organizational schemes has consistently shown the superiority of the latter versus the former approach in terms of learning benefits.[72]

Motor learning research that has compared various practice variability schedules has demonstrated the *contextual interference (CI) effect*. The term *contextual interference* refers to the interference (i.e., memory or performance disruption) that results from performing variations of skills or activities within the context of a practice session.[72,73] The "CI effect" is that higher amounts of CI during practice result in better learning than occurs with lower amounts. In terms of variable practice schedules, this effect translates into schedules that involve more interspersing of skill or activity variation within a practice session, which results in better learning than occurs with schedules that involve less interspersing of variations. The most commonly compared practice schedules have been *blocked* and *random* practice schedules, which are the two extremes of the types of schedules that can be organized within the CI framework.[73] Blocked practice schedules create the least amount of CI by engaging the learner in nonrepeated sets of practice trials (or amounts of time) for each skill or activity variation. In contrast, random practice schedules create the highest amount of CI by engaging the learner in performing all skill or activity variations in random order throughout the practice session.

An important characteristic of the CI effect is that performance of the skills or activities is qualitatively different when compared during practice sessions and transfer tests (i.e., performance trials that differ in some way from those experienced during practice sessions). Typically, people perform the skills or activities better during practice in a blocked practice schedule. But an opposite result occurs on transfer tests when people who followed a random practice schedule during practice show superior performance.

Although there is some controversy within the physical rehabilitation community about the applicability of the CI effect to rehabilitation contexts, it is important to note that research in these contexts has been sparse and typically limited to comparisons of only blocked and random schedules. Many alternative practice schedule variations induce different amounts of CI. Unfortunately, too few of these schedules have been investigated to determine the specific application limits for clinical situations.

Practice Specificity

The earlier discussion of the generalization of learning emphasized the importance of the degree of similarity between practice conditions and future performance situations. This relationship, which is often referred to as *practice specificity*, emphasizes the need for comparable conditions in both practice and future performance situations. The practice specificity hypothesis is one of the oldest principles of human learning, with origins that can be traced back to the early 1900s.[109,110] Motor learning researchers since that time have accumulated sufficient evidence to show that practice specificity is especially applicable to the sensory/perceptual characteristics of practice and future performance contexts. According to Proteau, motor skill learning is specific to the sources of sensory/perceptual information available during practice.[88] This conclusion is especially relevant to the availability of visual feedback. Because people use and rely on visual feedback when it is available, it can become a potential problem in practice settings. For example, the use of mirrors as a source of visual feedback to help people learn to move in specified ways can lead to a dependence on the mirrors for performing the skill or activity. When the mirrors are not available to perform the skill or activity, performance is typically poorer than if the mirror is available. In effect, the visual feedback from the mirrors becomes part of what is learned during practice.

The practice specificity and practice variability hypotheses may appear to be at odds with each other, but the two points are actually complementary. Both hypotheses propose that practice conditions can create a dependency on the availability of certain conditions during practice and future performance situations: the more specific the conditions during practice, the more dependent the person becomes on the availability of those conditions. And both hypotheses propose that varying conditions during practice can break this potential dependency.

Massed and Distributed Practice

Another practice structure issue concerns the amount of time to devote to various activities within and across sessions. Included in this issue are questions about the length of each session, the amount of active engagement in each activity within a session, and the amount of rest between activities within and between sessions. Each of these questions can be answered by determining whether to use massed or distributed practice conditions. The terms *massed* and *distributed* refer to the amount of time in which a person actively practices and rests between and during practice sessions. Researchers have not established objective definitions for these terms with respect to amount of time or number of trials. As a result, these terms are operationally defined with respect to the context in which they are used. Massed practice involves longer active practice and shorter rest periods than distributed practice.[72]

One application of massed and distributed practice relates to the *length and distribution of practice sessions*, that is, if a specified amount of time (or number of practice trials) should be devoted to practicing a skill or activity, is it better to schedule longer (and fewer) practice sessions or shorter (and more) practice sessions? In physical therapy settings, this question is often answered by limitations imposed by health care management and financing systems. But when the therapist can set these limits, he or she can make the decision on the basis of evidence from motor learning research. The general principle derived from this evidence is that shorter and more practice sessions are preferred to longer and fewer sessions.

The second application of massed and distributed practice relates to the *length of the rest intervals between trials*. For example, if a child is supposed to perform ten repetitions of an activity, how much time should the patient rest between repetitions to maximize the benefit of the repetitions? The answer to this question is not as straightforward as it was for determining the length and distribution of practice sessions. Although the traditional view has been that distributed practice is better than massed, recent research evidence indicates that distributed practice is better only for the learning of continuous skills, such as locomotion, cycling, and swimming activities, but massed practice is better for discrete skills, such as reaching and grasping, and limb positioning (e.g., range of motion exercises).[70] One of the factors influencing this effect of the type of skill is the role played by fatigue. Massed practice trials create fatigue problems for continuous skills more than for discrete skills.

Whole and Part Practice

Another of the many decisions the physical therapist must make in a therapy session concerns whether it is better to have the patient initially practice a skill or activity in its entirety or in parts. For example, if a child needs to learn to get out of bed and into a wheelchair, should the child initially practice the entire sequence of the parts of this activity as a whole, or should he or she practice the separate parts before trying the whole activity? One of the ways to determine an answer to this question is to analyze the skill in terms of its complexity and organization characteristics. As originally proposed by Naylor and Briggs, *complexity* refers to the number of parts of the skill, as well as the amount of attention demanded by the performer.[79] Complexity increases as the number of parts and the amount of attention demanded

increase. The *organization* of a skill is determined by the temporal and spatial relationships of the parts of the skill. Motor skills in which the parts are relatively independent in terms of temporal and spatial relationships between parts are considered to be low in organization. In contrast, skills in which the between-parts relationships are temporally and spatially interdependent have a high level of organization. According to the Naylor and Briggs complexity–organization model, skills that are low in complexity and high in organization should be practiced as whole skills, but skills that are high in complexity and low in organization should be practiced in parts.[79] To apply this model to the skills and activities in physical therapy, the clinician needs to analyze each skill in terms of its levels of complexity and organization before determining whether the child should initially practice the skill or activity as a whole or in parts.

Most of the functional skills and activities that a physical therapy patient must practice are relatively complex, which means that most of these skills should be practiced in parts before they are practiced as a whole skill. Now the question becomes which parts should be practiced separately and which should be combined? The answer is determined by the organization characteristic of the parts. Those parts that are temporally and spatially interrelated should be grouped together as a natural unit within the skill. For example, research has shown that the reach and grasp components of reaching for and grasping a cup to drink from it are temporally and spatially related, which would indicate a high level of organization for these two parts of the skill.[57] This relationship between these two parts suggests that they should be practiced together as a single natural unit of the skill.

A common strategy for engaging people in practicing individual parts is known as the *progressive part method*. Rather than have people practice each part of a skill separately before performing the whole skill, the progressive part method involves practicing the skill in increasing sizes of sequences of parts. The first part is practiced separately until a certain level of success is achieved and then the second part is added so that the first and second parts are practiced as one unit. Each part then gets progressively added until the whole skill is performed.

Reducing Difficulty of a Skill

For some skills or activities, it may be more desirable to reduce the difficulty of the skill and practice a modified version of the whole skill rather than to practice the skill by parts. The use of this approach to practicing a skill involves at least a two-step sequence. The first step is practicing the simplified version of the skill, which is followed by practicing the actual skill without the modification. Whether additional modifications are needed between these two steps will depend on the skill or activity and the person learning the skill or activity. Research has shown that several strategies effectively reduce a skill's difficulty and can be employed as an initial practice experience.[72] Each strategy relates to the characteristic of a skill or activity that makes it especially difficult to perform. In addition, each strategy simplifies the performance of the skill or activity in a way that allows the person to practice the skill's basic movement coordination pattern, which is essential to learn in the initial stage of learning. The following three strategies meet these requirements: (1) reduce the speed at which the skill is normally performed to a pace that allows attention to be given to the movement pattern; (2) reduce the difficulty of the object that must be manipulated while performing the skill or activity; and (3) reduce the attention demands required by the skill, such as by using the body weight support system for performing gait skills. Other effective methods for reducing the complexity and difficulty of skills include the use of virtual reality and simulators. Although physical therapists have increased their use of these devices in recent years, research concerning their use and effectiveness is lacking.

Mental Practice

The term *mental practice* refers to the cognitive or mental rehearsal of a physical skill in the absence of overt physical movement. When engaging in mental practice, people may think about the cognitive or procedural aspects of the skill or activity, or they may engage in visual and/or kinesthetic imagery in which they see and/or feel themselves actually performing the skill or activity. Research concerning the use of mental practice in motor skill learning has established its effectiveness in facilitating skill acquisition in adults and as a means of preparation just before performing a skill or activity.

As an aid to skill acquisition, mental practice is most effective when combined with actual physical practice of the skill or activity. In some research, the inclusion of mental practice can reduce the need for physical practice by 25% to 50%.[5] This means that 50 physical practice trials combined with 50 mental practice trials are as effective for learning a skill as 100 physical practice trials. Numerous research studies have reported the effectiveness of mental practice in physical rehabilitation settings.[72,81,103]

As a means of skill or activity performance preparation, mental practice involves the person visually and kinesthetically imaging himself performing the skill in the few minutes or seconds before actually performing the skill. An example in a physical rehabilitation setting would be a situation in which a child must stand up from a seated position. While seated, the child would visually see and kinesthetically feel himself or herself performing the entire sequence of movements required to perform the skill. After engaging in this brief mental imagery experience, the child would then physically perform the skill.

Why is mental practice effective for aiding motor skill learning and performance preparation? Researchers have proposed and provided evidence to support several hypotheses. One is the neuromuscular hypothesis, which states that the imaging or visualizing of motor skill performance creates electrical activity in the nerves and musculature involved in performing the skill.[22] Although this activity can be measured by electromyography (EMG), it does not reach a level of intensity that would produce the kind of muscle activity needed to produce observable movement. The brain activity hypothesis involves a similar notion of internal activity that simulates activity that occurs when the skill is actually performed. According to this hypothesis, which is based on the results of brain imaging studies, when a person imagines moving a body part, the brain activity is similar to what occurs when the person physically moves.[84] The third hypothesis, known as the cognitive hypothesis, proposes that mental practice engages the person in the type of cognitive processes in which a person engages before, during, and after physically performing a motor skill.[72] These processes may include cognitive activities such as decision making or developing strategies to correct performance errors. Together the research evidence supporting these three explanations for the effectiveness of mental practice establishes the potential roles that mental practice can play in physical therapy.

MOTOR LEARNING IN TYPICALLY DEVELOPING CHILDREN

Children learn motor skills with astonishing frequency. Functional activities (e.g., crawling, walking, grasping, manipulating), academic skills, and play increasingly involve complex, skilled actions that develop as various cognitive and social skills emerge. Thus not only do children undergo motor learning repeatedly, but this occurs as cognition and the physical constructs of their bodies change. Thus it is important to consider learning in the context of motor development of age-appropriate skills. Many of the principles derived from the adult studies outlined above most certainly hold true in children. Although oddly there is a paucity of motor learning studies in children, it is important to note that the nature and capacity of the learner may be quite different, and thus it is important to understand differences in motor learning between adults and children.

In this section of the chapter, we describe key differences between motor learning in children and in adults and discuss how many of the above described principles may or may not hold true in children.

CHILDREN ARE NOT SIMPLY LITTLE ADULTS

Perhaps the most important difference between children and adults is the concurrent changes in physical structure that provide the ability to learn and also force the child to relearn as his or her body changes. For example, learning to walk can occur only after suitable strength and balance capabilities emerge. Precision grasping can emerge only after the development of finger individuation, which depends on the maturation of the corticospinal tract.[40] That is not to say that learning and development are purely driven by maturation.

Rather, it is likely epigenetic, where both maturation of physical and neuronal structures and environmental cues and practice influence each other and guide development,[31] just as the person, task, and environment affect adult learning. Furthermore, as changes in body mass and limb length occur, the dynamics required to produce skilled action also change. Thus learning activities must be planned and occur continually in the context of the developing child (see Chapters 2 and 3), and motor learning at one time point may not directly transfer to another.

Equally important is the increasing capacity to process and store information. Adults have amazing cognitive processing capabilities, but these emerge slowly throughout development. Children are known to have decreased information processing capabilities compared with adults.[87] This limits the amount and type of information they can process. Children are slower processing such information and have decreased selective attention to do so. Limited processing and reduced object recognition capabilities affect their ability to copy images.[67] Higher-level attentional focus,[64,74] spatial working memories,[98] and verbal learning and memories[18] all differ between children and adults. This means that the amount of information (e.g., feedback) that children can process and the rate at which they may do so may be limited, and thus many of the principles of motor learning discussed so far may need to be adjusted according to age expectations, as well as any cognitive limitations.

Feedback Schedules

The above differences may also bring into question the applicability of some adult learning principles. In fact, in a number of cases, learning indeed has been shown to be quite different in children. One could imagine that slower feedback processing in children could result in information overload, which would interfere with learning, and thus like adults, they would benefit from intermittent feedback as described earlier. In contrast, however, such reduced feedback has been found to be *less* beneficial than feedback provided after every trial in children.[106] This can be seen in Figure 4-2, which shows variability during acquisition and retention of an arm movement task in adults (Figure 4-2, *A*) and children (Figure 4-2, *B*). Specifically, performance accuracy during acquisition was similar in adults regardless of whether or not feedback was reduced. In contrast, reduced feedback in children resulted in more error. This could be due to the reduced attentional capabilities described previously, but it may relate to the fact that children have increased error and movement variability,[7] whereby their signal-to-noise becomes much higher and intrinsic feedback is washed out. Errors may increase disproportionately as accuracy demands increase.[68] Children are also known to rely more on online adjustments during movement, and increased feedback may help calibrate these adjustments.[30,128] Children may require increased feedback to update internal representations, which may interact with information processing.

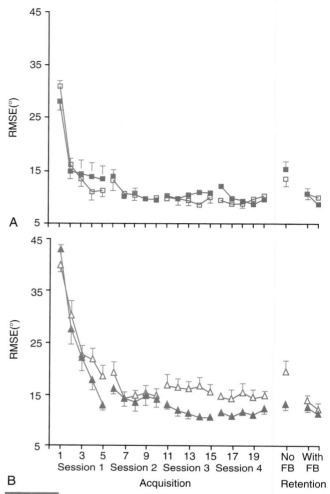

Figure 4-2   Block means (±SE) for root mean square error (RMSE) during acquisition, retention (no feedback), and reacquisition phases (with feedback) for young **(A)** adults and **(B)** children. *Filled symbols* denote feedback on all trials; *unfilled symbols* denote feedback on 62% of trials. (Modified with permission from Sullivan, K. J., Kantak, S. S., & Burtner, P. A. (2008). Motor learning in children: Feedback effects on skill acquisition. *Physical Therapy, 88,* 720–732.)

Early studies on feedback reduction suggested a similarity to adults whereby feedback fading was beneficial as learning progressed in children.[35,99] More recent evidence may suggest that fading of feedback beyond a critical point may in fact be detrimental to learning in children.[106] There may be a critical point in age or skill where feedback reduction interferes, and feedback may need to be withdrawn more gradually. Practice in children can be made more effective with feedback with optimal information without guiding to outcome.[78] Thus a key challenge to the therapist is to monitor how feedback is influencing performance and modify the frequency accordingly. Nevertheless even within a given patient, the optimal feedback frequency may vary, depending on the tasks being learned.

Types of Practice Schedules

The organization of practice variability to modulate contextual interference may also need to differ between children and adults. Some evidence suggests that for children, like adults, random practice is better for learning[62] and retention.[49,87] Yet blocked or mixed practice may be better for some tasks[48] and age groups.[127] Still other studies suggest no difference in practice schedules.[23,61] Blocked may be better for younger/less skilled learners for complex tasks.[52] In this case, random practice schedules may overload the system with too much information, given the reduced and slower information processing. Yet handwriting retention in elementary school kids was found to be better during random practice.[105] Thus the type of practice schedule that is most beneficial may in fact depend on age, task complexity, and skill level.[62,127]

Learning Occurs Over Considerable Time and Practice

An important consideration is that unlike many of the laboratory-based tasks used in published research, complex functional motor skills are not learned over short periods. Even in adults, expert typists,[9] chess players, musicians, and athletes[28] engaged in immense amounts of practice over long durations to acquire skill. Crawling infants have been shown to practice maintaining balance more than 5 hours per day, equal to approximately 3000 crawling steps; similarly, walking is practiced over 6 hours per day, equal to approximately 9000 steps.[1] Thus hundreds of thousands of trials are spread out over weeks or months during infant development of mobility skills. The naturalistic practice in which these infants and children engaged is not continually the same (blocked); actually a rich variety of events, locations, and surfaces are experienced over an extended time period. This can be considered an exaggerated version of random practice. Thus rather than practicing a solution, this random experience may construct new solutions and dissuade infants from relying on simple stimulus-response learning and instead promote "learning to learn."[1,2,51] This generalization strategy would promote broad transfer of learning within perception action systems (e.g., walking on various surfaces) and narrow specificity between them (walking versus crawling). Rest between learning sets during development of such skills is intermittent, which may promote the contextual interference effects described earlier in the chapter. Because in most cases physical therapists cannot be with patients over such long durations, promoting strategies that will generalize to home environments should be used to facilitate practice in that environment. An example is to use strategies involving active problem solving.[106] Thus the involvement of caregivers is a crucial component of continued learning.

MOTOR LEARNING IN PEDIATRIC REHABILITATION

Although much of pediatric rehabilitation focuses on learning of motor skills, little is known about the learning processes in children with physical or neurologic disabilities. Motor learning in this case is further complicated by the physical constraints involved, as well as by potential sensory impairments that may diminish feedback and affect the updating of internal models used for movement. In this section of the chapter, we provide some examples of learning in children with physical or neurologic disabilities with a focus on cerebral palsy, which is the most common type of childhood neurologic disability and the topic on which the majority of research in pediatric motor learning has been focused.

PRACTICE MAKES BETTER

Cerebral palsy (CP) is a developmental disorder of movement and posture that causes limitations in activity and deficits in motor skills (see Chapter 18). CP is attributed to nonprogressive disturbances in the developing fetal or infant brain. Spastic hemiplegia, characterized by motor impairments mainly affecting one side of the body, is among the most common subtypes, accounting for 30% to 40% of new cases.[53] Through much of the 20th century, the motor impairments, especially in the upper extremity (UE), were thought to be static, with little potential for habilitation. Thus therapy efforts were largely directed at minimizing impairment (e.g., reducing spasticity, preventing contractures). In fact, as recent as two decades ago, studies were suggesting that individuals with CP could reduce unwanted motor activity or spasticity with visual tracking or biofeedback, but that they had little ability to learn appropriate motor commands.[80,82] Early work studying prehensile force control reinforced this view, suggesting that children with CP retain infantile coordination strategies.[40] Subsequent studies, however, provided two separate lines of evidence that these impairments are not static, and instead improve with sufficient practice.

First, developmental studies of children with CP have shown that motor function does improve over the course of development. For example, gross motor function has been shown to improve as children with CP get older.[92] Development of hand function has also been observed. For example, Holmefur and colleagues studied the longitudinal development of bimanual UE use in children with hemiplegic CP.[55] Children were followed for 4 to 5 years with the Assisting Hand Assessment (AHA), a Rasch-based measure that describes how the affected UE is used as a nondominant assist during bimanual activities. Investigators found that bimanual proficiency improves during the course of development, but that the developmental rate and the subsequent plateau depend on the initial score at 18 months of age

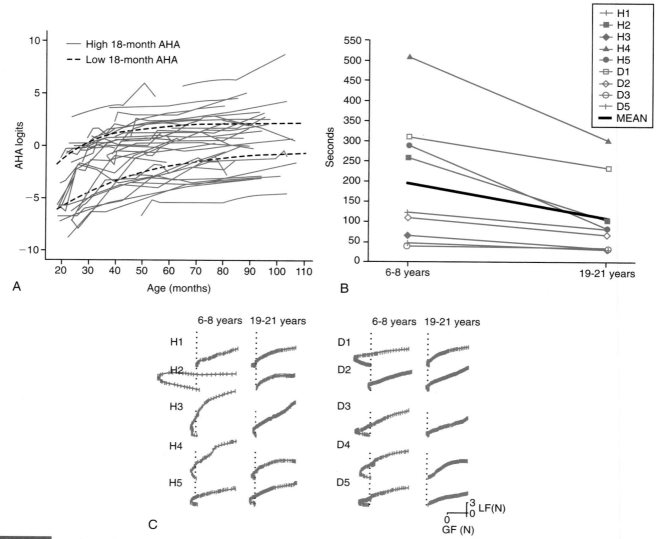

Figure 4-3 **A,** Observed and predicted Assisting Hand Assessment (AHA) development. Groups have high (n = 27) or low (n = 16) 18-month score (above or below −3 logits) on the AHA at age 18 months in children with CP. Higher scores mean better bimanual performance. **B,** Time to complete the six timed items (writing excluded) of the Jebsen-Taylor Test of Hand Function for individual participants, as well as mean *(bold line)* from the first (age 6 to 8 years) and second (age 19 to 21 years) data collection sessions. Faster times correspond to better performance. **C,** Mean grip-force/load-force trajectories for each subject *(A,* hemiplegic subjects; *B,* diplegic subjects) at the ages of 6 to 8 *(left)* and 19 to 21 *(right)* years. The *x*-axis corresponds to load force (LF), and the *y*-axis represents grip force (GF). *Straighter lines* indicate simultaneous increase in the two forces. *Dn,* Diplegic; *Hn,* hemiplegic. (**A,** From Holmefur et al., in press.) (**B, C,** From Eliasson et al., 2006.)

(Figure 4-3, *A*). Children with hemiplegia with higher bimanual function in early childhood developed bimanual skills faster and reached their limit earlier than children with lower bimanual function. It is interesting to note that the development of bimanual UE use differs from that of gross motor activities in CP,[92] where milder children reach their limit later. During a 13-year follow-up study starting at the age of 6 to 8 years, it was found that hand function in children with CP improves with age.[25] Specifically, time to complete items on the Jebsen-Taylor Test of Hand Function improved in all children, and grip force coordination during grasp improved (Figure 4-3, *B*). Thus both gross and fine motor functions do develop, although these two general types of skills seem to develop and reach plateaus differently.

A second line of evidence that motor function is not static in CP comes from systematic studies on the effects of extended practice that have demonstrated that motor performance can indeed improve with practice.[63] In one study, children with CP were asked to repeatedly lift an object of a given weight 25 times.[44] Even though motor learning was considerably slower than in typically developing children, impairments in fine manipulative capabilities and force regulation during grasp were partially ameliorated with this extended practice. This suggests that the initial impaired performance, at least in part, may be due to lack of use, and that many impairments in motor control previously documented may be due to the fact that insufficient practice was provided (i.e., early stages of motor learning rather than motor control capabilities were captured). Similarly, in-hand manipulation has been shown to improve with practice.[24] Such benefit of intensive training has also been documented in postural control in children with CP.[100] It is important to note that these findings suggest intensive practice may provide a window of opportunity for improvement. It is increasingly being recognized that reduction of unwanted tone (i.e., by the use of botulinum toxin) alone does not improve function,[89] and that functional or task-oriented approaches and physical conditioning provided with sufficient intensity have the potential to improve motor function in CP.[3,47,65,118] Unlike adults, children with CP may benefit more from concrete instructions than from movement outcome information.[117] Motor learning in this case may require providing careful feedback on knowledge of performance, as well as cognitive strategies to achieve better performance levels.[111]

Together, these lines of evidence contradict traditional clinical assumptions that motor impairments in CP are static. UE performance in children with CP may improve with practice and development. More important, this implies that hand function in particular may well be amenable to treatment.

So what type of practice schedules may be best for motor learning in children with CP? After a blocked practice schedule over several sessions, children with CP retain the ability to grade isometric grip force (using online visual feedback) after a 5-day delay.[116] Even within a single session of extended blocked practice, children with hemiplegic CP improved their ability to scale fingertip forces to the weight and texture of novel objects.[44] Similar to healthy adults, blocked practice resulted in better acquisition of force scaling to the grip of novel objects in children with CP than did random practice.[23] But both practice schedules resulted in similar retention (Figure 4-4). These findings suggest that children with CP can form and retain internal representations of novel objects for anticipatory control, irrespective of the type of practice schedule employed. It should be noted, however, that force scaling is a form of parameter learning as opposed to learning a new skill (such as how to grasp). In that sense, the findings are in line with the hypothesis that random

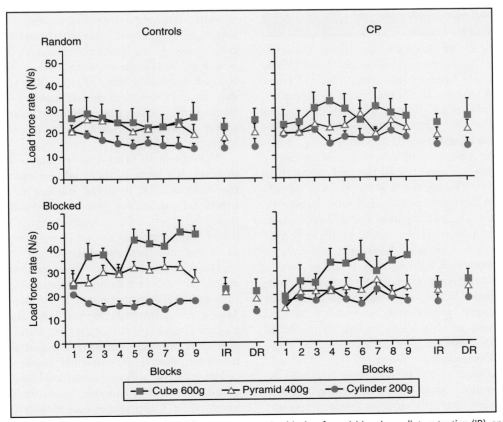

Figure 4-4   Mean ± standard error of the mean (SEM) load force rate across nine blocks of acquisition, immediate retention (IR), and delayed retention (DR) during lifts with cylinder *(circle)*, pyramid *(triangle)*, and *cube (square)* for control children *(left)* and children with hemiplegic cerebral palsy (CP) *(right)*. **Insets** show mean (SEM) single trials from first trial at immediate retention and first trial at delayed retention. Blocked practice resulted in better acquisition of force scaling, but retention was similar for both types of practice. (From Duff & Gordon, 2003.)

practice would not provide an advantage over blocked practice for parameter learning.[73] Thus it is unknown whether one form of practice is more beneficial than the other in this population, although random or mixed practice may resemble naturalistic learning to a greater extent. Nevertheless, it is clear that intensity of practice matters in rehabilitation.[8] An important point is that usual and customary therapy delivery schedules may not be sufficient for providing such intensity. For example, a study of physical therapy and occupational therapy sessions for adults with hemiparesis post stroke showed that the numbers of repetitions of UE movement observed were relatively small.[69] Although it is not known how many repetitions occur in pediatric therapies, one could imagine that this number would be even smaller given the requirement to maintain the interest and attention of children. In fact, one study of intensive constraint-induced movement therapy showed that 4- to 8-year-old children were engaged in tasks over less than 60% of a 6-hour day.[16] This effort is even less than it appears, as this number does not reflect time between trials and time taken to redirect focus as needed. It is interesting to note that children who required less redirection of focus improved to a greater extent than those who required a lot of redirection. Next we consider models for delivery of intensive practice schedules.

TASK-ORIENTED TRAINING

Unlike neuromuscular re-education approaches traditionally focused on impairment-level disablement (body functions/structures in International Classification of Functioning, Disability, and Health Resources [ICF] language), task-oriented training is a top-down approach that focuses on activity limitations (i.e., an important aspect of CP) rather than on remediation of impairments or correction of movement patterns. Task-oriented training can be considered a motor learning or goal-directed approach to rehabilitation.[11,113,121] The approach is based on integrated models of motor learning and control and behavioral neuroscience focusing on participation and skill acquisition. An important component is the active problem solving described earlier. The associated behavioral demands of the tasks and motor skill training may result in cortical reorganization[86] underlying concurrent functional outcomes. For optimal efficacy, task-oriented training must be challenging, must progressively increase behavioral demands, and must involve active participation. Skilled training in animals shows the plasticity of UE cortical representation, whereas unskilled training did not.[66] The tasks must also have salience to the performer to influence the person-task-environment triad. In fact there may not be a relationship between intensity and outcome unless the nature of training is considered.[123] Thus at least beyond a certain point, time on task may be less important than what is practiced.

The importance of task-oriented approaches was highlighted in a randomized trial of 55 children with CP comparing functional physical therapy versus a reference group whose therapy was based on the principle of movement normalization (including some aspects of neurodevelopmental treatment [NDT] and the Vojta method).[65] The functional therapy model consisted of the establishment of functional goals, repetitive practice of problematic motor abilities in a meaningful environment, active problem solving, and involvement of caregivers in goal setting, decision making, and implementation in daily life (i.e., many of the motor learning principles described earlier).

Gross motor abilities in a standardized environment were measured with the Gross Motor Function Measure (GMFM).[93] The GMFM is a standardized observational instrument for children with CP, developed to measure change in gross motor function, including lying and rolling, sitting, crawling and kneeling, standing, and walking, running, and jumping. Motor abilities in daily situations were measured using the Pediatric Evaluation of Disability Inventory (PEDI).[50] The PEDI is a judgment-based assessment that uses parent report through a structured interview. Two domains of the PEDI were measured: self-care and mobility. These include independent toileting, brushing teeth, dressing, etc.

Both measures were taken 6 months, 12 months, and 18 months after implementation of the training programs. Investigators found no group differences in improvement in basic gross motor abilities.[65] However, when examining functional skills in daily situations, they found that children in the functional therapy group improved more than children in the movement normalization group. Thus, functional training had the additional benefit of improving motor abilities in the daily environment identified to be important to caregivers.

The efficacy of functional training in CP using varying protocols has been documented by a number of additional investigators.[3,47,118] Treadmill training is another form of functional training that focuses on massed practice of locomotor behaviors. Efficacy in Down syndrome is well established[114]; however, it is not yet clear whether this holds true in CP and other pediatric disabilities.[19,77]

Although evidence for functional and task-oriented approaches is accumulating, evidence for other approaches such as NDT is more limited. An evidence report for the American Academy of Cerebral Palsy and Developmental Medicine concluded that as of 2001, "there was not consistent evidence that NDT changed abnormal motoric responses, slowed or prevented contractures, or that it facilitated more normal motor development or functional motor activities."[10] However, when applied with greater intensity, NDT approaches may provide greater benefit.[6] It should be noted, however, that NDT has been evolving beyond the original concepts introduced by the Bobaths shortly after the Second World War, and more recent NDT approaches appear to incorporate some principles of motor learning.[56]

The examples of task-oriented approaches described earlier highlight the importance of motor learning principles such as intensity, specificity, and task salience. Next we provide two examples of contemporary task-oriented approaches focusing on upper extremity that further incorporate motor learning approaches: constraint-induced movement therapy and functional bimanual training.

CONSTRAINT-INDUCED THERAPY

A rich history of theoretical constructs has been derived from the basic sciences (including neurosciences and motor learning) underlying the application of intensive practice-based models of rehabilitation. For example, it has long been noted that monkeys with unilateral lesions or deafferentation neglect to use their affected UE, but indeed will do so if forced by restraint of the contralateral unaffected UE, and that this forced use led to improved use of the affected UE.[107,112] The idea that "residual (masked) capability" could potentially be tapped into by forced use of the deafferentated or impaired limb drove the development of intensive practice-based therapies in humans. This line of research began with studies of forced use in adults with hemiparetic stroke by Wolf and colleagues nearly 30 years ago.[83,122] Subsequently, Taub and coworkers added 6 hours of structured activities using principles of behavioral psychology (shaping).[108] Shaping involves approaching motor activities in small steps by successive approximation to the movement goal and/or grading of task difficulty based on the patient's capabilities[85,101]; it is similar to part practice described earlier in this chapter. The active intervention involving restraint plus structured practice evolved to become known as *constraint-induced movement therapy (CIMT)*.[108] CIMT can be considered to be a special class of task-oriented training because the triad among person, task, and environment is very much applied, although functional arm use is promoted more than skill. Strong evidence of efficacy has been obtained in adult patients following stroke.[124,125] Although it would be easy to misinterpret this work as suggesting that it is the restraint that is essential, it is important to note that optimal efficacy depends on employing the motor learning principles described so far. A recent example of this has been found using an animal model of hemiplegia.[33] One hemisphere of the cat motor cortex is transiently inactivated with muscimol, and the cat wears a restraint on the unimpaired limb with no training or receives training for 1 hour per day, 5 days per week, for 4 weeks, along with the restraint (Figure 4-5). Early in training, aiming of the paw was variable in accuracy (left) but improved by the fourth (final) week of training. The lower panels in Figure 4-5, *A*, show the distribution of the terminal position of the paw tip during reaches. Intracortical microstimulation showed that in normal (no CP) cats, more than 60% of the motor map comprised sites

at which electrical stimulation produces movement of the digit, wrist, or multiple joints of the forelimb (Figure 4-5, *B*). Without training (CP/no training), the numbers of digit and multijoint sites were greatly reduced. Constraint and training (CP/training) resulted in a normal motor map, with a predominance of digit and multijoint sites. In normal cats, corticospinal tract terminations reside in the medial dorsal horn of the spinal cord. Without training (CP/no training), terminations were found in the sensory region of the dorsal horn (Figure 4-5, *C*). Constraint and training (CP/training) resulted in a normal distribution of corticospinal terminations. These results indicate that despite both groups of cats being forced to use the affected limb, only cats that receive active skilled training have normalization of functional and synaptic plasticity. Thus the ingredients of training matter.

Constraint-Induced Therapy in Children with Hemiparesis

CIMT has not been studied in the pediatric population nearly to the extent that it has in adults with stroke, nor is the level of evidence of efficacy nearly as strong because most studies were case studies or small sample projects. For CIMT to be conducted in children, the overall approach must be changed to focus on age-appropriate activities that sustain interest for long periods, as children are not as easily motivated to perform activities of daily living or part practice for sustained periods of time in the way that adults are. Often the duration of restraint wear must be modified along with the type of restraint. These studies differ in age of participants (ranging from 9 months to 18 years), inclusion criteria, duration and intensity of treatment (ranging from usual and customary care schedules to adult models of CIMT), restraint (gloves, mitts, slings, and casts), and outcome measures.[13,26,54] Although the evidence is not yet conclusive, all of these studies have reported positive outcomes, and as such, CIMT can be considered a promising therapeutic approach for use with children with hemiplegia.

An important point is that CIMT should not be viewed as a one-time opportunity whereby the less-affected UE is restrained as much as possible (e.g., with a cast) and the highest possible intensity is provided regardless of age. Despite the diversity of approaches, no evidence suggests that one type of restraint is more effective than another; thus comfort and safety should be a key factor in restraint selection. Furthermore, improvements in UE performance in young children have been noted with just 2 hours per day three times per week.[27] Perhaps most important, repeated doses of CIMT have been shown to have an additive effect (Figure 4-6).[15] This suggests that there is no advantage to maintaining the potentially invasive schedule and restraints, and instead, one could administer CIMT through repeated, and less intensive, bouts. Thus, overall, CIMT is just a task-oriented method to induce intensive practice; it can be considered as part of a child's long-term pediatric rehabilitative care.

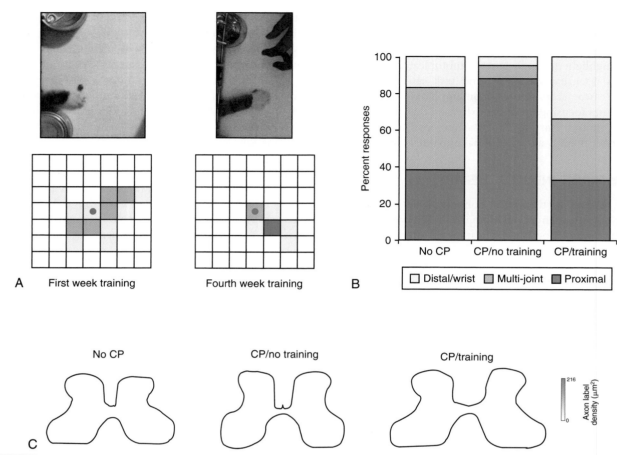

Figure 4-5 Constraint of the unimpaired forelimb and reach training of the impaired forelimb in a cat model of hemiplegic cerebral palsy. **A,** Reaching for cubes of meat on a horizontal surface. *Lower panels* show the trial distribution of the terminal position of the paw tip during reaches. **B,** Mapping of primary motor cortex using intracortical microstimulation. **C,** Distribution of corticospinal terminations in the lower cervical spinal cord. (Unpublished data courtesy of Dr. Kathleen Friel.)

CIMT utilizes a number of motor learning principles. These include use of both part and whole practice, modifying tasks to ensure success and progression of difficulty as success is achieved, active problem solving, optimal practice and feedback schedules, and the need to generalize learning to performance in everyday environments.

Despite the promise of CIMT, a number of conceptual problems have been noted in applying it to children that need consideration. First, CIMT was developed to overcome learned nonuse in adults with hemiplegia and to promote use over skill. These adults lost UE function and were often highly motivated to regain previously learned functional behaviors. Children, in contrast, must overcome *developmental disuse,* whereby they may have never learned how to effectively use their more affected extremity during many tasks and may need to learn how to use it for the first time. Thus, treatment must be developmentally focused and must take into account the principles of motor learning described earlier.

Second, restraining a child's less-affected extremity (especially with casts) is potentially psychologically and physically invasive, and thus should not be performed on young or severely impaired children with the same intensity as in adults. It must be remembered that use of the less-affected side is still developing in children. Neuroanatomic evidence in developing kittens indicates that refinement and maintenance of corticospinal terminations in the spinal cord are activity dependent.[76] Restriction of limb use on one side during a developmental critical period in early development reduces the topographic distribution, branch density, and density of presynaptic boutons on the side of restricted use.[45,75] This suggests that there may be a substantial risk of damage to the less affected UE if it is restrained for long periods at too early an age. Thus a greatly modified protocol is required in young children.

Finally, CIMT focuses on unimanual impairments, which do not greatly influence functional independence and quality of life in that children with hemiplegia have a well-functioning (dominant) hand.[102] Training it as a dominant hand while restrained likely will improve manual dexterity, although it lacks specificity of training for how the hand will be used once the restraint is removed, for example, as a

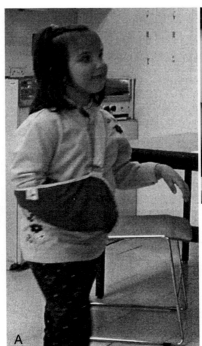

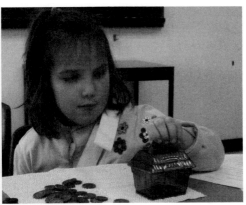

Figure 4-6 **A,** Schematic diagram of child with the less-affected upper extremity (UE) restrained with a cotton sling sewn shut, while the more affected UE practices placing coins in a coin bank. **B,** Mean ± SEM time to complete the six timed items (writing excluded) of the Jebsen-Taylor Test of Hand Function for eight children before and after 2 weeks of CIMT, 12 months later, and after a second dose of constraint-induced movement therapy (CIMT). Faster times correspond to better performance. The maximum allowable time to complete each item was capped at 120 seconds, resulting in a maximum score of 720 seconds. (Modified from Charles and Gordon, 2007.)

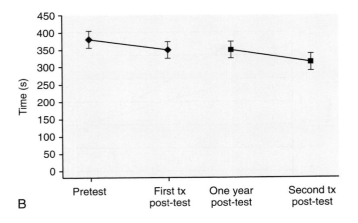

nondominant assisting hand during bimanual activities. Children with hemiplegia have impairments in spatial and temporal coordination of the two hands,[46,115] as well as global impairments in motor planning.[104] Constraint therapies cannot address these problems, and thus generalization of training may not apply.

UNCONSTRAINING THE CONSTRAINT: BIMANUAL TRAINING

Development of UE control is the consequence of activity-dependent competition between the two hemispheres, with the more active side winning out over the less active (damaged) side.[29,76] Balancing activity of the two hemispheres after unilateral brain damage may help restore motor function and may establish more normal anatomic organization of the corticospinal tract and motor representational

maps in the primary motor cortex.[34] One way to do this is by using repetitive transmagnetic stimulation (rTMS) or transcranial direct current stimulation (tDCS), both of which inhibit activation of ipsilateral pathways and enhance activation of contralateral pathways. Preliminary evidence suggests that such approaches may be promising in adult stroke rehabilitation[32] and may even facilitate motor learning.[90] From a functional perspective, principles of practice specificity would suggest that the best way to balance activity of the cerebral cortices and achieve improved bimanual control would be to directly practice bimanual coordination. Such bimanual training may be efficacious in adults with hemiparesis.[12,91] Recently, a child-appropriate form of task-oriented intensive functional training, hand-arm bimanual intensive therapy (HABIT) was developed, which aims to improve the amount and quality of involved UE use during bimanual tasks.[14] HABIT retains the two main elements of pediatric CIMT (intensive structured practice and child-friendliness), and similarly engages the child in bimanual activities 6 hours per day for 10 to 15 days in a day camp setting. It is important to note, however, that no physical restraint is used. Rather, bimanual UE coordination is elicited by modifying the environment. Similar to other functional training approaches often used in physical therapy and occupational therapy, HABIT involves task-oriented training to achieve meaningful goals. However, it differs from these approaches in that intensity is much greater, practice is far more structured, and children problem-solve and focus on how the UE performs at the *end point* of the movement. No effort to normalize movement is provided.

To date, two reports of efficacy have been documented. A small randomized control trial of HABIT was conducted on 20 children with hemiplegic CP between the ages of 3.5 and 14 years.[41] Children who received HABIT had improved scores on the Assisting Hand Assessment, while those in the no-treatment control group did not. Frequency of UE use increased for the children who received HABIT. Bimanual coordination, as determined by analysis of kinematics of a drawer-opening task,[58] showed that children improved temporal coordination of the movements of each extremity after receiving HABIT.

The above study provides preliminary evidence that task-oriented approaches directed at both UEs can improve bimanual UE use and coordination. Clearly, training without a restraint requires less intensive manipulative movements than CIMT because the more affected UE is being used as a nondominant assist. Is there a cost in treatment efficacy? Recent evidence suggests that there is not. The efficacy of CIMT was recently compared with that of bimanual training.[43] Similar significant improvements were demonstrated for each group from the pretest to the posttest on the Jebsen-Taylor Test of Hand Function and the Assisting Hand Assessment, and frequency of UE use was measured with accelerometers. Results indicate that the amount of improvement is not dependent on the use of a restraint. Ongoing work, however, suggests specificity of training in movement coordination. Specifically, during the task of opening a drawer with the less affected UE and reaching in and manipulating its content with the more affected UE (Figure 4-7, *A*), children who receive constraint-induced therapy or bimanual training (HABIT) both increase the overlap of use of their two UEs (Figure 4-7, *B*) and decrease the length of time between opening the drawer and manipulating its contents (Figure 4-7, *C*).[59] The HABIT group, however, improved in movement overlap and goal synchronization to a greater extent than the constraint group. Results support the notion of training specificity described earlier in the chapter and suggest that bimanual training may be more beneficial for improving spatial and temporal aspects of bimanual control. Furthermore, the HABIT group showed greater improvement in attainment of functional and play goals important to children and caregivers such as dressing, cutting food,

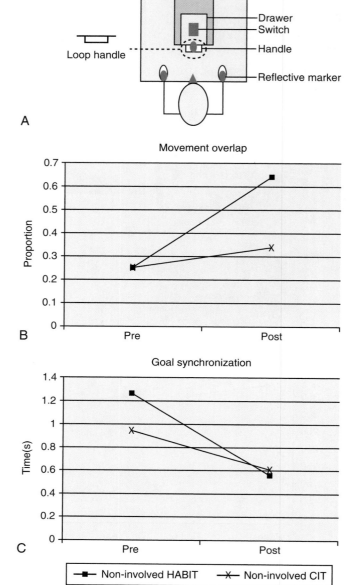

Figure 4-7 **A,** Task requiring opening a drawer with the less-affected hand and manipulating its contents with the more affected hand. The task was used to quantify the following measures before and after constraint-induced movement therapy (CIMT) and hand-arm bimanual intensive therapy (HABIT): **B,** Movement overlap of two hands, normalized as a proportion of total task completion time (higher values mean more overlap). **C,** Goal synchronization duration (time difference between two hands completing the tasks). Lower values mean better performance. (Hung, Casertano, Hillman, & Gordon, unpublished data.)

catching a ball, and dressing dolls. Thus the salience of the tasks trained must be considered.

SALIENCE OF MOTOR ACTIVITIES

For rehabilitation to remain effective in light of the importance of task salience (especially protocols involving long hours), it must constantly evolve to include activities that are meaningful and enjoyable, including video gaming. Children play video games on average 8 hours per week.[17] Actional immersion in a video/virtual environment can potentially allow individuals to produce movements that are not feasible in the real world as a result of their motor impairments (e.g., weakness, limited range of motion). This possibility therefore may have novel intriguing consequences and may enhance learning[20] for functional training, as it is therefore possible to provide positive KR for appropriate efforts.

The choice of video game platforms, consoles, and software needs to take into account (1) the initial abilities of the performer, (2) the specific motor impairments targeted, (3) the extent to which therapy is directed to one or both UEs, (4) the ability to attain progress in movement difficulty, and (5) the age and interest of the performer. Although use of virtual reality-based and video gaming protocols is indeed gaining momentum in rehabilitation,[21] presently there is insufficient evidence of the efficacy of gaming by itself. Like HABIT and CIMT, it is just one means of engaging task-oriented training, but one that is potentially beneficial in maintaining motivation and providing reward, which were shown earlier in the chapter to be important for motor learning and enhancing plasticity.

There are two general approaches to incorporating video-based or virtual reality (VR) training into pediatric rehabilitation protocols. The first is to develop game platforms that target specific impairments or elicit certain movements. This may be particularly useful for eliciting successful movements by altering the gain of required movement to virtual movement provided as feedback. Thus, specific impairments could be targeted (e.g., wrist extension) by creating games requiring such movement, again adjusting the gain of required to displayed movements. Such approaches are promising and will likely constitute an important part of pediatric rehabilitation in the future. To be successful, however, such forms of pediatric rehabilitation must adhere to the same principles described earlier (especially salience). A large limitation, meanwhile, is the expense of building and programming devices that are enjoyable and flexible and can progress training suitably with improvements to maintain sufficient challenge. Such activities must address an array of movement impairments across a wide variety of ages. Often there is considerable delay between development and testing and implementation in clinical environments. Even as robotic-assisted therapy becomes more available, the tasks that are employed (often center-out tasks where participants must move a cursor on a screen in a straight line to concentrically arranged targets) are still often unmotivating, and thus will not effectively maximize motor learning and generalization.

The second approach is to use or modify commercially available gaming systems (e.g., Nintendo Wii, Minami-ku Kyoto, Japan). Although commercially available motion capture VR systems have been tailored specifically for rehabilitation, the cost may prevent wide-scale application in the near future. Thus commercial, mainstream gaming consoles have the distinct advantage of constantly being updated by commercial game developers to maintain the interest of children and are familiar to most children; also, the initial financial investments are minimal compared with the diversity of devices and games available. A major limitation, however, is that these devices were not created to elicit specific movements that are necessarily impaired in children with disabilities and may not have sensors that are sensitive enough to translate subtle movement improvements into increases in game performance. During free play, children are likely to choose games or consoles that can be performed with one (nonparetic) UE or require minimal (stabilization) movement of the affected UE.

Paradoxically, because children often already engage in video gaming at home, simply continuing to perform what they do at home may be neither rewarding nor specific enough to elicit movement changes and improvement in gaming ability. Thus therapists must be creative about how the games are used to target movement impairment and elicit motor learning during game play. Rules about how each UE will be used and challenges that progress difficulty of movement beyond speed and accuracy requirements of the game must be considered (e.g., adding wrist weights to promote UE strength, challenging balance by having children sit on a yoga ball while playing). Given these limitations, gaming should be viewed as complementary to, but not as a replacement for, salient task-oriented activities in the real world.

CONSIDERATIONS

It is important to note that an overwhelming majority of motor learning studies in both adults and children have been conducted in carefully controlled laboratory environments. This allows researchers to parcel out important factors that may relate to learning, but has limitations in that we don't entirely know what aspects of training transfer to learning of functional complex tasks. Recent emphasis in adult motor learning has made use of technology to study center-out tasks or reaching perturbation studies, where subjects need to learn new movement gains. Such paradigms are useful for studying how subjects readapt learned patterns of movement under new conditions, but we do not know how they inform us about learning complex, skilled tasks, especially with the physical constraints present in pediatric patients.

SUMMARY

In this chapter, we have described a triad consisting of the person, the task, and the environmental context in which the child performs the task. We discussed this triad in relation to relevant motor learning principles derived from studies of adults without disabilities. This includes taxonomies of motor skills in relation to skill progression, types of knowledge gained during motor learning, different types and stages of learning, methods of instructions, feedback types and frequency, types of practice schedules, variability and specificity of training with whole and part practice, and benefits of mental practice. We highlighted important differences in motor learning between children and adults. We discussed the implications of reduced information-processing capabilities and processing/memory in children and the implications for feedback and the type and amount of practice, where we showed that skill emerges over enormous amounts of practice and extensive time periods. We demonstrated that although there are certainly many similarities, the way children learn may differ from the way adults learn. More research is required to parcel out these differences.

In the context of rehabilitation, we show that unlike in adults, learning in children must occur in the context of development, whereby age-appropriate skills are learned for the very first time. We showed that intensity of training matters, provided models of intensive, task-oriented approaches such as constraint-induced movement therapy and bimanual training, and discussed how tasks and the environment as part of the triad can be used to optimize learning. We showed the importance of training specificity and provided important clues from the neuroscience literature on how to take advantage of and maximize neuroplasticity. In particular, we showed that neuroplasticity is enhanced when the tasks are meaningful to the performer. Finally we provided an example of a recently salient task—playing video games targeting specific motor impairments. We discussed the limitations of existing knowledge and projected where pediatric rehabilitation research needs to be directed to fully incorporate motor learning into practice.

Motor learning approaches have been slow to gain popularity in pediatric rehabilitation. Although therapists may be implicitly applying motor learning principles in their treatment protocols, explicit application of these principles is required to determine if this approach is effective. A challenge in coming years to therapists who work with children will be to determine how the principles of motor learning described in this chapter may or may not differ from results of studies performed in adults and void of these characteristics. Although intensity of training is one important variable that surely will be an important factor in future task-oriented approaches, determining the key intervention ingredients to include in planning intensity will be all the more important.[97]

REFERENCES

1. Adolph, K. E. (2002). Babies' steps make giant strides toward a science of development. *Infant Behavior and Development, 25,* 86–90.

2. Adolph, K. E. (2008). Learning to move. *Current Directions in Psychological Science, 17,* 213–218.

3. Ahl, L. E., Johansson, E., Granat, T., & Carlberg, E. B. (2005). Functional therapy for children with cerebral palsy: An ecological approach. *Developmental Medicine and Child Neurology, 47,* 613–619.

4. Albert, F., Santello, M., & Gordon, A. M. (2009). Sensorimotor memory of object weight distribution during multidigit grasp. *Neuroscience Letters, 463,* 188–193.

5. Allami, N., Paulignan, Y., Brovelli, A., & Boussaoud, D. (2008). Visuo-motor learning with combination of different rates of motor imagery and physical practice. *Experimental Brain Research, 184,* 105–113.

6. Anttila, H., Autti-Rämö, I., Suoranta, J., Mäkelä, M., & Malmivaara, A. (2008). Effectiveness of physical therapy interventions for children with cerebral palsy: A systematic review. *BMC Pediatrics, 24,* 8–14.

7. Bo, J., Contreras-Vidal, J. L., Kagerer, F. A., & Clark, J. E. (2006). Effects of increased complexity of visuo-motor transformations on children's arm movements. *Human Movement Science, 25,* 553–567.

8. Bower, E., McLellan, D. L., Arney, J., & Campbell, M. J. (1996). A randomised controlled trial of different intensities of physiotherapy and different goal-setting procedures in 44 children with cerebral palsy. *Developmental Medicine and Child Neurology, 38,* 226–237.

9. Bryan, W. L., & Harter, N. (1899). Studies on the telegraphic language: The acquisition of a hierarchy of habits. *Psychological Review, 6,* 345–375.

10. Butler, C., & Darrah, J. (2001). Effects of neurodevelopmental treatment (NDT) for cerebral palsy: An AACPDM evidence report. *Developmental Medicine and Child Neurology, 43,* 778–790.

11. Carr, J., & Shepherd, R. B. (1989). A motor learning model for stroke rehabilitation. *Physiotherapy, 75,* 372–380.

12. Cauraugh, J. H., Coombes, S. A., Lodha, N., Naik, S. K., & Summers, J. J. (2009). Upper extremity improvements in chronic stroke: Coupled bilateral load training. *Restorative Neurology and Neuroscience, 27,* 17–25.

13. Charles, J., & Gordon, A. M. (2005). A critical review of constraint-induced movement therapy and forced use in children with hemiplegia. *Neural Plasticity, 12,* 245–261.

14. Charles, J., & Gordon, A. M. 2006. Development of hand-arm bimanual intensive training (HABIT) for improving bimanual coordination in children with hemiplegic cerebral palsy. *Developmental Medicine and Child Neurology, 48,* 931–936.

15. Charles, J. R., Gordon, A. M. (2007). A repeated course of constraint-induced movement therapy results in further improvement. *Developmental Medicine and Child Neurology, 49,* 770–773.

16. Charles, J., Wolf, S. L., Schneider, J. A., & Gordon, A. M. (2006). Efficacy of a child-friendly form of constraint-induced movement therapy in hemiplegic cerebral palsy: A randomized control trial. *Developmental Medicine and Child Neurology, 48,* 635–642.

17. Cummings, H. M., Vandewater, E. A. (2007). Relation of adolescent video game play to time spent in other activities. *Archives of Pediatrics and Adolescent Medicine, 161,* 684–689.

18. Czernochowski, D., Mecklinger, A., Johansson, M., & Brinkmann, M. (2005). Age-related differences in familiarity and recollection: ERP evidence from a recognition memory study

in children and young adults. *Cognitive, Affective, and Behavioral Neuroscience, 5,* 417–433.

19. Damiano, D. L., & DeJong, S. L. (2009). A systematic review of the effectiveness of treadmill training and body weight support in pediatric rehabilitation. *Journal of Neurologic Physical Therapy, 33,* 27–44.

20. Dede, C. (2009). Immersive interfaces for engagement and learning. *Science, 323,* 66–69.

21. Deutsch, J. E., Borbely, M., Filler, J., Huhn, K., & Guarrera-Bowlby, P. (2008). Use of a low-cost, commercially available gaming console (Wii) for rehabilitation of an adolescent with cerebral palsy. *Physical Therapy, 88,* 1196–1207.

22. Dickstein, R., Garzit-Grunwald, M., Plax, M., Dunsky, A., & Marcovitz, E. (2005). EMG activity in selected target muscles during imagery rising on tiptoes in healthy adults and post-stroke hemiparetic patients. *Journal of Motor Behavior, 37,* 475–483.

23. Duff, S. V., & Gordon, A. M. (2003). Learning of grasp control in children with hemiplegic cerebral palsy. *Developmental Medicine and Child Neurology, 45,* 746–757.

24. Eliasson, A. C., Bonnier, B., & Krumlinde-Sundholm, L. (2003). Clinical experience of constraint induced movement therapy in adolescents with hemiplegic cerebral palsy—A day camp model. *Developmental Medicine and Child Neurology, 45,* 357–359.

25. Eliasson, A. C., Forssberg, H., Hung, Y. C., & Gordon A. M. (2006). Development of hand function and precision grip control in individuals with cerebral palsy: A 13-year follow-up study. *Pediatrics, 118,* e1226–e1236.

26. Eliasson, A. C., & Gordon, A. M. (2008). Constraint-induced movement therapy for children with hemiplegia. In A. C. Eliasson, & P. Burtner (Eds.), *Improving hand function in children with cerebral palsy: Theory, evidence and intervention. Clinics in developmental medicine* (pp. 308–319). London: MacKeith Press.

27. Eliasson, A. C., Krumlinde-Sundholm, L., Shaw, K., & Wang, C. (2005). Effects of constraint-induced movement therapy in young children with hemiplegic cerebral palsy: An adapted model. *Developmental Medicine and Child Neurology, 47,* 266–275.

28. Ericsson, K. A., & Charness, N. (1994). Expert performance: Its structure and acquisition. *American Psychologist, 49,* 725–747.

29. Eyre, J. A. (2007). Corticospinal tract development and its plasticity after perinatal injury. *Neuroscience and Biobehavioral Reviews, 31,* 1136–1149.

30. Ferrel-Chapus, C., Hay, L., Olivier, I., Bard, C., & Fleury, M. (2002). Visuomanual coordination in childhood: Adaptation to visual distortion. *Experimental Brain Research, 144,* 506–517.

31. Forssberg, H. (1999). Neural control of human motor development. *Current Opinion on Neurobiology, 9,* 676–682.

32. Fregni, F., & Pascual-Leone, A. (2007). Technology insight: Noninvasive brain stimulation in neurology-perspectives on the therapeutic potential of rTMS and tDCS. *Nature Clinical Practice Neurology, 3,* 383–393.

33. Friel, K. M. Unpublished manuscript, 2010.

34. Friel, K. M., & Martin, J. H. (2007). Bilateral activity-dependent interactions in the developing corticospinal system. *Journal of Neuroscience, 27,* 11083–11090.

35. Gallagher, J. D., & Thomas, J. R. (1980). Effects of varying post-KR intervals upon children's motor performance. *Journal of Motor Behavior, 12,* 41–56.

36. Gentile, A. M. (1972). A working model of skill acquisition with application to teaching. *Quest Monograph, 17,* 3–23.

37. Gentile, A. M. (1987). Skill acquisition: Action, movement, and neuromotor processes. In J. H. Carr, R. B. Shepherd, J. Gordon, A. M. Gentile, & J. M. Hinds (Eds.), *Movement science: Foundations for physical therapy in rehabilitation* (pp. 93–154). Rockville, MD: Aspen.

38. Gentile, A. M. (1998). Implicit and explicit processes during acquisition of functional skills. *Scandanavian Journal of Occupational Therapy, 5,* 7–16.

39. Gentile, A. M. (2000). Skill acquisition: Action, movement, and neuromotor processes. In J. H. Carr, & R. B. Shepherd (Eds.), *Movement science: Foundations for physical therapy in rehabilitation* (2nd ed., pp. 111–187). Rockville, MD: Aspen.

40. Gordon, A. M. (2001). Development of hand motor control. In: A. F. Kalverboer, & A. Gramsbergen (Eds.), *Handbook of brain and behaviour in human development* (pp. 513–537). Dordrecht: Kluwer Academic Publishers.

41. Gordon, A. M., Charles, J., Schneider, J. A., & Chinnan, A. (2007). Efficacy of a hand-arm bimanual intensive therapy (HABIT) for children with hemiplegic cerebral palsy: A randomized control trial. *Developmental Medicine and Child Neurology, 49,* 830–838.

42. Gordon, A. M., Charles, J., & Wolf, S. L. (2005). Methods of constraint-induced movement therapy for children with hemiplegic cerebral palsy: Development of a child-friendly intervention for improving upper extremity function. *Archives of Physical Medicine and Rehabilitation, 86,* 837–844.

43. Gordon, A. M., Chinnan, A., Gill, S., Petra, E., Hung, Y. C., & Charles, J. (2008). Both constraint-induced movement therapy and bimanual training lead to improved performance of upper extremity function in children with hemiplegia. *Developmental Medicine and Child Neurology, 50,* 957–958.

44. Gordon, A. M., & Duff, S. V. (1999). Fingertip forces during object manipulation in children with hemiplegic cerebral palsy. I: Anticipatory scaling. *Developmental Medicine and Child Neurology, 41,* 166–175.

45. Gordon, A. M., & Friel, K. (2009). Intensive training of upper extremity function in children with cerebral palsy. In J. Hermsdoerfer, & D. A. Nowak (Eds.), *Sensorimotor control of grasping: Physiology and pathophysiology.* New York: Cambridge University Press. pp. 438–457.

46. Gordon, A. M., & Steenbergen, B. (2008). Bimanual coordination in children with cerebral palsy. In A. C. Eliasson, & P. Burtner (Eds.), *Improving hand function in children with*

cerebral palsy: Theory, evidence and intervention. Clinics in developmental medicine (pp. 160–175). London: MacKeith Press.

47. Gorter, H., Holty, L., Rameckers, E. E., Elvers, H. J., & Oostendorp, R. A. (2009). Changes in endurance and walking ability through functional physical training in children with cerebral palsy. *Pediatric Physical Therapy, 21,* 31–37.

48. Granda, J., Alvarez, J. C., & Medina, M. M. (2008). Effects of different practice conditions on acquisition, retention, and transfer of soccer skills by 9-year-old schoolchildren. *Perceptual & Motor Skills, 106,* 447–460.

49. Granda, J., Medina, M. M. (2003). Practice schedule and acquisition, retention and transfer of a throwing task in 6 year old children. *Perceptual & Motor Skills, 96,* 1015–1024.

50. Haley, S. M., Coster, W. J., Ludlow, L. H., et al. (1992). *Pediatric Evaluation of Disability Inventory (PEDI).* Boston, MA: New England Medical Center Hospitals.

51. Harlow, H. F. (1949). The formation of learning sets. *Psychological Review, 56,* 51–65.

52. Herbert, E. P., Landin, D., & Solmon, M. A. (1996). A comparison of three practice schedules along the contextual interference continuum. *Research Quarterly for Exercise & Sport, 68,* 357–361.

53. Himmelmann, K., Hagberg, G., Beckung, E., Hagberg, B., & Uvebrant, P. (2005). The changing panorama of cerebral palsy in Sweden. IX. Prevalence and origin in the birth-year period 1995–1998. *Acta Paediatrica, 94,* 287–294.

54. Hoare, B., Imms, C., Carey, L., & Wasiak, J. (2007). Constraint-induced movement therapy in the treatment of the upper limb in children with hemiplegic cerebral palsy: A Cochrane systematic review. *Clinical Rehabilitation, 21,* 675–685.

55. Holmefur, M., Krumlinde-Sundholm, L., Bergström, J., & Eliasson, A. C. (2010). Longitudinal development of hand function in children with unilateral cerebral palsy. *Developmental Medicine and Child Neurology, 52,* 352–357.

56. Howle, J. M. (2003). *Neuro-developmental treatment approach: Theoretical foundations and principles of clinical practice.* Laguna Beach, CA: Neuro-Developmental Treatment Association.

57. Hu, Y., Osu, R., Okada, M., Goodale, M. A., & Kawato, M. (2005). A model of coupling between grip aperture and hand transport during human prehension. *Experimental Brain Research, 167,* 301–304.

58. Hung, Y. C., Charles, J., & Gordon, A. M. (2004). Bimanual coordination during a goal-directed task in children with hemiplegic cerebral palsy. *Developmental Medicine and Child Neurology, 46,* 746–753.

59. Hung, Y. C., Casertano, L., Hillman, A., & Gordon, A. M. Unpublished manuscript, 2010.

60. Iacoboni, M., & Mazziotta, J. C. (2007). Mirror neuron system: Basic findings and clinical applications. *Annals of Neurology, 62,* 213–218.

61. Jarus, T., & Goverover, Y. (1999). Effects of contextual interference and age on acquisition, retention and transfer of motor skills. *Perceptual & Motor Skills, 88,* 437–447.

62. Jarus, T., & Gutman, T. (2001). Effects of cognitive processes and task complexity on acquisition, retention, and transfer of motor skills. *Canadian Journal of Occupational Therapy, 68,* 280–289.

63. Kantak, S. S., Sullivan, K. J., & Burtner, P. (2008). Motor learning in children with cerebral palsy: Implications for rehabilitation. In A. C. Eliasson, & P. Burtner (Eds.), *Improving hand function in children with cerebral palsy: Theory, evidence and intervention. Clinics in developmental medicine* (pp. 260–275). London: MacKeith Press.

64. Karatekin, C., Marcus, D. J., & Couperus J. W. (2007). Regulation of cognitive resources during sustained attention and working memory in 10-year-olds and adults. *Psychophysiology, 44,* 128–144.

65. Ketelaar, M., Vermeer, A., Hart, H., van Petegem-van Beek, E., & Helders, P. J. (2001). Effects of a functional therapy program on motor abilities of children with cerebral palsy. *Physical Therapy, 81,* 1534–1545.

66. Kleim, J. A., Barbay, S., & Nudo, R. J. (1998). Functional reorganization of the rat motor cortex following motor skill learning. *Journal of Neurophysiology, 80,* 3321–3325.

67. Lagers-van Haselen, G. C., van der Steen, J., & Frens, M. A. (2007). Copying strategies for patterns by children and adults. *Perceptual & Motor Skills, 91,* 603–615.

68. Lambert, J., & Bard, C. (2005). Acquisition of visual manual skills and improvement of information processing capabilities in 6 to 10 year-old children performing a 2D pointing task. *Neuroscience Letters, 377,* 1–6.

69. Lang, C. E., MacDonald, J. R., & Gnip, C. (2007). Counting repetitions: An observational study of outpatient therapy for people with hemiparesis post-stroke. *Journal of Neurology and Physical Therapy, 31,* 3–10.

70. Lee, T. D., & Genovese, E. D. (1989). Distribution of practice in motor skill acquisition: Different effects for discrete and continuous tasks. *Research Quarterly for Exercise and Sport, 59,* 277–287.

71. Magill, R. A. (2001). Augmented feedback in motor skill acquisition. In R. N. Singer, H. A. Hausenblaus, & C. M. Janelle (Eds.), *Handbook of research on sport psychology* (pp. 86–114). New York: John Wiley & Sons.

72. Magill, R. A. (2010). *Motor learning and control: Concepts and applications* (9th ed.). New York: McGraw-Hill.

73. Magill, R. A., & Hall, K. G. (1990). A review of the contextual interference effect in motor skill acquisition. *Human Movement Science, 9,* 241–289.

74. Mantyla, T., Carelli, M. G., & Forman, H. (2007). Time monitoring and executive functioning in children and adults. *Journal of Experimental Child Psychology, 96,* 1–19.

75. Martin, J. H., Choy, M., Pullman, S., & Meng, Z. (2004). Corticospinal system development depends on motor experience. *Journal of Neuroscience, 24,* 2122–2132.

76. Martin, J. H., Friel, K. M., Salimi, I., & Chakrabarty, S. (2007). Activity- and use-dependent plasticity of the developing corticospinal system. *Neuroscience and Biobehavioral Reviews, 31,* 1125–1135.

77. Mutlu, A., Krosschell, K., & Spira, D. G. (2009). Treadmill training with partial body-weight support in children with cerebral palsy: A systematic review. *Developmental Medicine and Child Neurology, 51*, 268–275.

78. Naka, M. (1998). Repeated writing facilitates children's memory for pseudocharacters and foreign letters. *Memory & Cognition, 26*, 804–809.

79. Naylor, J., & Briggs, G. (1963). Effects of task complexity and task organization on the relative efficiency of part and whole training methods. *Journal of Experimental Psychology, 65*, 217–244.

80. Neilson, P. D., O'Dwyer, N. J., & Nash, J. (1990). Control of isometric muscle activity in cerebral palsy. *Developmental Medicine and Child Neurology, 32*, 778–788.

81. Nilsen, D. M., Gillen, G., & Gordon, A. M. The use of mental practice to improve upper limb recovery post-stroke: A systematic review. *American Journal of Occupational Therapy*, In press.

82. O'Dwyer, N. J., & Neilson, P. D. (1988). Voluntary muscle control in normal and athetoid dysarthric speakers. *Brain, 111*, 877–899.

83. Ostendorf, C. G., & Wolf, S. L. (1981). Effect of forced use of the upper extremity of a hemiplegic patient on changes in function: A single-case design. *Physical Therapy, 61*, 1022–1028.

84. Page, S. J., Szaflarski, J. P., Eliassen, J. C., Pan, H., & Cramer, S. C. (2009). Cortical plasticity following motor learning during mental practice in stroke. *Neurorehabilitation and Neural Repair, 23*, 382–388.

85. Panyan, M. C. (1980). *How to use shaping.* Lawrence, KS: H & H Enterprises.

86. Plautz, E. J., Milliken, G. W., & Nudo, R. J. (2000). Effects of repetitive motor training on movement representations in adult squirrel monkeys: Role of use versus learning. *Neurobiology of Learning and Memory, 74*, 27–55.

87. Pollock, B. J., & Lee, T. D. (1997). Dissociated contextual interference effects in children and adults. *Perceptual & Motor Skills, 84*, 851–858.

88. Proteau, L. (1992). On the specificity of learning and the role of visual information for movement control. In L. Proteau & D. Elliott (Eds.), *Vision and motor control* (pp. 67–103). Amsterdam: North-Holland.

89. Rameckers, E. A., Speth, L. A., Duysens, J., Vles, J. S., & Smits-Engelsman, B. C. (2009). Botulinum toxin-a in children with congenital spastic hemiplegia does not improve upper extremity motor-related function over rehabilitation alone: A randomized controlled trial. *Neurorehabilitation and Neural Repair, 23*, 218–225.

90. Reis, J., Schambra, H. M., Cohen, L. G., Buch, E. R., Fritsch, B., Zarahn, E., et al. (2009). Noninvasive cortical stimulation enhances motor skill acquisition over multiple days through an effect on consolidation. *Proceedings of the National Academy of Sciences of the United States of America, 106*, 1590–1595.

91. Rose, D. K., & Winstein, C. J. (2004). Bimanual training after stroke: Are two hands better than one? *Topics in Stroke Rehabilitation, 11*, 20–30.

92. Rosenbaum, P. L., Walter, S. D., Hanna, S. E., Palisano, R. J., Russell, D. J., Raina, P., et al. (2002). Prognosis for gross motor function in cerebral palsy: Creation of motor development curves. *Journal of the American Medical Association, 288*, 1357–1363.

93. Russell, D., Rosenbaum, P. L., Gowland, C., et al. (1993). *Manual for the Gross Motor Function Measure.* Hamilton, Ontario, Canada: McMaster University.

94. Salimi, I., Frazier, W., Reilmann, R., & Gordon, A. M. (2003). Selective use of visual information signaling objects' center of mass for anticipatory control of manipulative fingertip forces. *Experimental Brain Research, 150*, 9–18.

95. Salimi, I., Hollender, I., Frazier, W., & Gordon, A. M. (2000). Specificity of internal representations underlying grasping. *Journal of Neurophysiology, 84*, 2390–2397.

96. Salmoni, A. W., Schmidt, R. A., & Walter, C. B. (1984). Knowledge of results and motor learning: A review and reappraisal. *Psychological Bulletin, 95*, 355–386.

97. Schertz, M., Gordon, A. M. (2009). Changing the model: A call for re-examination of intervention approaches & translational research in children with developmental disabilities. *Developmental Medicine and Child Neurology, 51*, 6–7.

98. Schumann-Hengsteler, R. (1996). Children's and adults' visuospatial memory: The game concentration. *The Journal of Genetic Psychology, 157*, 77–92.

99. Shapiro, D. C. (1977). Knowledge of results and motor learning in preschool children. *Research Quarterly, 48*, 154–158.

100. Shumway-Cook, A., Hutchinson, S., Kartin, D., Price, R., & Woollacott, M. (2003). Effect of balance training on recovery of stability in children with cerebral palsy. *Developmental Medicine and Child Neurology, 45*, 591–602.

101. Skinner, B. (1968). *The technology of teaching.* New York: Appleton-Century-Crofts.

102. Sköld, A., Josephsson, S., & Eliasson, A. C. (2004). Performing bimanual activities: The experiences of young persons with hemiplegic cerebral palsy. *American Journal of Occupational Therapy, 58*, 416–425.

103. Steenbergen, B., Crajé, C., Nilsen, D. M., & Gordon, A. M. (2009). Motor imagery training in hemiplegic cerebral palsy: A potentially useful therapeutic tool for rehabilitation. *Developmental Medicine and Child Neurology, 51*, 690–696.

104. Steenbergen, B., Verrel, J., & Gordon, A. M. (2007). Motor planning in congenital hemiplegia. *Disability Research, 29*, 13–23.

105. Ste-Marie, D. M., Clark, S. E., Findlay, L. C., & Latimer, A. E. (2004). High levels of contextual interference enhance handwriting skill acquisition. *Journal of Motor Behavior, 36*, 115–126.

106. Sullivan, K. J., Kantak, S. S., & Burtner, P. A. (2008). Motor learning in children: Feedback effects on skill acquisition. *Physical Therapy, 88*, 720–732.

107. Taub, E., & Shee, L. P. (1980). *Somatosensory deafferentation research with monkeys: Implications for rehabilitation medicine.* Baltimore/London: Williams & Wilkins.

108. Taub, E., & Wolf, S. L. (1997). Constraint-induced (CI) movement techniques to facilitate upper extremity use in stroke patients. *Topics in Stroke Rehabilitation, 3,* 38–61.

109. Thorndike, E. L. (1914). *Educational psychology: Briefer course.* New York: Columbia University Press.

110. Thorndike, E. L., & Woodworth, R. S. (1901). The influence of improvement in one mental function upon the efficiency of other functions. *Psychological Review, 8,* 247–261.

111. Thorpe, D. E., & Valvano, J. (2002). The effects of knowledge of performance and cognitive strategies on motor skill learning in children with cerebral palsy. *Pediatric Physical Therapy, 14,* 2–15.

112. Tower, S. S. (1940). Pyramidal lesion in the monkey. *Brain (London), 63,* 36.

113. Trombly, C. (1995). Clinical practice guidelines for post-stroke rehabilitation and occupational therapy practice. *American Journal of Occupational Therapy, 49,* 711–714.

114. Ulrich, D. A., Lloyd, M. C., Tiernan, C. W., Looper, J. E., & Angulo-Barroso, R. M. (2008). Effects of intensity of treadmill training on developmental outcomes and stepping in infants with Down syndrome: A randomized trial. *Physical Therapy, 88,* 114–122.

115. Utley, A., & Steenbergen, B. (2006). Discrete bimanual co-ordination in children and young adolescents with hemiparetic cerebral palsy: Recent findings, implications and future research directions. *Pediatric Rehabilitation, 9,* 127–136.

116. Valvano, J., & Newell, K. M. (1998). Practice of a precision isometric grip-force task by children with spastic cerebral palsy. *Developmental Medicine and Child Neurology, 40,* 464–473.

117. van der Weel, F. R., van der Meer, A. L., & Lee, D. N. (1991). Effect of task on movement control in cerebral palsy: Implications for assessment and therapy. *Developmental Medicine and Child Neurology, 33,* 419–426.

118. Verschuren, O., Ketelaar, M., Gorter, J. W., Helders, P. J., & Takken, T. (2009). Relation between physical fitness and gross motor capacity in children and adolescents with cerebral palsy. *Developmental Medicine and Child Neurology, 51,* 866–871.

119. Willingham, D. B. (1998). A neuropsychological theory of motor skill learning. *Psychological Review, 105,* 558–584.

120. Winstein, C. J., & Schmidt, R. A. (1990). Reduced frequency of knowledge of results enhances motor skill learning. *Journal of Experimental Psychology: Learning, Memory, and Cognition, 16,* 677–691.

121. Winstein, C. J., & Wolf, S. L. (2009). Task-oriented training to promote upper extremity recovery. In J. Stein, R. Harvey, R. Macko, C. J. Winstein, & R. Zorowitz (Ed.), *Stroke recovery and rehabilitation.* New York, NY: Demos Medical Publishing.

122. Wolf, S. L., Lecraw, D. E., Barton, L. A., & Jann, B. B. (1989). Forced use of hemiplegic upper extremities to reverse the effect of learned nonuse among chronic stroke and head-injured patients. *Experimental Neurology, 104,* 125–132.

123. Wolf, S. L., Newton, H., Maddy, D., Blanton, S., Zhang, Q., Winstein, C. J., et al. (2007). The Excite trial: Relationship of intensity of constraint induced movement therapy to improvement in the Wolf motor function test. *Restorative Neurology and Neuroscience, 25,* 549–562.

124. Wolf, S. L., Winstein, C. J., Miller, J. P., Taub, E., Uswatte, G., Morris, D., et al.; EXCITE Investigators. (2006). Effect of constraint-induced movement therapy on upper extremity function 3 to 9 months after stroke: The EXCITE randomized clinical trial. *Journal of the American Medical Association, 296,* 2095–2104.

125. Wolf, S. L., Winstein, C. J., Miller, J. P., Thompson, P. A., Taub, E., Uswatte, G., et al. (2008). Retention of upper limb function in stroke survivors who have received constraint-induced movement therapy: The EXCITE randomised trial. *Lancet Neurology, 7,* 33–40.

126. Wulf, G., Landers, M., Lewthwaite, R., & Töllner, T. (2009). External focus instructions reduce postural stability in individuals with Parkinson disease. *Physical Therapy, 89,* 162–168.

127. Wulf, G., & Shea, C. H. (2002). Principles derived from the study of simple skills do not generalize to complex skill learning. *Psychonomic Bulletin and Review, 9,* 185–211.

128. Yan, J. H., Thomas, K. T., Stelmach, G. E., & Thomas, J. R. (2003). Developmental differences in children's ballistic aiming movements of the arm. *Perceptual & Motor Skills, 96,* 589–598.

129. Zhang, W., Gordon, A. M., Fu, Q., & Santello, M. (2010). Manipulation after object rotation reveals independent sensorimotor memory representations of digit positions and forces. *Journal of Neurophysiology, 103,* 2953–2964.

5

Musculoskeletal Development and Adaptation

LINDA PAX LOWES, PT, PhD • MICHELLE SVEDA, PT • CARRIE G. GAJDOSIK, PT, MS • RICHARD L. GAJDOSIK, PT, PhD

Pediatric physical therapists routinely work with children whose clinical conditions influence the growth and development of the musculoskeletal system, either directly or indirectly. The musculoskeletal system demonstrates a remarkable ability to adapt to the physical demands, or lack of physical demands, placed on the system. Pathologic conditions may adversely influence the structure and function of any component of the system and may lead to impairments. For example, bone abnormalities due to congenital deformities, disease processes, or abnormal growth can disrupt the normal length/tension relationship of the muscle and result in weakness. Likewise, muscle pathology, such as Duchenne's muscular dystrophy (DMD), often leads to secondary adaptations and impairments such as joint contractures. The normal process of adaptation can either enhance function or lead to impairment, activity restriction, and participation limitation. The musculoskeletal system and the neurologic system are also intertwined. A neurologic insult such as cerebral palsy (CP) frequently leads to muscle contractures and skeletal changes. Conversely, when a person with an intact nervous system has a range of motion (ROM) limitation, the timing and sequencing of muscle activation can change. Therapeutic interventions are often designed to promote musculoskeletal adaptations in an effort to prevent or correct physical impairments with the hope of enhancing function and participation in daily life activities. Accordingly, knowledge of normal growth and development and of the principles of adaptation of the musculoskeletal system is essential for understanding the efficacy of interventions. The purposes of this chapter are to describe (1) the growth and development of muscle and bone, and (2) the adaptations of muscle and bone, including the effects of various interventions designed to promote desired adaptations.

MUSCULOSKELETAL DEVELOPMENT

Muscle tissue grows in length and width in response to stress. Tension results in longitudinal growth. This is illustrated as the rapid fetal bone growth passively stretches a muscle and stimulates it to grow longer at the same rate as the bone.[200] Muscle thickness, however, is produced by the active stress of exercise. Conversely, a lack of exercise results in muscle wasting.

MUSCLE HISTOLOGY

In the developing vertebrate embryo, two masses of mesoderm cells, called somites, form along the sides of the neural tube. Somites eventually differentiate into dermis (dermatome), skeletal muscle (myotome), and vertebrae (sclerotome). Because the sclerotome differentiates before the other two structures, the term *dermomyotome* refers to the combined dermatome and myotome. Progenitor cells (cells with the ability to differentiate into many types of cells) migrate from the dorsal medial lip of the dermomyotome and differentiate to form primary or secondary myotubes.[92] The primary myotubes are first observed at approximately 5 to 7 weeks' gestational age (GA), and most will eventually differentiate into type I (slow-twitch) fibers. Type II (fast-twitch) fibers primarily develop from the secondary myotubes and are observed at about 30 weeks of gestation.[81] The myofibers are long, cylindrical, multinucleated cells composed of actin and myosin myofibrils repeated as a sarcomere, the basic functional unit of the cell, which is responsible for the striated appearance of skeletal muscle.

A motor unit, consisting of a motoneuron and the muscle fibers it innervates, begins with the development of the neuromuscular junction. The primary myotubes are preferentially innervated first. By 8 weeks of gestation, acetylcholine receptors are dispersed within the myotubular membrane.[90] At this stage in development, multiple motor axons originating from different somites (precursor cells) innervate the developing end plates. These early motor units provide the earliest fetal movement, which is observed in the intercostal muscles. The presence of motor activity indicates that a viable connection between the neuromuscular junction and the motor axon has occurred. From 18 weeks' GA until several months post term, synaptic elimination occurs until each neuromuscular junction is innervated by only one axon.[116] Synaptic elimination occurs in both the central and peripheral nervous systems and is believed to be influenced by activity.[62] The adult pattern of one axon per muscle fiber permits a reproducible and predictable increase in force during performance of a task.[106] Why fetal muscles are innervated initially by several axons and later undergo the elimination of all but one axon is not well established. It does not appear that the reason is to ensure that every muscle fiber is innervated. In partially denervated muscles of animals, the

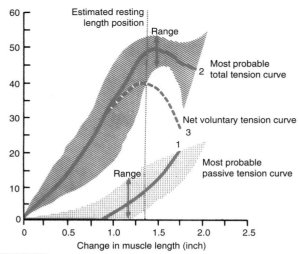

Figure 5-1 Classic length-tension curves for skeletal muscle. Net voluntary active tension is predicted by subtracting passive tension from total tension. (From Astrand, P., & Rodahl, K. [1977]. *Textbook of work physiology* (2nd ed., p. 102). New York: McGraw-Hill.)

few remaining muscle fibers still undergo synaptic elimination, thus further reducing the size of the motor unit.[28,204]

STRUCTURE AND FUNCTION OF THE NORMAL MUSCLE-TENDON UNIT

The normal muscle-tendon unit (MTU) comprises muscle fibers, two cytoskeletal systems within the muscle fibers (exosarcomeric and endosarcomeric), the supportive connective tissues within and around the muscle belly (endomysium, perimysium, and epimysium), and the dense regular connective tissue of the tendon that connects the muscle to the bone. Total muscle force production achieved by an MTU is influenced by many factors, including the size of the muscle fibers, the firing rate of the motor unit action potentials, recruitment and derecruitment patterns, muscle architecture, the angle of pull, the lever arm, and changes in the length of the muscle. A passive length-tension curve is developed on the basis of muscle tension that is produced as the muscle is stretched from its resting length to its maximal length. The initial take-up part of the curve (left part of the curve) represents the resting length, and the end point of the curve (right part of the curve) represents the maximal length.

This includes both active and passive components of the MTU, both of which are influenced by the length of the MTU. To determine the active force produced by the MTU, the passive force is subtracted from the total force (Figure 5-1). The force produced by the active component depends primarily on the amount of overlap of the actin and myosin filaments. The maximum isometric force is produced near the resting length of an isolated muscle; it decreases as the muscle is lengthened or shortened relative to the resting

length. This force-length relationship forms the basis of the sliding filament theory of muscle contraction.[77,97] At a muscle's resting length, the actin and myosin filaments are in a position of optimal overlap, which allows maximal isometric force (Figures 5-2 and 5-3). The force generated by the active component of the MTU also depends on the integrity of the central and peripheral nervous systems, the excitation-contraction coupling mechanism, and the cross-sectional area of the skeletal muscle tissues. In a completely relaxed skeletal muscle (i.e., when the central nervous system [CNS] is not intact, or when no artificial stimulation occurs), no active tension exists.

Passive resistance, which is the equivalent of resting muscle tone, increases exponentially as the muscle is lengthened. Gajdosik[71] provides an excellent summary of the muscle histology associated with passive resistance and clinical implications. Some of the information included in this article is presented here. When a resting muscle is passively stretched, the force produced by the passive component of the MTU is thought to be brought about by three mechanisms: (1) stretching stable cross-links between the actin and myosin filaments, (2) stretching proteins within the exosarcomeric and endosarcomeric cytoskeleton (series elastic component), and (3) deformation of the connective tissues of the muscle (parallel elastic component). The passive component accounts for the resistance felt during passive stretch of a fully relaxed muscle. Previously, passive tension was exclusively attributed to the resistance that arises from stretching stable cross-links between the actin and myosin filaments (filamentary resting tension hypothesis).[113] The stable bonds were believed to impart stiffness because the actin-myosin cross-bridges stretch a short distance from the stable position before slipping to reattach at other binding sites. Based on the results of more recent research methods, however, this theory is being revised. Intracellular and extracellular components are now thought to contribute to passive stiffness. Recent studies have indicated that much of the stiffness of a stretched relaxed muscle originates intracellularly from filamentous connections between the thick myosin filaments and the Z-discs of the sarcomere, particularly when the sarcomere is stretched beyond the actin and myosin overlap[71] (see Figure 5-3). These filamentous connections consist of very long, thin filaments of a giant protein named *titin* (also called "connectin"). The titin protein attaches into the M-line region (center of the myosin filament), runs the length of the sarcomere, and attaches into the Z-discs. The titin protein forms a major component of the endosarcomeric cytoskeleton. This protein is now believed to be the major subcellular component that resists passive lengthening of a relaxed muscle, thus contributing to passive stiffness.[69] Excessive muscle fiber stiffness is common in spastic muscles.[66] Previously, this excessive stiffness was attributable almost exclusively to a hyperactive stretch reflex.[63,64,157] Recently, the contribution of titin to excessive stiffness has been investigated. Different types of titin with different stiffness levels are found in different parts

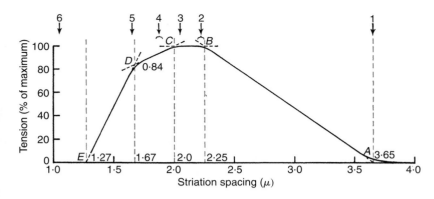

Figure 5-2 Schematic summary of tension changes in relation to sarcomere length changes. Arrows along the top are placed opposite the striation spacings for critical stages of actin and myosin filament overlap (see Figure 5-3). (From Gordon, A. M., Huxley, A. F., & Julian, F. J. [1966]. The variation in isometric tension with sarcomere length in vertebrate muscle fibers. *Journal of Physiology, 184,* 185.)

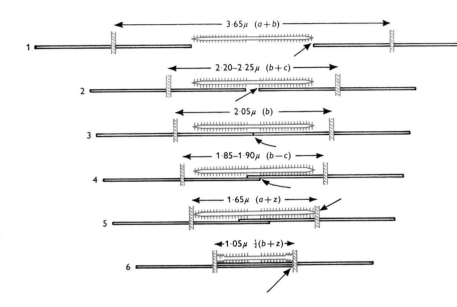

Figure 5-3 Critical stages in the increase of overlap between actin and myosin filaments as a sarcomere shortens. Numbers correspond to numbers in Figure 5-2. (From Gordon, A. M., Huxley, A. F., & Julian, F. J. [1966]. The variation in isometric tension with sarcomere length in vertebrate muscle fibers. *Journal of Physiology, 184,* 186.)

of the body. Titin has been shown to change its stiffness level after a heart attack. Perhaps a CNS lesion also signals titin to increase stiffness.

An intermediate-sized protein of the exosarcomeric cytoskeleton known as *desmin* (also called "skeletin") is thought to help reduce passive muscle stiffness. Desmin is the major subunit of the intermediate protein filaments forming the Z-discs. Desmin connects the Z-discs with many cell organelles and also extends longitudinally from Z-disc to Z-disc outside the sarcomere.[218] Because of this longitudinal orientation, desmin lengthens as the sarcomere is stretched. In animal studies, when desmin is removed from a muscle, passive stiffness increases dramatically.[5]

Nebulin is another giant protein that forms part of the endosarcomeric cytoskeleton but does not contribute to passive muscle stiffness. Nebulin is associated only with actin filaments within the I-band and is thought to provide structural support to the lattice array of actin[221] (Figure 5-4). Many proteins are present in a sarcomere, other than the three discussed here. Recent work has discovered that many

myopathies are caused by the absence or pathology of sarcomere protein.[113]

Recently researchers have been examining the relationship between the deep fascicle angle (angle at which fascicles arise from a deep aponeurosis) and stiffness. The fascicle angle of the gastrocnemii and rectus femoris muscles was reduced in CP compared with age-matched peers.[140,181] The authors hypothesize that this angulation contributes to muscle shortening.

In addition to the intracellular components, passive resistance may be influenced by lengthening of the connective tissues of the endomysium, perimysium, and epimysium of the muscle belly. The perimysium has a well-ordered three-dimensional crisscross array of crimped collagen fibers that become uncrimped as the muscle is lengthened. This change, combined with mechanical realignment of the perimysium, contributes to the exponentially increased resistance near the end of maximal passive muscle lengthening.[71]

In contrast, tendons, which are made up of dense regular connective tissue, are generally considered noncontributory

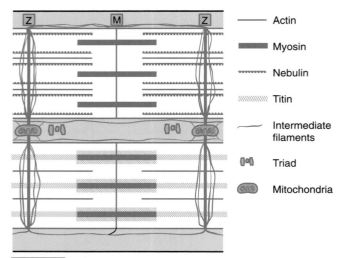

Figure 5-4 Schematic diagram of the proposed arrangement of cytoskeletal elements in and around the sarcomere. Both sarcomeres show the arrangement of intermediate filaments, composed mainly of the protein desmin, linking neighboring myofibrils both transversely and longitudinally at the Z-disc, and encircling the Z-disc. The upper sarcomere shows the arrangement of nebulin, running parallel to actin within the I-band. The lower sarcomere depicts the proposed location of titin, stretching the full length of the half sarcomere and attaching to myosin within the A-band. (Modified from Waterman-Storer, C. M. [1991]. The cytoskeleton of skeletal muscle: Is it affected by exercise? A brief review. *Medicine and Science in Sports and Exercise, 23,* 1243.)

to the overall passive length-tension relationships of the stretched MTU. Dense regular connective tissues present exceedingly high stiffness and therefore are unlikely to stretch.

Passive compliance is the reciprocal of passive stiffness and is defined as the "ease" with which the muscle lengthens. Passive compliance can be represented as the ratio of change in muscle length to change in muscle force.[24] To arrive at these measurements, however, requires invasive research methods not usually possible in humans. Clinically, therefore, passive compliance in humans is usually measured by the ratio of the change in the size of the joint angle to the change in the amount of passive torque.[74,201] Passive stiffness can be represented by the ratio of the change in passive torque to the change in the joint angle.

Despite all of the complex components associated with fetal muscle as outlined previously, during the first half of gestation 60% of muscle mass is made up of interstitial fluid. By 36 weeks' GA, this decreases to around 20%. During the last half of gestational growth, the number and size of muscle fibers increase so rapidly that most of the skeletal muscle fibers have developed by birth. This suggests that infants born very prematurely have different muscles from full-term babies.

Through the first year of life, muscle fibers continue to develop at a much slower rate than the increase seen prenatally. New muscle fibers now originate from either the division of existing cells or the differentiation of myoblasts into

secondary myotubes.[126] During the growing years, muscles increase in length and cross-sectional area through the addition of sarcomeres.[111] Their final size is dependent on many factors, including blood supply, innervation, nutrition, gender, genetics, and exercise.

The bulk associated with a mature muscle comes from the many multinucleated fibers. Next to these fibers, however, are quiescent satellite cells. Satellite cells are mononucleated, myogenic cells that proliferate in response to stress or injury to aid in muscle regeneration. The satellite cells themselves have the ability to regenerate after restoration of the damaged muscle fibers. In diseases such as DMD, the rate of muscle degeneration greatly exceeds the rate at which the satellite cells can repair tissue and regenerate themselves. This imbalance exhausts the supply of satellite cells, and muscle fibers can no longer be regenerated.[92] This, in turn, leads to progressive weakness.

ADAPTATIONS OF MUSCLE FIBERS

Muscle fiber types are susceptible to both internal and external influences. In normal muscle, fiber types are randomly distributed to form a mosaic pattern, and little variation in fiber size is noted. In the presence of disease or dysfunction, this pattern is altered and often well documented in adults. Evaluating muscle composition in children, however, is difficult because, unless the sample can be obtained as an adjunct to a surgery, a painful needle biopsy is required. This usually results in small sample sizes, which likely are a cause of the lack of consensus among reports. With this limitation in mind, the following information is presented.

Denervated muscles show atrophy of both major types of fibers, but type II (fast-twitch) fibers show more atrophy than type I (slow-twitch) fibers. When a muscle is reinnervated after denervation, one fiber type can become predominant and clump together, resulting in loss of the normal mosaic pattern.

Selective atrophy of type II fibers is also common when muscle strength is compromised by disuse. This is seen in adults with steroid-induced strength deficits.[167] This same pattern may be observed in children who receive steroids to treat diseases such as juvenile rheumatoid arthritis. Children with Prader-Willi syndrome also have atrophy of type II fibers.[187] It is believed that in malnourished children, type II fibers are converted to type I fibers.[220]

Selective atrophy of type I fibers has been documented in an array of childhood neuromuscular disorders, such as hypotonia,[6] congenital myotonic dystrophy,[61] and other congenital myopathies.[99] This was not the case in DMD when Imoto and Nonaka[99] found type I atrophy in only 2 of 280 cases, but excessive variability in fiber size has been documented in DMD.[25]

For children with spastic CP, muscle histopathology reports are inconsistent. Researchers agree that spastic muscles vary considerably from typical muscles.[64] The quality and quantity of these differences are disputable. This is due in part to the inability to dissect fibers out of a muscle for examination. Varying degrees of atrophy and hypertrophy of type I and type II fibers have been reported and appear to be dependent on muscle group, severity of CP, and age of the child.[25,37,100,165,166] Lieber[117,118,128] used a technique of intraoperative laser diffraction to look at small samples of flexor carpi ulnaris (FCU) muscles of children with CP and determined that sarcomere length was longer than in typical muscles. The muscles were similar to controls in total number of sarcomeres and in fiber length. Investigators also found a correlation, suggesting a relationship between longer FCU sarcomeres and greater degrees of contracture.

Moreau and colleagues[140] reported decreased cross-sectional area, muscle thickness, and fascicle length in children with CP compared with typically developing study participants. The same changes are observed with disuse and aging. Higher proportions of type I fibers, hypotrophy of both fiber types, and greater variability in fiber size are also commonly reported.[23,100,123] Booth[23] found excessive amounts of collagen and fibrous tissue in older children with CP. The author suggests that collagen and fibrous tissues are irreversible detriments to muscle performance.[23] It is not known whether this is a preventable change.

Why do pediatric physical therapists need to know about muscle fiber types and their responses to outside influences? This question is difficult to answer because the clinical significance is not well understood. One example, however, is the finding by Rose and colleagues[166] that children with spastic diplegia who had a predominance of type I fibers expended more energy and had more prolonged electromyograph (EMG) activity during walking than children with CP and a predominance of type II fibers.

Researchers speculate that spasticity may produce structural changes within the developing muscle.[66,100,166] If so, controlling spasticity in the very young child may be a method of promoting more normal muscle development, which, in turn, may allow more efficient expenditure of energy and better participation in daily activities. Additional studies of atypical fiber type distribution and its effects on activity level are needed. In the meantime, physical therapists should be aware that the two basic types of muscle fibers are influenced by exercise in different ways, that is, the effects of exercise on muscle fibers are training-specific. Endurance training enhances the performance of type I fibers, whereas strength training enhances the performance of type II fibers. The findings of Rose and colleagues[166] would further support the trend in physical therapy to include strength training as an integral component of a treatment plan for children with CP.

FORCE AND LENGTH ADAPTATIONS IN THE MUSCLE-TENDON UNIT

Experiments with numerous animal models have shown that anatomic and physiologic length adaptations of the MTU can be induced by immobilization, denervation, contraction produced by artificial stimulation (i.e., electrical stimulation), or a combination of these methods. Researchers have used length-tension curves to provide information about histologic and histochemical changes in muscles related to length and stiffness. After intervention, the position and steepness of the curve may change, indicating a change in muscle length or stiffness. For example, a shift of the curve to the left indicates a shorter muscle, and a shift to the right indicates a longer muscle. A steeper curve indicates that the muscle is less compliant (stiffer).

Animal studies report muscle atrophy, a loss of subcellular proteins (myosin, actin, titin, and desmin), and a decreased number of sarcomeres when a muscle is immobilized in shortened positions. These changes reduce the force and resting and maximal length of the muscle.[71,117] In very young immobilized mouse soleus muscles, the number of sarcomeres added postnatally was also reduced.[230] The remaining sarcomeres in a muscle immobilized in the shortened position adapt in length to maintain optimal actin and myosin overlap in response to the loss in the number of sarcomeres. When immobilization is discontinued, the muscles readapt to gain their original sarcomere number and length characteristics.

Although changes in muscle strength and resting length have been attributed to loss of sarcomeres, changes in stiffness demonstrated by changes in the steepness of the length-tension curves have been attributed to changes in the connective tissues of the muscles.[198,227] Early in shortened-position immobilization, an increase in the concentration of hydroxyproline occurs in relation to the total volume of the muscle, indicating an increase in connective tissue. Reorganization of the collagen fibers of the perimysium into more acute angles to the muscle fiber axis was also seen[228] (Figure 5-5). This resulted in greater tension per unit of passive elongation, otherwise known as increased stiffness. The passive length-tension curves were shifted to the left and appeared steeper, indicating that the muscles were shorter and stiffer after immobilization in the shortened position (Figure 5-6). The interrelationship of changes in the connective tissues and muscle proteins in light of changes in the form and position of length-tension curves is worthy of further study.

Conversely, animal research suggests that immobilization of muscles in lengthened positions can cause an increase in the number of sarcomeres and therefore in muscle length.[198,227,230] In animals, the number of sarcomeres will revert to the original number in 4 weeks.[195] The addition of sarcomeres was accompanied by muscle weight gain and increased protein synthesis after immobilization.[76] Similar to immobilization in a shortened position, the change in sarcomeres predominantly occurs at the ends of the muscle fibers, which appear to be the most responsive area, as most of the normal postnatal growth of young animals occurs here.[111,229] As with muscles immobilized in the shortened

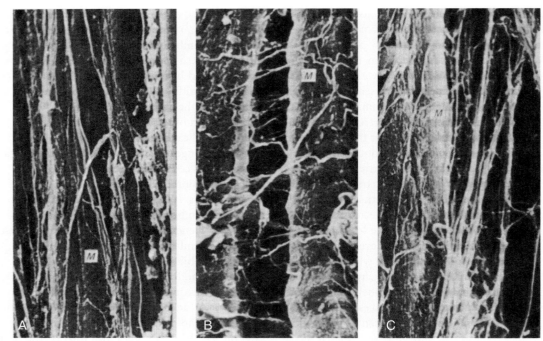

Figure 5-5 Scanning electron micrographs of collagen fibers in the perimysium. **A,** Normal muscle fixed in the lengthened position. **B,** Normal muscle fixed in the shortened position. **C,** Muscle immobilized for 2 weeks in the shortened position and then fixed in the same position. M = muscle fiber, ×1300. (From Williams, P. E., & Goldspink, G. [1984]. Connective tissue changes in immobilized muscle. *Journal of Anatomy London, 138,* 347. Reprinted with the permission of Cambridge University Press.)

Figure 5-6 Length-tension curves for young muscles **(A to D)** immobilized in the shortened position (o) and their controls (•). (From Williams, P. E., & Goldspink, G. [1978]. Changes in sarcomere length and physiological properties in immobilized muscle. *Journal of Anatomy London, 127,* 464. Reprinted with the permission of Cambridge University Press.)

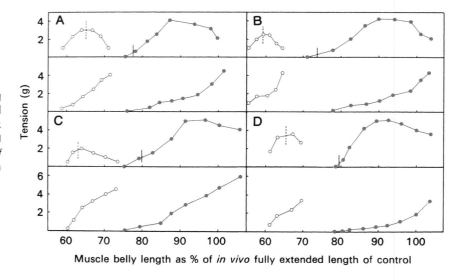

Muscle belly length as % of *in vivo* fully extended length of control

position, the sarcomere length adapts to maintain optimal actin and myosin overlap. Overall, animal research suggests that immobilization in a shortened position has a more profound change in sarcomeres (40% loss) than immobilization in the lengthened position (19% increase).[198]

Active and passive length-tension curves for adult muscles that were immobilized in the lengthened position were shifted to the right (indicating that they were lengthened) compared with those of adult controls (i.e., nonimmobilized muscle). In young mice, however, muscles immobilized in the shortened or lengthened position, resulted in an overall decreased muscle length, with a concomitant increase in tendon length.[227] This caused a shift in the length tension curve to the left indicating a decline in strength[227] (Figure 5-7). Evidence suggests that a tendon elongates more readily in young, growing animals than in adult animals. Although

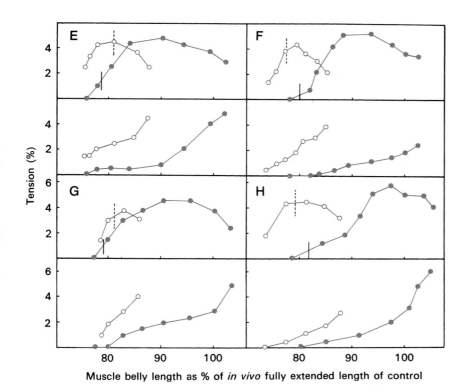

Figure 5-7 Length-tension curves for young animals **(E to H)** immobilized in the lengthened position (o) and their controls (●). (From Williams, P. E., & Goldspink, G. [1978]. Changes in sarcomere length and physiological properties in immobilized muscle. *Journal of Anatomy London, 127,* 464. Reprinted with the permission of Cambridge University Press.)

this work was performed in animals, it should still be considered with casting to increase ROM.

Studies of peripheral denervation of skeletal muscles have revealed gradual changes over a period of weeks to steeper length-tension curves and limited extensibility between their resting lengths and their maximal lengths.[192,205] Denervated animal muscles immobilized in shortened positions showed muscle belly shortening and increased stiffness that were essentially the same as those observed in innervated muscles. This suggests that length adaptations can result from myogenic changes alone. This idea that muscle length and associated physiologic changes may occur independent of neuronal control was supported by studies of muscles stimulated with tetanus toxin.[94,95]

Tetanus toxin injected into animal muscle produced a shift in the passive length-tension curve toward the left and a 45% decrease in sarcomere number, similar to that reported in previous immobilization studies.[95] The fact that a locally injected toxin had the same effect as immobilizing intact muscles may indicate that the length of muscles, not the tension, appeared to be the determining factor in sarcomere regulation.[94] Initial muscle tissue recovery from a toxin such as Botox is achieved by collateral sprouting from nerve terminals. Sprouting reaches a peak at around 8 weeks post injection. After 8 weeks, the original function of the neuromotor junction returns and synaptic elimination of excessive neurons begins. This process is similar to the synaptic elimination seen in postnatal development. In animals, the rate

of synaptic elimination is dependent on the amount of use the muscle receives.[47] If human muscle responds similarly, this may explain why the addition of Botox to serial casting frequently does not improve outcome.[104,106]

Although neural input is not required for muscle length changes, contraction of a shortened muscle may hasten sarcomere loss: Electrical stimulation of the sciatic nerve induced a 25% decrease in sarcomere numbers and increased stiffness within 12 hours,[199] whereas 5 days of shortening by immobilization in plaster casts alone was required to produce similar changes.[95]

Perhaps the mechanism that delays growth when a shortened muscle undergoes electrical stimulation also interferes with the growth of hypertonic muscles. Typically, muscle and bone grow at the same rate. Longitudinal growth of young, hypertonic mouse muscles, however, has been shown to increase in length at only 55% of the rate of growing bone in contrast to the expected 100%.[239]

Human Studies and Clinical Evidence

Studies of the length and stiffness adaptations of the MTU in humans are less common than such studies in animals, but a few attempts have been reported. Studies of children with CP and hypoextensible triceps surae muscles (gastrocnemius and soleus) showed that they have muscle shortening and increased stiffness compared with children with typical development.[201] In another study, nine children with hypoextensible triceps surae muscles were casted for 3 weeks with

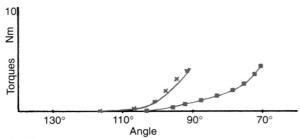

Figure 5-8 Results of successful progressive casting in child from group 2. × = passive torque curve before treatment; j = passive torque curve after treatment. The curve shifted to the right with increased passive compliance. (From Tardieu, G., Tardieu, C., Colbeau-Justin, P., & Lespargot, A. [1982]. Muscle hypoextensibility in children with cerebral palsy: II. Therapeutic implications. *Archives of Physical Medicine and Rehabilitation, 63,* 106.)

these muscles placed in the lengthened position.[202] Four children showed passive length-tension curves that were shifted to the right with decreased slopes, indicating longer muscles with decreased stiffness, whereas five children had curves that were shifted to the right without a change in steepness. In the same study, five children were casted in a shortened position. The passive length-tension curves shifted to the left with increased slopes in four of the five children, indicating increased stiffness.

In a follow-up study, children with CP and hypoextensible triceps surae muscles but no evidence of prolonged sustained contractions (group 1) were compared with children with CP and hypoextensible triceps surae muscles caused by an excessive triceps surae contractions (group 2).[201] Both groups were treated with progressive casting to lengthen the muscles. Group 1 showed a shift to the right of the passive length-tension curve without a change in the slope of the curve. Group 2 presented curves that were shifted to the right with decreased slopes, showing decreased stiffness (Figure 5-8). The authors suggested that the children in group 2 showed normal muscle adaptation because of the stiffness adaptation. These findings suggest that human muscles undergo adaptations that may be similar to those that have been reported for animals. This assumption is based on the association of the passive curves of animal and human muscles, measured by noninvasive methods, with the histologic and histochemical adaptations in animal muscles. Results of the study also elucidate the variability that can be expected in humans, particularly with regard to the possibility of different pathologic mechanisms underlying the adaptability of hypoextensible muscles in selected patient populations, such as children with CP.[201]

Clinical observations clearly provide evidence that the musculoskeletal system of humans undergoes adaptations in response to immobilization, disuse, postural disturbances, and muscle imbalances in relation to specific pathologic disorders. It is well known that the skeletal muscles of a limb

that is immobilized and is not used will atrophy as a result of protein degradation.[171] It is equally well known that normal muscle fibers respond to increased force and endurance demands through adaptive responses in structural, physiologic, and biochemical characteristics.[170] The presence of pathologic conditions that alter skeletal muscles directly (e.g., DMD) or indirectly through changes in neurologic activity to the skeletal muscles (e.g., hypotonia, hypertonia) may lead to postural contractures and deformities from muscle imbalances and chronic positioning.[31,177,201,203]

Many of the clinical manifestations of musculoskeletal disorders correlate well with the pathophysiologic conditions of the MTU described from experimental animal models. Abnormal shapes in the structures of the vertebral column (e.g., hemivertebra) are associated with adaptations of the MTU and other soft tissues of the back. If the lower limbs of a child with flaccid paralysis are held in a specific posture for an extended period (e.g., hip flexion, abduction, lateral rotation), the limbs adopt the characteristic position of the posture.[177] Recent evidence suggests that children with CP and spasticity may have increased collagen accumulation within the endomysium of muscle that may contribute to increased muscular stiffness.[23] Moreover, muscle fibers from upper extremity muscles of children with spastic CP have been shown to have shorter resting sarcomere lengths than normal muscle fibers.[66] This study provides support for intracellular and extracellular collagen remodeling that may contribute to increased resistance to passive stretch of muscles with spasticity.

Long-term conservative interventions, such as strengthening, stretching, and casting, may facilitate desired adaptations of the MTU and enhance activity, but much research is needed to examine these possibilities objectively. Inconsistent evidence that muscle activation patterns change after orthopedic surgery has been presented.[51,114,155,163] It is speculated that abnormal *muscle activation* before the operation can be related to a compensatory response in some patients, and this can be manipulated after surgery.[155] Studies that examine the combined influence of conservative and surgical interventions are clearly needed to determine the most efficacious methods of improving participation in daily activities.

Bone deformities and alterations in the MTU may result from abnormal skeletal growth, or both MTU and bone adaptations may be associated with abnormalities in muscle tonicity and muscle imbalances found in conditions such as CP. Numerous developmental changes in the musculoskeletal system have been associated with CP, and these changes correlate well with the presence of spasticity and imbalances in muscle force and muscle length. They include changes in the femur and acetabulum, resulting in medial femoral torsion and hip disorders, hip adduction contractures, and knee flexion contractures in spastic adductor and hamstring muscles, and severe equinus deformity caused by spasticity and shortening adaptations of the calf musculature.[141]

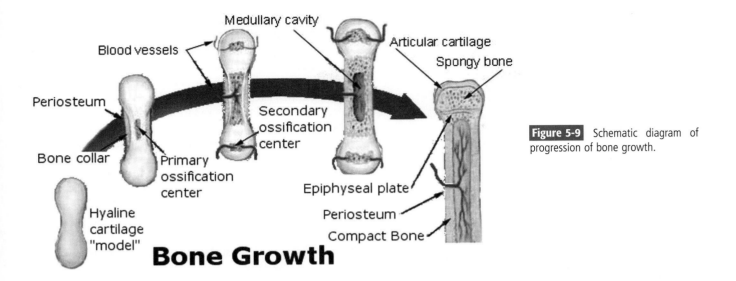

Figure 5-9 Schematic diagram of progression of bone growth.

SKELETAL AND ARTICULAR STRUCTURES

Like muscle tissue, both skeletal and articular tissues arise from the mesodermal layer of the embryo (Figure 5-9). Mesenchymal cells condense to form templates of the skeleton. From this point, two distinct processes of bone formation take place: (1) endochondral ossification, and (2) intramembranous ossification. All bones, with the exception of the clavicle, mandible, and skull, are formed by endochondral ossification (also called intracartilaginous ossification).[137,168,216] During the early embryonic period, collagenous and elastic fibers are deposited on the mesenchymal models and form cartilaginous models. Bone minerals are deposited on these new models and gradually replace the cartilage via the process of ossification. Intramembranous ossification occurs directly in the mesenchymal model. Mesenchymal cells differentiate into osteoblasts that deposit a matrix called osteoid tissue. This tissue is organized into bone as calcium phosphate is deposited. Ossification at the primary ossification centers, typically in the center of the diaphysis or body of the bone, commences at the end of the embryonic period (eighth fetal week).

Joint formation also begins as the cartilaginous models are formed. In a specialized area between cartilaginous bone models, the interzonal mesenchyme differentiates to form the joint. The basic structures of the joint are formed during the sixth to eighth weeks of gestation, but the final shape develops throughout early childhood under the influence of the forces of movement and compression.[55] In embryonic chicks, early joint formation occurred in the absence of mobility, but toward the end of the fetal period, cartilaginous bonds between the joint surfaces were present, and the articular surfaces were flattened and misshaped.[55] Examples of the relationship between joint formation and movement are also seen in children. Pearl and colleagues[156] examined 84 children between the ages of 7 months and 13½ years who

had obstetric brachial plexus palsy that resulted in medial rotation contractures of the shoulder. Sixty-one percent had extreme glenohumeral deformities, including flat glenoids, biconcave glenoids, pseudoglenoids, and flattened, oval humeral heads. The mechanical forces created by the unopposed medial rotators had a profound effect on the development of this joint.

Hip joint development is another good example of changes during the fetal period. At 12 weeks of GA, the acetabulum is extremely deep, and the head of the femur is quite round and well covered (Figure 5-10).[161] As the fetus increases in age, the relative depth of the acetabulum decreases as the head of the femur becomes more hemispheric. At birth, the acetabulum is so shallow that it covers less than one half of the femoral head; this results in a relatively unstable hip and is thought to allow for easier passage through the vaginal canal. Because of the combination of shallow acetabulum, flattened femoral head, high neck shaft angle, and a large amount of anteversion, the hip is especially vulnerable to dislocating forces during the third trimester.[161,178] The risk of dislocation is greatest if the child is delivered in single-breech position (i.e., hips flexed and knees extended).[195] "It was postulated that extreme hip flexion combined with knee extension caused the hamstrings to pull the head of the femur downward, stretching the compliant hip capsule. After birth, the femur may be dislocated by the upward pull of the iliopsoas muscle when infants are diapered and wrapped with the hips extended. This theory may explain why the incidence of congenital hip dislocation is increased among those Native American populations in which newborns are strapped onto cradle boards or wrapped with the legs in adduction and extension.[46,223]

During postnatal growth, the forces of compression and movement contribute to an increase in the depth of the acetabulum until the age of 8 years, when the adult level of femoral head coverage is reached.[14] The head of the femur

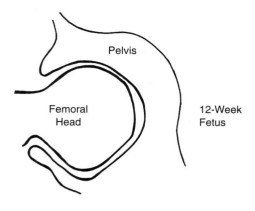

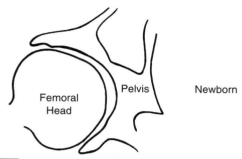

Figure 5-10 Schematic diagram of the fetal and newborn hip joint, illustrating changes in acetabular coverage of the femoral head. Coverage is extensive in the 12-week fetus, but is reduced in the newborn.

also becomes rounder, but it never achieves the roundness that it had during the early fetal period. Atypical pressures, such as those seen in children with obesity or spasticity, can deform the femur and component parts of the hip. Children with obesity are at increased risk of developing a flattened femoral head and a slipped capital epiphysis because of the excessive weight on the developing femoral head.[43,119] Children with spasticity are at risk for subluxation or dislocation from the asymmetrical pull of spastic muscles around the hip.[82,88,237]

Atypical changes in the shape of the acetabulum and femoral head have been reported in children with unstable or dislocated hips, such as children with congenitally dislocated hips, CP, or myelodysplasia. Buckley and colleagues[30] examined 33 unstable hips in children with these disabilities and found that all had significantly shallower acetabula compared with those of a control group; the hip was most shallow in children with CP. The percentage of coverage of the head of the femur also was less for these children compared with control groups of children without disabilities. The children with disabilities had thinly developed articular surfaces and small, shallow acetabula with poorly defined margins. Beals[14] reported that the acetabula of children with CP in his study

had appeared normal after birth, but that they did not increase in depth as expected by the age of 2 years. Nevertheless, acetabular depth was comparable with that of the typically developing population when the children were 8 years old. All but 1 of the 40 children included in this study were walking at this age, suggesting that the dynamic compressive forces of walking contributed to increased depth of the acetabulum. This relationship between hip stability and ambulation has been further supported in the literature by other studies.[1,214] Beals[14] also supported the use of a standing program to increase the depth of the hip joint.

Bone development progresses most rapidly in the prenatal period. By the time of birth, the diaphyses are almost ossified. If a child is born prematurely, however, osteopenia is frequently seen. In the very premature, it may result in bone fragility and must be considered if therapy is being provided to the very young neonate. After birth, long bones grow in length at the epiphyseal plate, which is between the diaphysis and the epiphysis. This cartilaginous plate rapidly proliferates on the diaphyseal side of the bone. The resultant chondrocytes, arranged in parallel columns, become enlarged and are then converted into bone by endochondral ossification.[129,164] Eventually, the epiphyseal plate is ossified, the diaphyses and epiphyses are joined, and the growth of the bone in length is considered complete. The timing of complete ossification varies with each particular bone. Most bones are fully ossified by 20 years of age, but for a few bones, the process can continue longer into adulthood.[137]

Bone is increased in width through appositional growth, which is the accumulation of new bone on bone surfaces. To keep the bone from becoming too thick and therefore too heavy, osteoblasts on the inside of the bone are reabsorbed as new bone is added on the surface. This results in an increase in thickness and density of the diaphysis without excess weight.

SKELETAL ADAPTATIONS

Although deformities can occur throughout the growing period, the skeleton is most vulnerable during the first few years of life (prenatal and postnatal), when the rate of growth is greatest.[35] Fetal position has been related to various deformities, especially those that occur toward the end of pregnancy. The incidence of tibial rotation and metatarsus adductus was reported to increase as the GA increased in preterm infants.[103] Many factors can cause prenatal deformities, including decreased amniotic fluid, the limited space in which the fetus can move in utero, multiple births, and external forces from tightly stretched uterine and abdominal walls. Associated deformities include congenital torticollis, plagiocephaly (asymmetrical head), and pelvic obliquity.[10,70,115,178]

The growth and resultant shape of the skeleton are affected by genetic coding, nutrition, and the combination of various mechanical forces that are imposed over time. The size, density, alignment, and trabecular arrangement of bone change as the forces of heredity and the environment play their roles. After initial development, bone shape can be changed through a process called modeling, which uses resorption of old or immature bone and formation of new bone to determine its shape. Wolff's law, first proposed in the 1870s, suggested that bones develop a particular internal trabecular structure in response to the mechanical forces that are placed on them.[67] The type of loading and stress (or force per bone area) in different situations affects bones differently.

Loading a bone longitudinally, parallel to the direction of growth, results in compression or tension. Either type of loading, applied intermittently with appropriate force, such as with weight bearing or muscle pull, stimulates bone growth. Intermittent compression forces appear to stimulate more growth than is stimulated by tension.[67] The Hueter-Volkmann principle describes the reaction of bone to excessive force and states that excessive static loading will cause bone material to decrease, which can be detrimental to bone integrity and strength.[67]

Shear forces, which run parallel to the epiphyseal plate, can lead to torsional or twisting changes in the bone. The columns of chondrocytes around the periphery of the plate veer away from the shear forces in a twisting pattern.[115] The normal pull of muscles around a joint contributes to the shear forces, resulting in normal torsional changes in the long bones. For example, at birth, the tibia exhibits 5° of medial torsion.[15] By the time of maturity, the longitudinal orientation of the tibia has changed to 18° to 47° of lateral torsion.[112]

Asymmetrical forces will lead to asymmetrical growth. Growth plates line up to be perpendicular to the direction of the forces. This can be advantageous during fracture healing. Bone is able to straighten some degree of malalignment though a process known as flexure drift. This remodeling mechanism describes a process whereby strain on a curved bone wall applied by repeated loading tends to move the bone surface in the direction of the concavity to straighten the bone.[67] Bone is resorbed from the convex side and is laid down on the concave side. This process is seen in the femur and tibia as a normal part of development of the position of the knee in the frontal plane.[41,87,169] At birth, the infant's knees are bowlegged (genu varum), but they gradually straighten until they reach a neutral alignment between the first and second years. The knee angulation then progresses toward genu valgum, reaching its peak between the ages of 2 and 4 years. After this time, the angle of genu valgum gradually decreases (Figure 5-11). The final knee angle may differ according to race and gender. Heath and Staheli[87] reported that by the age of 11 years, the mean knee angle of white boys and girls was 5.8° of valgus, and no child demonstrated genu varus. In contrast, Cheng and associates[38] found that Chinese children of both genders progressed to genu varus of less than 5° in the preteen years. Cahuzac and co-workers[32] studied European children and determined

that by the age of 16 years, girls maintained a valgus knee position and boys had developed a genu varus of 4.4°. The pediatric therapist should be aware that the presence of genu varus between the ages of 2 and 11 years may be considered atypical in white children,[87] but caution should be used when interpreting this finding in children of other races.

If the forces are directed unequally or abnormally across an epiphyseal plate, however, growth may be uneven, which may increase the malalignment. The spinal neural arch can experience asymmetrical growth. Six growth centers are present in the spinal neural arch, three within each half of the arch. Uneven growth of either half of the neural arch may be a significant factor in the later development of idiopathic scoliosis.[40,191] In the lower extremities, assymetrical growth can result in genu valgum ("knock-knees") or genu varum ("bowlegs"). Artificially applied asymmetrical compression by surgical stapling of the medial aspect of the epiphyseal plate of the proximal tibia retards growth on that side and can be used to correct these deformities.[134] For children with leg length differences, surgical staples are applied to both sides of the epiphyseal plate of the longer leg to slow its growth until the shorter leg catches up.[57] The Ilizarov and monolateral devices for limb lengthening use tension to facilitate bone growth.[183] With this technique, the diaphyseal cortex of the bone of the shorter leg is cut, and "gradual incremental distraction" is applied across the cut ends of the bone.[190] Osteogenesis occurs in the space between the two ends of the cut bone.

Normal developmental changes in the femur illustrate the impact of the muscular system on bone. To understand these changes, the terms *version* and *torsion* require discussion. Torsion refers to the normal amount of twist present in a long bone (Figure 5-12). Femoral torsion is the angle formed by an axis drawn along the head and neck of the femur and another through the femoral condyles. To visualize this angle, picture a femur with the posterior surfaces of the femoral condyles on a horizontal surface such as a table. When looking up toward the hip, you will notice that the head and neck of the femur are angled upward from the table approximately 15°. This is the angle of torsion.

Antetorsion occurs when the head and neck of the femur are rotated forward in the sagittal plane relative to the femoral condyles. If the head and neck of the femur are rotated posteriorly, the femur is said to be in retrotorsion. At birth, the femur has its maximum antetorsion at approximately 30° to 40°.[188] This angle decreases rapidly during the infant's first year, more slowly between 1 and 8 years, and then rapidly again through adolescence to a mean of 16° by age 14 to 16 years.[188] The femur is said to "untwist" through the process of growth, muscle action, reduction of the coxa valga angle, and reduction of the hip flexion contracture.[17] The femoral head, neck, and greater trochanteric areas are made of pliable cartilage and are attached to the rigid osseous diaphysis. As the infant develops, normal torsional forces

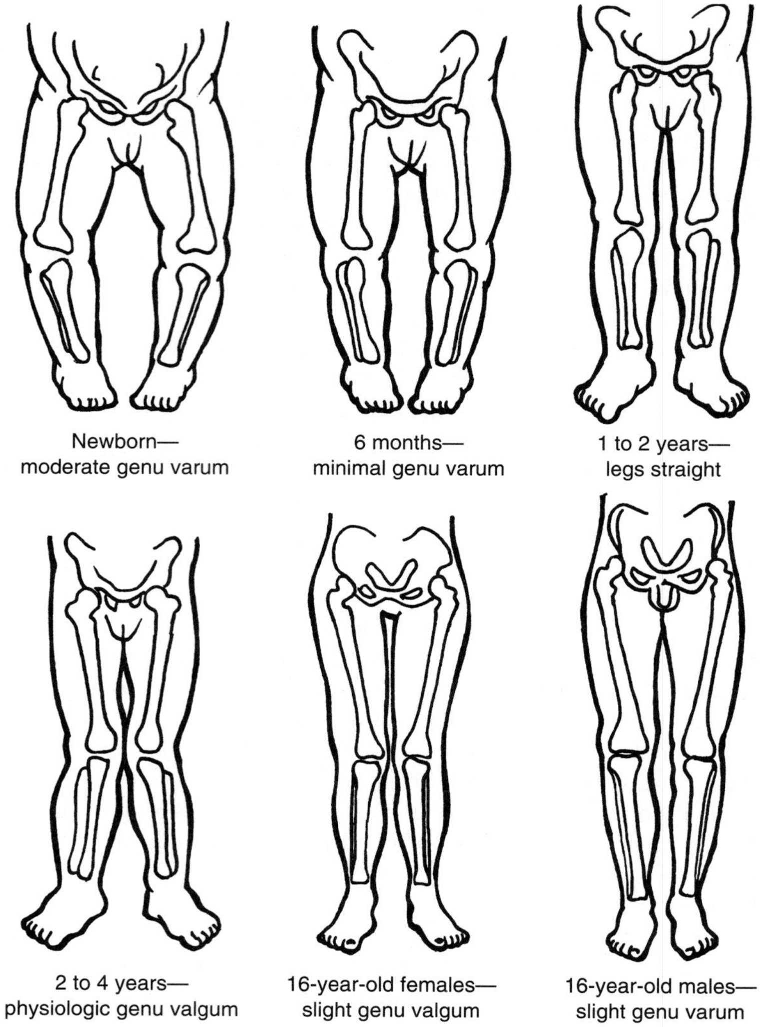

Figure 5-11 Physiologic evolution of lower limb alignment at various ages in infancy and childhood. (Redrawn from Tachdjian, M. O. [1972]. *Pediatric orthopedics* (2nd ed., p. 1463). Philadelphia: WB Saunders.)

Newborn— moderate genu varum

6 months— minimal genu varum

1 to 2 years— legs straight

2 to 4 years— physiologic genu valgum

16-year-old females— slight genu valgum

16-year-old males— slight genu varum

about this point of fixation cause a decrease in femoral antetorsion. Bleck[17] speculated that these forces are created by active external hip rotation and extension, and Fabeck and colleagues[59] calculated that forces created during walking have a major impact on developmental changes in femoral antetorsion. If active hip motions are minimal or walking is delayed, as is frequently observed in children with CP, the infantile femoral torsion does not decrease as it should.

Version refers to a position of a segment relative to a plane. Femoral version refers to the position of the head of the femur in the acetabulum (see Figure 5-12). When the pelvis is visualized in supine, the angle that the head and shaft create relative to the back of the pelvis aligned on the frontal plane is the amount of version. Anteversion positions the head of the femur anteriorly in the acetabulum and results in a position of thigh external rotation. Conversely, retroversion positions the head of the femur posteriorly in the acetabulum, which results in thigh internal rotation. At birth, a neonate has 40° to 60° of anteversion. This gradually

resolves over time to 15° to 20° by age 8 to 10 years and down to 12° in adulthood. The externally rotated posture seen in newborns is attributed to the high amount of anteversion. At birth, anteversion (60°) is greater than antetorsion (30°) with a net result of an externally rotated posture.[217]

Excessive or persistent fetal antetorsion can lead to an in-toed gait pattern. In-toeing becomes apparent as the amount of hip external rotation decreases with age. A majority of otherwise healthy children with persistent fetal antetorsion will improve as the hips spontaneously realign by age 10 years. In less than 1% of these children, antetorsion fails to resolve by age 10 years, and the children warrant treatment.[188] In children with CP, however, persistent fetal antetorsion is a causative factor in the development of hip instability. This is discussed in greater detail later in the chapter.

Another example of bone remodeling was seen in a child who was born without a tibia.[124] When the child reached 2 years of age, the fibula was surgically centered in relation to

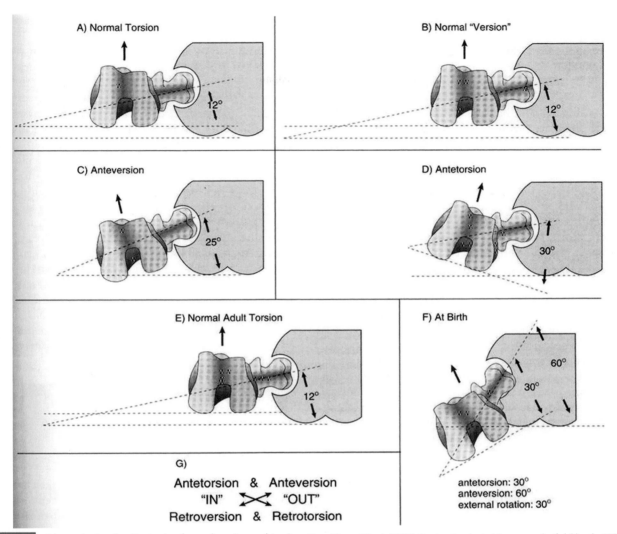

Figure 5-12 Schematic drawing illustrating femoral version and torsion. (From Effgen, S.K. ed. [2005] *Meeting the physical therapy needs of children* (p. 137) Philadelphia, Pa.: FA Davis.)

the femur to act as a tibia. Sixteen months later, the fibula looked like a tibia in terms of shape, size, and strength. The authors believed that mechanical stresses delivered in a functional weight-bearing manner induced changes in the bone.

Disuse adversely affects bone by delaying secondary ossification centers and causing the bone to reabsorb. Children with a reduced activity level due to conditions such as CP, myelodysplasia, or arthrogryposis multiplex congenita are at greater risk for fracture because of disuse atrophy of the bones. Researchers have attempted to predict which children with CP are most likely to sustain a fracture. Risk increases significantly with disability. In children with Gross Motor Function Classification System levels II through IV, the fracture rate was 4% which is more than double the rate of children who are typically developing, and 77% of the children had decreased bone density.[132] In this population, the ratio of the child's weight for age was the best

predictor of fracture risk. Feeding gastrostomy tubes and a previous history of fracture also increased the risk significantly.[98,190]

Disuse demineralization occurs quickly. One study found a 34% decrease in bone mineralization after non–weight-bearing immobilization following a fracture or surgery in only 4 to 6 weeks.[197] Studies have shown that weight bearing has a beneficial effect on fracture healing and improves the density and trabecular network of osteopenic bone when coupled with active exercise.[102,152]

Decreased bone mineralization is also seen in chronic conditions such as hemophilia,[12] leukemia,[225] symptomatic epilepsy,[179,180] long-term use of glucocorticoids,[185] growth hormone deficiency, and idiopathic scoliosis.[96] Likewise, bone density deficiencies accompany digestive system conditions such as Crohn's disease[84] and irritable bowel disorder.[196,215]

Fortunately, methods to promote healthy bone mineralization have been documented. Evidence suggests that calcium supplements can increase bone mineralization in healthy children[212] and in children with growth hormone deficiency.[238] Administering growth hormone to children with CP has also improved bone density and has promoted growth.[2] An increase in bone thickness and density is seen in athletes compared with nonathletes.[124] Nonathletes can, however, increase bone density by increasing their physical activity.[68,124] Numerous studies have demonstrated an increase in bone density in typically developing children with a consistent program of impact exercise,[91,128,213] but not in children who participated in non–weight-bearing exercise such as swimming.[80]

Weight-bearing programs also improve bone mineral density and promote hip modeling in children with CP. Mobile children with CP have greater bone mineral density when compared with their less mobile peers.[98,232] In a preliminary study, Stuberg[194] found that 60 minutes of standing four or five times a week increased the bone mineral density of nonambulatory children with severe to profound CP. Thirty minutes of standing, however, did not produce results. When the standing program was discontinued, bone mineral density decreased. In a review article, Pin[158] concluded that evidence supported the use of static standing programs for increasing bone density and temporarily reducing spasticity. Evidence was insufficient to support outcomes of improved communication, enhanced digestive function, and deepening of the acetabulum.

Intermittent weight bearing with movement was most beneficial to hip joint modeling.[194] Intermittent weight bearing with movement can be accomplished by partial-weight-bearing ambulation with the use of a treadmill or gait trainer. The Kaye Dynamic multipositional stander[1] also provides intermittent weight bearing by allowing movement within the base of support while the client is safely aligned in a standing position. Choosing an appropriate standing frame is also very important. Kecskemethy[105] and colleagues measured the percentage of a child's body weight that was being directed down to the stander and found that it ranged from 37% to 100%. If the goal is to provide weight bearing, than it would be logical to obtain as much weight as the child can tolerate during standing. The authors suggested that the Rifton supine stander positioned at an angle of 70° was an appropriate choice.[2] Weight bearing is an important part of physical therapy intervention for young children with neuromuscular diseases that delay the development of stance. The formation, growth, and integrity of articular cartilage are stimulated by compressive forces and movement between bone surfaces.[161] Intermittent joint loading leads to healthy, thick cartilage, but constant loading interrupts normal

nutrition, and the cartilage can eventually degenerate, leading to degenerative joint disease.[35,207]

Age and diet also affect bone mass and strength. Children are most at risk for distal forearm fractures during their pubertal growth spurt.[11,162] The rate of increase in the child's height and weight is greater than the rate of increase in the strength of the cortical bone at the radial metaphysis, which puts the bone at a mechanical disadvantage when an adolescent falls onto an outstretched arm.[162] Children who are obese have a higher bone mass density than children of appropriate weight, but not to the extent necessary to support their size.[79] Therefore obese children have a high incidence of upper extremity fractures compared with their lighter-weight peers.[78,226] The overall incidence of forearm fractures in childhood has increased over the past 30 years; this is postulated to result from the combination of vulnerable bone tissue with changes in diet (i.e., higher soft drink consumption and lower calcium intake) and increases in risky physical activity, such as skate boarding and inline skating.[109]

Changes in the muscular or skeletal system have interactive effects. Understanding the influences of these two systems on the development and final outcome of each system and recognizing the period when these systems are most mutable assist the therapist in designing effective treatment programs, as well as in knowing when to discontinue treatment procedures.

LONG-TERM EFFECTS OF ATYPICAL MUSCULOSKELETAL DEVELOPMENT

Many pathologic conditions of the musculoskeletal system have been identified in adults with developmental disabilities. Most commonly, these conditions develop during childhood and worsen during adulthood. Neurologic conditions such as CP frequently include a wide range of musculoskeletal issues such as scoliosis, hip dislocation, cervical neck dislocation, contracture, arthritis, patella alta, overuse syndrome, nerve entrapment, and fracture.[71] In neurologic or genetic diseases associated with developmental delay, the initial condition is considered nonprogressive, but the musculoskeletal impairments that frequently accompany these conditions typically worsen as the child grows. Discussed here are examples of common developmental musculoskeletal pathologies. More information on specific conditions mentioned can be found in subsequent chapters in this volume.

You have learned that the hip is unstable at birth but undergoes a great deal of normal developmental change, which increases stability. These normal developmental changes result from a combination of muscle pull and weight bearing. Children with CP typically have delayed walking, ROM limitations, and atypical muscular pull/spasticity. Hip subluxation and dislocation therefore are common problems in children with spastic CP, occurring in 30% to 60% of children with CP who are not walking independently at 5

---

years.[175] Over a lifetime, this equates to an incidence of 1% in children with spastic hemiplegia, 5% in those with diplegia, and up to 55% in those with quadriplegia.[145] Adequate ROM allows the hip to move into a stable well-covered position in the acetabulum. Children with CP tend to lose abduction range and to develop hip flexion contractures, both of which are detrimental to hip stability. Critical ROM values for hip stability include maintaining at least 30° of abduction and avoiding a hip flexion contracture of 20° to 25° or more.[135] Adequate hip abduction allows the head of the femur to move into the acetabulum. Hip abduction ROM is frequently limited in children with slipped capital femoral epiphysis and Legg-Calvé-Perthes disease.

Muscle contractures can interfere with sitting balance, hygiene, and activities of daily living.[17] For example, a hamstring contracture can pull the pelvis posteriorly and diminish sitting balance. Hamstring contractures also affect walking by causing a crouched gait pattern, limiting step length and heel strike, and may even appear as a valgus position of the knee. Hip flexor contractures can affect gait by limiting hip extension in stance phase, and hip adductor tightness can cause scissoring of the gait pattern, resulting in a narrow base of support.

Adults with CP frequently experience pain in the weight-bearing joints of the hip, knee, ankle, lumbar spine, and cervical spine.[101] Surveys of adults with CP report that between 53% and 82% of those interviewed have had one or more sites of chronic pain, with an average of three sites.[173,206] Pain can cause loss of function and deterioration of quality of life. In a study by Murphy, Molnar, and Lankasky,[146] about 75% of persons with CP who were ambulatory stopped walking by 25 years of age because of fatigue and inefficiency of movement. A smaller peak occurred around 45 years of age, when additional individuals stopped walking because of pain in the weight-bearing joints. It is therefore important that physical therapists consider the potential impact that long-term musculoskeletal malalignment can have on joints and address pain at early stages.[71]

A variety of idiopathic conditions are characterized by a disorder of endochondral ossification. The incidence of many of these conditions, which often result in a limp during walking, is increasing. This is most often attributed to the increased obesity rate in children.[39] Legg-Calvé-Perthes disease is a hip disorder that involves repeated episodes of transient synovitis of the hip, usually occurring in children between the ages of 3 and 12, with most cases affecting boys between the ages of 3 and 12.[34] The synovitis causes an increased joint pressure which interrupts blood flow in the vessels ascending the femoral neck. This typically results in pain, decreased hip abduction and internal rotation, and an atypical gait pattern, in which patients have a limp and a positive Trendelenburg sign. Slipped capital femoral epiphysis (SCFE) occurs when the growth plate of the proximal femoral physis is weak, resulting in displacement from the normal position. Patients with SCFE usually have an antalgic gait pattern and pain in the groin. Treatment for SCFE involves keeping the displacement to a minimum, maintaining ROM, and preventing degenerative arthritis. SCFE and Legg-Calvé-Perthes disease are childhood conditions that present a risk factor for the development of osteoarthritis and disability later in life.[7]

Lower extremity rotational and angular problems are common lower extremity abnormalities in children. Rotational problems include in-toeing and out-toeing. In-toeing is caused by metatarsus adductus, increased femoral anteversion, internal tibial torsion, or a combination of any of the three. Consequently, out-toeing is caused by the opposite factors for in-toeing. Internal tibial torsion is a normal finding in the newborn but may pose a problem at walking age if not corrected. Casting can correct metatarsus adductus, but conservative treatments for femoral anteversion and tibial torsion have not been shown to be effective. Angular problems such as genu varus and genu valgum are also common lower extremity abnormalities. Genu varus may lead to Blount's disease, which is a progressive deformity manifested by varus deformity and internal rotation of the tibia in the proximal metaphyseal region immediately below the knee. Blount's disease leads to irreversible pathologic changes at the medial portion of the proximal tibial epiphysis caused by growth disturbances of the subjacent physis.[39,231]

Patella alta is a condition in which the patella is positioned higher than expected on the femur. It frequently presents in early adolescence as anterior knee pain and progresses with age.[145] It is common in individuals who walk with flexed knees such as adults with CP or who have overactive quadriceps muscles. Maintaining adequate quadriceps and rectus femoris muscle length may help prevent patella alta.[145] With patella alta, quadriceps strength is compromised and terminal knee extension is difficult. Pain and weakness can result in functional losses during activities such as walking, climbing stairs, or getting out of a chair. In addition to maintaining adequate length and strength of the quadriceps and rectus femoris muscles, a neoprene patellar tracking sleeve may reduce symptoms in some individuals.[145]

A small study used magnetic resonance imaging to compare patellar movement in individuals with and without patella alta. The patella in those with patella alta had greater lateral displacement and less contact area. It is therefore not surprising that patella alta could lead to patellofemoral joint dysfunction.[219]

Feet are also subject to pathologic changes caused by an atypical musculoskeletal system; this can lead to complaints of pain in adults. Pes planus, or flat foot, is associated with a valgus heel and reduction in height of the longitudinal arch. Physiologic flat foot is flexible and is common in many typically developing individuals. Pathologic flat feet, however, have stiffness, often cause disability, and likely will require treatment.[188] Years of toe-walking and cavus foot deformities frequently result in pain in the metatarsal heads.

Obesity is now considered a pediatric epidemic that puts detrimental excessive weight on joints. Associated degenerative and inflammatory conditions such as osteoarthritis, rheumatoid arthritis, and spondyloarthropathy, are conditions that can affect the musculoskeletal system. Obesity increases the need for future joint replacement surgery.[4]

Arthrogryposis multiplex congenita (AMC) poses a variety of risks and challenges for individuals throughout all stages of life. Arthrogryposis is the presence of multiple contractures at birth. Joint deformities appear to be secondary to lack of movement during intrauterine development. Hip dislocations, arthritic changes in weight-bearing joints, overuse syndromes in muscles, carpal tunnel syndrome, and neuropathies can be commonly seen in adults with AMC as a result of lifelong malalignment.[16]

Adults with Down syndrome are at risk for developing hip disorders, such as subluxation, dislocation, and osteoarthritis.[44,45] Musculoskeletal disorders and orthopedic problems are believed to be acquired secondary to soft tissue laxity and muscle hypotonia.

Further study into the causes and prevention of secondary conditions is greatly needed to help guide the treatment of children with developmental disabilities. Pediatric therapists are appropriate professionals to educate parents and children about the lifelong attention that will need to be given to musculoskeletal problems, such as decreased strength and ROM. When appropriate, adolescents should be taught to be responsible for their physical and cardiopulmonary needs. Another role for pediatric therapists is educating their fellow orthopedic physical therapists who treat adults about the musculoskeletal problems in the neglected populations of adults with CP, myelodysplasia, and other developmental disabilities. Campbell[33] has written an excellent article on the issues surrounding secondary disabilities and how they can be addressed by pediatric therapists.

MEASUREMENT AND EFFECTS OF INTERVENTION

Fundamental goals of therapeutic intervention for physical disabilities include enhancing participation in daily activities and life roles by preventing or correcting the impairments that result from the underlying pathologic condition, or from the normal physiologic adaptations superimposed on the pathologic condition. Presumably activity and participation will be enhanced if impairments are prevented or corrected, although research is needed to justify this assumption. Achieving functional levels of ROM and strength are two fundamental goals of therapeutic intervention. Accurate assessments of ROM and strength are therefore important components of the physical therapy examination process.

Range of Motion Examination

A wide range of methods and instruments have been reported for examining the ROM about a joint or multiple joints, including simple visual estimation, use of various protractors and goniometers, measurements made from still photographs, and complex methods using computerized motion analysis systems. For most physical therapists, however, the universal goniometer (i.e., full-circle manual goniometer) remains the most versatile and widely used instrument in clinical practice. The design of the universal goniometer and procedures for its use have been described in detail in numerous publications. The articles by M.L. Moore[138,139] and the book by Norkin and White[150] are particularly comprehensive and should be consulted for complete descriptions.

The reliability of goniometry is based on the reproducibility or stability of ROM measurements in relation to (1) the time intervals between comparable measurements, or (2) the use of more than one rater. ROM measurements must be reliable to be adequately tested as valid. Many factors influence the reliability and validity of goniometric measurements. These factors include consistency of applied procedures, differences among joint actions and among the structure and function of body regions, passive versus active measurements, intrarater measurements (multiple measurements by one examiner) versus interrater measurements (multiple measurements by two or more examiners), normal day-to-day variations in ROM, and day-to-day variations in different pathologic conditions.[73]

Numerous studies have reported on the ROM characteristics and reliability of goniometry in adults, but reports on infants and children are more limited in number. Studies have demonstrated that full-term newborns present a limited range of hip and knee extension and greater dorsiflexion compared with adults.[56,222] These findings were attributed to the effects of intrauterine position and newborn flexor muscle tone. Consequently, clinicians should not use adult ROM values for comparison with limb ROM measurements of the newborn. Reference values for neonatal ROM are presented in Table 5-1.

Studies with normal healthy children have indicated that ROM can be measured reliably,[83] but studies of children with various pathologic conditions have shown that reliability varies with the number of raters and the pathologic problem. Pandya and colleagues[154] studied seven upper and lower extremity joint limitations in 150 children with DMD and reported that intrarater reliability was high (intraclass correlation coefficient [ICC] range, .81 to .91), but interrater reliability was lower, with wide variation from joint to joint (ICC range, .25 to .91). Although some reports suggest that ROM can be reliably measured in children with CP, most researchers have concluded that variances of ±10° to 28° (depending on the joint) in ROM over time do not signify a meaningful change in children with spastic CP.[13,86,110,127,193]

The hip is a particularly difficult joint for which to obtain reliable ROM measures. In a study of children who had a femoral fracture, Owen[153] concluded that only differences of 30° or more of hip rotation and 50° of flexion/extension should be concluded as reflecting true change. Bartlett and colleagues[13] compared four methods of measuring hip

TABLE 5-1 Central Tendency Values of Lower Extremity Range of Motion Reported in Degrees for Children Born Full Term, From Birth Through 5 Years Old

	Birth	6 Weeks	6 Months	1 Year	3 Years	5 Years
Hip extension limitation	34.2	19	7	7	7	7
Hip abduction	55			59	59	54
Hip adduction	6.4			30	31	24
Hip external rotation	90	48	53	58	56	39
Hip internal rotation	33	24	24	38	39	34
Popliteal angle	27		11	0	0	0

Handbook of pediatric physical therapy (1995) Long TM, Cintas HL, eds. Baltimore, MD 21202, Williams & Wilkins, (p. 81).

extension (by prone extension, Thomas test, Mundale method, and pelvic-femoral angle) in 15 children with spastic diplegia, 15 with meningomyelocele, and 15 with no known pathologic condition. They reported that the Thomas test was particularly difficult to apply to patients with spastic diplegia. The prone hip extension test[188] has been shown to have better reliability compared with the Thomas test in children with spastic diplegic CP.[13] For this test, the child is in the prone position on a table with the opposite leg hanging over the edge of the table. In this position, the lumbar spine is flattened. The examiner holds the pelvis down at the level of the posterior superior iliac spines and pulls the leg that is being examined into hip extension until the pelvis begins to move anteriorly. At that point, the angle between the femur and the surface is measured and reflects the degree of hip flexion contracture.[17] One limitation of this test is that it can be difficult to perform with large children because the therapist needs to hold the leg being tested while simultaneously holding the goniometer and measuring the angle.

The results of these few studies clearly indicate that the reliability of ROM measurements is influenced by the specific patient problem. Additional research is needed to clarify goniometric reliability among the many different types of patients treated by pediatric physical therapists. In the meantime, therapists are encouraged to do their own reliability studies to establish confidence intervals for recognizing changes in ROM that are clinically significant. Because intrarater reliability has generally been shown to be acceptable, another alternative would be to have one therapist with demonstrated rating consistency perform all goniometric measurements on one child. The impact of ROM on function is also unclear. In a study by Lowes et al.,[120] strength and to a lesser extent ROM were shown to be accurate predictors of balance and functional skills. Follow-up studies are needed to determine if daily skills require critical ROM values. In other words, can improved ROM guarantee an improved activity level?

Strength Examination

Accurate measurement of strength is important for identifying strength deficits and for documenting changes in strength

TABLE 5-2 Scaling Parameters Are Inserted Into the Formula Torque/ Mass Scaling Parameter to Normalize Strength Measurements of Children of Different Sizes

Joint Tested	Children Who Are Developing Typically	Children With CP
Hip abduction	1.32	1.66
Hip adduction	1.35	1.68
Knee extension	1.69	1.87
Knee flexion	1.33	1.59
Ankle dorsiflexion	1.49	1.47
Ankle plantar flexion	.75	1.32

that result from interventions. Numerous methods of measuring strength are available, including the traditional procedures of manual muscle testing and the use of various handheld force dynamometers[21] and computerized isokinetic testing systems.[107,167] Although manual muscle testing is probably the most versatile and widely used method, evidence indicates that handheld dynamometers may yield more precise measurements and are more sensitive to small changes in strength.[20] Isokinetic systems are effective for quantifying strength in adults, but it can be difficult to adjust the various components to fit children. Another concern is normalizing force measurements to account for differences in size. In adults, the force is normalized by dividing the force measurement by body mass. This method is not accurate in children. Wren and Engsberg (2009, 2007) have developed normalization coefficients for children who are typically developing and children with CP. Scaling coefficients are used in the equation torque/mass scaling coefficient. Please see Table 5-2 for a list of these coefficients.

In addition to normalizing measurements for size, a therapist must consider the reliability of methods of strength testing in different patient populations. Children must be able to understand the instructions and follow commands to produce accurate and reliable strength measurements. The reliability of the strength measurements may also vary with

TABLE 5-3 **Standardized Testing Positions for Handheld Dynamometry**

Muscle Group Patient Position	Limb Positions	Manually Stabilized Body Part	Dynamometer Placement
Wrist flexors Supine	Arm beside trunk, elbow flexed 90°, forearm in neutral supination, wrist in neutral flexion	Arm and forearm	Just proximal to metacarpophalangeal joints on extensor surface of hand
Wrist extensors Supine	As wrist flexors	As wrist flexors	Just proximal to metacarpophalangeal joints on flexor surface of hand
Elbow flexors Supine	As wrist flexors	Arm	Just proximal to wrist joint on radial surface of forearm
Elbow extensors Supine	As wrist flexors	Arm	Just proximal to wrist joint on ulnar surface of forearm
Shoulder internal rotators Supine	As wrist flexors	Arm	Just proximal to wrist joint on flexor surface of forearm
Shoulder external rotators Supine	As wrist flexors	Arm	Just proximal to wrist joint on extensor surface of forearm
Shoulder extensors Supine	Shoulder flexed 90°, shoulder in neutral horizontal adduction	Shoulder	Just proximal to elbow on extensor surface of arm
Shoulder flexors Supine	As shoulder extensors	Shoulder	Just proximal to elbow on flexor surface of arm
Shoulder adductors Supine	Elbow extended, shoulder abducted 45°	Trunk	Just proximal to elbow on medial surface of arm
Shoulder abductors Supine	As shoulder adductors	Trunk	Just proximal to elbow on lateral surface of arm
Ankle plantar flexors Supine	Hip and knee extended	Lower limb proximal ankle	Just proximal to metatarsophalangeal joints on plantar surface of foot
Ankle dorsiflexors Supine	As ankle plantar flexors	As ankle plantar flexors	Just proximal to metatarsophalangeal joints on dorsal surface of foot
Knee flexors Sitting	Knee and hip flexed to 90°	Thigh	Just proximal to ankle on posterior surface of leg
Knee extensors Sitting	Knee and hip flexed to 90°	Thigh	Just proximal to ankle on anterior surface of leg
Hip flexors Supine	Hip flexed to 90°, knee relaxed	Trunk	Just proximal to knee on extensor surface of thigh
Hip extensors Supine	As hip flexors	Trunk	Just proximal to knee on flexor surface of thigh
Hip abductors Supine	Knee extended, hip in neutral abduction	Contralateral lower extremity	Just proximal to knee on lateral surface of thigh
Hip adductors Supine	Knee extended, hip in neutral abduction	Contralateral lower extremity	Just proximal to knee on medial surface of thigh

Adapted from Bohannon, R. (1986). Test-retest reliability of hand-held dynamometry during a single session of strength assessment. *Physical Therapy, 66*(2), 206-209.

the time of day, particularly for patients who are fatigued by the end of the day and with the level of the child's enthusiasm; with the testing environment; and with the testing clinician's rapport with the child. Some children as young as 2 years old with typical development have produced consistent force with a handheld dynamometer,[72] and 6-year-olds have produced consistent force on isokinetic machines.[10,133] As with goniometry, standardized testing procedures are necessary for optimal reliability of strength measurements.

Standardized testing positions are listed in Table 5-3. Taking the average of two measurements rather than a maximum value also improves reliability.[210]

Several authors have reported good consistency when testing the strength of children with DMD using manual muscle testing,[63] isokinetic dynamometers,[186] a handheld dynamometer,[193] and an electronic strain gauge.[29] When strength was measured with a handheld dynamometer, children with meningomyelocele (9–17 years)[58] or with Down syndrome (7–15 years)[131] yielded highly reliable results. The reliability of the measurement of strength in children with CP can be more variable than in some other patient populations, but it is still a useful clinical tool. Van der Berg-Emons and associates[211] examined the intraday reliability of isokinetic muscle strength in 12 children with spastic CP and 39 children with typical development between the ages of 6 and 12 years. Using an isokinetic device, they measured quadriceps and hamstring muscle strength at three different speeds. Measures from the children with CP had lower levels of reliability than those from the comparison group, and as the speed increased, the reliability decreased. The authors concluded that at 30°/s, children with CP could produce consistent results, but at higher speeds, the measurements were not repeatable. In contrast, Ayalon and associates[9] reported excellent interday reliability when knee isokinetic strength was measured in 12 children with spastic CP. Several differences may be noted between the two studies. In the study by Ayalon and associates, strength was measured at a velocity of 90°/s, and data from twice as many trials were used to find an average strength value. In addition, 50% of the children had hemiplegic CP, but in the study by van der Berg-Emons and associates,[211] the children had a diplegic or a quadriplegic distribution. Recent studies using isometric testing with a handheld dynamometer have shown good reliability. Further study of the reliability of strength testing in children with CP is needed, especially with the variety of methods of measuring strength that are available to the pediatric therapist today.

In addition to the possibility of objectively measuring the voluntary force produced in spastic muscles, a combination of technologies may now permit objective assessments of the degree of underlying hypertonicity. Isokinetic passive movements at different velocities, combined with the recording of EMG activity of agonist and antagonist muscles, could permit quantification of hypertonicity because muscles with spasticity present a markedly increased velocity-dependent neuromuscular response to passive lengthening.[50,160] Rapid passive lengthening of spastic calf muscles through dorsiflexion ROM can yield an increase in the amount of passive resistance and EMG activity. For example, Boiteau and colleagues[22] passively stretched the calf muscles of 10 children with spastic CP at 10°/s and at 190°/s. They measured resistance to the stretch at 10° of dorsiflexion and attributed the passive force at 10°/s stretch to nonreflex components. The force at the 190°/s stretch was much greater because it included reflex muscle activation from the spasticity (documented with EMG). The study demonstrated that the reflex and nonreflex components of spastic hypertonia can be measured reliably. If change in the passive resistive force caused by the reflex and nonreflex components of spasticity can be assessed independently, the effects of specific therapeutic interventions that target each component can be determined and related to changes in activity and participation. These possibilities are particularly worthy of future study, and clinicians are encouraged to participate in research projects to help examine these possibilities.

EFFECTS OF INTERVENTION ON THE MUSCULOSKELETAL SYSTEM

Objective evidence of the effects of strengthening exercises for particular pediatric conditions is limited, but increasing. The recommendation of exercise in children with DMD and other degenerative muscle disorders has changed over the past 5 years. Early reports suggested that submaximal exercise has no negative effect[52,174] and may be of limited value in increasing strength in DMD.[52] Current research on animals, however, has documented an increased susceptibility to deformational exercise-induced stress to the muscle.[53] Eccentric contractions appear to have the most damaging effect on muscle.[50] These findings suggest that normal activities of daily living and social recreational programs provide sufficient exercise for children with degenerative muscular disease, and additional exercise programs are unnecessary and potentially harmful.

Several studies with children and adults with CP have shown that after participation in a resistive exercise program, values of their gait parameters improved[5,18,48,49,144] and scores on the Gross Motor Function Measure increased.[5,48,54,122,127] In a study by O'Connell and Barnhart,[151] three children with CP and three with meningomyelocele participated in a progressive circuit muscular strength training program. After 8 weeks, these children propelled their wheelchairs significantly farther during a 12-minute test period when compared with pretraining test results. Their speed, however, did not increase during a 50-meter wheelchair dash.

For individuals with CP, resistive strength training regimens have not been shown to adversely affect the level of spasticity,[5,151] and a positive outcome has been noted by adults with CP who perceived a decrease in lower extremity spasticity lasting for several hours after training.[5] Concerns that children with CP would co-contract the antagonist during resistive strength training regimens have been allayed by recent literature that has shown neither an increase in strength nor a decrease in ROM of the antagonist to the muscle being strengthened in individuals with CP.[5,48,49,93] Strength training should be an integral part of an intervention program for children with strength deficits, and we encourage clinicians to continue to document the relationship of strength changes to changes in the activity and participation levels of children.

Passive and active slow static stretching exercises are used routinely to address abnormally short MTUs. Despite the widespread use of stretching with children with CP, little is known about its efficacy. This is due in part to conflicting muscle histology literature. A review of published literature reported that evidence is insufficient to support manual stretching for lengthening muscles, reducing spasticity, or improving gait.[159]

Prolonged passive stretching (6 hours or longer) of MTUs in a state of severe contracture from long-term hypertonicity and shortening may promote lengthening adaptations and increased ROM in children with CP.[130] Serial casting and night splints employ the principles of lengthening and shortening adaptations within the MTU. As discussed earlier in this chapter, investigators have demonstrated that when hypoextensible, abnormally short muscles of children with CP were serially casted in lengthened positions, increased length and stiffness adaptations were enhanced.[201,202,203] In other words, the muscles were longer and more compliant. The researchers indicated that the adaptations resulted directly from changes in the MTU, but changes in the neurologic excitability of the muscles were not examined.

This proposal was also supported by the finding that splinting spastic muscles of patients with brain damage changed ROM without altering the integrated EMG activity of the muscles when compared with activity in muscles that were not splinted.[136] Another study examined the effects of 3 weeks of dorsiflexion serial casting on the reflex characteristics of spastic calf muscles of seven children with CP.[27] The authors reported that casting brought about increased dorsiflexion ROM, and that the angle of reflex excitability elicited by a rapid dorsiflexion stretch also was shifted toward increased dorsiflexion. The soleus and tibialis anterior co-activation EMG tracings, however, did not change as a result of the casting. More recently, Brouwer and co-workers[26] reported that 3 to 6 weeks of dorsiflexion serial casting for children with CP brought about decreased reflex excitability of the calf muscles when they were stretched rapidly. A study by Kay[104] revealed that the concurrent addition of Botox to a serial casting regimen led to earlier recurrence of spasticity, contracture, and equinus in gait by 6 months. An explanation of the results was that we as therapists need to strengthen the opposite muscle group to allow for balance. When Botox is combined with serial casting, strengthening cannot occur. A major problem in interpreting clinical reports of the effects of inhibitory casting is the confusing and variable definition of "tone." Is tone caused by central or peripheral influences, or by both? Knowledge of the interrelationships among length, tension, and stiffness of the MTU and of the neurologic excitability of the muscles of children with neurologic impairment and how these interrelationships are influenced by therapeutic interventions remains sparse.

Application of passive isokinetic movements combined with recording of EMG, as described earlier in this chapter, could be used to examine the effects of these interventions on spastic muscles. In the meantime, clinicians should maintain objective records of strength and ROM and should attempt to correlate these findings with specific therapeutic interventions and activity and participation outcomes.

The shape and size of the skeletal system are most susceptible to alteration during periods of rapid growth; hence undesirable forces, as well as appropriate corrective forces, are most influential during childhood. Many deformities that occur during the fetal or early postnatal period are more easily corrected in the infant than in the older child. For example, congenitally dislocated hips often readily respond to treatment with a Pavlik harness during the first year of life.[36,233,234] If, however, the dislocated hip is not diagnosed until after 12 months, surgery is often necessary. Serial casting for wrist deformities in children with distal arthrogryposis was very effective when applied during infancy.[184] When using serial casting for a knee flexion contracture, Westberry et al.[224] reported that younger children with CP had a better response than teenagers. Bracing for idiopathic scoliosis is most effective for preventing worsening of the curve during the preteen and teenage years.[8] After an individual has stopped growing, external support is no longer needed.

Orthotics for typically developing children with asymptomatic flexible flat feet are controversial. The medical literature supports that most young children with flat feet will naturally improve over time.[85] It is estimated that only 5% to 15% percent of leg abnormalities persist beyond skeletal maturity, which typically occurs in the teenage years.[17] If flexible flat feet in a typically developing child are producing pain or gait abnormalities it may be due to heelcord tightness.[85] The presence of risk factors, including ligamentous laxity, obesity, rotational deformities, tibial influence, pathologic tibia varum, equinus, presence of an os tibiale externum, and tarsal coalition, would require further foot evaluation. Prior to recommending long-term orthotics for flat feet, it is important to remember that cartilage needs movement to survive and repair itself, and joints that are stabilized too long frequently become rigid.

This leads to the question of what to do with asymptomatic flexible flat feet in children with hypotonia. Martin[125] studied 14 children with Down syndrome between the ages of $3\frac{1}{2}$ years and 8 years. Significant improvements on the Gross Motor Function Measure and the Bruinicks-Oseretsky Test of Motor Proficiency that could not be attributed solely to maturation were seen with supramalleolar orthoses. In 2001, Selby-Silverstein, Hillstrom, and Palisano used a gait analysis laboratory to study 16 children with Down syndrome and a control group of 10 children without disabilities, all ranging between 3 and 6 years of age.[176] Submalleolar (below ankle) bracing provided the children with Down syndrome a more neutral foot alignment, decreased toe-out position during walking, and a more controlled walking pattern. Speed, however, did not change.

In general, the decision to brace in the pediatric population is supported in five main areas of documented value: (1) prevention of deformity, (2) correction of deformity, (3) promotion of a stable base of support, (4) facilitating the development of skills, and (5) improving the efficiency of gait. Orthoses, however, can lead to the development of secondary deformities and disuse atrophy. Lusskin[121] reported two case studies of children with lower extremity paralysis resulting from poliomyelitis. Both children had marked tibial-fibular torsion and were braced in knee-ankle-foot orthoses with the knees and feet facing forward. As a result, a rotational force was placed at the ankle and foot, and these children developed severe metatarsus adductus and heel varus. Children who wear total contact ankle-foot orthoses for most of their growing years may be at risk for stunted growth of the foot and lower limb. Circumferential compressive forces and restriction in active movement can interfere with normal musculoskeletal growth. Pediatric physical therapists have an important responsibility to understand, document, and frequently reevaluate the effects of external devices on the growing child. While trying to solve one problem, intervention may inadvertently create another.

Movement has been reported to affect the formation and shape of joints in fetal animals.[55,147] Movement allows compressive forces to be spread throughout the joint surface rather than stay confined to a small area. Combining weight-bearing activities with movement would create more desirable forces for joint formation. Although no research has been reported on the effects on hip formation of stationary standing devices, such as prone boards or standing platforms, it appears reasonable to use caution when using these devices with very young children. Because remodeling of the bone and associated joints takes place most readily during the first few years of life, and because the acetabular shape is fairly well defined by the age of 3 years,[161] early intervention with weight-bearing activities may have a substantial influence on the shape and function of the joint. To help shape the joint, chronologic age and not developmental age may be more important when determining when to begin weight-bearing activities. Careful evaluation of the child's postural alignment when in equipment should be paramount.

For the young child with severe delays in motor development, in whom independent walking (with or without devices) is unlikely and hip dislocation is a risk, early and prolonged standing may be beneficial in developing a deeper hip joint. The shape of the acetabulum may not be appropriate for walking, but the hip may be more stable. Over time, this early standing may help prevent or decrease the severity of a dislocated hip. For children with milder delays, less stationary standing time and more weight bearing with movement may help to develop a more normally shaped hip socket. This may contribute to improved gait and a decreased risk of osteoarthritis in adulthood.

Treadmill training has become increasingly popular as an intervention for providing movement and weight-bearing opportunities for children with Down syndrome, spinal cord injury, and CP. Accelerated acquisition of walking was demonstrated in children with Down syndrome when a parent supported his infant on a treadmill for 8 minutes 5 days per week.[208,209] In a randomized, controlled study, 30 children received regular physical therapy, but half of them also received the in-home treadmill training program. The experimental group demonstrated the ability to pull to stand 60 days earlier than the control group, walked with help 73 days earlier than the control group, and walked independently 101 days earlier than the control group. Despite the documented efficacy of treadmill training in children with Down syndrome, the functional benefit of walking at 20 months versus 24 months is sometimes debated.

Because of the paucity of large, well-designed clinical trials to date, however, published evidence to support the efficacy of treadmill training for children with CP is inconclusive. This inconsistency might be due to the design of the intervention. Treatment intensity, frequency, and duration are critical to the success of a treadmill program. Traditional exercise training guidelines are quite explicit in the suggestion that, for fitness to improve, training must occur at a minimum of three times a week and must be sustained for 8 weeks or longer. Several small studies have reported improvements in gait, strength, and function.[38,42,148] Treadmill training can occur in a partial-weight-bearing (PWB) environment in which a therapist uses equipment that includes a harness, overhead support, and a motorized treadmill stimulus. The purpose of the PWB environment is to control body weight, posture, and balance while allowing the child the opportunity for prolonged periods of walking. This allows for strengthening and endurance improvements. Richards et al.[152] performed a feasibility study, "Early and intensive treadmill locomotor training for young children with CP." In this multiple case study design lasting for 17 weeks, 4 children with no independent ambulation at ages ranging from 1.7 to 2.3 years used the PWB system 4×/week. The children spent 20% to 30% of the time on the treadmill during a 45-minute treatment session. Support ranged from 40%, 20%, and 0% of body weight with speed ranging from 0.07 m/s to 0.70 m/s. As support decreased throughout the study, the treadmill speed was increased. At the conclusion of the training, two of the children walked independently, and the third with an assistive device. Despite the articles suggesting the potential benefits of PWB therapy for CP, more research is needed to determine the best protocols for frequency, duration, and patient selection.

Physical therapists sometimes use the application of neuromuscular electrical stimulation (NMES) as an intervention for the musculoskeletal system to provide sensory input and promote motor activity.[38] NMES is the application of current to innervated superficial muscles to stimulate sensory fibers, create muscle contractions, increase ROM, and increase sensory awareness. Evidence is insufficient to confidently conclude the efficacy of NMES because of the lack of high-quality studies,[3] but some evidence suggests that it may be a useful adjunct to strengthening in children who cannot tolerate an independent muscle strengthening program.[108]

Intramuscular injections of botulinum toxin A are used to reduce spastic muscle tone. The American Academy for

Cerebral Palsy and Developmental Medicine (AACPDM) performed a systematic review of the effect of Botox therapy (2006). The AACPDM concluded that the evidence for reduced spasticity was inconsistent. One large study found no change, and several smaller studies reported decreases in spasticity. No evidence was available to support that Botox enhances the results of serial casting. Low-level evidence suggests that strengthening and functional carryover may be enhanced in the upper extremity when therapy is combined with Botox. It was also suggested that ease of care was improved following Botox use in individuals with very high levels of spasticity.

Orthopedic surgery is not an option for managing spasticity. Instead, it is used to correct the secondary problems that occur with growth in the face of spastic muscles and poor motor control such as muscle contractures and bony deformities. Possible surgical procedures include muscle lengthening, transfer tenotomies, neurectomies, osteotomies, and fusions, which are beyond the scope of this chapter. The reader is referred to Lovell and Winters' *Pediatric Orthopedics*[143] or *Fundamentals of Pediatric Orthopedics*.[188]

SUMMARY

This chapter reviewed the normal growth and development of the musculoskeletal system, with emphasis on the adaptations of muscle and bone associated with pathologic conditions encountered by pediatric physical therapists. The microscopic and macroscopic structure and function of the normal MTU and the force and length adaptations to imposed physical changes, such as immobilization and denervation, have been well documented in nonhuman studies using invasive methods of investigation. The results of human studies using noninvasive methods of investigation indicate that the human MTU undergoes adaptations similar to those reported for animals. Clinical evidence for the musculoskeletal adaptations supports these research findings.

In the developing child, atypical changes in the MTU can exert forces on the skeletal system, resulting in bony deformities. Pediatric physical therapists routinely measure physical impairments and develop therapeutic interventions designed to promote musculoskeletal adaptations. To document therapeutic efficacy in relation to specific pediatric disorders, therapists are encouraged to use objective measures of ROM and strength during specific interventions for correlating changes in musculoskeletal impairment with levels of activity and participation. Additional research is needed to examine the efficacy of therapeutic strengthening and stretching programs and their interrelation with other approaches, such as surgical procedures, casting, and pharmacologic interventions. The application of new research technologies, such as isokinetic dynamometry and EMG, now permits objective measurement of the impairments associated with neuromuscular disorders and the effects of interventions designed to influence these disorders. Additional controlled studies will enhance the scientific basis for using physical therapy to promote participation in life activities.

REFERENCES

1. Abel, M. F., Wenger, D. R., Mubarak, S. J., & Sutherland, D. H. (1994). Quantitative analysis of hip dysplasia in cerebral palsy: A study of radiographs and 3-D reformatted images. *Journal of Pediatric Orthopedics, 14*, 283–289.
2. Ali, O., Shim, M., Fowler, E., Greenberg, M., Perkins, D., Oppenheim, W., et al. (2007). Growth hormone therapy improves bone mineral density in children with cerebral palsy: A preliminary pilot study. *The Journal of Clinical Endocrinology and Metabolism, 92*, 932–937.
3. Alon, G. (2006). Electrical stimulation in cerebral palsy: Are we asking clinically relevant questions? *Developmental Medicine and Child Neurology, 48*, 868.
4. Anandacoomarasamy, A., Fransen, M., March, L. (2009). Obesity and the musculoskeletal system. *Current Opinion in Rheumatology, 21*, 71–77.
5. Andersson, C., Grooten, W., Hellsten, M., Kaping, K., & Mattsson, E. (2003). Adults with cerebral palsy: Walking ability after progressive strength training. *Developmental Medicine and Child Neurology, 45*, 220–228.
6. Argov, Z., Gardner-Medwin, D., Johnson, M. A., & Mastaglia, F. L. (1984). Patterns of muscle fiber-type disproportion in hypotonic infants. *Archives of Neurology, 41*, 53–57.
7. Arkader, A., Sankar, W. N., Amorim, R. M. (2009) Conservative versus surgical treatment of late-onset Legg-Calve-Perthes disease: a radiographic comparison at skeletal maturity. *Journal of Childrens Orthopedics, 3*, 21–25.
8. Arlet, V., & Reddi, V. (2007). Adolescent idiopathic scoliosis. *Neurosurgery Clinics of North America, 18*, 255–259.
9. Ayalon, M., Ben-Sira, D., & Hutzler, Y. (2000). Reliability of isokinetic strength measurements of the knee in children with cerebral palsy. *Developmental Medicine and Child Neurology, 42*, 396–402.
10. Backman, E., & Oberg, B. (1989). Isokinetic muscle torque in the dorsiflexors of the ankle of children 6–12 years of age. *Scandinavian Journal of Rehabilitation Medicine, 21*, 97–103.
11. Bailey, D. A., Wedge, J. H., McCulloch, R. G., Martin, A. D., & Bernhardson, S. C. (1989). Epidemiology of fractures of the distal end of the radius in children as associated with growth. *Journal of Bone and Joint Surgery (American), 71*, 1225–1230.
12. Barnes, C., Wong, P., Egan, B., Speller, T., Cameron, F., Jones, G., et al. (2004). Reduced bone density among children with severe hemophilia. *Pediatrics, 114*, e177–e181.
13. Bartlett, M. D., Wolf, L. S., Shurtleff, D. B., & Staheli, L. T. (1985). Hip flexion contractures: A comparison of measurement procedures. *Archives of Physical Medicine and Rehabilitation, 66*, 620–625.
14. Beals, R. K. (1969). Developmental changes in the femur and acetabulum in spastic paraplegia and diplegia. *Developmental Medicine and Child Neurology, 11*, 303–313.
15. Bernhardt, D. B. (1988). Prenatal and postnatal growth and development of the foot and ankle. *Physical Therapy, 68*, 1831–1839.

16. Bevan, W. P., Hall, J. G., Bamshad, M., Staheli, L. T., Jaffe, K. M., & Song, K. (2007). Arthrogryposis multiplex congenita (amyoplasia): An orthopaedic perspective. *Journal of Pediatric Orthopedics, 27,* 594–600.

17. Bleck, E. E. (1987). *Orthopedic management in cerebral palsy.* Philadelphia: JB Lippincott.

18. Blundell, S. W., Shepherd, R. B., Dean, C. M., Adams, R. D., & Cahill, B. M. (2003). Functional strength training in cerebral palsy: A pilot study of a group circuit training class for children aged 4–8 years. *Clinical Rehabilitation, 17,* 48–57.

19. Bohannon, R. (1986). Test-retest reliability of hand-held dynamometry during a single session of strength assessment. *Physical Therapy, 66,* 206–209.

20. Bohannon, R. W. (1995). Measurement, nature, and implications of skeletal muscle strength in patients with neurological disorders. *Clinical Biomechanics, 10,* 283–292.

21. Bohannon, R. W., & Andrews, A. W. (1987). Inter-rater reliability of hand-held dynamometer. *Physical Therapy, 67,* 931–933.

22. Boiteau, M., Malouin, F., & Richards, C. L. (1995). Use of a hand-held dynamometer and the Kin-Com dynamometer for evaluating spastic hypertonia in children: A reliability study. *Physical Therapy, 75,* 796–802.

23. Booth, C. M., Cortina-Borja, M. J. F., Theologis, T. N. (2001). Collagen accumulation in muscles of children with cerebral palsy and correlation with severity of spasticity. *Developmental Medicine and Child Neurology, 43,* 314–320.

24. Botelho, S. Y., Cander, L., & Guiti, N. (1954). Passive and active tension-length diagrams of intact skeletal muscle in normal women of different ages. *Journal of Applied Physiology, 7,* 93–95.

25. Brooke, M. H., & Engel, W. K. (1969). The histographic analyses of human muscle biopsies with regard to fiber types: 4. Children's biopsies. *Neurology, 19,* 591–605.

26. Brouwer, B., Davidson, L. K., & Olney, S. J. (2000). Serial casting in idiopathic toe-walkers and children with spastic cerebral palsy. *Journal of Pediatric Orthopaedics, 20,* 221–225.

27. Brouwer, B., Wheeldon, R. K., & Stradiotto-Parker, N. (1998). Reflex excitability and isometric force production in cerebral palsy: The effect of serial casting. *Developmental Medicine and Child Neurology, 40,* 168–175.

28. Brown, M. C., Jansen, J. K. S., & Van Essen, D. (1976). Polyneuronal innervation of skeletal muscle in newborn rats and its elimination during maturation. *Journal of Physiology, 261,* 387–422.

29. Brussock, C. M., Haley, S. H., Munsat, T. L., & Bernhardt, D. B. (1992). Measurement of isometric force in children with and without Duchenne's muscular dystrophy. *Physical Therapy, 72,* 105–114.

30. Buckley, S. L., Sponseller, P. D., & Maged, D. (1991). The acetabulum in congenital and neuromuscular hip instability. *Journal of Pediatric Orthopedics, 11,* 498–501.

31. Bunch, W. (1977). Origin and mechanism of postnatal deformities. *Pediatric Clinics of North America, 24,* 679–684.

32. Cahuzac, J., Vardon, D., & Sales de Gauzy, J. (1995). Development of the clinical tibiofemoral angle in normal adolescents. *Journal of Bone and Joint Surgery (British), 77,* 729–732.

33. Campbell, S. K. (1997). Therapy programs for children that last a lifetime. *Physical and Occupational Therapy in Pediatrics, 17*(1), 1–15.

34. Canavese, F., & Dimeglio, A. (2008). Perthes' disease: Prognosis in children under six years of age. *The Journal of Bone and Joint Surgery (British) 90,* 940–945.

35. Carter, D. R., Orr, T. E., Fyhrie, D. P., & Schurman, D. J. (1987). Influences of mechanical stress on prenatal and postnatal skeletal development. *Clinical Orthopedics and Related Research, 219,* 237–250.

36. Cashman, J., Round, J., Taylor, G., & Clarke, N. (2002). The natural history of developmental dysplasia of the hip after early supervised treatment in the Pavlik harness. A prospective, longitudinal follow-up. *The Journal Of Bone And Joint Surgery. British Volume, 84,* 418–425.

37. Castle, M. E., Reyman, T. A., & Schneider, M. (1979). Pathology of spastic muscle in cerebral palsy. *Clinical Orthopedics, 142,* 223–232.

38. Cernak, K., Stevens, V., Price, R., & Shumway-Cook, A. (2008). Locomotor training using body-weight support on a treadmill in conjunction with ongoing physical therapy in a child with severe cerebellar ataxia. *Physical Therapy, 88,* 88–97.

39. Chan, G., & Chen, C. T. (2009). Musculoskeletal effects of obesity. *Current Opinion in Pediatrics, 21,* 65–70.

40. Chandraraj, S., & Briggs, C. A. (1991). Multiple growth cartilages in the neural arch. *Anatomical Record, 230,* 114–120.

41. Cheng, J. C. Y., Chan, P. S., Chiang, S. C., & Hui, P. W. (1991). Angular and rotational profile of the lower limb in 2,630 Chinese children. *Journal of Pediatric Orthopedics, 11,* 154–161.

42. Cherng, R., Liu, C., Lau, T., & Hong, R. (2007). Effect of treadmill training with body weight support on gait and gross motor function in children with spastic cerebral palsy. *American Journal of Physical Medicine & Rehabilitation/Association of Academic Physiatrists, 86,* 548–555.

43. Chung, S. M. K., Batterman, S. C., & Brighton C. T. (1976). Shear strength of the human femoral capital epiphyseal plate. *Journal of Bone and Joint Surgery (American), 58,* 94–105.

44. Cleve, S. N., & Cohen, W. I. (2006). Practice guidelines. Part 1: Clinical practice guidelines for children with down syndrome from birth to 12 years. *Journal of Pediatric Healthcare, 20,* 47–54.

45. Cleve, S. N., Cannon, S., & Cohen, W. I. (2006). Part II: Clinical practice guidelines for adolescents and young adults with Down syndrome: 12 to 21 years. *Journal of Pediatric Healthcare, 20,* 198–205.

46. Coleman, S. S. (1968). Congenital dysplasia of the hip in the Navajo infant. *Clinical Orthopedics and Related Research, 56,* 179–193.

47. Costanzo, E., Barry, J., & Ribchester, R. (2000). Competition at silent synapses in reinnervated skeletal muscle. *Nature Neuroscience, 3*(7), 694–700

48. Damiano, D. L., & Abel, M. F. (1998). Functional outcomes of strength training in spastic cerebral palsy. *Archives of Physical Medicine and Rehabilitation, 79*, 119–125.

49. Damiano, D. L., Kelly, L. E., & Vaughn, C. L. (1995). Effects of quadriceps femoris muscle strengthening on crouch gait in children with spastic diplegia. *Physical Therapy, 75*, 658–667.

50. Damiano, D. L., Quinlivan, B. F., Owen, B. F., Shaffrey, M., & Abel, M. F. (2001). Spasticity versus strength in cerebral palsy: Relationships among involuntary resistance, voluntary torque, and motor function. *European Journal of Neurology, 8*(Suppl. 5), 40–49.

51. Damron, T., Breed, A. L., & Roecker, E. (1991). Hamstring tenotomies in cerebral palsy: Long-term retrospective analysis. *Journal of Pediatric Orthopedics, 11*, 514–519.

52. de Lateur, B. J., & Giaconi, R. M. (1979). Effect on maximal strength of submaximal exercise in Duchenne muscular dystrophy. *American Journal of Physical Medicine, 58*, 26–36.

53. Deconinck, N., & Dan, B. (2007). Pathophysiology of Duchenne muscular dystrophy: Current hypotheses. *Pediatric Neurology, 36*, 1–7.

54. Dodd, J. K., Taylor, N. F., & Graham, H. K. (2003). A randomized clinical trial of strength training in young people with cerebral palsy. *Developmental Medicine and Child Neurology, 45*, 652–657.

55. Drachman, D. B., & Sokoloff, L. (1966). The role of movement in embryonic joint development. *Developmental Biology, 14*, 401–420.

56. Drews, J. E., Vraciu, J. K., & Pellino, G. (1984). Range of motion of the joints of the lower extremities of newborns. *Physical and Occupational Therapy in Pediatrics, 4*, 49–62.

57. Edmonson, A. D., & Crenshaw, A. H. (Eds.). (1980). Campbell's operative orthopaedics (vol. 2). St Louis: Mosby.

58. Effgen, S. K., & Brown, D. A. (1992). Long-term stability of hand-held dynamometric measurements in children who have myelomeningocele. *Physical Therapy, 72*, 458–465.

59. Fabeck, L., Tolley, M., Rooze, M., & Burny, F. (2002). Theoretical study of the decrease in the femoral neck anteversion during growth. *Cells Tissues Organs, 171*, 269–275.

60. Reference deleted in page proofs.

61. Farkas-Bargeton, E., Barbet, J. P., Dancea, S., Wehrle, R., Checouri, A., & Dulac, O. (1988). Immaturity of muscle fibers in the congenital form of myotonic dystrophy: Its consequences and its origin. *Journal of the Neurological Sciences, 83*, 145–159.

62. Favero, M., Massella, O., Cangiano, A., & Buffelli, M. (2009). On the mechanism of action of muscle fibre activity in synapse competition and elimination at the mammalian neuromuscular junction. *European Journal of Neuroscience, 29*, 2327–2334.

63. Florence, J. M., Pandya, S., King, W. M., Robison, J. D., Signore, L. C., Wentzell, M., & Province, M. A. (1984). Clinical trials in Duchenne dystrophy: Standardization and reliability of evaluation procedures. *Physical Therapy, 64*, 41–45.

64. Foran, J. R., Steinman, S., Barash, I., Chambers, H. G., & Lieber, R. L. (2005). Structural and mechanical alterations in spastic skeletal muscle. *Developmental Medicine and Child Neurology, 47*, 713–717.

65. Reference deleted in page proofs.

66. Friden, J., & Lieber, R. L. (2003). Spastic muscle cells are shorter and stiffer than normal cells. *Muscle and Nerve, 26*, 157–164.

67. Frost, H. M. (2004). A 2003 update of bone physiology and Wolff's Law for clinicians. *Angle Orthodontist, 74*, 3–15.

68. Fuchs, R. K., & Snow, C. M. (2002). Gains in hip bone mass from high-impact training are maintained: A randomized controlled trial in children. *Journal of Pediatrics, 141*, 357–362.

69. Fukuda, N., Granzier, H. L., Ishiwata, S., & Kurihara, S. (2008). Physiological functions of the giant elastic protein titin in mammalian striated muscle. *The Journal of Physiological Sciences: JPS, 58*, 151–159.

70. Fulford, G., & Brown, J. (1977). Position as a cause of deformity in children with cerebral palsy. *Developmental Medicine and Child Neurology, 18*, 305–314.

71. Gajdosik, C. G., & Cicirello, N. (2001). Secondary conditions of the musculoskeletal system in adolescents and adults with cerebral palsy. *Physical and Occupational Therapy in Pediatrics, 21*, 49–68.

72. Gajdosik C. G. (2005) Ability of very young children to produce reliable isometric force measurements. *Pediatric Physical Therapy, 17*251–17257.

73. Gajdosik, R. L., & Bohannon, R. W. (1987). Clinical measurement of range of motion: Review of goniometry emphasizing reliability and validity. *Physical Therapy, 67*, 1867–1872.

74. Gajdosik, R. L. (1991). Effects of static stretching on the maximal length and resistance to passive stretch of short hamstring muscles. *Journal of Orthopedic Sports and Physical Therapy, 14*, 250–255.

75. Gajdosik, R. L. (1991). Passive compliance and length of clinically short hamstring muscles of healthy men. *Clinical Biomechanics, 6*, 239–244.

76. Goldspink, D. F. (1977). The influence of immobilization and stretch on protein turnover of rat skeletal muscle. *Journal of Physiology, 64*, 267–282.

77. Gordon, A. M., Huxley, A. F., & Julian, F. J. (1966). The variation in isometric tension with sarcomere length in vertebrate muscle fibers. *Journal of Physiology, 184*, 170–192.

78. Goulding, A., Jones, I. E., Taylor, R. W., Manning, P. J., & Williams, S. M. (2000). More broken bones: A 4-year double cohort study of young girls with and without distal forearm fractures. *Journal of Bone and Mineral Research, 15*, 2011–2018.

79. Goulding, A., Taylor, R. W., Jones, I. E., McAuley, K. A., Manning, P. J., & Williams, S. M. (2000). Overweight and obese children have low bone mass and area for their weight. *International Journal of Obesity, 24*, 627–632.

80. Grimston, S., Willows, N., & Hanley, D. (1993). Mechanical loading regime and its relationship to bone mineral density in children. *Medicine And Science In Sports And Exercise*, *25*(11), 1203–1210.

81. Grinnell, A. D. (1995). Dynamics of nerve-muscle interaction in developing and mature neuromuscular junctions. *Physiological Reviews*, *75*, 789–834.

82. Gudjonsdottir, B., & Mercer, V. S. (1997). Hip and spine in children with cerebral palsy: Musculoskeletal development and clinical implications. *Pediatric Physical Therapy*, *9*, 179–185.

83. Haley, S. M., Tada, W. L., & Carmichael, E. M. (1986). Spinal mobility in young children: A normative study. *Physical Therapy*, *66*, 1697–1703.

84. Harpavat, M., Greenspan, S. L., O'Brien, C., Chang, C., Bowen, A., & Keljo, D. J. (2005). Altered bone mass in children at diagnosis of Crohn disease: A pilot study. *Journal of Pediatric Gastroenterology and Nutrition*, *40*, 295–300.

85. Harris, E. J. (2000). The oblique talus deformity. what is it, and what is its clinical significance in the scheme of pronatory deformities? *Clinics in Podiatric Medicine and Surgery*, *17*, 419–442.

86. Harris, S. R., Smith, L. H., & Krukowski, L. (1985). Goniometric reliability for a child with spastic quadriplegia. *Journal of Pediatric Orthopedics*, *5*, 348–351.

87. Heath, C. H., & Staheli, L. T. (1993). Normal limits of knee angle in white children—Genu varum and genu valgum. *Journal of Pediatric Orthopedics*, *13*, 259–262.

88. Heinrich, S. D., MacEwen, G. D., & Zembo, M. M. (1991). Hip dysplasia, subluxation, and dislocation in cerebral palsy: An arthrographic analysis. *Journal of Pediatric Orthopedics*, *11*, 488–493.

89. Henderson, R. C., Kairalla, J., Abbas, A., & Stevenson, R. D. (2004). Predicting low bone density in children and young adults with quadriplegic cerebral palsy. *Developmental Medicine and Child Neurology*, *46*, 416–419.

90. Hesselmans, L. F. G. M., Jennekens, F. G. I., Van Den Oord, C. J. M., Veldman, H., & Vincent, A. (1993). Development of innervation of skeletal muscle fibers in man: Relation to acetylcholine receptors. *Anatomical Record*, *236*, 553–562.

91. Hind, K., & Burrows, M. (2007). Weight-bearing exercise and bone mineral accrual in children and adolescents: A review of controlled trials. *Bone*, *40*, 14–27.

92. Hollway, G., & Currie, P. (2005). Vertebrate myotome development. Birth defects research. Part C. *Embryo Today: Reviews*, *75*, 172–179.

93. Hovart, M. (1987). Effects of a progressive resistance training program on an individual with spastic cerebral palsy. *American Corrective Therapy Journal*, *41*, 7–11.

94. Huet de la Tour, E., Tabary, J. C., Tabary, C., & Tardieu, C. (1979). The respective roles of muscle length and muscle tension in sarcomere number adaptation of guinea-pig soleus muscle. *Journal de Physiologie*, *75*, 589–592.

95. Huet de la Tour, E., Tardieu, C., Tabary, J. C., & Tabary, C. (1979). Decreased muscle extensibility and reduction of sarcomere number in soleus muscle following local injection of tetanus toxin. *Journal of the Neurological Sciences*, *40*, 123– 131.

96. Hung, V. W. Y., Qin, L., Cheung, C. S. K., Lam, T. P., Ng, B. K. W., Tse, Y. K., et al. (2005). Osteopenia: A new prognostic factor of curve progression in adolescent idiopathic scoliosis. *Journal of Bone and Joint Surgery (American)*, *87*, 2709– 2716.

97. Huxley, A. F., & Peachey, L. D. (1961). The maximum length for contraction in vertebrate striated muscle. *Journal of Physiology*, *156*,150–165.

98. Ihkkan, K. Y., & Yalcin, E. (2001). Changes in skeletal maturation and mineralization in children with cerebral palsy and evaluation of related factors. *Journal of Child Neurology*, *16*, 425–430.

99. Imoto, C., & Nonaka, I. (2001). The significance of type 1 fiber atrophy (hypotrophy) in childhood neuromuscular disorders. *Brain and Development*, *23*, 298–302.

100. Ito, J., Araki, A., Tanaka, H., Tasaki, T., Cho, K., & Yamazaki, R. (1996). Muscle histopathology in spastic cerebral palsy. *Brain and Development*, *18*, 299–303.

101. Jahnsen, R., Villien, L., Aamodt, G., Stanghelle, J. K., & Holm, I. (2004). Musculoskeletal pain in adults with cerebral palsy compared with the general population. *Journal of Rehabilitation Medicine*, *36*, 78–84.

102. Kato, T., Yamashita, T., Mizutani, S., Honda, A., Matumoto, M., & Umemura, Y. (2009). Adolescent exercise associated with long-term superior measures of bone geometry: A cross-sectional DXA and MRI study. *British Journal of Sports Medicine*, *43*(12), 932–935.

103. Katz, K., Naor, N., Merlob, P., & Wielunsky, E. (1990). Rotational deformities of the tibia and foot in preterm infants. *Journal of Pediatric Orthopedics*, *10*, 483–485.

104. Kay, R. M., Rethlefsen, S. A., Fern-Buneo, A., Wren, T. A. L., & Skaggs, D. L. (2004). Botulinum toxin as an adjunct to serial casting treatment in children with cerebral palsy. *Journal of Bone and Joint Surgery (American)*, *86*, 2377– 2384.

105. Kecskemethy, H. H., Herman, D., May, R., Paul, K., Bachrach, S. J., Henderson, R. C. (2008). Quantifying weight bearing while in passive standers and a comparison of standers. *Developmental Medicine & Child Neurology*, *50*, 520–523.

106. Keller-Peck, C., Walsh, M. K., Gan, W. B., Feng, G., Sanes, J. R., & Lichtman, J. W. (2001). Asynchronous synapse elimination in neonatal motor units: Studies using GFP transgenic mice. *Neuron*, *31*, 381–394.

107. Kendall, F. P., McCreary, E. K., Provance, P. G., Rodgers, M. M., Romani, W. M. (2005). *Muscles: Testing and Function, with Posture and Pain*. Lippincott Williams & Wilkins, Baltimore, Maryland.

108. Kerr, C., McDowell, B., Cosgrove, A., Walsh, D., Bradbury, I., & McDonough, S. (2006). Electrical stimulation in cerebral palsy: A randomized controlled trial. *Developmental Medicine and Child Neurology*, *48*, 870–876.

109. Khosla, S., Melton, L. J., Dekutoski, M. B., Achenback, S. J., Oberg, A. L., & Riggs, B. L. (2003). Incidence of childhood

distal forearm fractures over 30 years: A population-based study. *Journal of the American Medical Association, 290,* 1479–1485.

110. Kilgour, G., McNair, P., & Stott, N. S. (2003). Intrarater reliability of lower limb sagittal range-of-motion measures in children with spastic diplegia. *Developmental Medicine and Child Neurology, 45,* 391–399.

111. Kitiyakara, A., & Angevine, D. M. (1963). A study of the pattern of post-embryonic growth of *M. gracilis* in mice. *Developmental Biology, 8,* 322–340.

112. Kristiansen, L. P., Gunderson, R. B., Steen, H., & Reikeras, O. (2001). The normal development of tibial torsion. *Skeletal Radiology, 30,* 519–522.

113. Laing, N. G., & Nowak, K. J. (2005). When contractile proteins go bad: The sarcomere and skeletal muscle disease. *Bioessays: News and Reviews in Molecular, Cellular and Developmental Biology, 27,* 809–822.

114. Lespargot, A., Tardieu, C., Bret, M. D., Tabary, C., & Singh, B. (1989). Is tendon surgery for the knee flexors justified in cerebral palsy? *French Journal of Orthopedic Surgery, 3,* 446–450.

115. LeVeau, B. F., & Bernhardt, D. B. (1984). Effects of forces on the growth, development, and maintenance of the human body. *Physical Therapy, 64,* 1874–1882.

116. Lichtman, J. W., & Colman, H. (2000). Synapse elimination and indelible memory. *Neuron, 25,* 269–278.

117. Lieber, R. L., & Fridén, J. (2000). Functional and clinical significance of skeletal muscle architecture. *Muscle & Nerve, 23,* 1647–1666.

118. Lieber, R. L., & Friden, J. (2002). Spasticity causes a fundamental rearrangement of muscle-joint interaction. *Muscle & Nerve, 25,* 265–270.

119. Loder, R. T., & Greenfiled, M. V. H. (2001). Clinical characteristics of children with atypical and idiopathic slipped capital femoral epiphysis: Description of the age-weight test and implications for further diagnostic investigation. *Journal of Pediatric Orthopaedics, 21,* 481–487.

120. Lowes, L. P., Westcott, S. L., Palisano, R. J., Effgen, S. K., & Orlin, M. N. (2004). Muscle force and range of motion as predictors of standing balance in children with cerebral palsy. *Physical & Occupational Therapy in Pediatrics, 24,* 57–77.

121. Lusskin, R. (1966). The influence of errors in bracing upon deformity of the lower extremity. *Archives of Physical Medicine and Rehabilitation, 47,* 520–525.

122. MacPhail, H. E. A., & Kramer, J. F. (1995). Effect of isokinetic strength-training on functional ability and walking efficiency in adolescents with cerebral palsy. *Developmental Medicine and Child Neurology, 38,* 763–775.

123. Marbini, A., Ferrari, A., Cioni, G., Bellanova, M. F., Fusco, C., & Gemignani, F. (2002). Immunohistochemical study of muscle biopsy in children with cerebral palsy. *Brain & Development, 24,* 63–66.

124. Martin, A. D., & McCulloch, R. G. (1987). Bone dynamics: Stress, strain, and fracture. *Journal of Sports Sciences, 5,* 155–163.

125. Martin, K. (2004). Effects of supramalleolar orthoses on postural stability in children with down syndrome. *Developmental Medicine & Child Neurology, 46,* 406–411.

126. Mastaglia, F. L. (1974). The growth and development of the skeletal muscles. In J. A. Davis, & J. Dobbing (Eds.). *Scientific foundations of paediatrics* (pp. 348–375). Philadelphia: WB Saunders.

127. McDowell, B. C., Hewitt, V., Nurse, A., Weston, T., & Baker, R. (2000). The variability of goniometric measurements in ambulatory children with spastic cerebral palsy. *Gait and Posture, 12,* 114–121.

128. McKay, H. A., MacLean, L., Petit, M., MacKelvie-O'Brien, K., Janssen, P., Beck, T., et al. (2005). "Bounce at the bell": A novel program of short bouts of exercise improves proximal femur bone mass in early pubertal children. *British Journal of Sports Medicine, 39,* 521–526.

129. McKibbin, B. (1980). The structure of the epiphysis. In R. Owen, J. Goodfellow, & P. Bullough (Eds.). *Scientific foundations of orthopaedics and traumatology.* Philadelphia: WB Saunders.

130. McPherson, J. J., Arends, T. G., Michaels, M. J., & Trettin, K. (1984). The range of motion of long term knee contractures of four spastic cerebral palsied children: A pilot study. *Physical and Occupational Therapy in Pediatrics, 4,* 17–34.

131. Mercer, V. S., & Lewis, C. L. (2001). Hip abductor and knee extensor muscle strength of children with and without Down syndrome. *Pediatric Physical Therapy, 13,* 18–26.

132. Mergler, S., Evenhuis, H. M., Boot, A. M., De Man, S. A., Bindels-De Heus, K., Huijbers, W. A. R., et al. (2009). Epidemiology of low bone mineral density and fractures in children with severe cerebral palsy: A systematic review. *Developmental Medicine and Child Neurology, 51,* 773–778.

133. Merlini, L., Dell'Accio, D., & Granata, C. (1995). Reliability of dynamic strength knee muscle testing in children. *Journal of Sports Physical Therapy, 22,* 73–76.

134. Mielke, C. H., & Stevens, P. M. (1996). Hemiepiphyseal stapling for knee deformities in children younger than 10 years: A preliminary report. *Journal of Pediatric Orthopaedics, 16,* 423–429.

135. Miller, F., Cardoso, D. R., Dabney, K. W., Lipton, G. E., & Triana, M. (1997). Soft-tissue release for spastic hip subluxation in cerebral palsy. *Journal of Pediatric Orthopedics, 17*(5), 571–584.

136. Mills, V. M. (1984). Electromyographic results of inhibitory splinting. *Physical Therapy, 64,* 190–193.

137. Moore, K. L. (1988). *The developing human: Clinically oriented embryology* (4th ed.). Philadelphia: WB Saunders.

138. Moore, M. L. (1949). The measurement of joint motion: Part I. Introductory review of the literature. *Physical Therapy Review, 29,* 195–205.

139. Moore, M. L. (1949). The measurement of joint motion: Part II. The technique of goniometry. *Physical Therapy Review, 29,* 256–264.

140. Moreau, N. G., Teefey, S. A., & Damiano, D. L. (2009). In vivo muscle architecture and size of the rectus femoris and vastus lateralis in children and adolescents with cerebral palsy. *Developmental Medicine and Child Neurology, 51*, 800–806.

141. Morrell, D. S., Pearson, J. M., & Sauser, D. D. (2002). Progressive bone and joint abnormalities of the spine and lower extremities in cerebral palsy. *Radiographics: A Review, 22*, 257–268.

142. Reference deleted in page proofs.

143. Morrissy, R., & Weinstein, S. (Eds.). (2005). *Lovell and Winter's pediatric orthopedics* (6th ed.). Philadelphia: Lippincott Williams and Wilkins.

144. Morton, J. F., Brownlee, M., & McFadyen, A. K. (2005). The effects of progressive resistance training for children with cerebral palsy. *Clinical Rehabilitation, 19*, 283–289.

145. Murphy, K. P. (2009). Cerebral palsy lifetime care—Four musculoskeletal conditions. *Developmental Medicine and Child Neurology, 51*(Suppl. 4), 30–37.

146. Murphy, K. P., Molnar, G. E., & Lankasky, K. (1995). Medical and functional status of adults with cerebral palsy. *Developmental Medicine and Child Neurology, 37*, 1075–1084.

147. Murray, P. D. F., & Drachman, D. B. (1969). The role of movement in the development of joints and the related structures: The head and neck in the chick embryo. *Journal of Embryology and Experimental Morphology, 22*, 349–371.

148. Mutlu, A., Krosschell, K., & Spira, D. G. (2009). Treadmill training with partial body-weight support in children with cerebral palsy: A systematic review. *Developmental Medicine and Child Neurology, 51*, 268–275.

149. Reference deleted in page proofs.

150. Norkin, C. C., & White, D. J. (1985). *Measurement of joint motion: A guide to goniometry.* Philadelphia: FA Davis.

151. O'Connell, D. G., & Barnhart, R. (1995). Improvement in wheelchair propulsion in pediatric wheelchair users through resistance training: A pilot study. *Archives of Physical Medicine and Rehabilitation, 76*, 368–372.

152. O'Sullivan, M., Bronk, J., Chao, E., & Kelly, P. (1994). Experimental study of the effect of weight bearing on fracture healing in the canine tibia. *Clinical Orthopaedics And Related Research,* (302), 273–283

153. Owen, J., Stephens, D., & Wright, J. G. (2007). Reliability of hip range of motion using goniometry in pediatric femur shaft fractures. *Canadian Journal of Surgery, 50*, 251–255.

154. Pandya, S., Florence, J. M., King, W. M., Robison, J. D., Oxman, M., & Province, M. A. (1985). Reliability of goniometric measurements in patients with Duchenne muscular dystrophy. *Physical Therapy, 65*, 1339–1342.

155. Patikas, D., Wolf, S. I., Schuster, W., Armbrust, P., Dreher, T., & Döderlein, L. (2007). Electromyographic patterns in children with cerebral palsy: Do they change after surgery? *Gait & Posture, 26*, 362–371.

156. Pearl, M. L., Edgerton, B. W., Kon, D. S., Darakjian, A. B., Kosco, A. E., Kazimiroff, P. B., & Burchette, R. J. (2003). Comparison of arthroscopic findings with magnetic resonance imaging and arthrography in children with glenohumeral deformities secondary to brachial plexus birth palsy. *Journal of Bone and Joint Surgery (American), 85*, 890–898.

157. Pierce, S. R., Lauer, R. T., Shewokis, P. A., Rubertone, J. A., & Orlin, M. N. (2006). Test-retest reliability of isokinetic dynamometry for the assessment of spasticity of the knee flexors and knee extensors in children with cerebral palsy. *Archives of Physical Medicine and Rehabilitation, 87*, 697–702.

158. Pin, T. W. (2007). Effectiveness of static weight-bearing exercises in children with cerebral palsy. *Pediatric Physical Therapy, 19*, 62–73.

159. Pin, T., Dyke, P., & Chan, M. (2006). The effectiveness of passive stretching in children with cerebral palsy. *Developmental Medicine and Child Neurology, 48*, 855–862.

160. Price, R., Bjornson, K. F., Lehmann, J. F., McLaughlin, J. F., & Hays, R. M. (1991). Quantitative measurement of spasticity in children with cerebral palsy. *Developmental Medicine and Child Neurology, 33*, 585–595.

161. Ralis, Z., & McKibbin, B. (1973). Changes in shape of the human hip joint during its development and their relation to stability. *Journal of Bone and Joint Surgery (British), 55*, 780–785.

162. Rauch, F., Neu, C., Manz, F., & Schoenau, E. (2001). The development of metaphyseal cortex—Implications for distal radius fractures during growth. *Journal of Bone and Mineral Research, 16*, 1547–1555.

163. Reimers, J. (1990). Functional changes in the antagonists after lengthening the agonists in cerebral palsy: II. Quadriceps strength before and after distal hamstring lengthening. *Clinical Orthopedics and Related Research, 253*, 35–37.

164. Rodriguez, T. I., Razquin, S., Palacios, T., & Rubio, V. (1992). Human growth plate development in the fetal and neonatal period. *Journal of Orthopaedic Research, 10*, 62–71.

165. Romanini, L., Villani, C., Meloni, C., & Calvisi, V. (1989). Histological and morphological aspects of muscle in infantile cerebral palsy. *Italian Journal of Orthopaedics and Traumatology, 15*, 87–93.

166. Rose, J., Haskell, W. L., Gamble, J. G., Hamilton, R. L., Brown, D. A., & Rinsky, L. (1994). Muscle pathology and clinical measures of disability in children with cerebral palsy. *Journal of Orthopaedic Research, 12*, 758–768.

167. Rothstein, J. M., & Rose, S. J. (1982). Muscle mutability. Part 2, Adaptation to drugs, metabolic factors, and aging. *Physical Therapy, 62*, 1788–1798.

168. Royer, P. (1974). Growth of bony tissue. In J. A. Davis, & J. Dobbing (Eds.). *Scientific foundations of paediatrics.* Philadelphia: WB Saunders.

169. Salenius, P., & Vankka, E. (1975). The development of the tibiofemoral angle in children. *Journal of Bone and Joint Surgery (American), 57*, 259–261.

170. Salmons, S., & Hendriksson, J. (1981). The adaptive response of skeletal muscle to increased use. *Muscle and Nerve, 4*, 94–105.

171. Sargeant, A. J., Davies, C. T. M., Edwards, R. H. T., Maunder, C., & Young, A. (1977). Functional and structural changes

after disuse of human muscle. *Clinical Science and Molecular Medicine, 52,* 337–342.

172. Reference deleted in page proofs.

173. Schwartz, L., Engle, J. M., & Jensen, M. P. (1999). Pain in persons with cerebral palsy. *Archives of Physical Medicine and Rehabilitation, 80,* 1243–1246.

174. Scott, O. M., Hyde, S. A., Goddard, C., Jones, R., & Dubowitz, V. (1981). Effect of exercise in Duchenne muscular dystrophy. *Physiotherapy, 67,* 174–176.

175. Scrutton, D., Baird, G., Smeeton, N. (2001). Hip dysplasia in bilateral cerebral palsy: incidence and natural history in children aged 18 months to 5 years. *Developmental Medicine and Child Neurology, 43,* 586–600.

176. Selby-Silverstein, L., Hillstrom, H. J., & Palisano, R. J. (2001). The effect of foot orthoses on standing foot posture and gait of young children with Down syndrome. *NeuroRehabilitation, 16,* 183–193.

177. Sharrard, W. J. W. (1967). Paralytic deformity in the lower limb. *Journal of Bone and Joint Surgery (British), 49,* 731– 747.

178. Sherk, H. H., Pasquariello, P. S., & Watters, W. C. (1981). Congenital dislocation of the hip. *Clinical Pediatrics, 20,* 513–520.

179. Sheth, R. D., & Hermann, B. P. (2008). Bone in idiopathic and symptomatic epilepsy. *Epilepsy Research, 78,* 71–76.

180. Sheth, R. D., Binkley, N., & Hermann, B. P. (2008). Gender differences in bone mineral density in epilepsy. *Epilepsia, 49,* 125–131.

181. Shortland, A. P. (2008). In vivo gastrocnemius muscle fascicle length in children with and without diplegic cerebral palsy. *Developmental Medicine and Child Neurology, 50,* 339–340.

182. Reference deleted in page proofs.

183. Simard, S., Marchant, M., & Mencio G. (1992). The Ilizarov procedures: Limb lengthening and its implications. *Physical Therapy, 72,* 25–34.

184. Smith, D. W., & Drennan, J. C. (2002). Arthrogryposis wrist deformities: Results of infantile serial casting. *Journal of Pediatric Orthopaedics, 22,* 44–47.

185. Sochett, E. B., & Makitie, O. (2005). Osteoporosis in chronically ill children. *Annals of Medicine, 37,* 286–294.

186. Sockolov, R., Irwin, B., Dressendorfer, R. H., & Bernauer, E. M. (1977). Exercise performance in 6- to 11-year-old boys with Duchenne muscular dystrophy. *Archives of Physical Medicine and Rehabilitation, 58,* 195–200.

187. Sone, S. (1994). Muscle histochemistry in the Prader-Willi syndrome. *Brain and Development, 16,* 183–188.

188. Staheli, L. (2007). *Fundamentals of pediatric orthopedics* (4th ed.). Philadelphia: Lippincott Williams and Wilkins.

189. Stanitski, D., Shahcheraghi, H., Nicker, D., & Armstrong, P. (1996). Results of tibial lengthening with the Ilizarov technique. *Journal of Pediatric Orthopaedics, 16,* 168–172.

190. Stevenson, R. D., Conaway, M., Barrington, J. W., Cuthill, S. L., Worley, G., & Henderson, R. C. (2006). Fracture rate in children with cerebral palsy. *Pediatric Rehabilitation, 9,* 396–403.

191. Stokes, I. A. F. (2008). Mechanical modulation of spinal growth and progression of adolescent scoliosis. *Studies in Health Technology and Informatics, 135,* 75–83.

192. Stolov, W. C., Weilepp, T. B. Jr., & Riddell, W. M. (1970). Passive length-tension relationship and hydroxyproline content of chronically denervated skeletal muscle. *Archives in Physical Medicine and Rehabilitation, 51,* 517–525.

193. Stuberg, W. A., Metcalf, W. K. (1988). Reliability of quantitative muscle testing in healthy children and in children with Duchenne muscular dystrophy using a hand-held dynamometer. *Physical Therapy, 68,* 977–982.

194. Stuberg, W. A. (1992). Considerations related to weight-bearing programs in children with developmental disabilities. *Physical Therapy, 72,* 35–40.

195. Suzuki, S., & Yamamuro, T. (1986). Correlation of fetal posture and congenital dislocation of the hip. *Acta Orthopaedica Scandinavica 57*(no. 1), 81–84

196. Sylvester, F. A., Leopold, S., Lincoln, M., Hyams, J. S., Griffiths, A. M., & Lerer, T. (2009). A two-year longitudinal study of persistent lean tissue deficits in children with Crohn's disease. *Clinical Gastroenterology and Hepatology: The Official Clinical Practice Journal of the American Gastroenterological Association, 7*(4), 452–455.

197. Szalay, E. A., Harriman, D., Eastlund, B., & Mercer, D. (2008). Quantifying postoperative bone loss in children. *Journal of Pediatric Orthopedics, 28,* 320–323.

198. Tabary, J. C., Tabary, C., Tardieu, C., Tardieu, G., & Goldspink, G. (1972). Physiological and structural changes in the cat's soleus muscle due to immobilization at different lengths by plaster casts. *Journal of Physiology, 224,* 231–244.

199. Tabary, J. C., Tardieu, C., Tardieu, G., & Tabary, C. (1981). Experimental rapid sarcomere loss with concomitant hypoextensibility. *Muscle and Nerve, 4,* 198–203.

200. Taber L. A. (1998). Biomechanical growth laws for muscle tissue. Retrieved from http://search.ebscohost.com/login.aspx ?direct=true&db=mnh&AN=9714932&site=ehost-live

201. Tardieu, C., Huet de la Tour, E., Bret, M. D., & Tardieu, G. (1982). Muscle hypoextensibility in children with cerebral palsy: I. Clinical and experimental observations. *Archives of Physical Medicine and Rehabilitation, 63,* 97–102.

202. Tardieu, C., Tardieu, G., Colbeau-Justin, P., & Huet de la Tour, E. (1979). Trophic muscle regulation in children with congenital cerebral lesions. *Journal of the Neurological Sciences, 42,* 357–364.

203. Tardieu, G., Tardieu, C., Colbeau-Justin, P., & Lespargot, A. (1982). Muscle hypoextensibility in children with cerebral palsy: II. Therapeutic implications. *Archives of Physical Medicine and Rehabilitation, 63,* 103–107.

204. Thompson, W. J., & Jansen, J. K. S. (1977). The extent of sprouting of remaining motor units in partly denervated immature and adult rat soleus muscle. *Neuroscience, 2,* 523–535.

205. Thomson, J. D. (1955). Mechanical characteristics of skeletal muscle undergoing atrophy of degeneration. *American Journal of Physical Medicine, 34*, 606–611.

206. Tosi, L. L., Maher, N., Moore, D. W., Goldstein, M., & Aisen, M. L. (2009). Adults with cerebral palsy: A workshop to define the challenges of treating and preventing secondary musculoskeletal and neuromuscular complications in this rapidly growing population. *Developmental Medicine and Child Neurology, 51*(Suppl. 4), 2–11.

207. Trueta, T. (1974). The growth and development of bone and joints: Orthopedic aspects. In J. A. Davis, & J. Dobbing (Eds.). *Scientific foundations of paediatrics.* Philadelphia: WB Saunders.

208. Ulrich, D. A., Ulrich, B. D., Angulo-Kinzler, R. M., Yun, J. (2001). Treadmill training of infants with Down syndrome: Evidence-based developmental outcomes. *Pediatrics, 108*, e84.

209. Ulrich, D. A. (2008). Effects of intensity of treadmill training on developmental outcomes and stepping in infants with Down syndrome: A randomized trial. *Physical Therapy, 88*, 114–122.

210. van den Beld, W. A., van der Sanden, G. A. C., Sengers, R. C. A., Verbeek, A. L. M., & Gabreels, F. J. M. (2006). Validity and reproducibility of hand-held dynamometry in children aged 4–11 years. *Journal of Rehabilitation Medicine, 38*, 57–64.

211. van der Berg-Emons, R. J. G., van Baak, M. A., de Barbanson, D. C., Speth, L., & Saris, W. H. M. (1996). Reliability of tests to determine peak aerobic power, anaerobic power and isokinetic muscle strength in children with spastic cerebral palsy. *Developmental Medicine and Child Neurology, 38*, 1117–1125.

212. Vatanparast, H., & Whiting, S. J. (2006). Calcium supplementation trials and bone mass development in children, adolescents, and young adults. *Nutrition Reviews, 64*, 204–209.

213. Vicente-Rodriguez, G. (2006). How does exercise affect bone development during growth? *Sports Medicine (Auckland, N.Z.), 36*, 561–569.

214. Vidal, J., Deguillaume, P., & Vidal, M. (1985). The anatomy of the dysplastic hip in cerebral palsy related to prognosis and treatment. *International Orthopaedics, 9*, 105–110.

215. Viswanathan, A., & Sylvester, F. A. (2008). Chronic pediatric inflammatory diseases: Effects on bone. *Reviews in Endocrine & Metabolic Disorders, 9*(2), 107–122.

216. Walker, J. M. (1991). Musculoskeletal development: A review. *Physical Therapy, 71*, 878–889.

217. Wallach D. M., & Davidson, R. S. (2005). Pediatric lower limb disorders. In J. P. Dormans (Ed.). *Pediatric orthopaedics: Core knowledge in orthopaedics.* Philadelphia: Elsevier Mosby.

218. Wang, K., McCarter, R., Wright, J., Beverly, J., & Ramirez-Mitchell, R. (1993). Viscoelasticity of the sarcomere matrix of skeletal muscles: The titin-myosin composite filament is a dual-stage molecular spring. *Biophysical Journal, 64*, 1161–1177.

219. Ward, S. R., Terk, M. R., Powers, C. M. (2007). Patella alta: Association with patellofemoral alignment and changes in contact area during weight bearing. *Journal of Bone and Joint Surgery (American), 89*, 1749–1755.

220. Ward, S. S., & Stickland, N. C. (1991). Why are slow and fast muscles differentially affected during prenatal undernutrition? *Muscle and Nerve, 14*, 259–267.

221. Waterman-Storer, C. M. (1991). The cytoskeleton of skeletal muscle: Is it affected by exercise? A brief review. *Medicine and Science in Sports and Exercise, 23*, 1240–1249.

222. Waugh, K. G., Minkel, J. L., Parker, R., & Coon, V. A. (1983). Measurement of selected hip, knee, and ankle joint motions in newborns. *Physical Therapy, 63*, 1616–1621.

223. Weinstein, S. L. (1987). Natural history of congenital hip dislocation (CHD) and hip dysplasia. *Clinical Orthopedics and Related Research, 225*, 62–75.

224. Westberry, D. E., Davids, J. R., Jacobs, J. M., Pugh, L. I., & Tanner, S. L. (2006). Effectiveness of serial stretch casting for resistant or recurrent knee flexion contractures following hamstring lengthening in children with cerebral palsy. *Journal of Pediatric Orthopedics, 26*, 109–114.

225. White, J., Flohr, J. A., Winter, S. S., Vener, J., Feinauer, L. R., & Ransdell, L. B. (2005). Potential benefits of physical activity for children with acute lymphoblastic leukaemia. *Pediatric Rehabilitation, 8*, 53–58.

226. Whiting, S. J. (2002). Obesity is not protective for bones in childhood and adolescence. *Nutrition Reviews, 60*, 27–36.

227. Williams, P. E., & Goldspink, G. (1978). Changes in sarcomere length and physiological properties in immobilized muscle. *Journal of Anatomy (London), 127*, 459–468.

228. Williams, P. E., & Goldspink, G. (1984). Connective tissue changes in immobilized muscle. *Journal of Anatomy (London), 138*, 342–350.

229. Williams, P. E., & Goldspink, G. (1971). Longitudinal growth of striated muscle fibers. *Journal of Cell Science, 9*, 751–767.

230. Williams, P. E., & Goldspink, G. (1973). The effect of immobilization on the longitudinal growth of striated muscle fibers. *Journal of Anatomy (London), 116*, 45–55.

231. Wills, M. (2004). Orthopedic complications of childhood obesity. *Pediatric Physical Therapy, 16*, 230–235.

232. Wilmshurst, S., Ward, K., Adams, J. E., Langton, C. M., & Mughal, M. Z. (1996). Mobility status and bone density in cerebral palsy. *Archives of Disease in Childhood, 75*, 164–165.

233. Witt, C. (2003). Detecting developmental dysplasia of the hip. *Advances in Neonatal Care, 3*, 65–75.

234. Worley, G., & Henderson, R. C. (2006). Fracture rate in children with cerebral palsy. *Pediatric Rehabilitation, 9*, 396–403.

235. Wren, T. A., & Engsberg, J. R. (2007). Normalizing lower-extremity strength data for children without disability using allometric scaling. *Arch Phys Med Rehabil, 88*(11), 1446–1451.

236. Wren, T. A., & Engsberg, J. R. (2009). Normalizing lower-extremity strength data for children, adolescents, and young adults with cerebral palsy. *J Appl Biomech, 25*(3), 195–202.

237. Young, N. L., Wright, J. G., Lam, T. P., Rajaratnam, K., Stephens, D., & Wedge, J. H. (1998). Windswept hip deformity in spastic quadriplegic cerebral palsy. *Pediatric Physical Therapy*, *10*, 94–100.

238. Zamboni, G., Antoniazzi, F., Lauriola, S., Bertoldo, F., & Tato, L. (2006). Calcium supplementation increases bone mass in GH-deficient prepubertal children during GH replacement. *Hormone Research*, *65*, 223–230.

239. Ziv, I., Blackburn, N., Rang, M., & Koreska, J. (1984). Muscle growth in normal and spastic mice. *Developmental Medicine and Child Neurology*, *26*, 94–99.

6 Physical Fitness during Childhood and Adolescence

JEAN L. STOUT, PT, MS

The International Classification of Functioning, Disability and Health (ICF) emphasizes components of health as important factors related to participation in society.[279] According to its press release and using the ICF framework, the World Health Organization estimates that as many as 500 million healthy life years are lost each year because of disability associated with health conditions. This statistic includes children. Ensuring physical fitness is one aspect of primary prevention and health promotion upon which the practice of physical therapy is based[8] and is a construct that fits appropriately within the ICF model. As clinicians who design exercise programs and treat children with disabilities, we have a unique responsibility to understand and promote physical fitness as an aspect of those programs. It is a unique responsibility because we can have a great impact on the exercise lifestyle that children develop and carry with them throughout their lives. We also care for a group of children who might otherwise be physically inactive. Physical fitness is coming to the forefront of physical therapy practice as focus is directed toward prevention. A research summit devoted to the topic of physical fitness and prevention of secondary conditions for children with cerebral palsy (CP) and a presentation on the importance of physical activity and fitness for adults with CP underscores the attention and importance that the profession of physical therapy as a whole is placing on this topic.[98,249] Many believe that promotion of lifelong habits of physical activity in childhood will have direct and indirect effects on health and prevention of disease in adulthood.[30,118,228,239] Meanwhile studies based on fitness standards find fewer children are achieving the minimum criterion for activity.[204]

What defines *physical fitness* for able-bodied children? Are the criteria for physical fitness different in children with disabilities? How do we help children with physical disabilities incorporate physical fitness into the limitations of their disability? This chapter is designed to answer those questions and to provide the reader with an understanding of (1) physical fitness and the cardiopulmonary response to exercise in children of different ages who do not have disabling conditions; (2) the components of physical fitness (cardiorespiratory endurance, muscular strength and endurance, flexibility, and body composition) (Table 6-1); (3) the standards of fitness components consistent with good health; (4) the effects of training and conditioning on overall physical fitness; (5) the components of fitness in various special populations; and (6) guides for program planning. The chapter also includes a review of current physical fitness tests.

HEALTH, PHYSICAL ACTIVITY, AND PHYSICAL FITNESS

Physical fitness is difficult to define because it cannot be measured directly. Physical fitness is generally viewed as having two facets—health-related fitness and the more traditional motor fitness. Motor fitness generally includes physical abilities that relate to athletic performance, whereas health-related fitness includes abilities related to daily function and health maintenance. Physical activity is thought to be the path both to physical fitness and to good health, and therefore, is tightly coupled to fitness, but these are not synonymous terms. *Physical activity* refers to the amount of exercise in which an individual engages. Physical activity does not describe any "level" of physiologic function important to maintain health. Studies suggest that in adults, a positive correlation exists between regular physical activity, cardiovascular fitness, and reduced risk of mortality.[181] Just as in adults, physical inactivity is increasingly being implicated in the escalating "epidemic" of obesity and as a major risk factor for morbidity in children and adolescents.[49,150,165,205] The current consensus is that physical activity and physical fitness are reciprocally related and each exerts independent effects on health. Physical activity may improve physical fitness and health at the same time, but the improvement in health may be caused by biologic changes different from those responsible for improvement in physical fitness.[118] Some of the benefits from physical activity that are important to health and achievement have no relationship to what is defined as *physical fitness* per se.[112,172] One example is the importance of regular exercise to bone health and a reduced risk of osteoporosis; osteoporosis is related to health but not to the components of physical fitness.

Limited information is available regarding how much physical activity is necessary for health and fitness in children. The work of Strong and colleagues outlines the effects of physical activity on health and behavioral outcomes in school-aged youth and offers guidelines for the amount of exercise necessary.[240] "How much physical activity is

TABLE 6-1   **Health-Related Fitness Components and the Rationale for Importance to Health Promotion and Disease Prevention[194]**

Component	Rationale
Cardiorespiratory endurance	Improved physical working capacity
	Reduced fatigue
	Reduced risk of coronary heart disease
	Optimal growth and development
Muscular strength and endurance	Improved functional capacity for lifting and carrying
	Reduced risk of lower back pain
	Optimal posture
	Optimal growth and development
Flexibility	Enhanced functional capacity for bending and twisting
	Reduced risk of lower back pain
	Optimal growth and development
Body composition	Reduced risk of hypertension
	Reduced risk of coronary heart disease
	Reduced risk of diabetes
	Optimal growth and development

Adapted from Pate, P. R., & Shephard, R. J. (1989). Characteristics of physical fitness in youth. In C. V. Gisolfi, & D. R. Lamb (Eds.), *Perspectives in exercise science and sports medicine: Youth, exercise, and sport* (Vol. 2; pp. 1–45). Indianapolis, IN: Benchmark Press.

enough?" is not easily answered because it depends on so many factors. Assessing and understanding physical activity in preschool children relative to child development presents even more challenges.[79] Studies under way, such as the longitudinal LOOK project in Australia, which is investigating how early physical activity contributes to health and development, may also help to answer that question.[246]

The premise that physical activity is the path to both physical fitness and good health has become a primary focus in programs instituted by the United States (U.S.) Department of Health and Human Services. As early as 1985, the Centers for Disease Control put forth a specific activity plan for youth through old age to attain specific health fitness goals and achieve optimal health benefits. Developing lifelong physical activity patterns was one of the specific goals for children.[118] In 1990, Healthy Children 2000—a major federal planning document for health promotion and disease prevention for children—was introduced.[255] Originally, eight objectives were outlined to increase the physical activity and fitness levels of youth, with a target date of attainment by the year 2000. Every 10 years, through the Healthy People initiative, the Department of Health and Human Services develops the next iteration of the national objectives for promoting health and preventing disease, which include physical fitness. Draft objectives for Healthy People 2020 have been released for public comment.[257] http://www.healthypeople.gov/hp2020/Objectives/TopicArea.aspx?id=39&TopicArea=Physical+Activity+and+Fitness

Progress to targets has been slow ever since the year 2000 objectives were established. Many of the year 2000 targets were retained in the 2010 objectives, and most of the 2010 objectives remain in the 2020 objectives. Perhaps the greatest disappointment has been the lack of data available for children younger than high school age (grades K through 8).[256] As early as 1998, targets directed toward elementary-age and junior high–age children were dropped from the 2010 objectives. Fourteen objectives for physical activity and fitness are included in the Healthy People 2020 draft (Box 6-1). Of these 14 objectives, seven directly address adolescents (grades 9 through 12). Six include some aspect related to children from ages 5 to 15. Midcourse review of 2010 objectives indicated that two of the seven objectives are moving away from target (objectives 3 and 7), and two are moving toward target (objectives 4 and 8). No data are available for objective 2.[259]

Physical activity as the path to physical fitness is no less surprising than the relationship of physical activity to improved health and disease prevention. The content of the current nationwide objectives has been guided in part by the concept of health-related fitness. What is different may be the intensity of physical activity required to be physically fit compared with what is necessary to receive benefits to health. Regardless of intensity, both physical fitness and improved health begin with physical activity. Recently, the amount and intensity of physical activity were found to be the best predictors of vascular health and function in a group of 10- and 11-year-old children.[122] Evidence of the impact of physical activity and fitness in childhood on fitness, health, and prevention of disease in adulthood is mixed,[30,74,95,122,142,160,161,198,213,228,239,240] but any direct or indirect benefits for development of lifelong habits of physical activity and fitness in terms of health and disease prevention for able-bodied children should be no less true for children with physical disabilities. The concept of physical fitness becomes more important because as individuals become less active in adulthood, the decrease in activity level is more likely to result in loss of function, injury, or both.

DEFINITION OF PHYSICAL FITNESS

As defined previously, *health-related fitness* is a state characterized by (1) an ability to perform daily activities with vigor, and (2) traits and capacities that are associated with low risk of premature development of hypokinetic disease (i.e., physical inactivity).[192] Physical fitness is multidimensional. A combination of traits and capacities contributes to physical fitness, and the interaction among them creates true fitness. Each facet is a unique, independent characteristic or ability that is not highly correlated with other components. As the concept of health-related fitness has gained acceptance, four basic components have been identified: cardiorespiratory endurance, muscular strength and endurance, flexibility, and

BOX **6-1**   DRAFT OBJECTIVES HEALTHY PEOPLE 2020: PHYSICAL ACTIVITY AND FITNESS (PAF)

http://www.healthypeople.gov/hp2020/Objectives/TopicArea.aspx ?id=39&TopicArea=Physical+Activity+and+Fitness
  Goal: Improve health, fitness, and quality of life through daily physical activity.

OBJECTIVES FOR CHILDREN AND ADOLESCENTS

PAF HP2020-2 (retained from Healthy People 2010). Increase the proportion of the Nation's public and private schools that require daily physical education for all students.
  Target: 9.4%; baseline: 6.4% middle and junior high school
  Target: 5.8%; baseline: 14.5% senior high schools

PAF HP2020-3 (retained from Healthy People 2010). Increase the proportion of adolescents who participate in daily school physical education.
  Target: 50%; baseline: 29%

PAF HP2020-4 (retained from Healthy People 2010). Increase the proportion of adolescents who spend at least 50% of school physical education class time being physically active.
  Target: 50%; baseline: 38%

PAF HP2020-5 (retained from Healthy People 2010). Increase the proportion of the Nation's public and private schools that provide access to their physical activity spaces and facilities for all persons outside of normal school hours (i.e., before and after the school day, on weekends, and during summer and other vacations).
  Target: 50%

PAF HP2020-7 (retained but modified from Healthy People 2010). Increase the proportion of adolescents who meet current physical activity guidelines for aerobic physical activity and for muscle-strengthening activity.

PAF HP2020-8 (retained but modified from Healthy People 2010). Increase the proportion of children and adolescents who meet guidelines for television viewing and computer use.
  a. Increase the proportion of children age 0 to 2 years who view no television or videos on an average weekday.
  b. Increase the proportion of children and adolescents aged 2 years through 12th grade who view television or videos or play video games for no more than 2 hours a day.
    i. Children aged 2 to 5 years
    ii. Children aged 6 to 14 years
    iii. Adolescents in grades 9 through 12
  c. Increase the proportion of children and adolescents age 2 years to 12th grade who use a computer or play computer games outside of school (for nonschool work) for no more than 2 hours a day.
    i. Children aged 2 to 5 years
    ii. Children aged 6 to 14 years
    iii. Adolescents in grades 9 through 12

PAF HP2020-10b (retained but modified from Healthy People 2010). Increase the proportion of trips to school of 1 mile or less made by walking in children and adolescents age 5 to 15 years.
  Target: 50%; baseline 31%

PAF HP202-11b (retained but modified from Healthy People 2010). Increase the proportion of trips to school of 2 miles or less made by bicycling in children and adolescents age 5 to 15 years.
  Target: 5%; baseline 2.4%

PAF HP2020-13 (new to Healthy People 2020). Increase the proportion of school districts that require or recommend elementary school recess for an appropriate period of time.

From U.S. Department of Health and Human Services, Public Health Services. (2006). *Healthy People 2010 midcourse review: Physical activity and fitness.* Retrieved October 22, 2009, from http://www.healthypeople.gov/hp2020/Objectives/TopicAreas.aspx

body composition. The rationale for the importance of these parameters in day-to-day functional capacity, health promotion, and disease prevention, and therefore physical fitness, is presented in Table 6-1. The relative independence of the components from one another has been verified by low correlations between components. Of 60 possible correlation coefficients among test items for these components, only 6 were greater than 0.35.[209,212]

CARDIOPULMONARY RESPONSE TO EXERCISE

As in adults, the response of a child to exercise (a single event or repeated exercise) includes physiologic changes in the cardiovascular and pulmonary systems, as well as metabolic effects. In children, however, differences in physiologic changes are seen as growth and development occur.

Physiologic capacities depend on growth of the myocardium, skeleton, and skeletal muscle. Maturation and improved efficiency of the cardiovascular, pulmonary, metabolic, and musculoskeletal systems are also important. The physical work capacity of children increases approximately eightfold in absolute terms between the ages of 6 and 12 years, partially as a result of growth and maturation.[2] The absolute exercise capacity of children may be less than that of adults, but relative exercise capacity is similar.

Any exercise, in a child or an adult, increases the energy expenditure of the body. The energy for muscle contraction and exercise depends on splitting of adenosine triphosphate (ATP) at the cellular level. ATP is available in small quantities in resting muscle, but once contraction starts, additional sources are required if contraction is to be maintained. Three sources of ATP are available: (1) creatine phosphate (CPh),

(2) glycolysis, and (3) the tricarboxylic acid or Krebs cycle. It is beyond the scope of this chapter to describe these mechanisms in detail. The reader is referred to a standard textbook on exercise physiology.[45]

CPh and glycolysis as sources of ATP are referred to as anaerobic pathways because they do not require the presence of oxygen. CPh is found in the sarcoplasm of the muscle cell. During breakdown, it releases a high-energy phosphate bond that can be combined with adenosine diphosphate (ADP) to create ATP.

$$CPh \rightarrow C + P_i + Energy \qquad [1]$$

$$ADP + P_i + Energy \rightarrow ATP \qquad [2]$$

CPh breakdown together with ATP production provides enough energy for 10 to 15 seconds of exercise. Glycolysis, the other anaerobic pathway, breaks down glucose to produce pyruvic acid or lactic acid and ATP. This reaction takes place in the sarcoplasm of the cell. Together, glycolysis and CPh breakdown are methods of anaerobic energy production that can sustain energy for muscle contraction for 40 to 50 seconds.

Energy production by the tricarboxylic acid cycle is called an *aerobic pathway* because it requires oxygen. A supply of oxygen is required for sustained exercise and depends on the aerobic pathway. Most, if not all, activities use both aerobic and anaerobic pathways for supply of ATP, but often tasks are more highly dependent on one type of pathway than the other.

Because aerobic pathways must be used to sustain exercise, an index of maximal aerobic power is used to reflect the highest metabolic rate made available by aerobic energy. The most common index is maximal oxygen uptake (VO_{2max}), or the highest volume of oxygen that can be consumed per unit time. Oxygen supply to muscle is described by the Fick equation: oxygen uptake (VO_2) is equal to cardiac output (CO) times the difference in oxygen content between arterial (Cao_2) and mixed venous (Cvo_2) blood, or

$$VO_2 = CO \times (Cao_2 - Cvo_2)$$

Because CO is the product of heart rate and stroke volume, the following relationship is also true:

$$VO_2 = Heart\ rate \times Stroke\ volume \times Arteriovenous\ O_2\ difference$$

For VO_2 to increase, one or more of these factors must increase. During exercise, CO is elevated by increases in both heart rate and stroke volume. Elevated blood flow to the muscles increases the difference in oxygen content between arterial and venous blood.

VO_{2max} increases throughout childhood from approximately 1 L/min at age 5 years to 3 to 4 L/min at puberty.[41] These changes occur as a result of maturation of the cardiovascular, pulmonary, metabolic, and musculoskeletal systems. As a child grows, the cardiopulmonary and musculoskeletal systems are integrated so that oxygen flow during exercise optimally meets the energy demands of the muscle cells, regardless of body size.[59]

Cardiac Output

CO in children, as in adults, rises at the beginning of exercise or on transition from a lower to a higher level of exercise. CO increases by an increase in both stroke volume and heart rate. CO in children is similar to that in adults despite the fact that stroke volume in a 5-year-old is about 25% of the stroke volume in an adult.[107] Stroke volume increases as total heart volume increases. At all levels of exercise, stroke volume in boys is somewhat higher than in girls.[17] CO levels in children are similar to those in adults because of an increased heart rate throughout childhood. Maximal heart rates in children vary between 195 and 215 beats per minute (bpm) and decrease by 0.7 to 0.8 bpm per year after maturity.[41]

Arteriovenous Difference and Hemoglobin Concentration

At rest, the difference between arterial and mixed venous blood oxygen content is the same in children as in adults.[235] Research suggests, however, that children have a higher blood flow to muscles after exercise than do young adults, resulting in a higher arteriovenous oxygen difference.[137] Greater muscle blood flow facilitates increased oxygen transport to exercising muscles and thus a decrease in the oxygen content of the mixed venous blood.

Hemoglobin concentration is lower in children than in the average adult, and this affects the oxygen transport capacity of the blood in children.[139] Studies suggest that total hemoglobin concentration in 11- and 12-year-olds is approximately 78% of that in adults.[139]

Arterial Blood Pressure

Lower exercise blood pressure is seen in children than in adults—a finding consistent with lower CO and stroke volume. Blood pressure may also be reduced because of lower peripheral vascular resistance secondary to shorter blood vessels.[17]

Ventilation

Ventilation is the rate of exchange of air between the lungs and ambient air, measured in liters per minute. In absolute terms, ventilation increases with age. Ventilation normalized by body weight is the same for children and adults at maximal activity.[17] At submaximal exercise levels, ventilation is higher in children and decreases with age, suggesting that children have a lower ventilatory reserve than do adults. Studies suggest that children have less efficient ventilation than do adults (i.e., more air is needed to supply 1 L of oxygen in a child than in an adult).[17]

Vital Capacity

Vital capacity in a 5-year-old child is about 20% of that in an adult and increases with age. It is highly correlated with body size, particularly height,[107] and generally has not been found to be a limiting factor in exercise performance.

Respiratory Rate

Children have a higher respiratory rate than do adults during both maximal and submaximal exercise. A high rate of respiration compensates for decreased lung volume; respiratory rate decreases as lung volume increases.[17]

Blood Lactate

Blood and muscle lactate levels are lower in children than in adults.[11,84,83] It has been suggested but not confirmed that lactate production is related to testosterone production and therefore to sexual maturity in boys. Low lactate production in children could limit glycolytic capacity and thus contribute to reduced anaerobic capacity.

Table 6-2 summarizes comparisons between children and adults for various cardiopulmonary variables. Growth and maturation play a vital part in determining the values of these variables. Despite size differences between adults and children (which might lead one to believe that oxygen

transport in children is less efficient because they are smaller), optimal oxygen transport is maintained by highly integrated functions between the cardiopulmonary and musculoskeletal systems.

REVIEW OF TESTS OF PHYSICAL FITNESS

It has now been longer than 50 years since the first U.S. national youth fitness battery was published.[7] Once emphasizing motor fitness and the readiness of youth for military service, the transition of fitness testing to health-related fitness with a public health emphasis began in the 1970s. The National Children and Youth Fitness Study Tests I and II[209,211] remains the most recent effort to measure national youth fitness levels. The prevalence of national physical fitness testing in U.S. schools at the turn of the 21st century was approximately 65% across all school levels.[179,131] Comparison of nationally and regionally used health-related fitness tests can be found elsewhere.[102] The two national youth physical fitness tests recognized as a result of professional and scientific decisions over the past half century are the President's Challenge[200,201] and the FITNESSGRAM[178]/ACTIVITYGRAM.[60,61] A third program, Physical Best,[108] developed concurrently with the others, has since discontinued its assessment component.[179,180] Each test emphasizes health-related fitness components. The common President's Challenge and the FITNESSGRAM will be reviewed in relation to the National Children and Youth Fitness Studies. Most tests provide some information regarding interrater reliability. The validity of health-related fitness components has previously been reviewed.[125] A comparison of the tests and their components is presented in Table 6-3.

AAHPERD Physical Best Program

(http://www.aahperd.org/naspe/professionaldevelopment/physicalBest/index.cfm)

This program, originally designed to be both a physical fitness measure and an educational program to promote health and prevent disease, was developed by the American Alliance for Health, Physical Education, Recreation, and Dance (AAHPERD).[6] In 1993, AAPHERD adopted the FITNESSGRAM to measure physical fitness status and no longer uses its original fitness battery. The Physical Best Program remains active in its educational component to promote youth fitness.

FITNESSGRAM Program

(http://www.fitnessgram.net/overview/)

This test is a battery that uses criterion-referenced standards. The program was developed by the Cooper Institute for Aerobics Research.[60] Since its initial development, it has been revised twice, most recently in 2007.[60] Extensive information on the reliability and validity of the specific standards for all fitness components can be found in the test manual and has been published separately. Development of

TABLE 6-2   Cardiopulmonary Function Variables and Response to Exercise in Children

Function	Child vs. Adult Response	Sex Differences
Heart rate (max, submax)	Higher	M = F (max); F > M (submax)
Stroke volume (max, submax)	Lower	M > F
Cardiac output (max, submax)	Lower, similar	
Arteriovenous difference (submax)	Similar	
Blood flow to active muscle	Higher	M = F
Blood pressure	Lower	
Hemoglobin concentration	Lower	
Ventilation/kg body wt (max)	Similar	
Ventilation/ kg body wt (submax)	Higher	
Respiratory rate (max, submax)	Higher	
Tidal volume and vital capacity (max)	Lower	
Tidal volume and vital capacity (submax)	Lower	
Blood lactate levels (max, submax)	Similar/lower	M > F after puberty
	Lower	

Adapted from Bar-Or, O. (1963). *Pediatric sports medicine for the practitioner* (pp. 19, 31, 46). New York: Springer-Verlag.
max, Maximal exercise; *submax,* submaximal exercise.

TABLE 6-3 **Review of Current Physical Fitness Tests**

Test	Component of Fitness	Test Items	Standard	Reliability/ Validity
FITNESSGRAM (Cooper Institute for Aerobics Research, 1988, 2007)	Aerobic capacity Lower back flexibility Upper flexibility Upper body strength Abdominal strength Trunk strength Body composition	1-mile walk/run PACER* Walk test Sit and reach Shoulder stretch Modified pull-up Flexed arm hang 90° push-up Curl-up Trunk lift Skinfold measurement Body mass index *Progressive Aerobic Cardiovascular Endurance Run	Criterion	(Welk & Meredith, 2008)
National Child and Youth Fitness Study (Ross & Gilbert, 1985; Ross & Pate, 1987)	Cardiorespiratory endurance Lower back flexibility Upper body strength/endurance Abdominal strength/endurance Body composition	1-mile walk-run Half-mile walk-run Sit and reach Modified pull-up Bent knee sit-up Sum of skinfolds (triceps/subscapular/calf)	U.S. norms (for ages 6 to 18 yr)	(Ross, Katz, & Gilbert,1985; Ross et al., 1987)
President's Challenge (President's Council on Physical Fitness and Sports, 1987, 2009)	Cardiorespiratory endurance Lower back flexibility Upper body strength/endurance Abdominal strength/endurance Ability/power Body composition	1-mile walk-run V-sit Sit and reach Right-angle push-up Pull-up Curl-up Partial curl-up Shuttle run Body mass index	U.S. norms (for ages 6 to 18 yr)	General terms of validity reported; no specifics

the standards is also described.[274] All are based on rigorous use of scientific methods. For example, aerobic capacity standards development was based on determining (1) the lowest level of the laboratory standard for aerobic capacity (VO_{2max}) consistent with minimal risk of disease and adequate functional capacity; (2) the timing standards of the mile walk-run and progressive aerobic cardiovascular endurance run, consistent with the minimal VO_{2max}; and (3) a comparison of the standards with available national normative data to evaluate both consistency and accuracy. Standards using the FITNESSGRAM for individuals with disabilities are being developed, but progress has not been rapid.[223,278]

National Children, Youth, and Fitness Study (NCYFS) I and II

These tests were used in national studies undertaken to assess current levels of physical fitness of children and youth

in the United States and remain the most recent effort to assess national youth fitness levels.[193,208] Initiated by the U.S. Office of Disease Prevention and Health Promotion, the results have been used to set appropriate targets for improved health and fitness. NCYFS I produced normative data by sex and age and by sex and grade for children and youth age 10 to 18 years, and NCYFS II provided the same information for children age 6 to 9 years. Training procedures were developed for test administrators, and Pearson correlation interrater reliability estimates were found to be 0.99 for body composition measurements. Concurrent validity of the distance run and VO_{2max} for children of elementary school age had already been established.[126]

The President's Challenge
(http://www.presidentschallenge.org/)

This is a norm-referenced test created by the President's Council on Physical Fitness and Sports.[200,201] Standards continue to be based on data from the National Children, Youth, and Fitness Studies.[193,208] It remains the most commonly used fitness test among states in the United States that require fitness testing.[179]

COMPARISON OF TESTS

All tests measure similar components of health-related fitness. Each includes items for testing cardiorespiratory endurance, muscular strength and endurance, body composition, and flexibility. The tests differ in the reference standard used. Tests are either norm-referenced (performance is compared with that of a national U.S. sample of children taking the same test) or criterion-referenced (performance is compared with a preset standard consistent with fitness). The criterion for each item is independent of the performance of other children on the same test. The FITNESS-GRAM is the only criterion-referenced test.

Appropriate reliability and validity data are available for FITNESSGRAM, but not for the President's Challenge. Users must be cautious in interpreting scores and their meaning. Procedures for evaluating the reliability and validity of criterion-referenced tests are available.[215]

COMPONENTS OF PHYSICAL FITNESS

The components of health-related fitness, as mentioned earlier, are cardiorespiratory endurance, muscular strength and endurance, flexibility, and body composition. The following information will be reviewed for each component:
1. The criterion measure of the component
2. Laboratory measurement
3. Developmental aspects of the component and standards by age
4. Field measurement of the component and its validity in relation to the criterion measure
5. Standards by age as determined by the FITNESSGRAM program, a computer-scored fitness test with a health-related focus
6. Physical activities with high correlation to the particular fitness component
7. Response to training
8. Assessment of the component in children with disabilities

CARDIORESPIRATORY ENDURANCE

Criterion Measure

The most widely used criterion measure for cardiorespiratory endurance is directly measured VO_{2max}, or maximal oxygen uptake. This component measures the capabilities of the cardiovascular and pulmonary systems and is significant because oxygen supply to the tissues depends on the efficiency and capacity of these systems. VO_{2max} is the highest rate of oxygen consumed by the body in a given time period during exercise of a significant portion of body muscle mass.[139] It defines the limits of oxygen utilization by exercising muscle and serves as the fundamental marker of physiologic aerobic fitness.[213] Cardiorespiratory endurance is so important to overall fitness that many people view physical fitness as being synonymous with cardiorespiratory endurance.[228]

Laboratory Measurement

Laboratory measurement techniques include measurement of VO_{2max} with the use of an ergometer during progressive exercise to the point of exhaustion. This method is referred to as *direct determination of VO_{2max}*. Indirect determination methods predict VO_{2max} from submaximal exercise.

Direct Determination

An ergometer is a device that measures the amount of work performed under controlled conditions. The two devices commonly available are a cycle ergometer and a treadmill. The cycle ergometer has the advantage of being relatively inexpensive and portable, but compared with the treadmill it exercises a smaller total muscle mass. With the cycle ergometer, local fatigue develops (primarily in knee extensors), resulting in premature termination of the testing. Depending on the source, values of VO_{2max} are reported to be 5% to 30% lower on a cycle ergometer than on a treadmill.[17,41,139] For children, the coordination and rhythm, or cadence, required on a cycle ergometer are sometimes difficult to achieve. Both the treadmill and the cycle ergometer present problems when used to test populations with disabilities, in particular those with impairments of balance or coordination.

A variety of protocols for direct determination can be used with children. The most common protocol is one in which resistance, inclination, speed, or height is increased every 1 to 3 minutes without interruption until the child can no longer maintain the activity. In interrupted protocols, which are sometimes used, there is an interruption between each successive increment of exercise. Examples of some common direct determination protocols are given in Table 6-4. The main criterion for indicating that VO_{2max} has been achieved during a progressive protocol is that an increase in power load is not accompanied by an increased VO_2 (usually 2 mL/kg/min or higher).[139] Astrand,[11] however, reported that 5% of all children tested failed to reach a plateau in VO_2, even though evidence from secondary criteria suggested that exhaustion had been reached.

Despite the difficulty of determining attainment of VO_{2max}, studies suggest that the reliability of direct determination testing with children is high. Coefficients of variation of 3%, 5%, and 8% for VO_{2max} determined by treadmill walk-jogging, running, and walking, respectively, have been reported.[195] A mean variation of 4.5% was reported for children exercising to exhaustion on a cycle ergometer on 12 different occasions.[62]

TABLE 6-4 **Direct Determination All-Out Protocols**

Bruce Treadmill Protocol

Stage	Speed, mph	Grade, %	Duration, min
1	1.7	10	3
2	2.5	12	3
3	3.4	14	3
4	4.2	16	3
5	5.0	18	3
6	5.5	20	3
7	6.0	22	3

McMaster Progressive Continuous Cycling Test

Body Height, cm	Initial Load, watts	Increments, watts	Durations, min
<119.9	12.5	12.5	2
120-139.9	12.5	25.0	2
140-159.9	25.0	25.0	2
>160	25.0	25.0 (F) 50.0 (M)	2

Adapted from Bar-Or, O. (1983). Appendix II: Procedures for exercise testing in children. In O. Bar-Or (Ed.), *Pediatric sports medicine for the practitioner* (pp. 315–341). New York: Springer-Verlag.
watts, Joules per second.

TABLE 6-5 **Indirect Determination Protocols**

*Adams Submaximal Progressive Continuous Cycling Test**

Body Weight, kg	Stage, watts	Stage 2, watts	Stage 3, watts
30	16.5	33.0	50.0
30-39.9	16.5	50.0	83.0
40-59.9	16.5	50.0	100.0
>60	16.5	83.0	133.0

Stage duration = 6 min
Performance by W_{170}

Modified 3-Minute Step Test†

Stage	Duration, min	Ascent Rate, ascents/min
1	3	22
2	3	26
3	3	30

Step height dependent on height
Performance by recovery heart rate

*Adapted from Bar-Or, O. (1983). Appendix II: Procedures for exercise testing in children. In O. Bar-Or (Ed.), *Pediatric sports medicine for the practitioner* (pp. 315–341). New York: Springer-Verlag.
†Adapted and reprinted by permission from Francis, K., & Culpepper, M. (1989). Height adjusted, rate specific, single stage, step test for predicting maximal oxygen consumption. *Southern Medical Journal, 82*, 602–606.

Indirect Determination

Indirect determination methods use submaximal exercise to indirectly predict VO_{2max}. The child is not taken to his or her self-imposed maximum. Heart rate during one or more stages is the variable most commonly used to derive the index of VO_{2max}. Step tests for children are usually submaximal tests, with recovery heart rate used to predict VO_{2max}. Evidence suggests that height-specific step tests can be reliable predictors of VO_{2max}.[101] Important limitations exist, however, in predicting VO_{2max} from submaximal exercise data, and these should always be kept in mind.[280] Examples of test protocols are presented in Table 6-5.

The W_{170} is an index used to predict mechanical power in a submaximal test. Two or more measurements of heart rate are obtained at different powers or workloads, and heart rate is then extrapolated to 170 bpm. The corresponding power is W_{170}. This index, originally described by Wahlund,[271] is based on the assumption that heart rate is linearly related to power at 170 bpm or less. To minimize error, more than two heart rate measurements are taken, one of which is as close as possible to 170 bpm.

More recently, maximal power (as measured during a maximal exercise test on a cycle ergometer) has been advocated, used, and validated as a surrogate for direct measurement of VO_{2max}. This method has been used both in able-bodied children and in children with obesity.[72]

Developmental Aspects of Cardiorespiratory Endurance

Absolute maximal oxygen uptake, or VO_{2max}, increases with age throughout childhood and is slightly higher in boys than in girls.[139,214,226] Initial differences during early childhood are approximately 10%, increasing to 25% by age 14 years, and exceeding 50% by age 16.[139] The development of a greater muscle mass in boys and increasing differences in the amount of time spent in vigorous physical exercise are the most commonly given explanations. Overall, the physical working capacity of children increases approximately eightfold between the ages of 6 and 12 years. Few data are available on VO_{2max} for children younger than age 6.[2,213]

Relative to body weight, only a 1% change in VO_{2max} is noted between the ages of 6 and 16 years for boys (52.8 mL/kg/min at age 6; 53.5 mL/kg/min at age 16), whereas girls display a 12% reduction between the same ages (52.0 mL/kg/min at age 6; 40.5 mL/kg/min at age 16).[139,226] VO_{2max} is highly correlated with lean body mass. The decline in VO_{2max} in girls begins around age 10, when changes in body composition occur as girls develop a relatively increased amount of subcutaneous fat. When VO_{2max} is measured with reference to lean body mass, the difference in values between the sexes disappears.[41]

Although the increases in body dimensions of the heart, lungs, and exercising muscle are primarily responsible for the rise in VO_{2max} during the course of childhood, evidence indicates that other factors also contribute. When same-sex adolescents of different ages with identical body weight or body height are compared, the positive relationship with age remains.[236] Functional changes in cardiovascular, pulmonary, and musculoskeletal systems resulting in improved efficiency with maturity may play a role. Cooper and colleagues,[59] however, suggested that the functional components of body systems are integrated so that aerobic capacity is optimized throughout the growth process.

Measurement in the Field

The most common measure of cardiorespiratory fitness in the field is a long-distance run of various structures or lengths. All the physical fitness batteries reviewed previously have a distance run test, commonly a 1-mile run. Test-retest reliability of VO_{2max} during field testing has been shown to be between .60 and .95.[63,216] Construct and concurrent validity with VO_{2max} of 9- and 12-minute run tests in elementary children have also been established.[126,215] Estimation of peak oxygen consumption based on 1-mile run/walk performance is commonly used,[64] but a recent study has shown that this equation systematically underestimates peak oxygen consumption in endurance-trained children and adolescents with high peak oxygen consumption. This suggests than an alternate method should be applied to children in this category.[54]

The Progressive Aerobic Cardiovascular Endurance Run (PACER) is an alternative to the 1-mile walk/run test used in the FITNESSGRAM battery. Aerobic performance is estimated on a series of seven 20-meter runs of incrementally increased exercise intensity. Criterion-referenced reliability and equivalency of the PACER were found to be similar to the 1-mile walk/run test in a group of high school students.[24] When examined sequentially by repeated measures, aerobic performance using the PACER is noted to fluctuate over a 12-month period, likely the result of changing patterns of intensity and type of physical activity.[48]

Standards by Age

Standards of performance are determined by ranking a child's performance in relation to the performance of a group of children tested on the same test (norm-referenced standard) or against an established criterion found to be consistent with good health (criterion-referenced standard). One advantage of criterion-referenced standards is that they are independent of the proportion of the population that meets the standards. A ranking by a norm-referenced standard does not necessarily represent a desirable level of fitness or performance. The limitation of criterion-referenced standards,

however, is that they are somewhat arbitrary and that the criteria used in the current physical fitness tests differ from one another.[65] Establishing the validity of criterion-referenced standards for performance is in progress.

Cureton and Warren[65] described the procedures for development of criterion standards for the FITNESSGRAM Program. Validity coefficients for the FITNESSGRAM Program range from .73 to 1.00 when compared with the criterion standard of VO_{2max}. The actual percentage of VO_{2max} that is used during the walk/run test, however, is unknown, which makes evaluation of any or all values difficult. A comparison of walk/run standards by age is provided in Table 6-6.

Physical Activities

Activities that are highly correlated with development of cardiorespiratory endurance are boxing, running, rowing, swimming, cross-country skiing, and bicycling. The common component among these activities is a prolonged, sustained demand on the cardiorespiratory system that requires general stamina.

Response to Training

Debate exists over whether maximal aerobic power of prepubescence is a component that can be affected by training. Research results are equivocal. Those studies that report improvement in aerobic power with training suggest that the principles of training of children before puberty (i.e., frequency, intensity, and duration) are similar to those for adults.[228] The functional results of conditioning on the cardiorespiratory system include decreased heart rate, increased stroke volume, improved respiratory muscular endurance, and decreased respiration rate.[17,41] A more specific focus on conditioning and training will be found later in this chapter.

Assessment of Cardiorespiratory Endurance in Children with Disabilities

Children with disabilities often exhibit decreased or limited exercise capacity relative to their nondisabled peers. This can result from limited participation in exercise, which leads to deconditioning, or the specific pathologic factors of their disability that limit exercise-related functions. Regardless of the cause, children with disabilities often enter a cycle of decreased activity that precipitates loss of fitness and further decreases in activity levels.

Pathophysiologic factors that may limit cardiorespiratory endurance can sometimes be separated by the specific component of the Fick equation that they affect. This provides a convenient way to categorize conditions or diseases by the fitness components they affect most[19,21] (Figure 6-1). Studies suggest that maximal aerobic uptake is limited not only by central mechanisms of the cardiopulmonary system but also by peripheral mechanisms controlling blood flow, excitation processes in the muscle fiber, local fatigue, and enzyme availability.[219,241] When limitations or reductions in VO_{2max} in

TABLE 6-6   **One-Mile Walk/Run Standards**

Age, yr	Criterion* Standard		FITNESSGRAM† Field Standard		NCYFS I, II‡ Percentiles	
	M	**F**	**M**	**F**	**M**	**F**
5			§	§	–	–
6			§	§	–	–
7			§	§	–	–
8			§	§	15	15
9			§	§	20	20
10	42.0	39.0	11:30	12:30	25	35
11	42.0	38.0	11:00	12:00	20	40
12	42.0	37.0	10:30	12:00	30	30
13	42.0	36.0	10:00	11:30	20	35
14	42.0	35.0	9:30	11:00	35	50
15	42.0	35.0	9:00	10:30	25	55
16	42.0	35.0	8:30	10:00	20	50
17	42.0	35.0	8:30	10:00	30	50

Adapted from the Cooper Institute. (2007). *FITNESSGRAM/ACTIVITYGRAM test administration manual* (4th ed.). Champaign IL: Human Kinetics; Ross, J. G., Dotson, C. O., Gilbert, C. G., & Katz, S. J. (1985). The National Youth and Fitness Study I: New standards for fitness measurement. *Journal of Physical Education, Recreation and Dance, 56,* 62–66; Ross, J. G., Delpy, L. A., Christenson, G. M., Gold, R. S., & Damberg, C. L. (1987). The National Youth and Fitness Study II: Study procedures and quality control. *Journal of Physical Education, Recreation and Dance, 58,* 57–62.
*Criterion standard as set by FITNESSGRAM in ml/kg/min of oxygen uptake. Values reported are minimum for the Healthy Fitness Zone.
†Minutes required to complete a 1-mile walk-run. Times reported are minimum for the Healthy Fitness Zone.
‡Percentile rank of children performing this standard in National Children, Youth, and Fitness Study (NCYES) I, II.
§Completion of distance. Time standards not recommended.

children with disabilities are considered, both central and peripheral limitations must be considered.

Cerebral Palsy

Directly measured maximal aerobic capacity of children and adolescents with CP is 10% to 30% less than that of control subjects. The measurements have been shown to be reliable.[22,121,157,261] It seems that peripheral mechanisms related to the neuromuscular disorder itself are more likely to contribute to decreased capacity than are central cardiopulmonary mechanisms, although this has not been studied.

When indirectly assessed from submaximal heart rate, the aerobic capacity of adolescents was found to be reduced by 50%.[157] Low mechanical efficiency, however, creates disproportionately high submaximal heart rates in individuals with CP, making submaximal heart rate a poor predictor of maximal aerobic power.[18] Submaximal exercise tests, in general, underestimate aerobic capacity in poorly trained individuals.[11] Numerous studies suggest that heart rate is a good predictor or an appropriate substitute clinical measure of oxygen uptake because of its linear relationship to heart rate.[205,206] It is not a measure of maximal aerobic capacity, however, and therefore it is not an alternative measure of cardiorespiratory fitness.

An increase in blood flow to exercising muscles after conditioning is a response observed in children with CP but not seen in able-bodied children.[158] Spastic muscles of individuals with adult-onset brain damage exhibit subnormal blood flow during exercise.[143] Whether the rate of blood flow changes after conditioning in individuals with adult-onset brain injury is not known. One hypothesis to explain the increase in blood flow in conditioned individuals with CP is that it results from a decrease in spasticity. More rapid

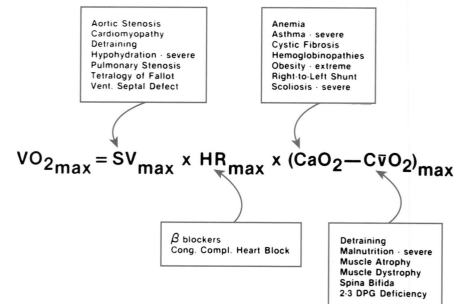

Figure 6-1 Maximal aerobic power (VO_{2max}) and pathology. The Fick equation and specific pathologic conditions that affect its variables and reduce VO_{2max} are shown. (From Bar-Or, O. [1983]. Exercise as a diagnostic tool in pediatrics. In O. Bar-Or [Ed.]. *Pediatric sports medicine for the practitioner* [p. 72]. New York: Springer-Verlag.)

deterioration of maximal aerobic uptake is seen after discontinuation of training in children with CP than in able-bodied children.[18]

Functional assessments that relate to the cardiorespiratory fitness of children with various disabilities are becoming more commonplace. The Pediatric Orthopedic Society of North America developed a functional outcomes questionnaire directed toward assessment of pediatric musculoskeletal conditions.[66] Within this questionnaire are queries regarding a child's ability to complete a 1-mile and a 3-mile walk. As more professionals caring for children with disabilities incorporate this assessment and others like it in daily practice, insight will be gained that may assist in determination of cardiorespiratory fitness. The 6-minute walk test has been used in children with CP as a submaximal test of capacity.[248] Standards for field testing aerobic capacity in individuals with CP using a long-distance run have been previously published for children age 10 to 17 years.[278] The manual for the Brockport Physical Fitness Test[277] includes standards for children with a variety of disabilities. Seaman and colleagues[223] present a review of alternative test items that can be used to assess aerobic capacity in children with various disabilities, including CP.

Juvenile Rheumatoid Arthritis

Maximal aerobic capacity measured by cycle ergometry in children with juvenile rheumatoid arthritis has been reported to be 15% to 30% lower than in their peers matched by age, sex, and body surface area.[105,106] No correlation was found between severity of articular disease and aerobic capacity, however. Children with juvenile rheumatoid arthritis have a shorter duration of exercise before exhaustion, which occurs at a lower than normal work rate with a lower peak heart rate. Deficient oxygen extraction from exercising muscles or low blood flow to exercising muscles has been postulated to occur in this population as a result of decreased activity levels.[18,21]

Scoliosis

Chest deformity, decreased lung size, and decreased physical activity are believed to contribute to the lower maximal aerobic capacity of children with advanced scoliosis. No functional or exercise-related deficits are found in children with minor or moderate scoliosis.[18] For those with advanced scoliosis, limitations of 50% to 70% in VO_{2max} have been reported. VO_2 and minute ventilation are decreased and pulmonary artery pressure increased at maximal exercise relative to able-bodied standards. Some improvements are seen with conditioning.

Mental Retardation

Most studies indicate that individuals with mental retardation display lower VO_{2max} scores than do their nondisabled peers[144]; however, significant variability has been reported among individuals with the same level of disability. Technical problems associated with testing individuals with mental retardation are encountered that create difficulties in establishing reliable and valid information. Treadmill testing appears to be the most reliable form of testing. Despite lower VO_{2max} scores, individuals with mental retardation without Down syndrome have been shown to exhibit similar age-related trends and changes as individuals without disability (i.e., decline with age).[23] Field test standards and alternative test items for aerobic capacity in individuals with mild or moderate mental retardation are available.[223,277]

Children with Obesity

The prevalence of obesity in children age 6 to 19 years designated as overweight by the National Health and Nutrition Examination Survey (1999–2002) was estimated at 16.5%, with 31.5% estimated to be at risk of overweight.[120] This is more than three times the target prevalence of the Healthy People 2010 objective. The prevalence of obesity in the United States has nearly doubled in the past two decades.[251] Although obesity is not considered a category of "disability" in traditional terms, public health concerns for this group of young people make it worthy of special attention. Field tests of cardiorespiratory endurance in obese youth using the 1-mile walk/run test demonstrate that they perform below typical standards for nonobese peers.[55,167] Only 34% of obese boys and 38% of obese girls tested fell within the Healthy Fitness Zone of the FITNESSGRAM 1-mile walk/run standards as compared with 73% and 61% of their nonobese counterparts, respectively. Estimation of peak oxygen uptake from the same 1-mile walk/run performance suggested similar results for VO_{2max}.[167] Recent evidence, however, suggests that VO_{2max} values from prediction equations or submaximal exercise tests overestimate actual VO_{2max} when measured on a maximal exercise test.[12] This suggests that the percentage of obese youth that fall within a zone of healthy fitness may actually be less. Racial differences in obese adolescents have also been reported. Black adolescents had significantly lower VO_{2max} and lower hemoglobin than did white adolescents with no differences in maximal heart rate or respiratory exchange ratio.[9]

MUSCULAR STRENGTH AND ENDURANCE

The second component of physical fitness is muscular strength and endurance. Strength is required for movement and has a direct impact on effective performance. Strength is also important for optimal posture and reduced risk of lower back pain, which is the criterion health condition to which this component of physical fitness is linked. Similar to cardiorespiratory endurance, positive relationships between musculoskeletal fitness and health status in adults have been demonstrated.[91,130] The theoretical link between fatigue-resistant trunk muscles (abdominal flexors and trunk extensors) and healthy low back function, however, is stronger than the research evidence between muscular strength and flexibility and the onset or recurrence of low back pain.[199] No critical level of strength or muscular endurance for good health has been identified.

Muscular strength, *muscular endurance*, and *muscular power* are not synonymous terms. Muscular strength refers to maximal contractile force. Muscular endurance is the ability of muscles to perform work and assumes some component of muscular strength. Muscular power refers to the ability to release maximal muscular force within a specified time. As velocity increases or time decreases (for maximal muscular force to be obtained), power increases. Because muscular endurance and muscular power have their basis in muscular strength, strength is the primary focus of this discussion.

Laboratory Measurement

The laboratory standard for muscular strength is measurement by dynamometry. Tests include isometric dynamometry, isokinetic dynamometry, and single-repetition maximal isotonic dynamometry. Most measurements are made on specific, selected muscles, and then results are extrapolated to give "whole body" strength. Unfortunately, a limitation for setting standards of strength is that force measurements depend on the type of dynamometer used.[32] The most commonly selected measures are hand grip, elbow flexion and extension, knee flexion and extension, and plantar flexion strength.

Isokinetic strength testing during childhood and adolescence is a relatively new area of study. The reliability of isokinetic testing in children presents unique issues because of the variability of muscle coordination and neuromuscular maturation. Coefficients of variation from 5% to 11% have been reported.[32] Children demonstrate the capacity to perform consistent maximal voluntary contraction under controlled conditions by age 6 to 7 years. The limited amount of research and the lack of available data do not allow definite conclusions on the effects of age and gender differences on isokinetic strength development. Body weight and muscle cross-sectional area, however, appear to correlate positively with isokinetic strength. Gender differences are minimal between ages 7 and 11. After age 13, boys tend to have greater isokinetic strength for the muscles tested than do girls.[14,245]

Developmental Aspects and Standards by Age

Grip Strength

Grip strength is the most commonly reported upper extremity strength measure in children. Absolute strength scores, however, are highly sensitive to the type of dynamometer used and to its positioning, making the results of studies difficult to compare. In general, single-hand grip strength increases from an average of approximately 5 kg for children at age 3 years to 45 kg for boys at age 17 and 30 kg for girls at age 17. Bilateral grip strength has been measured at a mean of 25 kg for children at age 7 years, increasing to an average

of 95 kg for boys and 50 kg for girls by age 17 years.[32,164] The rate of increase in strength for boys rises dramatically at puberty. This finding is confirmed in the Longitudinal Experimental Growth Study, where a marked acceleration of strength or a strength spurt was noted around the age of peak height velocity. The maximal increase in static strength occurs approximately 1 year later.[245] Absolute values of the developmental range of strength across childhood were measured to be slightly larger. Pearson correlations to static strength in adulthood were reported to be fair to high, depending on whether individuals were noted to be early, average, or late-maturing.

Elbow Flexion and Extension

Isometric elbow flexion strength is greater than isometric elbow extension strength throughout childhood and adolescence, and the difference between them increases with increasing age.[99] The extension/flexion strength ratio for boys is approximately 0.76 at the age of 7.5 years and decreases to 0.57 during late adolescence. No data are available for girls.

Shoulder Flexion and Extension

A single study has addressed isokinetic strength values for shoulder flexion and extension in children.[44] Twenty-four untrained, prepubescent boys with an average age of 11.7 years were tested on a Cybex II (Ronkonkoma, NY) at six different velocities. Mean values for peak torque for shoulder extension were relatively constant at speeds of between 60°/s and 150°/s (13.2 and 13.7 newton-meters); mean values for shoulder flexion increased as speed increased (12.5 to 24.3 newton-meters).

Knee Flexion and Extension

Isokinetic knee flexion strength and knee extension strength also increase throughout childhood. Results from Alexander and Molnar[3] and Molnar and Alexander[175] indicated that knee extension strength exceeds knee flexion strength for both sexes at all ages. Average knee flexion strength varies from 30% to 50% of average knee extension strength for girls and from 28% to 65% for boys. Boys have slightly greater strength than do girls before puberty but consistently greater strength from the age of 10 years onward.

Trunk Flexion and Extension

Few data are available for laboratory dynamometry standards for trunk strength in children. Clinical data have been collected for the ability of children to sustain isometric trunk flexion (actually a test of muscular endurance) between the ages of 3 and 7 years.[145] An isotonic test of the number of hook-lying sit-ups performed was also included in the study. Both the endurance for isometric trunk flexion and the ability to perform sit-ups improved with age. The greatest improvement occurred between the ages of 5 and 6 years, when average performance at least doubled. These results are important because the typical field test for muscular strength and endurance is performance of sit-ups or curl-ups.

Composite Strength

Composite strength provides a measure of overall or general strength and consists of a total strength score from several muscle groups. Usually, grip strength, thrust strength (shoulder girdle), and shoulder pull measures are included in composite strength scores.[55,90] Unfortunately, I can find no measures of composite strength that include lower extremity or trunk strength. The pattern of increase in composite strength during childhood is similar to that of grip strength.

Evoked Responses

A second method for muscular function assessment in the laboratory is by evoked responses from electrical stimulation. Muscle contractile characteristics, including force production, are studied with this method. Few data are available for children.[32,34]

Developmental Aspects of Muscular Strength and Endurance

A description of the development of the musculoskeletal system is found in Chapter 5 of this volume. Development of strength depends on the development of force production and is influenced by numerous factors, for example, the muscle's cross-sectional area.[186] Muscular strength in absolute terms increases linearly with chronologic age from early childhood in both sexes to approximately age 13 to 14 years. Increases in strength are closely related to increases in muscle mass during growth. Boys have greater strength than do girls at all ages (seen as early as age 3 years) and have larger absolute and relative amounts of muscle (kilogram of muscle per kilogram of body weight).[32,186,245] The sex difference in relative strength (per kilogram of body mass) before puberty is caused at least in part by a higher proportion of body fat in girls from midchildhood onward—a difference similar to the trend in cardiorespiratory endurance.[94,184] Rarick and Thompson[203] suggested that boys are 11% to 13% stronger than girls during childhood. This value reaches 20% by adulthood for strength per cross-sectional area of muscle.[168] Correlates and determinants of strength are thought to include age, body size, muscle size, muscle fiber type and size, muscle contractile properties, and biomechanical influences.

During adolescence, a marked acceleration in development of strength occurs, particularly in boys. Boys between the ages of 10 and 16 years who were followed longitudinally showed a 23% increase in strength per year. Peak growth in muscle mass occurred during and after peak weight gain, but maximal strength development occurred after peak velocity of growth in height and weight, suggesting that muscle tissue increases first in mass and then in strength.[52,160,245] Girls generally show peak strength development before peak weight gain.[90] Overall muscle mass increases more than five times in males from childhood to adulthood; the increase in females is 3.5 times.

Differentiation in strength between the sexes at puberty is caused, at least in part, by differences in hormonal concentrations, particularly testosterone. Hormones other than the male sex steroids also make an important contribution.[93] Unfortunately, no pediatric studies to date have correlated age-associated changes in endocrinologic function with muscle size and muscular strength.

Measurement in the Field

Field measurements of muscular strength usually entail movement of part or all of the body mass against gravity. The two common tests for muscular strength are the flexed arm hang and the curl-up. The curl-up has replaced the sit-up as the common field test item in recent years. All fitness tests previously reviewed include a curl-up test and a pull-up or flexed arm hang test. The FITNESSGRAM also includes a trunk lift test for back strength. The correlation between abdominal strength and endurance and shoulder girdle strength as measures of absolute strength for physical fitness is not well established. Although strength is considered an important part of physical fitness, the standards to meet minimal fitness requirements in this area are the least clear. This has resulted from lack of quantitative research in this area. Available data for reliability and validity of the curl-up and sit-up, tests of trunk extension, and upper arm and shoulder assessments are well outlined by Plowman. Results are variable. In some cases, such as for trunk extension, data on children are lacking.[199]

Curl-ups/Sit-ups

The exact relationship between curl-up performance and abdominal strength and endurance is unclear. How abdominal strength is related to a given number of curl-ups is unknown. Test-retest reliability estimates for sit-ups measured for 11- to 14-year-olds range from 0.64 to 0.94 for both boys and girls.[217]

Chin-ups and Flexed Arm Hang

Controversy exists concerning the validity of chin-ups and the flexed arm hang as measures of upper body strength. One of the difficulties encountered is that the musculature used for performance of a chin-up is different than that used for a modified pull-up, a flexed arm hang, or a 90° push-up. Hand position used can also alter muscle activity. Berger and Medlin[29] suggested that the number of chin-ups as a measure of absolute strength is not valid because body weight is inversely related to the number of chin-ups performed. Considine[58] demonstrated that pull-ups do not provide an indicator of shoulder girdle strength. The NCYFS II developed a modified pull-up test for 6- to 9-year-olds to overcome the problems associated with body weight.[193]

TABLE 6-7   **Field Standards for Strength**

Age, yr	FITNESSGRAM Curl-Ups, Number Completed		FITNESSGRAM Modified Pull-Ups, Number Completed		FITNESSGRAM Flexed Arm Hang, Seconds		FITNESSGRAM 90° Push-Ups, Number Completed	
	F	M	F	M	F	M	F	M
5	2	2	2	2	2	2	3	3
6	2	2	2	2	2	2	3	3
7	4	2	3	3	3	3	4	4
8	6	6	4	4	3	3	5	5
9	9	9	4	5	4	4	6	6
10	12	12	4	5	4	4	7	7
11	15	15	4	6	6	6	7	8
12	18	18	4	7	7	10	7	10
13	18	21	4	8	8	12	7	12
14	18	24	4	9	8	15	7	14
15	18	24	4	10	8	15	7	16
16	18	24	4	12	8	15	7	18

Data adapted from The Cooper Institute. (2007). *FITNESSGRAM/ACTIVITYGRAM test administration manual* (4th ed.). Champaign IL: Human Kinetics.

Standards by Age

The standards of performance for the FITNESSGRAM Program are listed in Table 6-7.

Branta and colleagues[42] assessed the performance of children on the flexed arm hang as part of a longitudinal study of age changes in motor skills during childhood and adolescence. A general increase in mean performance was noted throughout childhood in both sexes. The greatest gains occurred between the ages of 5 and 6 years and 12 and 13 years for girls and between 5 and 6, 7 and 8, and 13 and 14 years for boys. Both groups showed substantial improvements in performance at puberty. Sex differences were apparent by age 8 years. Relative gains across the age span were substantially higher for boys than for girls.

Physical Activities

Activities that have a high correlation with muscular strength are gymnastics, jumping, sprinting, weight lifting, and wrestling. Local muscular endurance is affected by cycling, figure skating, and middle-distance running.

Response to Training

Training-induced increases in strength can be influenced by numerous factors, including enhancement of motivation, improvement in coordination, increase in number of contractile proteins per cross-sectional area of muscle, and hypertrophy of muscle.[174] Gains in strength and muscle mass can be achieved by children with training at or after puberty. Prepubescent children also show improvements in force output with training but appear to have difficulty in increasing muscle mass.[19,218] Strength improvements in prepubescent children have thus been attributed to neurologic adaptations to training and improved motor unit activation rather than to increased cross-sectional area of muscle.[32,138] Direct evidence for the role of neurologic adaptation during strength training has been documented by increases in integrated electromyographic amplitudes and maximal isokinetic strength following an 8-week strength program.[189] Because the magnitude of change in neuromuscular activation is generally smaller than the observed increase in strength, it has been postulated that improved movement coordination is a contributor to strength gains, particularly in complex multijoint exercises.[34] Neuromuscular maturation in the prepubescent child is therefore an important contributor to strength and should not be underestimated.

Controversy has existed regarding the safety and efficacy of strength training programs for children and adolescents for a number of years. The American Academy of Pediatrics Council on Sports Medicine and Fitness has recently published new guidelines.[5] http://pediatrics.aappublications.org/cgi/content/abstract/121/4/835

Assessment of Muscular Strength and Endurance in Children with Disabilities

Muscular strength and endurance are crucial fitness components for walking, lifting, and performing most daily functions. Deficits of muscular strength in children with disabilities are a primary focus for the clinician in an attempt to improve (or maintain) maximum function. It is important to keep in mind, however, that strength as measured clinically is not simply the ability of a muscle to generate force. Strength as measured clinically is the effectiveness of the muscle force to produce movement of the joint. This encompasses both the ability of the muscle to generate force and appropriate skeletal alignment. In children with disabilities, strength deficits result from the muscles' inability to generate force, malalignment of the skeleton, or a combination of both.

Muscular Dystrophy

Strength measurements by dynamometry in children with Duchenne muscular dystrophy (DMD) exhibit progressive deterioration as compared with healthy children.[99] Failure of muscular strength to increase with growth is seen. The result is that the absolute strength in a child with DMD at the age of 16 years is similar to that of a typical 5-year-old.

Serial longitudinal measurements indicate that muscle strength decreases linearly with age approximately 0.25 manual muscle testing units per year from ages 5 to 13 years. Typically, by the time strength declines to grade 4 (manual muscle testing units), isometric strength measures are 40% to 50% of normal control values.[133,169]

Muscular endurance (the ability to sustain static or rhythmic contraction for long periods) is also affected in children with DMD. Ninety-two percent of the children tested by Hosking and colleagues[123] scored below the 5th percentile for strength in holding the head 45° off the ground. Measurement on the Wingate anaerobic cycling test indicates that both peak muscular power and mean muscular power output are significantly less than is typical.[21] The test-retest reliability of this test for various neuromuscular and muscular disease conditions has been established.[250]

Cerebral Palsy

Strength deficits in children with CP are common, and strength profiles for lower extremity muscle groups in children with spastic CP are available.[276] Children with spastic diplegia demonstrated strength values ranging from 16% to 71% of same-age peers depending on the muscle tested. The gluteus maximus and soleus muscles showed the greatest strength deficits. The involved side of children with hemiplegia exhibited values from 22% to 79% of strength values of same-age peers. The gluteus maximus and the anterior tibialis were the weakest muscles.

Inadequate joint moment and power production as measured by computerized gait analysis are seen in children with CP.[104,185,188] These measures provide indirect evidence in a functional context of decreased strength because strength is a prerequisite for moment and power production. Power production by the ankle plantar flexor muscles in terminal stance phase provides a key source of power for forward motion during the typical walking cycle. Power production in terminal stance phase is often reduced in children with CP. Occasionally, inappropriately timed power production results in excessive, but nonproductive, energy expenditure during gait[103] (Figure 6-2).

Muscular endurance is also decreased in CP. Performance on the Wingate anaerobic test in a group of children with CP resulted in averages that were 2 to 4 standard deviations below the mean.[21]

Little information is available regarding modification of lower extremity strength field test items in children with CP. Limited grip strength and flexed arm hang standards are available for upper extremity strength.[223] The United Cerebral Palsy Athletic Association uses functional abilities, including strength, to classify athletes for competition.[254]

Children with Obesity

Performance on field tests of abdominal and upper body muscle strength (curl-up and modified pull-up or flexed arm hang) is poorer for children identified as overweight (≥95% body mass index). Children who were overweight were three times less likely to pass the upper body strength test and 1.5

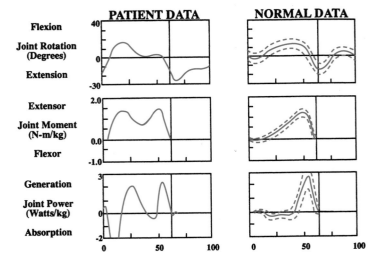

Figure 6-2 Sagittal plane joint rotation (kinematic), joint moment, and power (kinetics) of a child with cerebral palsy versus a normal child. The child's joint moment is biphasic, and the power graph indicates two distinct bursts of power generation instead of one. The first burst is abnormal and functions to drive the center of gravity upward, not forward, which is nonproductive energy expenditure. (From Gage, J. R. [1991]. *Gait analysis in cerebral palsy* [p. 145]. London: MacKeith Press.)

times less likely to pass the abdominal strength test than children who were not overweight.[134] The negative influences of biomechanical factors related to (1) increased body size such as the need to move fat tissue, which acts as an inert load; (2) weakened force production caused by increased mechanical work and moment of inertia due to a higher trunk mass; and (3) the fact that gravity itself may pull the trunk down; in certain tests, all likely contribute to impaired muscle strength and endurance performance.[94] The inverse relationship of obesity to fitness measures of strength is seen across cultures.[38,94,124] An increased incidence of musculoskeletal problems has been reported.[73,140,244]

FLEXIBILITY

The importance of flexibility as a component of health-related fitness is related to prevention of orthopedic impairments later in life, especially lower back pain.[257] Flexible muscles permit proper pelvic rotation, decrease disc compression, and avoid excessive stretch of musculature. Flexibility of the lower back, legs, and shoulders contributes to prevention of injury.[118] Limitations in spinal mobility can interfere with activities of daily living, such as dressing, turning, and driving. Restrictions in back mobility can also contribute to abnormalities in walking.

Criterion Measure

Joint range of motion (ROM) is the criterion used for standards of flexibility. Although ROM measures for adults are well established and can be found in various textbooks,[183] ROM information for the pediatric population correlated with changes in stature is limited. Upper extremity ROM data for children are not well documented. The typical measurement tool is the universal goniometer. A review of the reliability of goniometry is found in Chapter 5 of this text.

Laboratory Measurement and Developmental Aspects of Flexibility

Extremity Range of Motion

Lower extremity passive ROM measurements have been described in the newborn, infant, and toddler.[78,197,273] Newborn infants exhibit hypoextensibility of both hip and knee flexor muscles and increased popliteal angles consistent with the flexed posture in utero. Range increases in the first months of life. Ranges of hip abduction and rotation also differ from adult values. See Chapter 5 for information on ROM values for newborns.

Little to no information has been reported for ROM during childhood. Unpublished data from my laboratory on lower extremity ROM measurements in 140 children between the ages of 2 and 18 years suggest variation in some joints throughout childhood and relative stability in others[238,197] (Table 6-8). Test-retest reliability using Pearson correlations was 0.95, and interrater reliability was .90. Results suggested age and sex differences, with females exhibiting a trend toward greater flexibility at all ages. Greater flexibility of the hamstring muscles in females is especially apparent during the teenage years in straight leg raising and popliteal angle measurements.

Posture and Spinal Mobility

Spinal mobility has been measured in both young children and adolescents.[113,176] The technique of measurement of back mobility uses tape measure distance changes in bony landmark relationships before and after a standardized spinal movement. The concurrent validity of this measurement technique with anterior spinal flexion measured radiographically has been established.[159,176] Anterior spinal flexion appears to remain relatively stable throughout childhood and adolescence, but lateral flexion increases linearly with

TABLE 6-8 **Selected Range of Motion Measurements During Childhood**

Range of Motion Measure	2–5 Years		6–12 Years		13–19 Years	
	M	F	M	F	M	F
Straight leg raise	70	75	65	75	60	70
Popliteal angle (unilateral)*	15	10	30	25	40	25
Abduction†	60	60	50	55	45	50
Internal rotation‡	45	50	50	55	45	45
Femoral antetorsion§	10	15	7	7	0	0

*Supine position.
†Measured with hip extension.
‡Prone position.
§Prone position by lateral placement of the greater trochanter.
Note: All measurements in degrees.

age through adolescence and into early adulthood. Girls were significantly more flexible than boys in both anterior flexion and lateral flexion in the 5- to 9-year-old age group.[113]

The relationship of posture to physical fitness is not often addressed in today's emphasis on health-related fitness. Previous research discussing the relationship of posture to fitness included the importance of posture to trunk strength and the potential for imbalance, back pain, headache, foot pain, and orthopedic deformities.[56,132] Each aspect of posture may be important to mobility and cosmesis in children but becomes of greater importance in adulthood, when impairment can lead to further deformity and loss of function.

The New York State Physical Fitness Test

This test includes a posture assessment method consisting of three profiles of 13 posture areas. The test is used for children in grades 4 through 12. The 13 areas include head, shoulder, spine, hips, feet, and arches in the coronal plane and neck, chest, shoulders, upper back, trunk, abdomen, and lower back in the sagittal plane. The 50th percentile requires good posture scores on more than half the posture items.[57]

The Adams Forward Bending Test

This test is a commonly used screening test for scoliosis. The back is viewed as the individual bends the trunk forward to 90°. The classic sign of scoliosis is the presence of a posterior rib hump during this motion.[31] Although children with scoliosis often develop lack of spinal mobility if the scoliosis becomes severe, the Adams Forward Bending Test is not a test of trunk flexibility per se. Posture is often assessed in children with scoliosis for the presence of lordosis to assess hip flexibility; the presence of pelvic obliquity to assess flexibility of the hip adductors, abductors, and tensor fasciae latae; and the presence of a posterior pelvic tilt to assess hamstring muscle flexibility. For more information on scoliosis, see Chapter 8.

Gross Motor Performance Measure. This instrument, designed as a quality-of-movement companion instrument to the Gross Motor Function Measure, includes postural alignment as one of its performance attributes. A five-point scale of quality is used for assessment of the attribute. This instrument was developed specifically as an examination tool for children with CP.[39,40,110] Interobserver reliability as measured by intraclass correlation and the Kappa statistic has been reported as "fair to good" during patient evaluations and "good to excellent" using video recordings.[231,247] The reader is referred to Chapter 3 for more information.

Measurement in the Field

The field test for measurement of flexibility in tests of physical fitness is the sit and reach test or, more recently, the modified sit and reach test—a measure of hamstring muscle and lower back flexibility. The test measures the distance a child can reach forward (shoulders flexed to 90° and elbows extended) from a long-sit position. Starting position is with

the back straight, hips at 90°. No field test is available for assessment of low back flexibility. All physical fitness batteries used in the United States include some version of a sit and reach test. The intraclass correlation for test-retest reliability of the sit and reach test was found to be high; coefficients between .94 and .99 have been reported.[92,127,159] Jackson and Baker[127] assessed the criterion-related validity of the sit and reach test both for hamstring flexibility and for lower, upper, and total back flexibility. A moderate correlation with measurement of straight leg raising using a flexometer was found for hamstring flexibility (0.64). On the other hand, a low correlation with lower back flexibility (0.28) was found with this protocol developed by Macrae and Wright,[159] using tape measure distance changes in bony landmark relationships before and after a standardized spinal movement as the criterion measure (intraclass correlations). Upper back flexibility and total back flexibility were not correlated with the sit and reach scores. Recently, the criterion-related validity of the sit and reach test and the modified sit and reach test have been questioned.[53,115] Although both tests were found to be related to hamstring flexibility, the explained variance was low. The modified sit and reach test was found not to be a better method than the traditional sit and reach test as an assessment of hamstring flexibility.

Branta and colleagues[42] found sex differences in performance on the sit and reach test in children between 5 and 14 years of age, with girls showing better flexibility than boys at all ages. Girls showed little variability in flexibility from the ages of 5 to 11 years. Boys experienced a net loss of flexibility between the ages of 5 and 15. This is consistent with the goniometric measures of hamstring flexibility noted in my laboratory (Stout, J. L., Phelps, J. A., & Koop, S. E., unpublished data, 1991).

Standards by Age

The criterion standard of performance on the FITNESS-GRAM Program for the modified sit and reach test (back-saver sit and reach test) is 8 inches from the ages of 5 to 17 years in boys and 9 inches in girls. The FITNESSGRAM Program criterion is well below the average score obtained on the NCYFS I and II.[207,208,210]

Physical Activities

Activities that require a high degree of flexibility include figure skating, gymnastics, jumping (track and field), and judo. Stretching is an important part of any exercise program for general warm-up before vigorous activity and to reduce the potential for injury. Possible physiologic mechanisms for the benefits of stretching include increased blood flow to muscles, increased mechanical efficiency of muscle and tendon, and reduction of viscosity within the muscle.[17] Decreased resistance to extension of connective tissue leads to increased efficiency and power output by muscles. Much of this research is on the adult population, but the same principles are believed to apply to children.[19,141,281]

Assessment of Flexibility in Children with Disabilities

For clinicians involved in the rehabilitation (or habilitation) of children with musculoskeletal disorders, maintenance of flexibility or joint ROM is often a primary concern. Almost any musculoskeletal or neuromuscular disorder for which physical therapy is recommended includes treatment for loss of flexibility. Conditions such as CP, juvenile rheumatoid arthritis, muscular dystrophy (MD), or long bone fracture are common examples.

In Chapter 5, both measurement of and the effects of intervention on improving joint ROM in children were addressed. The interrater reliability, as measured by percentage agreement, of joint ROM measurements in children with spasticity has been found to be within the range of 0.50 to 0.85.[10,114] Similar results have been found in adults.[37,82] Because maintenance of flexibility is an important component of most physical therapy programs for children with disabilities, methods for more reliable assessment of joint ROM are needed.

Field test standards for the sit and reach test and suggested modifications for test administration have been published for children with visual impairment, mental retardation, and Down syndrome.[223,277]

Children with Obesity

Performance on field tests of flexibility (back-saver sit and reach test) is similar for children identified as overweight (≥95% body mass index) compared with typical weight or underweight peers.[134] This finding is supported for adolescents as well.[94,163]

BODY COMPOSITION

The term *body composition* is understood to mean total body content of water, protein, fat, and minerals, or the components that make up body weight.[71,109] The major contributors are muscle, bone, and fat content, along with organs, skin, and nerve tissue. In reference to health-related fitness, body composition is used as a measure of body fatness or obesity. Attainment of appropriate body weight for overweight individuals was an explicit objective of Healthy Children 2000 that has actually moved away from its target.[255,256] Healthy People 2020 has maintained objectives related to the nutritional health of adolescents and youth as one of its focus areas.[257] Large discrepancies continue to exist between current nutrition practices and projected targets.[182] Because of the clustering effects of obesity with other risk factors for coronary artery disease, hypertension, and diabetes mellitus, the relevance of obesity to a child's present and future health cannot be overemphasized. The prevalence of childhood and youth obesity is increasing worldwide. In the United States alone, the prevalence of children classified as overweight has increased from 10% in 1988–1994 to 14.4% by 1999–2000

to 16.5% by 2002.[120,184,269] Examination of the extent to which children exceed the overweight threshold indicates that the prevalence of overweight children getting heavier is increasing faster than the prevalence of children becoming overweight.[129] It has been suggested that regional distribution of abdominal fat is an important predictor of mortality, stroke, heart disease, and diabetes.[43]

Laboratory Measurement

The purpose of body composition measurement, whether in the laboratory or in the field, is to obtain a measure of fat-free or lean body mass. Chemical analysis is the only direct method to measure body composition.[136] Because this is expensive and impractical, even laboratory standards of measurement are from indirect assessment. Most standards rely on formulas and models of composition, which assume that fat and lean body mass are constant. Because infants and children exhibit variable, not constant, body composition throughout childhood,[36,116,152,233] numerous problems in determining body composition in children are encountered. Use of adult standards leads to overestimation or underestimation of body fatness, depending on the technique.[36] All methods presented have some limitations for use with children, but all have been used. There is no one "gold standard" for children.

Densitometry

More commonly referred to as underwater or hydrostatic weighing, densitometry determines the density of an individual by dividing actual body weight by the decrease in weight when the person is completely submerged in water. The densities of fat and lean body mass are assumed to be constant and can be calculated for an individual when the density of the whole body is known. Although it is considered the gold standard for measurement of body composition in adults, it has limited applicability to young children because of the requirement for submersion under water.

Total Body Water

The measurement of total body water is used as a means of estimating the nonfat portion of the body because neutral fat does not bind water. Stable isotopes of hydrogen or oxygen are administered orally and then measured to determine the amount of dilution in a body fluid.

Bioelectric Impedance Analysis

This method is based on the principle that impedance to electrical flow varies in proportion to the amount of lean tissue present. A weak electric current is passed through the body, and its impedance is measured.

Dual-Energy X-ray Absorptiometry (DXA)

Using DXA, the body's differential absorption of two low-dose x-rays at different energy levels is measured. The ratios are used to predict total body mass, lean body mass, and bone mineral density. It has fast become a reference standard for measurement of body composition. Despite its wide use, because of variability of software calculations and instrumentation, the continuous change in body composition of children as they grow suggest that DXA has not yet achieved sufficient reproducibility to be considered the gold standard in pediatric studies.[146,227] Cross-validation between DXA and bioelectric impedance analysis in children and adolescents suggests that the methods are not interchangeable but provide useful and complementary assessments of percent body fat. Less reproducibility is found when younger children are assessed.[80,148]

Developmental Aspects of Body Composition

From birth through adolescence, body composition is constantly changing. Part of this change is caused by chemical maturation as a result of increasing mineral mass and hydration of adipose tissue.[233] Chemical maturation occurs after adolescence, when the constants relating one component of body composition to another stabilize until the last decades of life.[35,36,152,230]

The four major components of body composition are water, protein, fat, and mineral. Reference models describe the body composition of these components in the child at various ages.[96,97,116,117,283] A composite of these reference models and changes with growth in males appears in Figure 6-3.

Fat is the most variable component of body composition during infancy and childhood. Increases begin in utero when fat content changes from 2.5% at 1 kg of body weight to 12% at term gestation.[233] The proportion of body fat rises from 12% to an average of 25% from birth to 6 months of age.

Fat content as a proportion of body weight decreases during early childhood as muscle mass increases. Sex differences are noted early in childhood; girls exhibit a greater percentage of fat content than do boys. At 6 to 8 years of age, the average fat content for boys is 13% to 15%, and for girls it is 16% to 18%.[153] During adolescence, fat content increases in girls so that between the ages of 14 and 16 years the mean percentage of fat content is 21% to 23%.

Water content of the body is approximately 89% of body weight at 24 weeks of gestation and drops to 75% at 40 weeks.[233] By 4 months of age, water content stabilizes at approximately 60% to 65% and remains at that level until puberty. Protein content as a proportion of body weight increases from approximately 13% at birth to 15% to 17% at age 10 years. Mineral content of the body rises from 3% at birth to 5% at age 18 years.

Differences between the sexes exist in each major component of body composition throughout childhood and are magnified at adolescence. Major changes during adolescence in both sexes consist of a decrease in the percentage of water and an increase in the percentage of osseous minerals.[116,155]

The influence of rapid growth in fetal and early infancy on fat mass percentage and body composition at 6 months of age has been investigated to gain a better understanding of predictions of obesity later in life. Findings suggest that factors and growth patterns as early as the third trimester of life in utero influence a higher fat mass percentage and body composition at 6 months of age.[13]

Measurement in the Field

Examination of body composition in the field is done by measurement of skinfold thickness. The validity of this measure is suspect, just as the validity of laboratory methods is in question. The major problem is that skinfold measurement is based on the assumption that body surface measures and body density relationships are stable throughout childhood.[151] Two other threats to the validity of this measurement are (1) that use of skinfold thickness implies that the subcutaneous fat layer reflects the total amount of fat in the body, and (2) that selected measurement sites reflect average thickness. These assumptions may not be true[136]; however, Lohman and colleagues[155] and Slaughter and colleagues[230] did not find large deviations in skinfold thickness distribution across sites.

Despite this controversy, measurement of body composition is an important part of almost all health-related fitness tests. Concurrent validity has been demonstrated consistently with moderately high correlations of 0.70 to 0.85 between measurements of skinfolds and densitometry or potassium spectrometry.[108]

Typical sites for measurement of skinfold thickness are over the triceps brachii, subscapular area, and calf. Usually these areas are measured in some combination. Lohman[153] has designed a series of charts for easy evaluation of skinfold thickness and percent body fatness based on either triceps

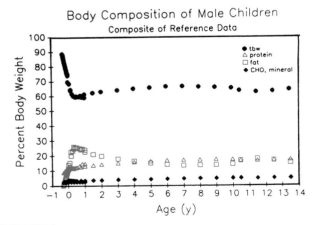

Figure 6-3   The normal body composition of male children as it changes with age. Derived from data found in descriptions of the reference fetus, infant, male child at 9 years, children from birth to 10 years, and adolescent male. *CHO,* Carbohydrate; *tbw,* total body water. (From Spady, D. W. [1989]. Normal body composition of infants and children. *98th Ross Laboratories Conference on Pediatric Research, 98,* 67–73. Used with permission of Ross Products Division, Abbott Laboratories, Columbus, OH 43216. ©1989 Ross Products Division, Abbott Laboratories.)

and subscapular or triceps and calf skinfold measures. The method of estimation of percent body fatness from skinfold measurements involves estimating density from skinfold measurements and then converting density to percent body fatness. The reader is referred to other sources for more detailed information.[151,152,184] A 3% to 5% error is reported for adults when body fatness is estimated from skinfold measurements.[151]

Although skinfold measurement remains the preferred method of assessing body composition, use of body mass index (BMI) has become more and more prevalent. The two national fitness tests, the FITNESSGRAM and the President's Challenge, now include standards for BMI. BMI is based on height and weight measurements, but the prediction error of the measurement is larger than that of skinfold measurement, and its use is not recommended.[109,154]

Standards by Age

The criterion values for ranges of body fatness conducive to optimal health in children are 10% to 25% for boys and 15% to 25% for girls.[153] Values higher than 25% in boys and 30% in girls are considered to place the child at risk for associated morbidity. This standard is consistent with the cutoffs at body composition of 32% for females and 25% for males set by the FITNESSGRAM Program.[30] Results from the NCYFS I and II studies suggest that children within the 40th to 50th percentiles on the test items fall within the optimal ranges described earlier.[207,208]

Response to Training

Conditioning and training programs alone may or may not affect body composition. If changes are to occur, the type of exercise must entail high-energy expenditure of intense effort. Appropriate activities include swimming, running, and weight training. Evidence of program effects on body composition is inconclusive in adults. Little information is available on children, but what is available indicates that percentage of body fatness can be reduced during training for specific sports but rises again when programs are discontinued.[191,270] Significant changes in body composition with structured physical activity programs are less likely than changes in bone mineral density in both obese and nonobese children.[16,112,173]

Assessment of Body Composition in Children with Disabilities

Premature Infants

Clinicians treat many children with disabilities who were born prematurely. Premature birth has been shown to affect body composition.[234] Compared with a "reference" fetus of similar weight, the infant who was born prematurely has a higher total fat content and a lower total body water content. These differences in composition are probably the result of living outside the womb and being faced with the necessity

of increasing body fat for temperature regulation. The implications of this altered body composition during growth have not been studied, nor has body composition been studied in premature infants who experience neonatal complications. There may or may not be effects of premature birth on composition throughout childhood and into adulthood. The previously described pattern of growth changes noted to influence fat mass percentage at 6 months of age may particularly influence children born prematurely, but again this has not been studied.[13]

Cerebral Palsy

Few studies have been conducted on body composition of individuals with CP.[15,28,263] All reported that adolescents with CP are shorter and typically weigh less than their age-matched peers. Resting metabolic rate was found to be lower than the norm in all studies. Contradictory findings were noted among the studies, however, which may or may not be related to differences in method. Results of the two older studies suggested that total body water as a percentage of body weight was higher in individuals with CP than in control subjects.[15,28] Findings in the later studies indicated the opposite, suggesting an increased percentage of body fat.[263] van den Berg–Emons and colleagues[263] postulated that children with CP may have proportionately more subcutaneous fat in the lower extremity skinfold sites because of disuse. Thus using skinfold measurements as an estimation of body fat may not be appropriate in this population. Correlations between methods (including DXA) was found to be excellent for determination of fat free body mass and moderate for determination of fat mass and percent body fat.[149] Subject numbers across all studies were relatively small and included children with a variety of types of CP and of functional levels. Both type of CP and functional level are likely to be important variables affecting body composition. The conflicting results of the studies cannot be resolved without further research.

Myelodysplasia

The study by Bandini and colleagues[15] also included individuals with myelodysplasia. This group, on average, showed decreased stature, reduced fat-free mass, and increased percentage of body fat as compared with able-bodied peers. The percentage of body fat was above the 95th percentile for all subjects with myelodysplasia. A significant correlation was not found between skinfold thickness and body composition, which suggests that fat distribution may be altered because of the type of paralysis. A previous study had also suggested that skinfold measurements and fat distribution may be altered in myelodysplasia.[119] Both studies indicate that children with myelodysplasia are at risk for obesity.

More recent studies confirm earlier studies indicating that the percentage of adolescents classified as obese ranged between 29% and 35% as measured by skinfold thickness and BMI.[46,47,260] Nonambulatory individuals had a higher percentage of body fat than those who were ambulatory. BMI, however, did not demonstrate a significant correlation with physical activity.

Muscular Dystrophy

Regional and whole body composition has been assessed in children with Duchenne muscular dystrophy (DMD) in comparison with able-bodied controls using DXA.[229] As noted in earlier studies, a decrease in lean tissue mass was noted. Body fat percentage was higher in children with DMD as well. In both cases, regional differences were noted. Trunk and lower leg lean tissue mass differences were not statistically different from those of able-bodied controls. Lean tissue mass was found to correlate well with the corresponding regional peak isometric strength for control subjects, but poor correlations were noted for individuals with DMD.[170,190,229]

CONDITIONING AND TRAINING

Whether the components of physical fitness can be affected by training programs is an important question, especially to clinicians who are designing programs for children with disabilities. Bar-Or[19] differentiated between the terms *conditioning* and *training*, which are often used interchangeably. *Physical conditioning* is defined as the process by which exercise, repeated over a specified duration, induces morphologic and functional changes in body systems and tissues. The tissues and systems can include skeletal muscles, the myocardium, adipose tissue, bones, tendons, ligaments, the central nervous system, and the endocrine system. Bar-Or[19] considered conditioning to consist of general exercise for overall physical fitness. *Training*, by contrast, is specific exercise designed to promote changes in performance of a particular type of activity. In the context of this chapter, training is discussed in relation to specific fitness components, but overall conditioning is discussed in reference to children with disabilities.

FITNESS COMPONENTS AND TRAINING IN CHILDREN

Many of the physiologic changes that result from training and conditioning in adults also take place during the process of growth and maturation in childhood. These naturally occurring changes make it difficult to study the specific effects of conditioning and training. The primary components of physical fitness of interest to trainers are cardiorespiratory endurance and physical strength.

Cardiorespiratory Endurance

Some controversy exists over whether maximal aerobic power or VO_{2max} can be increased by cardiorespiratory training in children.[19,139] Besides the improvements seen to occur naturally during growth and maturation, other problems in assessing the effects of training include seasonal differences in activity, difficulty in ensuring that a true VO_{2max} has been reached during the testing process, and the already high level of physical activity in young children.

Krahenbuhl and colleagues[139] as early as 1985 concluded that maximal aerobic power can be significantly increased after regular intensive training in children 8 to 14 years of age. A recent review of the influence of school-based programs continues to demonstrate the positive effects previously noted, especially in adolescence.[74] The long-term impact of such programs is unknown, and only one study reviewed used direct measurement of VO_{2max}.[50] Endurance exercise appeared more effective than intermittent exercise. General physical education programs alone were not effective in improving VO_{2max}. Effective activities included running, cycle ergometry, and swimming. Increases of 8% to 10% were measured in effective programs. Some studies reported little or no change in VO_{2max} despite improved long-distance running performance after training programs lasting 1 to 9 weeks.[19,62]

Less controversy exists over whether training is effective in improving cardiorespiratory endurance in adolescence. The effects of training in adolescents appear to be similar to those in adults. The functional and morphologic changes of the cardiovascular and pulmonary systems that take place as a result of training are listed in Table 6-9. Training effects usually include increases in myocardial mass, stroke volume, ventilation, and respiratory muscular endurance.

Muscular Strength and Endurance

Muscular strength is a component of fitness that can be affected by training, especially in children at or after puberty.

TABLE 6-9   Cardiorespiratory Function Variables and Response to Training in Children

Function Variable	Change with Training
Heart volume	Increase
Blood volume	Increase
Total hemoglobin	Slight increase
Stroke volume (max, submax)	Increase
Cardiac output (max, submax)	Increase, no change, or decrease
Arteriovenous difference (submax)	No change
Blood flow to active muscle	No change
Ventilation/kg body wt (max)	Increase
Ventilation/kg body wt (submax)	Decrease
Respiratory rate (submax)	Decrease
Tidal volume (max)	Increase
Respiratory muscle endurance	Increase

Adapted from Bar-Or, O. (1983). Physiologic responses to exercise in healthy children. In O. Bar-Or (Ed.), *Pediatric sports medicine for the practitioner*, p. 49. New York: Springer-Verlag.
max, Maximal exercise; *submax*, submaximal exercise.

Resistance strength training (RST) refers to training for improved muscular strength by repeatedly overcoming heavy resistance. The practice of resistance strength training is problematic in preadolescent children because controversy exists regarding (1) whether children can make gains in strength and muscle mass, (2) whether gains improve athletic performance, and particularly, (3) whether children are more susceptible to injury when participating in such training. Despite the controversy, RST has been shown to increase voluntary force production at all ages, may reduce the risk of injury during athletic participation, and may result in beneficial effects on important health-related indices such as cardiovascular fitness, body composition, and bone mineral density among others.[5,34,85,89,218]

Additionally, it has been reported that the risk of musculoskeletal injury in RST is no greater than for many other sports and recreational activities in which children and adolescents participate.[89] Just as in any exercise program, risks are minimized by appropriate program design, sensible progression, and careful selection of program equipment. Recommendations are available from the American Academy of Pediatrics Council on Sports Medicine and Fitness[5] (http://pediatrics.aappublications.org/cgi/content/abstract/121/4/835), the National Strength and Conditioning Association (http://www.nsca-lift.org/publications/posstatements.shtml),[89] and other sources.[162]

As previously described, the strength increases associated with growth are closely related to increases in muscle mass, including an increase in the numbers of sarcomeres and fibrils per muscle fiber.[160,164] The enhancement of muscular strength caused by growth is estimated to be approximately 1.5 kg per year from the age of 6 to 14 years.[174] In conjunction with muscular adaptations, neural adaptations associated with improved coordination and motor learning may play a role. For example, the increases in voluntary strength noted with training in prepubescent children have been found to be independent of increased muscle mass or hypertrophy such as that seen in postpubescent children or adults.[33,162,218] Improved motor unit activation and neural adaptations (including more appropriate co-contraction of synergist muscles and inhibition of antagonist muscles, as well as improvements in motor unit recruitment order and firing frequency within the prime movers) are believed to play a role in producing training effects in both adults and children.[138,162,177,202] It has been suggested that during the early stages of training, neural adaptation predominates in producing altered performance. Muscular adaptation contributes in the later stages of training[33,218] (Figure 6-4).

A compelling body of scientific evidence indicates that children and adolescents can significantly increase their strength above and beyond growth and maturation, provided the RST is of sufficient intensity, volume, and duration.[86,87,88,89,147,202,218,252,275] Children show a greater increase in strength than do adults when training-induced strength improvements are expressed as a percentage of change.

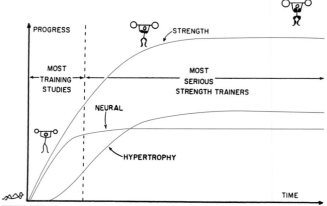

Figure 6-4   Relative roles of neural and muscular adaptation in strength training. Neural adaptation plays the biggest role in the early phase of training, which can last up to several weeks. Muscular adaptation predominates later and is limited by the extent to which muscles can hypertrophy. (From Sale, D. G. [1989]. Strength training in children. In C. V. Gisolfi, & D. R. Lamb [Eds.]. Perspectives in exercise science and sports medicine: Youth, exercise, and sport [Vol. 2] [p. 180]. Indianapolis, IN: Benchmark Press.)

During maximal voluntary contraction, children can develop the same force per unit of muscle cross-sectional area as adults despite differences in absolute strength and muscle size.

PRINCIPLES OF TRAINING

The principles of an effective training program include specificity, as well as guidelines for intensity, frequency, and duration of exercise. Rules for children are essentially the same as those for adults.

Specificity

The changes that take place in the body as a result of training are specific to the type of exercise performed and to the tissue involved. Myocardial tissue, for example, is affected by long-distance running but not by RST. The type of contraction (concentric, eccentric, or isometric), the number of repetitions performed, the velocity of muscle contraction, and the particular muscles exercised all influence the results of a strength training program. Different sports develop different components of fitness.

Intensity

Activity at a certain intensity is required to achieve conditioning or training effects. Intensity should be determined as a percentage of the individual's maximum because the same amount of activity can represent two entirely different levels of intensity for two different individuals. For example, a child with CP who walks at the same velocity as an able-bodied child may consume twice as much oxygen, so walking as a form of exercise for the child with CP is more intense.

An average 6- to 12-year-old walking at an average velocity consumes about 25% of VO_{2max}; for a child with CP, oxygen uptake can be as high as 75% to 90% of VO_{2max} (personal observation, 1998).

Intensity threshold refers to the intensity of exercise below which few or no training or conditioning effects are observed.[17] The intensity threshold of maximal aerobic power in adults required to produce a training effect is 60% to 70% of VO_{2max}. The threshold for strength is approximately 60% to 65% of maximal voluntary contraction. The principle of overload in strength training is in part related to the intensity threshold of exercise. *Overload* refers to a task that requires considerable voluntary effort to complete. No specific data are available for intensity thresholds for children, but they are thought to be at least equal to those of adults. Whether intensity thresholds for children with various disabilities are the same as those for able-bodied children is also unknown.

Frequency

The optimal frequency of training depends on the type of program, and frequency is interrelated with intensity and duration. Two or three times per week on nonconsecutive days is a general rule of thumb.[5,19,89]

Duration

Any program, whether a therapeutic program or a fitness program, requires a minimum implementation time before benefits are seen. Most effective conditioning programs last at least 6 to 8 weeks. The optimal duration of an exercise session depends on the type of program. In general, the session should consist of a warm-up phase of 10 minutes, an exercise phase above the exercise threshold for 15 to 30 minutes, and a 5- to 7-minute cool-down period. The warm-up phase has been shown to be important for increasing performance of both aerobic and anaerobic tasks in children.[5,19,89] The warm-up period should include (1) activities to raise core body temperature, (2) stretching exercises, and (3) activities specific to the exercise task. The American Academy of Pediatrics[5] recommends that strength training regimens for children include activities to provide strength training for all parts of the body to ensure balanced development (http://pediatrics.aappublications.org/cgi/content/abstract/121/4/835).

The duration of the exercise phase in strength training is sometimes associated with the goal of achieving maximal overload. This is usually done in one of two ways—by repeating brief maximal contractions or by repeating submaximal contractions to the point of fatigue.

Progression

A conditioning or training program must be progressive in its demands for continued improvement. The intensity threshold, the duration of exercise sessions, the number of repetitions performed during a session, or the frequency of exercise sessions may need to be increased. All contribute individually and collectively to the progression of the exercise program.

CONDITIONING IN CHILDREN WITH DISABILITIES

Cerebral Palsy

As children with CP approach and move through adolescence, an important aspect of function is the ability to maintain ambulation. Oxygen uptake during ambulation in preadolescent children with CP (ages 6 to 12 years) is more than twice that of able-bodied children walking at the same velocity.[234] If body weight and adiposity increase in adolescence without an increase in muscular strength, maximal aerobic capacity decreases, and the task of walking becomes more and more difficult. Growth in mass is a cubic function (volume), and growth in strength is a function of the square (cross-sectional muscle area). As previously mentioned, muscles increase first in mass, then in strength.[160] During the adolescent growth spurt, mass increases at a faster rate than does strength. For able-bodied children, this process occurs without noticeable deficit or loss of function, but for children with CP, loss of function sometimes occurs because the rate of increase in strength is inadequate to support the rate of increase in muscle mass. A major goal of physical therapy for adolescents with CP is maintenance of the ability to ambulate throughout the growth spurt. If a child has maximal strength and aerobic capacity on entering the growth spurt, function is also likely to be at maximal capacity. Conditioning in a child with CP could play a vital role in the process of maximizing the potential not only of the adolescent but of the preadolescent and school-aged child as well.

The ultimate goal of conditioning programs for children with CP is similar to that in all children—to promote life habits and physical health benefits. In addition, children with CP are often faced with deterioration of capacity during adolescence and adulthood. Children who lack the requisite fitness capacity may not be able to achieve their own maximum potential in gross motor activities. Daily physical activity has been found to correlate inversely with the energy cost of walking.[166] Verschuren and colleagues used field tests of physical fitness to assess gross motor capacity and found that performance-related fitness items and functional muscle strength exhibited higher correlations to gross motor capacity than aerobic capacity.[265] This finding supports previous research suggesting that short-term muscle power or anaerobic capacity is a better measure of gross motor capacity than aerobic capacity in children with CP.

Greater attention is now given to the benefits of strengthening in both children and adolescents with CP. Damiano and colleagues reported strength gains after a resistive exercise training program. Functional improvements in both gait and Gross Motor Function Measure scores were noted, as was decreased spasticity.[67–69] A recent systematic review of the literature evaluated 20 studies related to exercise programs for children with cerebral palsy.[267] Of the 20 evaluated, only five were randomized controlled trials, which provide the optimal design to test treatment (in this case, training) effects.[75,76,196,253,262] On the basis of the strength training programs that were reviewed, evidence exists supporting the view that progressive resistance exercise can increase the ability to generate force in children with CP.[267] The protocol for a randomized controlled trial of a functional progressive resistive exercise training program currently under way has recently been published.[221] Functional exercises combining aerobic capacity, anaerobic capacity, and muscle strength have demonstrated a 22% increase in strength in previous studies.[265a] Unfortunately, the benefits gained during training often are only partially maintained at follow-up.[265,262]

Aerobic capacity has been shown to improve by 35% to 38% after a training program.[262] Earlier studies had demonstrated that conditioning effects on aerobic capacity in the population of children and adolescents with CP are similar to those of children without disability.[22,27,158,157] In a longitudinal study of adolescents with CP, Lundberg[156] found that heart rate at a given power load increased an average of 10 bpm per year, implying decreasing efficiency with time.

Studies that addressed the issue of changes in body composition as a result of conditioning showed no change in the percentage of body fat after a 4-month program.[26,262]

Evidence suggests that neither regular physical education classes nor habitual activities are sufficient to induce conditioning changes in children with CP.[27,77] The program must increase in intensity beyond habitual exercise levels. The duration of the overall program should be longer than 6 weeks; results of 6-week training programs are equivocal.[81] Target heart rate was typically maintained for 15 to 30 minutes in most studies. Longer-duration protocols have been reported.[221] Activities in accordance with the child's ability were used; examples are cycle ergometry, swimming, running, and jogging.

Cystic Fibrosis

Results of studies in children and adolescents with cystic fibrosis (CF) that emphasized aerobic conditioning for 3 to 5 months suggest that VO_{2max}, endurance of respiratory muscles, and pulmonary function all show improvement.[186,282] Jogging, cycling, swimming, weight lifting, and calisthenics of various durations and combinations were used. Statistically significant increases in strength, balance, and submaximal aerobic exercise capacity have also been reported after a 4- to 6-week inpatient rehabilitation program emphasizing sporting-type activities.[111] Based on a growing body of research, it is now quite well accepted that exercise and exercise training programs are effective therapy methods to improve aerobic exercise capacity and strength as attributes of physical fitness and lung function in individuals with CF.[187,220,135,224,237]

In addition to the positive effects of conditioning on physical fitness, clinical benefits in the management of the disease have been reported.[20,111,282] Increased coughing and mucous clearance may reduce the need for chest therapy to manage secretions.[282]

The effects of exercise on children with CF and other clinical populations must be closely monitored to reduce or avoid potential detrimental effects. Particular concerns in the population with CF are dehydration (especially in high heat) and oxygen desaturation.[20] See Chapter 24 for more information on the management of CF.

Muscular Dystrophy

The effects of conditioning patients with DMD have been evaluated in numerous studies, which produced equivocal results.[1,70,100,268] Evaluation of the results must take into account that many of the studies were inadequately controlled for threats to internal validity. Results suggest that modest gains in strength can be made, or the rate of deterioration retarded. DeLateur and Giaconi[70] found no significant change in strength of the quadriceps femoris muscle after 6 weeks of a 6-month conditioning program of submaximal exercise. A modest, but not significant, increase in strength was found after 6 months. Each subject served as his or her own control. No deleterious effects of a strengthening program were found. Despite the lack of statistically significant effects, the increase in strength may be enough to delay future deterioration.

More recent research continues to cite these early studies, but a Cochrane review of strength and aerobic exercise training excluded most of these studies from their review because they were not randomized controlled trials.[264] A training program instituted for individuals with Becker muscular dystrophy demonstrated improvement in aerobic capacity without rendering patients susceptible to structural or mechanical damage to muscle.[242] There appears to be a consensus that low to moderate resistance and aerobic training may be helpful in patients with slowly progressive myopathic disorders.[4,222,242,243] Clearly, more work needs to be done in this area. See Chapter 12 for more information on the management of DMD and other types of dystrophies.

Children with Obesity

Although addressed elsewhere in this chapter, it is important to highlight known evidence regarding the influence of training and conditioning programs on children with obesity. Studies suggest that resistive training programs are safe and result in positive and significant changes in body composition, strength, and power.[25,171,225,232,272] Most studies found that an 8-week program was sufficient to achieve significant effects. Most resistive exercise programs or aerobic exercise programs did not demonstrate significant changes in peak oxygen uptake.[272,25] As in other areas, better-controlled randomized trials are needed to substantiate evidence.

SUMMARY

This chapter was designed to provide information on physical fitness and conditioning in the able-bodied child for promoting health and preventing disease. The components of fitness, how they are tested, and how they contribute to health were reviewed. An understanding of physical fitness, physical activity, and conditioning is valuable for appreciating the impact of disabling conditions on these variables, but health-related physical fitness is important for reducing future health risks in every child, regardless of the presence or absence of disability. Preadolescent fitness may be especially important to children with disabilities because of the effects particular disabilities may have on children as they enter puberty and adulthood. The design of exercise programs (their intensity, frequency, and duration) should encompass the minimal requirements for physical fitness, as well as incorporate therapeutic goals. Exercise programs should be designed so that the energy requirements for accomplishing day-to-day activities through the growth period are met. Meeting this goal is likely to require additional exercise beyond current therapy or physical education. One of our goals as pediatric therapists should be to ensure, to whatever extent possible, that our clients end their childhood at a fitness level suitable to a healthy adulthood. Research is needed to document the extent to which this goal can be met for specific populations and levels of disability.

Much research remains to be done in the able-bodied population as well. Reliability and validity studies must continue on criterion-based measures now being used to determine minimal fitness levels. Research must establish reliable, valid, and universal criteria, both in the laboratory and in the field. Continued identification of the relationship between childhood physical activity and fitness and health in adulthood is vital to our overall understanding of health-related fitness.

Research to benefit populations with disabilities or children with special needs has barely begun. With an inadequate base of research in children without disability, developing standards of fitness for specific disabled populations begins at a disadvantage. A question that remains to be answered is whether the fitness performance criteria for children without disabilities are valid for children with disabilities or special needs. Experience with development of testing and measurement tools for other purposes would suggest that they are not. Are children with disabilities such as CP more fit because they expend in walking an amount of energy equivalent to that of an able-bodied person walking up and down stairs all day long? Are the thresholds and target zones for fitness improvement the same for children with a variety of disabilities as for able-bodied children? How are conditioning and training programs best designed for children with disabilities? Do conditioning programs initiated before the onset of puberty help maintain fitness during and after puberty? What are the physiologic and behavioral factors that limit a child's capacity to improve fitness variables or to exercise? How much exercise is detrimental? How do presurgical strengthening programs affect the recovery of strength after surgery? Questions such as these represent only the beginning of our quest for understanding. The journey has just begun.

REFERENCES

1. Abrahamson, A. S., & Rogoff, J. (1952). Physical treatment in muscular dystrophy (abstract). In *Proceedings of the 2nd medical conference* (pp.123–124). New York: Muscular Dystrophy Association.
2. Adams, F. H. (1973). Factors affecting the working capacity of children and adolescents. In G. L. Rarick (Ed.), *Physical activity: Human growth and development* (pp. 89–90). New York: Academic Press.
3. Alexander, J., & Molnar, G. E. (1973). Muscular strength in children: Preliminary report on objective standards. *Archives of Physical Medicine and Rehabilitation, 54,* 424–427.
4. Ansved, T. (2003). Muscular dystrophies: The influence of physical conditioning on disease evolution. *Current Opinion in Clinical Nutrition and Metabolic Care, 6,* 455–459.
5. American Academy of Pediatrics Council on Sports Medicine and Fitness. (2008). Strength training by children and adolescents: Policy statement. *Pediatrics, 121,* 835–840.
6. American Alliance for Health, Physical Education, Recreation, and Dance. (1988). *The AAHPERD physical best program.* Reston, VA: American Alliance for Health, Physical Education, Recreation, and Dance.
7. American Association for Health, Physical Education, and Recreation. (1958). *AAHPER youth fitness test manual.* Washington, DC: American Association for Health, Physical Education, and Recreation.
8. American Physical Therapy Association. (2001). Guide to physical therapist practice. *Physical Therapy, 81,* 1–768.
9. Andreacci, J. L., Robertson, R. J., Dube, J. J., Aaron, D. J., Dixon, C. B., & Arslanian, S. A. (2005). Comparison of maximal oxygen consumption between obese black and white adolescents. *Pediatric Research, 58,* 478–482.
10. Ashton, B. B., Pickles, B., & Roll, J. W. (1978). Reliability of goniometric measurements of hip motion in spastic cerebral palsy. *Developmental Medicine and Child Neurology, 20,* 87–94.
11. Astrand, P. O. (1952). *Experimental studies of physical working capacity in relation to sex and age.* Copenhagen: Ejnar Munksgaard.
12. Aucouturier, J., Rance, M., Meyer, M., Isacco, L., Thivel, D., Fellmann, N., et al. (2009). Determination of the maximal fat oxidation point in obese children and adolescents: Validity of methods to assess maximal aerobic power. *European Journal of Applied Physiology, 105,* 325–331.
13. Ay, L., Van Houten, V. A. A., Steegers, E. A. P., Hofman, A., Witteman, J. C. M., Jaddoe, V. W. V., et al. (2009). Fetal and postnatal growth and body composition at 6 months of age. *Journal of Clinical Endocrinology and Metabolism, 94,* 2023–2030.
14. Baltzopoulos, V., & Kellis, E. (1998). Isokinetic strength during childhood and adolescence. In E. Van Praagh (Ed.), *Pediatric anaerobic performance* (pp. 225–240). Champaign, IL: Human Kinetics.

15. Bandini, L. G., Schoeller, D. A., Fukagawa, N. K., Wykes, L. J., & Dietz, W. H. (1991). Body composition and energy expenditure in adolescents with cerebral palsy or myelodysplasia. *Pediatric Research, 29*, 70–77.

16. Barbeau, P., Gutin, B., Litaker, M., Owens, S., Riggs, S., & Okuyama, T. (1999). Correlates of individual differences in body composition changes resulting from physical training in obese children. *American Journal of Clinical Nutrition, 69*, 705–711.

17. Bar-Or, O. (1983). Appendix II: Procedures for exercise testing in children. In O. Bar-Or (Ed.), *Pediatric sports medicine for the practitioner* (pp. 315–341). New York: Springer-Verlag.

18. Bar-Or, O. (1983). Neuromuscular diseases. In O. Bar-Or (Ed.), *Pediatric sports medicine for the practitioner* (pp. 227–249). New York: Springer-Verlag.

19. Bar-Or, O. (1983). Physiologic responses to exercise in healthy children. In O. Bar-Or (Ed.), *Pediatric sports medicine for the practitioner* (pp. 1–65). New York: Springer-Verlag.

20. Bar-Or, O. (1985). Physical conditioning in children with cardiorespiratory disease. *Exercise and Sport Sciences Reviews, 13*, 305–334.

21. Bar-Or, O. (1986). Pathophysiological factors which limit the exercise capacity of the sick child. *Medicine and Science in Sports and Exercise, 18*, 276–282.

22. Bar-Or, O., Inbar, O., & Spira, R. (1976). Physiological effects of a sports rehabilitation program on cerebral palsied and poliomyelitic adolescents. *Medicine and Science in Sports, 8*, 157–161.

23. Baynard, T., Pitetti, K. H., Guerra, M., Unnithan, V. B., & Fernhall, B. (2008). Age-related changes in aerobic capacity in individuals with mental retardation: A 20-year review. *Medicine and Science in Sports and Exercise, 40*, 1984–1989.

24. Beets, M. W., & Pitetti, K. H. (2006). Criterion-referenced reliability and equivalency between the PACER and the 1-mile run/walk for high school students. *Journal of Physical Activity and Health 3*(Suppl. 2), S21–S33.

25. Benson, A. C., Torode, M. E., & Fiatarone Singh, M. A. (2008). The effect of high-intensity progressive resistance training on adiposity in children: A randomized controlled trial. *International Journal of Obesity, 32*, 1016–1027.

26. Berg, K. (1970). Effect of physical activation and improved nutrition on the body composition of school children with cerebral palsy. *Acta Paediatrica Supplement, 204*, 53–69.

27. Berg, K. (1970). Effect of physical training of school children with cerebral palsy. *Acta Paediatrica Supplement, 204*, 27–33.

28. Berg, K., & Isaksson, B. (1970). Body composition and nutrition of school children with cerebral palsy. *Acta Paediatrica Supplement, 204*, 41–52.

29. Berger, R. A., & Medlin, R. L. (1969). Evaluation of Berger's 1-RM chin test for junior high school mates. *Research Quarterly, 40*, 460–463.

30. Blair, S. N., Clark, D. G., Cureton, K. J., & Powell, K. E. (1989). Exercise and fitness in childhood: Implications for a lifetime of health. In C. V. Gisolfi, & D. R. Lamb (Eds.), *Perspectives in exercise science and sports medicine: Youth, exercise, and sport* (Vol. 2; pp. 401–430). Indianapolis, IN: Benchmark Press.

31. Bleck, E. (1991). Adolescent idiopathic scoliosis. *Developmental Medicine and Child Neurology, 33*, 167–173.

32. Blimkie, C. J. R. (1989). Age and sex associated variation in strength during childhood: Anthropometric, morphologic, neurologic, biomechanical, endocrinologic, genetic, and physical activity correlates. In C. V. Gisolfi, & D. R. Lamb (Eds.), *Perspectives in exercise science and sports medicine: Youth, exercise, and sport* (Vol. 2; pp. 99–163). Indianapolis, IN: Benchmark Press.

33. Blimkie, C. J. R., Ramsay, J., Sale, D., MacDougall, D., Smith, K., & Garner, K. (1989). Effects of 10 weeks of resistance training on strength development in prepubertal boys. In S. Osteid, & K. H. Carlsen (Eds.), *Children and exercise XIII* (pp. 183–197). Champaign, IL: Human Kinetics.

34. Blimkie, C. J. R., & Sale, D. G. (1998). Strength development and trainability during childhood. In E. Van Praagh (Ed.), *Pediatric anaerobic performance* (pp. 193–224). Champaign, IL: Human Kinetics.

35. Boileau, R. A., Lohman, T. G., Slaughter, M. H., Ball, T. E., Going, S. B., & Hendrix, M. K. (1984). Hydration of the fat-free body in children during maturation. *Human Biology, 56*, 651–666.

36. Boileau, R. A., Lohman, T. G., Slaughter, M. H., Horswill, C. A., & Stillman, R. J. (1988). Problems associated with determining body composition in maturing youngsters. In E. W. Brown, & C. F. Branta (Eds.), *Competitive sports for children and youth: An overview of research and issues* (pp. 3–16). Champaign, IL: Human Kinetics.

37. Boone, D. C., Azen, S. P., Lin, C. M., Spense, C., Baron, C., & Lee, L. (1978). Reliability of goniometric measurements. *Physical Therapy, 58*, 1355–1360.

38. Bovet P., Auguste R., & Burdette H. (2007). Strong inverse association between physical fitness and overweight in adolescents: A large school-based survey. *International Journal of Behavioral Nutrition and Physical Activity 4*, 24 doi: 10.1186/1479-5868-4-24, 2007.

39. Boyce, W. F., Gowland, C., Hardy, S., Rosenbaum, P. L., Lane, M., Plews, N., et al. (1991). Development of a quality-of-movement measure for children with cerebral palsy. *Physical Therapy, 71*, 820–828.

40. Boyce, W. F., Gowland, C., Rosenbaum, P. L., Lane, M., Plews, N., Goldsmith, C. H., et al. (1995). The Gross Motor Performance Measure: Validity and responsiveness of a measure of quality of movement. *Physical Therapy, 75*, 603–613.

41. Braden, D. S., & Strong, W. B. (1990). Cardiovascular responses to exercise in childhood. *American Journal of Diseases of Children, 144*, 1255–1260.

42. Branta, C., Haubenstricker, J., & Seefeldt, V. (1984). Age changes in motor skills during childhood and adolescence. *Exercise and Sport Sciences Reviews, 12*, 467–520.

43. Bray, G. A., & Bouchard, C. (1988). Role of fat distribution during growth and its relationship to health. *American Journal of Clinical Nutrition, 47*, 551–552.

44. Brodie, D. A., Burnie, J., Eston, R. G., & Royce, J. A. (1986). Isokinetic strength and flexibility characteristics in preadolescent boys. In J. Rutenfranz, R. Mocellin, & F. Klimt (Eds.), *Children and exercise XII* (pp. 309–319). Champaign, IL: Human Kinetics.

45. Brooks, G. A., Fahey, T. D., & Baldwin, K. (2004). *Exercise physiology: Human bioenergetics and its applications* (4th ed.). New York: McGraw-Hill.

46. Buffart, L. M., Roebroeck, M. E., Rol, M., Stam, H. J., & van den Berg-Emons, R. J. G. (2008). Triad of physical activity, aerobic fitness, and obesity in adolescents and young adults in myelomeningocele. *Journal of Rehabilitation Medicine, 40,* 70–75.

47. Buffart, L. M., van den Berg-Emons, R. J. G., van Wijlen-Hempel, M. S., Stam, H. J., & Roebroeck, M. E. (2008). Health-related fitness of adolescents and young adults with myelomeningocele. *European Journal of Applied Physiology, 103,* 181–188.

48. Butterfield, S. A., & Lehnhrad, R. A. (2008). Aerobic performance by children in grades 4 to 8: A repeated-measures study. *Perceptual and Motor Skills, 107,* 775–790.

49. Caballero, B. (2007). The global epidemic of obesity: An overview. *Epidemiology Review, 29,* 1–5.

50. Carrel, A. L., Clark, R., Peterson, S. E., Nemeth, B. A., Sullivan, J., & Allen, D. B. (2005). Improvement in fitness, body composition, and insulin sensitivity in overweight children in a school-based exercise program—A randomized controlled study. *Archives of Pediatrics and Adolescent Medicine, 159,* 963–968.

51. Carrel, A. L., Sledge, J. S., Ventura, S. J., Clark, R., Peterson, S. E., Eickhoff, J. C., et al. (2008). Measuring aerobic cycling power as an assessment of childhood fitness. *Journal of Strength and Conditioning Research, 22,* 192–195.

52. Carron, A. V., & Bailey, D. A. (1974). Strength development in boys from 10–16 years. *Monographs of the Society for Research in Child Development, 39,* 1–37.

53. Castro-Pinero, J., Chillon, P., Ortega, F. B., Montesinos, J. L., Sjostrom, M., & Ruiz, J. R. (2009). Criterion-related validity of the sit-and-reach test and the modified sit-and-reach test for estimating hamstring flexibility in children and adolescents aged 6–17 years. *International Journal of Sports Medicine, 30,* 658–662.

54. Castro-Pinero, J., Mora, J., Gonzalez-Montesinos, J. L., Sjostrom, M., & Ruiz, J. L. (2009). Criterion-related validity of the one-mile run/walk test in children aged 8–17 years. *Journal of Sports Sciences, 27,* 405–413.

55. Chaterjee, S., Chaterjee, P., & Bandyopadhyay, A. (2005). Cardiorespiratory fitness of obese boys. *Indian Journal of Physiology and Pharmacology, 49,* 353–357.

56. Clarke, H. H. (1979). *Posture. Physical Fitness Research Digest, 9,* 1–23.

57. Clarke, H. H., & Clarke, D. H. (1987). *Application of measurement in physical education* (pp. 93–99). Englewood Cliffs, NJ: Prentice-Hall.

58. Considine, W. J. (1973). An analysis of selected upper body tasks as measures of strength (Abstract). *American Association of Health, Physical Education, and Recreation, 25,* 74.

59. Cooper, D. M., Weiler-Ravell, D., Whipp, B. J., & Wasserman, K. (1984). Growth-related changes in oxygen uptake and heart rate during progressive exercise in children. *Pediatric Research, 18,* 845–851.

60. Cooper Institute for Aerobics Research. (1988). *FITNESS-GRAM®.* Dallas, TX: Cooper Institute for Aerobics Research.

61. Cooper Institute for Aerobics Research. (2007). *FITNESS-GRAM®/ACTIVITYGRAM® test administration manual* (4th ed.). Champaign, IL: Human Kinetics.

62. Cumming, G. R., Goodwin, A., Baggley, G., & Antel, J. (1967). Repeated measurements of aerobic capacity during a week of intensive training at a youth track camp. *Canadian Journal of Physiology and Pharmacology, 45,* 805–811.

63. Cunningham, D. A., MacFarlane-VanWaterschoot, B., Paterson, D. H., Lefcoe, M., & Sangal, S. P. (1977). Reliability and reproducibility of maximal oxygen uptake in children. *Medicine and Science in Sports, 9,* 104–108.

64. Cureton, K. J., Sloniger, M. A., O'Bannon, J. P., Black, D. M., & McCormack, W. P. (1995). A generalized equation for prediction of VO2peak from 1-mile run/walk performance. *Medicine and Science in Sports and Exercise, 27,* 445–451.

65. Cureton, K. J., & Warren, G. L. (1990). Criterion-referenced standards for youth health-related fitness tests: A tutorial. *Research Quarterly for Exercise and Sport, 61,* 7–19.

66. Daltroy, L. H., Liang, M. H., & Fossel, A. H. (1998). The POSNA pediatric musculoskeletal functional health questionnaire: Report on reliability, validity, and sensitivity to change. *Journal of Pediatric Orthopaedics, 18,* 561–571.

67. Damiano, D. L., & Abel, M. F. (1998). Functional outcomes of strength training in spastic cerebral palsy. *Archives of Physical Medicine and Rehabilitation, 79,* 119–125.

68. Damiano, D. L., Kelly, L. E., & Vaughan, C. L. (1995). Effects of quadriceps muscle strengthening on crouch gait in children with spastic diplegia. *Physical Therapy, 75,* 668–671.

69. Damiano, D. L., Vaughan, C. L., & Abel, M. F. (1995). Muscle response to heavy resistance exercise in children with spastic cerebral palsy. *Developmental Medicine and Child Neurology, 37,* 731–739.

70. DeLateur, B. J., & Giaconi, R. M. (1979). Effect on maximal strength of submaximal exercise in Duchenne muscular dystrophy. *American Journal of Physical Medicine, 58,* 26–36.

71. Dell, R. B. (1989). Comparison of densitometric methods applicable to infants and small children for studying body composition. *Ross Laboratories Conference on Pediatric Research, 98,* 22–30.

72. Dencker, M., Thorsson, O., Karlsson, M. K., Linden, C., Wollmer, P., & Andersen, L. B. (2008). Maximal oxygen uptake versus maximal power output in children. *Journal of Sports Sciences, 26,* 1397–1402.

73. de Sa Pinto, A. L., de Barros Holanda, P. M., Radu, A. S., Villares, S. M. F., & Lima, F. R. (2006). Musculoskeletal findings

in obese children. *Journal of Paediatrics and Child Health, 42,* 341–344.

74. Dobbins, M., DeCorby, K., Robeson, P., Husson, H., & Tirilis, D. (2009). School-based physical activity programs for promoting physical activity and fitness in children and adolescents aged 6–18 (Review). *Cochrane Database of Systematic Reviews, 21(3),* CD007651.

75. Dodd, K. J., Taylor, N. F., & Graham, H. K. (2003). A randomized clinical trial of strength in young people with cerebral palsy. *Developmental Medicine and Child Neurology, 45,* 652–657.

76. Dodd, K. J., Taylor, N. F., & Graham, H. K. (2004). Strength training can have unexpected effects on the self-concept of children with cerebral palsy. *Pediatric Physical Therapy, 16,* 99–105.

77. Dresen, M. H. W. (1985). Physical and psychological effects of training on handicapped children. In R. A. Binkhorst, H. C. G. Kemper, & W. H. M. Saris (Eds.), *Children and exercise XI* (pp. 203–209). Champaign, IL: Human Kinetics.

78. Drews, J., Vraciu, J. K., & Pellino, G. (1984). Range of motion of the joints of the lower extremities of newborns. *Physical and Occupational Therapy in Pediatrics, 4,* 49–62.

79. Dwyer, G. M., Bauer, L. A., & Hardy, L. L. (2009). The challenge of understanding and assessing physical activity in preschool-age children: Thinking beyond the framework of intensity, duration, and frequency of activity. *Journal of Science and Medicine in Sport, 12,* 534–536.

80. Eisenmann, J. C., Keelan, K. A., & Welk, G. J. (2004). Assessing body composition among 3- to 8- year old children: Anthropometry, BIA, and DXA. *Obesity Research, 12,* 1633–1640.

81. Ekblom, B., & Lundberg, A. (1968). Effect of training on adolescents with severe motor handicaps. *Acta Paediatrica Scandinavica, 57,* 17–23.

82. Ekstrand, J., Wiktorsson, M., Oberg, B., & Gillquist, J. (1982). Lower extremity goniometric measurements: A study to determine their reliability. *Archives of Physical Medicine and Rehabilitation, 63,* 171–175.

83. Eriksson, B. O., Gollnick, P. D., & Saltin, B. (1973). Muscle metabolism and enzyme activities after training in boys 11–13 years old. *Acta Physiologica Scandinavica, 87,* 485–487.

84. Eriksson, B. O., Karlsson, J., & Saltin, B. (1971). Muscle metabolites during exercise in pubertal boys. *Acta Paediatrica Scandinavica Supplement, 217,* 154–157.

85. Faigenbaum, A. (2000). Strength training for children and adolescents. *Clinical Journal of Sports Medicine, 19,* 593–619.

86. Faigenbaum, A., Glover, S., O'Connell, J., LaRosa Loud, R., & Westcott, W. (2001). The effects of different resistance training protocols on upper body strength and endurance development in children. *Journal of Strength and Conditioning Research, 15,* 459–465.

87. Faigenbaum, A., Milliken, L., LaRosa Loud, R., Burak, B., Doherty, C., & Westcott, W. (2002). Comparison of 1 day and 2 days per week of resistance training in children. *Research Quarterly for Exercise and Sport, 73,* 416–424.

88. Faigenbaum, A., Milliken, L., Moulton, L., & Westcott, W. (2005). Early muscular fitness adaptations in children in response to two different strength training regimens. *Pediatric Exercise Science, 17,* 2337–2348.

89. Faigenbaum, A. D., Kaemer, W. J., Blimkie, C. J. R., Jeffreys, I., Micheli, L. J., Nitka, M., et al. (2009). Youth resistance training: Updated position statement paper from the National Strength and Conditioning Association. *Journal of Strength and Conditioning Research, 23*(Suppl. 5), S60–S79.

90. Faust, M. S. (1977). Somatic development of adolescent girls. *Society for Research in Child Development, 42,* 1–90.

91. FitzGerald, S. J., Barlow, C. E., Kampert, J. B., Morrow, J. R. Jr., Jackson, A. W., & Blair, S. N. (2004). Muscular fitness and all cause mortality: Prospective observations. *Journal of Physical Activity and Health, 1,* 7–18.

92. Flint, M. M., & Gudgell, J. (1966). Electromyographic study of abdominal muscular activity during exercise. *Research Quarterly, 36,* 29–37.

93. Florini, J. R. (1987). Hormonal control of muscle growth. *Muscle and Nerve, 10,* 577–598.

94. Fogelholm, M., Stigman, S., Huisman, T., & Metsamuuronen, J. (2008). Physical fitness in adolescents with normal weight and overweight. *Scandinavian Journal of Medicine and Science in Sports, 18,* 162–170.

95. Foley, S., Quinn, S., Dwyer, T., Venn, A., & Jones, G. (2008). Measures of childhood fitness and body mass index are associated with bone mass in adulthood: A 20-year prospective study. *Journal of Bone and Mineral Research, 23,* 994–1001.

96. Fomon, S. J. (1967). Body composition of the male reference infant during the first year of life. *Pediatrics, 40,* 863–867.

97. Fomon, S. J., Haschke, F., Ziegler, E. E., & Nelson, S. E. (1982). Body composition of reference children from birth to age 10 years. *American Journal of Clinical Nutrition, 35,* 1169–1173.

98. Fowler, E. G., Kolobe, T. H. A., Damiano, D. L., Thorpe, D. E., Morgan, D. W., Brunstrom, J. E., et al. (2007). Promotion of physical fitness and prevention of secondary conditions for children with cerebral palsy: Section on Pediatrics Research Summit Proceedings. *Physical Therapy, 87,* 1495–1507.

99. Fowler, W. M., & Gardner, G. W. (1967). Quantitative strength measurements in muscular dystrophy. *Archives of Physical Medicine and Rehabilitation, 48,* 629–644.

100. Fowler, W. M., Pearson, C. M., Egstrom, G. H., & Gardner, G. W. (1965). Ineffective treatment of muscular dystrophy with an anabolic steroid and other measures. *New England Journal of Medicine, 272,* 875–882.

101. Francis, K., & Feinstein, R. (1991). A simple height-specific and rate-specific step test for children. *Southern Medical Journal, 84,* 169–174.

102. Freedson, P. S., Cureton, K. J., & Health, G. W. (2000). Status of field-based fitness testing in children and youth. *Preventive Medicine, 31,* S77–S85.

103. Gage, J. R. (1991). *Gait analysis in cerebral palsy.* London: MacKeith Press.

104. Gage, J. R., & Stout, J. L. (2009). Gait analysis: Kinematics, kinetics, electromyography, oxygen consumption, and

pedobarography. In J. R. Gage, M. H. Schwartz, S. E. Koop, & T. F. Novacheck (Eds.), *The identification and treatment of gait problems in cerebral palsy* (pp. 260–284). London: MacKeith Press.

105. Giannini, M. J., & Protas, E. J. (1991). Aerobic capacity in juvenile rheumatoid arthritis patients and healthy children. *Arthritis Care and Research, 4,* 131–135.

106. Giannini, M. J., & Protas, E. J. (1992). Exercise response in children with and without juvenile rheumatoid arthritis: A comparison study. *Physical Therapy, 72,* 365–372.

107. Godfrey, S. (1981). Growth and development of the cardiopulmonary response to exercise. In J. A. Davis, & J. Dobbing (Eds.), *Scientific foundations in paediatrics* (pp. 450–460). London: William Heinemann Medical Books.

108. Going, S. (1988). Physical best: Body composition in the assessment of youth fitness. *Journal of Physical Education, Recreation and Dance, 59,* 32–36.

109. Going, S. B., Lohman, T. G., Falls, & H. B. (2008). Body composition assessment. In G. J. Welk, & M. D. Meredith (Eds.), *Fitnessgram/Activitygram reference guide* (pp. 121–128). Dallas, TX: Cooper Institute.

110. Gowland, C., Boyce, W. F., Wright, V., Russell, D. J., Goldsmith, C. H., & Rosenbaum, P. L. (1995). Reliability of the Gross Motor Performance Measure. *Physical Therapy, 75,* 597–602.

111. Gruber, W., Orenstein, D. M., Braumann, K. M., & Huls, G. (2008). Health-related fitness and trainability in children with cystic fibrosis. *Pediatric Pulmonology, 43,* 953–964.

112. Gutin, B., Barbeau, P., Lemmon, C. R., Bauman, M., Allison, J., Kang, H., et al. (2002). Effects of exercise on cardiovascular fitness, total body composition, and visceral adiposity of obese adolescents. *American Journal of Clinical Nutrition, 75,* 818–826.

113. Haley, S. M., Tada, W. L., & Carmichael, E. M. (1986). Spinal mobility in young children: A normative study. *Physical Therapy, 66,* 1697–1703, 1986.

114. Harris, S. R., Smith, L. H., & Krukowski, L. (1985). Goniometric reliability for a child with spastic quadriplegia. *Journal of Pediatric Orthopedics, 5,* 348–351.

115. Hartman, J. G., & Looney, M. (2003). Norm-referenced and criterion-referenced reliability and validity of the back-saver sit-and-reach. *Measurement in Physical Education and Exercise Science, 7,* 71–87.

116. Haschke, F. (1989). Body composition during adolescence. *Ross Laboratories Conference on Pediatric Research, 98,* 76–82.

117. Haschke, F., Fomon, S. J., & Ziegler, E. E. (1981). Body composition of a nine year old reference boy. *Pediatric Research, 15,* 847–850.

118. Haskell, W. L., Montoye, H. J., & Orenstein, D. (1985). Physical activity and exercise to achieve health-related fitness components. *Public Health Reports, 100,* 202–212.

119. Hayes-Allen, M. C., & Tring, F. C. (1973). Obesity: Another hazard for spina bifida children. *British Journal of Preventive and Social Medicine, 27,* 192–196.

120. Hedley, A. A., Ogden, C. L., Johnson, C. L., Carroll, M. D., Curtin, L. R., & Flegal, K. M. (2004). Prevalence of overweight and obesity among US children, adolescents, and adults, 1999–2002. *Journal of the American Medical Association, 291,* 2847–2850.

121. Hoofwijk, M., Unnithan, V., & Bar-Or, O. (1995). Maximal treadmill performance of children with cerebral palsy. *Pediatric Exercise Science, 7,* 305–313.

122. Hopkins, N. D., Stratton, G., Tinken, T. M., McWhannell, N., Ridgers, N. D., Graves, L. E. F., et al. (2009). Relationships between measures of physical fitness, physical activity, body composition and vascular function in children. *Atherosclerosis, 204,* 244–249.

123. Hosking, G. P., Bhat, U. S., Dubowitz, V., & Edwards, H. T. (1976). Measurement of muscle strength and performance in children with normal and diseased muscle. *Archives of Disease in Childhood, 51,* 957–963.

124. Huang, Y. C., & Malina, R. M. (2007). BMI and health-related fitness in Taiwanese youth 9–18 years. *Medicine and Science in Sports and Exercise, 39,* 701–708.

125. Jackson, A. S. (2006). The evolution and validity of health-related fitness. *Quest, 58,* 160–175.

126. Jackson, A. S., & Coleman, A. E. (1976). Validation of distance run tests for elementary school children. *Research Quarterly, 47,* 86–94.

127. Jackson, A. W., & Baker, A. A. (1986). The relationship of the sit and reach test to criterion measures of hamstring and back flexibility in young females. *Research Quarterly for Exercise and Sport, 57,* 183–186.

128. Jankowski, J. W. (1986). Exercise testing and exercise prescription for individuals with cystic fibrosis. In J. S. Skinner (Ed.), *Testing and exercise prescription for special cases.* Philadelphia: Lea & Febiger.

129. Jolliffe, D. (2004). Extent of overweight among US children and adolescents from 1971–2000. *International Journal of Obesity, 28,* 4–9.

130. Jurca, R., Lamonte, M. J., Barlow, C. E., Kampert, J. B., Church, T. S., & Blair, S. N. (2005). Association of muscular strength with incidence of metabolic syndrome in men. *Medicine and Science in Sports and Exercise, 37,* 1845–1855.

131. Keating, X. D., & Silverman, S. (2004). Teachers' use of fitness tests in school-based physical education programs. *Measurement in Physical Education and Exercise Science, 8,* 145–165.

132. Kendall, H. O., & Kendall, F. P. (1952). *Posture and pain* (p. 104). Baltimore: Williams & Wilkins.

133. Kilmer, D. D., Abresch, R. T., & Fowler, W. M. (1993). Serial manual muscle testing in Duchenne muscular dystrophy. *Archives of Physical Medicine and Rehabilitation, 74,* 1168–1171.

134. Kim, J., Must, A., Fitzmaurice, G. M., Gillman, M. W., Chomitz, V., Kramer, E., et al. (2005). Relationship of physical fitness to prevalence and incidence of overweight among school children. *Obesity Research, 13,* 1246–1254.

135. Klijn, P. H., Oudshoorn, A., van der Ent, C. K., van der Net, J., Klimpen, J. L., & Helders, P. J. (2004). Effects of anaerobic training in children with cystic fibrosis. *Chest, 125,* 1299–1305.

136. Klish, W. J. (1989). The "gold standard." *Ross Laboratories Conference on Pediatric Research, 98*, 4–7.

137. Koch, G. (1974). Muscle blood flow after ischemic work during bicycle ergometer work in boys aged 12. *Acta Pediatrica Belgica Supplement, 28*, 29–39.

138. Komi, P. V. (1986). Training muscle strength and power: Interaction of neuromotoric, hypertrophic, and mechanical factors. *International Journal of Sports Medicine, 7*(Suppl.), 10–15.

139. Krahenbuhl, G. S., Skinner, J. S., & Kohrt, W. M. (1985). Developmental aspects of maximal aerobic power in children. *Exercise and Sport Sciences Reviews, 13*, 503–538.

140. Krul, M., van der Wouden, J. C., Schellevis, F. G., van Suijlekom-Smit, L. W. A., & Koes, B. W. (2009). Musculoskeletal problems in obese and overweight children. *Annals of Family Medicine, 7*, 352–356.

141. Kuland, D. N., & Tottossy, M. (1985). Warm-up strength and power. *Clinics in Sports Medicine, 4*, 137–158.

142. Kvaavik, E., Knut-Inge, K., Tell, G. S., Meyer, H. E., & Batty, G. D. (2009). Physical fitness and physical activity at age 13 as predictors of cardiovascular disease risk factors at ages 15, 25, 33, and 40 years: Extended follow-up of the Oslo Youth Study. *Pediatrics, 123*, e80–e86.

143. Landin, S., Hagenfeldt, L., Saltin, B., & Wahren, J. (1977). Muscle metabolism during exercise in hemiparetic patients. *Clinical Science and Molecular Medicine, 53*, 257–269.

144. Lavay, B., Reid, G., & Cressler-Chaviz, M. (1990). Measuring the cardiovascular endurance of persons with mental retardation: A critical review. *Exercise and Sport Sciences Reviews, 18*, 263–290.

145. Lefkof, M. B. (1986). Trunk flexion in healthy children aged 3 to 7 years. *Physical Therapy, 66*, 39–44.

146. Leonard, C. M., Roza, M. A., Barr, R. D., & Webber, C. E. (2009). Reproducibility of DXA measurements of bone mineral density and body composition in children. *Pediatric Radiology, 39*, 148–154.

147. Lillegard, W., Brown, E., Wilson, D., Henderson, R., & Lewis, E. (1997). Efficacy of strength training in prepubescent to early postpubescent males and females: Effect of gender and maturity. *Pediatric Rehabilitation, 1*, 147–157.

148. Lim, J. S., Hwang, J. S., Lee, J. A., Kim, D. H., Park, K. D., Jeong, J. S., et al. (2009). Cross calibration of multi-frequency bioelectric impedance analysis with eight-point electrodes and dual-energy x-ray absorptiometry for assessment of body composition in healthy children ages 6–18 years. *Pediatrics International, 51*, 263–268.

149. Liu, L. F., Roberts, R., Moyer-Mileur, L., Samson-Fang, L. (2005). Determination of body composition in children with cerebral palsy: Bioelectrical impedance analysis and anthropometry vs. dual-energy x-ray absorptiometry. *Journal of the American Dietetics Association, 105*, 794–797.

150. Lobstein, T., Baur, L., & Uauy, R. (Eds.). (2004). Obesity in children and young people: A crisis in public health. Report to the World Health Organization. *Obesity Reviews, 5*(Suppl. 1), 4–104.

151. Lohman, T. G. (1982). Measurement of body composition in children. *Journal of Physical Education, Recreation and Dance, 53*, 67–70.

152. Lohman, T. G. (1986). Applicability of body composition techniques and constants for children and youth. *Exercise and Sport Sciences Reviews, 14*, 325–357.

153. Lohman, T. G. (1987). The use of skinfold to estimate body fatness on children and youth. *Journal of Physical Education, Recreation and Dance, 58*, 98–102.

154. Lohman, T. G., & Going, S. B. (1998). Assessment of body composition and energy balance. In I. Lamb, & R. Murray (Eds.), Perspectives in exercise science and sports medicine: Exercise, nutrition and control of body weight (*Vol. 22*). Carmel, IN: Cooper Publishing Group.

155. Lohman, T. G., Slaughter, M. H., Boileau, R. A., Bunt, J., & Lussier, L. (1984). Bone mineral measurements and their relation to body density in children, youth, and adults. *Human Biology, 56*, 667–679.

156. Lundberg, A. (1973). Changes in the working pulse during the school year in adolescents with cerebral palsy. *Scandinavian Journal of Rehabilitation Medicine, 5*, 12–17.

157. Lundberg, A., Ovenfors, C. O., & Saltin, B. (1967). The effect of physical training on school children with cerebral palsy. *Acta Paediatrica Scandinavica, 56*, 182–188.

158. Lundberg, A., & Pernow, B. (1970). The effect of physical training on oxygen utilization and lactate formation in the exercising muscle of adolescents with motor handicaps. *Scandinavian Journal of Clinical and Laboratory Investigation, 26*, 89–96.

159. Macrae, I., & Wright, V. (1969). Measurement of back movement. *Annals of the Rheumatic Diseases, 52*, 584–589.

160. Malina, R. M. (1986). Growth of muscle and muscle mass. In F. Falkner, & J. M. Tanner (Eds.), Human growth: A comprehensive treatise: Postnatal growth (*Vol. 2*; pp. 77–99). New York: Plenum Press.

161. Malina, R. M. (2001). Physical activity and fitness: Pathways from childhood to adulthood. *American Journal of Human Biology, 13*, 162–172.

162. Malina, R. M. (2006). Weight training in youth-growth, maturation, and safety: An evidenced base review. *Clinical Journal of Sports Medicine, 16*, 478–487.

163. Malina, R. M., Beunen, G. P., Classens, A. L., Lefevre, J., Vanden Eynde, B. V., Renson, R., et al. (1995). Fatness and physical fitness of girls 7–17 years. *Obesity Research*, 221–231.

164. Malina, R. M., Bouchard, C., & Bar-Or, O. (2004). *Growth, maturation, and physical activity*. Champaign, IL: Human Kinetics.

165. Malina, R. M., & Little, B. B. (2008). Physical activity: The present in the context of the past. *American Journal of Human Biology, 20*, 373–391.

166. Maltais, D. B., Pierrynowski, M. B., Galea, V. A., & Bar-Or, O. (2005). Physical activity level is associated with the O_2 cost of walking in cerebral palsy. *Medicine and Science in Sports and Exercise, 37*, 347–353.

167. Mastrangelo, M. A., Chaloupka, E. C., & Rattigan, P. (2008). Cardiovascular fitness in obese versus nonobese 8–11-year-old boys and girls. *Research Quarterly for Exercise and Sport, 79*, 356–362.

168. Maughan, R. J., Watson, J. S., & Weir, J. (1983). Strength and cross-sectional area of human skeletal muscle. *Journal of Physiology, 338*, 37–49.

169. McDonald, C. M., Abresch, R. T., Carter, G. T., Fowler, W., Jr., Johnson, E. R., & Kilmer, D. D. (1995). Profiles of neuromuscular diseases: Duchenne muscular dystrophy. *American Journal of Physical Medicine and Rehabilitation, 74*, S70–S92.

170. McDonald, C. M., Carter, G. T., Abresch, R. T., Widman, L., Styne, D. M., Warden, N., et al. (2005). Body composition and water compartment measurements in boys with Duchenne muscular dystrophy. *American Journal of Physical Medicine and Rehabilitation, 84*, 483–491.

171. McGuigan, M. R., Tatasciore, M., Newton, R. U., & Pettigrew, S. (2009). Eight weeks of resistance training can significantly alter body composition in children who are overweight or obese. *Journal of Strength and Conditioning Research, 23*, 80–85.

172. McKay, H., & Smith, E. (2008). Winning the battle against childhood physical inactivity: The key to bone strength? *Journal of Bone and Mineral Research, 23*, 980–985.

173. McWhannell, N., Henaghan, J. L., Foweather, L., Doran, D. A., Batterham, A. M., Reilly, T., et al. (2008). The effect of a 9-week physical activity programme on bone and body composition of children aged 10–11 years: An exploratory trial. *International Journal of Sports Medicine, 29*, 941–947.

174. Mersch, F., & Stoboy, H. (1989). Strength training and muscle hypertrophy in children. In S. Osteid, & K. H. Carlsen (Eds.), *Children and exercise XIII* (pp. 165–182). Champaign, IL: Human Kinetics.

175. Molnar, G. E., & Alexander, J. (1973). Objective, quantitative muscle testing in children: A pilot study. *Archives of Physical Medicine and Rehabilitation, 54*, 224–228.

176. Moran, H. M., Hall, M. A., Barr, A., & Ansell, B. (1979). Spinal mobility of the adolescent. *Rheumatology Rehabilitation, 18*, 181–185.

177. Moritani, T., & DeVries, H. A. (1979). Neural factors versus hypertrophy in the time course of muscle strength gain. *American Journal of Physical Medicine, 58*, 115–130.

178. Morrow, J. R., Jr., Falls, H. B., & Kohl, H. W., III (Eds.). (1993). *The Prudential FITNESSGRAM technical manual.* Dallas, TX: The Cooper Institute for Aerobic Research.

179. Morrow, J. R., Jr., Fulton, J. E., Brenar, N. D., & Kohl, H. W., III. (2008). Prevalence and correlates of physical fitness testing in U.S. schools—2000. *Research Quarterly for Exercise and Sport, 79*, 141–148.

180. Morrow, J. R., Jr., Weimo, Z., Franks, B. D., Meredith, M. D., & Spain, C. (2009). 1958–2008: 50 years of youth fitness testing in the United States. *Research Quarterly for Exercise and Sport, 80*, 1–11.

181. Myers, J., Prakash, M., Froelicher, V., Do, D., Partington, S., & Atwood, J. E. (2002). Exercise capacity and mortality among men referred for exercise testing. *The New England Journal of Medicine, 346*, 793–801.

182. Neumark-Sztainer, D., Story, M., Hannan, P. J., & Croll, J. (2002). Overweight status and eating patterns among adolescents: Where do youths stand in comparison with the Healthy People 2010 objectives? *American Journal of Public Health, 92*, 844–851.

183. Norkin, C. C., & White, D. J. (1985). *Measurement of joint motion: A guide to goniometry.* Philadelphia: FA Davis.

184. Ogden, C. L., Flegal, K. M., Carroll, M. D., & Johnson, C. L. (2002). Prevalence and trends in overweight among US children and adolescents, 1999–2000. *Journal of the American Medical Association, 288*, 1728–1732.

185. Olney, S. J., Boyce, W. F., & Wright, M. (1988). Lower extremity work patterns in gait of diplegic CP children (Abstract). *Physical Therapy, 68*, 847.

186. Orenstein, D. M., Franklin, B. A., Doershuk, H. K., Hellerstein, K. J., Germann, K. J., Horowitz, J. G., et al. (1981). Exercise conditioning and cardiopulmonary physical fitness in cystic fibrosis: The effects of a three-month supervised running program. *Chest, 80*, 392–398.

187. Orenstein, D. M., & Higgins, L. W. (2005). Update on the role of exercise in cystic fibrosis. *Current Opinions in Pulmonology and Medicine, 11*, 519–523.

188. Ounpuu, S. (2004). Patterns of gait pathology. In J. R. Gage (Ed.), *The treatment of gait problems in cerebral palsy* (pp. 217–237). London: MacKeith Press.

189. Ozmun, J. C., Mikesky, A. E., & Surburg, P. R. (1994). Neuromuscular adaptations following prepubescent strength training. *Medicine and Science in Sports and Exercise, 26*, 510–514.

190. Palmieri, M. D., Bertorini, M. D., Griffin, J. W., Igarashi, M., & Karas, J. G. (1996). Assessment of whole-body composition with dual-energy X-ray absorptiometry in Duchenne muscular dystrophy: Correlation of lean body mass with muscle function. *Muscle Nerve, 19*, 777–779.

191. Parizkova, J. (1977). *Body fat and physical fitness: Body composition and lipid metabolism in different regimens of physical activity* (pp. 152–156). The Hague: Martinus Nijhoff.

192. Pate, R. R. (1983). A new definition of youth fitness. *Physician and Sports Medicine, 11*, 77–83.

193. Pate, R. R., Ross, J. G., Baumgartner, T. A., & Sparks, R. E. (1987). The National Children and Youth Fitness Study II: The modified pull-up test. *Journal of Physical Education, Recreation and Dance, 58*, 71–73.

194. Pate, R. R., & Shephard, R. J. (1989). Characteristics of physical fitness in youth. In C. V. Gisolfi, & D. R. Lamb (Eds.), Perspectives in exercise science and sports medicine: Youth, exercise, and sport (*Vol. 2*; pp. 1–45). Indianapolis, IN: Benchmark Press.

195. Paterson, D. H., & Cunningham, D. A. (1978). Maximal oxygen uptake in children: Comparison of treadmill protocols at various speeds. *Canadian Journal of Applied Sport Sciences, 3*, 188.

196. Patikas, M., Wolf, S. I., Mund, K., Armbrust, P., Schuster, W., & Doderlein, L. (2006). Effects of a post-operative strength-training program on the walking ability of children with cerebral palsy: A randomized controlled trial. *Archives of Physical Medicine and Rehabilitation, 87,* 619–626.

197. Phelps, E., Smith, L. J., & Hallum, A. (1985). Normal ranges of hip motion of infants between 9 and 24 months of age. *Developmental Medicine and Child Neurology, 27,* 785–792.

198. Physical Activity Guidelines Advisory Committee. (2008). Physical Activity Guidelines Advisory Committee Report, 2008. *Nutrition Reviews, 67,* 114–120.

199. Plowman, S. A. (2008). Muscular strength, endurance and flexibility assessments. In G. J. Welk, & M. D. Meredith (Eds.), *Fitnessgram/Activitygram reference guide* (pp. 129–168). Dallas, TX: Cooper Institute.

200. President's Council on Physical Fitness and Sports. (1987). *The president's challenge.* Washington, DC: President's Council on Physical Fitness and Sports.

201. President's Council on Physical Fitness and Sports. (2008). The president's challenge: The health fitness test. Retrieved August 25, 2009, from http://www.presidentschallenge.org/educators/programs_details/health_fitness_test.aspx

202. Ramsay, J., Blimkie, C. J. R., Smith, K., Garner, S., Macdougall, J., & Sale, D. (1990). Strength training effects in prepubescent boys. *Medicine and Science in Sports and Exercise, 22,* 605–614.

203. Rarick, G. L., & Thompson, J. A. J. (1956). Roentgenographic measures of leg size and ankle extensor strength of 7 year old children. *Research Quarterly, 27,* 321–332.

204. Riddoch, C. J., & Boreham, C. A. G. (1995). Health related physical activity of children. *Sports Medicine, 19,* 86–99.

205. Rose, J., Gamble, J. G., Burgos, A., Medeiros, J., & Haskell, W. L. (1990). Energy expenditure index of walking for normal children and children with cerebral palsy. *Developmental Medicine and Child Neurology, 32,* 333–340.

206. Rose, J., Gamble, J. G., Medeiros, J., Burgos, A., & Haskell, W. L. (1989). Energy cost of walking in normal children and in those with cerebral palsy: Comparison of heart rate and oxygen uptake. *Paediatric Orthopaedics, 9,* 276–279.

207. Ross, J. G., Delpy, L. A., Christenson, G. M., Gold, R. S., & Damberg, C. L. (1987). The National Youth and Fitness Study II: Study procedures and quality control. *Journal of Physical Education, Recreation and Dance, 58,* 57–62.

208. Ross, J. G., Dotson, C. O., Gilbert, G. G., & Katz, S. J. (1985). The National Youth and Fitness Study I: New standards for fitness measurement. *Journal of Physical Education, Recreation and Dance, 56,* 62–66.

209. Ross, J. G., & Gilbert, G. G. (1985). The National Children and Youth Fitness Study: A summary of findings. *Journal of Physical Education, Recreation and Dance, 56,* 45–50.

210. Ross, J. G., Katz, S. J., & Gilbert, G. G. (1985). The National Youth and Fitness Study I: Quality control. *Journal of Physical Education, Recreation and Dance, 56,* 57–61.

211. Ross, J. G., & Pate, R. R. (1987). The National Children and Youth Fitness Study II: A summary of findings. *Journal of Physical Education, Recreation and Dance, 58,* 51–56.

212. Ross, J. G., Pate, R. R., Delpy, L. A., Gold, R. S., & Svilar, M. (1987). The National Children and Youth Fitness Study II: New health related fitness norms. *Journal of Physical Education, Recreation and Dance, 58,* 66–70.

213. Rowland, T. W. (2007). Evolution of maximal oxygen uptake in children. In G. R. Tominkinson, & T. S. Olds (Eds.), Pediatric fitness: Secular trends and geographic variability. *Medicine and Sports in Science, 50,* 200–209.

214. Rutenfranz, J., Macek, M., Lange-Anderson, A., Bell, R. D., Vavra, J., Radvansky, J., et al. (1990). The relationship between changing body height and growth related changes in maximal aerobic power. *European Journal of Applied Physiology, 60,* 282–287.

215. Safrit, M. J. (1989). Criterion-referenced measurement: Validity. In M. J. Safrit, & T. M. Wood (Eds.), *Measurement concepts in physical education and exercise science* (pp. 119–135). Champaign, IL: Human Kinetics.

216. Safrit, M. J. (1990). The validity and reliability of fitness tests for children: A review. *Pediatric Exercise Science, 2,* 9–28.

217. Safrit, M. J., & Wood, T. M. (1987). The test battery reliability of the health-related physical fitness test. *Research Quarterly for Exercise and Sport, 58,* 160–167.

218. Sale, D. G. (1989). Strength training in children. In C. V. Gisolfi, & D. R. Lamb (Eds.), Perspectives in exercise science and sports medicine: Youth, exercise, and sport (*Vol. 2*; pp. 165–222). Indianapolis IN: Benchmark Press.

219. Saltin, B., & Strange, S. (1992). Maximal oxygen uptake: Old and new arguments for a cardiovascular limitation. *Medicine and Science in Sports and Exercise, 24,* 30–37.

220. Schneiderman-Walker, J., Pollock, S. L., Corey, M., Wolkes, D. D., Canny, G. J., Pedder, L., et al. (2000). A randomized controlled trial of a 3-year home exercise program in cystic fibrosis. *Journal of Pediatrics, 136,* 304–310.

221. Scholtes, V. A., Dallmeijer, A. J., Rameckers, E. A., Verschuren, O., Tempelaars, E., Hensen, M., et al. (2008). Lower limb strength training in children with cerebral palsy—A randomized controlled trial protocol for functional strength training based on progressive resistance exercise principles. *BMC Pediatrics, 8,* 41–51.

222. Scott, O. M., Hyde, S. A., Goddard, C., Jones, R., & Dubowitz, V. (1981). Effect of exercise in Duchenne muscular dystrophy. *Physiotherapy, 67,* 174–176.

223. Seaman, J. A., & California Adapted Fitness Task Force. (1995). Test items and standards. In J. A. Seaman (Ed.), *Physical best and individuals with disabilities: A handbook for inclusion in fitness programs* (pp. 41–54). Reston, VA: The American Alliance for Health, Physical Education, Recreation, and Dance.

224. Selvadurai, H. C., Blimkie, C. J., Meyers, N., Mellis, C. M., Cooper, P. J., & Van Asperen, P. P. (2002). Randomized controlled study of in-hospital exercise training programs in children with cystic fibrosis. *Pediatric Pulmonology, 33,* 194–200.

225. Sgro, M., McGuigan, M. R., Pettigrew, S., & Newton, R. U. (2009). The effect of duration of resistance training interventions in children who are overweight or obese. *Journal of Strength and Conditioning Research, 23,* 1263–1270.

226. Shvartz, E., & Reibold, R. C. (1990). Aerobic fitness norms for males and females aged 6 to 75 years: A review. *Aviation Space and Environmental Medicine, 61,* 3–11.

227. Shypailo, R. J., Butte, N. F., & Ellis, K. J. (2008). DXA: Can it be used as a criterion reference for body fat measurements in children? *Obesity, 16,* 457–462.

228. Simons-Morton, B. G., O'Hara, N. M., Simons-Morton, D. G., & Parcel, G. S. (1987). Children and fitness: A public health perspective. *Research Quarterly for Exercise and Sport, 58,* 295–302.

229. Skalsky, A. J., Han, J. J., Abresch, R. T., Shin, C. S., & McDonald, C. M. (2009). Assessment of regional body composition with dual-energy X-ray absorptiometry in Duchenne muscular dystrophy: Correlation of regional lean mass and quantitative strength. *Muscle Nerve, 39,* 647–651.

230. Slaughter, M. H., Lohman, T. G., Boileau, R. A., Stillman, R. J., VanLoan, M., Horswill, C. A., et al. (1984). Influence of maturation on relationship of skinfolds to body density: A cross-sectional *study. Human Biology, 56,* 681–689.

231. Sorsdahl, A. B., Moe-Nilssen, R., & Strand L. I. (2008). Observer reliability of the Gross Motor Performance Measure and the Quality of Upper Extremity Skills Test, based on video recordings. *Developmental Medicine and Child Neurology, 50,* 146–151.

232. Sothern, M. S., Loftin, J. M., Udall, J. N., Suskind, R. M., Ewling, T. L., Tang, S. C., et al. (2000). Safety, feasibility, and efficacy of a resistance training program in preadolescent obese children. *American Journal of Medicine and Science, 319,* 370–375.

233. Spady, D. W. (1989). Normal body composition of infants and children. *Ross Laboratories Conference on Pediatric Research, 98,* 67–73.

234. Spady, D. W., Schiff, D., & Szymanski, W. A. (1987). A description of the changing composition of the growing premature infant. *Journal of Pediatric Gastroenterology and Nutrition, 6,* 730–738.

235. Sproul, A., & Simpson, E. (1964). Stroke volume and related hemodynamic data in normal children. *Pediatrics, 33,* 912–916.

236. Sprynarova, S., & Reisenauer, R. (1978). Body dimensions and physiological indicators of physical fitness during adolescence. In R. J. Shephard, & H. Lavallee (Eds.), *Physical fitness assessment* (pp. 32–37). Springfield, IL: Charles C Thomas.

237. Stanghelle, J. K., Hjeltnes, N., Bangstad, H. J., & Michaelsen, H. (1998). Effects of daily short bouts of trampoline exercise during 8 weeks on the pulmonary function and the maximal oxygen uptake of children with cystic fibrosis. *International Journal of Sports Medicine, 9,* 32–36.

238. Stout, J. L., & Koop, S. E. (2004). Energy expenditure in cerebral palsy. In J. R. Gage (Ed.), *The treatment of gait problems in cerebral palsy* (pp. 146–164). London: MacKeith Press.

239. Strong, W. B. (1990). Physical activity and children. *Circulation, 81,* 1697–1701.

240. Strong, W. B., Malina, R. M., Blimkie, C. J., Daniels, S. R., Dishman, R. K., Gutin, B., et al. (2005). Evidence based physical activity for school-age youth. *Journal of Pediatrics, 146,* 732–737.

241. Sutton, J. R. (1992). VO$_{2max}$—New concepts on an old theme. *Medicine and Science in Sports and Exercise, 24,* 26–29.

242. Sveen, M. L., Jeppesen, T. D., Hauerslev, S., Kober, L., Krag, T. O., & Vissing, J. (2008). Endurance training improves fitness in patients with Becker muscular dystrophy. *Brain, 131,* 2824–2831.

243. Sveen, M. L., Jeppesen, T. D., Hauerslev, S., Krag, T. O., & Vissing, J. (2007). Endurance training: An effective and safe treatment for patients with LGMD2I. *Neurology, 68,* 59–61.

244. Taylor, E. D., Theim, K. R., Mirch, M. C., Ghorbani, S., Tanofsky-Kraff, M., Adler-Wailes, D. C., et al. (2006). Orthopaedic complications of overweight in children and adolescents. *Pediatrics, 117,* 2167–2174.

245. Taeymans, J., Clarys, P., Abidi, H., Hebbelinck, M., & Duquet, W. (2009). Developmental changes and predictability of static strength in individuals of different maturity: A 30-year longitudinal study. *Journal of Sports Sciences, 27,* 833–841.

246. Telford, R. D., Bass, S. L., Budge, M. M., Byrne, D. G., Carlson, J. S., Coles, D., et al. (2009). The lifestyle of our kids (LOOK) project: Outline of methods. *Journal of Science and Medicine in Sport, 12,* 156–163.

247. Thomas, S. S., Buckon, C. E., Phillips, D. S., Aiona, M. D., & Sussman, M. D. (2001). Interobserver reliability of the Gross Motor Performance Measure: Preliminary results. *Developmental Medicine and Child Neurology, 43,* 97–102.

248. Thompson, P., Beath, T., Bell, J., Jacobson, G., Phair, T., Salbach, N. M., et al. (2008). Test-retest reliability of the 10-metre fast walk test and 6-minute walk test in ambulatory school-aged children with cerebral palsy. *Developmental Medicine and Child Neurology, 50,* 370–376.

249. Thorpe D. (2009). The role of fitness in health and disease: Status of adults with cerebral palsy. *Developmental Medicine and Child Neurology, 51*(Suppl. 4), 52–58.

250. Tirosh, E., Bar-Or, O., & Rosenbaum, P. (1990). New muscle power test in neuromuscular disease. *American Journal of Diseases of Children, 144,* 1083–1087.

251. Troiano, R. P., Flegal, K. M., Kuczmarski, S. M., Campbell, S. M., & Johnson, J. C. (1995). Overweight prevalence and trends for children and adolescents. *Archives of Pediatric and Adolescent Medicine, 149,* 1085–1091.

252. Tsolakis, C., Vagenas, G., & Dessypris, A. (2004). Strength adaptations and hormonal responses to resistance training and detraining in preadolescent males. *Journal of Strength and Conditioning Research, 18,* 625–629.

253. Unger, M., Faure, M., & Frieg, A. (2006). Strength training in adolescent learners with cerebral palsy. *Clinical Rehabilitation, 20,* 469–467.

254. United States Cerebral Palsy Athletic Association. (1996). *Classification system for athletes.* Trenton, NJ: USCPAA.

255. United States Department of Health and Human Services. (1990). *Healthy Children 2000: National health promotion and disease prevention objectives related to mothers, infants, children, adolescents, and youth.* Washington, DC: Public Health Service.

256. United States Department of Health and Human Services. (1995). *Healthy People 2000: Progress report for physical activity and fitness.* Washington, DC: Public Health Service.

257. United States Department of Health and Human Services. (2009). Healthy People 2020 objectives: Draft for public comment. Retrieved from http://www.healthypeople.gov/hp2020/Objectives/TopicArea.aspx?id=39&TopicArea=Physical+Activity+and+Fitness

258. United States Department of Health and Human Services. (2000). *Healthy People 2010.* Washington, DC: United States Department of Health and Human Services.

259. United States Department of Health and Human Services. (2006). *Healthy People 2010 mid course review: Physical activity and fitness.* Washington, DC: United States Department of Health and Human Services.

260. van den Berg-Emons, H. J. G., Bussmann, J. B. J., Meyerink, H. J., Roebroeck, M. J., & Stam, H. J. (2003). Body fat, fitness, and everyday physical activity in adolescents and young adults with myelomeningocele. *Journal of Rehabilitation Medicine, 35,* 271–275.

261. van den Berg-Emons, R. J. G., van Baak, M. A., deBarbanson, D. C., Speth, L., & Saris, W. H. M. (1996). Reliability of tests to determine peak aerobic power, anaerobic power, and isokinetic muscle strength in children with spastic cerebral palsy. *Developmental Medicine and Child Neurology, 38,* 1117–1125.

262. van den Berg-Emons, R. J. G., van Baak, M. A., Speth, L., & Saris, W. H. (1998). Physical training of school children with spastic cerebral palsy: Effects on daily activity, fat mass, and fitness. *International Journal of Rehabilitation Research, 21,* 179–191.

263. van den Berg-Emons, R. J. G., van Baak, M. A., & Westerterp, K. R. (1998). Are skinfold measurements suitable to compare body fat between children with spastic cerebral palsy and healthy controls? *Developmental Medicine and Child Neurology, 40,* 335–339.

264. van der Kooi, E. L., Lindeman, E., & Riphagen, I. (2005). Strength training and aerobic exercise training for muscle disease (Review). *Cochrane Database of Systematic Reviews, (1),* CD003907.

265. Verschuren, O., Ketelaar, M., Gorter, J. W., & Takken, T. (2009). Relation between physical fitness and gross motor capacity in children and adolescents with cerebral palsy. *Developmental Medicine and Child Neurology, 51,* 866–871.

265a. Verschuren, O., Ketelaar, M., Gorter, J. W., Helders, P. J. M., Uiterwaal, C. S. P. M., & Taaken, T. (2007). Exercise training program in children and adolescents with cerebral palsy: A randomized controlled trial. *Archives of Pediatric and Adolescent Medicine, 161,* 1075–1081.

267. Verschuren, O., Ketelaar, M., Takken, T., Helders, P. J. M., & Gorter, J. W. (2008). Exercise programs for children with cerebral palsy: A systematic review of the literature. *American Journal of Physical Medicine and Rehabilitation, 87,* 404–417.

268. Vignos, P. J., & Watkins, M. P. (1966). The effect of exercise in muscular dystrophy. *Journal of the American Medical Association, 197,* 843–848.

269. Vincent, S. D., Pangrazi, R. P., Raustorp, A., Michaud Tomson, L., & Cuddihy, T. F. (2003). Activity levels and body mass index of children in the United States, Sweden, and Australia. *Medicine and Science in Sports & Exercise, 35,* 1367–1373.

270. VonDobelin, W., & Eriksson, B. O. (1972). Physical training, maximal oxygen uptake and dimensions of the oxygen transporting and metabolizing organs in boys 11–13 years of age. *Acta Paediatrica Scandinavica, 61,* 653–657.

271. Wahlund, H. (1948). Determination of the physical working capacity. *Acta Medica Scandinavica Supplement, 215,* 5–108.

272. Watts, K., Jones, T. W., Davis, E., Green, D. (2005). Exercise training in obese children and adolescents: Current concepts. *Sports Medicine, 35,* 375–392.

273. Waugh, K. G., Minkel, J. L., Parker, R., & Coon, V. A. (1983). Measurement of hip, knee, and ankle joints in newborns. *Physical Therapy, 63,* 1616–1621.

274. Welk, G. J., & Meredith M. D. (Eds.). (2008). *FITNESSGRAM®/ACTIVITYGRAM® reference guide* (3rd ed.). Dallas, TX: The Cooper Institute.

275. Westcott, W., Tolken, J., & Wessner, B. (1995). School-based conditioning programs for physically unfit children. *Strength and Conditioning Journal, 17,* 5–9.

276. Wiley, M. E., & Damiano, D. L. (1998). Lower extremity strength profiles in spastic cerebral palsy. *Developmental Medicine and Child Neurology, 40,* 100–107.

277. Winnick, J. P., & Short, F. X. (1999). *The Brockport physical fitness test manual.* Champaign, IL: Human Kinetics.

278. Winnick, J. P., & Short, F. X. (1985). *Physical fitness testing of the disabled: Project UNIQUE* (pp. 101–104). Champaign, IL: Human Kinetics.

279. World Health Organization. (2001). *International classification of functioning, disability and health.* Geneva: World Health Organization.

280. Wyndham, C. (1976). Submaximal test for estimating maximal oxygen intake. *Canadian Medical Association Journal, 96,* 736–742.

281. Yamashita, T., Seiichi, I., & Isao, O. (1992). Effect of muscle stretching on the activity of neuromuscular transmission. *Medicine and Science in Sports and Exercise, 24,* 80–84.

282. Zach, M. S., Oberwalder, J., & Hausler, F. (1982). Cystic fibrosis: Physical exercise vs chest physiotherapy. *Archives of Disease in Childhood, 57,* 587–589.

283. Ziegler, E. E., O'Donnell, A. M., Nelson, S. E., & Fomon, S. J. (1976). Body composition of the reference fetus. *Growth, 40,* 329–334.

7

Juvenile Idiopathic Arthritis

PAUL J.M. HELDERS, PhD, MSc, PT, PCS • SUSAN E. KLEPPER, PhD, PT • TIM TAKKEN, PhD, MSc •
JANJAAP VAN DER NET, PhD, BSc(PT), PCS

Chronic arthritis in childhood can result from any one of a heterogeneous group of diseases, of which juvenile idiopathic arthritis (JIA) is the most common. The disease causes joint swelling, pain, and limited mobility and can significantly restrict a child's activities. Box 7-1 lists the common clinical manifestations of JIA. Other conditions that may cause childhood arthritis include juvenile psoriatic arthritis (JPsA), juvenile ankylosing spondylitis (JAS), and other enthesitis-related arthritides. Arthritis may also be a feature of juvenile scleroderma, systemic lupus erythematosus, and juvenile dermatomyositis.

This chapter provides an overview of the impairments, activity limitations, and participation restrictions common to JIA and describes the role of the physical therapist as a member of the rheumatology team in the examination, evaluation, and intervention for the child with arthritis. Outcome instruments appropriate for use in JIA, issues related to school and recreational activities, surgical procedures, and adherence to therapeutic regimens are discussed. A case study illustrates the therapeutic management of a child with JIA.

ROLE OF THE THERAPIST

Physical therapists (PTs) are essential members of the pediatric rheumatology team, which includes the pediatric rheumatologist, nurse, occupational therapist, pediatric ophthalmologist, pediatric orthopedist, and pediatrician. Other pediatric specialists, including dermatologists, cardiologists, orthotists, psychologists, and social workers, provide occasional consultation as needed. After a thorough history, the PT conducts a comprehensive examination to identify impairments relevant to physical therapy intervention and caused by the disease and determines their relationship to observed or reported activity and participation restrictions. Based on an evaluation of these findings, the PT develops a prioritized problem list and an intervention plan to reduce functional impairments, to prevent or minimize secondary problems, and to improve activity and participation levels. Therapists work with parents and the child to develop a home program that includes balanced rest and exercise. They provide guidelines for choosing physical activities and consult with school personnel to ensure the child's full participation in educational activities.

The role of the therapist varies based on stage and progression of the disease and the care setting; often more than one PT is involved in the child's care. Physical therapists working in a specialized pediatric rheumatology center may perform the initial assessment, set treatment goals, plan a home program, and monitor the child's status at routine clinic visits. Therapists within the child's home, school, or community usually provide direct services. The frequency of therapy varies widely and depends on the child's physical status, reimbursement for therapy services, and the availability of therapists. For children with JIA, the PT often serves an important role as a consultant to provide education, monitor the child's functional status, and maintain communication with other members of the rheumatology team.

DIAGNOSIS AND CLASSIFICATION

Three systems are used to diagnose and classify childhood arthritis: the American College of Rheumatology (ACR) criteria for juvenile rheumatoid arthritis (JRA),[9] the European League Against Rheumatism (EULAR) criteria for juvenile chronic arthritis (JCA),[22] and the International League of Associations for Rheumatology (ILAR) criteria for juvenile idiopathic arthritis (JIA).[81] The ILAR criteria are used in this chapter. Juvenile idiopathic arthritis is not a single disease, but a term that encompasses all forms of arthritis that begin before the age of 16 years, persist for longer than 6 weeks, and are of unknown cause.[82] The term represents, therefore, an exclusion diagnosis. Because there are no definitive laboratory tests for JIA, the diagnosis is primarily clinical and sometimes is undecided until a clear picture of the disease evolves. Table 7-1 shows the characteristics of the different disease types: systemic arthritis (sJIA), oligoarthritis, polyarthritis (polyJIA), enthesitis-related arthritis, and psoriatic arthritis. All are defined by the clinical signs and symptoms observed during the first 6 months of the disease.

An oligoarticular onset occurs in 27% to 56% of children with JIA, mostly girls between 2 and 4 years of age.[82] Disease signs include low-grade inflammation in four or fewer joints, most often the knee, followed in frequency by the ankles and elbows (Figure 7-1). The hip and small joints of the hand are usually spared. The joint is swollen and may be warm but is not always painful. Systemic signs such as skin rash or spiking fever are unusual, but about 30% of children develop iridocyclitis, an asymptomatic inflammation of the eye that may lead to functional blindness. These children must have their eyes examined by an ophthalmologist at diagnosis and depending

---

| Box 7-1 | PRIMARY (P) AND SECONDARY (S) CLINICAL MANIFESTATIONS OF JUVENILE IDIOPATHIC ARTHRITIS (JIA) |

PRIMARY

Joint swelling, pain, stiffness
Morning stiffness
Muscle atrophy; weakness; poor muscle endurance
Acute or chronic iridocyclitis (most common in oligoarticular JIA)
Systemic manifestations (may be severe in systemic JIA; mild to moderate in polyarticular JIA)

SECONDARY

Limited joint motion; soft tissue contracture
Fatigue
Decreased aerobic capacity; reduced exercise tolerance
Growth abnormalities (local and general)
Osteopenia; osteoporosis (increased risk with long-term use of oral corticosteroids)
Difficulties with activities of daily living
Possible activity/participation restrictions

PRIMARY AND SECONDARY

Gait deviations

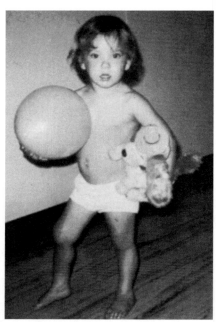

Figure 7-1   Oligoarticular juvenile idiopathic arthritis causing swelling and flexion contracture of the right knee in a 3-year-old girl with disease duration of 1 year. (From Cassidy, J. T., & Petty, R. E. [2001]. Juvenile rheumatoid arthritis. In J. T. Cassidy, & R. E. Petty [Eds.], *Textbook of pediatric rheumatology* [4th ed.; p. 231; Figure 12-8]. Philadelphia, WB Saunders.)

TABLE 7-1   **Frequency, Age at Onset, and Sex Distribution of the International League of Associations for Rheumatology (ILAR) Categories of Juvenile Idiopathic Arthritis**

	Frequency*	Onset Age	Sex Ratio
Systemic arthritis	4–17%	Throughout childhood	F = M
Oligoarthritis	27–56%	Early childhood; peak at 2–4 years	F >>> M
Rheumatoid-factor-positive polyarthritis	2–7%	Late childhood or adolescence	F >> M
Rheumatoid-factor-negative polyarthritis	11–28%	Biphasic distribution; early peak at 2–4 years and later peak at 6–12 years	F >> M
Enthesitis-related arthritis	3–11%	Late childhood or adolescence	M >> F
Psoriatic arthritis	2–11%	Biphasic distribution; early peak at 2–4 years and later peak at 9–11 years	F > M
Undifferentiated arthritis	11–21%	..	..

*Reported frequencies refer to percentage of all juvenile idiopathic arthritis.

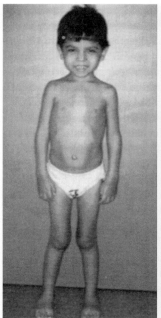
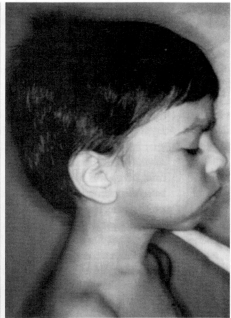
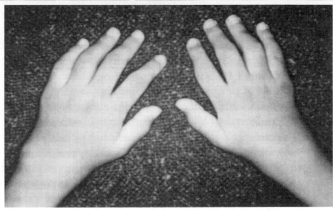

Figure 7-2 Symmetrical arthritis in large and small joints of the 6-year-old boy shown here is characteristic of polyarticular juvenile idiopathic arthritis. **A,** Flexion contractures are seen at the elbows, hips, and knees, and a slight valgus deformity is noted at the knees. The wrists and proximal interphalangeal joints are held in flexion. **B,** Loss of extension of the cervical spine. **C,** Symmetrical polyarthritis affects the metacarpophalangeal, proximal interphalangeal, and radiocarpal joints. (From Cassidy, J. T., & Petty, R. E. [2001]. Juvenile rheumatoid arthritis. In J. T. Cassidy, & R. E. Petty [Eds.], *Textbook of pediatric rheumatology* [4th ed.; p. 234; Figure 12-120]. Philadelphia: WB Saunders.)

on the risk every 3 to 4 or 6 to 12 months. Systemic or topical corticosteroids are used to control the inflammation.

Polyarticular JIA (Figure 7-2), subdivided into a rheumatoid factor (RF)-positive and an RF factor–negative polyarthritis and defined as arthritis in five or more joints, occurs in 2% to 28% of children with JIA, mostly girls. The RF factor–positive form has an early peak at 2 to 4 years and a later peak at 6 to 12 years, and RF factor–negative polyarthritis has an onset at late childhood or adolescence.[82] Onset is often insidious, with arthritis noted in progressively more joints. Arthritis is symmetrical, affects both large and small joints, and may include the cervical spine and temporomandibular joints. Joints are swollen and warm, but rarely red. Systemic symptoms are usually mild and include low-grade fever and mild to moderate hepatosplenomegaly and lymphadenopathy. About 19% develop iridocyclitis. The RF-positive group, mostly females with disease onset in late childhood or adolescence, follows a disease course similar to that seen in adults with rheumatoid arthritis. Individuals may have rheumatoid nodules on the elbows, tibial crests, and fingers and may develop erosive synovitis early in the disease course. Nodules are less common in children with RF-negative disease, and fewer joints are affected. Persistent arthritis may occur, causing juxta-articular osteopenia, muscle atrophy, weakness, contractures, and growth disturbances.

Systemic JIA occurs in 4% to 17% of cases. The disease arises as often in boys as in girls and does not know a preferential age onset. The diagnostic marker is a spiking fever of 39° C (102.2° F) or higher that occurs once or twice daily (afternoon or evening) for at least 2 weeks, with a rapid return to normal or below between spikes. The fever is accompanied by a typical evanescent rash (discrete, erythematous macules) that is most often found on the trunk or limbs, but may be seen on the face, palms, and soles of the feet (Figure 7-3). Other systemic signs include pleuritis, pericarditis, myocarditis, hepatosplenomegaly, and lymphadenopathy. Systemic disease may precede arthritis by several months or years. Fever, rash, and pericarditis often subside

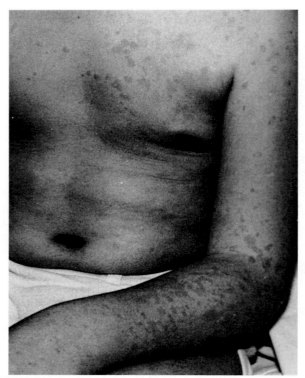

Figure 7-3 Typical rash of systemic-onset juvenile idiopathic arthritis in a 3-year-old boy. The rash is salmon-colored, macular, and nonpruritic. Individual lesions are transient, occur in crops over the trunk and extremities, and may occur in a linear distribution (Koebner's phenomenon) after minor trauma such as a scratch. (From Cassidy, J. T., & Petty, R. E. [2001]. Juvenile rheumatoid arthritis. In J. T. Cassidy, & R. E. Petty [Eds.], *Textbook of pediatric rheumatology* [4th ed.; p. 238; Figure 12-13]. Philadelphia: WB Saunders.)

after the initial disease period, but may recur during periods of exacerbation of the arthritis.[82]

INCIDENCE AND PREVALENCE

Studies reflecting mostly North American and European white populations place the incidence of JIA at between 2 and 20 per 100,000 at risk.[14] Based on a Mayo Clinic study, incidence in the United States decreased in recent years from 15 per 100,000 for the period from 1960 to 1969 to 7.8 per 100,000 for the years 1980 to 1993.[79] The reported prevalence of JIA varies from 16 to 150 per 100,000. Age at onset and gender distribution vary by disease type. In a study of 300 children with JIA, Sullivan and colleagues[92] reported that the peak age at onset was between 1 and 3 years for the total group and for girls, primarily those with oligoJIA and polyJIA. Disease onset for boys showed two peaks, one at 2 years, representing mostly boys with polyJIA, and another between 8 and 10 years of age that may partially represent children with JAS. Almost twice as many females as males develop JIA. The ratio of girls to boys is 3:1 for oligoJIA (5:1 for those with iridocyclitis) and 2.8:1 for polyJIA.[14]

ORIGIN AND PATHOGENESIS

The cause and pathogenesis of JIA are still poorly understood but seem to include both genetic and environmental components. The prevailing theory is that it is an autoimmune inflammatory disorder, activated by an external trigger, in a genetically predisposed host. A viral or bacterial infection often precedes disease onset. The notion that an infection triggers JIA in genetically susceptible individuals is attractive but still unproven.[82] Physical trauma may be associated with onset but may just draw attention to an already inflamed joint. The difference in onset types and disease course, the higher prevalence among girls, the narrow peak age periods of onset for all but systemic JIA, and the extensive immunologic abnormalities suggest that JIA may not be a single disease. Different etiologic vectors may be responsible for each onset type, or a single pathogen may cause distinct clinical patterns as it interacts with the host.

The role of the immune system in the pathogenesis and persistence of inflammation is evident in the altered immunity, abnormal immunoregulation, and cytokine production. The T-cell abnormalities and the pathology of the inflamed synovium suggest a cell-mediated pathogenesis. The presence of multiple autoantibodies and immune complexes and the complement activation indicate humoral abnormalities. The importance of genetic predisposition to JIA is not completely understood. Although few reports have described familial or multigenerational cases of JIA, studies of more than 3000 children with arthritis show concordance between siblings with JIA for age at onset, clinical manifestations, and disease course.[15] Many of the suspected genetic predispositions are within the major histocompatibility complex (MHC) region of chromosome 6, but the pathogenesis may involve the interactions of multiple genes. Recent studies indicate that correlations found between human leukocyte antigen (HLA) specificities and various types of JIA may have specific risks and protective effects that are age-related for each onset type and some course subtypes.[69]

MEDICAL MANAGEMENT

The goals of pharmacologic therapy in JIA are to control the arthritis, thereby preventing joint erosions, and to manage extra-articular manifestations. Children with severe or persistent disease often require a carefully orchestrated combination of sometimes aggressive drug therapies, started early in the disease. A core set of six outcome variables is often used in clinical trials to determine subjects' responses to medical therapy.[27] These include physician global assessment of disease activity, parent/patient assessment of overall health status, functional ability, number of joints with active arthritis, number of joints with limited motion, and erythrocyte sedimentation rate (ESR). A positive clinical response is defined as improvement of at least 30% from baseline in at least three of the six variables, with no more than one of the other variables worsening by more than 30%.

Nonsteroidal anti-inflammatory drugs (NSAIDs) are the most widely used first-line therapy. Naproxen, tolmetin, and ibuprofen are used most often, but other NSAIDs may be tried. The most common adverse effect is gastrointestinal irritation, although NSAIDs that selectively inhibit the cyclo-oxygenase 2 (COX-2) enzyme may limit this problem. However, experience with COX-2 inhibitors in children is scarce. NSAIDs reduce fever, pain, and inflammation but do not alter disease course. Methotrexate (MTX) is the most common disease-modifying antirheumatic drug (DMARD) prescribed for children with polyJIA and sJIA.[17] The drug is usually administered orally once a week, although subcutaneous injection is given if the response is inadequate or if the child experiences adverse effects with the oral dose, including gastrointestinal upset. Although liver toxicity in children taking MTX appears to be rare, physicians check blood counts and liver enzymes every 4 to 8 weeks. Data on the health risks associated with long-term use of MTX in children are not yet available.

Patients with a poor prognosis who fail to respond to MTX are treated with one of the so-called biological medications that target the tumor necrosis factor (TNF), a cytokine responsible for many of the effects of inflammation. These drugs include etanercept, infliximab, and adalimumab. In one clinical trial, children treated with etanercept showed significant improvement over placebo on standard outcome measures.[62] Other biologics being tested in adults with RA may prove useful in JIA. Sulfasalazine, another DMARD, has been shown to be effective in suppressing disease activity in some children, mostly in oligoJIA, but the risk for toxicity is high. Systemic glucocorticoid drugs are reserved for children, mostly those with sJIA who do not respond to other therapies. Although steroids have a potent anti-inflammatory effect, they do not alter disease course or duration. Serious adverse effects of long-term oral steroids include iatrogenic Cushing's syndrome, myopathy, growth disturbance, osteoporosis and fracture, diabetes mellitus, obesity, and increased susceptibility to infection. For children with refractory disease who are steroid-dependent, aggressive therapy with cyclosporin A or cyclophosphamide may provide some benefit.[17] Intra-articular injections of long-acting corticosteroids[17] are used successfully to treat severely inflamed and swollen joints. A recent study found that intra-articular steroid injections for lower extremity joints decreased the incidence of leg length discrepancies, a major cause of gait and postural abnormalities in children with JIA.[89]

PROGNOSIS

Studies assessing outcomes of JIA have provided inconsistent or conflicting results. Studies over the past 10 years have shown that only 40% to 60% of patients had inactive disease or clinical remission at follow-up. Despite long-term persistence of disease activity in most patients, a pronounced improvement in functional outcome has been documented in the past decade.[82] Poor articular and functional outcomes in sJIA and polyJIA are linked to the presence of hip involvement and polyarthritis in the first year of disease activity.[91] Children with oligoJIA have the best prognosis for joint preservation and function but may develop contractures during active disease and later degenerative arthritis. They also remain at high risk for inflammatory eye involvement. About 5% to 10% follow an extended disease course, adding multiple joints after the first 6 months. Those who are RF+ often follow a course similar to that of children with RF+ polyJIA, with persistent disease and poor functional outcomes. In contrast, outcome is usually good in boys with disease onset at 9 years of age or older, who are positive for the *HLA-B27* gene, and have arthritis mostly in the hip and sacroiliac joints.

Reports of long-term functional outcomes in JIA vary, possibly because of differences in study methods. Ruperto and colleagues[85] conducted a 15-year follow-up study of American and Italian patients with JIA. Subjects had favorable outcomes on measures of functional status, pain, overall well-being, and quality of life. However, in another study, adults with a history of JIA reported significantly greater pain, disability, and fatigue, as well as impaired physical function and perception of their health, compared with age- and gender-matched controls.[80] The inconsistencies in these reports illustrate the importance of early and effective treatment of the disease to prevent or minimize adverse outcomes.

PHYSICAL THERAPY EXAMINATION

When examining a child with JIA, the physical therapist has to consider the stage of the disease. In the acute phase, the child exhibits a great number of impairments, resulting in compensatory motor behavior that will change or disappear when the child is adequately medicated. It is important to know that physical therapy intervention will be significantly hampered when the child is not adequately medicated. Regular communication between rheumatologist and physical therapist during the acute phase is of utmost importance.

The approach to physical therapy examination in JIA must consider the child's age, motor development before disease onset, and cognitive and emotional development. By first gathering information about the child's activities and participation, the therapist is able to focus the physical examination on impairments that may contribute to the functional problems. However, the therapist must also closely monitor joint motion and integrity because loss of motion may be the first sign of joint damage and may signal an increased risk for functional decline. Appendix I lists standardized outcome instruments that provide quantitative data to guide intervention and evaluate change.

APPENDIX 1 OUTCOME MEASUREMENTS IN JUVENILE IDIOPATHIC ARTHRITIS			
OUTCOME	**LEVEL OF ICF**	**MEASUREMENT**	**REFERENCE**
Disease Activity			
Active joint count	Impairment	ACR joint count	Guzman et al., 1995
Morning stiffness	Impairment	Presence and duration of stiffness	Wright et al., 1996
Global ratings	Impairment	Physician rating on a VAS	Ruperto et al., 1999
Joint range of motion (AAROM or PROM)	Impairment	JC-LOM (ASS) pEPM-ROM GROMS/10-joint GROMS	Klepper et al., 1992; Len et al., 1999; Epps et al., 2002
Muscle strength	Impairment	MMT	Dunn, 1993;
		Handheld dynamometer	Wessel et al., 1999;
		Isokinetic dynamometer	Giannini & Protas, 1993
Grip strength	Impairment	Modified sphygmomanometer or handheld dynamometer	Dunn, 1993
Aerobic fitness	Impairment	Laboratory measures (VO$_2$peak)	Takken et al., 2002
		Standardized walk or run test	Klepper et al., 1992; Takken et al., 2001
Anaerobic fitness	Impairment	Laboratory measures (Wingate Anaerobic Test)	van Brussel et al., 2008
		50-meter sprint	Fan & Wessel, 1998
	Impairment/activity	Physical activity monitoring	Henderson et al., 1995
Gait			
Characteristics of gait pattern	Impairment	Observation	
Time/distance parameters and kinetic parameters	Impairment	Footprint analysis	Wright et al., 1996
		Instrumented gait lab tests	Lechner et al., 1987
Gross and fine motor	Activity	Developmental tests	Morrison et al., 1991; Van der Net et al., 2008
School function	Activity	School checklists	Szer & Wright, 2000
	Activity/participation	School function assessment	Coster et al., 1998
Pain behaviors	Activity	Observation	Jaworski et al., 1995
	Impairment	Child self-report	Beyer et al., 1992; Wong & Baker, 1988; Hester et al., 1990; Thompson & Varni, 1986
	Impairment/activity	Child self-report	Varni et al., 1996
Physical Function			
Parent/child report	Activity	CHAQ	Singh et al., 1994
		JAFAR	Howe et al., 1991
		JASI	Wright et al., 1992
Performance			
Performance	Participation	COPM	Law et al., 2005
Quality of life	Activity	JAFAS	Lovell et al., 1989
Parent/child report	Impairment/activity	JAQQ	Duffy et al., 1997
	Participation	PedsQL	Varni et al., 2002
		QOML scale	Feldman et al., 2000

ACR, American College of Rheumatology; *CHAQ,* Childhood Health Assessment Questionnaire; *COPM,* Canadian Occupational Performance Measure; *GROMS,* Global Range of Motion Scale; *ICF,* International Classification of Functioning, Disability, and Health; *JAFAR,* Juvenile Arthritis Functional Assessment Report; *JAFAS,* Juvenile Arthritis Functional Assessment Scale; *JAQQ,* Juvenile Arthritis Quality of Life Questionnaire; *JASI,* Juvenile Arthritis Functional Status Index; *JC-LOM,* (AS) Joint Count–Limitation of Motion, Articular Severity Score; *MMT,* manual muscle test; *PedsQL,* Pediatric Quality of Life Questionnaire; *pEPM-ROM,* Paediatric Escola Paulista de Medicina–Range of Motion Scale; *QOML,* Quality of MyLife Scale; *VAS,* visual analog scale; *VO$_2$peak,* peak oxygen uptake.

PARTICIPATION AND ACTIVITY RESTRICTIONS

The impact of JIA on a child's activities depends on the extent and duration of active disease, the child's developmental stage, resiliency, and desire to be independent, and expectations placed on the child by parents and others. Changes in motor activity could very well be the first notable sign of behavioral change in a child. For example, the first sign of wrist involvement in a toddler could be incomplete or compensated palmar support (e.g., when on "all fours"), limiting the ability to crawl during play activities on the floor. Another sign of wrist involvement may be a compensatory pattern of palmar support in which the child does not bear weight on the full palmar part of the hand, but only on the palmar part of the fingers, utilizing the ability to hyperextend the metacarpophalangeal (MCP) joints (which may have a detrimental effect on joint function later in life). A classic example of early impact on motor activities is the change in ambulation in a toddler with arthritis in the knee, leading to a change from walking to bottom shuffling. A child with oligoJIA may demonstrate few functional limitations, but one with severe polyJIA may need assistance with activities of daily living (ADLs) long past the time when other children of the same age are independent. They may have difficulty moving between standing and sitting on the floor, getting into and out of the bed or a bathtub, negotiating steps, and walking long distances. Even children with mild disease may be dependent for some self-care tasks, particularly if parents provide assistance that may be unnecessary. Children may fail to develop gross motor proficiency if parents discourage them from typical childhood activities, such as riding a bike, climbing on playground equipment, or other active play.[68] Most parents are confused as they tend to mix up juvenile idiopathic arthritis with the adult type of rheumatoid arthritis. A recent study showed that preschool age children display greater motor proficiency delays, whereas children at early school age face more delays in activity and participation development.[71]

The child's participation will also be affected by the extent and quality of supportive services available and utilized by the child and family. Many children who report problems with some aspect of their educational program do not receive related services recommended by the rheumatology team.[61,63] Tardiness as a result of morning stiffness and frequent absence due to illness or medical appointments may cause the child to miss academic time and social interactions with classmates. Children may feel different and somewhat isolated because they are unable to participate in the same activities as their classmates. Daily fluctuations in disease symptoms may also affect the child's mood and ability to cope.[86] Adolescents with JIA may be unable to gain the same level of independence as their peers because of physical limitations and the need for continued medical care.

Several standardized instruments examine the child's activities. The Childhood Health Assessment Questionnaire (CHAQ), a measure of physical function designed for children age 1 to 19 years, includes 30 activities organized into eight categories (Figure 7-4).[90] The respondent (parent or child 9 years or older) scores each item based on how much difficulty the child had performing the task during the past week (0 = without any difficulty; 1 = with some difficulty; 2 = with much difficulty; 3 = unable to do). An item is scored as "not applicable" if the child has difficulty because he is too young. The highest scored item in each section determines the score for that category. If the child needs an assistive device or help from another person to perform a task, the score for that category is at least 2. The Disability Index (DI), calculated as the average score for the eight categories, has a range of 0 to 3. Higher scores indicate greater disability. The CHAQ also includes a question about the presence and duration of morning stiffness and visual analog scales (VAS) to measure pain intensity and general health status. Recently, the CHAQ has been revised and extended with eight more physically demanding items to meet the challenges of a more physical active lifestyle in children with rheumatic conditions.[53]

Other questionnaires designed to measure physical function include the Juvenile Arthritis Functional Assessment Index (JASI)[112] and the Juvenile Arthritis Functional Assessment Report (JAFAR).[40] A school checklist can be used to examine school-related problems.[93] The School Function Assessment may also be useful.[16] Two other instruments measure both physical function and quality of life (QOL) in children with JIA. These are the Juvenile Arthritis Quality of Life Questionnaire (JAQQ)[18] and the Pediatric Quality of Life Questionnaire (PedsQL).[103] The only instrument that measures the child's actual performance is the Juvenile Arthritis Functional Assessment Scale (JAFAS) (Figure 7-5). The child is observed and timed while completing 10 tasks. The score is 0 if the time to complete the task is equal to or less than the criterion time, 1 if the time exceeds the criterion, and 2 if the child cannot perform the task. The test takes 10 minutes and requires a minimum of simple equipment.[64]

JOINT STRUCTURE AND FUNCTION

The cardinal signs of inflammation are swelling, end-range stress pain, stiffness, and loss of full range of joint motion. Swelling around a joint may be the result of intra-articular effusion, synovial hypertrophy, soft tissue edema, or periarticular tenosynovitis.[66] The joint may also be enlarged as a result of bony overgrowth due to increased blood supply to the inflamed area. Swelling and protective muscle spasm contribute to pain. This muscle spasm is referred to as a *contraction deformity*, in contrast with the more common *conception contracture*, which refers to a morphologic change in the periarticular soft tissue. Inactivity stiffness most noted upon awakening and after periods of prolonged sitting is a common indicator of disease activity.

In this section, we are interested in learning how your child's illness affects his/her ability to function in daily life. Please feel free to add any comments on the back of this page. In the following questions, please check the one response that best describes your child's usual activities (averaged over an entire day) *OVER THE PAST WEEK*. If your child has difficulty in doing a certain activity or is unable to do it because he/she is too young but NOT because he/she is RESTRICTED BY ARTHRITIS, please mark it as "Not Applicable." ONLY NOTE THOSE DIFFICULTIES OR LIMITATIONS THAT ARE DUE TO ARTHRITIS.

	Without ANY Difficulty	With SOME Difficulty	With MUCH Difficulty	UNABLE To Do	Not Applicable
DRESSING & GROOMING					
Is your child able to:					
• Dress, including tying shoelaces and doing buttons?	___	___	___	___	___
• Shampoo his/her hair?	___	___	___	___	___
• Remove socks?	___	___	___	___	___
• Cut fingernails/toenails?	___	___	___	___	___
ARISING					
Is your child able to:					
• Stand up from a low chair or floor?	___	___	___	___	___
• Get in and out of bed or stand up in crib?	___	___	___	___	___
EATING					
Is your child able to:					
• Cut his/her own meat?	___	___	___	___	___
• Lift a cup or glass to mouth?	___	___	___	___	___
• Open a new cereal box?	___	___	___	___	___
WALKING					
Is your child able to:					
• Walk outdoors on flat ground?	___	___	___	___	___
• Climb up five steps?	___	___	___	___	___

*Please check any AIDS or DEVICES that your child usually uses for any of the above activities.

_____ Cane   _____ Devices used for dressing (button hook, zipper pull, long-handled shoe horn, etc.)
_____ Walker   _____ Built-up pencil or special utensils
_____ Crutches   _____ Special or built-up chair
_____ Wheelchair   _____ Other (Specify:_____)

*Please check any categories for which your child usually needs help from another person BECAUSE OF ARTHRITIS:

_____ Dressing and Grooming   _____ Eating
_____ Arising   _____ Walking

	Without ANY Difficulty	With SOME Difficulty	With MUCH Difficulty	UNABLE To Do	Not Applicable
HYGIENE					
Is your child able to:					
• Wash and dry entire body?	___	___	___	___	___
• Take a tub bath (get in and out of tub)?	___	___	___	___	___
• Get on and off the toilet or potty chair?	___	___	___	___	___
• Brush teeth?	___	___	___	___	___
• Comb/brush hair?	___	___	___	___	___
REACH					
Is your child able to:					
• Reach and get down a heavy object such as a large game or books from just above his/her head?	___	___	___	___	___
• Bend down to pick up clothing or a piece of paper from the floor?	___	___	___	___	___
• Pull on a sweater over his/her head?	___	___	___	___	___
• Turn neck to look back over shoulder?	___	___	___	___	___
GRIP					
Is your child able to:					
• Write or scribble with pen or pencil?	___	___	___	___	___

Figure 7-4   Childhood Health Assessment Questionnaire: Disability and Discomfort Sections. (From Singh, G., Athreya, B., Fries, J., & Goldsmith, D. P. [1994]. Measurement of health status in children with juvenile rheumatoid arthritis. *Arthritis and Rheumatism, 37*, 1762–1764.)

	Without ANY Difficulty	With SOME Difficulty	With MUCH Difficulty	UNABLE To Do	Not Applicable
GRIP (*Continued*)					
• Open car doors?	_____	_____	_____	_____	_____
• Open jars that have been previously opened?	_____	_____	_____	_____	_____
• Turn faucets on and off?	_____	_____	_____	_____	_____
• Push open a door when he/she has to turn a door knob?	_____	_____	_____	_____	_____
ACTIVITIES					
Is your child able to:					
• Run errands and shop?	_____	_____	_____	_____	_____
• Get in and out of car or toy car or school bus?	_____	_____	_____	_____	_____
• Ride bike or tricycle?	_____	_____	_____	_____	_____
• Do household chores (e.g., wash dishes, take out trash, vacuuming, yardwork, make bed, clean room)?	_____	_____	_____	_____	_____
• Run and play?	_____	_____	_____	_____	_____

*Please check any AIDS or DEVICES that your child usually uses for any of the above activities:

_____Raised toilet seat   _____Bathtub bar
_____Bathtub seat   _____Long-handled appliances in reach
_____Jar opener (for jars opened previously)   _____Long-handled appliances in bathroom

*Please check any categories for which your child usually needs help from another person BECAUSE OF ARTHRITIS?

_____Hygiene   _____Gripping and Opening Things
_____Reach   _____Errands and Chores

We are also interested in learning whether your child has been affected by pain because of his or her illness.

*How much pain do you think your child has had because of his or her illness IN THE PAST WEEK?

Place a mark on the line below to indicate the severity of the pain.

No pain   Very severe pain
├──┤
0   100

HEALTH STATUS
1. Considering all the ways that arthritis affects your child, rate how your child is doing on the following scale by placing a mark on the line.

├──┤
0   100
Very well   Very poor
2. Is your child stiff in the morning?   _____Yes   _____No
   If YES, about how long does the stiffness usually last (in the past week)?
                        Hours/Minutes_____

Figure 7-4, cont'd

For each activity, please record how long the child took to perform the activity. If the activity was completed in less than or equal to the criterion time, then score the item as 0; if completed but requiring longer than the criterion time, score the item as 1; if unable to perform the activity, score the item as 2.

Activity	Criterion Time (seconds)	Observed Time (seconds)	Item Score 0	1	2
1. Button shirt/blouse	22.4	_____	___	___	___
2. Pull shirt or sweater over head	14.6	_____	___	___	___
3. Pull on both socks	27.2	_____	___	___	___
4. Cut food with knife and fork	12.8	_____	___	___	___
5. Get into bed	3.4	_____	___	___	___
6. Get out of bed	2.9	_____	___	___	___
7. Pick something up off of floor from standing position	2.4	_____	___	___	___
8. From standing position sit on floor, then stand up	4.0	_____	___	___	___
9. Walk 50 feet without assistance	15.1	_____	___	___	___
10. Walk up flight of 5 steps	3.7	_____	___	___	___
		TOTAL SCORE	_____		

Figure 7-5 Scoring for the Juvenile Arthritis Functional Assessment Scale. (From Lovell, D. J., Howe, S., Shear, E., Hartner, S., McGirr, G., Schulte, M., et al. [1989]. Development of a disability measurement tool for juvenile rheumatoid arthritis: The Juvenile Arthritis Functional Assessment Scale. *Arthritis and Rheumatism, 32*, 1393.)

Chronic inflammation causes abnormalities in joint structure and function. Increased production of synovial fluid stretches and weakens the joint capsule and adjacent structures, leading to ligamentous laxity and joint instability. Massive overgrowth of the synovium, called *pannus*, spreads over and invades the articular cartilage, releasing inflammatory enzymes into the synovial fluid. In some patients, erosions in the articular cartilage and subchondral bone cause irregularities in the joint surface, compromising alignment, congruency, and stability.[14] Early radiographs show periarticular swelling with widening of the joint space, juxtaarticular osteopenia, and periosteal new bone.[83] Radiographs of joints placed under physiologic strain (i.e., tested in function) provide a more precise indication of the quality of the periarticular soft tissue condition (e.g., laxity of wrist ligaments may be visualized in the translation of carpal bones).[35] General demineralization, thinning and loss of articular cartilage, marginal erosions, and osteophytes occur with persistent disease.[14] Nutritional deficiencies, low body weight, and decreased physical activity may result in low bone density and risk for fracture.[51] This is exacerbated by long-term use of systemic corticosteroids. Joint contractures usually result from intra-articular adhesions and fibrosis of adjacent tendons.

The therapist should be aware of possible patterns of joint restriction in JIA and their potential effects on function (Appendix II). Arthritis may occur in any joint, but the large joints are affected most often. Hip arthritis occurs in 30% to 50% of children, mostly those with sJIA and polyJIA.[91] Early signs of hip disease may include leg length inequality, pain in the groin, buttocks, medial thigh, or knee, and a gluteus medius limp. A child may compensate for a mild hip flexion contracture with increased lumbar lordosis. Children with oligoJIA may lose hip motion secondary to knee flexion contracture and leg length discrepancy. The knee is the joint most often affected in oligoJIA, but it is also involved in other disease types. Flexion contracture may result from intraarticular swelling, joint immobility, spasm of the hamstrings, and shortening of the tensor fasciae latae. Chronic synovitis, with overgrowth of the medial femoral condyle, results in a valgus deformity that is exaggerated by tightness in the iliotibial band (ITB) (see Figure 7-2). Ankle arthritis occurs in all disease types, but involvement of the small joints of the feet is more common in polyJIA. Problems may include loss of ankle dorsiflexion or, less often, of plantar flexion, metatarsalgia, subluxation of the metatarsophalangeal joints, hallux valgus, hallux rigidus, hammer toes, and overlapping toes. Arthritis of the subtalar joint may result in hindfoot valgus with forefoot pronation (Figure 7-6), although some children develop calcaneal varus and a forefoot cavus deformity.

The cervical spine and the temporomandibular joints are frequently involved. Early signs of neck involvement include pain and stiffness in the back of the neck, with loss of extension and limitations in rotation and lateral flexion. Atlantoaxial subluxation may occur early in the disease, placing the

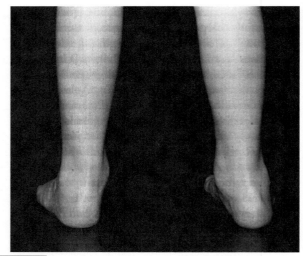

Figure 7-6   A common foot deformity is hindfoot valgus with pronation.

child at risk for injury from trauma or during intubation for surgery. Cervical spine ankylosis is sometimes seen and can cause similar problems during surgery.

Temporomandibular joint involvement includes difficulties in chewing food, loss of range of motion as shown by a restriction in mouth opening, and pain in the ear region. Chronic involvement of temporomandibular joints will lead to an overgrowth of the jaw or to micrognathia (undergrowth of the mandible) and difficulties in mouth closure. Even the joints of the larynx and the area of the vocal cords can be affected, leading to hoarseness of the voice.

Restrictions in shoulder rotation, flexion, and abduction may occur with arthritis in the glenohumeral joint, as well as in the acromioclavicular, sternoclavicular, and manubriosternal joints. Elbow flexion contractures occur early and may be accompanied by loss of forearm supination. Arthritis in the wrist and small joints of the hands is most common in polyJIA. The pattern and extent of involvement are related to disease type, the child's age, and maturation of the epiphyses at disease onset. Wrist malalignment associated with subluxation and undergrowth of the ulna, with ulnar deviation, occurs in children with disease onset at a young age. Those 12 years or older at onset have a pattern typical of adults, with radial deviation. The metacarpophalangeal (MCP) and proximal interphalangeal (PIP) joints are also involved, either directly by synovitis or indirectly as a result of inflammation in adjacent joints or tendon sheaths.

JOINT EXAMINATION

When examining the joints, the physical therapist has to consider the stage of the disease: acute, subacute, or chronic. Each stage of the disease has its typical joint expression. The acute or early phase of the disease is dominated by joint inflammation, joint effusion (can be felt and moved around), ligamentous laxity, and joint instability. In the subacute and

APPENDIX II PATTERNS OF JOINT AND SOFT TISSUE RESTRICTIONS AND CLINICAL ADAPTATIONS IN JUVENILE IDIOPATHIC ARTHRITIS (JIA)*	
CLINICAL MANIFESTATIONS	**RESTRICTIONS/ADAPTATIONS**
Cervical Spine	
In polyJIA and sJIA	Loss of EXT, rotation, side FLEX
Inflammation, narrowing, then fusion; observed first in C2-C3, but may progress to involve the entire cervical spine[†]	May develop torticollis if asymmetrical
	Intubation for anesthesia[†]
Dysplasia of vertebral bodies	Eye movements or turning body compensates for ↓ neck ROM
Odontoid process instability (less common than in adult RA)	
Temporomandibular Joint	
Common in polyJIA; less common in oligoJIA; often associated with cervical spine disease	Restriction in opening mouth; pain on chewing; may need orthodontia
Mandibular asymmetry if unilateral involvement	Greater functional restrictions if cervical spine is involved
Undergrowth of the mandible (micrognathia); malocclusion of the teeth	EXT is restricted
Shoulder Complex	
Most common in polyJIA[†]	Loss of active GL-H ABD and IR first limitations noted; limited FLEX, tightening of pectorals and scapular protractors; more dysfunction when elbow and wrist involved
Overgrowth of humeral head with irregular shape, shallow glenoid fossa	
Subluxation may occur	
Elbow	
Involved early in disease course[†]	EXT lost early; eventual limitation in FLEX and forearm rotation
Occurs in all types; symmetrical in polyJIA and sJIA; asymmetrical in oligoJIA[†]	Shoulder ROM initially compensates for ↓ supination; loss of >45° EXT restricts ability to push off from chair
Overgrowth of radial head restricts ROM	
Proximal radioulnar joint involved[†]	Wrist involvement accentuates loss of pronation and supination
Ulnar nerve entrapment possible	
Wrist	
All types; starts early; symmetrical in polyJIA and sJIA; unilateral in oligoJIA[†]	Rapid loss of EXT; weakness of extensors; FLEX contracture and volar subluxation
Accelerated carpal maturation	Rests in flexion and ulnar deviation with spasm of wrist flexors
Undergrowth of ulna; ulnar shortening; may migrate dorsally	In older-onset or RF+ polyJIA, tendency is toward radial deviation[†]
Radiocarpal and intercarpal fusion	Distal radioulnar disease causes loss of pronation and supination
Flexor tenosynovitis; carpal tunnel syndrome is rare; may occur late in disease	
Hand	
Premature epiphyseal fusion and growth abnormalities	PIP (especially 4th) more common than DIP contractures
Flexor tenosynovitis may be dramatic	Loss of MCP FLEX (especially 2nd digit); loss of MCP hyperextension
Involvement later in polyJIA and sJIA than in oligoJIA	Marked decrease in grip strength
MCP and CMP subluxation deformities	Boutonniere < swan neck
Thoracolumbar Spine	
Unusual site in JIA	Kyphosis in association with neck and shoulder involvement
Steroid drug therapy may cause osteoporosis, wedging of vertebral bodies, small compression fractures	Lumbar lordosis 2° to hip flexion contractures; scoliosis 2° to lower limb asymmetries
	Pain with compression fractures[†]
Hip	
Femoral head overgrowth	Flexion contractures, may be masked by lumbar lordosis
Osteoporosis	May present as pain in the groin, over buttocks, medial thigh, around knee[†]
Trochanteric growth changes	IR and ABD lost early 2° to pain and spasm of FLEXs and ADDs

Continued

APPENDIX II PATTERNS OF JOINT AND SOFT TISSUE RESTRICTIONS AND CLINICAL ADAPTATIONS IN JUVENILE IDIOPATHIC ARTHRITIS (JIA)*[2,4,5,20,49,107]—cont'd	
CLINICAL MANIFESTATIONS	**RESTRICTIONS/ADAPTATIONS**
Shallow acetabulum, ↓ femoral neck angle, especially if weight bearing limited	
Lateral subluxation of femoral head aggravated by tight adductors	May have marked pain on standing
Potential for protrusio acetabuli, avascular necrosis	Gluteus medius weakness may cause Trendelenburg gait deviation[†]
Primary cause of ↓ ROM and dysfunction	Secondary deformities of the contralateral hip, knees, and lumbar spine
Occurs in polyJIA and sJIA after a few years	
Potential for regeneration of articular cartilage with fibrocartilage if remission of synovitis[†]	Mobility and weight bearing improve cartilage repair[†]
KNEE	
Most common joint involved early in all types	Rapid development of flexion contracture
Overgrowth of distal femur may cause leg length discrepancy in unilateral disease	Rapid atrophy of quadriceps; loss of patellar mobility due to adhesions
Knee valgus aggravated by tight hamstrings and iliotibial band	Risk of femoral fracture associated with falling due to flexion and osteoporosis
Posterior tibial subluxation 2° to prolonged joint	Loss of flexion (often only to 90°)
Involvement or excessive correction of knee flexion contracture	Secondary hip flexion contracture
ANKLE/FOOT	
Altered growth causes bony changes in tarsals with potential fusion	Early loss of inversion, eversion
Hindfoot valgus/varus due to ankle joint arthritis or 2° to knee valgus	Later loss of D-FL and PL-FL, especially if ambulation is limited
MTP subluxation	Altered gait, loss of MTP hyperextension affects toe-off
Hallux valgus	Overlapping of IPs, especially with hallux valgus
IPs: growth changes due to premature epiphyseal closure	

*Data in this table are summarized from information published in Ansell, 1992; Atwood, 1989; Cassidy & Petty, 1990; Emery, 1993; Libby et al., 1991; Reed & Wilmot, 1991; Rhodes, 1991; White, 1990; and Cassidy, J. T., & Petty, R. E. (2001). Juvenile rheumatoid arthritis. In J. T. Cassidy, & R. E. Petty (Eds.), *Textbook of pediatric rheumatology* (4th ed.). Philadelphia: WB Saunders.
[†]The listing is not inclusive, but the features described are characteristic of juvenile arthritis.
ABD, abduction/abductors; *ADD,* adduction/adductors; *CMP,* carpometacarpal-phalangeal; *D-FL,* dorsiflexion; *DIP,* distal interphalangeal; *EXT,* extension; *FLEX,* flexion, flexors; *GL-H,* glenohumeral; *IP,* interphalangeal; *IR,* internal rotation; *MCP,* metacarpophalangeal; *MTP,* metatarsophalangeal; *polyJIA,* polyarticular JIA; *PL-FL,* plantar flexion; *ROM,* range of motion; *sJIA,* systemic JIA.
Adapted from Wright, F. V., & Smith, E. (1996). Physical therapy management of the child and adolescent with juvenile rheumatoid arthritis. In J. M. Walker, & A. Helewa (Eds.), *Physical therapy in arthritis* (p. 215; Table 12-6). Philadelphia: WB Saunders.

chronic phases, the inflammation has become prolonged (longer than 3 months), leading to joint swelling due to synovial hypertrophy (has a doughy feel) and loss of joint integrity, such as loss of normal joint physiology, erosive changes in cartilage, and loss of joint alignment. During joint examination, special attention should be paid to these typical disease expressions.

Joint counts for swelling (JC-S) and limitation of motion (JC-LOM) are recorded on a stick figure to document disease activity and joint restrictions (Figure 7-7). Figure 7-8 shows two methods of verifying a joint effusion by observing fluctuations of fluid from one area of the joint to another,

eliciting a bulge sign. To detect an effusion in the knee, the synovial pouch medial to the patella is emptied by stroking in an upward direction and then is refilled by stroking along the lateral border in an upward or downward direction.

Active joint motion can be estimated by watching the child perform a series of movements during various childhood activities, but goniometric measurement is necessary to document limited joint motion. Two standardized measures of the JC-LOM are the Articular Severity Score (ASS) and the Global Range of Motion Score (GROMS). The ASS scores global range of motion (ROM) for each joint, averaged for the right and left sides, on a 5-point scale (0 = no

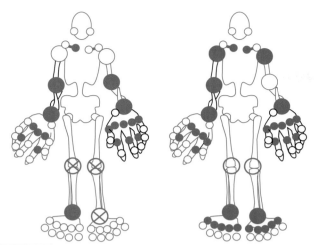

Figure 7-7   Example of active joint count in a child with polyarticular disease. There are 38 active joints. The *left figure* shows 22 with effusion (•) or soft tissue swelling (X). The *right figure* shows joints with stress pain or tenderness (•). (From Wright, F. V., & Smith, E. [1996]. Physical therapy management of the child and adolescent with juvenile rheumatoid arthritis. In J. M. Walker, & A. Helewa [Eds.], *Physical therapy in arthritis* [p. 215]. Philadelphia: WB Saunders.)

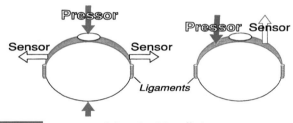

Figure 7-8   Two ways of detecting joint effusions. (From Smythe, H. A., & Helewa, A. [1996]. Assessment of joint disease. In J. M. Walker, & A. Helewa [Eds.], *Physical therapy in arthritis* [p. 133]. Philadelphia: WB Saunders.)

LOM; 1 = 25% LOM; 2 = 50% LOM; 3 = 75% LOM; and 4 = fused). In contrast, the GROMS provides a single score for global joint function. Each joint movement is weighted from 0 (least important) to 5 (essential), based on expert opinion of its functional importance. The examiner records the mean ROM in degrees for the right and left sides. The ratio of the measured value to the normative value is calculated to obtain the joint movement score. The total GROMS is calculated as the sum for all movements multiplied by 100 and divided by the number of movements (Table 7-2).

A reduced 10-joint version of the GROMS is also available that includes only those joint motions weighted as 5 (essential) on the original GROMS. The total score is calculated using the same method as the full scale. The Pediatric Escola Paulista de Medicina ROM Scale (pEPM-ROM)[57] also includes 10 essential joint movements but uses predetermined cutoff points for scoring (0 = full motion to 3 = severe limitation). The total score (0 to 3) for each side of the body is the sum of all joint scores divided by 10. Each scale demonstrates adequate concurrent validity with other measures of disease status and function in JIA.[21] Excellent test-retest

and intertester agreement are reported for the pEPM-ROM.[57] Testing of the 10-joint GROMS continues. Although a reduced JC-LOM saves time during the examination, it may not be appropriate for patients whose arthritis is extensive or does not affect any of the 10 joints measured.

MUSCULAR STRUCTURE AND FUNCTION

The different stages of the disease will show a difference in muscular structures and functions.

In the acute phase of the disease, periarticular musculature of the affected joints will show spasm and hypertonus, also referred to as *contraction deformity*.

In subacute and chronic stages of the disease, muscle atrophy and weakness are more pronounced, especially near the affected joints. This also may occur in distant areas and can persist long after remission of the arthritis.[19,27,30,38,59,60,75,105] Contributing factors to an altered muscle structure and function include alterations in anabolic hormones, production of inflammatory cytokines and high resting energy metabolism,[50] abnormal protein metabolism,[36] motor unit inhibition from pain and swelling, and disuse. Also a disease onset very early in life, with long periods of active arthritis, may negatively affect muscle development.[105]

PHYSICAL FITNESS

Health-Related Fitness

Physical fitness can be divided into various components, namely, health-related fitness (peak oxygen uptake [VO_2peak]) and performance-related fitness (muscle strength, anaerobic capacity). The VO_2peak is most frequently assessed using progressively graded exercise tests on a cycle ergometer with respiratory gas analysis in children with JIA,[95] although some researchers have used treadmill testing in children with JIA.[44]

A large body of evidence shows that the peak oxygen uptake of children and adolescents with JIA is lower than that in healthy peers. In the most recent studies in JIA, in the age between 6.7 and 18 years, VO_2peak (L/min) and VO_2peak corrected for body mass (VO_2peak/kg in ml/kg/min) were respectively 69.8% and 74.8% in children and 83% and 80% of predicted for adolescents with JIA.[5,10,55] These observations confirm the results of a previous meta-analysis showing that VO_2peak per kilogram body mass was on average 21.8% lower in children with JIA compared with healthy control subjects or reference values.[95]

Giannini and Protas[28,29] also found that children with JIA had a significantly lower peak work rate (amount of watt that a subject can generate on a cycle ergometer), peak exercise heart rate (HRpeak), and exercise time than healthy control subjects matched for age, gender, and body size. Unpublished observations in 98 children with JIA (Takken et al.) showed that children with JIA had on average an HRpeak of 182 ± 14.7 beats per minute, while healthy children have on

TABLE 7-2   Calculating a GROMS Using All Joint Movements Except the Lumbar and Thoracic Spine*

	A	B	C	D	E
Joint Movement	Measured	Normative	A ÷ B	Mode	C × D
Cx spine extension	30	45	0.66	4	2.64
Cx spine rotation	60	80	0.75	4	3
Shoulder flexion	142.5	180	0.79	4	3.16
Shoulder abduction	180	180	1.00	4	4
Shoulder ER	85	85	1.00	3	3
Shoulder IR	70	70	1.00	3	3
Elbow extension	145	145	1.00	3	3
Elbow flexion	145	145	1.00	5	5
R/U supination	90	90	1.00	4	4
R/U pronation	90	90	1.00	4	4
Wrist flexion	67.5	90	0.75	3	2.25
Wrist extension	27.5	90	0.31	5	1.55
MCP (2–5)	68.75	90	0.76	5	3.8
PIP (2–5)	72.5	100	0.73	5	3.65
DIP (2–5)	47.5	90	0.53	4	2.12
Thumb flexion	20	70	0.29	5	1.45
Thumb abduction	30	50	0.60	5	3
Thumb DIP 1	30	90	0.33	2	0.66
Hip flexion	135	135	1.00	5	5
Hip extension	150	155	0.97	5	4.85
Hip abduction	50	50	1.00	4	4
Hip IR	15	45	0.33	2	0.66
Hip ER	40	45	0.88	4	3.52
Knee flexion	145	145	1.00	5	5
Knee extension	145	145	1.00	5	5
Ankle dorsiflexion	20	20	1.00	4	4
Ankle plantar flexion	50	55	0.91	4	3.64

From Epps, H., Hurley, M., & Utley, M. (2002). Development and evaluation of a single value score to assess global range of motion in juvenile idiopathic arthritis. *Arthritis Care Research, 47,* 398. Reprinted by permission of Wiley-Liss Inc., a subsidiary of John Wiley & Sons, Inc.
*GROMS, Global Range of Motion Scale; *Mode* = weighted value for joint movement based upon experts' opinion of its functional importance.

$$\text{GROMS} = \frac{\text{Sum of E}}{\text{Sum of D}} \times 100 = \frac{88.95 \times 100}{110} = 80.86$$

Cx = cervical; ER = external rotation; IR = internal rotation; MCP = metacarpophalangeal; PIP = proximal interphalangeal; DIP = distal interphalangeal ; RU = radio-ulnar

average an HRpeak of 193 ± 7 beats per minute. Some of the children with JIA stopped the exercise test because of fatigue and/or musculoskeletal complaints—not because of a cardiopulmonary limitation. In addition, HR and VO_2 values during submaximal exercise were higher in subjects with JIA, suggesting that they worked at a higher percentage of their aerobic capacity than did control subjects during routine activities. Many centers do not have the equipment to perform respiratory gas analysis to measure VO_2peak. However, peak workload (Wpeak) during a graded bicycle test can be used as a surrogate measure for VO_2peak because an excellent correlation between Wpeak and VO_2peak ($r = 0.95$, $P < .0001$) has been observed in 92 children with JIA (Takken et al., unpublished observations). VO_2peak can

be predicted from Wpeak, weight, and gender using the following equation (Takken et al., unpublished observations):

$$VO_2\text{peak (L/min)} = (0.008 \times \text{Wpeak [Watt]}) + (0.005 \times \text{weight [kg]}) + (-0.138 \times \text{Gender} [1 = \text{boy}, 2 = \text{girl}]) + 0.588$$

Impaired aerobic capacity does not appear to be significantly related to the severity of joint disease but may be due to hypoactivity secondary to disease symptoms, especially in children with long-standing arthritis.[28,29] Physiologic factors, including anemia, muscle atrophy, generalized weakness, and stiffness, resulting in poor mechanical efficiency may also limit the child's performance. Klepper and colleagues[46] compared the aerobic performance of 20 children, age 6 to

11 years, with polyJIA and 20 matched control subjects (age, gender, body mass index) on the 9-minute run-walk test. Subjects with JIA scored significantly below control subjects and were not able to maintain a steady running pace.

Performance-Related Fitness

As mentioned above, performance-related fitness includes components like muscle strength and anaerobic capacity. Impairments in muscle strength include weakness in hip extension and abduction, knee extension, plantar flexion, shoulder abduction and flexion, elbow flexion and extension, wrist extension, and grip. Muscle bulk, strength, and endurance should be examined at disease onset and monitored regularly. Bilateral measurements of circumference quantify asymmetries in muscle bulk. Functional muscle strength can be estimated in young children by observing their performance of age-appropriate motor tasks or ADLs. In older children, manual muscle testing can be done to measure isometric strength, especially if the child has pain while moving the limb against resistance. Instrumented measurements using a handheld or isokinetic dynamometer or a modified sphygmomanometer[19,30,106] provide consistent and reliable information in individuals with arthritis.

Muscle strength testing in children with JIA, especially handheld dynamometry using the "break" technique, might be problematic in some cases because children might give way as a result of pain instead of the limits in muscle strength.

Dynamic muscle testing of functional muscle groups can be performed when there is no sign of joint inflammation or damage. The maximal weight the child can lift throughout the available ROM for 10 to 15 repetitions (6 to 10 Repetition Maximum (RM)) is usually sufficient to establish a baseline level of strength and monitor change.[52] An alternative method for children who have pain on movement is to measure isometric strength at multiple angles throughout the ROM. Muscular endurance can be measured by having the child perform as many repetitions as possible at a specified percentage (60% to 80%) of the 6 to 10 RM. A warm-up period of light activity should precede strength testing.

One study suggested that muscle weakness may contribute to activity restrictions in children with arthritis. Fan and colleagues[24] found a significant relationship between 50-meter run times and lower extremity CHAQ scores in girls with JIA.

Two recent studies investigating anaerobic capacity in children and adolescents with JIA reported significantly lower values of anaerobic capacity in subjects with JIA.[10,55] Anaerobic capacity was reduced to the same extent as aerobic fitness (VO_2peak). Previously, it was found that reduced anaerobic capacity was significantly correlated with CHAQ scores in 18 children with juvenile arthritis, age 7 to 14 years.[97] This is not surprising in that the typical physical activity behavior of children—short bursts of intense activity separated by periods of rest—is anaerobic in nature.[7] Given the apparently similar deficits in anaerobic capacity of

youth with JIA, exercise training of the anaerobic energy system (e.g., high-intensity interval training) might be equally as valuable as training of the aerobic system and therefore warranted in children with arthritis. However, this training modality has not yet been studied.

Another widely used performance-related fitness test is the 6-minute walk test (6MWT). In this test, children have to cover as much distance as they can in 6 minutes by walking (not running). This test is used in different patient groups such as JIA, spina bifida, cerebral palsy, and hemophilia.[34,87,101] Lelieveld et al. found a low correlation between walking distance and VO_2peak in children with JIA.[54] In addition, Paap et al. found that children with JIA were exercising at 80% to 85% of their HRpeak and VO_2peak during the 6MWT, indicating that it is an intensive, submaximal exercise test used to measure functional exercise capacity in children with JIA.[78] Furthermore, these data indicate that exercise intensity at the end of the 6MWT can be used for the programming of exercise intensity during aerobic exercise training in children with JIA because this intensity is sufficient to improve fitness levels.

ASSESSMENT OF PAIN

Pain is one of the causes of activity restrictions in JIA and is a predictor of the child's adjustment to the disease. Acute pain may result from inflammation and some medical procedures. The cause of chronic pain is less clear, but it may be due at least in part to abnormal joint loading during activity as a result of soft tissue restrictions and muscle imbalance. Older children, especially those with newly diagnosed JIA, report more pain than young children or those with longstanding disease, suggesting that pain perception and report are more closely related to age than to disease severity or duration.[33] Assessment of pain should be ongoing and should include a pain history, a self-report for children over the age of 4 years, a parent report, and behavioral observations. Validated pain behaviors in JIA include bracing, guarding, rubbing, rigidity, and flexing.[42] Self-report tools for young children include the Wong-Baker Faces Rating Scale[110] and the Oucher.[8] The child can also complete a body map, using different colors to represent pain intensity (Figure 7-9). Children over the age of 7 years can use a numeric rating scale, a horizontal word graphic scale, or a visual analog scale (VAS). The Varni/Thompson Pediatric Pain Questionnaire (PPQ)[100] provides a comprehensive assessment with both parent and child reports.

GROWTH DISTURBANCES AND POSTURAL ABNORMALITIES

Retardation of linear growth is associated with extended periods of active disease and is exacerbated by long-term use of systemic steroids. Accelerated growth may occur during remission if the epiphyses are still open. Puberty and the

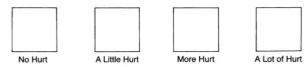

No Hurt   A Little Hurt   More Hurt   A Lot of Hurt

Pick the colors that mean *No Hurt, A Little Hurt, More Hurt,* and *A Lot of Hurt* to you and color in the boxes. Now, using those colors, color in the body to show how you feel. Where you have no hurt, use the *No Hurt* color to color in your body. If you have hurt or pain, use the color that tells how much hurt you have.

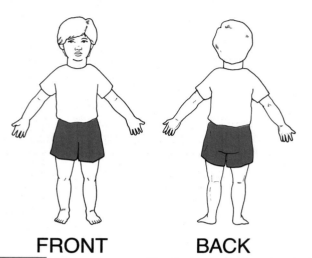

FRONT   BACK

Figure 7-9 Pain may be assessed by allowing the child to color a body map. Intensity of pain is matched with four different colors.

appearance of secondary sex characteristics may be delayed. Osteopenia, mainly in the appendicular skeleton, may be due to inadequate bone formation for age, low bone turnover, and depressed bone formation.[14] These circumstances may contribute to an increased risk of bone fracture. Increased blood supply to the inflamed joint early in the disease may cause accelerated growth of the ossification centers, resulting in bony overgrowth. Leg length discrepancies often occur as a result of unilateral knee arthritis. Growth discrepancies between ulnar and radial bones in wrist arthritis have been reported to contribute to instability and functional loss.[72] Premature closure of the growth plates may also occur. This may be widespread and symmetrical, as seen in the small hands and feet of some children with polyJIA, or isolated to a single digit.[14] Micrognathia may result from temporomandibular joint arthritis.

The therapist should observe the child's postural alignment in sitting and standing. Hip and knee flexion contractures, genu valgus, and foot deformities will affect the child's posture in standing. Children with asymmetrical cervical spine arthritis may present with torticollis (Grisel's syndrome). Children with leg length differences may develop a functional scoliosis. Small lifts of known thickness placed under the shorter leg with the child standing will level the pelvis and confirm or rule out a scoliosis.

INTERVENTION

The focus of physical therapy during the acute stage of the disease is different from that during the subacute and chronic stages. While in the acute phase, efforts are focused on maintaining and preserving joint function; in the subacute and chronic stages, the focus is on restoration and compensation of function and activities.

The overall goals of physical therapy are to maintain or improve function and to provide education and support to the child and family. Appendix III illustrates the physical therapy intervention in JIA. Intervention is geared to each child's physical, cognitive, and social development, and must also consider the family's cultural background. Physical activity and graded exercise are essential to manage the disease and maintain optimal health. Exercise in a warm pool, where the buoyancy of the water allows easier movement, is recommended. Most children with mild to moderate JIA can also participate in land-based exercise.

Adherence to the therapeutic regimen is extremely important. Home exercise programs are necessary, but are often a source of conflict between the parent and the child. The therapist can minimize the demands placed on the family by suggesting ways to incorporate the treatment into the child's daily routine. Giving the child some control over the exercise program, for example, choosing the time and place to exercise, may improve adherence. Older children can collaborate with the parent and therapist to set goals and plan intervention.

MANAGEMENT OF JOINT HEALTH

Physical measures used in the management of joint health include cold, exercise, and splinting. Rest, ice, compression, and elevation (RICE) reduces acute swelling and inflammation. There is no place for superficial or deep heat application in the management of arthritis. Studies have shown that intra-articular inflammation is increased when these modalities are used.[76,77] Ultrasound and short wave diathermy are not used in children. A study by Wiltink[108] et al. has suggested that these modalities may harm endochondral ossification and the proliferation of epithelial cells.

Balanced rest and exercise are important in managing joint health and function in JIA. Children who participate in group aquatic or land-based exercise programs report decreased pain.[6,25,47,94] Restful sleep helps to reduce morning stiffness and pain. Sleep time fragmentation is observed to have a negative effect on daytime performance.[115] Resting splints can support joints, may preserve function, and may relieve pain during the night.

A daily program of active ROM exercises is necessary to preserve joint motion and soft tissue extensibility. Active ROM is preferable, as several studies have shown that passive movement of inflamed joints evokes an increase in the release of the proinflammatory peptide substance P, resulting

APPENDIX III **INTERVENTIONS FOR JUVENILE IDIOPATHIC ARTHRITIS**

COORDINATION, COMMUNICATION, AND DOCUMENTATION

Anticipated Goals

- Care is coordinated with child, family, school, and other professionals.
- Insurance payer understands needed rehabilitation services.
- Need for modifications in school are determined.
- Available resources are maximally utilized.
- Decision making regarding child's health, wellness, and fitness needs is enhanced.

Specific Interventions

- Communication with community therapist, school personnel, and community resource providers
- Prescriptions and letters of medical necessity to support rehabilitation needs
- Individualized education plan (IEP); accommodations under Section 504 of Rehabilitation Act

PATIENT-RELATED INSTRUCTION

Anticipated Goals

- Awareness and use of community resources are increased.
- Behaviors that protect joints from secondary impairments are enhanced.
- Functional independence in activities of daily living (ADLs) is increased.
- Patient and family knowledge of the diagnosis, prognosis, interventions, and goals and outcomes is increased.

Specific Interventions

- Home exercise program
- Instruction regarding joint protection principles
- Information from the Arthritis Foundation regarding disease
- Referrals to other community resources

THERAPEUTIC EXERCISE

Anticipated Goals

- Ability to perform physical tasks related to self-care, home management, community and school integration, and leisure activities is increased.
- Aerobic capacity is increased.
- Gait is improved.
- Joint and soft tissue swelling, inflammation, or restriction is reduced.
- Joint integrity and mobility are improved.
- Pain is decreased.
- Postural control is improved.
- Strength, power, and endurance are improved.

Specific Interventions

- Aerobic conditioning
  - Aquatic exercise
  - Low-impact weight-bearing exercise
- Gait training
- Body mechanics training
- Postural training
- Strengthening, power, and endurance training
  - Active-assistive, active, and resistive exercise
  - Task-specific performance training
- Flexibility exercise
  - Muscle lengthening
  - Range of motion
  - Static progressive stretching
- Balance, coordination, and agility training

Continued

APPENDIX III   INTERVENTIONS FOR JUVENILE IDIOPATHIC ARTHRITIS—cont'd

FUNCTIONAL TRAINING IN SELF-CARE AND HOME MANAGEMENT

Anticipated Goals

- Ability to perform physical tasks related to self-care and home management is increased.
- Level of supervision required for task performance is decreased.
- Risk of secondary impairment is reduced.

Specific Interventions

- ADL training
- Assistive and adaptive device or equipment training
- Self-care or home management task adaptation
- Leisure and play recommendations
- Orthotic, protective, or supportive device or equipment training
- Injury prevention training

FUNCTIONAL TRAINING IN SCHOOL, PLAY, COMMUNITY, AND LEISURE INTEGRATION

Anticipated Goals

- School attendance is improved.
- Participation in peer groups for recreation and leisure activity is improved.
- Architectural barriers to access home, school, and community resources are removed.

Specific Interventions

- Appropriate transportation plan to school identified on IEP
- Modifications to school instruction identified on IEP
- ADL training
- Assistive and adaptive device or equipment training
- Adaptation of equipment to allow inclusion in recreation and leisure activity
- Home and school site visit to plan for accommodation of any architectural barriers

PRESCRIPTION, APPLICATION, AND FABRICATION OF DEVICES AND EQUIPMENT

Anticipated Goals

- Ability to perform physical tasks is increased.
- Deformities are prevented.
- Gait is improved.
- Joint stability is increased.
- Optimal joint alignment is achieved.
- Pain is decreased.
- Protection of body parts is increased.

Specific Interventions

- Adaptive devices or equipment
- Assistive devices or equipment (ambulation aids, wheelchairs, ADL equipment)
- Splints and orthotic devices (shoe inserts, resting splints, dynamic splints, braces)
- Protective devices (splints, taping, elbow or knee pads)
- Supportive devices (compression garments, cervical collars)

ELECTROTHERAPEUTIC MODALITIES

Anticipated Goals

- Muscle performance is increased.
- Pain is decreased.

Specific Interventions

- Biofeedback

APPENDIX **III**   INTERVENTIONS FOR JUVENILE IDIOPATHIC ARTHRITIS—cont'd

PHYSICAL AGENTS AND MECHANICAL MODALITIES

Anticipated Goals

- Pain is decreased.
- Soft tissue swelling, inflammation, or restriction is reduced.
- Tolerance to positions and activities is increased.
- Joint integrity and mobility are improved.

Specific Interventions

- Cryotherapy (RICE—rest, ice, compression, elevation)
- Hydrotherapy (aquatic therapy, whirlpool tanks)
- Continuous passive motion devices

Modified from Scull, S. (2000). Juvenile rheumatoid arthritis. In S. Campbell, D. Vander Linden, & R. Palisano (Eds.). *Physical therapy for children* (2nd ed.; p. 245). Philadelphia: WB Saunders.

in more pain and inflammation. The child can also be taught combination patterns cloaked in games that encourage motion in several joints at once. Commercial or custom splints for the wrists, hands, elbows, knees, and ankles rest the joint in an anatomically corrected position but should allow physiologic function.

Static progressive stretching (SPS), using serial splints or casts, extension orthoses, dynamic splints, or skin traction, can sometimes be used to resolve contractures.[65] Application of these passive corrective modalities demands careful consideration of the biomechanical forces that result from the application. Precautions should be taken not to induce a subluxation or to overload joint parts. Serial splints can be molded and easily modified by the therapist as the child gains motion. One drawback is that the child can remove the splint, decreasing its effectiveness. In contrast, serial casts provide a continuous low load stretch, usually for about 72 hours, after which they are removed and bivalved. During the next 1 to 2 weeks, the child wears the bivalved cast for 18 to 24 hours a day, removing it only for exercise sessions. A new cast is applied and the process repeated until optimal ROM is achieved.[113] Dynamic splints can be ordered to fit the child. The tension is set to the child's tolerance and is increased gradually as ROM improves. The child wears the splint for several 1-hour intervals during the day. Use throughout the night provides continuous stretching. Skin traction applied at night has also been shown to be effective in reducing hip and knee flexion contractures, although it may cause disturbed sleep with all known negative consequences on the disease course. One study, using a single subject design, reported that the combination of nighttime skin traction, daytime use of an extension orthosis during weight-bearing activities, and physical therapy twice a week was effective in reducing active and passive ROM deficits in several children with JIA.[26]

ORTHOPEDIC SURGERY AND THE ROLE OF THE PHYSICAL THERAPIST

Carefully planned orthopedic surgery in the young child is aimed at preserving joint health. In the older child with joint damage, reconstruction surgery may relieve pain and restore function. Staging the surgical procedures is important in a child with severe polyJIA. The first priority is to maintain or restore ambulation; this is followed by the need to improve the child's ability to perform ADLs. The choice of procedure depends on the child's age, disease activity, and functional status, and on the condition of the joint.

Synovectomy is hardly performed in children compared to adults. The procedure may be useful in children with nearly normal ROM and minimal evidence of articular damage who have not responded to medical therapies. The major postoperative complication is soft tissue contracture, although this may occur less often with arthroscopic surgery.[70] ROM exercises are begun soon after surgery to maintain preoperative joint motion. A continuous passive motion (CPM) machine is used for the elbow or knee. After discharge and wound healing, dynamic splints may be prescribed to preserve ROM. Arthrodesis is useful in advanced arthritis of the ankle and hindfoot, wrist, and interphalangeal (IP) joints, especially if there is a risk for ankylosis in an abnormal position. Postoperative care includes immobilization in a cast and exercise and positioning for adjacent joints. Protected weight bearing and ambulation with crutches or a walker follow lower limb surgery. Immobilization is maintained until there is radiographic evidence of successful fusion. Epiphysiodesis, or surgical arrest of the growth plate, may be used in some children with bony overgrowth. Osteotomy is considered when there is a severe valgus deformity at the knee if the articular cartilage is preserved and joint motion is normal. Postoperative care includes 4 to 6 weeks of immobilization.[70]

Total joint arthroplasty (TJA) is considered when there is irreversible joint damage and the child has significant pain and functional limitation. The procedure is most frequently performed at the hip and knee, although prostheses are available for other joints. Several factors are considered in the decision, including the child's age, skeletal maturity, general physical status, upper extremity function, and ability of the child to successfully complete the lengthy and intensive postoperative rehabilitation regimen. Customized computer-designed prostheses may be necessary to accommodate changes in joint anatomy, small bone size, and osteoporosis. The longevity of the prosthesis must also be considered, especially when TJA is performed in young children. Procedures are staged if the child requires extensive surgery to ensure the best functional outcome.

Postoperative care for total hip arthroplasty (THA) is influenced by the surgical approach and the type of implant.[70] Most surgeons require protected weight bearing for several weeks if an uncemented implant is used. With a posterior surgical approach, the child progresses from crutches or a walker to a cane. To protect the abductor muscle repair after an anterolateral approach, the child must use crutches or a walker for 6 to 8 weeks and avoid active hip abduction for 12 weeks.[70]

ROM active exercises should begin early, with precautions against hip flexion past 90° and hip adduction and internal rotation past neutral to avoid dislocation of the implant. A foam wedge placed between the legs is used to maintain hip abduction when lying in bed or sitting; periods of prone positioning help stretch the hip flexors. A CPM machine may be used to improve joint mobility. Active exercise and walking in chest-deep water can begin once the wound is healed. The child should also practice transfers, ambulation on level surfaces and stairs, and ADLs. Assistive equipment, including elevated toilet seats and dressing aids, should be used to avoid excessive hip flexion. These precautions are usually maintained for the first 2 to 3 postoperative months, although some surgeons prefer a longer period. Activities that cause high-impact loading on the joint, including running and jumping or carrying heavy objects, should be avoided.

Postoperative therapy following total knee arthroplasty begins with active and passive ROM exercises. The goal is to achieve complete extension and flexion greater than 90°. A CPM machine can be used immediately, with an extension splint worn at other times. Therapy includes isometric exercises for the quadriceps and hamstrings, straight leg raises, and limited arc knee extension. The child can bear weight, wearing a knee immobilizer. Gait training with crutches or a walker and protected weight bearing with a cane continue for about 6 weeks until there is adequate healing of the extensor mechanism. Stationary cycling may be included in the regimen if the bike has a range limiter applied to the pedal that allows the therapist to control the degree of knee flexion required during cycling.

FITNESS TRAINING

Aerobic Capacity

A recent Cochrane review identified only three published randomized controlled studies investigating the effects of exercise training for children with JIA.[99] None of these studies found improvements in VO2peak after the aerobic training program was completed. This lack of effect can be owed to a low exercise frequency (e.g., one time a week), a low exercise intensity (intensity of exercise has to be above the intensity of daily activities), or a low exercise adherence (children did often skip exercise sessions), or it may indicate that children did not perform the prescribed home exercises. However, aerobic fitness is important to improve the child's endurance for routine physical activities and play. In addition, aerobic fitness helps the recovery after intensive exercise. Based on the available literature, it is recommended that children with JIA and a deficit in aerobic fitness should train at least two times a week, with moderate to vigorous intensity (60% to 85% Heart Rate max), for 45 to 60 minutes per session for at least 6 to 12 weeks.[48,49,98] The specific mode of exercise appears to be less important than the intensity, duration, and frequency. However, weight-bearing exercise is necessary to maintain optimal bone growth and density. Low-impact activities to improve proprioceptive function, balance, and coordination can be incorporated into aerobic conditioning programs.

Anaerobic Capacity

In a recent study, van Brussel et al.[11] hypothesized that training of the anaerobic energy system (e.g., high-intensity interval training) might be equally valuable as training of the aerobic system and therefore warranted in children with JIA. Although this training modality has not yet been studied in children with JIA, improvements have been observed in function and fitness with anaerobic exercise training in children with other chronic conditions (e.g., cystic fibrosis, cerebral palsy).[45,104] Particularly in children with a larger reduction in anaerobic capacity compared with aerobic capacity, this training modality might be effective. In addition, children prefer this anaerobic type of exercise over the adult type of continuous endurance exercise. The suggested exercise set consists of 15 high-intensity cycling sprints (15 to 30 seconds all out), each sprint is followed by 1 to 2 minutes of active rest (cycling with low resistance). A training session could consist of three of these exercise sets, with 5 minutes of active rest for recovery between the three sets of interval training.

Muscle Strength

Little evidence suggests the effectiveness of strength training for children with JIA. Only one study, published in abstract form, studied muscle strength training in children with JIA. Fisher and colleagues[25] examined the effects of resistance exercise using isokinetic equipment in 19 children with JIA age 6 to 14 years, who trained as a group three times a week for 8 weeks. Each child's program was individualized and progressed on the basis of initial test results and response to training. Subjects showed significant improvement in quadriceps and hamstring strength and endurance, contraction speed of the hamstrings, functional status, disability, and performance of timed tasks. Control subjects with JIA who did not exercise had relatively no change to a slight decrease in muscle function during the same time period.[25]

Strengthening exercises target the muscles surrounding and supporting the joints with arthritis and adjacent areas. During acute joint inflammation, isometric exercise is recommended to maintain muscle bulk and strength. Prolonged maximal isometric contractions should be avoided because they may increase intra-articular pressure and constrict blood flow through the muscles.[41] The child is taught to perform and hold a submaximal contraction for approximately 6 seconds, exhaling during the contraction and inhaling during the relaxation phase. Five to 10 repetitions daily is sufficient.[67] EMG biofeedback may be helpful in training the child to regulate the intensity of the contraction. Isometric exercises performed at multiple points within the ROM may prepare the joint for dynamic exercise after active disease is resolved.

Dynamic exercise is added when joint inflammation subsides. Both concentric and eccentric exercises are included. External resistance, in the form of light hand or cuff weights or elastic bands, can be safely added once the child is able to correctly perform 8 to 10 repetitions of motion against gravity without pain.[67]

Clear directions and illustrations of the exercises are necessary, and training sessions should be supervised. Children should use lighter weights and perform 2 to 3 sets of 10 to 15 repetitions. A good starting point is to use the amount of resistance the child was able to lift 6 to 10 times without discomfort. Progression is based on periodic reassessment. Each training session should begin with light aerobic and flexibility activities and end with cool-down and stretching activities. Resistance exercises should be performed twice a week, allowing time between sessions for rest and recovery.[23]

ENCOURAGING ACTIVE-HEALTHY LIVING

Several studies have identified a hypoactive lifestyle of children with JIA.[36,56,96] A significant association has been reported between accelerometry-measured physical activity and health-related fitness (VO$_2$peak) in children with JIA,[96] suggesting a cause–effect relationship. In addition, no adverse effects of regular sport activity have been observed on joint scores in children with JIA.[43] The link between physical activity levels of children and motor performance[114] suggests that the physical activity levels of children with JIA might be enhanced by improvements in reduced motor proficiency observed in children with JIA.[71] Further, given the fact that

adult physical activity levels are established in youth, it is important to encourage children and families of children with JIA to participate in regular physical activity. Regular physical activity can help in the prevention of cardiovascular risk factors, obesity, and reduced bone health, as well as reduced health-related quality of life, in youth with JIA. Physical therapists should reassure parents and stimulate an active-healthy lifestyle as soon as possible after diagnosis.

SELF-CARE ACTIVITIES

A primary goal for every child with a chronic condition is to achieve independence in self-care within the home, school, and community. Expectations for independence differ at each age and stage of development. It has been reported that ambulation skills in children with JIA are delayed as early as 4 years of age.[71] This is in contrast with preschool age children, who show more limitations in motor proficiency and in the development of motor milestones.[71] Intervention for an infant with JIA may include suggestions to prevent contractures and facilitate function. A child with limited grasp may benefit from adapted toys. Functional wrist and hand splints can support the joint during hand use, and assistive devices can compensate for a weak grip and reduce hand pain and fatigue. Dressing and hygiene aids include Velcro closures on clothing and shoes, elastic shoelaces, a long-handled shoehorn, a dressing stick, a buttonhook, a zipper pull, and a long-handled bath brush. Built-up handles on grooming items, eating utensils, and writing implements are often necessary for optimal function and independence.

Some modifications within the home may be beneficial, including replacing knobs and faucets with levers, using a jar opener or an electric can opener, adding a raised toilet seat, and installing safety bars in the bathtub. More substantial modifications, including widening doorways and adding a ramp to the entrance, are needed for a child who must use a wheelchair. The therapist must consider the financial, physical, and emotional impact of these changes on the family. The device or adaptation must be affordable and must achieve the stated purpose, be easy to use, and be acceptable to the child and parent.

FUNCTIONAL MOBILITY

Weight bearing and ambulation are vital for optimal bone growth and density, joint health, and muscle development. Standing, cruising, and walking should be encouraged at the expected age, although the use of infant walkers should be avoided because they may promote an abnormal gait pattern and carry a high risk for injury. Toddlers and preschool age children should be encouraged to walk within the home and short distances outside. Shoes should support and cushion the joints of the feet and accommodate any deformities. Sneakers with a flexible sole, good arch support, and a high heel cup are good choices for most children. A wide, deep toe box may be necessary for a child with hallux valgus, hammer toes, or claw toes. A child with arthritis in the feet and toes should not wear high heels because of the excessive pressure on the metatarsophalangeal joints. A rocker-like addition to the sole of the shoe may provide a mechanical assist at toe-off for a child who has limited or painful toe hyperextension. A molded ankle-foot orthosis (AFO) may be necessary to support the ankle if pain and instability prevent weight bearing. Custom molded in-shoe orthoses can replace the standard insole to accommodate foot deformities and decrease pressure on those tender joints.

Few children with JIA require an assistive device for ambulation. However, if a child begins to show problems with weight bearing or difficulty walking, the cause should be determined and addressed immediately. Leg length differences can be accommodated by placing a lift inside the shoe or on the sole of the shoe on the shorter side. A child with unilateral lower extremity pain or weakness can use a cane on the opposite side to unload the involved limb and increase stability during ambulation. A walker or crutches may be needed if problems are bilateral. Platform attachments can be added if the child has upper limb impairments.

Some children may need to use a form of wheeled mobility for long distances within the school or community environment. A wagon or stroller with a firm seat and back is appropriate for toddlers or preschool age children. Older children can use a tricycle or a bicycle with training wheels to get around the community. A nonpowered two-wheeled scooter allows younger children to propel themselves with their feet without weight bearing. A powered scooter or lightweight wheelchair may be necessary for efficient mobility in school. Children with upper extremity arthritis often maneuver the wheelchair with their feet. Powered wheelchairs are usually reserved for children with severe impairments but may be necessary for a college student who must negotiate a large campus. Children who use a wheelchair should spend part of every day out of the chair, standing and walking to preserve bone health, prevent contractures, and maintain walking tolerance.

ISSUES RELATED TO SCHOOL

Children with JIA may need occasional modifications to their school program. These might include a second set of books for home, built-up or adapted writing tools, or an easel top for the desk in the classroom. Children with significant hand arthritis may need to record class notes on a tape recorder or word processor and take tests under untimed conditions. Modifications to the school schedule may include time out of the classroom to take medication or rest for brief periods during the day, extra time to travel between classes, or permission to use an elevator if the child is unable to negotiate stairs. Some schools provide these services voluntarily. In other situations, the child may need an

individualized educational plan (IEP) or accommodations specified under Section 504 of the Vocational Rehabilitation Act. Vocational counseling is often necessary to prepare adolescents for the transition to higher education and work. Although most states mandate transition planning, Lovell and colleagues[63] found that only 8% of children with JIA received vocational counseling.

Regular participation in physical education is encouraged. The instructor should be aware of the child's diagnosis and any activity restrictions or precautions. In general, the child should be allowed to monitor his/her own activity level, resting as needed. However, some activities are prohibited because of their potential for injury or joint damage. These prohibited activities include headstands and somersaults; handstands, push-ups, cartwheels, and other similar activities in a child with wrist and hand arthritis; and high-impact running or jumping in a child with spinal or lower extremity arthritis. The therapist can consult with the physical education instructor to modify activities as necessary.

RECREATIONAL ACTIVITIES

Recreational activities provide physical and psychosocial benefits. The choice of activities depends on the child's preferences, physical status, motor skills, and fitness level. Participation on any given day sometimes must be modified to accommodate disease symptoms. Scull and Athreya[88] provided a useful guide to help parents and children choose activities for a child with JIA. Swimming, water or low-impact weight-bearing aerobics, and bicycling provide good cardiovascular exercise. Activities that cause high-impact loading on inflamed or damaged joints should be avoided. Contact sports, including football, hockey, and boxing, and those with a high inherent potential for injury are discouraged. Competitive team sports may be physically and emotionally stressful, but each situation should be evaluated individually.

A physical conditioning program before participating in a sport prepares the child for the physical demands of the activity. Warm-up before each practice session or game and a cool-down period after the activity should be encouraged. Instruction in motor skills specific to the sport may be necessary. A sports orthosis or other adaptive equipment may improve joint alignment and stability.

SUMMARY

Juvenile idiopathic arthritis (JIA) is an autoimmune inflammatory disorder and the most common rheumatic disease of childhood. Although the exact cause is unclear, three major distinct onset types are recognized: systemic, polyarticular, and oligoarticular. With advances in the recognition and diagnosis of the disease and more effective medications to treat joint inflammation, most children with JIA do well with early diagnosis and appropriate treatment. However, for many children, JIA results in both short- and long-term problems, including chronic joint swelling, pain, and limited motion, as well as muscle atrophy and weakness, poor aerobic function, and impaired exercise tolerance. General and localized growth disturbances, postural abnormalities, and gait deviations occur with persistent disease. Activity and participation restrictions that result from the arthritis and extra-articular manifestations can negatively affect the child's quality of life. The long-term prognosis depends upon the child's age at disease onset, onset type, severity and duration of active inflammation, and quality and consistency of medical care and other resources available and utilized by the family. This chapter reviews the most common characteristics of JIA, standardized examination and outcome measures developed for use in children with arthritis, and current research findings regarding the effects of exercise and physical activity in individuals with chronic inflammatory arthritis. Physical therapists are vital members of the pediatric rheumatology team, providing examination, evaluation, intervention, and monitoring of a child with JIA. Therapists also serve as an important resource to parents or caregivers and school and community personnel to adapt activities so the child with JIA can participate fully in the home, school, and community environments.

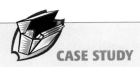

CASE STUDY

"Jason"

Client Description

Jason is a 13-year-old boy with polyarticular JIA of 8 years' duration. He lives in a single-family home with his parents and two siblings—an 18-year-old brother and a 16-year-old sister. He is in the 8th grade in a regional public junior high school and does well academically, but does not participate in any sports or other after-school activities. Jason's pediatrician provides routine medical care, and a pediatric rheumatology team at a specialized tertiary care center 2 hours from his home coordinates the care for his arthritis. His current medications include naproxen and methotrexate. He does not receive direct physical therapy, but has a home range of motion and strengthening exercise program prescribed by the rheumatology clinic PT. He also has wrist and hand splints fabricated by the clinic occupational therapist (OT). Jason sees both the OT and the PT at periodic intervals of 3 to 6 months during his regular rheumatology clinic appointment.

Medical History

Jason's arthritis was diagnosed when he was 5 years old, after several months of joint swelling and pain, lethargy, and mild systemic symptoms. At the time of diagnosis, he had active joint inflammation in knees, ankles, elbows, and wrists; more joints became involved over time.

Findings of Physical Therapy Examination

Primary Problems/Complaints

Jason's primary complaints during his clinic visit included morning stiffness lasting about 1 hour, low back pain during the day after sitting in his school desk for more than 20 minutes, neck pain when doing deskwork and riding in the school bus, foot pain, and general fatigue when walking around school and in the community. When asked about school and recreational activities, Jason stated his grades were good, but he has to work harder than other kids to make up material he misses when he is late or absent as a result of his arthritis. He stated that he feels different because he can't do some of the activities in physical education class and is not able to play any team sports at school or in the community. He missed a recent overnight school trip because his parents were afraid he would forget to take his medications and have problems getting up for early morning activities because of stiffness. Jason also stated he was concerned that his neck would hurt on the long bus ride. Jason's mother reported that he usually avoids family outings that involve hiking or other sports because he gets tired or his feet hurt. When asked about his home exercise program, Jason admitted he rarely did the prescribed exercises because they are boring and the instructions are a little confusing. He also stated that his hand splints hurt and caused an itchy rash on his forearms.

Jason's Goals

Jason stated that he wanted to be like other kids his age. Next year, he will transfer to a large 4-year high school and is concerned about his ability to keep up with the other kids. Specifically, he expressed a desire to have more energy so he could do the same physical activities as his classmates in school and play some type of recreational sport with his friends. He also stated that he would like to hike, bike, and ski with his family, when they take vacations.

Results of Tests and Measures

Participation and Activity

Three standardized instruments were chosen to assess Jason's quality of life, self-reported physical function, and gross motor proficiency, respectively: the Quality of My Life Scale, the visual analog version of the Childhood Health Assessment Questionnaire (VASchaq38), and the Bruininks-Oseretsky Test of Motor Proficiency, 2nd edition (BOT-2).

Continued

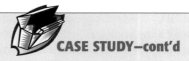

CASE STUDY—cont'd

EVIDENCE TO PRACTICE 7-1

CASE STUDY "JASON"

EXAMINATION DECISION

Quality of Life: Duffy and Lovell (2001), describing the hierarchy of outcomes in pediatric rheumatology, place quality of life (QOL) at the highest level, stating that health status is a complex construct, including physical, mental, and social well-being. Although several comprehensive QOL assessment tools have been designed for children with rheumatic disease, the Quality of My Life Scale (Feldman et al., 2000) is a simple to use self-report instrument requiring very little time or instruction to complete. It comprises two 10-centimeter visual analog scales measuring overall QOL and health-related QOL, where higher scores indicate a better QOL. Using a 5-point categorical scale, the child rates his QOL since the last clinic visit from "Much Better to Much Worse."

Physical Function: The original CHAQ is the most widely used measure of physical function in JIA and can be completed by a parent as proxy for a young child or by self-report in children 9 years of age and older. However, the test measures only disability and has demonstrated a ceiling effect in children with mild to moderate disease severity, with scores clustered at the lower end of the scale. A revised version of the CHAQ, the VASCHAQ38, includes eight additional items targeting more challenging activities and asks the child to compare his or her capabilities versus other children of the same age using a 10-cm VAS anchored on the left (0) by "Much worse than other kids my age" and on the right (10) by "Much better than other kids my age" (Lam et al., 2004). The new items ask the child about climbing and running activities, individual and team sports, balance abilities during rough play, and endurance during physical activity. The summary score is determined by averaging the score (0-10) for all 38 items, with higher scores indicating better function. The VASCHAQ38 provides a better view of the child's functional abilities and a more useful guide for clinical management than the original CHAQ. Although the sensitivity

of the VASCHAQ38 to change over time has not been reported in the literature, I have found it be responsive to change with intervention in individual children.

Gross Motor Proficiency: Two studies, using age-based reference values, reported delays or deficits in motor skill development in young children with JIA (Morrison et al., 1991; van der Net et al., 2008). These deficits are believed to result from general hypoactivity and limited experience in recreational or competitive sports in children with arthritis. Deficits in gross motor proficiency may limit a child's ability to safely and successfully participate in games and sports with peers, negatively affecting both physical health and social competence. Unlike most norm-referenced tests of motor development, the BOT-2 measures multiple components of gross motor proficiency (balance, bilateral coordination, speed, agility, and strength) and includes a wide age range (4.5 years to 21 years, 11 months). Although information on use of the BOT-2 in adolescents with JIA is limited, my clinical experience suggests the test is sensitive to changes in motor skills following task-specific training.

Duffy, C. M., & Lovell, D. J. (2001). Assessment of health status, function, and outcome. In J. T. Cassidy, & R. E. Petty (Eds.), Textbook of pediatric rheumatology (4th ed.; pp. 178–187). Philadelphia: WB Saunders.

Feldman, B. M., Grundland, B., McCullough, L., & Wright, V. (2000). Distinction of quality of life, health related quality of life, and health status in children referred for rheumatologic care. Journal of Rheumatology, 27, 226–233.

Lam, C., Young, N., Marwaha, J., McLimont, M., & Feldman, B. (2004). Revised versions of the Childhood Health Assessment Questionnaire (CHAQ) are more sensitive and suffer less from a ceiling effect. Arthritis and Rheumatism (Arthritis Care and Research), 51, 881–889.

Morrison, C. D., Bundy, R. C., & Fisher, A. G. (1991). The contribution of motor skills and playfulness to the play performance of preschoolers. American Journal of Occupational Therapy, 45, 687–694.

van der Net, J., van der Torre, P., Engelbert, R. H., Engelen, V., van Zon, F., Takken, T., et al. (2008). Motor performance and functional ability in preschool- and early school-aged children with juvenile idiopathic arthritis: A cross-sectional study. Pediatric Rheumatology Online Journal, 6.

Bruininks, R. H., Bruininks, B. D. Bruininks-Oseretsky test of motor proficiency (2nd ed.). Minneapolis, MN: Pearson Assessments.

Jason rated his life as about the same as during his last clinic visit 3 months ago. His scores on the QML Scale were 5/10 cm for Overall QOL and 4/10 cm for Health-Related QOL, suggesting that his health problems may influence his overall QOL. His VASchaq38 score of 5.35 indicated moderate activity limitations compared with those of other adolescents his age (median score for healthy community controls reported by Lam et al. was 6.44).[53] As expected, he rated his capabilities as most limited in sports and activities that require good balance, coordination, and endurance. His self-report is

supported by his performance on the Body Coordination and Strength and Agility composites of the BOT-2, where his standards scores were between −1 and −2 standard deviations from the mean, placing his performance in the Below Average category relative to others his age.

Impairments

Joint inflammation: Effusions were present in the wrists, MCPs and PIPs, ankles, and toes on both sides, indicating active arthritis in these joints.

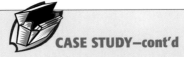

CASE STUDY—cont'd

Pain: Jason rates his overall pain intensity during the past week as 5 on a 10-cm VAS.

Passive range of motion (PROM): Bilateral hip flexion contractures of 10° were noted, along with limited abduction (0° to 15°) and internal rotation (0° to 30°) on the right side. Ankle dorsiflexion was 0° to 5° bilaterally with the knees extended; plantar flexion was full. Hindfoot inversion was full; eversion was 0° bilaterally. Both feet showed hallux valgus and hammer toe deformities. Cervical spine rotation and lateral flexion were limited by 50%; extension and flexion were within normal limits. Shoulder motion was full but painful at end range. Jason had bilateral elbow flexion contractures of 20°, and both wrists had limited extension (0° to 45°).

Muscle function: Grip strength measured on a Citec dynamometer (CIT Technics, BV Groningen, The Netherlands) was 160 Newtons.

Recently, reference values for grip strength were published[109] and show that his muscle strength was at the 3rd percentile for his age and gender. Arm strength was 3+/5. Leg strength was grossly 4/5 on manual muscle testing (MMT); however, his functional leg and trunk strength during activities on the BOT-2 (standing long jump, sit-ups, wall-sit, V-up, and knee push-ups) was classified as Well Below Average.

Aerobic function: His 6-minute walk distance (6MWD) was 630 meters, placing his performance between the 10th and 25th percentiles for his height compared with healthy children, but above the mean walk distance reported for 13-year-old children with JIA.

Anaerobic function: Jason's scale score on the Speed and Agility subtest of the BOT-2 was 6, placing his performance at the border between Below Average and Well Below Average compared with boys his age.

EVIDENCE TO PRACTICE 7-2

CASE STUDY "JASON"
EXAMINATION DECISION

Aerobic Function: The 6MWT is a reliable and valid performance measure of submaximal exercise capacity in children with JIA. Papp et al. (2005) examined physiologic responses in children with JIA during the 6MWT. Their findings indicate the test is a valid measure of intensive exercise performed at a submaximal level (80% to 85% of peak HR and VO₂) of aerobic capacity. The test requires minimal equipment and training, and standardized guidelines for administration are available (American Thoracic Society, 2002). One study of more than 1400 Chinese children presented height-referenced centile curves on the 6MWT for children between the ages of 7 and 16 years (Li et al., 2007). Although the responsiveness of the test to intervention in JIA has not been determined, it is reasonable to assume that Jason's walking speed and therefore 6MWD might improve with improvements in his aerobic and muscular fitness and a decrease in his self-reported foot pain during walking.

Anaerobic Function: Several studies provide evidence of impaired anaerobic fitness and its relationship to function in children and adolescents with JIA. Fan et al. (1998) reported that 15 of 20 young girls with polyarticular JIA and minimal functional disability according to their CHAQ score scored below the lowest performance level (bronze) on the 50-meter

sprint, a component of the Canada Fitness Award Program. They also found that lower limb strength was significantly related to running speed and to function on the CHAQ. Two studies (van Brussel et al., 2007; Lelieveld et al., 2007), using the Wingate Anaerobic Test (Want), reported significant deficits in anaerobic fitness in children and adolescents with JIA and found a strong negative correlation between anaerobic capacity and function as measured by the CHAQ Disability Index, pain, and overall well-being, suggesting that muscular fitness may contribute to overall well-being and decreased difficulty in performing daily activities.

American Thoracic Society. (2002). American Thoracic Society statement: Guidelines for the six-minute walk test. American Journal of Respiratory Care Medicine, 166, 111–117.

Papp, E., van der Net, J., Helders, P. J. M., & Takken, T. (2005). Physiologic response of the six-minute walk test in children with juvenile idiopathic arthritis. Arthritis Care and Research, 53, 351–356.

Fan, J., Wessel, J., & Ellsworth, J. (1998). The relationship between strength and function in females with juvenile rheumatoid arthritis. Journal of Rheumatology, 3, 1399–1405.

van Brussel, M., Lelieveld, O. T., van der Net, J., Engelbert, R. H., Helders, P. J. M., & Takken, T. (2007). Aerobic and anaerobic exercise capacity in children with juvenile idiopathic arthritis. Arthritis and Rheumatism, 57, 891–897.

Lelieveld, O. T., van Brussel, M., Takken, T., van Weert, E., van Leeuwen, M. A., & Armbrust, W. (2007). Aerobic and anaerobic exercise capacity in adolescents with juvenile idiopathic arthritis. Arthritis and Rheumatism, 57, 898–904.

Prognosis

Plan of Care

Problem: Poor Adaptation and Self-Efficacy in Managing the Diagnosis

Goal: Jason will assume increased responsibility for his own health care. The rheumatology team believes that poor adherence to the medical and therapeutic regimen contributes to Jason's problems. Team members agreed he should take a

Continued

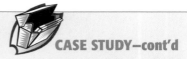

CASE STUDY—cont'd

more active role in setting goals and planning intervention, including the following:

- Explore the services provided by the Arthritis Foundation[3] and the JA Alliance, including teen support groups and local, regional, and national family retreats (http://www.arthritis.org/ja-alliance-main.php).
- Work with the rheumatology clinic team to develop a contract with Jason to enlist his adherence to the medical and exercise routine.
- Participate in a short course of direct PT and OT to increase Jason's self-efficacy for managing his arthritis.

Intervention Plan and Goals

Jason agreed to a 3-month contract with re-evaluation at his next clinic visit. The contract included taking his full medication dose each week, performing prescribed ROM exercises at night, and taking a warm bath upon arising to decrease the morning stiffness that has resulted in tardiness for school. A schedule of daily aerobic physical activity was developed, allowing Jason to choose among a number of activities. With the clinic's assistance, Jason's mother was able to obtain approval for several weeks of direct PT and OT twice a week. The clinic PT also worked with Jason to redesign his home exercise routine to fit into his daily schedule. The program included specific written instructions and illustrations for each exercise, as well as a plan for periodic testing and progression of exercise intensity and duration. He also agreed to try wearing a soft cervical collar on the school bus to decrease neck pain. Jason was referred to an orthotist for custom-molded in-shoe orthoses to decrease his foot pain when standing and walking.

Expected Outcomes

Improved exercise tolerance and decreased foot pain when walking resulting in increased 6MWD; improved endurance for physical activity with friends and family; decreased difficulty with physical activities as measured by the VASchaq38; improved ability to manage his health care, including increased adherence to medication and exercise prescription.

EVIDENCE TO PRACTICE 7-3

CASE STUDY "JASON"

PLAN OF CARE DECISION AND PATIENT

A study by Erhman-Feldman and colleagues (Erhman-Feldman D et al., 2007) found that moderate adherence to the medication regimen improved disease control, while moderate adherence to exercise recommendations was associated with positive short-term outcomes, including parent reports that their child had improved function and reduced pain, as well as the parents' perception of global improvement. Parents reported their preferences regarding exercise programs prescribed for their child. These included setting realistic goals that have meaning for the child, explaining how exercise will help the child meet his or her goals, providing written instructions and illustrations of exercises, and explaining how to recognize the difference between post-exercise soreness or stiffness and a disease flare and how to manage each situation. In addition, they wanted exercises that would engage their child's interest and challenge his abilities, include periodic reassessment and progression of the regimen, and provide rewards for adherence to the program.

Erhman-Feldman, D., De Civita, M., Dobkin, P. L., Malleson, P. N., Meshefedjian, G., & Duffy, C. M. (2007). Effects of adherence to treatment on short-term outcomes in children with juvenile idiopathic arthritis. Arthritis Rheumatism (Arthritis Care Res), 57, 905–912.

Problem: Slow and Inefficient Gait

Goal 1: Jason will decrease the time he currently requires to walk between classes and other areas in his school by 50% (to be achieved in 3 months).

Goal 2: Jason will increase his 6-minute walk distance to the 50th percentile for his height. Interventions for foot pain while walking (pain in the midfoot on loading and pain in MTP joints on push-off) include the following:

- Sneakers with a deep, wide toe box to accommodate toe deformities
- Evaluation for custom in-shoe orthoses to provide support for the cavus deformity and to reduce force on the metatarsophalangeal joints

Interventions to improve aerobic and anaerobic function:

- Jason will accumulate at least 30 minutes of moderately intense (60% to 70% of peak heart rate [HR]) aerobic activity throughout the day on most days of the week.
- Twice a week, Jason will perform more intense (80% to 85% of peak HR) aerobic exercise (treadmill or stationary bicycle, both available in his home) for at least 30 minutes.
- Jason's individual PT sessions twice a week will include speed training on a stationary bicycle or running pain to improve his anaerobic function.

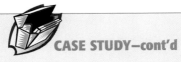

CASE STUDY—cont'd

EVIDENCE TO PRACTICE 7-4

CASE STUDY "JASON"
PLAN OF CARE DECISION AND PATIENT PREFERENCES

Low levels of physical activity (PA) are thought to be responsible at least in part for poor fitness in children with arthritis. One study found that adolescents with JIA spent more time sleeping or lying in bed and less time in recreational or competitive sports than healthy teens (Lelieveld et al., 2008). Only 23% of the JIA group, compared with 66% of the healthy control group, met recommended levels of PA. Higher levels of PA were significantly correlated with fitness and overall well-being, suggesting that increased PA may positively influence fitness and quality of life. Based on the available literature, it is recommended that children with JIA and a deficit in aerobic fitness train at a moderate to vigorous intensity (60% to 85% HRmax) for at least 30 to 45 minutes at least twice a week for at least 6 to 12 weeks (Klepper, 2003).

Klepper, S. (2003). Exercise and fitness in children with arthritis: Evidence of benefits for exercise and physical activity. Arthritis Care and Research, 49, 435–443.
Klepper, S. E. (2008). Exercise in pediatric rheumatic diseases. Current Opinions in Rheumatology, 20, 619–624.
Lelieveld, O. T., Armbrust, W., van Leeuwen, M. A., Duppen, N., Geertzen, J. H., Sauer, P. J, et al. (2008). Physical activity in adolescents with juvenile idiopathic arthritis. Arthritis Rheumatism (Arthritis Care Res), 59, 1379–1384.

Problem: Inability to Perform Activities in Physical Education (PE) Class and Participate in Recreational Sports
 Goal 1: Jason will participate in at least 80% of PE activities at each session to be achieved within 3 months.
 Intervention: PT to consult with PE instructor to integrate Jason more fully into activities
 Goal 2: Jason will participate in one family or community recreational sport (hiking, biking, or skiing) during the next 3 months.
 Intervention for poor exercise tolerance: see above for aerobic and anaerobic training
 Intervention for poor trunk and lower extremity muscle strength and endurance:

- Strengthening regimen twice a week for hip abductors, extensors, external rotators, quadriceps, and hamstrings. Begin with dynamic exercise against gravity. Add resistance in the form of Theraband or light cuff weights when Jason can perform 15 repetitions of each exercise with good form. Include training activities to improve core trunk control.
Intervention: Jason and his family will explore opportunities for community recreational sports clubs for adolescents, including recreational hiking and biking clubs. After choosing his preferred activity, Jason will investigate equipment and lessons for safe and enjoyable participation in the activity.

EVIDENCE TO PRACTICE 7-5

CASE STUDY "JASON"
PLAN OF CARE DECISION AND PATIENT PREFERENCES

Although there is little direct evidence to support the efficacy of strength training in children with JIA, there is general agreement on the importance of maintaining or improving muscle strength to support the joints and training to improve motor control. Faigenbaum et al. (2002) found that children could increase their muscle strength through a twice-weekly regimen of resistance exercises, performed at an intensity of 6 to 10 RM for 15 repetitions. Myer et al. (2005) also demonstrated the safety and benefits of specialized neuromuscular training, including resistance exercises, speed, and coordination drills, in a 10-year-old girl with inactive JIA who wished to participate in team sports.

 Participation in Sports: There is evidence to support the belief that long-term participation in sports does not increase joint scores (Kirchheimer et al., 1993). Most children whose disease is well controlled can play a sport, provided they have adequate training and use properly fitting equipment. Therapists should provide information to help the child and parents distinguish typical post-exercise muscle soreness from a joint flare. Activities that cause pain in joints with active disease should be stopped.

Faigenbaum, A. D., Milliken, L. A., Loud, R. L., Burak, B. T., Doherty, C. L., & Westcott, W. L. (2002). Comparison of 1 and 2 days per week of strength training in children. Research Quarterly for Exercise and Sport, 73, 416–424.
Myer, G. D., Brunner, H. I., Melson, P. G., Paterno, M. V., Ford, K. R., & Hewett, T. E. (2005). Specialized neuromuscular training to improve neuromuscular function and biomechanics in a patient with quiescent juvenile rheumatoid arthritis. Physical Therapy, 85, 791–802.
Kirchheimer, J. C., Wanivenhaus, A., & Engel, A. (1993). Does sport negatively influence joint scores in patients with juvenile rheumatoid arthritis: An 8-year prospective study. Rheumatology International, 12, 239–242.

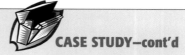

CASE STUDY—cont'd

Problem: Difficulty with Manipulative Activities at Home and School

Goal: Jason will report decreased hand pain and difficulty performing manipulative activities (improved VASchaq38 score for activities requiring hand use).

Interventions for weakness and pain in wrists and hands—consultation with OT:

- Revise resting splints; add liner to minimize skin irritation.
- Refer to occupational therapy for functional hand splints for use in school and adaptive equipment (jar opener, built-up utensils, Velcro closures, or elastic shoelaces).

Interventions for hand and neck pain when working at school desk: consult with school. Ask for evaluation and services under Section 504 of Rehabilitation Act.

- Use built-up writing tools, easel top for desk or laptop, and untimed conditions for tests.

Outcomes

Jason's progress toward his goals was re-evaluated at his regular 3-month rheumatology appointment. His mother reported that she contacted the school to ask that Jason be evaluated to determine if he is eligible for services and accommodations under Section 504 of the Rehabilitation Act. She was also able to find a PT to work with Jason in their home twice a week and to consult with the school PE

instructor to modify some activities so that Jason can participate more fully in the class. Jason reports that he performs the exercises 3 to 4 days a week. His activity log, with each entry co-signed by a parent, verifies his statement. Jason also states that he has been more consistent in taking his medication and admits to feeling better, with less morning stiffness. His hand splints were modified by clinic OT, and he now wears them for at least 4 to 5 hours a night. His progress toward the goals established at his last visit is described below.

1. Jason states that he participates in about 50% of each PE class. He and his family joined a local community ski club and Jason is taking lessons. The family is also planning to purchase bikes for outings. Jason's VASchaq38 is now 6.5—an improvement of 1.5 cm. He reports less difficulty moving between standing and sitting on the floor, running, and performing some manipulative tasks.

2. Jason's responses on the QOL scale show some improvement (overall QOL score is 7 cm and health-related QOL is 6 cm). He reports his health status since his last visit is better. Jason agreed to continue with his current therapy and physical activity program and to take his full medication dose and wear his hand splints every night. He continues to resist using a cervical collar when riding the school bus because he does not want to look different from the other students.

REFERENCES

1. American Physical Therapy Association. (2001). *Guide to physical therapist practice* (2nd ed.). Fairfax, VA: APTA.

2. Ansell, B. M., Rudge, S., & Schaller, J. G. (1992). *Color atlas of pediatric rheumatology* (pp. 13–75). London: Wolfe Publishing Limited.

3. Arthritis Foundation. (1998). *Raising a child with arthritis.* Atlanta, GA: Arthritis Foundation.

4. Atwood, M. (1989). Developmental assessment and integration. In J. Melvin (Ed.), *Rheumatic disease in adult and child: Occupational therapy and rehabilitation* (3rd ed.; pp. 188–214). Philadelphia: FA Davis.

5. Atwood, M. (1989). Treatment considerations. In J. Melvin (Ed.), *Rheumatic disease in adult and child: Occupational therapy and rehabilitation* (3rd ed., pp. 215–234). Philadelphia: FA Davis.

6. Bacon, M., Nicholson, C., Binder, H., & White, P. (1991). Juvenile rheumatoid arthritis: Aquatic exercise and lower extremity function. *Arthritis Care and Research, 4,* 102–105.

7. Bailey, R. C., Olson, J., Pepper, S. L., Porszasz, J., Barstow, T. J., & Cooper, D. M. (1995). The level and tempo of children's physical activities: An observational study. *Medical Science in Sports and Exercises, 27,* 1033–1041.

8. Beyer, J. E., Denyes, M. J., & Villarruel, A. M. (1992). The creation, validation, and continuing development of the

Oucher: A measure of pain intensity in children. *Journal of Pediatric Nursing, 7,* 335–346.

9. Brewer, E. J., Bass, J., Baum, J., Cassidy, J. T., Fink, C., Jacobs, J., et al. (1977). Current proposed revision of JRA criteria. *Arthritis and Rheumatism, 20*(Suppl.), 195–202.

10. van Brussel, M., Lelieveld, O. T., van der Net, J., Engelbert, R. H., Helders, P. J., & Takken, T. (2007). Aerobic and anaerobic exercise capacity in children with juvenile idiopathic arthritis. *Arthritis and Rheumatism, 57,* 891–897.

11. van Brussel, M., van Doren, L., Timmons, B. W., Obeid, J., van der Net, J., Helders, P. J., et al. (2009). Anaerobic-to-aerobic power ratio in children with juvenile idiopathic arthritis. *Arthritis and Rheumatism, 61,* 878–793.

12. Reference deleted in page proofs.

13. Reference deleted in page proofs.

14. Cassidy, J. T., & Petty, R. E. (2001). Juvenile rheumatoid arthritis. In J. T. Cassidy, & R. E. Petty (Eds.), *Textbook of pediatric rheumatology* (4th ed.; pp. 218–321). Philadelphia: WB Saunders.

15. Clemens, L. E., Albert, E., & Ansell, B. M. (1985). Sibling pairs affected by chronic arthritis of childhood: Evidence for a genetic predisposition. *Journal of Rheumatology, 12,* 108–113.

16. Coster, W., Deeney, T., Haltiwanger, J., & Haley, S. (1998). *School function assessment.* Boston, MA: Harcourt Brace & Co.

17. Cron, R. (2000). Current treatment for chronic arthritis in childhood. *Current Opinions in Pediatrics, 14,* 684–687.

18. Duffy, C. M., Arsenault, H. L., Duffy, K. N., Paquin, J. D., & Strawczynski, H. (1997). The Juvenile Arthritis Quality of Life Questionnaire—Development of a new responsive index for juvenile rheumatoid arthritis and juvenile spondyloarthritis. *Journal of Rheumatology, 24,* 738–746.

19. Dunn, W. (1993). Grip strength of children aged 3 to 7 years using a modified sphygmomanometer: Comparison of typical children and children with rheumatic disease. *American Journal of Occupational Therapy, 47,* 421–428.

20. Emery, H. M. (1993). The rehabilitation of the child with juvenile chronic arthritis. *Balliere's Clinical Pediatrics, 1,* 803–823.

21. Epps, H., Hurley, M., & Utley, M. (2002). Development and evaluation of a single score to assess global range of motion in juvenile rheumatoid arthritis. *Arthritis Care and Research, 47,* 398–402.

22. European League Against Rheumatism. (1977). *EULAR bulletin no. 4: Nomenclature and classification of arthritis in children.* Basel: National Zeitung AG.

23. Faigenbaum, A. D., Milliken, L. A., Loud, R. L., Burak, B. T., Doherty, C. L., & Westcott, W. L. (2002). Comparison of 1 and 2 days per week of strength training in children. *Research Quarterly for Exercise and Sport, 73,* 416–424.

24. Fan, J., Wessel, J., & Ellsworth, J. (1998). The relationship between strength and function in females with juvenile rheumatoid arthritis. *Journal of Rheumatology, 3,* 1399–1405.

25. Fisher, N. M., Venkatraman, J. T., & O'Neil, K. (2001). The effects of resistance exercises on muscle and immune function in juvenile arthritis. *Arthritis and Rheumatism, 44,* S276.

26. Fredriksen, B., & Mengshoel, A. M. (2000). The effect of static traction and orthoses in the treatment of knee contractures in preschool children with juvenile chronic arthritis: A single subject design. *Arthritis Care and Research, 13,* 352–359.

27. Giannini, E. J., Ruperto, N., Ravelli, A., Lovell, D. J., Felson, D. T., & Martini, A. (1997). Preliminary definition of improvement in juvenile arthritis. *Arthritis and Rheumatism, 40,* 1202–1209.

28. Giannini, M. J., & Protas, E. J. (1991). Aerobic capacity in juvenile rheumatoid arthritis patients and healthy children. *Arthritis Care and Research, 4,* 131–135.

29. Giannini, M. J., & Protas, E. J. (1992). Exercise response in children with and without juvenile rheumatoid arthritis: A case comparison study. *Physical Therapy, 72,* 365–372.

30. Giannini, M. J., & Protas, E. J. (1993). Comparison of peak isometric knee extensor torque in children with and without juvenile arthritis. *Arthritis Care and Research, 6,* 82–88.

31. Godges, J. J., MacRae, P. G., & Engelke, K. A. (1993). Effects of exercise on hip range of motion, trunk muscle performance, and gait economy. *Physical Therapy, 73,* 468–477.

32. Guzman, J., Burgos-Vargas, R., Duarte-Salazar, C., & Gomez-Mora, P. (1995). Reliability of the articular examination in children with juvenile rheumatoid arthritis: Interobserver agreement and sources of disagreement. *Journal of Rheumatology, 22,* 2331–2336.

33. Hagglund, K. J., Schopp, L. M., Alberts, K. R., Cassidy, J. T., & Frank, R. G. (1995). Predicting pain among children with juvenile rheumatoid arthritis. *Arthritis Care and Research, 8,* 36–42.

34. Hassan, J., van der Net, J., Helders, P. J., Prakken, B. J., & Takken, T. (2010). Six-minute walk test in children with chronic conditions. *British Journal of Sports Medicine, 44,* 270–274.

35. Helders, P. J., Nieuwenhuis, M. K., van der Net, J., Kramer, P. P., Kuis, W., & Buchanon, T. (2000). Displacement response of juvenile arthritic wrists during grasp. *Arthritis Care and Research, 13,* 375–381.

36. Henderson, C. J., Lovell, D. J., Specker, B. L., & Campaigne, B. N. (1995). Physical activity in children with juvenile rheumatoid arthritis: Quantification and evaluation. *Arthritis Care and Research, 8,* 114–119.

37. Reference deleted in page proofs.

38. Hendrengren, E., Knutson, L. M., Haglund-Akerlind, Y., & Hagelberg, S. (2001). Lower extremity isometric torque in children with juvenile chronic arthritis. *Scandinavian Journal of Rheumatology, 30,* 69–76.

39. Hester, N. O., Foster, R., & Kristensen, K. (1990). Measurement of pain in children: Generalizability and validity of the pain ladder and the poker-chip tool. In D. C. Tyler, & E. J. Kane (Eds.), *Advances in pain research and therapy* (pp. 79–84). New York: Raven Press.

40. Howe, S., Levinson, J., Shear, E., Hartner, S., McGirr, G., Schulte, M., et al. (1991). Development of a disability measurement tool for juvenile rheumatoid arthritis: The Juvenile Arthritis Functional Assessment Report for children and their parents. *Arthritis and Rheumatism, 34,* 873–880.

41. James, M. J., Cleland, L. G., Gaffney, R. D., Proudman, S. M., & Gibson, R. A. (1994). Effect of exercise on 99mTc-STPA clearance from knees with effusions. *Journal of Rheumatology, 21,* 501–504.

42. Jaworski, T. M., Bradley, L. A., Heck, L. W., Roca, A., & Alarcon, G. S. (1995). Development of an observation method for assessing pain behaviors in children with juvenile rheumatoid arthritis. *Arthritis and Rheumatism, 38,* 1142–1151.

43. Kirchheimer, J. C., Wanivenhaus, A., & Engel, A. (1993). Does sport negatively influence joint scores in patients with juvenile rheumatoid arthritis? An 8-year prospective study. *Rheumatology International, 12,* 239–242.

44. Keller-Marchand, L., Farpour-Lambert, N. J., Hans, D., Rizzoli, R., & Hofer, M. F. (2006). Effects of a weight bearing exercise program in children with juvenile idiopathic arthritis. *Medical Science in Sports and Exercises, 38*(5 Suppl.), S93–S94.

45. Klijn, P. H., Oudshoorn, A., van der Ent, C. K., van der Net, J., Kimpen, J. L., & Helders, P. J. (2004). Effects of anaerobic training in children with cystic fibrosis: A randomized controlled study. *Chest, 125,* 1299–1305.

46. Klepper, S., Darbee, J., Effgen, S., & Singsen, B. (1992). Physical fitness levels in children with polyarticular juvenile rheumatoid arthritis. *Arthritis Care and Research, 5,* 93–100.

47. Klepper, S. (1999). Effects of an eight-week physical conditioning program on disease signs and symptoms in children with chronic arthritis. *Arthritis Care and Research, 12,* 52–60.

48. Klepper, S. (2003). Exercise and fitness in children with arthritis: Evidence of benefits for exercise and physical activity. *Arthritis Care and Research, 49,* 435–443.

49. Klepper, S. E. (2008). Exercise in pediatric rheumatic diseases. *Current Opinions in Rheumatology, 20,* 619–624.

50. Knopps, K., Wulffraat, N., Lodder, S., Houwen, R., & de Meer, K. (1999). Resting energy expenditure and nutritional status in children with juvenile rheumatoid arthritis. *Journal of Rheumatology, 26,* 2039–2043.

51. Kotaniemi, A., Savolainen, A., Kroger, H., Kautiainen, H., & Isomaki, H. (1999). Weight-bearing physical activity, calcium intake, systemic glucocorticoids: Chronic inflammation and body constitution as determinants of lumbar and femoral bone mineral density in juvenile chronic arthritis. *Scandinavian Journal of Rheumatology, 28,* 19–26.

52. Kraemer, W., & Fleck, S. (1993). *Strength training for young athletes.* Champaign, IL: Human Kinetics.

53. Lam, C., Young, N., Marhawa, J., McLimont, M., & Feldman, B.M. (2004). Revised versions of the Childhood Health Assessment Questionnaire (CHAQ) are more sensitive and suffer less from a ceiling effect. *Arthritis and Rheumatism, 51,* 881–889.

54. Lelieveld, O. T., Takken, T., van der Net, J., & van Weert, E. (2005). Validity of the 6-minute walking test in juvenile idiopathic arthritis. *Arthritis and Rheumatism, 53,* 304–307.

55. Lelieveld, O. T., van Brussel, M., Takken, T., van Weert, E., van Leeuwen, M. A., & Armbrust, W. (2007). Aerobic and anaerobic exercise capacity in adolescents with juvenile idiopathic arthritis. *Arthritis and Rheumatism, 57,* 898–904.

56. Lelieveld, O. T., Armbrust, W., van Leeuwen, M. A., Duppen, N., Geertzen, J. H., Sauer, P., et al. (2008). Physical activity in adolescents with juvenile idiopathic arthritis. *Arthritis and Rheumatism, 59,* 1379–1384.

57. Len, C., Ferraz, M., Goldenberg, J., Oliveira, L. M., Araujo, P. P., Rodrigues, Q., et al. (1999). Pediatric Escola Paulista de Medicina range of motion scale: A reduced joint count score for general use in juvenile rheumatoid arthritis. *Journal of Rheumatology, 26,* 909–913.

58. Libby, A. K., Sherry, D. D., & Dudgeon, B. J. (1991). Shoulder limitation in juvenile rheumatoid arthritis. *Archives of Physical Medicine and Rehabilitation, 72,* 382–384.

59. Lindehammer, H., & Backman, E. (1995). Muscle function in juvenile chronic arthritis. *Journal of Rheumatology, 22,* 1159–1165.

60. Lindehammer, H., & Sandstedt, P. (1998). Measurement of quadriceps muscle strength and bulk in juvenile chronic arthritis: A prospective, longitudinal 2-year survey. *Journal of Rheumatology, 25,* 2240–2248.

61. Lineker, S. C., Badley, E. M., & Dalby, D. M. (1996). Unmet service needs of children with rheumatic diseases and their parents in a metropolitan area. *Journal of Rheumatology, 23,* 1054–1058.

62. Lovell, D. J., Giannini, E. J., Reiff, A., Cawkwell, G. D., Silverman, E. D., Nocton, J. J., et al. (2000). Etanercept in children with polyarticular juvenile rheumatoid arthritis. Pediatric Rheumatology Collaborative Study Group. *New England Journal of Medicine, 342,* 763–769.

63. Lovell, D. J., Athreya, B., Emery, H. M., Gibbas, D. L., Levinson, J. E., Lindsley, C. B., et al. (1990). School attendance and patterns, special services, and special needs in pediatric patients with rheumatic disease. *Arthritis Care and Research, 3,* 196–203.

64. Lovell, D. J., Howe, S., Shear, E., Hartner, S., McGirr, G., Schulte, M., et al. (1989). Development of a disability measurement tool for juvenile rheumatoid arthritis: The Juvenile Arthritis Functional Assessment Scale. *Arthritis and Rheumatism, 32,* 1390–1395.

65. Melvin, J., & Wright, F. V. (2000). Procedure for serial casting of contractures from juvenile arthritis. In J. Melvin, & F. V. Wright (Eds.), *Rheumatologic rehabilitation: Pediatric rheumatic diseases* (Vol. 3; pp. 295–297). Bethesda, MD: American Occupational Therapy Association.

66. Mier, R. J., Wright, F. V., & Bolding, D. J. (2000). Juvenile rheumatoid arthritis. In J. Melvin, & F. V. Wright (Eds.), *Rheumatologic rehabilitation: Pediatric rheumatic diseases* (Vol. 3; pp. 1–43). Bethesda, MD: American Occupational Therapy Association.

67. Minor, M., & Westby, D. (2001). Rest and exercise. In L. Robbins, C. Burckhardt, M. Hannan, & R. DeHoratius (Eds.), *Clinical care in the rheumatic diseases* (2nd ed.; pp. 179–184). Atlanta, GA: American College of Rheumatology.

68. Morrison, C. D., Bundy, R. C., & Fisher, A. G. (1991). The contribution of motor skills and playfulness to the play performance of preschoolers. *American Journal of Occupational Therapy, 45,* 687–694.

69. Murray, K. J., Moroldo, M. B., Donnelly, P., Prahalad, S., Passo, M. H., Giannini, E. H., et al. (1999). Age-specific effects of juvenile rheumatoid arthritis-associated HLA alleles. *Arthritis and Rheumatism, 42,* 1843–1853.

70. Nestor, B. J., Figgie, M. P., Wright, F. V., & Melvin, J. (2000). Surgical treatment of juvenile rheumatoid arthritis. In J. Melvin, & F. V. Wright (Eds.), *Rheumatologic rehabilitation: Pediatric rheumatic diseases* (Vol. 3; pp. 249–266). Bethesda, MD: American Occupational Therapy Association.

71. van der Net, J., van der Torre, P., Engelbert, R. H., Engelen, V., van Zon, F., Takken, T., et al. (2008). Motor performance and functional ability in preschool- and early school-aged children with juvenile idiopathic arthritis: A cross-sectional study. *Pediatric Rheumatology Online Journal, 6.*

72. Nieuwenhuis, M. K., van der Net, J., Kuis, W., Buchanon, T. S., & Helders, P. J. (1999). Assessment of wrist malalignment in juvenile rheumatoid arthritis. *Advances in Physiotherapy, 1,* 99–109.

73. Reference deleted in page proofs.

74. Reference deleted in page proofs.

75. Oberg, T., Karsznia, B., Gare, A., & Lagerstrand, A. (1994). Physical training of children with juvenile chronic arthritis. *Scandinavian Journal of Rheumatology, 23*, 92–95.

76. Oosterveld, F. G., Rasker, J. J., Jacobs, J. W., & Overmars H. J. (1992). The effect of local heat and cold therapy on the intra-articular and skin surface temperature of the knee. *Arthritis and Rheumatism, 35*, 146–151.

77. Oosterveld, F. G., & Rasker, J. J. (1994). Effects of local heat and cold treatment on surface and intra-articular temperature of arthritic knees. *Arthritis and Rheumatism, 37*, 1578–1582.

78. Paap, E., van der Net, J., Helders, P. J., & Takken, T. (2005). Physiologic response of the six-minute walk test in children with juvenile idiopathic arthritis. *Arthritis and Rheumatism, 53*, 351–356.

79. Petersen, L. S., Mason, T., Nelson, A. M., O'Fallon, W. M., & Gabriel, S. E. (1996). Juvenile rheumatoid arthritis in Rochester, Minnesota 1960–1993: Is the epidemiology changing? *Arthritis and Rheumatism, 39*, 1385–1390.

80. Petersen, L. S., Mason, T., Nelson, A. M., O'Fallon, W. M., & Gabriel, S. E. (1997). Psychosocial outcomes and health status of adults who have had juvenile rheumatoid arthritis. *Arthritis and Rheumatism, 40*, 2235–2290.

81. Petty, R. E., Southwood, T. R., Manners, P, et al. (2004). International League of Associations for Rheumatology classification of juvenile idiopathic arthritis, second revision, Edmonton 2001. *Journal of Rheumatology, 31*, 390–392.

82. Ravelli, A., Martini, A. (2007). Juvenile idiopathic arthritis. *The Lancet, 369*, 767–778.

83. Reed, M. H., & Wilmot, D. M. (1991). The radiology of juvenile rheumatoid arthritis: A review of the English language literature. *Journal of Rheumatology, 31*(Suppl.), 2–22.

84. Rhodes, V. J. (1991). Physical therapy management of patients with juvenile rheumatoid arthritis. *Physical Therapy, 71*, 910–919.

85. Ruperto, N., Ravelli, A., Migliavacca, D., Viola, S., Pistorio, A., & Duarte, C. (1999). Responsiveness of clinical measures in children with oligoarticular juvenile chronic arthritis. *Journal of Rheumatology, 26*, 1827–1830.

86. Schanberg, L. E., Sandstrom, M. J., Starr, K., Gil, K. M., Lefebvre, J. C., Keefe, F. J., et al. (2000). The relationship of daily mood and stressful events to symptoms in juvenile rheumatic disease. *Arthritis Care and Research, 13*, 33–41.

87. Schoenmakers, M. A., de Groot, J. F., Gorter, J. W., Hillaert, J. L., Helders, P. J., & Takken, T. (2009). Muscle strength, aerobic capacity and physical activity in independent ambulating children with lumbosacral spina bifida. *Disability and Rehabilitation, 104*, 657–665.

88. Scull, S., & Athreya, B. (1995). Childhood arthritis. In B. Goldberg (Ed.), *Sports and exercise for children with chronic health conditions* (pp. 136–148). Champaign, IL: Human Kinetics.

89. Sherry, D. D., Stein, L. D., Reed, A. M., Schanberg, L. E., & Kredich, D. W. (1999). Prevention of leg length discrepancy in young children with pauciarticular juvenile rheumatoid arthritis by treatment with intra-articular steroids. *Arthritis and Rheumatism, 42*, 2330–2334.

90. Singh, G., Athreya, B., Fries, J. F., & Goldsmith, D. P. (1994). Measurement of health status in children with juvenile rheumatoid arthritis. *Arthritis and Rheumatism, 37*, 1761–1769.

91. Spencer, C. H., & Bernstein, B. H. (2002). Hip disease in juvenile rheumatoid arthritis. *Current Opinions in Rheumatology, 4*, 536–541.

92. Sullivan, D. B., Cassidy, J. T., & Petty, R. E. (1975). Pathogenic implications of age of onset in juvenile rheumatoid arthritis. *Arthritis and Rheumatism, 18*, 251–255.

93. Szer, I. S., & Wright, F. V. (2000). School integration. In J. Melvin, & F. V. Wright (Eds.), Rheumatologic rehabilitation: Pediatric rheumatic diseases (*Vol. 3*; pp. 223–230). Philadelphia: WB Saunders.

94. Takken, T., van der Net, J. J., & Helders, P. J. (2001). Do juvenile idiopathic arthritis patients benefit from an exercise program? A pilot study. *Arthritis Care and Research, 45*, 81–85.

95. Takken, T., Hemel, A., van der Net, J. J., & Helders, P. J. (2002). Aerobic fitness in children with juvenile idiopathic arthritis: A systematic review. *Journal of Rheumatology, 29*, 2643–2647.

96. Takken, T., van der Net, J., & Helders, P. J. (2003). Relationship between functional ability and physical fitness in juvenile rheumatoid arthritis. *Scandinavian Journal of Rheumatology, 32*, 174–178.

97. Takken, T., Van der Net, J., Kuis, W., & Helders, PJ. (2003). Physical activity and health related physical fitness in children with juvenile idiopathic arthritis. *Annals of the Rheumatic Diseases, 62*, 885–889.

98. Takken, T. (2006). Exercise testing and training in children with juvenile idiopathic arthritis and dermatomyositis: State of the art. *Annals of the Rheumatic Diseases, 65*, 25.

99. Takken, T., van Brussel, M., Engelbert, R. H., van der Net, J., Kuis, W., & Helders, P. J. (2008). Exercise therapy in juvenile idiopathic arthritis: A Cochrane review. *European Journal of Physical and Rehabilitation Medicine, 44*, 287–297.

100. Thompson, K. L., & Varni, J. W. (1986). A developmental cognitive-behavioral approach to pediatric pain assessment. *Pain, 25*, 283–296.

101. Thompson, P., Beath, T., Bell, J., Jacobson, G., Phair, T., Salbach, N. M., et al. (2008). Test-retest reliability of the 10-metre fast walk test and 6-minute walk test in ambulatory school-aged children with cerebral palsy. *Developmental Medicine and Child Neurology, 50*, 370–376.

102. Varni, J. W., Waldron, S. A., Gragg, R. A., Rapoff, M. A., Bernstein, B. H., Lindsley, C. B., et al. (1996). Development of the Waldron/Varni pediatric pain coping inventory. *Pain, 67*, 141–150.

103. Varni, J., Seid, M., Smith Knight, T., Burwinkle, T., Brown, J., & Szer, I. S. (2002). The PedsQL in pediatric rheumatology: Reliability, validity, and responsiveness of the Pediatric Quality of Life Inventory generic core scales and rheumatology module. *Arthritis and Rheumatism, 46*, 714–725.

104. Verschuren, O., Ketelaar, M., Gorter, J. W., Helders, P. J., Uiterwaal, C. S., & Takken, T. (2007). Exercise training program in children and adolescents with cerebral palsy: A randomized controlled trial. *Archives of Pediatrics and Adolescent Medicine, 161,* 1075–1081.

105. Vostrejs, M., & Hollister, J. R. (1988). Muscle atrophy and leg length discrepancies in pauciarticular juvenile rheumatoid arthritis. *American Journal of Diseases of Childhood, 142,* 343–345.

106. Wessel, J., Kaup, C., Fan, J., Ehalt, R., Ellsworth, J., Speer, C., et al. (1999). Isometric strength measurements in children with arthritis: Reliability and relation to function. *Arthritis Care and Research, 12,* 238–246.

107. White, P. H. (1990). Growth abnormalities in children with juvenile rheumatoid arthritis. *Clinical Orthopedics and Related Research, 259,* 46–50.

108. Wiltink, A., Nijweide, P. J., Oosterbaan, W. A., Hekkenberg, R. T., & Helders, P. J. (1995). Effect of therapeutic ultrasound on endochondral ossification. *Ultrasound in Medicine and Biology, 21,*121–127.

109. Wind, A. E., Takken, T., Helders, P. J., & Engelbert, R. H. (2010). Is grip strength a predictor for total muscle strength in healthy children, adolescents, and young adults? *European Journal of Pediatrics, 169,* 281–287.

110. Wong, D. L., & Baker, C. M. (1998). Pain in children: Comparison of assessment scales. *Pediatric Nursing, 14,* 9–17.

111. Wright, F. V., Liu, G., & Milne, F. (1996). Reliability of the measurement of time-distance parameters of gait: A comparison in children with juvenile rheumatoid arthritis and children with cerebral palsy. *Physiotherapy Canada, 51,* 191–200.

112. Wright, F. V., Longo Kimber, J. L., Law, M., Goldsmith, C. H., Crombie, V., & Dent, P. (1996). The Juvenile Arthritis Functional Status Index (JASI): A validation study. *Journal of Rheumatology, 23,* 1066–1079.

113. Wright, F. V., & Smith, E. (1996). Physical therapy management of the child and adolescent with juvenile rheumatoid arthritis. In J. M. Walker, & A. Helewa (Eds.), *Physical therapy in arthritis* (pp. 211–244). Philadelphia: WB Saunders.

114. Wrotniak, B. H., Epstein, L. H., Dorn, J. M., Jones, K. E., & Kondilis, V. A. (2006). The relationship between motor proficiency and physical activity in children. *Pediatrics, 118,* 1758–1765.

115. Zamir, G., Press, J., Tal, A., & Tarasiuk A. (1998). Sleep fragmentation in children with juvenile rheumatoid arthritis. *Journal of Rheumatology, 25,* 1191–1197.

8

Spinal Conditions

HEIDI A. FRERE, PT, DPT • SUZANNE M. GREEN, PT • CHERYL R. PATRICK, PT, MBA

he spine is the framework for our posture and our movement. It supports our cranium, extremities, and spinal cord; allows for trunk flexibility; acts as a shock absorber; and provides structural support for normal chest and respiratory development. Orthopedic concerns arise when spinal alignment is altered by congenital or progressive changes, producing scoliosis, kyphosis, or lordosis.

Each one or a combination of these conditions, if left untreated, may affect a child's pulmonary function, psychosocial well-being, potential for back pain, and life expectancy. We, as physical therapists, play a vital role in the detection and treatment of spinal conditions. Two to four percent of the population of school-age children (7–18 years) is at risk for adolescent idiopathic scoliosis, the most common form of scoliosis.[82,87] The prevalence of other spinal conditions varies with the condition and the underlying disease process.[4,108] This chapter addresses the prevalence and natural history, identification, examination, and treatment of these spinal conditions. Specific case studies are presented to discuss impairments and restrictions in activity and participation of children with spinal conditions. Physical therapy intervention is emphasized, along with nonsurgical and surgical management of these spinal conditions.

DEVELOPMENT OF THE SPINE

Pathologic spinal conditions are discussed in this chapter, so it is necessary for the reader to have some knowledge of normal spinal development (Figure 8-1). Therefore, a discussion of development in the embryologic, fetal, and childhood stages follows.

Fetal development is divided into three stages. The first 3 weeks after fertilization is termed the pre-embryonic period. The embryonic period is next, lasting from week 3 to week 8 of gestation; during this stage, the organs of the body develop. The fetal period lasts from week 8 until term, and during this stage, maturation and growth of all structures and organs occur.[69]

Early development of the skeletal, muscular, and neural systems is related to the notochord. Cell proliferation occurs at approximately 3 weeks, forming a trilaminar structure with layers of ectoderm, mesoderm, and endoderm. Proliferation of the mesodermal tissue continues, forming 29 pairs of somites (a pair of block-like segments that give rise to

muscle and vertebrae, which are formed on each side of the notochord[104]) in the fourth week and the remainder (42–44 total) in the fifth week. Differentiation of the somites then occurs, producing 4 occipital, 8 cervical, 12 thoracic, 5 lumbar, 5 sacral, and 8 to 10 coccygeal somites. The occipital somites form a portion of the base of the skull and the articulation between the cranium and the cervical vertebrae, while the last 5 to 7 coccygeal somites disappear. Cervical, thoracic, lumbar, and sacral somites form the structures of the spine.[114]

Proliferation of the somites occurs, leading to the development of three distinct areas. Dorsally, the cells become dermatomes, giving rise to the skin. Medially to the dermatome, cells migrate deep to give rise to skeletal muscle. The ventral and medial cells migrate toward the notochord and the neural tube to form the sclerotome.[69,114]

The sclerotomal cells proliferate and differentiate, giving rise to rudimentary vertebral structures, including rib buds. Chondrification begins at the cervicothoracic level, extending cranially and caudally. Centers of chondrification allow for formation of the solid cartilage model of a vertebra with no line of demarcation between body, neural arch, or rib rudiments.[69]

Ossification occurs at primary and secondary centers. Ossification begins during the late fetal period and continues after birth. Primary centers of ossification extend to the spinous, transverse, and articular processes. Secondary ossification centers develop at the upper and lower portions of the vertebral body, at the tip of the spinous processes, and at each transverse process. These centers expand in late adolescence. Secondary ossification centers also develop in the ribs—one at the head of the rib and two in the tubercle. Ossification of the axis, atlas, and sacrum differs slightly from that of the other vertebrae. The atlas has two primary centers and one secondary center of ossification, and the axis has five primary and two secondary centers of ossification. Ossification of the axis begins near the end of gestation with fusion of the two odontoid centers and is completed in the second decade of life with fusion of the odontoid and centrum. Fusion of the sacrum begins in adolescence and is completed in the third decade of life.[69]

Spinal growth occurs throughout adolescence. Knowledge of spinal growth is essential in nonsurgical and surgical treatment of spinal deformities. Spinal growth does not

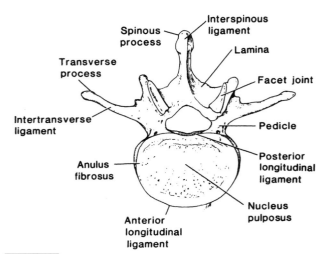

Figure 8-1 The L2 vertebra viewed from above. (From Moe, J. H., Winter, R. B., Bradford, D. S., Ogilvie, J. W., & Lonstein, J. E. [1987]. *Scoliosis and other spinal deformities* [2nd ed.; p. 8]. Philadelphia: WB Saunders.)

proceed in a uniform linear pattern.[101,102] Two periods of rapid spinal growth occur: The first from birth to age 3 years, and the second during the adolescent growth spurt. Between 3 years and the onset of puberty, growth is linear.

The spinal pubertal growth spurts occur at different chronologic and Tanner ages for females and males. In females, the growth spurt coincides with Tanner 2 or a chronologic age of 8 to 14 years, with maximum growth occurring at a mean of 12 years of age. The spurt lasts 2.5 to 3 years.[10] The growth spurt occurs later in males, at Tanner 3 or chronologic age 11 to 16 years, with maximum growth at age 14 years. These values are average values based on white Anglo-Saxon populations.[20]

A fused area of the spine does not grow longitudinally, as documented by Moe and colleagues.[68] The surgeon, therefore, considers the information on spinal growth potential for each individual case.

SCOLIOSIS

DETECTION AND CLINICAL EXAMINATION

Detection of scoliosis occurs primarily by identification of trunk, shoulder, or pelvic asymmetries. The American Academy of Pediatrics (AAP), American Academy of Orthopaedic Surgeons (AAOS), Scoliosis Research Society (SRS), and Pediatric Orthopaedic Society of North America (POSNA) commissioned a task force to investigate the effectiveness of scoliosis screening. They concluded that the literature does not provide sufficient evidence to merit scoliosis screening of asymptomatic adolescents. However, the societies do not support recommendations against scoliosis screening. The societies acknowledge the benefits of clinical screenings, including the potential to effect curve progression

by brace treatment, as well as earlier detection of severe deformities requiring operative correction.[85]

Children with asymmetries should be referred to an orthopedic surgeon with an interest in and knowledge of scoliosis for a baseline evaluation. An examination begins with a complete patient history to obtain information regarding curve detection, familial conditions, general health, and physical maturity. The examiner also evaluates signs and symptoms of any underlying disease and neurologic status. The physical examination includes assessment of general alignment, spinal alignment by forward bend test, shoulder and pelvic symmetry, trunk compensation using a plumb line, and leg length measurement. The magnitude of a rib hump is quantified using a scoliometer with the forward bend test.[69] The scoliometer, an inclinometer designed by Bunnell,[5] is placed over the spinous process at the apex of the curve to measure the angle of trunk rotation (ATR). The ATR correlates with the severity of the scoliosis.[87] A minimal measurement of at least 5° by the scoliometer is considered a good criterion for identifying lateral curvatures of the spine with Cobb angles of 20° or greater. Therefore, a scoliometer reading of 5° or greater warrants referral to an orthopedic physician for further evaluation[5] and is an indication for a radiograph.[96]

Radiographs (initially two views: lateral and anterior-posterior) are used to determine location, type, and magnitude of the curve, as well as skeletal age. Skeletal maturity is determined using the Risser sign, which quantifies the amount of ossification of the iliac crest, using grades 0 to 5. Grade 0 represents absence of ossification. Grades 1 to 4 are excursions from 25% to 100%, starting at the anterior-superior iliac spine. Grade 5 categorizes fusion of the iliac crest with the ileum.[121] Grades 0, 1, and 2 correlate with skeletal immaturity, grade 3 with progressing skeletal maturity, grade 4 with cessation of spinal growth, and grade 5 with cessation of increase in height (Figure 8-2).

The spinal curvature is measured using the Cobb method. To complete the measurement, one must first identify the end vertebrae. The end vertebrae are described as the most cephalad vertebra of a curve whose upper surface maximally tilts toward the curve's concavity and the most caudal vertebra with maximal tilt toward the convexity. Lines are drawn as extensions of the end vertebrae from end plate or pedicles. The degree of curvature is measured as the angle formed by the intersection of lines perpendicular to these end vertebral lines[16,28] (Figure 8-3). Magnetic resonance imaging, computed tomography, myelography, and bone scans can be used to identify subtle central nervous system abnormalities and to provide additional information as necessary to aid in diagnosis and detection of spinal conditions.

TERMINOLOGY

Scoliosis refers to a lateral curvature of the spine. To be considered a scoliosis, the curvature in the coronal plane must

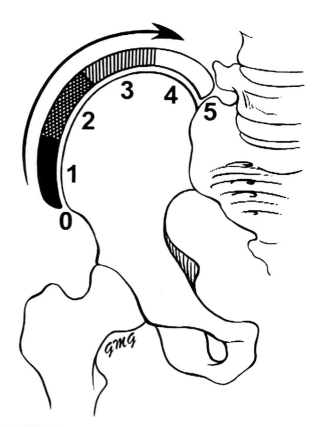

Figure 8-2 Risser sign, grades 0 to 5. (From Reamy, et al. [2001]. Adolescent idiopathic scoliosis: Review and current concepts. *American Family Physician, 64,* 111–116.)

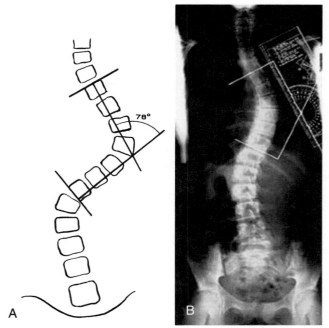

Figure 8-3 **A,** Cobb's method of measuring the angle of the curve in scoliosis (see text). **B,** The Cobb method of measuring the curve angle of scoliosis, as seen on a radiograph. (**A** from Tachdjian, M. O. [1990]. *Pediatric orthopedics* [2nd ed.; p. 2285]. Philadelphia: WB Saunders. **B** from Kim, H. J., et al. [2009]. Update on the management of idiopathic scoliosis. *Current Opinion in Pediatrics, 21,* 55–64.)

TABLE **8-1** **Classification of Spinal Curve Based on Location**

Cervical curve	C1-C6
Cervicothoracic curve	C7-T1
Thoracic curve	T2-T11
Thoracolumbar curve	T12-L1
Lumbar curve	L2-L4
Lumbosacral curve	L5-S1

be greater than 10° with a vertebral rotation component on the radiograph.[2,24] Spinal deformities are classified according to origin, location, magnitude, and direction. Curvatures may be idiopathic, neuromuscular, or congenital and may be further classified by the area of the spine in which the apex of the curve is located, as described in Table 8-1.

Magnitude is measured using the Cobb method. Direction of the curve is designated as right or left by the side of the convexity of the deformity.[35] Up to 90% of thoracic curves are right,[87] and if a left thoracic curve is discovered, more extensive evaluation is required to rule out tumors and other neurologic problems.[86,87,89] Left thoracic curves are not directly linked to a disease process, but merit further evaluation.[27,87] Schwend et al.[92] found 43 out of 95 patients had a left thoracic curvature, and of these 43, 10 (23%) had an intraspinal abnormality, compared with 4 (8%) of the 52 patients who had a different curve pattern.

Two major types of curvatures are known: structural and nonstructural. A nonstructural curve fully corrects clinically and radiographically on lateral bend toward the apex of the curve and lacks vertebral rotation. A nonstructural curve is usually nonprogressive and is most often caused by a shortened lower extremity on the side of the apex of the curve. It

is essential, however, to monitor nonstructural curves during growth because they may occasionally develop into structural deformities.

A structural curve cannot be voluntarily, passively, or forcibly fully corrected. Rotation of the vertebrae is toward the convexity of the curve. A fixed thoracic prominence or rib hump in a child with a thoracic deformity or a lumbar paraspinal prominence in a child with a lumbar curve is evidence of rotation when observed on clinical examination.[35]

IDIOPATHIC SCOLIOSIS

Idiopathic scoliosis denotes a lateral curvature of the spine of unknown cause and is the most common form of scoliosis in children. Lonstein and Carlson[55] identified three strong factors that correlate with curve progression for idiopathic scoliosis: curve magnitude, Risser sign, and the patient's chronologic age at the time of diagnosis.

Origin, Incidence, and Pathophysiology

Infantile idiopathic scoliosis develops in children younger than age 3, usually manifesting shortly after birth. This form of scoliosis accounts for less than 1% of all cases in North America.[63,66] Infantile idiopathic scoliosis occurs more frequently in male infants, and most curves are left. Eighty to ninety percent of these curves spontaneously resolve, but many of the remainder of cases will progress throughout childhood, resulting in severe deformity. Because infantile idiopathic scoliosis is common in England and northern Europe, but rare in the United States, environmental factors have been implicated in the development of the deformity.[35,63]

Juvenile idiopathic scoliosis develops between ages 3 and 9 years.[17] The most common curve is right thoracic, occurring in males and females with equal frequency.[12] It is most often recognized at around 6 years of age. Juvenile idiopathic curves have a high rate of progression and result in severe deformity if untreated. Charles et al.[12] found that curves greater than 30° at onset of the pubertal growth spurt increased rapidly and presented a 100% prognosis for surgery. Curves 21° to 30° also presented a 75% progression risk and would benefit from careful follow-up.

Adolescent idiopathic scoliosis (AIS) categorizes curves manifesting at or around the onset of puberty and accounts for approximately 80% of all cases of idiopathic scoliosis. The prevalence of idiopathic scoliosis is 2% to 4% of children ages 10 to skeletal maturity.[4,26,87] Three to nine percent of these children have curves greater than 10° and require intervention.[16,108] The overall female-to-male ratio for prevalence of AIS is 3.6:1. The female-to-male ratio is roughly equal (1.4:1) in curves of approximately 10°. With curve magnitude of 20° or greater, the female-to-male ratio increases to 5:1.[80,107,108] A greater percentage of curves will progress in the female patient—19.3% compared with 1.2% of males. A large number of AIS curvatures are structural at the time of detection, although flexibility and the progression of these curves vary. Structural curves have a greater tendency to progress throughout adolescence at an average rate of 1° per month if untreated, whereas nonstructural curves may remain flexible enough to avoid becoming problematic.[35]

Extensive research has been devoted to discovering the cause of idiopathic scoliosis, still the mechanics and specific origin are not clearly understood. A number of theories have been proposed to attempt to explain the mechanics of vertebral column failure and decompensation of the spine, as seen in idiopathic scoliosis. It is thought that the cause of scoliosis is multifactorial. Current researchers have investigated many areas, including, but not limited to, growth timing in

relationship to maturational changes; biomechanics; skeletal framework, specifically, spine slenderness; disproportionate growth of the anterior portion of the vertebrae compared with the posterior portion; melatonin; and genetics.[7] Data from studies by Wynne-Davies[119] and Cowell and colleagues[15] reflect the existence of a familial tendency. Janicki[42] also stated that a genetic component is included, noting that siblings of patients with scoliosis are diagnosed 7 times more often, and children of patients with scoliosis are diagnosed 3 times more often. Current research provides strong evidence for a genetic basis for idiopathic scoliosis; however, the specific mode or modes of heritability are still not clear. Understanding the genetic transmission of this disorder would be helpful in determining appropriate intervention approaches, particularly for those who might be at risk for severe disability.[67]

According to Wolff's law, bone responds to the loads applied to it. In accordance with the Hueter-Volkmann principle, compressive loading will hinder bone growth, and reduced loading will hasten it.[91] Asymmetrical loading of a growing spine will lead to asymmetrical bony growth, resulting in wedge-shaped vertebrae.[97] Associated changes are seen in the intraspinal canal and the posterior arch; these may cause angulation and stretch on the spinal cord but rarely cause functional disturbances. Cord compression and functional changes occur most often secondary to an unusually tight dura mater, as is seen in spines with marked dorsal kyphosis. Changes occurring on the concave side of the curvature include compression and degenerative changes of intravertebral discs and shortening of muscles and ligaments (Figure 8-4). Changes in the thoracic spine directly affect the rib cage. The translatory shift of the spine causes an asymmetrically divided thorax, producing decreased pulmonary capacity on the convex side and increased pulmonary capacity on the concave side. Severe curves in the thoracic spine associated with increased angulation of the ribs posteriorly further reduce aeration of the lung on the convex side, potentially causing abnormal stresses on the heart and disturbed cardiac function.[16,39] Structural changes cause cosmetic deformity that, in turn, affects appearance and may affect psychosocial well-being.

Some clinical studies have focused on the influence of balance control as related to scoliosis. O'Beirne et al.[75] found that balance dysfunction is characteristic of patients with progressive curves, regardless of origin, thereby implying that the dysfunction is a result of the curve, rather than the primary cause. Another study on standing stability and body parameters compared able-bodied girls versus those with AIS. Findings supported the concept of a primary or secondary dysfunction in the postural regulation system of girls with AIS.[72] Byl and Gray[6] reported decreased performance of adolescents with idiopathic scoliosis, particularly those with severe curves, on complex balance activities, especially when vision and proprioception were simultaneously challenged. The authors posed the question of whether balance

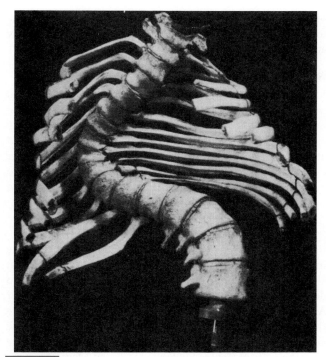

Figure 8-4 Anatomic specimen of the spine demonstrating structural changes of right thoracic scoliosis. Note vertebral wedging on the concave side and rotation of the vertebral bodies to the convexity of the curve. (From James, J. I. P. [1967]. *Scoliosis* [p. 13]. Baltimore: Williams & Wilkins. Copyright 1967, Williams & Wilkins.)

changes are due to structural impairment (scoliosis) or to an underlying sensory impairment. They strongly suggested the need for longitudinal studies to determine whether a predictive relationship exists between balance dysfunction and progressive scoliosis.

Natural History

A progressive curve is defined as a sustained increase of 5° or more on two consecutive examinations occurring at 4-to-6 month intervals. An untreated progressive curve has the potential to increase in magnitude in adult life. Following are the main factors that influence the probability of progression in the skeletally immature patient[108]:

1. The younger the patient at diagnosis, the greater the risk of progression.
2. Double-curve patterns have a greater risk for progression than single-curve patterns.
3. The lower the Risser sign, the greater the risk of progression.
4. Curves with greater magnitude are at greater risk to progress.
5. Risk of progression in females is approximately 10 times that in males with curves of comparable magnitude.
6. Greater risk of progression is present when curves develop before menarche.

CONGENITAL SCOLIOSIS

Origin, Incidence, and Pathophysiology

Congenital scoliosis curves are caused by anomalous vertebral development in utero. The term *congenital scoliosis* should not be confused with *infantile scoliosis*. Clinical manifestations of congenital scoliosis may not be apparent at birth, but the vertebral anomaly is present. Infantile scoliosis will not demonstrate vertebral anomalies upon radiography.[110] Congenital anomalies of the vertebrae can be attributed to failure of vertebral segmentation, failure of vertebral formation, or mixed defect, which is a combination of the two. Both pathologic processes are frequently seen in the same spine and may occur at the same or at different levels. Location of the pathologic process on the vertebrae (anterior, posterior, lateral, or a combination) determines the congenital deformity. Purely lateral deformity produces congenital scoliosis, and anterolateral and posterolateral deformities produce congenital kyphoscoliosis and lordoscoliosis, respectively.[114,115] The male-to-female ratio for congenital scoliosis is 1:1.4.[53]

A defect of segmentation is seen when adjacent vertebrae do not completely separate from one another, thereby producing an unsegmented bar, with no growth plate or disk between the adjacent vertebrae. A lateral, one-sided defect of segmentation produces severe progressive congenital scoliosis. Circumferential failure of segmentation produces en bloc vertebrae, an anomaly that results in loss of segmental motion and loss of longitudinal vertebral growth but no rotational or angular spinal deformity.[114]

Defects of formation may be partial or complete. Anterior failure of formation of all or part of the vertebral body produces a kyphosis. A partial unilateral defect of formation of a vertebra produces a wedge-shaped hemivertebra (Figure 8-5) with one pedicle and only one side with growth potential. A nonsegmented hemivertebra is completely fused to the adjacent proximal and distal vertebrae. A semisegmented hemivertebra is fused to only one adjacent vertebra and is separated from the other by a normal end plate and disc. A segmented hemivertebra is separated from proximal and distal vertebrae by a normal end plate and a disc. Hemivertebrae may be unbalanced, with the defect present on one side of the spine, or balanced, with different hemivertebrae present, with defects on opposite sides of the spine compensating for any curves.[114,115]

Abnormalities involving other organ systems have been found in as many as 61% of patients with congenital scoliosis.[34] Multiple organ systems develop while the sclerotomes are differentiating to form vertebral bodies during the embryonic period. Therefore, any noxious influence affecting the formation of vertebral structures may also have an adverse effect on the concomitant development of organ systems, including the heart, kidneys, trachea, and esophagus. Cardiac anomalies have been associated with congenital scoliosis of the thoracic spine, and kidney anomalies have been associated with lumbar scoliosis.[53]

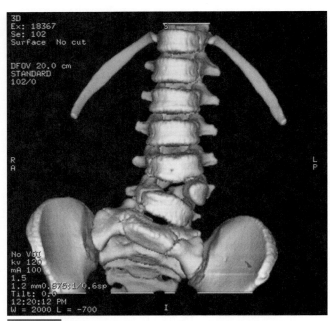

Figure 8-5 Computed tomography illustrating a hemivertebrae. (From Janicki, J. A., & Alman, B. [2007]. Scoliosis: Review of diagnosis and treatment. *Paediatric Child Health, 12,* 771–776.)

Other spinal anomalies or other organ system anomalies may be associated with congenital spinal malformations. According to Letts and Jawadi,[53] the occurrence of spinal dysraphism is high in patients with congenital scoliosis; investigators stated that the incidence of a dysraphic lesion was found to be approximately 40%. Clinical signs of a spinal dysraphism include a hair patch, unequal foot size, various foot deformities (e.g., cavus feet), and asymmetrical lower extremity circumference and strength. Other associated defects include urinary tract anomalies, hearing deficits, facial asymmetries, and Sprengel's deformity, which is a partially undescended scapula that may cause apparent webbing or shortening of the neck and limited shoulder range of motion.[114]

The risk of curve progression can be analyzed by examining the growth potential of the congenital anomaly. Many congenital curves become stable and do not progress. The highest risk of progression occurs when asymmetrical growth occurs, in which the convexity outgrows the concavity. This discrepancy usually occurs when the anatomy of the convex side is relatively normal and the concave side is deficient. A shortened trunk may be the main deformity if both convex and concave growth deficiencies occur over multiple levels.[115]

INTERVENTIONS FOR IDIOPATHIC AND CONGENITAL SCOLIOSIS

Treatment decisions are based on the skeletal maturity of the child, as measured by the Risser sign, the growth potential of the child, and the curve magnitude. In addition to surgical intervention, nonsurgical interventions that include exercise and orthotic treatment may be provided.

Nonsurgical Interventions

Idiopathic curves of less than 25°, curves of nonsurgical magnitude of any type in a skeletally mature patient, and nonprogressive congenital curves are evaluated by clinical examination every 4 to 6 months. Radiographs are obtained at each visit; however, unchanged results of a scoliometer examination may reduce the frequency of radiographs to every other visit, depending on individual physician and institution practice.

Exercise

Research is evaluating the potential for exercise to play a role in improvement of postural awareness and subsequent alignment. Negrini et al.[73] performed a literature review to determine whether exercise decreases the progression rate of AIS. The authors found that this review strengthened the theory that exercise may reduce the progression of AIS. The authors report that this evidence is level 1b in accordance with the Oxford Centre for Evidence-Based Medicine.

Generally speaking, a home exercise program designed to maintain or improve trunk and pelvic strength and flexibility is often prescribed for children with idiopathic or congenital scoliosis. Exercises include spinal stabilization, balance activities, core strengthening, and postural correction, including lateral shifts, flexibility exercises, and respiratory activities. Negrini et al.[74] investigated the Scientific Exercises Approach to Scoliosis (SEAS) protocol. In this approach, the patient actively corrects his own posture with a goal of maximal curve correction, and follows a specific exercise program designed to increase spinal stability, improve balance reactions, and retain physiologic sagittal spinal curvatures. Although research has supported the effectiveness of SEAS exercises in patients with AIS in decreasing the rate of brace prescription, further follow-up will be required because of stated study limitations.

The Schroth method, introduced in the 1930s, also utilizes a personalized exercise protocol tailored to each patient to achieve maximal postural correction. The Schroth method strives to decrease curve progression, reduce pain, increase vital capacity, and improve posture and appearance.[52] A 2003 study from Germany suggested that an intensive inpatient rehabilitative exercise program (at the Katharina Schroth Klinik) for 6 hours/day for a minimum of 4 to 6 weeks, including both group and individual therapy, has the potential to reduce the incidence of curve progression in children with idiopathic scoliosis. This study acknowledges the need for longer-term follow-up of participants, so the long-term effectiveness of the physical therapy program on the natural history of idiopathic scoliosis can be evaluated.[112]

These studies and others are preliminary works that require further investigation and long-term results. However, these trials do demonstrate that physical therapy may have the potential to effect positive change in individuals with idiopathic scoliosis.

Orthotic Management

The goal of orthotic management is to alter the natural history of curve progression in AIS. Correction of a frontal plane curvature involves application of force in directions opposite to the natural tendency of the curve. Forces are applied at the apex of the curvature, and opposing forces are applied both above and below it.[33]

The indication for orthotic use depends on curve type, magnitude, and location. Orthoses are typically prescribed for children with idiopathic scoliosis who are skeletally immature (with a Risser sign of 0, 1, or 2) and have a curve from 25° to 45°.[30,45,83] A curve with a greater magnitude at the time of detection has an increased risk of progression. Similarly, the effect of an orthosis on prevention of curve progression decreases as the magnitude of the curve increases.[46]

The Milwaukee brace or cervical-thoracic-lumbar-sacral orthosis (CTLSO) was the only spinal orthosis available until the 1970s, when the Boston bracing system was developed.[47,83] The Milwaukee brace is rarely used today in the United States, as the introduction of the thoracolumbosacral orthosis (TLSO) offers a low-profile option for the treatment of curves with an apex as high as T7.[40]

The Boston system (Figure 8-6) was designed to decrease costs, improve the acceptability of orthotic wear, and simplify construction.[21] An orthotist molds a prefabricated brace to the patient and customizes the orthosis by adding lumbar pads and relief areas to meet the individual's specific needs. The rigid shell provides a firm support, and the foam lining allows for comfort. A Boston brace is an example of a TLSO and best treats a thoracic curve with an apex of T7 or below.[110] A Boston brace may be modified by the addition of an extension on the concave side with lateral pressure from a convex pad to achieve improved control of curves with an apex at T7 to T9.[47,110]

Other TLSO types include the Wilmington and Charleston models. A Wilmington TLSO (Figure 8-7) is a total-contact, custom-molded orthosis that achieves maximal spinal correction by the tight contact and fit, not by pads and relief areas.[47] A Charleston orthosis is used for idiopathic curves and is worn only at night because it is fabricated in the position of maximum side-bend correction.[78] A long-term follow-up by Price and colleagues[79] found that 65 of 98 patients showed improvement or less than a 5° change in curvature, and only 17 patients progressed to the point of requiring surgery.

Using one type of TLSO over another has its benefits. Katz et al.[46] found that the Boston brace was more effective than the Charleston in preventing curve progression, specifically for patients with curves of 36° to 45°. The Charleston brace is most effective in the treatment of smaller, single thoraco-lumbar or lumbar curves.[46] Multiple articles suggest that restricting wear of the TLSO to nighttime, as with the Charleston brace, increases patient adherence and may be associated with decreased psychosocial stressors related to bracing.[22,29,43]

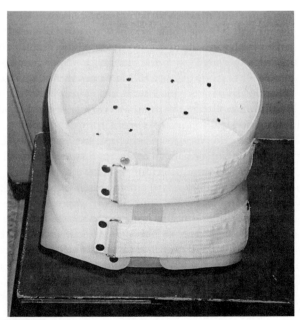

Figure 8-6   The Boston brace, underarm TLSO. Note pads for relief and pressure areas.

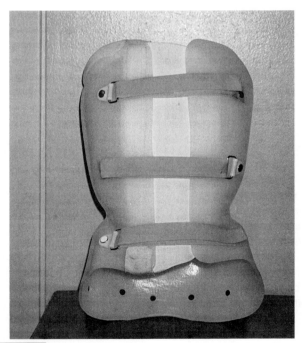

Figure 8-7   The Wilmington brace is a custom-molded, total-contact TLSO.

The active theory of orthotics is that curve progression is prevented by muscle contractions responding to the brace wear. A study by Wynarsky and Schultz,[118] however, showed no statistical difference between myoelectric activity during braced and unbraced states when female patients were treated with the Boston brace for idiopathic scoliosis. The passive theory is that curve progression is prevented by external forces of the brace on the spine.

Exercises to be performed while wearing the brace, such as pelvic tilts, thoracic flexion, and lateral shifts, are often taught to patients to improve the active forces. Carman et al.[11] showed no statistical difference in curve stability between those patients who complied with orthotic wear and exercises and those who complied only with orthotic wear. A physical therapist's main role is to encourage physical activity of the patient (e.g., physical education class, aerobics, dance) while wearing the orthosis to maintain balance, coordination, and strength and to develop good habits of achieving and maintaining cardiorespiratory fitness while promoting postural alignment. Specific trunk exercises, such as those for unbraced scoliosis, may be taught to the patient; these may be performed while out of the brace and are designed to maintain trunk strength and flexibility. Preliminary data from Margonato et al.[60] suggest that bracing appears to limit maximal exercise performance. These authors recommend moderate physical exercise during brace wear to offset the limitations of the cardiovascular, respiratory, and musculoskeletal systems associated with the brace encompassing the rib cage. This study, however, was limited by small sample size, thereby warranting further research.

Contrary to the traditional rigid braces previously discussed, the SpineCor brace, developed in the early 1990's, is dynamic and allows freedom of movement. It does not utilize the traditional three-point pressure technique for correction, as is seen in rigid bracing,[13] but rather it applies corrective forces by using a system of bands.[99] Recent research has evaluated the efficacy of the SpineCor dynamic brace and has found it to be effective in the treatment of AIS.[13,14,99] Szwed et al.[99] noted that further evaluation of long-term outcomes is necessary. Additional research is warranted to compare the efficacy of a dynamic versus a rigid bracing system.

Orthotic treatment continues until the curve is no longer controlled (usually at 40° to 45° or higher) or skeletal maturity occurs, at which time weaning may begin. Twenty to twenty-six percent of orthotically treated curves will progress enough to require spinal fusion.[45,77] High-risk factors include younger age at curve detection, higher magnitude, and low Risser sign, just as for untreated idiopathic scoliosis, although orthotic wear can positively influence the natural history of idiopathic scoliosis.[1,45,47]

The weaning process takes about 12 months from the time of skeletal maturity and consists of gradually decreasing the amount of time wearing the brace. An orthotic treatment is considered successful if the curve magnitude at the end of treatment is within 5° of the magnitude at the start of treatment.

Surgical Interventions

The major indication for spinal fusion is a documented progressive idiopathic curve with a Cobb angle that reaches 45° or greater in an immature spine. Curves greater than 40° are increasingly difficult to manage orthotically and have significant risk of progression after skeletal maturity.[50] The main objective of any scoliosis surgery is to obtain a solid arthrodesis because the fusion mass is ultimately what prevents further progression of the deformity.[18,50] The ideal correction system should provide correction in all three planes of the scoliosis, provide rigid fixation, and attain maximal correction with minimal fusion levels.[51]

A posterior surgical procedure, posterior spinal fusion (PSF) with instrumentation, is currently considered to be the gold standard used for spinal fusion.[81,117] Bone graft is packed around the lamina and facet joints of the vertebrae and instrumentation after surgical exposure and preparation (John Sarwark, MD, personal communication, October 5, 2009). The differences among posterior spinal fusion techniques lie with the instrumentation used to obtain correction and protect the fusion.

Spinal instrumentation has evolved since Harrington designed the first generation of posterior instrumentation for scoliosis. Harrington rods correct frontal plane deformities but do not allow for sagittal plane correction and do not address the rotatory components of scoliosis. Further, the placement of Harrington rods calls for postoperative bracing.[84]

The Cotrel-Dubousset (CD) posterior spinal instrumentation (Figure 8-8) was introduced in the early 1980s and strove for a three-dimensional correction of the spinal deformity while avoiding the need for postoperative bracing. A minimum of two parallel rods are used—one on either side of the spine and attached to the spine with hooks or screws. Selective compression or distraction forces may be applied on the rod at any level to correct the deformity.[19] Recent articles have questioned the rotational correction of scoliosis using conventional CD instrumentation.[51,71,98]

In 1999 a new model called direct vertebral rotation (DVR) was introduced. In a prospective study, Lee et al.[51] found improved curve correction as well as correction of apical vertebral rotation when patients with AIS underwent DVR as compared with simple rod derotation. The concept of DVR is to apply both a coronal and a rotational correction. Pedicle screw fixation allows a correcting force to be directed opposite the deformity. The addition of DVR provides the rotational plane correction of the deformity in idiopathic scoliosis.[51]

It is important to treat children with congenital scoliosis while they are still growing. These patients require surgical intervention because of rapid growth early in life, rapid curve progression, and/or large curve magnitude. Multiple

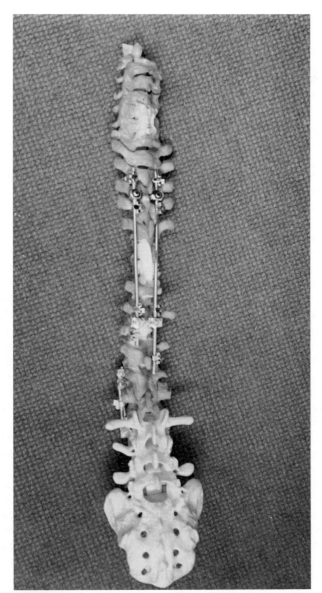

Figure 8-8   Cotrel-Dubousset instrumentation system implanted on a plastic spine.

factors are considered when determining if surgery to correct a congenital scoliosis is indicated. These factors include: attainment of spinal length, mobility, function of the thorax, performing the fewest surgeries possible, and risk of surgery. Expandable growing spinal rod technique surgery (GR) is indicated for children without bony anomaly of the vertebrae or rib cage and with curve flexibility. The mechanism of distraction yields increased growth of the spine and vertebral column. Serial lengthenings must be performed approximately every 6 months during the growing years. Another surgery performed for patients with congenital scoliosis with fused ribs or thoracic insufficiency syndrome is insertion of vertical expandable prosthetic titanium ribs

(VEPTR) with an expansion thoracotomy. In this procedure, one or more rib-to-rib or rib-to-spine configurations may be placed.[120] Campbell and Hell-Vocke[8] concluded that growth of the spine approached normal rates after the insertion of VEPTR, including those with bony bars. They believe that the distraction applied by the prosthesis unloads the concave side of the scoliosis, thereby facilitating growth by the Hueter-Volkmann principle. Smith et al.[95] found improvement in lung volume and density, suggesting consequential improved pulmonary function. This is of importance because the lungs are rapidly developing during childhood. A tenfold increase in the number of alveoli occurs by adulthood, but most form within the first 8 years of life.[40] Complications of VEPTR surgery may include brachial plexus injury and multiple outpatient subsequent lengthenings as the child grows.[120]

Postoperative Management

The postoperative use of an orthosis depends on the type of curve that was fused, the type of instrumentation used, and the postoperative alignment of the trunk. Postoperatively, an orthosis is worn until the fusion is solid as determined by radiograph, typically for 9 to 12 months.

The average length of a hospital stay for a posterior spinal fusion (or a one-stage procedure) is 5 to 7 days, with physical therapy initiated on the second postoperative day. A physical therapist's role after any spinal fusion procedure includes patient instruction in body mechanics for bed mobility, transfers, dressing, and ambulation. Trunk rotation is contraindicated; therefore the therapist must instruct the patient in log-rolling and in transitioning from a supine position to sitting without rotation. Shoes and socks are donned or removed with the legs in a "figure 4" seated position with negligible forward flexion (patient positioned sitting with the ankle of one leg supported on the distal thigh of the other leg, such that neither lower extremity exceeds hip flexion greater than 90°). If applicable, the therapist may also instruct the patient in donning or removing the orthosis while in bed, while from a sidelying to a supine position, or while standing with assistance (if not contraindicated by physician's orders). For the acute stage, donning or removing of the orthosis in bed is preferable. The patient is instructed in general range of motion and strengthening exercises (without resistance) for the extremities such as ankle pumps to promote circulation, isometric quadriceps contractions, supine hip abduction, heel slides, and isometric gluteal sets. Because the patient's functional activities for the first 2 postoperative weeks are limited to showering and walking, the therapist's role is to encourage ambulation. Not only does this enable the patient to experience fewer side effects from bed rest, it is also beneficial for the development of a strong, healthy fusion mass or arthrodesis.

Upon discharge from the hospital, the patient's postoperative activity remains restricted. In the early weeks and months after surgery, the activity guidelines are relatively similar for most patients with fusion of congenital and idiopathic curves, regardless of which instrumentation is used. At 6 weeks after surgery, the patient usually returns to school and can lift objects up to 5 pounds. At 3 months postoperatively, activity restrictions begin to differ according to the chosen method of surgical correction.[90] Pedicle screw and rod systems with DVR are more stable as compared with hook or hook-hybrid rod systems. For this reason, patients with pedicle screw and rod systems with DVR may return to noncontact sports in 4 to 6 months, as compared with 6 to 12 months for patients with hook or hook-hybrid systems (J. Sarwark, MD, personal communication, October 5, 2009).

OUTCOMES FOR PERSONS WITH IDIOPATHIC SCOLIOSIS

Most people with AIS live functional and normal lives and have a mortality rate similar to that of the general population.[109,111] However, Weinstein et al.[109] found that patients with untreated scoliosis not only reported an increased incidence of both chronic and acute back pain, but were found to have decreased body image as compared with people of similar age and gender without scoliosis. A Cobb angle greater than 50° at skeletal maturity was identified by Weinstein et al. (2003) as a strong predictor of decreased pulmonary function. A curvature with a thoracic apex is also associated with shortness of breath.[109] Severe thoracic curves, greater than 100°, have been shown to decrease pulmonary vital capacity to below 70% to 80% of the normal value.[111]

Merola et al.[64] studied patients status post surgical correction of AIS and found statistically significant improvements in general self-image, function from back condition, and level of activity domains as compared with preoperative status, but no significant correlation between magnitude of curve correction and outcome scores. Merola[64] suggests that successful outcomes may be correlated with patient perception, such as elimination of the rib hump or restoration of the waistline, rather than focusing on magnitude of curve correction alone.

The natural history of idiopathic scoliosis continues into adult life because curves can progress after skeletal maturity. Risk of progression depends on curve magnitude and location.[57] Curves of greater than 45° at the time of skeletal maturity have a higher risk of progressing and producing complications. Although both thoracic and lumbar curves can progress, progression in the thoracic region may cause more significant complications because of its effects on the cardiopulmonary system. Complications of untreated scoliosis include severe cosmetic deformity and major disability, which may include pain, respiratory insufficiency, or right-sided heart failure.[35] Indications for adult treatment include back pain, compromised pulmonary function, psychosocial effects, and an increased risk for premature death. The treatment plan is consistent with that for adolescent idiopathic scoliosis.[108]

NEUROMUSCULAR SCOLIOSIS

In comparison with idiopathic scoliosis, neuromuscular scoliosis has an onset at an earlier age, is associated with systemic or chronic diseases, and often has a rapid progression.[70] The direct cause of neuromuscular scoliosis is not understood; however, Berven and Bradford[2] identified asymmetrical paraplegia, mechanical forces, intraspinal and congenital anomalies, sensory feedback, and control of spinal balance by central pathways as possible contributors in children. Disruption in any one of these areas may lead to spinal deformity. The Scoliosis Research Society (SRS) divides neuromuscular scoliosis into two categories: neuropathic (i.e., cerebral palsy [upper motor neuron] or spinal muscular dystrophy [lower motor neuron]) and myopathic (i.e., Duchenne muscular dystrophy).[110] Neuromuscular curves tend to progress more rapidly than idiopathic curves and to have more disabling outcomes, such as decreased ability to sit, diminished hand function, or respiratory compromise due to intercostal muscle weakness.[110] Important health issues are associated with neuromuscular conditions that may be influenced by scoliosis. For example, energy consumption during activities of daily living such as transferring or ambulating is significantly higher in this population. Sitting balance may also become disrupted, and this may lead to the need for the child to use the upper extremities for support, decreasing his ability to perform bimanual tasks. Back pain related to compromised mechanics of the spine may also occur.[2] Variation in the curve pattern is seen among people with neuromuscular scoliosis, although the long C curve (Figure 8-9) is common, beginning in the thoracic region and extending into the sacrum.[110] Terjesen, Lange, and Steen[103] found that the severity of the curve correlated with pelvic obliquity. The highest prevalence of spinal deformities (90%–100%) occurs with a dystrophy diagnosis, such as spinal muscular atrophy or muscular dystrophy, and with spinal cord injuries that result in quadriplegia in infants or young children. A 60% prevalence of spinal deformity is seen in patients with myelomeningocele, as well as a 25% prevalence in patients with cerebral palsy.[56,110]

Interventions

Nonsurgical intervention for neuromuscular spinal curvatures includes clinical observation, radiographic examination, and orthotic management.[110] Clinical observation allows a thorough assessment of the child's present and potential function, level of comprehension, and ability to cooperate.[23] Research studies have not demonstrated that custom seating is effective in reducing or preventing progression of curves; however, it is an important part of the clinical intervention plan, in which the physical therapist plays a vital role. An appropriately designed and maintained postural support system allows the child to interact with peers and the environment. These children often have multiple disabilities, which are best addressed by the team approach,

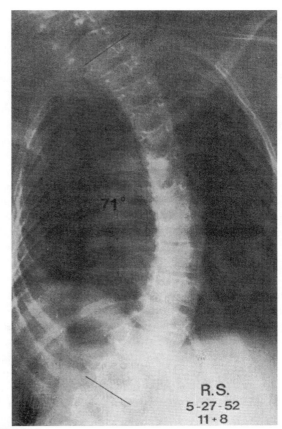

Figure 8-9 Severe neuromuscular scoliosis. (From Moe, J. H., Winter, R. B., Bradford, D. S., Ogilvie, J. W., & Lonstein, J. E. [1987]. *Scoliosis and other spinal deformities* [2nd ed.; p. 277]. Philadelphia: WB Saunders.)

including a physical therapist, an occupational therapist, a physician, an equipment vendor, and an orthotist. Please refer to the EVOLVE chapter, Assistive Technology, in this book regarding appropriate seating options for this population.

The child with a neuromuscular curvature managed by orthotics has special needs that must be considered when seating systems are ordered or fabricated. The orthosis eliminates the normal flexibility of the spine, which potentially reduces the child's ability to adjust the footrests, operate the brakes, and propel the chair. A child with a neuromuscular curve may demonstrate pelvic obliquity requiring specialized custom-molded seating to provide adequate support and pressure relief. Because these children may also require lower extremity orthotics, adequate clearance in the seating device is necessary to accommodate orthoses.

The goal of orthotic management in children with neuromuscular scoliosis differs from that with idiopathic scoliosis. With idiopathic scoliosis, the intention is to stabilize the curve and avoid the need for surgery; in neuromuscular scoliosis, the goal is to postpone surgery during growing years.[110] Studies have demonstrated that the use of a spinal

orthotic on a neuromuscular scoliosis does not have an impact on curve progression.[65] Terjesen, Lange, and Steen[103] found that despite this, many families and caregivers have remained pleased with the outcome following TLSO use for 2 years; improvements in sitting stability and overall function have been reported. Orthotic management might include the custom-molded, total-contact TLSO, the under-arm TLSO, or the Milwaukee brace.[56] Such orthoses are typically worn during all upright (i.e., sitting or standing) activities but usually are not worn at night.

The use of an orthosis must provide curve stabilization without limiting the child's functional abilities. For example, attempting to control the lordosis in an ambulating child with muscular dystrophy would eliminate compensatory functional posture and may result in earlier use of a wheelchair. An orthosis may be used to support the trunk before any measurable deformity is present. The use of a TLSO can improve head and upper extremity control. An orthosis should also be used to maintain alignment and provide trunk support for children with quadriplegic paralysis secondary to birth injuries or acquired spinal cord injuries. In these children, the use of an orthosis allows for upright orientation and may provide the support necessary for the child to operate a head switch or sip-and-puff mechanism to control an electric wheelchair.

Researchers have studied other methods to manage neuromuscular scoliosis. King et al.[49] evaluated the effects of daily corticosteroid use on orthopedic outcomes in 143 boys with Duchenne's muscular dystrophy. They found that those treated with steroids not only demonstrated a decreased prevalence of scoliosis, they also had decreased magnitude of curvatures as compared with the untreated group. However, 32% of the treated group suffered vertebral compression fractures, a serious adverse effect of corticosteroid therapy. Other researchers have studied the effects of intrathecal baclofen (ITB) on curve progression[93,94] and concluded that ITB does not have a significant effect on curve progression. Curve progression was found to increase compared with the expected natural history after insertion of ITB pumps in nonambulatory children with quadriplegic cerebral palsy and neuromuscular scoliosis.[25] Limited published research is available on the use of botulinum type A in the treatment of children with neuromuscular scoliosis. This may present an opportunity for research in the future.

If a neuromuscular scoliosis continues to progress, hygiene, functional abilities, pulmonary function, and life expectancy may be affected. Once again, a team approach is preferred for optimal management of children with neuromuscular disease.

Surgical Options

Surgical intervention for neuromuscular scoliosis is different from that for idiopathic scoliosis in several ways. Fusion to the sacrum is common because of pelvic obliquity or lack of sitting balance, blood loss is greater because of osteopenia, and the muscles are in poor condition; therefore time in surgery is longer. Also, the curve may require both anterior and posterior fusions with instrumentation. In the presence of a "long and stiff curve," anterior release is necessary to balance the spine over the pelvis. A posterior fusion with instrumentation may also be performed. The goal of surgery is to achieve a stable and compensated spine.[110]

An anterior surgical approach includes opening of the thoracic cavity, resection of a rib, and incision through the diaphragm to expose the necessary vertebrae. To obtain correction and protect the spinal fusion, Zielke or Dwyer screws are used on the vertebral bodies. Zielke screws are newer, provide control at each segment with a rod and screw, and prevent postinstrumentation kyphosis.[39] An anterior approach may be used to fuse a thoracolumbar or lumbar idiopathic scoliosis.

A two-stage procedure is used for higher-magnitude curves or severe kyphoscoliotic curves. An anterior approach is used for the release of anterior spinal ligaments, a discectomy, or a fusion with or without instrumentation. The procedure is completed by a posterior spinal fusion with instrumentation.[50]

An orthosis is almost always used postoperatively for support and immobilization of the fusion. The orthosis must be on the patient before out-of-bed mobility is initiated, unless otherwise specified by the physician. Orthotic use is most often discontinued when an x-ray reveals adequate arthrodesis.

The role of the physical therapist is similar to that for postoperative treatment of other curve types. The intervention may have to be modified to adjust to a patient's motor and cognitive abilities.

KYPHOSIS

A kyphosis is an abnormal posterior convexity of a segment of the spine; normal thoracic kyphosis measures 20° to 40°.[3] A spinal kyphosis may occur as the result of trauma, congenital conditions, or Scheuermann's disease, or it may be secondary to previous treatment of spinal tumors with laminectomy. Spinal kyphosis may also be found in children with osteochondrodystrophies, rickets, osteogenesis imperfecta, idiopathic juvenile osteoporosis, neurofibromatosis, myelomeningocele, and spondyloepiphyseal dysplasia. Spinal kyphosis should be differentiated from postural roundback.[35,116] The discussion in this section focuses on congenital kyphosis and Scheuermann's disease.

CONGENITAL KYPHOSIS

Congenital kyphosis occurs when the anterior part of the vertebra is aplastic or hypoplastic and the posterior elements of the vertebra form normally. An anterior unsegmented failure of formation, or unsegmented bar, leads to progressive kyphosis. Congenital kyphoscoliosis or lordoscoliosis is

the result when a combination of defective segmentation occurs at more than one location.[114,115]

The natural history of congenital kyphosis includes progression, cosmetic deformity, back pain, and neurologic deficit. Congenital kyphosis is the most common cause of spinal cord compression caused by a spinal deformity.[116] It is a potentially more debilitating deformity than congenital scoliosis without kyphosis. An anterior unsegmented bar at the thoracolumbar junction produces mild to moderate deformities but no reported paraplegia. Paraplegia is frequently noted with a progressive congenital kyphosis located in the upper thoracic spine when the posterior elements grow unaccompanied by anterior growth. The treatment of congenital kyphosis consists of surgery to prevent further progression.[114]

SCHEUERMANN'S DISEASE

Scheuermann's disease is a rigid form of postural kyphosis. It often is neglected, develops during childhood and adolescence, and usually is ascribed to poor posture.[110] Scheuermann's kyphosis is the most common type of kyphosis in the adolescent population, with a rate of incidence ranging from 1% to 8% in the literature, and with nearly equal incidence in males and females. Onset typically occurs just before puberty.[58] Diagnosis is made by these radiographic criteria: (1) Irregular vertebral end plates, (2) narrowing of the intervertebral disc space, (3) anterior wedging of 5° or greater for three or more contiguous vertebrae,[54,58] and (4) kyphosis greater than 40° that is uncorrected on active hyperextension. Schmorl's nodules are disc protrusions into the spongiosa seen on radiograph on either side of the disc; they may be the cause of end plate irregularity.[100] Scheuermann's disease can be found in the thoracic spine, producing an increased kyphosis; in the thoracolumbar and lumbar spine, producing a neutral appearance in the sagittal plane; and, more rarely, in the cervical spine.[35]

Further research on the origin of Scheuermann's kyphosis is needed. Studies demonstrate a strong genetic prevalence with a less significant environmental component.[58] Histologic studies have shown disorganized endochondral ossification, reduced amounts of collagen with thinner fibers, and increases in end plate mucopolysaccharides. Disc degeneration is present on magnetic resonance imaging (MRI) in half of patients with Scheuermann's kyphosis. One theory based on examination of the mechanical factors suggests that some kyphosis is likely present initially, which leads to vertebral wedging caused by anterior pressure exerted upon the vertebrae[110]—a reflection of the Hueter-Volkmann principle.

Clinical findings include tight pectoral and hamstring muscles,[100,110] increased thoracic kyphosis with a compensatory increased lumbar lordosis, and forward head posture. Further, 38% of patients with Scheuermann's kyphosis had pain and worked in lighter-duty jobs than controls.[58]

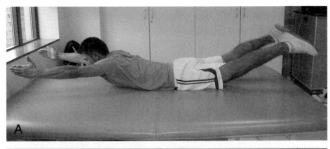

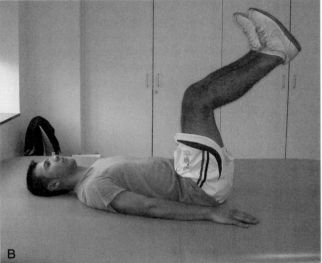

Figure 8-10 **A,** Active trunk extensor strengthening by prone lifts. **B,** Lower abdominal strengthening exercises.

Associated scoliosis is present in approximately 20% of children with Scheuermann's disease.[38]

Intervention

Treatment of patients with Scheuermann's disease includes exercise, orthotic management, and surgical management. The prescribed exercises are specific for active trunk extensor strengthening, general postural exercise, and hamstring stretches (Figure 8-10). Sports that have a trunk extensor component such as volleyball or swimming and aerobic exercise are recommended. The goals of physical therapy are to improve postural alignment and to increase flexibility and extensor strength.[110] Exercise as the sole treatment has not been established as effective, although it has been shown to be beneficial in conjunction with other methods of treatment in the early stages of Scheuermann's kyphosis.[39,69,110]

Orthotic treatment is used when the kyphosis is greater than 45° to 65°. A modified Milwaukee-type brace is used. The reported success rate is high in the skeletally immature patient; however, skeletally mature patients do not respond to this treatment.[38] The Milwaukee brace is worn full-time (22 hours per day) for 12 to 18 months. Once patients have reached skeletal maturity, it may be used part-time at night for maintenance. The brace works as a three-point dynamic system and promotes thoracic extension. Posterior pads apply pressure at the apex of the kyphosis, and pelvic pads stabilize the lumbar spine, decreasing the lordosis.[110] The procedure is considered to be successful when the kyphosis decreases and vertebral bodies appear less wedge-shaped on radiographs.[69] It has been observed that the anterior longitudinal ligament may thicken and partial reversal of vertebral wedging may occur with use of a brace.[110]

According to the Scoliosis Research Society, surgery is indicated when the curve continues to progress despite use of an orthotic during adolescence, when curves are greater than 65°, and when painful degenerative kyphoses are present. Surgical management of a less rigid curve often includes a posterior spinal fusion, although more rigid curves require an anterior in combination with a posterior fusion.[38]

Postural Roundback

Postural roundback may often be confused with Scheuermann's disease; however, the kyphosis of postural roundback is not fixed, and vertebrae show no end plate irregularity. Exercise alone, as described for the treatment of Scheuermann's disease, is the treatment of choice for this condition. If the kyphosis progresses to more than 60°, the patient may be treated with a Milwaukee brace to prevent permanent structural changes.[69]

LORDOSIS

An anterior convexity (or a posterior concavity) of a segment of spine is termed a *lordosis*. Congenital lordosis is the result of bilateral posterior failure of segmentation.[114] Lordosis, both fixed and flexible, may be found in children with a variety of diagnoses. Lordosis in children with myelomeningocele usually occurs in the lumbar spine secondary to use of a tripod gait pattern. A lordosis may develop in the thoracic vertebrae to compensate for an increased lumbar kyphosis.[35] Hahn et al.[32] stated that a lumbar lordosis facilitates balanced sitting in the DMD population. In Duchenne muscular dystrophy (DMD), the postural control muscles are weakened; therefore support for the vertebral column and upright control are affected. Hip flexion contractures, which are often present in the DMD population, mechanically pull the pelvis anteriorly, thereby leading to an increased lumbar lordosis. Kerr et al.[48] found that lordosis improved stability of the lumbar spine through locking of the articular facet joints.

Children without motor deficits may have an increased lumbar lordosis. Assessment includes testing of lower extremity ROM, spinal flexibility, trunk and lower extremity strength, posture, and gait. Interventions include abdominal strengthening (curls, crunches, and pelvic lifts), pelvic tilts in supine and standing positions, trunk extensor strengthening, and appropriate lower extremity stretching.

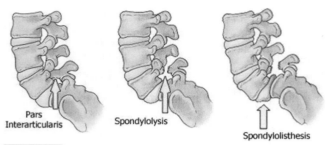

Figure 8-11 *Left,* The pars interarticularis is the bony segment between the inferior and superior articular facets in the lumbar spine. (Pugh, 2000.) *Center,* Illustration of a spondylolysis, depicting a fracture of the pars interarticularis. *Right,* Depiction of spondylolisthesis, anterior slippage of one vertebra on another. http://orthoinfo.aaos.org/topic.cfm?topic=a00053

SPONDYLOLYSIS AND SPONDYLOLISTHESIS

Spondylolysis is a defect of the pars interarticularis (Figure 8-11). Herman, Pizzutillo, and Cavalier[37] suggest that upright, bipedal position, genetic predisposition, and repetitive loading of the lumbar spine are possible causative factors. Athletes involved in sports with repetitive hyperextension and rotational loading on the lumbar spine, such as gymnastics and diving, are noted to have a higher incidence of spondylolyis and spondylolisthesis than the general population.[9,36] Spondylolisthesis is the forward translatory displacement of one vertebra on another, usually occurring at the fifth lumbar vertebra (see Figure 8-11). Multiple classification systems have been proposed for spondylolysis and spondylolisthesis; however, the Wiltse-Newman method remains the most widely utilized.[9] Five types of spondylolysis and spondylolisthesis have been classified by Wiltse and associates[113] as follows:

1. Dysplastic malformations develop secondary to congenital malformations of the sacrum and posterior vertebral arch of L5. These malformations may include hypoplasia of the superior surface of the body of S1, hypoplasia-aplasia of the facets, elongation of the pars interarticularis, and spina bifida. The malformations decrease the efficiency of the posterior stabilizing system.[113] The degree of slippage is usually severe and may produce neurologic deficits as the laminae of L5 are pulled against the dural sac.[39]

2. Isthmic describes slippage occurring secondary to an elongation of the pars interarticularis, a break in the pars interarticularis, or a combination of both, with the facets intact. A stress or fatigue fracture of the pars interarticularis is the basic pathologic occurrence. These pathogenic factors can cause elongation of the pars secondary to repeated microfractures that heal with the pars in an attenuated-elongated position. An isthmic spondylolisthesis may also be caused by an acute fracture of the pars.[39]

3. A degenerative type occurs in adults older than age 50 years and is caused by the structural destruction of the capsule and ligaments of the posterior joints producing hypermobility of the segment.

4. A traumatic type, more correctly defined as a fracture, is caused by a sudden fracture of the posterior arch of a vertebral segment. The fracture may occur at the pedicle, laminae, or facet, leaving the pars interarticularis intact.

5. Pathologic spondylolisthesis occurs most often secondary to an infectious disease that destroys the posterior arch of the vertebra.[113]

Dysplastic and isthmic spondylolisthesis types are the most common in the pediatric population. Spondylolisthesis is further described by degree of severity as characterized by percentage of slippage—grades I to IV. Grade I is the mildest slippage at less than 25%. Grade II is 25% to 50% slippage. Grade III is slippage of 50% to 75%, and grade IV is greater than 75% slippage.[39,113]

CLINICAL SYMPTOMS

A spondylolisthesis is often discovered on a radiograph taken for some other purpose. The clinical picture includes poor posture and increased lumbar lordosis in mild slippage. Higher-grade slippage may produce a flattened lumbar spine, a vertically oriented sacrum, and a visible or palpable step-off at the involved level[36,37] (Figure 8-12). Symptoms may include low back pain relieved by rest, sciatic-type pain, local tenderness, hamstring spasm or tightness, and, in severe cases, torso shortening.[39]

RISK OF PROGRESSION

The risk of progression of spondylolysis and low-grade spondylolisthesis is low, occurring in less than 3% of skeletally immature children or adolescents.[36] Clinically, adolescents who are symptomatic are at a higher risk for increased slippage during their growth spurt. Females are at greater risk than males, as are patients with increased ligament laxity, including those with Down syndrome or Marfan syndrome. Radiographically, dysplastic types or patients with a 50% slippage, with a slip angle greater than 55° in a skeletally immature patient (normal: −10° to 0° as identified by Mac-Thiong and Labelle[59]), or with bony instabilities or decreased anatomic stability of L5 and S1 are at greater risk for increased slippage.[39,69]

NONSURGICAL INTERVENTION

Observation is the treatment of choice with asymptomatic low-grade spondylolisthesis (less than 50% slippage). These children are routinely followed two times per year with clinical and radiographic examinations. Patients presenting with symptomatic spondylolysis or low-grade spondylolisthesis often respond well to activity restriction, physical therapy,

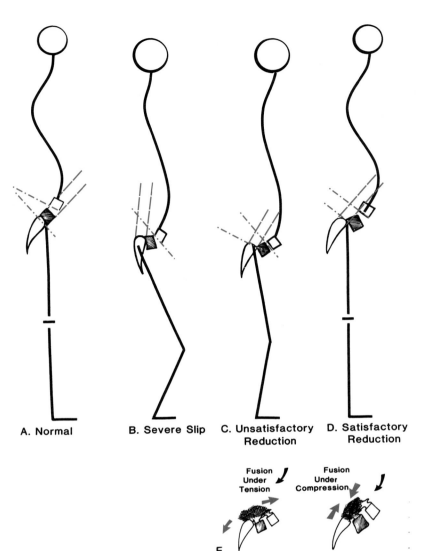

A. Normal   B. Severe Slip   C. Unsatisfactory Reduction   D. Satisfactory Reduction

Fusion Under Tension   Fusion Under Compression

E

Figure 8-12 **A,** Normal sagittal plane spinal alignment. **B,** Loss of alignment can be visualized after a severe L5 spondylolisthesis. The sacrum becomes vertical, and the resultant lumbosacral kyphosis "pushes" the lumbar spine forward. **C,** An unsatisfactory reduction occurs when L5 has little mobility and L4 lies anterior to the "anatomic zone" and is kyphotic in relationship to the sacrum. The fusion in this case will be under tension and less likely to hold. **D,** A satisfactory reduction occurs when L4 can be placed in the anatomic zone and oriented lordotic in relation to the sacrum. **E,** The more L4 can be positioned over the sacrum, the more posterior compressive forces will be directed across the fusion. In this position, sagittal plane alignment and hence deformity will be corrected. (From Moe, J. H., Winter, R. B., Bradford, D. S., Ogilvie, J. W., & Lonstein, J. E. [1987]. *Scoliosis and other spinal deformities* [2nd ed.; p. 418]. Philadelphia: WB Saunders.)

and spinal bracing.[36] Upon referral to physical therapy, patients learn lumbar stabilization exercises, in which they are taught to maintain pain-free, neutral alignment of the pelvis and lumbar spine while they vary their positions.[76] O'Sullivan et al.[76] emphasized the importance of strength training of the transverse abdominis, lumbar multifidus, and internal oblique muscles. They recommended incorporating co-contraction of these stabilizers into functional activities to support the lumbar spine and decrease low back pain in patients with spondylolysis and spondylolisthesis. Exercises may include bridging, wall squats, abdominal strengthening, prone gluteal strengthening, and other stabilization exercises in supine. A therapeutic exercise ball may be incorporated into the exercise session to allow patients to achieve and maintain neutral lumbar spine stabilization on a mobile surface.

Immobilization using a TLSO is indicated following a stress fracture of the pars or with a well-defined spondylytic defect, although the goals of treatment differ, namely, healing of the pars defect in the former and alleviation of symptoms in the latter. Brace wear ranges from 6 to 12 weeks, depending on the goal of treatment, and may continue for up to 6 months if radiographs reveal incomplete healing of the pars stress injury. Return-to-play guidelines for the young athlete include painless spinal mobility, resolved hamstring spasm and contracture, and return to activities without pain.[37] If symptoms persist, surgery is indicated.

SURGICAL INTERVENTION

Indications for surgery include persistent back pain despite conservative measures such as physical therapy, as well as gait deviations, greater than 50% slippage, marked instability of the defect with slip progression, neurologic deficit/radiculopathy, and hamstring contracture.[36,39] The goals of surgery are to prevent further slippage, immobilize the unstable segment, prevent further neurologic deficit, relieve any nerve root irritation, and correct clinical symptoms of poor posture, gait, and decreased hamstring length.[39]

Surgical options include posterolateral arthrodesis, anterior arthrodesis, decompression, and reduction and instrumentation. The surgical procedure most often performed is a bilateral posterolateral arthrodesis in situ. The fusion usually extends from L4 to S1 and is performed with an iliac bone graft.[31] Physical therapy is indicated for bed mobility, gait training, and activities of daily living and may be initiated to regain normal hamstring flexibility.

A neurologic deficit is the most common reason to perform a decompression. A decompression consists of removal of the bony anatomy that is causing nerve root irritation. The segments are then fused posteriorly to prevent further slippage.[105,106]

A reduction of the spondylolisthesis is indicated in cases in which the sacrum is in a vertical position, causing a severe lumbosacral kyphosis that displaces the lumbar spine anteriorly (see Figure 8-12). The result is a marked compensatory lumbar lordosis. An open reduction technique can be anterior or posterior, with or without instrumentation, or a combination of surgical approaches may be used. An anterior fibular strut graft may be used for severe slips.[41] Circumferential fusion may also be performed. This technique improves stability of the fusion and provides increased surface area for loading the joint surface.[59]

SUMMARY

Scoliosis, kyphosis, and lordosis are common pediatric orthopedic conditions of the spine. We, as pediatric physical therapists, often concentrate our therapy for many types of patients on the trunk for midline activities, symmetry, and stability for movement; therefore we can play a vital role in early detection of spinal deformities. We encourage children to become active to improve their cardiorespiratory function, muscle strength, and endurance. We can provide a referral source for families, instruction in home exercises, input for selecting appropriate adaptive equipment and seating, and rehabilitative intervention following injury or surgery. We address issues concerning the spine on a daily basis and play an important role in achieving and maintaining good health by maximizing proper alignment and function.

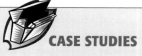

CASE STUDIES

"Noelle"

Noelle is a 15-year-old girl with a diagnosis of idiopathic scoliosis (curves measuring 48° right thoracic and 45° left lumbar), who has been followed by an orthopedic surgeon for 2 years. Noelle wears a Boston brace. The orthopedic surgeon recommended surgery, and Noelle underwent a posterior spinal fusion with direct vertebral rotation. Physical therapy was instituted on the second postoperative day, beginning with patient education regarding spinal fusion precautions and gentle bed exercises. The physical therapist gradually progressed Noelle's activities in accordance with spinal fusion precautions. Noelle was discharged home from the hospital after her parents demonstrated independence in assisting Noelle with functional mobility within her fusion precautions. Noelle was instructed to follow up with the orthopedic surgeon in 2 weeks, per protocol.

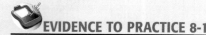

EVIDENCE TO PRACTICE 8-1

CASE STUDY "NOELLE"

EXAMINATION DECISION

The Boston brace is a TLSO and best treats a thoracic curve with an apex T7 or below.[110] The major indication for spinal fusion is a documented progressive idiopathic curve with a Cobb angle that reaches 45° or greater in an immature

EVIDENCE TO PRACTICE 8-1—cont'd

spine. Curves greater than 40° are increasingly difficult to manage orthotically and have significant risk of progression after skeletal maturity is reached.[50] A posterior surgical approach is currently considered to be the gold standard used for spinal fusion.[81,117] Direct vertebral rotation (DVR) offers correction of a tri-planar deformity in idiopathic scoliosis surgery. DVR has been found to improve curve correction and correction of apical vertebral rotation as compared with AIS in patients who underwent simple rod derotation.[51]

PLAN OF CARE DECISION

Patient education regarding spinal fusion precautions is a matter of high priority. Spinal fusion precautions are in place immediately postoperatively. Generally speaking, Noelle needs to avoid bending or twisting her back in the early postoperative phase. Activities are restricted until the physician notes evidence of bone healing. Recall that both Drummond (1991) and Kostuik (1990) found that the main objective of any scoliosis surgery is to obtain a solid

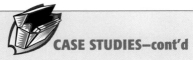

CASE STUDIES—cont'd

EVIDENCE TO PRACTICE 8-1—cont'd

arthrodesis, as the fusion mass is ultimately what prevents further progression of the deformity.[18,50]

PATIENT/FAMILY PREFERENCES

In this therapist's experience, it is important that Noelle's caregivers at home are trained on how to safely assist Noelle with her functional mobility within her fusion precautions. A physical therapist's role after spinal fusion includes patient instruction in body mechanics for bed mobility, transfers, dressing, ambulation, and stair climbing.

"Rick"

Rick is a 14-year-old boy who was recently seen in a scoliosis clinic and diagnosed with Scheuermann's kyphosis. He has a thoracic kyphosis measuring 53° with Schmorl's nodules present at thoracic levels seven through nine on radiograph, per report of the orthopedic physician. Rick will be fitted for a Milwaukee-type orthosis next week. He was also seen by a physical therapist in the clinic, who examined his posture, range of motion, and strength. Findings included forward head, rounded shoulders, protracted scapulae, overall rounded posture, and weight bearing through his sacrum in sitting; in standing, Rick demonstrated a posteriorly tilted pelvis. His pectoral and hamstring muscles were tight. He also exhibited decreased thoracic region paraspinal strength. Emphasis of treatment was on active and positional pectoral and hamstring stretches, trunk strengthening (abdominals, gluteals, and thoracic extensors), and postural training in sitting, standing, and during gait. Rick was also encouraged to swim 2 to 3 times per week. Over 4 weeks of physical therapy, Rick's hamstring length increased 10° bilaterally, and his paraspinal strength improved, as was seen by improved endurance to strengthening exercises and improved alignment. Rick's parents reported that he used a more erect posture throughout the day, and that they did not need to cue him to straighten out as often as they had in the past.

EVIDENCE TO PRACTICE 8-2

CASE STUDY "RICK"
EXAMINATION DECISION

Clinical findings include tight pectoral and hamstring muscles.[100,110] An increased thoracic kyphosis with a compensatory increased lumbar lordosis (Tachdjian, 1990) and forward head posture are seen.[100]

PLAN OF CARE DECISION

Herrera-Soto (2005) stated the Milwaukee brace is the most effective means of bracing and works well during the early

EVIDENCE TO PRACTICE 8-2—cont'd

phases of Scheuermann's kyphosis for patients who are skeletally immature.[38] The procedure is considered to be successful when the kyphosis decreases and vertebral bodies appear less wedge-shaped on radiographs. It has been observed that the anterior longitudinal ligament may thicken and there may be partial reversal of vertebral wedging with use of a brace.[110] The prescribed exercises are specific for active trunk extensor strengthening, general postural exercise, and hamstring stretches. Sports that have an extensor component such as volleyball or swimming and aerobic exercise are recommended. The goal of physical therapy is to improve postural alignment and to increase flexibility and extensor strength.[110] Exercise as the sole treatment has not been established as effective, although it has been shown to be beneficial in conjunction with other methods of treatment in the early stages of Scheuermann's kyphosis.[39,69,110] Herrera-Soto (2005) states that thoracic extension and postural exercises are considered to be the treatment of choice.[38]

PATIENT/FAMILY PREFERENCES

When families follow through with their home exercise program they have better outcomes than those who do not. Marker et al (2010) looked at 147 patients who underwent total hip resurfacing arthroplasty surgery to assess patient commitment to their rehabilitation and clinical outcomes.[61] They found that patients with an increased commitment to their rehabilitation had better outcomes.

"Nancy"

Nancy is a 14-year-old gymnast who presented to an orthopedic surgeon with c/o low back pain that has been gradually worsening over the past few months. She could not recall a specific injury or traumatic event. AP and lateral radiographs revealed a spondylolysis. The patient was prescribed a TLSO and was placed on activity restrictions. After 8 weeks of immobilization in the TLSO, Nancy was referred to physical therapy. Nancy gradually resumed activities over the next 6 to 8 weeks.

EVIDENCE TO PRACTICE 8-3

CASE STUDY "NANCY"
EXAMINATION DECISION

Good history taking is a must. Cavalier et al. (2006) and Herman and Pizzutillo (2005) found that athletes involved in

Continued

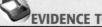 **CASE STUDIES—cont'd**

EVIDENCE TO PRACTICE 8-3—cont'd

sports with repetitive hyperextension and rotational loading on the lumbar spine are noted to have a higher incidence of spondylolysis and spondylolisthesis than the general population.[9,36]

Standing posteroanterior and lateral views of the spine, including the thoracic, lumbar, and sacral regions, are helpful in examining spinal alignment and in identifying spondylytic defects and spondylolisthesis. Other imaging studies, including a SPECT bone scan, are available if radiographs are inconclusive and spondylolysis is suspected.[37]

PLAN OF CARE DECISION

Patients presenting with symptomatic spondylolysis often respond well to activity restriction, physical therapy, and spinal bracing.[36] Immobilization using a TLSO is indicated after a stress fracture of the pars for a recommended period of 6 to 12 weeks. Herman, Pizzutillo, and Cavalier (2003)

 EVIDENCE TO PRACTICE 8-3—cont'd

report that bone healing is determined by using imaging such as a CT scan; this should be supported by clinical evidence of decreased sequelae.[37] Once Nancy was referred to physical therapy, she learned lumbar stabilization exercises and was taught to maintain pain-free neutral alignment of the pelvis and lumbar spine while varying her positions. Co-contracting the transverse abdominis, lumbar multifidus, and internal oblique muscles during functional activities will help stabilize the lumbar spine and decrease low back pain in patients with spondylolysis.[76]

PATIENT/FAMILY PREFERENCES

According to Herman, Pizzutillo, and Cavalier (2003), the athlete is permitted to return to competitive sports once he or she has full spinal ROM without complaints of pain or evidence of hamstring spasm, and after he or she has otherwise returned to full functional activities.[37]

REFERENCES

1. Basset, G. S., Burness, W. P., & MacEwen, G. D. (1986). Treatment of scoliosis with a Wilmington brace: Results in patients with 20–29 degree curves. *Journal of Bone and Joint Surgery (American), 68,* 602–605.

2. Berven, S., & Bradford, D. S. (2002). Neuromuscular scoliosis: Causes of deformity and principles for evaluation and management. *Seminars in Neurology, 22,* 167–178.

3. Betz, R. R. (2004). Kyphosis of the thoracic and thoracolumbar spine in the pediatric patient: Normal sagittal parameters and scope of the problem. *Instructional Course Lectures, 53,* 479–484.

4. Bleck, E. (1991). Annotation—Adolescent idiopathic scoliosis. *Developmental Medicine and Child Neurology, 33,* 167–176.

5. Bunnell, W. (1984). An objective criterion for scoliosis screening. *Journal of Bone and Joint Surgery (American), 66,* 1381–1387.

6. Byl, N. N., & Gray, J. M. (1993). Complex balance reactions in different sensory conditions: Adolescents with and without idiopathic scoliosis. *Journal of Orthopaedic Research, 11,* 215–227.

7. Burwell, R. G. (2003). Aetiology of idiopathic scoliosis: current concepts. *Pediatric Rehabilitation, 6,* 137–170.

8. Campbell, R. M., & Hell-Vocke, A. K. (2003). Growth of the thoracic spine in congenital scoliosis after expansion thoracoplasty. *Journal of Bone and Joint Surgery (American), 85,* 409–420.

9. Cavalier, R., Herman, M. J., Cheung, E. V., et al. (2006). Spondylolysis and spondylolisthesis in children and adolescents: I. Diagnosis, natural history, and nonsurgical management. *Journal of the American Academy of Orthopaedic Surgeons, 14,* 417–424.

10. Calvo, J. J. (1957). Observations on the growth of the female adolescent spine and its relationship to scoliosis. *Clinical Orthopedics, 10,* 40–47.

11. Carman, D., Roach, J. W., Speck, G., et al. (1985). Role of exercises in the Milwaukee brace treatment of scoliosis. *Journal of Pediatric Orthopedics, 11,* 65–68.

12. Charles, Y. P., Daures, J. P., deRosa, V., et al. (2006). Progression risk of idiopathic juvenile scoliosis during pubertal growth. *Spine, 31,* 1933–1942.

13. Coillard, C., Vachon, V., Circo, A. B., et al. (2007). Effectiveness of the SpineCor brace based on the new standardized criteria proposed by the Scoliosis Research Society for adolescent idiopathic scoliosis. *Journal of Pediatric Orthopaedics, 27,* 375–379.

14. Coillard, C., Circo, A., & Rivard, C. H. (2008). A new concept for the non-invasive treatment of adolescent idiopathic scoliosis: The corrective movement principle integrated in the SpineCor system. *Disability and Rehabilitation: Assistive Technology, 3,* 112–119.

15. Cowell, H. R., Hall, J. N., & MacEwen, G. D. (1972). Genetic aspects of idiopathic scoliosis. *Clinical Orthopedics, 86,* 121–132.

16. Dickson, R. A., Lawton, J. D., Archer, J. A., et al. (1984). The pathogenesis of idiopathic scoliosis. *Journal of Bone and Joint Surgery (British)*, 66, 8–15.

17. Dobbs, M. B., & Weinstein, S. L. (1999). Infantile and juvenile scoliosis. *Orthopedic Clinics of North America*, 30, 331–341.

18. Drummond, D. S. (1991). A perspective on recent trends for scoliosis correction. *Clinical Orthopedics and Related Research*, 264, 90–102.

19. Dubousset, J., & Cotrel, Y. (1991). Application technique of Cotrel-Dubousset instrumentation for scoliosis deformities. *Clinical Orthopedics and Related Research*, 264, 103–110.

20. Duval-Beaupere, G. (1972). The growth of scoliosis patients: Hypothesis and preliminary study. *Acta Orthopaedica Belgica*, 38, 365–376.

21. Farady, J. A. (1983). Current principles in the non-operative management of structural adolescent idiopathic scoliosis. *Physical Therapy*, 63, 512–523.

22. Federico, D. J., & Renshaw, T. S. (1990). Results of treatment of idiopathic scoliosis with the Charleston bending orthosis. *Spine*, 15, 866–867.

23. Fisk, J. R., & Bunch, W. H. (1979). Scoliosis in neuromuscular disease. *Orthopedic Clinics of North America*, 10, 863–875.

24. Giampietro, P. F., Blank, R. D., Raggio, C. L., et al. (2003). Congenital and idiopathic scoliosis: Clinical and genetic aspects. *Clinical Medicine and Research*, 1, 125–136.

25. Ginsburg, G. M., & Lauder, A. J. (2007). Progression of scoliosis in patients with spastic quadriplegia after the insertion of an intrathecal baclofen pump. *Spine*, 32, 2745–2750.

26. Glancy, G. L. (2007). Advances in idiopathic scoliosis in children and adolescents. *Advances in Pediatrics*, 54, 55–66.

27. Goldberg, C. J., Moore, D. P., Fogarty, E. E., et al. (1999). Left thoracic curve patterns and their association with disease. *Spine*, 24, 1228.

28. Goldstein, L. A., & Waugh, T. R. (1973). Classification and terminology of scoliosis. *Clinical Orthopedics*, 93, 10–22.

29. Green, N. (1986). Part-time bracing of adolescent idiopathic scoliosis. *Journal of Bone and Joint Surgery (American)*, 68, 738–742.

30. Green, N. E. (1986). Part-time bracing of adolescent idiopathic scoliosis. *Journal of Bone and Joint Surgery (American)*, 68, 738–742.

31. Grzegorzewski, A., & Kumar, S. J. (2000). In situ posterolateral spine arthrodesis for grades III, IV, and V spondylolisthesis in children and adolescents. *Journal of Pediatric Orthopedics*, 20, 506–511.

32. Hahn, F., Hauser, D., Espinosa, N., et al. (2008). Scoliosis correction with pedicle screws in Duchenne muscular dystrophy. *European Spine Journal*, 17, 255–261.

33. Heary, R. F., Bono, C. M., & Kumar, S. (2008). Bracing for scoliosis. *Neurosurgery*, 63, A125–A130.

34. Hedequist, D., & Emans, J. (2004). Congenital scoliosis. *Journal of the American Academy of Orthopaedic Surgeons*, 12, 266–275.

35. Herkowitz, H. N., Gardfin, S. R., Balderson, R. A., et al. (1999). *Rothman-Simeone: The spine*. Philadelphia: WB Saunders.

36. Herman, M. J., & Pizzutillo, P. D. (2005). Spondylolysis and spondylolisthesis in the child and adolescent: A new classification. *Clinical Orthopaedics and Related Research*, 434, 46–54.

37. Herman, M. J., Pizzutillo, P. D., & Cavalier, R. (2003). Spondylolysis and spondylolisthesis in the child and adolescent athlete. *Orthopedic Clinics of North America*, 34, 461–467.

38. Herrera-Soto, J. A., Parikh, S. N., Al-Sayyad, M. J., et al. (2005). Experience with combined video-assisted thoracoscopic surgery (VATS) anterior spinal release and posterior spinal fusion in Scheuermann's kyphosis. *Spine*, 30, 2176–2181.

39. Herring, J. A. (2002). *Tachdjian's pediatric orthopedics* (3rd ed., pp. 213–312, 323–349, 1279–1291). Philadelphia: WB Saunders.

40. Hsu, J. D., Michael, J. W., & Fisk, J. R. (2008). *AAOS atlas of orthoses and assistive devices* (4th ed.). Philadelphia: Mosby Elsevier.

41. Hu, S. S., Bradford, D. S., Transfeldt, E. E., et al. (1996). Reduction of high-grade spondylolisthesis using Edwards instrumentation. *Spine*, 21, 367–371.

42. Janicki, J. A., & Alman, B. (2007). Scoliosis: Review of diagnosis and treatment. *Paediatric Child Health*, 12, 771–776.

43. Jarvis, J., Garbedian, S., & Swamy, G. (2008). Juvenile idiopathic scoliosis: The effectiveness of part-time bracing. *Spine*, 33, 1074–1078.

44. Reference deleted in page proofs.

45. Katz, D. E., & Durrani, A. A. (2001). Factors that influence outcome in bracing large curve in patients with adolescent idiopathic scoliosis. *Spine*, 26, 2354–2361.

46. Katz, D. E., Richards, B. S., Browne, R. H., et al. (1997). A comparison between the Boston brace and the Charleston bending brace in adolescent idiopathic scoliosis. *Spine*, 22, 1302–1312.

47. Kehl, D. K., & Morrissy, R. T. (1988). Brace treatment in adolescent idiopathic scoliosis: An update on concepts and technique. *Clinical Orthopaedics and Related Research*, 229, 34–43.

48. Kerr, T. P., Lin, J. P., Gresty, M. A., et al. (2008). Spinal stability is improved by inducing a lumbar lordosis in boys with Duchenne muscular dystrophy: A pilot study. *Gait & Posture*, 28, 108–112.

49. King, W. M., Ruttencutter, R., Nagaraja, H. N., et al. (2007). Orthopedic outcomes of long-term daily corticosteroid treatment in Duchenne muscular dystrophy. *Neurology*, 68, 1607–1613.

50. Kostuik, J. P. (1990). Current concepts review operative treatment of idiopathic scoliosis. *Journal of Bone and Joint Surgery (American)*, 72, 1108–1113.

51. Lee, S. M., Suk, S. I., & Chung, E. R. (2004). Direct vertebral rotation: A new technique of three-dimensional deformity correction with segmental pedical screw fixation in adolescent idiopathic scoliosis. *Spine*, 29, 343–349.

52. Lehnert-Schroth, C. (1992). Introduction to the three-dimensional scoliosis treatment according to Schroth. *Physiotherapy, 78,* 810–815.

53. Letts, R. M., & Jawadi, A. H. (2009). Congenital spinal deformity. Retrieved from: http://emedicine.medscape.com/article/1260442-overview.

54. Lonner, B. S., Newton, P., Betz, R., et al. (2007). Operative management of Scheuermann's kyphosis in 78 patients: Radiographic outcomes, complications, and technique. *Spine, 32,* 2644–2652.

55. Lonstein, J. E., & Carlson, J. M. (1984). The prediction of curve progression in untreated idiopathic scoliosis during growth. *Journal of Bone and Joint Surgery (American), 66,* 1061–1071.

56. Lonstein, J. E., & Renshaw, T. S. (1987). *Neuromuscular spine deformities: Instructional course lectures* (Vol. 36; pp. 285–304). St Louis: Mosby.

57. Lonstein, J. E., & Winter, R. B. (1988). Adolescent idiopathic scoliosis. *Orthopedic Clinics of North America, 19,* 239–246.

58. Lowe, T. G., & Line, B. G. (2007). Evidence based medicine analysis of Scheuermann kyphosis. *Spine, 32,* S115–S119.

59. Mac-Thiong, J., & Labelle, H. (2006). A proposal for a surgical classification of pediatric lumbosacral spondylolisthesis based on current literature. *European Spine Journal, 15,* 1425–1435.

60. Margonato, V., Fronte, F., Rainero, G., et al. (2005). Effects of short term cast wearing on respiratory and cardiac responses to submaximal exercise in adolescents with idiopathic scoliosis. *Europa Medicophysica, 41,* 135–140.

61. Marker, D. R., Seyler, T. M., Bhave, A., et al. (2010). Does commitment to rehabilitation influence clinical outcome of total hip resurfacing arthroplasty? *Journal of Orthopaedic Surgery and Research, 5,* 20.

62. Reference deleted in page proofs.

63. Mehlman, C. T. (2008). Idiopathic scoliosis. Retrieved from: http://emedicine.medscape.com/article/1265794-overview.

64. Merola, A. A., Haher, T. R., Brkaric, M., et al. (2002). A multicenter study of the outcomes of the surgical treatment of adolescent idiopathic scoliosis using the Scoliosis Research Society (SRS) outcome instrument. *Spine, 27,* 2046–2051.

65. Miller, A., Temple, T., & Miller, F. (1996). Impact of orthoses on the rate of scoliosis progression in children with cerebral palsy. *Journal of Pediatric Orthopedics, 16,* 332–335.

66. Miller, N. H. (1999). Cause and natural history of adolescent idiopathic scoliosis. *Orthopedic Clinics of North America, 30,* 343–352.

67. Miller, N. H. (2007). Genetics of familial idiopathic scoliosis. *Clinical Orthopaedics and Related Research, 462,* 6–10.

68. Moe, J. H., Sundberg, A. B., & Gustlio, R. (1964). A clinical study of spine fusion in the growing child. *Journal of Bone and Joint Surgery (British), 46,* 784–785.

69. Moe, J. H., Winter, R. B., Bradford, D. S., et al. (1987). *Scoliosis and other spinal deformities* (2nd ed.; pp. 162–228, 237–261, 347–368, 403–434). Philadelphia: WB Saunders.

70. Murphy, N. A., Firth, S., Jorgensen, T., et al. (2006). Spinal surgery in children with idiopathic and neuromuscular scoliosis. What's the difference? *Spine, 26,* 216–220.

71. Muschik, M., Schlenzka, D., Robinson, P. N., et al. (1999). Dorsal instrumentation for idiopathic adolescent thoracic scoliosis: Rod rotation versus translation. *European Spine Journal, 8,* 93–99.

72. Nault, M. L., Allard, P., Hinse, S., et al. (2002). Relations between standing stability and body posture parameters in adolescent idiopathic scoliosis. *Spine, 27,* 1911–1917.

73. Negrini, S., Fusco, C., Minozzi, S., et al. (2008a). Exercises reduce the progression rate of adolescent idiopathic scoliosis: Results of a comprehensive systematic review of the literature. *Disability and Rehabilitation, 30,* 772–785.

74. Negrini, S., Zaina, F., Romano, M., et al. (2008b). Specific exercises reduce brace prescription in adolescent idiopathic scoliosis: A prospective controlled cohort study with worst-case analysis. *Journal of Rehabilitation Medicine, 40,* 451–455.

75. O'Beirne, J., Goldberg, C., Dowling, F. E., et al. (1989). Equilibrial dysfunction in scoliosis—Cause or effect? *Journal of Spinal Disorders, 2,* 184–189.

76. O'Sullivan, P. B., Twomey, L. T., & Allison, G. T. (1997). Evaluation of specific stabilizing exercise in the treatment of chronic low back pain with radiologic diagnosis of spondylolysis and spondylolisthesis. *Spine, 22,* 2959–2967.

77. Piazza, M. R., & Basset, G. S. (1990). Curve progression after treatment with the Wilmington brace for idiopathic scoliosis. *Journal of Pediatric Orthopedics, 10,* 39–43.

78. Price, C. T., Scott, D. S., Reed, F. R., Jr., et al. (1990). Nighttime bracing for adolescent idiopathic scoliosis with the Charleston bending brace: Preliminary report. *Spine, 15,* 1294–1299.

79. Price, C. T., Scott, D. S., Reed, F. R., Jr., et al. (1997). Nighttime bracing for adolescent idiopathic scoliosis with the Charleston bending brace: Long-term follow-up. *Journal of Pediatric Orthopedics, 17,* 703–707.

80. Pugh, M. B. (Ed.). (2000). *Stedman's medical dictionary* [27th ed.]. Baltimore: Lippincott Williams & Wilkins.

81. Puttlitz, C. M., Masaru, F., Barkley, A., et al. (2007). A biomechanical assessment of thoracic spine stapling. *Spine, 32,* 756–761.

82. Reamy, B. V., & Slakey, J. B. (2001). Adolescent idiopathic scoliosis: Review and current concepts. *American Family Physician, 64,* 111–116.

83. Renshaw, T. S. (1985). *Orthotic treatment of idiopathic scoliosis and kyphosis: Instructional course lectures* (Vol. 34; pp. 110–118). St Louis: Mosby.

84. Renshaw, T. S. (1988). The role of Harrington instrumentation and posterior spine fusion in the management of adolescent idiopathic scoliosis. *Orthopedic Clinics of North America, 19,* 257–267.

85. Richards, B. S., & Vitale, M. G. (2008). Screening for idiopathic scoliosis in adolescents: An information statement. *Journal of Bone and Joint Surgery (American), 90,* 195–198.

86. Rinsky, R. A., & Gamble, J. G. (1988). Adolescent idiopathic scoliosis. *Western Journal of Medicine, 148,* 183–191.

87. Roach, J. W. (1999). Adolescent idiopathic scoliosis. *Orthopedic Clinics of North America, 30*, 353–365.

88. Rogala, E., Drummond, D. S., & Gurr, J. (1978). Scoliosis: Incidence and natural history. *Journal of Bone and Joint Surgery (American), 60*, 173–176.

89. Sarwark, J. F., & Kramer, A. (1998). Pediatric spinal deformity. *Current Opinions in Pediatrics, 101*, 82–86.

90. Sarwark, J. F. (2006). Return to athletics after scoliosis surgery, unpublished.

91. Sarwark, J. F., & Aubin, C. E. (2007). Growth considerations of the immature spine. *Journal of Bone and Joint Surgery, 89*, 8–13. Retrieved from: http://www.schrothmethod.com.

92. Schwend, R. M., Hennrikus, W., Hall, J. E., et al. (1995). Childhood scoliosis: Clinical indications for magnetic resonance imaging. *Journal of Bone and Joint Surgery (American), 77*, 46–53.

93. Senaran, H., Shah, S. A., Presedo, A., et al. (2007). The risk of progression of scoliosis in cerebral palsy patients after intrathecal baclofen therapy. *Spine, 32*, 2348–2354.

94. Shilt, J. S., Lai, L. P., Cabrera, M. N., et al. (2008). The impact of intrathecal baclofen on the natural history of scoliosis in cerebral palsy. *Journal of Pediatric Orthopedics, 28*, 684–687.

95. Smith, J. T., Jerman, J., Stringham, J., et al. (2009). Does expansion thoracoplasty improve the volume of the convex lung in a windswept thorax? *Journal of Pediatric Orthopedics, 29*, 944–947.

96. Staheli, L. T. (2001). *Practice of pediatric orthopedics* (p. 160). Philadelphia: Lippincott Williams & Wilkins.

97. Stokes, I. (2007). Analysis and simulation of progressive adolescent scoliosis by biomechanical growth modulation. *European Spine Journal, 16*, 1621–1628.

98. Suk, S. I., Choon, K. L., Kim, W. J., et al. (1995). Segmental pedicle screw fixation in the treatment of thoracic idiopathic scoliosis. *Spine, 20*, 1399–1405.

99. Szwed, A., Kolban, M., & Jaolszewski, M. (2009). Results of SpineCor dynamic bracing for idiopathic scoliosis. *Ortopedia Traumatologia Rehabilitacja, 11*, 427–432.

100. Tachdjian, M. O. (1990). *Pediatric orthopedics* (*Vol. 4*, 2nd ed.). Philadelphia: WB Saunders.

101. Tanner, J. M., Whitehouse, R. H., & Takaisni, M. (1966). Standards from birth to maturity for height, weight, height velocity and weight velocity: British children, 1965. *Archives of Disease in Childhood, 47*, 454–471, 613–635.

102. Tanner, J. M., & Whitehouse, R. H. (1976). Clinical longitudinal standards for height, weight, height velocity and stages of puberty. *Archives of Disease in Childhood, 51*, 170–179.

103. Terjesen, T., Lange, J. E., & Steen, H. (2000). Treatment of scoliosis with spinal bracing in quadriplegic cerebral palsy. *Developmental Medicine & Child Neurology, 42*, 448–454.

104. Thomas, C. L. (Ed.). (1989). *Taber's cyclopedic medical dictionary* (16th ed.). Philadelphia: FA Davis.

105. Van Rens, T. G., & Van Horn, J. R. (1982). Long-term results in lumbosacral interbody fusion for spondylolisthesis. *Acta Orthopaedica Scandinavica, 53*, 383–392.

106. Verbeist, H. (1979). The treatment of lumbar spondyloptosis or impending lumbar spondyloptosis accompanied by neurologic deficit and/or neurogenic intermittent claudication. *Spine, 4*, 68–77.

107. Weinstein, S. L. (1994). Adolescent idiopathic scoliosis: Prevalence and natural history. In S. L. Weinstein (Ed.). *The pediatric spine* (pp. 463–478). New York: Raven Press.

108. Weinstein, S. L. (1989). *Adolescent idiopathic scoliosis: Prevalence and natural history: Instructional Course Lectures* (Chapter 6; *Vol. 38*). St Louis: Mosby.

109. Weinstein S. L., Dolan, L. A., Spratt, K. F., et al. (2003). Health and function of patients with untreated idiopathic scoliosis: A 50-year natural history study. *Journal of the American Medical Association, 289*, 559–567.

110. Weinstein, S. L. (2001). *The pediatric spine: Principles and practice* (2nd ed.). Philadelphia: Lippincott Williams & Wilkins.

111. Weinstein, S. L., Zavala, D. C., & Ponseti, I. V. (1981). Idiopathic scoliosis: Long-term follow-up and prognosis in untreated patients. *Journal of Bone and Joint Surgery (American), 63*, 702–712.

112. Weiss, H. R., Weiss, G., & Petermann, F. (2003). Incidence of curvature progression in idiopathic scoliosis patients treated with scoliosis inpatient rehabilitation (SIR): An age- and sex-matched controlled study. *Pediatric Rehabilitation, 6*, 23–30.

113. Wiltse, L. L., Newman, P. H., & MacNab, I. (1976). Classification of spondylolysis and spondylolisthesis. *Clinical Orthopedics, 117*, 23–29.

114. Winter, R. B. (1983). *Congenital deformities of the spine* (pp. 6–10, 43–49). New York: Thieme-Stratton.

115. Winter, R. B. (1988). Congenital scoliosis. *Orthopedic Clinics of North America, 19*, 395–408.

116. Winter, R. B., Moe, J. H., & Wang, J. F. (1973). Congenital kyphosis: Its natural history and treatment as observed in a study of one hundred and thirty patients. *Journal of Bone and Joint Surgery (American), 55*, 223–256.

117. Wong, H. K., Hee, H.-T., Yu, Z., et al. (2004). Results of thoracoscopic instrumented fusion versus convention posterior instrumented fusion in adolescent idiopathic scoliosis undergoing selective thoracic fusion. *Spine, 29*, 2031–2038.

118. Wynarsky, G. T., & Schultz, A. B. (1989). Trunk muscle activities in braced scoliosis patients. *Spine, 14*, 1283–1286.

119. Wynne-Davies, R. (1968). Familial (idiopathic) scoliosis. *Journal of Bone and Joint Surgery (British), 50*, 24–30.

120. Yazici, M., & Emans, J. (2009). Fusionless instrumentation systems for congenital scoliosis: Expandable spinal rods and vertical expandable prosthetic titanium rib in the management of congenital spine deformities in the growing child. *Spine, 34*, 1800–1807.

121. Zaouss, A. L., & James, J. I. P. (1958). The iliac apophysis and the evolution of curves in scoliosis. *Journal of Bone and Joint Surgery (British), 40*, 442–453.

9

Congenital Muscular Torticollis

KAREN KARMEL-ROSS, PT, PCS, LMT

ewborns may exhibit positional deformities at birth related to the intrauterine environment. One condition thought to be caused by in utero constraint is congenital muscular torticollis (CMT). CMT describes the posture of the head and neck from unilateral shortening of the sternocleidomastoid (SCM) muscle, causing the head to tilt toward and rotate away from the affected SCM muscle. The infant may exhibit asymmetric neck extension and a forward head posture because of upper cervical extension. The muscular torticollis is named for the side of the involved SCM muscle.

If the muscular torticollis has developed secondary to gestational fetal constraint (versus trauma to the SCM during labor and delivery), characteristics noted at birth may also include deformation of the craniofacial skeleton on the same side as the affected SCM. These skeletal changes are caused by compression of the anterior chest and shoulder against the face and the resultant impact of mechanical forces on otherwise normal tissue, causing associated positional deformation.[14,22,24,28,30,31,36,37,43,99]

The primary goal of intervention for CMT is to restore full neck movement as early as possible to help reverse or stop the progression of skull-based deformity, to prevent cranial facial asymmetry, and to prevent bony and postural changes that may cause asymmetric motor development. This chapter discusses the etiology and pathophysiology, examination, associated condition of deformational plagiocephaly, and intervention strategies and expected outcomes for CMT.

ETIOLOGY AND PATHOPHYSIOLOGY

There is little agreement on the etiology of congenital muscular torticollis. Theories include direct injury to the muscle, ischemic injury based on abnormal vascular patterns, rupture of the muscle, infective myositis, neurogenic injury, hereditary factors, and intrauterine compartment syndrome. The most often cited and most widely accepted theories are ischemia, birth trauma, and intrauterine malposition.[6,25,36,52,72,92,98] Davids and colleagues[28] postulated that head position in utero can selectively injure the SCM muscle, leading to the development of a perinatal compartment syndrome. In part, this theory may explain the upper extremity weakness one may observe on the same side as the involved

SCM muscle. Position of the head and neck in utero or during labor and delivery of forward flexion, lateral bending, and rotation may cause a compression injury of the ipsilateral SCM muscle and brachial plexus, resulting in ischemia, reperfusion, edema, and neurologic injuries.

Muscular torticollis is the third most common congenital musculoskeletal anomaly after dislocated hip and clubfoot, with reports of incidence varying from 0.3% to 16% of newborns.[17,18,26,31,52,62] Associated with muscular torticollis at birth are ipsilateral mandibular asymmetry, ear displacement, plagiocephaly, scoliosis, pelvic asymmetry, congenital dislocated hip, and foot deformity.[21,31,35,42,45,47,52,87,91,97]

The incidence of plagiocephaly has increased significantly since it was recommended that infants be placed on their backs to sleep to prevent sudden infant death syndrome (SIDS) in the 1992 "Back to Sleep" campaign.[1,5,48,50,53,76,79,93] More recently, the incidence of plagiocephaly has been reported to have increased to as high as 1 in 60 live births, which may be partially explained by infants sleeping on their backs.[1,5,53,93] In 2008, Stellwagon[88] reported that one in six, or 16%, of healthy newborns have torticollis, most newborns exhibit mild or moderate craniofacial asymmetries, and it is possible to detect torticollis early in life. In the study cohort, infants were identified by measuring neck rotation and neck lateral flexion (how far the ear tilted toward the ipsilateral shoulder), and by comparing left and right side neck mobility. Torticollis was defined as >15° difference when comparing the two sides. The study found that the newborn with torticollis generally can rotate the head to the shoulder but demonstrated restriction in lateral flexion when measured in supine.

Habal and colleagues[41] have suggested that a new syndrome, the "flathead" syndrome, is being introduced and may identify neurocognitive difference or delay disorders among patients who may have appeared normal before the change in sleep position. It is hypothesized that infants born with torticollis are at risk for developing deformational plagiocephaly, and this risk may be reduced by early intervention.[14,22,38,39] Plagiocephaly is reported as a coexisting impairment in 80% to 90.1% of children with congenital muscular torticollis.[17,19]

If cranial deformation begins in utero, the deformational forces on the occiput may continue after birth if the infant sleeps supine and also spends time in supine or semisupine during waking hours. In this case, the cranial deformation

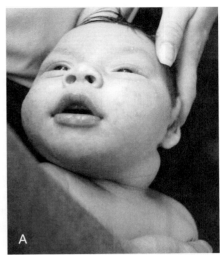

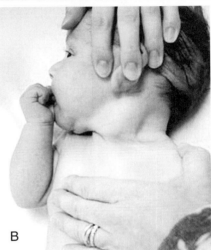

Figure 9-1 **A,** A 2-month-old infant with a fibrotic tumor in the left sternocleidomastoid (SCM) muscle involving the whole muscle. **B,** Same infant at 3 months of age.

may worsen after birth because the infant cannot yet move the head away from the supporting surface.

The risk factors for muscular torticollis and plagiocephaly are similar and include large birth weight, male gender, breech position, multiple birth, primiparous mother, difficult labor and delivery, use of vacuum or forceps assist, nuchal cord, and maternal uterine abnormalities.[5,22,31,43,62,87,88]

The typical history of congenital muscular torticollis includes the appearance of a fibrous tumor (usually 1 to 3 cm in diameter and spindle shaped) in the SCM muscle between 14 and 21 days after birth (Figure 9-1), although the first appearance can be as late as 3 months. The tumor disappears by the time the patient is 4 to 8 months of age. If the diagnosis is made within 2 to 6 weeks after birth, the term "pseudotumor of infancy" may be used.[52,98]

Biopsy of the tumor reveals the histologic appearance of a fibroma. The tumor is characterized by a deposition of collagen and fibroblasts around the individual muscle fibers, with an absence of normal striated muscle. The severity and distribution of the fibrosis, its location within the muscle, individual growth patterns, and the amount of atrophy of normal muscle tissue varies among patients. The nature of the fibrous tissue in the neonate suggests the disease may begin before birth and be related to in utero fetal positioning.[13,21,46,52,61,85,91] One may observe an associated head tilt because (1) the healthy myoblasts degenerate; (2) the remaining fibroblasts produce excess collagen, which results in a scarlike band and muscle contracture; or (3) the infant is unable to maintain a vertical head against gravity in static postures or during transitional movement.

Four subtypes of CMT have been identified:
- Sternomastoid tumor (SMT), in which a discrete mass is palpable within the SCM muscle and x-rays are normal
- Muscular torticollis (MT), in which there is tightness but no palpable mass within the SCM muscle and x-rays are normal
- Postural torticollis (POST), in which there is no SCM muscle tightness, no palpable mass, and x-rays are normal
- Postnatal muscular torticollis, which may be classified into the following:
  - Environmental-induced torticollis[5,50,65,78]
  - Plagiocephaly-induced torticollis[35a]
  - Positional preference-induced toritcollis[5]
    Late-onset muscular torticollis induced by inadequate muscle length of the injured muscle with growth and development[52]
  - CMT and other congenital birth problems such as CP, Myelodysplasia, Down syndrome[35]
  - OA (occiput-C1)somatic dysfunction resulting in CMT and Asymmetrical Human Movement Disorder of Infancy (AHMDI), a constellation of findings grouped together by the author based on clinical experience and osteopathic principles.[60a]

The causes of postural torticollis may be benign paroxysmal torticollis (BPT), congenital absence of one or several cervical muscles or of the transverse ligament, or contracture of other neck muscles.[18,21,25]

ANATOMY OF THE STERNOCLEIDOMASTOID MUSCLE

The SCM muscle may be called the sternocleido-occipitomastoid, as it comprises four distinct bands (Figure 9-2). A deep band, the cleidomastoid, runs from the medial third of the clavicle to the mastoid process, and three superficial bands form an "N" shape over the deep band. The three superficial bands are (1) the cleido-occipital, which overlies the bulk of the cleidomastoid and inserts into the lateral third of the superior nuchal line of the occiput, (2) the sterno-occipital, and (3) the sternomastoid.

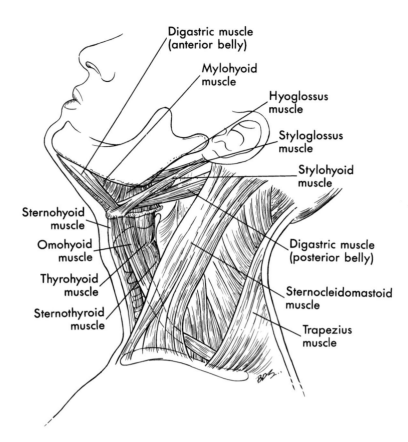

Figure 9-2 Sternocleidomastoid muscle and other muscles of the neck. (From Lingeman, R. E. [1998]. Surgical anatomy. In C. W. Cummings, F. M. Fredrickson, L. A. Harker, C. J. Krause, D. E. Schuller, & M. A. Richardson [Eds.], *Otolaryngology: Head and neck surgery* [3rd ed., Vol. 3, p. 1680]. St. Louis, MO: Mosby.)

Both of the latter two superficial bands arise from a common tendon attached to the superior margin of the sternum. The sterno-occipital inserts along with the cleido-occipital into the superior nuchal line, whereas the sternomastoid inserts into the superior and anterior borders of the mastoid. The SCM muscle is innervated by the second cervical nerve and the spinal portion of the accessory nerve, which also innervates the upper trapezius muscle. Infants with CMT as a result of uterine constraint often have involvement of the upper trapezius muscle on the same side as the involved SCM muscle. The trapezius is a synergist of the ipsilateral SCM muscle and has a similar action as the SCM muscle. The trapezius is also an important mover of the scapula. The contour of the lower part of the neck is formed by the fibers of the trapezius muscle, and the contour of the upper part of the neck is formed by the fibers of the SCM muscle.[54]

DIFFERENTIAL DIAGNOSIS

One in five children presenting with a torticollis posture has a nonmuscular etiology.[3] Nonmuscular causes may include skeletal abnormalities such as Klippel-Feil syndrome or neurologic causes such as brachial plexus injury. Because many lesions can masquerade as congenital muscular torticollis, the initial examination should include a detailed history and a thorough physical examination to determine if the lesion is congenital or acquired. Acquired nontraumatic torticollis may be caused by ocular lesions, Sandifer syndrome, benign paroxysmal torticollis, dystonic syndromes, posterior fossa pathology, postencephalitis syndromes, Arnold-Chiari malformation, and syringomyelia.[25,26]

CHANGES IN BODY STRUCTURE AND FUNCTION (IMPAIRMENTS)

In infants with CMT, neck range of motion is decreased for ipsilateral rotation, contralateral lateral flexion, and contralateral asymmetric flexion and extension. The infant is not able to maintain a midline alignment of the head with the torso in static postures or during movement because of the neck muscle imbalance and muscle contracture. Prolonged uncorrected head tilt caused by the underlying mechanism of imbalanced muscle pull acting on the growing spinal and craniofacial skeleton may worsen any scoliosis, skull and facial asymmetry, and influence compensatory movement patterns affecting motor control development.[34,55,83,86,99]

Facial and cranial characteristics often observed in infants are shown in Figure 9-3 and include the following:
- Asymmetry of the craniofacial skeletal structures
- Asymmetry of the masticatory and tongue muscles
- Underdevelopment of the ipsilateral jaw; canting of the mandible and gum line; elevation of the temporomandibular joint; dental occlusional problems

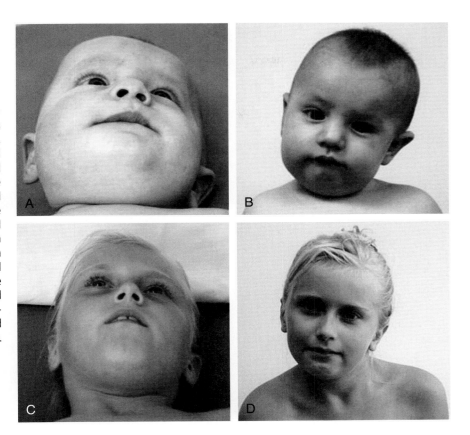

Figure 9-3 **A,** Submental view of an 8-month-old infant with left congenital muscular torticollis (CMT) and frontal deformational plagiocephaly. Note recession of the frontal bone, eyebrow, and zygoma on the ipsilateral side and inferiorly and posteriorly positioned ipsilateral ear. **B,** En face view shows hemihypoplasia of the face, decreased vertical facial height on the left, asymmetry of the eyes with the ipsilateral eye smaller, inferior orbital dystopia, canting of the mandible, and deviation of chin and nasal tip. **C,** Submental view of an 8-year-old with untreated left CMT and frontal deformational plagiocephaly demonstrating the same facial asymmetries as the 8-month-old infant. **D,** En face view of same 8-year-old demonstrates similar cranial facial asymmetries and shortening of the left sternocleidomastoid muscle.

- Inferiorly and posteriorly positioned ipsilateral ear; asymmetry of the ears with deformity of the ipsilateral ear, which may be cupped (bat ear)
- Asymmetry of the eyes with ipsilateral eye smaller; inferior orbital dystopia on the ipsilateral side
- Recessed eyebrow and zygoma on the ipsilateral side
- Deviation of the chin point and nasal tip
- Facial scoliosis (distorted craniofacial skeletal structures)
- Cranial base deformation, most prominent change occurring in the posterior cranial fossa.[15,34,44,45,48,83,97,99]

Yu and colleagues[99] found that cranial base deformity occurs as early as 1 month of age in infants with CMT. They also reported that gross facial deformity of jaw dysmorphology and occlusional tilting may worsen until 5 years of age and young adults with untreated CMT had asymmetric facial height and orbit size. Mandibular asymmetry was the most significant consistent finding of facial bone deformity. Ho and colleagues[43] found that 60% of those with CMT (13 of 22 patients) had mandibular hypoplasia at birth. They identified mandibular hypoplasia as an early sign of CMT.

Slate and colleagues[86] demonstrated a relationship between craniofacial asymmetry, congenital muscular torticollis, and cervical spine subluxation. They documented that 26 out of 30 patients with CMT had a C1–C2 subluxation with C1 rotated forward on C2. They suggested this finding

may help explain the residual asymmetric head and neck tilt observed in children even after extensive physical therapy intervention for CMT.

Other neck muscles may be involved either secondary to the SCM muscle tightness or without SCM tightness if the in utero position of the infant's head and neck posture was one of lateral flexion and rotation to the same side. Often observed with CMT is anterior neck muscle tightness affecting the platysma, scalenus, hyoids, tongue, and facial muscles, contributing to difficulty in the development of oral motor skills and development of head extension in the prone position (Figure 9-4).

Other musculoskeletal asymmetries may include trunk curvature toward the affected SCM, persistence of the asymmetric tonic neck reflex, and windswept hips with the hip joint markedly abducted on the facial side and adducted on the occipital side, causing the pelvis to tilt when the legs are brought together. When the infant acquires the ability to sit, a double spinal curve may develop as the infant compensates for the head tilt and tries to bring the center of gravity over the base of support and compensate for contracture of the hip and pelvic tilt. Jones[52] found that some children may elevate the shoulder, which allows the head to be in midline. Other children present with level shoulders but with a head tilt, which produces a lateral shift of the cervical spine leading to cervical spinal scoliosis.

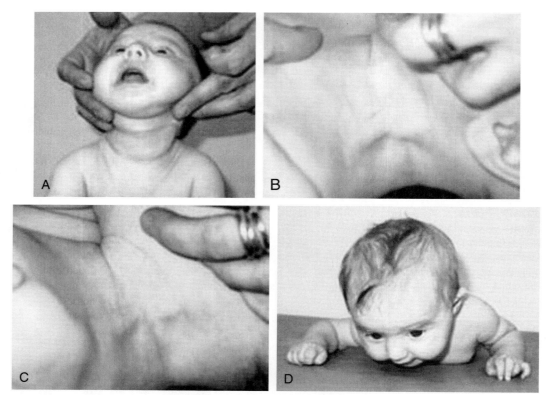

Figure 9-4 **A,** A 3-month-old with left congenital muscular torticollis (CMT) with multiple skin creases indicating tightness of the skin and anterior neck muscles. **B,** Same infant illustrating the tightness of lateral and posterior skin and neck muscles. **C,** Same infant with stretch of the left sterno-cleidomastoid and upper trapezius muscles revealing tightness of the scalenes and the lateral triangle of the neck. **D,** Anterior neck muscle tightness makes it difficult for the infant to extend the head in prone to clear the airway and rotate the head to the left or to the right.

TYPICAL ACTIVITY LIMITATIONS

The infant with CMT is unable to have purposeful symmetric movement of the head because of the neck muscle contracture and neck muscle strength imbalances. Impaired mobility may lead to persistent asymmetry of early reflexes and reinforcement of an asymmetric postural preference. This is turn may cause neglect of the ipsilateral hand; decreased visual awareness of the ipsilateral visual field; interference of symmetric development of head and neck righting reactions; delayed propping and rolling over the involved side; and limited vestibular, proprioceptive, and sensorimotor development. In the older child, this may result in asymmetric weight bearing in sitting, crawling, walking, and transitional movement skills as well as incomplete development of automatic postural reactions. If not addressed, these persistent postural asymmetries may result in structural deformities such as pelvic obliquity and scoliosis (Figure 9-5). Inability to turn the head and neck will cause the child to rotate the body to compensate, and inability to recruit lateral neck flexion with automatic reactions will cause the child to compensate with overuse of the torso muscles. Often the child with CMT may appear similar to a child with hemiplegic cerebral palsy.[4,55] Activity

limitations include difficulty in sustaining midline head posture in an upright position; regaining head midline posture in vertical, prone, or supine with weight shifts; and maintaining midline head posture during movement. Both the infant and child will have difficulty with upper extremity weight bearing on the involved side, reaching toward midline with forearm supination, shoulder external rotation and flexion, and full expression of upper extremity protective and equilibrium reactions. The infant will use compensatory maneuvers to perform a task such as hand clapping by crossing midline to bring the uninvolved side upper extremity toward the involved arm. The systems contributing to these activity limitations include the musculoskeletal system (limited cervical range of motion and muscle strength) and the sensory systems of vision, vestibular function, and somatosensation needed to regulate posture. These systems also influence adaptive and anticipatory responses to help control head position and anticipate postural adjustments by adapting head positions during weight shifts and active exploration.[84]

The infant with CMT responds to these imposed restrictions with self-initiated movements that include a pattern of head tilting to the ipsilateral side and rotation to the contralateral side of SCM muscle involvement. The infant with

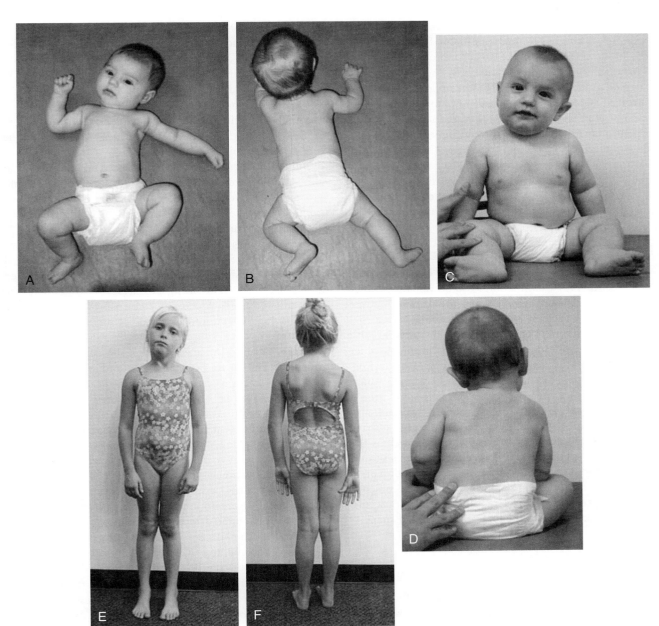

Figure 9-5   Characteristic asymmetric postural deformities shown in a 3-month-old infant (**A** and **B**), an 8-month-old infant (**C** and **D**), and an untreated 8-year-old child (**E** and **F**). All have left congenital muscular torticollis and deformational plagiocephaly. **A,** A 3-month-old in supine exhibiting characteristic asymmetric postural deformities including incurvation of the whole vertebral column, asymmetric tonic neck reflex, left arm abduction and internal rotation with forearm pronation, right hip abduction and external rotation, left hip adduction, and internal rotation. **B,** Same 3-month-old infant in prone. Note that there is little change in the postural alignment. **C,** Anterior view of 8-month-old in sitting exhibiting scoliosis, internal rotation and extension of the upper extremity with scapular elevation, abduction, anterior tilt, and upward rotation. **D,** Posterior view of same 8-month-old in sitting, exhibiting ipsilateral shortening of the posterior cervical muscles, shoulder elevation, extension of the humerus, and rotation of the thorax. **E,** Anterior view of untreated left 8-year-old in standing illustrates the long-term functional disturbances of CMT, molded baby syndrome, and DP. Patterns of dysfunction include sacral base declination to the right with compensatory rotoscoliosis, fascial bias, postural asymmetry, and somatic dysfunction. **F,** Posterior view of same 8-year-old. There is somatic dysfunction with FRSL of the OA joint and RL of C1-2, ERSL C3-7, and there are alternating compensatory rotational myofascial strain patterns at the transitional zones of muscular imbalance and fascial restrictions inhibiting movement and imposing functional restrictions: to the left at the craniocervical junction, to the right at the cervicothoracic junction, to the left at the thoracolumbar junction, and to the right at the lumbosacral junction. Note the relationship between pelvic rotation and foot postures. The longer left leg is pronated with the femoral head backward, hip abducted/externally rotated, and the shorter right leg is supinated with the femoral head forward, hip adducted/internally rotated. Frequently seen with this clinically is cephalad pubes dysfunction on the left, a posterior ilium on the left, an anterior ilium on the right, and a left on left sacral torsion.

CMT is therefore unable to adapt appropriately to the supporting surface and has limited kinesthetic feedback, which affects the development of the sensorimotor systems, postural organization, orientation, and body schema. The infant may demonstrate difficulty participating in activities toward the involved SCM muscle side while developing appropriate postural, motor, and visual control of the uninvolved side. The infant may not exhibit organized midline behavior as a result of the foregoing asymmetries. Motor milestones may develop atypically because the various subsystems (visual, vestibular, somatosensory, and musculoskeletal) are developing asymmetrically and the infant is not experiencing normal interactions of each system as growth and development occur.[55]

PHYSICAL THERAPY EXAMINATION

The physical therapy examination should evaluate the prenatal and birth history (vaginal or cesarean section delivery, use of vacuum or forceps assist, birth presentation, nuchal cord, birth order if multiple birth, birth weight, birth length), sex of the infant, side of SCM muscle involvement, other congenital anomalies, x-rays or other diagnostic testing, reports of previous subspecialists consulted, and age at diagnosis. The interview with the caregiver or parent should include questions about who provides care to the infant and the amount of time the child spends in infant seats, car seats, swings, and other infant positioning devices as well as the amount of time spent prone and supine. Questions should also be asked about sleeping position and head rotation preference when sleeping, sleeping surface, feeding problems, medications, previous physical therapy interventions, and present concerns regarding the torticollis and head shape.

FINDINGS IN CONGENITAL MUSCULAR TORTICOLLIS

The musculoskeletal system should be examined for restrictions in joint range of motion and muscle length with particular attention paid to ipsilateral neck rotation, contralateral lateral neck flexion, contralateral asymmetric flexion and extension, muscle and soft tissue extensibility, and skin creases about the neck (see Figure 9-4, A to C). Moving the head and neck passively through each motion allows the examiner to determine the infant's available range of motion. Gentle traction of the cervical spine may be used to assess the infant's ability to align the spinal vertebrae in neutral and eliminate the lateral glide position induced by the shortened SCM muscle. Gentle traction between the shoulder complex and the occiput combined with specific head and neck motions may be used to assess the tightness of the upper trapezius, scalene, and posterior neck muscles of the ipsilateral side. The infant's active and passive neck range of motion (ROM) should be assessed in prone with the head and neck free of the supporting surface because the infant may not

have enough ROM or strength to extend the head off the supporting surface and clear the airway. Having both adequate ROM and active movement for this task is important for providing safe playtime in prone (see Figure 9-4, D). Attention should also be directed toward the ipsilateral shoulder girdle and upper extremity to assess active movement toward midline with horizontal adduction and flexion, as well as ballistic shoulder movement. Movement of the forearm into supination and reach and grasp should also be examined. The trunk should be assessed for the ability to elongate with weight shifting. In addition, the pelvis and lower extremity on the ipsilateral side should be examined for ability to accept a weight-bearing load with proper biomechanical alignment.

Spinal motion should be assessed for restriction of extension, flexion, lateral flexion, and rotation.[40,56] Resting head posture and passive and active ROM should be documented in supine, prone, and sitting postures. Active ROM of the head and neck can be documented by using body landmarks while having the infant follow an object or person's face and voice or measured using goniometry.[55]

Examination of affected muscles should include palpation of the muscle for possible tumor and tonal quality. The affected muscles should also be examined for extensibility as well as function in a variety of postures. Developmental reflexes may be used to elicit automatic responses. Elicited voluntary movement should be documented as a response against gravity or with gravity eliminated, and the range through which active movement progresses is noted. Understanding motivational strategies and cultural differences and encouraging participation of the caregiver or parent during the examination are important. Examiners can interview the caregiver or parent to determine the infant's prior movement experiences. The infant's behavioral state during testing should be documented.

Hip asymmetry may be assessed by comparing leg lengths, assessing the thighs for extra skin folds, and measuring hip abduction. The incidence of hip dysplasia associated with muscular torticollis has been reported to be between 8% and 20% in children with CMT, most often occurring on the same side as the involved SCM muscle.[47,91,97] Infants with positive findings should be referred back to their primary care physician with a recommendation for an orthopedic consult.

PLAGIOCEPHALY AND FACIAL ASYMMETRY

Plagiocephaly (including head shapes of brachycephaly, scaphocephaly, and head shapes consistent with congenital syndromes) and facial asymmetry (facial scoliosis and hemihypoplasia) should be documented by photographs that include frontal, profile (left and right), posterior, vertex, and submental views that show head, shoulders, and torso. A tape measure is used to measure head circumference, and spreading or sliding calipers are used to document head asymmetry.

A narrative description of any noted asymmetries is used to document areas of occipital/parietal flattening; frontal/temporal flattening; head height differences; ear, orbit, and malar eminence alignment; bulging of parietal area; bossing of frontal area; eye size and alignment; canting of the mandible; narrowing of the temporal mandibular joint; alignment of the tongue and jaw with active movement or static posture; and any facial muscle asymmetry.[7,33,38,45,48,59,66,67]

In deformational plagiocephaly, the occiput and the frontal bone and the full face become deformed by molding forces induced by in utero constraint caused by compression of the fetal cranium between the maternal pelvic bone and lumbar sacral spine in the last trimester. The most common vertex presentation is left occipital anterior, which correlates with left CMT and right occipital/left frontal flattening. Plagiocephaly may be concordant (same side) or discordant (opposite side) to the muscular torticollis at birth. Acquired deformational plagiocephaly, which develops in the first 3 months of life, is always concordant with CMT.[52] The masticatory muscles are weaker on the affected SCM muscle side and may contribute to temporal mandibular joint dysfunction as it affects the formation of the joint.[11,15,34,44,49,58,59,83,89,97,99]

Associated risk factors that may predispose the infant to deformational plagiocephaly include oligohydramnios, uterine malformations, cephalohematoma, complication of the birth process, postnatal positioning, primiparity, male gender, and muscular torticollis.[6,7,27,75] In a cohort of 201 healthy infants, Peitsch and colleagues[78] reported the incidence of "localized" occipital cranial flattening (defined as transcranial asymmetry >4 mm) at 24 to 72 hours after delivery to be 13% in singleton births and 56% in twins, with greater frequency of occipital flattening observed on the right side. A significant associated finding was auricular deformation on the side of occipital flattening.

The progression of deformational plagiocephaly seems to halt around 6 months of age when intrinsic brain growth slows down and the infant begins to sit independently. However, a number of studies have demonstrated that cranial facial asymmetry present at 6 months of age has a high probability of persisting into adolescence and adulthood.[1,5,15,22,27,60,67,99] Bruneteau and Mulliken[7] and Mulliken and colleagues[75] reported muscular torticollis in 64% of infants with frontal deformational plagiocephaly and in 26% of infants with occipital deformational plagiocephaly.

Examination of infants with plagiocephaly should also include a screening assessment of vision, hearing, and infant vocalization. Automatic reactions, posture, and motor development should be thoroughly assessed using standardized tests. The Test of Infant Motor Performance (TIMP) is a good choice for infants from 32 weeks' gestational age through 4 to 5 months post term because a major construct assessed in this test is the infant's ability to independently control head position in a variety of spatial orientations.[10] The infant's primary behavior state during assessment, tolerance to stretching, and the ability to self-regulate should be

documented as well. Finally, referrals to other professionals should be made when appropriate.

PHYSICAL THERAPY INTERVENTIONS

Intervention is directed toward resolving each impairment or activity limitation identified in the physical therapy examination. Currently, most authors advocate conservative, nonoperative treatment for CMT. This conservative intervention typically consists of passive neck ROM exercises (Figure 9-6). It is equally important to include active assistive ROM, strengthening, and postural control exercises. Caregivers are instructed in how to carry and position the infant to promote elongation of the involved SCM as well as how to promote active contraction of the contralateral SCM. Caregivers are also instructed in developmental exercises (Figure 9-7) and how to reposition the child to prevent progression of deformational plagiocephaly (Figure 9-8).

Correct postural alignment and education about maintaining correct postural alignment are an integral part of rehabilitation, with the overall goals being to restore full joint and muscle ROM, to prevent occurrence of irreversible contractures, and to restore full muscle strength. Performing daily therapeutic exercises will also promote motor development. The duration of physical therapy intervention and outcomes of intervention depend on the cause of the torticollis, the initial deficit of passive neck rotation, and the age of the infant when intervention is initiated. Retrospective and prospective studies of passive neck ROM exercises have reported good to excellent results, with success rates ranging from 61% to 99% when intervention was initiated before 1 year of age.[12,14,16,17,18,19,20,29,32,73,98]

Published physical therapy intervention protocols for CMT vary considerably. They include neck stretching done twice daily, repeating each stretch five times with a 10-second hold;[32] manual stretching by physiotherapists three times a week, consisting of three repetitions of 15 manual stretches of the tight SCM, held for 1 second with a 10-second rest period combined with a prone sleeping home program;[18,21] two-person passive rotation neck stretching exercises carried out four to five times daily with at least 40 repetitions in each set;[29] and two-person neck stretching exercises of flexion, extension, rotation, and lateral flexion of 10 sets of each exercise with a 10-count hold for each repetition completed eight times each day.[12]

Contraindications for passive neck ROM include bony abnormalities, fracture, Down syndrome, myelomeningocele, a compromised circulatory or respiratory system, malignancy, osteomyelitis, tuberculosis, ruptured or lax ligaments, infection, shunt, or Arnold-Chiari malformation.[40] Caregivers providing ROM exercises should be instructed to observe for changes in vital signs, which may include color changes in the face, change in rate of breathing, eye rolling, perspiration, or nasal flaring and to stop exercises if any of these occur. Passive movement should be done slowly, and

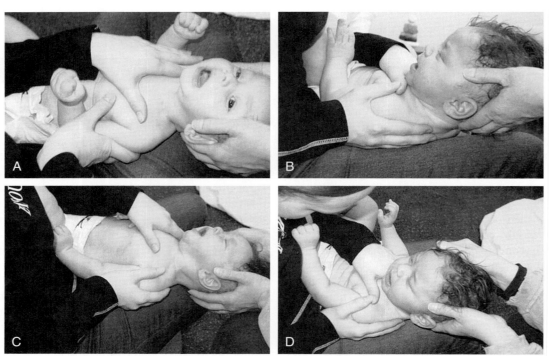

Figure 9-6   Two-person passive neck range of motion exercises for an infant with left congenital muscular torticollis. The shoulders are parallel to the pelvis, the pelvis is stabilized to prevent compensation during stretching by movement of the torso, and the shoulders are stabilized at the sternum, clavicle, ribs, and scapula by one person; the head and neck are free from the surface to allow for full neck motion; the second person holds under the occiput and applies a gentle traction to the cervical spine prior to performing neck motion to align the cervical spine in neutral and lengthen the muscles in the longitudinal axis. The holding hand on the left in the photos has been moved to show the tightness of the left sternocleidomastoid (SCM) muscle during the neck stretching exercises. **A,** Neck extension and asymmetric extension to the right to stretch the anterior neck muscles and left SCM muscle. **B,** Neck flexion and asymmetric flexion to the right to stretch the posterior cervical and left upper trapezius muscles. **C,** Neck lateral flexion right to stretch the left SCM muscle. **D,** Neck rotation left to stretch the left SCM muscle.

stretching should not be done against an infant actively resisting the stretch. Infants exhibiting discomfort may display avoidance behaviors including tense body posture, arching, facial grimacing, gaze aversion, crying, shutdown, or physiologic instability. Warm compresses, infant massage, and stretching after bath time may reduce infant stress. The use of a toy and setting up the environment can encourage the infant to look in the specific direction that promotes the desired neck muscle contraction and facilitate active stretch of the tight muscles.

BIOMECHANICS OF STRETCHING AND RECOMMENDED STRETCHING PROTOCOL

If one studies the origin and insertion of the SCM muscle and the biomechanics of this muscle, it will be clear that to properly stretch the SCM muscle, one should stabilize at the origin and insertion, moving the muscle into its elongated position. The elongated position can be attained with ipsilateral rotation, contralateral lateral flexion, and contralateral asymmetric extension from a starting point of neutral cervical spine alignment. The infant should be positioned supine with the head and neck free of the supporting surface

and with both shoulders stabilized and held parallel to a stable pelvis. The best stretching routine is done with two persons, especially when working with an older infant or toddler, in which one person stabilizes the shoulders and the other person stretches the neck (see Figure 9-6). Stretching should include all motions of the neck with particular attention to aligning the cervical spine with gentle traction prior to any motion. Anterior, posterior, and lateral neck muscles must all be stretched, and this can be done by including movements of rotation, lateral flexion, asymmetric flexion and extension, midline axial alignment rotation, lateral flexion, flexion, and extension. This stretching regimen should be done every 2 hours, if possible, for maximum benefit. Additional stretching exercises for the upper and lower extremities including the shoulder girdle and hip complex and the trunk should be included if impairments in shoulder and hip motion are present.[55,95]

To maintain the ROM, the infant must develop strength and active use of muscles that are antagonists to the involved SCM muscle to help develop good midline control. For example, the infant must be able to place the contralateral ear to the shoulder, flex and extend head toward the uninvolved side, and rotate the head and neck toward the involved

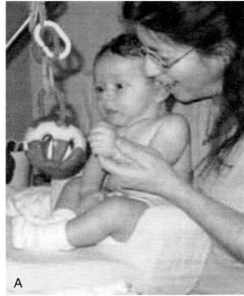

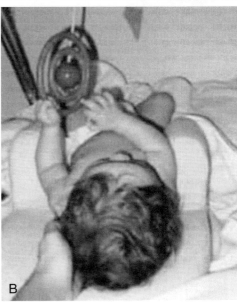

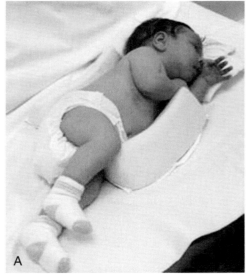

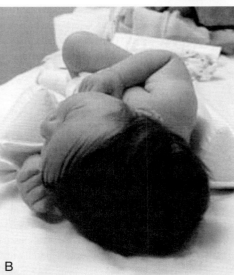

Figure 9-7 A 4-month-old infant with left congenital muscular torticollis. **A,** In a supported sitting position, the infant's head is prevented from tilting to the left and toy placement directs visual gaze to the left, promoting head rotation to the left while manual guidance is given to the ipsilateral upper extremity for forward flexion, external rotation, and forearm supination during reach and grasp. **B,** In a supine position, the toys are placed slightly to the left to promote rotation of the head to the left while the central axis alignment of head to body is maintained with sustained light traction on the occiput or base of the skull. The infant is exercising in an open kinetic chain to actively strengthen left upper extremity flexion, external rotation, elbow extension, horizontal abduction, and adduction, elbow extension, forearm supination, wrist and finger extension. It is important to establish normal resting muscle length and kinematic relationships of the thoracic spine, ribs, clavicle and movement between the scapulothoracic and glenohumeral area with growth and development.

Figure 9-8 A 2-month-old infant with left congenital muscular torticollis and deformational plagiocephaly (the left frontal region and the diagonal right occipital area are flattened, and the opposite areas are more full and bulging). **A,** Soft supports are placed anterior and posterior to the infant's trunk to allow the infant to be positioned in a three quarters side-lying position. **B,** A vertex view shows weight bearing of the calvarium on the fuller surface of the occiput while avoiding weight bearing on the already flattened area of the occiput.

side. By 15 months of age, the child can usually perform these movements with visual or verbal cueing if adequate passive neck ROM and strength are available.

ORTHOTIC DEVICES

Assistive devices that may be used to help obtain, maintain, or restrain motion include a fabricated to fit soft neck collar

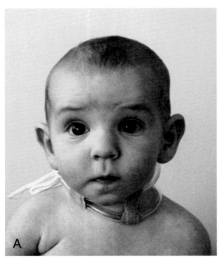

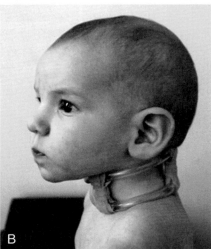

Figure 9-9   Five-month-old infant with left congenital muscular torticollis concordant with deformational plagiocephaly fitted with a tubular orthosis for torticollis (TOT Symmetric Designs Ltd., 125 Knott Place, Salt Spring Island, BC, Canada, V8K2M4). **A,** The anterior strut is shorter than the posterior strut and spans vertically from the anterior angle of the mandible to the midclavicle. **B,** The posterior strut is longer than the anterior strut and spans vertically from the occiput at the inferior nuchal line to the superior medial angle of the scapula where the levator scapulae muscle attaches.

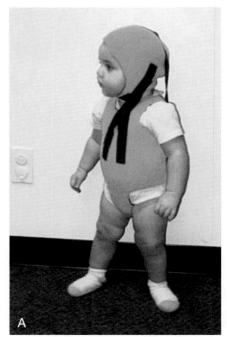

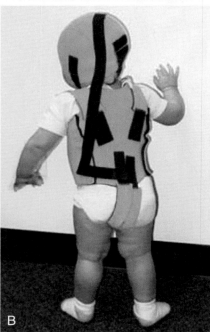

or a "tubular orthosis for torticollis" (TOT) collar (Figure 9-9). This collar was designed and developed at British Columbia's Children's Hospital. A contralateral torticollis postural positioning device may also be used (Figure 9-10).

Use of these devices is indicated for those infants or children who are 4 months of age or older, have a constant head tilt of 5° or greater for more than 80% of awake time, and perform all movement transitions and motor skills with a constant head tilt. In addition to these indications, children must have adequate passive ROM of the neck (at least 10° of lateral flexion toward the noninvolved side) or have lateral

Figure 9-10   A 15-month-old with right congenital muscular torticollis wearing a contralateral torticollis postural positioning device (CTPPD) consisting of a neoprene Velcro sensitive pediatric dynamic trunk orthosis and bathing cap (BENIK Corporation, 11871 Silverdale Way, NW, #107, Silverdale, Washington, 98383). The multiple strapping system was designed by and added by the author. **A,** The back strap simulates the pull of the contralateral upper trapezius muscle, and the front strap simulates the pull of the contralateral sternocleidomastoid muscle (preventing head tilt toward the side of the torticollis) and permits movement in the contralateral direction. **B,** The body vest provides stability to the shoulders and prevents ipsilateral shoulder elevation, whereas the strapping system provides a pull toward the contralateral side. This dynamic system promotes normal postural alignment, strength, and sensory motor development.

head righting reactions that demonstrate the ability to lift the head away from the involved side.[51]

The TOT collar should not be used as a passive support device. Possible complications include shoulder depression on the involved side, a shift in the shoulder girdle axis, and a lateral shift of the cervical spine. The infant should always be attended when using an orthotic device such as this and should never be allowed to wear these devices in a car seat or when sleeping. Vital signs should be observed at all times, and visual torticollis should be ruled out before these devices are used. The orthotics may be worn during awake time, and skin integrity should be checked when the orthosis is removed or at least every 2 hours.

INSTRUCTION TO CAREGIVERS

Reinforcing or improving neck ROM, strength, and postural control can be accomplished in any number of ways throughout the day. The caregiver should be taught how to carry and hold the infant, how to position the infant during sleep or nap time to create a prolonged stretch of the tight muscle and promote midline development, and how to present toys to the involved side to facilitate reaching in a horizontal and upward diagonal plane. The caregiver should also be taught to approach and feed the infant to promote looking toward the involved SCM muscle.[55] Home exercise programs can include eliciting balance reactions for strength development. Once an adequate amount of neck muscle strength is obtained, the exercises should be task specific so that the infant will use that strength to lift the head against gravity. This strengthening will promote development of transitional movements such as rolling and coming to sit from prone and supine.

MEDICAL MANAGEMENT

MANAGEMENT OF CONGENITAL MUSCULAR TORTICOLLIS

It is important for the physician, physical therapist, and family members to understand how CMT may progress over time because physical therapy intervention must be carried out consistently on a daily basis until all therapy goals are achieved. These goals include full passive neck muscle ROM with no regression during growth spurts over a continuous 3-month period. Once a child is discharged from physical therapy services, the child's pediatrician should include CMT and deformational plagiocephaly assessment in well-child follow-up visits to make sure there has been no regression of head tilt posture, loss of neck muscle ROM, changes in spinal alignment, or delay in motor skills.[79] Because deformational plagiocephaly may be disguised by hair, the pediatrician should palpate the head for volume asymmetries and note any abnormal dysplastic patterns of growth of the mandible as well as portions of the upper jaw and face related to

mastication and occlusal disharmonies. Referral to an orthodontist or oral facial surgeon may be necessary.

Surgical intervention may be considered for children who do not improve after 6 months of conservative intervention that includes manual stretching of the SCM muscle. Indications for surgical consideration include a residual head tilt, deficits of passive rotation and of lateral flexion of the neck greater than 15°, a tight muscular band or tumor of the SCM, hemihypoplasia, or a poor outcome to correction of the deformational plagiocephaly. Ultrasound studies can identify the type and extent of muscle fibrosis revealing the pathologic characteristics of the affected SCM muscle and whether surgical intervention would be helpful in relieving the persistent symptoms.[16,21,61,63,69,71,85]

The goals of surgery are to achieve a complete release of the shortened muscle and restore neck ROM and normal cervical spine mechanics, preserve neurovascular structures, and improve craniofacial asymmetry. Outcomes of surgical intervention are difficult to analyze because of the variety of surgical techniques used, the inconsistency in identifying homogeneous cohorts for type of SCM involvement (the site and extent of the disease within the muscle), and the variability in follow-up care including orthotics, physical therapy, and home exercise programs. Surgical procedures may include transection at one or more points of the SCM muscle body, total SCM excision, unipolar or bipolar releases at the tendinous attachments, functional SCM myoplasty, and more recently, endoscopic surgery. Common problems to each technique are damage to the facial, greater auricular, or spinal accessory nerves, visible scars, recurrent muscle band formation, loss of neck contour, and the recurrence of SCM contracture. Endoscopic surgery avoids many of these problems by allowing the surgeon to view the operative field directly with magnification, ensuring precise muscle fiber transection and preservation of the neurovascular structures. The best surgical outcomes have been reported in those children treated between 10 months and 5 years of age. Children who have releases before 1 year of age have the best chance of reversing their facial and skull deformities.[8,9,16,62,69,73]

PLAGIOCEPHALY

The key to successful management of deformational plagiocephaly associated with CMT is early diagnosis and intervention. Almost 80% of skull growth occurs before 12 months of age, affording only a small window of opportunity to provide nonsurgical treatment to correct the deformational plagiocephaly. A clinical pathway that includes the age of the infant at presentation, severity of the deformational plagiocephaly, resolution of the muscular torticollis, and response to conservative management (including an active repositioning program and neck exercises) will guide the practitioner in management of deformational plagiocephaly. These factors will also influence decisions regarding whether a cranial remodeling band may need to be prescribed.[23,57,66,67,68,79,80,82,96] To avoid postnatal progression of deformational plagiocephaly, Peitsch and colleagues[78] recommended that infants identified at birth or shortly thereafter with greater than 4 mm of cranial vault asymmetry be closely monitored and placed on an early sleep positioning program and supervised awake tummy time.

Caregivers and parents will need instruction and encouragement to help keep the infant from lying on the flattened areas of the skull. The ideal time for this active repositioning is in the first 3 months of life when the skull is most malleable and there is rapid intrinsic brain growth (see Figure 9-8). Repositioning may not be effective if the CMT persists, if the infant remains in a position of comfort that reinforces the plagiocephaly forces, or if the infant becomes too active during sleep to stay repositioned. Intrinsic brain growth slows at 5 to 6 months of age, and if plagiocephaly is still obvious at that time, the remaining plagiocephaly is unlikely to resolve without cranial remodeling band treatment.

The infant with plagiocephaly should undergo a reassessment for head shape on a monthly basis by the child's pediatrician or physical therapist (if the infant is having ongoing physical therapy). Changes in deformational plagiocephaly should be documented by use of anthropometric measures, photographs, and a written description. The child's head shape should be observed from multiple angles including from above (vertex view) as part of the standard examination, because observing the baby's face from a frontal (en face) perspective often fails to reveal the asymmetry. From a vertex position, the examiner can compare alignment of the orbits, zygoma, and ears in the frontal plane and assess the calvaria for frontal/temporal and contralateral occipital/parietal flattening. The skeletal structures may have a greater degree of asymmetry than the soft tissue drape that partially masks the underlying imbalances along with hair, which will cover the calvaria as the infant becomes older.[57,79]

The Dynamic Orthotic Cranioplasty® (DOC®) Band was the first approved Food and Drug Administration (FDA) class II neurology device generically known as a "cranial orthosis." It was developed as a proactive dynamic approach to treat deformational plagiocephaly in infants up to 24 months of age (Figure 9-11). The DOC Band is designed to redirect growth and thus improve craniofacial symmetry of the cranial vault, face, and cranial base by (1) applying an immediate mild holding pressure to the most anterior and posterior prominences of the cranium where growth is not desired and (2) allowing room for growth in the adjacent, flattened regions. Infants must be seen on a weekly to biweekly basis to make adjustments to the inner foam liner of the band. It is this process of continuously modifying the band and resultant corrective pressures that make the DOC Band treatment dynamic (Figure 9-12). This device offers a significant change from the original passive molding helmets in which the head grew into the helmet, taking on the shape of the helmet, with no change to the frontal deformation.

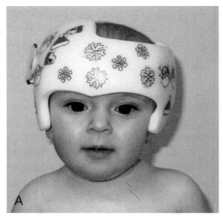

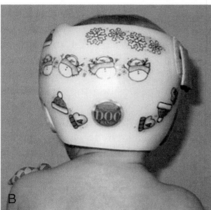

Figure 9-11 A 4-month-old infant with left congenital muscular torticollis and frontal deformational plagiocephaly wearing the DOC Band (Cranial Technologies, Inc., Phoenix, Arizona). **A,** En face view. **B,** Posterior view.

The DOC Band is worn 23 out of every 24 hours, with the exception of 1 hour for skin care and passive neck ROM exercises. The length of the treatment and the number of cranial bands necessary for correction will depend on the severity of the deformational plagiocephaly and the age at which treatment begins. The use of a cranial remodeling band has been reported to have excellent results in reshaping the heads of infants with deformational plagiocephaly and has a more effective outcome than repositioning.[22,67,82,96]

ANTICIPATED OUTCOMES OF PHYSICAL THERAPY INTERVENTION

Anticipated outcomes of physical therapy intervention are listed here in order of those more likely to be attained to those that are more difficult to attain:

- Full passive ROM of neck, trunk, and extremities (should be achieved before discharge from physical therapy)
- Active symmetric head rotation from midline to 80° left and right in supine, prone, sitting, and standing

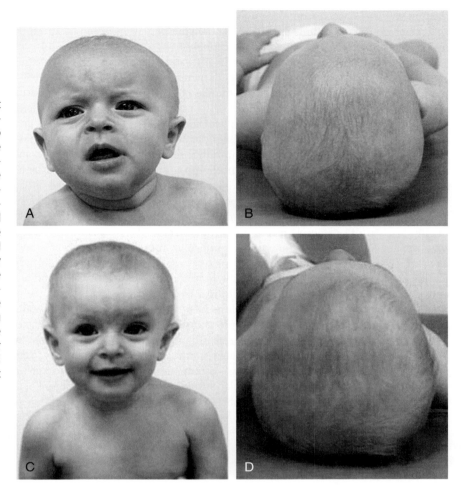

Figure 9-12 A 4-month-old infant with left congenital muscular torticollis and frontal deformational plagiocephaly. **A,** En face view prior to the start of DOC Band treatment. There is volume loss to the left frontal/temporal area and concordant right occipital/parietal area, recession of the left frontal and zygoma bones, posterior displacement of the ipsilateral ear, shortening of left vertical facial height, canting of the mandible, and developing hemihypoplasia. **B,** Vertex view before the DOC Band treatment showing the frontal and maxillary horizons with concordant asymmetry and flattening of the right occipital area. **C,** Same infant at 12 months of age after DOC Band treatment and endoscopic surgery at 10 months of age to release the left sternomastoid muscle showing improved cranial facial symmetry and neck muscle length. **D,** Vertex view at 12 months of age after DOC Band treatment showing symmetric frontal and maxillary horizons and fullness to the right occipital area.

- Active midline head-to-trunk alignment during static and dynamic play with only intermittent head tilts toward the involved side
- Normal antigravity trunk and neck strength with symmetry between uninvolved and involved sides
- Symmetry between left and right sides in righting and equilibrium reactions in both the horizontal and vertical planes
- Ability to assume head tilt toward the uninvolved side with or without rotation to the involved side during play activities involving either static or dynamic postures

Newborns are biologically constructed to develop symmetrically, although growth and development by design may cause different degrees of asymmetry to develop. This asymmetry may be partially compensated for or, conversely, made worse by activity, the environment, or internal structural restrictions. As an example, when the healthy full-term newborn infant is placed in the prone position with the elbows close to the trunk, with hips and knees flexed because of physiologic flexion, there is downward force on the shoulders, sternum, and clavicles, which actually helps to stabilize the attachment of the neck muscles anteriorly. As the infant lifts to extend and rotate the head to clear the airway, the infant is able to self-impose a stretch of anterior neck muscles, the SCM muscle, and the upper trapezius muscle. In the healthy infant, this self-initiated activity self-treats any neck tightness and facilitates symmetric development of the pelvis, trunk, shoulder, upper extremities, and neck. Early reflexes such as the asymmetric tonic neck reflex (ATNR) and Gallant and arm passage reflex help to reinforce both stretching and strengthening of the neck, shoulder girdle, and trunk. In the child with CMT, however, where there is neck motion restriction, these early reflexes can reinforce postural asymmetries of the pelvis, trunk, shoulder, upper extremities, and neck.

Other factors that may contribute to the persistence of asymmetry in the child with CMT are delays in motor development, back sleeping with no supervised tummy time to offset the constant supine positioning, and spending extended amounts of time semireclined in containment equipment such as car seats, infant seats, infant carriers, bouncy seats, or swings. Infants who do not spend time in prone and who spend too much time in containment equipment may have no opportunity to alter the surface against which their craniums lie, thus potentially perpetuating or imposing a deformational plagiocephaly as well as preventing development of neck strength and head control.[65,74] Other factors that may cause an increase in the head tilt with or without actual SCM muscle contracture are excessive spontaneous muscle fiber discharge in the SCM muscle, teething, ear infections, acquisition of new motor skills, crying, fatigue, stress, and illness. Faulty central nervous system (CNS) motor programming related to muscle tone, joint function, learned motor programs or autonomic reactions may also cause an increase in the torticollis posture. When the torticollis posture is not corrected, it may be due to unresolved SCM muscle contracture, rebound or sensory defensive positioning from overstretching, weakness of the antagonists, or abnormal muscle length-tension relationships.[55]

Infants with CMT may have atypical motor planning and execution because of movement disturbances and musculoskeletal imbalances that developed in utero or during the first year of life. The anatomic and physiologic bases for variability common to motor learning in the first postnatal year are restricted, causing neuromotor patterns of asymmetry to develop that may cause motor delays in the infant.[84,90,94] Understanding the relationship between movement disturbances and the associated effect of an abnormally shaped calvaria on the underlying cortex in children has been the focus of several recent studies.[2,4,41,70,77]

SUMMARY

This chapter discussed the management of congenital muscular torticollis and deformational plagiocephaly. A fibrotic and shortened SCM muscle is the most typical finding in CMT along with a head tilt toward the involved SCM muscle. The etiology and pathogenesis of CMT is not completely understood but may be related to breech presentation, birth trauma, in utero constraint, nuchal cord, or use of suction and forceps at birth. Sonography and physical examination can confirm the pathology of CMT. Most cases of infants with CMT can be successfully managed with conservative treatment utilizing passive and active neck stretching exercises, active repositioning, neck strengthening, and postural control exercises to encourage the head to turn toward the involved SCM muscle side. The severity of the neck rotation restriction, the amount and distribution of fibrosis in the SCM muscle, and the age of the infant at initiation of physical therapy intervention will influence the success rate of conservative management. Surgical intervention may be indicated for infants who do not respond to conservative treatment. A cranial remodeling band may be necessary to correct deformational plagiocephaly associated with CMT. Motor control and postural development as well as prevention and treatment of facial asymmetry and deformational plagiocephaly should be emphasized along with intervention of CMT.

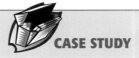

CASE STUDY

"Alex"

Alex was referred to physical therapy at the age of 3 months for left CMT and deformational plagiocephaly. She was born by cesarean section at 38 weeks' gestation. She was vertex presentation, and her mother remarked she had carried her low in her pelvis. Her parents became aware of their daughter's abnormal head shape a month after she was born and brought it to the attention of their pediatrician. Alex was a back sleeper with her head always rotated to her right. Her parents reported they tried to do as their pediatrician directed, to encourage her to look to her left. Alex would not stay repositioned and had no interest in looking to the left. When her parents determined that the head shape and neck mobility were not improving, their pediatrician referred Alex for physical therapy.

Upon the initial examination, the clinical findings revealed a 65% loss of passive and active neck ROM for right lateral flexion, left rotation, and asymmetric flexion/extension to the right of midline. The torso had limited rotation to the left and lateral flexion to the right, and the left upper extremity was limited in horizontal adduction, external rotation, shoulder flexion, forearm supination, and wrist extension. Alex was unable to maintain midline postural alignment in supine, prone, or sitting, and she did not demonstrate righting reactions of the head, neck, or trunk to her right side. She was unable to lift her head off the surface in prone to clear her airway. Alex's mother reported she did not like the prone position. Palpation of the neck

muscles revealed she had tightness throughout the left SCM muscle, hyoid muscles, left scalene muscles and left upper trapezius (see Figure 9-4). She had minimal reciprocal kicking, truncal curvature with convexity to the right, windswept hips, and no left upper extremity ballistic shoulder movement or movements toward the midline. The left upper extremity was postured in internal rotation, shoulder elevation, and forearm pronation, and the hand was fisted. She had a persistent asymmetric tonic reflex (see Figure 9-5). She was not able to bear any weight on her upper extremities or grasp a toy. A pacifier was used to help calm Alex, and her mother reported her as being "moody." She was being nursed, and the mother reported she had more difficulty with nursing her on the right breast. She was unable to track a toy or her mother's face to the left of midline in supine.

Alex had a deformational plagiocephaly with right occipital/parietal flattening, right anterior ear shift, right anterior orbit shift, flattening of the left frontal/temporal area, increased posterior head height, and left narrowed fissure. The anterior fontanel was open to palpation, and there was no suture ridging. Her cephalic index was 82.31% (1.92 standard deviations above the norm for her age and sex; the cephalic index is the relationship of the width of the head to the length of the head). She had 14 mm of cranial vault asymmetry, 3 mm of cranial base asymmetry, and 4 mm of facial asymmetry.

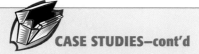

CASE STUDIES—cont'd

Physical therapy intervention began at 3 months of age and included passive and active neck ROM exercises, which the parents carried out on a daily basis. The parents were also instructed in how to position Alex during nap and sleep time to reduce the plagiocephaly. Her cranial vault asymmetry decreased by 4 mm with the positioning program by 5 months of age, but then no further decrease in asymmetry was measured. The frontal deformation was still apparent, and the family decided to pursue DOC Band treatment.

Alex was in the DOC Band for 4 months, from age 6 to 10 months. She had excellent correction of the cranial vault asymmetry at the completion of the DOC Band treatment, as shown in Figure 9-13.

The muscular torticollis required ongoing physical therapy with multiple visits each week when Alex was in growth spurts and losing neck ROM. Full passive neck ROM was achieved by 9 months of age, although this would regress with growth spurts. Alex still had an intermittent head tilt, poor sense of visual and postural midline, and

weakness of the right neck muscles. Once Alex completed the DOC Band treatment, a TOT collar, a contralateral torticollis posture bracing system (CTPBS), and taping were used to assist her with developing neck strength, midline postural control, and automatic reactions (Figure 9-14). The CTPBS prevented the left head tilt from continuing to occur as Alex developed transitional skills of pull to stand, squat to stand, cruising, creeping, walking, and stair climbing.

The parents carried out a daily exercise routine that included neck ROM exercises every 2 hours with diaper changes, neck-strengthening

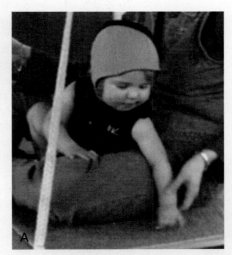

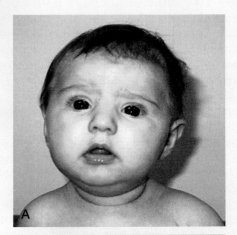

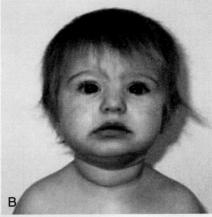

Figure 9-13   **A,** Alex at 3 months of age. She has left congenital muscular torticollis (CMT) and frontal deformational plagiocephaly and exhibits characteristic cranial facial asymmetries, tilted head posture left, and contralateral head rotation right. **B,** Alex at 12 months of age after DOC Band treatment and physical therapy intervention for left CMT.

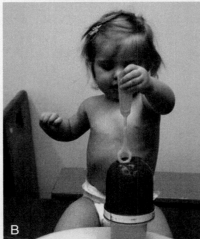

Figure 9-14   **A,** Alex wears a contralateral torticollis postural positioning device (CTPPD), consisting of a neoprene Velcro-sensitive pediatric dynamic trunk orthosis and bathing cap with multiple strapping system. The CTPPD maintains the correct postural alignment as she bears weight on an extended arm to the ipsilateral side. **B,** This play activity promotes correct alignment of the scapula, humerus, forearm, and wrist during reach and grasp. Placement of the toy on a supporting surface promotes downward gaze, elongating the neck extensors and strengthening the neck flexors in midline.

Continued

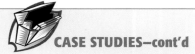

CASE STUDIES—cont'd

exercises (especially for the ability to lift the head off the surface using right neck muscles), and general ROM exercises with special attention to the left shoulder girdle, left upper extremity, torso for elongation of the left side, and ability to weight shift over the left hip. Other home program exercises included activities that encouraged Alex to look to her left and to look left and upward with reach, making sure she tilted her head to the right with rotation to the left. In addition, activities to promote balance reactions were carried out, and the parents carried and positioned her to prevent a left head tilt and shortening of the left side of her torso.

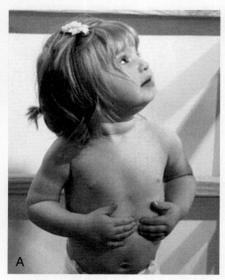

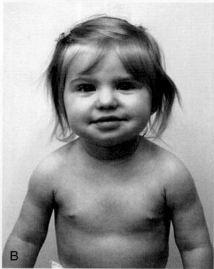

Figure 9-15 Alex was discharged from physical therapy at 15 months of age. **A,** Alex demonstrating an ability to adopt posture opposite of congenital muscular torticollis (CMT) posture as she is able to look left and upward with head tilt right. **B,** Alex exhibiting no apparent plagiocephaly, cranial facial asymmetries, head tilt, or other postural deformities associated with CMT.

At 15 months of age, Alex could imitate and follow directions to put her right ear to her shoulder. She still had a mild strength difference in her neck muscles with the left slightly more responsive than the right. She was age-appropriate with her motor skills and could maintain a midline head posture alignment. The timing and sequencing of her automatic reactions were appropriate except when she was fatigued. She was discharged from physical therapy at this time (Figure 9-15).

Alex's parents continue to carry out a home exercise program for Alex and will continue with physical therapy rechecks if any regression is observed in passive neck ROM.

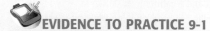

EVIDENCE TO PRACTICE 9-1

CASE STUDY "ALEX"

It is important to provide therapeutic strategies of physical therapy, orthotic devices, and surgical management in treatment of congenital muscular torticollis (CMT) and deformational plagiocephaly (DP). Preventive counseling of parents on positioning, handling, nursing, and bottle feeding is important to prevent or minimize the risks of rotational head preference and to diminish or correct deformational plagiocephaly. Generalized asymmetries in posture and movements (molded baby syndrome) and localized asymmetries of neck muscle imbalance (CMT) and misshapen head (DP) may lead to long-term functional asymmetry resulting in deformity of the musculoskeletal system.

Risk factors for DP identified at birth by van Vlimmeren et al. (2007) were male gender, firstborn birth rank, and brachycephaly and at 8 weeks; the risk factor included male gender, firstborn birth rank, positional preference when sleeping, head to the same side on chest of drawers, only bottle feeding, positioning to the same side during bottle feeding, tummy time when awake < 3 times per day, and slow achievement of motor skills.

Collett, B., Breiger, D., King, D., Cunningham, M., & Speltz, M. (2005). Neurodevelopment implications of deformational plagiocephaly. *Developmental and Behavioral Pediatrics, 26,* 379–389.

Sarwark, J., & Aubin, C. E. (2007). Considerations of the immature spine. *Journal of Bone and Joint Surg (American), 89,* 8–13.

van Vlimmeren, L. A., Helders, P. J. M., van Adrichem, L. N. A., & Engelbert, R. H. H. (2006). Torticollis and plagiocephaly in infancy: Therapeutic strategies. *Pediatric Rehabilitation, 9,* 40–46.

van Vlimmeren, L. A., van der Graaf, Y., & Boere-Boonekamp, M. M. (2007). Risk factors for deformational plagiocephaly at birth and at 7 weeks of age: A prospective cohort study. *Pediatrics, 119,* 408–418, 2007.

van Vlimmeren, L. A., van der Graaf, Y., Boere-Boonekamp, M. M., L'Hoir, M. P., Helders, P. J., & Engelbert, R. H. (2008). Effect of pediatric physical therapy on deformational plagiocephaly in children with positional preference: A randomized control trial. *Archives of Pediatrics and Adolescent Medicine, 162,* 712–718.

Wall, V., & Glass, R. (2006). Mandibular asymmetry and breastfeeding problems: Experience from 11 cases. *Journal of Human Lactation, 22,* 328–334.

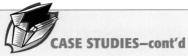

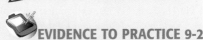 **CASE STUDIES—cont'd**

 EVIDENCE TO PRACTICE 9-2

CASE STUDY "ALEX"

The "gold standard" of care in treatment of CMT based on the current literature to assess the deficit of passive neck rotation–head rotation of the chin to reach the shoulder assumes that the sternocleidomastoid muscle has normal resting length. The treatment length is associated with the "type" of SCM presentation (sternomastoid tumor-SMT, muscular torticollis-MT, and postural torticollis-POST), passive rotation deficit of the SCM muscle and the age at presentation. There is no agreement in protocols of treatment or outcomes of the various studies.

Exercises for treatment of CMT should focus on active assistive exercises to facilitate muscle activity during functional activities, "corrective" program for the entire body to improve mobility of the spine, strengthen muscles, improve posture, promote circulation and ANS regulation, improve motor skills, balance, sensory motor integration, lessen craniofacial asymmetry, address oral-motor/feeding, speech language, social-emotional and cognitive learning problems. Attention should be placed to correcting a head rotation preference and improving tummy time skills.

Ohman et al. compared 82 infants with CMT and 40 healthy infants using the Alberta Infant Motor scale (AIMS) and found the risk of delay more strongly associated with little or no time in prone when awake than with CMT.

Ohman, A., Nillsson, S., & Lagerkvist, A. L. (2009). Are infants with torticollis at risk of a delay in early motor milestones compared with a control group of healthy infants? *Developmental Medicine and Child Neurology, 51,* 545–550.

Ohman, A. M., & Beckung, E. (2008). Reference values for range of motion and muscle function of neck in infants. *Pediatric Physical Therapy, 20,* 53–58.

Arbogast, K., Purushottam, B., Gholve, A., et al. (2007). Normal cervical spine range of motion in children 3-12 years old. *Spine, 10,* 309–315.

EVIDENCE TO PRACTICE 9-3

CASE STUDY "ALEX"

Reliability in method makes two-dimensional measurements a valid tool for daily physical therapy practice in measuring changes in craniofacial asymmetry in cases of deformational plagiocephaly to evaluate the effectiveness of therapy intervention. Anthropometric measurements should be done twice a month for infants 0 to 6 months of age and once a month for infants 6 to 24 months of age based on the growth and development of the growing craniofacial system. Measurements may be taken using a spreading or sliding caliper or by making a head ring using low-temperature plastic to mold the shape of the infant's head.

Klackenberg, E. P., Elfving, B., Haglunct-Akerlind, Y., & Carlberg, E. B. (2005). Intra-rater reliability in measuring range of motion in infants with congenital muscular torticollis. *Advances in Physiotherapy, 7,* 84–91.

Mortenson, P. A., & Steinbok, P. (2006). Quantifying positional plagiocephaly: Reliability and validity of anthropometric measurements. *Journal of Craniofacial Surgery, 17,* 413–419.

Ohman, A., & Beckung, E. (2005). Functional and cosmetic status in children treated for congenital muscular torticollis as infants. *Advances in Physiotherapy, 7,* 135–140.

Van Adrichem, L. N., van Vlimmeren, L. A., Cadanova, D., et al. (2008). Validation of a simple method for measuring cranial deformities. *Journal of Cranialfacial Surgery, 19,* 15–21

REFERENCES

1. Argenta, L. C., David, L. R., Wilson, J. A., & Bell, W. O. (1996). An increase in infant cranial deformity with supine sleeping position. *Journal of Craniofacial Surgery, 7,* 5–11.

2. Balan, P., Kushnerenko, E., Sahlin, P., Huotilainen, M., Naatanen, R., & Hukki, J. (2002). Auditory ERPs reveal brain dysfunction in infants with plagiocephaly. *Journal of Craniofacial Surgery, 13,* 520–525.

3. Ballock, R. T., & Song, K. M. (1996). The prevalence of non-muscular causes of torticollis in children. *Journal of Pediatric Orthopaedics, 16,* 500–504.

4. Binder, H., Eng, G. B., Gaiser, J. F., & Koch, B. (1987). Congenital muscular torticollis: Results of conservative management with long-term follow-up in 85 cases. *Archives of Physical Medicine and Rehabilitation, 68,* 222–225.

5. Boere-Boonekamp, M. M., & van der Linden-Kuiper, L. T. (2001). Positional preference: Prevalence in infants and follow-up after two years. *Pediatrics, 107,* 339–343.

6. Bredenkamp, J. K., Hoover, L. A., Berke, G. S., & Shaw, A. (1990). Congenital muscular torticollis. *Archives of Otolaryngology Head & Neck Surgery, 116,* 212–216.

7. Bruneteau, R. J., & Mulliken, J. B. (1992). Frontal plagiocephaly: Synostotic, compensational, or deformational. *Plastic and Reconstructive Surgery, 89,* 21–33.

8. Burstein, F. D., & Cohen, S. R. (1998). Endoscopic surgical treatment for congenital muscular torticollis. *Plastic and Reconstructive Surgery, 101,* 20–26.

9. Burstein, F. D. (2004). Long term experience with endoscopic surgical treatment for congenital muscular torticollis in infants and children: A review of 85 cases. *Plastic and Reconstructive Surgery, 114*, 491–493.

10. Campbell, S. K., Kolobe, T. H. A., Osten, E. T., Lenke, M., & Girolami, G. L. (1995). Construct validity of the Test of Infant Motor Performance. *Physical Therapy, 75*, 585–596.

11. Captier, G., Leboucq, N., Bigorre, M., Canovas, F., Bonnel, F., Bonnafe, A., & Montoya, P. (2003). Plagiocephaly: Morphometry of skull base asymmetry. *Surgery, Radiology and Anatomy, 25*, 226–233.

12. Celayir, A. C. (2000). Congenital muscular torticollis: Early and intensive treatment is critical, a prospective study. *Pediatric International, 42*, 504–507.

13. Chan, Y. L., Cheng, J. C. Y., & Metreweli, C. (1992). Ultrasonography of congenital muscular torticollis. *Pediatric Radiology, 22*, 356–360.

14. Chang, P. Y., Tan, C. K., Huang, Y. F., Sheu, J. C., Wang, N. L., Yeh, M. L., & Chen, C. C. (1996). Torticollis: A long term follow up study. *Acta Paediatrica Taiwanica, 37*, 173–177.

15. Chang, P. Y., Chang, N. C., Perng, D. B., Chien, Y. W., & Huang, F. Y. (2001). Computer-aided measurement and grading of cranial asymmetry in children with and without torticollis. *Clinical Orthodontics and Research, 4*, 200–205.

16. Cheng, J. C. Y., Tang, S. P., & Chen, T. M. K. (1999). Sternomastoid pseudotumor and congenital muscular torticollis in infants: A prospective study of 510 cases. *Journal of Pediatrics, 134*, 712–716.

17. Cheng, J. C. Y., & Au, A. W. Y. (1994). Infantile torticollis: A review of 624 cases. *Journal of Pediatric Orthopaedics, 14*, 802–808.

18. Cheng, J. C. Y., Wong, M. W. N., Tang, S. P., Chen, T. M. K., Shum, S. L. F., & Wong, E. M. C. (2001). Clinical determinants of the outcome of manual stretching in the treatment of congenital muscular torticollis in infants. *Journal of Bone and Joint Surgery, 83*, 679–687.

19. Cheng, J. C. Y., Tang, S. P., Chen, T. M. K., Wong, M. W. N., & Wong, E. M. C. (2000a). The clinical presentation and outcome of treatment of congenital muscular torticollis in infants: A study of 1,086 cases. *Journal of Pediatric Surgery, 35*, 1091–1096.

20. Cheng, J. C. Y., & Tang, S. P. (1999). Outcome of surgical treatment of congenital muscular torticollis. *Clinical Orthopaedics and Related Research, 362*, 190–200.

21. Cheng, J. C. Y., Metreweli, C., Chen, T. M. K., & Tang, S. P. (2000b). Correlation of ultrasonographic imaging of congenital muscular torticollis with clinical assessment in infants. *Ultrasound in Medicine & Biology, 26*, 1237–1241.

22. Clarren, S. K. (1981). Plagiocephaly and torticollis: Etiology, natural history, and helmet treatment. *Journal of Pediatrics, 98*, 92–95.

23. Clarren, S. K. (1979). Helmet treatment for plagiocephaly and congenital muscular torticollis. *Journal of Pediatrics, 94*, 43–46.

24. Clarren, S. K., & Smith, D. W. (1977). Congenital deformities. *Pediatric Clinics of North America, 24*, 665–677.

25. Cooperman, D. (1997). Differential diagnosis of torticollis in children. *Physical and Occupational Therapy in Pediatrics, 17*, 1–11.

26. Coventry, M. B., & Harris, L. E. (1959). Congenital muscular torticollis in infancy. *The Journal of Bone and Joint Surgery, 41*, 815–822.

27. Danby, P. M. (1962). Plagiocephaly in some 10 year old children. *Archives of Disease in Childhood, 37*, 500–504.

28. Davids, J. R., Wenger, D. R., & Mubarak, S. J. (1993). Congenital muscular torticollis: Sequela of intrauterine or perinatal compartment syndrome. *Journal of Pediatric Orthopaedics, 13*, 141–147.

29. Demirbilek, S., & Atayurt, H. F. (1999). Congenital muscular torticollis and sternomastoid tumor: Results of nonoperative treatment. *Journal of Pediatric Surgery, 34*, 549–551.

30. Dunn, P. M. (1976). Congenital postural deformities. *British Medical Bulletin, 32*, 71–76.

31. Dunn, P. M. (1974). Congenital sternomastoid torticollis: An intrauterine postural deformity. *Archives of Disease in Childhood, 49*, 824–825.

32. Emery, C. (1994). The determinants of treatment duration for congenital muscular torticollis. *Physical Therapy, 74*, 921–929.

33. Farkas, L. G., Posnick, J. C., & Hreczko, T. M. (1992). Anthropometric growth study of the head. *Cleft Palate-Craniofacial Journal, 29*, 303–308.

34. Ferguson, J. W. (1993). Surgical correction of the facial deformities secondary to untreated congenital muscular torticollis. *Journal of Cranio-Maxillo-Facial Surgery, 21*, 137–142.

35. Fulford, G. E., & Brown, J. K. (1976). Position as a cause of deformity in children with cerebral palsy. *Developmental Medicine and Child Neurology, 18*, 305–314.

35a. Golden K. A., Beals S. P., Littlefield T. R., Pomatto J. K. (1999). Sternocleidomastoid imbalance versus congenital muscular torticollis: their relationship to positional plagiocephaly. *Cleft Palate Cranioface J, 36*, 256–261.

36. Graham, J. M. (1988). *Smith's recognizable pattern of human deformation* (2nd ed.). Philadelphia: WB Saunders.

37. Graham, J. M. (1998). Craniofacial deformation. *Bailliere's Clinical Paediatrics, 6*, 293–316.

38. Graham, J. M., Kreutzman, J., Earl, D., Halberg, A., Samayoa, C., & Guo, X. (2005a). Deformational brachycephaly in supine-sleeping infants. *Journal of Pediatrics, 146*, 253–257.

39. Graham, J. M., Gomez, M., Halberg, A., Earl, D., Kreutzman, J., Cui, J., & Guo, X. (2005b). Management of deformational plagiocephaly: Repositioning versus orthotic therapy. *Journal of Pediatrics, 146*, 258–262.

40. Greenman, P. E. (1989). *Principles of manual medicine*. Baltimore: Williams & Wilkins.

41. Habal, M. B., Leimkuehler, T. L., Chambers, C., Scheuerle, J., & Guilford, A. M. (2003). Avoiding the sequela associated with deformational plagiocephaly. *Journal of Craniofacial Surgery, 14*, 430–437.

42. Hamanishi, C., & Tanaka, S. (1994). Turned head-adducted hip-truncal curvature syndrome. *Archives of Disease in Childhood, 70*, 515–519.

43. Ho, B. C. S., Lee, H. E., & Singh, K. (1999). Epidemiology, presentation and management of congenital muscular torticollis. *Singapore Medical Journal, 40,* 675–679.

44. Hidaka, J., Morishita, T., & Nakata, S. (1996). The relationship between cranial facial asymmetry and bilateral functional balance of the masticatory muscles. *Journal of the Japanese Orthodontic Society, 55,* 329–336.

45. Hollier, L., Kim, J., Grayson, B. H., & McCarthy, J. G. (2000). Congenital muscular torticollis and associated craniofacial changes. *Plastic and Reconstructive Surgery, 105,* 827–835.

46. Hsu, T. C., Wang, C. L., Wong, M. K., Hsu, K. H., Tang, F. T., & Chen, H. T. (1999). Correlation of clinical and ultrasonographic features in congenital muscular torticollis. *Archives of Physical Medicine and Rehabilitation, 80,* 637–641.

47. Hsieh, Y. Y., Tsai, F. J., Lin, C. C., Chang, F. C. C., & Tsai, C. H. (2000). Breech deformation complex in neonates. *Journal of Reproductive Medicine, 45,* 933–935.

48. Huang, M. H. S., Mouradian, W. E., Cohen, S. R., & Gruss, J. S. (1998). The differential diagnosis of abnormal head shapes: Separating craniosynostosis from positional deformities and normal variants. *Cleft Palate-Craniofacial Journal, 35,* 204–211.

49. Huang, M. H. S., Gruss, J. S., Clarren, S. K., et al. (1996). The differential diagnosis of posterior plagiocephaly: True lambdoid synostosis versus positional molding. *Plastic and Reconstructive Surgery, 98,* 765–774.

50. Huang, C. S., Cheng, H. C., Lin, W. Y., Liou, J. W., & Chen, Y. R. (1995). Skull morphology affected by different sleep positions in infancy. *Cleft Palate-Craniofacial Journal, 32,* 413–419.

51. Jacques, C., & Karmel-Ross, K. (1997). The use of splinting in conservative and post-operative treatment of congenital muscular torticollis. *Physical and Occupational Therapy in Pediatrics, 17,* 81–90.

52. Jones, P. G. (1968). *Torticollis in infancy and childhood.* Springfield, IL: Charles C Thomas.

53. Kane, A. A., Mitchell, L. E., Craven, K. P., & Marsh, J. L. (1996). Observations on a recent increase in plagiocephaly without synostosis. *Pediatrics, 97,* 877–885.

54. Kapandji, I. A. (1974). *The physiology of the joints, Vol 3. The trunk and vertebral column* (2nd ed.). London: Churchill Livingstone.

55. Karmel-Ross, K., & Lepp, M. (1997). Assessment and treatment of children with congenital muscular torticollis. *Physical and Occupational Therapy in Pediatrics, 17,* 21–67.

56. Kautz, S. M., & Skaggs, D. L. (1998). Getting an angle on spinal deformities. *Contemporary Pediatrics, 15,* 111–128.

57. Kelly, K. M., Littlefield, T. R., Pomatto, J. K., Ripley, C. E., Beals, S. P., & Aoba, T. J. (1999). Importance of early recognition and treatment of deformational plagiocephaly with orthotic cranioplasty. *Cleft Palate Craniofacial Journal, 36,* 127–130.

58. Kondo, E., & Aoba, T. (1999). Case report of malocclusion with abnormal head posture and TMJ symptoms. *American Journal of Orthodontics and Dentofacial Orthopedics, 116,* 481–493.

59. Kreiborg, S., Moller, E., & Bjork, A. (1985). Skeletal and functional craniofacial adaptations in plagiocephaly. *Journal of Craniofacial Genetics, 1,* 199–210.

60. Leung, Y. K., & Leung, P. C. (1987). The efficacy of manipulative treatment for sternomastoid tumors. *Journal of Bone and Joint Surgery, 69,* 473–478.

60a. Liebenson C. (Ed.). (2007). *Rehabilitation of the Spine: A. Practitioner's Manual* (2nd ed.). Philadelphia: Lippincott Williams and Wilkins.

61. Lin, J. N., & Chou, M. L. (1997). Ultrasonographic study of sternocleidomastoid muscle in the management of congenital muscular torticollis. *Journal of Pediatric Surgery, 32,* 1648–1651.

62. Ling, C. M. (1976). The influence of age on the result of open sternomastoid tenotomy in muscular torticollis. *Clinical Orthopaedics, 116,* 142–148.

63. Ling, C. M., & Low, Y. S. (1972). Sternomastoid tumor and muscular torticollis. *Clinical Orthopaedics, 86,* 144–150.

64. Lingeman, R. E. (1998). Surgical anatomy. In C. W. Cummings, F. M. Fredrickson, L. A. Harker, C. J. Krause, D. E. Schuller, & M. A. Richardson, (Eds.), *Otolaryngology: Head and neck surgery* (3rd ed., *Vol. 3,* p. 1680). St. Louis, MO: Mosby.

65. Littlefield, T. R., Kelly, K. M., Reiff, J. L., & Pomatto, J. K. (2003). Car seats, infant carriers, and swings: Their role in deformational plagiocephaly. *Journal of Prosthetics and Orthotics, 15,* 102–106.

66. Littlefield, T. R., Reiff, J. L., & Rekate, H. L. (2001). Diagnosis and management of deformational plagiocephaly. *BNI Quarterly, 17,* 18–25.

67. Littlefield, T. R., Beals, S. P., Manwaring, K. H., et al. (1998). Treatment of craniofacial asymmetry with DOC. *Journal of Craniofacial Surgery, 9,* 11–17.

68. Loveday, B. P. T., & de Chalain, T. B. (2001). Active counterpositioning or orthotic device to treat positional plagiocephaly. *Journal of Craniofacial Surgery, 12,* 308–313.

69. Maricevic, A., & Erceg, M. (1997). Results of surgical treatment of CMT. *Lijecnicki Vjesnik, 119,* 106–109.

70. Miller, R. I., & Clarren, S. K. (2000). Long term developmental outcomes in patients with deformational plagiocephaly. *Pediatrics, 105,* E26.

71. Minamitani, K., Inoue, A., & Okuno, T. (1990). Results of surgical treatment of muscular torticollis for patients 6 years of age. *Journal of Pediatric Orthopaedics, 10,* 754–759.

72. McDaniel, A., Hirsch, B. E., Kornblut, A., & Armbrustmacher, V. M. (1984). Torticollis in infancy and adolescence. *Ear, Nose and Throat Journal, 63,* 478–487.

73. Morrison, D. L., & MacEwen, G. D. (1982). Congenital muscular torticollis: Observations regarding clinical findings, associated conditions, and results of treatment. *Journal of Pediatric Orthopaedics, 2,* 500–505.

74. Monson, R. M., Deitz, J., & Kartin, D. (2003). The relationship between awake positioning and motor performance among infants who slept supine. *Pediatric Physical Therapy, 15,* 196–203.

75. Mulliken, J. B., Vander Woude, D. L., Hansen, M., LaBrie, R. A., & Scott, R. M. (1999). Analysis of posterior plagiocephaly: Deformational versus synostotic. *Plastic and Reconstructive Surgery, 103*, 371–380.

76. Najarian, S. P. (1999). Infant cranial molding and sleep position: Implications for primary care. *Journal of Pediatric Health Care, 13*, 173–177.

77. Panchal, J., Amirsheybani, H., Gurwitch, R., Cook, V., Francel, P., Neas, B., & Levine, N. (2001). Neurodevelopment in children with single-suture craniosynostosis and plagiocephaly without synostosis. *Plastic and Reconstructive Surgery, 108*, 1492–1498; discussion 1499–5000.

78. Peitsch, W. K., Keefer, C. H., LaBrie, R. A., & Mulliken, J. (2002). Incidence of cranial asymmetry in healthy newborns. *Pediatrics, 110*, 72–80.

79. Persing, J., James, H., Swanson, J., & Kattwinkel, J. (2003). Prevention and management of positional skull deformities in infants. *Pediatrics, 112*, 199–202.

80. Raco, A., Raimondi, A. J., De Ponte, F. S., et al. (1999). Congenital torticollis in association with craniosynostosis. *Child's Nervous System, 15*, 163–168.

81. Reference deleted in page proofs.

82. Ripley, L. E., Pomatto, J., & Beals, S. P. (1994). Treatment of positional plagiocephaly with dynamic orthotic cranioplasty. *Journal of Craniofacial Surgery, 5*, 150–159.

83. Shapiro, J. J. (1994). Relationship between vertical facial asymmetry and postural changes of the spine and ancillary muscles. *Optometry and Vision Science, 7*, 529–538.

84. Shumway-Cook, A., & Woollacott, M. (1985). The growth of stability; postural control from a development perspective. *Journal of Motor Behavior, 17*, 131–147.

85. Simon, F. T., Tang, M. D., Kuang-Hung, H., Wong, A. M. K., Hsu, C. C., & Chang, C. H. (2002). Longitudinal follow-up study of ultrasonography in congenital muscular torticollis. *Clinical Orthopaedics and Related Research, 403*, 179–185.

86. Slate, R. K., Posnick, J. C., Armstrong, D. C., & Buncic, R. (1993). Cervical spine subluxation associated with congenital muscular torticollis and craniofacial asymmetry. *Plastic and Reconstructive Surgery, 91*, 1187–1195.

87. Smith, D. W. (1981). *Recognizable patterns of human deformation*. Philadelphia: WB Saunders.

88. Stellwagon, L., Hubbard, E., Chambers, C., Lyons, K. J. (2008). Torticollis, facial asymmetry and plagiocephaly in normal newborns. *Arch Dis Child, 93*, 827–831.

89. St. John, D., Mulliken, J. B., Kaban, L. B., & Padwa, B. (2002). Anthropometric analysis of mandibular asymmetry in infants with deformational posterior plagiocephaly. *Journal of Oral and Maxillofacial Surgery, 60*, 873–877.

90. Thelen, E. (1995). Motor development, a new synthesis. *American Psychologist, 50*, 79–95.

91. Tien, Y. C., Su, J. Y., Su, G. T., Lin, G. T., & Lin, S. Y. (2001). Ultrasonographic study of the coexistence of muscular torticollis and dysplasia of the hip. *Journal of Pediatric Orthopaedics, 21*, 343–347.

92. Tom, L. W. C., Handler, S. D., & Wetmore, R. F. (1987). The sternocleidomastoid tumor of infancy. *International Journal of Pediatric Otorhinolaryngology, 13*, 245–255.

93. Turk, A. E., McCarthy, J. G., Thorne, C. H. M., & Wisoff, J. H. (1996). The "Back to Sleep Campaign" and deformational plagiocephaly: Is there cause for concern? *Journal of Craniofacial Surgery, 7*, 12–18.

94. Tscharnuter, I. (1993). A new therapy approach to movement organization. *Physical and Occupational Therapy in Pediatrics, 13*, 19–40.

95. Vandenburgh, H. H., Hatfaludy, S., Karlisch, P., & Shansky, J. (1989). Skeletal muscle growth is stimulated by intermittent stretch-relaxation in tissue culture. *American Journal of Physiology, 256*, C674–C682.

96. Vles, J. S. H., Colla, C., Weber, J. W., Beuls, E., Wilmink, J., & Kingma, H. (2000). Helmet versus non-helmet treatment in nonsynostotic positional posterior plagiocephaly. *Journal of Craniofacial Surgery, 11*, 572–574.

97. Watson, G. H. (1971). Relationship between side of plagiocephaly, dislocation hip, scoliosis, bat ears and sternomastoid tumors. *Archives of Disease in Childhood, 46*, 203–210.

98. Wei, J. L., Schwartz, K. M., Weaver, A. L., & Orvidas, L. J. (2001). Pseudotumor of infancy and congenital muscular torticollis: 170 cases. *Laryngoscope, 111*, 688–695.

99. Yu, C. C., Wong, F. H., Lo, L. J., & Chen, Y. R. (2003). Craniofacial deformity in patients with uncorrected congenital muscular torticollis: An assessment from three-dimensional computed tomography imaging. *Plastic and Reconstructive Surgery, 113*, 24–33.

10 Arthrogryposis Multiplex Congenita

MAUREEN DONOHOE, PT, DPT, PCS

Arthrogryposis multiplex congenita (AMC) is a non-progressive neuromuscular syndrome that is present at birth. AMC is characterized by severe joint contractures, muscle weakness, and fibrosis. Although the child's condition does not deteriorate as a result of the primary diagnosis, the long-term sequelae of AMC can be very disabling. Activity limitations in mobility and self-care skills can lead to varying degrees of participation restriction.

Working with children with AMC presents the physical therapist with a variety of challenges. Many children who have AMC are bright and motivated. Physical therapists must use their knowledge of biomechanics and normal development to maximize functional skills. Proper timing for therapeutic and medical interventions helps maximize the child's opportunities for independence. Creativity is needed to adapt equipment and the environment to allow the child with AMC to be able to participate in life roles to the fullest extent possible.

In this chapter, we address the pathophysiology of AMC, its management from a medical and surgical perspective, physical therapy examination and evaluation, and specific physical therapy and team interventions used for children with AMC from infancy to adulthood.

INCIDENCE AND ETIOLOGY

Arthrogryposis, which is defined by the presence of contractures in two or more body areas, is diagnosed in 1 of every 3000 to 6000 live births.[22,48] The cause of AMC is unknown; however, the insult is believed to occur during the first trimester of pregnancy.[12,20,64] It is believed that insults that occur early in the first trimester have the potential for creating greater involvement of the child than those that occur late in the first trimester. The basic pathophysiologic mechanism for multiple joint contractures appears to be lack of fetal movement.[57] With gene mapping, more than 65 different contracture syndromes have been mapped to specific genes.[21]

Various forms of arthrogryposis are known; amyoplasia is the most commonly recognized. Newborns with congenital contractures fall evenly into three groups: One consists of amyoplasia, the second is related to the central nervous system and is lethal, and the third is a heterogeneous group. The heterogeneous group includes neuromuscular syndromes, congenital anomalies, chromosomal abnormalities, contracture syndromes, and skeletal dysplasia. Distal arthrogryposis, which affects primarily the hands and feet and is highly responsive to treatment, has a genetic basis and is inherited as an autosomal dominant trait.[21,22] Gene mapping has been helpful in identifying those with arthrogryposis. Neuropathic arthrogryposis is found on chromosome 5 and can have survival motoneuron gene deletion.[8,49] Distal arthrogryposis type I maps to chromosome 9.[3,4]

AMC is associated with neurogenic and myopathic disorders in which motor weakness immobilizes the fetal joints, leading to joint contractures. It is not known whether all those with the neuropathic form of AMC have degeneration of the anterior horn cell, but of those studied post mortem, this is a consistent finding. A neurogenic disorder of the anterior horn cell is believed to cause muscle weakness with subsequent periarticular soft tissue fibrosis.[15,19,61,64] Because of failure of the muscle to function, the joints in the developing fetus lack movement, which probably explains the stiffness and deformities of the newborn's joints. The fetus may have an imbalance in strength of oppositional muscle groups, creating the tendency toward a certain posture. For example, the fetus with good strength in the hamstrings and triceps brachii but weakness in the quadriceps and biceps brachii will have a flexed knee and extended elbow posture in utero. Decreased amniotic fluid throughout the pregnancy, but especially during the last trimester when the fetus is largest, may further inhibit freedom of movement in utero.

Although the cause of AMC remains unknown, several factors have been implicated. Hyperthermia of the fetus is caused by a maternal fever greater than 37.8°C (100°F). Some mothers of children with AMC report having an illness with a fever for 1 to 2 days during the first trimester. Prenatal viral infection, vascular compromise of the blood supply between mother and fetus, uterine fibroid tumors, and a septum in the uterus have all been proposed as causes of AMC.[20,48,64]

PROGRESS IN PRIMARY PREVENTION

Arthrogryposis has been documented in artwork as early as the 1700s, although medical literature did not begin to address it until nearly the 1950s. Six major categories of problems can occur during a pregnancy that could precipitate the lack of movement associated with congenital contractures; these include maternal illness, fetal crowding, neurologic deficits, vascular compromise, connective tissue/skeletal defects, and muscle defects.[23] Given its nonspecific origin, little progress has been made in prevention of this rare disorder. However, significant improvements have been made in the management of children with AMC.

DIAGNOSIS

No definitive laboratory studies can diagnose AMC prenatally, unless a familial trait is documented. Some forms of arthrogryposis have been mapped to chromosomes 5, 9, or 11.[4,39,49] Most AMC cases occur sporadically with no known familial trait; therefore prenatal amniocentesis or chorionic villous sampling may be inconsequential. If a parent or physician suspects that something is amiss, a detailed level II ultrasound evaluation can be helpful in identifying anomalies and decreased fetal movements. Ultrasound studies that are real time lasting 45 to 60 minutes are most useful. Clues that are looked for include nuchal edema, thin undercalcified bones, small lungs, decreased movement time after 11 weeks of gestation, limitations in the diaphragm, and structural or space limitations.[21] If arthrogryposis is diagnosed during pregnancy, the mother can do some things to help exercise the baby as long as she is cleared by her physician from a health standpoint.[21] These activities include deep breathing, light exercise, and daily caffeine intake to help stimulate the baby.

During the first 6 months of life, an immunoglobulin study may identify evidence of a viral infection. After that time, an ophthalmologist can examine the eye for pigment clumps on the retina, called chorioretinitis. Chorioretinitis has no effect on vision but will establish whether the insult was the result of a prenatal viral process.

Muscle biopsy in AMC varies with the muscle under study. Histologic analysis reveals that relatively strong muscles appear virtually normal, and very weak muscles reveal fibrofatty changes but may have normal muscle spindles. Embryologically, the muscles are formed normally, but they are replaced by fibrous and fatty tissue during fetal development.[17,18,20] With electromyographic testing, neuropathic and myopathic changes can be seen in different muscles in the same patient.[45,51] Muscle biopsies along with blood tests and clinical findings rule out progressive and fatal disorders, while providing evidence to support the diagnosis of AMC.

CLINICAL MANIFESTATIONS

Clinical manifestations of AMC demonstrate great variability but generally include severe joint contractures and lack of muscle development or amyoplasia. The typical severely affected body parts in the AMC population include, in decreasing order of prevalence, the foot (78%–95%), the hip

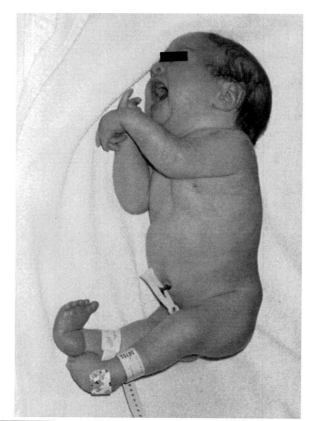

Figure 10-1 Infant with arthrogryposis multiplex congenita with flexed and dislocated hips, extended knees, clubfeet (equinovarus), internally rotated shoulders, flexed elbows, and flexed and ulnarly deviated wrists.

(60%–82%), the wrist (43%–81%), the knee (41%–79%), the elbow (35%–92%), and the shoulder (20%–92%).[47,48] One may see these percentages vary in the literature according to how the cases have been diagnosed (i.e., care centers will see different mixes based on their specialty).

Two commonly seen variations of AMC have been noted. In one type, the child has flexed and dislocated hips, extended knees, clubfeet (equinovarus), internally rotated shoulders, flexed elbows, and flexed and ulnarly deviated wrists (Figure 10-1). In another type, the child has abducted and externally rotated hips, flexed knees, clubfeet, internally rotated shoulders, extended elbows, and flexed and ulnarly deviated wrists (Figure 10-2). Parents often describe the legs in the first type as jackknifed, and in the second type as froglike. Because of the stiffness of the joints, extremity movements are described as wooden or marionette-like. The position of the upper extremities in the second type is described as the "waiter's tip" position owing to the internally rotated shoulder, extended elbow, pronated forearm, and flexed wrist. Common to both types are clubfeet, flexed and ulnarly deviated wrists, and internally rotated shoulders. Other associated characteristics may include scoliosis, dimpling of skin over joints, hemangiomas, absent or decreased finger creases, congenital heart disease, facial abnormalities, respiratory

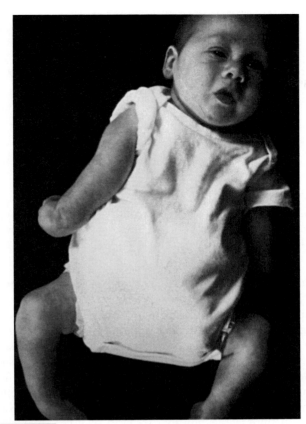

Figure 10-2 Infant with arthrogryposis multiplex congenita with abducted and externally rotated hips, flexed knees, clubfeet, internally rotated shoulders, extended elbows, and flexed and ulnarly deviated wrists.

problems, and abdominal hernias. Intelligence and speech are usually normal. Many arthrogrypotic syndromes occur that have the main characteristics of AMC but may also involve abnormal muscle tone, webbing at contracted joints, changes in cognition, seizure activity, feeding issues not related to muscle strength or jaw opening, and limited visual skills.[44,61]

MEDICAL MANAGEMENT

The main component of medical treatment includes well-timed surgical management.[19,42,55] Orthopedic treatment should be timed so that the child benefits optimally from the procedure. For example, clubfoot management with minimally invasive surgical techniques such as the Ponseti method should start approximately a month after the child is born. This allows the child to naturally stretch out and the family to become accustomed to the therapy routine before embarking on months of serial casting and positioning devices, allowing for plantigrade feet in time for developmentally appropriate upright activity.[5,31,38,60]

Some continue to have open surgical techniques such as the posteromediolateral release (PMLR) for clubfoot. The entire hindfoot is opened during surgery so as to shorten the lateral column, lengthen the medial column, and lengthen the tendo Achillis.[41,54] Occasionally, wires are used to realign the talus and the calcaneus. If the clubfoot recurs and does not respond to serial casting, a second PMLR involves shortening the cuboid bone to help improve forefoot alignment. If the foot is tight just in the hindfoot and no forefoot adductus is noted, a distal tibial wedge osteotomy is done to realign the foot in reference to the floor. Later in life, when the child is near the end of growth, a triple arthrodesis can be performed to prevent future inversion of the foot. This involves fusing the calcaneus to the cuboid, the talus to the navicular, and the talus to the calcaneus. Use of an external fixator such as an Ilizarov procedure to address recurrent clubfoot problems has had some promising results, although no data from long-term outcome studies are presently available.[7,10] Historically, in severe cases of equinovarus and in cases in which the Ilizarov procedure fails, a talectomy may be performed.[9,35] Salvage procedures to correct recurrent problems are difficult, however, when a talectomy has been previously performed.[34,41,54] Research supports that invasive surgical correction of feet results in stiff painful feet in adulthood.[28,34]

Children with AMC often have subluxed or dislocated hips. Dislocation is as frequently bilateral as unilateral. One dislocated hip is usually relocated to prevent secondary pelvic obliquity and scoliosis, unless the hip is extremely stiff.[45,53] Given that these hips tend to have poor acetabular development, if both hips are dislocated, they are not always surgically reduced because of the risk of continued unilateral dislocation even after open reduction. Careful evaluation of dislocated hips is necessary before surgical intervention is undertaken because if the hips are very tight into extension, limiting sitting ability, they will be even tighter after surgery. If the hips are dislocated high and posterior, with poor bony elements for the acetabulum, satisfactory surgical reduction may not be possible. Those who surgically reduce arthrogrypotic dislocated hips most commonly perform the surgery during the first year of life and use an anterolateral approach.[36,45,53,55,56] Szoke and colleagues[56] advocate early open reduction with a medial approach, as resultant hip stiffness was greater for those who were older at the initial surgery. Yau and colleagues[65] found that open reduction was necessary to have success in treating dislocated hips, as closed reduction in children with AMC was never successful. It may be more important to have mobile, painless, yet dislocated hips than to have very stiff but located ones. Prolonged immobilization following open or closed techniques can lead to the serious sequelae of fused or stiff hips.[1]

Moderate to severe contractures of the knee joint can be addressed surgically, but through the conservative approach, one waits until the child is ambulating comfortably before performing surgical correction. Knee flexion contractures are most commonly associated with capsular changes within the joint. Medial and lateral hamstring lengthening or

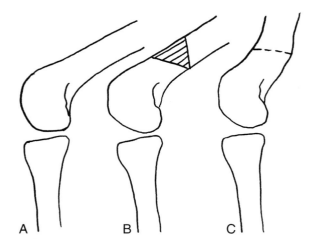

Figure 10-3   Diagram of a distal femoral wedge osteotomy performed to realign the contracted knee joint. **A,** Knee flexion contracture deformity before surgery. **B,** Distal femoral wedge osteotomy for reduction of the knee flexion deformity. **C,** Realignment after surgery.

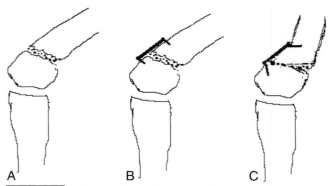

Figure 10-4   Diagram of guided growth for knee contracture management. **A,** Knee flexion contracture deformity before surgery. **B,** Distal femoral anterior epiphysiodesis for reduction of the knee flexion deformity. **C,** Realignment after surgery.

sectioning (if the muscle is fibrosed), along with a posterior capsulotomy of the knee joint, may be performed.[40,57] These contractures respond inconsistently to hamstring lengthening and posterior capsulotomy because subsequent loss of muscle strength and risk of scar tissue lead to further joint stiffness and recurrence of the contracture. A distal femoral osteotomy is more frequently successful in realigning the joint and changes the arc of motion without risk of increased scar tissue and loss of strength[13] (Figure 10-3). Growing children with moderate knee flexion contractures do well with distal femoral anterior epiphysiodesis. This procedure is done when the child is large enough to accept the surgical hardware but small enough to have adequate growth available, usually after the child is 5 years old but before 11 years of age. It allows the posterior aspect of the femur to continue to grow while the anterior aspect remains unchanged (Figure 10-4). The angle of the femur results in apparent knee straightening.[30,33,43] Severe knee flexion contractures are often addressed through the use of external fixators to distract the joint and slowly elongate the tissues.[7,27,59]

Knee extension contractures frequently have associated patellar subluxation.[6] Patellar realignment is done before the fifth birthday to allow the femoral groove to develop with growth.[6] Later in life, extension contractures are addressed by quadriceps lengthening if at least 25° of range of motion (ROM) is observed in the knee. Intra-articular procedures such as a capsulotomy may be necessary if the knee is stiff.[26] Some evidence suggests that surgery to address knee extension contractures results in better outcomes than surgery to address knee flexion contractures.[52] An important consideration before surgical intervention is determination of whether the limitation in ROM is creating problems with sitting or walking, and if so, if surgical intervention will likely improve the child's function. For example, if the legs extend straight out when sitting, this position may interfere with

activities such as sitting at school desks or riding in a car, and as a result may decrease participation at school and in the community. The child should participate in decisions regarding surgical interventions as appropriate for his or her age.

Restrictions in shoulder movement are rarely addressed through surgical interventions such as capsular or soft tissue release because the musculature is usually inappropriate for transfer. If adequate muscle strength and control are present, surgery may be indicated to place wrists and elbows in positions of optimal function. One scenario involves a child with symmetrical weakness or severe contractures of the upper extremities. In this case, a dominant arm can be identified for feeding (postured in flexion), and the other arm for hygiene care (postured in extension).[62] If both arms were postured in extension, surgery would be necessary to position one arm in a functional flexion position. Such surgical considerations would include a pectoralis or triceps brachii transfer to give a child active elbow flexion with a posterior capsulotomy to allow for elbow flexion.[2,57] The muscle under consideration for transfer would need to be strong before transfer with adequate passive elbow flexion could present. A consistent passive ROM and stretching program from birth is essential to maintain elbow motion for this type of surgery to be successful.

Wrists can be fused in positions for function if conservative splinting and stretching management have been unsuccessful. Wrists are fused in dissimilar positions. Before a surgical wrist fusion, casting of the wrist for 1 week in the position of the potential fusion is suggested. During this time, the child's functional ADL (activities of daily living) skills are assessed while the child is wearing the cast to ascertain the appropriateness of this potential surgery. Surgical management through carpectomies or dorsal wedge osteotomies of the carpal bones should be considered only if finger function will be enhanced.[2]

Scoliosis is frequently managed conservatively with bracing. In about one fifth of children and adolescents with AMC, a long C-shaped thoracolumbar scoliosis develops.[57]

If the curve continues to progress, surgical fusion should be considered. Those with a progressive congenital scoliosis have done well with the use of the vertical expandable prosthetic titanium rib implant for correcting scoliosis while allowing a significant amount of growth.[24] Most commonly, a posterior spinal fusion is performed when the child is close to puberty. On large stiff curves, an anterior release of structures limiting spinal mobility may be necessary before posterior spinal fusion to obtain satisfactory results.[66] The type of fixation used is based on the preference of the orthopedic surgeon (see Chapter 8).

BODY STRUCTURES AND FUNCTIONS

DIAGNOSIS AND PROBLEM IDENTIFICATION

The primary impairments in the child with AMC are limitations of joint movement and decreased muscle strength and bulk. Joint contractures are evident at birth, although a formal diagnosis of AMC may not be given at that time. In AMC, limitation of movement typically is seen in two or more joints in different body areas.[22] In the amyoplasia form of arthrogryposis, 85% have symmetrical presentation of contractures.[21]

Contractures can develop from an imbalance in muscle pull of agonist and antagonist muscles, but also occurs when symmetrical weakness is present on all sides of the joint, thus hindering movement. Theoretically, this may be indicative of the point in fetal development at which the insult occurs. For example, because flexors develop before extensors in the upper extremity, a child may develop elbow flexion contractures but does not develop the usual strength in either the biceps or the triceps brachii subsequent to the time of insult.

Decreased muscle bulk is evidence of muscle weakness secondary to decreased functioning motor units in a muscle. Histologic analysis of muscles reveals nonspecific changes in the muscle such as fibrofatty scar tissue. Weakened muscles often have a fat layer around the muscle with dimpling of the skin. A muscle with a contracture but of normal strength through its available ROM may not have normal muscle bulk secondary to its inability to be active throughout the entire ROM.

PROBLEM IDENTIFICATION BY THE TEAM

The team evaluation establishes a baseline from which to set realistic and functional goals. In addition to physical therapists, the primary intervention team consists of patients and their families and such medical professionals as orthopedists and geneticists, occupational therapists, and orthotists. Occasionally, speech pathologists, dentists or oral surgeons, neurologists, neurosurgeons, and ophthalmologists are consulted as well. One of the goals of the primary team is to educate the family about AMC. Families are taught that arthrogryposis is a nonprogressive disorder, but that without positioning, stretching, and strengthening, or possible surgery, the child's impairments could lead to further activity limitations and participation restrictions in later life (Table 10-1).

During the initial examination by the team, photographs and videos are taken of the child, illustrating the child's position of comfort and specific contractures such as clubfeet. This is an objective way to document changes that occur during growth and throughout splinting procedures and should be repeated every 4 months for the first 2 years.

In physical therapy, baseline goniometry is performed, documenting passive ROM and the resting position of each joint. ROM can be measured with a standard goniometer cut down to pediatric size. Active ROM is measured at the hips, knees, shoulders, elbows, and wrists. If possible, the same therapist consistently measures ROM for the child. Intratester and intertester reliability is determined for all therapists who evaluate children with AMC and should be checked annually. Functional active ROM is also assessed to assist with visualizing the whole composite of motions and evaluating functional abilities. For example, functional active ranges include assessment of hand to mouth, ear, forehead, top of head, and back of neck.

A formal manual muscle test is performed when appropriate. Muscle grades for infants and very young children are ascertained by using palpation, observation of the ability of extremities to move against gravity, and evaluation of gross motor function. The strength of the extensor muscles of the lower extremities is especially important in determining the appropriate level of bracing. Less than fair (grade 3/5) muscle strength in hip extensors will require bracing above the hip. Less than fair (grade 3/5) strength in knee extensors will require bracing above the knee. Corrected clubfeet require molded braces during growth to minimize problems of recurrent clubfeet. Children with poor upper extremity function and weak lower extremities may not be functional community ambulators as a result of decreased motor control and protective responses. Power mobility may be the most appropriate means of community locomotion.

Gross motor skills and functional levels of mobility and ADL are assessed. No current developmental tests have been designed specifically for children with AMC, but these children usually score lower than average on formal gross motor tests secondary to inadequate strength and ROM in their extremities. Certain gross motor skills may never be attained owing to physical limitations. For example, some developmental milestones such as creeping may not be attained, even though the child is able to stand and is beginning to walk. Cognitively, children with AMC tend to score average to above average in formal developmental tests.[45,51,63]

The physical therapist assesses the child for current and potential modes of functional mobility. This may include ambulation with assistive devices or the use of a manual or

TABLE 10-1   **International Classification of Functioning, Health, and Disability for Children With Arthrogryposis Multiplex Congenita**

Changes in Body Structure	Changes in Body Functions	Activity	Participation
Prenatal damage to the anterior horn cells, resulting in neurogenic and myopathic disorder	Multiple joint contractures Fibrotic joint capsule	Limited functional mobility skills, including rolling, creeping, and feeding, transitional movements, and high-level mobility skills	Limited opportunity for play with young peers
Decreased number of motor units within a muscle	Strength limitations, frequently imbalance of oppositional muscles with stronger muscles often shortened	Limited ability to transfer Dependence for transfers for ADL including toileting Limited independence in self-care skills, including dressing Limited ambulation Inability to manage uneven terrain	Inability to live independently Limited access to educational and work opportunities Need to learn how to adapt for new alignment once allowed to mobilize Limited access to a wide range of environments Health insurance may not pay for adaptive equipment necessary for
Scar tissue and fibrotic tissue do not grow and stretch to the same extent as healthy muscles.	Joint contractures can be progressive with growth.	Immobilization during periods of orthopedic management Increased limitations in mobility while immobilized Limited independence in wheelchair mobility without costly adaptations Decreased endurance	least restrictive mobility device. Limited participation in physical activities because of endurance and safety issues Social isolation

power wheelchair or mobility devices. The therapist evaluates movement patterns and muscle substitutions used to accomplish each motor task or ADL skill. Therapists should address a child with AMC from a biomechanical approach, because having limb segments aligned for mechanical advantage maximizes function and ultimately participation.

Following the examination, short-term and long-term goals are developed by the team related to splinting, stretching, developmental stimulation, orthopedic management including a surgical plan, and bracing. Incorporating the family early on as part of the team is important to maximize the child's independence in ADL and mobility.

PHYSICAL THERAPY IN INFANCY

Babies born with contracture syndromes have most significant involvement in the newborn period, as they have had limited mobility in utero, so benefit from early opportunities to stretch out and remold. It is important to be aware that a large population of newborns have early feeding issues caused by structural abnormalities at the jaw and tongue.[44]

Great variability can be seen in the presentation of contractures; however, two more common body types have been noted. One body type involves clubfeet, hip flexion contractures, knee extension contractures, shoulder tightness (especially internal rotation), and elbow and wrist flexion contractures. At birth, these children are commonly breech presentations. Another body type often associated with the amyoplasia type of AMC exhibits posturing of hips widely abducted, flexed, and externally rotated, flexed knees, clubfeet, internally rotated shoulders, extended and pronated elbows, and flexed wrists. Asymmetrical posturing of the extremities, which is especially problematic at the hip when dislocation of only one hip is present, occurs. The resulting asymmetry makes surgical correction the treatment of choice to relocate the hip and secondarily prevent pelvic obliquity and scoliosis. Children who are born with rocker-bottom feet and multiple contractures often have a syndrome with associated arthrogryposis and benefit from further genetic workup to possibly identify the specific contracture syndrome.

EXAMINATION

Formal assessment of an infant with arthrogryposis begins as soon as possible after birth. The assessment consists of goniometry of passive ROM with re-evaluation of ROM done on a monthly basis during this period. The therapist also documents the presence and strength of muscles based on observation of the child's movements and palpation of muscle contractions. Muscles of the trunk and upper and lower extremities are evaluated. Formal developmental assessment tools are used occasionally but reflect poorly on a child with contractures because strength and ROM limitations preclude the achievement of many motor milestones. Delayed motor milestones may result in activity limitations and participation restrictions when children with AMC are compared with healthy peers on standardized developmental tests.

Motor milestones in these children are often delayed or skipped. For example, good trunk control and balance, coupled with weak upper extremities in compromised positions, results in development of the ability to sit-scoot rather than creep for early floor mobility. Functional mobility and the mechanism used in attaining this mobility are more important to evaluate than is assignment of a developmental level or score. The therapist assesses rolling, prone tolerance, sitting control, scooting, creeping, crawling, transitional movements, and standing tolerance and upright mobility. Occupational therapy (OT) plays a key role in assessing feeding, ADL skills, and manipulation of objects. Physical therapists also assess the fit of any supportive or assistive devices that may be used. Another key role of therapists dealing with young children who have arthrogryposis is to track clubfoot alignment. Early recognition and aggressive treatment of clubfoot relapse may limit immobilization time.

Although it is not imperative to use formal scales in assessing motor development, some useful tests include the Alberta Infant Motor Scale, the Bayley Scales of Infant Development, and the Peabody Developmental Motor Scales. The Pediatric Evaluation of Disability Inventory and the WeeFIM (Functional Independence Measure for Children) may be used to measure activity and participation (see Chapter 2 for more information on these measurement tools).

Physical therapy goals for very young children include maximizing strength, improving ROM, and enhancing general sensorimotor development. Education of the family emphasizes instruction in proper positioning, stretching techniques, and the avoidance of potentially harmful activities that feed into deformity.

INTERVENTION STRATEGIES

Intervention strategies focus on improving alignment to maximize the biomechanical advantage for strengthening and reducing the joint contracture through stretching, serial casting, foot abduction braces, thermoplastic serial splinting, and positioning activities. Interventions address developmental skills, teaching compensatory strategies, especially in ADL and alternative modes of mobility, to maximize participation in age-appropriate activities.

DEVELOPMENT, STRENGTH, AND MOBILITY

Infants with the first type of AMC described earlier begin life with limited positioning options as a result of hip flexion contractures. Consequently, stretching hip flexors and prone positioning are encouraged within the first 3 months of life. Developmentally, these infants learn to roll or scoot on their bottoms as their primary means of floor mobility, because it is nearly impossible to comfortably assume the quadruped position without reinforcing a flexed posture of the upper extremities. Although delayed in their ability to attain sitting independently, they are often able to do so by 15 months of

age using trunk flexion and rotation. These children typically are able to stand when placed well before pulling to stand is initiated by the child. If the child has dislocated hips that have been surgically reduced in the first year, the child may have significant stiffness initially, limiting willingness to change position from sitting to standing. Usually, the child begins to walk with assistance, an assistive device, and lower extremity orthotics around 18 months of age; most are independent ambulators by the middle of their second year of life.

Initially, infants with the amyoplasia type of AMC have more positioning options due to their hip and knee flexion contractures. Some have difficulty with prone positioning because of elbow extension contractures that limit their ability to comfortably prop. A towel roll or wedge under the infant's chest assists with increasing tolerance for this position. Positioning the hips in neutral rotation and neutral abduction is encouraged. Towel rolls can be placed along the lateral aspect of the thighs when the infant is sitting, and a wide Velcro band can be strapped around the thigh when the child is lying supine to keep the legs in more neutral alignment (Figure 10-5).

Developmentally, these children tend to be a little slower in attaining rolling but faster in attaining sitting and scooting than children with the first type of posturing. Although assuming the quadruped position and creeping are often

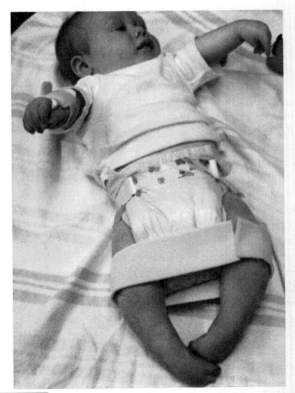

Figure 10-5 This child with arthrogryposis multiplex congenita is wearing a wide Velcro band strapped around the thigh to keep the legs in more neutral alignment.

feasible for this type of child, sitting and scooting are more energy efficient. Depending on muscle strength and the amount of bracing needed for standing, these children may never perform transitional movements from sitting on the floor to standing independently. They begin ambulating by the middle of their second year but require a significant amount of bracing for success. Independence with ambulation may take years and sometimes is not fully accomplished. Therapy focuses on addressing some key functional motor skills, such as rolling, sitting, sit-scooting, standing, and strengthening those muscles that assist in maintaining posture. The goal is to maximize mobility to enhance participation in age-appropriate activities, but with an eye toward skills necessary for lifelong independence.

Strengthening during the first 2 to 3 years is most frequently addressed through developmental facilitation and play. Dynamic strengthening of the trunk can be achieved by having the child reach for, swipe at, or roll toys in the positions of sitting and static standing, or while straddling the therapist's leg so that the child must rotate the trunk. These maneuvers incorporate stretching and strengthening into the therapeutic play activity. Aquatic therapy is often helpful for strengthening and developing functional mobility skills. If working on upright control in the pool, knee splints, specifically for use in the water, are helpful when bracing is needed on land, too. One way to determine whether functional training is having a strengthening effect is to ascertain the child's improved ability to perform the task.

Self-care skills, feeding, and manipulation of objects are dependent on hand function and elbow flexibility. Those children with limited upper extremity strength may have decreased ability to manipulate objects. Fortunately, these children tend to be resourceful in using other body parts, such as their feet or mouth, to manipulate objects when hands have inadequate strength and ROM. These skills are quite useful early in life but not as useful in an older child. If the child has adequate ROM but inadequate strength, the child learns to support the arm on a leg or a table to assist in bringing hand to mouth. If the child is unable to get hand to mouth, adaptive equipment may make it possible to do some self-feeding. For example, if shoulder strength is absent, overhead arm slings are fashioned out of polyvinyl chloride piping and added to the high chair to permit finger feeding. If the upper extremities are postured in elbow extension, a typical and effective method of grasping an object is with a hand cross-over maneuver, which affords some control and strength in holding or lifting an object. Electronic toys can be adapted so that the child can operate them via switches that can be activated by movement of the head, hand, or foot. These compensatory intervention strategies help to enhance skills needed for independence in ADL.

Standing is an important component of physical therapy during the first and second years. Families are encouraged to begin standing the child at approximately 6 months of age, as is normally done with children without physical limitations. If a child is in casts with knees flexed, upright positioning continues to be an important component of therapy, as it helps to strengthen the trunk for standing once casts are removed. Standing is best completely upright rather than angled toward supine or prone, as it helps develop skill in the biomechanical alignment necessary to stand without external support. During standing, splints can be used to maintain the lower extremities in adequate alignment. Shoes can be wedged to accommodate plantar flexion deformities and to allow the child to bear weight throughout the plantar surface of the foot.

Standing is initiated in a standing frame and progresses to independent static standing in the frame (Figure 10-6). A therapist may need to be creative to work on standing with a child who is wearing a foot abduction brace, but use of the brace should not limit work on standing skills. By 1 year of age, a child should be able to tolerate a total of 2 hours a day in the standing frame. This standing helps the child begin self-stretching of the feet and encourages emerging independent standing and walking skills. Use of a prone stander is usually avoided because this type of stander does not encourage dynamic trunk control, and therefore, the child is less likely to be working on the skills needed to stand outside the

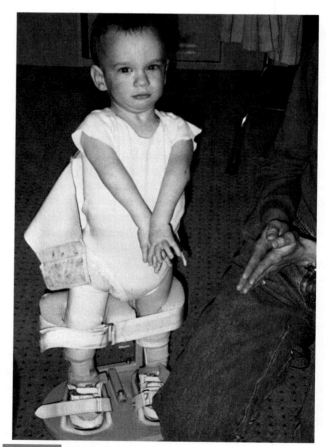

Figure 10-6 Child who has arthrogryposis multiplex congenita in a standing frame.

stander. Dynamic standing is encouraged through ball games such as kicking a soccer ball or batting a ball off a tee. Floor-to-stand activities usually do not begin to emerge until the child is ambulating securely, and sit-to-stand activities from a low chair usually begin to emerge when ambulation begins. Limitations in lower extremity strength and ROM can be addressed through splinting and bracing while the child is standing. Knee extension splints may be worn to compensate for weakness of knee extensors and mediolateral instability of the knees.

STRETCHING AND SPLINTING

Stretching programs for joint contractures are imperative and should be taught to parents and caregivers from the time of the initial examination. This intervention strategy addresses one of the primary impairments of AMC. A stretching program is divided into three to five sets a day with three to five repetitions during each set. Each stretch is held for 20 to 30 seconds. With the realization that this is a significant time commitment, families are taught to incorporate stretching into times when the child would normally have one-on-one time with the caregiver, such as performing lower extremity stretches during diaper changes and upper extremity stretches during feeding. Dressing and bath times also provide good opportunities for stretching, especially once the child is self-feeding and out of diapers. Stretching must be a daily lifelong commitment for a person with arthrogryposis, but consistent stretching is most critical during the growing years and especially within the first 2 years of life.[54]

To maintain the prolonged effect of the stretch, the extremity is maintained in a comfortable position of stretch with thermoplastic splints. Attempting to maintain the maximum stretch, rather than a comfortable position, over prolonged periods will cause skin breakdown and intolerance to splints. Splints are adjusted for growth and improvements in ROM, usually every 4 to 6 weeks during infancy. When ankle-foot orthoses (AFOs) are fabricated for clubfeet, the calcaneus must be aligned in a neutral position, because this will affect the position of the entire foot. If the calcaneus is allowed to move medially with respect to the talus, the forefoot will fall into an undesirable varus position. When the hindfoot and the forefoot are in a neutral position between varus and valgus, splinting can address insufficient dorsiflexion of the hindfoot rather than forefoot. This will prevent the potential problem of a midfoot break resulting in a rocker-bottom foot. To be maximally effective, AFOs are worn 22 hours per day.

Knee contractures are addressed early using splinting and stretching. For the first 3 to 4 months, anterior thermoplastic knee flexion splints for extension contractures or posterior knee extension splints for knee flexion contractures are worn up to 20 hours per day. For an older infant with knee extension contractures, it is advised that children not wear a knee flexion splint at greater than 50° of flexion for sleeping, because this may encourage hip flexion contractures. Older babies with knee extension contractures should use the knee flexion splints for activities that require flexion, such as sitting in the car seat or the high chair, or when positioned in prone, utilizing knee flexion and the splint to enhance the quadruped position. Knee extension splints, which control knee flexion contractures or medial-lateral instability, are initially worn up to 18 hours a day, especially during sleep. Once the child is older than 6 months of age, the knee extension splints can be used for standing activities, as they encourage optimal lower extremity alignment during upright activity. Splints to control knee flexion contractures should be off 6 hours a day to allow floor mobility in a child with emerging skills.

Newborns are provided with cock-up wrist splints, but splints for hands are generally provided only after 3 months of age. This allows the child to integrate the normal physiologic flexion before placing a stimulus across the palm. Two sets of hand splints are fabricated. For day use, the child wears dorsal cock-up splints with a palmar arch in a position of neutral deviation and a slight stretch into extension as tolerated. This allows the child to have fingers available to manipulate toys. For night wear, the splint is a dorsal cock-up splint with a pan to allow finger stretching when the child is sleeping.

When considering elbow splinting, note that function and independence in ADL are improved when one elbow is able to flex adequately to reach the mouth, and one elbow is in adequate extension to reach the perineum. Other factors to consider include available muscle strength and ROM, response to stretching, and potential future surgical procedures. Elbow extension splints are best worn while sleeping, but elbow flexion splints and elbow flexion-assist splints tend to be most functional when worn during the day. This allows the child to experiment with the hand in a more functional position for most play activities.[32]

Young children respond most readily to conservative treatment using serial splinting, frequent stretching, and proper positioning. In Figure 10-7, A, the infant's posture is shown without leg splints. In Figure 10-7, B, the infant's lower leg is held out of the deforming postures through molded thermoplastic knee and AFO splints. The key to successful intervention for contractures is family education. Family education begins during the initial evaluation, as caretakers not only are given general information about arthrogryposis but also receive information regarding their child's specific needs. Appropriate stretching exercises for involved joints are given with sketches or photographs to supplement the verbal instructions. Subsequent visits to the physical therapist allow work on splint fabrication and modification and positioning. Developmental play ideas are incorporated into the exercises to help the child progress developmentally. Physical therapists also work with the family to adapt age-appropriate toys to stimulate the child both physically and cognitively.

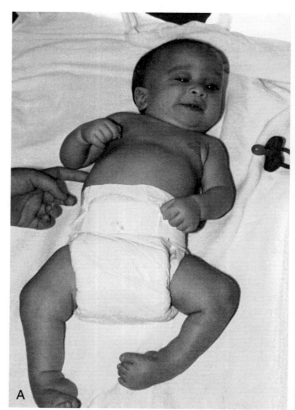
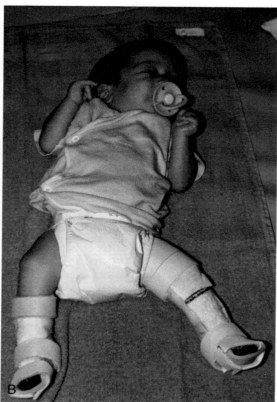

Figure 10-7 **A,** A child who has arthrogryposis multiplex congenita without leg splints. **B,** The same child's lower extremity is held out of the deforming positions through the use of molded thermoplastic knee splints and ankle-foot orthoses.

PHYSICAL THERAPY IN THE PRESCHOOL PERIOD

During the preschool period, the child's functional abilities and age-appropriate participation vary according to the degree of involvement. Poor upper extremity function from the contractures and lack of muscle strength may limit the child's independence in feeding, dressing, and playing, at a time when typical peers are relishing their independence. This may be particularly distressing for the parents, who become more aware of the magnitude of their child's limitations when the child is no longer an infant in whom dependency is expected.

Structural limitations impeding participation in age-appropriate activities during this stage are similar to those found in the younger child. Restriction in joint ROM continues to be a problem secondary to rapid growth changes. Independent ambulation is often limited by poor protective responses of the upper extremities.

EXAMINATION

Passive and active ROM continues to be closely monitored by the physical therapist and caregivers. Proper fit of orthotics and splints is imperative in providing adequate stretch and positioning to impede the development of further deformities.

Functional muscle strength is an important component in the preschooler because it determines to a great degree the extent of bracing necessary and the level of independence in self-care skills. Formal manual muscle testing[25,29] becomes more appropriate during this period because the child can comprehend verbal instructions. When testing strength, it is important to grade the resistance throughout the arc of motion because the child with AMC will frequently be strong in the midrange but unable to move the extremity to the shortened end range. This finding is significant because the end range is where the child needs to work the muscle to maintain stretch of the antagonist muscles.

Gait assessment should include distance, use of assistive devices (including braces and shoe adaptations, as well as upper extremity support), speed, symmetry of step length, gait deviations, and muscle activity. Some children ambulate as their primary means of locomotion; others rely on a stroller for community mobility. Despite research that supports powered mobility for the very young,[46,58] mobility with wheelchairs is not usually addressed until school age, when slow speed of ambulation, endurance, and safety concerns may preclude the child from interacting with peers. These children are bright and will often forgo ambulation for power mobility if it is presented too early. Forgoing ambulation early may limit standing for functional activities later in life.

GOALS

Ability rather than disability must be stressed, with a strong emphasis on assisting the child through problem solving rather than through physical assistance. The ultimate goals for this age are to reduce the disability and enhance independent ambulation and mobility with minimum bracing and use of assistive devices. Physical and environmental structural barriers may limit achievement of some fine and gross motor skills, but social skill attainment is paramount. Another goal is for the team to work together to improve the child's function in basic ADL skills.

INTERVENTION STRATEGIES

The team will work together during the preschool period to solve basic ADL challenges, such as independent feeding and toileting. For example, the use of a lightweight reacher may assist with dressing skills. Preschoolers usually can self-feed with adaptive equipment. These children are often toilet trained but lack the ability to perform the task independently. At times, orthopedic surgical intervention will be used to help gain better biomechanical alignment of joints. These surgeries initially may change the focus of the therapeutic intervention, but ultimately, the focus and the goal remain the same because surgical intervention is done to enhance position and function.

STRETCHING

The need for stretching at this age continues to be addressed despite the preschooler's decreased tolerance to passive stretching three to five times a day. Two times a day for the stretching program is more realistic and appears to maintain ROM adequately in most cases. Families report that the best time for this is during dressing and bathing, which incorporates the program into an automatic part of the daily routine. Children can be taught how to assist with stretching through positioning. The child is also encouraged to verbally participate in the program, for example, by counting the number of repetitions. AFOs and positional splints continue to be worn to maintain the achieved positions.

Independent mobility in a safe and efficient manner is important for the preschooler to achieve and enhance social skills, as well as allow functional mobility. Independent ambulation with supportive bracing and with as few assistive devices as possible is stressed. Children with adequate strength and ROM who do not require bracing to walk generally need an AFO to prevent recurring clubfoot deformities. Older preschoolers with AMC are generally at the level of bracing that will be continued throughout school age.

ORTHOTICS

Most orthotics are now fabricated from lightweight polypropylene and are more durable, less cumbersome, and more adjustable than the metal braces used previously. Children with knee extension contractures tend to require less bracing than those with knee flexion contractures. If there is any question about the child's ability to maintain an upright position without hip support, the child's first set of long leg braces, a hip-knee-ankle-foot orthosis, will include a pelvic band. This type of orthosis is used for several reasons. The family may perceive that the child is regressing if initially unsuccessful ambulating occurs without the pelvic band, and later a band is added for ambulation success. The pelvic band encourages neutral rotation and abduction of the lower extremities. The pelvic band can also facilitate full available hip extension, and the hips can be locked in that position for prolonged standing. Use of a pelvic band allows a pivot point for the trunk to move into extension to help with posterior weight shift on the stance side during gait. Once the child is ambulating with both hips unlocked, without jackknifing at the hips during stance, the pelvic band can be removed.

Maintaining hip strength, especially when the pelvic band is removed, continues to be important. One activity is to have the child begin static and dynamic standing on the tilt board. The child also begins taking steps forward, backward, and sideways. Strengthening, as with progressive resistive exercises, may be appropriate at this time. Clinical experience suggests that muscles may increase in strength by one half to a full muscle grade with exercise.

Ideally, the least amount of bracing is optimal, but if decreasing the bracing requires the child to use an assistive device that was previously unnecessary, increased bracing may be more appropriate. A child with strong extensors such as the gluteus maximus and quadriceps is more functional than a child who requires bracing as a functional substitute for the extensors. The child with a good deal of bracing has difficulty donning and removing braces and usually is dependent for locking and unlocking hip and knee joints for standing and sitting.

Those children who learn to walk may be limited in their independence if they do not have adequate strength and ROM to manipulate the assistive device, such as a walker, that is required to ambulate. Walkers are often heavy and cumbersome for the child, who may have inadequate protective responses in standing and upper extremity limitations. Thermoplastic material can be molded to the walker for forearm support when hand function is limited, affording the child added support and control (Figure 10-8). Many children prefer to walk with someone rather than use a walker while they are gaining confidence in ambulatory skills. When learning to stand and walk, it is of utmost importance that the child learns how to use the head and trunk to stand and balance, and then to weight shift for limb advancement. If a child uses a gait trainer and leans on the

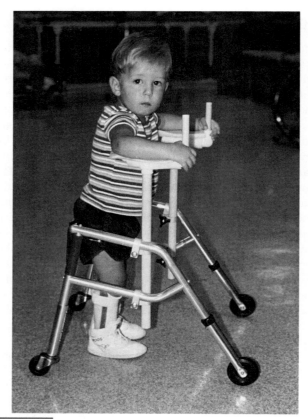

Figure 10-8 Thermoplastic forearm supports can be customized to the walker.

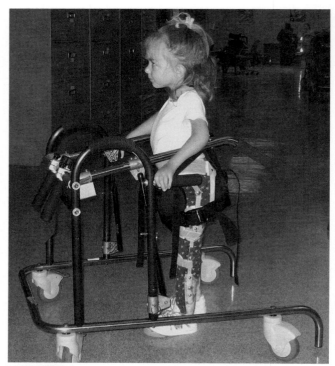

Figure 10-9 Child with arthrogryposis multiplex congenita wearing polypropylene hip-knee-ankle orthosis and using a gait trainer that allows dynamic weight shift.

device to move it, without regaining balance, he or she may not be training in the skills necessary to stand and balance for functional transfers for a lifetime. Use of a gait trainer that enhances the opportunity to stand upright and weight shift (Figure 10-9) while relying on the support as a "safety net," rather than leaning into it, may produce better long-term functional outcomes in upright for transfers and ADL. Careful evaluation of ambulation potential is needed when one is deciding on an assistive device for ambulation. Some walkers will give independence in exercise walking but will not translate into greater independence outside the walker.

Children with weak quadriceps and knee flexion contractures tend to ambulate with locked knee and ankle-foot orthoses. These braces can be fabricated with dial knee locks so that the knee position can be adjusted to coincide with the changing state of the knee flexion contracture. This will afford the ongoing opportunity to stretch out the contracture. Shoes may need external wedges to compensate for hip and knee flexion contractures that interfere with static standing. If the brace cannot stand in the wedged shoe, the child cannot be expected to balance in the brace with the shoes. The child should be able to comfortably balance with the feet plantigrade without upper extremity support.

Families may require assistance in identifying and removing environmental barriers that impede the child's independence both in the home and in the preschool environment.

Children in this age group are encouraged to participate in activities with children the same age in preschool, day care, and swimming classes, and in other peer group activities. They are encouraged to develop relationships with children who do not have disabilities, as well as with those who do. These early relationships help to enhance lifelong participation in integrated activities with peers. During the preschool period, many states mandate therapy services for children with special needs. Preschool services, as well as additional therapy services, are imperative for maximizing these children's skills for the demands they will encounter during school.

PHYSICAL THERAPY DURING THE SCHOOL-AGE AND ADOLESCENT PERIOD

The focus of physical therapy moves from the outpatient clinic into the classroom at this stage. Most children are enrolled in regular classrooms in their neighborhood schools, although they may have adaptive physical education, physical therapy, occupational therapy, and speech services to enhance the educational process.

Participation in school and classroom activities may be impeded by limitations in mobility. At school, children have increased demands to travel longer distances and move in groups under limited time frames. Alternative means of mobility such as a motorized wheelchair or a scooter may be needed to enhance independence while managing materials (such as books and personal effects) with minimal outside assistance. Efficient and independent dressing, feeding, and toileting abilities take on a more compelling nature. Joint contractures continue to be problematic, especially through the last few growth spurts. This is a time when the adolescent is becoming more independent in self-care, and adult monitoring of contractures tends to decrease.

EXAMINATION

The school therapist acts as a team member, addressing goals of the child and family with regard to enhancing the child's educational experience. The physical therapy examination determines what types of training and adaptive equipment are needed to achieve educational objectives. Functional ADL skills are assessed to ascertain how efficiency and independence can be improved. The School Function Assessment (SFA)[11,37] is a tool that is helpful in identifying functional skill levels in the school environment and in identifying activities for individualized educational plan (IEP) goals, so that physical therapy interventions can ultimately allow for greater participation of the child at school. The Activity Scale for Kids (ASK) is a self-report tool that may be helpful in defining where a child is having greatest limitations in functional skills at home and in the community.[67]

GOALS

During this period, the child with AMC must be responsible for self-care and for an exercise program to be performed to the best of the child's ability. If the child is physically unable to do these tasks, it is still important to be able to orchestrate care through verbal instructions to a caregiver. The family must also become more responsible for expecting and allowing the child to be more independent. The goal of independence in mobility and keeping up with friends is important in the development of peer relationships. Early school-based goals should include ability to independently participate in one to three playground activities during recess.

ROM is not an educational goal, but it continues to be a focus to maximize long-term function. The child with AMC will lose motion if he or she does not continue to stretch throughout the growing years. As sitting requirements for education increase, hip and knee flexion contractures also can increase if positioning options to enhance extension are not addressed. Final growth spurts, coupled with increased sitting requirements for education, can result in a significant loss of extension at the knees and the hips. If the school-age child is not conscientious about night splint use and positioning for stretch, the ability to walk may be lost during the

teen years. Surgical intervention to regain ambulation skill during the second decade of life is not always an option.

INTERVENTION STRATEGIES

Dressing, toileting, and feeding may require adaptive equipment or setup for the child to be independent. Children with AMC require some selective pieces of adaptive equipment for achieving independence, but most are adaptable and innovative in using compensatory strategies rather than relying on assistive devices to achieve their goals. Frequently, classroom chairs and tables must be at custom-made heights to accommodate rising from a chair without manipulating brace knee locks. The desktop may need to be adjusted so that the child, by using a mouth stick or a wrist aid to hold writing implements, can maneuver items on the desk or write (Figure 10-10). Assistive technology is quite helpful for those with limited hand function to perform school work on a computer, although management of the computer may be challenging for a child who changes classes. Implementation of ideas such as these limits disability by providing the child with successful compensatory strategies.

Continued adherence with the customized splinting and stretching program is expected. Children at this age may lose

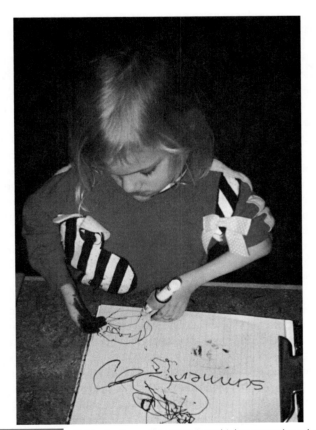

Figure 10-10 Child who has arthrogryposis multiplex congenita using a wrist aid to hold a crayon.

a few degrees of motion during growth, but further regression may result in loss of skills that previously were not a problem, when more motion was available. Surgical intervention is sometimes helpful for improving joint position. A self-stretching program, utilizing assistive straps, braces, and positioning, can be incorporated into the child's routine to promote independence in attaining goals. The adolescent must be permitted to help plan his or her schedule, or adherence can be expected to be poor. Adaptive physical education in school, as well as adaptive sports programs outside school, can be adjunctive to physical therapy for promoting strength, endurance, and mobility. Vocational rehabilitation may be a helpful adjunct in assisting those with physical limitations to access future employment opportunities.

Speed and safety in independent mobility are important in the development of peer relationships. Families may be advised during this time to consider powered mobility devices as an adjunct to manual mobility devices. Cumbersome bracing, inefficient gait, and poor upper extremity function can limit a child's ability to participate in playground or social activities.[14] Alternative modes of mobility may allow the child to participate safely. Use of alternative modes need not preclude ambulation but rather provides supplemental mobility for safety and energy conservation. Most children can achieve functional household ambulation but may require a wheelchair for efficient community mobility. The importance of standing and walking skills for maximal independence in the bathroom cannot be overstressed.

TRANSITION TO ADULTHOOD

Little has been published about the transition from childhood to adulthood for the person who has arthrogryposis. Sneddon[50] published the results of a survey of 100 adults with AMC regarding issues related to aging. Limitations in activities during adulthood were related to continued problems with ROM and strength that consequently limited independence in ADL, ambulation, and mobility. Those who required assistance with ADL during their school-age years continued to require assistance throughout their lifetime but were able to achieve a degree of independence with feeding, dressing, and grooming using selected assistive ADL devices. Those with severe joint involvement had long-term dependency on others for ADLs.[14,51]

Pain appears to be a significant issue that occurs with aging. Most respondents reported difficulty with back and neck pain and increased discomfort in other joints as well.[50] Those who have had surgical intervention for clubfeet can expect pain and stiffness to develop during the adult years.[28] Some specific problems that occur in adults include arthritic changes in weight-bearing joints and overuse syndromes in muscles and joints that are used for compensation or unique postures. Osteoarthritis, carpal tunnel problems, and neuropathies may develop as a result of prolonged joint constrictions and deformities. Increasing muscle weakness with increasing age has been found to occur, starting in early adulthood.[50] Mobility problems emerging later in life may stem from secondary degenerative changes and muscle overuse syndromes.[19] Manual or power wheelchairs may be used more commonly by adults than by adolescents and teenagers. Adults with AMC often use a wheelchair as their primary mode of mobility for long distances.

Advanced education is of utmost importance, so that the adult with AMC becomes trained in a specialized skill or field. The type of work chosen will depend on the degree of activity limitations, education, and marketable skills. Computer-related work and occupations that do not rely on manual labor should be considered as employment options. Advancements in technology allow those with arthrogryposis to have opportunities that enhance their freedom of mobility and their career options. Assistive technology, including computers and voice-activated equipment, can be of value in helping the individual safely and efficiently achieve work and leisure goals. Many people who have arthrogryposis who are artistically talented use their skills in painting and drawing for vocation and avocation.

Many of the barriers that the adult with AMC will meet are physical barriers. Although the Americans with Disabilities Act has helped, transportation continues to limit access to vocational and avocational activities. Those who live near strong public transportation systems or who have access to an automobile with proper adaptations have better opportunities for participation in activities outside the home. Adult rehabilitation facilities, although probably unfamiliar with AMC, owing to the small number of adults who have been given this diagnosis, can provide services regarding assistive technology and orthotics, as well as help in funding the equipment.

INTERVENTION STRATEGIES

Once skeletal growth has stopped, stretching is not as imperative, but maintaining flexibility and proper positioning is encouraged to impede the further development of deformities. Those with AMC who used orthoses during the school-age years typically continue to do so throughout adulthood. Those who used only ankle-foot orthoses for clubfoot control tend not to need these orthoses once growth is complete. Dressing and, most important, donning of shoes are often the last skills achieved, as abandoning bracing allows for easier dressing of the lower body.

Information about the long-term sequelae of AMC in relation to degenerative changes, mobility levels, and use of adaptive ADL devices is critical to providing the most effective therapy to persons with AMC. Joint conservation and addressing the secondary impairments resulting from degenerative changes that occur in adulthood are necessary to maximize long-term independence.

Research regarding the extent of independence of children, adolescents, and adults who have AMC is lacking in the areas of ADL, use of manual or power wheelchairs, and ambulation ability. This lack of data may be a result of the fact that children are followed early on within a medical model that addresses their primary orthopedic concerns, but when they transfer to the educational setting and require less medical intervention, they are lost to follow-up. To meet the objective of providing the most appropriate intervention to this population, a nationwide database on functional outcomes, mobility, and associated long-term problems should be established. Those who do enter the physical therapy system are often referred because of pain management issues. Pain is most likely due to overuse injuries, as well as to inefficient strategies for ADL. The emphasis of therapy should be placed on energy conservation, assistive devices to enhance efficiency, and the primary issue leading to the referral. As adults who have contracture syndromes age, they have secondary complications of being sedentary; therefore education on lifelong fitness opportunities needs to be investigated, to help with cardiovascular fitness and weight management.

SUMMARY

Arthrogryposis poses a variety of challenges for the health care team throughout the patient's lifetime. Although AMC is nonprogressive, its sequelae can limit participation in even basic ADLs. Variability in clinical manifestations has been noted, but severe joint contractures and lack of muscle development are hallmarks of the disease. Each

stage of development requires special attention for maximizing the child's function. An early goal of the team is to educate the family about AMC and to create the understanding that, without intervention, the child's body structure and functional skills could lead to further limitation in activity throughout a lifetime. Early medical and therapeutic management includes vigorous stretching, splinting, positioning, and strengthening, all of which will allow the child to develop optimal positions for functional ADL and will enhance motor skill development. Timing of surgical procedures is critical to minimize intervention while maximizing benefit.

Each age has challenges on which physical therapy can have a positive impact. During infancy, motor milestones are often delayed or skipped, and determining functional mobility is more important than ascribing a developmental level. Intervention strategies focus on maximizing postural alignment through serial splinting and strengthening and on facilitating developmental activities. Ambulation is a preliminary primary goal, but once the child reaches school age, the focus shifts toward more independent, functional, and safe mobility. During the school-age years, the child must become more responsible for stretching exercises because stretching is an integral part of the program throughout the growing years. The team emphasizes assisting the child with problem solving and working toward independent mobility. Adaptive equipment is often necessary to allow the child with AMC to be independent in mobility and self-care. A comprehensive and integrated team approach is critical in developing strategies to meet these challenges. Ultimately, the goal is to have the child who has arthrogryposis grow to be an adult who is as independent as possible and an active participant in the community.

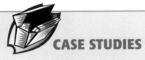

CASE STUDIES

"Will"

Will was initially referred to physical therapy (PT) at 12 days of age by the orthopedic department. During the initial evaluation, photographs were taken to document postural alignment and the position of his extremities. At the initial examination, the elbows were held in extension, the wrists were flexed and pronated, and the hips were in flexion, abduction, and external rotation (see Figure 10-2). Plain films revealed that the right hip was dislocated. ROM was measured using a goniometer.

The family was instructed in passive ROM of the lower extremities during diaper changes and of the upper extremities during feeding. The following week, therapists fabricated customized low-temperature thermoplastic splints. These included AFOs, knee extension splints, and dorsal hand splints. As an infant, Will was treated by medically based physical and occupational therapists every 3 to 4 weeks for splint adjustments and to monitor the home program. He also received weekly home-based early intervention services that emphasized developmental skills.

At 3 months of age, elbow flexion splints were fabricated and were worn 23 hours a day. To improve his hip alignment, his family used a wide Velcro strap to hold his legs in neutral alignment (see Figure

10-5). Hip flexion contractures were reduced from 85° at birth to 25° at 3 months, and the hips could be adducted to neutral. Knee flexion contractures were 30° on the right and 25° on the left. Forefoot abduction was 0° to 5° on the right and 0° to 10° on the left.

Muscle testing, determined by palpation, and observation of active movement revealed active hip flexion, extension, and abduction. The hamstrings were active against gravity. The contractions of the quadriceps and plantar flexors were palpable. No biceps brachii contraction was palpable. However, active shoulder flexion against gravity and at least fair strength of the pectoralis and triceps brachii were noted.

At 6 months of age, he began a standing program in AFOs with wedged sneakers and knee extension splints in a standing frame. At 7 months of age, he was able to sit independently when placed in sitting. At 10 months of age, he developed rolling as a means of locomotion and could crawl on his belly for short distances. He was able to straddle-sit on the floor and tolerate dynamic challenges to his balance. With his lower extremities stabilized, he was able to move from supine to sitting.

Will entered a center-based early intervention program at 12 months of age. He received PT three times a week with the goals of

Continued

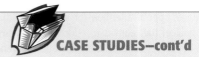

CASE STUDIES—cont'd

attaining independent mobility, improving ROM through stretching and positioning, and maximizing perambulation skills. He continued to be followed on a monthly basis in a medically based clinic to update the family's home program for Will, and to adapt and progress his splints as appropriate. His family was performing a stretching program two to three times a day. At this point, he began to explore the use of overhead slings for antigravity upper extremity activities such as feeding and table top play.

At 14 months of age, Will had the ability to move from prone to sitting by widely abducting his hips and using his arms to raise and lower his trunk. By 16 months of age, he could stand independently with knee splints, AFOs, and wedged sneakers, but his hips were widely abducted, so he relied on upper extremity support for success. Use of a figure eight strap on his thighs helped to control the excessive abduction of the hips, allowing him to step, but he required facilitation to weight shift.

By 20 months of age, Will was eager to stand and wanted to stand all the time. When supported through his axillae, he would walk. At 22 months of age, Will underwent bilateral posterior mediolateral releases for his clubfeet, which were subsequently placed in casts for 8 weeks. During this time, he used a cart for mobility. After cast removal, custom-made hip-knee-ankle-foot orthoses were fabricated, and ambulation training began. He started standing with a posterior walker with the braces unlocked at the hips and rapidly progressed to taking two steps with the walker. During this period, Will received PT three times per week, with concentration on independent standing and walking. He also participated in adaptive aquatics two times per week. By 27 months of age, he was able to stand independently with both hips unlocked and could take two steps without upper extremity support.

At 30 months, Will was able to walk 600 feet with a walker with unlocked hip joints. He could walk 6 feet without an assistive device. At that point, gait training without a pelvic band was initiated, requiring verbal cues for Will to control excessive abduction.

At 5 years of age, he had a triceps transfer and posterior elbow capsulotomy on the left upper extremity, followed by a left wrist fusion into neutral to allow for greater independence in ADL. At 6 years of age, Will had distal femoral osteotomies for persistent knee flexion contractures. He had a wrist fusion with a tendon transfer on his left hand at age 10 to improve his hand function on the arm that now has better elbow flexion. He had knee extension osteotomies revised when he was 11 years old. He ambulates unlimited distances with knee-ankle-foot orthoses (KAFOs) and is able to walk limited household distances without braces. He is able to toilet, dress, and feed himself independently. He has received medically based PT services for a brief period postoperatively to get him back on his feet or to a higher level of function. Whenever he gets new braces and shoes, he consults his medically based therapist for the brace checkout and shoe wedge measurement.

At the age of 13, he continued to receive weekly direct school-based therapy services. Emphasis of PT is on independent mobility within his educational environment. Stair ambulation continues to be challenging but necessary for fire drills. He independently managed his braces, including donning, doffing, and locking. He actively worked on a self-stretching program with emphasis on stretching his knees into extension. He continued to work on managing his books throughout the hallways and in the classroom. He received a power wheelchair when he was 10 years old but used it only for independence in the community with his peers, or when his braces had broken components. He continued to walk the entire school day in his KAFOs with wedged sneakers.

Now, Will is 18. He stopped receiving physical therapy services the year before graduation, as he had no mobility limitations that interfered with his educational process, and he had achieved adult height as documented on x-ray. He has graduated from high school and has a job working full time in a retail store doing customer service. He continues to use ambulation in his locked KAFOs with wedged shoes as his primary means of mobility. He is independent in self-care activities and is able to drive with hand controls and a steering wheel knob. At this point, he reports no desire to use power mobility, as he is happy with his ambulation endurance. He reports having an active social life with a wide variety of friends and a girlfriend he hopes to marry.

EVIDENCE TO PRACTICE 10-1

CASE STUDY "WILL"

EXAMINATION DECISION

Will is fully grown and perceives himself as completely independent. Considering his present age and the fact that he is functioning independently at this point is important, but he would benefit from some strategies to work on energy conservation.

PLAN OF CARE DECISION

Referral to Office of Vocational Rehabilitation. Recommend motorized mobility for long distances.

Patient/Family Preferences

Dillon, E. R., Bjornson, K. F., Jaffe, K. M., Hall, J. G., & Song, K. (2009). Ambulatory activity in youth with arthrogryposis: A cohort study. *Journal of Pediatric Orthopaedics, 29*, 214–217.

"Joseph"

Joseph is a 6-year-old male who is the third child in his family. His mother reported less activity during this pregnancy than during the previous two pregnancies but was not overly concerned. He was delivered by a planned cesarean section and presented in a frank breech position. He was diagnosed with AMC at birth and was subsequently transferred to a children's hospital for care.

PT was initiated before he was 2 days old. Posture was marked by hips so excessively flexed that his feet were positioned by his ears.

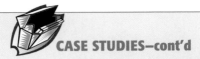

CASE STUDIES—cont'd

He had hyperextended knees, and his feet exhibited an equinovarus clubfoot deformity bilaterally. Torticollis with head rotation to the right was noted. The shoulders had what appeared to be normal passive range of motion. Joseph's elbows were flexed to 25°, his wrists were flexed and ulnarly deviated, and he had finger flexion contractures.

Photographs were taken to document posture and initial ROM. Goniometry was performed with a cut-down goniometer. Muscle strength was assessed through palpation and observation. Splinting of the feet and knees was initiated when he was 3 days old. Family and staff were educated on positioning to maximize hip extension. Joseph received passive ROM twice a day by a physical therapist, twice a day by nursing, and another one to two times a day by his dad, who stayed with him at the hospital. He was discharged from the hospital after 10 days. The extended stay was a result of feeding problems, which resolved before he was discharged. New splints were fabricated before discharge because of improvements made in ROM during his hospital stay. Home-based PT services were initiated when he returned home.

Joseph's health insurance plan had limited services for each lifetime condition. He qualified for 60 days of home-based PT services and 60 days of outpatient services. His family petitioned the insurance company, which agreed to pay for durable medical equipment past the 60 days, but no therapy once his benefit was exhausted.

Medically related home-based services began at 14 days of age and focused on maximizing lower extremity alignment with emphasis on hip extension, knee flexion, and neutral foot alignment. A stretching program was initiated to address the torticollis (see Chapter 12 for additional information on interventions for torticollis). Positioning, handling, and developmental skills were addressed during this time as well. The home-based physical therapist was able to adjust Joseph's foot and knee splints for increased girth. By 1 month of age, Joseph's hip flexion contractures had been reduced to 40°. Hips could be adducted to neutral, and his knees could be flexed to 120°. The forefeet could be brought to neutral, and the hindfeet corrected to −20° of dorsiflexion. Joseph exhibited a hypotonic trunk with poor head control, affecting prolonged positioning in his car seat and in prone. The car seat was padded with blanket rolls to allow neutral alignment of the head, trunk, and lower extremities. Adapted prone positions were addressed through football carries and prone positioning on mom's lap.

New foot splints were fabricated at 10 weeks of age. Knee splints were no longer needed at this time. Use of a strap to control excessive hip abduction was encouraged. He was seen every other week in a medically based PT clinic, where the physical therapist worked with the family on the long-term therapy plan of stretching and strengthening to maximize developmental skills. The long-term goal was independent ambulation with AFOs without an assistive device within the next 3 years.

Joseph's home-based PT benefit from his insurance was exhausted by the time he was 10 weeks old, but community-based early intervention (EI) services began at 14 weeks with weekly PT and occupational therapy. Emphasis of treatment was on trunk strengthening and head control activities, as well as on stretching.

He began a standing program in AFOs, wedged sneakers, and knee extension splints to help control his weak knees. This was initiated in a standing frame similar to the one shown in Figure 10-6. He progressed well with standing tolerance in the stander, and it was decided at 10 months to surgically correct his feet using posterior mediolateral releases. After 6 weeks of casting, he received KAFOs for day use and Dennis Brown shoes with a bar for night wear. Physical therapy services were increased to two times a week at this point. After 3 months, he was having difficulty with the Dennis Brown shoes and the bar, and they were replaced with AFOs for those times he was not in the KAFOs.

His EI physical therapist worked on standing and trunk strengthening for 5 months before it was decided that Joseph, at 15 months of age, would benefit from a pelvic band. He worked on standing and stepping with the HKAFOs for 6 weeks before starting postoperative medically based PT services at 17 months. In 8 weeks, he went from standing in HKAFOs to walking limited community distances with a posterior walker and KAFOs.

At 21 months, he was able to walk in AFOs with a posterior walker but has a significant amount of internal rotation from tibial torsion, putting excessive force across his knees. He could walk up to 20 steps in KAFOs without upper extremity support and would retrieve toys from the floor and return to upright with close supervision. At that time, he was working on safe falling techniques. By 24 months, he was walking in locked KAFOs without an assistive device and continued to get physical therapy services through his state's early intervention program.

At the age of 3 years, his physical therapy services transitioned to preschool-based services, for which the emphasis of care was on skills necessary for preschool participation. At that time, he also started walking with AFOs without an assistive device. He worked on playground skills, traveling through hallways while managing his personal items and classroom transitions, including floor-to-stand transfers. His family continued with a stretching program, but despite this, his feet started to get tight and painful.

He had 6 weeks of serial casting on his feet but ultimately needed a clubfoot revision with an anterior tibialis transfer on his feet to help with alignment at the age of 4 years, and a tibial derotation osteotomy on the right to correct excessive internal rotation at the age of 5 years.

Now at 7 years of age, Joe is an active second grader. He receives educationally based PT services on a consultative basis. He has few adaptations for his strength limitations during gym class but otherwise is able to keep up with his peers. He rides a bicycle with training wheels. Although Joe does not run as fast as his peers, he enjoys and participates in sports and group activities, especially his community little league baseball and soccer.

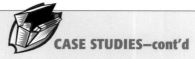

CASE STUDIES—cont'd

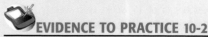

EVIDENCE TO PRACTICE 10-2

CASE STUDY "JOSEPH"

EXAMINATION DECISION

Joseph is a young man who is at risk for progression of contractures but who has few physical limitations to his preferred activity participation at this time. His present age should be considered, along with the fact that he is functioning independently in the educational environment and at a community level.

He would benefit from consultative therapy services addressing endurance, school mobility, strength, and changes in postural alignment with growth.

His family may need a support system to help work through strategies and adaptations necessary for strength limitations.

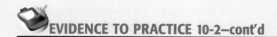

EVIDENCE TO PRACTICE 10-2—cont'd

PLAN OF CARE DECISION

Patient/Family Preferences[16]

Arthrogryposis Multiplex Congenita Support, Inc.: www.AMCsupport.org

Fassier, A., Wicart, P., Dubousset, J., & Seringe, R. (2009). Arthrogryposis multiplex congenita: Long-term follow-up from birth until skeletal maturity. *Journal of Child Orthopaedics, 3*, 383–390.

Coster, W. J., Deeney, T., Haltiwanger, J., & Haley, S. M. (1998). *School function assessment.* San Antonio, TX: The Psychological Corporation.

REFERENCES

1. Asif, S., Umer, M., Beg, R., Umar, M. (2004). Operative treatment of bilateral hip dislocation in children with arthrogryposis multiplex congenita. *Journal of Orthopedic Surgery, 12,* 4–9.

2. Axt, M. W., Niethard, F. U., Doderlein, L., & Weber, M. (1997). Principles of treatment of the upper extremity in arthrogryposis multiplex congenita type I. *Journal of Pediatric Orthopaedics Part B, 6,* 179–185.

3. Bamshad, M., Bohnsack, J. F., Jorde, L. B., & Carey, J. C. (1996). Distal arthrogryposis type 1: Clinical analysis of a large kindred. *American Journal of Medical Genetics, 65,* 282–285.

4. Bamshad, M., Watkins, W. S., Zenger, R. K., Bohnsack, J. F., Carey, J. C., Otterud, B., Krakowiak, P. A., Robertson, M., & Jorde, L. B. (1994). A gene for distal arthrogryposis type I maps to the pericentromeric region of chromosome 9. *American Journal of Genetics, 55,* 1153–1158.

5. Boehm, S., Limpaphayom, N., Alaee, F., Sinclair, M. F., & Dobbs, M. B. (2008). Early results of the Ponseti method for the treatment of clubfoot in distal arthrogryposis. *Journal of Bone and Joint Surgery (American), 90,* 1501–1507.

6. Borowski, A., Grissom, L., Littleton, A. G., Donohoe, M., King, M., & Kumar, S. J. (2008). Diagnostic imaging of the knee in children with arthrogryposis and knee extension or hyperextension contracture. *Journal of Pediatric Orthopaedics, 28,* 466–470.

7. Brunner, R., Hefti, F., & Tgetgel, J. D. (1997). Arthrogrypotic joint contracture at the knee and the foot: Correction with a circular frame. *Journal of Pediatric Orthopaedics, 6B,* 192–197.

8. Burglen, L., Amiel, J., Viollet, L., Lefebura, S., Burlet, P., Clermont, O., Raclin, V., Landriau, P., Verloes, A., Munnich, A., & Melki, J. (1996). Survival motor neuron gene deletion in arthrogryposis multiplex congenita—Spinal Muscular Atrophy Association. *Journal of Clinical Investigation, 98,* 1130–1132.

9. Cassis, N., & Capdevila, R. (2000). Talectomy for clubfoot in arthrogryposis. *Journal of Pediatric Orthopaedics, 20,* 652–655.

10. Choi, I. H., Yang, M. S., Chung, C. Y., Cho, T. J., & Sohn, Y. J. (2001). The treatment of recurrent arthrogrypotic club foot in children by the Ilizarov method. *Journal of Bone and Joint Surgery (British), 83B,* 731–737.

11. Coster, W. J., Deeney, T., Haltiwanger, J., & Haley, S. M. (1998). *School function assessment.* San Antonio, TX: The Psychological Corporation.

12. Darin, N., Kimber, E., Kroksmark, A., & Tulinius, M. (2002). Multiple congenital contractures: Birth prevalence, etiology, and outcome. *Journal of Pediatrics, 140,* 61–67.

13. DelBello, D. A., & Watts, H. G. (1996). Distal femoral extension osteotomy for knee flexion contracture in patients with arthrogryposis. *Journal of Pediatric Orthopedics, 16,* 122–126.

14. Dillon, E. R., Bjornson, K. F., Jaffe, K. M., Hall, J. G., & Song, K. (2009). Ambulatory activity in youth with arthrogryposis: A cohort study. *Journal of Pediatric Orthopaedics, 29,* 214–217.

15. Drummond, D. S., Siller, T. N., & Cruess, R. L. (1978). Management of arthrogryposis multiplex congenita. In *AAOS instructional lectures.* Montreal, Canada: American Academy of Orthopaedic Surgeons.

16. Fassier, A., Wicart, P., Dubousset, J., & Seringe, R. (2009). Arthrogryposis multiplex congenita: Long-term follow-up from birth until skeletal maturity. *Journal of Child Orthopaedics, 3,* 383–390.

17. Hall, J. G. (1981). An approach to congenital contractures (arthrogryposis). *Pediatric Annals, 10,* 249–257.

18. Hall, J. G. (1985). Genetic aspects of arthrogryposis. *Clinical Orthopedics, 194,* 44–53.

19. Hall, J. G. (1989). Arthrogryposis. *American Family Physician*, *39*, 113–119.

20. Hall, J. G. (1997). Arthrogryposis multiplex congenita: Etiology, genetics, classification, diagnostic approach, and general aspects. *Journal of Pediatric Orthopaedics Part B*, *6*, 157–166.

21. Hall, J. G. (2009). Genetics of multiple congenital contractures syndromes (arthrogryposes). Lecture at the Multidisciplinary Medical Approach to Managing Arthrogryposis, July 15, 2009, Wilmington, DE.

22. Hall, J. G. (2007). Arthrogryposes (multiple congenital contractures). In D. L. Rimoin, J. M. Connor, R. E. Pyeritz, & B. R. Kork (Eds.), *Emery and Rimoin's principle and practice of medical genetics* (Vol. 3, 5th ed.; Chap. 168; pp. 3785–3856). New York: Churchill Livingstone.

23. Hall, J. G. (1998). Overview of arthrogryposis. In L. T. Staheli, J. G. Hall, K. M. Jaffe, & D. O. Paholke (Eds.), *Arthrogryposis: A text atlas* (pp. 1–25). New York: Cambridge Press.

24. Hell, A. K., Campbell, R. M., & Hefti, F. (2005). The vertical expandable prosthetic titanium rib implant for the treatment of thoracic insufficiency syndrome associated with congenital and neuromuscular scoliosis in young children. *Journal of Pediatric Orthopaedics B*, *14*, 287–293.

25. Hislop, H. J., & Montgomery, J. (Eds.) (2007). *Daniels & Worthingham's muscle testing: Techniques of manual examination* (8th ed.). Philadelphia: Elsevier Science.

26. Ho C. A., & Karol, L. A. (2008). The utility of knee releases in arthrogryposis. *Journal of Pediatric Orthopaedics*, *28*, 307–313.

27. Hosny, G. A., & Fadel, M. (2008). Managing flexion knee deformity using a circular frame. *Clinical Orthopaedics and Related Research*, *466*, 2995–3002.

28. Ippolito, E., Farsetti, P., Caterini, R., & Tudisco, C. (2003). Long-term comparative results in patients with congenital clubfoot treated with two different protocols. *Journal of Bone and Joint Surgery (American)*, *85A*, 1286–1294.

29. Kendall, F. P., McCreary, E. K., & Provance, P. G. (2005). *Muscle testing and function* (5th ed.). Baltimore: Lippincott, Williams & Wilkins.

30. Klatt, J., & Stevens, P. M. (2008). Guided growth for fixed knee flexion deformity. *Journal of Pediatric Orthopaedics*, *28*, 626–631.

31. Kowalczyk, B., & Lejman, T. (2008). Short-term experience with Ponseti casting and the Achilles tenotomy method for clubfeet treatment in arthrogryposis multiplex congenita. *Journal of Child Orthopaedics*, *2*, 365–371.

32. Kozin, S. H. (2009). Congenital differences about the elbow. *Hand Clinics*, *91*, 277–291.

33. Kramer, A., & Stevens, P. M. (2001). Anterior femoral stapling. *Journal of Pediatric Orthopedics*, *21*, 804–807.

34. Legaspi, J., Li, Y. H., Chow, W., & Leong, J. C. (2001). Talectomy in patients with recurrent deformity in clubfoot. *Journal of Bone and Joint Surgery (British)*, *83B*, 384–387.

35. Letts, M., & Davidson, D. (1999). The role of bilateral talectomy in the management of bilateral rigid clubfeet. *American Journal of Orthopedics*, *28*, 106–110.

36. MacEwen, G. D., & Gale, D. I. (1983). Hip disorders in arthrogryposis multiplex congenita. In J. Katz, & R. Siffert (Eds.), *Management of hip disorders in children* (pp. 209–228). Philadelphia: J. B. Lippincott.

37. Mancini, M. C., Coster, W., Trombly, C. A., & Heeren, T. C. (2000). Predicting participation in elementary school of children with disabilities. *Archives of Physical Medicine and Rehabilitation*, *81*, 339–347.

38. Morcuende, J. A., Dobbs, M. B., & Frick, S. L. (2008). Results of the Ponseti method in patients with clubfoot associated with arthrogryposis. *Iowa Orthopaedic Journal*, *28*, 22–26.

39. Moynihan, L. M., Bundey, S. E., Heath, D., et al. (1998). Autozygosity mapping, to chromosome 11q25, of a rare autosomal recessive syndrome causing histiocytosis, joint contractures, and sensorineural deafness. *American Journal of Human Genetics*, *62*, 1123–1128.

40. Murray, C., & Fixsen, J. A. (1997). Management of knee deformity in classical arthrogryposis multiplex congenita (amyoplasia congenita). *Journal of Pediatric Orthopaedics Part B*, *6*, 186–191.

41. Niki, H., Staheli, L., & Mosca, V. S. (1997). Management of clubfoot deformity in amyoplasia. *Journal of Pediatric Orthopaedics*, *17*, 803–807.

42. Palmer, P. M., MacEwen, G. D., Bowen, J. R., & Matthews, P. A. (1985). Passive motion therapy for infants with arthrogryposis. *Clinical Orthopedics and Related Research*, *194*, 54–59.

43. Palocaren, T., Thabet, A., Rogers, K., Holmes, L., Donohoe, M., King, M., & Kumar, S. J. (2010). Anterior distal femoral stapling for correcting knee flexion contracture in children with arthrogryposis—Preliminary results. *Journal of Pediatric Orthopaedics*, *30*, 169–173.

44. Robinson, R. O. (1990). AMC: Feeding, language and other health problems. *Neuropediatrics*, *21*, 177–178.

45. Sarwark, J. F., MacEwen, G. D., & Scott, C. I. (1990). Amyoplasia (a common form of arthrogryposis). *Journal of Bone and Joint Surgery (American)*, *72*, 465–469.

46. Schiulli, C., Corradi-Scalise, D., & Donatelli-Schulthiss, M. L. (1988). Powered mobility vehicles as aides in independent locomotion for very young children. *Physical Therapy*, *68*, 997–999.

47. Scott, C. I., & Nicholson, L. (2003). Personal communication. Alfred I. duPont for Children, Genetics Department, Wilmington, *DE*.

48. Sells, J. M., Jaffe, K. M., & Hall, J. G. (1996). Amyoplasia, the most common type of arthrogryposis: The potential for good outcome. *Pediatrics*, *97*, 225–231.

49. Shohat, M., Lotan, R., Magal, N., Shohat, T., Fishel-Ghodsian, N., Rotter, J., & Jaber, L. (1997). A gene for arthrogryposis multiplex congenita neuropathic type is linked to D5S394 on chromosome 5qter. *American Journal of Human Genetics*, *61*, 1139–1143.

50. Sneddon, J. (1999). AMC & aging survey. *Avenues*, *10*, 1–3.

51. Sodergard, J., Hakamies-Blomqvist, L., Sainio, K., Ryoppy, S., & Vuorinen, R. (1997). Arthrogryposis multiplex congenital: Perinatal and electromyographic findings, disability, and

psychosocial outcome. *Journal of Pediatric Orthopaedics Part B*, 6, 167–171.

52. Sodergard, J., & Ryoppy, S. (1990). The knee in arthrogryposis multiplex congenita. *Journal of Pediatric Orthopedics, 10*, 177–182.

53. Staheli, L. T., Chew, D. E., Elliot, J. S., & Mosca, V. S. (1987). Management of hip dislocations in children with AMC. *Journal of Pediatric Orthopedics, 7*, 681–685.

54. Staheli, L. T., Hall, J. G., Jaffe, K. M., & Paholke, D. O. (1998). *Arthrogryposis: A text atlas.* New York: Cambridge Press.

55. St. Clair, H. S., & Zimbler, S. (1985). A plan of management and treatment results in the arthrogrypotic hip. *Clinical Orthopedics and Related Research, 194*, 74–80.

56. Szoke, G., Staheli, L. T., Jaffe, K., & Hall, J. (1996). Medial-approach open reduction of hip dislocation in amyoplasia-type arthrogryposis. *Journal of Pediatric Orthopedics, 16*, 127–130.

57. Tachdjian, M. O. (1990). Arthrogryposis multiplex congenita (multiple congenital contractures). In M. Tachdjian (Ed.), *Pediatric orthopedics* (pp. 2086–2114). Philadelphia: WB Saunders.

58. Tefft, D., Guerette, P., & Furumasu, J. (1999). Cognitive predictors of young children's readiness for powered mobility. *Developmental Medicine & Child Neurology, 41*, 665–670.

59. van Bosse, H. J., Feldman, D. S., Anavian, J., & Sala, D. A. (2007). Treatment of knee flexion contractures in patients with arthrogryposis. *Journal of Pediatric Orthopaedics, 27*, 930–937.

60. van Bosse, H. J., Marangoz, S., Lehman, W. B., & Sala, D. A. (2009). Correction of arthrogrypotic clubfoot with a modified Ponseti technique. *Clinical Orthopedics and Related Research, 467*, 1283–1293.

61. Vanpaelmel, L., Schoenmakers, M., van Nesselrooij, B., Pruijs, H., & Helders, P. (1997). Multiple congenital contractures. *Journal of Pediatric Orthopaedics Part B, 6*, 172–178.

62. Williams, P. F. (1973). The elbow in arthrogryposis. *Journal of Bone and Joint Surgery (British), 55*, 834–840.

63. Williams, P. (1978). The management of arthrogryposis. *Orthopedic Clinics of North America, 9*, 67–88.

64. Wynne-Davies, R., Williams, P. F., & O'Conner, J. C. B. (1981). The 1960s epidemic of arthrogryposis multiplex congenita. *Journal of Bone and Joint Surgery (British), 63*, 76–82.

65. Yau, P. W., Chow, W., Li, Y. H., & Leong, J. C. (2002). Twenty-year follow up of hip problems in arthrogryposis multiplex congenita. *Journal of Pediatric Orthopaedics, 22*, 359–363.

66. Yingsakmongkol, W., & Kumar, S. J. (2000). Scoliosis in arthrogryposis multiplex congenita: Results after nonsurgical and surgical treatment. *Journal of Pediatric Orthopaedics, 20*, 656–661.

67. Young, N. L., Williams, J. I., Yoshida, K. K., & Wright, J. G. (2000). Measurement properties of the Activities Scale for Kids. *Journal of Clinical Epidemiology, 53*, 125–137.

RESOURCES

Arthrogryposis Multiplex Congenita Support, Inc.: www.AMCsupport.org

Avenues: TAG: The Arthrogryposis Group: www.TAGonline.org/uk

11 Osteogenesis Imperfecta

MAUREEN DONOHOE, PT, DPT, PCS

Osteogenesis imperfecta (OI) is an inherited disorder of connective tissue. Other terms in the literature used to describe OI include fragilitas ossium and brittle bones. OI has an incidence of 1 in 10,000 individuals.[38,58] This disorder comprises a number of distinct syndromes and has great variability in its manifestations. The salient impairments of OI are lax joints, weak muscles, and diffuse osteoporosis, which result in multiple recurrent fractures. These recurring fractures, sustained from even minimal trauma, coupled with weak muscles and lax joints, result in major deformity. Additional impairments in OI with variable presentation include blue sclerae, dentinogenesis imperfecta, deafness, hernias, easy bruising, and excessive sweating. Dentinogenesis imperfecta is a defect in the dentin and the dentinoenamel junction of the tooth. Often the enamel is normal, but teeth initially look gray, bluish, or brown because of the dentin defect. These teeth have a higher incidence of cracking, wear, and decay as the enamel cracks away from the dentin. Primary teeth are often more affected than adult teeth.[63]

Without early and adequate intervention, these problems in children with OI may lead to irreversible deformities and disability. Physical therapy can have a positive impact on these children and their families. Therapists can accomplish this through strengthening exercises, conditioning activities, adapting the environment, educating caregivers, and encouraging activity participation across a lifetime. Early physical therapy and medical interventions help prevent deformities and long-term functional limitations.

Children and adolescents with OI are often overprotected as a result of recurring fractures, which can contribute to social isolation. Some have difficulty interacting in peer play, adjusting to regular school, and achieving an independence level necessary to accomplish vocational goals. Most children with OI have average or above-average intelligence and greatly benefit from a stimulating educational environment. These children become adults who are usually productive members of society. Management of their disabilities should be directed toward obtaining optimal independence, social integration, and educational achievement. The overall prognosis of OI and its long-term sequelae depend on the severity of the disease, which ranges from very mild to severe. Likewise, disability ranges from relatively mild with no deformities to extremely severe, with death occurring at birth or shortly thereafter.

In this chapter, we address the classification and pathophysiology of OI, medical and surgical interventions, physical therapy examination, evaluation, and interventions from infancy through adulthood. A case study of a child with OI is presented.

CLASSIFICATION

OI is a heterogeneous collection of impairments with varying severity, marked by fragility of bone. Clinically, many types of OI present similarly. Despite this, OI is not a single genetic disorder, but rather an array of different disorders based on a complement of information, including clinical presentation, genetic testing, and histologic analysis.

Historically, many classifications have been proposed to cover the diversity of clinical presentations.[28,68] Looser[43] classified OI into two types: OI congenital (OIC) and OI tarda (OIT). Seedorf[64] in 1949 further subclassified OI tarda into two types: tarda gravis (OIT type I) and tarda levis (OIT type II). The OI congenita and tarda classifications have clinical usefulness but do not reflect the scope of OI from a genetic or pathogenetic standpoint; however, the clinician will sometimes see these classifications referenced in the literature.

OIC has been known as the most severe and disabling form. It is characterized by numerous fractures at birth, dwarfism, bowing or deformities of the long bones, blue sclerae (80% of cases), and dentinogenesis imperfecta (80% of cases). Infants with OIC have a poor prognosis, with a high mortality rate resulting from intracranial hemorrhage at birth or recurring respiratory tract infections during infancy.[74]

OIT is considered the milder form of OI, in which fractures occur after birth. It has been subclassified on the basis of the degree of bowing of the extremities or the number of fractures.[74] The clinical characteristics of OIT type I include dentinogenesis imperfecta, short stature, and bowing of only the lower extremities. Most with OIT type I can ambulate but may need external support such as orthotics. Surgery is often indicated for correction of the long bone deformity. OIT type II is the least disabling form of OI, where fractures are not associated with bowing of the bones. Most of these children approach average height and have an excellent prognosis for ambulation.

In 1978, Sillence and Danks delineated four distinct genetic types of OI. This numeric classification system is based on clinical presentation, radiologic criteria, and mode of inheritance and is generally well accepted by clinicians, as well as basic scientists.[69] The Sillence Classification uses a numeric system that correlates with morphologic and biochemical studies of OI.[68] With the onset of gene mapping and better databases for tracking the OI population, Glorieux expanded the classification out to eight distinct categories.[7,33]

Autosomal recessive forms of OI make up less than 10% of cases.[32] Most of the first four types of OI are considered autosomal dominant in inheritance.[68-70] The first four types of OI are caused by a defect in type I collagen, which can be tracked back to a mutation in the genes *COL1A1* and *COL1A2* located on chromosomes 7 and 17. These genes are responsible for encoding the two alpha chains that make up type I collagen genes.[61] The other classifications of OI, types V through VIII, do not have a type I collagen defect but do have significant bone fragility and present clinically similar to types with the collagen defect.[32,34,62]

OI TYPE I

OI type I makes up 50% of the total OI population.[32] It is characterized by markedly blue sclerae throughout life, generalized osteoporosis with bone fragility, joint hyperlaxity, and presenile conductive hearing loss. Patients are generally short but are not as short as those with other forms of OI. At birth, weight and length are normal; short stature occurs postnatally. Dentinogenesis imperfecta is variably present. Those with OI type IA have normal teeth, and those with OI type IB have dentinogenesis imperfecta. Fractures may be present at birth (10%) or may appear at any time during infancy and childhood.[68] The frequency and development of skeletal deformity are also variable.

OI TYPE II

Based on the Sillence Classification, OI type II is not compatible with life, and infants may be stillborn or may die within a few weeks. Extreme bone fragility occurs with minimal calvarial mineralization. Marked delay of ossification of the skull and facial bones is noted, and the long bones are crumbled.[74] Infants are small for their gestational age and have characteristic short, curved, and deformed limbs.

OI TYPE III

According to the Sillence Classification, OI type III usually is autosomal dominant, but on the rare occasion it is recessive. This form is severe, with progressive deformity of the long bones, skull, and spine, resulting in very short stature.

Abnormal growth plate lines give the long bones a popcorn-like appearance.[54] Usually, severe bone fragility, moderate bone deformity at birth, multiple fractures, and severe growth retardation are noted. OI type III appears similar to OI type II, except that the lack of skull ossification is not as marked, and birth weight and length are within normal range. Sclerae in OI Type III have a variable hue, tending to be bluish at birth and becoming less so with age. Dentinogenesis imperfecta occurs in 45% of patients with OI type III, and hearing loss is common. As a result of the complications of severe kyphoscoliosis and resulting respiratory compromise, death may occur in childhood.

OI TYPE IV

OI type IV is characterized by mild to moderate deformity and postnatal short stature. Bone fragility and deformities of the long bones of variable severity are noted. Sclerae tend to be normal, but dentinogenesis imperfecta is common. Hearing loss is variable. The prognosis for ambulation in this population is excellent.[14]

OI TYPE V

In 2000, Glorieux first described the autosomal dominant OI type V. It is characterized by hypertrophic calcification of fractures and surgical osteotomies. Many patients have calcification of the interosseous membrane of the radius and ulna, ultimately limiting supination/pronation of the forearm. OI type V represents 5% of the moderate to severe cases of OI.[32,34,62]

OI TYPE VI

OI type VI is autosomal recessive and extremely rare, and presents with moderate to severe deformity, similar to OI type IV, but with normal teeth and sclera. No abnormality of calcium, phosphate, parathyroid hormone, vitamin D metabolism, or growth plate mineralization is noted.[32,34,62]

OI TYPE VII

OI type VII is presumed autosomal recessive and is associated with a gene defect mapped to chromosome 3p22-24.1. This mutation affects the translation of the collagen with mutations in the cartilage-associated protein gene *(CRTAP)* and the prolyl 3-hydroxylase-1 gene *(LEPRE1)*.[7,32] No type I collagen defect is noted in this form of OI, rather the defect involves how the collagen is translated to create bone.

With this gene defect, normal sclerae and dentin are noted, with moderate to severe bone fragility and shortening of the humerus and femur.[41] Those with partial expression of CRTAP have moderate bone dysplasia similar to OI type IV; all cases with absence of CRTAP have been lethal.[32]

OI TYPE VIII

OI type VIII is presumed autosomal recessive and caused by mutations of genes that affect the translation of the collagen with mutations in the cartilage-associated protein gene *(CRTAP)* and the prolyl 3-hydroxylase-1 gene *(LEPRE1)*.[7] No type I collagen defect is noted in this form of OI, rather the defect involves how the collagen is translated to create bone.

The absence or severe deficiency of prolyl-3-hydroxylase activity due to the *LEPRE1* gene results in lethal to severe osteochondrodystrophy. OI type VIII is clinically similar to OI types II and III. Those affected have white sclerae, flattened long bones, slender ribs without beading, and small to normal-sized head circumference. Severe growth deficiency and bone fragility are noted in those who survive into the teen years.[46,54]

With the rapid rate of gene mapping and the dedication of the Osteogenesis Imperfecta Foundation to maintaining a patient database, it is expected that new information on classification of OI will continue to grow. Many of the classifications defined beyond Sillence's initial four types resemble the first four types clinically, but molecularly, the bone fragility is vastly different (Table 11-1).[32]

PATHOPHYSIOLOGY

In the first four types of OI, a defect in collagen synthesis results from an abnormality in processing procollagen to type I collagen, apparently causing the bones to be brittle. This defect affects the formation of both enchondral and intramembranous bone. Collagen fibers fail to mature beyond the reticular fiber stage. Studies show that osteoblasts have normal or increased activity but fail to produce and organize the collagen.[60] Although similar bone fragility is found with OI types VI, VII, and VIII, the defect lies in how the normally developed type I collagen is translated into bone.[33] Histological variability is evident among the different types of OI. With OI type I, morphologic findings include an increased amount of glycogen in osteoblasts, mild hypercellularity of bone,[1] and no abnormality in collagen fiber diameter.[20] Those with OI type II have abnormally thin corneal and skin collagen fibers.[12] Bone histology reveals decreased trabeculae and cortical bone thickness.[62] In types III and IV, morphologic findings include an increased amount of woven bone, increased cellularity, an increased number of resorption surfaces, and wide osteoid seams.[27] Histologically, OI type V has lamellar organization in an irregular meshlike pattern.[62] OI type VI has a unique fish scale–like appearance of the lamellae. The appearance of a mineralization defect similar to osteomalacia is apparent with osteoid accumulation histologically, although no defects are associated with calcium, phosphate, parathyroid hormone, or vitamin D metabolism.[62]

OI type VII is histologically similar to OI type I, and it is not until analysis of the collagen and the genes is done that it can be differentiated. Both have decreased cortical width and trabecular number, with increased bone turnover.[76] The lethal form of OI type VIII is similar to OI type II, as bone histology has decreased trabeculae and cortical bone thickness.[62]

Persons who have inherited OI tend to have the same type of mutation through the family, although clinical manifestations within that type may be variable. First-generation OI tends to be caused by a novel mutation of the gene. This specific gene mutation can then be passed to offspring. Genetic counseling when OI is found gives parents an accurate estimate of the risk of recurrence and an understanding of clinical variability in the family.[57,78]

MEDICAL MANAGEMENT

No cure for OI is known. Historically, no consistently effective medications were available to strengthen skeletal structures and prevent fractures until the bisphosphonate class of drugs was introduced to this population in the late 1990s.[3,4,40] Since then, the direction of OI management has dramatically changed, especially for the population with moderate to severe bone fragility.[2]

Bisphosphonates are having promising effects. Positive results such as reducing fractures and improving bone density have been reported from such pharmacologic agents as bisphosphonates,[40] including pamidronate and alendronate.[26,49,57] Bisphosphonates work by reducing normal bone turnover. They inhibit osteoclast activity; therefore the osteoblasts are not destroyed as rapidly by the osteoclasts.

Despite significant improvements that have resulted from the use of bisphosphonates, great debate continues over long-term use and implications of use around the time of orthopedic surgery.[46,51,52,61,77]

Another aspect of care with OI is ensuring that the vitamin D level is adequate. Vitamin D allows the body to absorb calcium. Inadequate vitamin D limits the body's ability to form the hormone calcitriol. This in turn leads to insufficient calcium absorption from the diet; therefore the body must take calcium from the skeleton.[42] If vitamin D deficiency is established, vitamin supplementation, as well as calcium supplementation, is recommended.

Bone marrow transplant and stem cell therapy have been used sparingly. Transplantation of normal mesenchymal stem cells with the potential to differentiate into mature osteoblasts may result in significant improvement in bone collagen and mineral content. The therapeutic effect is possibly due to the selective growth advantage of normal cells over diseased host cells. Some research is being directed toward transplanting bone marrow cells with osteogenic potential with the collagen gene.[15,36,53,59]

The use of whole body vibration (WBV) is being researched as a minimally invasive technique to improve bone density and strength in children and adolescents with

TABLE 11-1   Classification of Osteogenesis Imperfecta

Classification	Inheritance	Genetic/Histologic Information	Clinical Features Fractures	Clinical Features Radiographic Features
Osteogenesis imperfecta type I (A, B)	Autosomal dominant	Lower than normal type I collagen, but structure of collagen is normal because of frameshift in *COL1A1*	Mild to severe bone fragility	Multiple fractures of long bones, compression fractures of vertebrae
Osteogenesis imperfecta type II (A, B, C)	New autosomal dominant mutation	Mutation in *COL1A1* and *COL1A2*, which encode for type I collagen	Extreme bone fragility	Absent or limited calvarial mineralization, flat vertebral bodies, crumpled long bones, beaded ribs
Osteogenesis imperfecta type III	Autosomal dominant (usual) Autosomal recessive (rare)	Mutation in *COL1A1* and *COL1A2*, which encode for type I collagen, reduced amounts of bone matrix	Variable bone fragility (often severe)	Progressive skeletal deformity (bowing), abnormal growth plates give long bones popcorn-like appearance
Osteogenesis imperfecta type IV	Autosomal dominant	Mutation in *COL1A1* and *COL1A2*, which encode for type I collagen, reduced amounts of bone matrix	Bone fragility	Variable deformity
Osteogenesis imperfecta type V	Autosomal dominant	No type I collagen defect, lamellae of bone have meshlike appearance, decreased cortical and cancellous bone	Moderate to severe bone fragility	Hypertrophic callus formation, calcification of the interosseous membrane between radius and ulna
Osteogenesis imperfecta type VI	Presumed autosomal recessive	No type I collagen defect, fishlike scales, appearance on the bone lamellae	Bone fragility, moderate severity	Variable deformity, vertebral compression fractures
Osteogenesis imperfecta type VII	Autosomal recessive	Mutation in gene for cartilage-associated protein (CRTAP) on chromosome 3p22-24.1	Bone fragility	Variable deformity, short humeri and femora, coxa vara common
Osteogenesis imperfecta type VIII	Autosomal recessive	Absence or severe deficiency of prolyl3-hydroxylase activity due to *LEPRE1* gene	Variable bone fragility (often severe)	Progressive skeletal deformity (bowing), may have popcorn calcifications on long bones

significant motor impairment. The child is on a vibrating platform on a tilt table. The best results in terms of increased bone density and improved function, based on the Brief Assessment of Motor Function, occurred when the subject was at a 35° angle during the vibration. Those who have telescoping rods and/or a history of joint subluxation are not good candidates for this treatment.[65-67]

Once a fracture occurs, the bone is more susceptible to re-fracture. The already weakened structure predisposes the child to limb deformities from bowing of the long bones. Immobilization to assist in setting the bone in proper alignment can cause disuse osteoporosis, which, in turn, puts these fragile bones at greater risk of fracture. Hence, a vicious circle is created: Osteoporosis leads to fracture, and immobilization secondary to fracture creates disuse osteoporosis, which leads to further fracture. The goal, then, is to limit immobilization of the extremities as much as possible to prevent exacerbation of osteopenia and risk of additional fractures.

Fractures in patients with OI generally heal within the normal healing time, although the resultant callus may be large but of poor quality. These fractures must be immobilized for pain relief and to promote healing in the correct alignment. Pseudarthrosis may occur when the fracture is not immobilized. Immobilization may occur in the form of splinting with thermoplastic materials, orthoses, hip spica posterior shells, or casting. With malunion of fractures, angulation and bowing of the long bones occur, frequently accompanied by joint contractures. The physis may be disrupted, resulting in asymmetrical growth and deformity. When angulation occurs, mechanical forces tend to increase the deformity, thus aggravating the overall problem.[1] The cartilaginous ends of the long bones are disproportionately large and have irregular articular surfaces. Fortunately, in nearly all patients with OI, the fracture rate diminishes near or after puberty.

The most successful means of fracture stabilization in long bones in OI is internal fixation with intramedullary

Clinical Features					
Stature	**Dentin**	**Sclerae**	**Hearing**	**Ambulation**	**Other**
Average or slightly shorter than average stature	Normal: IA Dentinogenesis imperfecta: IB	Blue	Hearing loss	Ambulation without assistive devices	50% of the total OI population. Trian Ular Face noted
Very short stature		Normal: IIA, IIB Blue: IIC		Nonambulatory	Lethal form of OI. Infants have low birth weight. Most have respiratory, swallowing problems. Some may have cardiac impairment
Very short stature	Variable dentin abnormality	Variable; blue at birth	Hearing loss	Nonambulatory to ambulation for exercise and transfers, usually relies on an assistive device for support	Rib fractures in infants can cause life-threatening breathing problems. Increasing scoliosis is noted with age. Loose joints and triangular face are present
Short stature	Normal/dentinogenesis imperfecta	Normal	Variable	Ambulatory but may use an assistive device	Triangular face and progressive scoliosis noted. Most fractures occur before puberty
Short stature	Normal	Normal		Ambulatory	5% of the moderate to severe cases of OI. Resembles type IV in clinical presentation
Short stature	Normal	Normal	Variable	Ambulatory but may use an assistive device	Extremely rare, resembles type IV in clinical presentation
Short stature	Normal/dentinogenesis imperfecta	Normal	Variable	Mild: ambulatory Severe: nonambulatory	Mild cases clinically resemble OI type IV, severe cases resemble OI type II and are lethal
Very short stature		Normal			Presents similarly to the lethal forms of OI type II or III

rods.[37] Consensus indicates that intramedullary rods are advantageous, although significant debate continues over the type of internal fixation to be used in terms of material (steel vs. titanium) and fixation (static rod vs. telescoping rod). Although use of the intramedullary rod is not without complications, it can be helpful in preventing long bones from bowing after fracture. The rod provides internal support to prevent additional fractures. Indications for stabilization with rods include multiple recurring fractures and increasing long bone deformity that is interfering with orthotic fit and impairing function. The age of the patient and the size of the bone determine the type and timing of surgery. Intramedullary rod fixation of the femur is best done after 4 or 5 years of age, when the thigh is not so short as to complicate surgery by compounding the technical difficulty. Surgical insertion of the rod in thin bones is also technically difficult.

The type of rod used depends on the type and severity of fracture. When a solid rod is used, bone growth may occur beyond the ends of the rods, necessitating subsequent surgery later for placement of a longer rod. Because children with severe OI are at greater than normal anesthetic risk from potential respiratory compromise, the number of operative procedures is best kept to a minimum. Special instrumentation has been designed that "elongates" with the child's growth, eliminating the need for multiple surgical revisions as the bone grows (Figure 11-1). These extensible intramedullary fixation devices were first introduced by Bailey and Dubow.[6] They are used most frequently in the femur but also may be used in the humerus, tibia, and forearm. A high incidence of complications associated with using the intramedullary rods has been reported.[37] Problems involve the control of rotation and migration when extensible rods are used; thus postoperative casting may be necessary. Orthoses may be needed after insertion of the rod for further external support. Early weight bearing with orthotic support is initiated as soon as possible. With internal fixation, a risk of osteopenia around the rod is present, especially with telescoping rods.

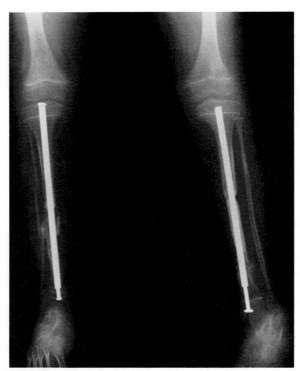

Figure 11-1 Extensible intramedullary fixation rods that elongate as the bone grows in a child with osteogenesis imperfecta.

Spinal deformities, including scoliosis and kyphosis, occur in 50% of patients with OI as a result of osteoporosis and vertebral compression fractures. Progressive spinal deformities such as scoliosis and pathologic kyphosis are more likely to occur in children with type III and IV OI than in those with type I OI.[22] Kyphoscoliosis can be disabling and may be present in 20% to 40% of patients.[74] Unlike in the typical population, kyphoscoliosis in those with OI can be progressive over a lifetime, which further compounds the patient's short stature. The most common curve is that of thoracic scoliosis. Scoliotic and kyphotic curves in patients with OI are not usually amenable to conservative bracing. In adolescents and adults with severe OI, the incidence of scoliosis is 80% to 90%. Surgical stabilization is often advocated for the management of these deformities, as the greater the curve, the greater difficulty is involved in meeting motor milestones.[25]

IMPAIRMENT

DIAGNOSIS AND PROBLEM IDENTIFICATION

In the most severe forms of OI, the infant is born with multiple fractures sustained in utero or during the birth process. The prognosis of OI depends on its type. In its most severe forms, multiple fractures that have occurred in utero and during birth are associated with a high mortality rate.

Prognostic indicators concerning survival and ambulation include the time of the initial fracture and the radiologic appearance of long bones and ribs at the time of the initial fracture. Spranger and associates[71] devised a scoring system for providing an accurate prognosis for newborns with OI. This system coded the degree of skeletal changes based on clinical and radiographic findings in 47 cases. These investigators found that newborns who had marked bowing of their lower extremities but less severe changes in the skull, ribs, vertebrae, and arms, and who had normal sclera, survived and had fewer fractures as they grew older. For the moderate and mild types, although the prognosis varies, a gradual tendency toward improvement has been noted when fracture incidence decreases after puberty.

If a family is known to be at risk of having a child with OI and the collagen defect, or if the genetic mutation has been identified in the parent, human chorionic villous biopsy can be done prenatally at 10 weeks of gestation to determine whether the child has the same defect. A prenatal ultrasound examination in the second trimester of pregnancy can be helpful in identifying skeletal dysplasia and associated fractures.[39]

The infant is usually of normal size at birth, but postnatal growth is impaired. Although no conclusive causative factors for this impaired growth are known, possible factors include the deformities themselves or abnormalities in the epiphyseal growth plates. The radiologic appearance of long bones associated with the most severe cases indicates bones with a thin radiolucent appearance. The malformed ribs affect respiratory function, which may lead to respiratory tract infection and reduced functional potential of the child.

Children with moderate OI are often identified after several fractures have resulted from seemingly slight trauma. An example is a fractured humerus caused by the child holding onto a car seat while the caretaker is trying to get the child out of the car. Those children who begin to have fractures of unknown origin at a young age can have collagen and biochemical studies done, usually from a skin biopsy. These tests can also be helpful in ruling out other disorders, such as idiopathic juvenile osteoporosis, leukemia, and congenital hypophosphatasia. Genetic testing can be done to identify if the child has one of the identified forms of OI, although not all forms of bone fragility have been specifically mapped at this time. Infants with large heads and short limbs may be initially misdiagnosed, as OI and achondroplasia are often confused. Radiographic reports, however, easily distinguish between the two.

Dual-energy x-ray absorptiometry (DEXA) is a helpful evaluation tool in the detection of low bone density. It is most useful in those children with milder forms of OI because it can detect changes more specifically than traditional radiographs.[50] DEXA scans are also helpful in tracking drug efficacy in gaining bone density.

Collagen and biochemical studies can assist in differentiating a battered infant from an infant with OI. Radiographic studies are helpful because fractures at the epiphysis are rare in OI but common in child abuse in which soft tissue trauma is also evident. Bruising is common to both the infant with OI and the battered infant, but the bruising will disappear when the battered infant is in a safe environment. Three of the most helpful radiographic views in diagnosing OI are those of the skull (wormian bones), the lateral view of the spine (biconcave vertebrae or platyspondyly), and the pelvis (the beginnings of protrusio acetabuli).[81]

In moderate to severe forms of OI, early childhood fractures lead to multiple recurring fractures caused by the already weakened structure. The child develops limb deformities from bowing, which leads to impairment of mobility and of other functional skills. In the least severe forms of OI, because the first pathologic fractures occur later in childhood, recurring fractures with associated long bone deformities are less likely, and the overall prognosis is improved.

Engelbert and colleagues,[23] in a cross-sectional study of 54 children with OI, analyzed range of motion (ROM) and muscle strength for different types of OI. In OI type I, generalized hypermobility of the joints occurred without a decrease in ROM. In OI type III, extremities, especially the lower extremities, were severely malaligned. In OI type IV, upper and lower extremities were equally malaligned. Muscle strength in OI type I was normal except in periarticular muscles at the hip joint. In OI type III, however, muscle strength was severely decreased, especially around the hip joint. In OI type IV, the proximal muscles of both upper and lower extremities were weak.

Team members other than physical therapists who have an important role in the management of OI include orthopedists, orthotists, occupational therapists, audiologists, dentists, and geneticists. Little progress has been made in the primary prevention of this disorder, but much improvement in medical management is evident in recent years.

EXAMINATION, EVALUATION, AND INTERVENTION

INFANCY

Typical participation restrictions for an infant with OI depend on the severity of the case. In severe cases, the most serious impairments are those of rib and skull fractures, which may compromise pulmonary status and neural status, respectively. Because of possible cardiopulmonary compromise, time may be spent in the neonatal intensive care unit; this could lead to decreased parental interaction and bonding. If OI is moderate to severe, parents have increased anxiety about holding the infant for fear of fracturing the infant's bones. This may result in minimal contact and may decrease the mutually nurturing interaction vital to both parent and child. Children with severe OI who have reduced mobility from skeletal deformities may be unable to achieve age-appropriate activities of daily living (ADLs) or to play in the normal peer environment.

Infants with OI are at a very delicate stage of life. They have special needs regarding handling, positioning, and playing. During this stage, the role of caregivers is paramount in minimizing fractures, thereby limiting further muscle weakness and joint laxity. This is accomplished primarily through a physical therapy home program and caregiver education involving proper positioning and handling, which begin as soon as the child has been recognized as an infant with fragile bones.

At birth the infant may be of normal size, but postnatal growth is almost always stunted. Typical deformities of the infant include a relatively large head with a soft and membranous skull, and bowed limbs, which usually are short in the more severe forms of OI. Other features include a broad forehead and faciocranial disproportion, which give the face a triangular shape. Radiographically, fractures present at birth may be at varying stages of healing. The bones of infants with severe OI are short and wide with thin cortices, and the diaphyses are as wide as the metaphyses. Crepitation can be palpated at fracture sites.

The physical therapist should be aware of the infant's medical history of past and present fractures and should know the types of immobilizations employed before beginning the examination. Assessing pain is important when working with this population, as it can establish baseline comfort and anticipated changes with intervention. The FLACC (face, legs, activity, cry, and consolability) Scale is an observational scale that is used to quantitatively assess pain behaviors in preverbal patients.[44,47]

Assessment of the caregiver's handling and positioning techniques during dressing, diapering, and bathing is necessary. Therapists can be helpful in identifying and modifying techniques that put the child at fracture risk. If the baby is hospitalized, it is imperative that all caregivers are educated in proper handling techniques.

Therapy assesses active, but not passive, ROM in the young child with OI, as passive stretching is contraindicated in most cases. A standard goniometer can be used for measuring active ROM but may need to be cut down to a size suitable for the infant. This active ROM can be translated to functional ROM, useful in visualizing the whole composite of motions needed in functional abilities. For example, functional active ranges include the extent to which the child can bring the hand to the mouth, reach hands to midline, and reach toward the top of the head. If possible, the same therapist measures ROM during reevaluations. Intrarater and interrater reliability of goniometry should be determined for therapists and should be checked annually if more than one therapist examines the child.

Muscle strength is assessed through observation of the infant's movements and palpation of contracting muscles, rather than with the use of formal muscle tests.

A gross motor developmental evaluation should also be performed because these children often have delayed development of gross motor skills secondary to fractures and muscular weakness. Delayed gross motor skills are manifested as activity limitations involving impaired achievement of motor milestones. Sitting by the age of 10 months is a good predictor of future walking ability.[18] Formal tests used include the Peabody Developmental Motor Scales, 2nd edition,[30] which is norm referenced and standardized; the Pediatric Evaluation of Disability Inventory,[35] which is designed to track progress and assess activity; and the Bayley Scales of Infant Development II[10] and the Brief Assessment of Motor Function, which can be used to obtain a quick description of gross, fine, and oral motor performance.[17,56] Finally, it is important to assess the appropriateness of equipment used for seating, transporting, and encouraging independent mobility of the infant.

Physical therapy includes early parent education on proper handling and positioning techniques. Safe bathing, dressing, and carrying of an infant with OI are critical to reduce the risk of fracture.[9] When handling the infant, it is important that forces not be put across the long bones; instead the head and trunk should be supported with the arms and legs gently draped across the supporting arm. Some parents feel most comfortable supporting the infant on a standard-sized bed pillow for carrying at home. It is important to have a repertoire of carrying positions for the infant, so the baby can develop strength by accommodating to postural changes. Holding and carrying positions that safely challenge head control are important in that head control is hallmark to function over time. Dressing and undressing can be facilitated by using loose clothing and front snaps, side snaps, or Velcro closures. Overdressing should be avoided to reduce excessive sweating. Proper diapering includes a technique of rolling the infant off the diaper and supporting the buttocks with one hand with the infant's legs supported on the caregiver's forearm, while the other hand positions the diaper. The infant should never be lifted by the ankles. Bathing is done in a padded, preferably plastic, basin. Infant carriers that are designed to safely support the head, trunk, and extremities are frequently used for household transporting. For the very fragile infant, the carrier can be customized, as with a one-piece molded thoracolumbosacral orthosis, which incorporates the legs so they will not dangle and sustain injury. This carrier minimizes stresses to the fragile bones while it aids in positioning and transporting the infant. Physical therapy can play a role in educating families on the proper car seat, even before the child is initially discharged from the hospital. Early on, an infant may need a car bed if a rear-facing infant seat is too large, or if the risk of fracture while getting into and out of the seat is too great during the first few months. Extra padding may have to be added between the child and the transportation device, allowing a snug fit without putting undue stress on the fragile child through the strap systems.

Families need to be trained on how to rearrange padding in the seat to accommodate the various devices the child may be placed in for immobilization of fracture sites. Given the low bone density and the high risk for fracture, the child should use a rear-facing car seat for as long as possible to maximize safety in the car.

Proper positioning is a critical component of the home program and management of the infant with OI. One position that offers good support is sidelying with towel rolls along the spine and extremities, so they are aligned and protected while allowing the child to be active (Figure 11-2).

Prone positioning should start with the baby on the caregiver, where the child is well supported and most comfortable when being challenged. As the child gains skill in prone, the baby can be positioned over a towel roll or with a soft wedge under the chest as an alternative. Prone positioning is helpful for improving head control, strengthening back extensors, and molding the anterior chest wall. When supine, the infant needs support for the arms, and the hips should be in neutral rotation with the knees over a roll (Figure 11-3). Positions should be changed frequently and should not restrict active spontaneous movement, as spontaneous movement enhances muscle strengthening and bone mineralization.[9] Positioning is useful not only for the purpose of protecting from fracture, but also for minimizing joint malalignment and deformities. Figure 11-4 shows an infant's legs being poorly positioned in an infant carrier. The same seat is modified with lateral leg pads to keep the infant's hips and legs in neutral alignment, along with lower leg molded plastic splints (Figure 11-5). Varying the position of the infant promotes the development of age-appropriate developmental skills.

Promotion of sensorimotor developmental skills is an ongoing component in the management of the infant and child. Identification of appropriate and safe toys for a child, and of comfortable play positions that promote development, is often addressed jointly by the occupational therapist

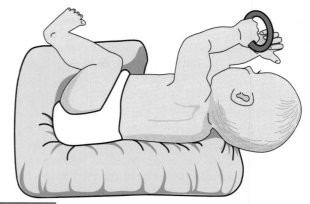

Figure 11-2 Infant positioned lying on side using rolls. Emphasis is on maintaining trunk alignment while allowing for active and spontaneous but safe movement.

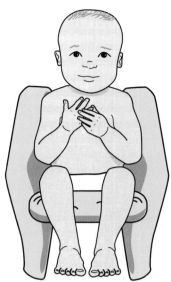

Figure 11-3   Infant positioned supine with hips in neutral rotation and knees flexed, and supported through the trunk.

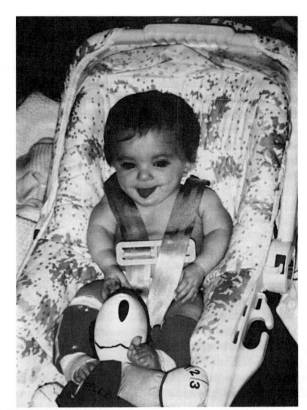

Figure 11-5   Child with improved positioning in an infant seat.

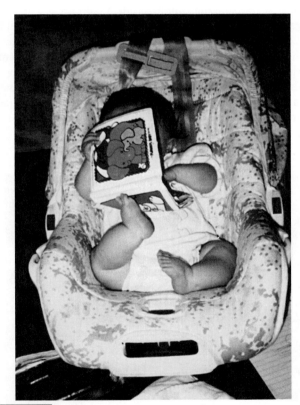

Figure 11-4   Child positioned poorly in an infant seat.

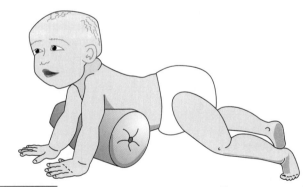

Figure 11-6   Infant positioned prone on a roll encourages weight bearing, extremity and trunk alignment, and strengthening of extensor musculature during developmental play.

and the physical therapist. For example, lying prone on a soft roll or over a parent's leg allows weight-bearing use of the arms with co-contraction of the shoulder musculature, which promotes active neck and back extensor muscle control (Figure 11-6). Increasing muscle strength and

support around the joint in activities such as this is especially important because the joint ligaments are lax. Prone positioning may be most comfortable over an elevated surface such as a wedge, a sofa cushion, or a roll, but just as important is lower extremity positioning with hips in neutral rotation and maximal hip extension.

Developmental activities such as rolling and supported sitting should be encouraged as tolerated by the child. When rolling is encouraged, the infant's arm is placed alongside his or her head, and then he or she attempts to roll over. Supported sitting is accomplished with seat inserts or corner chairs. Upright unsupported sitting can begin on the parent's lap with a pillow. When the child exhibits appropriate head control, short-sit and straddle activities can be done over the caregiver's leg or a roll but with avoidance of rotation across the lower extremity. These activities promote the development of protective and equilibrium responses and the beginning of protected weight bearing of the lower extremities. Many children with OI spend much time scooting on their buttocks before crawling is accomplished. Many children develop sitting skill and mobility in sitting long before they develop consistent ability to move from horizontal prone or supine to sitting. This fact is due to short arms in relation to body length and can be adapted for by giving a child a raised surface to push off of, such as a pillow, as the child is learning to move into a sitting position.

Proper handling while encouraging developmental skills is of key importance. For instance, a pull-to-sit maneuver is contraindicated when a distraction pull on the hands is used. Rather, this maneuver should be modified and facilitated by supporting the child around the shoulders while the child attempts to sit up. In working on trunk control over a ball, the therapist's hands are positioned on the pelvis and trunk, rather than supporting or facilitating movement from the legs. Parents should be cautioned against using devices that support a baby upright in standing such as baby walkers or jumping seats. These devices put unnecessary stress on the legs where the child fits through the sling, and if the baby has difficulty controlling the device, devastating torque to the bone may result. These devices do not foster proper positioning and weight bearing for these fragile children. Such upright activities can give parents a false sense that the infant is protected. Active, spontaneous activity and exercise are encouraged in sidelying and supine positions and in supported sitting, with the child reaching for, swiping at, rolling, and lifting lightweight toys of different textures. Pool exercises may begin as early as 6 months of age with the goals of promoting active exercise and weight bearing.[9] Extremity movement may occur unobstructed in the water as the child is supported in a flotation device accompanied by a parent or the therapist.

At this stage, goals include teaching safe handling and positioning techniques to caregivers and providing opportunities for development of age-appropriate skills. The intensity of treatment varies with the individual needs of the infant and family, but providing a home program and regular home visits by a physical therapist at least weekly is essential to ensuring that the environment is suitable for sensorimotor and cognitive development. The therapist can act as a resource and support for the caregivers as together they develop strategies to meet the challenges of safe caregiver handling, mobility, and developmental facilitation. Another important role for early intervention therapists in the home is to help families develop a repertoire of positioning and

activity options for the child. This is most important when the child recovers from fractures.

When fractures do occur, they may require splinting with a variety of materials such as thermoplastic materials or fiberglass. Ace wraps have been used to support and protect a limb in mild cases and in young infants. Fractures may heal within 2 weeks in the newborn and generally within the same time frame as other fractures in infancy (usually 6 weeks).

PRESCHOOL PERIOD

Bone fragility, joint laxity, and reduced muscle strength continue to be present in the preschool period but are now accompanied by secondary impairments of disuse atrophy and osteoporosis from fracture immobilization (Figure 11-7). At this point, if a child has had issues with recurrent fractures, treatment with bisphosphonates has begun to help decrease the fracture cycle. Structural changes and secondary impairments from fractures may limit mobility and subsequently restrict participation in play and socialization for the child with OI. This may affect the child's adjustment to regular school and may hinder academic progress. The temperament of the child with OI may play a role in his ability to adjust to his activity limitations and participation restrictions. Cintas and colleagues[17] demonstrated that the temperament of children with OI was comparable with that of children without disability, except for having lower activity scores. Temperament was significantly and positively related to motor performance in terms of persistence, approach, and activity.

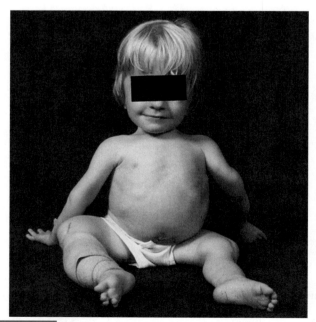

Figure 11-7   Child with osteogenesis imperfecta showing joint laxity and bony deformities: femoral anterolateral bowing and tibial anterior bowing.

At this stage, muscles are usually weakened and developmental motor skills are lagging as a result of frequent immobilization and relative disuse. Despite this, cognitive skills should be appropriate for the child's age. When a fracture is sustained, children with OI typically complain little of pain and usually have minimal soft tissue trauma.[82]

Microfractures may result from repeated trauma at the epiphyseal plates, leading to arrested growth and potential leg length discrepancy. In childhood, "popcorn calcifications" appear in the metaphyseal and epiphyseal areas of long bones.[54] It is postulated that these are fragments of the cartilaginous growth plate.

If the child begins to walk without adequate support, further bending of the long bones occurs as a result of abnormal stress on the weakened structure. Bowing occurs in the anterolateral direction in the femur and anteriorly in the tibia. In those children who do not walk, lack of normal weight-bearing stress leads to a honeycomb pattern of osteoporosis in the long bones.

Emphasis at this stage is on protected weight bearing and self-mobility for enhanced independence. Although proper positioning, handling, and transferring are still important, the emphasis shifts to the child's active participation in his or her care. During this period, the child with OI should have adequate upright control to begin bearing weight and, at the very least, should be held in a standing position, as early weight bearing appears to have some beneficial effect.[31] When radiographs of children with OI from the time of birth and several years later are compared, the changing levels of bone density suggest that progressive osteoporosis has been superimposed on the basic bone defect.[11] Upper extremity bones were frequently denser than those of the lower limbs and were less likely to fracture. This finding may be related to the use and stress placed on upper extremity bones during self-care and play activities.

For the preschool child, an evaluation of modes of mobility and adapted equipment is essential to promote supported sitting functional mobility and independence. Equipment requires constant updating because of changing positional needs related to mobilization-immobilization status. Splinting needs and adaptive ADL equipment are assessed for fit.

Developmental assessment tools that are appropriate include the Peabody Developmental Motor Scales II, the Brief Assessment of Motor Function, and the Pediatric Evaluation of Disability Inventory to assess gross motor function and activity limitations in children with OI. Pain should continue to be assessed in the preschool-age child. Appropriate pain assessments include the FLACC Behavioral Scale and the self-report Numeric or Wong-Baker Faces Scale.[44,79]

Active exercise continues to be emphasized to increase muscle strength of weakened muscles, most typically, hip extensor and abductor muscles. Active exercise can be achieved primarily through developmental play. One developmental activity to increase weight bearing and maintain or increase strength in the quadriceps and hip extensor

musculature involves having the child straddle a roll and come to stand, with the therapist supporting the child's pelvis (Figure 11-8). The therapist begins with the child sitting on a high roll that requires a small excursion of movement to go from sitting to standing and then gradually changes to using a lower roll. An active-resistive program graded for the patient's tolerance should be cautiously established. Use of light weights may be incrementally increased, but they should be attached close to large joints so as to avoid a long lever arm that increases the potential for fracture.

Early gym-related activities that can be introduced at this age may include scooter board activities, riding tricycles, and playground games such as Simon Says, Red Light Green Light, and Follow the Leader. Activities that encourage overhead reaching are helpful in maximizing trunk extension. These activities can include modified basketball activities when the ball is light and the child uses low-speed passing. Racket sports using a tethered tennis ball help to build upper body strength. All activities should be closely monitored by a responsible adult to ensure safety. If the child is attending preschool, all members of the team should have a basic emergency plan if fractures occur at school. This plan would include but is not limited to notification of family and splinting of involved extremities while awaiting supportive medical intervention.

An aquatic exercise program is excellent for the child with OI. It can be started at an early age and can continue for a lifetime. Aquatic therapy benefits include the opportunity to socialize with peers in a safe environment, a safe

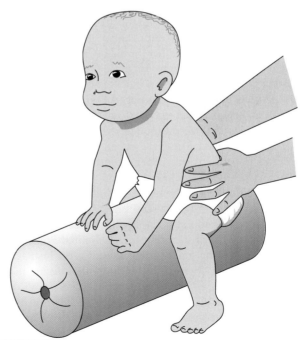

Figure 11-8 Straddle roll activity of supported sit-to-stand for lower extremity strengthening and weight bearing.

method of strengthening muscles through resistance and assistance of the water, and the opportunity to improve cardiovascular fitness and bear weight in a protected environment. The therapist can finely grade the progression of exercises in the pool by first using the buoyancy effect of the water to assist weak movements, then supporting the movements, and finally, using water to resist active movements. Exercises can be modified with floats by changing the length of the lever arm of the moving body part through the use of turbulence, and by altering the speed and direction of the movement.[21]

Pool exercises can enhance deep breathing to facilitate chest expansion and enhance overall respiratory function, which are especially important because chest deformities that compromise breathing capacity are common. Certain precautions should be taken when pool therapy is considered for the child with OI. The heat of the water creates a rise in body temperature and increases metabolism, which is frequently already elevated in these children. It is suggested, therefore, that time in the water, water temperature, and activity level be closely monitored for each child. Initially, pool sessions are generally limited to 20 to 30 minutes.[16]

Pool exercise therapy may interrupt the cycle of further disuse and secondary complications from immobilization. Not only is aquatic therapy an ideal therapeutic modality for the child with OI, it also can be a therapeutic, lifelong avocational activity that can ameliorate the effects of the disabling process.

One key goal and big challenge for the preschool child who has frequent fractures is safe, independent mobility. The aim is to prevent an activity limitation of reduced mobility resulting from the initial impairment. Research has linked limited mobility opportunities in the first few years with later life problem solving skill difficulties.[72] Opportunities for multiple safe modes of mobility should be explored to expand the child's repertoire of environmental experiences. A scooter for sitting propelled with legs or hands may be useful (Figure 11-9). Families should be encouraged to investigate ride-on toys that can be purchased at a toy store. It is often a challenge to get a device that accommodates the child's shortened femurs and shortened arms, yet gives enough weight-bearing surface to enhance trunk control. Sometimes handlebars need to be adapted to allow the child to steer effectively. A ride-on toy may give the child safe mobility without the rotational components of sit-scooting.

The degree of ambulation attainable varies for preschool children with OI. Those children with limited ambulatory skills may need formal gait training, as well as the instruction of family members. Interest in standing often occurs in the child's second year of life. Factors affecting the ability to stand and ambulate include the degree of bowing in the extremities and the muscle strength of the limbs. Ambulation is often introduced in the pool, for protected weight bearing. Because the buoyancy of water provides support for the body, weight bearing on weakened extremities and

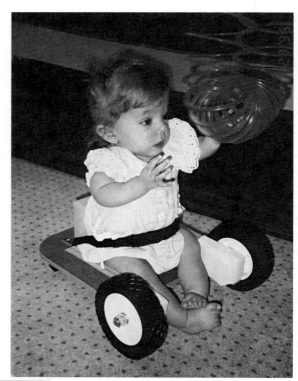

Figure 11-9 Scooter used for mobility that can be propelled by a child's legs or arms.

unstable joints can be gradually introduced without fear of causing trauma.

Weight relief depends on the proportion of the body that is below the water level. For maximum weight relief for ambulation, the child begins standing in the pool where the water level is at the child's neck. Over time, the child gradually progresses to bearing more weight in shallow water. If the child with OI is recovering from a fracture, it is recommended that thermoplastic splints be used to further protect the extremity while in the pool during early weight bearing. General guidelines for walking re-education in water according to Duffield[21] suggest that a patient start in parallel bars or a walking frame, with the therapist initially supporting the pelvis from the front. The patient practices weight shifts from side to side, forward, and backward and progresses to walking forward. The therapist cues the patient to lean slightly forward to counteract the upthrust of buoyancy, which tends to cause the child to overbalance backward. In this manner, protected walking for a child with OI can start much earlier than on a solid surface. Unsupported standing on solid ground is not recommended because it leads to rapid bowing of the long bones. When severe bowing of the extremities occurs, the child usually undergoes orthopedic surgery in the form of osteotomies. Age-appropriate lower extremity weight bearing is encouraged, although the child with moderate to severe OI needs external devices such as splints or braces to protect fragile long bones.

In moderate to severe OI, braces and splints are usually required to begin standing activities on solid surfaces. Use of orthotics provides the protected weight bearing needed to reduce the impact of stress on osteoporotic bony deformities. Braces or splints may be used first in conjunction with a standing frame if the child has significant lower extremity bowing and does not have standing skill.

The child who does not naturally embark on a standing program can use a standing device for support. An air splint can be used to prevent fractures and to temporarily manage fractures. Use of such a device may be a nice stepping stone between using a stander for weight bearing and standing freely without support.[63a] used these splints for instituting graded weight bearing and gait training in a child with OI. Drawbacks of air splints are that they may be bulky and hot, so the child may not always tolerate them well.

Once a child graduates from a stander, ambulation may be protected through the use of parallel bars or a walker. A walker that supports the majority of body weight through the trunk and pelvis is often used to assist in weight bearing during initial overland ambulation. This walker supports weight by means of a trunk support cuff and a padded pommel that is positioned between the child's legs. Rear-wheeled and four-point walkers followed by canes or crutches (depending on the type and severity of OI) also may be used. Forearm attachments to walkers or crutches afford a degree of weight bearing distributed throughout the forearm to reduce stress on the arm and wrist, as well as to relieve some weight bearing on the lower extremities. Older preschoolers who use a walker may benefit from a walker with a seat, so they can easily rest between walking activities and can fully participate in preschool-related play. Most children ambulate without braces when the fracture rate decreases. Although bracing of the lower extremity is not as prevalent as it had been before the use of bisphosphonates, many benefit from

orthotics in the shoe to support the longitudinal arch that often collapses as the result of ligamentous laxity.

Customized mobility carts may be fabricated to encourage independent mobility when the child is immobilized, enabling the child to explore his or her environment, gain some independence, and maintain strength in the upper extremities. When head and trunk control is good and the child can cognitively and safely handle a mobility device, power mobility may be an adjunct to preventing disability by allowing the child to keep up and interact with peers. These alternative mobility modes do not preclude ambulation but are useful additional mobility options. Regardless of the mode of mobility used, it is imperative to provide the child with a degree of functional independence in the home and in the preschool environment that will promote participation in social activities.

Physical therapists are often consulted on seating issues with children who have OI. Given that most states mandate child safety seats in cars for children younger than 8 years of age, it is important to assist families in proper seating choices once the child has outgrown the infant car seat. Children with the most severe forms of OI are safest in rear-facing seating devices for as long as possible. A five-point harness rather than a seat belt helps to distribute pressure from accidents more evenly. Booster seats should be used until the child meets the size restrictions for the seating; the age restrictions of the law should not be the only focus in these decisions.

SCHOOL AGE AND ADOLESCENCE

Due to reduced mobility and limited independence in ADLs, school-age children and adolescents often have limited ability to participate in peer-related activities (Table 11-2). Social skill development also may be hampered if the

TABLE 11-2   International Classification of Functioning, Health, and Disability for Children With Osteogenesis Imperfecta

Changes in Body Structure	Changes in Body Functions	Activity	Participation
Connective tissue disorder secondary to defect in collagen synthesis	Diffuse osteoporosis resulting in multiple recurrent fractures	Limited functional mobility skills, including rolling, creeping , transitional movements, and higher-level mobility skills	Limited participation in physical activities caused by endurance limitations and safety concerns
Brittle bones	Weak muscles	Limited ability to transfer	Limited peer play
	Joint laxity	Limited ambulation	Infantilization
	Bowing of long bones	Decreased endurance	Limited access to educational and work opportunities
	Scoliosis	Limited independence in self-care skills, including dressing and feeding	Limited access to wide range of environments
	Kyphosis	Limited ability for ambulation on uneven terrain	Limited independent living
		Limited independence in wheelchair mobility	Social isolation

school-age child has been overprotected by caregivers because of overwhelming fear and anxiety regarding fractures. This may have an impact on the school-age child's scholastic endeavors and future vocational achievements. Studies have shown that children with OI tend to have similar temperament to typically developing peers.[73] It is the child with negative behavior, such as generally negative mood and high intensity of expression, who influences a parent's perception of hassle. The severity of the child's disease does not have as heavy an impact on parental coping.[73] Parents and educators should encourage a positive attitude and excellence in school performance to prepare the child for a productive future.

At this age, the spine may exhibit varying degrees of deformity. Usually, scoliosis, kyphosis, or both are present, resulting from compression fractures of the vertebrae, osteoporosis, and ligamentous laxity. The child with moderate to severe OI typically has marked bowing of the long bones from multiple fractures and growth arrest at the epiphyseal plates. In the femur, the neck-shaft angle may be decreased with a coxa vara deformity and acetabular protrusion. The tibia is anteriorly angulated, which, in combination with the angulation of the femur, results in an apparent knee flexion contracture. The patellofemoral joint frequently dislocates, predisposing the patient to falls and fractures. Pes valgus frequently occurs at the ankle. In the upper extremities, the humerus is angulated laterally or anterolaterally and the forearms are limited in supination and pronation. The elbows often exhibit cubitus varus deformities, and elbow flexion contractures may be present.

The frequency of fracture tends to decrease markedly after puberty. Possible causes include hormonal changes, increased awareness of how to prevent fractures, improvement in coordination, and increasing bone strength.[32] Paradoxically, the adolescent who senses his or her increased stability and emerging independence may maximize involvement in activities, which increases the risk of more severe types of fractures. In an effort not to discourage these activities and independence, ongoing use of safe methods of mobility, caution, and responsible behavior should be stressed in patient instruction throughout childhood.

Physical therapy management at this stage involves other team members, including professionals in orthopedics, orthotics, occupational therapy, and rehabilitation engineering to maximize the child's independence in ADLs, mobility, endurance, problem solving, and adjustment to the school environment.

Children and adolescents should be encouraged to be active family members. They should have a share in home-related chores and responsibilities within their functional capacity. This is important because it helps the child learn a level of independence for a lifetime, allows the child to feel valued, and may lessen sibling rivalry.

In this period, physical therapy may be helpful in returning the child to premorbid mobility status after a series of immobilizations from prepubertal fractures. Weight management and physical activity are important at this age.

Management of scoliosis and kyphosis is usually addressed by a spinal fusion, but the long-term results in maintaining alignment are questionable. Orthotic devices such as orthoplast jackets have been deemed ineffective in controlling scoliosis and kyphosis.[8]

Along with occupational therapy, physical therapy can help to maximize the child's independence by identifying safe, energy-efficient positions in which the child can work. Adaptive equipment is imperative for those with severe involvement. Occupational therapists, physical therapists, and rehabilitation engineers work together to adapt wheelchairs and seating and mobility devices to accommodate skeletal deformity, scoliosis, and kyphosis. A variety of lightweight and easily maneuverable manual wheelchairs can be adapted with seating inserts for trunk control and proper positioning. Vinyl upholstery is usually unsatisfactory for the child with OI because of the propensity for excessive perspiration. Proper wheelchair positioning is critical for prevention of further disabling deformity and for protection of exposed extremities from trauma. Those who do rely on power mobility may benefit from a seat elevator and a motorized transfer arm to allow independence in transfers and ability to access all work surfaces in the home and at school.

Physical therapy continues with the adolescent to work on ambulation, endurance, and strength. Household ambulation is usually achieved with assistive devices if adequate upper extremity strength is present. Walkers with progression to canes or crutches may be used.

Many children with OI who have primarily used the wheelchair for mobility are now able to ambulate about the house without any special change in their program. It is important to emphasize the maintenance of adequate skeletal alignment and maximal muscular strength throughout childhood to prepare for this improved function as an adolescent and adult. Community ambulation, however, is not practical, given the patient's short stature, the energy expenditure required, and the reduced muscle power. Most school-age and older children with OI use wheelchairs for community ambulation.[11] Independence in mobility is paramount because it has been shown to correlate with the degree of adaptation to the community environment. Bachman[5] found that independence in travel away from home was the most important factor in an adolescent's ability to participate successfully outside the school environment.

Strengthening and endurance programs can be most successful when the child participates in developing a program that suits his or her interests and schedule. Of key importance at this age for the nonambulatory population is core strength and the ability to sit-scoot. Having adequate trunk strength will positively affect the child's ability to assist with transfer and self-care skills throughout adulthood. Programs can consist of progressive resistive exercises using incremental weights, aquatic activity, adaptive sport activities, or computer-assisted physical activity. Enjoyable avocational activities that incorporate functional strengthening and mobility also must be stressed at this age. Although contact sports, such as football, soccer, and baseball, must be avoided, customized athletic and fitness programs are vital for youngsters with OI. These adaptive physical education activities can assist in improving physical health, finding a competitive outlet, helping to discover one's potential, and providing an opportunity to make friends.[19] Sports and recreation activities should be encouraged as an adjunct to therapy. These activities will assist children to develop lifelong fitness interests. Adaptive sports that are available to the child who is interested include swimming, challenger baseball, cycling, boating, noncontact martial arts, adaptive dance, billiards, golf, wheelchair sports, racket sports, and even sled hockey. It is important to keep an open mind when helping a child develop fitness interests. Weigh the benefits against the risks when helping a child make choices. The physical therapist's role is to set appropriate parameters for participation, to provide precautions, and to upgrade the level of activity progressively. Volunteer jobs and social opportunities, such as Boy Scouts and Girl Scouts, encourage emotional growth and develop leadership skills. Experience in a volunteer capacity can be helpful to the adolescent when applying for employment in the future.[29]

TRANSITION TO ADULTHOOD

In the transition to adulthood, emphasis needs to be placed on the skills necessary for independent living. Identifying personal goals for education and employment is important for the physical therapist to establish a plan of care. Once personal goals are established, the therapist can assist the young adult in problem-solving aspects of the activity to allow participation. The mildly involved person with OI tends not to seek assistance; more involved individuals may need support to address specific goals such as transfers for toileting in public or gaining the skills necessary to run a household without outside assistance. Strategies need to be established to maximize independence with and without the presence of fractures. In the transition to adulthood, appropriate career placement is important, while taking into consideration the patient's intellectual capacity and physical constraints. Because most patients with OI become productive members of society, optimal academic, social, and physical development will enhance their opportunities to succeed in a competitive job market.[11]

In addition to functional independence, those who have OI need to participate in behaviors to enhance lifelong health. These involve regular exercise, weight management, a healthy calcium-rich diet, limited caffeine consumption, and avoidance of smoking tobacco. Therapists need to review how each aspect influences overall health and, more important, the management of osteoporosis.

Some encounter problems with deafness in adult life. Scoliotic curves may be severe and may continue to progress. The incidence of scoliosis approaches 80% to 90% in teenagers and adults.[1] Patients who have OI are especially susceptible to postmenopausal osteoporosis or the osteoporosis of immobilization[68] when more fractures may occur.[57] Adults with OI also report problems with arthritic changes and back pain.

By the time these children reach adulthood, most moderately involved persons use either manual or power wheelchairs for community mobility. Ambulation consists of household walking with an assistive device.

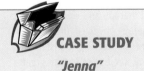

CASE STUDY

"Jenna"

Jenna is an 11-year-old girl who has been diagnosed with type III/IV OI. Jenna presents clinically with type III characteristics (see Table 11-1), but a skin biopsy exhibited cellular and collagen characteristics more consistent with type IV OI. She is the fourth child in her family, and no siblings have OI. At birth, she presented with five fractures despite delivery via cesarean section. Her family was initially trained in safe handling of their fragile child by nursing staff in the newborn nursery. She was discharged on day 5 and was referred to an OI clinic in the area. At 14 days of age, Jenna was examined at the OI clinic by members of an interdisciplinary team, including a physical therapist. She was transported to the clinic with the use of a car bed in the family car. At this initial examination, her parents preferred to have Jenna rest supine on a bed pillow while moving and holding her, to reduce the risk of fracture.

The initial comprehensive examination included an assessment of handling by the parents and positioning of Jenna, as well as an assessment of the transportation device used to transport Jenna to medical appointments. Postural alignment and motor skills were also observed, but formal goniometry was deferred because of fractures.

After the initial examination, the physical therapist worked with the family on a home program to promote proper positioning, handling, and facilitation of motor development within the context of daily activities. The parents were educated on how to safely change diapers and dress Jenna. They were shown how to safely hold Jenna in their arms rather than on a pillow, with encouragement toward the prone position when being held by the parents. The car bed was padded with rolled receiving blankets to protect Jenna's fragile limbs while she is being transported in the family car. The family was taught

Continued

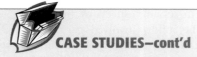

to follow positioning guidelines to protect the limbs from fracture and to facilitate proper skeletal alignment to minimize bony deformity. This included positioning the hips in a neutral position with extension whenever possible, as her preferred position was flexion, abduction, and external rotation at the hips. The family was taught how to fabricate thermoplastic splints and how to use the splints to protect limb segments when fractures were suspected. They were provided thermoplastic splinting materials so they could fabricate and apply the splints at home.

Jenna's family was given information on early intervention (EI) and began the process of getting physical therapy services in her natural environment. EI physical therapy services began when Jenna was 4 months old. When she was 12 weeks of age, Jenna began participation in a clinical trial using bisphosphonates to reduce fracture frequency. Jenna traveled every 8 to 10 weeks to a regional medical center for 3 days of intravenous pamidronate therapy until she was nearly a year old. At that point, she was old enough to receive the drug therapy closer to home. Before starting bisphosphonates, Jenna was sustaining fractures about every other week. After the drug therapy was begun, fracture frequency decreased to only a few a year.

Weekly early intervention (EI) physical therapy service initially concentrated on family education with emphasis on safe handling and play in Jenna's home environment. As Jenna's fracture frequency decreased and the family's comfort level increased, physical therapy then focused on strengthening the trunk and postural muscles. The physical therapist and the family worked closely together to design developmentally appropriate activities and safe handling in the context of her changing skills. They worked together on prone skills as well as rolling. As Jenna's trunk control improved, sitting skills were emphasized.

In addition to physical therapy services through the EI program, Jenna began an aquatic physical therapy program at 11 months of age. She was able to sit independently in waist deep water at 11 months of age, and was able to scoot in waist deep water at 18 months. She initiated walking in waist deep water with a walker at 18 months of age. Her family purchased a mobile hot tub, so Jenna could swim year round several times a week at home.

During this time, early intervention physical therapy services at home continued on a weekly basis as fractures allowed. At 18 months, she began standing activities in knee extension splints and an upright stander. Jenna began scooting on the floor in a sitting position at 20 months but that skill was put on hold for 8 weeks while she healed from femoral intramedullary rod surgery. At 23 months she was fitted with clam-shell hip-knee-ankle-foot orthoses (HKAFOs) and started walking in the braces at 28 months with a walker. At 30 months, Jenna achieved supine-to-sit, practicing it so often in the first 48 hours that she sustained an upper extremity fracture and was unable to use this newly developed motor skill for another 4 weeks. The supine-to-sit skill was delayed because of her short arms, which made it difficult for her to push into an upright position. At 34 months she was able to crawl on her belly on the floor.

At 3 years of age, Jenna started in an integrated preschool with her mother serving as a classroom aide. She received weekly school-based physical therapy services at the preschool, where wheelchair mobility was emphasized. She initially used a manual wheelchair temporarily until a power wheelchair became available when she was 3.5 years old. During this time, she continued to progress with her ambulation and was able to sit-to-stand from a small bench with ankle-foot orthoses (AFOs) and a walker.

At 4 years of age, it was discovered that Jenna had a C-2 migration cranially with compression of the foramen magnum and hydrocephalus. No medical intervention was indicated, and this condition continued to be monitored.

Jenna had continued to progress in her mobility skills, and when she was 4.5 years old, she participated in a Walk-a-Thon at school using a walker with a bench attached to it. This allowed Jenna to rest frequently and made it possible for her to participate in this school event with minimal adult assistance.

At 5 years of age, Jenna had a right tibial fracture and a suspected fracture of her left arm, which prevented her from walking with her walker for several weeks. Despite fractures, she continued to scoot on the floor for mobility and used her power wheelchair for mobility as well. When not immobilized, she continued to participate in an aquatics program with an emphasis on transitional mobility for prone and supine recovery in the water. She could walk 20 minutes in waist to chest deep water with a walker and stand independently with close supervision. In kindergarten, her mother again became her classroom aide, assisting with wheelchair and toilet transfers. School-based physical therapy was provided in the home because of multiple fractures, limiting school attendance that year.

As Jenna got more involved in her school career, she got a power wheelchair with a seat elevator and a transfer arm to allow greater independence in her self-care and transfers. In fourth grade, she continued to have weekly school-based therapy and weekly aquatic therapy. Much of the emphasis of therapy involved the strength and mobility needed for independent sit-scooting transfers. As she got more confident with her mobility, she began to take greater risks and therefore had a higher incidence of fractures, including arm fractures from scooting transfers and a femur fracture from a fall from a toilet, as she felt she could complete the transfer without help.

Now in fifth grade, Jenna has been fracture-free for 6 months. Through physical therapy in an aquatic medium, she is working on trunk strengthening to improve sitting balance for toilet transfers. She is doing some ambulation activities in waist deep water as she is preparing to embark on a walking program on land. In school-based therapy, she is working on upper body strengthening and avocational fitness activities to enhance participation in physical education classes, as well as recreational activities. For recreation, Jenna is on the cheerleading squad and is participating in interactive computer-based exercise activities with friends and family.

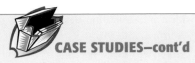

CASE STUDIES–cont'd

EVIDENCE TO PRACTICE 11-1

CASE STUDY "JENNA"

EXAMINATION DECISION

Jenna is a young lady who has participated in physical therapy most of her life. Considering her present age and the types of therapy she receives, the examination process is different between the school environment and the medically based aquatic environment.

School-based examination needs to tease out the gross motor skills necessary to maximize Jenna's educational opportunities.

In the medical environment, examination needs to look at orthopedic limitations and how they affect function.

PLAN OF CARE DECISION

Physical Training in Children With Osteogenesis Imperfecta[75]
Van Brussel, M., Takken, T., Uiterwaal, C., Pruijs, H. J., Van der Net, J., & Helders, P. J. M. (2008). Physical training in children with osteogenesis imperfecta. *Journal of Pediatrics, 152,* 111–116.

Patient/Family Preferences[24]
Engelbert, R. H., Gulmans, V. A., Uiterwaal, C. S., & Helders P. J. (2001). Osteogenesis imperfecta in childhood: Perceived competence in relation to impairment and disability. *Archives of Physical Medicine and Rehabilitation, 82,* 943–948.

ACKNOWLEDGMENTS

Many thanks to Debra Bleakney, Rebecca Zuck, and Nicole Defoe, who helped with research and edits.

REFERENCES

1. Albright, J. A. (1981). Management overview of osteogenesis imperfecta. *Clinical Orthopedics, 159,* 80–87.

2. Alharbi, M., Pinto, G., Finidori, G., et al. (2009). Pamidronate treatment of children with moderate-to-severe osteogenesis imperfecta: A note of caution. *Hormone Research, 71,* 38–44.

3. Astrom, E., & Soderhall, S. (1998). Beneficial effect of bisphosphonate during five years of treatment of severe osteogenesis imperfecta. *Acta Paediatrics, 87,* 64–68.

4. Astrom, E., & Soderhall, S. (2002). Beneficial effect of long term intravenous bisphosphonate treatment of osteogenesis imperfecta. *Archives of Disease in Childhood, 86,* 356–364.

5. Bachman, W. H. (1972). Variables affecting post school economic adaptation of orthopedically handicapped and other health-impaired students. *Rehabilitation Literature, 3,* 98.

6. Bailey, R. W., & Dubow, H. I. (1965). Experimental and clinical studies of longitudinal bone growth utilizing a new method of internal fixation crossing the epiphyseal plate. *Journal of Bone and Joint Surgery (American), 47,* 1669.

7. Basel, D., & Steiner, R. D. (2009). Osteogenesis imperfecta: Recent findings shed new light on this once well-understood condition. *Genetics in Medicine, 11,* 375–385.

8. Benson, D. R., & Newman, D. C. (1981). The spine and surgical treatment in osteogenesis imperfecta. *Clinical Orthopedics, 159,* 147–153.

9. Binder, H., Hawkes, L., Graybill, G., Gerber, N. L., & Weintrob, J. C. (1984). Osteogenesis imperfecta: Rehabilitation approach with infants and young children. *Archives of Physical Medicine and Rehabilitation, 65,* 537–541.

10. Black, M. M., & Matula, K. (1999). *Essentials of Bayley Scales of Infant Development II assessment.* New York: John Wiley & Sons.

11. Bleck, E. E. (1981). Nonoperative treatment of osteogenesis imperfecta: Orthotic and mobility management. *Clinical Orthopedics, 159,* 111–122.

12. Bluemcke, S., Niedorf, H. R., Thiel, H. J., & Langness, U. (1972). Histochemical and fine structural studies on the cornea in osteogenesis imperfecta. *Virchows Archives B Cell Pathology, 11,* 124–132.

13. Reference deleted in page proofs.

14. Byers, P. H. (1988). *Osteogenesis imperfecta: An update: Growth, genetics and hormones* (Vol. 4, Part 2). New York: McGraw-Hill.

15. Chamberlain, J. R., Schwarze, U., Wang, P. R., et al. (2004). Gene targeting in stem cells from individuals with osteogenesis imperfecta. *Science, 303,* 1198–1201.

16. Cintas, H. L. (2005). Aquatics, Chapter 5. In H. L. Cintas, & L. H. Gerber (Eds.). *Children with osteogenesis imperfecta: Strategies to enhance performance.* Gaithersburg, MD: Osteogenesis Imperfecta Foundation.

17. Cintas, H. L., Siegel, K. L., Furst, G. P., & Gerber, L. H. (2003). Brief assessment of motor function: Reliability and concurrent validity of the Gross Motor Scale. *American Journal of Physical Medicine and Rehabilitation, 82,* 33–41.

18. Daly, K., Wisbeach, A., Sampera, I. Jr., & Fixsen, J. A. (1996). The prognosis for walking in osteogenesis imperfecta. *Journal of Bone and Joint Surgery (British), 78,* 477–480.

19. Donohoe, M. (2005). Sports and recreation, Chapter 6. In H. L. Cintas, & L. H. Gerber (Eds.). *Children with osteogenesis imperfecta: Strategies to enhance performance.* Gaithersburg, MD: Osteogenesis Imperfecta Foundation.

20. Doty, S. B., & Matthews, R. S. (1971). Electronmicroscopic and histochemical investigation of osteogenesis imperfecta tarda. *Clinical Orthopedics, 80,* 191–201.

21. Duffield, M. H. (1983). Physiological and therapeutic effects of exercise in warm water. In A. T. Skinner, & A. M. Thomson (Eds.). *Duffield's exercise in water* (3rd ed.). London: Bailliere Tindall.

22. Engelbert, R. H. H., Gerver, W. J. M., Breslau-Siderius, L. J., van der Graaf, Y., Pruijs, H. E. H., van Doorne, J. M., Beemer, F. A., & Helders, P. J. M. (1998). Spinal complication in osteogenesis imperfecta: 47 patients 1–16 years of age. *Acta Orthopaedica Scandinavica, 69,* 283–286.

23. Engelbert, R. H., van der Graaf, Y., van Empelen, M. A., Beemer, A., & Helders, P. J. M. (1997). Osteogenesis imperfecta in childhood: Impairment and disability. *Pediatrics, 99,* E3.

24. Engelbert, R. H., Gulmans, V. A., Uiterwaal, C. S., Helders, P. J. (2001). Osteogenesis imperfecta in childhood: Perceived competence in relation to impairment and disability. *Archives of Physical Medicine and Rehabilitation, 82,* 943–948.

25. Engelbert, R. H., Uiterwaal, C. S., van der Hulst, A., Witjes, B., Helders, P. J., Pruijs, H. E. (2003). Scoliosis in children with osteogenesis imperfecta: Influence of severity of disease and age of reaching motor milestones. *European Spine Journal, 12,* 130–134.

26. Falk, M. J., Heeger, S., Lynch, K. A., DeCaro, K. R., Bohach, D., Gibson, K. S., & Warman, M. L. (2003). Intravenous biophosphate therapy in children with osteogenesis imperfecta. *Pediatrics, 111,* 573–578.

27. Falvo, K. A., & Bullough, P. G. (1973). Osteogenesis imperfecta: A histometric analysis. *Journal of Bone and Joint Surgery (American), 55,* 275–286.

28. Falvo, K. A., Root, L., & Bullough, P. G. (1974). Osteogenesis imperfecta: A clinical evaluation and management. *Journal of Bone and Joint Surgery (American), 56,* 783–793.

29. Fehribach, G. (1990). Independent living. Presented before the Osteogenesis Imperfecta Foundation National Convention, August 9, 1990, Pittsburgh, PA.

30. Folio, M., & Fewell, R. (1983). *Peabody Developmental Motor Scales and Activity Cards.* Allen, TX: DLM Teaching Resources.

31. Gerber, L. H., Binder, H., Weintrob, J., Grenge, D. K., Shapiro, J., Fromherz, W., Berry, R., Conway, A., Nason, S., & Marini, J. (1990). Rehabilitation of children and infants with osteogenesis imperfecta: A program for ambulation. *Clinical Orthopaedics and Related Research, 251,* 254–262.

32. Glorieux, F. (2007). *Guide to osteogenesis imperfecta for pediatricians and family practice physicians.* Bethesda, MD: National Institutes of Health Osteoporosis and Related Bone Diseases National Resource Center.

33. Glorieux, F. H., Rauch, F., Plotkin, H., Ward, L., Travers, R., Roughley, P., Lalic, L., Glorieux, D. F., Fassier, F., Bishop, N. J. (2000). Type V osteogenesis imperfecta: A new form of brittle bone disease. *Journal of Bone Mineralization Research, 15,* 1650–1658.

34. Glorieux, F. H., Ward, L. M., Rauch, F., Lalic, L., Roughley, P. J., Travers, R. (2002). Osteogenesis imperfecta type VI: A form of brittle bone disease with a mineralization defect. *Journal of Bone Mineralization Research, 17,* 30–38.

35. Haley, S. M., Faas, R. M., Coster, W. J., Webster, H., & Gans, B. M. (1989). *Pediatric Evaluation of Disability Inventory.* Boston: New England Medical Center.

36. Horwitz, E. M., Prockop, D. J., Gordon, P. L., et al. (2001). Clinical responses to bone marrow transplantation in children with severe osteogenesis imperfecta. *Blood, 97,* 1227–1231.

37. Jerosch, J., Mazzotti, I., & Tomasvic, M. (1998). Complications after treatment of patients with osteogenesis imperfecta with a Bailey-Dubow rod. *Archives of Orthopaedic Trauma Surgery, 117,* 240–245.

38. Kocher, M. S., Shapiro, F. (1998) Osteogenesis imperfecta. *Journal of the American Academy of Orthopedic Surgeons, 6,* 225–236.

39. Krakow, D., Alanay, Y., Rimoin, L. P., et al. (2008). Evaluation of prenatal-onset osteochondrodysplasias by ultrasonography: A retrospective and prospective analysis. *American Journal of Medical Genetics, 146,* 1917–1924.

40. Landsmeer-Beker, E. A. (1997). Treatment of osteogenesis imperfecta with the bisphosphonate olpadronate (dimethylaminohydroxypropylidene bisphosphonate). *European Journal of Pediatrics, 156,* 792–794.

41. Labuda, M., Morissette, J., Ward, L. M., et al. (2002). Osteogenesis imperfecta type VII maps to the short arm of chromosome 3. *Bone, 31,* 19–25.

42. Lips, P., Bouillon, R., van Schoor, N. M., Vanderschueren, D., Verschueren, S., Kuchuk, N., Milisen, K., & Boonen, S. (September 10, 2009). Reducing fracture risk with calcium and vitamin D. Clinical Endocrinology Online. accessed http://onlinelibrary.wiley.com/doi/10.1111/j.0300-0664.2009.03701.x/pdf

43. Looser, E. Zur Kenntnis der Osteogenesis imperfecta congenita und tarda (sogenannte idiopathische Osteopsathyrosis). *Mitteilungen Grenzgebieten Medizin und Chirurgie, 15,* 161, 1906. (Translation: Toward an understanding of osteogenesis imperfecta and tarda [also known as idiopathic osteopsathyrosis]. *Transactions of Frontiers of Medicine and Surgery.*)

44. Manworren, R. C., & Hynan, L. S. (2003). Clinical validation of FLACC: Preverbal patient pain scale. *Pediatric Nursing, 29,* 140–146.

45. Marini, J. C., Cabral, W. A., & Barnes, A. M. (2010). Null mutations in LEPRE1 and CRTAP cause severe recessive osteogenesis imperfecta. *Cell Tissues and Research, 339,* 59–70.

46. Marini, J. C. (2006). Should children with osteogenesis imperfecta be treated with bisphosphonates? *Nature Clinical Practice Endocrinology and Metabolism, 2,* 14–15.

47. Merkel, S., Voepel-Lewis, T., & Malviya, S. (2002). Pain assessment in infants and young children: FLACC scale. *American Journal of Nursing, 102,* 55–58.

48. Reference deleted in page proofs.

49. Montpetit, K., Plotkin, H., Pauch, F., Bilodeau, N., Cloutier, S., Rabzel, M., & Glorieux, F. H. (2003). Rapid increase in grip force after start of pamidronate therapy in children and

adolescents with severe osteogenesis imperfecta. *Pediatrics, 111,* 601–603.

50. Moore, M. S., Minch, C. M., Kruse, R. W., Harke, H. T., Jacobson, L., & Taylor, A. (1998). The role of dual energy x-ray absorptiometry in aiding the diagnosis of pediatric osteogenesis imperfecta. *American Journal of Orthopedics, 27,* 797–801.

51. Morris, C. D., & Einhorn, T. A. (2005). Bisphosphonates in orthopaedic surgery. *Journal of Bone Joint Surgery American, 87,* 1609–1618.

52. Munns, C. F., Rauch, F., Zeitlin, L., Fassier, F., & Glorieux, F. H. (2004). Delayed osteotomy but not fracture healing in pediatric osteogenesis imperfecta patients receiving pamidronate. *Journal of Bone and Mineral Research, 19,* 1779–1786.

53. Niyibizi, C., Wang, S., Mi, Z., & Robbins, P. D. (2004). Gene therapy approaches for osteogenesis imperfecta. *Gene Therapy, 11,* 408–416.

54. Obafemi, A. A., Bulas, D. I., Troendle, J., & Marini, J. C. (2008). Popcorn calcification in osteogenesis imperfecta: Incidence, progression, and molecular correlation. *American Journal of Medical Genetics Part A, 146A,* 2725–2732.

55. Reference deleted in page proofs.

56. Parks, R., Cintas, H. L., Chaffin, M. C., & Gerber, L. (2007). Brief Assessment of Motor Function: Content validity and reliability of the fine motor scale. *Pediatric Physical Therapy, 19,* 315–325.

57. Paterson, C. R. Clinical variability and life expectancy in osteogenesis imperfecta. *Clinical Rheumatology,* 14:228, 1995.

57. Poyrazoglu, S., Gunoz, H., Darendeliler, F., et al. (2008). Successful results of pamidronate treatment in children with osteogenesis imperfecta with emphasis on the interpretation of bone mineral density for local standards. *Journal of Pediatric Orthopedics, 28,* 483–487.

58. Primorac, D., Rowe, D. W., Mottes, M., Barisic, I., Anticevic, D., Mirandola, S., Gomez Lira, M., Kalajzic, I., Kusec, V., & Glorieux, F. H. (2001). Osteogenesis imperfecta at the beginning of bone and joint decade. *Croatian Medical Journal, 4,* 393–415.

59. Prockop, D. .J. (2004). Targetting gene therapy for osteogenesis imperfecta. *New England Journal of Medicine, 350,* 2302–2304.

60. Ramser, J. R., & Frost, H. M. (1966). The study of a rib biopsy from a patient with osteogenesis imperfecta: A method using in vivo tetracycline labeling. *Acta Orthopaedica Scandinavica, 37,* 229–240.

61. Rauch, F., & Glorieux, F. H. (2005). Bisphosphonate treatment in osteogenesis imperfecta: Which drug, for whom, for how long? *Annals of Medicine, 37,* 295–302.

62. Roughley, P. J., Rauch, F., & Glorieux, F. H. (2003). Osteogenesis imperfecta—Clinical and molecular diversity. *European Cells and Materials Journal, 5,* 41–47.

63. Schwartz, S. (2004). Dental care for children with osteogenesis imperfecta. In R. Chiasson, C. Munns, & L. Zeitlin (Eds.). *Interdisciplinary treatment approach for children with osteogenesis imperfecta* (pp. 137–150). Canada: Shriners Hospital for Children.

63a. Scott, E. F. (1990). The use of air splints for mobility training in osteogenesis imperfecta. *Clinical Suggestions, 2,* 52–53.

64. Seedorf, K. S. (1949). Osteogenesis imperfecta: A study of clinical features and heredity based on 55 Danish families comprising 180 affected members. *Opera ex Domo Biologiae Hereditariae Humanae Universitatis Hafniensis, 20,* 1–229.

65. Semler, O., Fricke, O., Vezyroglou, K., Stark, C., & Schoenau, E. (2007). Preliminary results on the mobility after whole body vibration in immobilized children and adolescents. *Journal of Musculoskeletal Neuronal Interaction, 7,* 77–81.

66. Semler, O., Fricke, O., Vezyroglou, K., Stark, C., & Schoenau, E. (2007). Improvement of individual mobility in patients with osteogenesis imperfecta by whole body vibration powered by Galileo-System. *Bone, 40,* S77.

67. Semler, O., Fricke, O., Vezyroglou, K., Stark, C., & Schoenau, E. (2008). Results of a prospective pilot trial on mobility after whole body vibration in immobilized children and adolescents with osteogenesis imperfecta. *Clinical Rehabilitation, 22,* 387–394.

68. Sillence, D. O. (1981). Osteogenesis imperfecta: Expanding panorama of variants. *Clinical Orthopaedics and Related Research, 159,* 11–25.

69. Sillence, D. O., & Danks, D. M. (1978). The differentiation of genetically distinct varieties of osteogenesis imperfecta in the newborn period. *Clinical Research, 26,* 178A.

70. Sillence, D. O., Senn, A., & Danks, D. M. (1979). Genetic heterogeneity in osteogenesis imperfecta. *Journal of Medical Genetics, 16,* 101–116.

71. Spranger, J., Cremin, B., & Beighton, P. (1982). Osteogenesis imperfecta congenita. *Pediatric Radiology, 12,* 21–27.

72. Stanton, D., Wilson, P. N., & Foreman, N. (2002). Effects of early mobility on shortcut performance in a simulated maze. *Behavioural Brain Research, 136,* 61–66.

73. Suskauer, S. J., Cintas, H. L., Marini, J. C., & Gerber, L. H. (2003). Temperament and physical performance in children with osteogenesis imperfecta. *Pediatrics, 111,* E153–E61.

74. Tachdjian, M. O. (Ed.). (2002). Pediatric orthopedics (*vol. 2,* 3rd ed.). Philadelphia: WB Saunders.

75. Van Brussel, M., Takken, T., Uiterwaal, C., Pruijs, H. J., Van der Net, J., & Helders, P. J. M. (2008). Physical training in children with osteogenesis imperfecta. *Journal of Pediatrics, 152,* 111–116.

76. Ward, L. M., Rauch, F., Travers, R., et al. (2003). Osteogenesis imperfecta type VII: An autosomal recessive form of brittle bone disease. *Bone, 31,* 12–18.

77. Weber, M., Roschger, P., Fratzl-Zelman, N., et al. (2006). Pamidronate does not adversely affect bone intrinsic material properties in children with osteogenesis imperfecta. *Bone, 39,* 616–622.

78. Widmann, R. F., Laplaza, F. J., Bitan, F. D., Brooks, C. E., & Root, L. (2002). Quality of life in osteogenesis imperfecta. *International Orthopedics, 26,* 3–6.

79. Wong, D., & Baker, C. (1988). Pain in children: Comparison of assessment scales. *Pediatric Nursing, 14,* 9–17.

81. Wynne-Davies, R., & Gormley, J. Clinical and genetic patterns in osteogenesis imperfecta. *Clinical Orthopedics and Related Research*, *159*:26–35, 1981.

82. Zack, P., Franck, L., Devile, C., & Clark, C. (2005). Fracture and non-fracture pain in children with osteogenesis imperfecta. *Acta Paediatrics*, *94*, 1238–1242.

RESOURCES

Osteogenesis Imperfecta Foundation
804 W. Diamond Avenue, Suite 210
Gaithersburg, M.D. 20878
www.oif.org

12 Muscular Dystrophy and Spinal Muscular Atrophy

WAYNE A. STUBERG, PT, PhD, PCS

Neuromuscular diseases include disorders of the motor neuron (anterior horn cells and peripheral nerves), neuromuscular junction, and muscle. Muscular dystrophy (MD) and spinal muscular atrophy (SMA) are two prevalent, progressive neuromuscular diseases that require physical therapy. Progressive weakness, muscle atrophy, contracture, deformity, and progressive disability characterize both diseases. No cure is available for either disease. *Incurable,* however, is not synonymous with *untreatable,* and the physical therapist can be influential in prevention of complications, preservation of function, and management of issues concerning quality of life.

The objective of this chapter is to present an overview of the childhood forms of MD and SMA and to discuss the role of the physical therapist as a member of the management team. The clinical presentation of the diseases is reviewed and examination procedures are presented to assist the clinician in identifying impairments and limitations in activities and participation associated with MD and SMA. Guidelines for physical therapy management are outlined and reflect my clinical experience and review of related literature.

ROLE OF THE PHYSICAL THERAPIST

As a member of the management team in the educational or medical setting, the physical therapist assists in identification and amelioration of impairments, as well as in promotion of activity and participation for persons with MD or SMA. The team often includes physician(s) (neurologist, orthopedist, or physiatrist), physical therapist, occupational therapist, speech therapist, educator, social worker, genetic counselor, psychologist, and orthotist. Because therapists typically maintain a higher frequency of contact with families, referral to and ongoing communication with other team members become an important part of maintaining continuity of care.

The team approach should be family centered with a focus on collaborative goal setting among individuals with the disorder, family members, and professionals, to ensure optimal care.[184] When care is provided using a family-centered philosophy, the pivotal role of the family is recognized and respected in the lives of persons with special health care needs.

Prevention is an important role of the physical therapist. Stress on the child/individual and family can be reduced and coping facilitated through accurate prognostic information and recognition of signs that portend changing status and a resultant increase in disability. Examples of status change are seen in the period before the loss of walking, before the need for architectural modifications to accommodate adaptive equipment for mobility, during transition from the educational to the vocational/avocational environment, and during the terminal stages of the disease, when the decision to use mechanical ventilation becomes a major issue for the family.

Providing information to family members, persons with MD or SMA, and other members of the team regarding physical limitations and expected participation restrictions is an important role of the physical therapist. Many resource materials are available online through the national Muscular Dystrophy Association (MDA) or through state chapter MDA offices.

PHYSICAL THERAPY EXAMINATION AND EVALUATION

Although the progression of MD and SMA is relatively well known, the clinician must carefully observe the child for changes that require intervention modifications. As stated by Thomas McCrae (1870–1935), "More is missed by not looking than by not knowing."[162] Ongoing dialogue with families is invaluable in identifying family-centered goals and the need for program modification.

The physical therapy examination is the initial step in management of the child with MD or SMA and should include those components identified in the *Guide to Physical Therapist Practice.*[2] Specifically, the following must be carefully examined:

1. History with family concerns
2. Aerobic capacity and endurance
3. Assistive and adaptive devices
4. Community and work (job/school/play) integration
5. Environmental, home, and job/school/play barriers
6. Gait, locomotion, and balance
7. Integumentary status (when using orthoses, adaptive equipment, or wheelchair)
8. Muscle performance
9. Neuromotor development
10. Orthotic, protective, and supportive devices
11. Posture

12. Range of motion
13. Self-care and home management
14. Ventilation/respiration

Systematic documentation of disease progression is essential for timing interventions during transitions from one functional status to another or during times of increased family need.

MUSCULAR DYSTROPHY

The origin of MD is genetic inheritance. The pathophysiology underlying the disease is progressive loss of muscle contractility caused by the destruction of myofibrils. The specific cellular mechanism behind the destruction in Duchenne's muscular dystrophy (DMD) and Becker's muscular dystrophy (BMD) has been partially identified and is discussed later in the chapter. The rate of progression of myofibril destruction is variable among the various forms of MD, giving evidence for the possibility of more than one cellular mechanism in the destructive process.

The diagnosis of MD is confirmed by clinical examination and laboratory procedures, including electromyography, muscle biopsy, DNA analysis, and assay of selected enzyme levels from blood samples.[89] Criteria for classification of the various forms of MD include mode of inheritance, age at onset, rate of progression, localization of involvement, muscle morphologic changes, and presence of a genetic marker if available. The MDA recognizes nine primary classifications of MD.[119] Table 12-1 lists the six most prevalent types that exhibit initial clinical signs in infancy, childhood, or adolescence. Emery-Dreifuss MD (humeroperoneal) is very rare and is discussed only briefly. Limb-girdle MD may exhibit signs in the teenage years, but the onset of symptoms more typically occurs in early adulthood; therefore, along with the adult-onset forms of MD, it is not discussed in this chapter.

The primary impairment in MD is insidious weakness secondary to progressive loss of myofibrils. In congenital forms of MD, the weakness is pronounced at birth and is easily recognizable. In DMD, the weakness becomes evident by age 3 to 5 years. In congenital and congenital myotonic MD, contractures present at birth also cause primary impairment. The incidence of intellectual disability is highest in congenital myotonic MD, but it is less frequently reported in DMD and the other childhood forms.

Secondary impairments in all forms of MD include the development of contractures and postural malalignment. Postural malalignment is seen in anti-gravity positions of sitting and standing and often includes development of scoliosis. Other secondary impairments include decreased respiratory capacity, easy fatigability, and, occasionally, obesity. Although significant intellectual impairment is not usual, IQ commonly averages 85; consequently, 30% of boys with DMD have an IQ below 70.[3] This finding has been related to a loss of dystrophin in the brain and, more specifically, to a disruption in gamma-aminobutyric acid (GABA) receptors in the central nervous system.[3] Learning difficulties are commonly reported in both DMD and BMD.[192]

With the progression of muscle weakness, increasing caregiver assistance is required for persons with MD to carry out activities of daily living (ADLs). Progressive disability is a hallmark of MD and requires multidisciplinary team management to maximize participation through the use of adaptive equipment and environmental adaptations.

Physical management is a key intervention in the treatment of MD because no drug or other therapy has been found to be curative.[115,121,173] Physical therapy has been used to prolong the child's independence, slow the progression of complications, and improve quality of life.

DYSTROPHIN-ASSOCIATED PROTEINS AND MUSCULAR DYSTROPHY

Over the past 10 years, significant advances have been made in the molecular genetics and biology of the muscular dystrophies. These advances have followed identification of the genetic defect behind DMD and the missing protein dystrophin. Many other proteins that are associated with dystrophin have been found to be defective or missing in other forms of MD. These proteins are termed *dystrophin-associated*

TABLE 12-1 **Classification of Muscular Dystrophy**

Type	Onset	Inheritance	Course
Duchenne's	1–4 years	X-linked	Rapidly progressive; loss of walking by 9 to 10 years; death in late teens
Becker's	5–10 years	X-linked	Slowly progressive; maintain walking past early teens; life span into third decade
Congenital	Birth	Recessive	Typically slow but variable; shortened life span
Congenital myotonic	Birth	Dominant	Typically slow with significant intellectual impairment
Childhood-onset facioscapulohumeral	First decade	Dominant/recessive	Slowly progressive loss of walking in later life; variable life expectancy
Emery-Dreifuss	Childhood to early teens	X-linked	Slowly progressive with cardiac abnormality and normal life span

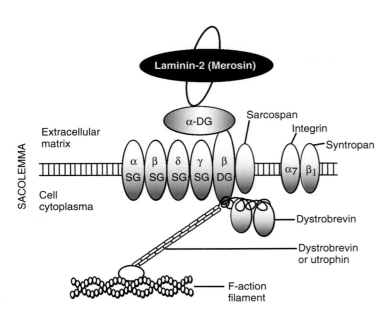

Figure 12-1 Dystrophin-associated protein complex. Cross section through muscle membrane with intracellular, transcellular, and extracellular proteins. *SG,* Sarcogylcan; *DG,* dystroglycan.

proteins (DAPs).[25] The DAPs form a complex of extracellular, transmembrane, and intracellular proteins, which are represented in Figure 12-1.

Dystrophin acts as an anchor in the intracellular lattice to enhance tensile strength. The other proteins are thought to act as a physical pathway for transmembrane signaling. Absence of any transmembrane protein, however, would result in faulty mechanics of the cell membrane. For example, sarcoglycan defects are present in adult forms of MD,[54] and merosin, alpha-dystroglycan, or integrin may be present in select forms of congenital MD.[70]

DUCHENNE'S MUSCULAR DYSTROPHY

DMD is the most common X-linked disorder known, with an incidence of about 1 in 3500 live male births.[119] The prevalence of DMD in the general population is reportedly 3 cases per 100,000.[53,119] Initial diagnosis in families without a genetic history typically occurs around 5 years of age, although symptoms are often seen as early as 2.5 years.[42] Longevity is variable, from the late teens to early twenties up to the end of the third decade, depending on the rate of disease progression, the presence of complications, and the aggressiveness of respiratory care, including the use of assisted ventilation (Finder et al., 2009).

Kunkel and associates[60a] identified the gene on the X chromosome *(Xp21)* that, when missing or defective, causes DMD and BMD; Hoffman and associates[83] then identified the protein (dystrophin) of the chromosome locus. Cloning of the dystrophin gene was the next major accomplishment, which provided a mechanism for prenatal or postnatal diagnosis and development of gene therapy.[95]

Muscle cell destruction in DMD and BMD is caused by abnormal or missing dystrophin and its effect at the muscle cell membrane. Mechanical weakening of the sarcolemma,

inappropriate calcium influx, aberrant signaling, increased oxidative stress, and recurrent muscle ischemia are all hypothesized as mechanisms associated with myofibril damage.[136]

The focus of research for the treatment of DMD is on exploring molecular, cellular, and pharmacologic therapies.[37,59,121] These interventions include myoblast transfer therapy, gene- and cell-based replacement therapy, attempts to increase production of other dystrophin-related sarcolemmal proteins such as utrophin, and use of drugs such as steroids. All therapies are in the experimental stage, and early clinical trial reports have described myoblast transfer therapy,[133] stem cell transplant,[174] and gene replacement therapy.[82] No trials on the use of utrophin in humans have begun.[135] Evidence for the use of steroids and creatine is growing.

In myoblast transfer therapy, embryologic precursor cells of the skeletal muscle (i.e., myoblasts) are obtained from a histocompatible donor. These stem cells are then injected into the muscle of the individual with DMD in the hope that the normal myoblasts will grow and mutate with surrounding cells that are lacking dystrophin, resulting in the development of dystrophin. Research in animals has shown that donor myoblast cells fuse with dystrophic cells to form a hybrid multinucleated cell that produces dystrophin.[128] Myoblast transfer therapy is currently showing low efficacy with limited production of dystrophin in early clinical trial results.[133,174]

Gene therapy research involves introduction of the dystrophin gene that is packaged in a modified adenovirus or retrovirus called a *vector,* or introduction of a vector that allows for splicing across the damaged DNA, with formation of at least partial dystrophin in the muscle. Lee and colleagues[100] produced an entire dystrophin gene, which has met with difficulty in clinical trials introducing the gene to muscle cells, except through injection. More recently, gene splicing using an oligonucleotide (moropholino), which allows "reading past" the gene defect, referred to as *exon skipping,* has shown promise in early clinical trials with boys with DMD.[94] The resultant dystrophin, although not complete, promises to improve the phenotype of the individual to shift to more of a Becker-type presentation than what is seen in DMD, where dystrophin is absent.

Utrophin is a muscle protein that has molecular similarity to dystrophin. Utrophin levels in the muscle are high in the fetus and newborn but gradually diminish, until utrophin is found primarily at the neuromuscular or musculotendinous junction in adults. Courdier-Fruh and colleagues[45] have demonstrated in vitro that utrophin levels can be increased through upregulation. It is hypothesized that utrophin might act as a substitute for abnormal or missing dystrophin. Upregulation of other compensatory proteins such as integrin and sarcospan has been reported in animal models, but human clinical trials have not yet begun.[121]

Medical management of DMD has included clinical trials of various drugs. Long-term steroid use (prednisone and deflazacort, and oxandrolone) has been shown to improve outcomes, including prolonged independent and assisted walking by up to 3 years, improved isometric muscle strength by 60% in the arms and 85% in the legs when compared with untreated control subjects, and improved pulmonary function.[20,22,26,115,190] Reported side effects, however, include weight gain (particularly with prednisone), growth suppression, and osteoporosis. Strict dietary controls to offset the side effects are recommended.[190] The use of creatine in a randomized double-blind study of 15 boys with DMD has demonstrated improved muscle strength and endurance and a reduction in joint stiffness.[103] Louis and colleagues also reported improved bone mineral density in boys who were wheelchair users, suggesting that the negative effects of steroids on bone mineral density might be offset by the use of creatine. However, a more recent clinical trial has not found similar evidence of improvements using creatine or glutamine.[58]

Although it is commonly agreed that the prevention of contractures and the preservation of independent mobility are primary goals of a physical management program,[176] the prolongation of ambulation through surgery or orthotics remains controversial. Some authors promote the use of surgery and lightweight bracing[11,16,79,85,117,172]; others express skepticism about prolonging the inevitable in a progressive disease, when the financial and emotional costs to the family may be very high.[66] Evidence is available that the use of steroids and supported walking and standing with knee-ankle-foot orthoses (KAFOs) are associated with reduced risk of scoliosis development and later onset of scoliosis.[93] A decreasing trend in the use of KAFOs from 69% of the MDA clinics surveyed in 1989 to 27% in 2000 has been reported[10] and would suggest a trend of less aggressive orthotic management in this population. Additional research in this area is needed for the clinician to develop consistent treatment recommendations regarding the use of KAFOs for prolonged walking or standing.

Surgical management has focused on control of lower extremity contractures, use of orthoses in conjunction with surgery to prolong ambulation, and spinal stabilization for control of scoliosis. Achilles tendon lengthening and fasciotomy of the tensor fasciae latae and iliotibial bands are two procedures commonly reported to be used in conjunction with orthotics and physical therapy to prolong ambulation.[11,85] Posterior tibialis transfer into the third cuneiform to reverse equinovarus deformity has also been reported.[85] Surgical management of scoliosis typically includes the use of spinal instrumentation with Luque rods.[109] Conservative management of scoliosis using orthoses remains prevalent[10]; however, 85% of boys with DMD develop severe scoliosis,[144] and orthotic management has not been shown to stop the progression of the curve,[80] nor to decrease the severity of the curve.[93]

Impairments, Activity Limitations, and Participation Restrictions

Examination of the 4- to 5-year-old child demonstrates the onset of classical clinical features of DMD and primary impairment of muscle weakness. The posterior calf is usually enlarged as a result of fatty and connective tissue infiltration, which corresponds to the term *pseudohypertrophic MD,* which is used for the eponym DMD. Pseudohypertrophy occasionally can be seen to affect the deltoid, quadriceps, or forearm extensor muscle groups. Initial weakness of the neck flexor, abdominal, interscapular, and hip extensor musculature can be noted, with a more generalized distribution with progression of the disease. Figure 12-2 demonstrates the trends of muscle strength decline up to age 16 years from a study by Brooke.[30] These data were obtained in a multiclinic study of 150 children with DMD over a follow-up period of 3 to 4 years. The data represent approximately 15 data points per boy, as recorded during follow-up visits. Similar findings on anthropometric data, range of motion, spinal deformity, pulmonary function, and functional skills were reported by McDonald and colleagues[112] in a cohort of 162 boys with DMD followed over a 3-year period.

Muscle strength can be documented using manual muscle testing (MMT), which has been reported to have acceptable intrarater reliability,[61] although it is not as accurate as using specialized devices such as a dynamometer. Instruments such as a handheld dynamometer[169] or strain gauge devices[33] can be used to obtain objective strength recordings in the older child to assist in prediction of disability, such as the loss of independent ambulation. Timed functional activities have also been shown to be closely correlated to muscle strength as another measure of strength.[19]

No limitations in range of motion (ROM) are typically noted before 5 years of age in DMD. Mild tightness of the gastrocnemius-soleus and tensor fasciae latae muscles usually occurs first. The normal lordotic standing posture is

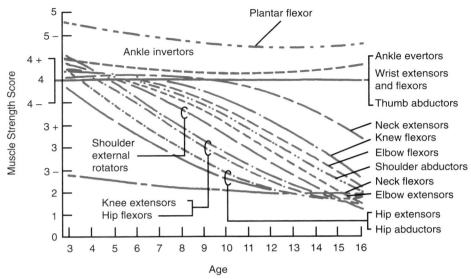

Figure 12-2 Muscle strength 50th percentile lines plotted against age of 150 children with Duchenne's muscular dystrophy. (Redrawn from Brooke, M. H. [1986]. *A clinician's view of neuromuscular diseases* [2nd ed.]. Baltimore: Williams & Wilkins.)

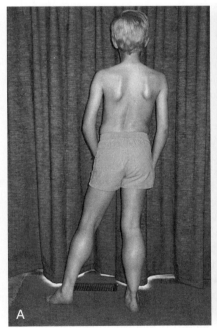
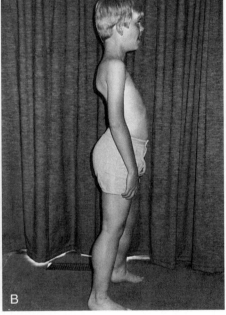

Figure 12-3 Typical standing posture of a 7-year-old boy with Duchenne muscular dystrophy. **A,** Posterior view; note the winging of the scapula, equinus contracture of the left ankle, and calf pseudohypertrophy. **B,** Lateral view; note the increased lumbar lordosis.

increased, and mild winging of the scapulae is then seen as compensation to keep the center of mass behind the hip joint to promote standing stability (Figure 12-3). Scoliosis typically develops just before or during adolescence.

Management Considerations

An international collaboration recently published a consensus document on the management of DMD.[35] More specific information related to physical therapy management by age and progression follows.

Infancy to Preschool-Age Period

No significant impairments, activity limitations, or participation restrictions are typically seen in the infant or toddler with DMD, although Gardner-Medwin[67] reported that half of children fail to walk until 18 months of age. Delay in walking, however, rarely leads to the diagnosis of DMD. Symptoms are seldom noted before age 3 to 5 years, unless the family history is positive and caregivers are looking for early signs. The mean age at diagnosis is usually reported to be around 5 years.[117]

Although no significant disability occurs in early childhood, many disability-related issues must be addressed. The family will have questions regarding peer interaction, routine activity level for the child, and the prognosis. The therapist must be aware of each family's coping response, goals, and needed supports, to provide family-centered care. This is the appropriate time to discuss with the family the social aspects of the disability and to answer questions without portraying a future without hope.

Early School-Age Period

Initial limitations in activity in DMD typically occur by age 5 years and include clumsiness, falling, and inability to keep up with peers while playing. The young child's gait pattern is only slightly atypical, with an increased lateral trunk sway (waddling). Attempts at running, however, accentuate the waddling progression, and neither running nor jumping is attained. Gowers' sign (using the arms to push on the thighs to attain standing) is usually present after one or repeated trials of assuming a standing position from sitting on the floor.

Stair climbing and arising to standing from the floor become progressively more difficult and signal the first significant functional limitation by age 6 to 8 years. Progressive changes in the gait pattern include deviations of an increased base of support, pronounced lateral trunk sway (compensated Trendelenburg), toe-walking, and retraction of the shoulders with lack of reciprocal arm swing. Toe-walking initially may be a compensation for weakness of the abdominal and hip extensor muscles, resulting in lordosis and forward shift of the body's center of mass, with later evidence of contracture of the posterior calf musculature.

Toe-walking caused by contracture of the posterior calf musculature, in-toeing with substitution of the tensor fasciae latae to compensate for weakness of the iliopsoas muscles, falls resulting from progressive weakness, and complaints of fatigue while walking become increasingly frequent from age 8 to 10 years. A restrictive pattern of pulmonary impairment and progressive decline in maximal vital capacity also becomes increasingly evident.[65]

Examination Considerations

An examination to document limitations in activity and participation is essential. Various formats have been reported[165,180] that are variations of the guidelines initially published by Swinyard and associates.[171] A classification system published by Vignos and colleagues[178] is outlined in Box 12-1. A more detailed examination format for DMD published by Brooke and associates[31] includes pulmonary function and timed performance of activities (Appendix I). Normative data for DMD have been published using the clinical protocol of Brooke and associates.[30] A similar assessment called the North Star Ambulatory Assessment has been devised and reliability established for use in multicenter clinical trials.[111] The assessment tool chosen will vary depending on the

---

Box 12-1 **VIGNOS FUNCTIONAL RATING SCALE FOR DUCHENNE MUSCULAR DYSTROPHY**

1. Walks and climbs stairs without assistance
2. Walks and climbs stairs with aid of railing
3. Walks and climbs stairs slowly with aid of railing (over 25 seconds for eight standard steps)
4. Walks, but cannot climb stairs
5. Walks assisted, but cannot climb stairs or get out of chair
6. Walks only with assistance or with braces
7. In wheelchair: Sits erect and can roll chair and perform bed and wheelchair ADLs
8. In wheelchair: Sits erect and is unable to perform bed and wheelchair ADLs without assistance
9. In wheelchair: Sits erect only with support and is able to do only minimal ADLs
10. In bed: Can do no ADLs without assistance

Data from Vignos, P. J., Spencer, G. E., & Archibald, K. C. (1963). Management of progressive muscular dystrophy. *Journal of the American Medical Association, 184*, 103–112. Copyright © 1963, American Medical Association.

---

diagnosis, as tools vary in their responsiveness depending on the rate of progression of the various types of muscular dystrophy.[104] Other functional assessment tools, such as the Pediatric Evaluation of Disability Inventory (PEDI),[76] the School Function Assessment (SFA),[44] the EK (Egen Klassifikation) Scale,[165] or the Barthel Index,[120] should also be considered to obtain more specific information on the child's functional skills. The EK Scale, which was recently validated for DMD and SMA, includes ordinal scoring of 10 categories, including items on mobility, transfers, ability to cough/speak, and physical well-being. The PEDI, the SFA, or the Vignos (Brooke) functional testing format can be used for diagnosis of other types of MD or SMA.

Muscle weakness is apparent in the school-age child by age 6 to 8 years and should be objectively documented using a handheld dynamometer,[169] electrodynamometer,[150] isokinetic dynamometer,[118,153] or other device. Use of a dynamometer in conjunction with manual muscle testing has been shown to provide reliable information on the progression of weakness in key muscle groups.[33,63,169] Contracture development should be documented using goniometry and a standardized protocol. Intrarater reliability of measurements has been shown to be acceptable in providing objective information for program planning when a standardized measurement protocol is used.[127]

A clinical estimate of respiratory function can be obtained through measurement of respiratory rate and chest wall excursion (using a tape measure) and by noting the child's ability to cough and clear secretions. A portable spirometer is recommended to obtain a more direct and objective

---

APPENDIX I   CLINICAL PROTOCOL FOR FUNCTIONAL TESTING IN DUCHENNE MUSCULAR DYSTROPHY*

A. Pulmonary
  1. Forced vital capacity.
  2. Maximum voluntary ventilation.
B. Functional grade (arms and shoulders). Select one.
  1. Starting with arms at the sides, the patient can abduct the arms in a full circle until they touch above the head.
  2. Can raise arms above head only by flexing the elbow (i.e., shortening the circumference of the movement) or using accessory muscles.
      If 1 or 2 is entered above, how many kilograms of weight can be placed on a shelf above eye level, using one hand?
  3. Cannot raise hands above head but can raise an 8 oz glass of water to mouth (using both hands if necessary).
  4. Can raise hands to mouth but cannot raise an 8 oz glass of water to mouth.
  5. Cannot raise hands to mouth but can use hands to hold pen or pick up pennies from the table.
  6. Cannot raise hands to mouth and has no useful function of hands.
C. Pulmonary.
  1. Maximum expiratory pressure.
D. Time to perform functions. Enter time in seconds. T = tried but failed to complete by time limit of 120 seconds.
  1. Standing from lying supine.
  2. Climbing four standard stairs (beginning and ending standing with arms at sides).
  3. Running or walking 30 feet (as fast as is compatible with safety).
  4. Standing from sitting on chair (chair height should allow feet to touch floor).
  5. Propelling a wheelchair 30 feet.
  6. Putting on a T-shirt (sitting in chair).
  7. Cutting a 3 × 3-inch premarked square from a piece of paper with safety scissors (lines do not need to be followed precisely).
E. Functional grade (hips and legs). Select one.
  1. Walks and climbs stairs without assistance.
  2. Walks and climbs stairs with aid of railing.
  3. Walks and climbs stairs slowly with aid of railing (over 12 seconds for four standard stairs).
  4. Walks unassisted and raises from chair but cannot climb stairs.
  5. Walks unassisted but cannot rise from chair or climb stairs.
  6. Walks only with assistance or walks independently with long leg braces.
  7. Walks in long leg braces but requires assistance for balance.
  8. Stands in long leg braces but is unable to walk even with assistance.
  9. Is in wheelchair.
  10. Is confined to bed.

(From Brooke, M.H., Griggs, R.C., Mendell, J.R., Fenichel, G.M., Shumate, J.B., & Pellegrino, R.J. (1981). Clinical trial in Duchenne dystrophy: I. The design of the protocol. *Muscle and Nerve, 4*:186–197.)

---

reading of expiratory capacity before formal pulmonary function testing is needed. Assessment of forced vital capacity is recommended; surgical intervention for scoliosis may not be possible for individuals when values fall below 30% of age norm values.[108]

Physical therapy management typically begins when the child is initially diagnosed at age 3 to 5 years. Goals of the program are to provide family support and education, obtain baseline data on muscle strength and ROM, and monitor for the progression of muscle weakness that will lead to limitations in activity and participation. Initial therapeutic input should not be burdensome to the child or family because the child is usually independent in all ADLs before the age of 5 years.

Information should be provided to the family pertaining to the therapist's role as a member of the management team. An appropriate activity level to avoid fatigue should be discussed with the family and school staff. Information on services available through the local MDA office should be provided, including identification of support groups or contact families.

Intervention Considerations

The role of exercise in the treatment of MD is controversial.[4,5,62,74,176] It is widely accepted that both overexertion[88,178] and immobilization[178] are detrimental. The use of graded resistive exercise has been reported to have a range of results from good[179] to limited[47a] to adverse.[4] Resistive exercise theoretically would be indicated with the disproportionate loss of type II (fast-twitch) muscle fibers in DMD.[52] However, the use of resistive exercise in the young school-age child should not be universally prescribed. Prescribing a submaximal exercise program early has been shown to have beneficial effects, but it should be offered only to families who have a specific desire to include it in the child's program. Consideration should be given to the fact that significant muscle weakness is not seen in the early stage of the disease, and the use of an exercise program may be burdensome to the child and family.

If exercise is initiated early, the key muscle groups to be included are the abdominal, hip extensor and abductor, and knee extensor groups. Abdominal exercises should include trunk curls as opposed to sit-ups, which primarily will strengthen the hip flexors. Assistance may be required for neck flexor weakness because the head typically cannot be flexed from a supine position. Cycling and swimming are excellent activities for overall conditioning and are often preferred over formal exercise programs.[5,67,176] Standing or walking for a minimum of 2 to 3 hours daily is highly recommended.[161,193] High resistance and eccentric exercise should be avoided.[4,5]

Breathing exercises have been shown to slow the loss of vital capacity and forced expiratory flow rate.[96,147] Game activities such as inflating balloons or using blow-bottles to maintain pulmonary function can easily be included in a home program and will decrease the severity of symptoms during episodes of colds or other pulmonary infections.

The use of electrical stimulation in DMD has also been suggested as a means of slowing the progression of weakness and improving function. Scott and co-workers[154] studied the effects of low-frequency electrical stimulation on the tibialis anterior muscle of 16 children with DMD. A 47% increase in maximum voluntary contraction was observed in younger children after a stimulation protocol was used for 8 weeks; little change was noted in older children. The authors concluded that the results were encouraging, and that further study on muscle groups used for functional activities was needed.

One of the primary considerations in the early management program of the young school-age child is to slow the development of contractures. Contractures have not been shown to be preventable, but their progression can be slowed with positioning and an ROM program.[86,152,155,191]

The initial ROM program should include stretching the gastrocnemius-soleus and tensor fasciae latae. Progressive contracture of the gastrocnemius-soleus and tensor fasciae latae corresponds to gait deviations of toe-walking and an increased base of support. Stretching for the gastrocnemius-soleus can be done using a standing runner's stretch. The child stands at a supportive surface, places one leg back at a time with the knee straight, and leans forward. The position also assists with maintenance of hip flexor flexibility; however, specific stretching for the hip flexors should be included when any limitation is noted. Having the child lie supine with one thigh off the edge of a mat or bed and the other held to the chest (Thomas test position) can be used to stretch the hip flexors initially. An alternative method is discussed later for use as progression of hip extensor weakness evolves. A standing stretch for the tensor is accomplished by having the child stand with one side toward the supportive surface with the feet away from the wall, and with the knee kept straight while leaning sideways toward the supportive surface.

A home ROM program should be emphasized for the young child, and the family should be instructed in the stretching activities. Agreement is lacking as to the frequency and duration of the stretching program. Suggested frequency of the program varies from once daily[67,117,152] to twice

daily,[178,193] and duration from 1 repetition up to 10.[178] Other authors have suggested a time frame of 10[191] to 20[67] minutes to complete the stretching exercises. As a general recommendation, each movement should be repeated for five repetitions with a 30-60-second hold in the stretched position. The stretch should be done slowly and should not be painful. Increased risk of muscle or tendon strain with the loss of myofibrils and replacement by connective tissue is present because of decreased muscle elasticity, and caution in using excessive passive force is advised. Reassessment of the contracture progression should be used as the final guide to stretching frequency and duration.

The ROM program can often be supplemented as part of the physical education program at school. Special instruction should be provided to the physical education teacher to develop an adapted program, particularly if the teacher does not have an adapted physical education endorsement. General physical education activities will require modification for the child's participation and should not be exhaustive. Physical fitness test activities such as push-ups, sit-ups, or timed running for long time periods should be modified or excluded to avoid fatigue or overwork weakness.

Night splints are helpful for slowing the progression of ankle contractures. Scott and associates[152] studied the efficacy of night splints and a home ROM program in a group of 59 boys diagnosed with MD and ranging in age from 4 to 12 years. Subjects were categorized into three groups on the basis of adherence with splint wear and use of stretching. The group that followed through on the daily passive stretching program and the use of below-knee splints over the 2 years of the study demonstrated significantly less progression of Achilles tendon contractures and less deterioration in functional skills, leading to a longer period of independent walking. Boys in the group that did not follow through on the stretching or splint program lost independent walking at a younger age. In a randomized study comparing the effects of ROM exercise versus ROM and night splints, the combined intervention was found to be 23% more effective than ROM alone in slowing the progression of posterior calf contracture.[86] Similar findings were reported in a study by Seeger and colleagues,[155] which compared the use of night splints, stretching, and surgery.

The use of prone positioning at night to slow the progression of hip and knee flexion contractures may be possible if tolerated by the child. The recommendation to have the child sleep prone with the ankles off the edge of the bed has not been shown to affect the progression of the contractures but theoretically is sound.

Scoliosis is not common when the child is ambulatory, but the spine should be checked routinely.[93] Kinali and associates[93] report an incidence of scoliosis ranging from 68% to 90% in boys with DMD, with onset typically seen after cessation of standing at around 12 years. Postural analysis using the forward bend test is recommended to monitor spinal alignment for scoliosis. The presence of a rib hump with the forward bend test verifies a structural versus functional curve of the spine. Amendt and colleagues[1] demonstrated that a rib hump measuring at least 5° of inclination with a scoliometer is a reliable method and can be correlated with radiographic assessment. However, the study by Amendt and colleagues[1] was not inclusive of children with DMD but demonstrates an objective method of performing noninvasive screening for scoliosis. Orthopedic referral is indicated if a rib hump is documented. Although the evidence for spinal stabilization surgery is limited, this option is routinely discussed with the family by orthopedists whenever a curve is noted.[39]

Falls and complaints of fatigue while walking become increasingly more frequent as the child reaches age 8 to 10 years. Guarding during stair climbing or during general walking should be considered to ensure safety as balance becomes tenuous. A manual wheelchair with appropriate fit and accessories will allow for limited mobility as walking becomes more difficult. As progression of weakness in the trunk and hip girdle begins to make walking difficult, a similar amount of weakness of the shoulder girdle musculature is also present, making propulsion of a manual wheelchair difficult, except on level and smooth surfaces such as linoleum. A motorized scooter should be considered to provide the child with independence, provided that access is available in the home and school (Figure 12-4).

Information should be made available to families concerning recreational activities provided through the local chapter of the MDA or other groups. Summer MDA camp is a wonderful experience for most children, and a support group is often developed for the child or family through participation in MDA and other group activities that provide both physical and emotional support.

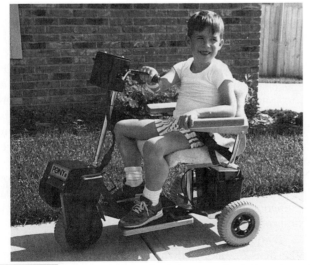

Figure 12-4 Motorized three-wheeled scooter for independence in distance mobility as an adjunct to walking.

Adolescent Period

Adolescence marks a time of significant progression that results from the combined impact of muscle weakness and development of contractures. Walking is lost as a means of mobility, and increasing difficulty in general mobility with transfers is seen. Use of a manual wheelchair or powered mobility becomes necessary during adolescence. If powered mobility is used, assistance with finances for the purchase of equipment or home modifications for access is typically needed, with coordination through a social worker or an MDA patient services coordinator. Changes in physical capacity such as muscle strength and pulmonary function using the EK Scale have been reported among adolescents by Steffensen and colleagues.[166] Muscle weakness leads to increasing difficulty with ADLs, including dressing, transfers, bathing, grooming, and feeding, and subsequent increasing involvement of the physical therapist and the occupational therapist. Possible surgical intervention may be considered for the management of scoliosis[39] or contractures or to prolong walking with the use of orthoses.[16]

As muscle weakness becomes more pronounced in the trunk and hip musculature, and as contractures of the hip flexors, tensor fasciae latae, and gastrocnemius-soleus progress, walking becomes increasingly difficult until cessation of independent walking occurs, usually by age 10 to 12. If orthoses are used to maintain a standing or walking program, they should be initiated before the child reaches the stage of being nonambulatory.

Various methods to predict the termination of walking have been reported, including 50% reduction in leg strength,[153,177] manual muscle test grade below grade 3 for hip extensors or below grade 4 for ankle dorsiflexors,[112] or inability to climb steps. Brooke and colleagues[30] reported the cessation of unassisted walking within 2.4 years (range, 1.2–4.1 years) when 5 to 12 seconds was required to climb four standard steps, or within 1.5 years (range, 0.6–2.2 years) when longer than 12 seconds was required. An alternative method, shown in Figure 12-5, has been suggested. The knee extension lag while sitting and the hip extension lag while prone are assessed to predict the cessation of independent walking. If the combined lag is greater than 90°, then termination of independent ambulation will occur within a few months. Monitoring and management of contractures becomes a key element in maintaining walking when the older child spends more time in a sitting position. Because the hip extensor musculature is significantly weak in the early stage of the disease and weakness of the quadriceps muscles becomes pronounced by age 8 to 10 years, inability to maintain the center of gravity behind the hip joint or in front of the knee joint during stance will lead to loss of the ability to stand.

Manual stretching may be discontinued at this point, as the contractures should be maintained through daily positioning and routine activities. They should continue to be

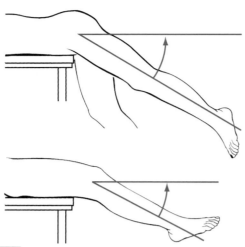

Figure 12-5 Prognostic method used by Siegel to determine cessation of independent walking caused by lack of anti-gravity hip and knee extensor torque. (Redrawn from Siegel, I. M. [1986]. *Muscle and its diseases: An outline primer of basic science and clinical method.* Chicago: Year Book Medical Publisher.)

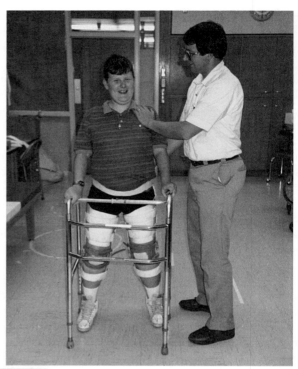

Figure 12-6 Polypropylene knee-ankle-foot orthosis and use of a reciprocating walker to promote walking for exercise in a 14-year-old boy with Duchenne's muscular dystrophy. The reciprocating walker allows progression without picking up the device.

monitored to ensure that they do not become an obstacle to routine ADLs.

Continuation of Standing or Walking

The use of orthoses for a standing program or continuation of supported walking is not appropriate for all individuals; in fact, this should be considered a personal rather than a therapeutic decision. Although a standing program may be useful to slow the progression of contractures, a braced walking program has little long-term functional or practical application because the child eventually will use a wheelchair. Continuation of standing through use of a standing frame, knee immobilizers, or KAFOs is a goal at our facility to address the issue of decreased bone mineral density[113] and subsequent increased risk of fracture.[21] Because surgery is often required in addition to orthotics for prolonged ambulation, the parents and the adolescent must agree on the management decision. Prolongation of ambulation through surgery and orthotics is not a common goal at our facility. More typically, limited resources are used for power mobility equipment, adaptive equipment, or environmental adaptations.

Prognostic factors for success that should be considered in making the decision to use orthoses to prolong walking include residual muscle strength (approximately 50%)[176]; absence of severe contractures; timely application of braces[11]; residual walking ability[177]; and motivation of the child and family.[27] The degree of mental impairment and obesity should also be considered. The timely use of orthoses has been shown to prolong walking[11,27,79] and to increase the child's longevity.[11,117,178]

If the decision to use orthoses to prolong standing or walking is made, KAFOs should be prescribed (Figure 12-6).[16,27] Ankle-foot orthoses (AFOs) are appropriate for

positioning but do not provide the knee stability required to avoid falls while walking. Although the use of AFOs to control equinus is common for other diagnoses such as cerebral palsy, with DMD the orthoses often interfere with the use of an ankle strategy and the preserved distal strength that is needed for standing balance and walking. A reciprocating or wheeled walker may be helpful when assistance for balance is needed. Assistive devices such as standard walkers, crutches, or canes are seldom functional because of the degree of proximal shoulder girdle and upper extremity muscle weakness that is present. Standby assistance should be provided when KAFOs are used, owing to the risk of injury from falls. Closer guarding and increased assistance will be needed as the weakness progresses. Transfers to and from standing are dependent because the knee joints of the KAFO must be locked to provide stability. KAFOs can be used for continuation of a standing program even after walking is no longer possible.

Surgical intervention is commonly needed in conjunction with the use of braced walking as contractures progress. Documented indications for surgery include ankle plantar flexion contractures greater than 10°, iliotibial band contractures greater than 20°, or knee-hip flexion contractures greater than 20° but less than 45°.[27] Subcutaneous tenotomy of the Achilles tendon and fasciotomy of the iliotibial bands are the most commonly reported surgical procedures.[11,27,85,176]

Transfer of the posterior tibialis tendon is occasionally used for correction of equinovarus foot posture.[85,151]

An intensive postoperative management program is essential to minimize the effects of immobilization.[162] Standing in the plaster casts can be done on the first or second postoperative day. Gait training is begun as tolerated, and general conditioning exercises for the hips, trunk, and upper extremities are recommended. Breathing exercises should also be stressed. A smooth transition from the casts to bracing is ensured by having the child fitted for the KAFOs before hospitalization for surgery.

Standing pivot transfers eventually must be replaced by one- or two-person lifts or use of equipment because of the development of knee and hip flexion contractures and pronounced weakness of the lower extremities. Transfers to and from the wheelchair, toilet, tub, car, and furniture usually become dependent by age 12 to 14. A sliding board, manual lift, or hydraulic lift can be used during transfers. Proper instruction for transfers is needed because the degree of trunk muscle weakness makes sitting balance tenuous by this stage. If the caregiver is using manual lifting for transfers, he or she should be observed for and instructed in proper body mechanics and safety. An hydraulic lift can be used for transfers to and from the wheelchair, particularly when the adolescent is large or obese, or when the caregiver cannot safely perform a manual lift. A U-style sling should be used with the lift to provide adequate head and trunk support during transfers. A tub lift or bath bench for bathing will be needed and a wheeled commode-shower chair should be considered, depending on bathroom accessibility.

Mobility and Spinal Alignment

A power scooter like the one shown in Figure 12-4 should be considered as an initial power wheelchair prescription for the child who is hesitant to use a power wheelchair when walking is no longer possible. The scooter is often more easily accepted by the child and may be used for transition to a standard power wheelchair. If a power scooter is used initially, transition to a power wheelchair will be necessary when the adolescent is seen propping on the arm rests for trunk control. Asymmetric sitting postures must be aggressively managed owing to the correlation of increased sitting time and poor sitting posture with the onset of scoliosis. When limited resources are an issue, which is typically the case for children in managed care, a power wheelchair should be acquired without consideration of a scooter.

A manual wheelchair will be needed if nonaccessible areas for a powered wheelchair are encountered in the usual environment. Architectural barriers in the home or inability to transport a power wheelchair may also necessitate the use of a manual wheelchair.

Fit of the wheelchair must be closely monitored to provide adequate support. The reader should refer to the Evolve Chapter, Assistive Technology, for information on wheelchairs and postural support systems. Special attention should be given to alignment of the spine and pelvis and to the need for customized accessories or modifications. Accessories to be considered for the manual or power wheelchair prescription should include a solid back and seat, lateral trunk supports, lumbar support, adductor pads, seat belt, and chest strap. The footrests should be modified to support the ankle in a neutral position. Additional items that may be appropriate include a tray; head support, if needed; or coated push rims, if the child has the strength to propel the wheelchair. A reclining back will allow a position change while sitting in the wheelchair and will help deter flexion contracture formation at the hip, or a tilt-in-space reclining option can be considered to allow for pressure relief. Midline placement of the control stick on a power wheelchair may be considered to assist in symmetrical trunk alignment. If a cushion is required, it should maintain the pelvis in a level position.

Maintaining the spine in a neutral or slightly extended position is essential to slow the formation of a scoliosis. The spine should be in slight extension to increase weight bearing through the facet joints, minimize truncal rotation and lateral flexion, and slow the progression of scoliosis formation.[68] Scoliosis is seen in approximately 15% to 25% of individuals before the cessation of walking.[112,116] Poor sitting posture, in addition to muscle weakness, has been shown to accelerate scoliosis formation and progression. The prevalence of scoliosis (Cobb angle >10°) is 50% between the ages of 12 and 15 years and 90% by the age of 17 years.[112] Spinal orthoses may also retard the progression of scoliosis, although they have not been shown to prevent development of a significant scoliotic curve.[36,43] Custom-molded seating inserts, corsets, and modular seating inserts are options to provide trunk support in an attempt to slow the progression of the scoliosis. However, studies comparing the three methods of spinal control in DMD have concluded that the progression of the curvature was not significantly changed by any of the three methods.[43,156]

Early surgical intervention is recommended for the control of scoliosis through the use of segmental spinal instrumentation with Luque rods or similar techniques.[109,116,158] Miller and associates[116] have reported improved quality of life, attainment of a balanced sitting posture, and more normal alignment following surgical intervention for scoliosis. Velasco and colleagues[175] have reported reduced rates of pulmonary function decline following spinal fusion as compared to no surgical intervention. Pulmonary complications are reported as minimal if forced vital capacity is at least 30% of normal age-predicted values.[6]

Exercise and Custom Equipment

With the cessation of walking in late childhood or early adolescence, the emphasis of an exercise program should shift from the lower extremities to active-assistive and active exercises of the upper extremities. More important, however, active exercise should be encouraged by having the adolescent assist as much as possible in ADLs such as grooming, upper body dressing, and feeding through consultation with an occupational therapist. Key muscle groups for maintenance of strength for transfers include the shoulder depressors and triceps. The shoulder flexor and abductor and elbow flexor muscle groups are key areas for exercises to maintain routine ADLs such as self-feeding and hygiene. Weakness of the upper arm musculature by 16 years of age makes ADLs such as dressing, feeding, or hygiene extremely difficult.

The ROM program will require further modification as the adolescent becomes nonambulatory. Gentle stretching of the aforementioned lower extremity joints should be continued if the child describes discomfort in the joints; stretching of the shoulder and elbow should be included as indicated. Limitations in shoulder flexion and abduction, elbow extension, forearm supination, and wrist extension are most common.

The family will need to consider additional equipment or home modifications as the child reaches adolescence. A van with a lift or ramp will be needed to transport a power wheelchair. Modification of the bathroom can significantly assist the family when a wheeled commode chair is used for toileting and a bath chair and handheld shower are used for bathing. A tub lift is a second option for bathing. A urinal should be available at home and at school to decrease the frequency of transfers to the toilet. Modifications of the bed are also frequently required because the adolescent is unable to change position. An airflow mattress, egg-crate foam cushion, and hospital bed are all possibilities to be considered. A positioning program to include position changes at night is necessary for adolescents who are thin to provide comfort and ensure against skin breakdown. Customized foam wedges fabricated by the therapist may also be helpful in positioning at night.

Transition to Adulthood

The transition to adulthood marks a time of continued progression of disability with greater reliance on assistive technology for environmental access and increased need for assistance to carry out routine ADLs.[168] Mobility using a power wheelchair is necessary because upper extremity and truncal weakness typically will not allow use of a motorized scooter. Assistance with ADLs, including dressing, transfers, and bathing, is now required. Hygiene about the face and feeding become increasingly difficult but usually remain manageable. Many social issues also arise with the completion of educational programming and transition to a prevocational, vocational, or home environment on a more full-time basis. Another major issue that requires thoughtful consideration by the family, individual, and management team is the utilization of assisted ventilation with progressive respiratory involvement at the terminal stage of the disease.

All transfers require assistance during late adolescence and by adulthood typically require use of a hydraulic or other type of mechanical lift. A high-backed sling seat is

indicated because head and trunk control is minimal with the progressive weakness.

A power recline feature on the power wheelchair may be desirable, depending on accessibility and family choice, if funding is available. If not, a regular schedule for pressure relief through lateral weight shifting with assistance is needed. A properly fitted and well-tolerated cushion to avoid skin breakdown becomes an important area of intervention with loss of the ability to weight shift in the wheelchair. Skin breakdown is not a typical problem in DMD, but a cushion should be considered. A Jay Medical cushion (Jay Medical, Boulder, CO) is often well tolerated and provides a firm base of support to control pelvic obliquity, yet the gel inserts can be adjusted to allow for adequate pressure distribution. A customized insert will be needed if deformity becomes severe (e.g., severe scoliosis without surgical stabilization). If the firmer cushion is not tolerated well, then use of a Roho cushion (The Roho Group, Belleville, IL) is recommended.

A ball-bearing feeder may be considered to assist arm movement when progression of upper extremity weakness makes independent feeding difficult.[41] The device can also be used to assist with general use of the arms in conjunction with activities at a table, such as when using a computer, but does not always work well depending on the individual. Trial use of a mobile arm support is recommended. Coordination of planning with an occupational therapist to address feeding and dressing issues is needed to identify solutions to increased dependence in the areas of feeding, dressing, and hygiene.

To maintain independence in environmental access, consideration should be given to using environmental control devices. An environmental control unit included on the power wheelchair can be used to independently access lights, telephone, television, motors on doors, or a computer, to name just a few applications. Computer access for vocational applications such as word processing or avocational activities such as games is available.

Breathing exercises, postural drainage, or intermittent pressure breathing treatments should be included in the management program based on results of pulmonary evaluation.[147] Specific tests of pulmonary function that document respiratory status include forced vital capacity (FVC = amount of air expired following a maximal inspiration) and peak expiratory flow rate (highest flow rate sustained for 10 ms during maximal expiration). Continuous positive airway pressure (CPAP) is recommended when FVC is below 30% of age-adjusted norm values.[105,166] Assisted ventilation with tracheostomy is recommended when respiratory insufficiency is present with abnormal blood gas levels during the day or night.[166] In addition to breathing exercises and assisted coughing, the family and caregivers should be instructed in the technique of postural drainage. For additional details, the reader should refer to the American Thoracic Society consensus statement on the care of individuals with DMD.[6]

Close monitoring of respiratory function should become routine with increasing age because respiratory failure or pulmonary infection is the major contributing factor to death in 75% of children with DMD.[69] Longevity in DMD can be significantly prolonged by assisted ventilation.[12,51] A 1997 survey of MDA-sponsored clinics reported that 88% of clinic directors offered noninvasive ventilatory aid for acute respiratory failure.[10] Bach and Chaudhry[10] stressed the need for health care professionals to explore attitudes toward mechanical ventilation because our perceived impression of patient desires may often be incorrect. The use of daytime intermittent positive-pressure ventilation via mask or nasal cannula, nocturnal bilevel positive airway pressure (BiPAP), CPAP, negative pressure ventilators, and suctioning should be considered for the chronic hypoventilation related to weakness of respiratory musculature.[10]

A power-controlled bed to allow elevation of the head for respiratory management should be considered. Use of a bed with elevating capability also allows for greater ease in transfers, and height adjustment promotes use of proper body mechanics by family members for activities that require assistance such as dressing. Mattress selection should also be reviewed with the family because an airflow mattress may be needed when increasing dependence for bed mobility is encountered. Use of an airflow mattress may decrease the frequency of need for turning and repositioning at night. If sitting in a wheelchair is no longer tolerated in the later stages of the disease, elevation of the head of the bed becomes beneficial for reading or watching television. An easel will be required for reading.

Although it may be assumed by care providers that the quality of life and therefore satisfaction are significantly reduced for severely disabled individuals with DMD, this notion may be incorrect. In a survey of 82 ventilator-assisted individuals with DMD, Bach and colleagues[9] concluded that a vast majority of individuals had a positive effect and were satisfied with life despite the physical dependence. Furthermore, it was found in a survey of 273 physically intact health care professionals that they significantly underestimated patient life satisfaction scores, and therefore they may make patient management recommendations based on their attitudes rather than on the patient's wishes. Bach and colleagues[9] strongly recommended that we as professionals need to constantly inquire and objectively assess family and individual needs when interacting to provide therapeutic programs. With the early use of steroids and intervention with ventilator assistance, longevity has been reported to increase from 19 years 9 months to 25 years 9 months.[6]

Respiratory insufficiency is a hallmark sign of the preterminal stage of DMD.[122] Progressive muscular weakness results in decreased ventilatory volumes caused by restriction of chest wall excursion. Coordination of care with the respiratory therapist is essential when clinical findings of respiratory muscle weakness, inability to cough, or chest wall restrictions are observed. Severe oxygen desaturation leading to a comatose state is evidence of the terminal stage of the disease.

Members of the team often become involved in answering questions regarding death. The physical therapist should be aware of the stages of disease progression and especially the preterminal signs to avoid making inappropriate comments concerning prognosis. Often little needs to be said, but rather a good listening ear is needed to help the family work through the crisis that is ever pending. It is often a comfort to individuals with DMD or family members that the end may come as sleep without wakening. The person with DMD and his family members may indicate the need for additional support, but if issues are not being resolved adequately by the support that is available, consideration for involvement by a psychologist, counselor, clergy member, MDA support group, or other trained professional is indicated. Literature is available through the MDA to comfort family members, and texts are available if the family is interested.[38,145]

BECKER'S MUSCULAR DYSTROPHY

BMD, a more slowly progressive variant of DMD, has an incidence of about 1 in 20,000 births and a prevalence of 2 to 3 cases per 100,000 population.[53] The impairments and participation restrictions of BMD closely resemble those of DMD; however, the progression is significantly slower, with a longevity into the forties.[55,69] The genetic defect for BMD is located on the same gene as that for DMD, only in a different area; therefore, dystrophin is present in reduced amounts or abnormal size rather than completely absent as in DMD, which may explain the slower progression of clinical symptoms.[101]

Initial clinical symptoms typically are not identified in boys with BMD before late childhood or early adolescence. Emery and Skinner[55] found the mean age at onset of symptoms to be 11 years, inability to walk at 27 years, and death at 42 years. The authors pointed out, however, that the range of walking cessation is very wide. Perhaps one of the best functional discriminators between BMD and DMD is that 97% of adolescents with DMD are using a wheelchair for mobility by age 11 years, whereas 97% of adolescents with BMD are still walking.[55] Another discriminator is the frequent complaint of muscle cramping in individuals with BMD that is rarely reported in DMD.[50]

The impairments of BMD are the same as in DMD, although less severe, and initial clinical signs include frequent falls and clumsiness in the mid to late teens. The exception is the increased presence of cardiac involvement in BMD. Dilated cardiac myopathy is more prevalent with BMD because of the longer life span, and routine cardiac screening is recommended.[92] The pattern of weakness is the same as in DMD, and pseudohypertrophy of the calves may be present. The incidence of contracture, scoliosis, and other skeletal deformities is lower in BMD. Although not as severe as in DMD, hip, knee, and ankle plantar flexor muscle contractures can be present when walking is no longer possible. The use of night splints to maintain ankle dorsiflexion ROM is often indicated, along with a home program of heel cord stretching. Significant disability will develop by the mid-twenties in most individuals, although this is variable. As weakness progresses, the use of power mobility will be required and the use of orthoses may be considered to maintain walking. KAFOs can also be used to prolong walking; however, braced ambulation will not be functional for community access but rather as a means of exercise. The general goals and management procedures outlined in the section on DMD are the same for BMD, including the progression from walking to use of power mobility. Although the general precautions against excessive fatigue and delayed-onset muscle soreness should be followed with BMD as with DMD, because of the variable involvement of individuals with BMD, endurance training has been found to be beneficial.[170] Sveen and colleagues reported on a cohort of 11 individuals with BMD who participated in a cycling program of fifty 30-minute sessions at 65% of their maximal oxygen uptake level over 12 weeks. The group demonstrated 47% improvement in maximum oxygen uptake and an 80% increase in maximal workload with no evidence of increased serum creatine phosphokinase levels and no presence of necrotic or increased numbers of central nuclei on muscle biopsy. The exercise group also demonstrated a significant increase in select leg musculature.

Because the person with BMD lives much longer than someone with DMD, transition planning following completion of school and assistance with living arrangements into adulthood become major issues. Longevity is commonly reported into the mid 40's, with complications from dilated cardiac myopathy being the limiting factor on longevity.[47] Vocational or avocational choices should be made with the disease progression and disability level in mind. Vocational rehabilitation services should be initiated before completion of high school to allow adequate time for evaluation. Governmental support through Medicaid, Social Security benefits, or other sources may be needed to offset expenses to allow for independent living because adaptive equipment and an attendant will be needed. Ongoing medical services are available through the MDA. No data are available regarding the number of individuals who go to college or become employed following high school, but with the assistive technology available to promote independence, either option can be explored.

CONGENITAL MUSCULAR DYSTROPHY

Congenital myopathies as a diagnostic category consist of many diseases, including congenital MD. Congenital MD is a heterogeneous group of muscle disorders with onset in utero or during the first year of life that are characterized by congenital hypotonia, delayed motor development, and early onset of progressive weakness.[140] Reported forms of congenital MD are (1) congenital MD with central nervous system (CNS) disease (Fukuyama syndrome, Walker-Warburg

disease, and muscle-eye-brain disease), (2) merosin-deficient congenital MD, (3) integrin-deficient congenital MD, and (4) congenital MD with normal merosin. Fukuyama, merosin-deficient, and normal merosin forms will be discussed. Congenital MD with complete merosin deficiency is the most common form, affecting approximately 50% of the children.[70] Onset is at birth, and children never attain the ability to walk in contrast to children with partial merosin deficiency, for which onset is during the first decade and children typically are able to walk by the age of 2 to 3 years. The reader should refer to the review article by Voit[181] for additional information. Other valuable resources for information are the Online Mendelian Inheritance of Man (OMIM) website of the National Center for Biotechnology (www.ncbi.nlm.nih.gov/omim) and GeneReviews (www.genereviews.org). The mode of inheritance in congenital MD is reported as autosomal recessive.[54,119] Although all forms are rare, the range of severity and disability varies significantly among types.

In congenital MD with associated CNS disease (Fukuyama type), intellectual disabilities and seizures are common, along with moderate to severe hypotonia at birth and the presence of contractures.[64] Magnetic resonance imaging reveals nonspecific cerebral malformations and occasionally lissencephaly as pathologic features of the CNS disease. Contractures typically involve the lower extremities (hips and knees) and elbows. Other commonly reported dysmorphic features include congenital dislocation of the hips, pectus excavatum, pes cavus, kyphoscoliosis, and an unusually long face. Weakness of the extraocular muscles, optic atrophy, and nystagmus have been reported.[140] Children with this type of MD rarely attain the ability to walk.[54,70] The genetic defect is at chromosome 9q31-q33 with the missing protein "fukutin."

The early management program in children with congenital MD with nervous system disease should focus on family instruction, developmental activities to address delays in gross motor skill development, and aggressive management of contractures. Attention to positioning is necessary to guard against secondary deformity resulting from gravitational effects on the trunk with the presence of moderate to severe hypotonia. Early intervention by an occupational therapist to address feeding and oral motor control issues is commonly coordinated with physical therapy. Impaired respiratory function and pulmonary complications are hallmark features of congenital MD. The family should be instructed in chest physical therapy, such as postural drainage, and consultation with a respiratory therapist may be needed on an ongoing basis.

Because many children with congenital MD and associated nervous system disease do not attain walking, maximizing functional skills in sitting becomes a primary goal of the physical therapy management program as the child ages. Therapeutic exercise to improve head and trunk control should be aggressively addressed with use of adaptive equipment to slow the progression of spinal deformity and contractures and to maximize access to the environment. Because intellectual disabilities are common, power mobility may not be an option. Additional management issues for children with significant hypotonia are discussed later in the chapter in the section on acute SMA.

In children with merosin-absent or -partial deficient MD, changes on MRI are reported, but with infrequent reduction in IQ. Thirty percent are reported to develop epilepsy.[81] Contractures and scoliosis are common, along with early breathing difficulties that may require assisted ventilation. Children with the merosin-deficient form of MD are reported to have cardiac involvement. In congenital MD with partial merosin deficiency, a delay in walking, with acquisition of walking ranging from 13 months to 6 years, is reported.[123]

Progressive contractures may be present, and in severe cases, the child may never walk. Longevity ranges from 15 to 30 years. Pegorago and associates[134] reported on a cohort of 22 children with merosin-deficient congenital MD. All children demonstrated severe floppiness at birth, normal intelligence, and delay in achievement of motor milestones. Merosin-deficient congenital MD is due to a defect at chromosome 6q22.

Muscle weakness and contractures are the primary impairment in merosin-deficient congenital MD, with scoliosis common in merosin-absent MD. Feeding delays are common with lesser involvement of the bulbar muscular than is generally observed with hypotonia of the trunk and axial musculature, requiring a feeding program that should be coordinated with occupational therapy. Contractures must be managed aggressively with a home ROM program that includes manual stretching, positioning, and splinting. Although children with merosin-deficient MD typically develop walking, ankle plantar flexion contractures that cannot be managed conservatively may require orthopedic intervention.

Activity limitations, such as delayed acquisition of gross motor skills, should be managed with an understanding of the natural progression of the diagnosis because a slower rate of skill progression is expected. Because these children vary in their rate of motor skill development, information can be provided to the family concerning probable rates of motor skill acquisition, but unrealistic therapeutic expectations should be avoided. Because children with congenital MD have a wide range of functional deficits, care must be taken in predicting functional gross motor outcomes or level of participation at home and school.

CHILDHOOD-ONSET FACIOSCAPULOHUMERAL MUSCULAR DYSTROPHY

Facioscapulohumeral MD is rare, with an incidence of 3 to 10 cases per million births, and typically demonstrates onset in adulthood, although an infantile form has been reported (FSHMD1A).[126,167] The disorder is inherited as autosomal dominant or recessive, with the genetic defect on chromosome 4q35. The disorder affects males and females equally.

Childhood-onset facioscapulohumeral MD typically results in the onset of clinical signs within the first 2 years but without significant impairment or disability until later in the first decade. Contractures are seldom a problem for mobility.

Infancy and Preschool-Age Period

The impairment of muscle weakness about the face and shoulder girdle is typically the only prominent feature of the disease during the infant and preschool-age period. Parents report that the child may sleep with the eyes partially open, and on physical examination weakness of the facial musculature is predominant. Children frequently are unable to whistle, and drinking with a straw may be difficult. When asked to purse the lips together and puff the cheeks out, the child is unable to maintain the cheeks out when even the slightest pressure is applied. The child's smile is also masked because of the weakness, thereby hindering communication as a result of inconsistency between what is spoken and the affect displayed.

Children with childhood-onset facioscapulohumeral MD typically develop independence in walking without significant delay. An excessive lordotic posture during walking is a classic clinical feature with progression of weakness. The scapulae are widely abducted and outwardly rotated, giving evidence of the degree of interscapular muscle weakness.

School-Age Period

Progressive disability occurs during the school-age period, with weakness becoming more generalized throughout the trunk, shoulder, and pelvic girdle musculature. Progression of childhood-onset facioscapulohumeral MD is more insidious than in the adult form, and independent walking may be lost by the end of the first decade.[67]

Severe winging of the scapula, a hallmark feature of the adult form of the disease, becomes more prominent with age in activities such as reaching overhead. Management should focus on instruction to the child and family on activities to avoid that may cause fatigue and on guarding against heavily resisted upper extremity activity. Studies of adults with facioscapulohumeral MD comparing dominant with nondominant arm strength have shown that overuse and perhaps just consistent use of the dominant arm play a significant role in progression of muscle weakness.[32,88]

As weakness of the hip and knee extensors progresses, the use of KAFOs should be considered for assisted walking and transfers. When walking becomes increasingly difficult, power mobility using a scooter or power wheelchair should be considered, because the degree of upper extremity weakness will not allow independence in propulsion of a manual wheelchair.

Transition to Adulthood

No specific prognostic information on the longevity of individuals with childhood-onset facioscapulohumeral MD is available; therefore transition planning from the educational environment should be a goal of the therapy program. If severe weakness is present and significant assistance from the family is needed, individuals may not desire to plan for living outside the family home. If independent living is desired, coordination of planning with an attendant will be necessary and accessibility issues will need to be evaluated. Assistance through vocational rehabilitation services should be coordinated with transition planning if vocational goals are identified.

CONGENITAL MYOTONIC MUSCULAR DYSTROPHY

Myotonic MD is the most common adult-onset neuromuscular disease, with an incidence of 1 in 8000 births.[78] Congenital myotonic MD is rare and demonstrates severe clinical features of the adult-onset diagnosis (see OMIM, myotonic MD type 1). Inheritance is reported as autosomal dominant with a genetic defect of chromosome 19q13.3 affecting males and females equally. More recently, a second form of myotonic MD (proximal myotonic myopathy, or PROMM) has been reported and linked to chromosome 3q21.[143]

Children with congenital myotonic MD are almost exclusively born to mothers with myotonic MD who have the chromosome 19 defect. Approximately 25% of children born to mothers with myotonic MD will have congenital myotonic MD.[24,78] Most children demonstrate severe hypotonia and weakness at birth; however, a few children first have only signs of intellectual disability by age 5 years and no significant motor impairment as infants. Because the children who initially have only intellectual impairment follow a progression of motor impairment similar to that of adult-onset myotonic MD, the infancy-onset form is discussed in this section of the chapter.

Intellectual disability in congenital myotonic MD is common, affecting 50% to 60% of the children. An average IQ of 65 is typically reported for children with cognitive impairment.[148,163] No evidence of progressive deterioration of cognitive function has been found. A study by Rutherford and co-workers[149] of 14 children provided prognostic information regarding survival and its relationship to mechanical ventilation at birth. No infant in the study who required mechanical ventilation survived for longer than 4 weeks.

Infancy

If the child survives the early weeks of life, the prognosis is one of steady improvement in motor function over the first decade, with most children developing independent walking.[79,87,148] A follow-up study by O'Brien and Harper[125] of 46 children reported only four children who died outside the neonatal period at ages 4, 18, 19, and 22 years. Four additional children demonstrated significant disability associated with a poor prognosis, and none was older than age 30 years. In a study of 115 children with congenital MD, Reardon and colleagues[139] reported that 25% of the children

lived to age 18 months, and of those who survived infancy, 50% lived into their mid 30s.

Severe weakness and partial paralysis of the diaphragm at birth are clinical features that often suggest the diagnosis of congenital myotonic MD. Myotonia (delay in relaxation after muscular contraction), a hallmark feature of adult myotonic MD, typically is not evident at birth in the congenital form but rather develops by 3 to 5 years of age. Myotonia in congenital myotonic MD typically is not considered to be a significant impairment or a cause of functional limitations in comparison with the degree of weakness that is present. The symptoms of myotonia, however, are increased with fatigue, cold, or stress. Typical facial features include a short median part of the upper lip, which gives the mouth an inverted-V shape. Facial movements are limited, with muscles innervated by the cranial nerves involved in the severe weakness pattern. Severe respiratory impairment is prominent in the newborn period, requiring resuscitation and assisted ventilation in most cases. Talipes equinovarus contractures are reported in more than 50% of children, and a general pattern of arthrogryposis occurs in less than 5%.[78]

Progressive improvement in gross motor skills can be expected if the child survives the newborn period. The presence and degree of intellectual impairment become a major factor in the progression of milestone acquisition. The development of hip abduction and external rotation contractures should be closely monitored if leg movement and habitual positioning favor the development of this secondary impairment.

Harper,[78] in a cohort of 70 children with congenital myotonic dystrophy, reported that hypotonia is rarely prominent beyond age 3 to 4 years. Children typically develop walking, but further motor impairment follows the clinical progression of adult-onset disease, although definitive data to document disease progression into adulthood are not available.

Consultation with a respiratory therapist on pulmonary care will be needed until the infant is weaned from assisted ventilation. Feeding may require the use of a nasogastric tube during the newborn period or early infancy, and initiation of a feeding program should be coordinated with an occupational therapist. A swallowing study may be indicated when the feeding program is initiated to evaluate potential for aspiration. If the newborn survives early respiratory difficulties, progressive improvement in pulmonary function is usually seen without the need for ongoing intervention.

Talipes equinovarus contractures should be aggressively managed in infancy with casting, taping, and exercise but may ultimately require orthopedic intervention because they have been shown to significantly delay walking.[139] Ankle-foot orthoses or night splints may be indicated on the basis of individual needs. In addition to home instruction for ROM activities to manage contractures, the family should be provided with a general program of activities to promote gross motor skill development. Because the natural progression of the disease consists of improved motor function,

TABLE 12-2   **Classification of Spinal Muscle Atrophy**

Type	Onset	Inheritance	Course
Childhood-onset, type I, Werdnig-Hoffmann (acute)	0–3 mo	Recessive	Rapidly progressive; severe hypotonia; death within first year
Childhood-onset, type II, Werdnig-Hoffmann (chronic)	3 mo–4 yr	Recessive	Rapid progression that stabilizes; moderate to severe hypotonia; shortened life span
Juvenile-onset, type III, Kugelberg-Welander	5–10 yr	Recessive	Slowly progressive; mild impairment

consultation rather than a direct service program is indicated, unless surgical intervention for contracture management is required.

School-Age Period

Consultation for development of adaptive physical education activities will be needed during the school-age period. Other physical therapy–related activities will depend on the use of orthoses and the progression of gross motor skill development. Specific therapeutic exercise programs for strengthening have not been reported but may be indicated, in addition to ROM activities.

Transition to Adulthood

The natural progression of myotonic MD is insidious weakness of the distal upper and lower extremity musculature and progressive increase in myotonia, leading to increasing disability. Children with congenital myotonic MD will demonstrate progression in the disease as described for adults, but typically at an earlier stage—usually by the middle of the second decade. The reader should refer to references on adult myotonic MD for further information on clinical course and management.[78]

EMERY-DREIFUSS MUSCULAR DYSTROPHY

Emery-Dreifuss MD1 (EDMD1) is inherited as an X-linked recessive disorder at gene locus Xq28 resulting in the absence of the protein emerin. Emery-Dreifuss MD2 (EDMD2) can also be inherited, but as an autosomal dominant or recessive disorder with a defect on chromosome 1q21.2 and a defect of the protein lamin (OMIM).

The clinical features of EDMD1 vary widely and include contracture of the posterior neck, elbow, and ankle joints. A humeroperoneal pattern of muscle weakness is observed with usual onset in the teen years, but ranging from neonatal to the third decade. Later progression of weakness to the legs with a peroneal weakness pattern is reported. Contracture is typically seen before the onset of weakness. The onset of EDMD2 is most common in the first or second decade, and a similar pattern of contracture to EDMD1 is seen. The humeroperoneal weakness is more prominent, especially affecting the elbow flexors. Cardiac abnormalities are more common in EDMD1, with sudden death (in persons ranging in age from 25 to 56 years) reported by Pinelli and colleagues[137] in a large family cohort with bradyarrhythmias.

Physical therapy management is limited during the childhood period because disability is not common. Independent walking is typically maintained into adulthood without significant disability. A ROM program for contracture prevention is advised, but orthopedic intervention is common to correct the Achilles tendon contractures.[159] Holter monitoring is advised when cardiac abnormalities are identified, and pacemakers are used to control rhythm.

SPINAL MUSCULAR ATROPHY

Classification of SMA into four groups is based on clinical presentation and progression (Table 12-2). Types I and II are commonly referred to as acute and chronic Werdnig-Hoffmann disease, respectively, type III as Kugelberg-Welander disease, and type IV as adult-onset SMA.

Standards of care have been developed but primarily deal with issues related to medical diagnostic procedures and respiratory care.[182] Functional status information on children with SMA is becoming prevalent.[40]

DIAGNOSIS AND PATHOPHYSIOLOGY

SMA represents the second most common group of fatal recessive diseases after cystic fibrosis.[157] The pathologic feature of SMA is abnormality of the large anterior horn cells in the spinal cord. The number of cells is reduced, and progressive degeneration of the remaining cells is correlated with loss in function.

The diagnosis of SMA is confirmed by clinical examination and laboratory procedures, including electromyography, muscle biopsy, and genetic testing.[106] Electromyographic findings include fibrillation and fasciculation potentials. Nerve conduction velocities are normal. Muscle biopsy demonstrates changes that are typical of a disease involving denervation (i.e., large groups of atrophic fibers are dispersed among groups of normal or hypertrophic fibers). The absence of fibrosis around the atrophic groups on muscle biopsy helps delineate SMA from DMD.

SMA is typically inherited as autosomal recessive with the genetic defect on chromosome 5q11.2-13.[157] The gene for SMA, termed *survival motor neuron* (SMN), was discovered on chromosome 5q13 in 1994 by MacKenzie and colleagues[106] and is responsible for the production of a protein bearing the same name. The SMN protein is involved in maintenance of the anterior horn cell and when missing results in a lack of survival of the cell, leading to apoptosis (programmed cell death). In addition to the SMN gene, another defect of the gene in a near locus results in the lack of formation of neuronal apoptosis inhibitory protein (NAIP), which has been shown to play a role in SMA. Variation in the amount of NAIP protein may explain the premature cell death seen in SMA, in association with the SMN gene defect.[146]

The incidence of Werdnig-Hoffmann disease is 1 in 10,000 live births,[157] and the incidence of Kugelberg-Welander disease is reported as 6 cases per 100,000 live births.[188] Reported incidence of the other forms is variable because of the inconsistency of applying classification criteria.

One criterion for classification of SMA is the level of functional ability.[49] Although this classification rubric is being questioned because SMA is now viewed more as a continuum of involvement without clear subtypes, this rubric will be used because it helps to clarify management goals. The more typical classification criteria are multifactorial and involve age at onset of the first clinical signs, pattern of muscle involvement, age at death, and genetic evidence.[138]

SMA is a heterogeneous disorder containing several different clinical presentations and rates of progression. Progressive SMA of early childhood (type I) was first reported by Werdnig and Hoffmann in the late 1800s.[84,185] A more slowly progressive form of SMA (type III) with onset usually between the ages of 2 and 9 years was reported by Kugelberg and Welander[97] and also by Wohlfart and colleagues.[189] Werdnig-Hoffmann disease and Kugelberg-Welander disease have therefore become the eponyms for early-onset and juvenile-onset SMA, with many authors preferring to use the numeric classification system as outlined in Table 12-2.

Pearn,[131] in a large multicenter study in England, reported SMA types II and III to be the most frequent, accounting for approximately 47% of the population. The next most prevalent forms were SMA type I at about 27% and adult-onset type IV at 8%; the other 18% had mixed classifications, including distal involvement, neurogenic SMA, SMA of adolescence with hypertrophied calf muscles, and childhood-onset SMA with cerebellar and optic atrophy.

No cure or treatment is available for SMA, but physical therapy is commonly advocated.[110,183] Poor prognosticators for long-term survival include early age at onset (before 4 months of age), which is often noted as weak fetal movement; fasciculations of the tongue in infancy; and severe, generalized weakness, particularly of the trunk and proximal musculature. More recent evidence has shown that children with severe onset of symptoms may survive up to their fifth birthday.[28]

ACUTE CHILDHOOD SPINAL MUSCULAR ATROPHY (TYPE I)

Impairments, Activity Limitations, and Participation Restrictions

The primary impairment in all forms of SMA is muscle weakness secondary to progressive loss of anterior horn cells in the spinal cord. Weakness is particularly pronounced in the acute and chronic childhood forms (types I and II) within the first 4 months. The cranial nerves are inconsistently involved in childhood-onset SMA, with rare involvement with juvenile onset. Contractures may be a primary impairment in acute-onset SMA, with reports of talipes equinovarus or other intrauterine deformities secondary to limited fetal movement. Muscle fasciculations, including fasciculations of the tongue, are most commonly reported in children with acute-onset SMA.[110] Unlike the faces of children with myotonic or facioscapulohumeral MD, children with acute childhood SMA appear alert and responsive. Respiratory distress is present early, and significant effort to augment breathing through use of the abdominal musculature is typical.

Secondary impairments in acute-onset SMA include the development of scoliosis and often contractures. It is widely reported in the literature that all children with SMA develop scoliosis, usually requiring surgical intervention.[73,102] Other secondary impairments include decreased respiratory capacity and easy fatigability. Because only the passage of time will allow differentiation of children with acute versus chronic childhood SMA, treatment should begin early with a focus on feeding, ROM, positioning, respiratory care, and selected developmental activities.

Infancy

In acute childhood SMA, weak or absent fetal movement during the last months of pregnancy is commonly reported by the mother. Significant weakness is present at birth or develops within the first 4 months; this manifests as inability to perform anti-gravity movements with the pelvic or shoulder girdle musculature and typical posturing in a gravity-dependent position (Figure 12-7).

The proximal musculature of the neck, trunk, and pelvic and shoulder girdles demonstrates the greatest weakness. Limited anti-gravity movement of distal upper and lower extremity musculature is present, and a positioning program is necessary in the newborn period or at the onset of symptoms. Use of wedges should be considered to avoid supine positioning in the presence of respiratory distress. If the supine position is used, rolled towels or bolsters are needed to keep the upper extremities positioned in midline and to prevent lower extremity abduction and external rotation. The sidelying position allows midline head and hand use for play without having to work against gravity. Prone positioning on wedges should be limited or not used, owing to the effort required for head righting to interact with the environment.

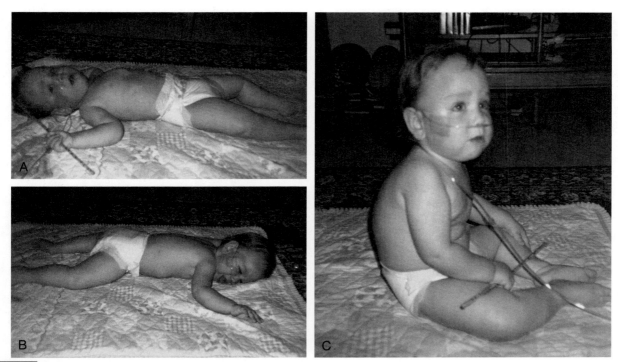

Figure 12-7 Typical postures seen in a young child with spinal muscular atrophy in supine **(A)**, prone **(B)**, and sitting **(C)** positions. Note the limited anti-gravity control and dependent posturing.

Respiratory care is a central focus of the therapy program in acute childhood SMA. Children frequently require intubation for respiratory distress and possible use of a tracheostomy, although use of noninvasive ventilatory support is being advocated so that children can develop language skills.[13,14] The use of ventilatory support with either tracheostomy or noninvasive mechanical ventilation has been shown to prolong survival in children with SMA type I.[13] Coordination with nurses and respiratory therapists on a program that includes suctioning, assisted coughing, and postural drainage is necessary. The use of supported sitting should be closely monitored for spinal alignment and respiratory response. An elastic binder around the abdomen in sitting may be useful for children who demonstrate a marked reduction in oxygen saturation when seated.

ROM exercises with proper positioning should be carried out to ensure maintenance of flexibility and comfort. Flexion contractures of the hips, knees, and elbows, hip abductors, ankle plantar flexors, and positional torticollis are deformities that can be avoided with a comprehensive ROM and positioning program.[23] The exercise program should also include limited activities for strengthening, such as lightweight toys or rattles with Velcro straps around the wrists or mobiles positioned close to the hands for easy access. The use of hammocks has also been advocated to provide the child with the opportunity for movement with only slight movements of the body.[56,57] Developmental activities such as the use of supported sitting for the development of head control should be of short duration to avoid fatigue.

Head control fails to develop or is significantly impaired in acute childhood SMA. The child is unable to lift the head from a prone position to clear the airway. Early developmental postures such as prone on elbows are not attained. The use of developmental exercise in acute childhood SMA is controversial but should be considered if the child tolerates the activities, because a few children with chronic childhood SMA exhibit clinical signs of weakness in the first year of life and as a result may be misdiagnosed as having acute SMA.

In conjunction with an occupational therapist, a feeding program that is safe and not excessively exhausting should be implemented. Small, frequent feedings may be necessary, and breast feeding may be difficult.[57] Special care with feeding is necessary to avoid aspiration and secondary respiratory problems.

Although death secondary to pneumonia or other respiratory complications is typical within a few months to a few years in acute childhood SMA, the child's death is usually not a struggle, owing to the degree of weakness and apnea.[57] The mean age of death is reported to be 6 months, with a range from 1 to 21 months reported by Merlini and associates.[114] However, with the use of ventilatory assistance, Bach and colleagues[8] have reported survival up to 42 months. Counseling and support for the parents and family is an extremely important component in the management of this condition.

CHRONIC CHILDHOOD SPINAL MUSCULAR ATROPHY (TYPE II)

Impairments, Activity Limitations, and Participation Restrictions

The onset of significant weakness in chronic childhood SMA usually appears within the first year, with the course of the disease widely variable. Pearn and colleagues[130] reported that of a cohort of 141 children, 95% demonstrated clinical signs before the age of 3 years. Forty-six percent never walked (even with orthotics), 38% were able to walk unaided at some stage, and the median age at death exceeded 10 years. More recently, muscle strength data on children and adults with SMA type II obtained by using handheld dynamometry,[60] manual muscle testing,[186] and qualitative muscle testing with a tensiometer[142] have been reported. Functional skills with a 2-minute walk test[142] and forced vital capacity[186] data are also available. Progressive loss of strength and pulmonary function is consistently reported. The Hammersmith Functional Motor Scale for Children with SMA has also been developed as a specific functional skills rating tool for children with SMA types II and III who have limited ambulation skills.[107]

Eng[57] has reported three separate subgroupings within type II based on the pattern of presentation and progression. In the most severely involved group, the children never developed the ability to sit alone, and respiratory capacity was significantly reduced. In the intermediate group, the children sat alone but never developed the ability to walk and demonstrated a regression of forced vital capacity to 45% by age 10 years. In the final group, independent walking was attained but half of the children lost this ability toward the end of the first decade. It is interesting to note that in the group of patients who remained ambulatory in the study by Eng,[57] forced vital capacity was maintained at 90% as compared with 65% for those who lost independent walking during the first decade. The results of the study led Eng to conclude that forced vital capacity may be a physiologic predictor of walking duration.

Contractures are infrequently an impairment in chronic SMA. The distribution of weakness is similar to acute childhood SMA with primary proximal involvement, but to a much less severe degree. Weakness is usually greatest in the hip and knee extensors and trunk musculature. Involvement of the distal musculature appears later in the course of the disease and is less severe than the proximal involvement. Involvement of the cranial nerves has been reported but is not considered to be a typical feature of SMA other than in the acute childhood form. Fasciculations of the tongue have been reported in approximately one half of the children.

Infancy

The clinical presentation and progression of chronic childhood SMA are highly variable, so the management program must address the major impairments, activity limitations,

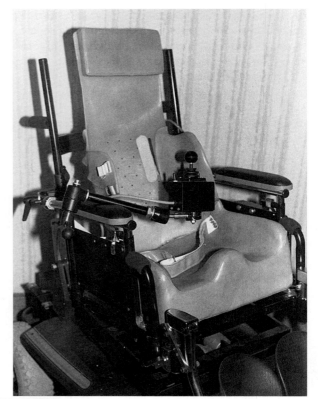

Figure 12-8 Custom-molded sitting-support orthosis to provide trunk support in sitting.

and participation restrictions as they are manifested. Approximately 15% of children have impairments within the first 3 months, and the remaining children have impairments by 18 months of age.[114,142] The program for the newborn with chronic SMA should be similar to that for children with acute SMA. Some children may develop the ability to stand, but few are able to use walking as a primary means of mobility.

Sitting posture is an area of primary concern in the management program for children who demonstrate significant weakness, requiring external head and trunk support in antigravity positions. A molded sitting support orthosis as shown in Figure 12-8 provides optimal contouring of the torso for support in sitting, or a thoracolumbosacral orthosis (TLSO, or "body jacket") can be used. Developmental activities provided on an ongoing basis are indicated to develop gross motor skills. Therapy sessions should be kept short to avoid fatigue and should emphasize selected developmental areas during each session because tolerance to handling in multiple positions is usually limited. Swimming has been reported to be beneficial in maintaining muscle strength and functional skills.[46] Instruction to the family in the use of adaptive equipment for proper positioning is crucial in slowing the deforming effects of gravity on the spine when the child is sitting or standing.

If the child is not standing by the age of 16 to 18 months, adaptive equipment for standing should be considered. The rate of fracture in SMA has been reported to range from 12% to 15%, and weight bearing has been shown to decrease the frequency of lower extremity fractures.[18] A supine stander is recommended for children without adequate head control. Orthopedic consultation for a corset or TLSO should be considered for use in standing to maintain trunk alignment if the adaptive equipment does not provide adequate control.

Preschool-Age and School-Age Period

In the toddler, orthotics for standing might be considered (lightweight KAFOs); however, the progression of weakness may make walking an unrealistic goal. In a report of promotion of walking in 12 children with intermediate SMA (ages 13 months to 3 years), Granata and associates[71] described success in attaining assisted ambulation, with 58% of the children using orthoses. Although only a small number of children were studied, these investigators also reported less severe scoliotic curves in the children who used the orthoses in comparison with a control group of children with SMA.

If a walking program is initiated, training in the parallel bars followed by use of a walker or other device to allow greater independence is desired. Close monitoring of safety with supported walking is necessary owing to the degree of weakness present and the potential for serious injury from a fall. The incidence of hip dislocation and contractures has also been reported as less when a supported walking program is used.[72]

Independence with mobility other than walking is a primary goal for the child who will not develop independence in walking, or when walking is no longer possible.[90] Because most power scooters do not provide adequate trunk control, use of a power wheelchair is indicated. If an orthopedic appliance is not used to support the trunk, close attention to fit is needed with use of lateral trunk supports and a trunk harness. Consideration should also be given to changing the side of the joystick every 6 months to avoid a pattern of leaning to one side. Prognosis for children with chronic childhood SMA is dependent on frequency and severity of pulmonary complications. Severe contractures as a result of prolonged sitting and progression of scoliosis are common, necessitating implementation of a consistent ROM program. Surgical intervention for spinal stabilization is an option if pulmonary function testing indicates a good prognosis for survival of the surgical intervention.

Transition to Adulthood

Survival into adulthood is extremely variable in chronic childhood SMA and depends on the progression of muscle weakness and secondary deformities. Because of the significant degree of muscle weakness, assistance is typically required for transfers and many ADLs. An attendant or family member is needed to provide assistance for general ADLs. Intelligence is rarely affected; therefore vocational goals in areas of interest should be explored through vocational rehabilitation services.

An aggressive program of pulmonary care is required, including breathing exercises and postural drainage. Forced vital capacity has been shown to decrease by about 1.1% per year, but mechanical ventilation is seldom needed.[166] The ROM program should also be continued to control progression of the contractures unless a pattern of stability is recorded.

JUVENILE-ONSET SPINAL MUSCULAR ATROPHY (TYPE III)

Juvenile-onset SMA may demonstrate symptoms of weakness within the first year of life in the proximal hip and shoulder girdle musculature, but more typically the onset is later in the first decade. Rarely are bulbar signs seen with the disease. Calf pseudohypertrophy is reported in approximately 10% of cases. Fasciculations are noted in about half of the patients, and minimyoclonus may be a primary impairment noted on examination, but it rarely interferes with function.[48]

Impairments, Activity Limitations, and Participation Restrictions

In a study by Dorscher and colleagues[48] reviewing the status of 31 patients with Kugelberg-Welander disease, proximal lower extremity weakness was the most common impairment reported. Secondary impairments included postural compensations resulting from muscle weakness, contractures, and, occasionally, scoliosis. An increased lumbar lordosis and compensated Trendelenburg gait pattern are common postural compensations for proximal muscle weakness of the lower extremities. Ankle plantar flexion contractures are occasionally reported but not with the frequency seen in DMD, which aids in differentiation of the two diseases. Scoliosis was reported in about 20% of patients by Dorscher and colleagues[48] but was reported in all patients by other researchers.[72] In adolescents with type III SMA, the incidence of scoliosis and its severity are related to the degree of weakness and functional status. Individuals who maintain independent walking have a lower incidence of scoliosis and less severe curves if scoliosis develops.

School-Age Period

A similar clinical presentation to DMD is seen in juvenile-onset SMA. The initial disability usually becomes apparent within the first decade and includes difficulty in arising from the floor, climbing stairs, and keeping up with peers during play. A waddling gait, which becomes more pronounced with attempts at running, will also be observed. Unlike DMD, no significant disability of upper extremity function is usually noted and proximal upper extremity strength is well preserved. Walking can usually be maintained lifelong as the primary means of ambulation. In those cases when weakness is noted before 2 years of age, however, a wheelchair or scooter may ultimately be required for mobility over long distances.

Management for the adolescent with juvenile-onset SMA is consistent with the concepts previously presented in this chapter. ROM exercises should be prescribed as appropriate, and selected strengthening exercises may be indicated to maintain functional skills. Adaptive equipment for mobility is not usually indicated, but a power scooter for long-distance mobility may be needed in certain cases. If performance of ADLs becomes a problem, collaboration with an occupational therapist to address concerns may be needed.

Transition to Adulthood

Difficulty in ADLs that require lifting of moderately heavy objects overhead can be expected, and vocational activities that involve manual labor are not recommended. Because the life span is not significantly shortened, vocational planning is needed. No significant disability requiring adaptive equipment or environmental access is usually required until later in adulthood.

SUMMARY

Muscle weakness and contracture are hallmark features of the childhood forms of muscular dystrophy and spinal muscle atrophy. Background knowledge of therapeutic exercise, functional use of orthoses and adaptive equipment, and strategies to minimize disabilities secondary to these impairments allow the physical therapist to bring unique information and skills to the management team.

Many of the disorders significantly reduce longevity. Therefore, the patient's quality of life and attention to how the family copes with the stress should be included in the team's intervention program. Providing the children and families with support and realistic expectations is an ongoing challenge. Support groups or contact with another family that has had a similar experience can often help the family work through crisis periods, particularly when extended family support is not available.

Through the combined perspectives and innovative solutions of team members, a comprehensive program can be provided that takes into consideration the multifaceted demands of each individual and family. A philosophy of using a family-centered approach to care will help ensure that needs are met to the best of the team's ability.

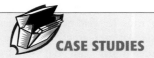 **CASE STUDIES**

Each of the two cases that are presented began before development of the *Guide to Physical Therapist Practice.*[2] However, the reports are presented with reference to the Guide to assist the practitioner in application of the Guide to clinical practice.

"Donald"

Donald is from a family with six siblings (three brothers and three sisters). Three of the four boys were diagnosed with DMD. No family history of neuromuscular disease had been reported previously, and diagnosis followed medical examination of Donald's older brother at age 5 years for clumsiness and frequent falls. Donald was 3 years of age at the time of diagnosis.

At the time of diagnosis, Donald's management program would be included in Musculoskeletal Practice Pattern C: Impaired Muscle Performance, in the *Guide to Physical Therapist Practice.*[2] He exhibited no significant gait deviations but had mild shoulder girdle and trunk flexor muscle weakness, evidence of Gowers' sign after the third attempt to rise to standing from the floor, and pseudohypertrophy of the posterior calf musculature.

A physical therapy examination at age 8 years revealed a gait pattern typical for DMD as previously described. No significant participation restrictions were noted, and impairments were only minimal. Donald was independent on stairs using a handrail but demonstrated a two-foot-per-step progression. Functional status corresponded to grade 2 on the scale published by Vignos and associates (see Box 12-1).[178] ROM was within normal limits, with the exception of mild limitation of ankle dorsiflexion with the knee in extension. Muscle strength was quantified with manual muscle testing and recorded as fair plus in the shoulder and hip girdle musculature, poor in the abdominals, and good minus in the intermediate and distal upper and lower extremities. A home program was provided that included daily ROM of the posterior calf musculature and instruction on general activities to avoid excessive fatigue. Services were coordinated by the local MDA clinic with a follow-up visit every 6 months.

Donald's initial disability was related to independent mobility with progressive loss of walking, which by age 12 involved inability to climb stairs and increased frequency of falls with attempts to walk on uneven surfaces. Furniture and walls were commonly used for balance. He was independent in scooting on the floor and used crawling for additional mobility at home. Although he was not able to stand from the middle of the floor, he was able to pull up to standing at a supportive surface. Night splints were initiated to augment the ROM program for the ankle plantar flexion contractures, and a manual wheelchair was provided for assistance with long-distance mobility.

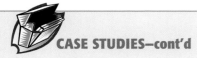

CASE STUDIES—cont'd

EVIDENCE TO PRACTICE 12-1

CASE STUDY "DONALD"
EXAMINATION DECISION

Progressive contracture of the posterior calf musculature is well documented as an impairment in Duchenne's MD and should be routinely screened (Brooke et al., 1983). Seeger and colleagues have documented a 0.4° per month progression rate in longitudinal data from boys with Duchenne's MD (Seeger et al., 1985). Limitations in posterior calf flexibility result in the inability of the individual to stand with a plantigrade foot, which then reduces the base of support and, along with progression of muscle weakness, leads to increased risk of falls and injury.

Muscle strength demonstrated progressive decline, with manual muscle testing measuring poor grades for the proximal hip and shoulder girdle musculature, fair plus grades for knee extension, and a Vignos scale rating of 5. Mild tightness of the iliotibial band was present, and limitation of full hip and knee extension was noted. The ROM program was expanded to include the additional areas of tightness. With the progression of impairments beyond muscle function,

PLAN OF CARE DECISION

The decision to use night splints to delay onset of posterior calf contractures is supported by research demonstrating a slower progression of contracture with use of the intervention (Scott, 1981; Seeger et al., 1985; Hyde, 2000). Scott demonstrated slowing in progression of posterior calf contracture when a combination of posterior calf stretching and night splints was used in the home program. Boys who used only the night splints consistently demonstrated greater posterior calf flexibility. Hyde (2000) demonstrated a 23% improvement in posterior calf flexibility in boys who used the night splints over use of a home program of stretching alone.

a shift in Musculoskeletal Practice Pattern C to D: Impaired Joint Mobility, Muscle Function, Muscle Performance, and Range of Motion Associated With Capsular Restriction would be indicated.

By age 15, Donald was walking only short distances, and primarily for mobility within the home. A three-wheeled motorized scooter was provided for distance mobility, and Donald was independent in all transfers from the scooter.

EVIDENCE TO PRACTICE 12-2

CASE STUDY "DONALD"
EXAMINATION DECISION

Progressive loss of strength and development of contracture lead to the inability to maintain walking in Duchenne's MD, typically by the age of 12 years (Brooke et al., 1983; Vignos, 1983; McDonald et al., 1995). The progression of upper extremity weakness along with proximal hip girdle weakness makes use of a manual wheelchair for mobility impractical, so that power mobility needs to be considered (Emery, 1993; Stuberg, 2001).

PLAN OF CARE DECISION

Limitation of endurance for distance walking, frequent falls, or limitation of general mobility due to fear of walking signals

the need for assistance with mobility. A motorized scooter should be initially considered, as a scooter is transportable by the family without use of a van and lift (Bach & Chaudhry, 2000; Stuberg, 2001). This choice, however, should include input from the school transportation system because some schools may have a policy in place that will not allow for transporting of a scooter and the child, as scooter frames are not crash tested and therefore are not safe for a student to be transported in the device. The child needs to transfer to the bus seat, where proper restraints can be used on both the scooter and the child for safety in transportation to and from school. Further progression of upper extremity weakness and inability of the scooter seat to provide adequate trunk control later require a change in power mobility to use of a power wheelchair (Stuberg, 2001).

A raised toilet seat and a tub bench were provided for the bathroom. He received adapted physical education and consultative physical therapy as a related service in the educational setting. He was followed through the MDA clinic, and Donald's home program was augmented by a school program, including standing using a prone stander, ROM exercises three times per week, and adaptive physical education activities for general mobility and upper and lower extremity strengthening.

Progressive weakness and flexion contractures at the hip and knee resulted in the loss of walking when Donald was 17. It should be noted that this is exceptionally late for the loss of walking because 10 to 11 years is more typically reported.[30] Because Donald's older brother had died following complications from a fracture resulting from a fall while wearing KAFOs, Donald and the family decided against continuation of a walking program using orthoses. A daily standing program at school was maintained until progression of the contractures

Continued

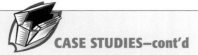

CASE STUDIES—cont'd

resulted in a need to discontinue the program because orthopedic intervention was not desired by the family.

At age 26, Donald was at stage 8 on the Vignos Functional Rating Scale (see Box 12-1). He was living in an apartment with a full-time home health aide. The scoliosis that was documented 6 years earlier had not progressed, nor was any intervention required. Donald used a power wheelchair with joystick control as shown in Figure 12-9 owing to progression of upper extremity weakness and a need to provide greater trunk support in sitting. Assistance was required for all transfers, for bathing, and for dressing. A tub bench was used. Donald was independent with eating and personal hygiene such as brushing his teeth. He required assistance for bed mobility. The sliding board transfer demonstrated in Figure 12-10 became too difficult at age 23, requiring use of a manual lift or Hoyer for all transfers.

Donald assisted as an aide for an art teacher at a school for children with multiple disabilities (Figure 12-11) until age 23, when his upper extremity weakness progressed to the point where he decided to stop working. He peacefully passed away at the age of 28 while sleeping at home following hospitalization for a bout of pneumonia.

"Derek"

Derek is 9 years, 3 months of age, with diagnosis of a dystrophinopathy and probable Duchenne's muscular dystrophy. History includes an unremarkable pregnancy and term birth. Derek weighed 8 lb 13 oz at birth and went home within 3 days. He has an older sister.

Derek's parents first began to have questions regarding his development at 17 months of age because of his delay in walking. His parents also reported what they perceived as clumsiness in his attempts to walk. Derek's pediatrician did not share the parents' concern regarding his delay or clumsiness in walking.

Following repeated expressions of concern by the family, Derek's pediatrician referred him for physical therapy services at age 5 because he was not able to keep up with peers, especially in activities that required running, jumping, or balance. He was seen by a physical therapist in a hospital setting for coordination and strengthening exercises. After almost 6 months of intervention, the physical therapist recommended further diagnostic testing as manual muscle test scores demonstrated a decline in strength despite the strengthening exer-

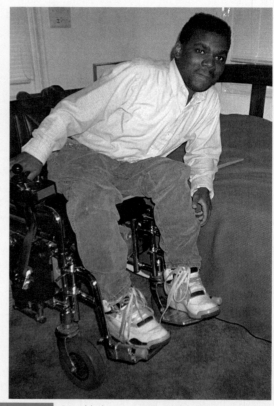

Figure 12-10 Donald demonstrating sliding board transfer technique used for chair-to-bed transfers.

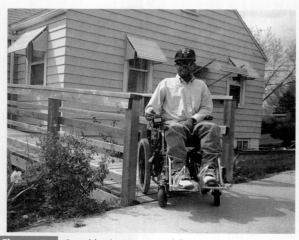

Figure 12-9 Donald using power mobility.

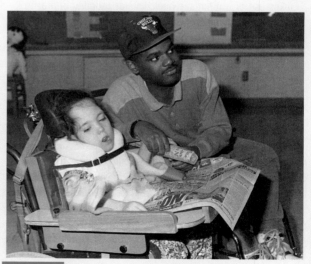

Figure 12-11 Donald assisting student in art class.

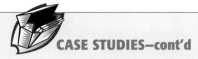

CASE STUDIES—cont'd

cises. He was subsequently referred to the local MDA-sponsored neuromuscular clinic for further examination.

At Derek's initial visit to the neuromuscular clinic, his standing posture was found to be mildly lordotic, his gait exhibited increased lateral trunk sway toward the stance phase leg, he had difficulty hopping on one foot, he exhibited a positive Gowers' sign when rising from the floor, and he needed to use a handrail when ascending or descending stairs. The physical examination found a pattern of mild proximal muscle weakness with most manual muscle test grades in the 4/5 range proximally and 5/5 distally. Creatine phosphate kinase testing resulted in a value of 20,009 IU/L (normal value, 25–204 IU/L). DNA analysis found a deletion of exon 45 of the X chromosome, which resulted in a diagnosis of dystrophinopathy. A muscle biopsy to test for the presence or absence of dystrophin has not yet been done to definitively differentiate between Duchenne's and Becker's muscular dystrophy.

Prednisone was prescribed for Derek following the initial clinic visit with a dosage of 15 mg/day that was increased to 20 mg/day at the age of 9 years. Night splints (Figure 12-12) and a home program for stretching of the posterior calf musculature were also initiated at the initial clinic visit with discontinuation of outpatient physical

therapy services. His ankle dorsiflexion range of motion, which was at neutral at the initial visit, has improved to 10° with the knee extended and has remained stable through use of the night splints and stretching program. Improved muscle strength was recorded following initiation of the prednisone regimen. Changes in muscle strength as documented with handheld dynamometry are shown in Table 12-3.

Currently, Derek is 9 years old and is in the fourth grade at his community elementary school. He receives consultative physical therapy at his school for input regarding his adapted physical education program and to address issues related to accessibility and fatigability during the school day. He is independently ambulatory with only mild gait deviations, which become more prominent when he attempts to run. He is independent in stair climbing using a handrail and is able to transfer from the floor to standing using a Gowers' maneuver. His home program of heelcord stretching (five repetitions of a standing runner's stretch carried out daily) (Figure 12-13) and night splint use is jointly monitored by the physical therapist at school and through the MDA clinic. At this point in time, he has no restriction on activity other than to avoid fatigue.

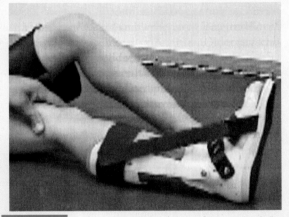

Figure 12-12 Night splints worn by Derek to maintain/improve ankle plantar flexor range of motion.

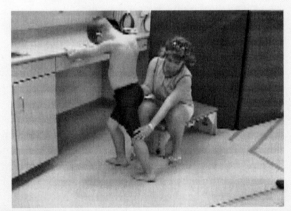

Figure 12-13 Runner's stretch used to stretch ankle plantar flexor muscles.

TABLE 12-3   **Handheld Dynamometry Scores Recorded with a Standardized Protocol with Isometric Contraction**

Measurement	Position	Right, lb		Left, lb	
		7 yr–2 mo	8 yr–4 mo	8 yr–4 mo	7 yr–2 mo
Hip flexion	Supine, 90°	9	15	7	13
Hip extension	Supine, 90°	28	26	29	28
Hip abduction	Supine, 0°	9	17	8	16
Knee flexion	Sitting, 90°	13	16	11	16
Knee extension	Sitting, 90°	20	23	19	23
Ankle dorsiflexion	Supine, 90°	10	9	9	12
Ankle plantar flexion	Supine, 90°	52	54	50	56

ACKNOWLEDGMENTS

My personal thanks goes to the children and their families who contributed to my knowledge of MD and SMA that made the writing of this chapter possible. Many challenges, accomplishments, disappointments, joys, and tears have paved the way. Special thanks to Donald and Derek and their families for sharing their stories, and to Becky, who first inspired me to take this path of clinical work.

REFERENCES

1. Amendt, L. E., Ause-Ellias, K. L., Eybers, J. L., Wadsworth, C. T., Nielsen, D. H., & Weinstein, S. L. (1990). Validity and reliability testing of the scoliometer. *Physical Therapy, 70,* 108–117.

2. American Physical Therapy Association (APTA). (2003). Guide to physical therapist practice. *Physical Therapy, 81,* 9–74.

3. Anderson, J. L., Head, S. I., Rae, C., & Morley J. W. (2002). Brian function in Duchenne muscular dystrophy. *Brain, 125,* 4–14.

4. Ansved, T. (2001). Muscle training in muscular dystrophies. *Acta Physiologica Scandinavica, 171,* 359–366.

5. Ansved, T. (2003). Muscular dystrophies: Influence of physical conditioning on the disease evolution. *Current Opinion in Clinical Nutrition & Metabolic Care, 6,* 435–439.

6. American Thoracic Society Documents. (2004). Respiratory care of the patient with Duchenne muscular dystrophy. *American Journal of Respiratory and Critical Care Medicine, 170,* 456–465.

7. Reference deleted in page proofs.

8. Bach, J. R., Baird, J. S., Plosky, D., Navado, J., & Weaver, B. (2002). Spinal muscular atrophy 1: Management and outcomes. *Pediatric Pulmonology, 34,* 16–22.

9. Bach, J. R., Campagnolo, D. I., & Hoeman, S. (1991). Life satisfaction of individuals with Duchenne muscular dystrophy using long-term mechanical ventilatory support. *American Journal of Physical Medicine and Rehabilitation, 70,* 129–135.

10. Bach, J. R., & Chaudhry, S. S. (2000). Standards of care in MDA clinics. *American Journal of Physical Medicine and Rehabilitation, 79,* 193–196.

11. Bach, J. R., & McKeon, J. (1991). Orthopaedic surgery and rehabilitation for the prolongation of brace-free ambulation of patients with Duchenne muscular dystrophy. *American Journal of Physical Medicine and Rehabilitation, 70,* 323–331.

12. Bach, J. R., O'Brien, J., Krotenberg, R., & Alba, A. S. (1987). Management of end stage respiratory failure in Duchenne muscular dystrophy. *Muscle and Nerve, 10,* 177–182.

13. Bach, J. R., Saltstein, K., Sinquee, D., Weaver, B., & Komaroff, E. (2007). Long-term survival in Werdnig-Hoffmann disease. *American Journal of Physical Medicine and Rehabilitation, 86,* 339–345.

14. Bach, J. R. (2008). The use of mechanical ventilation is appropriate in children with genetically proven spinal muscular atrophy type 1: The motion for. *Paediatric Respiratory Reviews, 9,* 45–50.

15. Reference deleted in page proofs.

16. Bakker, J. P., deGroot, I. J., Beckerman, H., deJong, B. A., & Lankhorst, G. J. (2000). The effects of knee-ankle-foot orthoses in the treatment of Duchenne muscular dystrophy: Review of the literature. *Clinical Rehabilitation, 14,* 343–359.

17. Reference deleted in page proofs.

18. Ballestrazzi, A., Gnudi, A., Magni, E., & Granata, C. (1989). Osteopenia in spinal muscular atrophy. In L. Merlini, C. Granata, & V. Dubowitz (Eds.), *Current concepts in childhood spinal muscular atrophy* (pp. 215–219). New York: Springer-Verlag.

19. Reference deleted in page proofs.

20. Beenakker, E. A., Fock, J. M., Van Tol, M. J., Maurits, N. M., Koopman, H. M., Brouwer, O. F., & Van der Hoeven, J. H. (2005). Intermittent prednisone therapy in Duchenne muscular dystrophy: A randomized controlled trial. *Archives of Neurology, 62,* 128–132.

21. Bianchi, M. L., Mazzanti, A., Galbiati, E., Saraifoger, S., Dubini, A., Cornelio, F., & Morandi, L. (2003). Bone mineral density and bone metabolism in Duchenne muscular dystrophy. *Osteoporosis International, 14,* 761–767.

22. Biggar, W. D., Gingras, M., Fehlings, D. L., Harris, V. A., & Steele, C. A. (2001). Deflazacort treatment of Duchenne muscular dystrophy. *Journal of Pediatrics, 138,* 45–50.

23. Binder, H. (1989). New ideas in the rehabilitation of children with spinal muscular atrophy. In L. Merlini, C. Granata, & V. Dubowitz (Eds.), *Current concepts in childhood spinal muscular atrophy* (pp. 117–128). New York: Springer-Verlag.

24. Bird, T. D. (2007). Myotonic muscular dystrophy type 1, GeneReview. Retrieved from: www.genereview.org.

25. Blake, D. S., Weir, A., Newey, S. E., & Davis, K. E. (2002). Function and genetics of dystrophia and dystrophia related proteins in muscle. *Physiological Review, 82,* 291–329.

26. Bonifati, M. D., Ruzza, G., Bonometto, P., Berardinelli, A., Gorni, K., Orcesi, S., Lanzi, G., & Angelini, C. (2000). A multicenter, double-blind, randomized trial of deflazacort versus prednisone in Duchenne muscular dystrophy. *Muscle and Nerve, 23,* 1344–1347.

27. Bowker, J. H., & Halpin, P. J. (1978). Factors determining success in reambulation of the child with progressive muscular dystrophy. *Orthopedic Clinics of North America, 9,* 431–436.

28. Borkowska, J., Rudhik-Schoneborn, S., Hausmanowa-Petrusewicz, I., & Zerre, K. (2002). Early infantile form of spinal muscle atrophy. *Folia Neuropathologica, 40,* 19–26.

29. Brooke, M. H., Fenichel, G. M., Griggs, R. C., Mendell, J. R., Moxley, R., Miller, J. P., & Province, M. A. (1983). Clinical investigation in Duchenne dystrophy: 2. Determination of the "power" of therapeutic trials based on the natural history. *Muscle Nerve, 6,* 91–103.

30. Brooke, M. H., Fenichel, G. M., Griggs, R. C., Mendell, J. R., Moxley, R., Florence, J., King, W. M., Pandya, S., Robinson, J., Schierbecker, J., Signnor, L., Miller, J. P., Gilder, B. F., Kaiser, K. K., Mandel, S., & Arfken, C. (1989). Duchenne muscular dystrophy: Patterns of clinical progression and effects of supportive therapy. *Neurology, 39,* 475–481.

31. Brooke, M. H., Griggs, R. C., Mendell, J. R., Fenichel, G. M., Shumate, J. B., & Pellegrino, R. J. (1981). Clinical trial in Duchenne dystrophy: I. The design of the protocol. *Muscle and Nerve, 4,* 186–197.

32. Brouwer, O. F., Paderg, G. W., Van Der Ploeg, R. J. O., Ruys, C. J. M., & Brand, R. (1992). The influence of handedness on the distribution of muscular weakness of the arm in facioscapulohumeral muscular dystrophy. *Brain, 115,* 1587–1598.

33. Brussock, C. M., Haley, S. M., Munsat, T. L., & Bernhardt, D. B. (1992). Measurement of isometric force in children with and without Duchenne's muscular dystrophy. *Physical Therapy, 72,* 105–114.

34. Burke, S. S., Grove, N. M., & Houser, C. R. (1971). Respiratory aspects of pseudohypertrophic muscular dystrophy. *American Journal of Diseases of Children, 121,* 230–234.

35. Bushby, K., Finkel, R., Birnkrant, D. J., Case, L. E., Clemens, P. R., Cripe, L., Kaul, A., Kinnett, K., McDonald, C., Pandya, S., Poysky, J., Shapiro, F., Tomezsko, J., & Constantin, C.; DMD Care Considerations Working Group. (2010). Diagnosis and management of Duchenne muscular dystrophy, part 2: Implementation of multidisciplinary care. *Lancet Neurology, 9,* 177–189.

36. Cambridge, W., & Drennan, J. C. (1987). Scoliosis associated with Duchenne muscular dystrophy. *Journal of Pediatric Orthopedics, 7,* 436–440.

37. Chakkalakal, J. V., Thompson, J., Parks, R. J., & Jasmin, B. J. (2005). Molecular, cellular, and pharmacological therapies for Duchenne/Becker muscular dystrophies. *FASEB Journal, 19,* 880–891.

38. Charash, L. I., Lovelace, R. E., Wolfe, S. G., Kutscher, A. H., Price, D., Leach, R., & Leach, C. F. (1987). *Realities in coping with progressive neuromuscular disease.* Philadelphia: Charles Press Publishers.

39. Cheuk, D. K., Wong, V., Wraige, E., Baxter, P., Cole, A., N'Diaye, T., & Mayowe V. (2007). Surgery for scoliosis in Duchenne muscular dystrophy. *Cochrane Database System Reviews, 24,* CD005375.

40. Chung, B. H., Wong, V. C., & Ip, P. (2004). Spinal muscular atrophy: Survival pattern and functional status. *Pediatrics, 114,* e548–e553.

41. Chyatte, S. B., Long, C., & Vignos, P. J. (1965). Balanced forearm orthosis in muscular dystrophy. *Archives of Physical Medicine and Rehabilitation, 46,* 633–636.

42. Ciafaloni, E., Fox, D. J., Pandya, S., Westfield, C. P., Puzhankara, S., Romitti, P. A., Mathews, K. D., Miller, T. M., Matthews, D. J., Miller, L. A., Cunniff, C., Druschel, C. M., & Moxley, R. T.(2009). Delayed diagnosis in Duchenne muscular dystrophy: Data from the Muscular Dystrophy Surveillance, Tracking, and Research Network (MD STARnet). *Journal of Pediatrics, 155,* 380–385.

43. Colbert, A. P., & Craig, C. (1987). Scoliosis management in Duchenne muscular dystrophy: Prospective study of modified Jewett hyperextension brace. *Archives of Physical Medicine and Rehabilitation, 68,* 302–304.

44. Coster, W., Deeney, T., Haltiwanger, J., & Haley, S. (1998). *School function assessment.* San Antonio, TX: Therapy Skill Builders.

45. Courdier-Fruh, I., Barman, L., Briguet, A., & Meier, T. (2002). Glucocorticoid-mediated regulation of utrophin levels in human muscle fibers. *Neuromuscular Disorders, 12*(suppl 1), S95–S104.

46. Cunha, M. C., Oliveira, A. S., Labronici, R. H., & Gabbai, A. A. (1996). Spinal muscular atrophy type II and III: Evolution of 50 patients with physiotherapy and hydrotherapy in a swimming pool. *Arquivos Neuro-Psiquiatria, 54,* 402–406.

47. Darras, B. T., Korf, B. R., & Urion, D. K. (1979). Dystrophinopathies. GeneReviews, www.genereviews.org. 2008.

48. Dorscher, P. T., Mehrsheed, S., Mulder, D. W., Litchy, W. J., & Ilstrup, D. M. (1991). Wohlfart-Kugelberg-Welander syndrome: Serum creatine kinase and functional outcome. *Archives of Physical Medicine and Rehabilitation, 72,* 587–591.

49. Dubowitz, V. (1989). The clinical picture of spinal muscular atrophy. In L. Merlini, C. Granata, & V. Dubowitz (Eds.), *Current concepts in childhood spinal muscular atrophy* (pp. 13–19). New York: Springer-Verlag.

50. Dubowitz, V. (1992). The muscular dystrophies. *Postgraduate Medical Journal, 68,* 500–506.

51. Eagle, M., Baudouin, S. V., Chandler, C., Giddings, D. R., Bullock, R., & Bushby, K. (2002). Survival in Duchenne muscular dystrophy: Improvements in life expectancy since 1967 and the impact of home nocturnal ventilation. *Neuromuscular Disorders, 12,* 926–929.

52. Edwards, R. H. T. (1980). Studies of muscular performance in normal and dystrophic subjects. *British Medical Bulletin, 36,* 159–164.

53. Emery, A. E. H. (1993). *Duchenne muscular dystrophy.* Oxford: Oxford University Press.

54. Emery, A. E. H. (2002). The muscular dystrophies. *Lancet, 359,* 687–695.

55. Emery, A. E. H., & Skinner, R. (1976). Clinical studies in benign (Becker-type) X-linked muscular dystrophy. *Clinical Genetics, 10,* 189–201.

56. Eng, G. D. (1989a). Therapy and rehabilitation of the floppy infant. *Rhode Island Medical Journal, 72*, 367–370.

57. Eng, G. D. (1989b). Rehabilitation of the child with a severe form of spinal muscular atrophy (type I, infantile or Werdnig-Hoffman disease). In L. Merlini, C. Granata, & V. Dubowitz (Eds.), *Current concepts in childhood spinal muscular atrophy* (pp. 113–115). New York: Springer-Verlag.

58. Escolar, D. M., Buyse, G., Henricson, E., Leshner, R., Florence, J., Mayhew, J., Tesi-Rocha, C., Gorni, K., Pasquali, L., Patel, K. M., McCarter, R., Huang, J., Mayhew, T., Bertorini, T., Carlo, J., Connolly, A. M., Clemens, P. R., Goemans, N., Iannaccone, S. T., Igarashi, M., Nevo, Y., Pestronk, A., Subramony, S. H., Vedanarayanan, V. V., & Wessel, H.; CINRG Group. (2005). CINRG randomized controlled trial of creatine and glutamine in Duchenne muscular dystrophy. *Annals of Neurology, 58*, 151–155.

59. Farini, A., Razini, P., Erratico, S., Torrente, Y., & Meregalli, M. (2009). Cell based therapy for Duchenne muscular dystrophy. *Journal of Cellular Physiology, 221*, 526–534.

60. Febrer, A., Rodriguez, N., Alias, L., & Tizzano, E. (2010). Measurement of muscle strength with a handheld dynamometer in patients with chronic spinal muscular atrophy. *Journal of Rehabilitation Medicine, 42*, 228–231.

60a. Finder J. D. A. (2009). perspective on the 2004 American Thoracic Society statement, "respiratory care of the patient with Duchenne muscular dystrophy". *Pediatrics*. 2009 May;*123*(Suppl 4), S239–S241.

61. Florence, J. M., Pandya, S., King, W. M., Robinson, J. D., Baty, J., Miller, J. P., Schierbecker, J., & Signore, L. C. (1992). Intra-rater reliability of manual muscle test (Medical Research Council Scale) grades in Duchenne's muscular dystrophy. *Physical Therapy, 72*, 115–122.

62. Fowler, W. M. (1982). Rehabilitation management of muscular dystrophy and related disorders: I. The role of exercise. *Archives of Physical Medicine and Rehabilitation, 63*, 208–210.

63. Fowler, W. M., & Gardner, G. W. (1967). Quantitative strength measurements in muscular dystrophy. *Archives of Physical Medicine and Rehabilitation, 48*, 629–644.

64. Fukuyama, Y., Osaw, M., & Suzuki, H. (1981). Congenital muscular dystrophy of the Fukuyama type: Clinical, genetic and pathological considerations. *Brain and Development, 3*, 1–29.

65. Galasko, C. S. B., Williamson, J. B., & Delany, C. M. (1995). Lung function in Duchenne muscular dystrophy. *European Spine, 4*, 263–267.

66. Gardner-Medwin, D. (1979). Controversies about Duchenne muscular dystrophy: II. Bracing for ambulation. *Developmental Medicine and Child Neurology, 21*, 659–662.

67. Gardner-Medwin, D. (1980). Clinical features and classification of the muscular dystrophies. *British Medical Bulletin, 36*, 109–115.

68. Gibson, D. A., Koreska, J., & Robertson, D. (1978). The management of spinal deformity in Duchenne's muscular dystrophy. *Clinical Orthopedics, 9*, 437–450.

69. Gilroy, J., & Holliday, P. (1982). *Basic neurology*. New York: Macmillan.

70. Gordon, E., Hoffman, E. P., & Pegoraro, E. (2006). Congenital muscular dystrophy overview, GeneReviews. Retrieved from www.genereviews.org.

71. Granata, C., Magni, E., Sabattini, L., Colombo, C., & Merlini, L. (1989a). Promotion of ambulation in intermediate spinal muscle atrophy. In L. Merlini, C. Granata, & V. Dubowitz (Eds.), *Current concepts in childhood spinal muscular atrophy* (pp. 127–132). New York: Springer-Verlag.

72. Granata, C., Marini, M. L., Capelli, T., & Merlini, L. (1989b). Natural history of scoliosis in spinal muscular atrophy and results of orthopaedic treatment. In L. Merlini, C. Granata, & V. Dubowitz (Eds.), *Current concepts in childhood spinal muscular atrophy* (pp. 153–164). New York: Springer-Verlag.

73. Granata, C., Merlini, L., Magni, E., Marini, M. L., & Stagni, S. B. (1989c). Spinal muscular atrophy: Natural history and orthopaedic treatment of scoliosis. *Spine, 14*, 760–762.

74. Grange, R. W., & Call, J. A. (2007). Recommendations to define exercise prescription for Duchenne muscular dystrophy. *Exercise and Sport Science Reviews, 35*, 12–17.

75. Reference deleted in page proofs.

76. Haley, S. M., Coster, W. J., Ludlow, L. H., & Haltiwanger, J. T. (1992). *Pediatric Evaluation of Disability Inventory (PEDI): Development, standardization and administration manual.* Boston: New England Medical Center Hospital.

77. Reference deleted in page proofs.

78. Harper, P. S. (1989). *Myotonic dystrophy: Major problems in neurology* (2nd ed.; *Vol. 21*). Philadelphia: WB Saunders.

79. Heckmatt, J. Z., Dubowitz, V., & Hyde, S. A. (1985). Prolongation of walking in Duchenne muscular dystrophy with light-weight orthoses: Review of 57 cases. *Developmental Medicine and Child Neurology, 27*, 149–154.

80. Heller, K. D., Forst, R., Forst, J., & Hengstler, K. (1997). Scoliosis in Duchenne muscular dystrophy. *Prosthetics and Orthotics International, 21*, 202–209.

81. Herrmann, R., Straub, V., Meyer, K., Kahn, T., Wagner, M., & Voit, T. (1996). Congenital muscular dystrophy with laminin alpha 2 chain deficiency: Identification of a new intermediate phenotype and correlation of clinical findings to muscle immunohistochemistry. *European Journal of Paediatrics, 155*, 968–976.

82. Hirawat, S., Welch, E. M., Elfring, G. L., Northcutt, V. J., Paushkin, S., Hwang, S., Leonard, E. M., Almstead, N. G., Ju, W., Peltz, S. W., & Miller, L. L.(2007). Safety, tolerability, and pharmacokinetics of PTC124, a nonaminoglycoside nonsense mutation suppressor, following single- and multiple-dose administration to healthy male and female adult volunteers. *Journal of Clinical Pharmacology, 47*, 430–444.

83. Hoffman, E. P., Brown, R. H., & Kunkel, L. M. (1987). Dystrophin: The protein product of the Duchenne muscular dystrophy locus. *Cell, 51*, 919–928.

84. Hoffmann, J. (1893). Ueber chronische spinale Muskelatrophie im Kindesalter, auf familiar Basis. *Deutsche Zeitschrift fur Nervenheilkunde, 3*, 427.

85. Hsu, J. D. (1995). Orthopedic approaches for the treatment of lower extremity contractures in the Duchenne muscular dystrophy patient in the United States and Canada. *Seminars in Neurology, 15*, 6–8.

86. Hyde, S. A., Floytrup, I., Glent, S., Kroksmark, A., & Salling, B. (2000). A randomized comparative study using two methods for controlling tendo Achilles contracture in Duchenne muscular dystrophy. *Neuromuscular Disorders, 10*, 257–263.

87. Joseph, J. T., Richards, C. S., Anthony, D. C., Upton, M., Perez-Atayde, A. R., & Greenstein, P. (1997). Congenital myotonic dystrophy pathology and somatic mosaicism. *Neurology, 49*, 1457–1460.

88. Johnson, E. W., & Braddom, R. (1971). Over-work weakness in facioscapulo-humeral muscular dystrophy. *Archives of Physical Medicine and Rehabilitation, 52*, 333–336.

89. Jones, K. J., & North, K. N. (1997). Recent advances in diagnosis of the childhood muscular dystrophies. *Journal of Paediatric Child Health, 33*, 195–201.

90. Jones, M. A., McEwen, I. R., & Hansen, L. (2003). Use of power mobility for a young child with spinal muscular atrophy. *Physical Therapy, 83*, 253–262.

91. Reference deleted in page proofs.

92. Kaspar, R. W., Allen, H. D., & Montanaro, F. (2009). Current understanding and management of dilated cardiomyopathy in Duchenne and Becker muscular dystrophy. *Journal of the American Academy of Nurse Practitioners, 21*, 241–249.

93. Kinali, M., Main, M., Eliahoo, J., Messina, S., Knight, R. K., Lehovsky, J., Edge, G., Mercuri, E., Manzur, A. Y., & Muntoni, F. (2007). Predictive factors for the development of scoliosis in Duchenne muscular dystrophy. *European Journal of Paediatric Neurology, 11*, 160–166.

94. Kinali, M., Arechavala-Gomeza, V., Feng, L., Cirak, S., Hunt, D., Adkin, C., Guglieri, M., Ashton, E., Abbs, S., Nihoyannopoulos, P., Garralda, M. E., Rutherford, M., McCulley, C., Popplewell, L., Graham, I. R., Dickson, G., Wood, M. J., Wells, D. J., Wilton, S. D., Kole, R., Straub, V., Bushby, K., Sewry, C., Morgan, J. E., & Muntoni, F. (2009). Local restoration of dystrophin expression with the morpholino oligomer AVI-4658 in Duchenne muscular dystrophy: A single-blind, placebo-controlled, dose-escalation, proof-of-concept study. *Lancet Neurology, 8*, 918–928.

95. Koenig, M., Hoffmann, E. P., & Pertelson, C. K. (1987). Complete cloning of the Duchenne muscular dystrophy (DMD) cDNA and preliminary genomic organization of the DMD gene in mouse and affected individuals. *Cell, 50*, 509–517.

96. Koessler, W., Wanke, T., Winkler, G., Nader, A., Toifl, K., Kurz, H., & Zwick, H. (2001). 2 years' experience with inspiratory muscle training in patients with neuromuscular disorders. *Chest, 120*, 765–769.

97. Kugelberg, E., & Welander, L. (1956). Heredofamilial juvenile muscular atrophy simulating muscular dystrophy. *Archives of Neurology and Psychiatry, 75*, 500.

98. Kunkel, L. M., Monaco, A. P., Middlesworth, W., Ochs, S. D., & Latt, S. A. (1985). Specific cloning of DNA fragments absent from the DNA of a male patient with an X chromosome deletion. *Proceedings of the National Academy of Science USA, 82*, 4778–4782.

99. Reference deleted in page proofs.

100. Lee, C. C., Pearlman, J. A., Chamberlain, J. S., & Caskey, C. T. (1991). Expression of recombinant dystrophin and its localization to the cell membrane. *Nature, 349*, 334–336.

101. Liechti-Gallati, S., Koenig, M., Kunkel, L. M., Frey, D., Boltshauser, E., Schneider, V., Braga, S., & Moser, H. (1989). Molecular deletion patterns in Duchenne and Becker type muscular dystrophy. *Human Genetics, 81*, 343–348.

102. Lonstein, J. E. (1989). Management of spinal deformity in spinal muscular atrophy. In L. Merlini, C. Granata, & V. Dubowitz (Eds.), *Current concepts in childhood spinal muscular atrophy* (pp. 165–173). New York: Springer-Verlag.

103. Louis, M., Lebacq, J., Poortmans, J. R., Belpaire-Dethiou, M. C., Devogelaer, J., Van Hecke, P., Goubel, F., & Francaux, M. (2003). Beneficial effects of creatine supplementation in dystrophic patients. *Muscle and Nerve, 27*, 604–610.

104. Lue, Y. J., Lin, R. F., Chen, S. S., & Lu, Y. M. (2009). Measurement of the functional status of patients with different types of muscular dystrophy. *Kaohsiung J Med Sci, 25*, 325–333.

105. Lyager, S., Steffensen, B., & Juhl, B. (1995). Indicators of need for mechanical ventilation in Duchenne muscular dystrophy and spinal muscular atrophy. *Chest, 108*, 779–785.

106. MacKenzie, A. E., Jacob, P., Surh, L., & Besner, A. (1994). Genetic heterogeneity in spinal muscle atrophy: A linkage analysis-based assessment. *Neurology, 44*, 919–924.

107. Main, M., Kairon, H., Mercuri, E., & Muntoni, F. (2003). The Hammersmith functional motor scale for children with spinal muscular atrophy: A scale to test ability and monitor progress in children with limited ambulation. *European Journal of Paediatric Neurology, 7*, 155–159.

108. Manzur, A. Y., Kinali, M., & Muntoni, F. (2008). Update on the management of Duchenne muscular dystrophy. *Archives of Disease in Childhood, 93*, 986–990.

109. Marchesi, D., Arlet, V., Stricker, U., & Aeibi, M. (1997). Modification of the original Luque technique in the treatment of Duchenne's neuromuscular scoliosis. *Journal of Pediatric Orthopaedics, 17*, 743–749.

110. Marshall, C. R. (1984). Medical treatment of spinal muscular atrophy. In I. Gamstorp, & H. B. Sarnat (Eds.), *Progressive spinal muscular atrophies: International Review of Child Neurology series* (pp. 163–171). New York: Raven Press.

111. Mazzone, E. S., Messina, S., Vasco, G., Main, M., Eagle, M., D'Amico, A., Doglio, L., Politano, L., Cavallaro, F., Frosini, S., Bello, L., Magri, F., Corlatti, A., Zucchini, E., Brancalion, B., Rossi, F., Ferretti, M., Motta, M. G., Cecio, M. R., Berardinelli, A., Alfieri, P., Mongini, T., Pini, A., Astrea, G., Battini, R., Comi, G., Pegoraro, E., Morandi, L., Pane, M., Angelini, C., Bruno, C., Villanova, M., Vita, G., Donati, M. A., Bertini, E., Mercuri, E. (2009). Reliability of the North Star Ambulatory Assessment in a multicentric setting. *Neuromuscular Disorders, 19*, 458–461.

112. McDonald, C. M., Abresch, R. T., Carter, G. T., Fowler, W. M., Johnson, E. R., Kilmer, D. M. D., & Sigford, B. J. (1995). Profiles of neuromuscular diseases: Duchenne muscular dystrophy. *American Journal of Physical Medicine and Rehabilitation, 74*(Suppl), S70–S92.

113. McDonald, D. G., Kinali, M., Gallagher, A. C., Mercuri, E., Muntoni, F., Roper, H., Jardine, P., Jones, D. H., & Pike, M. G. (2002). Fracture prevalence in Duchenne muscular dystrophy. *Developmental Medicine and Child Neurology, 44*, 695–698.

114. Merlini, L., Granata, C., Capelli, T., Mattutini, P., & Colombo, C. (1989). Natural history of infantile and childhood spinal muscular atrophy. In L. Merlini, C. Granata, & V. Dubowitz (Eds.), *Current concepts in childhood spinal muscular atrophy* (pp. 95–100). New York: Springer-Verlag.

115. Merlini, L., Cicognani, A., Malaspina, E., Gennari, M., Gnudi, S., Talim, B., & Franzoni, E. (2003). Early prednisone treatment in Duchenne muscular dystrophy. *Muscle and Nerve, 27*, 222–227.

116. Miller, F., Moseley, C. F., & Koreska, J. (1992). Spinal fusion in Duchenne muscular dystrophy. *Developmental Medicine and Child Neurology, 34*, 775–786.

117. Miller, G., & Dunn, N. (1982). An outline of the management and prognosis of Duchenne muscular dystrophy in Western Australia. *Australian Pediatric Journal, 82*, 277–282.

118. Molnar, G. E., & Alexander, J. (1973). Objective, quantitative muscle testing in children: A pilot study. *Archives of Physical Medicine and Rehabilitation, 54*, 224–228.

119. Muscular Dystrophy Association. (2010). *Facts about muscular dystrophy*. Tucson, AZ: Muscular Dystrophy Association.

120. Nair, K. P., Vasanth, A., Gourie-Devi, M., Taly, A. B., Rao, S., Gayathri, N., & Murali, T. (2001). Disabilities in children with Duchenne muscular dystrophy: A profile. *Journal of Rehabilitation Medicine, 33*, 147–149.

121. Nelson, S. F., Crosbie, R. H., Miceli, M. C., & Spencer, M. J. (2009). Emerging genetic therapies to treat Duchenne muscular dystrophy. *Current Opinion in Neurology, 22*, 532–538.

122. Newsom-Davis, J. (1980). The respiratory system in muscular dystrophy. *British Medical Bulletin, 36*, 135–138.

123. North, K. N., Specht, L. A., Sethi, R. K., Shapiro, F., & Beggs, A. H. (1996). Congenital muscular dystrophy associated with merosin deficiency. *Journal of Child Neurology, 11*, 291–295.

124. Reference deleted in page proofs.

125. O'Brien, T., & Harper, P. S. (1984). Course, prognosis and complications of childhood-onset myotonic dystrophy. *Developmental Medicine and Child Neurology, 26*, 62–67.

126. Reference deleted in page proofs.

127. Pandya, A., Florence, J. M., King, W. M., Robinson, J. D., Oxman, M., & Province, M. A. (1985). Reliability of goniometric measurements in patients with Duchenne muscular dystrophy. *Physical Therapy, 65*, 1339–1342.

128. Partridge, T. A., Grounds, M., & Sloper, J. C. (1978). Evidence of fusion between host and donor myoblasts in skeletal muscle grafts. *Nature, 273*, 306–308.

129. Reference deleted in page proofs.

130. Pearn, J. H. (1978). Autosomal dominant spinal muscular atrophy: A clinical and genetic study. *Journal of Neurologic Science, 38*, 263–275.

131. Pearn, J. H. (1980). Classification of spinal muscular atrophies. *Lancet, 1*, 919–922.

132. Reference deleted in page proofs.

133. Péault, B., Rudnicki, M., Torrente, Y., Cossu, G., Tremblay, J. P., Partridge, T., Gussoni, E., Kunkel, L. M., & Huard, J. (2007). Stem and progenitor cells in skeletal muscle development, maintenance, and therapy. *Molecular Therapy, 15*, 867–877.

134. Pegoraro, E., Marks, H., Garcia, C. A., Crawford, T., & Connolly, A. M. (1998). Laminin alpha2 muscular dystrophy: Genotype/phenotype studies of 22 patients. *Neurology, 51*, 101–110.

135. Perkins, K. J., & Davies, K. E. (2002). The role of utrophin in the potential therapy of Duchenne muscular dystrophy. *Neuromuscular Disorders, 12*, S78–S89.

136. Petrof, B. J. (2002). Molecular pathophysiology of myofiber injury in deficiencies of the dystrophin–glycoprotein complex. *American Journal of Physical Medicine and Rehabilitation, 81*, S162-S174, 2002.

137. Pinelli, G., Dominici, P., Merlini, L., DiPasquale, G., Granata, C., & Bonfiglioli, S. (1987). Cardiologic evaluation in a family with Emery-Dreifus muscular dystrophy. *Giornale Italiano di Cardiologia, 17*, 589–593.

138. Prior, T. W., & Russman B. S. (2006). Spinal muscular atrophy, GeneReviews. Retrieved from: www.genereviews.org.

139. Reardon, W., Newcombe, R., Fenton, I., Sibert, J., & Harper, P. S. (1993). The natural history of congenital myotonic muscular dystrophy: Mortality and long term clinical aspects. *Archives of Disease in Childhood, 68*, 177–181.

140. Reed, U. C. (2009). Congenital muscular dystrophy. Part I: A review of phenotypical and diagnostic aspects. *Arquivos de Neuro-Psiquiatria, 67*, 144–168, 2009.

141. Reference deleted in page proofs.

142. Rhodes, L. E., Freeman, B. K., Auh, S., Kokkinis, A. D., La Pean, A., Chen, C., Lehky, T. J., Shrader, J. A., Levy, E. W., Harris-Love, M., Di Prospero, N. A., Fischbeck, K. H. (2009). Clinical features of spinal and bulbar muscular atrophy. *Brain, 132*, 3242–3251.

143. Ricker, K. (2000). The expanding clinical and genetic spectrum of the myotonic dystrophies. *Acta Neurologica Belgium, 100*, 151–155.

144. Rideau, Y., Glorion, B., Delaubier, A., Tarle, O., & Bach, J. (1984). The treatment of scoliosis in Duchenne muscular dystrophy. *Muscle and Nerve, 7*, 281–286.

145. Ringel, S. P. (1987). *Neuromuscular disorders: A guide for patient and family.* New York: Raven Press.

146. Robinson, A. (1995). Programmed cell death and the gene behind spinal muscle atrophy. *Canadian Medical Association Journal, 153*, 1459–1462.

147. Rodillo, E., Noble-Jamieson, C. M., Aber, V., Heckmatt, J. Z., Muntoni, F., & Dubowitz, V. (1989). Respiratory muscle training in Duchenne muscular dystrophy. *Archives of Disease in Childhood, 64*, 736–738.

148. Roig, M., Balliu, P. R., Navarro, C., Brugera, R., & Losada, M. (1994). Presentation, clinical course and outcome of the congenital form of myotonic dystrophy. *Pediatric Neurology, 11*, 208–213.

149. Rutherford, M. A., Heckmatt, J. Z., & Dubowitz, V. (1989). Congenital myotonic dystrophy: Respiratory function at birth determines survival. *Archives of Disease in Childhood, 64*, 191–195.

150. Saranti, A. J., Gleim, G. W., & Melvin, M. (1980). The relationship between subjective and objective measurements of strength. *Journal of Orthopedic Sports and Physical Therapy, 2*, 15–19.

151. Scher, D. M., & Mubarak, S. J. (2002). Surgical prevention of foot deformity in patients with Duchenne muscular dystrophy. *Journal of Pediatric Orthopedics, 22*, 348–391.

152. Scott, O. M., Hyde, S. A., Goddard, C., & Dubowitz, V. (1981). Prevention of deformity in Duchenne muscular dystrophy: A prospective study of passive stretching and splintage. *Physiotherapy, 67*, 177–180.

153. Scott, O. M., Hyde, S. A., & Goddard, E. (1982). Quantification of muscle function in children: A prospective study in Duchenne muscular dystrophy. *Muscle and Nerve, 5*, 291–301.

154. Scott, O. M., Vrbova, G., Hyde, S. A., & Dubowitz, V. (1986). Responses of muscles of patients with Duchenne muscular dystrophy to chronic electrical stimulation. *Journal of Neurology, Neurosurgery and Psychiatry, 49*, 1427–1434.

155. Seeger, B. R., Caudrey, D. J., & Little, J. D. (1985). Progression of equinus deformity in Duchenne muscular dystrophy. *Archives of Physical Medicine and Rehabilitation, 66*, 286–288.

156. Seeger, B. R., Sutherland, A. D., & Clark, M. S. (1984). Orthotic management of scoliosis in Duchenne muscular dystrophy. *Archives of Physical Medicine and Rehabilitation, 65*, 83–86.

157. Semprini, L., Tacconelli, A., Capon, F., Brancati, F., Dallapiccola, B., & Novelli, C. (2001). A single strand conformation polymorphism-based carrier test for spinal muscle atrophy. *Genetic Testing, 5*, 33–37.

158. Sengupta, S. K., Mehdian, S. H., McConnell, J. R., Eisenstein, S. M., & Webb, J. K. (2002). Pelvic or lumbar fixation for the surgical management of scoliosis in Duchenne muscular dystrophy. *Spine, 27*, 2072–2079.

159. Shapiro, F., & Specht, L. (1991). Orthopaedic deformities in Emery-Dreifus muscular dystrophy. *Journal of Pediatric Orthopedics, 11*, 336–340.

160. Reference deleted in page proofs.

161. Siegel, I. M. (1978). The management of muscular dystrophy: A clinical review. *Muscle and Nerve, 1*, 453–460.

162. Siegel, I. M. (1986). *Muscle and its diseases: An outline primer of basic science and clinical method.* Chicago: Year Book Medical Publishers.

163. Spranger, M., Spranger, S., Tischendorf, M., Meinck, H. M., & Cremer, M. (1997). Myotonic dystrophy: The role of large triplet repeat length in the development of mental retardation. *Archives of Neurology, 54*, 251–254.

164. Reference deleted in page proofs.

165. Steffensen, B., & Hyde, S. (2001). Validity of the EK scale: A functional assessment of non-ambulatory individuals with Duchenne muscular dystrophy. *Physiotherapy Research International, 6*, 119–134.

166. Steffensen, B. F., Lyager, S., Werge, B., Rahbek, J., & Mattsson, E. (2002). Physical capacity in non-ambulatory people with Duchenne muscular dystrophy or spinal muscular atrophy: A longitudinal study. *Developmental Medicine and Child Neurology, 44*, 623–632.

167. Stevenson, W. G., Perloff, J. K., Weiss, J. N., & Anderson, T. L. (1990). Facioscapulohumeral muscular dystrophy: Evidence for selective, genetic electrophysiologic cardiac involvement. *Journal of the American College of Cardiology, 15*, 292–299.

168. Stuberg, W. A. (2001). Home accessibility and adaptive equipment in Duchenne muscular dystrophy: A case report. *Pediatric Physical Therapy, 13*, 169–174.

169. Stuberg, W. A., & Metcalf, W. M. (1988). Reliability of quantitative muscle testing in healthy children and in children with Duchenne muscular dystrophy using a hand-held dynamometer. *Physical Therapy, 68*, 977–982.

170. Sveen M. L., Jeppesen, T. D., Hauerslev, S., Køber, L., Krag, T. O., Vissing, J. (2008). Endurance training improves fitness and strength in patients with Becker muscular dystrophy. *Brain, 131*, 2824–2831.

171. Swinyard, C. A., Deaver, G. G., & Greenspan, L. (1957). Gradients of functional ability of importance in rehabilitation of patients with progressive muscular and neuromuscular diseases. *Archives of Physical Medicine and Rehabilitation, 38*, 574–579.

172. Taktak, D. M., & Bowker, P. (1995). Lightweight, modular knee-ankle-foot-orthosis for Duchenne muscular dystrophy: Design, development, and evaluation. *Archives of Physical Medicine and Rehabilitation, 76*, 1156–1262.

173. Tedesco, F. S., Dellavalle, A., Diaz-Manera, J., Messina, G., & Cossu, G. (2010). Repairing skeletal muscle: Regenerative

potential of skeletal muscle stem cells. *Journal of Clinical Investigation, 120,* 11–19.

174. Torrente, Y., Belicchi, M., Marchesi, C., Dantona, G., Cogiamanian, F., Pisati, F., Gavina, M., Giordano, R., Tonlorenzi, R., Fagiolari, G., Lamperti, C., Porretti, L., Lopa, R., Sampaolesi, M., Vicentini, L., Grimoldi, N., Tiberio, F., Songa, V., Baratta, P., Prelle, A., Forzenigo, L.,Guglieri, M., Pansarasa, O., Rinaldi, C., Mouly, V., Butler-Browne, G. S., Comi, G. P., Biondetti, P., Moggio, M., Gaini, S. M., Stocchetti, N., Priori, A., D'Angelo, M. G., Turconi, A., Bottinelli, R., Cossu, G., Rebulla, P., & Bresolin, N. (2007). Autologous transplantation of muscle-derived CD133+ stem cells in Duchenne muscle patients. *Cell Transplantation, 16,* 563–577.

175. Velasco, M. V., Colin, A. A., Zurakowski, D., Darras, B. T., & Shapiro, F. (2007). Posterior spinal fusion for scoliosis in Duchenne muscular dystrophy diminishes the rate of respiratory decline. *Spine, 32,* 459–465.

176. Vignos, P. J. (1983). Physical models of rehabilitation in neuromuscular disease. *Muscle and Nerve, 6,* 323–338.

177. Vignos, P. J., & Archibald, K. C. (1960). Maintenance of ambulation in childhood muscular dystrophy. *Journal of Chronic Diseases, 12,* 273–290.

178. Vignos, P. J., Spencer, G. E., & Archibald, K. C. (1963). Management of progressive muscular dystrophy. *Journal of the American Medical Association, 184,* 103–112.

179. Vignos, P. J., & Watkins, M. P. (1966). The effect of exercise in muscular dystrophy. *Journal of the American Medical Association, 197,* 121–126.

180. Vignos, P. J., Wagner, M. B., Karlinchak, B., & Katirji, B. (1996). Evaluation of a program for long-term treatment of Duchenne muscular dystrophy. *Journal of Bone and Joint Surgery (American), 78,* 1844–1852.

181. Voit, T. (1998). Congenital muscular dystrophies: 1997 update. *Brain Development, 20,* 65–74.

182. Wang, C. H., Finkel, R. S., Bertini, E. S., Schroth, M., Simonds, A., Wong, B., Aloysius, A., Morrison, L., Main, M., Crawford, T. O., Trela, A.; Participants of the International Conference on SMA Standard of Care. (2007). Consensus statement for standard of care in spinal muscular atrophy. *Journal of Child Neurology, 22,* 1027–1049.

183. Watt, J. M., & Greenhill, B. (1984). Commentary: Rehabilitation and orthopaedic management of spinal muscle atrophy. In I. Gamstorp, & H. B. Sarnat (Eds.), *Progressive spinal muscular atrophies: International Review of Child Neurology series.* New York: Raven Press.

184. Weidner, N. J. (2005). Developing an interdisciplinary palliative care plan for the patient with muscular dystrophy. *Pediatric Annals, 34,* 546–552.

185. Werdnig, G. (1894). Eine fruhinfantile progressive spinale Amyotrophie. *Archives fur Psychiatrie Nervenkrankheiten, 26,* 706–744.

186. Werlauff, U., Steffensen, B. F., Bertelsen, S., Fløytrup, I., Kristensen, B., & Werge, B. (2010). Physical characteristics and applicability of standard assessment methods in a total population of spinal muscular atrophy type II patients. *Neuromuscular Disorders, 20,* 34–43.

187. Reference deleted in page proofs.

188. Winsor, E. J., Murphy, E. G., Thompson, M. W., & Reed, T. E. (1971). Genetics of childhood spinal muscular atrophy. *Journal of Medical Genetics, 8,* 143–148.

189. Wohlfart, G., Fex, J., & Eliasson, S. (1955). Hereditary proximal spinal muscular atrophy: A clinical entity simulating progressive muscular dystrophy. *Acta Psychiatrica Neurologica Scandinavica, 30,* 395–406.

190. Wong, L. Y., & Christopher, C. (2002). Corticosteroids in Duchenne muscular dystrophy: A reappraisal. *Journal of Child Neurology, 17,* 184–190.

191. Wong, C. K., & Wade, C. K. (1995). Reducing iliotibial band contractures in patients with muscular dystrophy using custom dry floatation cushions. *Archives of Physical Medicine and Rehabilitation, 76,* 695–700.

192. Young, H. K., Barton, B. A., Waisbren, S., Portales Dale, L., Ryan, M. M., Webster, R. I., & North, K. N. (2009). Cognitive and psychological profile of males with Becker muscular dystrophy. *Journal of Child Neurology, 23,* 155–162.

193. Ziter, F. A., & Allsop, K. G. (1976). The diagnosis and management of childhood muscular dystrophy. *Clinical Pediatrics, 15,* 540–548.

13 Limb Deficiencies and Amputations

MEG STANGER, PT, MS, PCS • COLLEEN COULTER-O'BERRY, PT, DPT, PhD, PCS • BRIAN GIAVEDONI, MBA, CP, LP

The child with an amputation is defined as a person with an amputation who is skeletally immature because the epiphyses of the long bones are still open.[1] Amputations can be classified as congenital or acquired. Many different factors must be considered in the management of children with a limb deficiency or amputation. These factors differ from those involved in the management of adults with a limb deficiency or amputation because as children grow their musculoskeletal systems continue to develop. Children also are emotionally immature and variably dependent on adults for care and decision making regarding surgical and prosthetic issues.

In this chapter, the causes of limb deficiencies and amputations in children, surgical management, physical therapy intervention relative to a child's age and developmental function, and pediatric prosthetic options are discussed. Emphasis is on the aspects of management that differ from those encountered by adults with amputations. The role of the physical therapist includes education of parents of infants and children with limb deficiencies, development and progression of postoperative exercise programs, training in mobility and self-care skills, and providing input to both parents and the child or adolescent regarding prosthetic options. Studies have shown that children with limb deficiencies who participated in extensive rehabilitation programs have vocational skills with high employment potential.[80]

CONGENITAL LIMB DEFICIENCIES

CLASSIFICATION

Various classification systems of congenital limb deficiencies have been developed. Greek terminology has been used to describe various deficiencies but is often inaccurate and ambiguous.[16] Frantz and O'Rahilly[24] developed a classification system based on embryologic considerations and the absent skeletal portions. Swanson and colleagues[78] modified that system with a classification system of seven categories based on embryologic failure: (1) Failure of formation of parts (arrest of development), (2) failure of differentiation (separation of parts), (3) duplication, (4) overgrowth, (5) undergrowth (hypoplasia), (6) congenital constriction band syndrome, and (7) generalized skeletal deformities. The

International Society for Prosthetics and Orthotics (ISPO) made additional modifications to this classification system in 1973 and 1989. The classification developed by the ISPO has been published as an international standard, International Standards Organization (ISO) 8548-1:1989, "Method of Describing Limb Deficiencies Present at Birth."[16]

The ISO/ISPO classification of congenital limb deficiency is restricted to skeletal deficiencies described on anatomic and radiologic bases only; Greek terminology, such as *hemimelia* and *phocomelia*, is avoided because of its lack of precision and difficulty of translation into languages that are not related to Greek.[16] Deficiencies are described as transverse or longitudinal. In transverse deficiencies, the limb has developed normally to a particular level beyond which no skeletal elements exist, although digital buds may be present. A transverse deficiency is described by naming the segment in which the limb terminates and then describing the level within the segment beyond which no skeletal elements exist[16] (Figure 13-1).

In longitudinal deficiencies, reduction or absence of an element or elements occurs within the long axis of a limb. Normal skeletal elements may be present distal to the affected bones. A longitudinal deficiency is described by naming the bones affected in a proximal-to-distal sequence and stating whether each affected bone is totally or partially absent[16] (Figure 13-2).

One of the purposes of an international classification system is to provide a common language for accuracy when reporting statistics and research. However, because the ISO/ISPO system does not specifically characterize common clinical manifestations of limb deficiencies, other terminology persists, such as proximal femoral focal deficiency or fibular deficiency, and additional classifications exist to further define this broad spectrum of limb deficiencies. The additional classifications may be radiologically, anatomically, or functionally based and are often developed to guide medical interventions and decision making.

ORIGIN

To fully understand the causes of congenital limb deficiencies, a basic knowledge of embryonic skeletal development is necessary. Limb buds first appear at the end of the fourth week of embryonic development, arising from mesenchymal

385

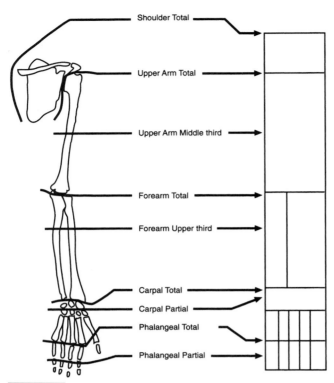

Figure 13-1 Examples of transverse deficiencies at various levels of the upper extremity. (From Day, H. J. [1992]. The ISO/ISPO classification of congenital limb deficiency. In J. H. Bowker, & J. W. Michael [Eds.], *Atlas of limb prosthetics: Surgical, prosthetic, and rehabilitation principles* [2nd ed.; p. 747]. St Louis: Mosby-Year Book.)

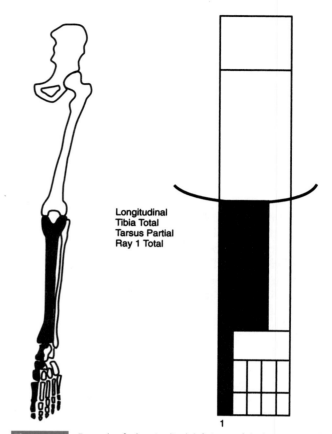

Figure 13-2 Example of a longitudinal deficiency of the lower extremity. (From Day, H. J. [1992]. The ISO/ISPO classification of congenital limb deficiency. In J. H. Bowker, & J. W. Michael [Eds.], *Atlas of limb prosthetics: Surgical, prosthetic, and rehabilitation principles* [2nd ed.; p. 748]. St Louis: Mosby-Year Book.)

tissue. During the next 3 weeks, the limb buds grow and differentiate into identifiable limb segments. Development of limb buds occurs in a proximodistal sequence, with upper limb development preceding lower limb development by several days. The mesenchymal tissue undergoes chondrification to become cartilaginous models of individual bones. By the end of the seventh week, a recognizable embryonic skeleton is present. The entire process of limb development is very complex and involves precise timing of events, which is often signalled by specific genes.[71]

Causative factors for congenital limb deficiencies include genetic, vascular, teratogenic, and amniotic bands, but for many children, the exact cause is unknown. A genetic link may be associated with a few limb anomalies, but most limb deficiencies are the result of sporadic genetic mutation.[40] Limb deficiencies, especially of the upper extremity, may be associated with other congenital anomalies such as Holt-Oram, Fanconi, Poland, thrombocytopenia-absent radius, and VATER syndromes. This association has led to the theory that disruption of the blood supply in the subclavian artery during early embryonic development may be the cause of some congenital limb deficiencies.[85] Several teratogenic factors (e.g., thalidomide, contraceptives, irradiation) have been indicated as possible causative factors for congenital

limb deficiencies but account for only 4% of cases in a study conducted by McGuirk.[50] A recent study by Robitaille et al. found that low maternal intake of riboflavin was associated with transverse limb deficiencies.[68] Teratogenic factors must be present at some time between the third and seventh weeks of embryonic development to produce a limb deficiency. McGuirk[50] reported that the cause of congenital limb deficiencies was unknown in 32% of cases.

LEVELS OF LIMB DEFICIENCY

The incidence of congenital limb deficiencies ranges from 2 to 7 per 10,000 live births. This rate has been relatively unchanged over time but varies slightly across geographic areas.[21] The clinical presentation of a child with a congenital limb deficiency depends on the type, level, and number of deficiencies. Almost any combination or variety of limb deficiency is possible, but some are more common, and these are discussed in this chapter in detail. The upper limb is involved in 58% of congenital limb deficiencies; a longitudinal deficiency of the hand is the most common presentation.

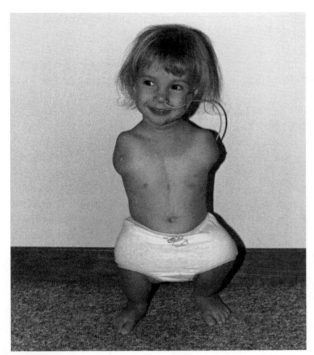

Figure 13-3 Child with multiple congenital limb deficiencies, including bilateral transverse upper arm deficiency and bilateral proximal femoral focal deficiency.

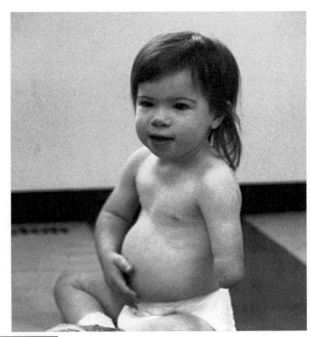

Figure 13-4 Child with congenital transverse forearm or below-elbow limb deficiency.

Approximately 20% of children present with limb deficiencies affecting more than one limb[17] (Figure 13-3).

Most transverse deficiencies are unilateral, with the transverse below-elbow limb deficiency being the most common[89] (Figure 13-4). Rudimentary finger vestiges called *nubbins* may be present. This type of deficiency occurs more frequently in females, with a left-sided predominance of almost 2:1.[72]

A complex lower extremity congenital limb deficiency has been termed *proximal femoral focal deficiency* (PFFD). Aitken[2] first described this deficiency, which includes absence or hypoplasia of the proximal femur with varying degrees of involvement of the acetabulum, femoral head, patella, tibia, and fibula. The deficiency may be unilateral or bilateral. If the deficiency is unilateral, the contralateral limb may exhibit subtle deficiencies such as hypoplasia of the femur that may not be initially recognized. Aitken described four classes of severity—A through D—with class A exhibiting the least involvement based on radiographic findings (Figure 13-5). Gillespie[29] has developed a classification system for PFFD based on the complexity of medical intervention. Children classified into group A may require only limb lengthening, and those in groups B and C may require some level of amputation or revision and prosthetic fitting.

The clinical manifestations of a child with PFFD are relatively consistent among children. They include a shortened thigh that is held in flexion, abduction, and external rotation; hip and knee flexion contracture; and severe leg length

discrepancy, with the foot often at the level of the opposite knee. These children also have instability of the knee joint secondary to absent or deficient cruciate ligaments and a 70% to 80% incidence of total longitudinal deficiency of the fibula. Fifteen percent of children with PFFD have bilateral involvement.[54] The incidence of PFFD is reported to be 1 per 50,000 live births, and it is usually of unknown origin.[54]

ACQUIRED AMPUTATIONS

Acquired amputations account for approximately 40% of childhood amputations. Of these, 70% to 85% can be attributed to trauma.[10] The remainder of acquired amputations in children are the result of disease (most frequently tumors, but also infection and vascular malformations). Ninety percent of acquired amputations involve only one limb, and the lower extremity is involved in 60% of cases.[18]

TRAUMATIC AMPUTATIONS

Males, especially in the adolescent age ranges, account for a larger percentage of traumatic amputations in children.[41,47]

Accidents involving farm machinery and household power tools are the leading cause of acquired amputations in the pediatric population, followed closely by vehicular accidents, gunshot wounds, and railroad accidents.[47] Incidences vary according to age and geographic location. When amputations of the digits are included in the data, the highest incidence of amputations is seen in the fingers of children younger than 2 years of age secondary to closing a door on

TYPE		FEMORAL HEAD	ACETABULUM	FEMORAL SEGMENT	RELATIONSHIP AMONG COMPONENTS OF FEMUR AND ACETABULUM AT SKELETAL MATURITY
A	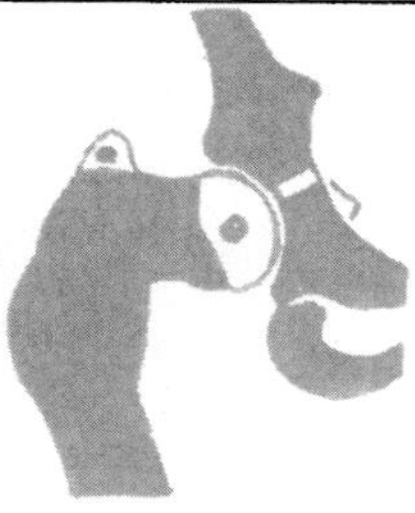	Present	Normal	Short	Bony connection between components of femur Femoral head in acetabulum Subtrochanteric varus angulation, often with pseudarthrosis
B	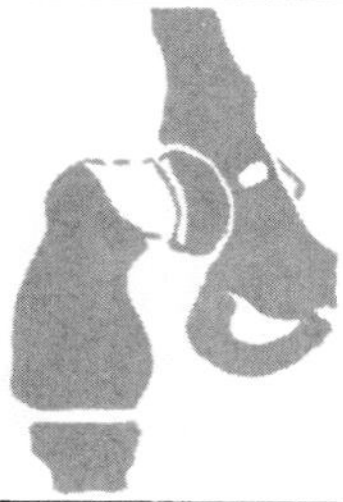	Present	Adequate or moderately dysplastic	Short, usually proximal bony tuft	No osseous connection between head and shaft Femoral head in acetabulum
C	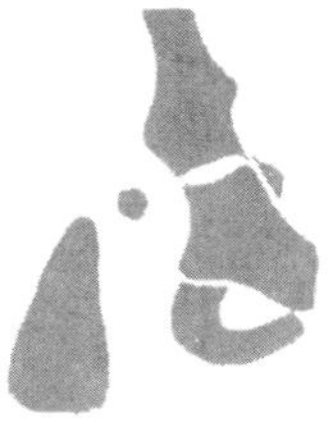	Absent or represented by ossicle	Severely dysplastic	Short, usually proximally tapered	May be osseous connection between shaft and proximal ossicle No articular relation between femur and acetabulum
D	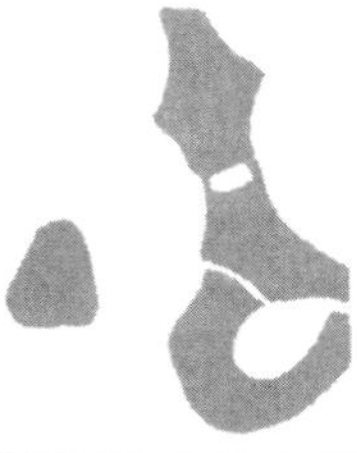	Absent	Absent Obturator foramen enlarged Pelvis squared in bilateral cases	Short, deformed	(none)

Figure 13-5   Aitken classification of proximal femoral focal deficiency. (From Herring, J. A. [Ed.]. [2002]. *Tachdjian's pediatric orthopedics* [3rd ed.; p. 1756]. Philadelphia: WB Saunders.)

the child's finger.[41] Vehicular accidents, farm machinery, gunshot wounds, and trains are more common causes of traumatic amputations in the older child.[47,82] Loder documented a seasonal trend with childhood amputations that could influence community prevention and education programs. It is no surprise that most traumatic amputations occur in the summer, with lawn mower injuries peaking in June, motor vehicle accidents in July, and farm machinery accidents in September.[47]

DISEASE-RELATED AMPUTATIONS

Sarcoma of Bone

Primary bone tumors are rare in children, accounting for only 6% of cancers in children younger than 20 years of age.

Osteosarcoma and Ewing's sarcoma are the most common of the primary bone tumors, with an annual incidence in the United States of 8.7 per million children younger than 20 years of age.[13]

Osteosarcoma

Osteosarcoma is a primary malignant tumor of bone derived from bone-forming mesenchyme in which the malignant proliferating spindle cell stroma produces osteoid tissue or immature bone. The peak incidence of osteosarcoma coincides with the pubertal growth spurt, and it occurs most frequently at the metaphyseal portion of the most rapidly growing bones in adolescence. As a result, the distal femur, proximal tibia, and proximal humerus are the most common sites for osteosarcoma. This finding supports the theory that these rapidly growing cells are susceptible to oncogenic agents or mitotic errors, and that osteosarcoma is the result of an aberration of the normal process of bone growth and remodelling.[46]

Ewing's Sarcoma Family of Tumors

The Ewing's sarcoma family of tumors (ESFT) includes a spectrum of neuroepithelial tumors ranging from the undifferentiated round cell tumor of Ewing's sarcoma of bone (ES) to the neural differentiated peripheral primitive neuroectodermal tumor (PNET). Ewing's tumors often involve both bone and soft tissue by the time of diagnosis, including infiltration into the medullary cavity and bone marrow. Ewing's tumors can occur in both flat and long bones with primary sites almost equally distributed between extremity (53%) and central axis (47%).[30] The most common primary sites are the pelvis, femur, ribs, humerus, and tibia.[33,34] Ewing's sarcoma is also seen during times of peak growth rates, with 50% of new patients diagnosed between 10 and 20 years of age.[30]

Diagnosis

The initial complaint for both osteosarcoma and Ewing's sarcoma is pain at the site of the tumor with or without a palpable mass. Localized swelling or the complaint of a palpable mass is seen with both osteosarcoma and Ewing's sarcoma. Systemic symptoms are rare in osteosarcoma unless widespread metastatic disease is present. On the other hand, systemic symptoms, most commonly fever and weight loss, are complaints with large Ewing's tumors.[38] Because the initial complaint for both osteosarcoma and Ewing's sarcoma is pain at the site of the tumor, diagnosis is often delayed. Children presenting to a physical therapist with a complaint of pain, which is often chronic, a negative history of injury, and no evidence of musculoskeletal abnormalities should be referred for further medical workup to rule out a malignant bone tumor.

The key to diagnosis of a bone tumor is radiologic evaluation. Plain-view radiographs will reveal evidence of a mass and bony destruction; however, a definitive diagnosis is made through biopsy and histologic examination. The extent of the tumor is more precisely defined through magnetic resonance imaging. To complete the workup, a radionuclide bone scan and chest computed tomography are performed to determine the extent of metastasis.[30,46]

MEDICAL MANAGEMENT OF MALIGNANCIES

Medical interventions for children with sarcomas typically include chemotherapy, surgery, and/or radiation therapy. Medical management of bony tumors and neoplasms is based on the following goals: (1) Complete and permanent control of the primary tumor, (2) control and prevention of microstatic and metastatic disease, and (3) preservation of

function to the greatest degree possible. Local control of the primary tumor is most often achieved through surgery and radiation therapy. Surgical options include amputation and limb-sparing procedures. The choice of surgical procedure depends on location and size of the tumor, extramedullary extent, presence or absence of metastatic disease, and the child's age, skeletal development, and lifestyle. Control of microstatic and metastatic disease is achieved through radiation therapy and chemotherapy.

Radiation Therapy

Osteosarcoma is generally unresponsive to radiation therapy. Osteosarcoma cells seem to repair themselves after radiation injury, whereas Ewing's sarcoma is highly responsive to radiation therapy.[46] Local control of Ewing's sarcoma may be achieved with moderately high doses of radiation directed at the local tumor; however, whole bone radiation is often recommended for tumors larger than 8 cm.[33]

The side effects of radiation therapy are related to tumor location, dose rate and duration, age of the patient, and use of chemotherapy. Acute side effects are seen in rapidly dividing tissues such as the skin, bone marrow, and gut. Common side effects are red and tender skin, mouth sores from irradiation to mucous membranes, and nausea and vomiting from irradiation to the abdomen.[79] Children receiving radiation therapy may exhibit a decreased activity level secondary to nausea and vomiting, poor appetite secondary to mouth sores, and generalized malaise. Their physical therapy sessions may need to be altered on a daily basis to accommodate their changing energy levels. Children wearing prostheses must be monitored closely for skin irritation and breakdown.

Late side effects of radiation include fibrosis of soft tissues, bony changes ranging from osteoporosis to fractures, and growth disturbances, including damage to the epiphyseal plate and bowing of the metaphysis. Butler and colleagues[12] reported that 77% of patients with Ewing's sarcoma who received radiation therapy developed a leg length discrepancy; in 58% of these patients, the leg length discrepancy was significant enough to require treatment. If possible, attempts are made to shield the epiphyseal plate at the opposite end of the involved bone to minimize radiation-linked growth retardation and still allow for some growth of the extremity. For some young children, an amputation may produce a more functional extremity than an extremity that is significantly shortened as a result of radiation therapy.

Chemotherapy

Chemotherapy is administered according to several principles, including the use of multiple drug combinations, administration of chemotherapy agents at maximally tolerated doses, and administration before the development of detectable micrometastatic disease (adjuvant chemotherapy). Most chemotherapy agents interfere with the function of DNA and RNA. However, these agents are nonselective and cause damage to both malignant and normal cells, resulting in undesirable and at times toxic side effects. Physical therapists working with children receiving chemotherapy should know the specific agents being used with the child and the side effects. Typical side effects of chemotherapy can include nausea and vomiting, hair loss, diarrhea, and constipation. Other potential side effects consist of blood-related concerns such as anemia, neutropenia, and thrombocytopenia or neurologic issues such as peripheral neuropathies. The physical therapy interventions may need to be altered or limited depending on the child's status and development of potentially serious side effects.[74]

Adjuvant chemotherapy, given preoperatively and postsurgically, has increased the survival rates for both osteosarcoma and Ewing's sarcoma. Survival rates are dependent upon age, location of the tumor, and the presence and location of metastatic disease at the time of diagnosis. Five-year event-free survival (EFS) rates for children with Ewing's sarcoma treated with a combination of radiation therapy, chemotherapy, and surgery have improved to 64% to 69% for patients with nonmetastatic disease. Overall survival rates for children with osteosarcoma treated with a combination of surgery and chemotherapy have also drastically improved from 20% in the 1970's to 60% to 65% more recently. Children with nonmetastatic osteosarcoma of the extremity are more likely to have a favorable outcome than children with more proximal tumors and the presence of metastatic disease.[32,52]

SURGICAL OPTIONS IN THE MANAGEMENT OF ACQUIRED AND CONGENITAL LIMB DEFICIENCIES

The goal of any surgical intervention is to improve the function of the child and, in the case of bone sarcoma, to not alter the child's chance of survival. Traditionally, amputation has been the typical approach for children with bone sarcoma. It has also been used to modify the lower extremities of children with congenital limb deficiencies for improved prosthetic fit and function. However, with improved survival rates of children with bone tumors, the long-term function and comfort of the child must also be considered. Limb-sparing procedures, including rotationplasty, are viable options for many children with congenital limb deficiencies and for those previously considered to be candidates for amputation secondary to a bone tumor. Each of these procedures offers advantages and disadvantages, and functional outcome, psychological impact, and long-term survival all must be considered in the surgical decision. This section discusses the surgical options of amputation, rotationplasty, and various limb-sparing procedures for children with congenital limb deficiencies, as well as those with a diagnosis of bone sarcoma.

AMPUTATION AS A GENERAL SURGICAL OPTION

Although most of the basic premises related to management of adults with amputations apply to children, important differences may be noted. First, skeletal immaturity and future growth are important factors when surgical alternatives are considered. Physes should be preserved whenever possible to ensure continued growth of the limb. For the upper extremity, most growth occurs in physes around the shoulder and wrist, whereas in the lower extremity the physes around the knee account for most of the growth.[39] If an amputation will result in a significant leg length difference, a limb-sparing procedure may offer better function and improved cosmesis for the child.

Second, the fact that amputation through long bones may result in terminal overgrowth is an important point that should not be overlooked. Terminal or bony overgrowth is a painful, spikelike prominence of new growth on the transected end of the residual limb. Significant pain can interfere with weight bearing and wearing of the prosthesis. The spikelike growth is not the result of growth from the proximal epiphysis but rather represents osteogenic activity of the periosteum.[28] Terminal overgrowth occurs most frequently in the humerus and fibula but is also seen in the tibia and femur. Surgical options include revisions and bone capping. The possibility of terminal overgrowth should not be a reason to elect higher-level amputation, such as a knee disarticulation rather than a below-knee amputation. As in adults, length of the lever arm, function of the extremity, and prosthetic fit remain important considerations when deciding on the level of amputation. Saving the child's life is, of course, the most important consideration, whether the amputation is the result of a malignancy or trauma.

Finally, wound healing in children is rarely a concern as it may be in adults with peripheral vascular disease. Skin grafts therefore may be used to close the amputation site in preference to performing a higher-level amputation for a child with a traumatic injury.

AMPUTATION TO REVISE CONGENITAL LIMB DEFICIENCIES TO IMPROVE FUNCTION

Amputation is rarely necessary with upper extremity limb deficiencies but may be indicated for some children with lower extremity limb deficiencies. Children with bilateral PFFD, however, may be more functional without any surgery. They will be of short stature but will walk quite well.[54] For cosmesis, extension prostheses may be an option.

The surgical treatment of a child with unilateral PFFD is case-specific. If the child has a stable hip and foot and a significant portion of normal femur is present, one of the limb-lengthening procedures may be appropriate. Most surgeons agree that 60% of predicted femoral length must be present for a lengthening procedure to be a viable alternative.[28,40] If limb lengthening is not an option, one of the surgical options for PFFD is a knee arthrodesis and foot amputation. Usually the Syme or Boyd amputation of the foot is recommended. A Syme amputation involves complete removal of the foot, including the calcaneus, but the Boyd amputation preserves the calcaneus. The Boyd procedure requires an arthrodesis of the calcaneus and the tibia, which adds length to the limb.[54] The knee is usually fused to form one long bone for fitting of an above-knee prosthesis[40,54] (Figure 13-6).

Amputation may also be an option for a child with a longitudinal tibial or fibular total deficiency in which a significant limb length difference exists along with deformity of the foot. Frequently, the foot is positioned in equinovarus or equinovalgus with absent rays. If the tibia is completely absent, a knee disarticulation and fitting with a prosthesis will provide a very functional lower extremity for the child. If the leg length difference is too significant for limb-lengthening techniques or epiphysiodesis of the uninvolved leg, or if the ankle is significantly unstable, a Syme or Boyd amputation may lead to a more functional lower extremity with the addition of a prosthesis for a child with partial absence of the fibula. When an amputation is being considered for a child, it is important that alternatives are discussed with the family and child, and that the ultimate lifestyle goals are known.

AMPUTATION IN THE MANAGEMENT OF TRAUMATIC INJURIES AND MALIGNANT TUMORS

Amputations secondary to trauma may result in a short residual limb if the child has significant growth remaining. This is especially true of an above-knee amputation in which the distal physes around the knee have been resected. It may be possible to increase the length of a residual limb in older children by using one of the limb-lengthening techniques (see Chapter 14). Lengthening of a short residual limb may increase the efficiency of gait and promote a better prosthetic fit.[20]

The traditional approach for malignant bone tumors has been amputation of the limb in which the tumor is found. The surgical margin for an amputation is usually 6 to 7 cm above the most proximal medullary extent of tumor as defined by magnetic resonance imaging. This level of surgical margin allows for removal of microscopic tumor and skip lesions, while allowing for the greatest amount of residual limb length for the individual. Local recurrence rates using this level of surgical margin are less than 5%.[46]

For those tumor sites that are in the proximal humerus or femur, amputation results in severe loss of function. For example, a tumor of the proximal humerus treated by amputation would leave the patient with severely diminished function as a result of loss of the hand. Therefore most surgeons elect not to perform an amputation, if possible, for

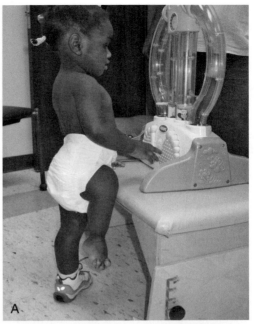

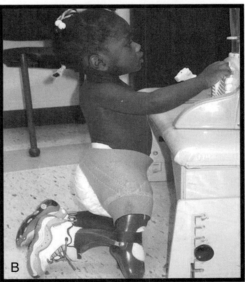

Figure 13-6 **A,** Child with unilateral proximal femoral focal deficiency (PFFD) without any surgical modifications to her leg. **B,** Same child wearing a prosthesis to equalize limb lengths for weight bearing. Initial surgery has not yet occurred.

tumors of the upper extremity. Amputation for tumors of the pelvis or proximal femur also results in complete loss of the limb or a very short residual limb, which makes functional ambulation with a prosthesis difficult. Limb-sparing procedures may result in a more functional extremity than a proximal amputation without decreasing the expected rate of survival for the child. The decision regarding an amputation is based on expectations regarding control of the primary tumor, survival of the child, and functional use of the extremity.

ROTATIONPLASTY

Rotationplasty, or a turnabout procedure, is a typical option for children with congenital limb deficiencies, specifically PFFD, as well as for those with bony tumors of the proximal tibia or distal femur. This procedure involves excision of the distal femur and proximal tibia; 180° rotation of the residual lower limb, including the distal femur and proximal tibia, ankle joint, foot, and neurovascular supply; and reattachment to the proximal femur (Figure 13-7). The ankle then functions as a knee joint, with ankle plantar flexion used to extend the "knee," and ankle dorsiflexion to flex the "knee"[45] (Figure 13-8). Rotationplasty requires a functioning hip joint and ankle joint. In the case of malignant tumors, the tumor cannot have invaded the surrounding soft tissue, especially the neurovascular supply. For children with PFFD, the residual foot must be normal with minimal alignment problems for a rotationplasty to be a functional surgical option. If the fibula is absent, alignment of the foot may not be adequate for a successful rotationplasty.

The advantages of a rotationplasty include increased limb length, improved prosthetic function with the ankle serving as a knee joint, improved weight-bearing capacity, and elimination of the problems of terminal overgrowth and pain from neuromas or phantom limb sensations.[44] Weight is borne through the heel, which is more suitable for weight bearing than the end of a residual limb. Rotationplasty also allows for some growth of the leg. With an appropriate

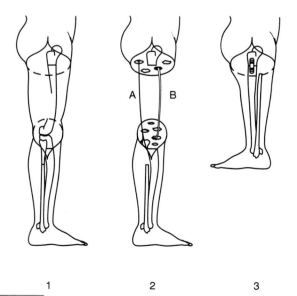

Figure 13-7 A schematic illustration of a rotationplasty procedure. Neurovascular structures (**A** and **B**) are left intact and are wrapped into the existing space when the tibia is reattached to the femur.

prosthesis, children who have had a rotationplasty procedure can run, jump, and play with their peers.

Disadvantages are cosmesis and derotation of the foot. Critics of rotationplasty cite poor cosmesis and psychological issues as a deterrent to the procedure. In my experience with children who underwent a rotationplasty for a tumor or for congenital PFFD, cosmesis was not a complaint from the child or the child's parents. Krajbich and Bochmann[44] cite their experience of 27 children with osteosarcoma who underwent a rotationplasty. Twenty-two of these children are alive with no evidence of metastatic disease. No long-term complications related to cosmesis and psychological decompensation were reported; in fact, virtually all of the children with a rotationplasty now actively participate in sports and other activities with their peers. When a rotationplasty is being considered as a surgical option, it may be helpful for parents and the child to meet another child who has had the rotationplasty performed. Certainly, the cosmetic disadvantages must be discussed. Additional studies have shown that children with PFFD who underwent a rotationplasty demonstrated a higher walking speed with less oxygen consumption and fewer compensatory gait deviations than children who underwent a foot amputation and foot and knee arthrodesis.[23,57]

When the procedure is performed on young children, derotation of the foot may occur, requiring re-rotation of the limb. The limb may derotate secondary to the spiral pull of the muscles proximal and distal to the osteotomy.[40] Both Krajbich[45] and Gillespie[28] discussed surgical options to limit derotation of the limb after a rotationplasty. Derotation is more common in children younger than 10 years of age and is most frequently seen in children when a rotationplasty is performed at 3 or 4 years of age.[28] Concern has also been raised about the long-term consequences of the altered weight bearing on the ankle joint. A study by Akahane[4] assessed 21 patients at a mean follow-up of 13.5 years post rotationplasty and found no evidence at that point of joint arthrodesis or degenerative joint changes.

LIMB-SPARING PROCEDURES

With the use of chemotherapy, improvements in diagnostic imaging to determine tumor margins, and new techniques of reconstruction, amputation is not always the treatment of choice for children with bony malignancies. Limb-sparing or limb-salvage procedures may be an alternative to amputation for some children with malignant bone tumors. Limb-sparing procedures involve resection of the tumor and reconstruction of the limb to preserve function without amputation of the limb. Reconstruction of the limb may include excision of bone without replacement of the excised area or replacement with an allograft or endoprosthetic implant.

Appropriate selection of children for limb-sparing surgery is critical. The goal of saving the limb should never

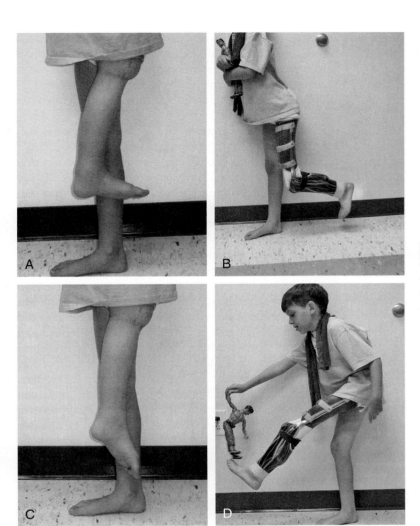

Figure 13-8 An 11-year-old boy who underwent a rotationplasty procedure. **A,** Ankle dorsiflexion. **B,** Ankle dorsiflexion produces prosthetic knee flexion. **C,** Ankle plantar flexion. **D,** Ankle plantar flexion produces prosthetic knee extension.

compromise the goal of removing all gross and microscopic tumor.[46] Limb-sparing surgery is contraindicated if the tumor has invaded the surrounding soft tissue to a large extent, if it involves the neurovascular supply, or if the tumor has invaded the intramedullary cavity.[46] In addition, limb-sparing surgery for the lower extremity of a young child may not be beneficial when the child is skeletally immature and may be left with a severe leg length discrepancy and a nonfunctional lower extremity. In these cases, amputation may be a better choice than limb-sparing surgery.

Autologous grafts are rarely appropriate because long segments of bone usually must be excised. Replacement of the excised bone with a near-equal length of noninvolved bone from another portion of the body often is not possible. Cadaver osteoarticular allografts are another option. They involve resection of the tumor and surrounding bone and implantation of a section of cadaver bone. Osteoarticular allografts can preserve some growth plates, especially those of the distal femur and proximal tibia, if the tumor resection involves the proximal femur. The grafts are stabilized with

plates or intramedullary rods until osteosynthesis has occurred. Once osteosynthesis has occurred and the child's bone has formed a latticework within the implanted bone, the graft is very stable and does not loosen over time.[46] In addition, osteoarticular allografts have fewer complications (infections, nonunion, and fractures) over time than metallic endoprosthetic implants. Infections and nonunions are early-onset complications that are seen with greater frequency in children receiving chemotherapy. When fractures occur, they are typically seen later, occurring 3 to 8 years after the procedure. Nonunions and significant infections are serious complications that can ultimately lead to an amputation. Allografts are a viable surgical alternative for children nearing skeletal maturity or for those children requiring only excision of a portion of the shaft of the bone. For a child who is skeletally immature, the implanted bone can be cut 1 to 2 cm longer than the portion removed to accommodate some growth. As is true with most limb-sparing procedures, high-intensity activities such as athletic participation are limited for the child with an osteoarticular allograft.

At times a tumor may be excised without replacing the excised bone. The proximal fibula may be resected if the soft tissue involvement is minimal and the peroneal nerve is not included in the soft tissue involvement. The biceps femoris tendon and the fibular collateral ligament are reattached to the lateral condyle of the tibia.[39] After healing, full knee motion and a normal gait pattern can be expected. The Tikhoff-Linberg procedure has been successfully used for tumors involving the proximal humerus when the brachial plexus is not included in the soft tissue involvement. With this procedure, the proximal humerus is excised and is not replaced. The remaining muscles of the upper arm are reattached to the trapezius and pectoralis muscles to suspend the remaining portion of the humerus.[75] The shoulder is unstable, but the elbow and hand are functional. Endoprosthetic devices may be implanted to provide stability and function to the shoulder. In either case, the functional outcome is superior to that following amputation of the entire upper extremity.

Endoprosthetic devices are ultimately an extension of joint arthroplasty procedures. These manufactured devices consist of modular components that are implanted in the area of the excised bone such as the proximal humerus, elbow, proximal and distal femur, and proximal tibia. Potential problems include infection and mechanical issues such as loosening of the prosthesis and mechanical failure of the device.[83] Children and adolescents may be very active, and this may create vigorous stresses on prosthetic implants that lead to failure and the need for replacement of the devices over time. Implants may not be appropriate for the young, skeletally immature child because these devices are limited in the amount of growth that can be accommodated.

Endoprosthetic designs often incorporate a telescoping unit that can be expanded to accommodate growth. Expansion of the prosthesis typically involves a surgical procedure at periodic intervals. Complications of expansion include loosening of the prosthesis, infection after lengthening procedures, mechanical failure, and fracture. The need for repeat surgical procedures to expand or grow the device is costly and inconvenient for the child, and the risk for infection is increased with each procedure. Some clinics have begun using an endoprosthesis that can be expanded with the use of an external electromagnetic field. Exposure of the limb to the electromagnetic field unlocks an energy-stored spring and allows for controlled lengthening without a surgical procedure.[88] Preliminary studies are showing decreased rates of infection and more frequent but smaller adjustments in length that are less disruptive to gait and possible range of motion (ROM) complications.[7,56]

A review by Eckardt and colleagues[19] of 32 patients with expandable prostheses included patients ranging from 3 to 15 years of age. Fourteen of the 32 patients had no complications. Eighteen patients had 27 complications, including infection, loosening of the device, mechanical failure, fracture, knee flexion contracture, and prosthetic shoulder joint

subluxation, and one patient died of a pulmonary embolism. The authors stressed the need for strong family participation during rehabilitation to avoid knee flexion contractures in skeletally immature patients.[19] Effective growth of the child's limb of 7 to 9 cm with the use of an endoprosthetic device has been reported.[19]

Several studies have reported comparable long-term survival rates between groups undergoing amputation versus a limb-sparing procedure.[69] Limb-sparing procedures may also result in improved function, but these procedures are plagued by higher complication rates than are seen in amputation surgery.[46,66]

Limb-sparing surgery is as effective in controlling the tumor as amputation when adjuvant chemotherapy is used, and when particular attention is given to patient selection, surgical margins, and surgical techniques. A limb-sparing procedure involving the distal femur and/or proximal tibia may result in a significant leg length difference in a child 10 years of age or younger because growth will be lost with excision of the growth plates around the knee. Futani and colleagues[25] retrospectively assessed 40 children younger than 11 years who underwent a limb-sparing procedure secondary to a bone sarcoma. They determined that a limb-sparing procedure could provide good functional outcomes in this younger population. The authors did caution that the functional outcome often was the result of multiple procedures and revisions, including limb lengthenings for expandable prostheses.[25] A long-term complication of lower extremity limb-sparing procedures is reduced ROM, especially at the knee.[11] The range of motion deficits, specifically at the hip and knee, that are frequently seen after a limb-sparing procedure are correlated with deficits in mobility.[49] Children with knee flexion range of motion deficits exhibited greater difficulty with timed up and down stairs, timed up and go, and a 9-minute run-walk distance.

Lifestyle of the child is another important presurgical consideration because many limb-sparing procedures such as osteoarticular allografts and endoprosthetic implants will limit participation in competitive physical activities. Limb-sparing procedures for the upper extremity clearly result in improved function for the patient when compared with amputation and use of a prosthesis. Limb-sparing procedures such as rotationplasty and limb lengthening are increasingly used with children with congenital limb deficiencies to avoid an amputation and often result in excellent function for the child.

COMPARISON OF SURGICAL OPTIONS

With improved survival rates of children with bone sarcomas since the 1970's and the increased use of limb-sparing procedures, it is important to assess the functional outcomes of the various surgical options and to understand the role of physical therapy in successful rehabilitation of these children. Limb-sparing procedures were developed to provide alternatives that spare the child's limb and minimize the functional limitations associated with high-level amputations. However, most of the outcome studies have not demonstrated the marked advantage of limb-sparing procedures that was expected because of some of the complications associated with these procedures.

To compare outcomes, it is best to differentiate between below- and above-knee amputations, as well as between femur and tibia limb-sparing procedures. Ginsberg et al.[31] compared functional outcomes and quality of life among children who had an amputation, limb-sparing, or rotation-plasty procedure. They utilized a newer assessment tool, the Functional Mobility Assessment (FMA), which measures pain, timed up and down stairs, timed up and go, use of ambulation supports, satisfaction of walking quality, participation in work and sports, and endurance.[48] Adolescents and young adults who underwent a femur limb-sparing surgery scored significantly higher on the FMA than those who had an above-knee amputation. However, those who underwent a below-knee amputation scored higher on quality of life measures than those patients who had a limb-sparing procedure of the tibia. Pardasaney[58] and colleagues found that individuals who had undergone an above-knee amputation used an assistive device and walked with a limp more frequently and had higher anxiety levels than those had a femur limb-sparing procedure. However, employment status and ability to participate in sports were not significantly different between the two groups. Researchers also reported that no significant physical functioning or psychological differences were noted between individuals who had a below-knee amputation and those who had a tibia limb-sparing procedure.

LIMB REPLANTATION

For children with traumatic amputations, limb replantation may be a surgical option. As with other surgical options, the goal of replantation is directed not only at preserving the amputated limb but also at restoring pain-free function to the extremity that is superior to the function obtained with a prosthesis. For an upper extremity replantation to be considered successful, function of the elbow and hand and distal sensation must be restored. Replantation of a lower extremity must provide a painless, sensate extremity capable of bearing weight during normal daily activities.[8]

Distal replantations of an upper extremity usually result in a more favorable outcome than proximal replantations. Proximal replantations are often associated with a violent mechanism of injury that results in damage to the nerves, blood vessels, and muscles. A proximal replantation also necessitates a longer distance for the nerves to regenerate for functional use of the hand. Children often achieve better functional results than adults with upper extremity limb replantation, making limb replantation a viable surgical option for some children.[9]

Physical therapy is indicated for these children for wound care, control of edema, joint ROM, strengthening, gait training, and self-care activities. Rehabilitation will include close communication with the physician regarding precautions and progression of activities and family instruction while the child is in the hospital and is treated as an outpatient.

OSSEOINTEGRATION

Osseointegration is the direct attachment of a prosthesis to the end of the bone of the residual limb. The prosthesis attaches to an abutment that has been surgically attached to the bone and protrudes through the skin. The concept of directly attaching a prosthesis to the bone is not new, but the technology to enable the interface of a foreign material with the bone and yet protrude through the skin has expanded the clinical application of this technique. Osseointegration is a long process that requires multiple surgical procedures. The first surgical stage involves the implant of a threaded cylinder directly into the end of the residual bone. At least 6 months later, a metal abutment is threaded onto the existing cylinder at the second surgical stage. The metal abutment protrudes through the skin at the distal end of the residual limb and will eventually receive the prosthesis. During the last but lengthy stage, weight-bearing loads on the abutment are gradually increased through the use of a temporary and then a permanent prosthesis. To allow for secure integration of the abutment with the skeleton, this last stage of gradually increasing weight-bearing loads can take well over a year.[59,67]

The purported advantages of osseointegration are the elimination of a socket and the inherent problems associated with poorly fitting sockets and suspension methods. Because the prosthesis is directly attached to the bone through the abutment, some sensation is preserved such as the ability to perceive stepping on a stone or an uneven surface.[59] This procedure is still in its infancy stages and is not indicated at this time for children or adolescents who are skeletally immature.

PHANTOM LIMB SENSATIONS

Phantom limb sensations are an occurrence in many adults with amputations, but fewer reports are available concerning children with phantom limb sensations. Some persons may believe that if young children do not complain of phantom limb pain, they therefore must not have any pain. Simmel[73] reported that the incidence of phantom limb sensations increases with the age of the child, such that all children older than 8 years of age reported some degree of phantom limb sensation. Melzack and colleagues[51] reported that 20% of individuals with a congenital limb deficiency and 50% of those with an acquired amputation before 6 years of age experienced phantom limb sensations. However, most of the individuals reporting phantom limb sensations reported not

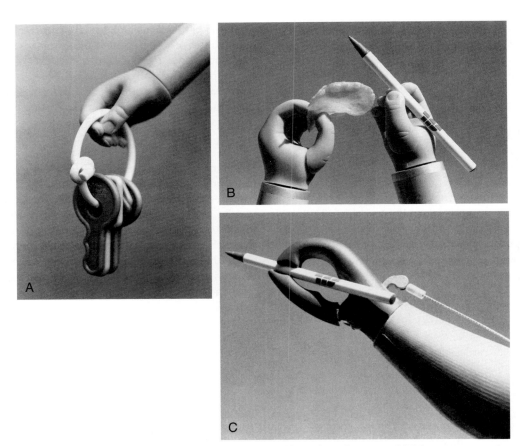

Figure 13-9 Terminal device options: **A,** Passive Infant Alpha Hand (TRS, Boulder, CO). **B,** L'IL E-Z Hand (TRS) promotes grasping when the thumb is moved. **C,** ADEPT voluntary closing hand (TRS).

pain, but rather the perceived ability to voluntarily move the phantom limb.[51]

The phantom limb sensations and pain of adolescents can become intense. If left untreated, phantom limb sensations can become debilitating and interfere with prosthetic wear and daily activities. Some teenagers are able to control the sensations through rubbing or massaging the uninvolved limb at similar points to those in which they are experiencing the phantom limb sensations of the amputated limb. Others feel more in control by keeping a daily log of their sensations and reporting the pain intensity on one of a variety of pain scales. For some adolescents, the use of analgesics may be beneficial. If available, a referral to a pain management team should be instituted for children undergoing amputations.

OVERVIEW OF PROSTHETICS

UPPER EXTREMITY PROSTHETICS

Upper extremity prosthetic systems may be body powered or externally powered. Externally powered prosthetic devices are typically referred to as myoelectric devices. Body-powered components include a terminal device, a wrist unit,

possibly an elbow unit, and a socket, and are operated by a harness and cable system. With a myoelectric system, a muscle contraction by the child activates an electrode inside the shaft of the device, which generates electrically controlled movement of the terminal device, wrist, or elbow. Children may also utilize a prosthesis that is a combination of body-powered and externally powered components. For example, the child may operate the elbow using a body-powered cable system and operate the hand with a myoelectric system.[22]

Terminal devices range from the passive hand or fist to a myoelectric hand. Terminal devices often used in pediatrics include the passive fist or hand, the CAPP (Child Amputee Prosthetics Project [Hosmer Dorrance, Campbell, CA]), various hooks, including the Dorrance and ADEPT (Anatomically Designed-Engineered Polymer Technology [Therapeutic Recreation Systems, Boulder, CO]) models, and myoelectric hands such as the Otto Bock Electrohand (Otto Bock Orthopedic, Plymouth, MN) and the New York Mechanical Hand (Hosmer Dorrance) (Figure 13-9). The child's age and size, as well as the parents' and child's desires and functional goals, determine the appropriate terminal device. The wrist unit allows forearm pronation and supination and accommodates the terminal device.

As a child's activities change, different terminal devices may be needed. Various recreational terminal devices are available to allow participation in a variety of sports activities.[15,22] Teenagers may desire a cosmetic hand for social activities and a functional terminal device for daily activities.

Suspension systems generally fall into two categories. The first is a harnessed system that is used to suspend a prosthesis or to control a terminal device. Both above-elbow and below-elbow amputation levels can use this type of suspension. The figure eight and the chest strap are two harness configurations that can be used to suspend and/or control a terminal device.

The figure eight harness and chest strap fit over the shoulder of the involved limb and around the chest to secure the prosthesis without limiting shoulder movement. The figure eight harness securely anchors the prosthesis, so the child may activate the cable system of an above-elbow prosthesis. Self-suspending sockets are available for young children. A simple self-suspending socket may be all that is necessary to suspend a below-elbow prosthesis of an infant or toddler. If additional suspension is required, a small silicone sleeve can be rolled over the prosthesis and onto the humeral area. This affords added suspension without any additional restriction of movement. When the cable for the terminal device is added to the prosthesis, a triceps pad or cuff to secure the cable can be incorporated. A shoulder disarticulation prosthesis is secured with a chest strap. A prosthesis at this level is often very difficult to fit and now is most commonly restricted to myoelectric or hybrid control.

With recent developments in upper extremity research, an increasing number of options are becoming available to the child amputee. Electrodes embedded into silicone liners allow the prosthesis to be both self-suspending and myoelectrically controlled. Recent technological enhancements to electrodes now allow the fitting of children with heavy scarring or weak signal strength so they can benefit from a myo-controlled prosthesis.

LOWER EXTREMITY PROSTHETICS

The fact that children are growing and may be facing several surgical interventions makes fitting a child with a prosthesis very different from fitting an adult with a prosthesis. In addition, angular deformities associated with various congenital deficiencies result in gait and alignment challenges not generally seen in the adult traumatic population. Consequently, many prosthetists will fit a child with a prosthesis that accommodates some growth, stage the introduction of components, and utilize components that can be replaced as the child grows. The variety of components available to the pediatric population continues to expand but does not yet compare with the wide variety available for the adolescent or adult population.

The SACH (Solid Ankle Cushion Heel [Otto Bock Orthopedic]) foot has long been the mainstay for pediatric prosthetic feet and continues, in various forms, to be used for young toddlers. The L'IL foot (TRS Industries, Fargo, ND) is a variation of the SACH foot. The entire foot is made of a more flexible plastic that allows a better response during kneeling and pulling to stand. However, young children can now be fitted with dynamic response or energy storing feet (Figure 13-10). In two separate retrospective analyses, Anderson found that parents and children preferred the cosmetic appearance of dynamic response feet and stated that these feet improved their child's endurance and possibly stability.[3]

The shank of a lower extremity prosthesis has either an exoskeletal or an endoskeletal design. Exoskeletal shanks are fabricated of a rigid polyurethane foam and are laminated to form a hard outer covering. Endoskeletal shanks consist of a pylon made of ultralight material, such as graphite or titanium, and covered with foam. Teenagers often prefer endoskeletal shanks because of their cosmesis and decreased weight. The durability of exoskeletal shanks is often more appropriate for the younger child. Exoskeletal shanks can then be finished with various patterns or designs that are appropriate for the younger amputee.

A wider variety of prosthetic knees are now available for the pediatric population, including toddlers just beginning to pull to stand. A single-axis constant-friction knee is set to function at a certain walking speed. If the speed of walking increases, the prosthesis lags behind because the shank cannot swing through as quickly as the uninvolved limb. In addition, this type of knee is not very stable and buckles quickly if the ground reaction force is not anterior to the knee joint.[53] When the young toddler who is only beginning to stand is fitted, the socket is aligned anterior to the knee center to increase stability. Another type of knee joint available for the pediatric population is a polycentric knee with a four-bar linkage mechanism (Figure 13-11). A polycentric knee mimics the anatomic knee joint to increase stability. The axis of motion is posterior during stance to provide added stability and anterior during swing to shorten the shank and assist with clearance. A lower extremity prosthesis with a polycentric knee is shown in Figure 13-12. Polycentric knees are now available for use with toddlers, leading some centers to incorporate a prosthetic knee into a child's first prosthesis.

A larger variety of knee units are available for teenagers, including hydraulic, pneumatic, and microprocessor-controlled knees. Hydraulic and pneumatic knee units are variable-friction units that allow variable walking and running speeds. Variable-friction units are equipped with a swing control mechanism that sets the drag of the shank through swing phase and a stance control unit that permits knee flexion during stance without collapse of the leg. Swing and stance control mechanisms are excellent options for active teenagers, especially those engaged in physical

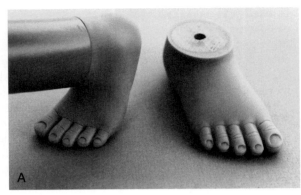

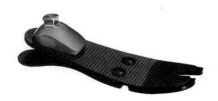

B

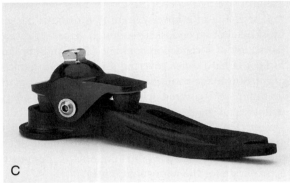

C

Figure 13-10 Prosthetic feet options: **A,** Little Feet (TRS, Boulder, CO). **B,** Flex-Foot Junior (Össur Americas, Foothill Ranch, CA). **C,** TruPer Foot (College Park Industries, Fraser, MI). (**B,** Photo courtesy Össur of North America.)

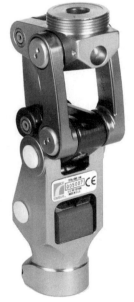

Figure 13-11 Total Knee Junior (Össur Americas, Foothill Ranch, CA) is a polycentric knee that provides stability and aids in the initiation of a smooth gait pattern. (Photo courtesy Össur of North America.)

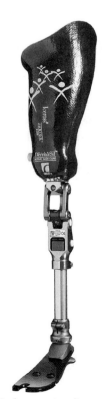

Figure 13-12 Pediatric lower extremity prosthetic system, including socket, Total Knee Junior (Össur Americas, Foothill Ranch, CA), and Flex-Foot Junior (Össur). (Photo courtesy Össur of North America.)

activities. Drawbacks of hydraulic and pneumatic knees are the added weight to the prosthesis, cost, and the intricacy of adjustments. Recent advances in technology have reduced the size and weight of hydraulic systems, resulting in a more functional option for the child amputee.

Like adult sockets, pediatric socket design has changed over the past 15 years. Children with a transfemoral amputation can be fitted with a narrowed medial-lateral ischial containment socket or an anatomically correct socket design. The narrowed medial-lateral socket with ischial containment more evenly distributes weight-bearing pressures and allows less lateral movement of the distal femur, thereby providing greater stability during stance. Adolescents with a below-knee or transtibial amputation may be fitted with the standard patellar-tendon-bearing socket or total surface-bearing design. However, younger children may require a supracondylar socket that offers greater suspension. Because most congenital deficiencies result in disarticulations, the Syme prosthesis is the most common lower extremity socket design in the pediatric population. The bulbous end present in most Syme revisions allows for a suspension point just proximal to the distal end. The bladder or segmented socket design is then used to increase independence and eliminate additional suspension systems. These designs are often referred to as self suspending.

Infants and toddlers will require some type of suspension to secure their prosthesis. A Silesian belt or total elastic suspension (TES) belt works well for younger children with an above-knee amputation or PFFD, and preschoolers can become independent in their use (Figure 13-13). Neoprene sleeves and silicone liners with a locking mechanism are additional suspension methods commonly used with young children. The silicone liner is rolled on the residual limb, and the pin on the end of the sleeve is threaded into the prosthesis and locked in place. To remove the prosthesis, the pin is released by pushing a button on the distal end of the socket[15] (Figure 13-14).

Suction sockets are appropriate for the older child who is not growing rapidly or is undergoing weight fluctuations secondary to chemotherapy treatment. Suction sockets utilize negative pressure as air is expelled through a distal valve and surface tension between the skin and socket to maintain the suspension.[15]

Children with a rotationplasty use a prosthesis that incorporates the plantarflexed foot in the socket. The socket is essentially a below-knee socket with a thigh cuff attachment and external hinges for the knee joint. A Silesian or TES belt may be needed for suspension.

Children of all ages with a limb deficiency or amputation should be encouraged to participate in activities with their peers. Many children may want to participate in sports at a recreational or a competitive level (Figure 13-15). Many prosthetic options are available that promote participation in various sports. Recreational prosthetics options are too numerous to mention for this discussion, and the reader is

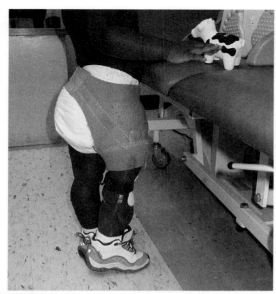

Figure 13-13 Toddler with a right proximal femoral focal deficiency fitted with a prosthesis before any surgical procedures were performed to modify her leg. A Neoprene total elastic suspension belt is used as the suspension method to secure the prosthesis.

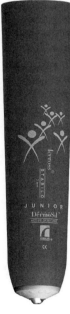

Figure 13-14 Suspension systems may utilize a silicone liner that is rolled onto the residual limb and attached to the distal end of the socket with a pin-locking mechanism.

referred to other resources.[64] Ultimately, any prosthesis for a child must have some cosmetic appeal and be more functional than the limb without a prosthesis (Figure 13-16). Decision making for infants' and toddlers' prosthetic needs should include the parents, orthopedist, prosthetist, and physical therapist. The older child should be included in the decision-making process.

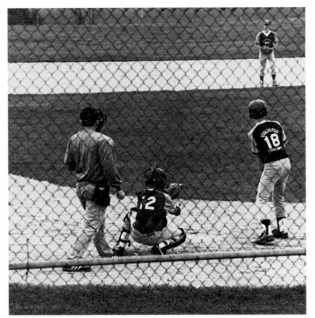

Figure 13-15 Catcher is an adolescent with a left below-knee amputation.

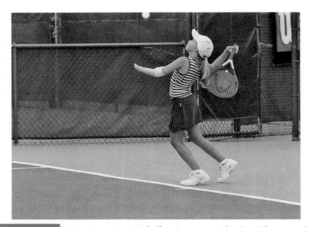

Figure 13-16 Tossing a tennis ball using a prosthesis with a passive hand.

Appropriate prosthetic components are costly, and a full prosthesis must be replaced at least every 12 to 18 months for growing children and adolescents. If an adolescent chooses to participate in sports or swimming activities, an additional prosthesis or components may be required. Third-party payers are reluctant to pay for multiple prostheses or myoelectric devices. Currently, some health maintenance organizations will pay for only one prosthesis in a lifetime.

Studies are beginning to examine the cost-effectiveness of surgical procedures and various prosthetic options. Grimer and colleagues[35] compared long-term costs of limb-sparing procedures versus amputation with a prosthesis. Limb-sparing procedures are more costly initially, but amputations

for children or adolescents are very costly over time because of the need for multiple and sophisticated prostheses.

PHYSICAL THERAPY INTERVENTION FOR THE CHILD WITH A LIMB DEFICIENCY OR AN ACQUIRED AMPUTATION

The parents are an integral part of the rehabilitation team for a child with an amputation or a limb deficiency. The rehabilitation team should also include an orthopedist, a prosthetist, and a physical therapist, who are experienced in the management of children with amputations. This may often mean traveling to a major medical center for periodic assessments and prosthetic adjustments. Physical therapy can be delivered in the local community if available, but the therapist must be in communication with the managing rehabilitation team.

The overall goals of physical therapy are to facilitate as normal a sequence of development as possible for the child and to prevent or minimize the development of impairments, activity limitations, and participation restrictions. Impairments can include joint contractures and weakness with resultant activity limitations of reduced mobility and a lack of independence in self-care skills. Physical therapy goals are directed toward preventing joint contractures, minimizing muscle strength imbalances, preventing skin breakdown, and developing independence with mobility and self-care skills. Ideally these goals are accomplished through physical therapy intervention for the child, child or parent instruction, and follow-up of a child's progress and functional outcomes. The child's age, type of limb deficiency, or level of amputation, as well as other medical factors, will influence the intensity of physical therapy needed.

The physical therapy examination should follow the components listed in the *Guide to Physical Therapist Practice*.[5] A thorough examination of joint integrity and mobility and range of motion is important for the child with a limb deficiency. Some children with a congenital limb deficiency may have other associated musculoskeletal impairments, as well as other syndromes that affect the integrity of the musculoskeletal system. Integumentary integrity will be important post surgery and for the child with a prosthesis. Examination of gait and balance, neuromotor development, aerobic capacity and endurance, community and work integration, and self-care will begin to highlight the child's functional abilities.

Functional outcomes can be assessed using current assessment tools. However, these assessment tools may not be able to determine the functional effectiveness of various prosthetic options. Third-party payers and state-funded programs will opt for the prosthetic options that are less costly if outcomes are not present to justify the more expensive options. Pruitt and colleagues (1996) developed and tested an outcome measure for children with limb deficiencies.

The Child Amputee Prosthetics Project–Functional Status Inventory (CAPP-FSI) assesses 40 activities on two scales to determine whether the child performs the activity with or without a prosthesis. The child is also rated for the severity of his or her limb loss. Internal reliability for the two scales that compose the CAPP-FSI was 0.96.[61] The CAPP-FSIP and the CAPP-FSIT were developed to assess the functional outcomes of preschoolers age 4 to 7 years and toddlers age 1 to 4 years, respectively.[62,63] The Functional Mobility Assessment (FMA) is a more recently developed functional outcome measure that has been validated for children and young adults with bone sarcomas. The FMA comprises six categories: (1) pain, (2) function as measured by the timed up and down stairs (TUGS) and the timed up and go (TUG), (3) use of supports or assistive devices, (4) satisfaction with quality of walking, (5) participation in work, school, and sports, and (6) endurance as measured by a 9-minute walk/run test.[48]

INFANCY AND TODDLER PERIOD

An infant with a limb deficiency should be referred for an initial examination by a pediatric orthopedist and a physical therapist shortly after birth. Monitoring by the physical therapist with suggestions to parents regarding positioning and ROM exercises may be all that is needed initially. The motor development of children with multiple limb deficiencies or upper extremity deficiencies may become delayed or impaired owing to their inability to use their arms for such activities as pushing up to sit, crawling, and pulling to stand. Physical therapy is necessary to monitor the infant's developmental progress, ROM, and strength needed for later prosthetic use. The physical therapist should also teach the parent or caregiver how to incorporate physical therapy goals into the child's daily activities. This can be accomplished through periodic physical therapy examinations and evaluations, optimally at 1-month intervals, with updated parent instruction provided.

Generally, infants with limb deficiencies do not develop contractures after birth, but ROM should be carefully monitored according to individual needs. The parents of a child with a PFFD may benefit from instruction to decrease the hip flexion and abduction contractures that are typically noted at birth and will later interfere with prosthetic fit. Most children with upper extremity limb deficiencies will maintain ROM and strength through their developmental activities.

Careful monitoring of the developing infant is necessary to evaluate ROM, functional strength, weight-bearing capabilities, and posture while prone, sitting, and standing. Often a child with a limb deficiency will tend to bear weight asymmetrically in prone and during sitting activities. Some children will take increased weight on their limb-deficient side to free their uninvolved side for reaching and movement. Other children may take more weight through their uninvolved side because of weight-shifting and balance difficulties. Suggestions may be given to the parents and therapy provided to encourage weight-shifting activities to improve symmetry. For the child with an upper limb deficiency, this will encourage co-contraction of the shoulder musculature as needed later for prosthetic use. For the child with a lower limb deficiency, this encourages assumption of an erect trunk with normal balance reactions. Shifting weight to the limb-deficient side is also important for the preprosthetic training needed for standing and ambulation activities.

If an infant is not progressing developmentally, physical therapy intervention may be warranted to provide alternative methods of achieving the normal developmental sequence. For example, a child with bilateral upper extremity limb deficiencies may need assistance to learn to stand from sitting or to safely learn to balance in standing.

A child is usually fitted with a prosthesis at a developmentally appropriate age. A child with a lower extremity deficiency therefore will be fitted for a prosthesis when weight bearing is appropriate and the child is beginning to pull to stand (between 8 and 10 months of age depending on the child's developmental progress). A child with a unilateral PFFD may have a Syme or Boyd amputation and be fitted with a prosthesis before or after the surgery.[54] A child with an upper extremity limb deficiency may be fitted with a prosthesis to assist with early playing skills in sitting, or even as early as 3 months to assist with weight-bearing skills while prone. Children are typically fitted with an upper extremity prosthesis between 5 and 7 months, when they are able to sit independently.[70]

When a child first receives a prosthesis, the fit and alignment as well as the overall function of the prosthesis are assessed. The initial session is spent on instructing the parents in properly donning the prosthesis, checking the skin, and developing a wear schedule. The initial goal is to have the infant or toddler wear the prosthesis comfortably for as many hours a day as possible and for the parents to be comfortable in donning and removing the prosthesis. The prosthesis may be removed for naps and should be removed when the child sleeps at night.

A child with an upper extremity prosthesis may initially ignore it. The focus of therapy should be on having the child wear the prosthesis while playing and to begin to use it for bimanual play such as manipulating and holding large toys, and during gross motor activities such as pushing up to sitting or quadruped, protective reactions, and propping in sitting.

The child's first upper extremity prosthesis may have one of several terminal device options (see Figure 13-9). A young infant may have a passive hand that is cosmetically appealing but has limited function (Figure 13-17). As the child begins to engage in bimanual play and reaching activities, the decision to use a body-powered or an externally powered myoelectric device is made. Body-powered devices may be a

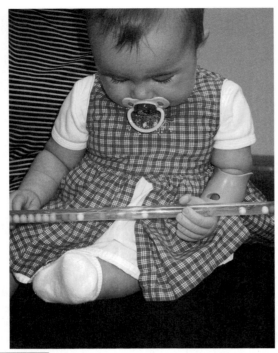

Figure 13-17   Toddler holding a toy in the passive hand of her prosthesis.

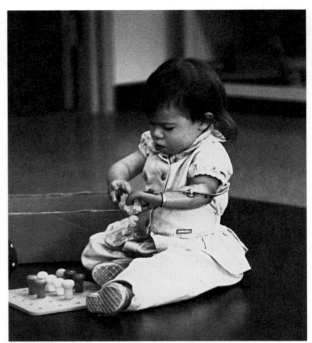

Figure 13-18   Child engaging in bimanual play wearing a forearm prosthesis with an ADEPT voluntary closing hook (Therapeutic Recreation Systems, Boulder, CO).

simple split hook terminal device or a CAPP voluntary opening device. The split hook is similar to that used with adult prosthetics, except it is smaller. The CAPP was designed specifically for children, is cosmetically more appealing than a hook terminal device, is safer than a hook for a young child, and provides an efficient grip without requiring great operating force. The goal for the young child at this time is to adjust to the weight of a prosthesis, to begin to use it to manipulate larger toys, and to shake or remove toys placed in the terminal device by an adult.

Children are not expected to begin to operate the terminal device until 18 months of age or later, when they understand simple commands and cause and effect.[70] Training to operate the terminal device is dependent on the child's developmental level. Generally, children are taught to open the terminal device, place objects in it, and then release them, in that order. This corresponds with the normal developmental sequence of learning to grasp before learning to release objects.[60] The therapist must be familiar with the mechanism that controls the terminal device because this can differ from child to child, depending on the design of the device. The CAPP and Hosmer Dorrance hook are voluntary-opening terminal devices; forward reaching of the arm pulls the cable tight and activates opening of the terminal device. Children with a transverse deficiency of the upper arm will need to use scapular abduction to activate opening of the terminal device with the elbow locked; control of the prosthetic elbow comes at a later age. The ADEPT hook is a voluntary-closing terminal device designed to mimic forward reaching to grasp

or close on an object (Figure 13-18). If the decision is made to fit the child with an externally powered prosthesis, the New York Hand (Hosmer Dorrance) or the Otto Bock Electrohand is commonly used with young children. Children typically are fitted initially with a myoelectric hand with only one electrode. When this electrode is activated through muscle contraction, the hand opens. When the child relaxes the muscle, the hand closes. Typically by 3 to 4 years of age, the child's myoelectric device can be converted to two electrodes so that opening and closing the hand are controlled by the child[15,42] (Figure 13-19).

Children younger than 2 years of age with a lower limb deficiency or above-knee amputation are typically fitted with a prosthesis without a knee. The goal is to begin weight-bearing and ambulation activities and to progress to learning control of a prosthetic knee when they are closer to 3 years of age. The rationale for this decision is that the articulated knee components are often too large to fit into the small prosthetic shaft required with a small child, and that the fixed knee extension of the prosthesis provides stability for early gait training and confidence in the use of a prosthesis. With the development of smaller pediatric prosthetic components, several clinics have begun to use articulated prosthetic knees in the initial prosthesis with toddlers. The principle for fitting a young child with a knee component is that knee flexion during gait simulates a more normal gait pattern and may therefore eliminate some of the gait deviations that develop and become ingrained after ambulating with a fixed prosthesis. In addition, the prosthetic knee

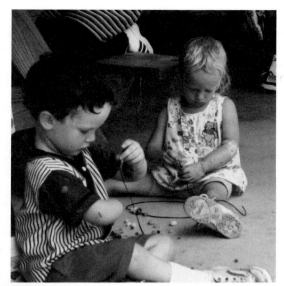

Figure 13-19 Young girl using her myoelectric single-site prosthesis to complete a bimanual activity.

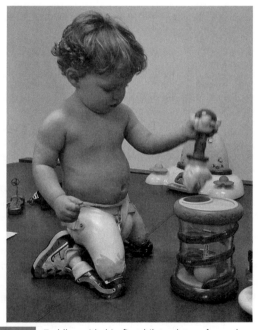

Figure 13-20 Toddler with his first bilateral transfemoral prostheses with knee joint to promote age-appropriate ambulation skills and play activities on the floor.

allows other typical movements seen in young children such as crawling, squatting, and kneeling (Figure 13-20).[14,87] When toddlers are fitted with a lower extremity prosthesis, normal stance and gait patterns for their developmental age should be kept in mind. Children 1 year of age stand and walk with a wide base of support and exhibit increased hip external rotation during the swing phase.[77] For this reason,

a toddler's prosthesis may need to be aligned with greater hip abduction than is provided to an older child.

Because a goal of physical therapy is symmetry of posture and movement during developmental activities, proper alignment and controlled weight-shifting and balance activities are emphasized for children with a lower limb prosthesis. Many children with a lower limb prosthesis do not require an assistive device for ambulation; however, initial gait training with an assistive device promotes a reciprocal gait pattern and an erect trunk. As the child develops balance and is able to control weight shifting, he or she will naturally discard the assistive device when comfortable with independent ambulation.

PRESCHOOL- AND SCHOOL-AGE PERIOD

When a child attends a preschool or kindergarten class for the first time, many anxieties may resurface for the parents of a child with a limb deficiency. Parents will worry that their child may not fit in or will look different from his or her peers. This is also an age by which typical children have achieved independence with ADL skills such as eating and dressing, and their social relationships with peers increase. The preschool years should emphasize development of independence in self-care skills and mobility, and acquisition of school skills such as coloring, cutting, and writing. If these skills are achieved during the preschool years, the child will enter school with minimal or no activity limitations or participation restrictions.

The child with an upper limb deficiency should be able to activate the terminal device of the prosthesis by this age. Children using above-elbow prostheses can begin to learn to control the elbow by 3 or 4 years of age. Most above-elbow prostheses have a dual cable system that allows the child to control elbow flexion and extension and forearm pronation and supination. With control of the elbow and forearm, the terminal device of the prosthesis becomes more functional in a variety of positions.

Emphasis should always be on assisting the child to learn skills that are appropriate for his or her age. Play skills involving manipulation of smaller objects, using the prosthesis to hold and turn paper for coloring and cutting activities, holding the handlebars of a tricycle, and self-dressing and feeding skills are important. A child with a unilateral upper limb prosthesis will always use it as a helper hand and not as the dominant hand.

For those children with bilateral upper limb deficiencies, the use of a prosthesis should be carefully monitored. These children should always be allowed to use their feet or mouth for play and self-care activities. A prosthesis may aid these children for only some periods of the day and may actually limit their function during some activities. Children with a lower limb deficiency, including those children with unilateral PFFD, should be functional ambulators at this age. A child with a below-knee limb deficiency should be wearing a prosthesis for most of the day and engaging in normal activities with peers. The child with an above-knee limb deficiency should be ready to begin ambulation with a prosthesis with a knee joint by around age 3 years. Initially, children usually are given a constant-friction knee joint. They may need a short period of physical therapy to learn control of the knee joint and weight-shifting activities without falling.

During the preschool years, some surgery is usually necessary for the child with a unilateral PFFD. Arthrodesis of the knee joint, usually performed between 2.5 and 4 years of age, increases the lever arm of the thigh and eliminates any knee instability.[28,54] Femoral or tibial epiphysiodesis may be performed at the time of knee arthrodesis. The ultimate goal is for limb length on the prosthetic side to be 5 cm shorter than on the contralateral femur. This enables the prosthetic knee joint to be at approximately the same level as the contralateral knee joint at maturity. Placement of the prosthetic knee joint at the same level as the contralateral knee joint allows for improved cosmesis and improved gait.

For the child with an acquired lower extremity amputation, an immediate-fit prosthesis is usually used. This may not be the case if significant trauma to the surrounding tissue was present, or if skin grafting was necessary after the injury. The physical therapy examination and evaluation focuses on sensitivity of the residual limb, active movement, strength, bed mobility, transfers for toileting and getting out of bed, and ambulation. The goals of postoperative physical therapy are similar to those for an adult with an amputation.

Children are more likely than an adult to move about after an amputation, so contractures are less likely to occur. However, some children undergoing chemotherapy are extremely ill and weak and may tend to lie in bed with their residual limb propped on pillows. They must be monitored for developing contractures, and parents and nursing staff must be instructed in ROM exercises and positioning of the residual limb.

Gait training should begin as soon as cleared by the physician. Young children can safely learn to ambulate with an immediate-fit prosthesis using a walker or crutches. If a child has been hospitalized for a period of time, strengthening exercises for the uninvolved leg and the residual limb may be necessary.

After removal of the immediate-fit prosthesis, the child is fitted with a permanent prosthesis. The exception to this would be a child who is undergoing chemotherapy. These children tend to have weight fluctuations secondary to side effects of the medications. They are better fitted with a socket that allows for weight fluctuations, such as one with Velcro closures, or any inner socket that can be removed or added to accommodate changes in size of the residual limb. Children with above-knee amputations should be fitted with a prosthesis with a knee joint. Most children with an above-knee amputation will require a suspension method to help

hold the prosthesis in place. Instruction must be given to both the parents and the child in donning and removing the prosthesis, care of the prosthesis, skin checks, and wear schedule.

For the child who undergoes a rotationplasty, the surgical leg is usually casted to allow healing of the bone. The cast may incorporate a pylon to permit the shortened leg to contact the ground for safe ambulation when a walker or crutches are used. After the cast is removed and the bone has healed, the child with a rotationplasty must work on increasing ROM at the ankle joint, which functions as the child's knee. For ambulation and sitting, 0° to 20° of ankle dorsiflexion is more than adequate. Some children will be able to achieve 30° of ankle dorsiflexion, which will allow for some squatting activities and facilitate bike riding. Maximal plantar flexion will allow for greater extension of the leg in stance. Optimal plantar flexion ROM is at least 45° to 50°; the prosthetist can align the prosthesis to achieve an additional few degrees of plantar flexion for stance. Exercises should begin gently and progress to active and resistive exercises.

The child who undergoes a rotationplasty is fitted with a custom-made prosthesis that incorporates the foot in a position of maximum plantar flexion and allows it to act as a knee joint. An external knee hinge joint must be used with an attached thigh cuff. The prosthesis is usually held in place with a pelvic strap.

A child who has had a limb-sparing procedure will also require physical therapy after surgery. Lower extremity procedures usually require a period of non–weight bearing. Rehabilitation for children with a limb-sparing procedure to the upper or lower extremity includes exercise through active movement with progression to strengthening exercises. The progression of the intervention is dictated by the procedure that was performed, the surgeon's protocols, and the amount of bone replaced. Children who have had a limb-sparing procedure involving the femur will also frequently require physical therapy after a lengthening procedure of the endoprosthetic implant. ROM of the knee often becomes restricted, similar to what is seen with children who undergo limb-lengthening techniques (see Chapter 14).

Gait training for all children at this age will focus on symmetry and the normal characteristics of gait, such as stride length, step length, and velocity, as well as all skills that the child needs to participate in play and games with other children. When initially learning to ambulate or after a surgical procedure, most children will use an assistive device. As balance and ambulation speed improve and postsurgical limitations are lifted, many children will begin to discard the assistive device. The assistive device should be discarded, however, only if the child's ambulation is safe and speed is functional to keep pace with the child's peers.

During the school-age years, the physical therapist should instruct the child in running techniques so that he or she may participate in play and games with her or his peers. This is the age at which the child may also show an interest in participating in various sports or recreational programs designed for persons with amputations.

When attending school for the first time, the child will be questioned about the prosthesis and assistive devices. This is especially true of a child with an upper limb deficiency. A meeting before the beginning of school with the child and his or her parents, the child's teacher, and perhaps the child's physical therapist may be helpful to allay any concerns and to answer or develop a way to answer the questions of the child's peers. The child with a unilateral limb deficiency or amputation should succeed in school with minimal adaptations.

The child with bilateral upper limb deficiencies may need to use a tape recorder or computer to assist with writing skills. In school, a child with bilateral upper limb deficiencies may be able to carry papers or books in the classroom between the chin and shoulder. The child may use the mouth for manipulating and holding objects such as pencils. Whether the child uses his or her feet in school for manipulation or grasping is something that should be clearly discussed with the child, parents, and teacher before school entrance. Many children opt not to use their feet for grasping objects in public as they get older; however, this can limit their independence, especially with toileting and feeding. If a child is adept with the use of his or her feet and is independent and chooses to use the feet, this should not be discouraged. If the teacher displays a supportive attitude toward the child's use of the feet, the child's classroom peers will soon view this as usual procedure in their classroom. The ultimate outcome is for the child to be functional in our society as an adult; this may mean use of the feet or a combination of use of the feet and prostheses.

ADOLESCENCE AND TRANSITION TO ADULTHOOD

Adolescence, with its hallmark concerns of appearance and acceptance by peers, relationships with the opposite sex, career decisions, and the struggle for independence, can be a trying time for anyone. Restrictions on participation for the child with a limb deficiency may become more apparent during adolescence. Most teenagers with a congenital limb deficiency have been adjusting both functionally and emotionally from birth. At this point in their lives, they are part of a social network of friends, realize the support of their families, and have attempted and succeeded at various activities in school and the community. They will be dealing with these adolescent issues right alongside their peers, although increased fears concerning dating and social acceptance can be typical at this time, and participation in school athletic activities may be limited. A higher percentage of children and adolescents with congenital limb deficiencies exhibit greater behavioral and emotional problems and lower social competence than their peers without a disability.[84]

Amputation of a limb during the adolescent years adds quite an emotional burden to a teenager, who must deal with the loss of a body part and the grieving process and may be facing the possibility of death. Added to the physical appearance difficulties are possible side effects such as hair loss from chemotherapy. A teenager who is facing a possible amputation as the result of cancer should be included, if he or she desires, in discussions of treatment options, including surgical options. Obviously, this is not possible if the amputation is the result of sudden trauma.

The immediate postoperative concerns and physical therapy interventions for adolescents undergoing an amputation or a limb-sparing procedure are similar to those described for school-age children. If an immediate-fit prosthesis is not used, teenagers are more likely to develop edema of their residual limb following surgery. In this case, wrapping of the residual limb or fitting with a shrinker sock should be instituted.

Teenagers who sustain a lower extremity amputation are fitted with a prosthesis when the residual limb has stabilized. They should be involved in the fitting of the prosthesis and in deciding on the design of the socket and the type of knee joint and foot to be used. For most teenagers, a large variety of prosthetic options are available. These should be fully discussed with the teenager and parents, and the choice should complement the lifestyle of the user. Both the teenager and his or her family should be cautioned that the prosthesis will not function and will not look exactly like the contralateral limb.

Many teenagers with a high above-knee amputation will attempt to ambulate with a prosthesis but will ultimately opt for no prosthesis and crutches, as ambulation with crutches is faster and more energy efficient. The decision to use or not to use a prosthesis should be the child's and should not be based on society's idea of the most appropriate physical appearance. Some teenagers use a prosthesis for certain activities and not for others. The ultimate outcome is for them to be comfortable with their peers and to interact socially with their peers at school and in the community.

The use of prosthetics varies for teenagers with upper limb deficiencies. Those who have become adept with a prosthesis since early childhood probably will continue to use their prosthesis. The teenager who has an upper limb amputation may learn to operate a body-powered above- or below-elbow prosthesis. To become functional with the prosthesis requires much practice, and the teenager may opt not to use one. An outcome study assessed the function and quality of life of 489 children with a transverse below-elbow limb deficiency, comparing 321 children who wore a prosthesis and 168 who did not wear a prosthesis. Researchers found small differences between the two groups, but they were not significant enough to meet the definition of a clinically important difference in the Pediatric Quality of Life Inventory.[43]

One major milestone for teenagers is the acquisition of a driver's license. Nearly all teenagers with a limb deficiency or amputation can learn to drive. Hand controls can be used for the teenager with bilateral PFFD or with bilateral lower extremity amputation as the result of trauma. For the teenager with a unilateral upper limb deficiency or amputation, minimal adjustments will be necessary. Driving can be done by using the sound hand, or a driving ring can be attached to the steering wheel. The prosthetic terminal device, preferably a hook, slips into the ring to assist with controlling the steering wheel and easily slips out of the ring in emergencies. Driving becomes more difficult for the teenager with bilateral upper limb deficiencies or amputations. A driving ring may be used by the dominant limb. Controls such as light switches or turn signals may need to be moved to the dominant side and within reach of the limb or can be operated by the driver's knee. Unless specifically trained in the area of driver education, physical therapists should assist the teenager and his or her parents to seek information and driver training from a local rehabilitation center.

Career and college decisions are also made during adolescence. Some teenagers may work at a part-time job during high school. Most teenagers with limb deficiencies or amputations eventually seek employment. At times, adjustments must be made to a prosthesis, such as a specific terminal device, to assist the young adult in his or her particular career area. Going to college is a true test of independence with self-care skills. Some individuals with bilateral upper limb deficiencies or multiple limb deficiencies will always require some degree of assistance with self-care activities. Toileting, especially wiping after defecation, and dressing, specifically managing underpants and bras, are self-care activities for which it is difficult for anyone with bilateral upper limb deficiencies or short above-elbow amputations to achieve total independence. This does not preclude

attending college or independent living, but an aide or other arrangements may be needed. Creativity, experimentation, and talking with other teenagers or adults with limb deficiencies can often produce strategies for accomplishing difficult tasks. High employment rates, active lifestyles, and marriage are reported for adults who underwent an amputation as a child or adolescent.[55,80] However, survivors of childhood bone tumors are more likely to have a physical limitation than those from other groups of childhood cancer, and those survivors with physical limitations are less likely to be employed, married, and/or earning an annual income greater than $20,000.[56a]

SUMMARY

The origin and classification of congenital limb deficiencies and the causes of acquired amputations were reviewed in this chapter. An overview of the medical and surgical management of congenital limb deficiencies and amputations was presented. Treatment of a child with a congenital limb deficiency or amputation is complex and must involve a team of professionals who recognize the impact of various treatment options on the child's functioning in both home and school environments and ultimately as an independent adult. Careful planning and thoughtful discussions with the family regarding expected outcomes, goals of physical therapy, surgical options, and prosthetic options, are necessary. Each child must be assessed as an individual, with consideration given to the child's age and musculoskeletal development and immediate and long-term functional abilities, the family's and child's activity level and lifestyle choices, and prosthetic and physical therapy interventions needed to meet the child's goals.

The continued proliferation of prosthetic designs and materials available to the pediatric population has opened up many options for recreation and sports, vocation, and self-care, as well as early fitting of infants and toddlers with prostheses.

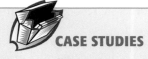

CASE STUDIES

"Becca"

Child with PFFD (Proximal Focal Femoral Deficiency)

Becca is a 7-year-old girl with a congenital right PFFD, Aitken type C (see Figure 13-5). A radiologic assessment shortly after birth revealed an absence of the right proximal head of the femur, dysplastic acetabulum, and a short proximally tapered femoral segment. The right leg was approximately 50% shorter than the left, making the right foot at the level of the left knee. The right knee was proximal, close to the right hip. Becca was attempting to pull to stand and cruise by 11 months of age but was having challenges accommodating for the leg length difference. Up until transitioning into upright and supported standing, Becca met all of her developmental milestones. At

this point, she was fitted with an unconventional prosthesis that accommodated the anatomic foot by placing an Otto Bock 3R 80 single-axis knee under the prosthetic socket to allow knee flexion function for age-appropriate gross motor development. The prosthetic socket was designed to control and contain the hip impairment. A TES (total elastic suspension) belt was used for suspension, and a TRS infant foot was provided (see Figure 13-6, B). Becca learned to control the prosthetic knee and began to walk independently by 15 months of age. She walked with a limp with decreased stance on the right and limited right hip flexion due to the degree of right hip and femur impairment.

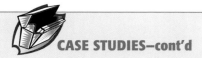

CASE STUDIES–cont'd

Physical therapy was initiated at 1 month of age when first diagnosed with PFFD and focused on assessment of age-appropriate developmental skills and instruction of the family in ROM activities to decrease contractures of the hip and foot typically seen in infants with PFFD. Once pulling to stand and after prosthetic fitting, physical therapy incorporated transitions into and out of upright standing, cruising, and walking. Initial gait training utilized pushing toys and progressed to walking without assisted devices.

Becca was followed by a pediatric orthopedic surgeon every 6 months to monitor the development of the right femur and hip and deformity of the right foot. Appointments with the prosthetist took place every 4 months to monitor prosthetic fit and function. Becca required a new prosthesis every year to assure adequate containment of the proximal hip, femur, and knee. By 4 years of age, Becca's hip and proximal femur development did not change, and the proximal femoral deficiency was confirmed to be Aitken C. The foot remained dorsiflexed and everted in spite of the parents' daily stretching. A Symes amputation of the right foot with femoral osteotomy and right knee fusion was performed. Becca was placed in a body spica cast for 6 weeks postop to allow for healing of the right knee fusion and femoral osteotomy. Prosthetic fitting was initiated at 10 weeks postop following a 4-week period of Ace wrapping for shaping of the residual limb and edema control once the cast was removed.

Becca's prosthesis after surgery consisted of a high proximal socket with a TES belt, a total multi-axis prosthetic knee, and a College Park TruPer prosthetic foot (College Park Industries, Fraser, MI) to promote smooth transitions into upright through ½ kneel and kneeling, standing, and weight shifting. Postoperatively and after cast removal, physical therapy focused on preprosthetic management of the residual limb to include the skin and incisions; scar massage; Ace wrapping for edema control and shaping; hip ROM and strengthening; and functional activities to regain independent sitting and transitions upright. After prosthetic fitting, gait training was resumed to instruct Becca on how to control the multi-axis stance control prosthetic knee.

At the end of 8 weeks of physical therapy, Becca was ambulating independently without an assistive device and was able to kick a ball with her noninvolved leg. By 6 months after surgery, Becca was trying to run step over step. Becca's running speed was slower than her peers with asymmetrical step lengths because of the right hip dysplasia. Both Becca and her family appeared pleased with her progress and ability to participate in activities with her pre-kindergarten class and her siblings.

Presently, Becca is in third grade in her community school. She wears her prosthesis throughout the day and continues to ambulate independently, runs and climbs with her peers at recess, and is learning to ride a bicycle. She has been independent with donning and removing the prosthesis. Before the start of the year in school, Becca and her parents met with school administrators, the teacher, and the PE teacher to discuss her limb difference, use of a prosthesis, and

her functional ability. It was decided that accommodations only for running and high-impact activities were required, and a 504 plan was formulated to document these accommodations at this time. Becca did not require extra help in class or at school other than in certain PE activities. As she gets older, her activity limitations include decreased running speed and single-limb stance and balance compared with her peers. This may limit her ability to participate in sports at a competitive level. Becca may benefit from running instruction provided by a physical therapist with expertise in development of higher-level gross motor skills for individuals with an amputation. Becca continues to be followed at 6-month intervals in a pediatric amputee clinic by the orthopedist, the prosthetist, and a physical therapist. It is possible that Becca will require a right distal tibial epiphysiodesis at age 9 or 10 years to ensure that knee joints are at equivalent height at maturity.

EVIDENCE TO PRACTICE 13-1

CASE STUDY "BECCA"

Infants with PFFD typically present with hip flexion and abduction contractures of the involved leg. Initial physical therapy consists of stretching exercises and parent education to reduce the contractures for optimal prosthetic fitting when the child begins to pull to stand. The initial prosthesis will incorporate her foot, which is near the level of the knee of her uninvolved leg. The initial prosthesis will promote weight bearing, cruising, and walking, now that her leg lengths will be near equal with the use of a prosthesis. If space is adequate, a prosthetic knee joint should be incorporated in the prosthesis to assist in upright transitions and floor play appropriate for her age (Coulter-O'Berry, 2009).

"Andrew"

Child with Cancer, Osteosarcoma Right Distal Femur

Andrew is a 6-year-old boy who was diagnosed with osteosarcoma of the right distal femur at 3 years of age. He had no metastases at the time of diagnosis. Andrew underwent a course of preoperative chemotherapy to shrink the tumor and prevent any micrometastatic disease. Physical therapy at the time of diagnosis consisted of instruction in non–weight-bearing 3-point gait training using a front-wheeled walker and progressed to axillary crutches once Andrew demonstrated adequate balance and coordination. Weight bearing on the right leg needed to be limited to prevent pathologic fracture through the tumor.

Surgical options, including limb sparing, amputation, and rotationplasty, were discussed with the family. At his young age, an amputation would result in a very short above-knee residual limb by the time of skeletal maturity. Limb-sparing procedures were not

Continued

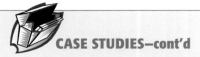

CASE STUDIES—cont'd

possible because of his young age, significant skeletal immaturity, and limitations of available technology for an expandable endoprosthesis for a very young child. A rotationplasty was chosen because it afforded below-knee function and created a longer residual limb with better function than an above-knee amputation.

Once the surgical decision for the rotationplasty was made, Andrew and his family met with another child and family who had had a rotationplasty because of cancer, to obtain firsthand education about the surgical decision, what to expect after surgery, prosthetics, rehabilitation, and impact on day-to-day activities.

Postoperatively, Andrew was placed in a hip spica cast with his right ankle incorporated at approximately 45° of plantar flexion. He was fitted with a reclining rental wheelchair. Daily physical therapy was provided while an inpatient with the goals of transfers, bed mobility, positioning with the spica cast, ambulation with a walker for short household distances, and maintenance of upper body strength. Andrew was discharged home able to transfer and walk short distances with a walker in the hip spica cast. Chemotherapy was resumed 4 weeks after surgery. The cast was removed 8 weeks postoperatively, and active-assisted ROM to the right hip and ankle was initiated. Impairments assessed immediately after cast removal included a long, thick adherent scar; a 15° right ankle plantar flexion contracture; and limitations in all active and passive hip ranges. Strength was limited in the hip and ankle, measuring 2+/5 bilaterally, with right ankle plantar flexor strength of 3/5 and right ankle dorsiflexion strength of 2/5. When not in the hospital for chemotherapy, Andrew attended outpatient physical therapy with goals of achieving increasing right ankle dorsiflexion to 20° and improving strength of the hip and ankle musculature to 5/5 bilaterally with progression to gait training with a prosthesis. His parents were instructed in a home program of ROM and strengthening exercises. Four weeks after cast removal, right ankle motion was as follows: dorsiflexion 0° to 15° and plantar flexion 0° to 50°. Andrew could actively move his foot through available ranges, and resistive exercises were added.

Cosmetically, Andrew exhibited no problems in looking at or manipulating his foot. His mother often expressed the feeling that dealing with the appearance of a "backward foot" was nothing compared with dealing with Andrew's cancer and unknown fate. Twelve weeks after cast removal, Andrew had been fitted with a prosthesis. The socket held the foot in maximum plantar flexion with single-axis external knee hinges attached to a leather custom-molded thigh cuff.

Family goals related to physical therapy were for Andrew to walk independently and engage in play activities with his older siblings. Andrew's parents were instructed in donning the prosthesis, wearing schedule, increasing wearing time, skin checks, and gait training for Andrew using a walker. The parents were able to incorporate wearing of the prosthesis into Andrew's daily routine and readily encouraged ambulation for functional activities within their home.

Andrew discarded the walker on his own for independent ambulation.

Presently, Andrew attends fourth grade in his neighborhood school. He runs, climbs on playground equipment, and rides a skateboard. Andrew is monitored for recurrence of his cancer and is followed at an amputee clinic at 4-month intervals. During the summer, he goes to the community pool with his family and swims without the prosthesis. He has also participated in Little League within his community. He performs well academically in school and is becoming skilled on the computer. To date, Andrew's mother states that he has not expressed any anger at the appearance of his leg. She has noticed stares from persons at the pool, but they quickly accept Andrew once they are aware of his medical history.

EVIDENCE TO PRACTICE 13-2

CASE STUDY "ANDREW"

Significant future skeletal growth is expected with a 3-year-old child. An above-knee amputation for a distal femur osteosarcoma in a young child would result in a very short residual limb with minimal potential for future growth of the leg. An endoprosthetic device would require multiple operative procedures for lengthening and yet would not be able to achieve the required limb length at skeletal maturity for functional ambulation. A rotationplasty would offer increased limb length, including some potential future growth, for functional use of a prosthesis. Akahane (2007) assessed 22 patients 1 year after an amputation, a limb-sparing procedure, or a rotationplasty. Subjects who underwent a rotationplasty exhibited higher scores on the Musculoskeletal Tumor Assessment and the health-related quality of life measure (SF-36).

EVIDENCE TO PRACTICE 13-3

CASE STUDY "ANDREW"

After a rotationplasty, the child's ankle now must function as a knee. Optimal ankle dorsiflexion range of motion will promote improved flexion for sitting as well as prosthetic knee function for gait. The ability to achieve ankle plantar flexion of 50° to 60° will streamline the position of the foot in the prosthesis to mimic knee extension. Once adequate range of motion is achieved, strengthening of the ankle and toe musculature will optimize the power available at the knee joint for a smoother and faster walking pattern (Coulter-O'Berry, 2004; Stanger, 2008).

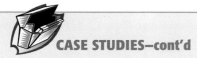

CASE STUDIES—cont'd

"Anthony"

Child With Traumatic Amputation

Anthony is a 14-year-old boy who sustained a mutilating injury to his left leg when he was hit by a train. He was attempting to jump onto a moving freight train with his friends, but he slipped and his leg was crushed by the train. Replantation or limb-sparing procedures were not viable options owing to the extent of the crush injuries and the warm ischemia time. A left transfemoral amputation was performed, and a soft dressing was applied for the first week. A rigid cast dressing with pylon and a prosthetic foot were applied after the first week to control edema and promote early weight bearing. As an inpatient, Anthony received physical therapy on a daily basis for gentle ROM exercises, transfer training, and education for positioning and compression wrapping of his residual limb. Physical therapy included gait training after week 1 and progressed to weight bearing as tolerated and began to incorporate strengthening exercises. Focus of strengthening was on core muscles for stability and hip extensors and abductors.

EVIDENCE TO PRACTICE 13-4

CASE STUDY "ANTHONY"

Unfortunately, no evidence is available to guide our physical therapy intervention with children with acquired amputations. Much of what is practiced has been gained by experience and is based on the long-term theory of rehabilitation of individuals with an amputation. Experienced clinicians base their interventions for early mobility on the fact that children who do not get out of their bed or move during their initial inpatient stay may become debilitated and develop secondary impairments such as hip flexion contractures of the residual limb and weakness. Edema control and shaping of the residual limb can also be affected by decreased adherence with use of compression wrapping and rigid dressings (Gailey, 2004; Coulter-O'Berry, 2004). These secondary problems eventually will affect the timing of prosthetic fitting and may slow the rehabilitation process, influencing eventual outcomes.

After 6 weeks, Anthony was fitted for a permanent prosthesis. Outpatient physical therapy goals included increasing hip extension ROM, increasing strength of residual muscles with an emphasis on hip extensors and hip abductors, and improving strength of upper extremities and the right lower extremity. Long-term goals included independent mobility in his school and community settings and a return to school and active participation in peer and family activities.

Prosthetic components of the permanent prosthesis included a narrowed medial-lateral containment socket, a silicone liner with locking pin, a four-bar linkage knee, and an energy-storing prosthetic foot. Physical therapy intervention included weight-shifting and balance activities, gait training, endurance activities, and education for skin care and donning and doffing the prosthesis.

EVIDENCE TO PRACTICE 13-5

CASE STUDY "ANTHONY"

No studies have supported or refuted the types of physical therapy interventions used with children after an amputation. Reports of clinical experiences support the decision to begin standing weight-shift and balance activities (Gailey, 2004; Coulter-O'Berry, 2004). One study of 58 men found that an intensive physical therapy program showed greater gains on a 2-minute walk test, physiologic cost index (PCI) scores, and weight bearing through the prosthesis compared with a control group that underwent the standard level of physical therapy for that center (Rau, 2007).

Anthony was able to develop the skills to ambulate independently at school using his prosthesis but often did not use his prosthesis when at home. Participation restrictions included difficulty running to participate in activities with his friends and in long-distance walking with his prosthesis to keep up with his friends. Therefore, Anthony will often ambulate using crutches and no prosthesis when hanging out with his friends.

EVIDENCE TO PRACTICE 13-6

CASE STUDY "ANTHONY"

Ambulation without a prosthesis: Children with a transfemoral amputation and prosthesis ambulate at slower speeds and at greater physiologic cost compared with their peers. Hagberg and colleagues found that the physiologic cost index (PCI) was higher in middle-age adults ambulating with a transfemoral prosthesis than in peers without an amputation. In addition, adults with the transfemoral amputation ambulated at a slower comfortable walking speed and walked shorter distances outdoors compared with their peers (Hagberg, 2007). In an earlier study of 56 children with lower limb amputations, Ashley and colleagues found that the children with amputations were highly functional and often participated in sports, but they ambulated more slowly and had higher heart rates compared with their peers (Ashley, 1992). Even though children with transfemoral amputations may be very active and may ambulate independently with a prosthesis, they do so at a higher physiologic cost than their peers. Therefore they may choose at times to not use their prosthesis and preserve energy.

REFERENCES

1. Aitken, G. T. (1963). Surgical amputation in children. *Journal of Bone and Joint Surgery (American), 45,* 1735–1741.

2. Aitken, G. T. (1969). Proximal femoral focal deficiency: Definition, classification, and management. In *Proximal femoral focal deficiency: A congenital anomaly.* Washington, DC: National Academy of Sciences.

3. Anderson, T. F. (1998). Aspects of sports and recreation for the child with a limb deficiency. In J. A. Herring, & J. G. Birch (Eds.), *The child with a limb deficiency.* Rosemont, IL: American Academy of Orthopedic Surgeons.

4. Akahane, T., Shimizu, T., Isobe, K., Yoshimura, Y., Fujioka, F., & Kato, H. (2007). Evaluation of postoperative general quality of life for patients with osteosarcoma around the knee joint. *Journal of Pediatric Orthopedics, 16,* 269–272.

5. American Physical Therapy Association (APTA). (2003). *Guide to physical therapist practice, revised second edition.* Alexandria, VA: APTA.

6. Ashley, R. K., Vallier, G. T., & Skinner, S. R. (1992). Gait analysis in pediatric lower extremity amputees. *Orthopaedic Review, 21,* 745–749.

7. Beebe, K., Song, K. J., Ross, E., Tuy, B., Patterson, F., & Benevenia, J. (2009). Functional outcomes after limb-salvage surgery and endoprosthetic reconstruction with an expandable prosthesis: A report of 4 cases. *Archives of Physical Medicine & Rehabilitation, 90,* 1039–1047.

8. Beris, A. E., Soucacos, P. N., Malizos, K. N., Mitsionis, G. J., & Soucacos, P. R. (1994). Major limb replantation in children. *Microsurgery, 15,* 474–478.

9. Beris, A. E., Soucacos, P. N., & Malizos, K. N. (1995). Microsurgery in children. *Clinical Orthopedics and Related Research, 314,* 112–121.

10. Bryant, P. R., & Pandian, G. (2001). Acquired limb deficiencies in children and young adults. *Archives of Physical Medicine and Rehabilitation, 82*(Suppl 1), S3–S8.

11. Buchner, M., Zeifang, F., & Bernd, L. (2003). Medial gastrocnemius muscle flap in limb-sparing surgery of malignant bone tumors of the proximal tibia: Mid-term results in 25 patients. *Annals of Plastic Surgery, 51,* 266–272.

12. Butler, M. S., Robertson, W. W., Rate, W., D'Angio, G. J., & Drummond, D. S. (1990). Skeletal sequelae of radiation therapy for malignant tumors. *Clinical Orthopedics and Related Research, 251,* 235–239.

13. Caudill, J. S., & Arndt, C. A. (2007). Diagnosis and management of bone malignancy in adolescents. *Adolescent Medicine: State of the Art Reviews, 18,* 62–78.

14. Coulter-O'Berry, C. (2005). Physical therapy. In D. G. Smith, J. W. Michael, & J. H. Bowker (Eds.), *Atlas of limb amputations and limb deficiencies* (3rd ed.; pp. 831–840). Rosemont, IL: American Academy of Orthopedic Surgeons.

15. Cummings, D. R. (2000). Pediatric prosthetics, current trends and future possibilities. *Physical Medicine and Rehabilitation Clinics of North America, 11,* 653–679.

16. Day, H. J. B. (1991). The ISO/ISPO classification of congenital limb deficiency. *Prosthetics and Orthotics International, 15,* 67–69.

17. Dillingham, T. R., Pezzin, L. E., & MacKenzie, E. J. (2002). Limb amputation and limb deficiency: Epidemiology and recent trends in the United States. *Southern Medical Journal, 95,* 875–883.

18. Dormans, J. P., Erol, B., & Nelson, C. B. (2004). Acquired amputations in children. In D. G. Smith, J. W. Michael, & J. H. Bowker (Eds.), *Atlas of limb amputations and limb deficiencies* (3rd ed.; pp. 841–852). Rosemont, IL: American Academy of Orthopedic Surgeons.

19. Eckhardt, J. J., Kabo, J. M., Kelley, C. M., Ward, W. G., Asavamongkolkul, A., Wirganowics, P. Z., Yang, R. S., & Eilber, F. R. (2000). Expandable endoprosthesis reconstruction in skeletally immature patients with tumors. *Clinical Orthopedics and Related Research, 373,* 51–61.

20. Eldridge, J. C., Armstrong, P. F., & Krajbich, J. I. (1990). Amputation stump lengthening with the Ilizarov technique. *Clinical Orthopedics and Related Research, 256,* 76–79.

21. Ephraim, P. L., Dillingham, T. R., Sector, M., Pezzin, L. E., & MacKenzie, E. J. (2003). Epidemiology of limb loss and congenital limb deficiency: A review of the literature. *Archives of Physical Medicine and Rehabilitation, 84,* 747–761.

22. Farnsworth, T. (2003). The call to arms, overview of upper limb prosthetic options. *Active Living, Health and Activity for the O & P Community, 12,* 43–45.

23. Fowler, E., Zernicke, R., & Setoguchi, Y. (1996). Energy expenditure during walking by children who have proximal femoral focal deficiency. *Journal of Bone and Joint Surgery (American), 78,* 1857–1862.

24. Frantz, C. H., & O'Rahilly, R. (1961). Congenital skeletal limb deficiencies. *Journal of Bone and Joint Surgery (American), 43,* 1202–1204.

25. Futani, H., Minamizaki, T., Nishimoto, Y., Abe, S., Yabe, H., & Ueda, T. (2006). Long-term follow-up after limb salvage in skeletally immature children with a primary malignant tumor of the distal end of the femur. *Journal of Bone and Joint Surgery (American), 88,* 595–603.

26. Gailey, R. S., & Clark, C. R. (2004). Physical therapy. In D. G. Smith, J. W. Michael, & J. H. Bowker (Eds.), *Atlas of limb amputations and limb deficiencies* (3rd ed.; pp. 589–619). Rosemont, IL: American Academy of Orthopedic Surgeons.

27. Reference deleted in page proofs.

28. Gillespie, R. (1990). Principles of amputation surgery in children with longitudinal deficiencies of the femur. *Clinical Orthopedics and Related Research, 256,* 29–38.

29. Gillespie, R. (1998). Classification of congenital abnormalities of the femur. In J. A. Herring & J. G. Birch (Eds.), *The child with a limb deficiency* (pp. 63–72). Rosemont, IL: American Academy of Orthopedic Surgeons.

30. Ginsberg, J. P., Woo, S. Y., Johnson, M. E., Hicks, M. J., & Horowitz, M. E. (2002). Ewing's sarcoma family of tumors: Ewing's sarcoma of bone and soft tissue and the peripheral primitive neuroectodermal tumors. In P. A. Pizzo, & D. G.

Poplack (Eds.), *Principles and practice of pediatric oncology* (4th ed.; pp. 973–1016). Philadelphia: Lippincott Williams & Wilkins.

31. Ginsberg, J. P., Rai, S. N., Carlson, C. A., Meadows, A. T., Hinds, P. S., Spearing, E. M., Zhang, L., Callaway, L., Neel, M. D., Rao, B. N., & Marchese, V. G. (2007). A comparative analysis of functional outcomes in adolescents and young adults with lower-extremity bone sarcoma. *Pediatric Blood Cancer, 49,* 964–969.

32. Goorin, A. M., Schwartzentruber, D. J., Devidas, M., Gebhardt, M. C., Ayala, A. C., Harris, M. B., Helman, L. J., Greier, H. E., & Link, M. P. (2003). Presurgical chemotherapy compared with immediate surgery and adjuvant chemotherapy for nonmetastatic osteosarcoma: Pediatric oncology group study pog-8651. *Journal Clinical Oncology, 21,* 1574–1580.

33. Granowetter, L., & West, D. C. (1997). The Ewing's sarcoma family of tumors: Ewing's sarcoma and peripheral primitive neuroectodermal tumor of bone and soft tissue. In D. O. Walterhourse, & S. L. Cohn (Eds.), *Diagnostic and therapeutic advances in pediatric oncology* (pp. 253–308). Boston: Kluwer Academic Publishers.

34. Grier, H. E. (1997). The Ewing family of tumors; Ewing's sarcoma and primitive neuroectodermal tumors. *Pediatric Clinics of North America, 44,* 991–1004.

35. Grimer, R. J., Carter, S. R., & Pynsent, P. B. (1997). Cost-effectiveness of limb salvage for bone tumors. *Journal of Bone and Joint Surgery (British), 79,* 558–561.

36. Reference deleted in page proofs.

37. Hagberg, K., Haggstrom, E., & Bronemark, R. (2007). Physiological cost index (PCI) and walking performance in individuals with transfemoral prostheses compared to healthy controls. *Disability & Rehabilitation, 29,* 643–649.

38. Heare, T., Hensley, M. A., & Dell'Orfano, S. (2009). Bone tumors: Osteosarcoma and Ewing's sarcoma. *Current Opinion in Pediatrics, 21,* 365–372.

39. Herring, J. A. (Ed.). (2002a). Growth and development. In *Tachdjian's pediatric orthopedics* (3rd ed.; pp. 3–21). Philadelphia: WB Saunders.

40. Herring, J. A. (Ed.). (2002b). Limb deficiencies. In *Tachdjian's pediatric orthopedics* (3rd ed.; pp. 1745–1810). Philadelphia: WB Saunders.

41. Hostetler, S. G., Schwartz, L., Shields, B. J., Xiang, H., & Smith, G. A. (2005). Characteristics of pediatric traumatic amputations treated in hospital emergency departments: United States, 1990–2002. *Pediatrics, 116,* 667–674.

42. Hubbard, S. A., Kurtz, I., Heim, W., & Montgomery, G. (1998). Powered prosthetic intervention in upper extremity deficiency. In J. A. Herring, & J. G. Birch (Eds.), *The child with a limb deficiency* (pp. 405–416). Rosemont, IL: American Academy of Orthopedic Surgeons.

43. James, M. A., Bagley, A. M., Brasington, K., Lutz, C., McConnell, S., & Molitor, F. (2006). Impact of prostheses on function and quality of life for children with unilateral congenital below-the-elbow deficiency. *Journal of Bone and Joint Surgery (American), 88,* 2356–2365.

44. Krajbich, J. I., & Bochmann, D. (1992). Van Nes rotation-plasty in tumor surgery. In J. H. Bowker, & J. W. Michael (Eds.), *Atlas of limb prosthetics: Surgical, prosthetic, and rehabilitation principles* (2nd ed.; pp. 885–899). St Louis: Mosby.

45. Krajbich, J. L. (1998). Rotationplasty in the management of proximal femoral focal deficiency. In J. A. Herring, & J. G. Birch (Eds.), *The child with a limb deficiency* (p. 87). Rosemont, IL: American Academy of Orthopedic Surgeons.

46. Link, M. P., Gebhardt, M. C., & Meyers, P. A. (2002). Osteosarcoma. In P. A. Pizzo, & D. G. Poplack (Eds.), *Principles and practice of pediatric oncology* (4th ed.; pp. 1051–1089). Philadelphia: Lippincott Williams & Wilkins.

47. Loder, R. T. (2004). Demographics of traumatic amputations in children. *Journal of Bone and Joint Surgery (American), 86,* 923–928.

48. Marchese, V. G., Rai, S. N., Carlson, C. A., Hinds, P. S., Spearing, E. M., Zhang, L., Callaway, L., Neel, M. D., Rao, B. N., & Ginsberg, J. P. (2007). Assessing functional mobility in survivors of lower-extremity sarcoma: Reliability and validity of a new assessment tool. *Pediatric Blood Cancer, 49,* 183–189.

49. Marchese, V. G., Spearing, E., Callaway, L., Rai, S. N., Zhang, L., Hinds, P. S., Carlson, C. A., Neel, M. D., Rao, B. N., & Ginsberg, J. P. (2006). Relationships among range of motion, functional mobility, and quality of life in children and adolescents after limb-sparing surgery for lower-extremity sarcoma. *Pediatric Physical Therapy, 18,* 238–244.

50. McGuirk, C. K., Westgate, M. N., & Holmes, L. B. (2001). Limb deficiencies in the newborn infants. *Pediatrics, 108,* E64.

51. Melzack, R., Israel, R., Lacroix, R., & Schultz, G. (1997). Phantom limbs in people with congenital deficiency or amputation in early childhood. *Brain, 120,* 1603–1620.

52. Meyers, P. A., & Gorlick, R. (1997). Osteosarcoma. *Pediatric Clinics of North America, 44,* 973–989.

53. Michael, J. W. (1999). Modern prosthetic knee mechanisms. *Clinical Orthopedics and Related Research, 361,* 39–47.

54. Morrissy, R. T., Giavedoni, B. J., & Coulter-O'Berry, C. (2006). The limb-deficient child. In R. T. Morrissy, S. L. Weinstein (Eds.), *Lovell & Winter pediatric orthopedics* [6th ed.; pp. 1333–1382]. Philadelphia: Lippincott Williams & Wilkins.

55. Nagarajan, R., Neglia, J. P., Clohisy, D. R., Yasui, Y., Greenberg, M., Hudson, M., Zevon, M. A., Tersak, J. M., Ablin, A., & Robison, L. L. (2003). Education, employment, insurance, and marital status among 694 survivors of pediatric lower extremity bone tumors. *Cancer, 97,* 2554–2564.

56. Neel, M. D., Wilkins, R. M., Rao, B. N., & Kelly, C. M. (2003). Early multicenter experience with a noninvasive expandable prosthesis. *Clinical Orthopedics and Related Research, 415,* 72–81.

56a. Ness, K.K., Hudson, M. M, Ginsberg, J. P., Nagarajan, R., Kaste, S. C., Marina, N., Whitton, J., Robison, L. L., & Gurney, J. G. (2009). Physical performance limitations in the childhood cancer survivor study cohort. *Journal of Clinical Oncology, 27,* 2382–2389.

57. Oppenheim, W. L., Setoguchi, Y., & Fowler, E. (1998). Overview and comparison of Syme amputation and knee fusion with the Van Nes rotationplasty in proximal femoral focal deficiency. In J. A. Herring, & J. G. Birch (Eds.), *The child with a limb deficiency* (pp. 73–86). Rosemont, IL: American Academy of Orthopedic Surgeons.

58. Pardasaney, P. K., Sullivan, P. E., Portney, L. G., & Mankin, H. J. (2006). Advantage of limb salvage over amputation in proximal lower extremity tumors. *Clinical Orthopedics and Related Research, 444,* 201–208.

59. Parente, M. A., & Geil, M. (2006). In the future: Surgical and educational advances and challenges. In K. Carroll, & J. E. Edelstein (Eds.), *Prosthetics and patient management: A comprehensive clinical approach* (pp. 233–241). Thorofare, NJ: Slack Publishing.

60. Patton, J. G. (2004). Occupational therapy. In D. G. Smith, J. W. Michael, & J. H. Bowker (Eds.), *Atlas of limb amputations and limb deficiencies* (3rd ed.; pp. 813–830). Rosemont, IL: American Academy of Orthopedic Surgeons.

61. Pruitt, S. D., Varni, J. W., & Setoguchi, Y. (1996). Functional status in children with limb deficiency: Development and initial validation of an outcome measure. *Archives of Physical Medicine and Rehabilitation, 77,* 1233–1238.

62. Pruitt, S. D., Varni, J. W., Seid, M., & Setoguchi, Y. (1998). Functional status in limb deficiency: Development of an outcome measure for preschool children. *Archives of Physical Medicine and Rehabilitation, 79,* 405–411.

63. Pruitt, S. D., Seid, M., Varni, J. W., & Setoguchi, Y. (1999). Toddlers with limb deficiency: Conceptual basis and initial application of a functional status outcome measure. *Archives of Physical Medicine and Rehabilitation, 80,* 819–824.

64. Radocy, R. (2004). Prosthetic adaptations in competitive sports and recreation. In D. G. Smith, J. W. Michael, & J. H. Bowker (Eds.), *Atlas of limb amputations and limb deficiencies* (3rd ed.; pp. 327–338). Rosemont, IL: American Academy of Orthopedic Surgeons.

65. Rau, B., Bonvin, F., & de Bie, R. (2007). Short-term effect of physiotherapy rehabilitation on functional performance of lower-limb amputees. *Prosthetics and Orthotics International, 31,* 258–270.

66. Renard, A. J., Veth, R. P., Schreuder, H. W., van Loon, C. J., Koops, H. S., & van Horn, J. R. (2000). Function and complications after ablative and limb-salvage therapy in lower extremity sarcoma of bone. *Journal of Surgical Oncology, 73,* 198–205.

67. Robinson, K. P., Branemark, R., & Ward, D. A. (2004). Future developments: Osseointegration in transfemoral amputees. In D. G. Smith, J. W. Michael, & J. H. Bowker (Eds.), *Atlas of limb amputations and limb deficiencies* (3rd ed.; pp. 841–852). Rosemont, IL: American Academy of Orthopedic Surgeons.

68. Robitaille, J., Carmichael, S. L., Shaw, G. M., & Olney, R. S. (2009). Maternal nutrient intake and risks for transverse and longitudinal limb deficiencies: Data from the national birth defects prevention study, 1997–2003. *Birth Defects Research (Part A), 85,* 773–779.

69. Rougraff, B. T., Simon, M. A., & Kneisel, J. S. (1994). Limb salvage compared with amputation for osteosarcoma of the distal end of the femur: A long-term oncological, functional and quality of life study. *Journal of Bone and Joint Surgery (American), 163,* 1171–1175.

70. Shaperman, J., Landsberger, S. E., & Setoguchi, Y. (2003). Early upper extremity prosthesis fitting: When and what do we fit. *Journal Prosthetics and Orthotics, 15,* 11–17.

71. Shimizu, H., Yokoyama, S., & Asahara, H. (2007). Growth and differentiation of the developing limb bud from the perspective of chondrogenesis. *Development, Growth, & Differentiation, 49,* 449–454.

72. Shurr, D. G., & Cook, T. M. (1990). *Prosthetics and orthotics* (pp. 183–193). East Norwalk, CT: Appleton & Lange.

73. Simmel, M. L. (1962). Phantom experiences following amputation in childhood. *Journal of Neurology, Neurosurgery, and Psychiatry, 25,* 69–78.

74. Sparreboom, A., Evans, W. E., & Baker, S. D. (2007). Chemotherapy in the pediatric patient. In S. H. Orkin, D. E. Fisher, A. T. Look, et al (Eds.), *Oncology of infancy & childhood* (pp. 175–207). Philadelphia: Saunders Elsevier.

75. Springfield, D. S. (1991). Musculoskeletal tumors. In S. T. Canale, & J. H. Beatty (Eds.), *Operative pediatric orthopedics* (pp. 1073–1113). St Louis: Mosby.

76. Stanger, M. (2008). Orthopedic management. In J. S. Tecklin (Ed.), *Pediatric physical therapy* (4th ed.; pp. 417–450). Philadelphia: Lippincott Williams & Wilkins.

77. Sutherland, D. H. (1984). *Gait disorders in childhood and adolescence* (pp. 14–27). Baltimore: Williams & Wilkins.

78. Swanson, A. B., Barsky, A. J., & Entin, M. A. (1968). Classification of limb malformations on the basis of embryological failures. *Surgical Clinics of North America, 48,* 1169–1179.

79. Tarbell, N. J., & Kooy, H. M. (2002). General principles of radiation oncology. In P. A. Pizzo, & D. G. Poplack (Eds.), *Principles and practice of pediatric oncology* (4th ed.; pp. 369–380). Philadelphia: Lippincott Williams & Wilkins.

80. Tebbi, C. K. (1993). Psychological effects of amputation in sarcoma. In G. B. Humphrey, H. S. Koops, W. M. Molenaar, & A. Postma (Eds.), *Osteosarcoma in adolescents and young adults* (pp. 39–44). Boston: Kluwer Academic.

81. Reference deleted in page proofs.

82. Trautwein, L. C., Smith, D. G., & Rivara, F. P. (1996). Pediatric amputation injuries: Etiology, cost and outcome. *Journal of Trauma: Injury, Infection and Critical Care, 41,* 831–838.

83. Unwin, P. S., & Walker, P. S. (1996). Extendible endoprosthesis for the skeletally immature. *Clinical Orthopedics and Related Research, 322,* 179–193.

84. Varni, J. W., & Setoguchi, Y. (1992). Screening for behavioral and emotional problems in children and adolescents with congenital or acquired limb deficiencies. *American Journal of Diseases in Childhood, 146,* 103–107.

85. Weaver, D. D. (1998). Vascular etiology of limb defects: The subclavian artery supply disruption sequence. In J. A. Herring, & J. G. Birch (Eds.), *The child with a limb deficiency* (pp.

25–38). Rosemont, IL: American Academy of Orthopedic Surgeons.

86. Reference deleted in page proofs.

87. Wilk, B., Karol, L., Halliday, S., Cummings, D., Haideri, N., & Stephenson, J. (1999). Transition to an articulating knee prosthesis in pediatric amputees. *Journal of Prosthetics and Orthotics, 11,* 69–74.

88. Wilkins, R. M., & Soubeiran, A. (2001). The Phoenix expandable prosthesis: Early American experience. *Clinical Orthopedics and Related Research, 382,* 51–58.

89. Wright, P. E., & Jobe, M. T. (1991). Congenital anomalies of the hand. In S. T. Canale, & J. H. Beatty (Eds.), *Operative pediatric orthopedics* (pp. 253–330). St Louis: Mosby.

14 Orthopedic Conditions

MARY WILLS JESSE, PT, DHS, OCS • JUDY LEACH, PT

Physical therapists working with the pediatric population may not frequently treat patients with a primary orthopedic diagnosis; however, general knowledge of orthopedics is important throughout the intervention process. This becomes even more challenging in the pediatric population as the musculoskeletal system grows and changes with age. What may be considered "typical" at one age may be significantly atypical at another.

Additionally, as physical therapist practice becomes more autonomous, we are challenged to identify problems that may be outside the scope of our practice and make appropriate referrals for care. We have a responsibility as therapists to have the knowledge base to determine these conditions in children.

Space in this chapter will not allow an exhaustive review of all the orthopedic conditions that affect children. Many references are provided throughout the text for further study, however. This chapter presents information on conditions commonly seen; specific areas of concern to the physical therapist will be highlighted to provide a basic framework for the practicing clinician.

TORSIONAL CONDITIONS

A chief complaint of in-toeing or out-toeing is probably the most common reason for elective referral of a child to an orthopedist. Even though these rotational conditions in the lower extremities usually do not require any treatment, they are often a source of significant concern for parents and other family members. Concern often escalates with comments from neighbors, teachers, and strangers on the street: "Why does your child walk funny?" This group of children has been described by Dr. Mercer Rang as "the worried well," a phrase that indicates the strong concern of the family and others involved with the child over alignment conditions that are often part of the spectrum of normal musculoskeletal development.

Numerous differences of opinion exist on how to define torsional conditions, how to measure them, and especially how to treat them, or if they should be treated at all. Most treatment with special shoes, casts, or braces has no proven efficacy, and many orthopedists believe that persistent deformity beyond skeletal maturity is unusual and significant functional disability is rare.[24] Less than 1% of femoral and tibial torsional deformities fail to resolve and may require operative correction in late childhood.[188] Unfortunately, the term *torsional deformities* is used in the literature, at national meetings, and in verbal discussions. Patients and parents hear the term *deformity*, and their worst fears are validated. For this reason, terminology should be used correctly in describing and classifying a child's condition. Version describes the position of the femoral head in the frontal plane. If the head lies anterior to the plane, it is anteverted, but a head that is positioned posterior to the frontal plane is retroverted.[38] Torsion describes the osseous position of a bone in its longitudinal axis, or "twist." It is measured by the angle formed at the intersection of the axis of the head and neck and the axis of the femoral condyles.[38]

Once neuromuscular dysfunction or other serious conditions have been ruled out, it is important to spend sufficient time educating the parents about the current reason for their child's condition and why it may not need treatment. Anticipatory guidance about future possibilities should be provided. For example, a 2-year-old child's in-toeing may resolve as his internal tibial torsion (ITT) resolves, but in-toeing may reappear at age 4 to 6 years as the result of femoral anteversion (FA).

OBTAINING A HISTORY

A specific history provides a wealth of information regarding possible causative factors and indications for possible treatment. Specific information obtained may also direct the examiner to expand the examination to rule out other, more severe conditions that may initially produce a chief complaint of in-toeing or out-toeing. Relevant information to be elicited from the parents includes the following:

1. **Birth history.** Was the infant full-term or premature? Was it a vaginal or cesarean delivery? Was oligohydramnios (deficiency of amniotic fluid) present? How many times has the mother been pregnant? What is the birth order of the parent? Many of the torsional problems seen in infants are "packaging" defects (i.e., caused by a restricted intrauterine environment). It is easy to imagine that an infant's lower limbs may "grow" into a particular position if one visualizes a full-term 9-pound fetus in the womb of a gravida 1, para 1 mother.

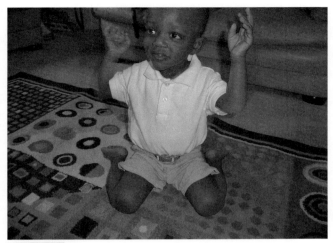

Figure 14-1   This is a child in the "W"-sitting position.

2. **Age when in-toeing or out-toeing was noted.** Has it improved or worsened since first noted? Was any previous treatment provided? For the walking child, at what age did the child start to walk independently? In the differential diagnosis, the index of suspicion should be increased when a child has a history of prematurity, difficult birth, or delayed motor milestones or has significant in-toeing or out-toeing that is worsening with time or is very asymmetrical. Children with mild spastic diplegia may have in-toeing, and children with Duchenne's muscular dystrophy may have out-toeing and flat feet. Conditions such as these must be ruled out.
3. **Family history.** In many cases, a positive family history for in-toeing or out-toeing is reported, and this should be noted, especially if treatment was undertaken for other family member(s).
4. **Sleeping and sitting positions.** Sleeping prone and sitting on feet encourages internal tibial torsion.[175] Sitting in a W-sit position may encourage the persistence of femoral anteversion (Figure 14-1).

CLINICAL EXAMINATION AND INTERVENTIONS

Clinical examination of the child with in-toeing and out-toeing should include documentation of the foot progression angle during walking, hip rotation ROM, the thigh-foot angle, and alignment of the foot. These four components provide the information necessary to establish the level and severity of any torsional problem.[188] Means and ranges for these components have been established throughout the stages of development.[188]

Foot Progression Angle

Foot progression angle (FPA), or "the angle of gait," is defined as the angular difference between the axis of the foot and the line of progression.[188] The child is observed while walking, and a value is assigned to the angle of both the right and the left foot (Figure 14-2). This is a subjective determination and represents an average of the angles noted on multiple steps. Various footprint techniques can be used to measure FPA, but these are time-consuming and may not be practical in the clinical situation. In-toeing is expressed as a negative value (e.g., −30°), and out-toeing is expressed as a positive value (e.g., +20°). This angle gives an overall view of the degree of in-toeing or out-toeing in the walking child. The FPA can also be assessed in supported stance for the child who is not yet walking independently. FPA is variable during infancy. During childhood and adult life, it shows little change, with a mean of +10° and a normal range of −3° to +20°.[190] In-toeing of −5° to −10° is mild, −10° to −15° is moderate, and more than −15° is severe.[188]

Hip Rotation, Femoral Anteversion, and Retroversion

Clinical Examination

Hip rotation ROM is measured most accurately in the prone position, with the hip in a position of neutral flexion/extension. (An extremely frightened, crying young child can be examined more easily by having the parent stand up and hold the child against the chest, facing the parent. This allows the child's hips to hang into neutral flexion/extension, and the examiner can then bend the child's knees and evaluate the hip rotation range.) This hip rotation measurement will be a reflection of the flexibility of the soft tissues and the version of the femur.

Torsion is defined by the position of the proximal reference axis (axis of the head and neck) compared with the distal reference axis (axis of the femoral condyles) when the distal reference axis is placed in the frontal plane.[38] Antetorsion in indicated if the femoral head lies anterior to the frontal plane, and retrotorsion is indicated if the femoral head lies less than 10° to 12° anterior to the frontal plane.[38] Norms have been defined for the magnitude of torsion (Figure 14-3). When the hip is in anteversion (or "anteverted") because of the femoral head being positioned on the frontal plane, the patient will usually have more hip internal rotation (IR) than external rotation (ER) ROM, assuming no soft tissue tightness. If hip IR is measured at 70° and ER at 25°, for example, the child is said to have FA and may in-toe when walking. In retroversion, the femoral head is positioned posterior to the frontal plane when the knee is aligned straight ahead, and the patient will have greater ER range. These describe positions in the child who matures without neurologic disorders such as cerebral palsy. The neonatal biomechanics and typical skeletal maturational changes in the child are presented in greater detail in Chapter 5.

Femoral and tibial torsion can be measured by computed tomography (CT), ultrasound, conventional radiography, and clinical examination.[79,110] Although use of diagnostic equipment may be helpful in some situations, clinical measurements have shown good accuracy when compared with CT and ultrasound findings.[79,110] Clinical measurements,

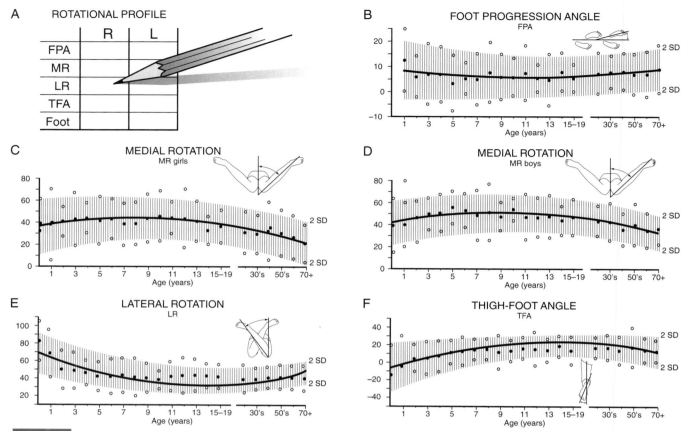

Figure 14-2   The foot progression angle from birth to maturity is depicted graphically. The graph includes two standard deviations from the mean. (Redrawn from Morrissy, R. T., & Weinstein, S. L. [Eds.]. [2006]. *Lovell and Winter pediatric orthopaedics* [6th ed., p. 1160]. Philadelphia: Lippincott Williams & Wilkins.)

therefore, are sufficient for documentation in most children with benign rotational problems.

Internal rotation measuring between 70° and 90° is evidence of femoral torsion.[161] True femoral retroversion in an infant is rare; it is usually tightness in the hip external rotation muscles and capsular ligaments that is producing the externally rotated position, masking the femoral anteversion.[156] The tightness of the hip soft tissues gradually stretches out, and the true anteversion of the femur becomes apparent. This process is often described incorrectly as "femoral anteversion increases"; the amount of femoral version is actually decreasing, but it is more easily visualized because the muscle tightness of the external rotators is decreasing. The FA becomes increasingly more apparent clinically as the child approaches 5 to 6 years of age, as the soft tissue tightness resolves. Studies have shown a gradual decrease in FA with age: 40° at birth to between 15° and 20° by 8 to 10 years of age.[210] Femoral antetorsion is mild if internal hip rotation is 70° to 80°, moderate if 80° to 90°, and severe if 90° plus in childhood.[188] By mid-childhood, the femoral head and neck have usually assumed a relatively more neutral position in relationship to the femoral shaft, and children typically have approximately equal amounts of hip IR and ER (Figure 14-4). This is measured by using the Ryder test in which the

child is positioned prone or supine with the knee flexed to 90°. The examiner holds the leg proximal to the ankle and rotates the hip while palpating the anterior and posterior borders of the greater trochanter. When the trochanter is at the most lateral position of the arc, the femoral neck and head are considered to be aligned in the frontal plane. Hip rotation is measured in this position and is used as the angle of torsion. It is important to remember that this test underestimates the true value of the medial twist of the femur that would be measured by CT scan by approximately 20°.[197]

Femoral Anteversion: Intervention

Many types of interventions have been tried to correct FA, including braces, twister cables, and special shoes. These have not proved effective.[52,210] Anecdotal findings may note the efficacy of these conservative methods, although spontaneous improvement does naturally occur in most cases. One reasonable recommendation is to have the child avoid W-sitting (reverse tailor sitting) and to encourage tailor sitting in maximum ER. If significant FA is still present at age 10 to 14 years and is resulting in cosmetically unappealing in-toeing, surgical correction in the form of femoral derotation osteotomies may be considered, although the possible risks of the operation may outweigh the benefits of

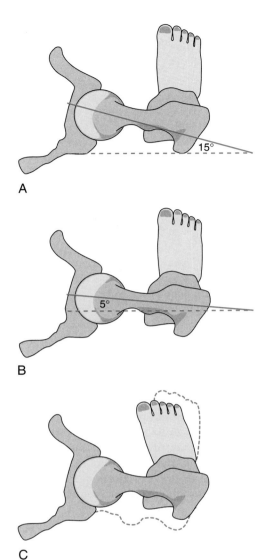

Figure 14-3 In the femur, version is the angular difference between the transcondylar axis of the knee *(the horizontal line in this drawing)* and the axis of the femoral neck. These two lines form an angle and document whether the femur is in anteversion or retroversion. **A,** Normal anteversion: With this small amount of anteversion, the individual can walk comfortably with the foot pointed straight ahead (i.e., a neutral angle of foot progression). **B,** Excessive anteversion with in-toeing: When a large amount of anteversion is present, the individual must internally rotate the femur to seat the femoral head in the acetabulum and achieve improved joint congruity. This results in a negative foot progression angle, and the foot is pointed in during gait (in-toeing). **C,** Retroversion: In this drawing, significant reduction can be seen in the angle formed between the two axes, depicting retroversion. If this were excessive, the individual would need to externally rotate the femur to seat the femoral head in the acetabulum and would have a positive angle of foot progression (out-toeing). (From Neumann, D. A. [2002]. *Kinesiology of the musculoskeletal system* [p. 395]. St Louis: Mosby.)

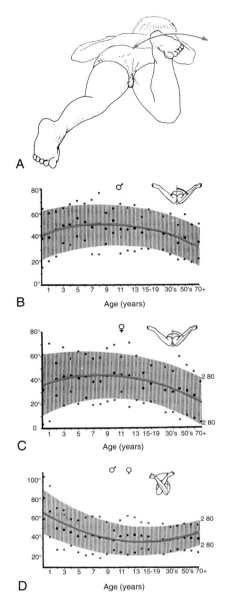

Figure 14-4 Hip rotation is measured with the patient prone, knee flexed to 90°. Means for hip rotation in mid-childhood and in older subjects. **A,** Medial rotation in males: 50° (range, 25°–65°). **B,** Medial rotation in females: 40° (range, 15°–60°). **C,** Lateral rotation: 45° (range, 25°–65°), with no gender difference. (From Staheli, L. T., Corbett, M., Wyss, C., & King, H. [1985]. Lower extremity rotational problems in children. *Journal of Bone and Joint Surgery* [American], *67*, 41–42.)

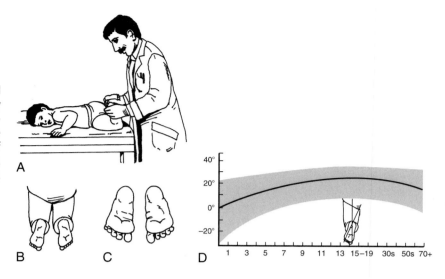

Figure 14-5 The rotational status of the tibia and the foot is best evaluated in the prone position. By allowing the foot to fall into its natural resting position **(A)**, the thigh-foot axis **(B)** and the shape of the foot **(C)** can be determined. The normal range of motion can be seen in graphic form **(D)**. (From Staheli, L. T. [2006]. *Practice of pediatric orthopedics* [2nd ed., p. 89]. Philadelphia: Lippincott Williams and Wilkins.)

realignment. In the adult, femoral antetorsion does not cause degenerative arthritis and rarely causes any disability.[188] Surgical intervention may be warranted and has proved successful in children with severe symptomatic torsional malalignment with excessive FA or external tibial torsion (ETT) associated with patellofemoral pathology, when conservative treatment has failed.[25]

Thigh-Foot Axis, Tibial Torsion

Clinical Examination

The alignment of the lower leg can be measured by documenting the thigh-foot axis, which is a reflection of the version of the tibia. Tibial torsion is assessed using the thigh-foot angle, the angular difference between the longitudinal axes of the thigh and foot, as measured in the prone position with the knee flexed (Figure 14-5). Some examiners measure tibial torsion with the child sitting and the knee flexed to 90°. Tibial torsion can also be described as the angle formed by the axis of the femoral condyles and the axis through the medial and lateral malleoli. This is called the transmalleolar axis. By convention, internal tibial torsion (ITT) is expressed as a negative value, such as "tibial torsion of −30 degrees." External tibial torsion (ETT) is expressed as a positive value. Another reliable method that can be used to measure the transmalleolar axis is the footprint method. In this test, the patient sits with his hip and knee at 90° of flexion with the hip in neutral rotation and the tibial tubercle facing forward. The foot is set on a piece of lined paper so that the lines are parallel to the knee axis. The footprint is traced and two marks are made vertically below the centers of the malleoli. A line drawn between this line and any line on the paper will provide the transmalleolar axis.[69] Changes in tibial torsion throughout childhood to skeletal maturity are described in Chapter 5.

ITT in infancy often is not apparent to the parents or the casual examiner because the hips have external rotation muscle contractures and the infant's legs tend to assume an abducted and externally rotated position. The ITT may become noticeable only as the hip contractures stretch out, resulting in a more neutral position of the hip, especially when the child begins to walk independently.

Internal Tibial Torsion: Intervention

Controversy exists regarding appropriate treatment of ITT, as it does in FA. Many orthopedists believe that it should not be treated at all because the natural history of the condition is gradual improvement. The very small percentage of children who do not improve and who have a significant functional deficit as a result of ITT can be treated surgically at a later date with external rotational osteotomy of the tibia and fibula. A different school of thought relies on natural improvement up to about 18 months of age, and at that age advocates treating persistent ITT with a Friedman counter splint (a flexible leather strap) or a Denis Browne bar (a metal bar) for night wear, usually for about 6 months. These devices attach to shoes and hold the feet in an externally rotated position. The Denis Browne bar is an uncomfortable treatment that because of this adherence is sometimes limited. Also, with the knees extended, the torque applied by the bar may be directed to the hips because the knees are extended. The Wheaton brace with an upper component has also been developed to isolate the correction to the tibia, not to apply torque to the hip. With this device, the knee is flexed to 90°, and improved comfort with this device may improve adherence.

Complications at the knee have been associated with abnormal values of ITT and ETT. Weidow et al.[213] found that subjects with medial knee osteoarthritis had 9° more external tibial torsion than controls, and those with lateral knee osteoarthritis had 6° less external tibial torsion. Also reported has been an increased incidence of osteochondritis dissecans in those with higher external tibial torsion.[18] Increased ETT may be a predisposing factor in the onset of Osgood-Schlatter syndrome in male athletes, especially on the side preferentially used for jumping and sprinting.[58] However, in-toeing in certain sports may be beneficial. Fuchs and Staheli[56] studied high school students (50 sprinters and 50 control subjects) and found that the sprinters tended to have low normal thigh-foot angles and in-toed when sprinting.

Surgical correction is a supported option when a child is at least 8 years of age, has significant or functional deformity, and has a thigh-foot angle greater than three standard deviations beyond the mean.[189] Successful approaches have included same level distal tibial and fibular osteotomies with crossed Kirschner wires,[41] and the Haas procedure involving multiple longitudinal bicortical osteotomies with fixation by a long cast or pins-in-plaster.[43]

Metatarsus Adductus

The infant foot is malleable, making it susceptible to deformation and compression from intrauterine positioning. Alterations in alignment of the foot can be divided into two categories: (1) positional or "packaging" problems caused by a restricted intrauterine environment and (2) "manufacturing" defects or true congenital abnormalities such as talipes equinovarus. Metatarsus varus, also called metatarsus adductus (MTA), is one of the most commonly seen positional conditions in infants (occurs in 1 per 1000 live births).[210] Observable deformities that have been noted with MTA by researchers have included abnormal insertions of the tibialis anterior or posterior tendons, an abnormal shape of the medial cuneiform, and medial obliquity of the first cuneiform–first metatarsal joint.[23,103,131,163] These may be primary causes or adaptive changes.[211]

In MTA the forefoot is curved medially, the hindfoot is in the normal slight valgus position, and full dorsiflexion ROM is noted. The degree of MTA can be graded as (I) flexible with the ability to correct beyond the midline, (II) moderately flexible with the ability to correct to midline, or (III) severe with the inability to achieve midline.[14] Having the child stand on the glass plate of a photocopy machine and copying the feet is an easy, quick way to document the amount of metatarsus (Figure 14-6). Also present in some cases is a dynamic deformity seen only during the child's gait, called "searching great toe." The foot appears straight at rest, but forefoot varus as a result of muscle action occurs with medial motion of the great toe. This usually corrects spontaneously.[188]

Treatment is rarely required for mild cases (grade I), which usually resolve on their own by about 4 to 6 months. Moderate cases (grade II) may be treated with stretching exercises and corrective shoes (straight-last or reverse-last shoes or both). A recommended stretching technique is to face the child, cup the heel of the foot with the left hand (if right foot MTA), and abduct the foot with the right hand while keeping the heel in varus. Pressure should be applied gently across the metatarsals.[210] Severe cases may be treated with manipulation and serial casting, followed by corrective shoes. Surgery is not considered before 4 years to allow for

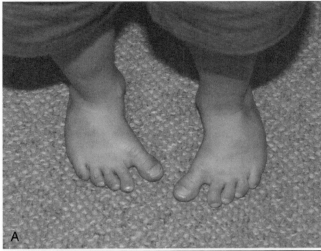
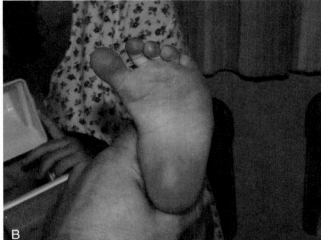
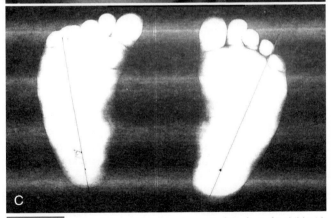

Figure 14-6   Clinical view of the dorsal aspect of the feet of a child with metatarsus adductus **(A)** is shown in standing. The plantar aspect of the same child's feet is shown in a non–weight-bearing position **(B)**. A photocopy of a child's feet with metatarsus adductus is used for documentation **(C)**. (From Wallach, D. M., & Davidson, R. S. [2005]. Pediatric lower limb disorders. In J. P. Dormans [Ed.]. *Pediatric orthopaedics: Core knowledge in orthopaedics* [p. 207]. Philadelphia, Elsevier Mosby.)

spontaneous resolution.[210] Although surgery should be used selectively, correction may be important in prevention of further problems as the child reaches adulthood. Theodorou et al.[201] described an increased risk of stress fractures in those with metatarsus adductus. Patients (ages 25 to 61 years) who experienced metatarsal fractures had a forefoot adductor angle of 21° to 37° (normal range, 8° to 14°).[201]

Calcaneovalgus

Calcaneovalgus is a common positional foot problem in newborns, and more than 30% of neonates have bilateral calcaneovalgus.[198] This is another example of an intrauterine "packaging" deformity. The ankle is in excessive dorsiflexion, the forefoot is curved out laterally, and the hindfoot is in valgus. The dorsum of the foot may actually be touching the anterior surface of the leg at birth. The positional calcaneovalgus foot corrects spontaneously and does not require treatment. It must be distinguished from more severe conditions, such as a congenital calcaneovalgus foot caused by a vertical talus. In this more uncommon condition, the talus is vertically oriented and the navicular is displaced onto the dorsal surface of the talus. The forefoot is dorsiflexed but the hindfoot is plantarflexed, and the foot bends at the instep. This characteristic position is described as a "rocker-bottom" deformity of the foot, and the foot is much more rigid than the typical calcaneovalgus foot. Idiopathic or congenital vertical talus is rare and is more commonly associated with other conditions such as neural tube defects, neuromuscular disorders, or congenital malformation syndromes.[105,210] Without treatment, this leads to progressive foot pain in all sensate ambulators.[210] Nonambulators can be treated with shoes that accommodate their deformity, as surgery is considered the only corrective treatment.[210]

Foot Alignment Problems: Summary

Table 14-1 is a decision matrix that provides a quick and easy way to categorize foot conditions.[217]

TORSIONAL PROFILE

The components that may contribute to in-toeing are femoral anteversion, internal tibial torsion, and metatarsus adductus. Those that may contribute to out-toeing are external rotation contractures of the hip (and, rarely, femoral retroversion), ETT, and calcaneovalgus. The foot progression angle can be viewed as the "summation" of the rotational alignment of the three segments of the lower limb: the hip and femur, the lower leg, and the foot. For example,

significant femoral anteversion at the hip may be balanced by ETT with a straight foot (no MTA or calcaneovalgus). The foot progression angle would be 0°/0° (right/left) with the feet pointing straight ahead. When a child toes in or toes out, the condition is usually bilateral, but occasionally one sees "windswept" lower extremities, with one limb toeing in and the other limb toeing out.

A typically developing 8-month-old infant supported in upright might have a torsional profile as follows:

	Right	Left
Foot progression angle (not yet standing)	–	–
Internal rotation of hip	20°	20°
External rotation of hip	90°	90°
Thigh-foot angle	0°	0°
Foot	Neutral	Neutral

In this example, the legs are positioned in external rotation, the usual position for the lower extremities in infancy.

The torsional profile of a 5-year-old child with in-toeing might look like this:

	Right	Left
Foot progression angle	−40°	−30°
Internal rotation of hip	70°	70°
External rotation of hip	20°	20°
Thigh-foot angle	−10°	+15°
Foot		

From this discussion, it is clear that one must determine which component(s) of the lower extremity is causing the torsional condition and intervene at that level, if indicated. For example, using heavy, high-topped orthopedic shoes will not correct femoral anteversion. In fact, the child will probably be clumsier and stumble more frequently. The concept of a natural history of improvement over time is also pivotal. It is important not to extol the virtues of various treatments too vigorously, because it is difficult to differentiate benefits obtained from the treatment versus benefits that occurred simply with the passage of time as a result of skeletal maturation. In summary, however, in-toeing is usually attributable to MTA in the infant, ITT in the toddler, and femoral anteversion in the child up to 10 years old.[114]

In children with neuromuscular disorders such as cerebral palsy (CP), the basic examination format described

TABLE 14-1 Decision Matrix for Foot Deformity

	Metatarsus Varus	Clubfoot	Calcaneovalgus
Side view (Can foot dorsiflex?)	Yes	No	Yes
Foot shape (viewed from bottom)	Kidney-shaped (deviated medially)	Kidney-shaped	Banana-shaped (deviated laterally)
Heel position	Valgus	Varus	Valgus

previously is useful in helping to delineate the child's problem with gait. This assessment mainly addresses bony alignment. One must also document muscle tone, muscle strength, and motor control. Abnormalities in any of these areas can cause in-toeing or out-toeing, alone or in conjunction with skeletal malalignment. An example would be a child with CP who ambulates with a foot progression angle of −40°/−30°. This may be due to a combination of FA, ITT, MTA, and spasticity in the hip adductors, medial hamstrings, and posterior tibialis muscles. Bobroff et al.[15] studied 147 patients (267 hips) with CP, comparing FA and neck-shaft angle (NSA) versus those in children without CP. As age increased, those with CP showed little change in FA (FA decreased in the control group) and an increase in NSA compared with the control group. By contrast, a child with Duchenne's muscular dystrophy may ambulate with an in-toeing gait at age 6 because of FA and then gradually develop an out-toeing gait by age 10, resulting from resolution of the FA and increasing weakness of the gluteus maximus and quadriceps muscles, plus tightness in the iliotibial band and plantar flexors.

Another area of assessment and treatment in which this multilevel concept is useful involves measurement of other gross motor activities, such as sitting. Many children with increased tone, as well as children with hypotonia, will W-sit. This postural preference is frequently ascribed to problems with spasticity, or it is thought of as a compensatory mechanism to achieve better sitting balance. However, a more detailed examination might reveal that the child has, in addition to spasticity or poor balance, significant FA that simply does not allow comfortable sitting with the hips in external rotation.

ANGULAR CONDITIONS

Genu varum (bowlegs) and genu valgum (knock-knees) are similar to torsional conditions in that they are commonly seen in typically developing children, and a specific natural history has been described that results in normal skeletal alignment at maturity (Figure 14-7). This is described in greater detail in Chapter 5.

GENU VARUM

Clinical Examination

The child must be undressed with diaper removed for accurate documentation of genu varum. The child is placed with the medial malleoli approximated. The distance between femoral condyles is measured. Some clinicians use the distance between the knees at the knee joint line. A plastic triangle with centimeters marked on both sides is useful, allowing the examiner to easily obtain accurate measurements, especially of a wiggling child. Infants usually have ITT and genu varum, and this combination tends to make the child look "bowlegged and pigeon-toed," causing many

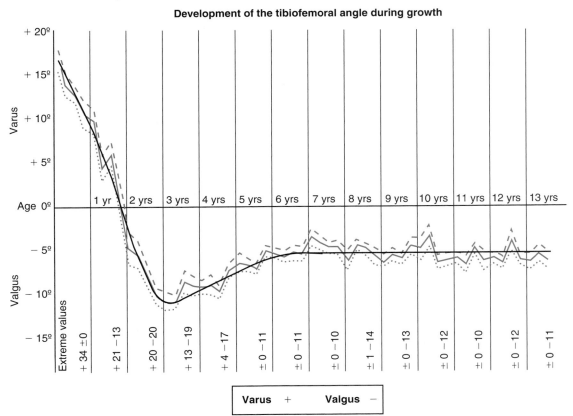

Development of the tibiofemoral angle during growth

Figure 14-7 Graphic representation of the development of the tibiofemoral angle during growth. (Redrawn from Salenius, P., & Vankka, E. [1975]. The development of the tibiofemoral angle in children. *Journal of Bone and Joint Surgery* [American], *57*, 260.)

parents and others great concern. Even when the genu varum has resolved and the child may actually have developed genu valgum, the presence of ITT may make the child look bowlegged.

Differential Diagnosis

When a child develops severe genu varum, especially after 4 years of age or worsening over time, systemic disorders such as vitamin D–resistant rickets, achondroplasia, renal osteodystrophy, and osteogenesis imperfecta must be ruled out, along with a variety of skeletal dysplasias and other conditions that cause genu varum.[13,21] Radiographs are used to rule out idiopathic tibia vara, also known as Blount's disease.

Physiologic (normal) genu varum in the infant must also be distinguished from pathologic anterolateral bow of the tibia, usually noted at birth.[188] In this extremely serious condition, radiographs demonstrate a tibia with a narrowed, sclerotic intramedullary canal, which puts the tibia at severe risk of fracture in the first year of life. In these cases, both tibia and fibula may fail to unite; hence the term "pseudarthrosis of the tibia" is used to describe this condition. Protective bracing and surgical treatment may be helpful, but may eventually require amputation because of persistent pseudarthrosis.[188]

Intervention

"Physiologic" genu varum does not usually require intervention unless it persists after age 2 years and either shows no tendency to correct or is actually worsening. This latter condition may require bracing in hip-knee-ankle-foot orthoses (HKAFOs) or knee-ankle-foot orthoses (KAFOs) with no knee joint or a hinged knee joint that can be locked. Surgical correction is sometimes required, although this is rare.

GENU VALGUM

Like genu varum, genu valgum can occasionally persist beyond the age range when one expects the legs to become generally straight. Many of the children with persistent genu valgum are overweight and have an out-toeing foot progression angle, an awkward gait, and flat feet. Genu valgum can be measured by documenting the intermalleolar distance in supine or standing, with the medial aspects of the knees lightly touching each other.

Children with significant femoral anteversion may often appear knock-kneed. Once again, a clear understanding of the three-level concept of torsional conditions and the angular conditions of genu varum and genu valgum is necessary to define the specific problem(s). Athletes have been noted to be predisposed to developing overuse injuries from both extrinsic factors (e.g., training errors) and intrinsic or anatomic factors, such as malalignment of the lower extremities.[127] Genu varum or valgum, along with torsional malalignment, may predispose athletes to knee extensor mechanism injuries, iliotibial band syndrome, stress fractures, and plantar fasciitis. Some adolescents with genu valgum present with anterior knee pain, patellofemoral instability, circumduction gait, and difficulty running.[195] Genu valgum can also be seen in multiple epiphyseal dysplasia.[129] Asymmetrical genu valgum may result from trauma or fracture of the lateral distal femoral epiphysis.

If severe, physiologic genu valgum can be safely and effectively corrected in the teenage years by stapling of the medial femoral growth plate, and genu varum by leg stapling of the lateral growth plate.[127] This allows the unstapled side of the femoral growth plate to continue growing, and the leg gradually grows into better alignment. A second option for surgical treatment is femoral osteotomy.

FLAT FOOT

Flat foot is a common condition seen in the orthopedic clinic, with incidence ranging from 7% to 22%.[11] The medial longitudinal arch of the foot is not present at birth, and the area of the arch consists of fatty tissue.[145] Normally, the arch will develop in the first decade of life, with progression of this seen between 2 and 6 years of age.[145] The critical age of development of the arch is 6 years of age, and evaluation before this age may overestimate the problem.[145] At walking age, an arch may be present in sitting but disappear upon standing, which is referred to as flexible flat foot.[145] Although this condition rarely causes problems, parents are often concerned about the abnormal appearance.

The most common cause of flexible flat foot is ligamentous laxity, which allows the foot to flatten with weight bearing.[31] Children often will also demonstrate hypomobility of other joints as well, such as hyperextension of the fingers, elbows, and knees.[31,145] In these cases, the child can form an arch when asked to stand on tiptoe.[31] The heels roll into a varus position, and good strength of the ankle and foot muscles is measurable[158] (Figure 14-8).

Another factor that may influence the prevalence of flat foot is the wearing of shoes.[31,158,171] In a study of 2300 children between the ages of 4 and 13 years, flat foot was most common in children who wore closed-toe shoes (13.2%), less common in those who wore sandals (6.0%) or slippers (8.2%), and least in the unshod (2.8%).[158] The incidence among those who wore shoes was even higher in those with ligament laxity.[158] Others have found an association between being overweight and the prevalence of flat foot diagnosed in 4- and 5-year-olds.[11,42] Treatment of the flexible flat foot generally is not necessary.[31,145,176,188] Another study found that boys had a significantly greater tendency for flat foot than girls in a population of 3- to 6-year-olds, and that overweight and obese children were at higher risk.[154] Shoe modifications or inserts have been used, although studies have not shown these to be beneficial.[31,188,218]

It has been widely documented that a low arch usually is less of a problem in adulthood than high-arched (cavus) feet. Michelson et al.[126] studied 196 college athletes with flat feet, who had 227 episodes of lower extremity injury. Pes planus

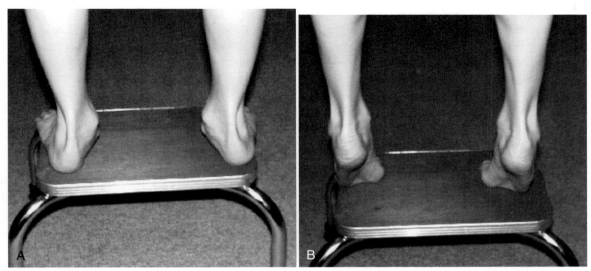

Figure 14-8   Flexible flat foot with heel rolling into varus when standing on toes. (From Dormans, J. P. [2005]. *Pediatric orthopaedics: Core Knowledge in orthopaedics.* Philedelphia: Elsevier Mosby.)

was not a risk factor for any lower extremity injury, therefore the use of orthotics to prevent further injury was discouraged.[126] In a retrospective study of 97,279 military recruits, mild pes planus resulted in no greater incidence of anterior knee pain or intermittent low back pain when compared with controls.[106]

Most pediatric orthopedists who now counsel parents regarding the natural history of improvement in flat feet through childhood advise the use of a lightweight running shoe as the only recommendation. Using shoes with an arch support and a strong counter will not correct the flat foot but can help decrease wear on the medial border of the shoes, thereby decreasing the expense of frequent shoe purchases.

Flat foot can occur secondary to other diagnoses, and these should be considered. A tendo Achillis contracture can produce a secondary flat foot. Examples of conditions in which this may occur are cerebral palsy, congenital or familial tight heel cords, and muscular dystrophy. A fixed valgus of the hindfoot causing symptoms such as pain, callus, ulceration, poor brace tolerance, and excessive shoe wear can be relieved by tendo Achillis lengthening and other soft tissue and osseous procedures.[132,218]

Children occasionally have an extra ossicle located at the medial border of the navicular, called an accessory navicular, frequently associated with flat feet. This condition may become symptomatic in late childhood or early adolescence, resulting in pain over the ossicle and along the medial arch, and can be corrected surgically.

Some children with flat foot have a rigid, painful foot with limited subtalar motion. Some of these children carry the diagnosis of peroneal spastic flat foot because of clonus in the peroneal muscles, and may be referred for physical therapy.[99] These children deserve further diagnostic scrutiny and a workup for tarsal coalition (a congenital fibrous, cartilaginous, or osseous union of two or more tarsal bones).

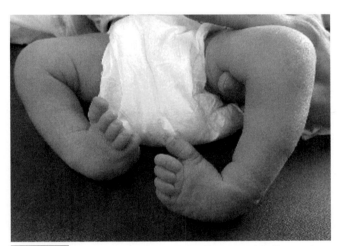

Figure 14-9   Child with clubfoot with hindfoot varus, hindfoot equinus, and forefoot varus. (From Wallach, D. M., & Davidson, R. S. [2005]. Pediatric lower limb disorders. In J. P. Dormans [Ed.]. *Pediatric orthopaedics: Core knowledge in orthopaedics* [p. 257]. Philadelphia: Elsevier Mosby.)

CLUBFOOT

Clubfoot, also referred to as talipes equinovarus (TEV), is a congenital deformity that includes components of forefoot adductus, hindfoot varus, and ankle equinus (Figure 14-9). Severe cases of metatarsus adductus may be confused with this, but the equinus component differentiates the diagnosis. The foot appears smaller as the result of a flexible, softer heel caused by the hypoplastic calcaneus.[65] Ankle valgus may evolve with growth and may be mistaken for "overcorrected clubfoot," or hindfoot valgus.[196] The talus is smaller in clubfoot than a normal foot and has a flattened superior surface with consequent decreases in talocalcaneal angle.[223] The subtalar joint facets are misshapen, and the navicular is oriented more downward and medial than in the normal foot.[223] Deformities of the tarsal bones are considered to be the primary cause while ligament and joint capsule changes adjust to the distorted position.[223] The ligaments are generally thickened and the muscles hypoplastic, resulting in generalized hypoplasia of the limb with shortening of the foot and smallness of the calf.[188]

Disagreement concerning the increased presence of femoral, tibial, and total limb torsion in limbs with clubfoot exists. Decreased ETT[107,162] and increased IR of the hip have been documented by some.[77] Others have described these findings as insignificant, however, and have noted that ETT increased with age and FA decreased with age.[37,162] Therefore, rotational malalignment should be assessed and monitored, although operative correction generally is not recommended until after 7 years of age, as alignment may spontaneously correct with growth.[162]

The cause of clubfoot is considered to be a combination of genetic and environmental factors.[188,210] A genetic influence is suggested, as siblings have up to 30 times the risk of developing clubfoot deformity.[188,210] Others have established an intrauterine disruption that affects the normal development of the foot.[53,165] Incidence is 1 to 2 per 1000 live births, with a higher incidence in Hispanics and a lower incidence in Asians.[65,188] Males are affected twice as often as females.[188,210] The condition is bilateral in half the cases.[188] Histologic anomalies have been identified in every tissue in the clubfoot, including muscle, nerve, vessels, tendon insertions, ligaments, fascia, and tendon sheaths.[85] In addition, Loren et al.[117] found congenital muscle fiber type disproportion or fiber size variation in 50% of peroneus brevis muscle biopsies performed at the time of posteromedial release, and those feet with such muscle variation had a significantly greater incidence of recurrent equinovarus deformity.

The goal of treatment of clubfoot is to correct the deformity and retain mobility and strength.[188] The foot needs to be plantigrade and must have a normal load-bearing area.[188] Also included in the objectives are the ability to wear normal shoes, satisfactory appearance, and avoidance of unnecessary complicated or prolonged treatment.[188] Extrinsic clubfoot (severe positional or soft tissue deformity that is supple) can often be successfully treated with serial casting,[85] which should be started as soon as after birth as possible.[210] Casts are changed semiweekly or weekly, and the foot should be positioned to correct the foot in an orderly sequence by first correcting the cavus, rotating the foot from under the talus, and finally correcting the equinus.[188] In cases of intrinsic (rigid) clubfoot, manual reduction and surgery may be required.[65] Surgical techniques include Z lengthening of the Achilles and posterior tibiotalar and talocalcaneal capsulotomy to correct equinus, posteromedial talocalcaneal capsulotomy and/or subtalar release to correct hindfoot varus, release of the abductor hallucis and talonavicular joint for midfoot adduction, and plantar fascia release for cavus deformity.[210]

The Ponseti approach has become the standard approach to treatment in the last decade.[188,210] This is a program of approximately four to six weekly foot manipulations and castings, followed by a percutaneous tenotomy.[210] This is followed by bracing for 3 months, then nighttime splinting for 2 to 4 years.[210] About 30% may then need an anterior tibialis transfer laterally to improve balance.[188,210] Colburn and Williams[33] documented successful treatment in 54 of 57 subjects treated with infantile clubfoot.

BLOUNT'S DISEASE/TIBIA VARA

Tibia vara, or Blount's disease, is a growth disorder of the medial aspect of the proximal tibial growth plate.[188] Increased compressive forces across the medial knee cause suppression of growth and resultant bowleg deformity.[202]

Blount's disease can be classified by age of presentation as follows: infantile (0 to 4 years old), juvenile (5 to 10 years old), and adolescent (11 years old to maturity).[210] Risk factors for infantile Blount's disease include early weight bearing and weight greater than 95% for age.[210] Also at greater risk are African Americans and those with affected family members.[188] Individuals who develop adolescent (late-onset) Blount's disease are thought to have excessive loads caused by body weight and preexisting genu varum that inhibits proximal medial physeal growth.[210] In addition, the angle at the knee in weight bearing related to soft tissue at the proximal thigh in the obese adolescent affects weight distribution at the knee.[40] Other risk factors include ligamentous instability and postural asymmetry.

In children younger than 2 years of age, it sometimes is difficult to distinguish between physiologic genu varum and Blount's disease.[210] Physiologic genu varum will be demonstrated by angular deformity from the femur and the tibia, and infantile Blount's disease involves deformity isolated to the proximal tibia.[210] Radiographic findings will show varus angulation centered at the knee, mild metaphyseal beaking (appearance similar to a bird's beak), thickening of the medial tibial cortices, and tilted ankle joints. Six stages of infantile Blount's disease (from 1 through 6, least to more involved) have been described on the basis of their radiographic appearance[188,210] (Figure 14-10). Also useful in the diagnosis and treatment of infantile Blount's disease is the metaphyseal-diaphyseal angle.[188,210] This angle is used as a predictor for the development of infantile Blount's disease.[188,210] If the angle exceeds 16°, Blount's disease is likely to develop.[188] Radiographs are followed every 3 to 6 months, and improvement will be seen with physiologic varus after the child's second birthday; however, Blount's disease will progress and show metaphyseal changes.[188] In adolescent Blount's disease, the distal femur may also be angulated and radiographs will demonstrate medial physeal and epiphyseal hypoplasia of the proximal tibia.[210] Also, a lateral or varus thrust during gait may be seen.[210]

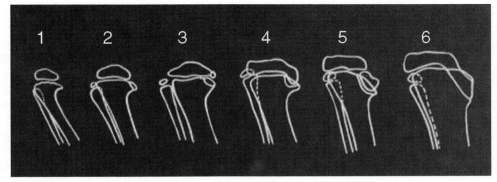

Figure 14-10 Langenskiold classification system describes six stages of infantile Blount's disease. (From Micheli, L. J., & Kocher, M. [2006]. *The pediatric and adalescent knee* [1st ed]. Philadelphia: Saunders.)

Treatment is based on the stage of tibia vara and the age of the child.[188] In children younger than 3 years of age, observation is very important, with bracing prescribed in the presence of a lateral thrust[188] or in stages 1 and 2.[210] Bracing consists of HKAFOs worn 23 hours per day.[88] Surgery is recommended if the tibia vara progresses or is initially seen in stage 3 or 4.[188] This option is considered if conservative treatment has failed by the fourth birthday.[210] Surgery may be needed to correct the varus deformity, correct the internal tibial torsion, restore normal joint congruity, and prevent or correct limb length discrepancy.[3] Best outcomes are seen if surgery is performed before permanent physeal damage has occurred.[75] Also noted is lesser recurrence in those who undergo surgery before 4.5 years.[210] Late-onset Blount's disease is treated surgically with proximal tibial osteotomy and/or lateral physeal hemiepiphysiodesis (selective closure of half of the growth plate to allow the contralateral portion of the physis to correct with growth).[210]

DEVELOPMENTAL DYSPLASIA OF THE HIP

The term *developmental dysplasia of the hip (DDH)* has replaced the term *congenital dysplasia of the hip*. The term *DDH* is also used as an abbreviation for developmental dislocation of the hip. The term *developmental dysplasia* includes hips that may have been normal, or were believed to be normal at birth but subsequently were documented to have dysplasia. Ilfeld et al.[82] noted that delayed diagnosis of dislocation is not evidence that these hips were "missed" by inadequate examinations. They describe a separate entity of the delayed subluxed or dislocated hip, possibly the result of a dynamic process caused by an increased acetabular index.

The term *dysplasia* describes abnormal development or growth. Normal muscle balance and a femoral head that is concentric, congruent with, and seated deep within the acetabulum are necessary prerequisites for normal hip development. The concave acetabulum develops in response to a spherical femoral head, and the depth normally increases with growth.

The incidence of hip dysplasia in the United States is 1 per 100 persons for dysplasia or subluxation[35,47,160,188] and 1 to 1.5 cases of dislocation per 1000 newborns.[35] Prompt recognition and treatment of DDH, preferably in the newborn period, provide the best chance for subsequent optimal hip development and a normal hip at skeletal maturity. Because the pathologic processes leading to hip dysplasia may not be present or identifiable at birth, however, periodic examination until the child is 1 year old is recommended.[49]

The origin of DDH is thought to be multifactorial. The Subcommittee on Developmental Dysplasia of the Hip of the American Academy of Pediatrics[35] has identified four periods during which the hip is at risk. If a dislocation occurs as the fetal lower limb rotates medially during the 12th week of gestation, all elements of the hip joint develop abnormally.[35] During the 18th gestational week, the hip muscles are developing, and neuromuscular problems occurring at this time, such as myelodysplasia and arthrogryposis, can lead to dislocation.[35] During the final 4 weeks of pregnancy, dislocation can occur as the result of mechanical forces.[35] Most noted in this time frame is breech positioning, as DDH occurs in as many as 23% of breech presentations.[35] The breech position puts the child at high risk by placing the hip in flexion and the knee in extension.[35] In the postnatal period, positioning such as swaddling, combined with ligament laxity, can have a role.[35] Girls are more susceptible to the maternal hormone relaxin, which may contribute to ligament laxity[35] and possibly account for the five times higher frequency in females.[160] Also of interest is the reduced incidence of DDH among cultures in which infants are routinely carried with their hips in flexion and wide abduction in cloth slings on the mother's back or astride her hips.[49] The left hip is involved three times more often than the right hip because of intrauterine positioning with the left hip positioned posteriorly against the mother's spine, potentially limiting abduction.[35,93] Also, approximately 60% of affected infants are firstborn.[160] Because mechanical factors can act to restrict the position of the head, neck, and feet of the developing fetus, as well as the hips, the rate of association of DDH with other intrauterine molding abnormalities, such as torticollis and metatarsus adductus, is high.[49,208]

CLINICAL EXAMINATION

Because different examination processes are used for diagnosis of DDH, the true incidence cannot be determined. Physical examination, ultrasonography, and plane radiography are useful tools in identifying a problem.

Clinically, newborn hips can be classified as follows[135]:
1. Normal—no instability noted.
2. Subluxatable (9.8/1000)[204]—the femoral head is in the socket but can be partially displaced out to the acetabular rim.
3. Dislocatable (1.3/1000)[204]—the femoral head is reduced but can be dislocated with a Barlow maneuver.
4. Dislocated but reducible (1.2/1000)[204]—the femoral head is out of the acetabulum at rest but can be reduced with an Ortolani maneuver.
5. Dislocated but not reducible—seldom encountered in the newborn to 2-month-old age group. (When seen, this type of dislocation is usually teratologic, occurring before birth, typically from a neuromuscular or musculoskeletal abnormality such as myelomeningocele or arthrogryposis.)

Clinical examination includes documentation of the ROM of hip abduction in flexion. Most infants have 75° to 90° of abduction. Significant limitation or an asymmetry of even 5° to 10° may indicate hip dysplasia, warranting further workup. Other clinical findings may include asymmetrical thigh folds, pistoning, apparent (not true) femoral shortening with uneven knee heights (positive Galeazzi sign), and positive Barlow or Ortolani signs (Figure 14-11). Hip "clicks" usually are not clinically significant. The experienced examiner can distinguish between hip clicks and the characteristic

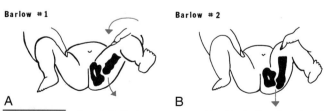

Figure 14-11 **A** and **B**, Barlow maneuver: The hip is first flexed and abducted, then is gradually adducted, with pressure exerted in a posterior direction. Dislocation of the femoral head over the posterior acetabular rim indicates an unstable hip. The head may slide to the edge of the socket (subluxatable) or may dislocate out of the acetabulum (dislocatable). Ortolani test: In the Ortolani-positive hip, the hip is dislocated in a position of flexion and adduction. Gentle flexion, abduction, and slight traction (the Ortolani maneuver) reduce the hip. A positive Ortolani sign indicates a more unstable hip than a positive Barlow sign. (From Mubarak, S. J., Leach, J. L., & Wenger, D. R. [1987]. Management of congenital dislocation of the hip in the infant. *Contemporary Orthopedics, 15*, 29.)

"clunk" felt during the Barlow maneuver as a hip dislocates. Kane and associates[92] studied 171 infants with 193 clicking hips and found that those with hip clicks and a normal hip ultrasound examination on initial assessment had a normal radiograph at 6 months of age.

The infant must be completely relaxed for the Barlow and Ortolani maneuvers to have reliable diagnostic value. Even slight muscular contraction around the hip can obscure the instability and negate the examination. These two signs of hip instability usually will disappear by 2 to 3 months of age, because the hip may improve in stability and may stay in the socket or become fixed in a dislocated position. Often, limited hip abduction is the only clinical sign of hip dysplasia in the infant older than 1 month. It continues to be the most reliable clinical finding in older infants and toddlers with dysplasia. Additional diagnostic studies are warranted if these are positive findings on clinical examination, and even with a normal clinical examination but a high index of suspicion, because of multiple risk factors, such as female firstborn child with breech presentation and a family history of DDH.

Ultrasonography to examine newborn hips and classification according to the Graf index are now widely used in the United States and Europe.[166] The Graf index classifies hips into one of 10 categories, each of which has a specific treatment recommendation to avoid residual acetabular dysplasia and, therefore, premature osteoarthritis.[166] Ultrasonography is more accurate and helpful than radiography in diagnosing DDH in infants. It is most useful in the newborn and in infants up to 3 to 6 months of age, before the femoral head starts to ossify and obscure the structures deep to it. Harcke[67] demonstrated usefulness of ultrasonography in detecting DDH in children up to 1 year of age. The secondary ossification center is present in 80% of children at age 6 months.[178] Ultrasonography allows assessment of the cartilaginous structures not visualized on plain radiographs and allows stress testing (to document instability), with the additional advantage of no radiation exposure. It is a useful tool not only in the diagnosis, but also in the management of DDH, documenting reduction of the dislocated hip in the Pavlik harness[200] and providing information on the status of the hip to aid decisions on altering or stopping treatment. Ultrasonography is superior to radiography for assessing hip position in the harness. Song and Lapinsky[186] found that hip ultrasound findings agreed with clinical examination in 100% of hips in their study. Therefore, ultrasonography is recommended as an adjunct to clinical evaluation for clarifying a physical finding, assessing a high-risk infant, and monitoring DDH as it is observed or treated.[35]

Radiographs rather than ultrasound are used for older infants (4 to 6 months). Because of the need for a radiograph of the uninvolved side for comparison, and because of the frequency of bilateral involvement, the standard radiograph is an anterior-posterior view of the pelvis. Many parameters of hip development can be measured on hip radiographs.[70]

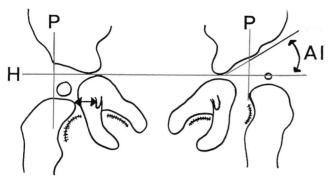

Figure 14-12 Radiographic parameters of hip development involve use of the Hilgenreiner line (H) and Perkin's line (P) to document proximal lateral migration of the femoral head, with disruption of Shenton's line *(cross-hatched line)*. The acetabular index (AI) of the left hip is increased, documenting acetabular dysplasia, and Shenton's line is broken, indicating subluxation of the left hip. (From Mubarak, S. J., Leach, J. L., & Wenger, D. R. [1987]. Management of congenital dislocation of the hip in the infant. *Contemporary Orthopedics, 15,* 29.)

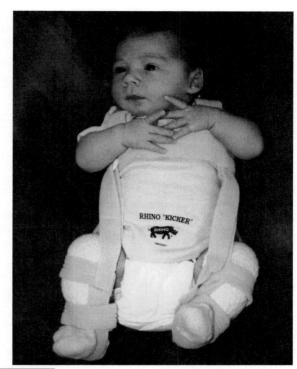

Figure 14-13 The Pavlik harness can be used to reduce a dislocated hip, to stabilize a lax hip, and to treat acetabular dysplasia.

Scoles and colleagues[178] studied 50 boys and 50 girls at each of six age levels: 3, 6, 9, 12, 18, and 24 months. They documented a decrease in acetabular index with age and concluded that this was a helpful parameter in following hip development (Figure 14-12). J.T. Smith and colleagues[185] proposed that appearance of the teardrop is the earliest radiographic sign that a stable, concentric reduction of the hip has been achieved. Hips can be classified radiographically as acetabular dysplasia (without subluxation or dislocation); subluxated, with associated acetabular dysplasia; and dislocated.

Between 18 and 24 months of age, children with hip dislocation usually have an abnormal gait. With unilateral dislocation, the child will limp, demonstrating a positive Trendelenburg sign on the involved side in the stance phase of gait. With bilateral dislocation, the child will have a waddling gait.

INTERVENTION

Birth to 9 Months

The Pavlik harness is the primary method of treating DDH during infancy. The Pavlik harness was first described by Dr. Arnold Pavlik, who originally called his treatment device "stirrups." Modifications have been made in the design of the device, but the principles of treatment and the requirements of the harness remain essentially the same as described by him over 50 years ago.[151] Pavlik stressed that one of the main advantages of the harness over casts is that it allows active motion, thereby decreasing the incidence of avascular necrosis (AVN) of the femoral head.[152]

The Pavlik harness restricts hip extension and adduction and allows the hips to be maintained in flexion and abduction—the "protective position" (Figure 14-13). Studies

with newborn pigs found that maintaining the hips in extension precipitated hip dislocation.[172] The position of flexion and abduction enhances normal acetabular development, and the kicking motion allowed in this "human" position (not as radical as the "frog" position) stretches the contracted hip adductors and promotes spontaneous reduction of the dislocated hip. Because of the biologic plasticity of growing bone, positioning the hip in flexion/abduction can promote acetabular development.

Complications of use of the Pavlik harness include AVN of the femoral head, femoral nerve palsy, inferior dislocation, and erosion of the posterior rim of the acetabulum. Essentially all these complications can be avoided by using a Pavlik harness of proper design, educating the caregiver to apply it correctly, and monitoring the status of the hip carefully over the entire treatment period.[136] The prognosis with Pavlik harness treatment is excellent, with 90% to 95% success in cases of subluxation and dysplasia, and approximately 85% success in cases of dislocation (Figure 14-14). The overall success rate has been described as 91.5% at a minimum of 14 years' follow-up.[138] Triple diapering is no longer recommended.[35]

If a brief trial (up to 3 years) of the Pavlik harness is not successful in reducing a dislocated hip, surgical treatment is indicated. This may include a period of 2 to 3 weeks of traction to reduce the incidence of AVN of the femoral head. Home traction is a safe, effective, and much less expensive

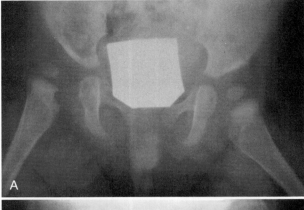

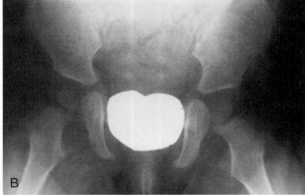

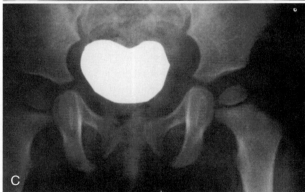

Figure 14-14   **A,** Age 4 months: Right hip dislocated, severe acetabular dysplasia. **B,** Age 7 months: Treated with a Pavlik harness for 3 months full time. Right hip is reduced; continued acetabular dysplasia. Patient continued Pavlik harness treatment for 3 more months, part time (night and naps only). **C,** Age 15 months: Both hips centered in the acetabula with good acetabular development bilaterally.

alternative to the 2- to 3-week admission required for hospital traction.[134] Surgery includes an arthrogram to define the anatomic landmarks of the femoral head and acetabulum and to detect the presence of soft tissue (pulvinar) interposition between the head and acetabulum; adductor tenotomy; closed or (if necessary) open reduction of the hip; and application of a spica cast. Luhmann and colleagues[118] reported that delaying reduction of a dislocated hip until the

appearance of an ossification nucleus more than doubled the need for additional reconstructive procedures.

Age 9 Months and Older

In infants older than 9 months of age who are beginning to walk independently, an abduction orthosis should be considered as an alternative to the Pavlik harness for treatment of acetabular dysplasia with or without subluxation. This orthosis should be designed so the child can walk while in the orthosis. For dislocatable or dislocated hips diagnosed in the 6- to 18-month age group, surgical treatment in the form of closed reduction is usually required. Treatment falls into a gray zone in the 18- to 24-month age group, when open or closed reduction may be used. Failure to achieve a stable hip with a closed reduction indicates the need for open reduction.[49] Failure may be evident at the time of the initial closed reduction, or it may become apparent when dislocation occurs later (perhaps while in a plaster cast).[49]

The diagnosis of hip dislocation in the child age 2 years or older is generally considered to mandate open reduction, because the results of closed reduction are not predictable in these older children. For those 2 to 3 years of age, preliminary traction may be used before open reduction and femoral shortening.[49] Children older than 3 years generally need a femoral shortening procedure (removal of a segment of the femoral shaft) to reduce the compressive forces on the femoral head once it is reduced back into the acetabulum.[49] Older children with continuing acetabular dysplasia will benefit from a pelvic osteotomy, as the remodeling potential of the acetabulum decreases with age. Children 3 to 8 years of age can be treated with an acetabular reshaping osteotomy (e.g., a Pemberton or San Diego osteotomy). In the 8- to 10-year-old group, a triple innominate osteotomy is usually indicated. After age 14 to 15 years, when the triradiate cartilage is closed, the Ganz periacetabular osteotomy is effective.[216] Three-dimensional computed tomographic analysis (3D-CT) helps define the nature and degree of acetabular and femoral deformity and can be used to evaluate the results of the surgery.[100,184]

A number of children with acetabular dysplasia are never diagnosed as infants or toddlers. With mild dysplasia, they will walk without a limp, will have essentially normal hip ROM, and can actively participate in all childhood activities, including sports. However, the hip is like a tire that is out of alignment—you can drive on it for quite a few miles, but uneven wear will occur. The dysplastic hip, especially the one with subluxation, also develops uneven wear with subsequent articular cartilage damage. The person may develop degenerative arthritis, hip pain, and limp as early as the late teens. Very mild dysplasia may go undetected for many decades and may be diagnosed later in life when the patient develops degenerative hip joint disease. The age at symptom onset in untreated patients with subluxation is variable, with the mean in the mid-30s for women and the mid-50s for men.[214] Many middle-age adults requiring total hip

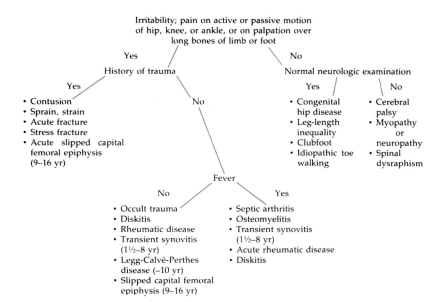

Irritability; pain on active or passive motion
of hip, knee, or ankle, or on palpation over
long bones of limb or foot

Yes / No

History of trauma — Normal neurologic examination

Yes / No — Yes / No

• Contusion
• Sprain, strain
• Acute fracture
• Stress fracture
• Acute slipped capital femoral epiphysis (9–16 yr)

• Congenital hip disease
• Leg-length inequality
• Clubfoot
• Idiopathic toe walking

• Cerebral palsy
• Myopathy or neuropathy
• Spinal dysraphism

Fever

No / Yes

• Occult trauma
• Diskitis
• Rheumatic disease
• Transient synovitis (1½–8 yr)
• Legg-Calvé-Perthes disease (–10 yr)
• Slipped capital femoral epiphysis (9–16 yr)

• Septic arthritis
• Osteomyelitis
• Transient synovitis (1½–8 yr)
• Acute rheumatic disease
• Diskitis

Figure 14-15 A clinical decision tree for children with a limp. (From Scoles, P. V. [1988]. *Pediatric orthopedics in clinical practice* [2nd ed., p. 21]. Chicago: YearBook.)

replacement had DDH that was never diagnosed and treated or was treated in childhood without full resolution. A number of studies have documented the association of osteoarthritis (OA) in adults who have residual hip dysplasia[125,170] and the increased technical difficulties of total hip arthroplasty with high acetabular component failure rates.[87]

CAUSES OF LIMPING IN CHILDREN

The acute onset of limp in a child is a condition that warrants evaluation. In this section, chronic causes of limp, such as those due to muscle weakness, will not be addressed. Orthopedic conditions that can result in acute limping will be reviewed. Although some of these are transitory and benign, some can result in lifelong impairments, especially if not treated promptly and effectively. The clinical decision tree in Figure 14-15 is useful in the identification of conditions that need immediate medical or surgical attention. Especially for those treating in a direct access situation, attention to the history and systemic symptoms are important in the determination of referral to other professionals.

HISTORY AND PHYSICAL EXAMINATION

When a child has a limp, a complete and thorough evaluation is recommended. A detailed history should be taken and should include a description of any recent illness or injury that may be a contributory factor. The clinician should be aware, however, that children do fall frequently, and a fall could be related to the onset of the limp or other injury, even though it may be incidental and unrelated.

Physical examination should include an observational gait analysis. This should allow the clinician to determine which leg is involved and perhaps the location within the leg. Gait analysis can provide much assistance in the direction of further testing. The algorithm in Figure 14-16 demonstrates

the process of generally categorizing the gait by observation with further physical examination and diagnostic testing used as confirmation.

The physical examination should also include a complete assessment of the spine, hips, thighs, knees, lower legs, ankles, and feet, including the uninvolved side for comparison. Objective measurements of ROM and strength should be taken, as should observations of the presence of muscle atrophy, swelling, redness, and difference in temperature between limbs. Also, the child's subjective response of pain with palpation and with movement and muscle contraction is important. Much information can be gathered from the way a child performs functional activities, which is especially important when a child's cooperation might limit a formalized evaluation. Observation of the child moving from the floor to standing or crawling or achieving a comfortable sitting position can provide usable information. For example, a child may refuse to walk because of pain but may crawl easily, indicating that the problem is probably evident in the lower part of the leg, rather than in the hip or knee. A child might also demonstrate the use of his hands to "walk" up his body to rise to standing from the floor (Gowers' sign) because of hip and thigh muscle weakness, which could be related to neurologic disorders or other conditions causing proximal muscle weakness. Discitis may also present as a patient's refusal to walk and difficulty with changing position.[22]

OTHER DIAGNOSTIC TESTS

In addition to a careful clinical examination, other tests are often indicated. Radiographs can document fractures or other bony abnormalities, although some occult fractures are not identifiable on radiography until 10 to 14 days after onset, when a repeat radiograph may document formation of callus. Laboratory examination of blood samples provides

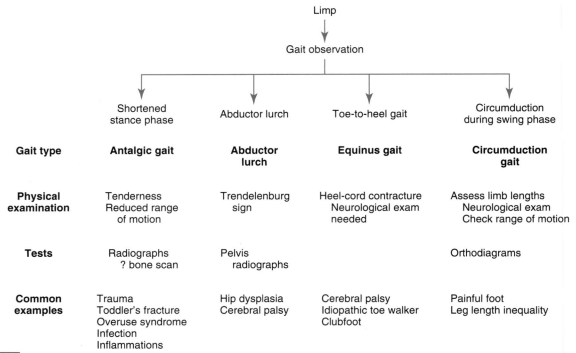

	Limp			
	Gait observation			
	Shortened stance phase	Abductor lurch	Toe-to-heel gait	Circumduction during swing phase
Gait type	**Antalgic gait**	**Abductor lurch**	**Equinus gait**	**Circumduction gait**
Physical examination	Tenderness Reduced range of motion	Trendelenburg sign	Heel-cord contracture Neurological exam needed	Assess limb lengths Neurological exam Check range of motion
Tests	Radiographs ? bone scan	Pelvis radiographs		Orthodiagrams
Common examples	Trauma Toddler's fracture Overuse syndrome Infection Inflammations	Hip dysplasia Cerebral palsy	Cerebral palsy Idiopathic toe walker Clubfoot	Painful foot Leg length inequality

Figure 14-16 Algorithm used for evaluation of limping. A general category can be determined by observation with physical examination and tests used to confirm the problem. (From Staheli, L. T. [2006]. *Practice of pediatric orthopedics* [2nd ed., p. 78]. Philadelphia: Lippincott Williams and Wilkins.)

information regarding the presence of infection or other acute processes. The erythrocyte sedimentation rate (ESR) and C-reactive protein (CRP) can indicate the presence of acute inflammation, as well as response to treatment. More complex diagnostic studies may also be needed to define the problem or evaluate treatment efficacy. These studies include bone scans, magnetic resonance imaging (MRI) (for soft tissue), and CT (for bony structures).

The cause of a limp in a child may be as simple as a foreign object in the shoe or as complex as osteogenic sarcoma. Therefore, generalizations regarding management should not be made, and a diagnosis should be established as quickly as possible. Many cases may be easily treated, and some require no treatment beyond observation. Many causes of limp are associated with specific age groups, specifically one of three groups: birth to 5 years, 5 to 10 years, and 10 to 15 years. Soft tissue injuries (i.e., contusions, ligaments, and tendon injuries) and fractures are found in all age groups. Spine injury or disease can also be a factor in a child's limp, at any age, with discitis being the most common pediatric spinal infection.[59]

COMMON DIAGNOSES BY AGE GROUP

Birth to Age 5 Years

Osteomyelitis

Osteomyelitis is an infection in bone that occurs most frequently in children, with the overall prevalence rated as high as 1 case per 5000 children.[121] The most common causative

bacterial organism is *Staphylococcus aureus*, although other organisms may be involved.[39,227] Most of these infections are caused by spread of bacteria through the bloodstream, or occasionally by entry of organisms through an open wound, either by puncture or by spreading of infection from adjacent tissue.[39] In some instances, a history of recent respiratory infection, otitis media, or an infected wound is reported, but most often acute haematogenous osteomyelitis begins spontaneously in a healthy child.[39] Trauma to the bone may cause local edema and may alter the blood flow; the formation of a hematoma may provide a good environment for bacterial proliferation.[221] When the infection extends to the adjacent joint, septic arthritis may result. Perlman et al.[153] have reported that 33% of those with osteomyelitis also have septic arthritis.

The onset of osteomyelitis is generally sudden, and the rapid progression can cause permanent damage and later consequences in the child.[39] The most common sites of osteomyelitis are the rapidly growing ends of long bones; the condition is more common in the lower extremity.[39] Therefore, the metaphyses of the distal femur and of the proximal tibia are the most common sites of infection.[123,153]

The signs and symptoms of acute hematogenous osteomyelitis are variable, according to factors such as age of the patient, site of infection, resistance of the child, and virulence of the affecting organism.[39] Generally, however, onset is sudden, with localized bone tenderness, swelling, and pain over the metaphysis of the involved bone.[39] A high fever and chills are often present, and the patient is often unwilling to use the affected limb.[39] Frequently, the child will refuse to walk when the lower extremity is affected.[39] Neonates often do not demonstrate signs of systemic illness, and signs of pseudoparalysis and pain with passive motion are difficult to detect.[39]

Laboratory testing should include complete blood cell count, ESR, and CRP.[39] The white blood cell count is usually increased. ESR and CRP are usually elevated, and the values normalize after successful treatment.[39] The CRP value declines and returns to normal in 7 to 10 days, while the ESR normalizes after 3 to 4 weeks.[39]

Blood cultures acquired by aspiration from the site of infection should be obtained before antibiotic treatment is begun.[39] Blood cultures are positive in 30% to 50% of cultured cases.[121] Sonography is useful in early diagnosis, as it helps to identify subperiosteal abscess formation[62] or intra-articular fluid collection before radiographic changes are evident.[62] A bone scan will show the site of osteomyelitis much sooner than plain radiographs but is nonspecific in the differential diagnosis between infection, tumor, and trauma.[39] It is helpful, however, in detecting multiple locations of infection.[39] Radiographs show the inflammatory response of the infection; osseous changes are not visible until 7 to 14 days after onset.[39] By this time, mottling of bone density is visible, and if untreated, cortical erosion follows and the sequestrum and the involucrum become radiologically visible.[39] An MRI can provide further information about the extent of the infection and the localization of abscess formation.[62,194]

The recommended treatment for a typical case of acute hematogenous osteomyelitis is 5 to 7 days of intravenous antibiotics followed by 3 to 4 weeks of oral antibiotics.[199] Treatment should be individualized; the duration of the antibiotic therapy correlates with the severity of the infection, the time elapsed between onset of the disease and initiation of treatment, the extent of bone involvement, and laboratory responses after the initial treatment.[139]

In quickly progressing and extreme cases, acute hematogenous osteomyelitis can be fatal as a result of overwhelming septicemia, and treatment must be instituted on an emergency basis. Treatment consists of aspiration, antibiotics, and immobilization of the affected part, and possibly surgical decompression if gross purulence is identified. Surgical drainage usually is required when the diagnosis is delayed. Delayed treatment may control the septicemia and may be lifesaving, but it may not be effective in controlling the progression of the pathologic process within the bone.

Subacute osteomyelitis is a classification used to describe an infection lasting longer than 3 weeks, but it may have symptoms that present for one to several months.[60] Chronic osteomyelitis is generally a progression of an untreated or insufficiently treated osteomyelitis. Chronic recurrent multifocal osteomyelitis (CRMO) specifically describes an autoinflammatory osteopathy that predominantly affects children.[128] Although most children with CRMO have resolution of symptoms postpubertally,[128] long-term studies

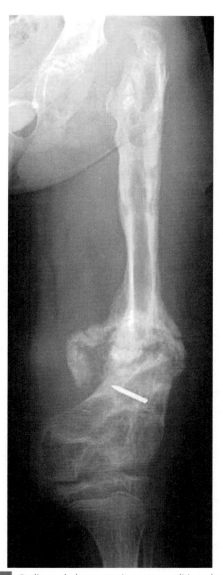

Figure 14-17 Radiograph demonstrating osteomyelitis and septic arthritis. Consequent problems include destruction of the hip joint and the presence of a pathologic fracture. (From De Boeck, H. [2005]. Osteomyelitis and septic arthritis in children. *Acta Orthopaedica Belgica, 71,* 512.)

have shown that up to 25% have persistent disease, with complications including risk of permanent bone deformities, poorer quality of life, and difficulty in achieving vocational goals.[76,78,122,155] Pathologic fracture can be one complication in a difficult case[39] (Figure 14-17).

Septic Arthritis

Septic arthritis (pyogenic arthritis) is defined as an infection of a joint caused by bacterial organisms. This is an extremely threatening condition, because a joint may be destroyed within 48 hours of onset of symptoms. Septic arthritis causes destruction of articular cartilage and long-term growth arrest. The resulting deformities may be permanent and may have a wide-ranging, lifelong impact, affecting the person's gait, participation in sports, and choice of occupation and leisure activities.

Staphylococcus aureus is the most common organism.[30,39,212,230] *Haemophilus influenzae* has virtually been eliminated[123] through vaccination.[128] *Neisseria gonorrhoeae* is found in sexually active teenagers or is transmitted to newborns from their mothers during birth.[121] Salmonella septic arthritis may also develop during the course of Salmonella bacteremia in infants.[212] Other incidence rates that should be considered are the higher incidence in children who are HIV-positive[80] and the higher incidence and severity in children with community-associated methicillin-resistant *Staphylococcus aureus* (MRSA).[7] The organism enters the joint by hematogenous spread (e.g., from an ear infection), direct spread (from adjacent osteomyelitis), or direct inoculation (from a foreign body, needle, or surgical penetration of a joint). In infants, vascular channels allow progression of infection through the growth plate and into the epiphysis and joint space.[39] Specifically, in the hip, vessels cross the proximal growth plate until approximately 18 months of age, allowing infection to spread from the metaphysis of the femur to the hip joint.[121] Approximately 75% of cases of septic arthritis occur before the age of 3 years.[121] Any joint may be affected, but about 80% of cases are located in the lower extremity, with the hip (in the young child) and the knee (in the older child) being the most common locations.[64,93,123]

Septic arthritis generally causes a rapid inflammatory response.[39] The synovial membrane responds with a hyperemia followed by excessive production of fluid and pus.[39] Pus contains enzymes that rapidly destroy articular cartilage, causing irreversible joint damage.[39] Permanent joint destruction can result in as little as 3 days.[39] In a newborn, the cartilaginous femoral head can be completely destroyed, requiring salvage procedures later in life. Damage to the epiphysis may cause trochanteric overgrowth and leg length discrepancy when the growth plate is damaged.[39] Other cases can cause increased intra-articular pressure that occludes the blood supply to the femoral head, causing avascular necrosis.

The diagnosis of septic arthritis is based on clinical findings. Generally, the disease has an acute onset of irritability, fever to 104°F (40°C), and anorexia.[121] When the lower extremity is involved, the child will limp and refuse to bear weight, and passive ROM is painful. When the hip is affected, the child typically will hold the joint in a position of flexion, abduction, and external rotation as the intracapsular pressure increases.[121] In peripheral joints, swelling, redness, warmth, and local tenderness are present early.[39] For other joints, including the hip joint, these signs manifest late and can delay diagnosis.[39] In neonates and infants, these usual signs of inflammation generally are not present, and the child may not demonstrate a fever or signs of sickness.[39] The most common clinical sign is absence of spontaneous movement of the involved limb (pseudoparalysis).[39]

Laboratory test results will show elevated white blood-cell count of >12,000 mm,[153] with 40 percent to 60 percent polymorphonuclear leukocytes, and ESR of >50 mm/hr.[121] The CRP is also generally elevated but is nonspecific.[121] These levels may be normal, however, in the neonate with septic arthritis.[39]

Radiographs are useful to show soft tissue swelling, capsular distention, joint space widening, or radiologic signs of adjacent osteomyelitis.[39] Ultrasonography is helpful to identify small joint effusions and can guide joint aspiration.[39] A bone scan may also help diagnostically to determine diffuse uptake within the joint in the early phase or a rise in intra-articular pressure.[39]

Joint aspiration is imperative for the diagnosis and should not be delayed if septic arthritis is suspected.[39,121] The aspirated fluid should be cultured, and drainage and intravenous antibiotics should be started immediately.[39,121] Intravenous antibiotic therapy is recommended until improvement in clinical signs is seen; at such time oral antibiotics may be used.[121]

Transient Synovitis

Transient synovitis is a common cause of painful hip in children younger than 10 years of age. Both transient synovitis and septic arthritis initially present as an atraumatic, acutely irritable hip in a child who has a limp or difficulty bearing weight, and who has limited motion, joint effusion, and abnormal laboratory findings on evaluation of the blood and joint fluid.[104] For this reason, differential diagnosis is necessary, as transient synovitis will generally resolve in 7 days with conservative treatment and observation, while septic arthritis can progress quickly and have many complications.[104,119] Males are affected more than females, with one study showing 73% of subjects with transient synovitis being male.[119] The cause is unclear, but often a history can be elicited of a recent upper respiratory infection or other illness.[109] Treatment generally is symptomatic, consisting of limitation of activity, bed rest, and use of crutches if the child is able to manage them. Children sometimes have recurrent problems with hip synovitis, and a small percentage will develop Legg-Calvé-Perthes disease.[109,206]

Occult Fractures

Occult fracture is usually a benign condition, causing an acute limp in children. The most common sites of involvement for these fractures in infants and toddlers are the tibia/fibula and femur, although cases have been found in the pelvis and metatarsals.[144] The child usually refuses to walk or walks with a limp, has no history of significant trauma, and has no signs of infection. Laboratory data are normal, and radiographs of the painful area are usually normal initially. The child can be treated with a splint or cast for comfort and observed closely for signs of incipient infection. If an occult fracture is present, radiographs will not show evidence of callus (new bone formation) 10 to 14

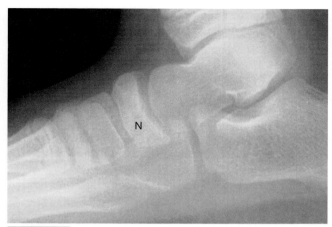

Figure 14-18   Kohler syndrome demonstrated on radiograph by sclerosis of the navicular. (From Weissman, B. M. [2009]. *Imaging of arthritis and metabolic bone disease.* St. Louis: Mosby.)

days later. Therefore, the diagnosis generally is confirmed retrospectively.

Kohler Syndrome

Kohler syndrome is an osteochondrosis affecting the navicular bone, usually occurring in children between ages 3 and 8 years.[205] It was first described by Alban Kohler, a German radiologist.[219] This condition occurs when the navicular bone temporarily loses its blood supply. The child usually has localized pain in the area of the navicular bone and a limp. Radiographic changes are characteristic, with the navicular being sclerotic and small compared with the opposite side (Figure 14-18). All these cases resolve with time, with no clinical and radiologic abnormalities seen in adulthood.[180] Children with limited ambulation as a result of severe pain may be best treated with a brief period of casting.[29]

Additional Causes of Limp

Other orthopedic conditions that can cause an acute limp in children from birth to age 5 years include juvenile rheumatoid arthritis (see Chapter 9), nonaccidental trauma (fractures or soft tissue injuries), hemophilia (for more information, refer to the Evolve website), discitis, discoid meniscus, popliteal cysts, foreign bodies, and bone tumors.

Ages 5 to 10 Years

Various types of osteochondroses are common causes of limp in the 5- to 10-year-old group and in the 10- to 15-year-old age group. The osteochondroses represent a group of diseases of children and adolescents in which localized tissue death (necrosis) occurs, usually followed by full regeneration of healthy bone tissue.[47] During the years of rapid bone growth, blood supply to the epiphyses (growing ends of bones) may be compromised, resulting in necrotic bone, usually near joints.[47] Because bone is undergoing a

continuous rebuilding process, the necrotic areas are often self-repaired over a period of weeks or months.[47] Osteochondrosis is generally divided into three locations: physeal, articular, and nonarticular.[47] Physeal osteochondrosis (Scheurmann's disease) occurs at the intervertebral joints.[47] Articular diseases occur at the joints (articulations), with common forms occurring at the hip, foot, and elbow.[47] Nonarticular osteochondrosis occurs at any other skeletal location, with one example being Osgood-Schlatter disease, which occurs at the tibia.[47] Many cases are idiopathic although stress-related; repetitive trauma and infection are noted causes, and occurrence generally is more frequent at times of rapid growth of the epiphysis.[47]

Legg-Calvé-Perthes Disease

Legg-Calvé-Perthes disease (LCPD) is a condition that occurs in children, who may receive referrals for physical therapy for treatment of resulting muscle weakness, ROM limitations, and gait deviations. It was initially described in the early 1900s by three separate authors: Arthur T. Legg in the United States, Georg Perthes in Germany, and Jacques Calvé in France. Generally, LCPD has been described as ischemic necrosis of the center of ossification of the femoral head.[215] The medial femoral circumflex artery is the principal vessel in the complex vascular distribution in the neck and head of the femur. Further examination of affected femurs has shown the epiphyseal cartilage to contain high proteoglycan content, a decrease in structural glycoproteins, and different-size collagen fibrils compared with normal tissue, suggesting that the disease could be a localized expression of a generalized transient disorder responsible for delayed skeletal maturation.[215] These abnormalities can be primary or secondary to the ischemia, but collapse and necrosis of the femoral head could result from the breakdown and disorganization of the matrix of the epiphyseal cartilage, followed by abnormal ossification.[215] The exact cause is unknown, but it occasionally follows repeated episodes of transient synovitis of the hip. Increased joint pressure secondary to synovitis may be one of the pathologic processes that causes an interruption of blood flow in vessels ascending the femoral neck.

LCPD usually occurs in children between ages 4 and 8, although it has been reported in patients from 2 to 12 years.[49] It is most commonly seen in boys, with the male-to female ratio being 4 or 5 to 1.[49] These children generally have been described as small for their age with delayed bone age,[45,108,116] although some have disputed this.[95] This relation to short stature has been described by some as an underlying metabolic or endocrine deficiency, but reports on this have not been conclusive.[95,116] Kealey et al.[95] described relative normal stature in younger children (4-, 5-, and 6-year-olds) but relative short stature in older children (ages 10, 11, and 12 years), with no differences seen in the length of time since diagnosis.[95] Crofton et al.[36] have described a normal symmetrical stature at onset, but a later decline in relative height values at 2-year follow-up. Leg length was not significantly different at follow-up but was asymmetrical upon initial presentation.[36] Their theory, developed from this finding, is that the limp associated with acute onset of Perthes' disease increases weight bearing and therefore stimulates increased linear growth on the unaffected side.[36] Cessation of lower leg growth is then seen between weeks 2 and 6, which reflects the time period during which weight bearing is limited by traction and bed rest, wheelchair confinement, or reduced physical activity.[36] By 3 months after the initial presentation, most children were mobilized, and growth of both lower legs was similar and normal.[36]

Socioeconomic status has also been associated with the incidence of Perthes' disease.[63,95,96] This has been related to dietary issues, as well as to increased second-hand smoke exposure.[96] Kealey et al.[96] found that 64.9% of 208 patients with Perthes' disease lived in households where one or both parents smoked, which was considerably higher than the rate of 38.9% of exposure to passive smoking found in control children.[96] Both nutrition and smoke exposure have also been related to small stature and delayed bone age in children.[95] Learning disability[108] and attention deficit disorder[96] have been identified at a higher rate in those with Perthes' disease.[108] Other factors related to the incidence of LCPD include an increase in blood viscosity, disturbances in the clotting mechanism, and abnormal venous drainage of the femoral head and neck.[47] Furthermore, Gaughan et al.[57] found that, similar to adults with HIV, who have an increased risk of osteonecrosis of the hip, children with perinatal HIV infection also have an increased risk for LCPD, and attention should be given to a limp or to hip pain in this group.

The disease is bilateral in 10% of cases, but the femoral heads are usually in different stages of collapse.[49] About 35% of children with unilateral Perthes' disease also demonstrate changes in the unaffected proximal femur on radiographs, including small epiphysis, flattening of the epiphysis, contour irregularities, and changes in the growth plate.[91] Recurrent cases of LCPD have been noted and generally will have a poor prognosis, as the entire femoral head is generally involved and recurrence occurs when the child is older.[215]

LCPD is a self-limiting disorder with complete revascularization of the avascular epiphysis occurring almost invariably, over a period of time.[90] Generally, the time frame from initiation to complete healing is a median of 2.8 years.[90] Many progress through the stages of this disease without complications in later life, although deformation of the epiphysis can occur during the process of revascularization, resulting in degenerative arthritis in later years.[90] Prognostic factors include age at onset (younger children tend to do better),[52,89] extent of the disease, the amount of femoral head deformity, and the amount of incongruity between the femoral head and the acetabulum,[187,215] because hip joint growth and development depend on a well-located, centered, and spherical femoral head.[215]

Symptoms of LCPD can be attributed to synovitis that goes with LCPD.[26] The most common symptom of LCPD is a limp for varying periods.[49] A painful limp, or antalgic gait, may be present and is characterized by a shortened stance phase on the affected side. A Trendelenburg gait, or abductor lurch, is seen with hip abductor weakness and is characterized by lateral shoulder sway toward the affected side.[188] Limited hip ROM is noted, especially in hip abduction and internal rotation. Pain complaints are usually related to activity, and pain may be present in the groin and/or referred to the anteromedial thigh or knee region. Failure to recognize the thigh or knee pain as referred may result in delayed diagnosis and inappropriate treatment of the knee.[49] Careful clinical examination and observational gait analysis usually provide the information needed to localize the problem at the hip.

Radiographic studies will demonstrate the four stages of LCPD.[49] These can be described as follows:

- *Initial stage:* Early signs include lateralization of the femoral head with widening of the medial joint space and a decreased size ossification center. Later signs include subchondral fractures and physeal irregularity.
- *Fragmentation stage:* Epiphysis is fragmented and acetabulum contour is more irregular.
- *Reossification (healing) stage:* New bone formation is seen on the femoral head.
- *Residual stage:* Femoral head is fully reossified, with gradual remodeling of the head shape until skeletal maturity.

Three commonly used methods of grading femoral head changes radiographically are the Catterall grouping,[27] the Salter and Thompson grouping,[174] and the Herring lateral pillar classification,[72] which is the most widely used.[49]

The best course of treatment for LCPD is a subject of controversy. Because the new bone of the revascularizing epiphysis is "biologically plaster" and therefore susceptible to irreversible deformation, weight-bearing forces and muscular stresses transmitted across the acetabular rim can deform the femoral epiphysis.[90] The focus of current methods of treatment, therefore, is to prevent deformation of the femoral head by ensuring that the anterolateral part of the avascular capital femoral epiphysis is contained within the acetabulum,[90] as well as to maintain hip ROM.[49] During the active stage of the disease, the goal is to keep the femoral head contained within the acetabulum.[90] Full abduction to 45° is needed for containment.[26] This can be done through the use of an abduction orthosis, such as the Atlanta Scottish Rite orthosis, and should be continued until subchondral reossification is visible on anteroposterior radiographs.[49] Non–weight-bearing use of orthoses is recommended in more severe cases.[215] Other conservative treatment methods include bed rest, traction, nonsteroidal anti-inflammatory drugs, and reduction in weight-bearing status to minimize pain.[49] If the entire femoral head cannot be contained with these methods, maintaining and improving ROM is still important, especially hip abduction, to avoid hinge abduction caused by the deformed femoral head impinging on the lateral margin of the acetabulum during abduction of the hip.[49] Recent studies have compared long-term outcomes in those treated conservatively and those treated surgically. Arkader et al.[6] found that those with late-onset LCPD had no statistical differences in outcome when treated surgically or conservatively, although a trend toward better radiographic outcomes was described when varus derotational osteotomy was performed early in the disease process. Herring et al.[71] further described that the lateral pillar classification and age at onset of the disease determined outcome, rather than the course of treatment. In the conservative group, those who were braced and those who had no treatment showed no significant difference in outcome. The effectiveness of physical therapy, specifically ROM, stretching, strengthening, and balance training, has not been noted radiographically.[19] However, significant improvements in articular ROM, muscular strength, and articular dysfunction have been described in those receiving physical therapy.[19]

Surgical containment is an option for LCPD.[49] Proximal femoral varus derotation osteotomy (VDRO) decompresses the femoral head, centers it more deeply in the acetabulum when the limb is in the weight-bearing position, and allows long-term remodeling.[44,220] A pelvic osteotomy may be used alone or combined with VDRO for certain patients (e.g., with a femoral head so large or subluxated that femoral osteotomy alone will not contain the head). A prophylactic trochanteric arrest is often performed to prevent trochanteric overgrowth and resulting hip abduction muscle weakness.[124] Kim and Wenger[101,102] described the concept of "functional retroversion" and "functional coxa vara" of the deformed femoral head in severe LCPD and discussed the use of valgus-flexion-internal rotation femoral osteotomy and acetabuloplasty for correction. Bankes and colleagues[9] described the use of valgus extension osteotomy as a salvage procedure for "hinge abduction" to relieve pain and correct deformity. The best outcomes will occur in those who experience the least deformity during the time the softened structure exists.[47] In some cases, surgical treatment may be the best option to assist this. Arkader et al.[6] found in a retrospective study that in children with disease onset after 8 years of age, better radiographic outcomes (10 years post) were observed in those who had various derotational osteotomies performed early in the disease process.[6]

Discoid Lateral Meniscus

The lateral meniscus is generally circular in shape and covers a larger portion of the tibial plateau than the medial side.[32] A discoid lateral meniscus is a common abnormal variant in children, occurring in 1% to 3% of the pediatric population, with bilateral incidence in 10% to 20%.[192] This is thought to be a congenital deviation or hypermobility due to lack of sufficient posterior attachments.[97] The more firmly attached medial meniscus rarely develops the discoid shape. Unlike the normal C-shaped appearance of the meniscus, a discoid

meniscus has a completely filled-in central area or a very small void in the central area.[68] The outer rim is also much thicker than a normal meniscal rim.[68] The thickened cartilage is more prone to tear with activities, and the abnormal mechanics can cause hypertrophy and irregularity of the cartilage.[68]

Clinically, children between the ages of 5 and 10 years present with a snapping knee joint, which may coexist with any combination of pain, giving way to effusion, quadriceps atrophy, limitation of motion, clicking, or locking.[159] Additional signs and symptoms related to a tear may include pain, knee locking, and inability to put weight on the affected extremity.[68] Many children remain asymptomatic and require no treatment.[68] For those with symptoms, arthroscopic debridement, partial meniscectomy, and repair are the treatments used with good results.[68]

Sever Disease

Sever disease, or calcaneal apophysitis, is an osteochondrosis of the calcaneus, generally related to mechanical overuse due to repetitive impact pressure and shear stresses.[143] This results in involvement at the Achilles tendon insertion at the calcaneus or in the retrocalcaneal bursa that lies between the skin and the tendon.[205] Traction of the Achilles tendon results in fragmentation or avulsion of cartilage at the point of attachment, disruption of chondrogenesis, reparative callus, fibrosis, and ossification.[182] This is generally seen in children 7 to 10 years of age[205] but can be present from ages 10 to 14 years as well.[61] The presenting complaint is pain in the heel, especially after activity, with consequent development of a limp.[61,205] Local tenderness at the posterior aspect of the heel, at the calcaneal apophysis, is present,[61,205] and pain may be reproduced with resistance of plantar flexion, such as when standing on tiptoes, because of the pull of the insertion on the Achilles tendon.[61] The condition is usually self-limiting. Conservative treatment is recommended and includes rest, ice, heel cups, heel lifts, reduced activity, and Achilles tendon stretching exercises. In cases of severe pain, a short leg walking cast may be helpful.

Growing Pains

"Growing pains" is the most common form of episodic musculoskeletal pain, primarily affecting children between the ages of 3 and 12 years.[207] The prevalence has been reportedly as high as 37% in children aged 4 to 6 years.[51] Clinical characteristics of the pain have been described as follows.[207]

- Pain is nonarticular. In two thirds of children, pain is located in the shins, calves, thighs, or popliteal fossa and is almost always bilateral.
- Pain occurs late in the day or is nocturnal, often waking the child. Mornings are almost always pain-free.
- Pain has a duration ranging from minutes to hours and can be mild or severe.
- The condition is episodic with pain-free intervals from days to months but can occur daily in severe cases.

No signs of inflammation are noted on physical examination. Possible relationships have been identified with periods of rapid growth and joint hypermobility.[50] The diagnosis of growing pains is based on the clinical signs and symptoms, and more serious conditions must be ruled out. Reassurance, symptomatic treatment using massage, nonsteroidal antiinflammatory medications, and muscle stretching, and time usually resolve the symptoms.[50]

Ages 10 to 15 Years

Slipped Capital Femoral Epiphysis

Ambroise Paré first described slipped capital femoral epiphysis (SCFE) in 1572. SCFE (also called epiphysiolysis) occurs when the growth plate of the proximal femoral physis is weak and becomes displaced ("slips") from its normal position. This disorder is classified into three subtypes:

1. *Acute:* Occurs with significant trauma and causes immediate, severe pain and restricted hip abduction and internal rotation.
2. *Acute-on-chronic:* The patient has already experienced some aching in the hip, thigh, or knee for weeks or even months as a result of a chronic slip. Then, with significant trauma, the epiphysis suddenly slips farther, and acute symptoms are noted.
3. *Chronic:* In this most common form, the child has a history of limp and pain, often for weeks or months, and loss of hip motion, especially internal rotation and abduction.

The cause is unclear but is likely a combination of mechanical and endocrine factors.[49] Mechanical factors that may influence the occurrence of SCFE include a decrease in femoral anteversion, retroversion of the femoral neck, and a more oblique orientation of the physeal plate during adolescence, all of which generate an increased shear force at the proximal femoral physeal plate.[49] Also, the decrease in mechanical strength of the physeal perichondral ring, the stabilizer of the physeal plate during the growth years, influences the mechanical strength of the physis.[49] Evidence of an association between endocrine dysfunction and SCFE has been identified with systemic abnormalities of hypothyroidism, hyperthyroidism, hypogonadism, and renal osteodystrophy.[49] Because growth hormone increases the physiologic activity of the physes during puberty, rapid longitudinal growth of the physis and a widened and weakened proximal femoral growth plate may allow a negative impact by shear forces, resulting in SCFE.[49]

In the United States, the incidence rate has been found to be 10.80 per 100,000,[112] compared with 2 per 100,000 globally.[49] Also noted is a 3.94 times higher incidence in African American children and a 2.53 times higher incidence in Hispanic children than in Caucasian children.[112] Climate was also found to be a factor, with an increased incidence of SCFE north of 40° latitude during the winter.[112] Suggested reasons for this seasonal increase include seasonal changes

in activity, seasonal patterns of growth and weight gain in adolescence, and vitamin D deficiency caused by decreased cutaneous synthesis during the winter.[115] Boys were at greater risk (13.35 cases/100,000 children) than girls (8.07 cases/100,000 children).[112] SCFE is related to puberty, with 78% of cases occurring during the adolescent growth phase.[49] Therefore, the age range for presentation is most often between 10 and 16 years in males and between 9 and 15 years in females.[49] SCFE may be bilateral in as many as 60% of cases, although involvement is usually not symmetrical and is more common in younger patients.[49] Obesity is a factor in the development of SCFE, with reports of two thirds of patients being over the 90th percentile in weight-for-age profiles,[49] and others reporting 76.6% above the 90th percentile for body weight.[113] The rise in childhood obesity in past years may help provide an explanation for the increasing incidence of SCFE.[137]

Patients with SCFE usually have complaints of pain in the groin with referred pain to the anteromedial aspect of the thigh and knee.[49] Pain may be noted in the thigh or knee only.[47,49] Evaluation of the hip in the obese child with knee pain is important. The child generally remains ambulatory but demonstrates an antalgic gait.[49] Consistently noted is a limitation in internal rotation of the hip, with the affected limb generally positioned in an externally rotated and shortened position.[49] When the hip is flexed, the thigh will rotate into external rotation and flexion will be limited.[49] In acute conditions, the reported complaint involves sudden onset of severe, fracture-like pain in the affected hip region, usually after a minor fall or twisting injury.[49] If SCFE is suspected, the rehabilitation professional should recommend limited weight bearing, especially impact activities, until further evaluation can be scheduled with a physician.

Conventional radiographs in anteroposterior and lateral views can be used to evaluate SCFE.[49,188] The anteroposterior radiograph usually shows widening of the growth plate and rarefaction of the adjacent metaphysis.[188] The head lies above and lateral to a line drawn along the superior margin of the neck.[188] On the lateral radiograph, any slipping will disrupt the alignment.[188] The severity of SCFE is then graded according to the amount of displacement.[188] The frog-leg lateral view will demonstrate posterior displacement and step-off of the epiphysis on the femoral neck, but this position is not advised in the acute or unstable presentation because of the potential for increasing physeal displacement during positioning[49] (Figure 14-19). MRI can help in early diagnosis of SCFE when plain radiographs and CT scans appear normal.[49] The CT scan is useful in confirming closure of the proximal femoral physis, which is difficult to view on plain radiographs.[49]

The goals of treatment are to keep the displacement to a minimum, maintain motion, and delay or prevent premature degenerative arthritis. Recommended treatment of the unstable/acute SCFE case includes in situ pinning after positioning of the femur.[130] Fixation is often adequate with one

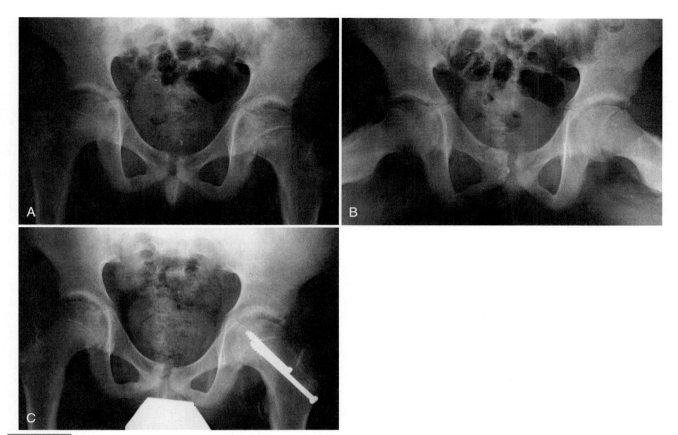

Figure 14-19 **A,** Twelve-year-old boy with a 4-month history of hip pain, exacerbated by jumping off a picnic table 2 days previously. The slipped capital femoral epiphysis is not clearly identified on the anterior-posterior view. **B,** Frog view demonstrates a slipped capital femoral epiphysis on the left, thought to be an acute-on-chronic slip by history. **C,** Treatment with percutaneous pin fixation was successful.

pin if good position is achieved.[188] Early decompression and fixation reduces the risk of avascular necrosis.[188] The acute case should be protected with non–weight bearing until callus is seen radiographically.[188] In the stable SCFE case, percutaneous pinning is advised, followed by walking as tolerated.[188] Prophylactic pinning of the contralateral hip is also a consideration.[177] Physical therapy is useful following surgery to increase strength and progress gait as weight bearing allows. Most will return to normal activity within 3 to 6 months postoperatively.

Two complications of SCFE are avascular necrosis and chondrolysis.[49,188] Avascular necrosis of the femoral head is more frequently associated with acute and unstable slips and is most likely due to vascular injury associated with the initial femoral head displacement, with more severe steps exhibiting greater involvement of the vascular supply.[188] Additional problems can occur with aggressive manipulation of the femoral head or penetration of the fixation device in the posterior cortex of the femoral head or articular surface.[188] Treatment should be directed at maintaining motion and preventing collapse by decrease weight bearing until healing occurs.[188] Chondrolysis is an acute dissolution of articular cartilage in association with rapid progressive

joint stiffness and pain.[188] Although this can occur in the untreated hip,[49,188] it has been most often found with manipulative reduction, prolonged immobilization, realignment osteotomies, and pin penetration of the femoral head.[188] The rate of these problems has decreased significantly in recent years with improved screw placement.[188] The joint space narrows, hip motion decreases, and an abduction contracture may develop.[49] Treatment should include modification of activities, use of crutches, gentle ROM to maintain motion, and anti-inflammatory medications.[188] Physical therapy may be helpful during this time to keep the patient mobile. A combination of avascular necrosis and chondrolysis is extremely devastating and usually results in hip fusion.[49]

Hips with SCFE are characterized by degenerative changes in later life, even when surgically stabilized.[2] These changes can occur along with avascular necrosis and chondrolysis. Abraham et al.[2] described premature development of osteoarthritis in the adult hip joint in patients with SCFE. This was related to hip impingement caused by loss of the head-neck offset and reorientation of the articular cartilage of the femoral head.[2] Their study showed that patients with SCFE undergoing total hip arthroplasty were 11 years younger than those with primary osteoarthritis.[2] This demonstrates how a developmental condition in childhood can cause disability later in life. This disability may influence the individual's choice of adult occupation and recreational activities and can cause secondary impairments, including hip pain.

Osgood-Schlatter Syndrome

Osgood-Schlatter disease, or syndrome, is characterized by activity-related pain and swelling at the insertion of the patellar tendon on the tibial tubercle caused by minor degrees of separation of the tibial tubercle.[173] Several causes have been suggested, including trauma, local alterations of the chondral tissue,[46] and mechanical overpull by the extensor muscles of the knee, which can result in patella alta and traction apophysitis,[5,86] eccentric muscle pull and muscle tightness,[81] reduced width of the patellar angle,[179] and increased external tibial torsion.[58] Unlike SCFE, Osgood-Schlatter syndrome is not thought to be an abnormality of physeal development or structure.[225] It may manifest as acute, severe pain, causing a child to limp, or may be noted by the child over a period of months as low-grade discomfort, usually brought on by running or participating in sports. Treatment consists of application of ice and rest, decreasing activity, and avoidance of all squatting and jumping activities. Use of a supportive brace may be helpful. Severe cases may require cast immobilization initially. The condition is usually self-limiting and resolves when the tubercle fuses to the main body of the tibia, usually at around 15 years of age.

Osteochondritis Dissecans

The term *osteochondritis dissecans (OD or OCD)* describes the separation of subchondral bone from the articular surface. It is characterized by a localized necrosis of the subchondral bone, which later revascularizes, reabsorbing and reossifying the bone necrosis.[28] Joint damage may occur because these lesions are adjacent to articular cartilage.[47] The fragment of bone can also detach, becoming a loose body in the joint.[47] Many patients have no history of trauma, but repetitive microtrauma, including shear and compressive forces, leads to subchondral bone stress, especially in athletic persons.[142] Other factors such as genetic predisposition, ischemia that may be caused by vascular spasm, fat emboli, infection thrombosis, and abnormal ossification seem to play a causative role.[74] Patients are typically 12 to 20 years of age and are often active in sporting activities.[74] The male-to-female ratio is 2:1.[164] The most commonly affected areas (in decreasing order of frequency) are the femoral condyles, the talar dome, and the capitellum of the humerus.[55] In the distal femur, the most commonly affected area is the lateral surface of the medial femoral condyle, but it may occur in areas such as the femoral capital epiphysis as well.[224] Joint pain is usually the primary complaint, although swelling or locking at the joint may occur if loose bodies are present.[47] Weight bearing with joint involvement also results in an antalgic gait. OCD is diagnosed radiologically with a radiolucent area identified

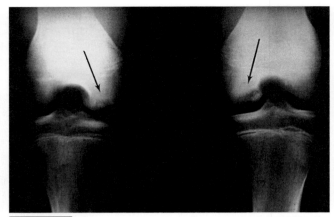

Figure 14-20 A notch, or tunnel, view of the distal femurs demonstrates the osteochondritis dissecans lesions, noted by arrows.

at the area of the lesion. An anteroposterior film may not visualize lesions on the posterior aspect of the medial femoral condyle, and a notch, or tunnel, view may be needed[74] (Figure 14-20). MRI is the most accurate method for staging lesions and is important for clinical management and determination of the need for conservative or surgical treatment.[74,141] In mild to moderate cases, treatment may consist of cast immobilization and then graduated activity with quadriceps strengthening exercises. Most cases of OCD of the distal femur are self-limiting and heal without surgical intervention. Yoshida et al.[228] reported that resting from sporting activities was adequate for healing in 81% of cases. About one half of lesions resolve over a period of 10 to 18 months with conservative measures.[74] If a fragment is free within the joint as a loose body, surgical treatment is effective in removal or fixation of the loose body.[47] For other marginal lesions, bone grafting or drilling of the necrotic fragment to promote more rapid vascular ingrowth and replacement is helpful.[47,74]

Tarsal Coalition

Tarsal coalition is a failure of segmentation between adjoining tarsal bones. Coalitions may exist between all of the tarsal bones, but talocalcaneal and calcaneonavicular coalitions are the most common.[188,210] Coalitions are often familial, may be unilateral or bilateral, and occur in both sexes equally.[188] Tarsal coalition usually produces symptoms between ages 8 and 12, when the abnormal cartilaginous bar begins to ossify. The resulting fusion imposes increased stress on adjacent joints and consequently may result in degenerative arthritis, pain, and peroneal spasm.[188] Because the coalitions may be fibrous (syndesmosis), cartilaginous (synchondrosis), or osseous (synostosis), limitation of motion at the subtalar joint is usually found, with inversion commonly limited.[210] This would present as a rigid flat foot. The coalition may be seen on plain radiographs of the foot (oblique views); however, CT or MRI provides the most definitive information about the site of the bridging, allowing differentiation of osseous from nonosseous coalitions and defining the extent of joint involvement, as well as secondary degenerative changes.[140] Symptomatic coalitions can be treated conservatively with a short leg walking cast.[188,210] Surgical resection is an option for those with persistent problems.[188,210]

Freiberg Disease

Freiberg disease or infraction is an idiopathic segmental avascular necrosis of the head of a metatarsal.[188] Most commonly, this occurs in adolescent girls, 13 to 18 years of age, and involves the second metatarsal.[188] This is generally a result of repetitive stress, such as running, with microfractures occurring at the junction of the metaphysic and growth plate, causing consequent inadequate circulation to the epiphysis.[210] Clinical presentation generally consists of pain in the forefoot, localized to the head of the second metatarsal, and localized swelling and limitation of motion in the metacarpophalangeal (MP) joint.[188,210] In the early stages, a bone scan will show increased uptake; later radiographs will show the stages of irregularity of the articular surface, sclerosis, fragmentation, and finally re-formation.[188,210] Initial treatment includes proper footwear with a metatarsal pad placed beneath the involved bones and limitation of activity for 4 to 6 weeks.[188,210] With severe symptoms, a short leg walking cast may ease the symptoms.[188,210] In most severe cases, surgical resection of the metatarsal heads can be performed.[188,210]

Accessory Navicular

Accessory navicular is an accessory or extra bone that develops on the medial side of the tarsal navicular, either within the posterior tibial tendon or as a separate bone.[188] This occurs in about 10% of the population.[188] Classification consists of three types:

- Type I is a small oval to round ossicle within the posterior tibialis tendon that is seldom symptomatic.[188,210]
- Type II is a larger lateral projection from the medial aspect of the navicular with a clear separation from the navicular.[210] This is often painful because of disruption of the synchondrosis.[188] These disruptions commonly occur during adolescence in relation to repetitive trauma, resulting in pain and tenderness.[188]
- Type III results in a prominence that, if too large, may cause irritation of the overlying skin.[188,210]

Pain will occur in type II lesions with midfoot dorsiflexion stresses in a planovalgus foot, direct pressure on the area, and motion between the navicular and accessory navicular.[210] Treatment is directed toward relief of symptoms, including a short leg walking cast and custom orthoses and eventual surgical removal for persistent cases.[188,210]

Additional Causes of Limp

Patellofemoral pain and recurrent patellar subluxation or dislocation are two common causes of limp in this age group

(see Chapter 15 for a detailed discussion). Monoarticular inflammatory arthritis and gonococcal arthritis also can cause acute onset of limp in a child.

Many types of neoplasms and related bone lesions can cause a child to limp. Commonly seen conditions include osteoid osteoma, unicameral bone cyst, osteochondroma (single or multiple), enchondroma, aneurysmal bone cyst, eosinophilic granuloma, and nonossifying fibroma. Symptoms may include limp, pain, and pathologic fracture through the lesion.[188,210]

HEMANGIOMA/VASCULAR MALFORMATION

A hemangioma is an abnormal proliferation of blood vessels that may occur in any vascularized tissue. Hemangiomas that affect the musculoskeletal system are more accurately termed *vascular malformations*. These are rare congenital lesions that are caused by a defect during vascular embryogenesis. By definition, they are always present at birth, but are not always clinically evident until later in life.[48] Skeletal changes are commonly seen with vascular malformations, although they are rarely seen with hemangiomas.[16]

At birth, vascular formations are fully formed, although the lesion may not be clinically apparent.[120] This type of lesion may appear later because of vessel dilation or hematoma formation, resulting in rapid enlargement.[120] Although this swelling and dilation may occur, vascular formations do grow in proportion to the patient.[120] Males and females are equally affected.[120] Vascular malformations can be subclassified by the predominant type of vessels found within the lesion (i.e., venous, arterial, lymphatic, capillary, or mixed) and by blood flow within the lesion (i.e., high flow vs. low flow).[120] Venous malformations often remain asymptomatic, although complications may include pain secondary to vessel dilation, bleeding, and hematoma formation, as well as intra-articular involvement, hemarthrosis, and pathologic fractures of bone.[120] They may also result in skeletal and soft tissue undergrowth or overgrowth in an affected limb.[120] Deep arteriovenous malformations can progress to distal ischemia, pain, and necrosis, with consequent risk for fracture, related to arterial steal of the bone.[20,120] The increased blood flow can also cause soft tissue and bone hypertrophy that can result in leg length discrepancy.[20,120] Overall, patients with vascular malformations of the limbs have been found to have bony involvement in 20% to 31% of cases.[16,20]

Diagnostically, ultrasonography, Doppler flow imaging, and magnetic resonance imaging are the most informative methods, revealing the extent of tissue involvement and differentiating fast-flow from slow-flow anomalies.[48] Epiphysiodesis may be required in cases of skeletal overgrowth to correct for leg length discrepancy, and further surgical intervention may be needed when involvement of muscle or bone has resulted in pain, functional impairment, or pathologic fracture.[120] Conservative treatment includes compression stockings and analgesia.[20]

MISCELLANEOUS CONDITIONS

BACK PAIN

In past years, reports of low back pain (LBP) in children have been considered carefully because they often indicated serious disease in children.[12] These conditions might include spondylosis, spondylolisthesis, infection (e.g., discitis, vertebral osteomyelitis), and benign or malignant tumors. Caution should especially be taken and appropriate consultations sought for those who have pain persisting for longer than 1 to 2 weeks, and for those whose pain is accompanied by fever, neurologic signs, or night pain, or inability to walk without a limp.[54]

Over the past two decades, epidemiologic studies have shown that the prevalence of nonspecific LBP in children is high.[12] In one study of elementary school children, 83% of 749 students reported occurrence of back pain in the past 3 months.[167] Although body weight was not considered in this study, one might question whether the rise in obesity among youth could be a factor, because a review of 65 epidemiologic studies of LBP did report that 32% of the 65 reviewed studies showed a statistically positive link between weight and LBP.[111] A detailed review of spinal conditions may be found in Chapter 8.

IDIOPATHIC TOE-WALKING

A number of children tend to toe-walk some of the time when first walking independently. A smaller subset persist in toe-walking, yet have no history of prematurity or difficult delivery and no evidence of hypertonicity or abnormal developmental reflexes that might lead to a diagnosis of cerebral palsy. This "idiopathic toe-walking" (ITW) usually responds well to a conservative treatment program of therapeutic exercise to stretch the gastrocnemius and soleus muscles and strengthen the ankle dorsiflexors. With significant tendo Achillis contractures, patients may require serial casting, perhaps with short leg cutout casts to encourage active dorsiflexion. Operative treatment is rarely required and carries the risk of over-lengthening, which can cause a serious functional deficit. Generally, nonsurgical treatment does not seem to have long-term results, and most cases do resolve spontaneously.[73] Surgical treatment should be reserved for those with a fixed ankle joint contracture.[73]

Differences in knee and ankle kinematics between patients with ITW and those with spastic diplegia can be documented on gait analysis.[98] Children with ITW may have "soft" neurologic signs, such as mild residual asymmetrical tonic neck reflexes in the quadruped position. Shulman and colleagues[181] also identified an association between persistent toe-walking and speech or language deficits (10 of 13 subjects), fine motor delays (4 of 13 subjects), and gross motor delays (3 of 13 subjects). Also, a family history of toe-walking can be documented in a group of idiopathic toe-walkers. This is an

autosomal dominant pattern described by Katz and Mubarak.[94]

ACHONDROPLASIA

Achondroplasia (dwarfism) is the most common of a large group of conditions known as the osteochondrodysplasias, a heterogeneous group of disorders characterized by abnormal growth and remodeling of cartilage and bone, affecting from 2 to 4.7 per 10,000 individuals.[8] The disorder is an autosomal dominant trait, but 80% of cases are the result of a random mutation.[47] Orthopedic manifestations of this condition include frontal bossing, cuboid-shaped vertebral bodies that may cause narrowing of the spinal canal and cord compression, with short pedicles, lumbar lordosis, short tubular bones, and short trident-shaped hands. Tibia vara is usually present, with the fibula longer than the tibia.[191] The incidence of neurologic complications secondary to spinal abnormalities ranges from 20% to 47%, although frequently the symptoms are subtle.[169] Persons with achondroplastic dwarfism have abnormal length ratios of limbs to trunk, with more shortening of the proximal limb segments, in contrast to persons classified as midgets, who have proportionate limb and trunk ratios. Some centers advocate surgical lengthening of the lower extremities for children with dwarfism.[226]

Many infants with achondroplasia demonstrate hypotonia with transient kyphotic deformity. In 10% to 15% of children, this may result in fixed angular kyphosis with serious neurologic sequelae later in life. Discouraging early unsupported sitting is effective, and bracing can also be used.[150]

LEG LENGTH INEQUALITY

Leg length inequality (LLI) may also be called leg length discrepancy (LLD) and is often defined as a 2.5 cm or greater difference in leg length. Differences smaller than this tend not to cause clinical problems. Differences in leg length may be due to relative overgrowth or shortening.

ORIGIN

The origin of LLI is divided into a number of categories: trauma; congenital, neuromuscular, or acquired diseases; infections causing physeal growth arrest; tumors; and vascular disorders. Types of trauma include epiphyseal and diaphyseal injuries. Epiphyseal injuries with growth plate closure may be asymmetrical, as in fracture involving the medial epiphysis of the distal femur. This type of injury can result in an angular deformity (varus), as well as shortening of the femur.

Congenital disorders include hemihypertrophy, in which one half of the body (the arm and leg) is larger than the other. Conversely, in hemiatrophy, one half of the body is smaller than the other. These sometimes can be difficult to distinguish, necessitating a decision on which arm and leg best "match" the rest of the body. Proximal focal femoral deficiency, congenital coxa vara, fibular and tibial hemimelia, and other focal dyplasias are additional causes of LLI (see Chapter 13). DDH can also cause a leg length discrepancy, as the result of an apparent femoral shortening noted when the hip is dislocated or actual shortening caused by femoral head AVN. Surgical treatments for DDH can change the leg length; these include use of a varus derotation osteotomy (VDRO), which shortens the femur, and pelvic osteotomies, which may add up to 1 inch to the height of the pelvis.

Neuromuscular disorders can cause asymmetrical growth of lower extremity bones. Decreased growth in the affected leg may be due to decreased muscle forces in weak or paralyzed muscles. Examples include myelodysplasia, poliomyelitis, and hemiplegia caused by congenital or acquired cerebral palsy. However, not all cases of LLI should be corrected. A child with hemiplegia can have a short lower limb on the affected side. With weakness and spasticity in that leg, foot clearance may be difficult as a result of decreased hip and knee flexion and equinus. The shortness of the leg makes foot clearance in swing easier.

Acquired conditions such as LCPD and SCFE can also result in shortened lower extremity, usually as a result of AVN of the femoral head, or occasionally as the result of surgical treatment. Fibrous dysplasia and tumors, including benign bone cysts and malignant neoplasms, can change leg length by interfering with growth centers or secondarily as a result of fracture or surgical treatment.

IMPAIRMENTS

The effects of LLI vary widely among patients because of the actual amount of difference and how well the patient physically compensates for it, the possibility of progression of the inequality, the patient's perception of the problem, and the overall picture of muscle strength, motor control, and ROM. If the discrepancy is marked or compensation is limited, poor cosmesis may be evident, and a significant increase in energy expenditure may be required to walk. Musculoskeletal adaptations and compensations may result. These secondary impairments include pelvic obliquity with changes in spinal alignment that can cause a functional scoliosis and rotation of the pelvis,[229] or low back pain, although pain is not something found to carry into adulthood[188] or to be a major complaint in those 15 years of age or younger.[203] Other musculoskeletal adaptations may be observed at the hip, knee, and ankle, including pelvic tilt, contralateral knee flexion, and ipsilateral equinus. These problems may be significant but easily accommodated because of the inherent energy and motivation usually present in children. In adulthood, however, factors of increased size and weight, increased energy expenditure to walk, increased sensitivity regarding the poor cosmesis of a lurching gait, and long-term effects

of asymmetrical lumbosacral spinal alignment may combine to significantly reduce the person's ability to walk and even render him or her nonambulatory.

CLINICAL EXAMINATION

The physical therapy examination for patients with LLI starts with obtaining a complete history, including any previous treatment. The physical examination incorporates the following elements:

- Measurement of ROM, joint stability, and muscle strength of the trunk, hips, knees, ankles, and feet
- Sensation of the lower extremities
- Anthropometric measurement: sitting and standing height, weight, and arm span; girth of thighs and calves; leg lengths
- Functional activities, such as rising from a chair to standing and moving down to the floor and back up
- Clinical analysis of posture and gait, including observation of the spine and lower extremity alignment and substitution patterns; observation of the patient with and without assistive devices and shoe lift during gait on level ground, ramps, and stairs.

Two options are available for clinical measurement of leg lengths. One is to level the pelvis in standing, using blocks under the short leg, and then to measure the height of the blocks. The other is to measure the legs using various landmarks, with the patient in the supine position: anterior-superior iliac spine to medial malleolus, anterior-superior iliac spine to lateral malleolus, anterior-superior iliac spine to heel pad, and umbilicus to heel pad. In a patient without significant lower extremity contractures, leveling the pelvis in standing with blocks may be the most accurate and reproducible method. Caution should be used when correcting LLI of less than 5 mm when only clinical assessment methods have been used, because of the inaccuracy and lack of reliability of the techniques.[17] Radiographic measurement of leg lengths is usually done with scanograms. The patient is positioned on the x-ray table with a ruler alongside the legs, and three radiographs are taken on the same cassette, at the level of the hips, knees, and ankles, with the patient held motionless. These three views with the ruler markings next to them allow the examiner to measure the length of the femur and tibia and combine them for the total leg length. Landmarks commonly used are the top of the femoral head, the bottom of the medial femoral condyle, and the tibial plafond. A film of the left wrist and hand should be performed in conjunction with the scanogram. This allows determination of the skeletal age of the patient, using the standard reference established by Greulich and Pyle.[66]

Measurement error is present in any of these techniques, making both clinical and radiographic leg length determinations an inexact science. Validity of the measurement is affected by hip and knee flexion contractures that "shorten" the leg. Determination of bone age is somewhat subjective.

Determining the percentage of growth inhibition assists in estimating the eventual discrepancy at skeletal maturity. For example, a 10% inhibition of growth in the short leg may result in minor discrepancy when the child is quite young. When the leg is 20 cm long, a 10% shortening is only 2 cm. However, as the child matures, when the unaffected leg is 70 cm long, a 10% inhibition of growth on the involved side will result in a shortening of 7 cm, which is significant.

If the patient can be followed with serial measurements over time, scanogram measurements of total length of both the long and the short leg and skeletal age at the time of each scanogram can be plotted on the Moseley graph, which depicts past growth and predicts future growth[133] (Figure 14-21). Timing of epiphysiodesis is based on the predicted LLD at skeletal maturity. The effects of surgery can also be plotted on the graph to predict alteration in leg lengths and the eventual impact on discrepancy at skeletal maturity. Paley et al.[148] have developed a mathematical formula that allows these predictions to be accurately based on as few as one or two measurements (Table 14-2).

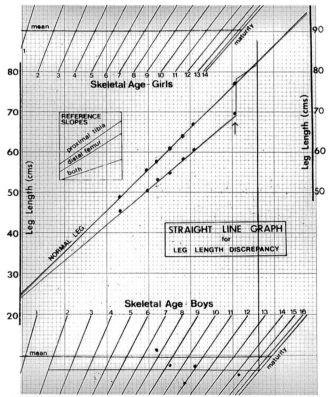

Figure 14-21 An example of the use of the Moseley graph to plot a patient's serial scanogram measurements and bone ages to determine the discrepancy at maturity and the possibilities for surgical intervention. Growth of the short leg is depicted by the line below the normal leg line. The increase in the length of the short leg (arrow) shows the effects of a leg-lengthening procedure. The two legs are approximately equal at skeletal maturity.

TABLE 14-2 Lower-Limb Multipliers for Boys and Girls Used to Predict the Limb Length Discrepancy and the Amount of Growth Remaining

Age (yrs + mos)	Multiplier	
	Boys	Girls*
Birth	5.080	4.630
0 + 3	4.550	4.155
0 + 6	4.050	3.725
0 + 9	3.600	3.300
1 + 0	3.240	2.970
1 + 3	2.975	2.750
1 + 6	2.825	2.600
1 + 9	2.700	2.490
2 + 0	2.590	2.390
2 + 3	2.480	2.295
2 + 6	2.385	2.200
2 + 9	2.300	2.125
3 + 0	2.230	2.050
3 + 6	2.110	1.925
4 + 0	2.000	1.830
4 + 6	1.890	1.740
5 + 0	1.820	1.660
5 + 6	1.740	1.580
6 + 0	1.670	1.510
6 + 6	1.620	1.460
7 + 0	1.570	1.430
7 + 6	1.520	1.370
8 + 0	1.470	1.330
8 + 6	1.420	1.290
9 + 0	1.380	1.260
9 + 6	1.340	1.220
10 + 0	1.310	1.190
10 + 6	1.280	1.160
11 + 0	1.240	1.130
11 + 6	1.220	1.100
12 + 0	1.180	1.070
12 + 6	1.160	1.050
13 + 0	1.130	1.030
13 + 6	1.100	1.010
14 + 0	1.080	1.000
14 + 6	1.060	NA
15 + 0	1.040	NA
15 + 6	1.020	NA
16 + 0	1.010	NA
16 + 6	1.010	NA
17 + 0	1.000	NA

From Paley, D., Bhave, A., Herzenberg, J. E., & Bowen, J. R. (2000). Multiplier method for predicting limb-length discrepancy. *Journal of Bone and Joint Surgery (American), 82,* 1440.
*NA = not applicable.

TABLE 14-3 Percentage of Growth for Each Growth Center in the Femur and Tibia

Growth Center	For Entire Leg	Total Length of Femur	Total Length of Tibia
Proximal femur	15%	30%	–
Distal femur	35%	70%	–
Proximal tibia	30%	–	60%
Distal tibia	20%	–	40%

TREATMENT

Treatment of LLI can be conservative or surgical. Conservative treatment consists of observation only or use of a shoe lift. Surgical treatment is directed at either shortening the long leg or lengthening the short leg. Some patients need both limbs addressed to achieve equality at maturity. Shortening the long leg in the growing child is achieved by epiphysiodesis, the surgical physical arrest of one or more growth centers in the long leg, which allows the short leg to "catch up" in length. This can be done percutaneously or with an open procedure, although the percutaneous method has good outcomes and a quicker recovery.[4,84] The contribution to growth varies with each growth center, and this must also be considered (Table 14-3).

Timing of the epiphysiodesis is obviously crucial. Future growth of each leg must be predicted and the surgery performed at a time when the amount of growth denied the long leg will match the amount of growth still available in the short leg, allowing them to be approximately equal in length at skeletal maturity. If epiphysiodesis is performed too early, the long leg may actually become the short leg, with an obviously less than optimal surgical result. Another option for shortening the long leg is a shortening osteotomy, usually considered in a skeletally mature patient who is not a candidate for epiphysiodesis.

Epiphysiodesis can also be performed on only the medial or lateral growth part of the growth plate to correct angular deformities. For example, a fracture of the distal femur may cause damage to the medial aspect of the distal femoral growth plate. The lateral part of the growth plate continues to function normally, and the leg grows into varus, which also produces a functional shortening.

If the medial portion of the growth plate is still open, stapling of the lateral portion can allow the femur to gradually grow out of varus. This type of surgery may include resection of a bony bar on the involved side of the growth plate.

LIMB LENGTHENING

Surgical lengthening of the short leg has appeal because the surgery is performed on the affected leg, not the "normal" leg, and opportunity exists for correction of discrepancies of

much greater magnitude. Criteria for leg lengthening include a discrepancy of greater than 4 to 6 cm, adequate soft tissue mobility available to allow correction, and a stable joint above and below, although unstable joints can be protected with an external frame. A decision must be made whether to lengthen the femur or the tibia or both. Ideally the final result at maturity will be fairly equal leg lengths and equal knee heights in standing. If the discrepancy is too large to be amenable to these procedures, as in some cases of proximal focal femoral deficiency, amputation of the distal segment to allow the use of a prosthesis would be considered the most practical alternative (see Chapter 13). Another option is rotationplasty of the affected limb.[222]

Limb lengthening was first reported in the literature by Dodivilla in Italy in 1905.[34] Two biologic approaches to lengthening may be used: (1) lengthening through bone, and (2) lengthening by physeal distraction. Physeal distraction includes the option of subacute epiphysiolysis, initially described by Monicelli and Spinelli and called chondrodiastasis.[34] It consists of gradual distraction of the growth plate using a circular fixator, leading to a sudden rupture of the growth plate 3 to 4 days after the procedure begins. This is rarely used except for adolescent limb lengthening near the end of the patient's growth, because it may lead to premature closure of the growth plate.

A number of devices have been developed for lengthening bone, including diaphyseal lengthening devices (Wagner, unilateral frame) and metaphyseal lengthening devices, such as the Ilizarov (circular frame). The Wagner technique for lengthening through bone involved an osteotomy of the bone followed by rapid distraction, with cancellous bone grafting and planting of the distraction gap.[209]

Dr. Gavriil Abramovich Ilizarov first developed his technique and device in Russia to treat World War II veterans and later widened the applications.[83] The Ilizarov method of slow distraction does not use bone grafting of the distraction gap. The circular design and the custom fitting of the external fixator allow simultaneous correction of rotational and angular deformities, in addition to achieving lengthening.[193] The standard rate of distraction is usually four times per day (0.25 mm each time). After the desired correction has been achieved, the fixator is left in place to allow consolidation of new bone. One study documented that consolidation will occur at the rate of 26 days for each centimeter of extension with the Ilizarov technique.[1] The Ilizarov technique is used for both adult and pediatric disorders, including limb length discrepancy, angular deformities such as adolescent Blount's disease, congenital tibial pseudarthrosis, resistant or recurrent clubfeet, correction of forearm or humeral shortening and deformity due to trauma or infection, and others.[157] Another, more controversial indication for leg lengthening is its bilateral use in patients with achondroplasia to achieve a more normal height.[146]

Alternate methods allow for less time in the external fixator and resulting shorter times needed for bone healing and protection against refracture.[168] One method has the intramedullary (IM) nail inserted concomitantly with the external fixator,[149] and the other method has the IM nail inserted during the consolidation phase.[168] Both methods allow earlier removal of the external fixator and therefore earlier rehabilitation.

As defined by Paley,[147] "problems" following lengthening procedures represent difficulties that do not require operative intervention, "obstacles" require operative intervention, and true "complications" include all problems that do not resolve by the end of treatment. Difficulties that may be encountered during lengthening procedures include the following:

- *Bone:* angulation, delayed union or nonunion, fractures, pin tract infections, osteomyelitis
- *Joint:* cartilage degeneration, stiffness, subluxation, dislocation
- *Nerves:* transient or permanent stretch paralysis
- *Muscle:* weakness, contracture, ischemia
- *Vascular:* transient hypertension, probably due to stretching of the sciatic nerve, although this has not been well documented.

Barker et al.[10] studied 35 patients undergoing femoral lengthening by the Ilizarov method. They found that 92% of patients regained their knee flexion by 12 months, and 97% by 18 months. Significant loss of knee flexion occurred in the period before lengthening, in response to application of the fixation device, and investigators stressed the need for active physical therapy intervention when the fixation device is first applied. Historical guidelines recommend limiting the amount of lengthening to 10% to 20% of the length of the segment before surgery. However, Yun et al.[231] undertook 35 lengthenings in 31 patients and achieved a mean gain of 33% with only a 0.9% complication rate by Paley's classification. Also, gait characteristics significantly improve after limb lengthening.[203]

Children undergoing leg lengthening must adjust to the pain of the procedure, which can be significant and extended.[229] The child may experience frustration, anger, and fear because of the temporary loss of independence inherent in the procedure. Difficult behavior may require intervention by a psychologist to assist the child and family in developing appropriate coping strategies. Candidates for surgical lengthening must be extremely motivated, with a supportive and committed family. Successful limb lengthening also mandates a comprehensive medical care system, with knowledgeable, experienced physicians, nurses, and therapists to guide the patient and family through the process.

ROLE OF PHYSICAL THERAPY IN LIMB LENGTHENING

An excellent description of preoperative and postoperative physical therapy goals and interventions for patients undergoing limb lengthening has been provided by Simard and colleagues.[183] The preoperative phase includes the following:

- Comprehensive physical therapy examination
- Crutch fitting and instruction in restricted weight bearing on the involved leg
- Instruction in home exercise and postoperative positioning and splinting in conjunction with the patient, parents, and other caregivers
- Stretching and strengthening exercises to use in preparation for surgery

The greatest challenges for the physical therapist treating children in the postoperative phase include promoting weight bearing in the presence of significant pain, maintaining the child's ROM, and motivating the child to continue with the program both in the hospital and at home over the long period of treatment. Significant difficulty may be associated with obtaining funding for physical therapy, an example of an environmental factor that can affect the success of the surgery. Insurance carriers require documentation of improved function during the treatment period. For the patient undergoing leg lengthening by the Ilizarov technique, the goal is to maintain ambulation, joint ROM, and strength while undergoing the lengthening, with a long-term goal of improved function after the device is removed.

The postoperative phase includes instruction in functional activities, active assistive and isometric exercise, proper positioning of the extremity, gait training with progressive weight bearing as tolerated, and pin care. Modalities such as ice or transcutaneous electrical nerve stimulation (TENS) may be useful for pain management. Dynamic splinting may be used in the limb-lengthening stage to provide low-intensity, prolonged stretch to joints with significantly limited ROM. Exercise techniques that may be useful throughout the Ilizarov lengthening include closed- and open-chain exercises for strengthening and active-assistive or passive exercises for ROM. A stationary bicycle and a treadmill may be used. After removal of the fixator, the patient may require additional gait training, monitoring, and adjusting of the exercise program, and possibly refitting and retraining, with orthotic or prosthetic devices worn preoperatively. Throughout the course of treatment, children are encouraged to participate in their usual school and leisure activities to the fullest extent possible.

SUMMARY

The pediatric orthopedic conditions presented in this chapter represent a wide range of problems that may be encountered by physical therapists in children referred to them for a specific problem (e.g., clumsy gait), or perhaps a specific complaint that turns out to be a "red herring." An example of this is a child referred to physical therapy for intervention for knee pain, who in fact has a slipped capital femoral epiphysis. Alternatively, a child might be referred from a primary care physician or a neurologist to a physical therapist with one diagnosis (e.g., gross motor developmental delay), but also may be under treatment by an orthopedist for developmental dysplasia of the hip. In all these various scenarios, it is essential that the physical therapist be knowledgeable about various pediatric orthopedic conditions, including their signs, symptoms, differential diagnoses, and interventions. Physical therapists must be well informed regarding when to refer to other practitioners, such as the orthopedist surgeon in the case of a child with a suspected acute SCFE. As physical therapists,

we often have the advantage of following a child intensively over a period of time, as opposed to a physician's visit once every 6 months, and thereby have unique insights into the child's condition and the family dynamics surrounding it. The well-informed physical therapist can often serve to bridge the gap that sometimes occurs between various specialists following a child, including primary care physicians, orthopedists, neurologists, and physiatrists.

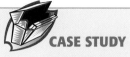

CASE STUDY

"David"

David was seen by his primary care provider at age 12, when pain in his left heel became significant enough that he could not continue his normal activities at school, including marching in the band and playing soccer. He was referred to a podiatrist at that time for further consultation. After an MRI was obtained, the diagnosis of Sever disease was made by the podiatrist, and the patient was then referred for physical therapy.

On the initial visit to physical therapy, David rated his pain as 8 on a scale of 10. Activities that aggravated his pain included standing, walking, and generally any weight-bearing activities. He was able to completely relieve his pain with ice, rest, and taking weight off the feet. Ibuprofen had been used sporadically for pain, as the parents did not want it to be used routinely. At the time of evaluation, David had not participated in soccer, physical education classes, or marching band practice for 1 week. The podiatrist had started him on a short-term steroid regimen that began on the day of the evaluation and would continue through 5 days.

Evaluation of David showed the classic signs of Sever disease with pain in the heel that was aggravated by activity and relieved with rest,

tenderness at the Achilles tendon insertion region, pain with resisted ankle plantar flexion, decreased active dorsiflexion to −10 degrees, and a gradual progression of symptoms leading to cessation of activity.

During the evaluation process, several other conditions were ruled out that can cause heel pain in children, including plantar fasciitis, Achilles tendinitis, retrocalcaneal bursitis, and calcaneal stress fracture. Radiology testing also helped to rule out tarsal coalition, calcaneal osteomyelitis, heel fat pad syndrome, and tumor.

Intervention for David's care was consistent with traditional interventions for a patient with Sever disease. Iontophoresis with dexamethasone was applied to the area of the calcaneal apophysis. The patient also received a heel lift to decrease the stress placed on the Achilles tendon and was instructed in the application of ice with activity. Iontophoresis treatments were used only four times, with the pain significantly decreasing. The patient was also able to advance with the therapeutic exercise to achieve 15° active dorsiflexion without pain. Strengthening activities were then pursued further to progress plantar flexor strength without an increase in pain. Heel cups were provided, as he returned to marching band activities within 3 weeks.

EVIDENCE TO PRACTICE 14-1

CASE STUDY "DAVID"

EXAMINATION DECISION

The evaluation techniques used to evaluate this patient included testing procedures specific for Sever disease, as well as other procedures to rule out other conditions.[61,205]

Plan of care decision: Conservative treatment is generally attempted initially and is usually effective.[61,143,205]

PATIENT/FAMILY PREFERENCES

Parents were involved in all aspects of the treatment plan. The risks and benefits of each aspect of care were discussed, as was the effectiveness of conservative treatment that has been well documented.[61,143,205]

REFERENCES

1. Aaron, A. D., Eilert, R. E. (1996). Results of the Wagner and Ilizarov methods of limb-lengthening. *Journal of Bone and Joint Surgery (American)*, 78, 20–29.

2. Abraham, W. R., Gonzalez, M. H., Pratap, S., Amirouche, F., Atluri, P., & Simon, P. (2007). Clinical implications of anatomical wear characteristics in slipped capital femoral epiphysis and primary osteoarthritis. *Journal of Pediatric Orthopaedics*, 27, 788.

3. Accadbled, F., Laville, J. M., & Harper, L. (2003). One-step treatment of evolved Blount's disease: Four cases and review of the literature. *Journal of Pediatric Orthopaedics*, 23, 747.

4. Alzahrani, A. G., Behairy, Y. M., Alhossan, M. H., Arab, F. S., & Alammari, A. A. (2003). Percutaneous versus open epiphysiodesis. *Saudi Medical Journal*, 24, 203.

5. Aparicio, G., Abril, J. C., Calvo, E., & Alvarez, L. (1997). Radiologic study of patellar height in Osgood-Schlatter disease. *Journal of Pediatric Orthopaedics*, 17, 63.

6. Arkader, A., Sankar, W. N., & Amorin, R. M. (2009). Conservative versus surgical treatment of late-onset Legg-Calve-Perthes disease: A radiographic comparison at skeletal maturity. *Journal of Children's Orthopaedics, 3*, 21.

7. Arnold, S. R., Elias, D., Buckingham, S. C., et al. (2006). Changing patterns of acute hematogenous osteomyelitis and septic arthritis: Emergence of community-associated methicillin-resistant *Staphylococcus aureus*. *Journal of Pediatric Orthopaedics, 26*, 703.

8. Baitner, A. C., Maurer, S. G., Gruen, M. B., & DiCesare, P. E. (2000). The genetic basis of the osteochondroplasias. *Journal of Pediatric Orthopaedics, 20*, 594.

9. Bankes, M. J., Catterall, A., Hashemi-Nejad, A. (2000). Valgus extension osteotomy for 'hinge abduction' in Perthes' disease: Results at maturity and factors influencing the radiological outcome. *Journal of Bone and Joint Surgery (British), 82*, 548.

10. Barker, K. L., Simpson, A. H. R. W., & Lamb, S. E. (2001). Loss of knee range of motion in leg lengthening. *Journal of Orthopaedic & Sports Physical Therapy, 31*, 238.

11. Barry, R. J., & Scranton, P. E. Jr. (1983). Flat feet in children. *Clinical Orthopaedics and Related Research, 181*, 68.

12. Bejia, I., Abid, N., Ben-Salem, K., et al. (2005). Low back pain in a cohort of 622 Tunisian schoolchildren and adolescents: An epidemiological study. *European Spine Journal, 14*, 331.

13. Berkowitz, C. D. (2008). Angular deformities of the lower extremity: Bowlegs and knock-knees. In C. D. Berkowitz (Ed.). *Berkowitz's pediatrics: A primary care approach* (3rd ed.). Elk Grove Village, IL: American Academy of Pediatrics.

14. Bleck, E. E. (1983). Metatarsus adductus: Classification and relationship to outcomes of treatment. *Journal of Pediatric Orthopaedics, 3*, 2.

15. Bobroff, E. D., Chambers, H. G., Sartoris, D. J., Wyatt, M. P., & Sutherland, D. H. (2000). Femoral anteversion and neck-shaft angle in children with cerebral palsy. *Clinical Orthopaedics and Related Research, 364*, 194.

16. Boyd, J. B., Mulliken, J. B., Kaban, L. B., Upton, J. III, Murray, J. E. (1984). Skeletal changes associated with vascular malformations. *Plastic and Reconstructive Surgery, 74*, 789.

17. Brady, R. J., Dean, J. B., Skinner, T. M., & Gross, M. T. (2003). Limb length inequality: Clinical implications for assessment and intervention. *Journal of Orthopaedic and Sports Physical Therapy, 33*, 221.

18. Bramer, J. A., Maas, M., Dallinga, R. J., te Slaa, R. L., & Vergroesen, D. A. (2004). Increased external tibial torsion and osteochondritis dessicans of the knee. *Clinical Orthopaedics and Related Research, 422*, 175.

19. Brech, G. C., & Guarnieiro, R. (2006). Evaluation of physiotherapy in the treatment of Legg-Calve-Perthes disease. *Clinics (Sao Paulo), 61*, 521–528.

20. Breugem, C. C., Maas, M., Breugam, S. J. M., Schaap, G. R., & van der Horst, C. M. A. M. (2003). Vascular malformations of the lower limb with osseous involvement. *Journal of Bone and Joint Surgery (British), 85*, 399.

21. Brooks, W. C., & Gross, R. H. (1995). Genu varum in children: Diagnosis and treatment. *Journal of the American Academy of Orthopedic Surgery, 3*, 326.

22. Brown, R., Hussain, M., McHugh, K., Novelli, V., & Jones, D. (2001). Discitis in young children. *Journal of Bone and Joint Surgery (British), 83*, 106.

23. Browne, R. S., & Paton, D. F. (1979). Anomalous insertion of the tibialis posterior tendon in congenital metatarsus varus. *Journal of Bone and Joint Surgery (British), 61*, 74.

24. Bruce, R. W. Jr. (1996). Torsional and angular deformities. *Pediatric Clinics of North America, 43*, 867.

25. Bruce, W. D., & Stevens, P. M. (2004). Surgical correction of miserable malalignment syndrome. *Journal of Pediatric Orthopedics, 24*, 392.

26. Carney, B. T., & Minter, C. L. (2004). Nonsurgical treatment to regain hip abduction motion in Perthes disease: A retrospective review. *Singapore Medical Journal, 97*, 485.

27. Catterall, A. (1971). The natural history of Perthes' disease. *Journal of Bone and Joint Surgery (British), 53*, 37.

28. Cepero, S., Ullot, R., & Sastre, S. (2005). Osteochondritis of the femoral condyles in children and adolescents: Our experience over the last 28 years. *Journal of Pediatric Orthopaedics B, 14*, 24.

29. Chambers, H. (2003). Ankle and foot disorders in skeletally immature athletes. *Orthopedic Clinics of North America, 34*, 445–459.

30. Chang, W. S., Chiu, N. C., Chi, H., Li, W. C., & Huang, F. Y. (2005). Comparison of the characteristics of culture-negative versus culture-positive septic arthritis in children. *Journal of Microbiology, Immunology, and Infection, 38*, 189.

31. Churgay, C. A. (1993). Diagnosis and treatment of pediatric foot deformities. *American Family Physician, 47*, 883.

32. Clark, C., & Ogden, J. (1983). Development of the menisci of the human joint: Morphologic changes and their potential role in childhood meniscal injury. *Journal of Bone and Joint Surgery (American), 65*, 538.

33. Colburn, M., & Williams, M. (2003). Evaluation of the treatment of idiopathic clubfoot by using Ponseti method. *Journal of Foot and Ankle Surgery, 42*, 259.

34. Coleman, S. S., & Scott, S. M. (1991). The present attitude toward the biology and technology of limb lengthening. *Clinical Orthopaedics and Related Research, 76*, 264.

35. Committee on Quality Improvement, Subcommittee on Developmental Dysplasia of the Hip. (2000). Clinical practice guideline: Early detection of developmental dysplasia of the hip. *Pediatrics, 105*, 896.

36. Crofton, P. M., MacFarlane, C., Wardhaugh, B., et al. (2005). Children with acute Perthes' disease have asymmetrical lower leg growth and abnormal collagen turnover. *Acta Orthopaedica, 76*, 841.

37. Cuevas de Alba, C., Buille, J. T., Bowen, J. R., & Hareke, H. T. (1998). Computed tomography for femoral and tibial torsion in children with clubfoot. *Clinical Orthopaedics and Related Research, 353*, 203.

38. Cusick, B. D., & Stuberg, W. A. (1992). Assessment of lower-extremity alignment in the transverse plane: Implications for management of children with neuromotor dysfunction. *Physical Therapy, 72,* 13.

39. De Boeck, H. (2005). Osteomyelitis and septic arthritis in children. *Acta Orthopaedica Belgica, 71,* 505.

40. Dietz, W. H., Gross, W. L., & Kirkpatrick, J. A. (1982). Blount disease (tibia vara): Another skeletal disorder associated with childhood obesity. *Journal of Pediatrics, 101,* 735.

41. Dodgin, D. A., deSwart, R. J., Stefko, R. M., Wenger, D. R., & Lo, J. Y. (1998). Distal tibial/fibular derotation osteotomy for correction of tibial torsion: Review of technique and results in 63 cases. *Journal of Pediatric Orthopedics, 18,* 95.

42. Dowling, A. M., Steele, J. R., & Baur, L. A. (2001). Does obesity influence foot structure and plantar pressure patterns in pre-pubescent children? *International Journal of Obesity Related Metabolic Disorders, 25,* 845.

43. Dror, L., Alan, A., & Leonel, C. (2007). The Haas procedure for the treatment of tibial torsional deformities. *Journal of Pediatric Orthopedics, 16,* 120.

44. Eckerwall, G., Hochbergs, P., Wingstrand, H., & Egund, N. (1997). Magnetic resonance imaging and early remodeling of the femoral head after femoral varus osteotomy in Legg-Calve-Perthes disease. *Journal of Pediatric Orthopedics B, 6,* 239.

45. Eckerwall, G., Wingstrand, H., Hagglund, G., & Karlberg, J. (1996). Growth in 110 children with Legg-Calve-Perthes disease: A longitudinal infancy childhood puberty growth model study. *Journal of Pediatric Orthopedics B, 5,* 181.

46. Ehrenberg, G., & Engfeldt, B. (1961). Histologic changes in the Osgood-Schlatter lesion. *Acta Chirurgica Scandinavica, 121,* 328.

47. Eilert, R. E. (2005). Orthopedics. In W. W. Hay, Jr., M. J. Levin, J. M. Sondheimer, & R. R. Deterding (Eds.). *Current pediatric diagnosis and treatment* (17th ed.). Chicago: Lange Medical Books/McGraw-Hill.

48. Enjolras, O., & Mulliken, J. B. (1993). The current management of vascular birthmarks. *Pediatric Dermatology, 10,* 311.

49. Erol, B., & Dormans, J. P. (2005). Hip disorders. In J. P. Dormans (Ed.). *Pediatric orthopaedics: Core knowledge in orthopaedics* (1st ed.). Philadelphia: Mosby.

50. Evans, A. M. (2008). Growing pains: Contemporary knowledge and recommended practice. *Journal of Foot and Ankle Research, 1,* 4.

51. Evans, A. M., & Scutter, S. D. (2004). Prevalence of "growing pains" in young children. *Journal of Pediatrics, 145,* 255.

52. Fabry, K., Fabry, G., & Moens, P. (2003). Legg-Calve-Perthes disease in patients under 5 years of age does not always result in a good outcome: Personal experience and meta-analysis of the literature. *Journal of Pediatric Orthopedics B, 22,* 222.

53. Farrell, S. A., Summers, A. M., Dallaire, L., Singer, J., Johnson, J. A., & Wilson, R. D. (1999). Clubfoot, an adverse outcome of early amniocentesis: Disruption or deformation? Canadian Early and Mid-Trimester Amniocentesis Triad. *Journal of Medical Genetics, 36,* 843.

54. Fernandez, M., Carrol, C. L., & Baker, C. J. (2000). Discitis and vertebral osteomyelitis in children: An 18-year review. *Pediatrics, 105,* 1299.

55. Fisher, D. R., & DeSmet, A. A. (1993). Radiologic analysis of osteochondritis dissecans and related osteochondral lesions. *Contemporary Diagnostic Radiology, 16,* 1.

56. Fuchs, R., & Staheli, L. T. (1996). Sprinting and intoeing. *Journal of Pediatric Orthopedics, 16,* 389.

57. Gaughan, D. M., Mofeson, L. M., Hughes, M. D., Seage, G. R. III, Ciupak, G. L., & Oleske, J. M. (2002). AIDS Clinical Trials Group Protocol 219 Team. Osteonecrosis of the hip (Legg-Calve-Perthes disease) in human immunodeficiency virus-infected children. *Pediatrics, 109,* E74-4.

58. Gigante, A., Bevilacqua, C., Bonetti, M. G., & Greco, F. (2003). Increased external tibial torsion in Osgood Schlatter disease. *Acta Orthopaedica Scandinavica, 74,* 431.

59. Glazer, P. A. (1996). Pediatric spinal infections. *Orthopedic Clinics of North America, 27,* 111.

60. Gledhill, R. B. (1973). Subacute osteomyelitis in children. *Clinical Orthopedics, 96,* 57.

61. Goel, K., & Watt, G. F. (2002). Paediatric podiatry. In D. L. Lorimer, G. French, M. O'Donnell, J. G. Burrow (Eds.). *Neale's disorders of the foot: Diagnosis and management* (6th ed.). St Louis: Churchill Livingstone.

62. Goergens, E. D., McEvoy, A., Watson, M., & Barrett, I. R. (2005). Acute osteomyelitis and septic arthritis in children. *Journal of Paediatrics and Child Health, 41,* 59.

63. Gordon, J. E., Schoenecker, P. L., Osland, J. D., Dobbs, M. B., Szymanski, D. A., & Luhmann, S. J. (2004). Smoking and socio-economic status in the etiology and severity of Legg-Calve-Perthes disease. *Journal of Pediatric Orthopedics B, 13,* 367.

64. Gordon, J. E., Wolff, A., Luhman, S. J., et al. (2005). Primary and delayed closure after open irrigation and debridement of septic arthritis in children. *Journal of Pediatric Orthopedics B, 14,* 101.

65. Gore, A. I., & Spencer, J. P. (2004). The newborn foot. *American Family Physician, 69,* 865.

66. Greulich, W. W., & Pyle, S. I. (1950). *Radiographic atlas of skeletal development of the hand and wrist.* Stanford, CA: Stanford University Press.

67. Harcke, H. T. (1992). Imaging in congenital dislocation and dysplasia of the hip. *Clinical Orthopaedics and Related Research, 281,* 22.

68. Hart, E. S., Kalra, K. P., Grottkau, B. E., Albright, M., & Shannon, E. G. (2008). Discoid lateral meniscus in children. *Orthopaedic Nursing, 27,* 174.

69. Hazelwood, M. E., Simmons, A. N., Johnson, W. T., et al. (2007). The footprint method to assess transmalleolar axis. *Gait Posture, 25,* 597–603.

70. Hensinger, R. H., & Jones, E. T. (1981). Neonatal orthopaedics. In T. K. Oliver (Ed.). *Monographs in neonataology.* New York: Grune and Stratton.

71. Herring, J. A., Kim, H. T., & Browne, R. (2005). Legg-Calve-Perthes disease. Part II: Prospective multicenter study of the

effect of treatment on outcome. *Journal of Bone and Joint Surgery (American), 87,* 1164.

72. Herring, J. A., Neustadt, J. B., Williams, J. J., Early, J. S., & Browne, R. H. (1992). The lateral pillar classification of Legg-Calve-Perthes disease. *Journal of Pediatric Orthopedics, 12,* 143.

73. Hirsch, G., & Waagner, B. (2004). The natural history of idiopathic toe-walking: A long-term follow-up of fourteen conservatively treated children. *Acta Paediatrica, 93,* 196.

74. Hixon, A. L., & Gibbs, L. M. (2000). Osteochondritis dissecans: A diagnosis not to miss. *American Family Physician, 61,* 151.

75. Hofmann, A., Jones, R. E., & Herring, J. A. (1982). Blount's disease after skeletal maturity. *Journal of Bone and Joint Surgery (American), 64,* 1004.

76. Holden, W., & David, J. (2005). Chronic recurrent multifocal osteomyelitis: Two cases of sacral disease responsive to corticosteroids. *Clinical Infectious Diseases, 40,* 616.

77. Howlett, J. P., Mosca, U. S., & Bjornson, K. (2009). The association between idiopathic clubfoot and increased hip internal hip rotation. *Clinical Orthopaedics and Related Research, 467,* 1231.

78. Huber, A. M., Lam, P. Y., Duffy, C. M., et al. (2002). Chronic recurrent multifocal osteomyelitis: Clinical outcomes after more than five years of follow-up. *Journal of Pediatrics, 141,* 198.

79. Hudson, D. (2008). A comparison of ultrasound of goniometric and inclinometer measurements of torsion in the tibia and femur. *Gait & Posture, 28,* 708.

80. Hughes, L. O., & Aronson, J. (1994). Skeletal infections in children. *Current Opinion in Pediatrics, 6,* 90.

81. Ikeda, H., Yamauchi, Y., Saluraba, K., & Kim, S. (1996). Etiologic factor of Osgood-Schlatter disease in young sports players. In Proceedings of the 20th Congress of the SICOT, Amsterdam, The Netherlands.

82. Ilfeld, F. W., Westin, G. W., & Makin, M. (1986). Missed or developmental dislocation of the hip. *Clinical Orthopaedics and Related Research, 203,* 276.

83. Ilizarov, G. A., & Ledyaev, V. I. (1969). The replacement of long tubular bone defects by lengthening distraction osteotomy of one of the fragments. *Vestnik Khirurgii, 6,* 78. (Translated by Schwartzman, V. [1992]. *Clinical Orthopaedics and Related Research, 280,* 7.)

84. Inan, M., Chan, G., Littleton, A. G., Kubiak, P., & Bowen, J. R. (2008). Efficacy and safety of percutaneous epiphysiodesis. *Journal of Pediatric Orthopedics, 28,* 648.

85. Ippolito, E., & Panseti, I. V. (1980). Congenital clubfoot in the human fetus: A histological study. *Journal of Bone and Joint Surgery (American), 62,* 8.

86. Jakob, R. P., von Gumppenberg, S., & Engelhardt, P. (1981). Does Osgood-Schlatter disease influence the position of the patella? *Journal of Bone and Joint Surgery (British), 63,* 579.

87. Jasty, M., Anderson, M. J., & Harris, W. H. (1995). Total hip replacement for developmental dysplasia of the hip. *Clinical Orthopaedics and Related Research, 311,* 40.

88. Johnston, C. E. (1990). Infantile tibia vara. *Clinical Orthopaedics and Related Research, 255,* 13.

89. Joseph, B., Mulpuri, K., & Varghese, G. (2001). Perthes' disease in the adolescent. *Journal of Bone and Joint Surgery (British), 83,* 715.

90. Joseph, B., Varghese, G., Mulpuri, K., Rao, N., & Nair, N. S. (2003). Natural evolution of Perthes disease: A study of 610 children under 12 years of age at disease onset. *Journal of Pediatric Orthopedics, 23,* 590.

91. Kandzierski, G., Karski, T., & Kozlowske, K. (2003). Capital femoral epiphysis and growth plate of the asymptomatic hip joint in unilateral Perthes disease. *Journal of Pediatric Orthopedics B, 12,* 380.

92. Kane, T. P., Harvey, J. R., Richards, R. H., Burby, N. G., & Clarke, N. M. (2003). Radiological outcome of innocent infant hip clicks. *Journal of Pediatric Orthopedics B, 12,* 259.

93. Kao, H. C., Huang, Y. C., Chiu, C. H., et al. (2003). Acute hematogenous osteomyelitis and septic arthritis in children. *Journal of Microbiology, Immunology, and Infection, 36,* 260.

94. Katz, M. M., & Mubarak, S. J. (1984). Hereditary tendo Achillis contractures. *Journal of Pediatric Orthopedics, 4,* 711.

95. Kealey, W. D. C., Lappin, K. J., Leslie, H., Sheridan, B., & Cosgrove, A. P. (2004). Endocrine profile and physical stature of children with Perthes disease. *Journal of Pediatric Orthopedics, 24,* 161.

96. Kealey, W. D. C., Moore, A. J., Cook, S., & Cosgrove, A. P. (2000). Deprivation, urbanization and Perthes' disease in Northern Ireland. *Journal of Bone and Joint Surgery (British), 82,* 167.

97. Kelly, B. T., & Green, D. W. (2002). Discoid lateral meniscus in children. *Current Opinion in Pediatrics, 14,* 54.

98. Kelly, I. P., Jenkinson, A., Stephens, M., & O'Brien, T. (1997). The kinematic patterns of toe-walkers. *Journal of Pediatric Orthopedics, 17,* 478.

99. Kelo, M. J., & Riddle, D. L. (1998). Examination and management of a patient with tarsal coalition. *Physical Therapy, 78,* 518.

100. Kim, H. T., & Wenger, D. R. (1997). "Functional retroversion" of the femoral head in Legg-Calve-Perthes disease and epiphyseal dysplasia: Analysis of head-neck deformity and its effect on limb position using three-dimensional computed tomography. *Journal of Pediatric Orthopedics, 17,* 240.

101. Kim, H. T., & Wenger, D. R. (1997). Surgical correction of "functional retroversion" and "functional coxa vara" in late Legg-Calve-Perthes disease and epiphyseal dysplasia: Correction of deformity defined by new imaging modalities. *Journal of Pediatric Orthopedics, 17,* 247.

102. Kim, H. T., & Wenger, D. R. (1997). The morphology of residual acetabular deficiency in childhood hip dysplasia: Three dimensional computed tomographic analysis. *Journal of Pediatric Orthopedics, 17,* 637.

103. Kite, J. H. (1967). Congenital metatarsus varus. *Journal of Bone and Joint Surgery (American), 49,* 388.

104. Kocher, M. S., Mandiga, R., Zurakowski, D., Barnewolt, C., & Kasser, J. R. (2004). Validation of a clinical prediction rule for

the differentiation between septic arthritis and transient synovitis of the hip in children. *Journal of Bone and Joint Surgery (American)*, 86, 1629.

105. Kodros, S. A., & Dias, L. S. (1999). Single-stage surgical correction of congenital vertical talus. *Journal of Pediatric Orthopedics*, 19, 42.

106. Kosashvili Fridman, T., Backstein, D., Safir, O., & Bar Ziv, Y. (2008). The correlation between pes planus and anterior knee pain or intermittent low back pain. *Foot & Ankle International*, 29, 910.

107. Krishna, M., Evans, R., Sprig, A., & Taylor, J. F. (1991). Tibial torsion measured by ultrasound in children with talipes equinovarus. *Journal of Bone and Joint Surgery (British)*, 73, 207.

108. Lahdes-Vasama, T. T., Sipila, I. S., Lamminranta, S., et al. (1997). Psychosocial development and premorbid skeletal growth in Legg-Calve-Perthes disease: A study of nineteen patients. *Journal of Pediatric Orthopedics B*, 6, 133.

109. Landin, L. A., Danielsson, L. G., & Wattsgard, C. (1987). Transient synovitis of the hip. *Journal of Bone and Joint Surgery (American)*, 69, 238.

110. Lang, L. M., & Bolpe, R. G. (1998). Measurement of tibial torsion. *Journal of the American Podiatric Medical Association*, 88, 160.

111. Leboeuf-Yde, C. (2000). Body weight and low back pain. *Spine*, 25, 226.

112. Lehmann, C. L., Arons, R. R., Loder, R. T., & Vitale, M. G. (2006). The epidemiology of slipped capital femoral epiphysis: An update. *Journal of Pediatric Orthopedics*, 26, 286.

113. Lim, Y. J., Kagda, F., Lam, K. S., et al (2008). Demographics and clinical presentation of slipped capital femoral epiphysis in Singapore: Comparing the East with the West. *Journal of Pediatric Orthopedics B*, 15, 289.

114. Lincoln, T. L., & Suen, P. W. (2003). Common rotational variations in children. *Journal of the American Academy of Orthopedic Surgeons*, 11, 312.

115. Loder, R. T. (1996). A worldwide study on the seasonal variation of slipped capital femoral epiphysis. *Clinical Orthopedics*, 322, 28.

116. Loder, R. T., Farley, F. A., Herring, J. A., Schork, M. A., & Shyr, Y. (1995). Bone age determination in children with Legg-Calve-Perthes disease: A comparison of two methods. *Journal of Pediatric Orthopedics*, 15, 90.

117. Loren, G. J., Karpinski, N. C., & Mubarak, S. J. (1998). Clinical implications of clubfoot histopathology. *Journal of Pediatric Orthopedics*, 18, 765.

118. Luhmann, S. J., Bassett, G. S., Gordon, J. E., Schootman, M., & Schoenecker, P. L. (2003). Reduction of a dislocation of the hip due to developmental dysplasia: Implications for the need for future surgery. *Journal of Bone and Joint Surgery (American)*, 85, 239.

119. Luhman, S. J., Jones, A., Schootman, M., Gordon, J. E., Schoenecker, P. L., & Luhmann, J. D. (2004). Differentiation between septic arthritis and transient synovitis of the hip in children with clinical prediction algorithms. *Journal of Bone and Joint Surgery (American)*, 86, 956.

120. McCarron, J. A., Johnston, D. R., Hanna, B. G., et al. (2001). Evaluation and treatment of musculoskeletal vascular anomalies in children: An update and summary for orthopaedic surgeons. *University of Pennsylvania Orthopedic Journal*, 14, 15.

121. McCarthy, J. J., Dormans, J. P., Kozin, S. H., & Pizzutillo, P. D. (2004). Musculoskeletal infections in children: Basic treatment principles and recent advancements. *Journal of Bone and Joint Surgery (American)*, 86, 850.

122. Manson, D., Wilmot, D. M., King, S., & Laxer, R. M. (1989). Physeal involvement in chronic recurrent multifocal osteomyelitis. *Pediatric Radiology*, 20, 76.

123. Maraqa, N. F., Gomez, M. M., & Rathore, M. H. (2002). Outpatient parenteral antimicrobial therapy in osteoarticular infections in children. *Journal of Pediatric Orthopedics*, 22, 506.

124. Matan, A. J., Stevens, P. M., Smith, J. T., & Santora, S. D. (1996). Combination trochanteric arrest and intertrochanteric osteotomy for Perthes' disease. *Journal of Pediatric Orthopedics*, 16, 10.

125. Michaeli, D. A., Murphy, S. B., & Hipp, J. A. (1997). Comparison of predicted and measured contact pressures in normal and dysplastic hips. *Medical Engineering & Physics*, 19, 180.

126. Michelson, J. D., Durant, D. M., & McFarland, E. (2002). The injury risk associated with pes planus in athletes. *Foot & Ankle International*, 23, 629.

127. Mielke, C. H., & Stevens, P. M. (1996). Hemiepiphyseal stapling for knee deformities in children younger than 10 years: A preliminary report. *Journal of Pediatric Orthopedics*, 16, 423.

128. Miettunen, P. M. H., Wei, X., Kaura, D., Reslan, W. A., Aguirre, A. N., & Kellner, J. D. (2009). Dramatic pain relief and resolution of bone inflammation following pamidronate in 9 pediatric patients with persistent chronic recurrent multifocal osteomyelitis (CRMO). *Pediatric Rheumatology*, 7, 2.

129. Miura, H., Naguchi, Y., Mitsuyasu, H., et al. (2000). Clinical features of multiple epiphyseal dysplasia expressed in the knee. *Clinical Orthopaedics and Related Research*, 380, 184.

130. Mooney, J. F. III, Sanders, J. O., Browne, R. H., et al. (2005). Management of unstable/acute slipped capital femoral epiphysis. *Journal of Pediatric Orthopedics*, 25, 162.

131. Morcuende, J. A., & Ponsetti, I. V. (1996). Congenital metatarsus adductus in early human fetal development: A histologic study. *Clinical Orthopedics*, 333, 261.

132. Mosca, V. S. (1995). Calcaneal lengthening for valgus deformity of the hindfoot: Results in children who had severe, symptomatic flatfoot and skewfoot. *Journal of Bone and Joint Surgery (American)*, 77, 500.

133. Moseley, C. F. (1977). A straight-line graph for leg-length discrepancies. *Journal of Bone and Joint Surgery (American)*, 59, 174.

134. Mubarak, S. J., Beck, L., & Sutherland, D. (1986). Home traction in the management of congenital dislocation of the hips. *Journal of Pediatric Orthopedics*, 6, 721.

135. Mubarak, S. J., Leach, J. L., & Wenger, D. R. (1987). Management of congenital dislocation of the hip in the infant. *Contemporary Orthopedics*, 15, 29.

136. Mubarak, S. J., Gargin, S. R., Vance, R., McKinnon, N. B., & Sutherland, D. (1981). Pitfalls in the use of the Pavlik harness for treatment of congenital dysplasia, subluxation, and dislocation of the hip. *Journal of Bone and Joint Surgery (American)*, *63*, 1239.

137. Murray, A. W., & Wilson, N. I. (2008). Changing incidence of slipped capital femoral epiphysis: A relationship with obesity? *Journal of Bone and Joint Surgery (British)*, *90*, 92.

138. Nakamura, J., Kamegaya, M., Saisu, T., Someya, M., Koizumi, W., & Moriya, H. (2007). Treatment for developmental dysplasia of the hip using the Pavlik harness: Long-term results. *Journal of Bone and Joint Surgery (British)*, *89*, 230.

139. Nelson, J. D. (1997). Toward simple but safe management of osteomyelitis. *Pediatrics*, *99*, 883.

140. Newman, J. S., & Newberg, A. H. (2000). Congenital tarsal coalition: Multimodality evaluation with emphasis on CT and MR imaging. *Radiographics*, *29*, 321.

141. O'Connor, M. A., Palaniappan, M., Khan, N., & Bruce, C. E. (2002). Osteochondritis dissecans of the knee in children. *Journal of Bone and Joint Surgery (British)*, *84*, 258.

142. Obedian, R. S., & Grelsamer, R. P. (1997). Osteochondritis dissecans of the distal femur and patella. *Clinical Sports Medicine*, *16*, 157.

143. Ogden, J. A., Ganey, T. M., Hill, J. D., & Jaakkola, J. I. (2004). Sever's injury: A stress fracture of the immature calcaneal metaphysic. *Journal of Pediatric Orthopedics*, *24*, 488.

144. Oudjhane, K., Newman, B., Oh, K. S., Young, L. W., & Girdany, B. R. (1988). Occult fractures in preschool children. *Journal of Trauma*, *28*, 858.

145. Ozlem, E. I., Akcali, O., Losay, C., et al (2006). Flexible flatfoot and related factors in primary school children: A report of a screening study. *Rheumatology International*, *26*, 1050.

146. Paley, D. (1988). Current techniques of limb lengthening. *Journal of Pediatric Orthopedics*, *8*, 73.

147. Paley, D. (1990). Problems, obstacles, and complications of limb lengthening by the Ilizarov technique. *Clinical Orthopaedics and Related Research*, *250*, 81.

148. Paley, D., Bhave, A., Herzenberg, J. E., & Bowen, J. R. (2000). Multiplier method for predicting limb-length discrepancy. *Journal of Bone and Joint Surgery (American)*, *82*, 1432.

149. Paley, D., Herzenberg, J. E., Paremain, G., & Bhave, A. (1997). Femoral lengthening over an intramedullary nail. *Journal of Bone and Joint Surgery (American)*, *79*, 1464.

150. Pauli, R. M., Breed, A., Horton, V. K., Glinski, L. P., & Reiser, C. A. (1997). Prevention of fixed, angular kyphosis in achondroplasia. *Journal of Pediatric Orthopedics*, *17*, 726.

151. Pavlik, A. (1950). Stirrups as an aid in the treatment of congenital dysplasias of the hip in children. *LeKarskeListy*, *5*, 81. (Translated by Bialik, V., & Reis, N. D. [1989]. *Journal of Pediatric Orthopedics*, *9*, 157.)

152. Pavlik, A. (1957). The functional method of treatment using a harness with stirrups as the primary method of conservative therapy for infants with congenital dislocation of the hip. *Zeitschrift fur Orthopadie und Ihre Grenzgeneit*, *89*, 341.

(Translated by Peltier, L. F. [1992]. *Clinical Orthopaedics and Related Research*, *281*, 4.)

153. Perlman, M. H., Patzakis, M. J., Kumar, P. J., & Holton, P. (2000). The incidence of joint involvement with adjacent osteomyelitis in pediatric patients. *Journal of Pediatric Orthopedics*, *20*, 40.

154. Pfeiffer, M., Kotz, R., Ledl, T., Haruse, G., & Sluga, M. (2006). Prevalence of flat foot in preschool-aged children. *Pediatrics*, *118*, 634–639.

155. Piddo, C., Reed, M. H., & Black, G. B. (2000). Premature epiphyseal fusion and degenerative arthritis in chronic recurrent multifocal osteomyelitis. *Skeletal Radiology*, *29*, 94.

156. Pitkow, R. B. (1975). External rotation contracture of the extended hip. *Clinical Orthopaedics and Related Research*, *110*, 139.

157. Rajacich, N., Bell, D. F., & Armstrong, P. F. (1992). Pediatric applications of the Ilizarov method. *Clinical Orthopaedics and Related Research*, *280*, 72.

158. Rao, U. B., & Joseph, B. (1992). The influence of footwear on the prevalence of flat foot. *Journal of Bone and Joint Surgery (British)*, *74*, 525.

159. Rebello, G., Grottkau, B., Albright, M., & Patel, D. (2006). Discoid lateral meniscus: Anatomy and treatment. *Techniques in Knee Surgery*, *5*, 64.

160. Redjal, H. R., & Zamorano, D. P. (2008). Developmental hip dysplasia. In C. D. Berkowitz (Ed.). *Berkowitz's pediatrics: A primary care approach* (3rd ed.). Elk Grove Village, IL: American Academy of Pediatrics.

161. Redjal, H. R., & Zamorano, D. P. (2008). Rotational problems of the lower extremity: In-toeing and out-toeing. In C. D. Berkowitz (Ed.). *Berkowitz's pediatrics: A primary care approach* (3rd ed.). Elk Grove Village, IL: American Academy of Pediatrics.

162. Reikeras, O., Kristiansen, L. P., Gunderson, R., & Steen, H. (2001). Reduced tibial torsion in congenital clubfoot. *Acta Orthopaedica Scandinavica*, *72*, 53.

163. Reimann, I., & Werner, H. H. (1975). Congenital metatarsus varus: A suggestion for a possible mechanism and relation to other foot deformities. *Clinical Orthopedics*, *110*, 223.

164. Robertson, W., Kelly, B. T., & Green, D. W. (2003). Osteochondritis dissecans of the knee in children. *Current Opinion in Pediatrics*, *15*, 38.

165. Rodgveller, B. (1984). Talipes equinovarus. *Clinical Podiatry*, *1*, 477.

166. Roposch, A., & Wright, J. G. (2007). Increased diagnostic information and understanding disease: Uncertainty in the diagnosis of developmental hip dysplasia. *Radiology*, *242*, 355.

167. Roth-Isigkeit, A., Thyen, V., Stoven, H., Schwarzenberger, J., & Schmucker, P. (2005). Pain among children and adolescents: Restriction in daily living and triggering factors. *Pediatrics*, *115*, 152.

168. Rozbruch, S. R., Kleinman, D., Fragomen, A. T., & Ilizarov, S. (2008). Limb lengthening and then insertion of an intermedullary nail: A case-matched comparison. *Clinical Orthopaedics and Related Research*, *466*, 2923.

169. Ruiz-Garcia, M., Tovar-Baudin, A., Del Castillo-Ruiz, V., et al: (1997). Early detection of neurological manifestations in achondroplasia. *Child's Nervous System, 13*, 208.

170. Russell, M. E., Shivanna, K. H., Grosland, N. M., & Pederson, D. R. (2006). Cartilage contact pressure elevations in dyplastic hips: A chronic overload model. *Journal of Orthopedic Surgery, 1*, 6.

171. Sachithananandam, V., & Joseph, B. (1995). The influence of footwear on the prevalence of flat foot: A survey of 1846 skeletally mature persons. *Journal of Bone and Joint Surgery (British), 77*, 254.

172. Salter, R. B. (1968). Etiology, pathogenesis and possible prevention of congenital dislocation of the hip. *Canadian Medical Association Journal, 98*, 933.

173. Salter, R. B., & Harris, W. R. (1963). Injuries involving the epiphyseal plate. *Journal of Bone and Joint Surgery (American), 45*, 587.

174. Salter, R. B., Thompson, G. H. (1984). Legg-Calve-Perthes' disease: The prognostic significance of the subchondral fracture and a two-group classification of the femoral head involvement. *Journal of Bone and Joint Surgery (American), 66*, 479.

175. Sass, P., & Hassan, G. (2003). Lower extremity abnormalities in children. *American Family Physician, 68*, 461.

176. Scherl, S. A. (2004). Common lower extremity problems in children. *Pediatric Reviews, 25*, 52.

177. Schultz, W. R., Weinstein, J. N., Weinstein, S., & Smith, B. G. (2002). Prophylactic pinning of the contralateral hip in slipped capital femoral epiphysis. *Journal of Bone and Joint Surgery (American), 84*, 1205.

178. Scoles, P. V., Boyd, A., & Jones, P. K. (1987). Roentgenographic parameters of the normal infant hip. *Journal of Pediatric Orthopedics, 7*, 656.

179. Sen, R. K., Sharma, L. R., Thakur, S. R., & Lakhanpal, V. P. (1989). Patellar angle in Osgood-Schlatter disease. *Acta Orthopaedica Scandinavica, 60*, 26.

180. Sharp, R. J., Calder, J. D., & Saxby T. S. (2003). Osteochondritis of the navicular: A case report. *Foot & Ankle International, 24*, 509.

181. Shulman, L. H., Sala, D. A., Chu, M. L., McCoul, P. R., & Sandler, B. J. (1997). Developmental implications of radiopathic toe walking. *Journal of Pediatrics, 130*, 541.

182. Siffert, R. S. (1981). Classification of the osteochondroses. *Clinical Orthopaedics and Related Research, 158*, 10.

183. Simard, S., Marchant, M., & Mencio, G. (1992). The Ilizarov procedure: Limb lengthening and its implications. *Physical Therapy, 72*, 25.

184. Smith, B. G., Millis, M. G., Hey, L. A., Jaramillo, D., & Kasser, J. R. (1997). Post-reduction computed tomography in developmental dislocation of the hip. Part II: Predictive value for outcome. *Journal of Pediatric Orthopedics, 17*, 631.

185. Smith, J. T., Matan, A., Coleman, S. S., Stevens, P. M., & Scott, S. M. (1997). The predictive value of the development of the acetabular teardrop figure in developmental dysplasia of the hip. *Journal of Pediatric Orthopedics, 17*, 165.

186. Song, K. M., & Lapinsky, A. (2000). Determination of hip position in the Pavlik harness. *Journal of Pediatric Orthopedics, 20*, 317.

187. Sponseller, P. D., Desai, S. S., & Millis, M. B. (1989). Abnormalities of proximal femoral growth after severe Perthes' disease. *Journal of Bone and Joint Surgery (American), 71*, 610.

188. Staheli, L. T. (2006). *Practice of pediatric orthopedics* (2nd ed.). Philadelphia: Lippincott Williams and Wilkins.

189. Staheli, L. T. (1989). Torsion—Treatment indications. *Clinical Orthopedics, 247*, 61.

190. Staheli, L. T., Corbett, M., Wyss, C., & King, H. (1985). Lower extremity rotational problems in children. *Journal of Bone and Joint Surgery (American), 67*, 39.

191. Stanley, G., McLoughlin, S., & Beals, R. K. (2002). Observations in the cause of bowlegs in achondroplasia. *Journal of Pediatric Orthopedics, 22*, 112.

192. Stanitski, C. L. (2002). Knee disorders. In P. D. Sponseller (Ed.). *Orthopaedic knowledge update: Pediatrics.* Rosemont, IL: American Academy of Orthopaedic Surgeons.

193. Stanitski, D. F., Shaheheraghi, H., Nicker, D. A., & Armstrong, P. F. (1996). Results of tibial lengthening with the Ilizarov technique. *Journal of Pediatric Orthopedics, 16*, 168.

194. Steer, A. C., & Carapetic, J. R. (2004). Acute hematogenous osteomyelitis in children: Recognition and management. *Paediatric Drugs, 6*, 333.

195. Stevens, P. M., Maguire, M., Dales, M. D., & Robins, A. J. (1999). Physeal stapling for idiopathic genu valgum. *Journal of Pediatric Orthopedics, 19*, 645.

196. Stevens, P. M., & Otis, S. (1999). Ankle valgus and clubfeet. *Journal of Pediatric Orthopedics, 19*, 515.

197. Stuberg, W. A., Koehler, A., Wichita, M., et al. (1989). Comparison of femoral torsion assessment using goniometry and computerized tomography. *Pediatric Physical Therapy, 3*, 115.

198. Sullivan, J. A. (1999). Pediatric flatfoot: Evaluation and management. *Journal of the American Academy of Orthopedic Surgeons, 7*, 44.

199. Syrogiannopoulos, G. A., &Nelson, J. D. (1988). Duration of antimicrobial therapy for acute suppurative osteoarticular infections. *The Lancet, 1*, 37.

200. Taylor, G. R., & Clarke, N. M. (1997). Monitoring the treatment of developmental dysplasia of the hip with the Pavlik harness: The role of ultrasound. *Journal of Bone and Joint Surgery (British), 79*, 719.

201. Theodorou, D. J., Theodorou, S. J., Boutin, R. D., et al. (1999). Stress fractures of the lateral metatarsal bones in metatarsus adductus foot deformity: A previously unrecognized association. *Skeletal Radiology, 28*, 679.

202. Thompson, G. H., & Carter, J. R. (1990). Late onset tibia vara (Blount's disease). *Clinical Orthopaedics and Related Research, 255*, 24.

203. Tjernstrom, B., & Rehnberg, L. (1994). Back pain and arthralgia before and after lengthening: 75 patients questioned after 6 (1–11) years. *Acta Orthopaedica Scandinavica, 65*, 328.

204. Tredwell, S. J., & Bell, H. M. (1981). Efficacy of neonatal hip examination. *Journal of Pediatric Orthopedics, 1*, 61.

205. Trott, A. W. (1991). Developmental disorders. In M. H. Jahss (Ed.). *Disorders of the foot and ankle.* Philadelphia: WB Saunders.

206. Uziel, Y., Butbul-Aviel, Y., Barash, J., et al. (2006). Recurrent transient synovitis of the hip in childhood: Longterm outcome among 39 patients. *Journal of Rheumatology, 33,* 810.

207. Uziel, Y., & Hashkes, P. J. (2007). Growing pains in children. *Pediatric Rheumatology, 5,* 5.

208. von Heideken, J., Green, D. W., Burke, S. W., et al. (2006). The relationship between developmental dysplasia of the hip and congenital muscular torticollis. *Journal of Pediatric Orthopedics, 26,* 805–808.

209. Wagner, H. (1978). Operative lengthening of the femur. *Clinical Orthopaedics and Related Research, 136,* 125.

210. Wallach, D. M., & Davidson, R. S. (2005). Pediatric lower limb disorders. In J. P. Dormans (Ed.). *Pediatric orthopaedics: Core knowledge in orthopaedics.* Philadelphia: Elsevier Mosby.

211. Wan, S. C. (2006). Metatarsus adductus and skewfoot deformity. *Clinical Podiatric Medicine and Surgery, 23,* 23.

212. Wang, C. L., Wang, S. M., Yang, Y. J., Tsai, C. H., & Liu, C. C. (2003). Septic arthritis in children: Relationship of causative pathogens, complications, and outcome. *Journal of Microbiology, Immunology, and Infection, 36,* 41.

213. Weidow, J., Tranberg, R., Saari, T., & Karrholm, J. (2006). Hip and knee joint rotations differ between patients with medial and lateral knee osteoarthritis: Gait analysis of 30 patients and 15 controls. *Journal of Orthopedic Research, 24,* 1890.

214. Weinstein, S. L. (1992). Congenital hip dislocation: Long range problems, residual signs and symptoms after successful treatment. *Clinical Orthopaedics and Related Research, 281,* 69.

215. Weinstein, S. L. (2000). Long-term follow-up of pediatric orthopedic conditions. *Journal of Bone and Joint Surgery (American), 82,* 980.

216. Wenger, D. R., & Bomar, J. D. (2003). Human hip dysplasia: Evolution of current treatment concepts. *Journal of Orthopedic Science, 8,* 264.

217. Wenger, D. R., & Leach, J. (1986). Foot deformities in infants and children. *Pediatric Clinics of North America, 33,* 1411.

218. Wenger, D. R., Mauldin, D., Speck, G., Morgan, D., & Lieber, R. L. (1989). Corrective shoes and inserts as treatment for flexible flatfoot in infants and children. *Journal of Bone and Joint Surgery (American), 71,* 800.

219. Wenger, D. R., & Rang, M. (1993). *The art of pediatric orthopaedics.* New York: Raven Press.

220. Wenger, D. R., Ward, W. T., & Herring, J. A. (1991). Current concepts review: Legg-Calve-Perthes disease. *Journal of Bone and Joint Surgery (American), 73,* 778.

221. Whalen, J. L., Fitzgerald, R. H. Jr., & Morrisy, R. T. (1988). A histological study of acute hematogenous osteomyelitis following physeal injuries in rabbits. *Journal of Bone and Joint Surgery (American), 70,* 1383.

222. Wick, J. M., & Alexander, K. M. (2006). Rotationplasty—A unique surgical procedure with a functional outcome. *Association of periOperative Registered Nurses (AORN J), 84,* 190.

223. Windisch, G., Ander Huber, F., Haldi-Brandle, V., & Exner, G. U. (2007). Anatomical study for an update comprehension of clubfeet. Part I: Bones and joints. *Journal of Child Orthopedics, 1,* 69.

224. Wood, J. B., Klassen, R. A., & Peterson, H. H. (1995). Osteochondritis dissecans of the femoral head in children and adolescents: A report of 17 cases. *Journal of Pediatric Orthopedics, 15,* 313.

225. Yashar, A., Loder, R. T., & Hensinger, R. N. (1995). Determination of skeletal age in children with Osgood-Schlatter disease by using radiographs of the knee. *Journal of Pediatric Orthopedics, 15,* 298.

226. Yasui, N., Kawabata, H., Kajimoto, H., et al. (1997). Lengthening of the lower limbs in patients with achondroplasia and hypochondroplasia. *Clinical Orthopaedics and Related Research, 344,* 298.

227. Yeh, T. C., Chiu, N. C., Li, W. C., Chi, H., Lee, Y. J., & Huang, F. Y. (2005). Characteristics of primary osteomyelitis among children in a medical center in Taipei, 1984–2002. *Journal of the Formosan Medical Association, 104,* 29.

228. Yoshida, S., Ikata, T., Takai, H., et al. (1998). Osteochondritis dissecans of the femoral condyle in the growth stage. *Clinical Orthopedics, 346,* 162.

229. Young, R. S., Andrew, P. D., & Cummings, G. S. (2000). Effect of simulating leg length inequality on pelvic torsion and trunk mobility. *Gait Posture, 11,* 217.

230. Yuan, H. C., Wu, K. G., Chen, C. J., Tang, R. B., & Hwang, B. T. (2006). Characteristics and outcome of septic arthritis in children. *Journal of Microbiology, Immunology, and Infection, 39,* 342.

231. Yun, A. G., Severino, R., & Reinker, K. (2000). Attempted limb lengthening beyond twenty percent of the initial bone length: Results and complications. *Journal of Pediatric Orthopedics, 20,* 151.

15

Sports Injuries in Children

MARK V. PATERNO, PT, MS, MBA, SCS, ATC • LAURA C. SCHMITT, PT, PhD(PT) • DONNA BERNHARDT BAINBRIDGE, PT, EdD, ATC

Youth participation in sports is growing at an exponential rate. Current estimates suggest greater than 30 million to 45 million youths between the ages of 5 and 17 years of age participate in community-sponsored athletic programs.[2,247] This represents an increase from roughly 5 million participants in 1970. More than 6.5 million teenagers regularly participate in competitive high school team sports.[37] Half of all males and one fourth of all females aged 8 to 16 years (approximately 7 million) were reported to be engaged in competitive, organized school sports.[304] Heath and colleagues[135] reported that approximately 37% of all students in grades 9 to 12 engaged in vigorous physical activity for at least 20 minutes three or more times per week according to the 1990 Youth Risk Behavior Survey. By 1997, participation had increased to 63.8%.[266] Participation remained higher for males than for females (72.3% versus 53.5%).

Participation in athletics is a means for our youth to remain physically active and reap the many advantageous health benefits of activity. The Surgeon General[312] has reported the incidence of obesity in our youth is reaching epidemic proportions as approximately 15% of children ages 6 to 19 years old are classified as obese and 30% are classified as overweight.[237] This has resulted in a health care expense in excess of $117 billion.[342]

Current estimates from the Centers for Disease Control and Prevention (CDC) suggest fewer than 65% of adolescents participate in regular physical activity and fewer than 45% are enrolled in a physical education class at their school. Participation in sports likely increases physical activity levels, which is critical to the long-term health of our youth. In addition, participation in athletics provides children with an opportunity to enhance their physical abilities and skills as well as for social interaction with their peers. Participation in sports is linked to positive aspects of individual development and academic performance including higher grade point averages, lower school absentee rates, and overall better behavior.

Coinciding with increased participation is the potential for increases in sports-related injury in children. Emergency room data acquired since the later 1990s suggests more than 3.5 million children between the ages of 5 and 14 years old require medical attention for acute, sports-related injuries. More concerning is the fact that more than 50% of sports-related injuries in children are likely overuse injuries[227] and

would not be included in these data. Furthermore, the progression of many children to become specialized in a singular sport early in their life has raised concerns from the American Academy of Pediatrics and other health care organizations about the safety of year-round participation in a single sport with infrequent rest periods and a lack of diversity in activity.[7] Attention must be placed on the management of unique injuries in this population. However, the child cannot be considered simply a small adult. Children have different structural and physiologic components that must be specifically addressed.[305] This chapter provides an extensive overview of sports medicine in children and youth for the pediatric physical therapist. The purposes of the chapter are to review the elements of injury prevention/risk reduction and to discuss those factors that increase risk for sports-related injury in children with and without disabilities. The chapter addresses the types and sites of sports injuries unique to the child and provides considerations for rehabilitation.

INCIDENCE OF INJURY

Appreciating the true incidence of sports-related injuries in a young, active population is a challenge because of the varying methodologies in current research. Injury incidence is defined as the number of new cases of a disease (or injury) during a specific period of time, such as an athletic season or a year.[159] Incidence can be further subdivided into clinical incidence, which reports the percentage of new cases within a defined population and incidence rate, which describes the rate of injuries per unit of exposure to activity.[53] Incidence rate is a much more powerful descriptor of the risk of injury in a population or within a certain activity and is necessary to accurately compare the rate of injury, normalized to exposure, between populations. Unfortunately, the prevalence of these data in the pediatric sports medicine literature is lacking. Varying methodologies and definitions of injury have hindered development of broad epidemiologic data accurately reporting the incidence of injuries in this population. In addition, many sports with high participation rates have little or no epidemiologic reports in the literature, which limits the ability to assess a documented risk in sports participation.

A summary of studies reporting incidence rates for males and females, separated by sport, is listed in Tables 15-1 and 15-2. The highest rate of injuries in males per 1000 hours of

453

TABLE 15-1 Summary of Incidence Rates in Boys' Sports

Study	Study Design[a] / Country	Data Collection[b]	Duration of Injury Surveillance	Team Type or Age(s)	Number of Injuries	Number of Exposures (Hours)	Number of Exposures (AEs)[c]	Rate: Number of Injuries per 1000 Hours	Rate: Number of Injuries per 1000 AEs	95% CI (Low/High)
Baseball										
Knowles et al	P (United States)	DM	3 years	HS	94				0.95	0.61/1.47
Comstock et al	P (United States)	DM	1 year	HS					1.19	
Radelet et al	P (United States)	Q	2 years	7–13 years	128		6913		17.0	
Powell and Barber-Foss	P (United States)	Q	3 seasons	HS	861		311,295		2.8	
Basketball										
Knowles et al	P (United States)	DM	3 years	HS	186				2.32	1.45/3.71
Comstock et al	P (United States)	DM	1 year	HS					1.89	
Powell and Barber-Foss	P (United States)	DM	3 seasons	HS	1933		444,338		4.8	
Messina et al	P (United States)	DM	1 season	HS	543	169,885		3.2		
Cross-country running										
Rauh et al	P (United States)	DM	1 season	HS	159		10,600		15.0	
Rauh et al	P (United States)	DM	15 seasons	HS	846		77,491		10.9	
Football										
Knowles et al	P (United States)	DM	3 years	HS	909				3.54	2.86/4.37
Comstock et al	P (United States)	DM	1 year	HS					4.36	
Malina et al	P (United States)	DM	2 seasons	Youth	259				10.4	9.2/11.8
				4th–5th grades	58				6.6	5.1/8.6
				6th grade	61				9.8	7.6/12.7
				7th grade	90				13.4	10.8/16.5
				8th grade	50				16.2	12.2/21.5
Turbeville et al	P (United States)	DM	2 seasons	HS	132				3.2	2.7/3.8
Turbeville et al	P (United States)	DM	2 seasons	MS	64				2.0	
Radelet et al	P (United States)	Q	2 years	7–13 years	129		8462		15.0	
Powell and Barber-Foss	P (United States)	DM	3 seasons	HS	10,557		1,300,446		8.1	
Gymnastics										
Bak et al	P (Denmark)	Q	1 year	Club	26			1.0		
Ice hockey										
Emery and Meeuwisse	P (Canada)	DM	1 season	All minor	296			4.13		3.67/4.62
				Atom	14			1.12		0.61/1.87
				Pee Wee	53			3.32		2.49/4.34
				Bantam	73			4.16		3.26/5.23
				Midget	156			6.07		5.16-7.1
Smith et al	296 P (United States)	DM	1 season	HS	27			34.4		
Gerberich et al	R (United States)	Q	1 season	HS				5		

Study	Design[a]	Data collection[b]	Duration	Age/Level	No. of subjects	No. of AE[c]	Injury rate	Injury rate	Practice/Game
Rugby									
McManus and Cross	P (Australia)	DM	1 season	Junior Elite	84		13.3		
Garraway and Macleod	P (United Kingdom)	DM	1 season	Less than 16 years	26		3.4		2.1/4.8
				16–19 years	72		8.7		6.5/10.8
Roux et al	P (France)	Q	1 season	HS	495		7.0	1.6	
Soccer									
Knowles et al	P (United States)	DM	3 years	HS	252			2.81	2.03/3.90
Comstock et al	P (United States)	DM	1 year	HS				2.43	
Le Gall et al	P	DM	10 seasons	All	1152		4.8		
				U16	371		5.2		
				U15	361		4.6		
				U14	420		4.9		
1152									
Kucera et al	P (United States)	Q	3 years	U12–18	467	109,957		4.3	3.9/4.7
Emery et al	P (Canada)	DM	1 season	Overall				5.5	
				U18	16	2030		3.2	
				U16	16	2817		5.7	
				U14	7	2177		7.9	
16									
Radelet et al	P (United States)	Q	2 years	7–13 years	47	2799		17	
Junge et al	P (Europe)	DM	1 year	14–18 years Alsace					
				Czech Republic	57		2.3		
				14–18 years	130		2.6		
Powell and Barber-Foss	P (United States)	DM	3 seasons	HS	1765	385,443		4.6	
Backous et al	P (United States)	Q	1 week	6–17 years				7.3	
Wrestling									
Knowles et al	P (United States)	DM	3 years	HS	154			1.49	0.85/2.62
Comstock et al	P(United States)	DM	1 year	HS				2.5	
Pasque and Hewett	P (United States)	I, Q	1 season		219			6.0	
Powell and Barber-Foss	P (United States)	DM	3 seasons	HS	2910	522,608		5.6	
Hoffman and Powell	P (United States)	DM	2 seasons			36,262		7.6	

From Caine, D., Maffulli, N., & Caine, C. (2008). Epidemiology of injury in child and adolescent sports: injury rates, risk factors and prevention. *Clinics in Sports Medicine, 27,* 22–25.
a, Design: P, prospective cohort; R, retrospective cohort. b, Data collection: DM, direct monitor; HS, high school; IR, insurance records; MS, middle school; Q, questionnaire; RR, record review. c, AE is one athlete participating in one practice or game in which the athlete is exposed to the possibility of athletic injury.

TABLE 15-2 Summary of Incidence Rates in Girls' Sports

Study	Study Design[a]	Data Collection[b]	Duration of Injury Surveillance	Team Type or Age(s)	Number of Injuries	Number of Exposures (Hours)	Number of Exposures (AEs)[c]	Rate: Number of Injuries per 1000 Hours	Rate: Number of Injuries per 1000 AEs	95% CI (Low/High)
Basketball										
Knowles et al	P (United States)	DM	3 years	HS	151				1.28	0.88/1.86
Comstock et al	P (United States)	DM	1 year	HS					2.01	
Powell and Barber-Foss	P (United States)	DM	3 seasons	HS	1748		394,143		4.4	
Messina et al	P (United States)	DM	1 season	HS	543		120,751	3.6		
Gomez et al	P (United States)	DM	1 year	HS	436	107,353		4.1		
Cross-country Running										
Rauh et al	P (United States)	DM	1 season	HS	157		8008		19.6	
Rauh et al	P (United States)	DM	15 seasons	HS	776		46,572		16.7	
Field Hockey										
Powell and Barber-Foss	P (United States)	DM	3 seasons	HS	510		138,073		3.7	
Gymnastics										
Caine et al	P (United States)	DM	3 years	All levels	192	76,919.5	22,584	2.5	8.5	
				Top	125	36,040.0		3.5		
				Beginning	67	40,879.5		1.6		
Kolt and Kirkby	PR (Australia)	Q	18 months	All levels	349	105,583		3.3		
				Elite	151	57,383		2.6		
				Subelite	198	48,200		4.1		
Kolt and Kirkby	R (Australia)	Q	1 year	All levels	321	163,920		2.0		
				Elite	111			1.6		
				Subelite	210			2.2		
Bak et al	P (Denmark)	Q	1 year	Club	41			1.4		
Lindner and Caine	P (Canada)	QI	3 seasons	Club	90	173,263		0.5		
Caine et al	P (United States)	IR	1 year	All levels	147	40,127		3.7		
				Top	83	22,536		3.7		
				Middle	64	20,591		3.1		

Study	Design (Country)	Data collection	Duration	Setting						
Soccer										
Knowles et al	P (United States)	DM	3 years	HS	121				2.35	1.55/3.55
Comstock et al	P (United States)	DM	1 year	HS	320				2.36	
Kucara et al	P (United States)	Q	3 seasons	12–18 years		60,166	5.3			4.7/6.0
Emery et al	P (Canada)	DM	1 season	Overall			5.6			
				U14	20	2526	7.9			
				U16	14	2440	5.7			
				U18	5	1976	2.5			
Soderman et al	P (Sweden)	DM	1 season	14–19 years	79		6.8			
Radelet et al	P (United States)	Q	2 years	Community	16	1637		23.0		
Powell and Barber-Foss	P (United States)	DM	3 seasons	HS	1771	355,512		5.3		
Backous et al	P (United States)	Q	1 week	6–17 years			10.6			
Softball										
Knowles et al	P (United States)	DM	3 years	HS	71			.96		0.61/1.42
Comstock et al	P (United States)	DM	1 year	HS				1.13		
Radelet et al	P (United States)	Q	2 years	Community	37	3807		10.0		
Powell and Barber-Foss]	P (United States)	DM	3 seasons	HS	910			3.5		
Volleyball										
Comstock et al	P (United States)	DM	1 year	HS	601			1.64		
Powell and Barber-Foss	P (United States)	DM	3 seasons	HS		359,547		1.7		

From Caine, D., Maffulli, N., & Caine, C. (2008). Epidemiology of injury in child and adolescent sports: injury rates, risk factors and prevention. *Clinics in Sports Medicine, 27,* 26–28.
a, Design: P, prospective cohort; R, retrospective cohort. b, Data collection: DM, direct monitor; HS, high school; IR, insurance records; Q, questionnaire; RR, record review. c, AE is one athlete participating in one practice or game in which the athlete is exposed to the possibility of athletic injury.

exposure occurs in ice hockey, rugby, and soccer. Females experience the highest rate of injury per 1000 hours of exposure in basketball and gymnastics. Interestingly, when injury data is normalized to the number of athletic exposures rather than hours of exposure, higher incidence rates are noted in cross-country running for males and soccer and cross-country running for females.[54] With respect to age and participation level, young males appear to experience higher rates of injury as they age.[53] Authors theorized that as males grow in body mass, strength, and speed, they have the ability to create greater forces and increase the risk of injury.[53,54] Interestingly, injury data related to age and development in females are more controversial.

ANATOMIC LOCATION

In regard to anatomic location, the incidence of lower extremity injury in children is greatest across many sports, including basketball, football, gymnastics, soccer, and track and field.[53] Other sports, such as baseball,[53] snowboarding,[131] judo,[258] and tennis,[156] result in a greater incidence of upper extremity injuries. Still others, such as wresting, result in a higher incidence of head injuries.[141] Collectively, the anatomic location with the greatest incidence of injury in children is the lower extremity, particularly the knee and ankle.[53]

INCIDENCE OF ACUTE INJURIES

Acute injuries, often from emergency room visit data, have been reported in the epidemiologic literature for years. Taylor and Attia[314] reviewed all sports-related injuries in children between 5 and 18 years of age seen in an emergency room over a 2-year period. They reported 677 injuries, 71% in males. Sports most commonly implicated were basketball (19.5%), football (17.1%), baseball/softball (14.9%), soccer (14.2%), inline skating (5.7%), and hockey (4.6%). Sprains and strains were the most frequent types of injuries, followed by fracture, contusions, and lacerations; and these accounted for 90% of all injuries. The National Health Interview Survey estimated that the sports-related injury rate for 5- to 24-year-olds was 42% higher than the estimates based on emergency room visits. The highest rate (59.3%) was for 5- to 14-year-olds.[73] Lenaway and colleagues[179] noted that middle school/junior high students had the highest injury rate, followed by elementary school students and then high school students. Sports, which accounted for 53% of all injuries, were an increasing cause of injury as grade level increased. Location of injury was the playground for elementary ages, the athletic field for middle school students, and the gym for high school students.

INCIDENCE OF OVERUSE INJURIES

Of more recent concern is the rising incidence of overuse injuries in the pediatric population. Once thought to be a rare occurrence in children, overuse injuries are now estimated to make up more than 50% of injuries in this population.[227] This measure is likely a conservative estimate as, unlike acute injuries, which often require immediate medical attention and facilitates data tracking, overuse injuries are often self-managed and as a result are typically underreported. Micheli and Nielson[212] reported the mechanism behind this increase in overuse injury is likely due to increased participation in sports and more specifically, a tendency toward sports specialization in greater numbers of children. Other factors may include an increase in complexity and duration of training at a young age, hence increasing stress to a growing body and a lack of appropriate coaching and skill training. Specific risk factors for stress fractures and other overuse injuries typically seen in a younger, athletic population are outlined later in this chapter.

ALTERNATIVE SPORTS

Children and adolescents are becoming more involved in extreme variations of sports as well as increased risk-taking with everyday sports. Various authors have noted significant injury rates with cycling[115,340]; exer-cycling,[29] riding in all-terrain vehicles[44,47]; diving[38]; snowboarding and skiing[90,292,293]; and inline skate, skateboard, or scooter use.[169,193,229,241,262,263] Although many of these injuries are contusions, fractures, and sprains/strains, authors noted significant numbers of abdominal trauma with damage to the kidney, pancreas, or liver; head and neck injury; and hand trauma. Schmitt and Gerner[283] noted that sports and diving caused 6.8% and 7.7% of 1016 cases of spinal cord injury, respectively, in persons aged 9 to 52 years. The sports implicated were alpine skiing, horseback riding, air sports (hang gliding and para-gliding), gymnastics, and trampoline in decreasing order of incidence. Smith and Shields,[296] who documented 214 trampoline injuries in 1995 through 1997, noted that these children were supervised in 55.6% of the injury occasions.

CATASTROPHIC INJURIES

The incidence of catastrophic injuries and fatalities in high school has been documented for the years 1977 through 1998.[61] Of 384 reported incidents, there were 118 fatalities, 200 nonfatal but permanent cervical injuries with severe neurologic disability, and 66 permanent cerebral injuries. Most cervical injuries occurred with tackling. Attention to the causes of severe injuries or deaths (i.e., proper education about game fundamentals, close monitoring of fair play, higher equipment standards, and improved medical care) have led to a 27% reduction in permanent spinal cord injury since the mid-1980s.[62] Brown and Brunn[46] noted that 27% of cervical injuries seen in a trauma center were related to sports, and football accounted for 29% of those cervical injuries. Head and neck injuries accounted for 23% of all injuries in youth ice hockey players (9 to 15 years old), with 86% caused by body checking.[49] Baseball also has significant injury potential; the U.S. Consumer Product Safety Commission reported 88 deaths related to baseball between 1973 and 1995. These deaths resulted from impact from the bat, or direct ball contact to chest, head, neck, or throat.[173]

GENDER DIFFERENCES IN INJURY RATES

Significant attention has been directed to differences in types and rates of injuries in males and females. Some researchers[1,16,50,185,205] compared boys and girls in similar sports and reported no difference in overall injury rates. Other researchers have noted differences in specific injury type or in injury rates for targeted joints. A study by de Loes and colleagues[86] reported that the risk of knee injury was significantly higher for women ages 14 to 20 years than men of the same age in cross-country and downhill skiing, gymnastics, volleyball, basketball, and handball. Hosea and colleagues[144] reported increased risk for grade 1 ankle sprains in women basketball players.

Several studies have noted an increased incidence of anterior cruciate ligament (ACL) injuries in females.[21,196,298] The relative risk ranged from 2.1 in recreational and elite youth soccer players[86] to 9.5 in intramural soccer players at the Naval Academy.[130] Gomez and colleagues[120] reported that ACL injuries accounted for 69% of severe knee injuries in basketball. Soderman and colleagues[300] reported that 38% of soccer players with ACL injuries had sustained the injury before the age of 16 years. In addition, Shea et al.[289] noted the greatest incidence of ACL injuries occurred at approximately 16 years old. Although research has yet to conclusively define the reasons for this increased risk, prevailing theories include (1) anatomic differences such as recurvatum, navicular drop, and excessive pronation;[188] (2) hormonal status;[142] and (3) neuromuscular control and biomechanical differences including differences in landing mechanics and muscle strength.[138]

PREVENTION OF INJURIES

The key to management of sports injuries in children is prevention. As discussed in Chapter 6, children need proper physiologic conditioning, strength, and flexibility to participate safely in an organized or recreational athletic endeavor. Although lack of fitness, strength, and flexibility does not preclude participation, remediation must be built into conditioning and training programs to decrease the risk of injury. The major elements in the process of injury risk management are preparticipation examination, conditioning and training, proper supervision, protection of the body, and environmental control.[298]

PREPARTICIPATION EXAMINATION

The preparticipation examination (PPE) is the initial step in the process of injury prevention. The American Medical Association Committee on Medical Aspects of Sports constructed a Bill of Rights for the Athlete, one part of which is a thorough preseason history and medical examination. The underlying goal of a PPE is to ensure the safety and health of athletes during training and athletic participation.[294] Specifically, the PPE attempts to (1) determine the general health of the athlete and detect conditions that place the participant at additional risk, (2) identify relative or absolute medical contraindications to participation, (3) identify sports that may be played safely, (4) assess maturity and overall fitness, and (5) educate the athlete. These examinations are also necessary to meet legal and insurance requirements in many states.[23] Several successful studies have demonstrated the usefulness of these screenings.[42,89,107,118,121,171,183,189,194,273]

Most states require either an individual examination or a multistation screening. The merits and disadvantages of these methods have been evaluated. The primary physician performing an individual examination knows or has access to the athlete's health records, can discuss sensitive health or personal issues, and may be most qualified to oversee any necessary follow-up care. The time and cost are a disadvantage of the individual examination. Additionally, disparate knowledge and interest among physicians regarding sports and the requirements to participate may hinder effective evaluation for all participants. The multistation approach to PPE is more cost and time efficient and provides a thorough and appropriate screening for all potential participants. Professional experts assess each athlete in the area of her or his specialization (Table 15-3), increasing the probability of detection of abnormalities.[111,297] North Carolina has adopted a PPE for its specific needs based on questions that have shown significant yield.[98] The use of a web-based examination has also been reported.[253]

The frequency of the PPE is often debated. Although annual evaluations are most traditional,[264] many clinicians

TABLE 15-3   Multistation Preparticipation Examination

Station	Personnel
Sign-in/instructions	Ancillary personnel/coach
Height/weight/vital signs	Nurse, exercise physiologist, athletic trainer, or physical therapist
Visual examination	Nurse or coach
Medical examination	Internist or family practitioner
Orthopedic evaluation	Physician or physical therapist
Flexibility assessment	Physical therapist or athletic trainer
Strength evaluation	Physical therapist, athletic trainer, or exercise physiologist
Body composition	Exercise physiologist, physical therapist, or athletic trainer
Speed, agility, power, balance, endurance	Exercise physiologist, coach, or athletic trainer
Assessment/clearance	Physician

advocate evaluation before each season.[121] A complete entry-level examination and evaluation, followed by annual reevaluation that includes a brief physical examination, a physical maturity assessment, and an examination/evaluation of all new problems, is one such recommendation.[42] The American Academy of Pediatrics[5] has recommended a biannual complete evaluation followed by an interim history before each season. The schedule that meets the primary objectives of the academy, however, is a complete entry-level evaluation followed by a limited annual reevaluation that includes a brief physical examination (to evaluate height, weight, blood pressure, and pulse; perform auscultation; examine the skin; and test visual acuity), a physical maturity assessment if previous level was less than Tanner stage IV, and an evaluation of all new problems.[261]

The components of the PPE are the medical history; the physical examination, including cardiovascular and eye examinations; a musculoskeletal assessment; body composition and height and weight determination; specific field testing; and readiness, both physical and psychologic. Research has identified alterations in movement mechanics, landing patterns, and functional performance that are associated with increased risk of sports-related injuries.[248] As such, dynamic functional performance assessments may be implemented into PPE, although this is not standard practice. The PPE should be completed 6 weeks before the practice season to allow adequate time for further evaluation or for correction of any problems.[111,187] The components of the examination should be tailored to the specific demands of the sport.

History

The medical history is the cornerstone of the medical evaluation[187] and identifies the majority of problems affecting athletes.[121,273] Short forms that are easy to complete, written in lay terms, and understandable to young athletes are preferable. Forms should be completed and signed by the athlete and parent or legal guardian. Content areas that should be particularly noted include exercise-induced syncope or asthma; family history of heart disease or sudden death; history of loss of consciousness, concussion, or neurologic conditions; history of heat stroke; medications; allergies; history of musculoskeletal dysfunction; dates of hospitalizations or surgery; absence or loss of a paired organ; and immunizations. A Preparticipation Physical Evaluation Form is available at the American Academy of Pediatrics website (www.aap.org/profed.html).

Physical Examination

The physical examination is used to evaluate areas of concern identified in the history.[10] The minimally sufficient examination includes cardiovascular and eye examinations, a maturity assessment, and a review of all body systems. Blood pressure should be measured using appropriately sized sphygmomanometer cuffs.[187] Blood pressure is most accurately predicted by gender and percentile of height in those under the age of 18 years.[226] The 95th percentile upper limit values for normal blood pressure are 110/75 mm Hg below age 6, 120/80 mm Hg for 6- to 10-year-olds, 125/85 mm Hg for 11- to 14-year-olds, and 135/90 mm Hg for 15- to 18-year-olds.[74] A diagnosis of hypertension requires three abnormal readings. If blood pressure is elevated, repeat measures should be taken later in the examination or the next day.[95] High blood pressure requires further evaluation for clearance to participate in sports.[187] The remainder of the cardiovascular screening evaluation assesses peripheral pulses and heartbeat for symmetry and rate. Auscultation of the heart should be performed with the young person both seated and supine.[187] Because as many as 85% of youths have benign heart murmurs, various maneuvers such as squat to stand, Valsalva, and deep inspiration can differentiate functional from pathologic murmurs. Arrhythmias are not abnormal in children, but increases in premature ventricular contractions with exercise require further assessment.[107,118] Paroxysmal supraventricular tachycardia needs to be evaluated but is not a reason for disqualification.[189,194,273]

Visual acuity is tested using a Snelling chart and should be correctable to 20/200. Any inequality of pupil diameter or reactivity should be noted so responses after potential injury can be compared with this baseline value. Uncorrectable legal blindness (acuity less than 20/200 or absence of an eye) requires counseling regarding participation in collision or contact sports. The importance of protective eyewear for athletes who wear glasses or have unilateral vision should be stressed.[23]

Pulmonary status is determined by symmetry of diaphragmatic excursion and breath sounds. Children with asthma, including exercise-induced asthma, should be allowed to participate in activities if the condition is properly controlled with medication.[187,333] Abdominal assessment determines rigidity, tenderness, organomegaly, or the presence of masses. Participation by any athlete with organomegaly is restricted until further tests determine the cause of the enlarged organ.[23]

Careful examination of the skin is vital in examination of all persons, but it is particularly important for those who will participate in contact sports. Participation in these sports should be deferred for children with evidence of any communicable skin disease, such as impetigo, carbuncles, herpes, scabies, and louse or fungal infections.[24,187]

Genitourinary examination of males is used to assess the child for testicular presence, descended testicles, and possible inguinal hernia. The genital examination is deferred in girls unless a history of amenorrhea or menstrual irregularity warrants referral. A maturational index should be determined for all athletes so that appropriate matching of age and sport can occur.[23] Guidelines for staging of secondary sexual characteristics are reliable, proven, and practical (Table 15-4).

TABLE 15-4 **Maturity Staging Guidelines**

Male		
Pubic Hair	**Penis**	**Testis**
None	Preadolescent	
Slight, long, slight pigmentation	Slight enlargement	Enlarged scrotum, pink slight ruga
Darker, starts to curl, small amount	Longer	Larger
Coarse, curly, adult type, but less quantity	Increase in glans size and breadth of penis	Larger, scrotum darker
Adult—spread to inner thighs	Adult	Adult

Female	
Pubic Hair	**Breasts**
Preadolescent (none)	Preadolescent (no germinal button)
Sparse, lightly pigmented, straight medial border of labia	Breast and papilla elevated as small mound; areolar diameter increased
Darker, beginning to curl, increased	Breast and areola enlarged; no contour separation
Coarse, curly, abundant, but less than adult	Areola and papilla form secondary mound
Adult female triangle and spread to medial surface	Mature, nipple projects, areola part of general breast contour

From McKeag, D. (1985). Preseason physical examination for the prevention of sports injuries. *Sports Medicine, 2,* 425.

The musculoskeletal screening examination should include assessment of posture with particular attention to atrophy, spinal asymmetry, pelvic level, discrepancy of leg lengths, and lower extremity deformities such as genu valgus or varus, patellar deformities, and pes planus. Gait should be examined with the child walking and running, as well as walking on toes and heels. Passive range of motion and two-joint musculotendinous flexibility should be screened. Muscle strength can be assessed using a manual muscle test, handheld dynamometer, or isokinetic device. Special stability testing of the shoulders, knees, and ankles should be conducted if the child has had a previous injury or if the current assessment indicates that instability may be present.[111,264] Dynamic functional performance assessments may also be implemented to identify potential injury risk.

Body Composition

Height and weight should be assessed and results compared with standard growth charts. A body mass index (BMI) should also be calculated. Children are considered underweight if calculated BMI-for-age is below the 5th percentile, in the normal range if between the 5th and 85th percentile, at risk for overweight if between the 85th and 95th percentile, and overweight if BMI-for-age is over the 95th percentile.[67] Because weight alone gives no specific assessment of the percentage of lean mass and fat tissue, assessment of subcutaneous body fat provides a more specific evaluation of body composition, although fat thickness varies from birth to adolescence (see Chapter 6). The most practical method for screening is skinfold measurement. This method has demonstrated correlations of 0.70 to 0.85 with hydrostatic weighing if performed by an experienced examiner.[119]

Although the criterion ranges for body fatness related to optimal health are 15% to 25% for girls and 10% to 25% for boys,[186] 20% for girls and 12% for boys are ideal for most activities. Elevated body fat levels may indicate the need for weight reduction. Low weight or low body fat warrants a thorough evaluation of eating habits, weight loss, and body image to rule out the possibility of an eating disorder. High weight and very low body fat could signal use of anabolic steroids, growth hormone, or other performance-enhancing drugs.[187,198] Because of unorthodox weight loss methods, nutritional content and patterns should also be evaluated, especially in those athletes who must "make weight."[256]

The PPE can be utilized to screen for involvement in risky health behaviors such as tobacco and alcohol use, use of recreational drugs or ergogenic aids,[150] and unsafe sexual practices.[9,234] In addition to questions, the examiner should be alert for loss of attention, irritability, reported changes in behavior, poor grades, and change in weight.[9]

A meta-analysis of the literature in which athletes reported drug use documented an overall doping prevalence of 3% to 5% among athletes 18 years or younger.[177] Risk factors for substance abuse include poor or single parent family situation, poor health perception, other drug consumption, antisocial behavior, depression, and clumsiness, and good communication with a parent, academic achievement, regular sports participation, serious and organized personality, and mother at home were cited as protective.[68,124,254,311]

From 3% to 12% of adolescent males and 1% to 2% of females report having used steroids.[17,343] In addition to the risk factors noted for general use of drugs, attempts to increase strength added another risk for use of steroids.[91,105] The most compelling reasons for taking steroids are to increase body weight and muscle mass, decrease fatigue, and increase aggressive behavior. The adverse effects, including hypertension, hepatitis, testicular atrophy, loss of libido, hepatic carcinoma, and premature epiphyseal closure, far outweigh the benefits of these drugs.[37,176,279,306] Warning signs of steroid abuse include irritability; sudden mood swings; puffiness in face, upper arms, and chest; sudden increases in blood pressure and weight; yellowish coloration around the fingernails and eyes; hirsutism; and deepening of voice and acne in girls.[23,198,306]

Other substances that have been utilized to increase muscle performance include DHEA (dehydroepiandrosterone), branched chain and essential amino acids, creatine, growth hormone, and dietary supplements containing nandrolone and testosterone.[13,22,82,168,323] Most recently, designer steroids have been introduced to provide the effects of steroid use, but avoid detection. Other dietary substances including ephedra and carnitine have been utilized to increase energy and endurance, suppress appetite, and promote weight loss.[27,132,136] These natural elements have been touted in popular literature as aids for growth, performance, immunity, and healing and are used by both high school and college athletes, as well as professional athletes.[228,338] Research has not supported the efficacy of these substances for performance enhancement with the exception of creatine[287] and carnitine.[165] The research that exists has examined these substances in young adults; no research has been done in the pediatric population under the age of 18 years. Research has reported potential risk and harm with ingestion of substantial amounts of several substances including steroids and nandrolone, ephedra, and branched chain amino acids. The use of ephedrine-containing compounds has been banned by most professional and collegiate sports organizations, as well as the National Federation of State High School Associations.

Diuretics are frequently used to "make weight" for an event or to mask drug usage.[122] Performance may, however, decrease as a result of dehydration or electrolyte losses.[37,122,198] Likewise, stimulants, such as caffeine and amphetamines, are commonly abused in an effort to increase performance in sports. They serve only to mask normal fatigue and to increase aggression, hostility, and uncooperativeness and can lead to addiction and death.[329]

The use of barbiturates, antidepressants, and beta-blockers has been noted in sports in which fine control is required, such as shooting and archery. Although they do calm the nervous system and lower heart rate, even therapeutic doses may cause bronchospasm, hypotension, and bradycardia.[215]

The use of recreational drugs, including nicotine, smokeless tobacco, alcohol, marijuana, cocaine, and even heroin, is increasing among youth.[299] Symptoms including agitation, restlessness, insomnia, difficulty with short-term memory or concentration, and decline in performance might signal behavior indicative of substance abuse.[70,123]

The Food and Drug Administration (FDA) has not approved dietary supplements, so actual ingredients are not listed on the label, nor are safety and effectiveness validated. The few protections offered to the consumer include a USP (United States Pharmacopeia) label, a nationally known manufacturer, and appropriate and accurate claims supported by research. Overdosage of both fat- and water-soluble vitamins can cause damage to the liver and kidneys.[215]

Specific Field Tests

Field testing is done to assess specific athletic potential in a specific sport. The components assessed are muscle strength, muscle power, endurance, speed, agility and flexibility, and cardiovascular performance.[24] Field test performance has been shown to identify deficits from previous injury that standard physical examination may not define.[224]

General muscle strength can be assessed with a maximal activity pertinent to the sport, such as bench presses, pull-ups, or push-ups for the upper extremities and leg presses or sit-ups for the lower extremities. Endurance can be assessed by performing as many repetitions of the task as possible. Muscle power can be evaluated with vertical jumping, performing a standing long jump, or throwing a medicine ball, as appropriate.

Speed is evaluated using a 40- or 50-yard dash, and agility can be assessed with the Vodak agility test[108] or a similar battery of tests. The most common, standardized methods of assessing flexibility are the sit and reach test, which has norms for children, and active knee extension performed in a supine position with the hips flexed to 90°.[145] Cardiovascular performance is most easily assessed using a submaximal test on an appropriate device, such as a cycle ergometer, treadmill, or upper-body ergometer. A field test for cardiovascular performance is the 12-minute run or the timed 1.5-mile run.[23,51,175] Field tests that involve jumping and sprinting have been correlated to laboratory results.[20]

Despite efforts to create a thorough and comprehensive PPE, it is not without limitations. The PPE is designed to identify life-threatening contraindications to sports participation. In addition, the PPE is able to identify various static musculoskeletal deficiencies. However, often some PPE settings do not address more dynamic risk factors. More concerning is the lack of follow-up that may occur if deficits are identified. McKeag et al.[204] reported that 10% of athletes receiving a PPE present with a musculoskeletal disorder; however, others have noted that only 1% to 3% of athletes are referred for intervention following a PPE.[297] Although many athletes are identified with musculoskeletal deficits, the deficits are often not addressed. Future work should focus on increasing the ability of the PPE to identify dynamic risk factors for injury and create a more seamless approach to recommend intervention to those athletes who are identified at risk.

The outcome of the PPE determines the level of clearance to participate in sports. Clearance can be unrestricted for any sport or restricted to specific types of sports in the following manner: (1) no collision (violent, direct impact) or contact (physical touching), (2) limited contact or impact, or (3) noncontact only. The American Academy of Pediatrics has developed a classification system for sports activities and recommendations for restriction of participation that are excellent guides in making decisions for individual athletes.[7] All decisions or recommendations for further evaluation should be thoroughly discussed with the athletes and their parents.[23,264]

TRAINING PROGRAM

The preseason examination clearly defines the individual athlete's areas of strength and limitations (Figure 15-1). The next appropriate step in prevention is the development of an individualized training plan designed to address the particular problems of the athlete as they relate to the requirements of the sport(s). This program could be developed by a sports physical therapist, athletic trainer, or exercise physiologist involved in the preseason screening. Once developed, it should be taught to the athlete, the parent, and the coach.

The training program should be a systematic, progressive plan to address the athlete's weaknesses and to maximally condition the athlete for participation. Training consists of off-season, preseason, in-season, and postseason programs for year-round conditioning and for development of appropriate peak performance. Components should include energy training (aerobic foundation and anaerobic training), muscle training (strength, endurance, flexibility, and power), speed, and proper nutrition. A well-developed, variable, and well-paced program will help the young athlete to avoid boredom and potential overuse injury. The psychologic effects of year-round training, or exercise in general, are controversial and not well documented. The risk-benefit ratio, however, tends to favor exercise for improvement of mood, self-concept, and work behavior when competition is sensibly controlled.[211]

Energy Training

The basis of energy training, a strong aerobic base, should be developed during the off-season. Good training consists of low-intensity, long-duration activity with natural intervals of low- and moderate-intensity work that is sport-specific. Swimming would be a good choice for the field athlete, and cycling or running is appropriate for those in track, soccer, and football. Training on hills or performance of similar resistance efforts should be done once weekly. Children exhibit less efficient movement patterns and a lower maximal acidosis level. Their greater surface area to body mass ratio facilitates greater heat gain on hot days and greater heat loss on colder days. Children produce less sweat and less total evaporative heat loss. Children produce more metabolic heat per pound of body weight during exercises, such as walking and running. Finally, although children can

acclimatize, they do so at a slower rate than adults.[14,23] Consequently, intense training in the extreme heat and hard training involving long durations should be minimized until puberty. This avoidance of excessive exercise also helps avert early burnout.[288]

Anaerobic training programs consist of exertion at 85% to 90% of maximal heart rate for short periods. Anaerobic drills develop a person's ability to tolerate the production of excess lactic acid. Twice-weekly anaerobic training should be performed for maximal benefit. Methods including interval training, fartlek (speed play, or alternate fast and slow running in natural terrain), and pace training are variations of the anaerobic method. Sport-specific anaerobic skills should be developed during preseason and early-season activities.[288] Young children are less able to use muscle glycogen and produce lactic acid, so this training is difficult for young athletes and has only minor fitness benefits until they mature. Some training should be used, however, to achieve relaxation and mechanical efficiency at these levels.

Resistance Training (Strength Training)

The use of resistance training (strength training) in prepubertal children has been controversial. Historically, clinicians and researchers believed individuals with growing bones and open growth plates should not participate in resistance training as it could potentially place the open growth plates at risk for injury. In 1983, the American Academy of Pediatrics issued a position statement, which suggested that resistance training in a prepubescent athlete may not only be a high risk activity but also may have little ability to result in a significant increase in strength because of the lack of circulating androgens in this population.[4] Importantly, recent evidence suggests both of these fears are unfounded, and several professional organizations now advocate appropriately implemented resistance training as an intervention for young athletes.

With regard to efficacy of resistance training, several research studies have demonstrated that strength can be improved by systematic overload of muscle in postpubescent athletes with results similar to training in adults.[34,211] The mechanism of this gain in strength is likely related to neural adaptations in the muscle and not secondary to an increase in cross sectional area or hypertrophy of muscle tissue.[164] Similar to an adult who initiates a resistance training program, initial gains in strength in the first 4 to 6 weeks after onset of training are due to neural adaptations in the muscle. Only after this initial neuromuscular change do adults see a change in their muscle diameter, which may result in continued progression of strength. Children have the potential to experience a similar neuromuscular adaptation, which can increase strength despite the absence of circulating androgens, once thought to be necessary to see any increase in strength.[93,128]

Safety during resistance training is a priority in a population of young athletes. Initial epidemiology data regarding

Athletic fitness scorecard for boys

	0	1	2	3	4
Test	**Below average**	**Above average**	**Good**	**Very good**	**Excellent**
Strength Pull-ups (no)	Fewer than 7	7 to 9	10 to 12	13 to 14	15 or more
Power Long jump (in)	Fewer than 85	85 to 88	89 to 91	92 to 94	95 or more
Speed 50-yd dash (sec)	Slower than 6.7	6.7 to 6.4	6.3 to 6.0	5.9 to 5.6	5.5 or less
Agility 6-c agility (c)	Fewer than 5-5	5-5 to 6-3	6-4 to 7-2	7-3 to 8-1	8-2 or more
Flexibility Forward flexion (in)	Not reach ruler	1 to 2	3 to 5	6 to 8	9 or more
Muscular endurance Sit-ups (no)	Fewer than 38	38 to 45	46 to 52	53 to 59	60 or more
Cardiorespiratory endurance 12-min run (mi)	Fewer than 1½	1½	1¾	2	2¼ or more

YOUR SCORE

	Strength	Power	Speed	Agility	Flexibility	Muscular endurance	Cardiorespiratory endurance
Your Score							
Rating (0–4)							

Athletic fitness scorecard for girls

	0	1	2	3	4
Test	**Below average**	**Above average**	**Good**	**Very good**	**Excellent**
Strength Pull-ups (no)	Fewer than 2	2 to 3	4 to 5	6 to 7	8 or more
Power Long jump (in)	Fewer than 63	63 to 65	66 to 68	69 to 71	72 or more
Speed 50-yd dash (sec)	Slower than 8.2	8.2 to 7.9	7.8 to 7.1	6.9 to 6.0	5.9 or less
Agility 6-c agility (c)	Fewer than 3-5	3-5 to 4-3	4-4 to 5-2	5-3 to 6-2	6-3 or more
Flexibility Forward flexion (in)	Fewer than 3	3 to 5	6 to 8	9 to 11	12 or more
Muscular endurance Sit-ups (no)	Fewer than 26	26 to 31	32 to 38	39 to 45	46 or more
Cardiorespiratory endurance 12-min run (mi)	Fewer than 1¼	1¼	1½	1¾	2 or more

YOUR SCORE

	Strength	Power	Speed	Agility	Flexibility	Muscular endurance	Cardiorespiratory endurance
Your Score							
Rating (0–4)							

Figure 15-1 Athletic Fitness Scorecards for Boys and Girls. (Reproduced with permission from Gaillard, B., Haskell, W., Smith, N., & Ogilvie, B. [1988]. *Handbook for the young athlete.* Boulder, CO: Bull Publishing.)

injuries during resistance training suggested a high incidence of injury in a population of young individuals. Evidence suggests the incidence of injury is relatively low and, with certain precautions, this risk can be reduced even further.[221] Many of the injuries reported by Myer and colleagues identify accidentals as the primary cause of injury in the weight room with a young population. As a result current guidelines regarding resistance training in young athletes suggest appropriate supervision be present at all times to minimize the chance of these accidental injuries. In fact, professional organizations such as the American College of Sports Medicine, the National Strength and Conditioning Association, and the American Academy of Pediatrics suggest that resistance training is a safe and effective intervention in young athletes.[94] Furthermore, resistance training has also been shown to be effective in reducing various lower extremity injuries.[180]

Through the joint contributions of these professional organizations, a general consensus on the safe initiation of resistance training in a young population has been issued.[221] These recommendations suggest a young athlete should have sufficient emotional maturity to accept and follow directions prior to initiating a resistance training program. Appropriate supervision should be available at all times to reduce the risk of accidental injuries and also to provide regular feedback regarding "technique" of each lift. A primary goal of the onset of a resistance training program is to develop good lifting technique at an early age. Supervision is necessary to insure this development. Finally, a dynamic warm-up is always recommended and an appropriate volume and intensity of each activity should be initiated and monitored. Specifically, young athletes should avoid executing 1 maximum repetition and should focus on the use of lighter weight with higher sets and repetitions rather than using lower sets and striving to gain power. Together, these factors have resulted in a more safe and efficacious algorithm for resistance training participation by young athletes.

Speed

Because the proportion of fast twitch fibers in muscle is inherited, speed is "born" in the child.[288] All athletes, however, can train the intermediate fibers and improve the components of reaction and movement time. Faster reactions are taught in sport-specific practice drills such as starts, acceleration drills, or play drills that gradually narrow choice. Movement time is enhanced from a base of flexibility and strength with ballistic motions, sprint loading (explosive jump or throw), overspeed, or resisted sprinting.[288]

Nutrition

Many general articles have been written on nutritional requirements for athletes[25,69] with recent revisions for pediatric and adolescent athletes.[74,197,257,281] The preparticipation screening includes components of a nutritional assessment: skinfold measurements, height, and weight. Skinfold standards for the triceps and calf in children allow one to determine whether the child is overfat.[74] The body fat percentage can be matched to the approximated body fat values developed for various sports, although percentages are not well standardized for younger athletes.[158]

Caloric requirements for children are age dependent and vary directly with body weight and surface area. Generally, a young child requires more calories than an adolescent or adult—36 to 40 calories (kcal) per pound per day.[74,257] An additional caloric load is necessary depending on the level of energy output. An approximation for energy expenditure, based on a child weighing 100 lb, is 4 kcal/minute for low-intensity activities, 4 to 7 kcal/minute for moderate-intensity activities, and greater than 7 kcal/minute for high-intensity activities.[257] A more complex, but also more accurate, method is to multiply ideal weight in pounds times 10 for basal calories. Basal activity calories are then calculated by multiplying weight in pounds times 3 for sedentary activity, times 5 for moderate activity, and times 10 for vigorous activity. The additional requirements of the sports activity are determined by adding 10 to 14 kcal/minute for boys and 9 to 12 kcal/minute for girls.

Protein requirements of the preadolescent and adolescent athlete approximate those of the adult, but younger athletes have increased protein needs for growth. Small children have special iron needs, as do females after menarche.[257,281] Recommended dietary allowances for children are available online.[321]

The training diet of the young athlete should routinely consist of 50% to 55% carbohydrate, 15% protein, and 30% to 35% fat, of which only 10% is saturated. Smaller, growing muscles cannot store glycogen as efficiently as larger, strong muscles, so more complex carbohydrates may be necessary if the child complains of fatigue.[257] The basic food groups should be included in these plans with attention to total caloric intake.[103] Additional supplements are not necessary if the diet is adequate and may even be dangerous in the growing child.[70] Glycogen loading, or increased amounts of glycogen to increase muscle stores above their normal levels, is not recommended in young children or in early adolescence because of the side effects of muscle stiffness and water retention, but they can be used with caution by teenagers.[37,306]

Dietary recommendations differ during the four phases of training and competition. In the postseason and off-season periods, the athlete should receive all nutritional and caloric needs for optimal weight; during the preseason and in-season periods, optimal weight and performance should guide the nutritional balance and caloric load. The pregame meal should be eaten 2 to 3 hours before competition to guarantee digestion in the stomach and upper intestine. The meal should be easy to digest; be low in fat, protein, salt, and bulk; and have abundant liquid content and complex carbohydrates for adequate energy and hydration. Examples are waffles, pasta, sandwiches, or liquid meals. The goal during competition is maintenance of adequate hydration (and glycogen for endurance events). Postcompetition meals should immediately replenish glycogen stores and restore fluid balance. Two 8-oz cups of water should be consumed for each pound of body weight lost.[69,122,257]

Alterations in weight can and should be made carefully. If a special nutrition program and counseling for weight loss or gain is indicated, it should be supervised by a nutritionist or nurse. Difficulties with excess leanness and eating disorders are being identified more frequently in the preadolescent population. Weight gain diets should have a similar composition to the training diet but include additional calories. An added 1000 kcal a day will result in a gain of 2 lb weekly. This gain will occur in lean body tissue if the child is moderately active. Determination of whether an athlete is overfat or overweight must be made before recommendation of a diet for weight loss. If the athlete is excessively fat or has too great a percentage of body fat in relation to total body composition, careful structure of a training plan can decrease fat mass and increase lean muscle mass. If an athlete is also overweight, a weight loss diet of composition similar to that of the normal athlete but with 1000 fewer kcal per day should be constructed. This will result in a safe loss of 2 lb weekly. Additional exercise will hasten weight loss and maintain firmness of body tissue.[257]

PROPER SUPERVISION

The first in the series of supervisors is the coach, the key to a successful sports program. However, 2.5 million adult volunteers with varying levels of expertise coach approximately 20 million children. The American Academy of Pediatrics has stated that coaches should encourage preparticipation screenings every 1 to 2 years, enforce use of warm-up procedures, require suitable protective equipment, and enforce rules concerning safety. In addition, it recommends completion of a certification program that covers teaching techniques, basic sports skills, fitness, first aid, sportsmanship, enhancement of self-image, and motivational skills.[5]

Qualified officials and professional medical personnel at games and practices are the second level of supervision. These individuals provide game control and immediate injury containment onsite. Medical personnel could include physicians, physical therapists, or athletic trainers who have certification in basic first aid and cardiopulmonary resuscitation techniques in addition to their medical skills.[5,268]

PROTECTION

Outfitting the child athlete with proper equipment should be mandated and enforced for the protection of the participants. Equipment must be appropriate for the sport. High quality and proper fit are essential to correct function.[304] Proper footwear with adequate cushioning, rearfoot control, and sole flexibility for the sport should be required.[211,286] Protective padding in contact or kicking sports, such as shoulder and shin pads, should be required.

Protective headgear for contact and collision in football, baseball, and hockey is necessary to limit the number of head and neck injuries. Schuller and colleagues[285] have demonstrated a lower risk of auricular damage in wrestlers wearing headgear (26% incidence) versus those with no headgear (52% incidence). Helmets should be approved by the National Operating Committee on Standards for Athletic Equipment and the American National Safety Institute.[122,235]

Eye injuries have been on the increase, particularly in racquet sports, baseball, and basketball.[225,309,310] An estimated 100,000 sports-related eye injuries occur yearly and are the most common cause of eye trauma in children younger than age 15 years (Box 15-1).[309] Eye protectors that dissipate injury to a wider area without reducing visual field should be required in racquet sports, ice hockey, baseball, basketball, and football and during use of air-powered weapons. They should be cosmetically and functionally acceptable and made of impact-resistant material. Polycarbonate is the most impact- and scratch-resistant material. A list of high-risk sports and recommended protection is given in Table 15-5. All eye protectors should be approved by either the Canadian Standards Association or the American Society for Testing and Materials.

Studies have highlighted the incidence of oral and facial injuries in many sports, particularly football, hockey, baseball, basketball, wrestling, and boxing.[112,190] Youth baseball generated the greatest number of head and face injuries in 1980.[19,66,85,255] Before mandatory use of mouthguards, oral trauma constituted 50% of all football injuries.[206] The mandatory use of mouthguards has cut the injury rate of oral trauma in football to fewer than 1% of all injuries.[155] The mouth protector serves to prevent injury to the teeth and lacerations of the mouth. Because it absorbs blows to the oral and facial structures, it also prevents fractures, dislocations, and concussions. It should position the bite so the condyles of the mandible do not contact the fossae of the joints. These mouthguards should be inexpensive, strong, and easy to

---

| Box **15-1** | SPORTS ASSOCIATED WITH EYE INJURY AT VARIOUS AGES |

CHILDREN (5 TO 12 YEARS OF AGE)
Baseball
Basketball
Soccer
BB gun injuries

ADOLESCENTS (13 TO 21 YEARS OF AGE)
Basketball
Football
Ice hockey
Soccer

ADULTS (21 YEARS OF AGE AND OLDER)
Racquetball
Squash
Tennis
Badminton

From Stock, J., & Cornell, M. (1991). Prevention of sports-related eye injury. *American Family Practice, 44,* 516; published by the American Academy of Family Physicians.

TABLE 15-5 Risk Level for Eye Injury with Recommendations for Protective Eyewear

Risk	Sport	Protective Wear
Unacceptable	Boxing	Not applicable
Very high	Ice hockey	Helmet with full visor
	Squash	Polycarbonate sports protector
	Badminton	Polycarbonate sports protector
	Basketball	Polycarbonate sports protector
	Men's lacrosse	Helmet with full visor
High	Racquetball	Polycarbonate sports protector
	Baseball	Polycarbonate sports protector
	Cricket	Helmet with full visor
	Field hockey	Helmet with full visor
	Rugby football	Debatable
	Soccer	Debatable
	Water polo	Polycarbonate goggles
	Shooting	Polycarbonate sports protector
	Women's lacrosse	Helmet with full visor
Moderate	Tennis	Plastic lens spectacles
	American football	Helmet with polycarbonate visor
Low	Golf	Sports protector if one-eyed
	Volleyball	Sports protector if one-eyed
	Skiing	UV filter goggles ± helmet
	Cycling	Sports protector ± helmet
	Fishing	Polycarbonate protector if one-eyed
	Swimming	Goggles if in water for long periods
	High diving	Not feasible
	Track & field	None required

From Jones, N. (1989). Eye injury in sport. *Sports Medicine, 7,* 178.

TABLE 15-6 Recommended Fluid Intake and Availability for a 90-Minute Practice

Weight Loss		Minutes between Water Break	Fluid per Break	
Lb	Kg		Oz	Ml
8	3.6	*		
7.5	3.4	*		
7	3.2	10	8–10	266
6.5	3.0	10	8–9	251
6	2.7	10	8–9	251
5.5	2.5	15	10–12	325
5	2.3	15	10–11	311
4.5	2.1	15	9–10	281
4	1.8	15	8–9	251
3.5	1.6	20	10–11	311
3	1.4	20	9–10	281
2.5	1.1	20	7–8	222
2	0.9	30	8	237
1.5	0.7	30	6	177
1	0.5	45	6	177
0.5	0.2	60	6	177

From Peterson, M., & Peterson, K. (1988). *Eat to compete: A guide to sports nutrition* (p. 182). Chicago: Year Book Medical.
*No practice recommended.

clean and should not interfere with speech or breathing. They should be used alone in field hockey, rugby, wrestling, basketball, and other field events and used in conjunction with face protectors in football, ice hockey, baseball, and lacrosse.[122]

ENVIRONMENTAL CONTROL

Assessment and control of the environment is also vital to the safety of the child athlete. The playing area should be well lighted and maintained for safety. Surfaces should be free from obstacles and smooth and even, with good shock-absorbing qualities (wood as opposed to concrete). Modifications of equipment that have been shown to decrease injury (e.g., breakaway bases) should be installed. Sports equipment and playing environments should be scaled down to the size of the athlete.[211,225,306]

Ambient temperature and humidity should be carefully monitored. During exercise, children require more fluid replacement per kilogram of body weight than adults to avoid dehydration. Children have a greater surface area per body weight, so their rate of heat exchange is greater with lower ability to endure exercise in climatic extremes. They also have a distinctly deficient ability to perspire, so they carry a larger heat load. They acclimatize less efficiently and require more "exposures" for acclimatization to occur.[23,303] Exercise should be modified if the wet bulb temperature (an index of climatic heat stress) is above 75°F.[6]

Dehydration can be avoided by drinking plenty of liquid before, during, and after play. Thirst is not a valid indicator of the amount of water needed, so every pound (16 oz) lost should be replaced with two cups (16 oz) of water.[257] The American College of Sports Medicine[8] recommends that 400 to 500 mL of water be ingested before distance running. It further recommends water intake every 35 to 45 minutes of football practice and nude weighing before and after practice. If residual weight loss from day to day exceeds 2 to 3 lb, practice is restricted until water is replenished. Recommendations for hydration include prehydration of 3 to 12 oz (3 to 6 oz for <90 lb; 6 to 12 oz for >90 lb weight) 1 hour before activity, and 3 to 6 oz just prior to activity. During activity 3 to 9 oz (3 to 5 oz for <90 lb; 6 to 9 oz for >90 lb) should be ingested every 10 to 20 minutes relative to the temperature and humidity. Eight to 12 oz should be consumed for each pound of weight lost in 2 to 4 hours following activity (Table 15-6).[65]

Children will not ingest enough plain water to remain hydrated or to rehydrate following activity. However, if flavor is added to the water, volume of intake is improved substantially.[149,246] Sports drinks have been shown to improve energy both in intensive as well as endurance exercise.[28,82,110,322,334] In addition to flavor, well-constituted sports drinks have a simple low-carbohydrate content that provides energy, speeds fluid absorption, and provides sodium to stimulate the thirst mechanism.[246,275,291]

Successful hydration programs involve not only fluid intake, but also fluid availability. Cool fluids infuse into the system more readily, so accessible liquids should be chilled or ice provided. Education of everyone involved with the activity, including parents and participants, is of paramount importance to ensure continued compliance. Knowledge of the common signs of dehydration—irritability, headache, nausea, dizziness, weakness, cramps, abdominal distress, and decreased performance—assist those involved with early recognition and intervention.[65]

RISK FACTORS FOR INJURY

Injury can be the result of a single macrotrauma or of repetitive microtrauma.[212] Seven risk factors for repetitive trauma, or "overuse," have been identified: (1) training errors; (2) musculotendinous imbalances of strength, flexibility, or bulk; (3) anatomic malalignment of the lower extremity; (4) improper footwear; (5) faulty playing surface; (6) associated disease states of the lower extremity such as old injury or arthritis; and (7) growth factors.[191,209,313]

TRAINING ERROR

Training error is frequently the cause of overuse injuries in children, as it is in adults. Dramatic increases in the total volume of activity, an increase in the rate of progression of training or an attempt to participate at a level above the capacity of the athlete are often identified as mechanisms of overuse injury.[2,212] The evolution of sports specialization has contributed to this phenomenon as more children are attempting to participate in several seasons of a single sport throughout the year. This results in few rest periods throughout a year and an increased focus on intense training. A sudden transition from casual play to 6 or 8 hours of intense participation, as may occur in a camp setting has also contributed to the increased incidence of overuse injury in children.

MUSCLE-TENDON IMBALANCE

Muscle-tendon imbalance can occur in strength, flexibility, or training. Until recently, little attention was paid to conditioning in children. This position may have been appropriate for free play activities but not for organized sport. The repetitive, often predictable, demands of a sport may result in imbalances of muscle and tendon unless the child is on a well-designed training plan. For example, a baseball pitcher or swimmer who does breast stroke might develop a loose anterior capsule and a tight posterior capsule, a situation that could lead to impingement or excessive anterior shoulder laxity and even subluxation. Repetitive running creates strength and tightness in the quadriceps femoris and triceps surae muscles with relatively weaker hamstrings. This could be problematic if pace and hence stride length are increased.

ANATOMIC MALALIGNMENT

Anatomic malalignment, such as leg length difference or abnormal frontal and rotational plane alignments, can be a factor in the occurrence of injury. Anatomic malalignments may result in compensations for abnormally high forces created by the altered alignment under the demands of a sport. For example, femoral anteversion in a young dancer can cause compensatory excessive tibial external rotation and ankle pronation as substitutes for natural hip external rotation. Hyperlordosis of the spine or hyperextension of the knee creates abnormal loading on portions of the joint, leading to pain and increased risk of injury. Pes planus can increase the valgus moment at the knee, as well as allowing the weight of the body to land on a flexible foot. This malalignment can cause pain and abnormal wear on the medial knee joint and foot.

IMPROPER FOOTWEAR AND PLAYING SURFACE

Well-fitting shoes with a firm heel counter, slight heel lift, and flexible toe box are essential for the young athlete. Inadequate footwear that does not support the structures of the foot can lead to a number of foot and lower extremity problems. The shoe should compensate for changes in alignment and shock absorption. Likewise, improper playing surfaces can predispose the child to knee pain, shin splints, or stress fractures. These symptoms have been associated with playing on hard, banked surfaces or synthetic courts, as opposed to clay and hardwood surfaces.[211]

ASSOCIATED DISEASE STATES

Associated disease has the potential to result in compensatory movement patterns during physical activity that may predispose athletes to overuse injuries. Conditions such as a history of Legg-Calvé-Perthes disease or juvenile rheumatoid arthritis may result in abnormal lower extremity alignment or abnormal movement patterns during dynamic activities or exacerbate joint pain or synovitis. Evaluation of dynamic movement patterns is an appropriate screening in these athletes to attempt to determine their risk for future injury.[222]

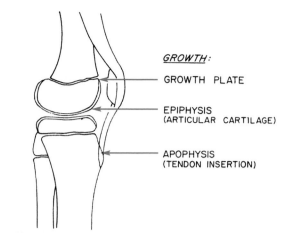

GROWTH:

GROWTH PLATE

EPIPHYSIS
(ARTICULAR CARTILAGE)

APOPHYSIS
(TENDON INSERTION)

Figure 15-2 Sites of susceptibility of the growth cartilage. (From Micheli, L. [1983]. Overuse injuries in children's sports: The growth factor. *Orthopedic Clinics of North America, 14,* 341.)

GROWTH FACTORS

The first aspect of growth that is a factor in overuse injuries is the articular cartilage (Figure 15-2). Clinical and biomechanical evidence suggests that growing cartilage has low resistance to repetitive loading, resulting in microtrauma to either the cartilage or the underlying growth plate. Damage may result in osteoarthritis or growth asymmetry.[114,209]

Growing articular cartilage is also less resistant to shear, particularly at the elbow, knee, and ankle. Repetitive shear has been implicated in osteochondritis dissecans of the capitellum in Little League pitchers and of the proximal and distal femur and talus in runners. Debate exists in the literature as to the etiology of osteochondritis dissecans; however, some authors postulate that a segment of subchondral bone becomes avascular and separates with its articular cartilage from the surrounding bone to become a loose body.[191,238] Shear stress has also been implicated in epiphyseal displacement.[116]

The final site of growth cartilage weakness is the apophysis. The apophysis is a point of attachment of the tendon to the bone and represents an ossification center of the bone. Apophysitis is inflammation secondary to microavulsions at the bone-cartilage junction caused by repetitive motion and overuse at times of rapid growth. The apophysis will ultimately fuse as the child matures; however, until this time it is vulnerable to overuse injuries.[35] Increasing evidence suggests that traction apophysitis, such as Osgood-Schlatter disease, Sever disease, and irritation of the rectus femoris or sartorius muscle origins, is the result of degeneration of the growth center with tiny avulsion fractures and associated healing.[79,191,210,242,247]

The second element of growth involved in overuse injury is abnormal stress created by longitudinal growth. Long bone, longitudinal growth occurs initially in the bones, with secondary elongation of the soft tissues. During periods of rapid bone growth ("growth spurts") the musculotendinous structures tighten and cause loss of flexibility. A coincidence of overuse injury and growth spurt has been noted.[79,209]

The biomechanical properties of bone also change with growth and maturation. As bone becomes less cartilaginous and stiffer, the resistance to impact decreases. Sudden overload may cause the bone to bow or buckle. The epiphysis, defined as the area of growth in the long bones, is more susceptible to injury and may shear or fracture. Examples of this process include avulsion fracture of the anterior cruciate ligament, avulsion fracture of the ankle ligament, and growth plate fractures. Because fractures through the epiphysis can be difficult to visualize on radiographs, any injury to the epiphyseal area is considered a fracture and is treated as such in order to avoid potential growth disturbance.[71,192,214] Growth plate fractures are typically classified with a Salter-Harris classification system. Salter-Harris I fractures represent a traction injury to the growth plate. Although more significant Salter-Harris II–V fractures involve additional portions of the bone and may represent more significant injuries that may affect growth.[280]

TYPES OF INJURIES

Although injuries in children have some similarity to those in adults, several are unique to the growing child. These specific injuries fall into three categories: (1) fractures, (2) joint injuries, and (3) muscle-tendon unit injuries.[116,209]

FRACTURES

A relatively new injury in children is the stress fracture, which usually results from repetitive microtrauma or poor training. Repetition causes cancellous bone fractures as opposed to cortical bone fatigue in adults.[71,191] These cancellous bone fractures are often imperceptible on radiographs until 6 to 8 weeks after the onset of pain. Clinical signs and symptoms indicative of a stress fracture can be confirmed by imaging tools, such as a bone scan or magnetic resonance imaging (MRI), to appropriately diagnose this condition. Stress fractures cause persistent, activity-related pain that can be reproduced by indirect force to the bone.

Growth plate or epiphyseal fractures are unique to the child. The cartilaginous growth plate is less resistant to shear or tensile-deforming force than either the ligament or bony cortex, so mechanical disruption frequently occurs through the plate itself, usually in the zone of hypertrophy.[191] This disruption can be caused by a single macrotrauma, such as jumping, or by repetitive microtrauma as in distance running. The potential for problems from epiphyseal fracture depends on the specific plate involved and on the extent of the injury. Decreased limb length, angular deformity, joint incongruity, and premature closure are frequent sequelae.[191,209] Shaft fractures are more common in the older child who is approaching adult status.[102]

JOINT INJURIES

Joint injuries in the young athlete include ligamentous sprains, internal derangement, and musculotendinous insertional injuries. These can result from a single discrete injury or from repetitive trauma. The diagnosis of sprain must be made carefully in the child. During a growth spurt, ligaments may be stronger than the growth plate, so excessive bending or twisting forces cause the plate rather than the ligament to yield. Severe ligamentous injuries can occur, and careful examination is necessary to differentiate among these injuries.[116,209] Repetitive microtrauma of the joint articular cartilage may result in softening, followed by frank shredding and thinning of the surface.

MUSCLE-TENDON UNIT INJURIES

Another area at particular risk of injury in the growing child is the insertion of the musculotendinous unit into the bone through the apophyseal cartilage. Growth occurs at the apophyseal growth plate, where tendons and ligaments are attached. During growth spurts the increased tension on the attachments often leads to detachment of the structure at the apophysis (avulsion fracture). Tendonitis occurs much less frequently in the child than in the adult because the insertion becomes symptomatic before the tendon.[2,209]

Irritation of the insertional area of the musculotendinous unit, the enthesis, can cause pain and inflammation. This area is highly vascular and metabolically active. During exercise, when blood is diverted to the active muscle, these areas may suffer periods of ischemia.[191] The symptoms cause inhibition of muscle activity with resultant weakness and loss of flexibility. The weakness and tightness then lead to greater irritation and pain.[240]

Children can overuse muscles, resulting in strain, just like adults. The increase in muscle volume during exercise may cause exertional compartment syndromes. Muscle hernias, however, occur in children secondary to tight fascial or musculotendinous structures.[320]

SITES OF INJURY

Mechanism, presentation, and management of injuries in children are often unique when compared to adult populations secondary to their developing anatomy and periods of rapid growth. The following sections will discuss the unique aspects of these various conditions in the pediatric and adolescent athlete.

CONCUSSIONS

Concussion was defined at the Third International Conference on Concussion as "a complex pathophysiologic process affecting the brain, induced by traumatic biomechanical forces."[203] Generally, a concussion results from either compression, tensile or shearing forces imposed on the brain.[127] The term "mild traumatic brain injury" has been used synonymously in the literature with concussion; however, this is a misnomer as any insult to the brain represents a serious injury.[208] The incidence of concussion is relatively high, as more than 300,000 injuries occur yearly, often in the young population.[318] These injuries can potentially result in long-term impairments.

Attempts to classify the severity of concussions have been controversial as these approaches are often dependent on loss of consciousness and amnesia. These two symptoms have recently been shown to be poor predictors of injury severity.[127] In general, three classification approaches exist in the literature. One method focuses on grading the severity at the time of injury based on the presenting signs and symptoms. The American Academy of Neurology's scale is based on this approach (Table 15-7). A second approach grades the severity based on the presence and duration of symptoms after the injury. The Cantu Evidenced Based grading system is based on this approach (Table 15-8).[58] The third approach is focused on the rate of recovery rather than the presenting symptoms. In the presence of more evidence-based classification schemes, prior attempts to classify the severity of concussions into simple and complex have been abandoned at the International Conference on Concussion, as these descriptors inadequately describe the condition.[203] These authors do agree, however, that 80% to 90% of concussions in adults will resolved in a 7- to 10-day time frame.[203]

Once a concussion occurs, evaluation of the injury becomes a multifactorial process. The initial assessment of the injury should occur on the field or at the time of injury. Signs of an acute concussion include headache, cognitive changes (i.e., feeling "in a fog"), emotional lability, irritability, slowed reaction times, and, in some cases, loss of consciousness and amnesia.[203] A thorough history in addition to serial assessments of these symptoms is critical to document the progression of the injury over time. The Graded Symptom Checklist (GSC) (Table 15-9) is a convenient tool to accomplish this task. In addition, a sideline assessment of cognitive function should be implemented, such as the Standardized Assessment of Concussion (SAC)[201,202] or another comparable assessment tool. Finally, an assessment of an athlete's postural stability is indicated using a standard test, such as a Rhomberg test or the Balance Error Scoring System (BESS).[127] Once the athlete is referred to either an emergency room or a physician's office, additional evaluation should include a detailed neurologic evaluation, an assessment of mental status and cognitive functioning, and an assessment of gait and balance. Objective measures of postural stability and neuropsychologic assessments have been identified as key components to a comprehensive concussion evaluation.[203] Neuroimaging may be indicated to evaluate the presence of intracerebral structural lesions, but it has not been shown to be effective in evaluating the severity of the concussion.

TABLE 15-7 American Academy of Neurology Concussion Grading Scale

Grade	Description
Grade 1/Mild	Transient confusion; no loss of consciousness; symptoms and mental status abnormalities resolve in less than 15 minutes
Grade 2/Moderate	Transient confusion; no loss of consciousness; symptoms and mental status abnormalities last more than 15 minutes
Grade 3/Severe	Any loss of consciousness

Adapted from Practice parameter: The management of concussion in sports (summary statement). (1997). Report of Quality Standards Subcommittee of the American Academy of Neurology. *Neurology, 48*, 581–585.

TABLE 15-8 Cantu Evidence-Based Grading System for Concussion

Grade	Description
Grade 1/ Mild	No loss of consciousness; posttraumatic amnesia less than 30 minutes; postconcussion signs and symptoms other than amnesia less than 24 hours
Grade 2/ Moderate	Loss of consciousness less than 1 minute OR posttraumatic amnesia less than or equal to 30 minutes but less than 24 hours OR postconcussion signs and symptoms other than amnesia less than or equal to 24 hours but less than 7 days
Grade 3/ Severe	Loss of consciousness greater than or equal to 1 minutes OR posttraumatic amnesia greater than or equal to 24 hours OR postconcussion signs and symptoms other than amnesia greater than or equal to 7 days

Data from Cantu, R. C. (2001). Posttraumatic retrograde and anterograde amnesia: Pathophysiology and implications in grading and safe return to play. *Journal of Athletic Training, 36*, 244–248.

Life-threatening complications from concussion include intracranial hemorrhage such as epidural and subdural hematoma. The leading cause of death from head injury is intracranial hemorrhage. Cantu and Mueller[63] reported that 86% of brain-injury deaths resulted from subdural hematoma. The most rapidly progressing and universally fatal disorder if missed is the epidural hematoma. Symptoms include initial preservation of consciousness with increasingly severe headache, lethargy, and focal neurologic signs. An acute subdural hematoma is the most common fatal head injury and should always be considered as a possible diagnosis in the athlete who loses and does not regain consciousness. A chronic subdural hematoma should be suspected in the athlete who is demonstrating abnormal behavior for days or weeks after a head injury. Signs may include headache or mild mental, motor, or sensory signs and symptoms.[18] These conditions represent medical emergencies, and these patients should be immediately transported to emergency medial facilities.

Once a concussion has been evaluated, initial management should focus on rest until symptoms resolve. After symptom resolution, a gradual return to activity program should be implemented to allow a progressive return to activity while monitoring the patient's symptoms (Table 15-10). If symptoms arise during this progression, modification should be made to allow the symptoms to resolve. Return-to-activity recommendations after a concussion are controversial. Many suggest the absence of symptoms in addition to a minimum 7-day rest before returning to sports after an initial concussion.[127] This may allow enough time for the majority of individuals who suffer an initial concussion to have resolution of symptoms before their return to activity. In addition, this may reduce the incidence of repeat injury, which typically occurs in the first 7 to 10 days after the initial concussion.[127] Because of the occurrence of second impact syndrome, in which a series of insults can lead to excessive cerebral damage beyond the effect of a single impact, conservative management is critical.[59,72] Return-to-activity evaluations should be a multifactorial process, inclusive of symptoms, medical evaluation, neurologic exam, neurocognitive assessment, balance assessment, and a consideration of history and desired return to play activity. Special consideration should be made to the individual who has suffered multiple concussions and the potential for disqualification should be considered.

Young athletes represent a unique population in the presence of concussions. The brain of a young athlete is still developing, and as a result the effect of a concussion in this population is still unknown.[127] General consensus in the literature does suggest that a more conservative approach to concussion management be implemented in this younger population.[203] Therefore, advancement through rehabilitation including time to return to play is often progressed slower in this population. In addition, return to play requires that no symptoms be present before release. Future research needs to focus on better understanding the effects of concussion on a developing brain and developing more evidence-based guidelines related to management and return to activity following a concussion in a young athlete.

CERVICAL INJURIES

The incidence of central nervous system injury in children is low, varying from 1% to 5% of sports-related injuries, but these cases constitute 50% to 100% of the deaths from injury. Cervical spine injuries result in 30% to 50% of cases of childhood quadriplegia.[48] The rate of spinal cord injuries in children younger than age 11 years is low, but it escalates dramatically in the 15-to-18-year-old age bracket. Because the brain and spinal cord are largely incapable of regeneration, these injuries take on a singular importance.[57]

TABLE 15-9   **Graded Symptoms Checklist (GSC)**

Symptom	Time of Injury	2–3 Hours Postinjury	24 Hours Postinjury	48 Hours Postinjury	72 Hours Postinjury
Blurred vision					
Dizziness					
Drowsiness					
Excess sleep					
Easily distracted					
Fatigue					
Feel "in a fog"					
Feel "slowed down"					
Headache					
Inappropriate emotions					
Irritability					
Loss of consciousness					
Loss or orientation					
Memory problems					
Nausea					
Nervousness					
Personality change					
Poor balance/ coordination					
Poor concentration					
Ringing in ears					
Sadness					
Seeing stars					
Sensitivity to light					
Sensitivity to noise					
Sleep disturbance					
Vacant stare/glassy eyed					
Vomiting					

From Guskiewicz, K. M., et al. (2006). Research based recommendation on management of sport related concussion. *British Journal of Sports Medicine, 40,* 6–10. NOTE: The GSC should be used not only for the initial evaluation but for each subsequent follow-up assessment until all signs and symptoms have cleared at rest and during physical exertion. In lieu of simply checking each symptom present, the ATC can ask the athlete to grade or score the severity of the symptom on a scale of 0–6, where 0 = not present, 1 = mild, 3 = moderate, and 6 = most severe.

TABLE 15-10   **Return to Activity Program**

Rehabilitation Stage	Functional Exercise at Each Stage of Rehabilitation	Objective of Each Stage
No activity	Complete physical and cognitive rest	Recovery
Light aerobic exercise	Walking, swimming or stationary cycling keeping intensity <70% MPHR. No resistance training.	Increase HR
Sport-specific exercise	Skating drills in ice hockey, running drills in soccer. No head impact activities.	Add movement
Non-contact training drills	Progression to more complex training drills (e.g., passing drills in football and ice hockey). May start progressive resistance training).	Exercise, coordination, cognitive load
Full contact practice	Following medical clearance, participate in normal training activities	Restore confidence, assessment of functional skills by coaching staff
Return to play	Normal game play	

(From McCrory, P., et al. [2009]. Consensus statement on concussion in sport: The 3rd International Conference on Concussion in Sports Held in Zurich, November 2008. *JAT, 44*(4), 434–448.)

Participation in several sports carries a particularly high risk for head and neck injuries. Football accounts for 40% of all concussion injuries in school sports. Although 69% of deaths between 1945 and 1999 were from brain injuries, the incidence of serious head injuries has decreased since the late 1980s.[63] Fatalities in children younger than age 12 have not been reported, but the mortality rate is 0.44 per 100,000 participants in tackle football. The incidence of serious head injury is still 0.75 to 1.5 per 100,000 participants per season, with a mortality rate of 0.5 to 1.09 per season.[48] Sosin and colleagues[301] documented 247 deaths from traumatic brain injury of the 140,000 head injuries in those younger than 18 years between 1989 and 1992.

Severe spinal injuries may result in paralysis and total disability. A population-based study over 7 years identified 32 children younger than 15 years of age who sustained spinal fracture, dislocation, or severe ligamentous injury; sports were the cause of all injuries in children over the age of 10 years.[99] Rugby, a popular collision sport outside the United States, has head and neck injury rates similar to those of American football. Wrestling has the second highest injury rate of all high school sports, although the central nervous system injury rate is low. The rate of catastrophic wrestling injuries (cervical ligament injury, spinal cord contusion, severe head injury, or herniated disk) is 2.11 per year (1 per 100,000 participants) as a result of direct blows or falls.[39] Baseball accounts for a large number of concussions secondary to collision with the bat, other players, or the ball, although exact incidence figures have not been reported. Diving accounts for 3% to 21% of all cervical spine injuries in young people.[38] Noguchi[230] noted that swimming and gymnastics accounted for 51% and 22.8%, respectively, of all spinal injuries in persons younger than 30 years of age.

Most neck injuries are caused by hyperflexion or hyperextension. Hyperflexion injuries, the most common, result from spearing (Figure 15-3). Because of the poorly developed musculature in young athletes and the commonly associated fracture, hyperflexion injury can be serious. Hyperextension injuries often occur even in the absence of severe force because the anterior neck musculature is weaker than the posterior musculature. Common causes are face or head tackling (Figure 15-4). Hyperextension injury with a rotatory component is the most common cause of nerve root damage.[37,306] Evaluation of these injuries should always include radiographs of the cervical spine. In the adolescent, the second cervical vertebra is normally displaced posteriorly over the third secondary to hypermobility. This pseudosubluxation is normal and not the result of injury[57] but should be referred for assessment.

Another common injury is a "burner," which is a traction injury to the brachial plexus. It is caused by a forceful blow to the head from the side creating lateral deviation of the head or from depression of the shoulder while the head and neck are fixed. Repeated injuries may cause weakness of the deltoid, biceps, and teres major muscles, which should be

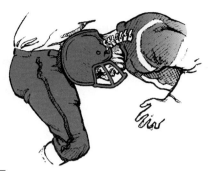

Figure 15-3 Hyperflexion damage from head butting. (From Birrer, R., & Brecher, D. [1987]. *Common sports injuries in youngsters.* Oradell, NJ: Medical Economics, p. 36.)

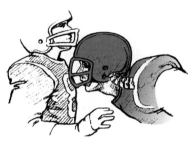

Figure 15-4 Hyperextension injury from face blocking. (From Birrer, R., & Brecher, D. [1987]. *Common sports injuries in youngsters.* Oradell, NJ: Medical Economics, p. 38.)

resolved with strengthening exercises. If the use of a collar or a change in technique or neck strength does not solve the problem, cessation of participation is warranted.[56] Return to play in a collision or contact sport following any type of cervical injury should be closely monitored.[60]

THORACIC AND LUMBAR SPINAL INJURIES

Back injuries in children are different from those in adults and require careful evaluation.[113,166,330] Spinal injuries can occur in both the thoracic and the lumbar areas, although thoracic injuries are rare. Costovertebral injury secondary to compression of the rib cage in a pile-up in football or from a forceful takedown in wrestling can injure the costovertebral articulations. Complaints include pain and muscle spasm along the associated rib. Axial compression forces on a preflexed spine, as in sledding or tobogganing, can fracture the vertebrae, particularly at the vulnerable T12-L1 level. These injuries can cause pain but are frequently asymptomatic.[37,306]

The most common injuries in the lumbar spine are spondylolysis and spondylolisthesis. One study of 3132 competitive athletes ages 15 to 27 years noted an incidence of spondylolysis of 12.5%.[276] Repeated hyperflexion and hyperextension in football blocking, clean and jerk lift, diving, pole vaulting, wrestling, high jump, or gymnastic maneuvers can place excessive forces on the pars interarticularis and cause a stress fracture. Spondylolisthesis, or fracture and slippage of one vertebra on another, usually L5 over S1, is most common at ages 9 to 14 years. Loading of a bilateral spondylolysis, in which there is a defect in the bony connection of the posterior arch with the vertebral body, can cause a spondylolisthesis, as can traumatic or repetitive bilateral loading of a normal spine. The slippage is graded from 1 to 4, depending on the degree of slippage. Athletes with grade 2 or greater slippage should be counseled against participation in weight lifting, baseball, diving, gymnastics, or wrestling. Participation in basketball or football is permissible with use of a brace.[83,87,166,207] The growth spurt in the spine causes lumbar lordosis secondary to the enhanced anterior growth with posterior tethering by the heavy lumbodorsal fascia. This biomechanical situation increases the tendency of posterior element failure at the pars and perhaps at the disk.[214] Athletes with spondylolysis are managed in a brace until healing occurs. Physical therapy is indicated to maintain flexibility in the lumbosacral spine and the spinal and hip musculature and to improve trunk and abdominal muscle strength while braced. Surgery is indicated only in cases of unstable lesions or nerve root compression.[37,106,236]

The incidence of disk lesions in young athletes is unknown, but several studies have demonstrated that disk herniation can occur. Although acute trauma may cause this condition, degenerative changes of the vertebral bodies and intervertebral joints may be the contributing factors, with trauma being the acute precipitating incident.[191]

SHOULDER INJURIES

Specific shoulder injuries can be predicted based on the biomechanics of the sport and the age of the athlete.[146,160] Participation in football, wrestling, and ice hockey may increase the likelihood of upper extremity fractures and dislocations, and sports with repeated overhead activities, such as volleyball and baseball, are more likely to result in overuse injuries.[1] The hyperelasticity of juvenile joints, particularly the shoulder, makes them vulnerable to passive and dynamic instability patterns that can predispose the shoulder to injury.[146,249]

Acromioclavicular sprains may occur in the immature athlete without clavicular fracture; however, it is more common in skeletally mature athletes. The most common mechanism is direct force from a fall or blow to the lateral aspect of the shoulder or a fall on an outstretched arm.[37,106,160,209] Grade I and II sprains are more common in the athlete whose skeleton is immature. Grade III sprains commonly rupture the dorsal clavicular periosteum, but the acromioclavicular and coracoclavicular ligaments remain intact.[160,249] These lesions are treated symptomatically with rest, ice, compression, and elevation (RICE) in a sling. Exercises are often necessary to increase scapulothoracic and glenohumeral mobility and strength after the sprain is healed.

Fractures are most common in the middle third of the clavicle from a direct blow. These can be actual fractures in the older child or greenstick fractures in the youngster. They are managed with a figure-of-eight strap until healed.

The proximal humerus is an area of bone growth in children and is typically not as strong as the surrounding capsule and ligamentous structures. Therefore, fractures are more common in children than in adults, who are more prone to dislocation. Epiphyseal displacements occur in the younger child, and metaphyseal fractures are more common in the older child or adolescent.[209] Once bony healing is identified, therapeutic intervention to normalize mobility and strength of the scapular, shoulder, and elbow muscles is frequently indicated.[249]

Little League shoulder, a relatively common injury in young pitchers and catchers, involves a fracture of the proximal humeral growth plate secondary to rotatory torque. A skeletally immature athlete who complains of proximal shoulder pain in the absence of trauma should be suspected of having an epiphyseal fracture until proved otherwise. The athlete should not do any throwing until the pain subsides[146,160,249]; however, strengthening of the parascapular and core musculature is indicated to facilitate a more smooth transition back to sports once the pain has subsided.

Frank anterior subluxation and dislocation of the glenohumeral joint is rare in children but common in adolescents. Because of the laxity of juvenile joints, a blow or forceful maneuver in abduction, external rotation, or extension can dislodge the head of the humerus.[37,106,249,306] This condition is common in contact sports, gymnastics, and overhead throwing sports. Patients with posterior glenohumeral instability respond better to conservative strengthening of appropriate musculature than those with anterior instability, although a program of scapular and shoulder muscle strengthening in a biomechanically correct range of motion should be attempted. Motion should be limited to ranges that prevent chronic subluxation. Surgery is more often an option with anterior or multidirectional instability but may occur in the case of posterior instability.[160,249] Debate exists in the literature regarding the most appropriate timing of arthroscopic stabilization following first time shoulder dislocations in adolescent athletes.[84,167] Future research will need to identify if immediate surgical stabilization is indicated after first time dislocation or if a trial of conservative management would be successful in some athletes.

Rotator cuff tears are not as common in the skeletally immature athlete as in the older athlete. They occur in throwing and racquet sports, as well as from direct contact blows in collision sports. These tears can be treated successfully with arthroscopic surgery and rehabilitation that includes strength and endurance training for all scapular and shoulder muscles, as well as training with correct biomechanical movements of the shoulder complex.[160]

Rotator cuff impingement syndrome (Figure 15-5) is a frequent injury in athletes younger than 25 years of age.

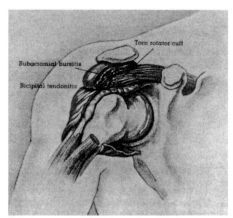

Figure 15-5   Common causes of impingement. (From Birrer, R., & Brecher, D. [1987]. *Common sports injuries in youngsters.* Oradell, NJ: Medical Economics, p. 61.)

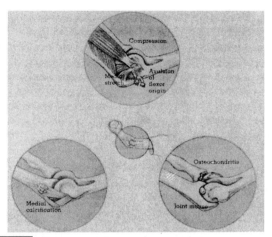

Figure 15-6   Little League elbow. (From Birrer, R., & Brecher, D. [1987]. *Common sports injuries in youngsters.* Oradell, NJ: Medical Economics, p. 74.)

More than 50% of swimmers aged 12 to 18 years complain of shoulder pain.[37,106,306] Unlike adults who typically present with impingement resulting from a mechanical compression in the subacromial space (primary impingement), children often present with impingement symptoms caused by excessive laxity or mobility in the shoulder joint complex described as secondary impingement. This may be due to a laxity of the static stabilizers in the shoulder with an inability of the dynamic shoulder stabilizers to compensate appropriately. Others theorize altered arthrokinematics of the shoulder may be due to a contracture around the shoulder with loss of internal rotation at 90° of abduction and with increased external rotation in all positions of abduction. This might reflect a tightened posterior and a loosened anterior capsule, suggesting a tendency to translate anteriorly during functional movement patterns. Conservative physical therapy with a focus on improved strength and muscle activation of the dynamic shoulder stabilizing musculature, along with normalization of mobility and dynamic movement patterns, has been successful at addressing the underlying instability.[160,209,249] All positions of impingement (anterior, lateral, or overhead) should be modified until the athlete is pain-free.

ELBOW INJURIES

Supracondylar fracture of the humerus is the second most common fracture in the skeletally immature client. Most of these fractures occur in the age group of 5 to 10 years. They are often the result of significant forces into extension. Avulsion fractures of the medial epicondyle are also common in the population and are associated with elbow dislocations or throwing injuries. Anatomic reduction is indicated with internal fixation, when appropriate. Loss of motion is a common impairment following these injuries; therefore, early protected range of motion to avoid loss of extension is critical.[116,160] Subsequent to healing, normalization of mobility and strength of the shoulder, elbow, and forearm are necessary for full function.

Repetitive microtrauma from pitching may result in epiphyseal fracture of the radial head. Loss of extension and supination with a history of repetitive compressive loading of the radiocapitellar joint may indicate a fracture. A radial head fracture is treated with rest.[80,146] Forcefully pulling the arm of a child younger than 7 years old can subluxate the radial head because of the poor development of the annular ligament. The child positions the injured arm in flexion and pronation, dangling it at the side of the body.[37,106,160,306]

Elbow dislocation is seen in contact sports secondary to a fall on an abducted, extended arm. Early reduction will avoid neurovascular damage, and further evaluation and radiographs are necessary to assess the presence of associated fracture. Early protected mobility is necessary to preserve normal elbow motion.[37,106,160] Physical therapy to normalize elbow and forearm mobility and to improve strength at the elbow, forearm, and hand is appropriate.

Little League elbow commonly results from the extreme valgus stress placed on the epicondyles during the acceleration phase of pitching (Figure 15-6). If this is not recognized and regular throwing continues, mild separation of the medial epicondyle with hypertrophy, irregularity, fragmentation, and avulsion can occur. The most serious damage is the jamming of the radial head against the capitellum on the lateral side, a finding that occurs in 8% to 10% of young pitchers. This jamming can result in osteochondritis of the capitellum, avascular necrosis of the radial head, and loose bodies within the joint. Treatment is RICE and rest from throwing.[37,106,116,236] Eventual alteration of throwing technique may be necessary.

Tennis elbow is seen in a variety of racquet sports as a result of repeated injury to the lateral epicondyle. A faulty stroke initiates the process. The resulting friction between the extensor muscles, the lateral epicondyle, and the radial head causes irritation, microtears in the extensor muscle origin, and adhesions between the annular ligament and the joint capsule. Using tightly strung racquets, racquets with small handles, and old tennis balls will aggravate the situation. Rehabilitation to decrease irritation, reduce adhesions, and strengthen the forearm and hand musculature is required. Alteration of technique and equipment, such as enlargement of the racquet grip area or reduction of string tension, is helpful.[106,116,146]

WRIST AND HAND INJURIES

Because of the inherent complexity of the anatomy of the wrist joint, potentially serious injuries may be missed or underdiagnosed. Careful diagnosis using knowledge of biomechanics of the wrist and hand is crucial.[37,116,160,306]

Fractures about the wrist follow an age-related pattern. In the young child a torus, or buckle fracture, of the distal radial epiphysis is common after a fall. Clinical signs are minimal pain and tenderness, so careful radiologic examination is necessary. Simple splinting is adequate for healing.[37,55,160,236] Metaphyseal fractures of the distal radius and ulna are more common in the child. Often displaced, they require reduction with the use of anesthesia. In the younger adolescent, fractures through the growth plate are common, again from falls, and require operative reduction to minimize trauma to the growth plate.[160] Rehabilitation to regain normal forearm and wrist mobility as well as wrist and grip strength is desirable. Posttraumatic arthritis of the wrist and hand has been documented in active children. Management requires careful monitoring with nonoperative techniques to permit extensive remodeling, although occasionally surgery is necessary.[252] Stress injuries to the distal radial epiphysis have been noted in athletes such as gymnasts who bear weight on their hands. Complaints of pain with wrist dorsiflexion and of wrist stiffness are common. Radiographs demonstrate a widened epiphysis, cystic changes, and breaking of the distal metaphysis. Management consists of cessation of gymnastics with or without casting.[160]

Although fracture of most carpal bones is rare, fracture of the navicular or scaphoid bone is common in children from 12 to 15 years of age. This fracture results from a fall on the dorsiflexed hand of an outstretched arm. Although the fracture may not be initially visible on a radiograph, early diagnosis is important because of the high incidence of avascular necrosis and nonunion. If tenderness in the anatomic snuffbox occurs with a high degree of suspicion of fracture, use of a short-arm spica cast will be adequate management.[37,106,117,306]

Because the hand and fingers are so essential in most sports, the small structures absorb tremendous forces of initial contact, and therefore injuries to the hand and fingers are common.[37,236,306] Dislocations are uncommon in the child's hand because the forces necessary to produce these injuries are usually dissipated by production of a fracture. If dislocations do occur, it is usually in the adolescent and in patterns similar to those in an adult. Thus, the most common dislocation occurs at the carpometacarpal joint of the thumb,

usually secondary to axial compression forces on the thumb tip in contact sports. Although reduction is easy, maintenance is not, and chronic instability can result. The thumb is put in a short-arm thumb spica, and participation in sports should be avoided for 6 weeks. A short opponens splint is advisable for the initial 6 weeks of reentry to play.[26,55,160]

Dorsal dislocation of the thumb metacarpophalangeal joint is the most common dislocation in the hand of a child. A fall or forceful contact hyperextends the metacarpophalangeal joint. If the proximal phalanx is parallel to the metacarpal, the volar plate has been avulsed and surgical reduction is necessary. Cast immobilization for 3 weeks with sports participation permitted is adequate for healing. Physical therapy may be indicated to normalize thumb mobility and strength following casting. Metacarpophalangeal dislocations in the fingers are rare except for those that affect the index finger. After this injury is reduced, splinting in flexion for 3 weeks with immediate mobilization after splint removal is the treatment of choice.[26,37,106,306]

Joint injuries are common in ball sports and skiing. The metacarpophalangeal joint of the thumb is the most commonly injured joint in skiers. The majority of these injuries in youth are bony gamekeeper's thumb in which the ulnar collateral ligament avulses a segment of bone, as compared with the purely ligamentous injury in adults. If the bony fragment lies close to its origin, good results are obtained with use of a short-arm thumb spica cast for 6 weeks, followed by exercises to normalize mobility and strength. Athletic participation may continue in some cases and can be facilitated by the use of a custom molded splint to protect the healing tissues. If the radiograph is negative, integrity of the ulnar collateral ligament must be established by assessing radial deviation in extension and 30° of flexion. Deviation of greater than 30° indicates at least a partial tear. No firm end point in full extension or greater than 45° of deviation in flexion indicates full ligamentous tear with volar plate injury, which will require surgical repair.[26,37,160,306] Hand therapy is necessary to regain normal mobility, strength, and pinch.

Jammed fingers are common injuries in all age groups. Axial compression force to the fingertips causes distal interphalangeal flexion with proximal interphalangeal hyperextension. Reduction is easily accomplished by distal traction. Buddy taping will allow the athlete to return to play.[26,67,306] Caution should be exhibited, however, because fractures through the growth plate of the phalanx are common. These intraarticular, or neck, fractures have a great tendency to displace and then require open reduction with internal fixation.[55,209] In the absence of a fracture or dislocation, damage to the collateral ligaments can occur and is managed in similar fashion. Jamming at the distal interphalangeal joint can result in "mallet finger," or tearing of the terminal extensor tendon with or without a bony fragment. This injury is easily managed with use of a dorsal extension splint for 6 to

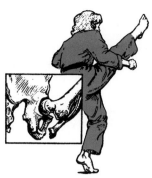

Figure 15-7   Avulsion of the ischial tuberosity. (From Birrer, R., & Brecher, D. [1987]. *Common sports injuries in youngsters.* Oradell, NJ: Medical Economics, p. 101.)

8 weeks. If active and passive extension ranges are equal at 6 weeks, active flexion can be initiated. If not, splinting is continued for another month. Participation is allowed with the splint in place.[37,106,160,306]

PELVIS AND HIP INJURIES

Because the hip and pelvis have complex ossification patterns and fuse late in childhood, the potential for injury is high. The acetabulum has three sections joined by triradiate cartilage. Likewise, three ossification centers exist on the femoral head: the capital femoral epiphysis, the greater trochanter, and the lesser trochanter. The circular vascularity of the femoral head and neck also creates risk for injury in the growing child.[244,331]

Fractures are uncommon but can occur in the epiphyseal plate, the femoral neck, or the subtrochanteric area. Slipped capital femoral epiphysis (SCFE) is not caused by sports but must be suspected in any athlete with persistent hip or knee pain and a limp. SCFE typically occurs during the period of rapid growth in adolescence in either obese or very thin males, but it can occur in females as well. Surgical reduction with internal fixation is necessary (see Chapter 14). Hip dislocations, usually posterior, are uncommon but serious; these can be resolved with few long-term consequences if managed carefully.[133]

Fractures of the neck or subtrochanteric area are rare but can be the result of severe trauma, usually incurred during contact sports such as football and rugby. Surgical reduction is necessary to maintain position.[331] More common are avulsion fractures from a sudden violent muscular contraction or excessive muscle stretch. The most common sites are the anterior-superior iliac spine (origin of the sartorius), the ischium (hamstring origin) (Figure 15-7), the lesser trochanter (insertion of the iliopsoas), the anterior-inferior iliac spine (rectus femoris origin), and the iliac crest (abdominal insertion).[217] These injuries are classic in sprinting, jumping, soccer, football, and weight lifting. Rest with gradual increase of excursion to full mobility followed by progressive resistance exercise and reintegration to play is the treatment sequence.[37,213,306,331] One less traumatic overuse parallel of

avulsion is iliac apophysitis, which usually affects adolescent track, field, or cross-country athletes or dancers. Repeated contraction of the tensor fasciae latae, rectus femoris, sartorius, gluteus medius, and oblique abdominal muscles causes nonspecific pain and tenderness over the iliac crest. Rest helps this problem,[37,106] but often exercises to increase strength and normalize two-joint muscle flexibility are required.

Stress fractures and osteitis pubis are being diagnosed more frequently as a result of repetitive microtrauma in runners or athletes who have suddenly increased their involvement in jumping or kicking activities. Persistent pain and tenderness in the groin with limited mobility and activity-related increases in pain could signal either of these conditions. Radiographs showing inflammation, demineralization, and sclerosis confirm the diagnosis of osteitis pubis, but a bone scan is necessary to diagnose a stress fracture. Stress fractures have been seen in the pelvis at the junction of the ischium and pubic ramus and in the femoral neck and shaft.[37,306,331] Relative rest, use of crutches, and restriction from percussive activities (running and jumping) are required for resolution of these disorders.

Snapping hip syndrome is an overuse problem noted in gymnasts, dancers, and sprinters. The term "snapping hip syndrome" can refer either to irritation of the iliotibial band over the greater trochanter with hip motion or to tenosynovitis of the iliopsoas tendon near its femoral insertion. Usually, relative rest, use of appropriate modalities, stretching, and improved muscle strength overcome these symptoms.[209,331]

A serious condition seen in the young athlete age 5 to 12 years is avascular necrosis of the femoral head. Activity can irritate the synovium, leading to joint effusion and reduction of the blood supply to the femoral head. The initial complaint is nonspecific hip pain, but radiographs demonstrate periosteal rarefaction followed by sclerosis and irregular collapse of the femoral head. Bracing or surgery may be required, depending on the degree of progression of the problem (see Chapter 14).[106,209,306]

Contusions are common, but the most frequent is the hip pointer. This iliac crest contusion, occurring typically in football or hockey, is caused by a driving blow by a helmet. The overlying muscle is damaged with a resultant subperiosteal hematoma. RICE and padding will resolve this problem with time.[106,306] Occasionally, use of ultrasound and soft tissue mobilization with stretching may be necessary.

KNEE INJURIES

As the largest joint in the body and one with minimal anatomic protection, the knee is the focal point of stress forces applied along the tibia and femur. Consequently, it is not only the site of macrotrauma but also the most frequent site of overuse injury.[148,170,305]

Fractures about the knee, although not frequent, are significant for their possible influences on growth.[316,344] Distal femoral epiphyseal fractures occur in the young athlete as a consequence of twisting injuries. Careful open anatomic reduction with internal fixation is necessary to avoid subsequent growth disturbances.[308] Physical therapy is usually necessary for children who sustain distal femoral or proximal tibial epiphyseal fractures. Either open reduction with internal fixation or casting causes loss of knee and ankle mobility and decreased thigh and calf muscle strength. Rehabilitation to reverse these effects and retrain the child in balance and agility skills is necessary.

Fractures of the proximal tibial epiphysis are rare but can be treacherous because of associated popliteal artery damage and compartment syndrome. More common is fracture of the tibial tuberosity alone or in association with the proximal tibia. These are most common at the end of adolescence in jumping sports such as basketball and track. These fractures can be managed with immobilization if minimal displacement has occurred or with internal fixation if displaced. Growth disturbances are rare because of the late occurrence of the fracture.[106,211] Stress fractures were rare but are being reported more commonly in the tibias of runners. Reduction of the loading stress of the involved limb is recommended until healing occurs.[308] Ligament injuries are becoming more common in the young athlete, with one study reporting medial collateral ligament injury in children as young as 4 years of age.[211] All ligament injuries should be assessed for coincident physis fractures. Medial collateral ligament tears in youth can include both the superficial and the capsular components of the ligament. Nonoperative treatment with splinting and avoidance of valgus stress has been successful in adolescents, so it may be possible to obtain equally good results in younger children.[106] Physical therapy to improve lower extremity strength and retrain coordination is often needed.

Anterior cruciate ligament tears in the preteen group are occurring with increased frequency and may represent either avulsion fractures at the tibial insertion or midsubstance tears of the ligament.[3,12] The fracture of the tibial spine usually occurs through the cancellous bone, demonstrating avulsion of the tibial spine on a radiograph. The mechanism of injury is typically an accident or fall in preteens and a contact sport in adolescents. Casting in 30° of knee flexion is accepted practice for minimally displaced fractures, but internal fixation is needed for full displacement of the fragment. Midsubstance tears of the anterior cruciate ligament are most common in the adolescent but are occurring more frequently in children under 15 years of age.[337] Traditional reconstructive procedures are avoided in the adolescent under the age of 15 years because of fear of injury to the growth plate with the proximal tibial drill hole.[129,163] Alternate surgical options that include modified procedures that avoid the growth plate have recently been utilized to provide mechanical stability to the knee and reduce the risk of secondary injury to the surrounding articular cartilage and meniscus during physical activity.[11,161] Classic conservative

management includes functional bracing and development of muscular strength and balance for knee stability.[162]

Internal derangement of the knee joint can be either juvenile osteochondritis dissecans or meniscal injury. The etiology of juvenile osteochondritis dissecans is still an enigma. Compression of the tibial spine against the medial femoral condyle, interruption of the vascularity, anatomic variations in the knee, and abnormal subchondral bone are all possible causes. The most common sites of involvement are the lateral side of the medial femoral condyle and the lateral femoral condyle in the weight-bearing region or posteriorly. The condition usually causes pain, recurrent swelling, or catching in the knee. Pain is usually evident as the tibia rotates internally and the knee extends from a flexed position.[106,211,306] Because these lesions have a poor prognosis after skeletal maturity, every attempt should be made to gain healing before growth plate closure. In the child younger than 15 years of age, diminished activity to the point of not bearing weight is suggested. Drilling of the condyles with removal of fragments is recommended in children older than 15 years of age.[52] This procedure usually necessitates restriction of running and jumping for at least 6 weeks with concomitant intensive rehabilitation to regain strength, balance, and agility in the lower extremity.[106,122]

The challenge of meniscal injuries in the young athlete is accurate diagnosis.[219] Often the initial incident is forgotten and clinical testing is less diagnostic than in the adult. Arthroscopic excision or repair is the treatment of choice if conservative management fails. Excision necessitates physical therapy to regain mobility and strength deficits. Meniscal repair requires further limitations of knee mobility and weight bearing while healing occurs.[41] Discoid lateral meniscus can create joint line tenderness, decreased joint mobility, effusion, and, most notably, a prominent snap in the lateral compartment as the knee is extended.[308] Normal menisci do not go through a discoid stage during development. The complete type of discoid meniscus, producing symptoms in late adolescence, is distinguished by intact peripheral attachments. Good results are obtained with saucerization of the meniscus. The Wrisberg type of discoid meniscus, which is more common in the pediatric group, has an attachment only through the ligament of Wrisberg and can be resolved by cutting the ligament and removing the portions with no peripheral attachments.[216,231,308] As in adults, meniscal tear in the presence of anterior cruciate ligament injury can occur and should be carefully evaluated and managed.[337]

The most common knee conditions in children are disorders of the patellar mechanism.[30,308,324] Macrotrauma, repetitive microtrauma, and growth all can contribute to the disorders of the patellofemoral joint. Patellofemoral pain is the most frequent problem in the young athlete. Malalignment of the patellofemoral joint is the major cause of this pain. Several factors can cause or contribute to this malalignment. Anatomic factors such as patella alta, large Q angle, hip anteversion, flattened lateral femoral condyle, shallow

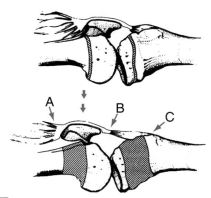

Figure 15-8 Tension resulting from growth. Pain may occur at the patella **(A)**, lower pole of the patella **(B)**, or patellar tendon insertion on the tibia **(C)**. (From Micheli, L. [1983]. Overuse injuries in children's sports: The growth factor. *Orthopedic Clinics of North America, 14*, 353.)

femoral groove, or pes planus and hyperpronation can cause abnormal tracking of the patella during knee motion.[317] Acquired factors such as weakness of the medial quadriceps or hip external rotators, tension in the lateral retinaculum and lateral soft tissues, or ligamentous laxity can affect patellar alignment and tracking (Figure 15-8). The malalignment of the patella in relation to the femoral groove can be the result of a more laterally positioned patella or a more internally rotated femur.[265] The source of pain has been postulated to be the increased stress on the subchondral bone from abnormal patellar stresses, increased tension in the lateral retinaculum, or formation of synovitis from articular cartilage degeneration.[317] Management of patellofemoral pain can be conservative or surgical. Conservative management consists of early relative rest, balancing of muscle strength and length, and correction of abnormal lower extremity biomechanics.[341] Surgical options include arthroscopic management of the articular cartilage, lateral retinacular release, and patellar realignment.[209,307]

Apophysitis, or degeneration of the ossification centers where tendons attach with chronic inflammation and microavulsion, is common in the knee in girls between ages 8 and 13 years and in boys between 10 and 15 years. These can result from longitudinal traction with bone growth or from repetitive activity of sports participation. The most common apophysitides are Osgood-Schlatter disease of the tibial tubercle and Sinding-Larsen-Johansson disease at the inferior pole of the patella. Careful differential diagnosis is necessary to correctly identify these disorders (see Chapter 14). Relative rest, maintenance of quadriceps muscle strength with pain-free exercise, and possible extension splinting are treatment options.[37,191,209,295,306]

Infrapatellar tendinitis or traction irritation at the inferior pole, otherwise known as jumper's knee, is noted most frequently in the older adolescent. The etiology includes involvement in sports that require running, jumping,

climbing, or kicking.[30] RICE with subsequent strengthening of the knee musculature is important in treatment. Assessment of two-joint muscle length is vital because tightness of the hamstring muscles or iliotibial band may increase the flexion moment at the knee.[30,37]

Patellar subluxation or dislocation can be seen in young athletes secondary to the stresses of sports requiring cutting and twisting such as soccer, dancing, cheerleading, gymnastics, and track jumping events or as a result of a direct blow to the knee. Imbalance of the length or strength of the extensor muscles, the hamstrings, the retinaculum, or the iliotibial band, as well as anatomic malalignments such as genu valgus, patella alta, or shallow condylar cup, can be etiologic factors. Management of patellar instability may include bracing in conjunction with physical therapy to normalize length-strength relationships. Failure of conservative management, although the exception, may necessitate surgical intervention to realign the patella by release of the tight structures or by alteration of the line of pull of the infrapatellar tendon.[122,209]

ANKLE AND FOOT INJURIES

Because of the peculiarities of their growing skeleton and their penchant for ingenious physical activity, children suffer from foot and ankle problems that may not have counterparts in the adult.[195,282] Injuries to the distal tibial and fibular growth plates are common in the young athlete. Gregg and Das[125] have classified growth plate injuries into a clinically useful system (Figure 15-9). The most common fractures to the ankle in the skeletally immature athlete are the Salter-Harris type 1 and 2 injuries to the distal fibula. Although these fractures can occur with adduction and abduction injury to the distal tibia, they frequently occur alone as a result of inversion injury. The Ottawa rules for prediction of need for radiograph to rule out fracture have been validated in children.[182] The Ottawa rules state that an ankle series is indicated only for patients with pain in the malleolar zone and bone tenderness at the posterior edge of either the medial or lateral malleolus or inability to bear weight immediately after injury and take four steps in the emergency room. The rules further state that a foot series is only required with midfoot pain and bone tenderness at the base of the fifth metatarsal or bone tenderness at the navicular or inability to bear weight immediately and in the emergency room. Treatment with immobilization in a short leg cast for 4 to 6 weeks is suggested, although the fracture will usually heal even if untreated.[152] Physical therapy after casting to increase ankle and foot mobility and strength and to improve balance may be indicated. Increasing incidence of osteochondral defects of the talar dome has necessitated a review of surgical options for treatment.[319]

Type 2 injury of the distal tibia is a result of ankle pronation and eversion. Common in football and soccer players, this injury is frequently associated with greenstick fracture

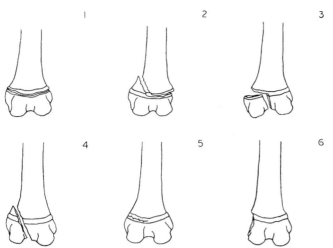

Figure 15-9 Modified Salter-Harris classification of growth plate injuries: 1, Disruption entirely confined to the growth plate; distraction or slip injury. 2, Fracture line runs partially through the growth plate then extends through the metaphysis. 3, Fracture line runs partially through the growth plate then extends through the epiphysis. 4, Combined disruption of metaphysis, growth plate, and epiphysis. 5, Crush or compression injury of growth plate. 6, Abrasion, avulsion, or burn of the perichondral ring of the growth plate. (From *Gregg, J., & Das, M. [1982]. Foot and ankle problems in the preadolescent and adolescent athlete. Clinics in Sports Medicine, 1, 133.*)

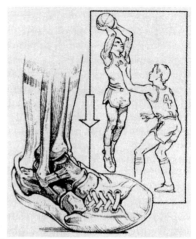

Figure 15-10 Plantar flexion-inversion injury. (From *Birrer, R., & Brecher, D. [1987]. Common sports injuries in youngsters.* Oradell, NJ: Medical Economics, p. 120.)

of the distal fibula. Care must be taken to reduce these fractures and immobilize them in a long leg cast with knee flexion to prevent impaction of the tibial metaphysis into the growth plate. The results of this type of fracture are unpredictable; occasionally angulation or premature closure of the plate occurs.[106,282] The most common mechanism of injury in type 3 and 4 fractures of the medial malleolus is ankle supination or inversion. Adduction injuries appear in approximately 15% of these injuries and are characterized by medial displacement of part or all of the distal tibial epiphysis. The affected children are usually young, so the incidence of growth disturbance is higher. Internal fixation with restoration of ankle joint congruity is critical.[181]

Because of the porosity of the bones of the foot in a child, stress fractures are common in the metatarsals in all jumping and distance running activities. If suspected by local tenderness that is aggravated with activity, these injuries should be casted for 3 weeks. After casting, one can progressively and slowly increase activities to former levels over 3 more weeks.[106,282]

Several types of ischemia can occur in the bones of the child's foot. Freiberg infarction, or avascular necrosis of the metatarsal epiphysis, occurs in those who walk or perform on their toes. Initial synovitis is followed by sclerosis, resorption, plate fracture and collapse, and bone re-formation. It does not affect children younger than 12 years of age. Most

commonly affected is the second metatarsal head. Treatment consists of cessation of toe-walking, wearing high-heeled shoes, and jumping. A negative-heel shoe is fitted. Kohler's disease is seen in active boys age 3 to 7 years who have a tendency to cavus feet (see Chapter 14). Focal tenderness and swelling around the navicular bone are noted clinically. The radiograph reveals sclerosis and irregular rarefaction indicative of ischemia. Conservative treatment calls for use of a walking cast for 6 to 8 weeks followed by use of an arch support and limitation of activity for another 6 weeks.[211]

Although ankle sprains can occur in the young athlete, epiphyseal fractures are more common. Sprains occur in the older adolescent near the end of growth. The common cause of injury is landing on the lateral border of a plantar-flexed foot (Figure 15-10). Management is similar to that in adults. Quinn and colleagues[269] have noted a decrease in ankle sprains with external support. Surgery is indicated only in multiple sprains with gross instability.

Sever disease, or apophysitis of the calcaneus, is an Osgood-Schlatter syndrome of the foot (Figure 15-11). It is seen most frequently in basketball and soccer players with complaint of heel pain on running. The usual age of occurrence is 8 to 13 years. Frequently, tight heel cords, a tendency toward in-toeing, and forefoot varus are noted. Treatment consists of heel cord stretching and initial use of a heel lift in well-constructed shoes (see Chapter 14).[106]

REHABILITATION AND RETURN TO PLAY

In adults, rehabilitation following common sports injuries and subsequent medical treatment (i.e., anterior cruciate ligament injury and reconstruction) is described in the literature. Commonly, rehabilitation guidelines that are accepted practice in adults are often applied to children and

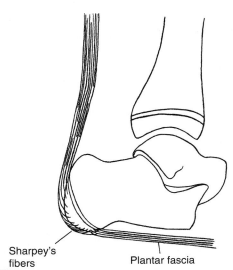

Figure 15-11   Insertion of Sharpey's fibers from the Achilles tendon into the calcaneal apophysis. (From Gregg, J., & Das, M. [1982]. Foot and ankle problems in the preadolescent and adolescent athlete. *Clinics in Sports Medicine, 1,* 140.)

Sharpey's fibers

Plantar fascia

adolescents. However, rehabilitation in a child or adolescent requires age-appropriate modifications, specifically related to relevant anatomy, surgical procedures/modifications performed (if applicable), protection and preservation of future bone growth, as well as the unique psychosocial aspects of the pediatric or adolescent patient.

Children and adolescents require supervised rehabilitation programs that begin with first aid on the field of play.[304] The goal of first aid is to contain the extent of injury and reduce any possibility of further harm. Following, or in conjunction with medical management of the injury, the long-term goal of rehabilitation is return to play in a safe manner with minimal risk of further injury. In healthy individuals, studies indicate that comprehensive training programs utilizing components of strength, balance and core stability training, as well as biomechanical technique and plyometric training induce changes in movement mechanics that are associated with reducing injury risk.[137,138,140,222] Similar principles are utilized when establishing a rehabilitation program for individuals following injury. Following injury, successful rehabilitation that advances toward unrestricted activity and sport participation requires a comprehensive, progressive, and criterion-based plan of physical therapy care.

A comprehensive rehabilitation program and individualized plan of care maximizes outcomes. The physical therapy plan of care will vary based on the individual's unique characteristics and attributes within the context of their injury and relevant anatomy (i.e., open versus closed epiphyseal "growth" plates). Physical characteristics, such as anatomic alignment, skeletal age, body mass, severity of impairments and injury history, are considered in rehabilitation

planning.[272,336] Also considered are psychosocial attributes, such as motivation, maturity level, patient/family goals, kinesthetic awareness, and demonstration of fear avoidance or kinesiophobic movement patterns. The young athlete's specific goals, as well as the magnitude of his or her impairments and functional limitations, will guide the specific interventions and pace of rehabilitation progression. For the young athlete, communication among the health care providers, as well as with the patient, family, coaches, and other involved personnel, will ensure effective collaboration with the recommended plan of care. Given the limited information available regarding injuries in young individuals, the rehabilitation specialist plays a large role in the education of the patient, patient's family, and the teaching and coaching staff involved with the young athlete.

Successful physical therapy management requires adherence to a systematic and criterion-based progression of interventions and considerations for the unique psychosocial and anatomic aspects of a young patient. This approach to rehabilitation will protect injured tissues, promote healing, maximize outcomes, and ultimately preserve long-term tissue and joint integrity.[272,336] A rehabilitation program that is developed and advanced based on criterion-based decision making, rather than time-based decision making, is advocated to ensure adequate tissue healing and adequate accommodation of the injured tissues to the forces associated with activity.[272,336] A thorough history and clinical examination is important to establish accurate differential diagnosis and to develop an individual plan of care based on severity of impairments and functional limitations.

ACUTE AND INTERMEDIATE PHASES OF REHABILITATION

Protecting the injured tissue or joint during the early phases of healing is important for successful outcome. Adherence to necessary activity modifications may be a challenge for young, active patients. Patient and family education is important for effective cooperation with the plan of care. Resolution of impairments and progression toward functional activities is the goal of these phases of rehabilitation. Each patient's specific goals, as well as the magnitude of their impairments and functional limitations, will guide the specific interventions and pace of rehabilitation progression.

ADVANCED STAGES OF REHABILITATION

The long-term goal of rehabilitation is a safe transition and reintegration into sport following injury. The objective of the return to activity phase of rehabilitation is successful transition from advanced rehabilitation to safe participation in sports with minimal risk of injury. Criterion-based progression through the advanced stages of rehabilitation depends on achievement of clinical milestones with consideration of the participation demands for the activity and position for which the individual desires to return (i.e., the amount of cutting/pivoting, amount of overhead throwing, amount of contact, and level of activity [elite versus recreational]). Advanced stages of rehabilitation should realize resolution of pain, effusion, range of motion, and joint loading or weight-bearing restrictions. During the advanced stages of rehabilitation, the young athlete should be progressed through a functional program (based on activity- and position-specific demands) that optimizes strength and muscle performance in terms of intensity, frequency, and duration of activity.[223] Functional activities that progress neuromuscular control, including plyometric and technique training, should also be implemented.[223]

Return to Activity

Determination of timing for return to desired sports activities following injury should be based on objective measures during a comprehensive functional evaluation.[172,223] Patient reintegration into sport and activities are considered when there is demonstration of adequate tissue healing, resolution of impairments (such as pain, effusion, range of motion), adequate muscle strength and performance, and acceptable levels of functional performance necessary for the demands of the desired activity. Muscle strength should be objectively measured (via dynamometry), and recommended criterion for return to activity is involved muscle strength that is 85% to 90% of the contralateral muscle.[153,172,218,233,277]

Patient-reported outcome tools and performance-based functional assessments are also utilized in physical therapy clinical decision making.[100] A number of region-specific patient-reported outcome measures are valid and reliable measures of function during activities of daily living, recreational activities, and sport activities, although most measures were developed based on adult patient populations. A recent study[284] demonstrated the internal consistency and validity of the International Knee Documentation Committee (IKDC) Subjective Knee Evaluation Form in young individuals, ages 6 to 18 years. Measures of general health assessment, such as the Pediatric Quality of Life Inventory 4.0 Generic Core Scales (PedsQL),[326,327] are valid, responsive and reliable measures of health-related quality of life in children and adolescents (age 2 to 18 years). In addition to patient-reported measures of function, performance-based assessments are often used to determine readiness for return to sport and activity. Physical performance is often evaluated via jumping, hopping, or cutting tasks, depending on the demands of the activity of which the patient desires to return. Single limb hop tests (such as the single hop, triple hop, crossover hop, and 6-meter timed hop[232]) are often used because of their convenience and reliability.[40,45,271] Recommended criteria for return to sport are performance of involved limb that is at least 85% to 90% of the uninvolved limb.[172] Additional performance measures may also be

useful. Performance on the Star Excursion Balance Test has been associated with risk of lower extremity injury,[157,260] and a composite reach distance of >94 is recommended to reduce injury risk.[157,260] Altered movement patterns and neuromuscular control have been associated with increased risk of injuries,[139] and movement and technique assessment during high-level activities is important for safe return to activity. The drop vertical jump task has been used repeatedly as an assessment tool of lower extremity biomechanics during a plyometric task.[92,104,139,220,239,243] The Tuck Jump exercise has been advocated as another clinician-friendly and reliable tool to identify lower extremity landing technique faults during a plyometric activity.[221,223]

For young athletes participating in overhead sports, such as baseball, softball, volleyball, a progressive return to overhead activity or throwing program is warranted following resolution of identified impairments and limitations. For overhead and throwing athletes, analysis of appropriate technique and addressing identified deviations is important to prevent further injury.[278,335] During the advanced and return to sport stages of rehabilitation, adherence to a progressive return to throwing or overhead activity program[15,335] will maximize performance and mitigate risk of further injury.

The clinical-decision making for reintegration into sport activities utilizes a comprehensive and criterion-based approach that includes assessment of impairments as well as functional performance. A rehabilitation plan that culminates with a progressive reintegration of the young individual into the desired activity is advocated. Using a progressive approach toward unrestricted activity participation may be initiated with modification of activity participation, such as time of participation and demands of participation. Appropriate communication among the health care team and with the patient, family, and other involved persons (i.e., coaches) is important during the advanced stages of rehabilitation to ensure collaboration with the progressive plan of care.

THE YOUNG ATHLETE WITH A PHYSICAL DISABILITY

Children with a disability have the same activity needs as their able-bodied peers.[174] With the approval in the United States of Public Law 94-142, the Rehabilitation Act of 1973, and the Americans with Disabilities Act in 1991, a variety of physical activity and sports programs are available to those with disability.[32,64,199,332] In a survey of 100 persons with lower extremity amputations, 60% were active in sports. Persons with disabilities of both genders were most active when they are younger.[154] Of a group of 67 individuals with spinal cord injury, 72% participated in sports at least once weekly. These sports included basketball, swimming, weight lifting, road racing, and boating. The group included 19 athletes currently involved in competition.[78]

Both psychologic and physiologic benefits of sports participation have been demonstrated in individuals with disabilities. Self-concept and self-acceptance were shown to be equal or greater in athletes of various ages with disabilities when compared with control subjects who were able bodied.[81,134,250,290] Wheelchair basketball players had significantly better mental profiles than players who were able bodied and nonathletes.[251] When novice and veteran wheelchair athletes were compared, the novice group had lower perceived social adequacy and lower self-perception, suggesting that sports participation might change these perceptions in a positive way.[250] Among children with limb deficiencies, athletic competence was one predictor of higher perceived physical appearance and lower levels of depression and higher self-esteem.[325]

Disability often causes reduction of overall fitness relative to the general population.[97,126,259,270,274] Several research studies have demonstrated that individuals who participate in fitness training can reverse the reduction of physiologic fitness status. In classic studies by Zwiren and Bar-Or[345] and others, the physiologic capabilities of athletes who participated in wheelchair sports were shown to be only 9% lower than those of athletes without disabilities and fully 50% greater than those of sedentary individuals who used wheelchairs. Other studies have confirmed these findings.[31,81] Decreases in body fat and increases in muscle strength and endurance, often beyond that of individuals without disabilities, have also been documented.[81] In a comparison of the health and functional status of athletes and nonathletes with spinal cord injuries, the athletes had an average of only 2.4 physician visits per year compared with 6.7 physician visits for the nonathletes. Although they were involved in sports significantly more hours per week (10.2 ± 9.6 hours for athletes; 4.9 ± 4.1 hours for nonathletes), the athletes on average had fewer hospitalizations, decubitus ulcers, medical complications, and hours of required attendant care. The researchers concluded that the medical risks associated with intense sports activity for those with spinal cord injuries were minimal.[78]

RISK OF INJURY

Little information has been gathered on the incidence and type of sports injuries that occur in persons with a disability. Although several studies have appeared in the literature, they have had small sample sizes and select groups of individuals with specific disabilities. An exception was a survey distributed to 1200 athletes in regional wheelchair competition during 1981. One hundred two male and 27 female athletes responded. The group represented 32 sports. Seventy-two percent of all athletes had sustained at least 1 injury, with some reporting as many as 14 injuries. The most prevalent injuries were soft tissue trauma (33%), blisters (18%), and lacerations or abrasions (17%). The majority of the injuries occurred in the upper extremity. Most of

the injuries were associated with track (26%), basketball (24%), and road racing (22%).[77] A survey of the 1990 Junior National Wheelchair Games demonstrated injury rates of 97% in track, 22% in field events, and 91% in swimming among 83 athletes.[339] A 1995 study by Taylor and Williams[315] in the United Kingdom reported a similar overall rate of injury.

The largest study, a retrospective survey of 426 athletes participating in the 1989 competitions of the National Wheelchair Athletic Association (NWAA), the United States Association for Blind Athletes (USABA), and the United States Cerebral Palsy Association (USCPA), demonstrated that 32% of the respondents had at least one time-loss injury. Twenty-six percent of all injuries were from the NWAA, with 57% of this total at the shoulder and elbow. Fifty-three percent of all USABA athletes' injuries were in the lower extremity. The injuries in the USCPA athletes were noted in all areas. Injury rates were the same for athletes with or without disabilities.[96] Data from the International Flower Marathon showed that 19 athletes experienced 20 medical problems, many caused by climate and spills. Problems were more frequent in groups with disabilities caused by paraplegia and poliomyelitis. Thirteen medical problems were classified as injuries: five were ulcers and abrasions and eight were soft tissue injuries.[143] A study of the injuries at the Special Olympic games demonstrated that 3.5% of the athletes required care for an injury or illness. Track and field events consumed the least time but had the greatest injury rate.[200] The Connecticut State Special Olympics Games in 1994 through 1996 noted that the most frequent injuries were sprains/strains to the lower extremities, followed by fractures and dislocations. They also noted a six-fold increase in heat-related dehydration in 1996.[109] Data from the 2001 Special Olympics World Winter Games documented 1081 total incidents (58% mild to moderate and 41% moderate to severe). These injuries were 49.5% orthopedic and 49.8% medical with 6% requiring a hospital visit and 2% requiring admission.[302] Because limited data are available documenting the occurrence or management of injuries in the athlete with a disability, more research is needed.

PREPARTICIPATION EXAMINATION

Preparticipation assessment of a young person with a disability is similar to that of someone without a disability and can be conducted in a multistation fashion. Several areas, however, must be more thoroughly addressed. The personnel performing the assessment must understand not only the physical, physiologic, and psychologic requirements of the sport but also the potential medical risks of participation. The athlete may be prone to additional injury or illness secondary to the disability.[298] In addition, the physician may be involved in classification of the athlete depending on the type and severity of the disability and must be aware of international and national classification systems.[33,81]

The history should include the date of the onset of disability. Description and dates of all medical problems, hospitalizations, and operations before and after the onset of disability should be included. Releases for participation from all attending physicians are required. Thorough documentation of medications for comparison with lists of permissible drugs is necessary.[33]

Physical examination must include documentation of level of understanding, vocalization, communication abilities, and hearing. Flexibility should be evaluated because greater than normal muscle length may be required for certain activities (e.g., flexible hips for positioning in sports wheelchair). Special consideration should be given to instability in specific disability groups, such as the propensity for cervical instability and subluxation in Down syndrome.[43,267] Complete assessment of all sensory systems is required for classification and safety. Documentation of the presence of abnormal muscle tone and primitive, protective, or pathologic reflexes is critical for participation in sports such as archery, horseback riding, and swimming. Assessment of integrity and toughness of the skin and documentation of any history of skin problems are vital in any athlete with sensory impairment.[33]

The level of sitting and standing posture and balance as it pertains to the sport is critical for effective and safe participation. The athlete who skis while seated or rides horseback must have adequate balance to perform these activities. The athlete can be placed in a mock-up situation for assessment if necessary. Assessment of gait is mandatory in all clients who are ambulatory. The pattern and efficiency, as well as assistive devices needed, must be reviewed. Estimation of locomotor endurance is helpful.

The assessment of gross and fine motor skills should be performed in tasks similar to those required by the sport. Bilateral comparisons and timing and quality should be noted.[33] Muscle strength and endurance should be assessed, if possible, with either manual or mechanical methods. Although this area has received little attention, dominant hand grip force can be used as a partial predictor of upper body strength.[81,151] Davis[81] has also shown that a good relationship exists between upper body isokinetic strength and habitual activity.

Physiologic assessment should include nutritional analysis, body composition measurement, and exercise testing. Exercise testing may be advisable for assessment of cardiopulmonary functional capacity or the efficacy of medications. Testing must often be adjusted for the disability, such as arm crank, wheelchair, or single leg ergometry.[31,33,36,88,245] Field testing can be completed as long as standard testing principles are followed.[101,178] Although maximal oxygen consumption is the best single indicator of cardiovascular fitness, submaximal testing can be performed as an estimation of maximal capacity.

For many athletes with a disability, equipment is part of their participation. Specially designed wheelchairs, skiing outriggers, ergonomic racquet handles, rotation platforms for field events, and custom prostheses are but a few of the technologic advances that have made sports more accessible. The examiner should check the equipment for function, fit, safety, and conformity to rules of competition or participation.[33]

TRAINING PROGRAMS

Persons with disabilities should be placed on training programs in a manner similar to those without disabilities (Figure 15-12).[31,32,75,76] Several studies have evaluated the efficacy of these training programs in various disability groups. Research on wheelchair training demonstrated increases in maximal oxygen uptake, decreases in exercise and resting heart rate, and increases in maximal work capacity. Documented increases in muscle force and endurance and peak force have been noted after strength training.[147,184,328]

SUMMARY

Young athletes are not small adults. They have unique issues in sports participation that must be specifically addressed. Recognition of these unusual qualities is necessary for effective prevention and management of sports-related injuries.

Physical therapists should play a significant role in the total management of the child athlete. The broad-based and eclectic medical background of physical therapists makes them ideal professionals for the assessment and rehabilitation of sports injuries in athletes with full or altered physical capabilities. Depending on advanced experience or certification in sports physical therapy, athletic training, or exercise physiology, they may be the primary medical professionals to administer total management, from prevention to return to participation after injury.

A physical therapist is an important part of the comprehensive medical team that manages sports-related injuries in young athletes. Physical therapists may work with certified athletic trainers or exercise physiologists to provide comprehensive sports safety management. The certified trainer is appropriately skilled to assist with preparticipation screenings and to provide onsite coverage of practices and games with immediate triage and injury management. The exercise physiologist plays an integral part in the preseason screening and in conditioning and training programs. The physical therapist can provide assessment and total rehabilitation of sports injuries and aid in phasing the athlete back to play with appropriate progression, supportive devices, or medical limitations. The certified trainer or the exercise physiologist often works with the physical therapist in the return-to-play planning and follow-up.

The goal of these programs is to promote the health and safety of the young athlete. All those involved should work in a manner appropriate to their education, skills, and practice statutes as members of a team, including coaches and parents, toward the goal of safe, rewarding, and successful participation in sport and recreation.

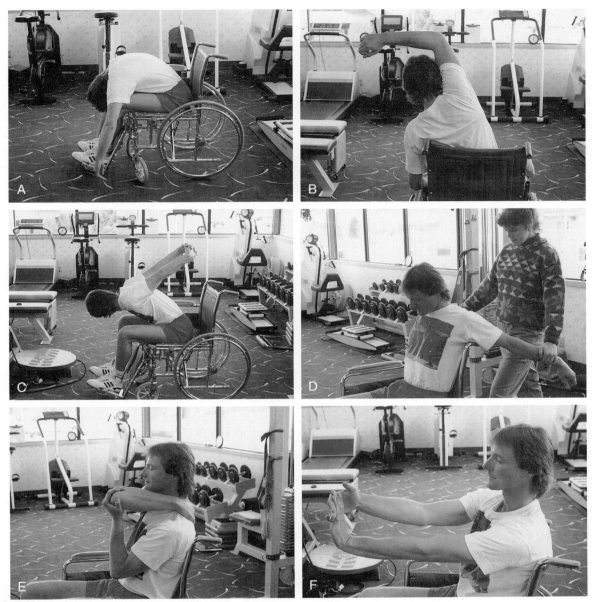

Figure 15-12 Stretching exercises for the athlete in a wheelchair. **A,** Low back stretch. Exhale; lean forward to touch ground. **B,** Shoulder and lateral trunk muscles stretch. Lift one arm over head and lean to side. Repeat on opposite side. **C,** Anterior chest and wrist stretch. Exhale, clasp hands, lean forward, and lift arms high in back. **D,** Partner anterior chest muscle stretch. Pull arms to side with palms facing forward. Pull back with elbows straight. **E,** Scapular and posterior shoulder muscle stretch. Bend arm across chest. Reach for opposite shoulder blade. Push on elbow. Repeat on opposite side. **F,** Wrist and finger flexor muscle stretch. Straighten elbow. Push wrist and fingers back. Repeat for opposite side.

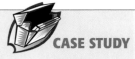

CASE STUDY

"John"

John is a 10-year-old boy who regularly participates in play activities with his friends and the local YMCA basketball team. He was referred to physical therapy following insidious onset of right knee pain with a medical diagnosis of a small (100 mm²) stable osteochondritis dissecans lesion in the medial femoral condyle. Imaging revealed no disruption of the articular cartilage.

The initial physical therapy examination is consistent with medial diagnosis. John reports right knee pain 3 out of 10 that increases with activity to 5 out of 10. Examination shows bilateral hip muscle weakness, right quadriceps muscles weakness (80% of uninvolved) and unloading of the right lower extremity during a double leg squat. Initial score on the IKDC is 80. The initial phase of rehabilitation focuses on joint protection including activity modification and progressive resistive exercise targeting the core, hip, thigh, and calf musculature.

Rehabilitation is progressed to include functional strengthening activities and neuromuscular reeducation activities. Patient and family education has been ongoing throughout rehabilitation to ensure collaboration with the plan of care. Following medical clearance and resolution of impairments, plyometric activities with focus on appropriate technique are initiated and progressed. In preparation for return to recreational activities, functional examination is performed and John demonstrates normalized hip muscle strength, quadriceps strength that is 94% of the uninvolved, appropriate technique during a double-leg squat, and performance on single leg hop tests range from 93% to 98% of the uninvolved. His score on the IKDC is 94. A progressive return to recreational basketball was conducted without return of symptoms, and John was discharged from physical therapy.

EVIDENCE TO PRACTICE 15-1: "JOHN"

CASE STUDY "JOHN"

EVIDENCE DECISION

John was diagnosed with a stable osteochondritis dissecans (OCD) lesion of the medial femoral condyle of the knee. The current evidence is limited with respect to the optimal medical management of these lesions. Limited evidence from Wall et al. does suggest that in the presence of a small lesion (<208 mm²) with intact articular cartilage in a skeletally immature knee, a course of conservative management is indicated before surgical intervention.

PLAN OF CARE DECISION

Because of the size of John's lesion, the patient was referred for conservative management of his OCD lesion of his knee to include limited weight bearing active and passive range of motion, and physical therapy to initiate conservative management of the OCD lesion.

Wall, E. J., Vourazeris, J., Myer, G. D., et al. (2008). The healing potential of stable juvenile osteochondritis dissecans knee lesions. *Journal of Bone and Joint Surgery (American), 90*, 2655–2664. doi:10.2106/JBJS.G.01103

EVIDENCE TO PRACTICE 15-2: "JOHN"

CASE STUDY "JOHN"

EVIDENCE DECISION

This patient presented to physical therapy with impaired quadriceps strength on his involved leg as indicated by an 80% limb symmetry index on an isokinetic assessment. Although strength deficits have not been investigated specifically in patients with OCDs of the knee, lower extremity strength deficits have been shown to persist long after surgery or injury to the lower extremity (Mattacola et al., 2002). In addition, some authors have demonstrated altered movement patterns in the lower extremity with dynamic movements in the presence of these deficits (Ernst et al., 2000; (Schmitt et al., 2009). Altered movement patterns could, in turn result in high-risk movements that predispose to future injury (Paterno et al., 2010).

PLAN OF CARE DECISION

A progressive resistive exercise program was initiated to focus on targeted impairments. The primary impairment identified

at the time of the evaluation was a significant strength deficit as demonstrated by an 80% limb symmetry index. The most recent evidence suggests these deficits could lead to altered movement patterns. Therefore, targeted interventions were initiated with focus on core and hip strength with a planned progression to initiate more dynamic training once this impairment resolved.

Ernst, G. P., Saliba, E., Diduch D. R., et al. (2000). Lower extremity compensations following anterior cruciate ligament reconstruction. *Physical Therapy 80*(3), 251–260.

Mattacola, C. G., Perrin, D. H., Gansneder B. M., et al. (2002). Strength, functional outcome, and postural stability after anterior cruciate ligament reconstruction. *Journal of Athletic Training, 37*(3), 262–268.

Paterno M.V. Schmitt L.C., Ford K.R. et al (2010). Biomechanical measures during landing and postural stability predict second anterior cruciate ligament injury after ACL reconstruction. *American Journal of Sports Medicine* (in press 10/2010)

Schmitt, L. C., Paterno, M. V., & Hewett, T. E. (2009). Functional performance at the time of return to sport following ACL reconstruction: The impact of quadriceps strength asymmetry. *Journal of Orthopaedic and Sports Physical Therapy, 39*(1), A103.

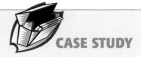

CASE STUDY

"Sarah"

Sarah was a star basketball player in her junior year of high school. She landed off balance during a midseason game and fell, twisting her right knee. Immediate field examination revealed tenderness over the medial joint line. She demonstrated +2 laxity on a Lachman test and could not bear weight on her leg. Follow-up 2 days later by her orthopedist confirmed the probability of anterior cruciate ligament (ACL) injury. An magnetic resonance imaging (MRI) scan demonstrated both an ACL tear and medial meniscal damage. She was referred for preoperative rehabilitation and scheduled for surgery.

Initial physical therapy examination showed a positive Lachman test, a positive pivot-shift test, and medial joint line tenderness, consistent with the MRI findings. Further examination revealed an edematous knee with some bruising. Her gait was antalgic with decreased heel strike and push-off, limited knee motion, and minimal comfortable weight bearing. Knee range of motion was −12° extension to 80° flexion. Her pain level was 5 on a scale of 10, and she had difficulty sleeping. Volitional quadriceps muscle activation was reduced, and she was unable to perform a straight leg raise.

Before surgery, she began a program to reduce edema, increase knee range of motion, promote quadriceps muscle activation, improve lower extremity muscle strength, and normalize gait. Therapeutic activities included progressive resistive exercise targeted at the core, hip, thigh, and calf musculature; neuromuscular electrical stimulation to the quadriceps muscles; edema and pain management; and gait training. The goals for this rehabilitation period were to minimize edema, restore knee range of motion, and maximize volitional quadriceps muscle activation and strength. Education regarding the injury and rehabilitation following the surgical procedure was ongoing. At her final preoperative visit, she was instructed in the use of crutches and a postsurgical home exercise program including quadriceps

setting, assisted straight leg raises, appropriate range of motion activities, and edema management.

Outpatient rehabilitation following the ACL reconstruction with patellar tendon bone-tendon-bone autograft and meniscus repair was initiated 5 days following surgery. Following clinical examination and assessment, the rehabilitation program was initiated with a focus on joint protection and acute management of impairments. Her rehabilitation program consisted of exercise for cardiovascular fitness; progressive resistive exercise targeted at the core, hip, thigh and calf musculature; neuromuscular electrical stimulation to the quadriceps muscles, edema, and pain management; and gait training with weight bearing to tolerance using bilateral axillary crutches. The use of crutches was discontinued when she demonstrated appropriate range of motion, appropriate volitional quadriceps muscle activation, appropriate weight-shift onto involved limb, and no change with pain or effusion with increased joint loading.

Her rehabilitation program progressed to incorporate functional muscle strength and endurance and neuromuscular reeducation activities. During the advanced stages of rehabilitation, plyometric activities were initiated and advanced with emphasis on appropriate technique and minimizing compensation patterns. A jogging program was initiated and progressed. In preparation for reintegration into basketball activities, a functional assessment was performed. Sarah demonstrated knee range of motion comparable to contralateral knee, quadriceps strength that was 91% of the contralateral muscle, a score of 87 on the IKDC Subjective Knee Form, and performance on single leg hop tests that ranged from 90% to 92% of the uninvolved limb. A progressive return to basketball was conducted in collaboration with her coach. She returned for functional evaluation 1 month following full participation in basketball and at that time was discharged from physical therapy.

REFERENCES

1. Aagaard, H., & Jorgensen, U. (1996). Injuries in elite volleyball. *Scandinavian Journal of Medicine & Science in Sports*, 6, 228–232.

2. Adirim, T. A., & Cheng, T. L. (2003). Overview of injuries in the young athlete. *Sports Medicine*, 33, 75–81.

3. Aichroth, P. M., Patel, D. V., & Zorrilla, P. (2002). The natural history and treatment of rupture of the anterior cruciate ligament in children and adolescents: A prospective review. *Journal of Bone and Joint Surgery (British)*, 84, 38–41.

4. Reference deleted in page proofs.

5. American Academy of Pediatrics. (1989). American Academy of Pediatrics. Organized athletics for preadolescent children. *Pediatrics*, 84, 583–584.

6. American Academy of Pediatrics. (2000). Climatic heat stress and the exercising child and adolescent. American Academy

of Pediatrics. Committee on Sports Medicine and Fitness. *Pediatrics*, 106, 158–159.

7. American Academy of Pediatrics Committee on Sports Medicine and Fitness. (2001). Medical conditions affecting sports participation. *Pediatrics*, 107, 1205–1209. Available at http://aappolicy.aappublications.org/cgi/reprint/pediatrics;107/5/1205. Accessed September 26, 2005.

8. American College of Sports Medicine. Inter-Association Task Force on exertional heat illnesses consensus statement, 2003.

9. American Medical Association. (1993). Ensuring the health of the adolescent athlete. *Archives of Family Medicine*, 2, 446–448.

10. Anderson, S. J. (2002). Lower extremity injuries in youth sports. *Pediatric Clinics of North America*, 49, 627–641.

11. Reference deleted in page proofs.

12. Andrish, J. T. (2001). Anterior cruciate ligament injuries in the skeletally immature patient. *American Journal of Orthopedics*, 30, 103–110.

13. Armsey, T. D., Jr., & Green, G. A. (1997). Nutrition supplements: Science vs. hype. *Physician and Sports Medicine, 25,* 77–92.

14. Armstrong, L. E., Maresh, C. M., Riebe, D., et al. (1995). Local cooling in wheelchair athletes during exercise-heat stress. *Medicine & Science in Sports & Exercise, 27,* 211–216.

15. Axe, M. J., Snyder-Mackler, L., Konin, J. G., & Strube, M. J. (1996). Development of a distance-based interval throwing program for Little League-aged athletes. *American Journal of Sports Medicine, 24*(5), 594–602.

16. Backx, F. J., Erich, W. B., Kemper, A. B., & Verbeek, A.L. (1991). Sports injuries in school-aged children: An epidemiological study. *American Journal of Sports Medicine, 17,* 234–240.

17. Bahrke, M. S., Yesalis, C. E., & Brower, K. J. (1998). Anabolic-androgenic steroid abuse and performance-enhancing drugs among adolescents. *Child and Adolescent Psychiatric Clinics of North America, 7,* 821–838.

18. Bailes, J. E., & Cantu, R. C. (2001). Head injury in athletes. *Neurosurgery, 48,* 26–45.

19. Bak, M. J., & Doerr, T. D. (2004). Craniomaxillofacial fractures during recreational baseball and softball. *Journal of Oral and Maxillofacial Surgery, 62,* 1209–1212.

20. Baker, J. S., & Davies, B. (2002). High intensity exercise assessment: Relationships between laboratory and field measures of performance. *Journal of Science in Medicine and Sport, 5,* 341–347.

21. Baker, M. M. (1998). Anterior cruciate ligament injuries in female athletes. *Journal of Women's Health, 7,* 343–349.

22. Balsom, P. D., Soderlund, K., & Ekblom, B. (1994). Creatine in humans with special reference to creatine supplementation. *Sports Medicine, 18,* 268–280.

23. Bar-Or, O. (1995a). *Child and adolescent athlete* (Vol. 6). Malden, MA: Blackwell.

24. Bar-Or, O. (1995b). The young athlete: Some physiological considerations. *Journal of Sports Science, 13,* S31–S33.

25. Bauman, M. (1986). Nutritional requirements for athletes. In Bernhardt, DB (Ed.). *Sports Physical Therapy* (pp. 89–105). New York: Churchill Livingstone, 1986.

26. Beatty, E., Light, T. R., Belsole, R. J., & Ogden, J. A. (1990). Wrist and hand skeletal injuries in children. *Hand Clinics, 6,* 723–738.

27. Bell, D. G., McLellan, T. M., & Sabiston, C. M. (2002). Effect of ingesting caffeine and ephedrine on performance. *Medicine & Science in Sports & Exercise, 34,* 1399–1403.

28. Below, P. R., Mora-Rodriguez, R., Gonzalez-Alonso, J., & Coyle, E. F. (1995). Fluid and carbohydrate ingestion independently improve performance during 1 h of intense exercise. *Medicine & Science in Sports & Exercise, 27,* 200–210.

29. Benson, L. S., Waters, P. M., Meier, S. W., Visotsky, J. L., & Williams, C. S. (2000). Pediatric hand injuries due to home exercycles. *Journal of Pediatric Orthopedics, 20,* 34–39.

30. Bergstrom, K. A., Brandseth, K., Fretheim, S., Tvilde, K., & Ekeland, A. (2001). Activity-related knee injuries and pain in athletic adolescents. *Knee Surgery, Sports Traumatology, and Arthroscopy, 9,* 146–150.

31. Bernhardt, D. B. (1985a). Exercise testing and training for disabled populations: The state of the art. In D. B. Bernhardt (Ed.). *Recreation for the disabled child* (pp. 3–25). New York: Haworth Press.

32. Bernhardt, D. B. (1985b). The competitive spirit. In D. B. Bernhardt (Ed.). *Recreation for the disabled child* (pp. 77–86). New York: Haworth Press.

33. Bernhardt, D. B. (1991). The physically challenged athlete. In R. C. Cantu & L. J. Micheli (Eds.), *ACSM's guidelines for the team physician* (pp. 242–251). Philadelphia: Lea & Febiger.

34. Bernhardt, D. T., Gomez, J., Johnson, M. D., et al. (2001). Strength training by children and adolescents. *Pediatrics, 107,* 1470–1472.

35. Bernhardt, D. T., Landry, G. L. (1995). Sports injuries in young athletes. *Advances in Pediatrics, 42,* 465–500.

36. Bhambhani, Y. N., Holland, L. J., & Steadward, R. D. (1993). Anaerobic threshold in wheelchair athletes with cerebral palsy: Validity and reliability. *Archives of Physical Medicine and Rehabilitation, 74,* 305–311.

37. Birrer, R. B., Griesemer, B. A., & Cataletto, M. B. (2002). *Pediatric sports medicine for primary care.* Philadelphia: Lippincott Williams & Wilkins.

38. Blanksby, B. A., Wearne, F. K., Elliott, B. C., & Blitvich, J. D. (1997). Aetiology and occurrence of diving injuries. A review of diving safety. *Sports Medicine, 23*(4), 228–246.

39. Boden, B. P., Lin, W., Young, M., & Mueller, F. O. (2002). Catastrophic injuries in wrestlers. *American Journal of Sports Medicine, 30,* 791–795.

40. Bolgla, L. A., & Keskula D. R. (1997). Reliability of lower extremity functional performance tests. *Journal of Orthopaedic and Sports Physical Therapy, 26*(3), 138–142.

41. Boyd, K. T., & Myers, P. T. (2003). Meniscus preservation: Rationale, repair techniques and results. *Knee, 10,* 1–11.

42. Bratton, R. L. (1997). Preparticipation screening of children for sports. Current recommendations. *Sports Medicine, 24,* 300–307.

43. Brockmeyer, D. (1999). Down syndrome and craniovertebral instability: Topic review and treatment recommendations. *Pediatric Neurosurgery, 31,* 71–77.

44. Brogger-Jensen, T., Hvass, I., & Bugge, S. (1990). Injuries at the BMX Cycling European Championship, 1989. *British Journal of Sports Medicine, 24,* 269–270.

45. Brosky, J. A., Jr., Nitz, A. J., Malone, T. R. et al. (1999). Intrarater reliability of selected clinical outcome measures following anterior cruciate ligament reconstruction. *Journal of Orthopaedic and Sports Physical Therapy, 29*(1), 39–48.

46. Brown, R. L., Brunn, M. A., & Garcia, V. F. (2001). Cervical spine injuries in children: A review of 103 patients treated consecutively at a level 1 pediatric trauma center. *Journal of Pediatric Surgery, 36,* 1107–1114.

47. Brown, R. L., Koepplinger, M. E., Mehlman, C. T., Gittelman, M., & Garcia, V. F. (2002). All-terrain vehicle and bicycle crashes in children: Epidemiology and comparison of injury severity. *Journal of Pediatric Surgery, 37,* 375–380.

48. Bruce, D. A., Schut, L., & Sutton, L. N. (1982). Brain and cervical spine injuries occurring during organized sports activities in children and adolescents. *Clinical Sports Medicine, 1,* 495–514.

49. Brust, J. D., Leonard, B. J., Pheley, A., & Roberts, W. O. (1992). Children's ice hockey injuries. *American Journal of Diseases of Childhood, 146,* 741–747.

50. Brynhildsen, J., Ekstrand, J., Jeppsson, A., & Tropp, H. (1990). Previous injuries and persisting symptoms in female soccer players. *International Journal of Sports Medicine, 11,* 489–492.

51. Bunc, V. (1994). A simple method for estimating aerobic fitness. *Ergonomics, 37,* 159–165.

52. Cain E. L., Clancy W. G. (2001). Treatment Algorithm for Osteochongral injuries of the knee. *Clin Sports Med.,* 321–342.

53. Caine, D. J., DiFiori, J., & Maffulli, N. (2006). Physeal injuries in children's and youth sports. Reasons for concern? *British Journal of Sports Medicine, 40,* 749–760.

54. Caine, D., Maffulli, N., & Caine, C. (2008). Epidemiology of Injury in Child and Adolescent Sports: Injury Rates, Risk Factors and Prevention. *Clinics in Sports Medicine, 27,* 19–50.

55. Campbell, R. M., Jr. Operative treatment of factures and dislocations of the hand and wrist region in children. *Orthopedic Clinics of North America, 21,* 217–243, 1990.

56. Cantu, R. C. (1998). Return to play guidelines after a head injury. *Clinics in Sports Medicine, 17,* 45–60.

57. Cantu, R. C. (2000). Cervical spine injuries in the athlete. *Seminars in Neurology, 20,* 173–178.

58. Cantu, R. C. (2001). Posttraumatic retrograde and anterograde amnesia: Pathophysiology and implications in grading and safe return to play. *Journal of Athletic Training, 36,* 244–248.

59. Cantu, R. C. (2003). Recurrent athletic head injury: Risks and when to retire. *Clinics in Sports Medicine, 22,* 593–603.

60. Cantu, R. C., Bailes, J. E., & Wilberger, J. E., Jr. (1998). Guidelines for return to contact or collision sport after a cervical spine injury. *Clinics in Sports Medicine, 17,* 137–146.

61. Cantu, R. C., & Mueller, F. O. (2000). Catastrophic football injuries: 1977–1998. *Neurosurgery, 47,* 673–675.

62. Cantu, R. C., & Mueller, F. O. (2003a). Catastrophic spine injuries in American football, 1977–2001. *Neurosurgery, 53,* 358–362.

63. Cantu, R. C., & Mueller, F. O. (2003b). Brain injury-related fatalities in American football, 1945–1999. *Neurosurgery, 52,* 846–852.

64. Carek, P. J., Dickerson, L. M., & Hawkins, A. (2002). Special Olympics, special athletes, special needs? *Journal of Southern Connecticut Medical Association, 98,* 183–186.

65. Casa, D. J., Armstrong, L. E., Hillman, S. K., et al. (2000). National Athletic Trainers' Association position statement: Fluid replacement for athletes. *Journal of Athletic Training, 35,* 212–224.

66. Castaldi, C. R. (1986). Sports related oral and facial injuries in the young athlete: A new challenge for the pediatric dentist. *Pediatric Dentistry, 8,* 311–316.

67. CDC. BMI for Children and Teens. Available at www.cdc.gov/nccdphp/dnpa/bmi/bmi-for-age.htm. Accessed September 26, 2005.

68. Challier, B., Chau, N., Predine, R., Choquet, M., & Legras, B. (2000). Associations of family environment and individual factors with tobacco, alcohol, and illicit drug use in adolescents. *European Journal of Epidemiology, 16,* 33–42.

69. Clark, N. (1991). Nutrition: Pre-, intra-, and post-competition. In R. C. Cantu & L. J. Micheli (Eds.), *ACSM's guidelines for the team physician* (pp. 58–65). Philadelphia: Lea & Febiger.

70. Clarkson, P. M. (1996). Nutrition for improved sports performance. Current issues on ergogenic aids. *Sports Medicine, 21,* 393–401.

71. Coady, C. M., & Micheli, L. J. (1997). Stress fractures in the pediatric athlete. *Clinics in Sports Medicine, 16,* 225–238.

72. Collins, M. W., Lovell, M. R., Iverson, G. L., Cantu, R. C., Maroon, J. C. & Field, M. (2002). Cumulative effects of concussion in high school athletes. *Neurosurgery, 51,* 1175–1179.

73. Conn, J. M., Annest, J. L., & Gilchrist, J. (2003). Sports and recreation related injury episodes in the US population, 1997–1999. *Injury Prevention, 9,* 117–123.

74. Cooper, K. (1991). *Kid fitness.* New York: Bantam Books.

75. Curtis, K. A. (1981a, July/August). Wheelchair sports medicine: II. Training. *Sports "n" Spokes,* pp. 16–19.

76. Curtis, K. A. (1981b, September/October). Wheelchair sport medicine: III. Stretching. *Sports "n" Spokes,* pp. 16–18.

77. Curtis, K. A. (1981b, January/February). Wheelchair sports medicine: IV. Athletic injuries. *Sports "n" Spokes,* pp. 20–24.

78. Curtis, K. A., McClanahan, S., & Hail, K. M. (1986). Vocational and functional status in spinal cord injured athletes and nonathletes. *Archives of Physical Medicine and Rehabilitation, 67,* 862–865.

79. Dalton, S. E. (1992). Overuse injuries in adolescent athletes. *Sports Medicine, 13,* 58–70.

80. DaSilva, M. F., Williams, J. S., Fadale, P. D., Hulstyn, M. J. & Ehrlich, M. G. (1998). Pediatric throwing injuries about the elbow. *American Journal of Orthopedics, 27,* 90–96.

81. Davis, G. M. (1981). Cardiorespiratory fitness and muscle strength in lower-limb disability. *Canadian Journal of Applied Sports Science, 6,* 159–165.

82. Davis, J. M., Welsh, R. S., & Alerson, N. A. (2000). Effects of carbohydrate and chromium ingestion during intermittent high-intensity exercise to fatigue. *International Journal of Sport Nutrition and Exercise Metabolism, 10,* 476–485.

83. Debnath, U. K., Freeman, B. J., Gregory, P., de la Harpe, D., Kerslake, R. W., & Webb, J. K. (2003). Clinical outcome and return to sport after the surgical treatment of spondylolysis in young athletes. *Journal of Bone and Joint Surgery (British), 85,* 244–249.

84. Deitch, J., Mehlman, C. T., Foad, S. L., Obbehat, A., & Mallory, M. (2003). Traumatic anterior shoulder dislocation in adolescents. *American Journal of Sports Medicine, 31*(5), 758–763.

85. Delibasi, C., Yamazawa, M., Nomura, K., Iida, S., & Kogo, M. (2004). Maxillofacial fractures sustained during sports played

with a ball. *Oral Surgery Oral Medicine Oral Pathology Oral Radiology and Endodontics*, 97, 23–27.

86. deLoes, M., Dahlstedt, L. J., & Thomee, R. (2000). A 7-year study on risks and costs of knee injuries in male and female youth participants in 12 sports. *Scandinavian Journal of Medicine & Science in Sports*, 10, 90–97.

87. d'Hemecourt, P. A., Gerbino, P. G., 2nd, & Micheli, L. J. (2000). Back injuries in the young athlete. *Clinics in Sports Medicine*, 19, 663–679.

88. Draheim, C. C., Laurie, N. E., McCubbin, J. A., & Perkins, J. L. (1999). Validity of a modified aerobic fitness test for adults with mental retardation. *Medicine & Science in Sports & Exercise*, 31, 1849–1854.

89. Drezner, J. A. (2000). Sudden cardiac death in young athletes: Causes, athlete's heart and screening guidelines. *Postgraduate Medicine*, 108, 37–44, 47–50.

90. Drkulec, J. A., & Letts, M. (2001). Snowboarding injuries in children. *Canadian Journal of Surgery*, 44, 435–439.

91. DuRant, R. H., Escobedo, L. G., & Heath, G. W. (1995). Anabolic-steroid use, strength training, and multiple drug use among adolescents in the United States. *Pediatrics*, 96, 23–28.

92. Ekegren, C. L., Miller, W. C., Celebrini, R. G., Eng, J. J., & Macintyre, D. L. (2009). Reliability and validity of observational risk screening in evaluating dynamic knee valgus. *Journal of Orthopaedic and Sports Physical Therapy*, 39(9), 665–674.

93. Faigenbaum, A. D., Milliken, L. A., Loud, R. L., Burak, B. T., Doherty, C. L., & Westcott, W. L. (2002). Comparison of 1 and 2 days per week of strength training in children. *Research Quarterly of Exercise & Sports*, 73, 416–424.

94. Faigenbaum, A. D., Kraemer, W. J., Cahill, B., et al. (1996). Youth tesistance training: Position statement paper and literature review. *Strength and Conditioning*, 18(6), 62–75.

95. Feld, L. G., Springate, J. E., & Waz, W. R. (1998). Special topics in pediatric hypertension. *Seminars in Nephrology*, 18, 295–303.

96. Ferrara, M. S., Buckley, W. E., McCann, B. C., Limbird, T. J., Powell, J. W., & Robl, R. (1992). The injury experience of a competitive athlete with a disability: Prevention implications. *Medicine & Science in Sports & Exercise*, 24, 184–188.

97. Field, S. J., & Oates, R. K.(2001). Sports and recreation activities and opportunities for children with spina bifida and cystic fibrosis. *Journal of Science & Medicine in Sport*, 4(1), 71–76.

98. Fields, K. B. (1994). Clearing athletes for participation in sports: The North Carolina Medical Society Sports Medicine Committee's recommended examination. *North Carolina Medical Journal*, 55, 116–121.

99. Finch, G. D., & Barnes, M. J. (1998). Major cervical spine injuries in children and adolescents. *Journal of Pediatric Orthopedics*, 18, 811–814.

100. Fitzgerald, G. K., Lephart S. M., Hwang J. H., et al. (2001). Hop tests as predictors of dynamic knee stability. *Journal of Orthopaedic and Sports Physical Therapy*, 31(10), 588–597.

101. Fletcher, G. F., Lloyd, A., Waling, J. F., & Fletcher, B. (1988). Exercise testing in patients with musculoskeletal handicaps. *Archives of Physical Medicine and Rehabilitation*, 69, 123–127.

102. Flynn J. M., Skaggs D. L., Sponseller P. T., et al. (2003). The surgical management of pediatric fractures of the lower extremity. *Instr Course Lect 52*, 647–659.

103. Food Guide Pyramid. (1992). Washington, DC: US Department of Agriculture.

104. Ford, K. R., Myer, G. D., & Hewett, T. E. (2003). Valgus knee motion during landing in high school female and male basketball players. *Medicine and Science in Sports and Exercise*, 35(10), 1745–1750.

105. Forman, E. S., Dekker, A. H., Javors, J. R., & Davison, D. T. (1995). High-risk behaviors in teenage male athletes. *Clinical Journal of Sport Medicine*, 5, 36–42.

106. Fu, F. H. (2001). *Sports injuries: Mechanisms, prevention, and treatment* (2nd ed.). Philadelphia: Lippincott Williams & Wilkins.

107. Fuller, C. M., McNulty, C. M., Spring, D. A., et al. (1997). Prospective screening of 5,615 high school athletes for risk of sudden cardiac death. *Medicine & Science in Sports & Exercise*, 29, 1131–1138.

108. Gaillard, B. (1978). *Handbook for the young athlete*. Palo Alto, CA: Bull Publishing.

109. Galena, H. J., Epstein, C. R., & Lourie, R. J. (1998). Connecticut State Special Olympics: Observations and recommendations. *Connecticut Medicine*, 62, 33–37.

110. Galloway, S. D., & Maughan, R. J. (2000). The effects of substrate and fluid provision on thermoregulatory and metabolic responses to prolonged exercise in a hot environment. *Journal of Sports Science*, 18, 339–351.

111. Garrick, J. G. (1990). Orthopedic preparticipation screening examination. *Pediatric Clinics of North America*, 37, 1047–1056.

112. Gassner, R., Tuli, T., Hachl, O., Rudisch, A., & Ulmer, H. (2003). Cranio-maxillofacial trauma: A 10 year review of 9,543 cases with 21,067 injuries. *Journal of Craniomaxillofacial Surgery*, 31, 51–61.

113. Gerbino, P. G., 2nd, & Micheli, L. J. (1995). Back injuries in the young athlete. *Clinics in Sports Medicine*, 14, 571–590.

114. Gerrard, D. F. (1993). Overuse injury and growing bones: The young athlete at risk. *British Journal of Sports Medicine*, 27, 14–18.

115. Gerstenbluth, R. E., Spirnak, J. P., & Elder, J. S. (2002). Sports participation and high grade renal injuries in children. *Journal of Urology*, 168, 2575–2578.

116. Gill, T. J., 4th, & Micheli, L. J. (1996). The immature athlete: Common injuries and overuse syndromes of the elbow and wrist. *Clinics in Sports Medicine*, 15, 401–423.

117. Gillon, H. (2001). Scaphoid injuries in children. *Accident and Emergency Nursing*, 9, 249–256.

118. Glover, D. W., & Maron, B. J. (1998). Profile of preparticipation cardiovascular screening for high school athletes. *Journal of the American Medical Association*, 279, 1817–1819.

119. Going, S. (1998). Physical best: Body composition in the assessment of youth fitness. *Journal of Physical Education, Recreation, and Dance, 59*, 32–36.

120. Gomez, E., DeLee, J. C., & Farney, W. C. (1996). Incidence of injury in Texas girls' high school basketball. *American Journal of Sports Medicine, 24*(5), 684–687.

121. Grafe, M. W., Paul, G. R., & Foster, T. E. (1997). The preparticipation sports examination for high school and college athletes. *Clinics in Sports Medicine, 16*, 569–591.

122. Grana, W. A., & Kalenak, A. (1991). *Clinical sports medicine.* Philadelphia: WB Saunders.

123. Green, G. A. (1990). Drugs, athletes, and drug testing. In Sanders, B. (Ed.). *Sports physical therapy* (pp. 95–111). Norwalk, CT: Appleton & Lange.

124. Green, G. A., Uryasz, F. D., Petr, T. A., & Bray, C. D. (2001). NCAA study of substance use and abuse habits of college student-athletes. *Clinical Journal of Sport Medicine, 11*, 51–56.

125. Gregg, J. R., & Das, M. (1982). Foot and ankle problems in the preadolescent and adolescent athlete. *Clinics in Sports Medicine, 1*, 131–147.

126. Greydanus, D. E., & Patel, D. R. (2002). Sports doping in the adolescent athlete: The hope, hype and hyperbole. *Pediatric Clinics of North America, 49*, 829–855.

127. Guskiewicz, K. M., Bruce S. L., Cantu R. C. et al. (2004). National Athletic Trainers' Association position statement: Management of sport-related concussion. *Journal of Athletic Training, 39*(3), 280–297.

128. Guy, J. A., & Micheli, L. J. (2001). Strength training for children and adolescents. *Journal of American Academy of Orthopedic Surgery, 9*, 29–36.

129. Guzzanti, V. (2003). The natural history and treatment of rupture of the anterior cruciate ligament in children and adolescents. *Journal of Bone and Joint Surgery (British), 85*, 618–619.

130. Gwinn, D. E., Wilckens, J. H., McDevitt, E. R., Ross, G., & Kao, T. C. (2000). The relative incidence of anterior cruciate ligament injury in men and women at the United States Naval Academy. *American Journal of Sports Medicine, 28*, 98–102.

131. Hagel, B. (2005). Skiing and snowboarding injuries. In J. Caine & N. Maffulli (Eds.), Epidemiology of Pediatric Sports Injuries. *Individual Sports. Med Sport Sci* (pp. 74–119). *vol. 48.* Basel: Karger.

132. Haller C. A., Benowitz N. L. (2000). Adverse cardiovascular and central nervous system events associated with dietary supplements containing ephedra alkaloids. *N Engl J Med, 343*(25), 1833–1888.

133. Hamilton, P. R., & Broughton, N. S. (1998). Traumatic hip dislocation in childhood. *Journal of Pediatric Orthopedics, 18*, 691–694.

134. Hanson, C. S., Nabavi, D., & Yuen, H. K. (2001). The effect of sports on level of community integration as reported by persons with spinal cord injury. *American Journal of Occupational Therapy, 55*, 332–338.

135. Heath, G. W., Pratt, M., Warren, C. W., & Kann, L. (1994). Physical activity patterns in American high school students. Results from the 1990 Youth Risk Behavior Survey. *Archives of Pediatric & Adolescent Medicine, 148*, 1131–1136.

136. Heinonen, O. J. (1996). Carnitine and physical exercise. *Sports Medicine, 22*, 109–132.

137. Hewett, T. E., Ford, K. R., & Myer, G. D. (2006). Anterior cruciate ligament injuries in female athletes: Part 2, a meta-analysis of neuromuscular interventions aimed at injury prevention. *American Journal of Sports Medicine, 34*(3), 490–498.

138. Hewett, T. E., Lindenfeld, T. N., Riccobene, J. V., & Noyes, F. R. (1999). The effect of neuromuscular training on the incidence of knee injury in female athletes. A prospective study. *American Journal of Sports Medicine, 27*, 699–706.

139. Hewett, T. E., Myer, G. D., & Ford, K. R. (2005). Reducing knee and anterior cruciate ligament injuries among female athletes: A systematic review of neuromuscular training interventions. *Journal of Knee Surgery, 18*(1), 82–88.

140. Hewett, T. E., Myer, G. D., & Ford, K. R. (2006). Anterior cruciate ligament injuries in female athletes: Part 1, mechanisms and risk factors. *American Journal of Sports Medicine, 34*(2), 299–311.

141. Hewett, T. E., Pasque, C., Heyl, R., & Wroble, R. (2005). In D. J. Caine & N. Maffulli (Eds.), *Epidemiology of Pediatric Sports Injuries. Individual Sports. Med Sport Sci* (pp. 152–178). *vol. 48.* Basel: Karger.

142. Hewett, T. E., Zazulak, B. T., & Myer, G. D. (2007). Effects of the menstrual cycle on anterior cruciate ligament injury risk: A systematic review. *American Journal of Sports Medicine, 35*(4), 659–668. Epub 2007 Feb 9.

143. Hoeberigs, J. H., Debets-Eggen, H. B., & Debets, P. M. (1990). Sports medical experiences from the International Flower Marathon for disabled wheelers. *American Journal of Sports Medicine, 18*(4), 418–421.

144. Hosea, T. M., Carey, O. C., & Harrer, M. F. (2000). The gender issue: Epidemiology of ankle injuries in athletes who participate in basketball. *Clinical Orthopedics, 372*, 45–49.

145. Hunter, S. C., Etchison, W. C., & Halpern, B. (1985, Fall). Standards and norms of fitness and flexibility in the high school athlete. *Journal of Athletic Training*, 210–212.

146. Hutchinson, M. R., & Ireland, M. L. (2003). Overuse and throwing injuries in the skeletally immature athlete. *Instructional Course Lectures, 52*, 25–36.

147. Hutzler, Y., Ochana, S., Bolotin, R., & Kalina, A. (1998). Aerobic and non-aerobic arm-cranking outputs of males with lower limb impairments: Relationship with sport participation intensity, age, impairment with functional classification. *Spinal Cord, 36*, 205–212.

148. Iobst, C. A., & Stanitski, C. L. (2000). Acute knee injuries. *Clinics in Sports Medicine, 19*, 621–635.

149. Iuliano, S., Naughton, G., Collier, G., & Carlson, J. (1998). Examination for the self-selected fluid intake practices by junior athletes during a simulated diathlon event. *International Journal of Sport Nutrition, 8*, 10–23.

150. Iven, V. G. (1998). Recreational drugs. *Clinics in Sports Medicine, 17*, 245–259.

151. Jackson, R. W., & Davis, G. M. (1983). The value of sports and recreation for the physically disabled. *Orthopedic Clinics of North America, 14*, 301–315.

152. Kay, R. M., & Matthys, G. A. (2001). Pediatric ankle fractures: Evaluation and treatment. *Journal of American Academy of Orthopedic Surgery, 9*, 268–278.

153. Keays, S. L., et al. (2003). The relationship between knee strength and functional stability before and after anterior cruciate ligament reconstruction. *Journal of Orthopaedic Research, 21*(2), 231–237.

154. Kegel, B., & Webster, J. C., & Burgess, E. (1980). Recreational activities of lower extremity amputees. *Archives of Physical Medicine and Rehabilitation, 61*, 258–264.

155. Kerr, I. L. (1986). Mouth guards for the prevention of injuries in contact sports. *Sports Medicine, 5*, 415–427.

156. Kibler, W. B., & Safran, M. (2005). Tennis injuries. In D. J. Caine & N. Maffulli (Eds.), Epidemiology of Pediatric Sports Injuries. Individual Sports. Med Sport Sci (pp. 120–137). *vol. 48*. Basel: Karger.

157. Kinzey, S. J., & Armstrong, C. W. (1998). The reliability of the star-excursion test in assessing dynamic balance. *Journal of Orthopaedic and Sports Physical Therapy, 27*(5), 356–360.

158. Klish, W. J. (1995). Childhood obesity: Pathophysiology and treatment. *Acta Pediatrica Japan, 37*, 1–6.

159. Knowles, S. B., Marshall, S. W., Guskiewicz, K. M. (2006). Issues in estimating risks and rates in sports injury research. *Journal of Athletic Training, 41*(2), 207–215.

160. Kocher, M. S., Waters, P. M., & Micheli, L. J. (2000). Upper extremity injuries in the paediatric athlete. *Sports Medicine, 30*, 117–135.

161. Kocher, M. S., Garg, S., Micheli, L. J. (2006). Physeal sparing reconstruction of the anterior cruciate ligament in skeletally immature prepubescent children and adolescents. Surgical technique. *Journal of Bone and Joint Surgery (American), 88*(Suppl 1 Pt 2), 283–293.

162. Kocher M. S., Saxon H. S., Hovis W. B., Hawkins R. J. (2002). Management and complications of anterior cruciate ligament injuries in skeletally immature patients: survey of the Herodicus Society and the ACL Study Group. *J Pediatr Orthop, 22*(4), 452–457.

163. Kouyoumjian, A., & Barber, F. A. (2001). Management of anterior cruciate ligament disruptions in skeletally immature patients. *American Journal of Orthopedics, 30*, 771–774.

164. Kraemer, W. J., Duncan, N. D., & Volek, J. S. (1998). Resistance training and elite athletes: Adaptations and program considerations. *Journal of Orthopaedic and Sports Physical Therapy, 28*(2), 110–119.

165. Kraemer, W. J., Voleck, J. S., French, D. N., et al. (2003). The effects of L-Carnitine tartrate supplementation on hormonal responses to resistance exercise and recovery. *Journal of Strength and Conditioning Research, 17*, 455–462.

166. Kraft, D. E. (2002). Low back pain in the adolescent athlete. *Pediatric Clinics of North America, 49*, 643–653.

167. Kraus, R., Pavlidis, T., Heiss, C., Kilian, O., & Schnettler, R. (2010, March 9). Arthroscopic treatment of post-traumatic shoulder instability in children and adolescents. *Knee Surgery, Sports Traumatology, Arthroscopy*. [Epub ahead of print] PMID: 20217390.

168. Kreider, R. B., Ferriera, M., Wilson, M., et al. (1998). Effects of creatine supplementation on body composition, strength, and sprint performance. *Medicine & Science in Sports & Exercise, 30*, 73–82.

169. Kubiak, R., & Slongo, T. (2003). Unpowered scooter injuries in children. *Acta Paediatrica, 92*, 50–54.

170. Kujala, U. M., Taimela, S., Antti-Poika, I., Orava, S., Tuominen, R., & Myllynen, P. (1995). Acute injuries in soccer, ice hockey, volleyball, basketball, judo and karate: Analysis of national registry data. *British Medical Journal, 311*, 1465–1468.

171. Kurowski, K., & Chandran, S. (2000). The preparticipation athletic evaluation. *American Family Physician, 61*, 2696–2698.

172. Kvist, J. (2004). Rehabilitation following anterior cruciate ligament injury: Current recommendations for sports participation. *Sports Medicine, 34*(4), 269–280.

173. Kyle, S. B. (1996). *Youth baseball protective equipment project: Final report*. Washington, DC: US Consumer Product Safety Commission.

174. Lai, A. M., Stanish, W. D., & Stanish, H. I. (2000). The young athlete with physical challenges. *Clinics in Sports Medicine, 19*, 793–819.

175. Larsen, G. E., George, J. D., Alexander, J. L., Fellington, G. W., Aldana, S. G., & Parcell, A. C. (2002). Prediction of maximum oxygen consumption from walking, jogging, or running. *Research Quarterly in Exercise & Sport, 71*, 66–72.

176. Laseter, J. T., & Russell, J. A. (1991). Anabolic steroid-induced tendon pathology: A review of the literature. *Medicine & Science in Sports & Exercise, 23*, 1–3.

177. Laure, P. (1997). Epidemiologic approach of doping in sport: A review. *Journal of Sports Medicine and Physical Fitness, 37*, 218–224.

178. Leger, L. A., Mercier, D., Gadoury, C., & Lambert, J. (1988). The multistage 20 meter shuttle run for aerobic fitness. *Journal of Sports Science, 6*, 93–101.

179. Lenaway, D. D., Ambler, A. G., & Beaudoin, D. E. (1992). The epidemiology of school-related injuries: New perspectives. *American Journal of Preventive Medicine, 8*, 193–198.

180. Lehnhard, R. A., Lehnhard, H. R., Young R., & Butterfield S. A. (1996). Monitoring injuries on a college soccer team: The effect of strength training. *Journal of Strength and Conditioning Research, 10*, 115–119.

181. Letts, M., Davidson, D., & McCaffrey, M. (2001). The adolescent pilon fracture: Management and outcome. *Journal of Pediatric Orthopedics, 21*, 20–26.

182. Libetta, C., Burke, D., Brennan, P., & Yassa, J. (1999). Validation of the Ottawa ankle rules in children. *Journal of Accidental and Emergency Medicine, 16*, 342–344.

183. Linder, C. W., DuRant, R. H., Seklecki, R. M., & Strong, W. B. (1981). Preparticipation health screening of young athletes. *American Journal of Sports Medicine, 9,* 187–193.

184. Lintunen, T., Heikinaro-Johansson, P., & Sherrill, C. (1995). Use of Perceptual Physical Competence Scale with adolescents with disabilities. *Perceptual Motor Skills, 80,* 571–577.

185. Lodge, J. F., Langley, J. D., & Begg, D. J. (1990). Injuries in the 14th and 15th years of life. *Journal of Paediatrics and Child Health, 26,* 316–322.

186. Lohman, T. G. (1992). *Advances in body composition assessment.* Champaign, IL: Human Kinetics.

187. Lombardo, J. A. (1991). Preparticipation examination. In Cantu, R. C., & Micheli, L. J. (Eds.), *ACSM's guidelines for the team physician* (pp. 71–94). Philadelphia: Lea & Febiger.

188. Louden, J. K., Jenkins, W., & Louden, K. L. (1996). The relationship between static posture and ACL injury in female athletes. *Journal of Orthopedic & Sports Physical Therapy, 24,* 91–97.

189. Lyznicki, J. M., Nielsen, N. H., & Schneider, J. F. (2000). Cardiovascular screening of student athletes. *American Family Physician, 62,* 765–774.

190. Maestrello-deMoya, M. G., & Primosch, R. E. (1989). Orofacial trauma and mouth-protector wear among high school varsity basketball players. *ASDC Journal of Dentistry in Children, 56,* 36–39.

191. Maffulli, N. (1990). Intensive training in young athletes. *Sports Medicine, 9,* 229–243.

192. Maffulli, N., & Bruns, W. (2000). Injuries in young athletes. *European Journal of Pediatrics, 159,* 59–63.

193. Mankovsky, A. B., Mendoza-Sagaon, M., Cardinaux, C., Hohlfeld, J., & Reinberg, O. (2002). Evaluation of scooter-related injuries in children. *Journal of Pediatric Surgery, 37,* 755–759.

194. Maron, B. J. (2002). The young competitive athlete with cardiovascular abnormalities: Causes of sudden death, detection by preparticipation screening, and standards for disqualification. *Cardiology and Electrophysiological Review, 6,* 100–103.

195. Marsh, J. S., & Daigneault, J. P. (2000). Ankle injuries in the pediatric population. *Current Opinions in Pediatrics, 12,* 52–60.

196. Marshall, S. W., Padua, D., McGrath M. (2007). Incidence of ACL Injury. In T. E. Hewett, S. J. Shultz & L. Y. Griffin (Eds.), *Understanding and Preventing Noncontact ACL Injuries* (pp. 5–30). Champaign: Human Kinetics.

197. Maughan, R. (2002). The athlete's diet: Nutritional goals and dietary strategies. *Proceedings of the Nutrition Society, 61,* 87–96.

198. McArdle, W. D., Katch, F. I., & Katch, V. L. (2001). *Exercise physiology: Energy, nutrition, and human performance.* Philadelphia: Lippincott, Williams & Wilkins.

199. McCormick, D. (1985). Handicapped skiing. In D. B. Bernhardt (Ed.), *Recreation for the disabled child* (pp. 27–44). New York: Haworth Press.

200. McCormick, D. P., Niebiehr, V. N., & Risser, W. L. (1990). Injury and illness surveillance at local Special Olympic Games. *British Journal of Sports Medicine, 24,* 221–224.

201. McCrea, M., Kelly, J., Randolph, C., et al. (1998). Standardized assessment of concussion (SAC): On-site mental status evaluation of the athlete. *Journal of Head Trauma Rehabilitation, 13*(2), 27–36.

202. McCrea, M., Kelly, J., Randolph, C. (2000). *The Standardized Assessment of Concussion (SAC): Manual for administration, scoring and interpretation* (3rd ed.). Waukesha, WI: Comprehensive Neuropsychological Services.

203. McCrory, P., Meeuwisse W., Johnston K., et al. (2009). Consensus Statement on Concussion in Sport: The Third International Conference on Concussion in Sports Held in Zurich, November 2008. *Journal of Athletic Training, 44*(4), 435–448.

204. McKeag, D. (1985). Preseason physical examination for prevention of sports injuries. *Sports Medicine, 2,* 413–431.

205. McLain, L. G., & Reynolds, S. (1989). Sports injuries in a high school. *Pediatrics, 84,* 446–450.

206. McNutt, T., Shannon, S. W., Wright, J. T., & Feinstein, R. A. (1989). Oral trauma in adolescent athletes: A study of mouth protectors. *Pediatric Dentistry, 11,* 209–213.

207. McTimoney, C. A., & Micheli, L. J. (2003). Current evaluation and management of spondylolysis and spondylolisthesis. *Current Sports Medicine Reports, 2,* 41–46.

208. Meehan, W. P., & Bachur, R. G. (2009). Sports-Related Concussions. *Pediatrics, 123,* 114–123.

209. Micheli, L. J. (1995). Sports injuries in children and adolescents. Questions and controversies. *Clinics in Sports Medicine, 14,* 727–745.

210. Micheli, L. J., & Fehlandt, A. F., Jr. (1992). Overuse injuries to tendons and apophyses in children and adolescents. *Clinics in Sports Medicine, 11,* 713–726.

211. Mitchell, L. J., & Jenkins, M. (2001). *Sports Medicine Bible for Young Athletes.* Naperville, IL: Sourcebooks, Inc.

212. Micheli, L. J., & Nielson, J. H. (2008). Overuse Injuries in the Young Athlete: Stress Fractures. In H. Hebestreit & O. Bar-or (Eds.), *The young athlete* (pp. 151–163). MA: Blackwell.

213. Micheli, L. J., & Smith, A. D. (1982). Sports injuries in children. *Current Problems in Pediatrics, 12,* 1–54.

214. Micheli, L. J., & Wood, R. (1995). Back pain in young athletes. Significant differences from adults in causes and patterns. *Archives of Pediatric and Adolescent Medicine, 149,* 15–18.

215. Millar, A. L. (1990). Ergogenic aids. In B. Sanders (Ed.). *Sports physical therapy* (pp. 79–93). Norwalk, CT: Appleton & Lange.

216. Mintzer, C. M., Richmond, J. C., & Taylor, J. (1998). Meniscal repair in the young athlete. *American Journal of Sports Medicine, 26,* 630–633.

217. Moeller, J. L. (2003). Pelvic and hip apophyseal avulsion injuries in young athletes. *Current Sports Medicine Reports, 2,* 110–115.

218. Moller, E., Forssblad, M., Hansson, L., et al. (2001). Bracing versus nonbracing in rehabilitation after anterior cruciate ligament reconstruction: A randomized prospective study with 2-year follow-up. *Knee Surgery, Sports Traumatology, Arthroscopy, 9*(2), 102–108.

219. Moti, A. W., & Micheli, L. J. (2003). Meniscal and articular cartilage injury in the skeletally immature knee. *Instructional Course Lectures, 52,* 683–690.

220. Myer, G. D.; Ford, K. R., Brent, J. L., & Hewett, T. E. (2007). Differential neuromuscular training effects on ACL injury risk factors in "high-risk" versus "low-risk" athletes. *BMC Musculoskeletal Disorders, 8,* 39.

221. Myer, G. D., Ford, K. R., & Hewett, T. E. (2008, September). Tuck jump assessment for reducing anterior cruciate ligament risk. *Athletic Therapy Today,* 39–44.

222. Myer, G. D., Ford, K. R., Palumbo, J. P., & Hewett, T. E. (2005). Neuromuscular training improves performance and lower-extremity biomechanics in female athletes. *Journal of Strength and Conditioning Research, 19*(1), 51–60.

223. Myer, G. D., Paterno, M. V., Ford, K. R., Quatman, C. E., & Hewett, T. E. (2006). Rehabilitation after anterior Cruciate ligament reconstruction: Criteria-based progression through the return-to-sport phase. *Journal of Orthopaedic and Sports Physical Therapy, 36*(6), 385–402.

224. Nadler, S. F., Malanga, G. A., Feinberg, J. H., Rubanni, M., Moley, R., & Foye, P. (2002). Functional performance deficits in athletes with previous lower extremity injury. *Clinical Journal of Sport Medicine, 12,* 73–78.

225. Napier, S. M., Baker, R. S., & Sanford, D. G. (1996). Eye injuries in athletics and recreation. *Survey Ophthalmologia, 41,* 229–244.

226. National Institutes of Health. (1996). *Update on the Task Force report on high blood pressure in children and adolescents.* National Institutes of Health Publication 96–3790.

227. National Safe Kids Campaign: Injury Facts. Available at www.safekids.org/ [Accessed on July 31, 2004].

228. Naylor, A. H., Gardner, D., & Zaichkowsky, L. (1996). Drug use patterns among high school athletes and nonathletes. *Adolescence, 36*(144), 627–639.

229. Nguyen, D., & Letts, M. (2001). In-line skating injuries in children: A ten year review. *Journal of Pediatric Orthopedics, 21,* 613–618.

230. Noguchi, T. (2001). A survey of spinal cord injuries resulting from sport. *Paraplegia, 32,* 170–173.

231. Noyes, F. R., & Barber-Westin, S. D. (2002). Arthroscopic repair of meniscal tears extending into the avascular zone in patients younger than twenty years of age. *American Journal of Sports Medicine, 30,* 589–600.

232. Noyes, F. R., Barber, S. D. & Mangine, R. E. (1991). Abnormal lower limb symmetry determined by function hop tests after anterior cruciate ligament rupture. *American Journal of Sports Medicine, 19*(5), 513–518.

233. Noyes, F. R., Berrios-Torres, S., Barber-Westin, S. D., et al. (2000). Prevention of permanent arthrofibrosis after anterior cruciate ligament reconstruction alone or combined with associated procedures: A prospective study in 443 knees. *Knee Surgery, Sports Traumatology, Arthroscopy, 8*(4), 196–206.

234. Nsuami, M., Elie, M., Brooks, B. N., Sanders, L. S., Nash, T. D., Makonnen, F., Taylor, S. N., & Cohen, D. A. (2003). Screening for sexually transmitted diseases during preparticipation sports examination of high school adolescents. *Journal of Adolescent Health, 32,* 336–339.

235. Objective testing group certifies head protection. (1988, March). *Occupational Health and Safety,* 18–20.

236. Ogden, J. A. (2000). *Skeletal injury in the child.* New York: Springer-Verlag.

237. Ogden, C. L., Flegal, K. M., Carroll, M. D., et al. (2002) Prevelance and trends in overweight among US children and adolescents 1999–2000. *JAMA 288*(14), 1728–1732.

238. Omey M. L., & Micheli L. J. (1999) Foot and Ankle problems in the young athlete. *Med Sci Sports Exerc, 31,* S470–486.

239. Onate, K., Cortes, N., Welch, C., Van Lunen, B. L. (2010). Expert versus novice interrater reliability and criterion validity of the landing error scoring system. *Journal of Sports Rehabilitation, 19*(1), 41–56.

240. O'Neill, D. B., & Micheli, L. J. (1988). Overuse injuries in the young athlete. *Clinics in Sports Medicine, 7,* 591–610.

241. Osberg, J. S., Schneps, S. E., DiScala, C., & Li, G. Skateboarding: More dangerous than roller skating or in-line skating. *Archives of Pediatrics and Adolescent Medicine, 52,* 985–991, 1998.

242. Outerbridge, A. R., & Micheli, L. J. (1995). Overuse injuries in young athletes. *Clinics in Sports Medicine, 14,* 503–516.

243. Padua, D. A., Marshall, S. W., Boling, M. C., Thigpen, C. A., Garrett, W. E. Jr., & Beutler, A. L. (2009). The Landing Error Scoring System (LESS) is a valid and reliable clinical assessment tool of jump-landing biomechanics: The JUMPACL study. *American Journal of Sports Medicine, 37*(10), 1996–2002. Epub 2009 Sep 2.

244. Paletta, G. A., Jr., & Andrish, J. T. (1995). Injuries about the hip and pelvis in the young athlete. *Clinics in Sports Medicine, 14,* 591–628.

245. Pare, F., Noreau, L., & Simard, C. (1995). Prediction of maximal aerobic power from a submaximal exercise test performed by paraplegics on a wheelchair ergometer. *Paraplegia, 31,* 584–592.

246. Passe, D. H., Horn, M., & Murray, R. (1995). Impact of beverage acceptability on fluid intake during exercise. *Appetite, 35*(3), 219–229.

247. Patel, D. R., & Nelson, T. L. (2000). Sports injuries in adolescents. *Medical Clinics of North America, 84,* 983–1007.

248. Paterno, M. V., Schmitt, L. C., Ford, K. R., et al. (2010, in press). Biomechanical Measures during Landing and Postural Stability Predict Second Anterior Cruciate Ligament Injury after ACL Reconstruction and Return to Sport. *American Journal of Sports Medicine.*

249. Paterson, P. D., & Waters, P. M. (2000). Shoulder injuries in the childhood athlete. *Clinics in Sports Medicine, 19,* 681–692.

250. Patrick, G. D. (1984). Comparison of novice and veteran wheelchair athletes' self-concept and acceptance of disability. *Rehabilitation Counseling Bulletin, 27,* 186–188.

251. Paulsen, P., French, R., & Sherrill, C. (1991). Comparison of mood states of college able-bodied and wheelchair basketball players. *Perceptual Motor Skills, 73,* 396–398.

252. Peljovich, A. E., & Simmons, B. P. (2000). Traumatic arthritis of the hand and wrist in children. *Hand Clinics, 16,* 673–684.

253. Peltz, J. E., Haskell, W. L., & Matheson, G. O. (1999). A comprehensive and cost-effective preparticipation exam implemented on the World Wide Web. *Medicine & Science in Sports & Exercise, 31*(12), 1727–1740.

254. Peretti-Watel, P., Guagliardo, V., Verger, P., Pruvost, J., Mignon, P., & Obadia, Y. (1995). Sporting activity and drug use: Alcohol, cigarette and cannabis use among elite student athletes. *Addiction, 98,* 1249–1256.

255. Perkins, S. W., Dayan, S. H., Sklarew, E. D., Hamilton, M., & Bussell, G. S. (2000). The incidence of sports-related facial trauma in children. *Ear Nose Throat Journal, 79,* 632–638.

256. Perriello, V. A., Jr., Almquist, J., Conkwright, D., Jr., et al. (1995). Health and weight control management among wrestlers. A proposed program for high school athletes. *Virginia Medical Quarterly, 122,* 179–183.

257. Peterson, M., & Peterson, K. (1988). *Eat to compete: A guide to sports nutrition.* Chicago: Year Book Medical.

258. Pieter W. (2005). Martial arts injuries. In D. J. Caine & N. Maffulli (Eds.), Epidemiology of Pediatric Sports Injuries. Individual Sports. Med Sport Sci (pp. 59–73). *vol. 48.* Basel: Karger.

259. Pitetti, K. H., Rimmer, J. H., & Fernhall, B. (1993). Physical fitness and adults with mental retardation: An overview of current research and future directions. *Sports Medicine, 16,* 23–56.

260. Plisky, P. J., Rauh, M. J.; Kaminski, T. W., & Underwood, F. B. (2006). Star Excursion Balance Test as a predictor of lower extremity injury in high school basketball players. *Journal of Orthopaedic and Sports Physical Therapy, 36*(12), 911–919.

261. Powell, E. C. (1997). Protecting children in the accident and emergency department. *Accidents and Emergency Nursing, 5,* 76–80.

262. Powell, E. C., & Tanz, R. R. (2000). Tykes and bikes: Injuries associated with bicycle-towed child trailers and bicycle-mounted child seats. *Archives of Pediatric & Adolescent Medicine, 154,* 351–353.

263. Powell, E. C., & Tanz, R. R. (2000). Cycling injuries treated in emergency departments: Need for bicycle helmets among preschoolers. *Archives of Pediatric & Adolescent Medicine, 154,* 1096–1100.

264. Powell, J. (1987). 636,000 injuries annually in high school football. *Athletic Trainer, 22,* 19–22.

265. Powers, C. M. (2003). The influence of altered lower-extremity kinematics on patellofemoral joint dysfunction: A theoretical perspective. *Journal of Orthopaedic and Sports Physical Therapy, 33*(11), 639–646.

266. Pratt, M., Macera, C. A., & Blanton, C. (1999). Levels of physical activity and inactivity in children and adults in the United States: Current evidence and research issues. *Medicine & Science in Sports & Exercise, 31,* S526–S533.

267. Pueschel, S. M. (1998). Should children with Down syndrome be screened for atlantoaxial instability? *Archives of Pediatric & Adolescent Medicine, 152,* 123–125.

268. Puffer, J. C. (1991). Organizational aspects. In R. C. Cantu & L. J. Micheli (Eds.), *ACSM's guidelines for the team physician* (pp. 95–100). Philadelphia: Lea & Febiger.

269. Quinn, K., Parker, P., de Bie, R., Rowe, B., & Handoll, H. (1990). Interventions for preventing ankle ligament injuries. *Cochrane Database Systems Review, 2,* CD000018.

270. Regan, K. J., Banks, G. K., & Beran, R. G. (1995). Therapeutic recreation programmes for children with epilepsy. *Seizure, 2,* 195–200.

271. Reid, A., Birmingham, T. B., Stratford, P. N. et al. (2007). Hop testing provides a reliable and valid outcome measure during rehabilitation after anterior cruciate ligament reconstruction. *Physical Therapy, 87*(3), 337–349.

272. Reinold, M. M., Wilk, K. E., Macrina, L. C., et al. (2006). Current concepts in the rehabilitation following articular cartilage repair procedures in the knee. *J Orthop Sports Phys Ther, 36,* 774–794.

273. Rifat, S. F., Ruffin, M. T., 4th, & Gorenflo, D. W. (1995). Disqualifying criteria in a preparticipation sports evaluation. *Journal of Family Practice, 41,* 42–50.

274. Rimmer, J. H. (2001). Physical fitness levels of persons with cerebral palsy. *Developmental Medicine and Child Neurology, 43*(3), 208–212.

275. Rivera-Brown, A. M., Gutierrez, R., Gutierrez, J. C., Frontera, W. R., & Bar-Or, O. (1997). Drink composition, voluntary drinking, and fluid balance in exercising, training, heat-acclimatized boys. *Journal of Applied Physiology, 86,* 78–84.

276. Rossi, F., & Dragoni, S. (1990). Lumbar spondylolisthesis: Occurrence in competitive athletes. *Journal of Sports Medicine and Physical Fitness, 30,* 450–452.

277. Roi, G. S., Creta D., Nanni G., et al. (2005). Return to official Italian First Division soccer games within 90 days after anterior cruciate ligament reconstruction: A case report. *Journal of Orthopaedic and Sports Physical Therapy, 35*(2), 52–61; discussion, 61–66.

278. Rudzki, J. R., Paletta, G. A. (2004). Jr. Juvenile and adolescent elbow injuries in sports. *Clinics in Sports Medicine, 23*(4), 581–608, ix.

279. Sachtelben, T. R., Berg, K. E., Elias, B. A., Cheatham, J. P., Felix, G. L., & Hofschire, P. J. (1993). The effects of anabolic steroids on myocardial structure and cardiovascular fitness. *Medicine & Science in Sports & Exercise, 25,* 1240–1245.

280. Salter, R. B., & Harris, W. R. (1963). Injuries Involving the Epiphyseal Plate. *Journal of Bone and Joint Surgery, 45-A,* 587–622, and *Joint Surgery, 45-A,* 587–622.

281. Sanders, B. (Ed.). *Sports physical therapy.* Norwalk, CT: Appleton & Lange, 1990.

282. Santopietro, F. J. (1993). Foot and foot-related injuries in the young athlete. *Clinics in Sports Medicine, 7,* 563–589.

283. Schmitt, H., & Gerner, H. J. (1993). Paralysis from sport and diving accidents. *Clinical Journal of Sport Medicine, 11,* 17–22.

284. Schmitt, L. C., Paterno, M. V., Huang, S. (in press). Validity and Internal Consistency of the International Knee Documentation Committee Subjective Knee Form in Children and Adolescents. *American Journal of Sports Medicine.*

285. Schuller, D. E., Dankle, S. K., Martin, M., & Strauss, R. H. (1993). Auricular injury and the use of headgear in wrestlers. *Archives of Otolaryngological Head Neck Surgery, 115,* 714–717.

286. Segesser, B., & Pforringer, W. (Eds.). *The shoe in sport.* Chicago: Year Book Medical, 1989.

287. Selsby, J. T., Beckett, K. D., Kern, M., & Devor, S. (2003). Swim performance following creatine supplementation in division III athletes. *Journal of Strength & Conditioning, 17*(3), 421–424.

288. Sharkey, B. (1991). Training for sports. In R. C. Cantu & L. J. Micheli (Eds.), *ACSM's guidelines for the team physician* (pp. 34–47). Philadelphia: Lea & Febiger.

289. Shea, K. G., Pfeiffer, R., Wang J. H., et al. (2004). Anterior cruciate ligament injury in pediatric and adolescent soccer players: An analysis of insurance data. *Journal of Pediatric Orthopedics, 24*(6), 623–628.

290. Sherrill, C., Hinson, M., Gench, B., Kennedy, S. O., & Low, L. Self-concepts of disabled youth athletes. *Perceptual Motor Skills, 70,* 1093–1098, 1990.

291. Shi, X., Summers, R. W., Schedl, H. P., Flanagan, S. W., Chang, R., & Gisolfi, C. V. (1995). Effects of carbohydrate type and concentration and solution osmolarity on water absorption. *Medicine & Science in Sports & Exercise, 27,* 1607–1615.

292. Shorter, N. A., Mooney, D. P., & Harmon, B. J. (1999). Snowboarding injuries in children and adolescents. *American Journal of Emergency Medicine, 17,* 261–263.

293. Skokan, E. G., Junkins, E. P., Jr., & Kadish, H. (2003). Serious winter sports injuries in children and adolescents requiring hospitalization. *American Journal of Emergency Medicine, 21,* 95–99.

294. Small, E. (2008). The preparticipation physical evaluation. In H. Hebestreit & O. Bar-or (Eds.), *The young athlete* (pp. 191–202). Boston: Blackwell.

295. Smith, A. D. (2003). The skeletally immature knee: What's new in overuse injuries. *Instructional Course Lectures, 52,* 691–697.

296. Smith, G. A., & Shields, B. J. (1998). Trampoline-related injuries to children. *Archives of Pediatric & Adolescent Medicine, 152,* 694–699.

297. Smith, J., & Laskowski, E. R. (1998). The preparticipation physical examination: Mayo Clinic experience with 2,739 examinations. *Mayo Clinic Proceedings, 73,* 419–429.

298. Smith, J., & Wilder, E. P. (1999). Musculoskeletal rehabilitation and sports medicine. *Archives of Physical Medicine and Rehabilitation, 80,* S68–S89.

299. Sobal J., Marquart L. F. (1994) Vitamin/Mineral supplement use among high school athletes. *Adolescence, 29,* 835–843.

300. Soderman, K., Pietila, T., Alfredson, H., & Werner, S. (2002). Anterior cruciate ligament injuries in young females playing soccer at senior levels. *Scandinavian Journal of Medicine and Science in Sports, 12,* 65–68.

301. Sosin, D. M., Sacks, J. J., & Webb, K. W. (1996). Pediatric head injuries and deaths from bicycling in the United States. *Pediatrics, 98*(5), 868–870.

302. Special Olympics inquiry data. (2001). Washington, DC: World Winter Games.

303. Squire, D. L. (1990). Heat illness. Fluid and electrolyte issues for pediatric and adolescent athletes. *Pediatric Clinics of North America, 37,* 1085–1109.

304. Stanitski, C. (1989). Common injuries in preadolescent athletes. *Sports Medicine, 7,* 32–41.

305. Stanitski, C. L. (1997). Pediatric and adolescent sports injuries. *Clinics in Sports Medicine, 16,* 613–633.

306. Stanitski, C. L., Delee, J. C., & Drez, D. (1994). *Pediatric and adolescent sports medicine.* Philadelphia: WB Saunders.

307. Reference deleted in page proofs.

308. Steiner, M. E., & Grana, W. A. (1988). The young athlete's knee: Recent advances. *Clinics in Sports Medicine, 7,* 527–546.

309. Stock, J. G., & Cornell, F. M. (1991). Prevention of sports-related eye injury. *American Family Practice, 44,* 515–520.

310. Strahlman, E., Elman, M., Daub, E., & Baker, S. (1990). Causes of pediatric eye injuries. A population-based study. *Archives of Ophthalmology, 108,* 603–606.

311. Stronski, S. M., Ireland, M., Michaud, P., Narring, F., & Resnick, M. D. (2000). Protective correlates of stages in adolescent substance use: A Swiss National Study. *Journal of Adolescent Health, 26*(6), 420–427.

312. Surgeon General. Call to action to prevent and decrease overweight and obesity. Washington, D. C., 2001. Available at www.surgerongeneral.gov/topics/obesity. Accessed September 26, 2005.

313. Taimela, S., Kujala, U. M., & Osterman, K. (1990). Intrinsic risk factors and athletic injuries. *Sports Medicine, 9,* 205–215.

314. Taylor, B. L., & Attia, M. W. (2000). Sports-related injuries in children. *Academy of Emergency Medicine, 7,* 1376–1382.

315. Taylor, D., & Williams, T. (1995). Sports injuries in athletes with disabilities: Wheelchair racing. *Paraplegia, 33,* 296–299.

316. Tepper, K. B., & Ireland, M. L. (2003). Fracture patterns and treatment in the skeletally immature knee. *Instructional Course Lectures, 52,* 667–676.

317. Thomee, R., Renstrom, P., Karlsson, J., & Grimby, G. (1995). Patellofemoral pain syndrome in young women: A clinical analysis of alignment, pain parameters, common symptoms, and functional activity level. *Scandinavian Journal of Medicine & Science in Sports, 5,* 237–244.

318. Thurman, D. J., Branche, C. M., & Sniezek, J. E. (1998). The epidemiology of sports-related traumatic brain injuries in the United States: Recent developments. *Journal of Head Trauma Rehabilitation, 13,* 1–8.

319. Tol, J. L., Struijs, P. A., Bossuyt, P. M., Verhagen, R. A., & van Dijk, C. N. (2000). Treatment strategies in osteochondral defects of the talar dome: A systematic review. *Foot Ankle International, 21,* 119–126.

320. Trepman, E., & Micheli L. J. (1998). Overuse injuries in sports. *Seminars in Orthopedics, 3,* 217–222.

321. USDA/ARS Children's Nutrition Research Center at Baylor College of Medicine. Available at www.bcm.tmc.edu/cnrc/consumer/archives/percentDV.htm. Accessed September 26, 2005.

322. Utter, A., Kang, J., Nieman, D., & Warren, B. (1997). Effect of carbohydrate substrate availability on ratings of perceived exertion during prolonged running. *International Journal of Sport Nutrition, 7,* 274–285.

323. Van Hall, G., Raaymakers, J. S. H., Saris, W. H. M., & Wagenmakers, A. J. M. (1995). Ingestion of branched-chain amino acids and tryptophan during sustained exercise in man: Failure to affect performance. *Journal of Physiology, 486,* 789–794.

324. Van Mechelen, W. (1992). Running injuries: A review of the epidemiological literature. *Sports Medicine, 14,* 320–335.

325. Varni, J. W., & Setoguchi, Y. (1991). Correlates of perceived physical appearance in children with congenital/acquired limb deficiencies. *Journal of Developmental and Behavioral Pediatrics, 12,* 171–176.

326. Varni, J. W., Seid, M., & Kurtin, P. S. (2001). PedsQL 4.0: Reliability and validity of the Pediatric Quality of Life Inventory version 4.0 generic core scales in healthy and patient populations. *Medical Care, 39*(8), 800–812.

327. Varni, J. W., Seid, M., & Rode, C. A. (1999). The PedsQL: Measurement model for the pediatric quality of life inventory. *Medical Care, 37*(2), 126–139.

328. Veeger, H. E., Hadj Yahmed, M., van der Woude, L. H., & Charpentier, P. (1991). Peak oxygen uptake and maximal power output of Olympic wheelchair-dependent athletes. *Medicine & Science in Sports & Exercise, 23,* 1201–1209.

329. Wagner, J. C. (1991). Enhancement of athletic performance with drugs. An overview. *Sports Medicine, 12,* 250–265.

330. Waicus, K. M., & Smith, B. W. (2002). Back injuries in the pediatric athlete. *Current Sports Medicine Reports, 1,* 52–58.

331. Waters, P. M., & Millis, M. B. (1988). Hip and pelvic injuries in the young athlete. *Clinics in Sports Medicine, 7,* 513–526.

332. Webster, J. B., Levy, C. E., Bryant, P. R., & Prusakowski, P. E. (2001). Sports and recreation for persons with limb deficiency. *Archives of Physical Medicine and Rehabilitation, 82*(3), S38–S44.

333. Wiens, L., Sabath, R., Ewing, L., Gowdamarajan, R., Portnoy, J., & Scagliotti, D. (1992). Chest pain in otherwise healthy children and adolescents is frequently caused by exercise-induced asthma. *Pediatrics, 90,* 350–353.

334. Wilk, B., & Bar-Or, O. (1996). Effect of drink flavor and NaCl on voluntary drinking and hydration in boys exercising in the heat. *Journal of Applied Physiology, 80,* 1112–1117.

335. Wilk, K. E., Reinold, M. M., & Andrews, J. R. (2004). Rehabilitation of the thrower's elbow. *Clinics in Sports Medicine, 23*(4), 765–801, xii.

336. Wilk, K. E., Briem, K., Reinold, M. M., Devine, K. M., Dugas, J., & Andrews, J. R. (2006). Rehabilitation of articular lesions in the athlete's knee. *Journal of Orthopaedic and Sports Physical Therapy, 36*(10), 815–827.

337. Williams, J. S., Jr., Abate, J. A., Fadale, P. D., & Tung, G. A. (1996). Meniscal and nonosseous ACL injuries in children and adolescents. *American Journal of Knee Surgery, 9,* 22–26.

338. Williams, M. H. (1994). The use of ergogenic aids in sports: Is it an ethical issue? *International Journal of Sports Nutrition, 4,* 120–131.

339. Wilson, P. E., & Washington, R. L. (1993). Pediatric wheelchair athletics: Sports injuries and prevention. *Paraplegia, 31,* 330–337.

340. Winston, F. K., Weiss, H. B., Nance, M. L., Vivarelli, O., Neill, C., Strotmeyer, S., Lawrence, B. A., & Miller, T. R. (2002). Estimates of the incidence and costs associated with handlebar-related injuries in children. *Archives of Pediatric & Adolescent Medicine, 156,* 922–928.

341. Witvrouw, E., Lysens, R., Bellemans, J., Cambier, D., Cools, A., Danneels, I., & Bourgois, J. (2002). Which factors predict outcome in the treatment program of anterior knee pain? *Scandinavian Journal of Medicine & Science in Sports, 12,* 40–46.

342. Finkelstein E. A. Fiekbelkorn I. C., & Wang G. (2003). National Medical spending attributable to overweight and obesity: how much and who's paying? *Health Aff, W3,* 219–226.

343. Yesalis, C. E., & Bahrke, M. S. (2000). Doping among adolescent athletes. *Baillieres Best Practices Research in Clinical Endocrinology Metabolism, 14,* 25–35.

344. Zoints, L. E. (2002). Fractures around the knee in children. *Journal of American Academy of Orthopedic Surgery, 10,* 345–355.

345. Zwiren, L., & Bar-Or, O. (1975). Response to exercise of paraplegics who differ in conditioning level. *Medicine and Science in Sports, 7,* 94–98.

16 Developmental Coordination Disorder (DCD)

LISA RIVARD, PT, BSc(PT), MSc • CHERYL MISSIUNA, PhD, OTReg(Ont) • NANCY POLLOCK, MSc, OTReg(Ont) •
KATHRYN STEYER DAVID, PT, MS, PCS

Pediatric physical therapists evaluate and manage care for children presenting with a variety of motor challenges. They observe children's movement skills and ask key questions about children's motor abilities and development to differentiate among motor behaviors that are characteristic of particular conditions. This differentiation guides their selection of a course of intervention. Some of the children whom physical therapists observe are quite a "puzzle" to figure out. These children frequently trip over their feet and bump into others with clumsy, awkward movements. They may have an unusual gait pattern, or a unique way of "fixing" or stabilizing their joints. Despite these differences, they are often observed to reach their motor milestones within normal age limits. Many of these children appear to have difficulty generalizing learned motor skills across settings or transferring skills to other contexts. Each child with motor difficulties such as these presents a little differently from the others, making it difficult to develop and apply a treatment approach. The children who are captured by this description are those who have developmental coordination disorder (DCD).[4]

Approximately 5% to 6% of school-age children have movement difficulties, unrelated to specific neurologic conditions or cognitive impairment, that limit their potential and affect their long-term academic achievement.[4] Recently, the prevalence rate for the most significantly impaired children in a United Kingdom (U.K.) birth cohort of 6990 children aged 7 to 8 years was close to 2% of the population.[115] These children struggle with everyday functional tasks such as dressing, throwing and catching balls, and learning to ride a bicycle.[10,64,129,135,136] They experience daily frustration with activities that are effortless for their peers, and, as a consequence of their motor problems, they may demonstrate additional difficulties, including poor perceived competence, social isolation, low self-worth, anxiety, and depressive symptoms, even at early ages.[60,163–165,194,195,204,212,217] These

difficulties are characteristic features of developmental coordination disorder (DCD), a condition in which poorly developed fine and/or gross motor coordination has a substantial impact on motor skill performance with far-reaching consequences for daily life activities and scholastic achievement.[4] Although it was once believed that these difficulties would diminish with time and maturation, compelling evidence now suggests that DCD is a lifelong condition,[25,39,49,56,119] making this disorder one that warrants significant attention.

Physical therapists have a unique service to offer children with DCD and their families. Therapists' understanding of normal and abnormal motor control, motor learning, and motor development can be used to identify and evaluate the condition, and to plan programs for children with DCD. Through education of children with DCD and their families, teachers, and others in the community, physical therapists can help children with DCD become more active and successful participants in their home, school, and community life.

The information presented in this chapter is intended to increase awareness, recognition, and understanding of children with DCD. The complex nature of DCD and its challenges for clinical management are described. The role of the physical therapist in managing children with this disorder and intervention approaches shown to be effective with children with DCD are explored. Evidence is presented to support the need for a multidisciplinary assessment, and tailored, family-centered intervention with collaborative consultation is emphasized. Three case studies conclude the chapter and serve to illustrate the heterogeneity of the disorder—a factor that greatly influences the decision-making process and strategies employed in the management of a child with DCD. Resources available for children with DCD and their families, as well as health professionals involved in their care, are provided on the Evolve website.

HISTORICAL BACKGROUND

A disorder of "clumsiness" whose key feature is poor motor coordination has been recognized and described for over a century. Much of our current understanding of DCD, however, has resulted from an explosion of research in the field over the past two decades.[124] DCD is a childhood disorder that is of interest to numerous professionals in the medical, rehabilitation, and education fields. Clinicians and researchers, each adopting various perspectives on the condition, have utilized diverse theoretical frameworks in their study of children with DCD. This wide-reaching interest in DCD has provided fertile ground for the development of knowledge about the condition. Historically, however, this diversity in perspectives has also led to a lack of consensus, impacting the progression of research in the field. Different labels have been ascribed to children with DCD, including the clumsy child syndrome,[76] the physically awkward child,[237] developmental dyspraxia,[31] sensory integrative dysfunction,[7] disorder of attention, motor and perception (DAMP),[71] and minor coordination dysfunction,[242] each reflecting the perspectives of professionals who work with these children.[143] In 1994 an international consensus exercise was undertaken,[174] and the term *DCD* was adopted to unify descriptions of children with significant motor incoordination. This decision, in part, was grounded in the recognition that DCD had become an officially recognized movement skills disorder.[3] Recently, a second international consensus conference recommended maintaining use of the term *DCD*.[225] Although *DCD* is the term most widely used in the literature, other terms continue to appear, highlighting the diverse perspectives of researchers who study children with motor difficulties.

DEFINITION AND PREVALENCE

DCD is a chronic condition involving impairment in gross motor, postural, and/or fine motor performance that affects a child's ability to perform the skilled movements necessary for daily living, including the performance of academic and self-care tasks. By definition, DCD is not attributable to a known neurologic or medical disorder.[4] The manifestation of the disorder varies across children, with a spectrum of severity. DCD would be included under the *Guide to Physical Therapist Practice*[2] diagnostic group 5C: Impaired Motor Function and Sensory Integrity Associated With Nonprogressive Disorders of the Central Nervous System—Congenital Origin or Acquired in Infancy or Childhood.

Research performed in many countries around the world has confirmed that large numbers of children are affected by this childhood motor disorder.[58,69,95,102,115,261] Although DCD is highly prevalent in school-age children, it has only recently received worldwide recognition.[4] Attention is increasingly being paid to this disorder because of the impact of children's primary motor limitations on everyday life. The American Psychiatric Association (APA) estimates that DCD affects 5% to 6% of school-age children. Although it is commonly accepted that boys with DCD outnumber girls by a 2:1 ratio,[4] recent population-based studies of children with DCD would suggest that more equal numbers of boys and girls may be affected.[24] The prevalence of DCD appears to be substantially higher than average in preterm populations.[37,43,73,93,251,259] It has also been noted that, over time, preterm/low birth weight infants tend to exhibit poor coordination and many of the physical consequences associated with DCD such as decreased aerobic fitness, strength, and physical activity levels.[190]

DIAGNOSIS

DCD is present when (1) motor impairment and/or motor skill delay significantly impacts a child's ability to perform age-appropriate complex motor activities, (2) adequate opportunities for experience and practice have been provided, and (3) no other explanation can be offered for the motor impairment.[198] In most states and provinces, a diagnosis of DCD can be made only by a physician because it is critical to rule out any other underlying neurologic or medical reasons for the observed motor impairment. Four distinct criteria must be met for a diagnosis of DCD to be given, as outlined in the *Diagnostic and Statistical Manual of Mental Disorders* (Box 16-1)[4]: (A) The motor impairment

---

Box **16-1** DIAGNOSTIC CRITERIA FOR DEVELOPMENTAL COORDINATION DISORDER (DCD)

- Performance in daily activities that require motor coordination is substantially below that expected, given the person's chronologic age and measured intelligence. This may be manifested by the following:
  - Marked delays in achieving motor milestones (e.g., walking, crawling, sitting)
  - Dropping things
  - "Clumsiness"
  - Poor performance in sports
  - Poor handwriting
- The disturbance significantly interferes with academic achievement or activities of daily living.
- The disturbance is not due to a general medical condition (e.g., cerebral palsy, hemiplegia, muscular dystrophy) and does not meet criteria for a pervasive developmental disorder.
- If mental retardation is present, motor difficulties are in excess of those usually associated with it.

American Psychiatric Association (APA). (2000). *Diagnostic and statistical manual of mental disorders, fourth edition, text revision (DSM IV-TR)*. Washington, DC: American Psychiatric Association.

must be substantial and discrepant from other abilities, (B) it must have an impact on academic achievement or activities of daily living (ADLs), (C) it must not meet the criteria for a pervasive developmental disorder (PDD) (see Chapter 17 on children with cognitive and motor impairment); and, (D) if accompanied by cognitive difficulties, it must be greater than what would be accounted for by that cognitive impairment.[4] Recently, it has been recommended that if the criteria for diagnosis of PDD are met, both diagnoses should be given.[225] Physical therapists have an important role to play in facilitating a diagnosis of DCD by assisting physicians with confirmation of whether a child meets both criteria A and B of the DCD diagnostic criteria. This will be discussed in greater detail later in this chapter.

DCD usually is not considered to be present if (1) recent head injury or trauma has occurred, (2) progressive deterioration in previously acquired skills is evident, or (3) increased or fluctuating muscle tone is present. DCD also would not be suspected routinely where there is a history of headaches or blurred vision, when evidence of asymmetrical tone or strength is observed, or when musculoskeletal abnormalities or Gowers' sign are present (Box 16-2).[77,138] If children do not show any of these signs but demonstrate uncoordinated movements and motor abilities below those expected for their age, they may have DCD, and it is important for these children to be seen by a physician. A medical practitioner can rule out other possible causes for poor coordination, including genetic causes (e.g., Down syndrome), neurologic disorders (e.g., cerebral palsy), degenerative conditions (e.g., muscular dystrophy, brain tumors),

musculoskeletal abnormalities (e.g., Legg-Calvé-Perthes disease), physical impairments (e.g., impaired visual acuity), cognitive impairment (e.g., developmental delay), pervasive developmental disorder (e.g., autism), and head injury (e.g., traumatic brain injury) (Box 16-3).[77,138] See respective chapters in this volume for further information on these other conditions.

CO-OCCURRING CONDITIONS

Strong associations have been demonstrated between DCD and attention deficit hyperactivity disorder (ADHD), speech/articulation difficulties (specific language impairment [SLI]), and language-based learning disabilities (LDs) (in particular, reading disability).[47,61,89,99,101,166,168,181,230,244] When a child has any of these conditions, the likelihood that DCD is also present is at least 50%. When criteria for more than one disorder are met, more than one diagnosis should be given.[4,225] It is recognized that the presence of co-occurring conditions may increase the probability of negative outcomes.[12,181,204] In particular, children who have DCD in addition to ADHD have a significantly poorer outcome in terms of academic achievement and mental health than children with ADHD alone.[83,181,230] It is important to determine whether or not motor coordination problems are present, and whether they are occurring in combination with another recognized condition. Knowledge of a child's complete profile (including associated conditions) will assist in the identification process and will help to determine intervention and management strategies. The frequently documented association between other developmental disorders and DCD underscores the need for a multidisciplinary assessment.

Box **16-2** DEVELOPMENTAL COORDINATION DISORDER (DCD)—DIFFERENTIAL DIAGNOSIS

Coordination difficulties are likely not DCD when a history of any of the following is reported:
- Recent head injury or trauma
- Deterioration in previously learned or acquired skills
- Headaches, eye pain, blurred vision
- Global developmental delays
- Increased muscle tone, fluctuating tone, or significant hypotonia
- Asymmetrical tone or strength
- Musculoskeletal abnormality
- Neurocutaneous lesion
- Avoidance of eye contact, unwillingness to engage socially
- Gowers' sign (difficulty rising to a standing position)
- Ataxia, dysarthria
- Absence of deep tendon reflexes
- Dysmorphic features
- Visual impairment (untreated)

From Missiuna, C., Gaines, R., & Soucie, H. [2006]. Why every office needs a tennis ball: A new approach to assessing the clumsy child. *Canadian Medical Association Journal, 175,* 471–473.

Box **16-3** DEVELOPMENTAL COORDINATION DISORDER

Medical and neurologic disorders that can be associated with motor incoordination must be excluded before a formal diagnosis of DCD is made. These include the following:
- Genetic disorders (e.g., Down syndrome)
- Neurologic disorders (e.g., cerebral palsy)
- Degenerative conditions (e.g., Duchenne's muscular dystrophy, brain tumor)
- Musculoskeletal disorders (e.g., Legg-Calvé-Perthes disease)
- Physical impairments (e.g., impaired visual acuity)
- Cognitive impairments (e.g., developmental delay)
- Pervasive developmental disorders (e.g., autism)
- Injuries (e.g., traumatic brain injury)
- Environmental contaminants (e.g., lead, pesticides)

From Missiuna, C., Gaines, R., & Soucie, H. [2006]. Why every office needs a tennis ball: A new approach to assessing the clumsy child. *Canadian Medical Association Journal, 175,* 471–473.

LONG-TERM PROGNOSIS

Longitudinal research clearly demonstrates that, without intervention, children with DCD do not "grow out of" the disorder. Strong evidence indicates that the motor problems of childhood persist into adolescence and adulthood.[25,39,49,56,119] In fact, children with DCD are at risk of developing serious negative physical, social, emotional, behavioral, and mental health consequences that are not limited to the presenting motor difficulties. Multiple studies have shown that, over time, children with DCD are more likely to demonstrate poor social, academic, and physical competence, social isolation, academic and behavior problems, poor self-esteem, low self-efficacy, victimization, and higher rates of psychiatric and mental health problems.[26,34,53,65,119,163,167,181,194,204,212,217]

Children with DCD engage in less vigorous play and spend significantly more time away from the playground area than their peers.[12] They spend more time alone on the playground and spend less time in formal and informal team play.[217] Many researchers have shown that they are less likely to be physically fit or to participate voluntarily in motor activity, predisposing them to an inactive lifestyle.[12,156,183,241] Their reduced physical activity participation and the associated risks for long-term obesity and poor cardiovascular health are now being documented.[19–22,54,81,207] Although this picture of the numerous consequences associated with motor impairment appears dire, the potential exists for positive trajectories and pathways of resilience.[146] The long-term outcome of the disorder is influenced not only by the severity of impairment and co-occurring conditions, but also by the presence of supportive environments and the strengths of individuals with DCD, including their coping mechanisms. It is possible to "tip the scale" in favor of more positive

outcomes,[141] and physical therapists can be instrumental in preventing secondary impairments, which often become areas of greater focus as children mature.

The increased risk for children with DCD of secondary health issues and academic failure highlights the need to identify children with DCD as early as possible.[149] Early identification may facilitate the education of teachers and parents about how to make tasks easier and how to ensure that activities are matched to children's capabilities. In this way, children with DCD can be provided with optimally challenging situations that emphasize mastery and avoid multiple failed attempts.[150]

DESCRIBING CHILDREN WITH DCD

The International Classification of Functioning, Disability, and Health (ICF) provides a useful framework for understanding and describing the difficulties experienced by children with DCD.[260] In the ICF model, observable sensory/perceptual and motor impairments, at the level of body structure and function, can lead to difficulties with skill acquisition, and task performance or activity limitations. These activity constraints, in turn, can place limitations on participation in the many aspects of daily life, conceptualized in the ICF framework as participation restrictions. In addition, personal and environmental factors are seen as important mediating factors at each of these levels (Table 16-1).

BODY STRUCTURE AND FUNCTION

Any description of children with DCD is influenced by the heterogeneity of the condition. The presentation of DCD is somewhat age dependent, is highly variable across children,

TABLE 16-1 **Relationships Among Body Structures and Function, Activity, and Participation for a Child With Developmental Coordination Disorder (DCD)**

Health Condition	Body Structure and Function	Activity Limitations	Participation Restrictions— Environmental Factors	Participation Restrictions— Personal Factors
Unknown/possibly heterogeneous nervous system insult (of prenatal, perinatal, or postnatal origin)	Soft signs: Poor strength Poor coordination Jerky movements Poor visual perception Joint laxity Poor spatial organization Inadequate information processing Poor sequencing Poor feedback and feed forward motor control Poor short- and long-term memory	Awkward, slow gait Delayed and poor quality of fine and gross motor skills, such as hopping, jumping, ball skills, and writing Delayed oral-motor skills	Doors too heavy to open Physical education is competitive and skill oriented Late to class because passing time is too short Time to dress and undress reduces participation in recess and readiness for home and community activities Slow and messy written communication in class limits academic performance Peers don't wait to try to understand conversations	Depression Quit trying to participate, unmotivated Low self-esteem Poor fitness Activities performed without concern for time restrictions Vocational anxiety

TABLE 16-2   **Impairments of Body Structure and Function Identified in Children With Developmental Coordination Disorder (DCD)**

Body Function	Reference
Visual-perceptual, visual-spatial, and visuomotor impairment	Mon-Williams et al., 1999[153]; O'Brien et al., 1988[157]; Wilson & McKenzie, 1998[257]
Inefficient use of visual feedback in fast, goal-directed arm movements	van der Meulen et al., 1991[232]
Impaired visual memory	Dwyer & McKenzie, 1994[52]
More dependent on visuospatial rehearsal to memorize	Skorji & McKenzie, 1997[213]
Difficulty with visual and motor sequencing tasks requiring short- and long-term recall	Murphy & Gliner, 1988[154]
Impairments of size-constancy judgments, spatial position, and visual discrimination	Lord & Hulme, 1987[117]
Slow performance related to reliance on information feedback rather than feed forward programming	Missiuna et al., 2003[149]; Rosblad & van Hofsten, 1994[193]; Smyth, 1991[220]
Slow reaction time and movement time related to impaired response selection	Raynor, 1998[182]; Van Dellan & Geuze, 1988
Prolonged response latency related to the process of searching for and retrieving the correct responses with reliable timing	Henderson et al., 1992[86]
Poor timing, rhythm, and force control	Lundy-Ekman et al., 1991[120]; Volman & Geuze, 1998[236]; Williams et al., 1992[250]
Impaired performance on kinesthetic acuity, linear positioning, and weight discrimination	Hoare & Larkin, 1991[92]
Prolonged burst of agonist activity and delayed onset of antagonist activity	Huh et al., 1998[94]
Reduced power and strength	Raynor, 2001[183]
Reduced ability to successfully inhibit an action	Mandich et al., 2002[125]

and is complicated by the possible presence of co-occurring conditions. This variability in presentation has led investigators to examine multiple sensory and motor processes that contribute to the development of motor coordination. In a recent review of research into possible underlying mechanisms for DCD, primary impairments at the level of body structure and function have been proposed in the sensory, motor, and sensorimotor domains (Table 16-2).[235]

Primary Impairments

Sensory/Perceptual Deficits

Early research on children with DCD focused on possible impairments in visual, kinesthetic, and proprioceptive processing. Children with DCD were shown to have difficulties with visual-spatial processing, including determining object size and position, as well as with visual memory. Children with DCD have also demonstrated a limited ability to use visual rehearsal strategies.[52,257] More recent research suggests that in children with DCD, visual feedback is managed differently and is processed more slowly than in typically developing children.[255,264] Children with movement problems have also shown deficiencies in kinesthetic processing, have poor proprioceptive function,[111,221] and demonstrate a heavy reliance on visual feedback to guide task performance.[86,134,171,263] This predominant use of vision to control movement is observed well beyond the age at which typically developing children would rely on vision.[134,213,219] As a result, children with DCD lack automation in their movements and remain at an early stage of motor learning for much longer.

Because both visual and kinesthetic perceptual deficits have been demonstrated in groups of children with DCD, it has been suggested that the deficit may not be confined to one specific sensory modality, but may be multisensory in nature.[252] This seems plausible given that fluent, coordinated movements require multiple processes to plan, execute, and, when necessary, correct motor activity. Further, the motor impairments could be accounted for by impaired perception-action coupling or poor integration of the senses, including poor "mapping" of visual and proprioceptive information with the motor system.[153,191,210,218,264]

Research examining different profiles, or subtypes, of children with motor impairment has contributed to understanding in the area of possible sensory/perceptual deficits. Although studies have differed on the specific clusters of children identified and the individual characteristics of the subgroups, there appears to be general agreement that there is a group of children who demonstrate a generalized, and often significant, perceptual deficit, including both visual and kinesthetic difficulties.[46,91,122,151] Questions remain, however, in that these specific perceptual deficits have not been shown to be present in all subgroups with motor impairment. This again serves to underscore the heterogeneity of the condition and suggests that different profiles of motor coordination problems may exist in children with DCD with varying sensory/perceptual impairments.

Motor Deficits

Children with DCD move awkwardly and slowly, with a rigid, jerky quality to their movements.[5,103,247] They frequently bump into objects and people and have a tendency to trip and fall.[107] Poor balance, especially pronounced during single-leg stance, and difficulty maintaining postures are often noted (see video of Bill for an example of a child with similar problems).[247] To compensate for their instability, children with DCD may demonstrate many associated movements.[107] On physical examination, decreased muscle tone and neurologic soft signs can often be observed. This constellation of physical signs, combined with the possible sensory deficits outlined previously, have led many to hypothesize that the origins of the motor impairments seen in children with DCD may lie in faulty motor control and motor learning processes.

Motor Control Deficits

Children with DCD demonstrate inappropriate and ineffective neuromuscular strategies, both in muscular activation and in sequencing. This is particularly evident in their use of atypical postural control strategies,[92,247] including when their balance is challenged.[249] An increased level of muscle co-contraction has also been described, in which children with DCD demonstrated a much less effective method of muscular organization than their peers, which did not improve with age.[183] Children with movement difficulties tend to "fix" or stabilize their joints during task performance.[183,209] The deliberate stabilization of their joints in this way leads to lack of fluency in their movements[149] and contributes to their stiff, awkward, and clumsy appearance[209]; it also increases the time it takes them to adapt to changes in their movement environment.[134] Fixing can be thought of as a strategy to control the multiple degrees of freedom of joints and muscles for efficient functioning. Children with DCD who "fix" their joints during task performance are more likely to fatigue[161] and to demonstrate inconsistency in task performance.[134,209] Overall, the postural fixation and atypical muscular activation and sequencing seen in children with DCD result in less efficient movement patterns and reflect a less skilled stage of movement acquisition than is typical of age peers.

When performing reaching tasks, children with DCD use different neuromuscular strategies than their typically developing age-matched peers, contributing to their slower and more variable movement and reaction times, as well as their movement inaccuracy. These findings have been consistently described in the literature.[68,86,97,120,121,221,232,233,236,245,247,250] Children with DCD display gait differences, which have also been suggested to be a result of their movement variability.[197] Decreased and variable force control and difficulties with temporal precision (both movement production and time perception) have also been noted in the motor control literature.[63,86,97,236,245,248,250]

As can be seen from extensive motor control research, in comparison with their typically developing peers, children with DCD demonstrate variations in movement speed, timing, and force across a series of different tasks, resulting in qualitative differences in their movement and motor control patterns.

Motor Learning Deficits

In addition to poorly controlled movements, children with DCD exhibit limited movement repertoires, lacking both adaptability and flexibility in their motor behavior.[110] This, along with the variability and inconsistency seen in their motor performance, suggests difficulties in motor learning processes.[6,68] Evidence from subtyping and other research would suggest that, although some children with DCD exhibit problems primarily in execution and control of movements, others have difficulties related to motor planning processes.[64,67,216,220]

As has been previously described, children with DCD demonstrate movements that are inaccurate and lack fluency, as they are unable to accurately correct their movement patterns through error detection or feedback. Although these children may achieve motor milestones within normal time limits, they have difficulty learning new motor skills.[85,134] They fail to see the similarities between motor tasks and thus are unable to transfer learned skills from one activity to a closely related activity. They also experience difficulty generalizing from one context or situation to another. Both of these processes reflect an early, more cognitive stage of motor learning (see Chapter 4 for more information on motor learning).[72,134,139,140] According to motor learning theory, as skills are learned, feedback requirements lessen and change, with proprioceptive and kinesthetic feedback relied on more than visual input.[55] Children with DCD continue to rely predominantly on visual information, as if they were still in the early stages of motor learning. As a result, their motor performance is sometimes more similar to that of younger children than to that of age peers.[117,118,239]

Children with coordination difficulties have also been described as repeating tasks the same way over and over again, regardless of their success with the task.[85,128] They appear to have difficulty understanding the demands of a task and its component parts, interpreting environmental cues, and selecting the best motor response for a task.[72] As a result, they do not effectively use the feedback originating from knowledge of their past performance to prepare for upcoming actions (anticipatory preparation), and they have difficulty adapting to situational demands.[67,72,134,139] It has been postulated that children with DCD might attend to the wrong cues and not to the more salient aspects of available feedback.[72] Others have suggested that the problem might lie in the failure of children with DCD to use anticipatory control strategies for motor tasks[247]; as a result, they might have to rely heavily on a feedback or closed loop strategy to control movement.[191,193,216]

In summary, children with DCD have difficulties with error detection and movement correction during the execution of motor skills. This is especially evident when motor tasks are complex and involve spatial uncertainty.

Secondary Impairments

Physical

Although slow, awkward movements are typical of children with DCD and are easy to casually observe (e.g., see video of Bill), what is less evident is the extra effort that motor skills seem to require and the struggle that children have in making adaptations and in "fine-tuning" movements.[28] Secondary impairments related to primary motor coordination difficulties are of considerable concern and include lack of energy and fatigue, as well as decreased strength, power, and endurance.[156,183] Children with DCD complain of being tired more easily than their peers and are often exhausted by the end of the day as they must exert more effort during motor-based activities at school and at home.[107] Maintaining their posture for extended periods of time is fatiguing for these children, so they may try to lean against the wall or on other children when standing or may assume a slouched posture when sitting (Figure 16-1). Recent strong empirical evidence indicates a progressive decrease in strength and power in children with DCD over time, which is already apparent between the ages of 6 and 9 years.[183] Obesity in children with DCD and the relationship between their motor difficulties and cardiovascular risk factors have begun to be studied in greater detail.[20,54] As will be discussed later in this chapter, these secondary sequelae are precursors for participation restrictions in sporting and/or leisure activities, reduced opportunities for social interaction, and diminished physical fitness across the life span. Secondary impairments in children with DCD may be preventable and are appropriate targets for physical therapy.

Social/Emotional/Behavioral

Often children with DCD demonstrate associated behavioral problems that become the focus of concern, especially in the classroom.[187] Children with DCD may be quiet and withdrawn at school, with avoidance of schoolwork and frequent "off-task" behaviors.[32,33,136] Alternatively, children may act out in class, disrupting the teacher and/or others.[129] Learning new skills in physical education is a continuous challenge (e.g., see video of Bill), and children may try to avoid these classes with complaints of illness or problem behaviors. Avoidance of written work can result in "behaviors" such as needing to sharpen the pencil multiple times, talking and asking questions, attention seeking, and interference with other children. Low frustration tolerance, decreased motivation, and poor self-esteem are commonly observed.[204,212] Children with movement difficulties give up on tasks easily, which occasionally leads to angry, aggressive classroom behavior. Task initiation and task completion are often major issues, both at home and at school.[136]

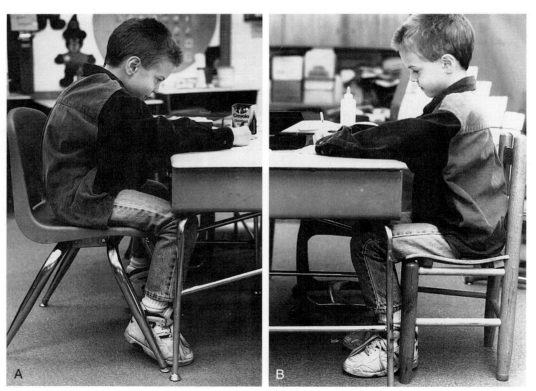

Figure 16-1 **A,** This child demonstrates poor posture that interferes with fine motor classroom activities. **B,** A different desk and chair improve this child's posture and improve the precision of his fine motor activities.

Like the physical impairments outlined previously, these associated social, emotional, and behavioral difficulties can be significant but are not inevitable. All efforts should be made through early identification and management to prevent their occurrence.

ORIGIN AND PATHOPHYSIOLOGY

Although much has been learned regarding the body structure and function deficits of children with DCD and the potential sensory, motor control, and motor learning processes affected, the origin of the disorder remains poorly understood.[235,265] Currently, no specific pathologic process or single neuroanatomic site has been definitively associated with DCD, but many behavioral studies, in particular studies on co-occurring conditions and possible subtypes of DCD, have led researchers to speculate as to the underlying mechanism(s) involved in DCD. Some researchers have postulated that diffuse, rather than distinct, areas of the brain may be affected, resulting in the variable expression of the disorder and the different profiles seen in children with DCD (including co-occurring conditions).[104] This would imply that the specific combination of co-occurring disorders depends on the location and severity of neurologic insult. This theory, however, does not take into account cases where developmental disorders occur alone.[235] Other researchers highlight the strong association between motor, attention, and perceptual processes[70] and point to the possible role of neuroanatomic structures such as the cerebellum and basal ganglia.

Research studies employing a dual-task paradigm indicate a lack of automatization of motor actions in children with DCD when attentional demands increase.[35,113] These findings implicate the cerebellum as a possible site of pathophysiology in children with DCD, given its known role in the automatization and learning of motor tasks.[27,108,200] The thinking behind the interference seen in dual-task paradigms is that performance of one task will be negatively affected by the second if both tasks need to make use of the same "pool" of resources, including visual and cognitive resources. Concurrent work examining motor adaptation, or the ability of children with DCD to adapt their performance to changing environmental contexts, comes to a similar conclusion with respect to the potential role of the cerebellum in children with DCD. In these studies, children with motor difficulties show poor adaptation to gradual changes in environmental stimuli.[13,27] Given the rapid growth and vulnerability of the developing cerebellum to external events in the first year of life, theories regarding the possible link between cerebellar involvement and motor impairments are plausible.[74] Although the proposed link between motor coordination difficulties and the role of the cerebellum appears to be strong,[265] especially in situations of co-occurring conditions,[158,166] testing of causal models will be necessary to confirm these hypotheses.

Another avenue of research includes the investigation of motor imagery deficits in children with DCD. Understanding in this area has led to a proposal that impaired feed forward models could be a potential mechanism underlying DCD (efference-copy-deficit hypothesis).[256,258] In this theory, motor imagery deficits seen in children with DCD are related to difficulties in generating efference copies of motor commands through feed forward models, pointing to the possible involvement of the posterior parietal cortex.[256]

Recently, increasing interest in the possibility of impaired internal models can be seen in the DCD literature.[103] Internal models are neural representations of the visual-spatial coordinates of intended motor actions.[131] It has been hypothesized that children with motor impairment may have inadequate forward modeling of movements and are unable to form, access, or update their internal models, which results in poor "online" error correction and ultimately affects motor learning.[216] It is believed that internal models are located in the cerebellum.[265] Parallel work investigating the role of "mirror neurons" (which are housed in the ventral premotor and posterior parietal cortices) has shed additional light on how motor representations are formed not only during the performance, but also in the observation, of movements.[131,188] Mirror neurons in the posterior parietal cortex may work in concert with internal models in the cerebellum through extensive neural projections between these two brain structures to code and update movement.[131]

Taken together, behavioral studies suggesting involvement of the cerebellum, research investigating motor imagery deficits in children with DCD, and the recent discovery and understanding of the role of mirror neurons suggest that a complex and shared interplay may occur between different neuroanatomic regions of the brain when learning, executing, and correcting movements. Research studies employing neurodiagnostic technologies such as functional magnetic resonance imaging and electroencephalography are becoming more prevalent in the literature investigating possible mechanisms involved in DCD.[159,266] Combined with behavioral research, these experimental studies will likely shed more light on the potential neuroanatomic sites involved in the pathophysiology of DCD.

In the end, why are there so many plausible theories regarding the origin of DCD and so many proposed sites of neurologic abnormality? The production of well-coordinated, smooth motor movements is a complex process requiring multiple levels of information processing, each of which requires different abilities such as sensory acuity, memory, decision making, attention, perception, feedback, and feed forward mechanisms. It is likely that children with DCD may have impairments in one or more of these functions and in related brain areas, and that different groups of children may have abnormalities in different neural correlates.[74,96,265] Other possible influencing factors have already been alluded to earlier in this chapter. The heterogeneity of the disorder and the presence of co-occurring conditions give rise to different profiles of impairment, which may indeed have different underlying neural mechanisms.

ACTIVITY LIMITATIONS

How do the proposed body structure and function deficits manifest themselves in a practical sense? Children with DCD tend to have the greatest difficulty with skills that must be taught. In particular, skills requiring accuracy and refined eye-hand coordination and that require constant monitoring of feedback pose significant challenges for the child with DCD.[140,225] Children with DCD may experience difficulty with fine motor activities, gross motor activities, or both (see video of Bill).[123] These activity limitations are readily observable in the classroom, on the school playground, and at home.[32,136]

Fine Motor Activity Limitations

Self-Care

The ability of children with DCD to perform self-care activities such as doing up snaps, zippers, and buttons, tying shoelaces, opening snack containers, and managing juice boxes is poorer than expected for their age. Tying shoelaces is an example of a skilled activity required at school by the time a student is in first grade. Children with impairments in sequencing skills cannot correctly sequence the steps in shoe tying, even though they may have practiced it many times before. When children with DCD make a mistake in one step of the sequence, they have to start over again rather than simply redo the last step. Or they might omit a different step in the sequence each time they try to tie their shoes (Figure 16-2). At home, parents notice difficulties when children are using cutlery, and there is a tendency to spill liquid from drinking glasses or when pouring from a container. Parents also describe problems with grooming such as bathing, combing hair, and brushing teeth.[129,136,228] At school, children with movement difficulties are often the last to get snowsuits, jackets, and boots on, or to get their knapsacks organized to go home at the end of the day.

Academic

Classroom fine motor difficulties include problems with printing and handwriting (Figure 16-3).[9,132,136] Written work is illegible and inconsistent in sizing and requires great effort.[160,161] Frequent erasures of work, inaccurate spacing of words, and unusual letter formation are evident.[107] Pencil/crayon grasps are awkward, and written work is not well aligned. Pencils may be dropped frequently and pencil leads broken or paper torn as the result of excessive pressure on the page.[28,107] Because of this, teachers and parents often note that children with DCD have difficulty finishing academic tasks, including homework, on time. Children with these

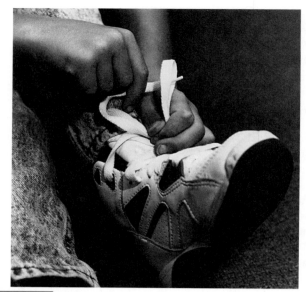

Figure 16-2 This 8-year-old boy still cannot independently tie his shoes. His verbal cues were "loop around and go through." He forgot to "loop around" and forgot to make a second loop.

difficulties tend to rush through tasks or may be unusually slow (see video of Bill). Academic tasks that have a motor component require extra effort and attentional resources. Children with DCD can become fatigued and frustrated, as they work harder than children their age to complete the same activity. Teachers often describe a large discrepancy between their oral and written work. Copying from the board and other fine motor tasks such as completing puzzles and turning door handles or washroom taps are also affected. Many children with DCD tend to avoid art projects and craft activities that require coloring, cutting, and pasting.[129,142] In addition, they may be intolerant of sensations such as those encountered at rice, sand, and water tables, or during finger painting activities.[105]

Overall, children with DCD, in comparison with typically developing children of the same age, have been noted to require more support and assistance from those around them to complete motor-based self-care and academic tasks at home and at school.[137,228]

Gross Motor Activity Limitations

Lacking good balance and postural control, children with DCD often have difficulties with the flexibility and adaptability required for gross motor activities. They may show delays each time they learn a novel skill such as riding a push toy, learning to ride a tricycle or bicycle, and pumping a swing.[107,129,136] They demonstrate poorly coordinated running, skipping, hopping, and jumping and may have difficulty managing stairs, especially when they must maneuver around others (Figure 16-4).[9,32,42] Coordination of eyes and hands at a whole body level is problematic, so children with

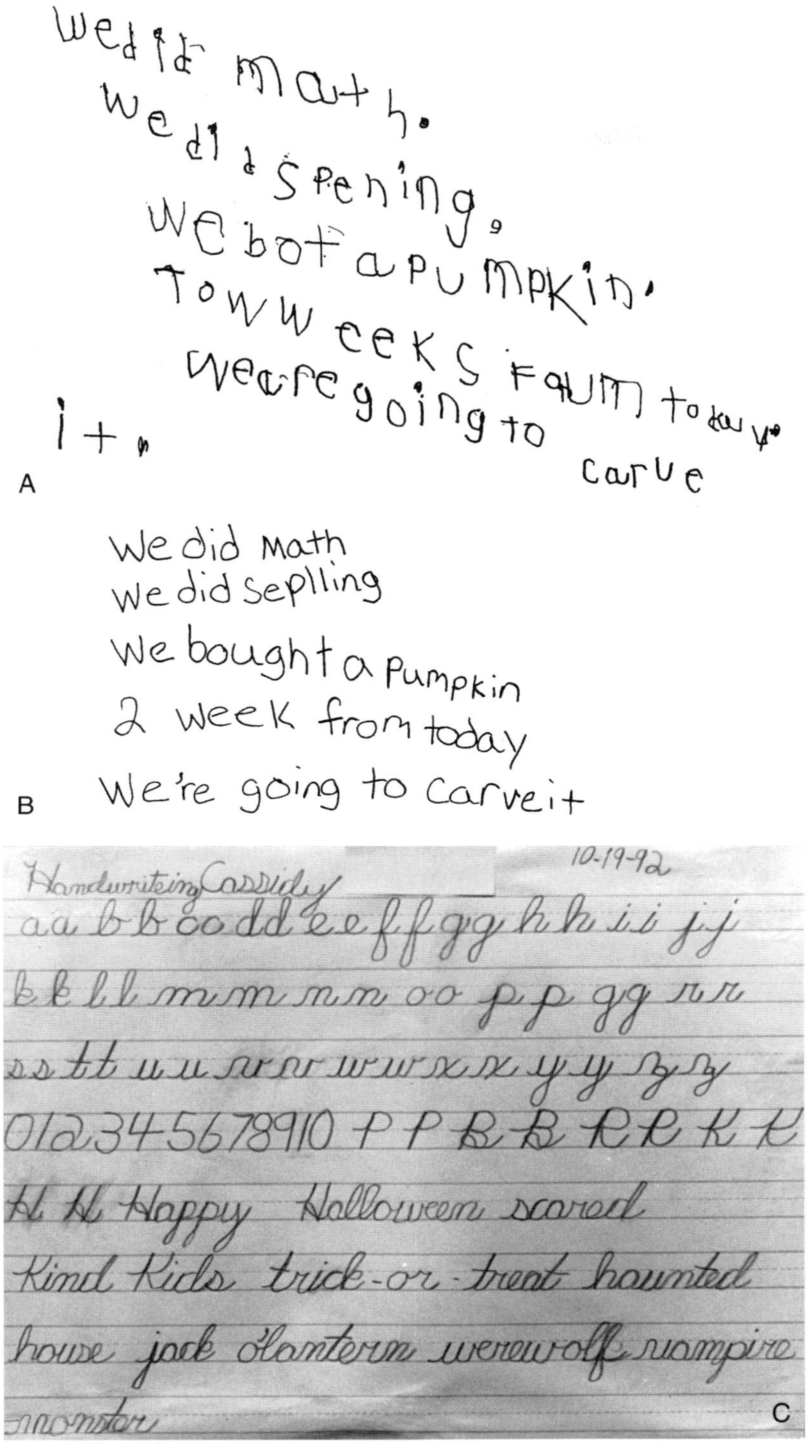

we did math.
we did spening,
we bot a pumpkin,
Tow weeks faum today
we are going to
i t ,
carve

A

We did Math
We did Seplling

We bought a Pumpkin
2 week from today

We're going to carve it

B

Figure 16-3   **A,** Handwriting sample of a third grade child with developmental coordination disorder and a learning disability. **B,** Handwriting sample obtained for comparison from a randomly selected third grade peer without motor difficulties. **C,** Sample of cursive writing from another peer without motor difficulties demonstrates an even more advanced expectation of third grade students.

10-19-92

Handwriting Cassidy

a a b b c c d d e e f f g g h h i i j j

k k l l m m n n o o p p q q r r

s s t t u u v v w w x x y y z z

0 1 2 3 4 5 6 7 8 9 10 P P B B R R K K

H H Happy Halloween scared

Kind Kids trick-or-treat haunted

house jack o'lantern werewolf vampire

monster

C

DCD have difficulty with throwing, catching, and kicking a ball accurately.[6,27,136] When kicking or throwing a ball, the child with DCD may have trouble judging the amount of force required to throw the ball,[107] with resulting performance on these tasks being more like that of a younger child (see www.cmaj.ca/cgi/content/full/175/5/471, and click on "videos" in right-hand menu; also see video of Bill). Children with DCD have more difficulty with gross motor activities that require constant changes in body position or adaptation to changes in the environment, such as when playing baseball or tennis or jumping rope.[136,226] Activities that require the coordinated use of both sides of the body

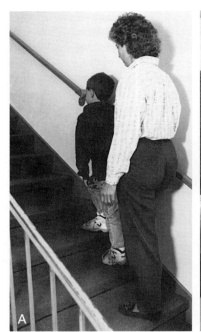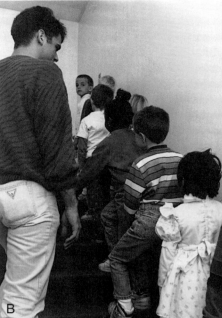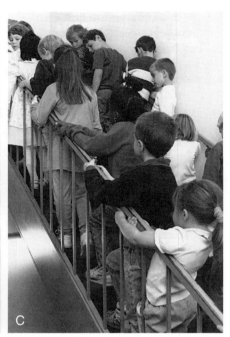

Figure 16-4 **A,** Managing stairs can be challenging for children with developmental coordination disorder (DCD), given their difficulties with posture and balance. **B** and **C,** Stair climbing is made more challenging when children with DCD must maneuver around others in a crowded environment.

are difficult (e.g., stride jumps, swinging a bat, handling a hockey stick).[136]

The fine and gross motor activity limitations of children with DCD can be understood in the context of associated body structure and function deficits, according to the ICF model (Table 16-3). An appreciation of the link between underlying deficits and their expression in ADLs can be instrumental when planning effective and targeted interventions.

PARTICIPATION RESTRICTIONS

In the context of the ICF framework, the fine and gross motor activity limitations seen in children with DCD in their school and home environments can lead to participation restrictions that prevent them from having opportunities for optimal physical, social, and cognitive development. When parents of children with DCD are asked what their concerns are, they frequently identify restricted participation.[189,208] As a result of their motor difficulties, children with DCD have reduced interest in physical activities and usually begin to withdraw from, and avoid, motor and sports activities at an early age.[12,29,136,238,241] Because of their difficulties with self-care tasks at school, they are often slow to get to the playground for recess, restricting their physical participation and further diminishing their opportunities for physical and social interactions.

Complicating their physical challenges, children with motor difficulties often do not know how to play physical

games, nor do they understand the rules of the game,[107] limiting both physical and social participation with peers. They are often the last to "get picked" for teams and are not sought out to play with others.[129,241] As a result, these children can quickly become isolated from their peer group.[107] Difficulties in relating to their peers have been noted in children with DCD.[107] This may be the result of not being chosen to participate in motor-based activities, or because their clumsy, less predictable movements may disrupt their play with others.[129] Typically, children with DCD tend to watch more than play, preferring to wander the playground periphery or talk to teachers rather than engage in active play with others and socialize with their peers; this may be related to decreased self-confidence.[179] With fewer opportunities for social interaction, they often appear not to have learned the "intuitive" rules of social situations.[107]

PERSONAL FACTORS

Children with DCD often self-impose restrictions on their participation. They perceive themselves to be less competent than their peers and have lower self-worth and greater anxiety.[212] When poor gross motor skills lead to inactivity and avoidance of physically challenging games, the child with DCD becomes less fit and further avoids physical activity. Avoidance of games requiring fine motor skill leads to decreased opportunities for practice, preventing ongoing academic skill development. Parents have reported that the more difficulty their children had with motor skills, the less

TABLE 16-3 **Examples of Activity Limitations and Related Body Structure and Function Deficits in Children With Developmental Coordination Disorder (DCD)**

Activity Limitations	Related Body Structures and Functions
SELF-CARE ACTIVITIES	
Eating:	
Frequent spills, messy eating	Poor body awareness
Leaning on the table	Poor postural tone
Poor use of cutlery when spreading/cutting	Difficulties with in-hand manipulation
Dressing:	Difficulties judging force and distance, targeting
Slow and disorganized	Poor use of dominant-assistant hands
Trouble with fasteners (buttons, zippers)	Poor body awareness and proprioception
Clothes twisted or on backward	Lack of balance
Shoes on wrong foot	Poor finger dexterity and strength
	Difficulties with touch perception, sequencing
ACADEMIC ACTIVITIES	
Printing/handwriting:	Muscle tone and postural issues
Slow, poor legibility	Poor fine motor control
Awkward grasp	Over-reliance on vision
Reduced volume of work	Use of attentional resources to maintain posture
Frequent erasures	Language and learning issues
Avoidance behaviors	Low muscle tone, fatigue
Sitting at a desk/in circle time:	Decreased postural control
Slumped posture	Poor body awareness
Holding head	Need for boundaries, increased sensory feedback
Leaning on others, lying down	Need to move to maintain muscle activity
Wiggling	
Falling out of chair	
SPORTS AND LEISURE ACTIVITIES	
Ball-related activities:	Poor management of multiple degrees of freedom
Miss the ball, get hit by the ball	Timing issues
Slow to react	Difficulties correcting errors, poor generalization
Can't keep up	Difficulties attending to body position
Fatigue	Passivity response a coping mechanism
Passive—watch rather than play	Need to avoid failure, possibility of humiliation
Interact with adults rather than with peers	

willing they were to engage in physical activity.[170] Self-imposed isolation becomes a self-perpetuating cycle of poor skill development, limited skill practice, poor performance, and further isolation.[177]

ENVIRONMENTAL FACTORS

With younger children, the environment tends to be more accepting of motor difficulties because of the wide range of normal variation. Early signs of incoordination may be viewed as part of normal developmental awkwardness or normal but slower maturation. As preschoolers become elementary school children, however, peers, parents, teachers, and/or communities may create unwarranted restrictions, artificial barriers, or rigid expectations.[180] If a physical education class or a community recreation program strictly adheres to performance criteria for group activities such as

baseball, basketball, or dance class, a child with DCD can be prevented from participating with peers. If parents restrict their child's outdoor play to certain environments or to certain activities because they are afraid the child will get hurt, then another barrier is established and peer relationships are potentially limited. If a family feels uncomfortable eating out at a restaurant or with relatives and friends because of a child's messy eating and restricts these opportunities to certain environments, social interactions will be unduly limited. Indoor manipulative play can pose just as much of a problem. When limitations exist in fine motor skills of coloring, cutting, and stacking objects, imaginative play with paper, small toy people, or building blocks is very difficult. When children are not allowed to play with modified toys, or when individualized expectations are not acceptable, a child's experiences can be artificially limited.

ROLE OF THE PHYSICAL THERAPIST

Physical therapists are skilled in the observation of gross motor task performance and can help to identify children whose poor motor performance leads to activity limitations and participation restrictions. Physical therapists can observe the lack of adaptive flexibility, the lack of pre-movement organization, and the "fixing" that is so characteristic of children with DCD in the early years.[149] These observations can facilitate early identification, which can help to prevent the development of secondary impairments. Physical therapists can provide education and guidance that will encourage the engagement of children with DCD in the typical activities of childhood, thereby reducing the risks of decreased physical health, as well as decreased self-esteem, self-efficacy, and social participation, that have been noted at an early age.[109]

IDENTIFICATION AND REFERRAL TO PHYSICAL THERAPY

The recognition of DCD will depend on the extent to which physical, social, and attitudinal factors have influenced motor skill acquisition. Although DCD must be considered at least theoretically to be present from birth, children differ with respect to the apparent age of onset, as the developmental progression will vary depending upon the environmental and task demands placed upon the child in the early years. Because DCD is a disorder that has an impact on the development of movement skills, children with motor impairments often do not display the full extent of their functional difficulties until they are of school age. Limitations observed in the preschool years may be seen as "slow development" or temperamental differences. However, poor performance on everyday activities is tolerated less and less as children with DCD reach school age. Their coordination difficulties may not be easy to observe until they reach the point at which they attempt to learn and perform skills that require adaptations in speed, timing, and grading of force. As has been mentioned, the presence of secondary impairments and co-occurring conditions can complicate the identification process.

Typically, children with motor difficulties are identified and referred to physical therapy via one of two principal routes—through the health care system or through the educational system. In the medical pathway, children with motor difficulties may have been investigated for possible musculoskeletal, orthopedic, or neurologic concerns. These may include concerns regarding ligament laxity, low tone, or an unusual gait pattern, or the results of regular monitoring after premature birth or low birth weight.[162] In the education system, referrals are usually made when poor motor performance affects academic functioning. Sources of initial identification within each of these pathways are varied and may include primary care physicians, community and developmental pediatricians, and hospital and infant programs, as well as classroom, physical education, and resource teachers, educational psychologists, and occupational therapists (OTs). Although some children are identified by the health care system, a significant number of the children referred to physical therapy for investigation of motor problems are referred through the educational route.

Although parents are often keenly aware early on of their child's activity limitations and participation restrictions,[1,189] classroom and special education teachers may be the initial source of referral to rehabilitation professionals when they notice poor skill development interfering with classroom work and overall academic performance.[227] Often, the structured demands of the classroom with expectations of increasingly precise motor skills and shorter time frames for performance stress a child with DCD to his or her limit. In fact, children with DCD are commonly underrecognized until academic failure begins to occur[59,77,132,223] and often are not identified before age 5.[132] In addition, teachers have many opportunities to compare the performance of children with poor motor coordination with that of their more typically developing peers. At school age, poor written communication is frequently the first activity limitation that educators identify, so children with incoordination are most often referred to OTs for handwriting difficulties. This is often, however, just the "tip of the iceberg," as children commonly experience other challenges at school, on the playground, and at home. In the school setting, children with motor impairments may be referred to physical therapists for assistance with physical education programming and for safety concerns, as well as for strength and endurance issues. A physical therapist working in an educational setting has the advantage of screening children in natural environments while the children participate in everyday, functional activities. Immediate collaborative consultation with the classroom and/or physical education teacher can occur, to gather information regarding the nature and extent of the motor concerns. After this, an appropriate physical therapy examination allows more comprehensive observation of function and functional difficulties in the classroom, at recess, and in physical education class. When children with possible DCD are referred and examined in a clinic setting, in-depth interviewing of parents and teachers regarding their motor difficulties, as well as observation of functional activities, is needed to accurately identify concerns related to body structure and function and activity limitations.

EXAMINATION AND EVALUATION

Given the heterogeneous nature of DCD, it is important for a physical therapy assessment to utilize multiple sources of information and types of examinations.[144] The *Guide to Physical Therapist Practice*[2] recommends the collection of historical information, including a developmental and medical history (pregnancy, delivery, and past and current health status); results of previous musculoskeletal and neuromuscular examinations; and a history of current functional status from the family and from school personnel. As part of the examination and evaluation process, physical therapists must differentiate the motor behaviors of children with DCD from those of other movement disorders. Children referred in the early years with poor coordination and/or motor delay may have disorders such as cerebral palsy, muscular dystrophy, global developmental delay, or DCD. Physical therapists must make evaluation hypotheses regarding the origin of the coordination difficulties. Some key questions may help therapists focus on differentiating among each of these patterns of motor behavior. In a young child, it would be important to ask these questions: (1) Is there evidence of increased or fluctuating tone? (Observed alterations in muscle tone might be suggestive of a condition such as cerebral palsy.) (2) Are the delays more global in nature, rather than occurring in the motor domain alone—a situation in which global developmental delay might be suspected? (With a preschool- or school-age child, questions might center around the history of the poor coordination.) (3) Have the difficulties been present from an early age? (4) Are the motor concerns appearing to worsen over time? (5) Has there been a loss of previously acquired skills? (If so, this might be suggestive of a condition like muscular dystrophy.) (See chapters in this volume on specific conditions for further information on differential diagnosis.)

The following example suggests the process used in the examination of a young child who is demonstrating movement difficulties. A typical initial referral in a school-based service delivery environment might be made by a physical education teacher regarding a 5-year-old kindergarten student who is falling often. Initial hypotheses concerning why Sarah is falling more often than her peers might include the following: (1) She has mild cerebral palsy, spastic diplegia, or hemiplegia; (2) she has early symptoms of muscular dystrophy; (3) she has DCD; (4) she has characteristic symptoms of ADHD, and as a result she is impulsive and distracted to the extent that she bumps into people and objects; (5) her shoes are too big and she trips over the laces; or (6) she has a perceptual or visual impairment. If hypothesis 4 or 6 seems likely based on physical examination and observation, referral to another health care service provider would be warranted.

Direct observation of Sarah on the playground and during physical education class could rule out falling related to improperly fitting shoes (hypothesis 5) or significant impulsivity and distractibility possibly related to ADHD (hypothesis 4). Additional observation could identify a positive Gowers' sign and large calf muscles, suggesting further medical referral for possible muscular dystrophy (hypothesis 2). Observation of movement patterns during play may suggest typical symmetrical synergies of hip adduction and internal rotation with knee flexion and ankle plantar flexion (more suggestive of cerebral palsy, spastic diplegia; hypothesis 1), or unilateral shoulder retraction, internal rotation

and adduction, elbow flexion with forearm pronation, wrist and finger flexion, and hip adduction and internal rotation with knee flexion and plantar flexion (indicative of cerebral palsy, hemiplegia; hypothesis 1). If none of these observations is made, then the likelihood increases that Sarah has DCD (hypothesis 3).

Direct observation of functional activities in naturally occurring situations is an important part of the physical therapy assessment. If observations and examinations must be performed in a hospital or clinic setting, then behavior might have to be observed in a noisy, distracting, fast-paced environment such as a busy waiting room or a children's play area. Putting a coat on while surrounded by 25 other 7-year-old children, all struggling in a small space to get dressed and get outside for recess first, is much different from putting on a coat in a quiet room with one adult giving positive encouragement.

Additional information obtained from parent and teacher interviews is vital. A parent may describe her daughter as having a pattern of general incoordination with delayed speech, messy eating, and general clumsiness present from a young age but without a medical diagnosis related to a neurologic impairment (suggesting hypothesis 3). If you suspect that a child is demonstrating the characteristics of DCD, you might want to ask parents about other developmental concerns (fine motor, self care, leisure). It will be important to inquire whether or not difficulties are observed at home, such as struggling with buttons, using eating utensils, or tying shoelaces. Parents can provide information on the amount of effort required to complete motor tasks and whether their child participates in organized sports or other physical activities. The parent interview combined with information from a teacher can confirm the presence of a significant problem with academic achievement or ADLs—a key diagnostic finding in DCD (again suggesting hypothesis 3). However, if the parent describes a pattern of typical motor development followed by a recent decrease in strength and the loss of ability to climb stairs independently, the hypothesis of muscular dystrophy (2) would be supported.

Direct examination by the physical therapist might identify muscle hypertonicity that increases with faster movements (possible cerebral palsy; hypothesis 1). On the other hand, if direct examination suggests low muscle tone with shoulder, elbow, and knee hyperextension, DCD again becomes a valid hypothesis (3). If muscle testing reveals a weak gastrocnemius and pseudohypertrophy, the hypothesis of muscular dystrophy (2) would be supported. During direct examination, the therapist may be able to relate the most striking activity limitations to difficulties in following directions when asked to perform a motor task or to poor attention to task. Children with DCD often cannot imitate body postures or follow two- or three-step motor commands. Frequent demonstration and actual physical assistance may be needed to accomplish items on standardized tests.

Clinical Assessment Tools for DCD

Initial Screening

To identify children with motor challenges so that early and effective interventions can be implemented, the use of reliable and valid screening instruments is critical. To meet this need, several screening tools have been developed to elicit parent, teacher, and child perceptions of children's motor concerns.

Parent Report

Parents know their children's developmental history, have observed their functioning in multiple environments, and can provide important diagnostic information during screening for potential DCD.[58] The Developmental Coordination Disorder Questionnaire (DCDQ)[254] is a parent-report screening tool (at the ICF activity level) that measures the functional impact of a child's motor coordination difficulties. The DCDQ has recently been revised as the DCDQ'07.[253] Originally intended for use with parents of children 8 to 14 years of age, this 15-item tool has now been extended to include children 5 through 15 years old. Each item of the DCDQ describes tasks that are often of concern with children with motor impairment (e.g., catching a ball, riding a bicycle, writing), and parents are asked to compare their child's coordination to that of children the same age by choosing ratings on a 5-point scale. Percentiles are provided to assist the clinician in determining definite motor difficulties, "suspect" for motor difficulties, and no motor difficulties. The DCDQ is quick to complete and can provide valuable information regarding the impact of motor coordination difficulties on activities of daily life (i.e., Criterion B of the DSM-IV).[4] Research performed on the original version of the DCDQ provides evidence of internal consistency of the test items, construct validity, and concurrent validity with both the Movement Assessment Battery for Children (MABC) test of motor impairment[87] and the Bruininks-Oseretsky Test of Motor Proficiency (BOTMP),[15] as well as high sensitivity and specificity for identification of risk for DCD versus no DCD in populations of children in several different countries.[36,40,75,203,254] The new version of the DCDQ'07 was developed with a population-based sample from Alberta, Canada, and validated with typically developing children, as well as children with, or likely to have, coordination difficulties. The new DCDQ'07 was again noted to have high sensitivity and specificity, as well as construct and concurrent validity.[253] Findings from more recent studies of the criterion-related psychometric properties of the DCDQ are conflicting.[23,116] This may relate, in part, to the fact that the DCDQ measures the functional impact of poor coordination, whereas several of the criterion standards to which the DCDQ has been compared measure difficulties in skill performance directly. The DCDQ'07 is available online at no charge (http://www.dcdq.ca/pdf/DCDQ_Administration_and_Scoring.pdf).

Teacher Checklists

Although teachers identify some children who have DCD, they have been shown to be inaccurate in some cases.[51,100,167] In one study of children 9 to 11 years of age, classroom teachers were able to identify only 25% and physical education teachers identified only 49% of the children with DCD.[167] This discrepancy is partially explained by the different environments on which the two types of teachers based their observations and may also be related to the fact that teachers may not be able to observe all functional tasks included in checklists. The popular teacher checklist (ICF activity level) used in this study, the Movement Assessment Battery for Children Checklist (MABC-C),[87] is also limited as it is somewhat lengthy, making it time-consuming for teachers to complete. With regard to studies of the psychometric properties of this checklist, the results have been mixed. The MABC-C has been shown to demonstrate internal consistency, construct validity, and concurrent validity when measured against the Movement Assessment Battery for Children (MABC)[87] test of motor impairment.[206] However, the checklist has been noted to have poor sensitivity, meaning that many of the children at risk for motor problems may not be identified.[100] The MABC checklist has recently been revised (MABC Checklist-2)[88] and includes fewer items, along with a new standardization sample of 395 children. Determination of the new checklist's psychometric properties will be important to determine whether the issues raised above have been addressed.

Recently, the Children Activity Scale for Teachers (ChAS-T) has been developed for younger children 4 to 8 years of age.[196] In addition, the Motor Observation Scale for Teachers (MOQ-T) (previously known as the Groningen Motor Observation Scale) has been revised and new norms developed.[201] This checklist is intended for use with teachers of 5- to 11-year-old children. Only preliminary work has been conducted to examine the reliability and validity of these tools.[196,202] Until further validation studies have been done on these teacher checklists, caution should be exercised when relying only on the judgment of classroom or physical education teachers to identify children with DCD.

Child Report

The Children's Self-Perceptions of Adequacy in, and Predilection for, Physical Activity Scale (CSAPPA)[80] is a brief 19-item child self-report measure of self-efficacy with regard to physical activity. It is intended for use with children aged 9 to 16 years. Specifically, the CSAPPA is a participation measure of children's perceptions of their adequacy in performing, and their desire to participate in, physical activity. It contains three subscales: perceived adequacy, predilection to physical activity, and enjoyment of physical education class. The CSAPPA uses a structured alternative choice format wherein children choose from two statements the one that best describes them (i.e., "some kids are among the last to be chosen for active games" vs. "other kids are usually picked to play first") and then indicate whether the statement is true or very true for them. The tool has been shown to have high test-retest reliability, as well as predictive and construct validity.[80] The CSAPPA tool has been used in screening large groups of school-age children, primarily for research purposes, and scores on the CSAPPA have compared well with scores on a standardized test of general motor ability.[81] Several research studies suggest that the tool may be useful in the clinical setting for identification purposes.[23,81,82] Although it is possible to use only the subscales when screening for motor impairment, the use of additional sources of information on motor performance has been recommended to increase the specificity of the tool.[23]

Regardless of the type of screening tool used (parent, teacher, or child report), it should be noted that screening tools are just the first step in identifying potential DCD. Children identified through these tools as having possible motor impairment should undergo a more detailed assessment intended for use with children with DCD to confirm their motor difficulties (Criterion A).[225] When multiple measures are employed to confirm motor impairment (such as a checklist or questionnaire for initial screening followed by a test of motor ability), it should also be remembered that different tools may measure different constructs, including a child's capability (what the child can do, as measured by a standardized assessment) and the child's actual performance (what the child does do in everyday life and in multiple contexts or environments).[36] It is important to know a tool's strengths and limitations and to use a tool suited for the examination purpose. Each of these different tools can provide valuable information in understanding the complete picture of a child's difficulties.

Evaluation of Motor Impairment

One of the DSM-IV discriminating criteria for DCD is that motor coordination is markedly below expected levels for the child's chronologic age.[4] To distinguish DCD from a developmental motor delay, standardized tests of developmentally sequenced gross and fine motor items can be used. Currently, there is no widely accepted standard for the assessment of children with DCD,[40,84,104,123,144,254] in part because of the heterogeneous nature of DCD and the frequent presence of co-morbidities. It is important to note that studies have reported inconsistencies in the numbers and types of children identified using different assessment tools specifically designed for children with DCD.[40,123] Without a gold standard to identify these children, researchers have often used more than one assessment tool to confirm the identity of children with movement problems in research study samples.[261] It has been recommended that any examination of children with DCD should include information from a number of sources, including standardized tests, functional task analysis, and examination of tasks in natural environments.[40,123,144] The next sections describe a number of tests that are used with children with DCD. Further

information on standardized tests can be found in Chapters 2 and 3.

Young Children

In the early years, identification of children who may be at risk for DCD is critical[148] and can be achieved through the use of descriptive measures designed for this purpose. As has been described previously, when DCD is suspected, it is important to confirm that a motor impairment is present and to determine the impact of that impairment on activity. Standardized assessments developed for very young children often examine activities by measuring the achievement of developmental skills but do not usually focus on impairment in the qualitative aspects of movement. Identification of a motor skill delay in the young child indicates the need for ongoing monitoring, intervention, or an assessment of motor impairment at a later age.[149]

One tool used to assess early motor skills is the Peabody Developmental Motor Scales–Second Edition (PDMS-2).[57] Popular among clinicians, the PDMS-2 is clinically relevant, with high test-retest reliability and internal consistency. The PDMS-2 has been shown to demonstrate construct validity and concurrent validity with the previous version of the tool.[57] A diagnostic and an evaluative measure, the PDMS-2 is an appropriate choice for assessment of the young child with characteristics of DCD. Given that the PDMS-2 has evaluative properties, it could also be used as a preintervention and postintervention measure to evaluate whether change has occurred.

Older Children

Two popular assessment tools used for older children with DCD are the Bruininks-Oseretsky Test of Motor Proficiency (BOTMP)[15] and the Movement Assessment Battery for Children (MABC).[87] Both of these assessment tools have been recently revised from their original versions as the BOT-2[16] and the MABC-2,[88] respectively.

The BOTMP (original version) has been reported as one of the most frequently used assessments with school-age children $4\frac{1}{2}$ to $14\frac{1}{2}$ years of age.[17,18,184] It is a standardized, norm-referenced discriminative and evaluative measure of the construct of motor ability (fine motor and gross motor) and is available in short or long form. Of concern for the DCD population, the BOTMP does not measure impairment in terms of quality of movement but, rather, measures only the ability to perform a given activity. It has been shown that children with DCD may achieve performance criteria on an activity but still have such poor quality of movement and reduced speed that their performance is not functional.[144] The diagnostic validity of the original version has previously come under scrutiny in the research literature[18,40,79,229,246,254] with speculation that the BOTMP may fail to identify some children with motor impairment when compared with the MABC.[40,229] This inability to identify children with motor impairment was not alleviated even when more stringent cutoff scores were adopted.[229] The BOTMP became outdated in its normative data and was in need of revision and re-standardization after 25 years.[229]

The newest version, the BOT-2,[16] has an expanded age range from 4 to 21 years, and items have been added and modified. This revision consists of 4 motor area composites (fine manual control, manual coordination, body coordination, and strength and agility), with 2 subtests in each composite, and, like its predecessor, both long and short forms of the test are available. The instructions are less standardized in the newer version, allowing greater flexibility for testing. New norms based on a representative, stratified, random sample of 1520 children and youth in the United States were developed. As reported in the manual, the BOT-2 has good interrater reliability, with evidence of test-retest reliability for the total motor composite and short form (reliability is variable, however, when one looks specifically at the composites and subtests, and a practice effect has been noted).[16] Internal consistency is high for the total motor composite and acceptable for the short form (except in the case of 4- to 8-year-olds) and borderline to high for the subtests. In addition, the developers of the tool indicate that the BOT-2 demonstrates construct validity and concurrent validity with the BOTMP and the PDMS-2.[16] With respect to its clinical use, although the items in the newer version are more functionally relevant and the norms are current, some practical issues and limitations remain.[44] The scoring system is noted to be lengthy and prone to error, and some issues have been noted with regard to the stability or reliability of subtest scores, necessitating that total scores be used. The use of total scores may pose problems in cases where children have poor motor skills in a single area only (e.g., poor gross motor skills but adequate fine motor skills)——a situation that has been known to occur with some children with DCD. Using a total score, these children may score well overall despite having significant difficulties in one area of their motor performance. Because of the inclusion of children with disabilities in the new normative sample, cutoffs previously used with the original version may no longer apply, as using the previous cutoffs may under-identify children with motor difficulties. In addition, the BOT-2 does not assess handwriting—a skill that is frequently problematic for the DCD population. Despite its wide usage, the BOT-2 may not be the most appropriate clinical assessment to identify children with DCD, given these concerns.

The MABC-2[88] is based upon the earlier MABC,[87] which has been translated into several languages and is used internationally to identify children with motor impairment. The MABC-2 is a norm-referenced examination that was normed on a stratified sample of 1172 children representative of the U.K. population. The MABC-2 (ICF activity level) contains three sections, and each section includes eight items for each of three age bands: 3 to 6 years, 7 to 10 years, and 11 to 16 years. Items are divided into manual dexterity (three items), aiming and catching (two items), and balance (three items) and include activities such as threading beads, putting pegs in a pegboard, catching and throwing a beanbag, balancing on one leg, jumping, hopping, and heel-to-toe walking. The total score is used to determine if performance is within normal ranges, if motor performance is borderline or at risk, if a motor impairment is present, and if the motor impairment is significant.

The original version of the MABC has been shown to demonstrate good test-retest reliability and concurrent validity with the BOTMP.[40,41,87] In addition, numerous studies conducted worldwide have demonstrated that the MABC identifies children with DCD at the same prevalence rates as would be predicted,[192,214,261] and the body of evidence examining the use of the MABC has been steadily growing. After a literature review of 176 publications, Geuze and colleagues[66] concluded that the MABC is the best assessment tool for DCD in spite of the fact that it omits tasks related to handwriting—an important task to assess.[225] With regard to the newer MABC-2, two studies undertaken by the test developers demonstrate acceptable test-retest reliability (the tool was less reliable when the younger age band was used); information regarding other forms of reliability, however, is not available.[88] Although recent investigations of pilot versions of the lower and upper age bands of the updated MABC-2 provide some evidence of interrater, intrarater, and test-retest reliability, issues related to translation of the test items into other languages, cross-cultural examination, and use of single bands of the assessment tool in these studies have all been identified as issues influencing these results.[14] To date, evidence of the new tool's construct and concurrent validity has not yet been firmly established.[14] Additional studies regarding these properties are emerging and include research on the concurrent validity of the MABC-2 with the MABC-C and the BOT-2, factor analytic validation, and further investigation of test-retest reliability.[8,215,234]

The MABC-2 has several advantages over other assessment tools. The age bands for this instrument cover from 3-0 to 16-0 years, but testing time is short as the assessor presents only activities appropriate for that child's age. The original version has been shown to identify more children with coordination difficulties than the BOTMP[48] and appears to identify more readily those children who have additional learning or attention problems.[40] One of the key contributions of the tool to the assessment of children with DCD is its inclusion of qualitative descriptors of motor behavior (i.e., impairment level descriptions) that the therapist can focus on during the administration of each test item. The MABC-2 also contains a behavioral checklist that can provide insight into the effects of motivation on assessment results and overall compliance with testing. Each of these unique features of the MABC-2 is of value to the clinician in identifying children with, or suspected of having, motor impairment. Although the MABC-2 demonstrates many clinical benefits, given that the psychometric properties of the MABC-2 have yet to be firmly established, therapists are encouraged to make use of several sources of information, including the MABC-2, in their clinical decision making.[14]

Additional Assessment Tools

Although initial tests of motor impairment can screen for, and confirm the presence of, significant motor difficulties, these tools do not provide a complete profile of a child's motor functioning,[98] an understanding of which is important for program planning and intervention.[243] In addition, the definition of DCD,[4] with its emphasis on the impact of motor coordination difficulties on daily life functioning, implies that a comprehensive assessment of the child with DCD will include some examination of the child's ability to perform functional, everyday tasks in natural environments. Only a few assessment measures are available that include this functional and contextual emphasis, such as the Vineland Adaptive Behavior Scale, Second Edition (VABS).[222] When secondary impairments are also present, it may be important to perform additional examinations at a body structure and function level (e.g., strength, physical fitness measures) to plan interventions to address these secondary issues specifically.[58]

FACILITATING A DIAGNOSIS OF DCD

It is not within the scope of practice of physical therapists to formally diagnose DCD. Nevertheless, physical therapists, through their examination and evaluation of test results, are in an ideal position to recognize the motor and behavioral characteristics of potential DCD, and they can provide useful information to the child's physician regarding Criteria A and B of the diagnostic criteria in particular.[4] Criterion A of the DSM-IV indicates that a significant impairment in motor coordination must be present, which can be difficult to determine in a physician's office.[4] Physical therapists can observe and test for motor impairment and provide information to both the family and the physician. The DSM-IV Criterion B states that the motor impairment must interfere with academic achievement and/or ADLs. The therapist can gather information from parents, teachers, and the child about what tasks are difficult for the child to perform and can relay this information to the physician.

Although health professionals may be hesitant to label the observed difficulties as DCD, a strong case can be made for the need to identify and recognize the disorder and for the role of the therapist in facilitating formal recognition of the motor difficulties.[146] DCD has a significant impact not only on the child, but on the entire family.[141,142,228] Parental concerns are not often heard or acknowledged,[1,189] and parents are often frustrated with the health care and educational systems as they pursue answers to their concerns.[58] Significant family stress can occur regarding daily activities at home and around schoolwork. Parents not only are aware of the

difficulties their child experiences from an early age,[1,189] but are searching for answers and access to resources and are often relieved once they have a greater understanding of their children's difficulties. Recent research has shown that in pursuing answers to their concerns, parents are often involved with multiple education and/or health professionals before a diagnosis is made.[1,142]

Facilitating a diagnosis is critically important for the prevention of secondary consequences, in particular, self-esteem issues for the child. A diagnosis can help to initiate education, intervention, and accommodations for the child and allows parents to access resources. Equally important, recognition of the impairment can help to facilitate a long-term relationship with the family's primary care physician. This is critical for follow-up of potential secondary issues that may develop as the child matures and for identifying other developmental conditions that often coexist with DCD (e.g., expressive and receptive language difficulties, attention deficit disorder). Referral to other health care providers for assessment can then be made as appropriate. If DCD is suspected, the physical therapist should encourage the family to have the child seen by their primary care physician.

REFERRAL TO OTHER DISCIPLINES

As has already been discussed in this chapter, it should not be assumed that DCD is an isolated motor problem. An examination performed by any of the following individuals may be needed: (1) a family physician or neurologist when neuromuscular or musculoskeletal concerns are identified; (2) an OT when fine motor, self-help, or motor planning areas need further examination; (3) a speech and language pathologist when speech, oral-motor dysfunction, or possible cognitive-linguistic problems are observed; (4) a psychologist when intellectual or behavioral issues have surfaced; or (5) an adapted physical education teacher when more thorough gross motor skill training is needed.

INTERVENTION

DIRECT INTERVENTION APPROACHES

According to the ICF model, physical therapy interventions can be directed toward remediating impairment, reducing activity limitations, and/or improving participation.[260] In the past, treatment interventions used with children with DCD were aimed primarily at changing body structure and function impairments by trying to improve either the child's sensory processing abilities (vision, kinesthesis) or the difficulties in individual motor components (balance, strength) that were believed to contribute to poor performance. These interventions have been referred to as "bottom-up" interventions, as they tend to address movement problems by emphasizing the building of foundational skills.[126] Examples of bottom-up interventions include perceptual-motor training, process-oriented approach, sensory integration (SI), and neurodevelopmental therapy (NDT). These interventions reflect more traditional theories of motor development and are based on the theoretical belief that, by changing these underlying deficits, task performance will be improved.[126] Some of these bottom-up interventions are still employed by therapists today when working with children with DCD, but several recent and comprehensive systematic reviews on the effectiveness of these approaches have found them to produce minimal change in functional outcomes and to offer no clear advantage of one approach over the other.[58,90,126,152,172,173] When gains are seen after the use of these approaches, the question has been posed as to whether they may be more a function of the skill of the therapists or application of general learning principles than of the treatment itself.[152,211,224] Physical therapists are challenged to re-think the importance of implementing intervention strategies for children with DCD that serve only to change primary impairments.

Dynamic systems theorists have proposed that improvement in functional tasks relies on many variables and tends to be environment-specific.[231] This way of thinking emphasizes that intervention must be contextually based, with intervention occurring in everyday situations and being of significance to the individual child. More recent interventions for children with DCD reflect these beliefs and now tend to emphasize the development of specific skills rather than underlying skill components alone. These have been referred to as "top-down" interventions,[126] which focus on motor learning principles in combination with other theories that emphasize the role of cognitive processes in the learning of new movement skills.[139] Top-down interventions include task-specific interventions and cognitive approaches. See Chapter 4 for more information on motor learning and task-specific intervention.

When selecting an intervention approach for children with DCD, physical therapists need to consider the motor learning difficulties that are particularly evident in this population such as the inability to transfer and generalize skills and learn from past performance. It would seem reasonable from a motor learning perspective that giving feedback at the right stage of learning as well as opportunities to solve movement problems are instrumental guiding principles for interventions with children with movement difficulties.[139] It is likely that interventions that directly target the transfer and generalization of new skills and that emphasize motor learning will be the most successful. Many techniques to foster motor learning can be incorporated into intervention; these include providing verbal instructions, positioning, handling, and providing opportunities for visual or observational learning. Physically demonstrating or modeling movement sequences as well as helping children to learn strategies for managing feedback and organizing their bodies so they can attend to the most salient environmental cues may also be helpful, especially when intervening with young children. The use of frequent practice, practice in variable settings, and consistent provision of feedback should be key elements in any intervention approach for children with DCD. It is important to create practice opportunities in a variety of environments so that each repetition of the action goal becomes a new problem-solving opportunity.[139]

Task-Specific Approaches

A growing body of research demonstrates the value of task-specific interventions.[169,185,211] Movement educators have found task-specific intervention to be a useful way to teach children with DCD specific gross motor skills[185]; they also emphasize its indirect effect in enhancing general participation in physical activity.[110]

Task-specific interventions have as their focus the direct teaching of functional skills in appropriate environments with the intended goal of reducing activity limitations and, by implication, increasing participation levels. Task-specific interventions are individualized approaches that attempt to increase the efficiency of movement by optimizing the way in which skills are performed, given the constraints within each of the several systems that interact during task performance—the child, the task itself, and the environment.[110] As children attempt to solve a movement problem, they may discover several ways to complete a motor task (Figure 16-5). Children explore a variety of solutions to motor problems and are encouraged to experience the resulting effects of using different aspects of their bodies or the environment. The therapist guides the child in choosing which of these different ways of performing represents the most efficient, optimal way for him individually, and in a specific environment.

In task-specific interventions, the therapist is directive, providing verbal instructions, visual prompts, or physical assistance by guiding and directing movement so that children can appreciate the "feel" of efficient movement. Based on tasks that the child needs or wants to perform, the goal of task-specific instruction is to teach "culturally normative tasks in mechanically efficient ways" (p. 238)[110] with the result that children will be less clumsy and will derive more enjoyment from the performance of tasks that were previously performed poorly.[185] Neuromotor Task Training[205] is one example of a task-oriented intervention that emphasizes components of motor learning such as verbal feedback and variable practice. Although there is good evidence that children learn the tasks that are taught through a task-oriented approach (and since they are culturally normative skills, this is important), there is not much evidence for transfer or generalization in this approach.[152,185] The latter are significant considerations when choosing an effective intervention for the child with DCD; more research is needed on how to best achieve these effects.

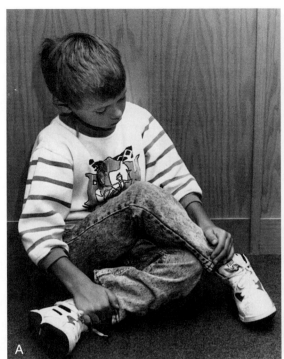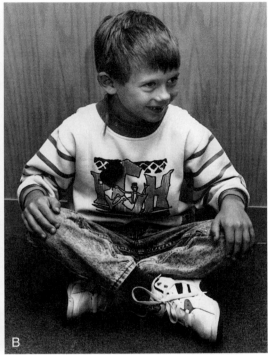

Figure 16-5 **A,** After many therapy sessions with verbal and physical prompts, this child is still unable to sit on the floor and cross his legs independently. **B,** After being reminded of the verbal cues he needs to say to himself, he now successfully crosses his legs.

Cognitive Approaches

Like the task-oriented approaches described previously, interventions employing cognitive approaches also address activity and participation goals. Cognitive approaches, based on theoretical frameworks from cognitive and educational psychology as well as motor learning principles, use direct skill teaching in their approach but differ in their unique problem-solving framework that attempts to help children develop cognitive strategies, acquire tasks, and generalize from the learning of one skill to the next.[140] Cognitive approaches are based on the premise that children with DCD may be deficient in what has been termed their "declarative knowledge" related to motor tasks, that is, they lack knowledge of how to approach a task, how to determine what is required for the task, and how to develop strategies to use when learning and performing a motor task. Intervention approaches using cognition stress the importance of children learning to monitor their performance and use self-evaluation. Mediation is used wherein children are guided to discover problems, generate solutions, and evaluate their success independently.[150]

Preliminary evidence has been shown for the effectiveness of a cognitive approach known as Cognitive Orientation to Daily Occupational Performance (CO-OP).[176] This approach guides the child in discovering verbally based strategies that help him problem-solve in new movement situations.[127,133,175,199] CO-OP emphasizes a child-centered approach with goals that are ecologically valid and performed in a realistic setting. Practice focuses on the child's ability to select, apply, evaluate, and monitor task-specific cognitive strategies with emphasis on facilitating transfer and generalization of the newly learned strategies (for a more in-depth review of the specific CO-OP protocol and the essential components of this approach, including the development of global and task-specific cognitive strategies, the reader is referred to Polatajko, Mandich, Missiuna, Miller, Macnab, Malloy-Miller & Kinsella, 2001).[176] This cognitive approach was shown to be effective in a research clinic setting and, of note, demonstrated some generalization and transfer of skills in children with DCD.[175] Additional research studies have begun to investigate its suitability for use with younger children in clinical settings.[11,240]

The way in which cognitive intervention approaches are used by physical therapists will depend on the age of the child. For younger children, a participatory or consultative approach may be most effective. Using the principles of motor learning, it is important to provide appropriate feedback to children with DCD and to help them to focus on the salient aspects of a given activity by modeling and/or providing them with verbal guidance as they proceed through it. For older children, direct intervention with a more cognitive approach can be used to encourage them to think independently through motor problems. Whether a direct or consultative method of intervention is used, increasing a child's self-efficacy should be a major aim of therapy.[223]

Tools for Goal Setting and Measuring Intervention Effectiveness

Depending upon the target of intervention, several measures can be used to set collaborative goals and evaluate the efficacy of intervention. Whenever possible, goals should be child- and family-centered, as well as environmentally referenced to a problem related to participation in real-life situations.[58] OTs frequently use the Canadian Occupational Performance Measure (COPM)[114] as both a goal setting and outcome measure, and this tool would be similarly applicable to identifying and measuring physical therapy intervention goals. This semistructured interview is used before intervention to have the child and/or family identify areas of functional difficulty (i.e., activity limitations or participation restrictions) and to rate the child's current performance of, and satisfaction with, each task. After intervention, the rater is asked to reflect upon his performance and satisfaction for each targeted goal, and a change score can be generated. The COPM is best suited for use with children older than 8 or 9 years of age. With children younger than this, the Perceived Efficacy and Goal Setting System (PEGS)[147] may be a more appropriate goal-setting tool. In this pictorial measure, children reflect on and indicate their competence in performing 24 tasks that they need to do every day. They then identify any other activities that are difficult for them and select and prioritize tasks as goals for therapy. Using the PEGS, young children have been shown to be able to rate their competence at performing motor tasks and set goals for intervention.[145,148] The PEGS includes companion questionnaires that can be completed by caregivers and teachers. Research evidence indicates that children's goals often differ from those of their parents and teachers, so the views of both may need to be solicited.[50,145]

Goal attainment scaling (GAS) is increasing in usage as a rehabilitation outcome measure with regard to both program evaluation and assessment of individualized client outcomes.[106] With GAS, five possible levels of specific functional attainment are developed for a child to create a criterion-referenced individualized measurement. To date, its use with children with DCD has been described mainly at a programmatic level. In this population, GAS that focuses on the levels of activity and/or participation, not on primary impairment, is warranted.

A measure that can be used to describe or evaluate activity and/or participation is the School Function Assessment (SFA).[38] The SFA evaluates a child's participation in six school-related settings (Participation Scale) and also examines the amount of assistance and/or the types of adaptations required for the child to perform essential school tasks (Task Support Scale). A third scale is very detailed and focuses on the performance of specific activities. In addition to more typical classroom tasks, a section of this scale focuses on the child's mobility and ability to maintain and change positions, manipulate objects, and move on recreational equipment. The SFA requires observation of functional performance over time, so it is usually completed by the therapist through interview of the teacher and others familiar with the child. The SFA has been used to describe the participation patterns of children with DCD,[262] but its use in a pre- to postintervention study of change has not been reported.

EDUCATION AS INTERVENTION

An important, perhaps even primary, benefit of an evaluation for DCD is the follow-up consultation that allows the physical therapist the opportunity to discuss restrictions in activity and participation with the child, the parents, and school personnel.[48] Education and consultation with the family, school personnel, and the community lessen the impact of environmental and personal-contextual factors that may restrict participation.[58] Family members and school personnel are key players in improving outcomes for children with DCD. The physical therapist should always provide parents and school personnel with information about the disorder and its impact on functional activities, and should provide additional resources regarding DCD tailored to the child's and family's needs, including print and web-based educational materials (see resources provided on Evolve website). After collaborative goal setting and intervention planning, written recommendations for home and school would also be helpful for families and school staff. When working toward the acquisition of specific skills, meaningful learning takes place over time and in multiple environments. Daily environmental modifications and task adaptations are critical for improved performance and motor learning for the child with DCD.[48,69]

Helping parents to understand their child's strengths and limitations is an important component of secondary prevention and risk management.[149] Family and cultural expectations can be inconsistent with a child's motor abilities. Expecting proficiency in competitive sports or dance or valuing perfect penmanship can lead to frustration and stress for everyone. Physical therapists can help families and children match interests and skills with expectations that lead to success. When parents are able to look at a play situation in their neighborhood or community recreation program and understand which motor skills are interfering with their child's ability to participate, the play situation can be adapted to maximize the child's participation and help prevent the imposition of societal limitations on full participation in community activities. Consultation with parents and teachers regarding promoting physical activity participation in children with DCD is addressed specifically in a later section in this chapter.

Communication with other disciplines is also an important component of physical therapy intervention for children with DCD.[58] DCD is a multifaceted disability, and more than one service provider may be involved with a child at any given time. If delays in speech and poor social language skills are associated with developmental incoordination, intervention by a speech/language pathologist may be appropriate. If oral-motor impairment is present, goals may be directed at improving articulation and fluency of speech.

Occupational therapists (OTs) are able to contribute in a variety of ways when children are experiencing difficulties with self-care, academic performance, and social participation. Assessments typically conducted by OTs will provide useful information about diagnostic Criterion B.[146] OTs are frequently asked to assist teachers and to provide assessments and interventions related to handwriting. OTs can also address classroom and home modifications that may remediate problems related to organization and spatial orientation in changing environments.[136]

Adapted physical education teachers can consult with regular physical education teachers to help modify the curriculum so that the child with DCD can participate and experience success. As has been discussed, children with DCD have a lower activity level than their peers,[12] have decreased anaerobic power, and have decreased muscle strength.[156,183] For example, if a child cannot run fast enough or safely without falling, then games such as baseball can be modified so that a designated runner is used or players are grouped into teams for all activities with one person hitting and one person running or one person catching and one person throwing. In addition, peer helpers can be identified to help the child with DCD practice basic motor skills such as hopping, jumping, or skipping .

If distractibility and attending to task are identified problems, a school psychologist can assist the physical therapist in managing disruptive or otherwise negative behaviors that interfere with learning motor skills. When concerns regarding distractibility and hyperactivity arise, a referral to a physician should be considered for evaluation of possible attention deficit disorder, or ADHD. Many children with ADHD but not DCD will appear clumsy. If they attend poorly, they will bump into and trip over objects in their environment. When ADHD is associated with DCD, the term DAMP (dysfunction of attention, motor control, and perception) has been used.[70] If behavioral and/or emotional problems such as poor self-esteem, depression, and anxiety become apparent, follow-up by the child's primary care physician is important. If the level of depression or anxiety is serious, psychiatric intervention, medication, and/or counseling might be needed. Physical and mental health complaints should be taken seriously, and previously unidentified medical conditions should be ruled out before other approaches to deal with the symptoms are implemented.

Recently, innovative service delivery models have begun to be explored, incorporating therapists in primary care settings (physician's office) as part of a multidisciplinary team. These service delivery models have the potential to increase awareness of DCD in the community, facilitating accurate and early identification and referral of children with DCD.[62] These new methods of service delivery provide models to enhance collaboration among the many health care professionals involved in the management of children with DCD.

CONSULTATION REGARDING PHYSICAL ACTIVITY

Task-specific and cognitive approaches target intervention at the level of activity limitation. To increase participation levels, a key role for the physical therapist lies in early consultation with physical educators about strategies for the school environment and education for families about appropriate leisure activities that will likely be most successful for children with DCD.[58] These strategies emphasize participation without the risk of injury and are aimed at preventing the physical effects of inactivity.[9,149] In so doing, it may be possible to prevent many of the detrimental consequences that have been documented in children with DCD, including decreased activity, participation, strength, and fitness as well as poor self-competence and self-esteem.[12,45,112,130,155,156,183,204,252] Although it may not be possible to change or "fix" the primary impairments of the child with DCD (such as low tone), the decrease in strength and fitness that can result from avoidance of physical activity is not inevitable and might be improved through promotion of an active lifestyle at home, at school, and in the community.[177]

Physical Education Class

Although teachers can often modify or adapt academic activities in which motor performance is not the primary focus, it may not be as easy to decrease the motor requirements in physical education class. Strategies can be used, however, to encourage children with DCD to make progress within their own range of abilities, to foster self-esteem, and to promote the value of physical activity for long-term fitness and health. As a general strategy, teachers can learn how to "MATCH" tasks to fit the needs of individual children with DCD to encourage maximal participation.[150] With the MATCH strategy, teachers are encouraged to Modify the task, Alter their expectations, Teach strategies, Change the environment, and Help by understanding. (The reader is referred to the *CanChild* Centre for Childhood Disability website at http://www.canchild.ca for downloadable educator resources by grade level. These resources provide examples of different ways to adjust, i.e., MATCH, a task to improve fit with the abilities of a child with DCD.)

When physical activities are taught to children with DCD, emphasis should always be placed on encouraging fun, effort, and participation rather than proficiency. Noncompetitive games in which goals are measured against one's own performance and not that of other children may be helpful.[178] Another strategy is to divide the class into smaller groups when practicing skills, as fewer obstacles will need to be avoided. When a new skill is taught to the class, children with

DCD can be models while instructions are given so that they have an opportunity to experience the movement in addition to observing.[136] With ball skills, modifying the equipment will decrease the risk of injury and increase the likelihood of successful participation; beanbags, nerf balls, and large balls can all be used effectively.

The School Playground

For outside play, introducing children with movement difficulties to playground equipment on an individual basis and teaching them how to use the equipment when in a relaxed environment will increase their motivation to try independently. Children with DCD often avoid playground apparatus from an early age and have not had the experience of discovering how the equipment can be used.[241] The addition of moving objects (in this case, other children) increases the complexity of the environment significantly. Guiding them toward activities where they are more likely to have success (e.g., running or tag instead of ball games) will foster positive self-esteem and reward participation.

Sports and Leisure Activities

From what is now understood about the specific body structure and function impairments of children with DCD, it is possible to predict those types of functional tasks that are more likely to be problematic and to understand why certain sports and leisure activities may be more or less successful for them. It is important, first, to make the distinction between two types of motor behaviors. Early milestones such as sitting, crawling, and grasping (which are considered basic motor abilities) appear to develop relatively spontaneously in these children without any teaching (although milestones sometimes may be delayed and movement quality may not be optimal). Coordination difficulties appear to be much more evident when skills have to be purposefully learned. These skills include such things as catching or kicking a ball and playing baseball. Children with DCD experience particular difficulty with skills that require greater precision, continuous adaptability, and eye-hand coordination.[139] It is also important to appreciate the requirements of individual tasks. Some require constant monitoring of feedback during task performance, and others, once learned, do not require adaptations in response to environmental feedback. As one might expect, tasks with a heavy reliance on integrating feedback from the senses will be difficult for children with DCD.[139]

The type of task, as well as the degree of teaching involved, need to be taken into account when recommendations about sporting and leisure activities are made for children with DCD. Activities like swimming, skating, skiing, and cycling require some initial teaching of the skill and may pose a challenge for children with DCD during early learning of the skill because all novel skills are difficult for them and they do not generalize easily from previous learning.[186] Without encouragement and individualized attention, children with DCD may express dissatisfaction with these activities. Children with DCD, as well as their parents, can be helped to understand that, because these sports contain a sequence of movements that are very repetitive, and these activities do not require constant monitoring of feedback during their performance, children with DCD can become very successful with these activities.[78,149] These are important "lifestyle" sports that individuals with DCD can continue to participate in throughout their lifetime. As well, since many of these sports tend to be taught through verbal guidance, they may be easier for children with DCD to learn. In contrast, activities such as hockey, baseball, football, and basketball (and other ball-related sporting activities) contain a high level of unpredictability. When the environment is changing or variable, the child not only has to learn the movement but also must continuously monitor the environment to adapt to change. Any time a player is required to hit or catch a baseball, contact a hockey stick to a puck, or move quickly around other players, changes must be made in the direction, force, speed, and distance of the movement. Even when the skill is learned, children must continue to adapt to changes in the environment and their place in it. Activities with a high degree of spatial and temporal uncertainty or unpredictability are likely to be challenging for the child with DCD.[82] The need for ongoing adaptation to changes in the environment is always a consideration; running on a smooth surface like a road or track, for example, will be much easier for a child with DCD than running on a forest trail.[149]

Parents of children with DCD have found that their child's involvement in organized sports is greatly enhanced if coaches are flexible about the child's role (e.g., having the child with DCD be the goalie).[142] Self-esteem is promoted through participation in organized sporting activities, and children appreciate when effort and personal mastery are emphasized.[30] Resources regarding ways to promote increased participation in community sports and leisure activities are available for parents, service providers, coaches, and community leaders on the CanChild website (http://www.canchild.ca).

TRANSITION TO ADULTHOOD AND LIFELONG MANAGEMENT OF DCD

High school classes, learning to drive a car, and vocational exploration present new challenges for the adolescent with DCD. It is now apparent that issues related to DCD are lifelong for many, if not all, individuals with DCD. Physical therapy re-examination needs to include discussion of the prevention of secondary problems in adolescents with DCD. Identification of strategies to prevent impairments in body function from limiting activity or restricting participation can be one of the most important outcomes of physical therapy. Musculoskeletal or neuromuscular problems that would signal the need for future physical therapy care should be discussed, as the changing environment and variables related to growth may place new demands on these systems. Preventive initiatives are needed, as adults with DCD often have decreased strength, experience pain, and have poor aerobic capacity and endurance. Appropriate leisure activities that foster strength, endurance, and joint protection should be encouraged. The physical therapist can assist the individual with DCD to identify and participate in appropriate community fitness programs. Goals for life-long leisure and recreational activity should be discussed with young adults. Activities should minimize competition and the need for quick motor responses. Swimming is likely to be more fun and more successful than playing tennis, and therefore more likely to provide health benefits. Singing in a community choir may be a better choice than playing in a community basketball league. Riding a bike for exercise and enjoyment would be more appropriate than participating in a volleyball competition. Additional practical suggestions have been outlined in books for adolescents[107] and adults.[49]

Vocational choices are important decisions for individuals with DCD. Jobs that minimize the need for changing motoric and environmental expectations should be emphasized. Based on Henderson and Sugden's four-level categorization of motor skill difficulty, vocations that involve skills in which neither the individual nor the environment is moving or changing would be top choices.[87] Vocations in which the individual is moving and the environment is changing would be more challenging for the young adult with DCD (Table 16-4).

SUMMARY

DCD is a chronic condition affecting approximately 5% to 6% of the regular school-age population. A motor impairment disorder, its impacts are seen in academic underachievement and poor performance of everyday motor-based tasks. The exact origin and pathophysiology are unknown, but DCD appears to have both motor production and cognitive-linguistic components. Physical therapists have an important role to play both in identifying the impairments of body function and the activity limitations associated with DCD and in providing intervention to prevent or minimize the participation restrictions related to the person and the environment that might otherwise occur. DCD is a lifelong disability that presents challenges for adults, as well as for children and adolescents. Physical therapists function as members of the comprehensive team needed to manage the multiple ramifications of DCD and its many associated learning and medical problems.

TABLE 16-4   Examples of Occupations Categorized by Motor Skill Difficulty

Individual	Environment	
	Stable	**Changing**
STATIONARY	Secondary school and college teaching	Air traffic controller
	Managerial occupations	Preschool and early elementary teaching
	Psychologist	Taxi driver in urban areas
	Data processor	
	Budget analyst	
MOVING	Custodian	Fire fighter
	Mail carrier	Physical education teacher
	Gardener	
	Nurse	Athlete in competitive sports
	Restaurant waiter	

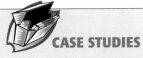

CASE STUDIES

The case studies that follow describe several typical presentations of DCD. They are presented here to demonstrate the variable nature of DCD and the different challenges that arise for physical therapy management.

"Daniel Dreads School"

Daniel, age 5 years, is in kindergarten. Daniel's school has initiated an evaluation for special education services and, as part of this, has made a referral to you as the school-based physical therapist, indicating "fine and gross motor delay" and requesting assistance for the classroom teacher with physical education programming. A referral has also been made to the school-based OT regarding Daniel's fine motor concerns. Daniel's parents have provided permission for you to observe and evaluate Daniel in the classroom and have provided input to the school-based team that is assessing the need for special education services.

Physical Therapy Examination

School Concerns

You use the MABC checklist to guide your interview with Daniel's classroom teacher in identifying specific classroom concerns. When you speak with the teacher, the teacher reports that Daniel slouches when sitting at a table, and when participating in circle time, he tends to lean on nearby walls or classmates and sometimes lies down on the floor. The teacher notes that when printing his name, his work is labored and that he struggles with cutting and pasting activities.

Continued

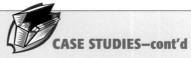

CASE STUDIES—cont'd

Daniel is usually the last one to get ready for recess or to organize his backpack to go home. In physical education class, he is able to throw a tennis ball with direction, but cannot catch one that is thrown to him (see video of Bill for an example of a child with similar problems). Daniel is able to hop only twice on one foot before losing his balance, and tends not to participate in activities that the class is doing (see videos Skip, Hop, Gallop, Jump, and Hopping Strategy Development in a 6-year-old child from Chapter 2 for comparison with typical development of hopping).

Family Concerns

Daniel's parents report that Daniel seems reluctant to go to school, often complaining that his stomach hurts. Getting dressed is always a struggle, so his mother ends up helping him to get him to school on time. On days that he is at home, he is far happier, preferring solitary play with books or on the computer. Daniel's parents are worried that something is wrong. Although they don't feel that anything has deteriorated in his development, they haven't seen much progress or have noted very slow progress in his motor skills. Daniel's parents are also concerned that Daniel's younger brother is catching up to him and worry about how Daniel will feel about himself if his brother overtakes him.

Developmental History

Daniel's birth and early childhood health history are unremarkable. He achieved motor milestones at the expected age, and his parents describe him as an easy child with a gentle temperament. When Daniel started to attend preschool, his parents noticed that he seemed to be a bit behind the other children in self-help skills and did not enjoy some preschool activities. His teachers encouraged them to spend time at home on fine motor activities to encourage Daniel, but he was fairly resistant to working on these tasks, preferring to watch TV, look at books, and play with his robot toys. These play patterns have persisted and strengthened as he has become older.

Medical History

Daniel's hearing and vision have been tested and are normal. At his mother's request, Daniel has been seen by the family doctor for investigation of the family's concerns. Although the doctor does note slightly decreased muscle bulk overall with low postural tone, he is not overly concerned about Daniel's health or his development. He assures Daniel's parents that Daniel will eventually grow out of his difficulties.

Observation at School

You observe that Daniel likes sharing stories with his teacher and class and playing at the sand and water centers. You notice that he has trouble using scissors and avoids drawing or printing letters. Daniel seems to like listening to the teacher when reading books, but often has difficulty sitting quietly at circle time; he usually ends up getting in trouble, as he leans on other children or lies down on the floor. In outdoor play, Daniel is cautious and frequently spends time walking around the perimeter of the playground or walking and talking with the teachers. You spend some time talking with Daniel about things he likes to do and about things he would like to learn how to do. Daniel shares with you that he wants to learn how to catch a ball, as his peers are often engaged in playing catch at recess and lunch time and he is starting to feel left out because he has trouble joining in. You observe Daniel's throwing and catching abilities and you note that he demonstrates immature catching and throwing patterns (see www.cmaj.ca/cgi/content/full/175/5/471; click on "videos" in the right-hand menu).

Standardized Examination

You ask Daniel's parents to complete the Developmental Coordination Disorder Questionnaire (DCDQ'07) to obtain some initial screening information about Daniel's motor difficulties (see Examination Decision in Evidence to Practice Box). You use the framework of the Movement Assessment Battery for Children Checklist (MABC-C) to guide your interview with the teacher to determine the nature of concerns about Daniel at school. You complete a standardized assessment (the Movement Assessment Battery for Children [MABC-2]) to document the nature and extent of Daniel's difficulties. For a summary of Daniel's scores on the MABC-2, see Table 16-5.

TABLE 16-5 **Summary of MABC-2* Scores for Case Study "Daniel Dreads School"**

Component	Component Score	Standard Score	Percentile
Manual dexterity	9	3	1
Aiming and catching	12	5	5
Balance	19	6	9
Total test score	40	3	1

*MABC-2, Movement Assessment Battery for Children, 2nd edition (Henderson & Sugden, 2007).

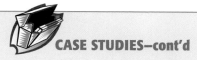

CASE STUDIES—cont'd

EVIDENCE TO PRACTICE 16-1

CASE STUDY "DANIEL DREADS SCHOOL": EXAMINATION, EVALUATION, AND PLAN OF CARE DECISION MAKING

Examination Decision: Parents' perspectives are critical when gathering information related to motor difficulties. Parents can provide useful information about the impact of motor coordination problems on functional, everyday tasks—a necessary diagnostic criterion for the identification of developmental coordination disorder (DCD). The decision to use the Developmental Coordination Disorder Questionnaire (DCDQ'07) is supported by its strong psychometric properties, including its ability to differentiate between children with and without coordination difficulties. The newest version of the questionnaire is appropriate for a child 5 years of age.

Evaluation Decision: Although physical therapists are in an ideal position to observe movement impairments characteristic of DCD, it is not within the scope of practice of physical therapists to formally diagnose DCD. Other underlying medical or neurologic causes for the motor impairment may be present, and when DCD is suspected, it is important that the child be seen by his primary care physician to rule out other explanations for the motor difficulties. Where it would be appropriate (given local regulations), referral directly to a neurologist or physiatrist with expertise in DCD may be beneficial.

Plan of Care Decision: When goals for intervention are set, a collaborative approach is recommended. This approach emphasizes gathering child, parent, and teacher perspectives on priorities for goal setting. The Perceived Efficacy and Goal Setting System (PEGS) facilitates the setting of goals that are child- and family-centered and is environmentally referenced to real-life situations. Using the PEGS, young children with movement impairment have been shown to be able to judge their performance on everyday tasks and are capable of planning appropriate intervention goals.

1. Wilson, B. N., Crawford, S. G., Green, D., Roberts, G., Aylott, A., & Kaplan, B. J. (2009). Psychometric properties of the revised Developmental Coordination Disorder Questionnaire. *Physical & Occupational Therapy in Pediatrics, 29,* 184.
2. Wilson, B. N., Kaplan, B. J., Crawford, S. G., Campbell, A., & Dewey, D. (2000). Reliability and validity of a parent questionnaire on childhood motor skills. *The American Journal of Occupational Therapy, 54,* 484–493.
3. Schoemaker, M. M., Flapper, B., Verheij, N. P., Wilson, B. N., Reinders-Messelink, H. A., & de Kloet, A. (2006). Evaluation of the Developmental Coordination Disorder Questionnaire as a screening instrument. *Developmental Medicine & Child Neurology, 48,* 668–673.
4. American Psychiatric Association. (2000). *Diagnostic and statistical manual of mental disorders* (4th ed.). Washington, DC: Author.
5. Hamilton, S. S. (2002). Evaluation of clumsiness in children. *American Family Physician, 66,* 1435–1440.
6. Sugden, D. A., Chambers, M., & Utley, A. (2006). *Leeds consensus statement 2006.* Retrieved July 28, 2009, from www.dcd-uk.org/consensus.html
7. Dunford, C., Missiuna, C., Street, E., & Sibert, J. (2005). Children's perceptions of the impact of developmental coordination disorder on activities of daily living. *The British Journal of Occupational Therapy, 68,* 207–214.
8. Missiuna, C., Pollock, N., & Law, M. (2004). *Perceived Efficacy and Goal Setting System (PEGS).* San Antonio, TX: Psychological Corporation.
9. Missiuna, C., Pollock, N., Law, M., Walter, S., & Cavey, N. (2006). Examination of the Perceived Efficacy and Goal Setting System (PEGS) with children with disabilities, their parents, and teachers. *American Journal of Occupational Therapy, 60,* 204–214.
10. Forsyth, K., Howden, S., Maciver, D., Owen, C., Shepherd, C., Rush, R., et al. (2007). *Developmental co-ordination disorder: A review of evidence and models of practice employed by allied health professionals in Scotland—Summary of key findings.* Retrieved from NHS Quality Improvement Scotland Web site: www.nhshealthquality.org

Physical Therapy Evaluation, Diagnosis, and Prognosis

Results of your examination indicate that Daniel seems to be demonstrating motor difficulties that would be characteristic of DCD (see American Physical Therapy Association [APTA] Guide to Physical Therapist Practice Pattern 5C–Impaired Motor Function and Sensory Integrity Associated With Nonprogressive Disorders of the Central Nervous System–Congenital Origin or Acquired in Infancy or Childhood2). Daniel is experiencing significant motor difficulties, and the impact of his motor challenges is already apparent, as his teacher and family report both his dislike of school and his avoidance of physical activity. You are concerned about the development of additional secondary consequences, both physical and social/emotional. You would like to have input from Daniel's physician to rule out any other possible reasons for his difficulties (see Evaluation Decision in Evidence to Practice Box). In addition, you feel it would be important to provide some services to Daniel and assistance to the teacher with physical education programming, and you outline your evaluation recommendations to the school team.

Plan of Care/Intervention

The team has reviewed your evaluation recommendations and has decided that special education services are needed; an individual

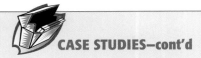

CASE STUDIES—cont'd

education plan (IEP) is developed. As part of the IEP, you have indicated that you will do the following:

- Provide general and tailored information/resources on children with motor difficulties to people involved with Daniel at home and in school.
- Encourage Daniel's parents to follow up with their primary care physician regarding motor concerns at home and in the classroom, and/or initiate a direct referral to other health care professionals such as a neurologist or a physiatrist familiar with the disorder (if appropriate within local regulations).
- Establish some tasks that Daniel wishes to accomplish by having Daniel complete the Perceived Efficacy for Goal Setting system (PEGS) (see Plan of Care Decision in Evidence to Practice Box).
- Encourage the teacher and parents to complete the PEGS to identify tasks for work on generalization of function within the classroom and at home; collaboratively set goals for intervention.
- Work on acquisition of Daniel's chosen tasks to build initial success using motor learning principles and modeling combined with verbal guidance to develop strategies (e.g., "helper hand, doer hand" strategy for tasks that require dominant/assistant use of upper extremities).
- Identify tasks at home and school for transfer and generalization of the strategies ("helper hand/doer hand" is a useful strategy for catching a ball [one of Daniel's goals], holding paper while cutting with scissors [teacher's goal], and using a knife and fork to cut food [parents' goal]); encourage home and school to use mediation techniques to help Daniel develop his problem-solving abilities.
- Make recommendations to Daniel's parents about activities within the community in which he is likely to be successful, and discuss the importance of promoting physical activity and building overall strength for long-term health.
- Make recommendations to the classroom teacher regarding accommodations for the classroom, the physical education class, and the playground.

Outcome

To determine whether any functional gains have been made in Daniel's chosen goals (and to see whether gains have been sustained), you re-administer the PEGS in 6 months' time with Daniel, his teacher, and his parents. You discuss strategies for long-term management with Daniel's teacher and parents, encouraging them to continue to use a mediational approach when new motor problems are identified and to foster Daniel's independence in using problem-solving strategies. You also encourage the use of accommodations and adaptations of the environment to reduce participation restrictions whenever possible.

"Katie Can't Keep Up"

Katie is an 8-year-old girl who was referred by her family physician to the local children's treatment center where you work because of concern regarding her gross motor difficulties.

Physical Therapy Examination

Family Concerns

Katie's parents are concerned about her lack of strength, endurance, and overall coordination. In particular, she seems to have trouble participating in, and sustaining, physical activities. When she and her family go out for a hike, they often have to come back early because she complains of being physically tired. Katie's parents report that at school Katie has trouble sitting on the floor for long periods without something to lean on and has difficulty carrying her knapsack to school. Her parents have also noted Katie's tendency to lean on her desk while doing her homework. She has difficulty with her balance, especially when she is required to stand on one foot, including while dressing (pants in particular) and in managing stairs. Katie's parents note that she was delayed in achieving some of her milestones and has not yet learned to ride a bicycle. Katie's lack of endurance has caused her parents to wonder if perhaps she is anemic. She has difficulties with bowel control, which also concerns her parents. Hoping to improve her overall strength and endurance, her parents enrolled her in dance lessons. Katie was so frustrated with regular dance classes that her parents decided to register her in a musical theater class. Katie is often anxious and her parents are worried about the effect that her incoordination is having on her overall motivation and self-esteem.

Developmental History

Katie is an only child, and she is reported by her parents to have been slower in her motor development than other children of her age. They report that she was a "floppy" child in infancy. Her gross motor skills were acquired slowly, and they had hoped that she would outgrow her delays. A review of Katie's chart indicates that the pregnancy, birth, and developmental history are unremarkable, other than the delays evident in gross motor development.

Medical History

Katie's physical and neurologic exams are unremarkable, with the exception of mildly decreased tone in the extremities and trunk. Overall, Katie shows decreased strength in all extremities. Katie is slightly overweight for her age. Medical investigations regarding the issue of incontinence and lab (bloodwork) results were all normal.

Observation

Katie attends your treatment center. You observe Katie performing several gross motor skills (e.g., throwing and catching, running and skipping) on an informal basis. Her movements are generally slow,

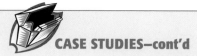

CASE STUDIES—cont'd

and she appears somewhat stiff when moving, particularly when running. She has limited success in catching a small ball and is unable to skip rope (see www.cmaj.ca/cgi/content/full/175/5/471; click on "videos" in right-hand menu). Katie appears to be shy and reserved during the visit and needs quite a bit of encouragement to try the activities.

Standardized Examination

You administer the MABC-2 to Katie and her total score is at the 2nd percentile, with an equal distribution of impairment scores across

categories (see Examination Decision in Evidence to Practice Box). Katie moves very slowly during the manual dexterity items, and although she completes the tasks, she takes too long. During the ball skill activities, you notice that she does not use any consistent patterns of movement, but instead changes her strategy with every trial and never really finds a successful strategy. Her balance difficulties are most evident in the static balance item (see video of Bill for an example of a child with similar problems). She comments a few times during the testing that she is "kind of a klutz."

EVIDENCE TO PRACTICE 16-2

CASE STUDY "KATIE CAN'T KEEP UP": EXAMINATION, EVALUATION, AND PLAN OF CARE DECISION MAKING

Examination Decision: Young children observed to have movement difficulties may be demonstrating characteristics of developmental delay or motor impairment. To determine if motor impairment is present, it is important to use a standardized tool intended for this purpose. The Movement Assessment Battery for Children-2 is a norm-referenced examination that incorporates test items that are difficult for children with development coordination disorder (DCD) (manual dexterity, ball skills and balance). Studies of the psychometric properties of the MABC-2 are emerging. The original version of the MABC is believed to be a valid and useful tool that has several advantages over other assessment tools, including the wide age range it covers and its ability to identify children with DCD and co-occurring learning or attention problems. The test also includes qualitative descriptors of motor behavior and a behavioral checklist, both of which would be extremely helpful to the physical therapist.

Evaluation Decision: Strong evidence suggests that children with motor difficulties do not outgrow the condition and that, over time, they are at significant risk of developing numerous negative secondary consequences unrelated to their primary impairment. When a physical therapist observes movement impairment that is suggestive of DCD, it is important to encourage the family to follow up with their primary care physician. Facilitating this relationship is critical, as the primary care physician can monitor for the development of physical, social, emotional, and behavioral difficulties and can initiate referrals to other health care providers as appropriate. Children with movement difficulties may also have unrecognized co-occurring conditions. Early identification of these difficulties can lead to appropriate interventions and may reduce the potential for negative long-term outcomes.

Plan of Care Decision: Adoption of a task-based intervention approach to address Katie's difficulties is supported by the research literature. Task-specific intervention is ecologically valid because it involves the direct teaching of functional tasks in natural environments. The approach fits well with contemporary thinking about motor development and performance and has been shown to be a successful way to teach children with DCD specific motor skills that they need or want to perform in their everyday lives. In turn, the skills acquired through a task-based approach can enhance physical and social participation, both of which are particularly important for children with DCD. Children with DCD tend to withdraw from physical activity at an early age, limiting their physical and social interactions.

See also Chapter 4 on task-based motor learning programs.

1. Henderson, S., & Sugden, D. (2007). *The Movement Assessment Battery for Children* (2nd ed.). London: Pearson Assessment.
2. Crawford, S. G., Wilson, B. N., & Dewey, D. (2001). Identifying developmental coordination disorder: Consistency between tests. *Physical & Occupational Therapy in Pediatrics, 20,* 29–50.
3. Geuze, R. H., Jongmans, M. J., Schoemaker, M. M., & Smits-Engelsman, B. C. M. (2001). Clinical and research diagnostic criteria for developmental coordination disorder: A review and discussion. *Human Movement Science, 20,* 7–47.
4. Croce, R. V., Horvat, M., & McCarthy, E. (2001). Reliability and concurrent validity of the Movement Assessment Battery for Children. *Perceptual Motor Skills, 93,* 275–280.
5. Losse, A., Henderson, S. E., Elliman, D., Hall, D., Knight, E., & Jongmans, M. (1991). Clumsiness in children—Do they grow out of it? A 10-year follow-up study. *Developmental Medicine and Child Neurology, 33,* 55–68.
6. Cairney, J., Hay, J. A., Faught, B. E., & Hawes, R. (2005). Developmental coordination disorder and overweight and obesity in children aged 9–14 y. *International Journal of Obesity, 29,* 369–372.
7. Skinner, R. A. & Piek, J. P. (2001). Psychosocial implications of poor motor coordination in children and adolescents. *Human Movement Science, 20,* 73–94.

Continued

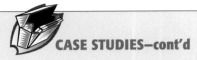

CASE STUDIES—cont'd

EVIDENCE TO PRACTICE 16-2—cont'd

8. Rasmussen, P., & Gillberg, C. (2000). Natural outcome of ADHD with developmental coordination disorder at age 22 years: A controlled, longitudinal, community-based study. *Journal of the American Academy of Child and Adolescent Psychiatry, 39,* 1424–1431.
9. Missiuna, C., Moll, S., King, S., King, G., & Law, M. (2007). A trajectory of troubles: Parents' impressions of the impact of developmental coordination disorder. *Physical and Occupational Therapy in Pediatrics, 27,* 81–101.
10. Pless, M., & Carlsson, M. (2000). Effects of motor skill intervention on developmental coordination disorder: A meta-analysis. *Adapted Physical Activity Quarterly, 17,* 381–401.
11. Revie, G., & Larkin, D. (1993). Task specific intervention for children with developmental coordination disorder: A systems view. *Adapted Physical Activity Quarterly, 10,* 29–41.
12. Larkin, D., & Parker, H. (2002). Task-specific intervention for children with developmental coordination disorder: A systems view. In S. Cermak & D. Larkin (Eds.), *Developmental coordination disorder* (pp. 234–247). Albany, NY: Delmar.

Physical Therapy Evaluation, Diagnosis, and Prognosis

Clinically Katie is showing a movement impairment pattern that is suggestive of developmental coordination disorder (see APTA Guide to Physical Therapist Practice Pattern 5C—Impaired Motor Function and Sensory Integrity Associated With Nonprogressive Disorders of the Central Nervous System—Congenital Origin or Acquired in Infancy or Childhood). Although your professional expertise allows you to identify the motor and activity limitations that Katie has, it is not within your scope of practice to diagnose the medical condition (see Evaluation Decision in Evidence to Practice Box). You believe it is important to have additional medical input regarding the clinical issues you are observing to rule out alternative diagnoses (e.g., see Box 16-3). Katie has a motor coordination impairment that is affecting her ability to participate fully in activities of daily living, a condition that can be addressed with physical therapy. She is at high risk for physical, emotional, and social problems as secondary consequences of her movement difficulties.

Plan of Care/Intervention

- Discuss your findings with the parents to help them understand the role that DCD is likely playing in Katie's difficulties.
- Talk with Katie about DCD, using child-friendly language so she has an understanding of why she is struggling.
- Encourage Katie's parents to return to the family physician for further diagnostic workup and to develop a bowel management program.
- Provide individualized task-based physical therapy procedural interventions to address Katie's performance difficulties with an additional focus on building core skills such as strength, endurance, balance, and stability (see Plan of Care Decision in Evidence to Practice Box). Establish baseline strength and fitness measurements preintervention for future comparison to evaluate change. Have

Katie complete the COPM to establish child-centered goals for intervention and to measure progress.
- Provide consultation to Katie's parents regarding ways to incorporate/transfer and generalize tasks learned during intervention to daily activities and how to encourage Katie's participation in regular physical activities, including those available within the community.
- Encourage Katie's parents to share with her dance teacher educational materials designed for community leaders and coaches (http://www.canchild.ca).
- Speak to the parents about making a referral to the center-based OT to assess potential fine motor difficulties.

Outcome

As you progress toward achieving Katie's goals, you re-administer the COPM and repeat measurements of strength and overall fitness. As necessary, you make modifications to your intervention, including progressing strengthening activities as necessary. You have a follow-up visit with Katie's teachers in a few weeks to see how things have been working at school and provide additional information/resources to the teacher as necessary. You continually monitor Katie's progress and goals to establish or revise intervention frequency and duration.

"Aidan Acts Out"

Aidan is a 13-year-old boy who has ADHD and a history of behavior problems at school. You have a pediatric private practice and receive a call from Aidan's family. Aidan's parents think something is not "quite right" but can't seem to pinpoint the specific origin of his difficulties.

Physical Therapy Examination

Family and School Concerns

Aidan's parents are aware and have been dealing with his ADHD since kindergarten, but believe there is more going on with him. He is

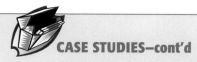

CASE STUDIES—cont'd

frequently in trouble and sent to the office and has been suspended from school several times. Aidan's parents indicate that he is currently receiving special education services at his school and has an IEP. He has very poor written expression, rarely completes tasks independently, and is disruptive in class. Homework completion is a huge problem and is placing a lot of stress on the family. He is taking medication, which has helped with his attention, but teachers report that he continues to act out, particularly during physical education class and when he is expected to write. He has recently been given greater access to assistive technology for writing, and this has been a positive step, but the school has expressed concerns about his readiness for moving on to high school, and staff members also wonder if they aren't missing something. Aidan's mother describes him as awkward-looking and "gangly" and says that he covers up his difficulties by clowning around. Aidan's mother reports a history of withdrawal from organized physical activities, with frequent sign-ups and then dropouts. He tends to spend all his time at home on the computer. Recently, Aidan's parents have become increasingly concerned about Aidan being socially rejected by his friends, especially given some issues with bullying in the earlier grades. Aidan is spending most of his time alone, and his parents can see his mood deteriorating.

Developmental History

Aidan was born prematurely but has had few health concerns since. His development was monitored at regular intervals because of his prematurity. Although Aidan often seemed slow in his development, he did manage to meet all of his motor milestones in a timely fashion. He was diagnosed with ADHD in his early school years.

Medical History

Aidan does not have any current health issues and takes medication for his ADHD.

Observation

You observe Aidan informally and notice that his movements are awkward and have a rigid quality to them. His ability to jump, hop, and maintain balance are less than what you would expect for his age. Aidan is reluctant to demonstrate his motor skills to you, and you observe frequent "off-task" behaviors during your assessment.

Standardized Examination

You have Aidan complete the CSAPPA to get more information about Aidan's perceptions of his abilities (see Examination Decision in Evidence to Practice Box). You also administer the MABC-2, which suggests that Aidan has motor difficulties in addition to his attention difficulties (see video of Bill for an example of a child with similar problems).

EVIDENCE TO PRACTICE 16-3

CASE STUDY "AIDAN ACTS OUT": EXAMINATION AND PLAN OF CARE DECISION MAKING

Examination Decision: The Children's Self-Perceptions of Adequacy in, and Predilection for, Physical Activity Scale (CSAPPA) provides information regarding a child's self-efficacy toward physical activity. Use of this scale is supported by the research evidence and would be particularly helpful in this case scenario. The tool is age-appropriate and would provide valuable information about Aidan's desire, and his perceived ability, to participate in physical activity. He is reluctant to demonstrate his motor abilities. The CSAPPA can provide information about his physical participation levels, which can be useful to you as you plan intervention. As he has already begun to withdraw from participation, you hope to focus your intervention on physical activities in which he can achieve success and build his confidence, and that he can continue for his lifetime. The CSAPPA has demonstrated construct validity, and it has been suggested it may be useful to clinicians in screening for motor impairment.

Plan of Care Decision: Children with developmental coordination disorder (DCD) can become successful

participants in physical activity and receive the long-term health and social benefits that regular physical activity provides. The key to encouraging participation in children with DCD lies in matching children's abilities with activities that promote success. Consultation with children, family, and others about activities that are likely to be successful in children with DCD is an important role for the physical therapist and should be part of the intervention process. Parents, teachers, and others in the community can be helped to understand the role of physical activity participation for positive social and physical health.

Plan of Care Decision: Children with DCD may have difficulties in both fine and gross motor skills, leading to activity limitations and participation restrictions. Consultation and collaboration with other health care providers may be necessary, as a variety of motor performance issues may need to be addressed with the child with DCD. Each health care provider brings area-specific expertise and can be instrumental in facilitating appropriate environmental accommodations and adaptations for success at home and in the classroom.

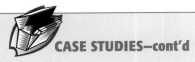

CASE STUDIES—cont'd

EVIDENCE TO PRACTICE 16-3—cont'd

1. Hay, J. (1992). Adequacy in and predilection for physical activity in children. *Clinical Journal of Sport Medicine, 2,* 192–201.
2. Hay, J. A., Hawes, R., & Faught, B. E. (2004). Evaluation of a screening instrument for developmental coordination disorder. *Journal of Adolescent Health, 34,* 308–313.
3. Hay, J., & Missiuna, C. (1998). Motor proficiency in children reporting low levels of participation in physical activity. *Canadian Journal of Occupational Therapy, 65,* 64–71.
4. Cairney, J., Veldhuizen, S., Kurdyak, P., Missiuna, C., Faught, B. E., & Hay, J. A. (2007). Evaluating the CSAPPA sub-scales as potential screening instruments for developmental coordination disorder. *Archives of Disease in Childhood, 92,* 987–991.
5. Barnhart, R. C., Davenport, M. J., Epps, S. B., & Nordquist, V. M. (2003). Developmental coordination disorder. *Physical Therapy, 83,* 722–731.
6. Forsyth, K., Howden, S., Maciver, D., Owen, C., Shepherd, C., Rush, R., et al. (2007). *Developmental co-ordination disorder: A review of evidence and models of practice employed by allied health professionals in Scotland—Summary of key findings.* Retrieved from NHS Quality Improvement Scotland Web site: www.nhshealthquality.org

7. Poulsen, A. A., & Ziviani, J. M. (2004). Can I play too? Physical activity engagement of children with developmental coordination disorders. *Canadian Journal of Occupational Therapy, 71,* 100–107.
8. Forsyth, K., Howden, S., Maciver, D., Owen, C., Shepherd, C., Rush, R., et al. (2007). *Developmental co-ordination disorder: A review of evidence and models of practice employed by allied health professionals in Scotland—Summary of key findings.* Retrieved from NHS Quality Improvement Scotland Web site: www.nhshealthquality.org
9. Missiuna, C. (2003). *Children with developmental coordination disorder: At home and in the classroom (booklet).* McMaster University, ON: CanChild (Online).
10. Missiuna, C., Pollock, N., Egan, M., DeLaat, D., Gaines, R., & Soucie, H. (2008). Enabling occupation through facilitating the diagnosis of developmental coordination disorder. *Canadian Journal of Occupational Therapy, 75,* 26–34.

Physical Therapy Evaluation, Diagnosis, and Prognosis

You believe that Aidan's poorly developed motor abilities may be consistent with developmental coordination disorder, and that these difficulties are present in addition to his attention issues (see APTA Guide to Physical Therapist Practice Pattern 5C—Impaired Motor Function and Sensory Integrity Associated With Nonprogressive Disorders of the Central Nervous System—Congenital Origin or Acquired in Infancy or Childhood). You are concerned about Aidan, given his motor difficulties, his co-occurring ADHD, and the fact that he is already demonstrating physical and social participation withdrawal.

Plan of Care/Intervention

- Help Aidan to understand the nature of his attention and motor difficulties and the combined impact that these are having on his physical and social participation.
- Speak to Aidan's parents and obtain permission to observe Aidan in the classroom and meet with school personnel; coordinate with general education personnel at Aidan's school and the special education teacher. Determine if Aidan has a school-based physical therapist currently working with him at school, and coordinate services as appropriate.

- Consult with Aidan's parents and teachers by providing resources and information; suggest some physical activities that might "MATCH" his abilities and interests, and promote his physical participation both at school and in the community (see Plan of Care Decision in Evidence to Practice Box).
- Discuss with school personnel and Aidan's parents upcoming high school courses that might be challenging (e.g., music, shop); make recommendations/provide input for his IEP regarding possible accommodations and/or adaptations that could be put in place.
- Reinforce the need for accommodations regarding writing assignments and access to a laptop at school.
- Suggest a referral to OT for any additional recommendations regarding writing issues (see Plan of Care Decision in Evidence to Practice Box).

Outcome

You plan to continue to assist Aidan and his family as they make the transition to high school. You help Aidan and his parents to proactively problem-solve as new issues arise. You follow up with Aidan and his family several months after he has settled in to high school, monitoring the need for referral to other health care service providers for social, emotional, and behavioral issues.

ACKNOWLEDGMENTS

The authors are grateful to Doreen Bartlett, PhD, PT (University of Western Ontario, London, Ontario, Canada), for her valuable contributions to the ideas presented in this chapter, and to Jennifer Siemon for her assistance in editing and preparing the bibliographic citations.

REFERENCES

1. Ahern, K. (2000). Something is wrong with my child: A phenomenological account of a search for a diagnosis. *Early Education & Development, 11,* 188–201.

2. American Physical Therapy Association. (2001). *Guide to physical therapist practice* (2nd ed.). Alexandria, VA: American Physical Therapy Association.

3. American Psychiatric Association. (1994). *Diagnostic and statistical manual of mental disorders.* Washington, DC: Author.

4. American Psychiatric Association. (2000). *Diagnostic and statistical manual of mental disorders* (4th ed.). Washington, DC: Author.

5. Astill, S., & Utley, A. (2006). Two-handed catching in children with developmental coordination disorder. *Motor Control, 10,* 109–124.

6. Astill, S., & Utley, A. (2008). Coupling of the reach and grasp phase during catching in children with developmental coordination disorder. *Journal of Motor Behavior, 40,* 315–323.

7. Ayres, A. J. (1972). Types of sensory integrative dysfunction among disabled learners. *American Journal of Occupational Therapy, 26,* 13–18.

8. Barnett, A., Henderson, S., Sugden, D., & Schulz, J. (2009, June). *Validity of the Movement ABC Test* (2nd ed.). Paper presented at the DCD VIII Developmental Coordination Disorder International Conference, Baltimore, MD.

9. Barnhart, R. C., Davenport, M. J., Epps, S. B., & Nordquist, V. M. (2003). Developmental coordination disorder. *Physical Therapy, 83,* 722–731.

10. Benbow, M. (2002). Hand skills and handwriting. In S. Cermak & D. Larkin (Eds.), *Developmental coordination disorder* (pp. 248–279). Albany, NY: Delmar.

11. Bernie, C., & Rodger, S. (2004). Cognitive strategy use in school-aged children with developmental coordination disorder. *Physical and Occupational Therapy in Pediatrics, 24,* 23–45.

12. Bouffard, M., Watkinson, E. J., Thompson, L. P., Causgrove Dunn, J. L., & Romanow, S. K. E. (1996). A test of the activity deficit hypothesis with children with movement difficulties. *Adapted Physical Activity Quarterly, 13,* 61–73.

13. Brookes, R. L., Nicolson, R. I., & Fawcett, A. J. (2007). Prisms throw light on developmental disorders. *Neuropsychologia, 45,* 1921–1930.

14. Brown, T., & Lalor, A. (2009). The Movement Assessment Battery for Children–Second edition (MABC-2): A review and critique. *Physical and Occupational Therapy in Pediatrics, 29,* 86–103.

15. Bruininks, R. H. (1978). *Bruininks-Oseretsky Test of Motor Proficiency.* Circle Pines, MI: American Guidance Service.

16. Bruininks, R., & Bruininks, B. (2005). *Bruininks-Oseretsky Test of Motor Proficiency* (2nd ed.). Circle Pines, MN: AGS Publishing (American Guidance Services).

17. Burton, A. W., & Miller, D. E. (1998). *Movement skill assessment.* Champaign, IL: Human Kinetics.

18. Burtnor, P., McMain, M., & Crowe, T. (2002). Survey of occupational therapy practitioners in Southwestern schools: Assessments used and preparation of students for school-based practice. *Physical & Occupational Therapy in Pediatrics, 22,* 25–39.

19. Cairney, J., Hay, J. A., Faught, B. E., Flouris, A., & Klentrou, P. (2007). Developmental coordination disorder and cardiorespiratory fitness in children. *Pediatric Exercise Science, 19,* 20–28.

20. Cairney, J., Hay, J. A., Faught, B. E., & Hawes, R. (2005). Developmental coordination disorder and overweight and obesity in children aged 9–14 y. *International Journal of Obesity, 29,* 369–372.

21. Cairney, J., Hay, J., Faught, B., Mandigo, J., & Flouris, A. (2005). Developmental coordination disorder, self-efficacy toward physical activity, and play: Does gender matter? *Adapted Physical Activity Quarterly, 22,* 67–82.

22. Cairney, J., Hay, J. A., Faught, B. E., Wade, T. J., Corna, L., & Flouris, A. (2005). Developmental coordination disorder, generalized self-efficacy toward physical activity, and participation in organized and free play activities. *Journal of Pediatrics, 147,* 515–520.

23. Cairney, J., Missiuna, C., Veldhuizen, S., & Wilson, B. (2008). Evaluation of the psychometric properties of the Developmental Coordination Disorder Questionnaire for Parents (DCD-Q): Results from a community based study of school-aged children. *Human Movement Science, 27,* 932–940.

24. Cairney, J., Veldhuizen, S., Kurdyak, P., Missiuna, C., Faught, B. E., & Hay, J. A. (2007). Evaluating the CSAPPA sub-scales as potential screening instruments for developmental coordination disorder. *Archives of Disease in Childhood, 92,* 987–991.

25. Cantell, M., & Kooistra, L. (2002). Long-term outcomes of developmental coordination disorder. In S. Cermak & D. Larkin (Eds.), *Developmental coordination disorder* (pp. 23–38). Albany, NY: Delmar.

26. Cantell, M., Smyth, M. M., & Ahonen, T. (1994). Clumsiness in adolescence: Educational, motor and social outcomes of motor delay detected at 5 years. *Adapted Physical Activity Quarterly, 11,* 115–129.

27. Cantin, N., Polatajko, H. J., Thach, W. T., & Jaglal, S. (2007). Developmental coordination disorder: Exploration of a cerebellar hypothesis. *Human Movement Science, 26,* 491–509.

28. Case-Smith, J., & Weintraub, N. (2002). Hand function and developmental coordination disorder. In S. Cermak, & D.

Larkin (Eds.), *Developmental coordination disorder* (pp. 157–171). Albany, NY: Delmar.

29. Causgrove Dunn, J., & Watkinson, E. J. (1996). Problems with identification of children who are physically awkward using the TOMI. *Adapted Physical Activity Quarterly, 13,* 347–356.

30. Causgrove Dunn, J., & Watkinson, E. J. (2002). Considering motivation theory in the study of developmental coordination disorder. In S. Cermak & D. Larkin (Eds.), *Developmental coordination disorder* (pp. 185–199). Albany, NY: Delmar.

31. Cermak, S. (1985). Developmental dyspraxia. *Advances in Psychology, 23,* 225–248.

32. Cermak, S., Gubbay, S., & Larkin, D. (2002). What is developmental coordination disorder? In S. Cermak & D. Larkin (Eds.), *Developmental coordination disorder* (pp. 2–22). Albany, NY: Delmar.

33. Cermak, S., & Larkin, D. (2002). Families as partners. In S. Cermak & D. Larkin (Eds.), *Developmental coordination disorder* (pp. 200–208). Albany, NY: Delmar.

34. Chen, H. F., & Cohn, E. S. (2003). Social participation for children with developmental coordination disorder: Conceptual, evaluation and intervention considerations. *Physical & Occupational Therapy in Pediatrics, 23,* 61–78.

35. Cherng, R. J., Liang, L. Y., Chen, Y. J., & Chen, J. Y. (2009). The effects of a motor and a cognitive concurrent task on walking in children with developmental coordination disorder. *Gait & Posture, 29,* 204–207.

36. Civetta, L. R., & Hillier, S. L. (2008). The Developmental Coordination Disorder Questionnaire and Movement Assessment Battery for Children as a diagnostic method in Australian children. *Pediatric Physical Therapy, 20,* 39–46.

37. Cooke, R. W. I., & Foulder-Hughes, L. (2003). Growth impairment in the very preterm and cognitive and motor performance at 7 years. *British Medical Journal, 88,* 482–487.

38. Coster, W., Deeney, T., Haltiwanger, J., & Haley, S. (1998). *School function assessment.* San Antonio, TX: Psychological Corporation.

39. Cousins, M., & Smyth, M. M. (2003). Developmental coordination impairments in adulthood. *Human Movement Science, 22,* 433–459.

40. Crawford, S. G., Wilson, B. N., & Dewey, D. (2001). Identifying developmental coordination disorder: Consistency between tests. *Physical & Occupational Therapy in Pediatrics, 20,* 29–50.

41. Croce, R. V., Horvat, M., & McCarthy, E. (2001). Reliability and concurrent validity of the Movement Assessment Battery for Children. *Perceptual & Motor Skills, 93,* 275–280.

42. David, K. S. (2006). Developmental coordination disorders. In S. K. Campbell (Ed.), *Physical therapy for children* (3rd ed., pp. 559–589). Philadelphia: W. B. Saunders.

43. Davis, N. M., Ford, G. W., Anderson, P. J., Doyle, L. W., & Victorian Infant Collaborative Study Group. (2007). Developmental coordination disorder at 8 years of age in a regional cohort of extremely-low-birthweight or very preterm infants. *Developmental Medicine and Child Neurology, 49,* 325–330.

44. Deitz, J. C., Kartin, D., & Kopp, K. (2007). Review of the Bruininks-Oseretsky Test of Motor Proficiency (BOT-2). *Physical & Occupational Therapy in Pediatrics, 27,* 87–102.

45. Denckla, M. B. (1984). Developmental dyspraxia: The clumsy child. In M. D. Levine & P. Satz (Eds.), *Middle childhood: Development and dysfunction* (pp. 245–260). Baltimore, MD: University Park Press.

46. Dewey, D., & Kaplan, B. J. (1994). Subtyping of developmental motor deficits. *Developmental Neuropsychology, 10,* 265–284.

47. Dewey, D., Kaplan, B. J., Crawford, S. G., & Wilson, B. N. (2002). Developmental coordination disorder: Associated problems in attention, learning, and psychosocial adjustment. *Human Movement Science. Special Current Issues in Motor Control and Coordination, 21,* 905–918.

48. Dewey, D., & Wilson, B. N. (2001). Developmental coordination disorder: What is it? *Physical & Occupational Therapy in Pediatrics, 20,* 5–27.

49. Drew, S. (2005). *Developmental coordination disorder in adults.* West Sussex, UK: Whurr Publishers Ltd.

50. Dunford, C., Missiuna, C., Street, E., & Sibert, J. (2005). Children's perceptions of the impact of developmental coordination disorder on activities of daily living. *The British Journal of Occupational Therapy, 68,* 207–214.

51. Dunford, C., Street, E., O'Connell, H., Kelly, J., & Sibert, J. R. (2004). Are referrals to occupational therapy for developmental coordination disorder appropriate? *Archives of Disease in Childhood, 89,* 143–147.

52. Dwyer, C., & McKenzie, B. E. (1994). Impairment of visual memory in children who are clumsy. *Adapted Physical Activity Quarterly, 11,* 179–189.

53. Elliott, J. G., & Place, M. (2004). *Children in difficulty: A guide to understanding and helping* (2nd ed.). London: Routledge-Falmer.

54. Faught, B. E., Hay, J. A., Cairney, J., & Flouris, A. (2005). Increased risk for coronary vascular disease in children with developmental coordination disorder. *The Journal of Adolescent Health, 37,* 376–380.

55. Fitts, P. M., & Posner, M. I. (1967). *Human performance.* Belmont, CA: Brooks/Cole Publishing.

56. Fitzpatrick, D. A., & Watkinson, E. J. (2003). The lived experience of physical awkwardness: Adults' retrospective views. *Adapted Physical Activity Quarterly, 20,* 279–297.

57. Folio, M. R. & Fewell, R. R. (2000). *Peabody Developmental Motor Scales–2* (2nd ed.). Austin, TX: Pro-Ed.

58. Forsyth, K., Howden, S., Maciver, D., Owen, C., Shepherd, C., Rush, R., et al. (2007). Developmental co-ordination disorder: A review of evidence and models of practice employed by allied health professionals in Scotland—Summary of key findings. Retrieved from NHS Quality Improvement Scotland Web site: www.nhshealthquality.org.

59. Fox, A. M., & Lent, B. (1996). Clumsy children: Primer on developmental coordination disorder. *Canadian Family Physician, 42,* 1965–1971.

60. Francis, M., & Piek, J. P. (2003). *The effects of perceived social support and self-worth on depressive symptomatology in*

children with and without developmental coordination disorder (DCD). Presented at the 38th APS Annual Conference, Perth, Western Australia.

61. Gaines, R., & Missiuna, C. (2007). Early identification: Are speech/language-impaired toddlers at increased risk for developmental coordination disorder? *Child: Care, Health, and Development, 33*, 325–332.

62. Gaines, R., Missiuna, C., Egan, M., & McLean, J. (2008). Interprofessional care in the management of a chronic childhood condition: developmental coordination disorder. *Journal of Interprofessional Care, 22*, 552–555.

63. Geuze, R. H. (2003). Static balance and developmental coordination disorder. *Human Movement Science, 22*, 527–548.

64. Geuze, R. H. (2005). Motor impairment in DCD and activities of daily living. In D. Sugden & M. Chambers (Eds.), *Children with developmental coordination disorder* (pp. 19–46). London, England: Whurr Publishers Ltd.

65. Geuze, R. H., & Borger, H. (1993). Children who are clumsy: Five years later. *Adapted Physical Activity Quarterly, 10*, 10–21.

66. Geuze, R. H., Jongmans, M. J., Schoemaker, M. M., & Smits-Engelsman, B. C. M. (2001). Clinical and research diagnostic criteria for developmental coordination disorder: A review and discussion. *Human Movement Science, 20*, 7–47.

67. Geuze, R. H., & Kalverboer, A. (1987). Inconsistency and adaptation in timing of clumsy children. *Journal of Human Movement Science, 13*, 421–432.

68. Geuze, R. H., & Kalverboer, A. (1994). Tapping a rhythm: A problem of timing for children who are clumsy and dyslexic? *Adapted Physical Activity Quarterly, 11*, 200–213.

69. Gillberg, C. (1998). Hyperactivity, inattention and motor control problems: Prevalence, comorbidity and background factors. *Folia Phoniatrica Logopaedica, 50*, 107–117.

70. Gillberg, C. (2003). Deficits in attention, motor control, and perception: A brief review. *Archives of Disease in Childhood, 88*, 904–910.

71. Gillberg, I. C., & Gillberg, C. (1989) Preschool children with minor neurodevelopmental disorders. IV: Behaviour and school achievement at age 13. *Developmental Medicine and Child Neurology, 30*, 3–13.

72. Goodgold-Edwards, S. A., & Cermak, S. A. (1990). Integrating motor control and motor learning concepts with neuropsychological perspectives on apraxia and developmental dyspraxia. *American Journal of Occupational Therapy, 44*, 431–439.

73. Goyen, T. A., & Lui, K. (2008). Developmental coordination disorder in 'apparently normal' school children born extremely preterm. *Archives of Disease in Childhood, 94*, 298–302.

74. Gramsbergen, A. (2003). Clumsiness and disturbed cerebellar development: Insights from animal experiments. *Neural Plasticity, 10*, 129–140.

75. Green, D., Bishop, T., Wilson, B., Crawford, S., Hooper, R., Kaplan, B., et al. (2005). Is questionnaire-based screening part of the solution to waiting lists for children with developmental coordination disorder? *British Journal of Occupational Therapy, 68*, 2–10.

76. Gubbay, S. S. (1975). *The clumsy child: A study of developmental apraxia and agnosic ataxia.* Philadelphia: W. B. Saunders.

77. Hamilton, S. S. (2002). Evaluation of clumsiness in children. *American Family Physician, 66*, 1435–1440.

78. Hands, B., & Larkin, D. (2002). Physical fitness and developmental coordination disorder. In S. Cermak & D. Larkin (Eds.), *Developmental coordination disorder* (pp. 172–184). Albany, NY: Delmar.

79. Hattie, J., & Edwards, H. (1987). A review of the Bruininks-Oseretsky test of motor proficiency. *British Journal of Educational Psychology, 57*, 104–113.

80. Hay, J. (1992). Adequacy in and predilection for physical activity in children. *Clinical Journal of Sport Medicine, 2*, 192–201.

81. Hay, J. A., Hawes, R., & Faught, B. E. (2004). Evaluation of a screening instrument for developmental coordination disorder. *Journal of Adolescent Health, 34*, 308–313.

82. Hay, J., & Missiuna, C. (1998). Motor proficiency in children reporting low levels of participation in physical activity. *Canadian Journal of Occupational Therapy, 65*, 64–71.

83. Hellgren, L., Gillberg, I. C., Bagenholm, A., & Gillberg, C. (1994). Children with deficits in attention, motor control and perception (DAMP) almost grown up: Psychiatric and personality disorders at age 16 years. *Journal of Child Psychology and Psychiatry, 35*, 1255–1271.

84. Henderson, S., & Barnett, A. (1998). The classification of specific motor coordination disorders in children: Some problems to be solved. *Human Movement Science, 17*, 449–469.

85. Henderson, S. E., & Henderson, L. (2002). Toward an understanding of developmental coordination disorder. *Adapted Physical Activity Quarterly, 19*, 12–31.

86. Henderson, L., Rose, P., & Henderson, S. (1992). Reaction time and movement time in children with developmental coordination disorder. *The Journal of Child Psychology and Psychiatry, 33*, 895–905.

87. Henderson, S., & Sugden, D. A. (1992). *Movement Assessment Battery for Children.* San Antonio, TX: Psychological Corporation.

88. Henderson, S., & Sugden, D. (2007). *The Movement Assessment Battery for Children–2* (2nd ed.). London: Pearson Assessment.

89. Hill, E. L. (2001). Non-specific nature of specific language impairment: A review of the literature with regard to concomitant motor impairments. *International Journal of Language and Communication Disorders, 36*, 149–171.

90. Hillier, S. (2007). Intervention for children with developmental coordination disorder: A systematic review. *The Internet Journal of Allied Health Sciences and Practice, 5*, 1–11.

91. Hoare, D. (1994). Subtypes of developmental coordination disorder. *Adapted Physical Activity Quarterly, 11*, 158–169.

92. Hoare, D., & Larkin, D. (1991). Kinaesthetic abilities of clumsy children. *Developmental Medicine & Child Neurology, 33*, 671–678.

93. Holsti, L., Grunau, R. V. E., & Whitfield, M. F. (2002). Developmental coordination disorder in extremely low birth weight children at nine years. *Journal of Developmental & Behavioral Pediatrics, 23,* 9–15.

94. Huh, J., Williams, H., & Burke, J. (1998). Development of bilateral motor control in children with developmental coordination disorders. *Developmental Medicine & Child Neurology, 40,* 474–484.

95. Iloeje, S. O. (1987). Developmental apraxia among Nigerian children in Enugu, Nigeria. *Developmental Medicine and Child Neurology, 29,* 502–507.

96. Ivry, R. B. (2003). Cerebellar involvement in clumsiness and other developmental disorders. *Neural Plasticity, 10,* 141–153.

97. Johnston, L. M., Burns, Y. R., Brauer, S. G., & Richardson, C. A. (2002). Differences in postural control and movement performance during goal directed reaching in children with developmental coordination disorder. *Human Movement Science, 21,* 583–601.

98. Johnston, L., & Watter, P. (2006). Clinimetrics: Movement assessment battery for children. *Australian Journal of Physiotherapy, 52,* 68.

99. Jongmans, M. J., Smits-Engelsman, B. C. M., & Schoemaker, M. M. (2003). Consequences of comorbidity of developmental coordination disorders and learning disabilities for severity and pattern of perceptual-motor dysfunction. *Journal of Learning Disabilities, 36,* 528–537.

100. Junaid, K., Harris, S., Fulmer, K., & Carswell, A. (2000). Teachers' use of the MABC checklist to identify children with motor coordination difficulties. *Pediatric Physical Therapy, 12,* 158–163.

101. Kadesjo, B., & Gillberg, C. (1998). Attention deficits and clumsiness in Swedish 7-year-old children. *Developmental Medicine & Child Neurology, 40,* 796–804.

102. Kadesjo, B., & Gillberg, C. (1999). Developmental coordination disorder in Swedish 7-year-old children. *Journal of the American Academy of Child and Adolescent Psychiatry, 38,* 820–828.

103. Kagerer, F. A., Bo, J., Contreras-Vidal, J. L., & Clark, J. E. (2004). Visuomotor adaptation in children with developmental coordination disorder. *Motor Control, 8,* 450–460.

104. Kaplan, B. J., Wilson, B. N., Dewey, D., & Crawford, S. G. (1998). DCD may not be a discrete disorder. *Human Movement Science, 17,* 471–490.

105. Kimball, J. (2002). Developmental coordination disorder from a sensory integration perspective. In S. Cermak & D. Larkin (Eds.), *Developmental coordination disorder* (pp. 210–220). Albany, NY: Delmar.

106. King, G., McDougall, J., Tucker, M., Gritzan, J., Malloy-Miller, T., Alambets, P., et al. (1999). An evaluation of functional, school-based therapy services for children with special needs. *Physical & Occupational Therapy in Pediatrics, 19,* 5–29.

107. Kirby, A. (2001). *Dyspraxia: The hidden handicap.* London, UK: Souvenir Press.

108. Konczak, J., & Timmann, D. (2007). The effect of damage to the cerebellum on sensorimotor and cognitive function in children and adolescents. *Neuroscience & Biobehavioural Reviews, 31,* 1101–1113.

109. Larkin, D., & Parker, H.E. (1998). Physical activity profiles of adolescents who have experienced motor difficulties. In D. Drouin, C. Lepine, & C. Simard (Eds.), *Proceedings of the International Symposium for Adapted Physical Activity.* Quebec City, Canada: International Federation of Adapted Physical Activity.

110. Larkin, D., & Parker, H. (2002). Task-specific intervention for children with developmental coordination disorder: A systems view. In S. Cermak & D. Larkin (Eds.), *Developmental coordination disorder* (pp. 234–247). Albany, NY: Delmar.

111. Laszlo, J. I., Bairstow, P. J., Bartrip, J., & Rolfe, U. T. (1989). Process-oriented assessment and treatment of children with perceptuo-motor dysfunction. *British Journal of Developmental Psychology, 7,* 251–273.

112. Laszlo, J. I., Bairstow, P. J., Bartrip, J., & Rolfe, V. T. (1988). Clumsiness or perceptuo-motor dysfunction? In A. M. Colley & J. R. Beech (Eds.), *Cognition and action in skilled behaviour* (pp. 293–310). Amsterdam: North Holland.

113. Laufer, Y., Ashkenazi, T., & Josman, N. (2008). The effects of a concurrent cognitive task on the postural control of young children with and without developmental coordination disorder. *Gait & Posture, 27,* 347–351.

114. Law, M., Baptiste, S., Carswell, A., McColl, M., Polatajko, H., & Pollock, N. (1998). *Canadian occupational performance measure* (3rd ed.). Ottawa: CAOT Publications.

115. Lingam, R., Hunt, L., Golding, J., Jongmans, M., & Emond, A. (2009). Prevalence of developmental coordination disorder using the DSM-IV at 7 years of age: A UK population based study. *Pediatrics, 123,* e693–e700.

116. Loh, P. R., Piek, J. P., & Barrett, N. C. (2009). The use of the Developmental Coordination Disorder Questionnaire in Australian children. *Adapted Physical Activity Quarterly, 26,* 38–53.

117. Lord, R., & Hulme, C. (1987). Kinesthetic sensitivity of normal and clumsy children. *Developmental Medicine & Child Neurology, 29,* 720–725.

118. Lord, R., & Hulme, C. (1988). Visual perception and drawing ability in normal and clumsy children. *British Journal of Developmental Psychology, 6,* 1–9.

119. Losse, A., Henderson, S. E., Elliman, D., Hall, D., Knight, E., & Jongmans, M. (1991). Clumsiness in children—Do they grow out of it? A 10-year follow-up study. *Developmental Medicine and Child Neurology, 33,* 55–68.

120. Lundy-Ekman, L., Ivry, R. B., Keele, S., & Woollacott, M. (1991). Timing and force control deficits in clumsy children. *Journal of Cognitive Neuroscience, 3,* 367–376.

121. Mackenzie, S. J., Getchell, N., Deutsch, K., Wilms-Floet, A., Clark, J. E., & Whitall, J. (2008). Multi-limb coordination and rhythmic variability under varying sensory availability conditions in children with DCD. *Human Movement Science, 27,* 256–269.

122. MacNab, J. J., Miller, L. T., & Polatajko, H. J. (2001). The search for subtypes of DCD: Is cluster analysis the answer? *Human Movement Science, 20,* 49–72.

123. Maeland, A. F. (1992). Identification of children with motor coordination problems. *Adapted Physical Activity Quarterly, 9,* 330–342.

124. Magalhaes, L., Missiuna, C., & Wong, S. (2006). Terminology used in research reports of developmental coordination disorder. *Developmental Medicine and Child Neurology, 48,* 937–941.

125. Mandich, A., Buckolz, E., & Polatajko, H. (2002). On the ability of children with developmental coordination disorder (DCD) to inhibit response initiation: The Simon effect. *Brain Cognition, 50,* 150–162.

126. Mandich, A. D., Polatajko, H. J., MacNab, J. J., & Miller, L. T. (2001). Treatment of children with developmental coordination disorder: What is the evidence? *Physical and Occupational Therapy in Pediatrics, 20,* 51–68.

127. Mandich, A. D., Polatajko, H. J., Missiuna, C., & Miller, L. T. (2001). Cognitive strategies and motor performance in children with developmental coordination disorder. *Physical and Occupational Therapy in Pediatrics, 20,* 125–143.

128. Marchiori, G. E., Wall, A. E., & Bedingfield, E. W. (1987). Kinematic analysis of skill acquisition in physically awkward boys. *Adapted Physical Activity Quarterly, 4,* 305–315.

129. May-Benson, T., Ingolia, P., & Koomar, J. (2002). Daily living skills and developmental coordination disorder. In S. Cermak & D. Larkin (Eds.), *Developmental coordination disorder* (pp. 140–156). Albany, NY: Delmar.

130. McKinlay, I. (1987). Children with motor difficulties: Not so much a syndrome—A way of life. *Physiotherapy, 73,* 635–637.

131. Miall, R. C. (2003). Connecting mirror neurons and forward models. *NeuroReport, 14,* 2135–2137.

132. Miller, L. T., Missiuna, C. A., MacNab, J. J., Malloy-Miller, T., & Polatajko, H. J. (2001). Clinical description of children with developmental coordination disorder. *Canadian Journal of Occupational Therapy, 68,* 5–15.

133. Miller, L. T., Polatajko, H. J., Missiuna, C., Mandich, A. D., & MacNab, J. J. (2001). A pilot trial of a cognitive treatment for children with developmental coordination disorder. *Human Movement Science, 20,* 183–210.

134. Missiuna, C. (1994). Motor skill acquisition in children with developmental coordination disorder. *Adapted Physical Activity Quarterly, 11,* 214–235.

135. Missiuna, C. (2002). Poor handwriting is only a symptom: Children with developmental coordination disorder. *OT Now (Consumer Special Issue),* Sept/Oct, 4–6.

136. Missiuna, C. (2003). *Children with developmental coordination disorder: At home and in the classroom (booklet).* McMaster University, ON: CanChild (Online). Retrieved from www.canchild.ca.

137. Missiuna, C., Gaines, B. R., & Pollock, N. (2002). Recognizing and referring children at risk for developmental coordination disorder: Role of the speech-language pathologist. *Journal of Speech-Language Pathology & Audiology, 26,* 172–179.

138. Missiuna, C., Gaines, R., & Soucie, H. (2006). Why every office needs a tennis ball: A new approach to assessing the clumsy child. *Canadian Medical Association Journal, 175,* 471–473.

139. Missiuna, C. & Mandich, A. (2002). Integrating motor learning theories into practice. In S. Cermak & D. Larkin (Eds.), *Developmental coordination disorder* (pp. 221–233). Albany, NY: Delmar.

140. Missiuna, C., Mandich, A. D., Polatajko, H. J., & Malloy-Miller, T. (2001). Cognitive orientation to daily occupational performance (CO-OP): Part I—Theoretical foundations. *Physical Occupational Therapy in Pediatrics, 20,* 69–81.

141. Missiuna, C., Moll, S., King, S., King, G., & Law, M. (2007). A trajectory of troubles: Parents' impressions of the impact of developmental coordination disorder. *Physical and Occupational Therapy in Pediatrics, 27,* 81–101.

142. Missiuna, C., Moll, S., Law, M., King, S., & King, G. (2006). Mysteries and mazes: Parents' experiences of children with developmental coordination disorder. *Canadian Journal of Occupational Therapy, 73,* 7–17.

143. Missiuna, C., & Polatajko, H. (1995). Developmental dyspraxia by any other name: Are they all just clumsy children? *American Journal of Occupational Therapy, 49,* 619–627.

144. Missiuna, C., & Pollock, N. (1995). Beyond the norms: Need for multiple sources of data in the assessment of children. *Physical & Occupational Therapy in Pediatrics, 15,* 57–71.

145. Missiuna, C., & Pollock, N. (2000). Perceived efficacy and goal setting in young children. *Canadian Journal of Occupational Therapy, 67,* 101–109.

146. Missiuna, C., Pollock, N., Egan, M., DeLaat, D., Gaines, R., & Soucie, H. (2008). Enabling occupation through facilitating the diagnosis of developmental coordination disorder. *Canadian Journal of Occupational Therapy, 75,* 26–34.

147. Missiuna, C., Pollock, N., & Law, M. (2004). *Perceived efficacy and goal setting system (PEGS).* San Antonio, TX: Psychological Corporation.

148. Missiuna, C., Pollock, N., Law, M., Walter, S., & Cavey, N. (2006). Examination of the perceived efficacy and goal setting system (PEGS) with children with disabilities, their parents, and teachers. *American Journal of Occupational Therapy, 60,* 204–214.

149. Missiuna, C., Rivard, L., & Bartlett, D. (2003). Early identification and risk management of children with developmental coordination disorder. *Pediatric Physical Therapy, 15,* 32–38.

150. Missiuna, C., Rivard, L., & Pollock, N. (2004). They're bright but can't write: Developmental coordination disorder in school aged children. *Teaching Exceptional Children Plus, 1,* Article 3.

151. Miyahara, M. (1994). Subtypes of students with learning disabilities based upon gross motor functions. *Adapted Physical Activity Quarterly, 11,* 368–382.

152. Miyahara, M. (1996). A meta-analysis of intervention studies on children with developmental coordination disorder. *Corpus, Psyche et Societas, 3,* 11–18.

153. Mon-Williams, M. A., Wann, J. P., & Pascal, E. (1999). Visual-proprioceptive mapping in children with developmental coordination disorder. *Developmental Medicine and Child Neurology, 41*, 247–254.

154. Murphy, J., & Gliner, J. (1988). Visual and motor sequencing in normal and clumsy children. *Occupational Therapy Journal, 8*, 89–103.

155. Njiokiktjien, C. (1988). Developmental dyspraxia. In C. Njiokiktjien (Ed.), *Pediatric behavioural neurology: Volume 1—Clinical principles* (pp. 266–228). Amsterdam: Suyi Publishers.

156. O'Beirne, C., Larkin, D., & Cable, T. (1994). Coordination problems and anaerobic performance in children. *Adapted Physical Activity Quarterly, 11*, 141–149.

157. O'Brien, V., Cermak, S., & Murray, E. (1988). The relationship between visual-perceptual motor abilities and clumsiness in children with and without learning disabilities. *American Journal of Occupational Therapy, 42*, 359–363.

158. O'Hare, A., & Khalid, S. (2002). The association of abnormal cerebellar function in children with developmental coordination disorder and reading difficulties. *Dyslexia, 8*, 234–248.

159. Pangelinan, M., Hatfield, B. & Clark, J. (2009, June). *Differences in electro-cortical activity during movement planning in children with DCD.* Paper presented at the DCD VIII Developmental Coordination Disorder International Conference, Baltimore, MD.

160. Parush, S., Levanon-Erez, N., & Weintraub, N. (1998). Ergonomic factors influencing handwriting performance. *Work, 11*, 295–305.

161. Parush, S., Pindak, V., Hahn-Markowitz, J., & Mazor-Karsenty, T. (1998). Does fatigue influence children's handwriting performance? *Work, 11*, 307–313.

162. Peters, J. M., Henderson, S. E., & Dookun, D. (2004). Provision for children with developmental co-ordination disorder (DCD): Audit of the service provider. *Child: Care, Health & Development, 30*, 463–479.

163. Piek, J. P., Barrett, N. C., Allen, L. S., Jones, A., & Louise, M. (2005). The relationship between bullying and self-worth in children with movement coordination problems. *British Journal of Educational Psychology, 75*, 453–463.

164. Piek, J. P., Bradbury, G. S., Elsley, S. C., & Tate, L. (2008). Motor coordination and social–emotional behaviour in preschool-aged children. *International Journal of Disability, Development and Education, 55*, 143–151.

165. Piek, J. P., Dworcan, M., Barrett, N., & Coleman, R. (2000). Determinants of self-worth in children with and without developmental coordination disorder. *The International Journal of Disability Development and Education, 47*, 259–271.

166. Piek, J. P., & Dyck, M. J. (2004). Sensory-motor deficits in children with developmental coordination disorder, attention deficit hyperactivity disorder and autistic disorder. *Human Movement Science, 23*, 475–488.

167. Piek, J. P., & Edwards, K. (1997). The identification of children with developmental coordination disorder by class and physical education teachers. *British Journal of Educational Psychology, 67*, 55–67.

168. Pitcher, T. M., Piek, J. P., & Hay, D. A. (2003). Fine and gross motor ability in males with ADHD. *Developmental Medicine and Child Neurology, 45*, 525–535.

169. Pless, M., & Carlsson, M. (2000). Effects of motor skill intervention on developmental coordination disorder: A meta-analysis. *Adapted Physical Activity Quarterly, 17*, 381–401.

170. Pless, M., Carlsson, M., Sundelin, C., & Persson, K. (2002). Preschool children with developmental coordination disorder: A short-term follow-up of motor status at seven to eight years of age. *Acta Paediatrica, 91*, 521–528.

171. Polatajko, H. (1999). Developmental coordination disorder (DCD): Alias the clumsy child syndrome. In K. Whitmore, H. Hart, & G. Willems (Eds.), *A neurodevelopmental approach to specific learning disorders* (pp. 119–133). London: Mac Keith Press.

172. Polatajko, H., & Cantin, N. (2005). Attending to children with developmental coordination disorder: The approaches and the evidence. *The Israel Journal of Occupational Therapy, 14*, E117–E150.

173. Polatajko, H. J., & Cantin, N. (2006). Developmental coordination disorder (dyspraxia): An overview of the state of the art. *Seminars in Pediatric Neurology, 12*, 250–258.

174. Polatajko, H., Fox, M., & Missiuna, C. (1995). An international consensus on children with developmental coordination disorder. *Canadian Journal of Occupational Therapy, 62*, 3–6.

175. Polatajko, H. J., Mandich, A. D., Miller, L. T., & MacNab, J. J. (2001). Cognitive orientation to daily occupational performance (CO-OP): Part II—The evidence. *Physical and Occupational Therapy in Pediatrics, 20*, 83–106.

176. Polatajko, H. J., Mandich, A. D., Missiuna, C., Miller, L. T., MacNab, J. J., Malloy-Miller, T., et al. (2001). Cognitive orientation to daily occupational performance (CO-OP): Part III—The protocol in brief. *Physical & Occupational Therapy in Pediatrics, 20*, 107–123.

177. Poulsen, A. A., & Ziviani, J. M. (2004). Can I play too? Physical activity engagement of children with developmental coordination disorders. *Canadian Journal of Occupational Therapy, 71*, 100–107.

178. Poulsen, A. A., Ziviani, J. M., & Cuskelly, M. (2006). General self-concept and life satisfaction for boys with differing levels of physical coordination: The role of goal orientations and leisure participation. *Human Movement Science, 25*, 839–860.

179. Poulsen, A. A., Ziviani, J. M., & Cuskelly, M. (2008). Leisure time physical activity energy expenditure in boys with developmental coordination disorder: The role of peer relations self-concept perceptions. *Occupation, Participation and Health, 28*, 30.

180. Poulsen, A. A., Ziviani, J. M., Cuskelly, M., & Smith, R. (2007). Boys with developmental coordination disorder: Loneliness and team sports participation. *The American Journal of Occupational Therapy, 61,* 451–462.

181. Rasmussen, P., & Gillberg, C. (2000). Natural outcome of ADHD with developmental coordination disorder at age 22 years: A controlled, longitudinal, community-based study. *Journal of the American Academy of Child and Adolescent Psychiatry, 39,* 1424–1431.

182. Raynor, A. J. (1998). Fractional reflex and reaction time in children with developmental coordination disorder. *Motor Control, 2,* 114–124.

183. Raynor, A. J. (2001). Strength, power and co-activation in children with developmental coordination disorder. *Developmental Medicine and Child Neurology, 43,* 676–684.

184. Reid, D. (1987). Occupational therapists' assessment practices with handicapped children in *Ontario. Canadian Journal of Occupational Therapy, 54,* 181–188.

185. Revie, G., & Larkin, D. (1993). Task specific intervention for children with developmental coordination disorder: A systems view. *Adapted Physical Activity Quarterly, 10,* 29–41.

186. Rivard, L., & Missiuna, C. (2004). Encouraging participation in physical activities for children with developmental coordination disorder. Retrieved June 30, 2009, from http://dcd.canchild.ca/en/EducationalMaterials/community.asp

187. Rivard, L.M., Missiuna, C., Hanna, S., & Wishart, L. (2007). Understanding teachers' perceptions of the motor difficulties of children with developmental coordination disorder (DCD). *British Journal of Educational Psychology, 77,* 633–648.

188. Rizzolatti, G., Fogassi, L., & Gallese, V. (2006). Mirrors of the mind. *Scientific American, 295,* 54–61.

189. Rodger, S., & Mandich, A. (2005). Getting the run around: Accessing services for children with developmental co-ordination disorder. *Child: Care, Health and Development, 31,* 449–457.

190. Rogers, M., Fay, T. B., Whitfield, M. F., Tomlinson, J., & Grunau, R. E. (2005). Aerobic capacity, strength, flexibility, and activity level in unimpaired extremely low birth weight ($\leq$800 g) survivors at 17 years of age compared with term-born control subjects. *Pediatrics, 116.*

191. Rosblad B. (2002). Visual perception in children with developmental coordination disorder. In S. Cermak & D. Larkin, (Eds.), *Developmental coordination disorder* (pp. 104–116). Albany, NY: Delmar Thomson Learning.

192. Rosblad, B., & Gard, L. (1998). The assessment of children with developmental coordination disorders in Sweden: A preliminary investigation of the suitability of the Movement ABC. *Human Movement Science, 17,* 711–719.

193. Rosblad, B., & von Hofsten, C. (1994). Repetitive goal-directed arm movements in children with developmental coordination disorder: Role of visual information. *Adapted Physical Activity Quarterly, 11,* 190–202.

194. Rose, B., Larkin, D., & Berger, B. G. (1997). Coordination and gender influences on the perceived competence of children. *Adapted Physical Activity Quarterly, 12,* 210–221.

195. Rose, E., & Larkin, D. (2002). Perceived competence, discrepancy scores, and global self-worth. *Adapted Physical Activity Quarterly, 19,* 127–140.

196. Rosenblum, S. (2006). The development and standardization of the Children Activity Scales (ChAS-P/T) for the early identification of children with developmental coordination disorders. *Child: Care, Health and Development, 32,* 619–632.

197. Rosengren, K. S., Deconinck, F. J., Diberardino, L. A. 3rd, Polk, J. D., Spencer-Smith, J., De Clercq, D., et al. (2009). Differences in gait complexity and variability between children with and without developmental coordination disorder. *Gait & Posture, 29,* 225–229.

198. Sanger, T. D., Chen, D., Delgado, M. R., Gaebler-Spira, D., Hallett, M., Mink, J. W., et al. (2006). Definition and classification of negative motor signs in childhood. *Pediatrics, 118,* 2159–2167.

199. Sangster, C. A., Beninger, C., Polatajko, H. J., & Mandich, A. (2005). Cognitive strategy generation in children with developmental coordination disorder. *Canadian Journal of Occupational Therapy, 72,* 67–77.

200. Saywell, N., & Taylor, D. (2008). The role of the cerebellum in procedural learning—Are there implications for physiotherapists' clinical practice? *Physiotherapy Theory and Practice, 24,* 321–328.

201. Schoemaker, M. M. (2003). *Manual of the motor observation questionnaire for teachers.* Groningen: Internal Publication, Center for Human Movement Sciences (Dutch).

202. Schoemaker, M. M., Flapper, B. C., Reinders-Messelink, H. A., & de Kloet, A. (2008). Validity of the motor observation questionnaire for teachers as a screening instrument for children at risk for developmental coordination disorder. *Human Movement Science, 27,* 190–199.

203. Schoemaker, M. M., Flapper, B., Verheij, N. P., Wilson, B. N., Reinders-Messelink, H. A., & de Kloet, A. (2006). Evaluation of the developmental coordination disorder questionnaire as a screening instrument. *Developmental Medicine & Child Neurology, 48,* 668–673.

204. Schoemaker, M. M. & Kalverboer, A. (1994). Social and affective problems of children who are clumsy: How early do they begin. *Adapted Physical Activity Quarterly, 11,* 130–140.

205. Schoemaker, M. M., Niemeijer, A. S., Reynders, K., Smits-Engelsman, B. C. (2003). Effectiveness of neuromotor task training for children with developmental coordination disorder: A pilot study. *Neural Plasticity, 10,* 155–163.

206. Schoemaker, M. M., Smits-Engelsman, B. C., & Jongmans, M. J. (2003). Psychometric properties of the M-ABC checklist as a screening instrument for children with a developmental co-ordination disorder. *British Journal of Educational Psychology, 73,* 425–441.

207. Schott, N., Alof, V., Hultsch, D., & Meermann, D. (2007). Physical fitness in children with developmental coordination disorder. *Research Quarterly for Exercise & Sport, 78,* 438–450.

208. Segal, R., Mandich, A., Polatajko, H., & Cook, J. V. (2002). Stigma and its management: A pilot study of parental perceptions of the experiences of children with developmental coordination disorder. *American Journal of Occupational Therapy, 56,* 422–428.

209. Sellers, J. S. (1995). Clumsiness: Review of causes, treatments and outlook. *Physical & Occupational Therapy in Pediatrics, 15,* 39–55.

210. Sigmundsson, H., Hansen, P. C., & Talcott, J. B. (2003). Do 'clumsy' children have visual deficits. *Behavioural Brain Research, 139,* 123–129.

211. Sigmundsson, H., Pedersen, A. V., Whiting, H. T., & Ingvaldsen, R. P. (1998). We can cure your child's clumsiness! A review of intervention methods. *Scandinavian Journal of Rehabilitation Medicine, 30,* 101–106.

212. Skinner, R. A. & Piek, J. P. (2001). Psychosocial implications of poor motor coordination in children and adolescents. *Human Movement Science, 20,* 73–94.

213. Skorji, V., & McKenzie, B. (1997). How do children who are clumsy remember modelled movements? *Developmental Medicine and Child Neurology, 39,* 404–408.

214. Smits-Engelsman, B. C. M., Henderson, S. E., & Michels, C. G. J. (1998). The assessment of children with developmental coordination disorder in the Netherlands: Relationship between the Movement Assessment Battery for children and the Korperkoordinations Test Fur Kinder. *Human Movement Science, 17,* 699–709.

215. Smits-Engelsman, B. C. M., Niemeijer, A. & Van Waelvelde, H. (2009, June). *Reliability of the outcomes of the Movement Assessment Battery for Children, second edition (MABC-2): Are 3-year-old children ready for formal testing?* Paper presented at the DCD VIII Developmental Coordination Disorder International Conference, Baltimore, MD.

216. Smits-Engelsman, B. C. M., Wilson, P. H., Westenberg, Y., & Duysens, J. (2003). Fine motor deficiencies in children with developmental coordination disorder and learning disabilities: An underlying open-loop control deficit. *Human Movement Science, 22,* 495–513.

217. Smyth, M. M. & Anderson, H. I. (2000). Coping with clumsiness in the school playground: Social and physical play in children with coordination impairments. *British Journal of Developmental Psychology, 18,* 389–413.

218. Smyth, M. M., Anderson, H. I., & Churchill, A. (2001). Visual information and the control of reaching in children: A comparison between children with and without development coordination disorder. *Journal of Motor Behavior, 33,* 306–320.

219. Smyth, M. M., & Mason, U. C. (1997). Planning and execution of action in children with and without developmental coordination disorder. *Journal of Child Psychology and Psychiatry, 38,* 1023–1037.

220. Smyth, T. R. (1991). Abnormal clumsiness in children: A defect of motor programming? *Child: Care, Health and Development, 17,* 283–294.

221. Smyth, T. R. (1994). Clumsiness in children: A defect of kinaesthetic perception? *Child: Care, Health & Development, 20,* 27–36.

222. Sparrow, S. S., Cicchetti, D. V., & Balla, D. A. (2005). *Vineland adaptive behavior scales* (2nd ed.). Circle Pines, MN: American Guidance Service.

223. Stephenson, E., McKay, C., & Chesson, R. (1991). The identification and treatment of motor/learning difficulties: parents' perceptions and the role of the therapist. *Child: Care, Health and Development, 17,* 91–113.

224. Sugden, D. A., & Chambers, M. E. (1998). Intervention approaches and children with developmental coordination disorder. *Pediatric Rehabilitation, 2,* 139–147.

225. Sugden, D. A., Chambers, M., & Utley, A. (2006). Leeds consensus statement 2006. Retrieved July 28, 2009, from www.dcd-uk.org/consensus.html

226. Sugden, D. A., & Sugden, L. (1990). *The assessment and management of movement skill problems.* Leeds: School of Education.

227. Sugden, D. A., & Wright, H. C. (1998). *Motor coordination disorders in children.* Thousand Oaks, California: Sage Publication, Inc.

228. Summers, J., Larkin, D., & Dewey, D. (2008). Activities of daily living in children with developmental coordination disorder: Dressing, personal hygiene, and eating skills. *Human Movement Science, 27,* 215–229.

229. Tan, S. K., Parker, H. E., & Larkin, D. (2001). Concurrent validity of motor tests used to identify children with motor impairment. *Adapted Physical Activity Quarterly, 18,* 168–182.

230. Tervo, R. C., Azuma, S., Fogas, B., & Fiechtner, H. (2002). Children with ADHD and motor dysfunction compared with children with ADHD only. *Developmental Medicine and Child Neurology, 44,* 383–390.

231. Thelen, E. (1995). Motor development: A new synthesis. *American Psychologist, 50,* 79–95.

232. van der Meulen, J. H., Denier van der Gon, J. J., Gielen, C. C., Gooskens, R. H. J. M., & Willemse, J. (1991). Visuomotor performance of normal and clumsy children: Fast goal-directed arm movements with and without visual feedback. *Developmental Medicine & Child Neurology, 33,* 40–54.

233. van der Meulen, J. H., Denier van der Gon, J. J., Gielen, C. C., Gooskens, R. H. J. M., & Willemse, J. (1991). Visuomotor performance of normal and clumsy children: Arm-tracking with and without visual feedback. *Developmental Medicine & Child Neurology, 33,* 118–129.

234. van Waelvelde, H., Peersman, W., Debrabant, J., & Smits-Engelsman, B. C. M. (2009, June). *Factor analytical validation of the Movement Assessment Battery for Children—Second edition.* Paper presented at the DCD VIII Developmental

Coordination Disorder International Conference, Baltimore, MD.

235. Visser, J. (2003). Developmental coordination disorder: A review of research on subtypes and comorbidities. *Human Movement Science, 22,* 479–493.

236. Volman, M., & Geuze, R. H. (1998). Relative phase stability of bimanual and visuomanual rhythmic coordination patterns in children with a developmental coordination disorder. *Human Movement Science, 17,* 541–572.

237. Wall, A. E. (1982). Physically awkward children: A motor development perspective. In J. P. Das, R. F. Mulcahy, & A. E. Wall (Eds.), *Theory and research in learning disabilities* (pp. 253–284). New York: Plenum Press.

238. Wall, A. E., Reid, G., Paton, J. (1990). The syndrome of physical awkwardness. In G. Reid (Ed.), *Problems in movement control* (pp. 284–316). Amsterdam: Elsevier Science.

239. Wann, J. P., Mon-Williams, M., & Rushton, K. (1998). Postural control and coordination disorders: The swinging room revisited. *Human Movement Science, 17,* 491–513.

240. Ward, A., & Rodger, S. (2004). The application of cognitive orientation to daily occupation performance (CO-OP) with children 5–7 years with developmental coordination disorder. *British Journal of Occupational Therapy, 67,* 256–264.

241. Watkinson, E. J., Causgrove Dunn, J., Cavaliere, N., Calzonetti, K., Wilhelm, L., & Dwyer, S. (2001). Engagement in playground activities as a criterion for diagnosing developmental coordination disorder. *Adapted Physical Activity Quarterly, 18,* 18–34.

242. Watter, P. (1996). Physiotherapy management—Minor coordination dysfunction. In Y. R. Burns & J. MacDonald (Eds.), *Physiotherapy and the growing child* (pp. 415–432). Toronto, Canada: W. B. Saunders.

243. Watter, P., Rodger, S., Marinac, J., Woodyatt, G., Ziviani, J., & Ozanne, A. (2008). Multidisciplinary assessment of children with developmental coordination disorder: Using the ICF framework to inform assessment. *Physical & Occupational Therapy in Pediatrics, 28,* 331–352.

244. Webster, R. I., Majnemer, A., Platt, R. W., & Shevell, M. I. (2005). Motor function at school age in children with a preschool diagnosis of developmental language impairment. *Journal of Pediatrics, 146,* 80–85.

245. Whitall, J., Chang, T-Y., Horn, C. L., Jung-Potter, J., McMenamin, S., Wilms-Floet, A., et al. (2008). Auditory-motor coupling of bilateral finger tapping in children with and without DCD compared to adults. *Human Movement Science, 27,* 914–931.

246. Wiart, L. & Darrah, J. (2001). Review of four tests of gross motor development. *Developmental Medicine and Child Neurology, 43,* 279–285.

247. Williams, H. (2002). Motor control in children with developmental coordination disorder. In S. Cermak & D. Larkin (Eds.), *Developmental coordination disorder* (pp. 117–137). Albany, NY: Delmar.

248. Williams, H. G., Fisher, J. M., & Tritschler, K. A. (1983). Descriptive analysis of static postural control in 4, 6, and 8 year old normal and motorically awkward children. *American Journal of Physical Medicine, 62,* 12–26.

249. Williams, H., & Woollacott, M. (1997). Characteristics of neuromuscular responses underlying postural control in clumsy children. *Motor Development: Research and Reviews, 1,* 8–23.

250. Williams, H. G., Woollacott, M. H., & Ivry, R. (1992). Timing and motor control in clumsy children. *Journal of Motor Behavior, 24,* 165–172.

251. Williams, J., Anderson, P., & Lee, K. (2009, June). *The prevalence of DCD in children born preterm: A systematic review.* Paper presented at the DCD VIII Developmental Coordination Disorder International Conference, Baltimore, MD.

252. Willoughby, C., & Polatajko, H. J. (1995). Motor problems in children with developmental coordination disorder: Review of the literature. *American Journal of Occupational Therapy, 49,* 787–794.

253. Wilson, B. N., Crawford, S. G., Green, D., Roberts, G., Aylott, A., & Kaplan, B. J. (2009). Psychometric properties of the revised Developmental Coordination Disorder Questionnaire. *Physical & Occupational Therapy in Pediatrics, 29,* 184.

254. Wilson, B. N., Kaplan, B. J., Crawford, S. G., Campbell, A., & Dewey, D. (2000). Reliability and validity of a parent questionnaire on childhood motor skills. *The American Journal of Occupational Therapy, 54,* 484–493.

255. Wilson, P. H., Maruff, P., Butson, M., Williams, J., Lum, J., & Thomas, P. R. (2004). Internal representation of movement in children with developmental coordination disorder: A mental rotation task. *Developmental Medicine and Child Neurology, 46,* 754–759.

256. Wilson, P. H., Maruff, P., Ives, S., & Currie, J. (2001). Abnormalities of motor and praxis imagery in children with DCD. *Human Movement Science, 20,* 135–159.

257. Wilson, P. H., & McKenzie, B. E. (1998). Information processing deficits associated with developmental coordination disorder: A meta-analysis of research findings. *Journal of Child Psychology and Psychiatry, 39,* 829–840.

258. Wilson, P. H., Thomas, P. R., & Maruff, P. (2002). Motor imagery training ameliorates motor clumsiness in children. *Journal of Child Neurology, 17,* 491–498.

259. Wocadlo, C., & Rieger, I. (2008). Motor impairment and low achievement in very preterm children at eight years of age. *Early Human Development, 84,* 769–776.

260. World Health Organization. (2001). *The international classification of functioning, disability and health (ICF).* Geneva: World Health Organization.

261. Wright, H. C., & Sugden, D. A. (1996). A two-step procedure for the identification of children with developmental co-ordination disorder in Singapore. *Developmental Medicine and Child Neurology, 38,* 1099–1105.

262. Wynn, K. (2003). *Exploring the participation of children with disabilities in school.* Unpublished master's thesis, McMaster University, Hamilton, Ontario, Canada.

263. Zaichkowsky, L. D., & Fuchs, C. Z. (1986). *The psychology of motor behavior: Development, control and learning.* Ithaca, NY: Movement Publications.

264. Zoia, S., Castiello, U., Blason, L., & Scabar, A. (2005). Reaching in children with and without developmental coordination disorder under normal and perturbed vision. *Developmental Neuropsychology, 27,* 257–273.

265. Zwicker, J. G., Missiuna, C., & Boyd, L. A. (2009). Neural correlates of developmental coordination disorder: A review of hypotheses. *Journal of Child Neurology, 24,* 1273–1281.

266. Zwicker, J. G., Missiuna, C., Harris, S. R., & Boyd, L. A. (2009, June). *Motor learning of children with developmental coordination disorder: An fMRI study.* Paper presented at the DCD VIII Developmental Coordination Disorder International Conference, Baltimore, MD.

17 Children With Motor and Intellectual Disabilities

IRENE R. MCEWEN, PT, DPT, PhD, FAPTA • MARY J. MEISER, PT, MS • LAURA H. HANSEN, PT, MS

Children with intellectual disabilities often have secondary or associated delays in motor development and may have problems with motor learning and motor control. This is especially true of children whose intellectual functioning is moderately or severely limited. Some children's motor problems are minimal, requiring little, if any, physical therapy. Other children have cerebral palsy and other neurologic, musculoskeletal, and cardiopulmonary impairments that require considerable attention by physical therapists and other members of service delivery teams.

Many of the physical therapy examination and intervention methods used with children who have intellectual disabilities differ little from approaches used with any child who has similar motor characteristics, as described in other chapters of this volume. The learning characteristics of children with intellectual disabilities, however, can make it necessary to modify or supplement these approaches. These aspects of examination and intervention, along with current evidence-based and "best" practices for children with intellectual disabilities, are the foci of this chapter. This chapter will cover the definition, incidence, prevalence, origin, pathophysiology, and prevention of intellectual disabilities in children; team assessment; determining goals; interventions to reduce impairments and activity limitations, prevent secondary complications, and promote participation; and considerations for transition to adulthood. The chapter ends with three case examples that illustrate the chapter content. One case also illustrates application of the *Guide to Physical Therapist Practice*.[4]

DEFINITION OF INTELLECTUAL DISABILITIES

The definition of intellectual disabilities and the means by which children are identified as having intellectual disabilities are, and have been, highly controversial.[138] Much of the controversy surrounds the risk of inappropriately classifying children of cultural and linguistic minorities as having intellectual disabilities. The validity of this concern is supported by overrepresentation of children from cultural and linguistic minorities among children who have been identified as having intellectual disabilities and children placed in special education.[114,178]

Children with motor and sensory impairments also are at risk for being identified as having intellectual limitations when they do not, or for being classified as having a greater degree of intellectual disability than actually exists.[29] This is especially true if an examiner uses tests that require motor and spoken responses or has neither experience nor skill in examining children who require alternative input modes, such as manual signs, or alternative response modes, such as a communication board.

In the United States, organizations and educational and social service agencies often use the term *mental retardation* to refer to the condition of people whose intellectual disabilities were acquired before age 18. The term *intellectual disability*, however, is being used increasingly instead, for instance, by the American Association on Intellectual and Developmental Disabilities (AAIDD), formerly known as the American Association on Mental Retardation (AAMR).[138] Regardless of the term used, the definition has evolved over the years from a primary emphasis on intelligence test scores to an emphasis on individual functioning within natural environments. AAMR has proposed the most widely accepted definitions, which have served as a basis for many other definitions, including those used by school districts for placement of students in special education.[3]

In 2002, the AAMR board of directors adopted a definition of *mental retardation* (the term used in 2002) that was intended to help change the way people with intellectual disabilities are viewed. This definition is based on the supports people need within their own environments, rather than on an intelligence quotient (IQ)-derived level of intellectual functioning, and incorporates the dimension of participation:

> Mental retardation is a disability characterized by significant limitations both in intellectual functioning and in adaptive behavior as expressed in conceptual, social, and practical adaptive skills. This disability originates before age 18. The following five assumptions are essential to the application of this definition: (1) limitations in present functioning must be considered within the context of community environments typical of the individual's age, peers, and culture; (2) valid assessment considers cultural and linguistic diversity as

well as differences in communication, sensory, motor, and behavioral factors; (3) within an individual, limitations often coexist with strengths; (4) an important purpose of describing limitations is to develop a profile of needed supports; (5) with appropriate personalized supports over a sustained period, the life functioning of the person with mental retardation generally will improve[3] (p. 1).

Although an IQ of 70 to 75 or below still is required for a diagnosis of intellectual disability, the definition also includes adaptive skills, participation, interactions and social roles, health, and context consistent with the International Classification of Function, Disability, and Health (ICF).[173] The 2002 definition emphasizes identification of the changing supports one needs over a lifetime to live successfully in the community, rather than simply on classification of the individual. Children identified as having intellectual disability who require supports to learn in school settings, for example, may not be labeled in adulthood when participating independently in home, work, and social roles.[3] AAIDD plans to publish a new edition of the definition, classification, and supports manual in 2011.[1]

Other definitions of intellectual disability or mental retardation have coexisted with the AAMR definition, including those used in the United States to qualify students for special education and for services for individuals with developmental disabilities. In the United States, Public Law 98-527, the Developmental Disabilities Act of 1984, authorized states to provide habilitation, medical, and social services for children and adults with intellectual disabilities and, in some states, for people with other disabilities. The term *developmental disabilities* was defined in the most recent version of the Developmental Disabilities Assistance and Bill of Rights Act of 2000 (Public Law 106-402) as "a severe, chronic disability that is attributable to a physical or mental disability that is likely to continue throughout the person's life and results in functional limitations in three or more areas of life activities" (Sec. 102[8][A]). The only important difference between this definition and the AAMR definition of mental retardation is that the definition of developmental disability has no IQ requirement and the age of onset can be as high as 22 years.[3]

Because of varying definitions of intellectual disability or mental retardation and eligibility criteria, confusion can exist both within and between states as to who is considered to have intellectual disability and who qualifies for which services. For this reason, physical therapists often need to seek information about programs in their own areas to determine the criteria for eligibility and who is qualified to classify a child as having an intellectual disability. Some programs provide wheelchairs, orthoses, and other equipment for children with intellectual disabilities; other programs pay for services, such as physical therapy, respite care, and recreational activities.

For any child, a label of intellectual disability primarily is useful as a "passport" to early intervention, special education, and other educational, social, and medical programs. Such a label provides little, if any, insight into the strengths of the individual or the services that are needed[3] and may limit a child's opportunities if the label causes others to have inappropriate or inadequate expectations of the child's capabilities.

INCIDENCE AND PREVALENCE OF INTELLECTUAL DISABILITIES

Reported estimates of the incidence and prevalence of intellectual disabilities vary widely. These differences are thought to be due to a number of factors, including variations in the definition; the methods employed; the sex, age, and communities of the samples; and the sociopolitical factors affecting the design and interpretation of the studies.[82] Larson and colleagues[82] used data from the 1994 and 1995 Disability Supplement of the National Health Interview Survey to estimate the prevalence of intellectual disabilities and developmental disabilities among community-dwelling people in the United States. They estimated the prevalence of mental retardation to be 7.8 per 1000 people and the prevalence of developmental disability to be 11.3 per 1000 people. The combined prevalence of intellectual disabilities and/or developmental disabilities was 14.9 per 1000 people. Others have criticized the study because data were collected using a telephone survey, and respondents may have underreported disability.[159] School districts reported approximately twice as many school-age children classified as having mental retardation (one of the 13 categories of disability under the Individuals with Disabilities Education Act) as were identified by the telephone survey.[159] The U.S. Department of Education report theorized that cultural differences in the concept of disability might be the reason for some of the discrepancies. People with intellectual disabilities may also function independently in home settings, where they are familiar with routines and expectations, yet require support for more challenging environments such as school and work. A study of the incidence of intellectual disability among a birth cohort of children in Minnesota found a rate of children with intellectual disability similar to that reported by the U.S. Department of Education Report.[64] Using IQ scores from school records as the only criterion, these authors found the cumulative incidence of intellectual disability (IQ < 70) by age 8 to be 9.1 per 1000 children. The prevalence of children with severe intellectual disability, defined as an IQ score of 50 or below, was 4.9 per 1000 children in this study, and the prevalence of children with mild mental intellectual disability, defined as an IQ of 51 to 70, was 4.3 per 1000 children. Of 6.1 million school-age children receiving special education and related services, 9.3% have been identified for reporting purposes as having mental retardation, 2.2% as having multiple disabilities, and 2.7% as having autism.[160] About 70% of people with autism spectrum disorders have intellectual disabilities,[51] and children with chromosomal or other birth defects, regardless of the type, are 27 times more likely to have intellectual disabilities than children without birth defects.[68]

ORIGIN AND PATHOPHYSIOLOGY OF INTELLECTUAL DISABILITIES

Multiple causes of intellectual disabilities exist, many of which have been identified and many of which have not. Shevell[140] reviewed retrospective and prospective studies and concluded that causes could be identified for approximately 50% of intellectual disabilities in children. Understanding the origin of a child's intellectual disability may assist physical therapists and others to better predict current or future needs for support and life planning, and to identify other health-related problems that might be associated with a given diagnosis.[3]

More than 350 causes for intellectual disabilities have been identified that can be broadly categorized into prenatal, perinatal, and postnatal causes. Prenatal causes have been further classified as chromosomal disorders, genetic syndromes, inborn errors of metabolism, developmental disorders of brain formation, and environmental influences (for more information, see the Genomics and Genetic Syndromes Affecting Movement chapter on the Evolve website). Perinatal causes include intrauterine disorders and neonatal disorders. One meta-analysis of 15 studies that examined intellectual outcomes of children born prematurely provides evidence that prematurity alone may be associated with reduced scores on intellectual tests.[14] Pooled data demonstrated that test scores of children born at full gestation were significantly higher than scores of children born prematurely. Classifications of postnatal causes of intellectual disability include head injuries, infections, demyelinating disorders, degenerative disorders, seizure disorders, toxic-metabolic disorders, malnutrition, environmental deprivation, and hypoconnection syndrome.[3]

Movement dysfunction is more often associated with some causes than with others, and in general, children with more severe intellectual disabilities are likely to have more severe motor delays and disabilities.[5,31] Years ago, Ellis[43] proposed that the relatively poor motor performance of people with intellectual disabilities is the result of their limited capacity to process information and the rapid decay of that information over time. Others have supported this notion,[5] proposing that intellectual deficits impede motor learning, leading to the slow and clumsy movements that children with intellectual disabilities often have, even when they do not have cerebral palsy or another movement-related diagnosis. Many children also have associated problems, such as vision and hearing disabilities, cerebral palsy, low levels of arousal, seizure disorders, cardiopulmonary dysfunction, and various other medical problems that can further negatively influence motor development, motor learning, and motor performance.

PREVENTION

Some forms of intellectual disability and associated disorders can now be prevented, such as those resulting from phenylketonuria, rubella, and lead poisoning. In addition, amniocentesis, ultrasound, and other techniques have enabled prenatal diagnosis of many conditions, which may help decrease morbidity, such as delivery of a child with myelodysplasia by cesarean section. Genetic counseling also can be offered.

Although the factors known to cause intellectual disabilities may be present in a given child, complex and powerful interactions between those factors and later environmental events can alter the actuality or the severity of intellectual limitations and associated impairments. In a review of research and theories on the development of intelligence, DiLalla[37] suggested that about half of a person's IQ may be influenced by environmental factors. Some infants, for example, who have severe medical problems during the postnatal course, with documented neuroanatomic pathology during this period, have few if any sequelae. On the other hand, children with no known pathology but who experience one or more environmental risk factors may eventually be classified as having intellectual disability. Two of the most common environmental causes of intellectual disability are early severe psychosocial deprivation and antenatal exposure to toxins, such as drugs or alcohol.[140]

In the United States, the family-centered services directed by Part C of the Individuals With Disabilities Education Act (IDEA), described in Chapters 29 and 30 of this volume, reflect a belief in the power of early social and physical environments to influence a child's development. Part C regulations also imply confidence in the capability of physical therapists and other service providers to assist families in providing environments that both help to prevent unnecessary disability and promote the achievement of a child's potential.

PRIMARY IMPAIRMENT

The time at which impairments in intellectual functioning and movement become recognized varies widely, both within and between medical diagnoses. In some cases, prenatal or neonatal diagnosis can predict disabilities that may not yet be apparent, such as with children with Down syndrome or myelodysplasia. In other cases, a medical diagnosis will not be made until after impaired functioning is noted, perhaps not until months or years after birth.

DIAGNOSIS/PROBLEM IDENTIFICATION

Delay in achievement of developmental motor milestones or abnormal motor behaviors may be an early indication of intellectual disability that was present prenatally or perinatally. This is particularly true for children with severe intellectual disabilities.[170] Some children, such as those with Rett syndrome or Tay-Sachs disease, will appear to develop normally for a period of time and then regress. In these cases, too, motor manifestations of the condition may be the first indication of a more global developmental problem.[42] Many children with autism have intellectual disabilities,[51] and analysis of motor behaviors of infants who by age 3 years were diagnosed with autism showed varying types of movement abnormalities at age 4 to 6 months.[152]

Neuromotor Impairments of Children with Intellectual Disabilities

The movement impairments of children with limited intellectual functioning are as diverse as the causes of their primary and associated conditions. Many of these movement problems, however, have their bases in central nervous system pathology that can lead to impairments in flexibility (too much or too little), force production, coordination, postural control, balance, endurance, and efficiency. Cardiopulmonary and musculoskeletal impairments also may contribute to movement problems.

About 10% of people with mild intellectual disability have motor impairments, and about 20% of those with severe intellectual disability have motor impairments. Among children with cerebral palsy, approximately 50% have intellectual disability,[165] and among children with autism, 50% to 73% have motor delays compared with normative data.[123]

Although the type and degree of movement and related problems vary greatly, certain medical diagnoses are likely to be associated with specific constellations of neuromuscular, musculoskeletal, and cardiopulmonary impairments. Table 17-1 summarizes impairments that are common among children with selected diagnoses who often receive physical therapy. Box 17-1 summarizes common motor, cognitive, language, and medical characteristics of children with Down syndrome. Other characteristics of people with Down syndrome are summarized in the Genomics and Genetic Syndromes Affecting Movement chapter on the Evolve website. A source of good information, including growth charts for children with Down syndrome, is the National Down Syndrome Society at http://www.ndss.org/. The National Association for Down syndrome also has useful information at http://www.nads.org/. Box 17-2 summarizes common motor, communication, social, and other characteristics of children with autism spectrum disorders. The Oklahoma Autism Network has a useful list of online resources related to autism spectrum disorders at http://www.okautism.org/.

Physical therapy examination of the movement impairments of children who have intellectual impairments is similar to that of other children who have problems addressed by physical therapists. Observation, criterion-referenced instruments, norm-referenced tests, and other formats are used, depending on the age of the child, the problem being assessed, and the purpose of the assessment (see chapters on

Understanding Motor Performance in Children and chapters on specific disabilities in other sections of this volume).

Although the same examination methods and tools may be used for children with and without intellectual impairments, recognizing that a child's intellectual impairment may affect performance of motor activities is important. This is especially the case when a child has to follow directions or perform motor tasks that have major intellectual components. Examination of infants and young children may be less affected by intellectual abilities than that of older children and adolescents, and intellectual disability may require more modification of methods to examine activity or participation than to measure impairments.

Learning in Children with Intellectual Impairments

By definition, *impaired learning* is what distinguishes children with intellectual impairments from other children. Although their motor problems often are similar to those of children without intellectual impairments, and they respond to intervention based on the same physical therapy principles, the application of those principles must be sensitive to the children's learning characteristics. Research demonstrating that physical therapy is less effective with children who have intellectual disability[118] may at least partially relate to inadequate modification of therapeutic approaches to enhance their learning.

The degree and types of learning disabilities of children with intellectual limitations vary considerably, but several common learning characteristics have been identified. Compared with typically developing children, children with intellectual disabilities have been found (1) to be capable of learning a lesser number of things; (2) to need a greater number of repetitions to learn; (3) to have greater difficulty generalizing skills; (4) to have greater difficulty maintaining skills that are not practiced regularly; (5) to have slower response times; and (6) to have a more limited repertoire of responses.[113] People with mild intellectual disabilities learn at about 50% to 66% the rate of people without intellectual disabilities, people with moderate intellectual disabilities at about 33% to 50% the rate, those with severe intellectual disabilities at about 24% to 33% the rate, and those with profound intellectual disabilities at about 25% the rate of people without intellectual disabilities.[165] Implications of these learning characteristics for physical therapy are described in later sections of this chapter.

TEAM ASSESSMENT

The complex problems of children with both intellectual and motor disabilities usually require a team approach for assessment and for planning, implementation, and evaluation of intervention.[113,126] The team always will include the child's family or another caregiver, with other team members as required by the nature and severity of the child's problems, the child's age, and the service delivery setting. Many

TABLE 17-1   **Common Neuromuscular, Musculoskeletal, and Cardiopulmonary Impairments of Children With Intellectual Disabilities Caused by Selected Conditions***

Condition	Neuromuscular	Musculoskeletal	Cardiopulmonary
Cri du chat syndrome[35] A rare chromosomal disorder (1 in 50,000 live births) caused by loss of chromosomal material from region 5p (5p12)[34]	Hypotonia in early childhood, sometimes hypertonia later	Facial and minor upper extremity anomalies, scoliosis	Congenital heart disease is common
Cytomegalovirus (prenatal)[85] One of the most common causes of prenatal infections in developed countries, with incidence estimated to be between 0.15% and 2.0%[53]	Cerebral palsy, seizure disorder, microcephaly (hearing problems)	Secondary to neuromuscular problems	Pulmonary valvular stenosis, mitral stenosis, atrial septal defect
Cornelia deLange syndrome[70] Caused by mutations in the *NIPBL, SMC1A,* and *SMC3* genes; estimated to affect 1/10,000 to 30,000 newborn infants[106]	Spasticity, intention tremor, seizure disorder (10%–20%), microcephaly	Severe growth retardation; decreased bone age, small stature, small hands and feet, short digits, proximal thumb placement, clinodactyly of fifth fingers, other arm and hand defects, limited elbow extension	Neonatal respiratory problems, congenital heart disease, recurrent upper respiratory infections
Fetal alcohol syndrome[104] Caused by prenatal exposure to alcohol, the estimated prevalence of fetal alcohol syndrome is about 1%[58]	Fine motor and visual motor deficits, balance deficits	Minor facial abnormalities, joint anomalies with abnormal position or function, maxillary hypoplasia, poor growth	Heart defects
Fragile X syndrome[36] The most common form of inherited mental retardation, it is primarily caused by expansion of a sequence in the *FMR1* gene of the X chromosome[117]	Poor coordination and motor planning, seizures	Connective tissue abnormalities, which may lead to congenital hip dislocation in infancy and later to scoliosis and pes planus	Mitral valve prolapse
Hurler's syndrome[70] Autosomal recessive storage disorder with lack of lysosomal hydrolase α-L-iduronidase[70]	Hydrocephalus	Joint contractures, clawlike deformities of hands, short fingers, thoracolumbar kyphosis, shallow acetabular and glenoid fossae, irregularly shaped bones	Cardiac deformities, cardiac enlargement because right ventricular hypertension is common, death frequently due to cardiac failure
Lesch-Nyhan syndrome[70] Caused by a genetic deficiency of hypoxanthine-guanine phosphoribosyltransferase located on the X chromosome[86]	Hypotonia followed by spasticity and chorea, athetosis, or dystonia; compulsive self-injurious behavior	Secondary to neuromuscular problems	
Prader-Willi syndrome[28] A chromosomal microdeletion disorder that occurs in 1:10,000 to 15,000 live births. It is the leading genetic cause of obesity[28]	Severe hypotonia and feeding problems in infancy, excessive eating (usual onset 1–6 years) and obesity in childhood, poor fine and gross motor coordination, average age of sitting 12 months and walking 24 months	Small hands and feet with sometimes tapering fingers; scoliosis, kyphosis, or both are common; hip dysplasia in 10%; osteoporosis is frequent	Upper airway obstruction, sleep apnea, and oxygen desaturation are common

Continued

TABLE 17-1 **Common Neuromuscular, Musculoskeletal, and Cardiopulmonary Impairments of Children With Intellectual Disabilities Caused by Selected Conditions*—cont'd**

Condition	Neuromuscular	Musculoskeletal	Cardiopulmonary
Rett syndrome[121] Definitive diagnosis is accomplished by mutation analysis on leukocyte DNA for the gene *MECP2*.[121] A study in Texas estimated prevalence of 1/22,800	Deceleration in rate of head growth in infancy, gradual loss of acquired skills after 6 to 18 months of age, loss of purposeful hand skills, stereotypic hand movements (clapping, wringing, clenching), apraxia, teeth grinding, seizure disorder	Scoliosis/kyphosis, growth failure, bone demineralization	Breathing irregularities, such as hyperventilation and breath holding
Williams (elfin facies) syndrome[102] Caused by mutation or deletion of the *elastin* gene at 7q11.23; it occurs in 1/20,000 live births[102]	Mild neurologic dysfunction, hypotonia, hyperreflexia, cerebellar dysfunction	Facial abnormalities, slow and abnormal growth, connective tissue abnormalities, radioulnar stenosis, spinal deformities, joint hyperextension when young, contractures when older	Supravalvar aortic stenosis, hypertension, peripheral pulmonic stenosis, and mitral valve prolapse

*Not all children with each condition exhibit all impairments.

Box **17-1** COMMON CHARACTERISTICS OF CHILDREN WITH DOWN SYNDROME

MOTOR DEVELOPMENT

- Hypotonia[131]
- Hyperflexibility[64]
- Oral motor and feeding delays[64]
- Problems with postural control and balance[141]
- Delayed gross motor development[116,131]
- Gross motor development begins to level off after age 3 years.[116]
- Motor development may be below mental age.[64,69]
- Delayed fine motor skills[33]
- Usually follow sequence of typical motor development[116]
- Require more time to learn movements as complexity increases[116]
- Atypical patterns of movement to maintain postural stability[163]
- Reduced strength[163]
- Better motor performance with visual than verbal instructions[97]
- Perceptual-motor deficits in perception of complex visual motion cues[97]
- Slower reaction times during movement[64]

COGNITIVE DEVELOPMENT

- Usually moderate to severe intellectual disability, although some have been reported to be within typical range[163]
- Intelligence test scores progressively decrease with age[120]

- Early onset (4th decade) of dementia is common[164,166]
- Motivation may be low[163]

LANGUAGE DEVELOPMENT

- Usually poor; below other areas of development and when compared with typical children or children with other causes for intellectual disabilities of the same mental age[163]
- Impairment of verbal memory skills and other verbal processing abilities[166]
- Language comprehension less impaired than expressive language[163]

MEDICAL PROBLEMS[131,132]

- Congenital heart disease (66%)
- Vision deficit (60%)
- Hearing impairments (60%–80%)
- Obesity (60%) and low levels of physical fitness
- Skin conditions (50%)
- Seizure disorder (6%)
- Atlantoaxial instability (subclinical 14%; symptomatic 1%)
- Hypothyroidism (subclinical 30%–50%; overt 7%)
- Periodontal disease

OTHER

- Perhaps increased incidence of autism spectrum disorders[147]

Approximately 70% of people with autism spectrum disorders have intellectual disabilities.[51] The following characteristics are common, but are not universal.

MOTOR DEVELOPMENT

- Impaired performance of skilled motor tasks and gestures (most common motor finding)[81]
- Delayed gross and fine motor development[57,123]; rate of development often slows at age 2 to 3 years[115]
- Muscle tone and reflex abnormalities (especially hypotonia when young)[90,100]
- Impaired motor imitation[67,172]
- Generalized deficit in praxis (in addition to imitation)[7,90,103]
- Poor balance and coordination[2]
- Unusual gait patterns, such as toe-walking[90]
- Repetitive and stereotypic movements of body, limbs, and fingers[90]
- Delayed learning of complex motor skills, such as tricycle riding[81]
- Lack of anticipation during movement preparation phases[7]

COMMUNICATION AND SOCIAL DEVELOPMENT[107]

- Deficits in joint attention (coordinating attention between people and objects)
  - Orienting and attending to a communication partner
  - Shifting gaze between people and objects
  - Sharing affect or emotional state with another person
  - Following the gaze and point of another person
  - Sharing experiences by drawing another person's attention to objects or events
- Difficulty learning conventional or shared meaning for symbols, such as conventional gestures, conventional meanings for a word, and pretend play
- Some have limited ability to use speech for communication; most who can speak go through a period of echolalia.
- Some have idiosyncratic or unconventional means of communication, including behaviors that others perceive as problems.
- Low rates of initiation of interaction with others and response to them
- Less attention to others' emotions than other children

OTHER

- Unusual responses to sensory input[7]
- Cerebellar abnormalities[2]
- Attention deficits and hyperactivity[2]
- Visual-spatial skills often more advanced than other areas[7]
- Oral-motor problems, feeding problems, and limited food preferences[7,48]
- Sleep disturbances, particularly of sleep-wake cycles[48]

children need the services of two or more teams at the same time, such as a clinically based health care team and an early intervention or public school team. Usually, the health care team is primarily responsible for assessment of the child's body functions and structures, with the early intervention or school-based team responsible for addressing activity limitations and ongoing efforts to promote the highest possible level of family and community participation. When the teams have mutual responsibilities and concerns, overlapping or conflicting services can result, with confusion for the family and unnecessary expenditure of limited resources. To avoid such problems, the teams must communicate well and the roles and responsibilities of the members of each team must be clear to all.[126]

MODELS OF TEAM FUNCTIONING

Each team must decide on a model of service delivery that will enable comprehensive evaluation of a child's abilities and disabilities and provide the most effective intervention. The transdisciplinary model of service delivery, developed in the mid-1970s by the United Cerebral Palsy National Collaborative Infant Project,[158] is often recommended as best practice in early intervention programs and in special education programs for children with severe and multiple disabilities.[113,126,146]

The transdisciplinary model permits greater coordination of comprehensive services for individuals with complex health, educational, and social needs than many other approaches. Two of the distinguishing features of the model are that assessments are conducted collaboratively by team members and that a single, discipline-free service plan is developed to meet the highest-priority needs of the child and the family. This mode of operation contrasts with other service delivery models in which service providers conduct separate assessments and develop separate, discipline-referenced intervention plans.[96]

Another distinguishing feature of the transdisciplinary model is that one team member is designated as the primary service provider,[125] usually the person who spends the greatest amount of time with the child or the person who has the skills necessary to address the child's greatest areas of need.[113] The primary service provider will change over time as the child's needs and environments change. A parent or physical therapist may be the primary service provider for an infant or young child, a teacher the primary service provider for an older child, and a personal care assistant the primary service provider for a young adult.

When using a transdisciplinary approach, team members are responsible for determining which of their own disciplinary knowledge and skills are needed by the child, for consulting with and teaching the necessary knowledge and skills to the primary service provider, and for monitoring outcomes. The primary service provider incorporates the knowledge and strategies of other disciplines into ongoing intervention with the child. In effect, team members "release" part of their roles to the primary service provider.[113]

ASSESSMENT OF ACTIVITY AND PARTICIPATION

Assessment of a child's activities and participation is best conducted in the environments in which the child actually participates or in environments in which children of similar age and social background participate. Assessment in natural environments is increasingly advocated for all children who have disabilities, but especially for children with intellectual disabilities, who have difficulty generalizing skills from one setting to another. Intervention based on environmental assessment is far more likely to result in improved abilities to participate in everyday activities and in age-appropriate life roles than assessment that takes place in an isolated or clinical setting, is based on a normal development sequence, or focuses primarily on identification of impairments, such as range of motion, postural responses, or retention of reflexes.[95,126]

The same tools described in other chapters of this volume that commonly are used to measure activity among children with other types of disabilities can be used with children with intellectual impairments. These tools include the functional skills scales of the Pediatric Evaluation of Disability Inventory,[62] the Peabody Developmental Motor Scales,[34] the Gross Motor Function Measure,[137] and the Daily Activities of Infants Scale,[11] among others.

Tools are becoming increasingly available to measure aspects of participation of children with disabilities. The Children's Assessment of Participation and Enjoyment (CAPE) and Preferences for Activities of Children (PAC),[76] for example, measure participation of children and youth age 6 to 21 in recreation and leisure activities outside of school. The CAPE measures the diversity, intensity, enjoyment, and context of the activities. The PAC measures preferences for involvement in activities. The Caregiver Assistance Scale of the Pediatric Evaluation of Disability Inventory[62] measures participation and activities related to mobility, self-care, and social function in the home environment. The School Function Assessment[35] measures participation, activities, and necessary task supports in the school environment of children in kindergarten through sixth grade.

ASSESSMENT OF BODY STRUCTURES AND FUNCTIONING

Assessment of body structures and functions can help to identify reasons for identified activity and participation limitations. A child with Down syndrome, for example, is likely to have low muscle tone and joint hyperextensibility. Methods for assessing body structures and functions of children described in other chapters of this volume are applicable to children with intellectual disabilities.

ASSESSMENT OF INTELLECTUAL FUNCTIONING

Determining if a child has an intellectual disability requires a standardized, norm-referenced measure of intelligence, which usually is administered by a psychologist or psychometrist. Even though most physical therapists do not administer intelligence tests, they are often able to promote an environment in which children with motor disabilities can perform optimally, such as by providing positioning to enhance a child's communication and eye and hand use[143] or by assisting the examiner to determine alternative response modes for use by children who have motor impairments.

Assessment of Infants

Physical therapists may be involved in the administration of tests designed to assess the intellectual abilities of infants, because many of these tests focus on an infant's perceptual-motor development, such as accomplishment of motor developmental milestones or coordination of vision and hearing with body movement.[29,56] These tests include instruments described in Chapters 2 and 3 of this volume.

Unfortunately, perceptual-motor–based infant evaluations are poor predictors of intellectual ability at later ages, with little, if any, relationship found between scores on infant tests and children's subsequent scores on intelligence tests for preschool or school-age children.[44,142] The most common error is identification of infants as having intellectual delays who later demonstrate normal intelligence.[92] Better predictability has been found with children who have severe intellectual delays and multiple disabilities,[78] with most children who have severe intellectual delays identified before they are 2 years old.[73] Gibbs[56] proposed that this is a result of the limited capacity of infants with severe disabilities to be influenced by positive environmental circumstances; thus, their range of possible outcomes is more restricted and their test scores are more stable over time.

Some tests of infant intellectual abilities attempt to measure infants' intellectual functioning through evaluation of their information-processing capacity rather than their perceptual-motor skills. These tests use infants' responses to novel and previously presented stimuli to assess their visual or auditory memory and their ability to discriminate among stimuli.[61] These tests are based on the tendency of infants, almost from birth, to respond for shorter periods of time to stimuli to which they have been previously exposed. Thus, if an infant has a longer response to a new stimulus than to one presented previously, memory for the familiar stimulus and discrimination of the two stimuli are demonstrated. Visual attention to stimuli is often assessed, as with the Fagan Test of Infant Intelligence (FTII),[45] but changes in heart rate, smiling, and other responses can also indicate an infant's processing of information.[177]

One advantage of information-processing tests for infants is that they are essentially motor- and language-free, making them more appropriate for infants with motor and hearing impairments than many other tests.[44] Another advantage is that their predictive validity is much better than that of tests that focus on perceptual-motor behaviors; they may be most predictive when infants are tested at around 9 to 10 months corrected age.[61] This probably is so because they tap information-processing capacities that are more similar to requirements of intelligence tests for older children than are the qualities assessed by perceptual-motor–based tests.[29,56]

Assessment of Children

According to the AAMR,[3] the most widely used IQ tests for children are the Stanford-Binet Intelligence Scale IV,[154] which was updated in 2003,[130] and the Wechsler Intelligence Scale for Children III,[168] which was updated in 2004.[72] Standardized administration of these and most other intelligence tests requires spoken and motor responses that seriously limit their usefulness with children who have communication and motor impairments.

A few intelligence tests have been developed that require children only to indicate a choice from among an array of alternatives. The Columbia Mental Maturity Scale[18] is one such test; it was developed specifically to assess the intelligence of children with cerebral palsy. This test requires no oral response, and the only motor response required is to indicate which pictures are unrelated to others.

Raven's Progressive Matrices,[128] which requires selection of missing elements of abstract designs, and the Leiter International Performance Scale–Revised[133] are other non–language-based tests with minimal motor requirements. They may, however, suggest spuriously low intellectual abilities in children who have visual-perceptual deficits or visual impairments. It is also important to be aware that all tests with limited motor and language requirements sample only a narrow range of abilities compared with more traditional tests of intelligence, so they may overestimate or underestimate more global aspects of a child's intelligence.[29] For children with profound multiple disabilities, whose intellectual abilities are the most difficult to assess, tests of visual memory, similar to those developed for evaluation of infants, could provide some elusive information about their capacities to store and process information.[148]

ASSESSMENT OF ADAPTIVE BEHAVIORS

Although examiners often emphasize intelligence test scores in the diagnosis of intellectual disability, adaptive behaviors are also central in the assessment of intellectual disability.[3] Nihira[110] defined adaptive behavior as a person's effectiveness in coping with environmental demands. Assessment of adaptive behavior relies heavily on professional judgment, in both the selection of means to assess adaptive behaviors and in their interpretation. Physical therapists often can provide information about a child's adaptive behaviors, such as self-help and mobility skills, and may also be instrumental in providing assistive devices that can improve a child's adaptive skills.

Instruments to measure adaptive behaviors have been developed, but they are of more recent vintage than many of the intelligence tests and are fewer in number. The Pediatric Evaluation of Disability Inventory (PEDI)[62] described in Chapter 2 was developed to measure self-care, mobility, and social function in children age 6 months to 7.5 years with physical or combined physical and intellectual disabilities. This tool is divided into two parts: functional skills and caregiver assistance. Tests that are commonly used for older children include the AAMR Adaptive Behavior Scale-School (ABS-S:2)[79] and the Vineland Adaptive Behavior Scales, Second Edition (VABS-II).[145] The ABS-S:2 was designed for assessment of adaptive behaviors and for assistance in program planning.[69] This tool is divided into two parts: personal independence and social behavior. The tool yields scores in five areas, including personal self-sufficiency, community self-sufficiency, personal-social responsibility, social adjustment, and personal adjustment. Results of a validity study of the ABS-S:2 indicated that the personal independence and social behavior scales of the tool demonstrated the largest difference between typical children and children with intellectual disabilities.[167] The results of this study suggested that these two sections of the tool, rather than scores in all five areas, should be used when children are assessed for intellectual disabilities. The VABS-II is administered as a questionnaire or rating form that asks about activities of daily living, cognition, language, play, and social competency. The authors estimated test-retest reliability to be between 0.88 and 0.92 and interrater reliability to be between 0.71 and 0.81 across domains.

ASSESSMENT OF CONTEXTUAL FACTORS

The AAMR definition of *intellectual disability* requires consideration of function within context. Similarly, the ICF views outcomes as resulting from interactions between health conditions and contextual factors. Contextual factors include both personal and environmental factors.[173] Environmental factors outside the child can profoundly affect child development, test scores, and intervention planning.[98] Brooks-Gunn and colleagues[16] found, for example, that differences between IQ test scores of African American and Caucasian children at age 5 years were nearly eliminated after adjustments were made for poverty and home environment. Physical therapists may not be able to change the effects of environmental factors on test scores but should consider the effects of physical, social, and attitudinal environments on test performance. Participation in everyday activities is considered important for typical child development, and children with combined physical and intellectual disabilities are at increased risk for less participation in all settings.[75] Some evidence suggests that intervention focused on expanding existing natural learning opportunities in everyday settings can have a positive effect on children's participation.[39] Assessment of environmental factors related to activity and participation is necessary for development of interventions that can promote improved participation.

Physical therapists are often involved in assessing the physical environment and a child's interaction with it. Many years ago, Brown and associates[17] described an ecologic approach to assessment that others have subsequently promoted as a means to determine functional outcomes and to plan programs for people who have intellectual disabilities and for children in early intervention programs.[113,126] An ecologic assessment is an approach or format, rather than a specific assessment instrument.[113] Orelove and Sobsey[113] described four major steps in an ecologic assessment:

1. Determine the domains to be included in the child's program. Four domains are considered to be primary: home, community (e.g., school, stores, church), vocational, and recreation-leisure. Certain critical skills, such as mobility, communication, and hand use, are required for functioning in all domains.

2. Determine the environments and subenvironments within each domain in which the child currently functions or could function in the future. A child's team might identify the home, school, and restaurant as especially important. Subenvironments could be the bedroom at home, the cafeteria at school, and the restroom in a restaurant.

3. Determine the activities the child needs to function in each of the subenvironments. Activities could include getting out of bed at home, obtaining and eating lunch at school, and using the toilet in a restaurant.

4. Determine the skills the child needs for each activity. Skills are determined through task analysis of the activities and by identifying the components the child needs to be able to do to accomplish each of them. To get out of bed, for example, one child may need to respond to the alarm, remove the covers, assume a sitting position, and transfer to a wheelchair. A child with less ability could learn to do other components of the task, such as rolling over to sit up after the covers have been removed, and assisting with the transfer.

An example of an ecologic assessment is included in the case study of Jeff at the end of the chapter.

Physical therapists often have less experience examining the social and attitudinal aspects of the environment than the physical aspects. Children rarely function alone in their environment, however, so social and attitudinal factors need to be considered. Young children are a part of their families, and older children spend their time in classrooms, in after-school activities, and in the community with their peers, family, and other community members. Successful physical therapy services depend on more than developing intervention focused on the physical aspects of a task. Rather, successful intervention often depends on opportunities to practice within supportive social and attitudinal environments.

Personal Factors

In the ICF model, personal factors include those aspects of a person that are not part of the health condition, such as gender, race, coping styles, and those things that are intrinsically motivating.[173] Physical therapists need to consider such personal factors to effectively promote children's chosen activities and participation within the context of family, school, and community. A tool that is helpful for identifying the level of supports that adolescents and adults with intellectual disabilities and other developmental disabilities need for quality participation in society is the Supports Intensity Scale (SIS).[1] The tool was normed with people age 16 to over 70 years and measures the supports needed in daily life activities and exceptional medical and behavioral support needs. A supplemental protection and advocacy scale also is included. A version of the scale for children age 5 to 15 years with intellectual disabilities is being developed.[1]

INTELLECTUAL REFERENCING

Intellectual referencing is an assessment approach that has been used to determine whether children are eligible for services, especially for physical therapy, occupational therapy, and speech pathology, in public schools.[26] The approach is based on an assumption that children's potential for gains in motor and communication development is related to their intellectual abilities, and that children whose intellectual abilities are lower than or equal to their motor or communication abilities would not benefit from services, so they are not eligible for them. Obviously, many children with intellectual disabilities could be declared ineligible for physical therapy services under such an assumption, so the use of intellectual referencing has been highly controversial. Critics have been supported by at least one study that examined the association between IQ scores and progress in occupational therapy or physical therapy over the course of one school year.[6] Children were divided into two groups based on their IQ scores, and their motor skills were tested before and after 1 year's intervention. Children received approximately 40 minutes of occupational therapy or physical therapy per week. Both groups showed significant change in their age-equivalence scores, but the researchers found no significant correlation between IQ and change in motor test scores. The U.S. Department of Education, Office of Special Education Programs (OSEP), declared intellectual referencing to be an unlawful means of determining whether a child should receive related services in public schools.[124] The OSEP statement supported the authority of each child's educational team to decide on the services necessary for that child to meet individualized educational goals. When goals of children with intellectual and neuromotor impairments focus on reducing activity limitations and improving

TOP-DOWN APPROACH

BOTTOM-UP APPROACH

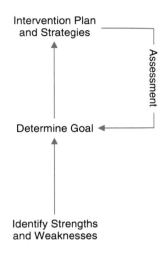

A

B

participation, some type of physical therapy often is needed, as determined through coordination and communication with the family and other team members.

DETERMINING INTERVENTION GOALS AND OUTCOMES

Functional goals have been emphasized for many years in special education and physical therapy.[95,126,127] Functional skills have been defined as age-appropriate activities or tasks that someone else will have to do if the child does not,[17] and that reflect the needs and interests of the child and family.[113] Some children can learn to complete a task or activity, whereas others will be capable of learning to carry out only a part of it. Partial participation, or completion of only part of a task, is a legitimate outcome for some children who have severe disabilities.[47] A child may, for example, be unable to transfer independently but can learn to unbuckle a seat belt and support weight in standing. Another child may be unable to put a DVD into a player but can learn to turn it on using a switch.

Outcomes of interventions to improve a child's abilities to participate in life must represent specific functional skills that the child will acquire. Team members cannot assume that interventions directed toward remediation of impairments, such as improving postural responses, range of motion, or strength, or toward reducing the degree of activity limitation indicated by failed items on a developmental test, will necessarily lead to meaningful outcomes.[95,126,127]

This is especially true of children with intellectual disabilities who need many repetitions to learn, who forget easily, and who generalize poorly. These characteristics make it difficult or impossible for a child with intellectual disabilities to synthesize isolated activities or components of movement into meaningful skills.

Campbell[22] proposed a "top-down" approach to determining outcomes, in which the desired functional outcomes are determined first, then obstacles to their accomplishment are identified, and then intervention to overcome the obstacles is planned and implemented (Figure 17-1). This process in similar to the decision-making process of the hypothesis-oriented algorithm for clinicians (HOAC II),[135] in which a person's goals for intervention are identified first, then the person is examined to generate a hypothesis about why the goals can or cannot be met at the present time.

As described earlier as a component of an ecologic assessment, functional outcomes can be anything that are of high priority and meaningful to the child and family, are age-appropriate, and are, or could be, a home, community, recreation-leisure, or vocational activity. Giangreco and colleagues[55] proposed five valued life outcomes for all children, including those with severe disabilities:

1. Having a safe, stable home in which to live now or in the future
2. Having access to a variety of places and engaging in meaningful activities
3. Having a social network of personally meaningful relationships

4. Having a level of personal choice and control that matches one's age
5. Being safe and healthy

Teams usually have the most difficulty determining meaningful outcomes for children with profound multiple disabilities, who often have extremely limited repertoires of behavior. Even these children, however, can accomplish outcomes that require active behavioral changes, such as indicating a choice of food or activity or using body movements to activate switches. Such active outcomes lead to acquisition of skills that increase participation and are in contrast to passive activities that are done to the child, such as sensory stimulation, range of motion exercises, and positioning (often stated as something the child will "tolerate"). Passive activities may be part of the intervention to help a child accomplish a skill, but only the child's active behavior can increase true participation.

One helpful tool for assisting families to identify meaningful outcomes and to measure whether they have been accomplished is the Canadian Occupational Performance Measure (COPM).[83] The COPM was designed as an individualized measure of performance and satisfaction in self-care, productivity (work, household management, play/school), and leisure. Although the COPM was intended for occupational therapists, it is an equally useful tool for physical therapists. Another tool that is useful for children with receptive language at the 5-year level is the Perceived Efficacy and Goal Setting System (PEGS).[101] The PEGS uses a questionnaire format to help children rate their competence in everyday tasks and to select goals important to them. This chapter's section on Evaluation of Outcomes gives more information about the tools.

When desired outcomes are determined first, they are discipline-free, that is, they describe the skills the child will accomplish without regard for discipline-related concerns. Only after team members identify the highest-priority outcomes do they decide which disciplines will be needed to help the child accomplish each one.[126] This team-oriented process for determining outcomes is not necessarily inconsistent with processes described in the HOAC II[135] or the *Guide to Physical Therapist Practice* (Guide),[4] although both the HOAC II and the Guide describe primarily a unidisciplinary approach in which the physical therapist makes decisions in collaboration with the patient and perhaps the patient's family. When working with children whose complex problems require teams of professionals, the process must include other professionals as well. Amy's case history at the end of this chapter provides an example of application of the Guide to the decision-making process of a school-based team.

INTERVENTION

During planning and implementation of intervention for children with intellectual disabilities, it is important to keep in mind what are widely regarded as best practices for working with children who have intellectual disabilities and other developmental disabilities. Some of these practices have been discussed previously and include families and children as full and equal team members, assessment in natural environments, and emphasis of functional outcomes with active participation by children.[95]

Other considerations that influence intervention for children with intellectual disabilities include interventions to limit impairments and promote activity and participation, use of teaching methods that are most likely to result in acquisition of skills by children with intellectual disabilities, and the role of physical therapists in promoting development in nonmotor domains. Each of these considerations, which are discussed in the following sections, involves one or more of the three components of intervention included in the *Guide to Physical Therapist Practice*[4]: coordination, communication, and documentation; patient/client-related instruction; and procedural interventions.

LIMITING IMPAIRMENTS, MINIMIZING ACTIVITY LIMITATIONS, AND PREVENTING SECONDARY IMPAIRMENTS

Early identification of neuromuscular, musculoskeletal, and cardiopulmonary problems, at whatever age they occur, allows for intervention designed to limit the impairments, thus restricting the development of secondary impairments and activity limitations. Specific intervention will depend on the identified problems and on consequences that can be predicted to follow from the natural history of the condition. Children with Down syndrome and other relatively mild movement impairments, for example, often benefit from activities designed to enhance postural control and force production and accomplishment of motor milestones.[131] Other children with more severe impairments may benefit from positioning and other activities designed to maintain flexibility, prevent musculoskeletal malalignments and deformities, and enhance motor development and control. Such intervention is described in other chapters of this volume. As examples, Box 17-3 provides recommendations for physical therapy for children with Down syndrome from infancy through school age, and Box 17-4 provides considerations for physical therapy for children with autism.

LIMITING INTELLECTUAL, COMMUNICATION, AND PSYCHOSOCIAL AND FUNCTIONAL LIMITATIONS

Children who have motor impairments that restrict or prevent exploration of their environments may be at risk for secondary delays in domains that are not primarily affected, especially cognition, communication, and psychosocial

BOX 17-3   PHYSICAL THERAPY FOR CHILDREN WITH DOWN SYNDROME

Interventions for children with Down syndrome should be targeted to helping children achieve measurable goals[33,64] identified with the parents and with the child when the child is old enough to have an opinion. Children's need for physical therapy and specific interventions change as children age. Interventions are likely to be direct and more intensive for infants and toddlers, and then involve more consultation than direct therapy as the child attends preschool and school.

INFANTS AND TODDLERS (AGE BIRTH TO 3 YEARS)

- Early intervention services from the time the infant is medically stable to provide the parents with information about resources,[131] the development of children with Down syndrome, and methods to promote their child's motor development and development of functional skills[64]
- Arrange access to parent-to-parent support.[104]
- Attempt to prevent compensatory movements.
- Consider treadmill training starting at about 10 months, which research has shown can reduce delay in walking and may promote developmental benefits of independent locomotion.[157]
- When the child starts to stand, consider flexi supramalleolar orthoses to improve postural stability.[91]
- Coordination and communication with other team members of the early intervention team, such as speech/language pathologists, for strategies to promote communication development. Consider manual signs.[166]
- Structure environments so the child can participate, such as provide adaptive seating to compensate for lack of postural control to facilitate reaching and hand function.
- Facilitate parent–child interactions.

- Promote early perceptual-motor competencies such as eye gaze and joint attention to people, objects, and the environment.[164]
- Coordinate and communicate with any day care or preschool providers.

PRESCHOOL

- Coordinate and consult with preschool teachers about how to include the child in motor activities that will continue to promote motor development.
- Consult with parents to involve child in active play, such as trike riding, swimming, etc.
- Consider the need for orthoses to improve stability as necessary for development of higher-level motor skills.
- Consider orthoses to enhance stability.[91]
- Consider manual signs for communication.[166]

SCHOOL AGE[69]

- Prevention of problems associated with aging is important.[10]
- Coordinate and consult with physical education teachers and parents to include the child in activities that:
  - Teach skills necessary to participate in a variety of fun physical activities that involve continuous movement and promote physical fitness, such as gymnastics, cycling, walking, and swimming
  - Involve in organized programs that culminate in Special Olympics or inclusive events
  - Develop and practice activities that promote body and space awareness, balance, timing, and effort in movement
  - Teach the rules of games and sportsmanship
  - Teach enjoyable physical activities that can be lifelong

BOX 17-4   PHYSICAL THERAPY FOR CHILDREN WITH AUTISM SPECTRUM DISORDERS

Although children with autism spectrum disorders commonly have motor delays or deficits, no consistent research exists to support the effectiveness of interventions designed to improve motor function.[7,107] Recommendations, therefore, are based on best practice principles for examination and intervention with children with autism and other developmental disabilities.

The motor function and postural control of children with autism spectrum disorders should be examined as part of a comprehensive developmental assessment to identify each child's unique strengths and weaknesses.[7,123] Interventions should be targeted to helping children achieve measurable functional goals identified with the parents and with the child when the child is old enough to have an opinion.

General recommendations for intervention with children with autism spectrum disorders include the following:
- Be aware of the difficulty many children have with imitation.[7]
- Individualize interventions to accomplish functional goals.

- Integrate interventions into functional activities within daily routines in natural environments.[107]
- Focus on activities that are meaningful to the child and are a match with overall goals for the child.[8]
- Provide short duration interventions with frequent and systematic documentation of progress.[7,8]
- Measure outcomes in the three components of the ICF: sensory and motor function, specific activities, and participation.[8]
- Modify interventions if the child is not making progress toward functional goals.[7]
- Assess and structure the physical and sensory environments to accommodate a child's sensory and motor function.[7]

development.[71] Campos and Bertenthal[23] suggested that independent mobility is an organizer of psychological changes in typically developing infants, especially developmental changes in social understanding, spatial cognition, and emotions. They also proposed theoretical links between independent mobility and the growth of brain structures, self-awareness, attachment to others, and ability to cope with the environment.

Most of the theoretical links have not been examined empirically, but relations between mobility and spatial cognition have received considerable research attention. Several studies have demonstrated that locomotion, not age per se, is related to changes in such spatial intellectual tasks as recognition of heights,[13] retrieving hidden toys,[12] and performance on Piagetian spatial search tasks by typical infants and infants with meningomyelocele.[74,153] Results of the individual studies were supported by a meta-analysis, which found that self-produced locomotion has an effect on spatial cognitive performance in typical children.[174] Self-produced locomotion also has been shown to influence social-communicative behaviors of infants,[60] and the proposed theoretical link between mobility and development of brain structures has been supported by studies demonstrating that experience shapes the brains of animals (for a review, see Kolb et al.[77]). Imaging techniques have shown similar effects of experience on the structure of infants' brains.[30]

Although much of the research has demonstrated an association between motor and intellectual development, other research suggests that the links are indirect, with motor and intellectual abilities facilitating each other but capable of relatively independent development. One study, for example, found that the object permanence task performance of children with cerebral palsy was more closely related to their mental age than to the severity of their motor impairments.[41] This finding is consistent with the well-known capacity for some people to develop average or superior mental abilities in spite of severe motor impairments.

Further research is needed to determine the relative contributions of innate mental capability and sensorimotor experiences on various aspects of intellectual development. It may be that the inborn intelligence of some children enables them to compensate for their motor limitations, thus making them less vulnerable to effects of sensorimotor deprivation than children whose intellectual capacities are more limited.

If it is assumed that exploration and manipulation of the environment do influence intellectual, communication, and social-emotional development, physical therapy has an obvious role in the development of these nonmotor domains of children who have motor impairments. One means is through intervention strategies designed to improve motor performance, as described in other chapters of this volume. Another potentially important strategy is to provide alternative means of mobility when children's motor impairments prevent exploration of the environment at an age when other children are crawling and walking. In addition, the use of postural support systems to promote interaction with the environment is important when adaptive equipment and powered mobility are used.

Use of Power Mobility to Prevent Activity Limitations

Butler[19] asserted that self-produced locomotion can have such a powerful impact on development that functional means of mobility should be provided for all young children who have mobility restrictions, regardless of whether or not the child is expected to walk eventually. Aided mobility is not seen as "giving up" on walking for young children, but as providing critical assistance at a time when it is needed to promote age-appropriate activity and participation.

Several reports have demonstrated that very young children can learn to use power mobility devices. Zazula and Foulds[176] reported that an 11-month-old child with congenital limb deformities learned to activate the controls of a motorized cart within 4 hours and controlled all aspects of the cart by 17 months of age. In another study, 12 of 13 children between ages 20 and 37 months, with various disabilities, became competent motorized wheelchair users within their homes after an average of 16.4 days of practice.[20] More recently, a case report described the development of independent power mobility in a 20-month-old child with spinal muscular atrophy within 6 weeks of the time she received a power wheelchair.[71]

Although these young children were believed to have normal intelligence, other studies have demonstrated that children with intellectual disabilities also can become independent users of power mobility devices.[162] Certain intellectual abilities may be necessary to achieve independent power-aided mobility, but the specific abilities that are necessary and the means to assess them have not been determined. Because typically developing children learn to crawl and become independently mobile well before their first birthday, and because children have become independently mobile using power mobility devices before age 2, children with intellectual disabilities who have adequate vision and the intellectual skills typical of an 18-month-old (or perhaps younger) are likely to be capable of learning to use powered means of mobility, given appropriate equipment, instruction, and opportunities. Tefft and colleagues[151] investigated intellectual predictors associated with young children who learn to use power mobility independently after six training sessions in a clinical setting. They found spatial relations and problem-solving abilities were better among children who learned to maneuver a chair than in those who did not. Children with poorer spatial relations and problem-solving abilities may be able to learn to use power mobility, however, if practice occurs in their everyday settings and if they have adequate opportunities for practice.

Use of Assistive Positioning to Promote Environmental Interaction

Seating and other assistive positioning devices, as described in the chapter on Assistive Technology on the Evolve website, also can influence children's interactions with their physical and social environments through their effects on such variables as hand function,[111] communication,[93] and respiration.[112] One of the most important environmental interactions is communication with others because this affects not only a child's communication development but also his intellectual and social-emotional development.[21]

To learn to communicate, children must have opportunities to communicate. One study found that teachers initiated interactions at higher rates when children were positioned in wheelchairs than when they were in sidelyers or supine on a mat.[93] Observations suggested that wheelchairs promoted interaction by placing students nearer the normal interaction level of adults than positioning them on the floor. The adults who participated in the study rarely sat on the floor to interact with children unless they were involved in structured programming—a finding that is consistent with other investigations.[66]

In addition to providing opportunities for interaction with other persons in the environment, research suggests that positioning can influence children's own communicative behaviors. Typically developing 3- to 6-month-old infants looked at their mothers for longer periods of time when they were supine than when reclined 45° or seated upright.[50] Similarly, children with profound intellectual disabilities and physical disabilities interacted with attentive teachers and classroom assistants for longer periods of time when they were in the supine position than when they were seated in their wheelchairs or in a sidelyer.[93] The reason for these findings is not known, although the environment might have been less distracting when children were in a supine position, or, in the case of children with disabilities who had inadequate head control, the supine position might have provided head support necessary for them to maintain eye contact and interact. Because a supine position may be socially isolating and physically detrimental, it should be monitored carefully and used only while the child is actively engaged in social interaction.

Positioning also may influence children's interactions with their environments through the effect of position on their behavioral state or arousal. Low levels of arousal and behavioral states that interfere with attention to environmental stimuli are common among children with the most severe intellectual and motor disabilities.[59] Guess and colleagues[59] found that when children with multiple disabilities were positioned upright, their behavioral states were more compatible with learning than when they were placed in recumbent positions. Similarly, Landesman-Dwyer and Sackett[80] found that children's activity levels and receptivity to environmental stimuli were improved when intervention included an upright position. Other studies suggested that oxygenation is improved in the upright position,[108] and inadequate oxygenation has been proposed as a factor contributing to the lethargy of children with profound multiple disabilities.[59]

Although research concerning effects of positioning with children who have multiple disabilities is limited, it does suggest that positioning may influence children's interactions with their environments through a variety of mechanisms. The upright position is more likely to enhance children's opportunities for interaction with the environment than recumbent positions,[21,93] although the supine position might facilitate the development of interaction in some children with the most severe disabilities when they have the one-on-one attention of a communicative partner.

ENHANCING PARTICIPATION OF CHILDREN WITH INTELLECTUAL AND MOTOR IMPAIRMENTS

A major way to enhance the participation of children with intellectual and motor impairments is to provide them with the supports necessary to be fully involved with family, friends, and peers in least restrictive environments. The concept of least restrictive environments has its roots in the U.S. Constitution, which affirms that the government shall intrude into peoples' lives in the least restrictive manner possible.[150] Since the 1960s, this concept has been incorporated into state and federal laws affecting services for people with intellectual disabilities, mandating that, to the extent possible, people with disabilities will go to school, live, and work in environments with people who do not have disabilities.

The definition of the *least restrictive environment* for people with intellectual disabilities has been moving steadily away from segregated services and toward full inclusion in community-based settings, as evidenced by closure of many institutions for people with intellectual disabilities and court-ordered inclusion of children with intellectual disabilities in general education classrooms. In 1992, for example, a judge of the U.S. Court for the District of New Jersey ordered a New Jersey school district to develop a plan to include an 8-year-old boy with Down syndrome in his neighborhood elementary school, with any needed supplementary aids and services. One of the court's findings was that "school districts ... must consider placing children with disabilities in regular classroom settings, with the use of supplementary aids and services ... before exploring other, more restrictive, alternatives."[149] The IDEA amendments of 2004 placed additional emphasis on the need for individualized education program (IEP) teams to consider whether a child's needs could be addressed in the general education classroom with supplementary aids and services. Physical therapists often are involved in coordination and communication with other team members to decide on a child's educational placement.

Physical therapy is one of the services that must follow children with disabilities as they move into their communities and neighborhood schools. Physical therapists often must provide all three components of intervention described in the *Guide to Physical Therapist Practice*[4] (coordination, communication, and documentation; student-related instruction; and procedural interventions) to promote children's accomplishment of outcomes that will enable them to participate as successfully as possible in inclusive environments.[126] Giangreco and colleagues[55] have written a helpful "how-to" manual for inclusion of children with severe disabilities in general education classrooms that addresses provision of physical therapy and other related services. In their book, Downing and associates[38] have given practical and creative suggestions for including children with severe disabilities in typical classrooms.

TEACHING AND LEARNING CONSIDERATIONS

Much of what physical therapists do is teach children to move more effectively and efficiently. Educational researchers have identified a number of teaching strategies that optimize the learning of students with intellectual disabilities; these may be helpful to physical therapists when designing and implementing intervention plans. Although most of these strategies were designed for educational programming of students with intellectual disabilities, they can be applied to motor learning, as well as academic learning. Many of the strategies are closely related to current motor learning principles (see Chapter 4 on Motor Learning). Physical therapists should coordinate and communicate with other team members to identify opportunities for students to practice motor skills and should show parents and teachers how to promote learning during those opportunities. Physical therapists also may apply the principles during direct intervention with children.

Instruction in Natural Environments

One strategy that has received considerable attention over the past two decades and is intended to address several of the learning problems of students with intellectual disabilities, especially severe intellectual disabilities, is a focus on teaching functional skills in natural environments.[17,46] Because students with intellectual disabilities may take a long time to learn a few things, and because they have difficulty generalizing and maintaining skills, traditional curricula that build sequentially on fundamental nonfunctional skills have not generally led to meaningful gains.[38] Children are often unable to generalize such nonfunctional activities as putting pegs in pegboards, for example, to functional activities such as putting coins in a machine to get a soft drink. Practicing "prerequisite" skills, such as writing the letters of the alphabet, also often fails to result in such functional outcomes as the ability to sign one's name or select the correct restroom in a public place.

Children with severe motor impairments encounter similar difficulties when nonfunctional or presumed prerequisite skills are the focus of physical therapy. Research has largely failed to support children's generalization (carryover) of skills demonstrated during physical therapy sessions to other settings, or synthesis of presumed components and prerequisites of movement into measurable functional motor activities.[65]

When the emphasis is on acquisition of specific functional skills in natural environments, generalization is unnecessary or less difficult, and skills are likely to be maintained by natural reinforcers and ongoing occasions for practice.[113] If several people work with the child on the same skills, learning may be enhanced by providing more opportunities to learn (repetitions) and by varying the stimulus conditions under which the skill is practiced, thus promoting generalization. These principles serve as a basis for integrated models of service delivery that have been advocated for physical therapists and occupational therapists working in early intervention and public school programs.[113,126] Although limited research has been conducted to support the effectiveness of teaching motor skills in natural environments, research in other areas, such as life skills, language, and social interaction, has suggested that such an approach would be valuable.[139]

Behavioral Programming Intervention

Behavioral programming is based on the assumption that behaviors are learned through interactions with social, physical, and biologic environments; by manipulating such environments, behaviors can be taught.[15] After a review of research on the effectiveness of motor skills instruction for children with neuromotor impairments, Horn[65] concluded that physical therapists and occupational therapists should develop procedures to incorporate behavioral techniques into their intervention programs. This recommendation was made based on the relative success of interventions using behavioral techniques compared with the neuromotor and sensory stimulation techniques that occupational therapists and physical therapists commonly use. By incorporating behavioral techniques into other intervention strategies, physical therapists not only may be able to increase the rate at which children with intellectual disabilities acquire motor skills and the number of skills they acquire, but also may promote generalization and maintenance of motor behaviors.

Positive Reinforcement

A child is positively reinforced by a stimulus if a behavior that preceded the stimulus increases.[119] Possible reinforcing stimuli are unlimited, ranging from tangible items, such as food and toys, to social reinforcers, such as attention or descriptive praise, and activity reinforcers, such as watching a video.[119] With children who have intellectual disabilities, especially severe or profound intellectual disabilities, common reinforcers such as praise, access to activities, and food often fail to lead to increases in behaviors, and identification of reinforcers can be a challenge.[113] To identify potential reinforcers, Haney and Falvey[63] suggested (1) identifying natural consequences of the behavior, such as playing in water as a consequence of walking to the sink; (2) surveying the child's likes and dislikes by observing the child, or asking the child, parents, or teachers; and (3) offering paired choices to determine which of several potential reinforcers the child considers to be the most desirable. Reinforcers must not be overused because children can become satiated, and the stimuli will no longer have reinforcement value.[100]

Reinforcers, such as use of music as biofeedback to increase an erect head position,[89] and a combination of music and food to increase the distance that a child walked independently, have been effective in increasing motor behaviors.[27] A common limitation of such studies, however, is that few have examined generalization to nonexperimental settings or maintenance of behaviors beyond the period of intervention. Also, reinforcement has not been shown to result in acquisition of behaviors not previously in the child's repertoire. A combination of reinforcement with antecedent techniques and modification of consequences has, however, resulted in new behavioral responses.[65,144]

Antecedent Techniques

The first step in shaping a new behavior is to prompt the desired behavior or an approximation by providing instructions, models, cues, or physical prompts.[144] Instructions can take a variety of forms, such as verbal or gestural instructions (e.g., "Reach for the toy") or verbal instructions paired with models, cues, or physical prompts (e.g., "Reach for the toy," paired with facilitation of movement at the shoulder). Modeling provides a demonstration of a behavior that the child attempts to imitate. Cues direct a child's attention to a task that can result in the desired behavior, without a physical prompt. To cue the child to reach for the toy, the toy could be tapped on the table or held above the child to encourage an erect posture, reaching, or assuming a standing position. Many of the handling techniques used by physical therapists provide physical prompts for motor behaviors.

For optimal learning to occur, the type and amount of prompting must be matched to the skills of the child, with the least amount of help necessary being the most conducive to the child's learning.[144] Prompting should be faded as the child responds, so that natural cues eventually provide the stimulus for response. A natural cue is the least intrusive prompt (e.g., the presence of a friend serving as a cue for a child to lift the head) and is the level of prompt required for independent behaviors. Physical prompts, often used by physical therapists, are the most intrusive.

Providing Consequences

Once a behavior has been prompted, it can be improved or expanded through shaping or chaining techniques. Shaping

and chaining can also be used to build new behaviors through reinforcement of behaviors that successively approximate the desired behavior.[144]

New behaviors can be shaped by reinforcing behaviors that are increasingly similar to the target behavior, such as reinforcing components of standing up from a chair, or chaining to link standing, walking, opening doors, and other behaviors necessary to accomplish a goal of walking to lunch. Backward chaining, in which the last step in the sequence is learned first, is often a useful technique because children receive the reward of task completion, often a natural reinforcer, throughout the process of learning the skill.[144]

Behavioral intervention is one of the areas in which physical therapists should take advantage of the expertise of other members of service delivery teams, such as teachers and psychologists. Physical therapy educational prerequisites and curricula rarely provide more than superficial information about behavioral strategies, and this limits the extent to which many physical therapists can use them effectively to promote the development of motor skills by children with intellectual disabilities.

Positive Behavior Support

Positive behavior support is another approach to intervention for children with developmental disabilities, including intellectual disabilities, who may lack knowledge, communication, or the social skills necessary to function effectively in their everyday environments. Lucyshyn and colleagues[87] hypothesized that children with these limitations may develop unwanted behaviors as a means of getting their needs and wants met, and for limiting events that they find aversive. Positive behavior support interventions involve the use of methods to redesign children's social and attitudinal environments, and sometimes their physical environments, to enhance their ability to enjoy life with behaviors that are more acceptable to others. Intervention is aimed at replacing problem behaviors with more socially acceptable behaviors and making problem behaviors ineffective and undesirable.[25] Positive behavior support shows promise as an intervention that encourages participation in everyday routines without limiting children's personal preferences. The interventionist begins by observing the child in the child's everyday environments to look for antecedents that may be triggering a problem behavior, and identifying any environmental influences on the behavior.[24] The interventionist must work closely with family members or other primary care providers to develop hypotheses about causes of problem behaviors, learn what motivates the child, and develop a plan that is acceptable for the people in the environments in which the child spends time.[87] An effective plan redirects the child before the problem behavior occurs by adapting the task, the environment, or the demands.

Case studies have described the use of positive behavior support in a variety of everyday environments.[32,161] Vaughn and colleagues,[161] for example, examined positive behavior support intervention to decrease problem behaviors that a 7-year-old with intellectual disability exhibited while eating out with his family. The authors videotaped and used task analysis of the family's routines while eating out to determine any recurring antecedents and consequences of the child's behavior. With the child's mother, they developed hypotheses about the causes and functions of the behaviors, and determined activities the child most enjoyed doing that could be used as positive reinforcers while eating out. The mother, for example, theorized that the child engaged in disruptive behaviors while standing in line to order because he did not want to wait for a soft drink, which is what he wanted most when they ate out. As an intervention to reduce disruptive behavior while standing in line, the mother took a cup from home and filled it with his favorite soft drink, so he could have it while they waited to order. With the assistance of the authors, the mother also identified and used reinforcers to decrease the child's disruptive behaviors associated with other aspects of eating out, such as staying at the table to finish eating and leaving the playground equipment when it was time to go home. As measured by direct observation, the interventions were associated with both a decrease in disruptive behavior and an increase in the child's engagement. Using a similar approach, Cole and Levinson[32] found that providing choice in aspects of unpleasant tasks (such as where to stand in line) reduced occurrence of problem behaviors in two children with developmental disabilities.

Although no randomized controlled studies have examined positive behavior support, the case studies suggest that positive behavior support has promise to assist families, teachers, and other care providers in helping children with intellectual disabilities participate more successfully in everyday routines. As members of teams, physical therapists may participate in task analysis, developing an intervention plan, and using the intervention while working with children. One important aspect of positive behavior support is promoting children's communication abilities so they can express desires and needs in behaviorally acceptable ways.

PROMOTING CHILDREN'S COMMUNICATION DEVELOPMENT

When working with children who have intellectual disabilities, all team members are responsible for promoting development in areas often not considered part of their disciplinary domains. One of the most effective ways physical therapists can contribute to the overall development of children with intellectual disabilities is to assist efforts to improve their communication abilities. At its most basic level, communication enables children to influence their social and physical environments to control what happens to them. All children, even those with the most profound multiple disabilities, can communicate.[105] Some communicate in many of the same ways as infants, such as by looking at a person, crying, or smiling; others can learn to communicate using

signs, communication boards, or electronic voice-output communication aids (see also the chapter on Assistive Technology on the Evolve website). Having the ability to control what happens to themselves is often said to be the key to prevention or reduction of these children's pervasive passivity or "learned helplessness," a condition that can result in difficulty with problem solving and mastering tasks.[175]

The importance of communication and the need for all team members to participate in communication development were recognized by creation in the United States of the National Joint Committee for the Communicative Needs of Persons With Severe Disabilities. Representatives of seven organizations, including the American Physical Therapy Association, served on the joint committee and developed guidelines that cross traditional disciplinary boundaries and reflect a "shared commitment to promoting effective communication by persons with severe disabilities, thus providing a common ground on which the disciplines of the member organizations can unite their efforts to improve the quality of life of such persons" (p. 1).[105] This means that physical therapists are responsible for promoting effective communication, not only through such traditional means as positioning and improving motor skills to enable access to communication aids but also through provision of environments that acknowledge and address the Communication Bill of Rights (Figure 17-2) of children who have communication disabilities.[105]

EVALUATION OF OUTCOMES

Because children and young adults with intellectual disabilities, particularly those with severe disabilities, often progress slowly, using evaluation methods that are responsive to small changes is important. This is necessary not only to determine if progress is being made but also to prevent expenditure of time and effort on intervention strategies that are not leading to meaningful outcomes. Three related methods that are especially useful for assessing outcomes of physical therapy for children with intellectual disabilities are (1) accomplishment of behavioral objectives and goal attainment scaling, (2) use of the Canadian Occupational Performance Measure,[83] and (3) single-subject research methods.

Use of Behavioral Objectives and Goal Attainment Scaling

Assessment of outcomes can be relatively straightforward if functional goals and behavioral objectives leading to them are identified before intervention. As described by Randall and McEwen,[127] the components of behavioral objectives should enable therapists to monitor a child's progress toward accomplishment of a goal, determine if it is necessary to modify an intervention, and determine when and if goals have been met. Once a goal, such as "David will go to the kitchen and make himself a peanut butter sandwich," has been identified, behavioral objectives leading to achievement

All persons, regardless of the extent or severity of their disabilities, have a basic right to affect, through communication, the conditions of their own existence. Beyond this general right, a number of specific communication rights should be ensured in all daily interactions and interventions involving persons who have severe disabilities. These basic communication rights are as follows:

1. The right to request desired objects, actions, events, and persons and to express personal preferences or feelings.
2. The right to be offered choices and alternatives.
3. The right to reject or refuse undesired objects, events, or actions, including the right to decline or reject all proffered choices.
4. The right to request, and be given, attention from and interaction with another person.
5. The right to request feedback or information about a state, an object, a person, or an event of interest.
6. The right to active treatment and intervention efforts to enable people with severe disabilities to communicate messages in whatever modes and as effectively and efficiently as their specific abilities will allow.
7. The right to have communication acts acknowledged and responded to, even when the intent of these acts cannot be fulfilled by the responder.
8. The right to have access at all times to any needed augmentative and alternative communication devices and other assistive devices and to have those devices in good working order.
9. The right to environmental contexts, interactions, and opportunities that expect and encourage persons with disabilities to participate as full communicative partners with other people, including peers.
10. The right to be informed about the people, things, and events in one's immediate environment.
11. The right to be communicated with in a manner that recognizes and acknowledges the inherent dignity of the person being addressed, including the right to be part of communication exchanges about individuals that are conducted in his or her presence.
12. The right to be communicated with in ways that are meaningful, understandable, and culturally and linguistically appropriate.

Figure 17-2 Communication bill of rights. (From National Joint Committee for the Communication Needs of Persons with Severe Disabilities. [1992]. *Guidelines for meeting the communication needs of persons with severe disabilities.* Atlanta, GA: Author.)

of the goal can be developed by comparing David's abilities with the goal's requirements. Although the Individuals with Disabilities Education Act amendments of 2004 no longer require teams to write objectives, breaking goals down into behavioral objectives helps team members to determine if children with intellectual disabilities, who tend to change slowly, are making progress.

Behavioral objectives have five components: (1) Who will do (2) what, (3) under what condition, (4) how well, and (5) by when.[127] These components permit a measurable evaluation of whether the goal is being met within the projected time frame. One of David's behavioral objectives, leading to the sandwich-making goal, might be to move himself from the living room to the kitchen, which could be written, "David will walk using his reverse walker from the living room to the kitchen in less than 1 minute on four of five consecutive days after school by December 14, 20__." Assessing whether this objective, or part of it, is accomplished, regardless of the intervention methods used, should not be difficult.

To allow detection of smaller gains, objectives can be scaled using goal attainment scaling (GAS).[156] Starting with the objective that the child is expected to achieve, four additional objectives are determined—two that exceed the objective and two that fall below it. By identifying objectives above and below a child's anticipated achievement, a range of outcomes related to a general goal can be assessed.

As an example, David's objective (above) could be scaled by modifying the distance that he will walk, the time he takes to walk, or both. A score of 0 would represent achievement of the anticipated objective. A score of −2 would represent achievement of an objective two steps below the anticipated objective, such as "David will walk from the dining room to the kitchen in less than 2 minutes on four of five consecutive days after school by December 14, 20__." An objective one step below the anticipated objective might include walking from the living room to the kitchen in less than 2 minutes. Similarly, objectives could be written to represent accomplishments one and two steps above the anticipated objective. With five objectives, GAS has a 5-point scale (−2 to +2), which can yield a T-score that may be useful for examining the effectiveness of interventions.[156]

Canadian Occupational Performance Measure

The COPM[83] was designed to help identify and measure individually meaningful goals for people in the areas of self-care, productivity (work, household management, and play/school), and leisure. An interviewer asks patients or caregivers to think about a typical day to identify activities in these areas that they want to do, need to do, or are expected to do. The interviewer then asks which of the activities the person is able to do satisfactorily and to rate the importance of these activities on a 10-point scale. Using the importance ratings, the interviewer asks the patient or caregiver to select the five problems that seem to be the most important and asks if the activities should be the focus of intervention. After the patient or caregiver selects activities for intervention, the person rates the current performance of each on a 10-point scale, from "not able to do it at all" to "able to do it extremely well," and rates satisfaction on a 10-point scale, from "not satisfied at all" to "extremely satisfied." Performance, satisfaction, and total scores are then calculated for each activity. Following a period of intervention, outcomes can be measured by asking the patient or caregiver to again rate performance and satisfaction of each activity, and change scores can be calculated. Change scores are a useful measure of change across all goals for one child or as a measure of change across children.

Single-Subject Research Methods

Single-subject research methods are another useful means of assessing intervention outcomes in clinical, educational, and other service settings. These methods can be used to assess the outcomes for a single child or can assess effects of intervention across several children. Unlike case reports, single-subject research designs have controls that allow identification of cause–effect relationships among interventions and outcomes.[94] Several types of single-subject designs exist, including A-B, withdrawal, alternating treatment, and multiple baseline.[122] Although the designs differ, they all have certain characteristics, such as repeatedly measuring and graphing the outcome variable over time and comparing data in adjacent phases, such as baseline and intervention phases, or phases when two or more treatments are alternated.[122] Graphed data usually are first analyzed visually by comparing stability, levels, and trends in adjacent phases. Statistical analyses specific to single-subject designs also can be used, such as the two standard deviation bandwidth method and testing the significance of trends in adjacent phases using the split-middle line.[122]

Many examples of single-subject research exist in rehabilitation literature. Meiser and McEwen,[99] for example, used an A-B-A single-subject design to compare the effect of ultralight and lightweight wheelchairs on the preference and propulsion of two young girls with myelodysplasia. Nearly all of the measured propulsion variables favored the ultralight wheelchairs, and the children and their mothers preferred them. Thorpe and Valvano[155] used a single-subject multiple baseline design across 13 children with cerebral palsy to examine effects of application of motor learning principles on the children's performance of a novel task. Fragala and colleagues[52] used an A-B design across seven children to determine the effect of botulinum toxin A injections on children's passive range of motion, Modified Ashworth Scale scores, and the COPM. Reid and colleagues[129] used an A-B-A (withdrawal) design with six children to identify the effect of a wheelchair-mounted rigid pelvic stabilizer (RPS) compared with a traditional wheelchair lap belt on task performance and satisfaction with performance as measured by the COPM. Textbooks and research articles are good resources for anyone interested in using single-subject research methods to measure outcomes of intervention. The classic text by Barlow and Hersen[9] and the chapter on single-subject methods in the text by Portney and Watkins[122] are excellent resources.

TRANSITION TO ADULTHOOD

Some people with intellectual disabilities, especially those with severe and profound multiple disabilities, may receive physical therapy throughout their childhood years and during their transition to adulthood. Others will receive short episodes of physical therapy services as their abilities and needs change over time. The types of services provided, the intensity of services, and the model of service delivery should be individualized to the needs of the person. Therapists working in public schools are especially likely to be involved in the transition to adulthood because Part B of IDEA requires that transition planning begin by at least age 16 for all students with disabilities. The role of physical therapists, along with other IEP and interagency team members, should be to enable students to function meaningfully and as independently as possible in their current and possible future environments. See Chapter 32 for more information.

The transition to adulthood is difficult for many young people, regardless of their abilities or disabilities. Until recently, most young adults with intellectual and neuromotor impairments had few options available to them, and the greater their intellectual disabilities, the fewer options they had. Employment options did not exist or were limited to sheltered workshops or activity centers. Residential options usually included staying at home with aging parents or moving into a large residential facility. Young people also had few choices about how they spent their time, with whom they spent time, or where they could go.

In recent years, more employment and community life options have become available for people with severe intellectual disabilities, including those with the most severe multiple disabilities. To be able to take full advantage of these options, young people need to prepare for transition to adult life throughout their years in school, and then should continue to receive support as the transition takes place and the new life begins. Physical therapy often can make a difference in the options available to young people with both intellectual and neuromotor disabilities as they make the transition to adult life and in the success of their transitions. Self-determination and employment are particularly important for most young people.

SELF-DETERMINATION

Youth with disabilities often have difficulty achieving goals that their peers without disabilities achieve relatively easily, such as independent living, higher education, and employment. Teaching and supporting self-determination have been proposed to be important for improving outcomes for youth with disabilities, including youth with intellectual disabilities. Wehmeyer and Bolding[170] defined self-determination at the personal level as "having control over one's life and destiny" (p. 372). Self-determination has four parts: freedom, control over one's own life, support, and responsibility. Each of these parts is defined in Box 17-5.

People exhibit self-determination by making everyday decisions and life decisions for themselves.[170] In a review of the self-determination literature, Malian and Nevin[88] found six curricula for teaching self-determination skills that have been field-tested. Overall, the studies suggested that direct instruction in self-determination skills can lead to positive changes in the knowledge, attitudes, and behaviors associated with self-determination. Wehmeyer and Schwartz[171] examined the relationship between scores on a self-determination rating scale and outcomes of youth with mental retardation or learning disabilities 1 year after leaving school. In their sample of 80 participants, students with higher scores on a self-determination rating scale were more likely to be employed and earn more per hour than students who achieved lower scores on the self-determination rating scale.

Wehmeyer and Bolding[169,170] also studied the relationship between environment and self-determination. In one study, they matched adults by intelligence, age, and gender to examine the relationship between living and working environments and self-determination. They found that those living or working in general community-based settings reported greater self-determination and autonomous function than matched peers living or working in segregated community-based settings or non–community-based segregated settings. This study suggested that environments and, in particular, inclusive community environments were important for greater self-determination and autonomy for people with intellectual disabilities. Wehmeyer and Bolding[170] also studied change in self-determination with changes in work or living environments. When 31 people moved from

Box 17-5   SELF-DETERMINATION

Self-determination is the ability for people to control their lives, reach goals they have set, and take part fully in the world around them. Self-determination has four basic rights and responsibilities:

Freedom. Freedom for Americans with disabilities is like freedom for any American. It means deciding for oneself about how to work, live, and love; direct one's life; and give to the community; as well as deciding what kinds of services and supports to use (if any).

People who experience disability do not have to accept segregated schooling, institutional placement, service slots, or forced treatment of any kind.

Authority or control of own life. Americans with disabilities have the right to direct their lives. This includes having control over how to spend their money, having the right to vote, being able to sign legal contracts, and being able to decide how funds available for support services will be spent.

Support agreements must be developed together by individuals and funders. Funds must be assigned to individuals rather than slots. People with disabilities must be allowed to use those funds to purchase the supports they require. They also must be able to personally select (hire) and direct people who provide support or assistance.

Support. People with disabilities may desire support/assistance to care for themselves and be an active part of their communities.

Each person who experiences disability can determine the supports that work for him or her. People with disabilities (together with those they trust, if they want) have the right to figure out their life goals, what kinds of supports might work, and how to make and keep track of plans and budgets.

Those who assist people with disabilities will work toward bringing support and access to life opportunities at the highest potential.

Independent brokers must be available to assist people in designing, setting up, and managing their supports. Fiscal intermediaries must be available to assist with employment paperwork and bill paying. Both must work at the direction of the person with a disability and must be free from conflicts of interest.

Responsibility. People with disabilities have the responsibility to fulfill the ordinary obligations of citizenship like voting, obeying laws, directing their own lives, and participating in community life.

Policy barriers must be removed when they prevent people who earn money from receiving health insurance, personal assistance, or other needed supports.

From The Oregon Health & Science University Center on Self-Determination. Retrieved from http://www.selfdeterminationohsu.org/about/ index.html a restrictive environment (such as a nursing home or sheltered workshop) to a less restrictive environment, self-determination increased when compared with pre-move test scores.

Physical therapists can help children with intellectual disabilities to develop self-determination. This is best accomplished through a team approach that identifies priorities for the child and family and considers the environments in which the child does or will spend time. Self-determination is something that does not start in adolescence. It needs to begin early, with young children being offered opportunities to make choices in any way they are able to indicate preferences. Older children should be expected to be responsible for their choices, and young adults should be expected to thoughtfully decide what is best for them, and then others should support their choices.

EMPLOYMENT

Employment options in the United States for people with intellectual disabilities and multiple disabilities have expanded greatly over the past several years, particularly in some parts of the country. Many places still offer primarily sheltered workshop and activity center alternatives, but progress is being made nationwide as federal, state, and other public and private initiatives support development and expansion of employment opportunities for people with disabilities.[31]

Supported employment, one model of employment services, has been responsible for increasing the employment options for many people who have severe disabilities. Rather than working on prerequisite or prevocational skills in sheltered settings until they are "ready" for a job, people in supported employment learn real jobs while they are doing them, with ongoing support from team members to learn and maintain the job.[49]

Since the early 1980s, supported employment has been gaining credibility as a viable employment option and has received significant support from the Vocational Rehabilitation Act Amendments of 1986 (PL 99-506), which authorized new funds for states to provide supported employment services to people with severe disabilities. As yet, however, few communities offer a supported employment alternative to sheltered workshops and day activity centers for those with the most severe disabilities. The economic value of supported employment was documented by Cimera,[31] who studied the cost-efficiency of supported employment programs and found that (1) supported employment is a cost-efficient way to serve people with severe intellectual and multiple disabilities; (2) supported employment is cost-efficient from the cost-accounting perspective of the client, the taxpayer, and society; and (3) projections of lifelong benefits suggested that all individuals, regardless of the severity or number of disabilities, can be served cost-effectively in supported employment.

Physical therapists often have a pivotal role in the successful employment of individuals who have both intellectual disabilities and limited motor skills. Physical therapists can assist employment specialists to assess an individual's abilities to perform job-related motor skills and to identify jobs that are compatible with those skills. They can also identify assistive technology and environmental modifications that may enable the person to perform a job that might not be possible otherwise. Physical therapists can also help develop training for job-related motor skills and for self-care and mobility during working hours.

SUMMARY

Regardless of their medical diagnoses, children with intellectual disabilities have learning characteristics that physical therapists need to consider for effective physical therapy management. Compared with typically developing children, children with intellectual disabilities have been shown, for example, to be able to learn a lesser number of things, to need a greater number of repetitions for learning to occur, to have greater difficulty generalizing skills from one environment to another, to have greater difficulty maintaining skills that are not practiced regularly, to have slower response times, and to have a more limited repertoire of responses. Physical therapy intervention strategies that address these learning characteristics and that promote communication, inclusion, and self-determination can have an important role in the meaningful participation of people with intellectual and motor disabilities in the lives of their families and communities. Whatever the future of children with intellectual and neuromotor disabilities, physical therapy services can often help expand the options, ease the transition, and promote independence within the community-based environments in which people choose to live and work.

CASE STUDIES

"Liz"

Liz is a 6-year-old girl with Down syndrome. She lives in an upstairs apartment with her 3-year-old sister and her mother. Liz was born eight weeks prematurely and had heart surgery to correct a septal defect at 5 months of age. She had a gastrostomy tube placed because of feeding difficulties and poor weight gain; Liz was removed at 18 months of age. Liz is again scheduled for heart surgery at the end of this school semester for valve repair.

Liz received early intervention services from infancy until she was 18 months of age. She received services under the transdisciplinary model; a developmental specialist came to the home on a weekly basis with programming structured to include communication, feeding, social, and motor development.

Liz entered an early childhood program at her local public school when she turned 3 years. Her first school experience was in a classroom with other children who had similar disabilities. She received speech therapy with her classroom group, and a physical therapist and an occupational therapist consulted with her mother and teacher about activities to improve gross and fine motor skills.

Liz now attends a general education kindergarten classroom for 2 hours a day, with the rest of her 7-hour school day spent in a self-contained special education classroom. She does not receive physical therapy at school, but participates with her peers in a structured motor group twice a week. Recently, her mother became concerned with her frequent falling, difficulty with stairs, and poor endurance. Because she believes it is important for Liz to spend her time at school on academics and socialization, she has arranged for Liz to receive physical therapy in her home after school, provided by a private agency.

Liz walks independently, can climb on and off furniture, and runs for short distances when playing. She falls when trying to increase her running speed and when running distances greater than 25 yards. Liz has hypotonia, poor strength, and hypermobility/laxity in most joints. Her gait pattern is with lumbar lordosis, a wide base of support, and poor foot clearance during the swing phase. Liz is easily distracted and falls frequently outdoors when activity, noises, or people divert her attention.

The physical therapist assessed Liz in her home to establish a baseline of current abilities and functioning and to determine a plan of care and recommendations (refer to video). The therapist used the Gross Motor Function Measure (GMFM),[137] which is an observation-based, criterion-referenced, standardized tool that yields a percentage score, with 100% being motor skill acquisition of a typical 5-year-old child. The GMFM was developed for children with cerebral palsy, but has been shown to be responsive to change in children with Down syndrome.[136] The GMFM was administered with distractions present, in a small living room in the family apartment. The items were given out of sequence to maximize her interest and cooperation, as Gemus et al.[54] recommended for testing children with Down syndrome. Liz needed frequent directions and demonstration to complete the tasks on the test. The test measures skills in the following five domains (Liz's scores are in parentheses): Lying and Rolling (98%), Sitting (95%), Crawling and Kneeling (83%), Standing (79%), the Walking, Running, and Jumping (71%). Liz's scores reflect her achievement of motor skills in lower positions and her difficulty with motor skills that require increased strength, balance, and motor coordination. Her summary score of 85% is close to the predicted maximum of 86% to 88% outlined by Palisano et al.[116] in an analysis of motor development curves for children with Down syndrome.

EVIDENCE TO PRACTICE 17-1

EXAMINATION DECISION

Two examination tools were chosen for Liz. The decision to use the Gross Motor Function Measure (GMFM) was supported by a study that Russell and colleagues conducted.[5] They used the GMFM with children with Down syndrome and found test-retest and interrater reliability to be >0.90. They also found the GMFM to be responsive to change in children with Down syndrome when incorporating parent report of children's skills into the scoring and not requiring the examiner to observe every skill. Pearson product moment correlations between total GMFM scores and judgments of change by parents, intervenors, and videotaped analysis were between 0.16 (parents) and 0.29 (video analysis) when scores were based on observation only. When parent report was incorporated into scoring, correlation coefficients increased to between 0.30 (intervenor) and 0.34 (video analysis). For this reason, the researchers recommended incorporating parent report into scoring when using the GMFM with children with Down syndrome. The researchers also administered the Bayley Scales of Infant Development-II and found that the GMFM was more responsive to change.[5]

The testing procedure incorporated modifications as outlined by Gemus and colleagues,[2] who found the test to be reliable when administration was modified to enhance testing for children with Down syndrome. Strategies included using imitation as a supplement to simple verbal instructions, incorporating parent feedback, and giving credit for lower items on the scale that required the same motor behaviors as a higher item.

Continued

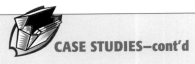

CASE STUDIES—cont'd

EVIDENCE TO PRACTICE 17-1—cont'd

The Pediatric Evaluation of Disability Inventory (PEDI)[3] was chosen as an additional tool to provide information on Liz's capabilities and performance in routine daily activities. The decision to use the PEDI is supported by numerous studies examining the internal consistency, test-retest, and discriminative validity of the PEDI.[1,4] Moreover, the PEDI provides normative standards for children ages 6 months to 7.5 years. The PEDI, given in an interview format with Liz's mother, helped identify areas of concern.

Plan of Care Decision: The plan of care for Liz was guided by multiple factors. Her mother's concerns about safety on apartment stairs and inability to manage community environments influenced the decision to provide physical therapy to establish a home program directed at underlying impairments and increasing participation. Motor development curves created by Palisano and colleagues[9] indicated that Liz is close to achieving expected motor abilities, supporting the decision to establish a home program rather than provide ongoing physical therapy. Research evidence to support specific treatment protocols to address Liz's identified needs is not available. Given Liz's age and cognitive abilities, incorporating strengthening and practice into everyday, routine activities[6] would provide her with multiple opportunities to develop the necessary components to manage stairs and uneven environments.

An additional component to the plan of care is helping Liz's mother access community resources. An increasing body of literature suggests use of community recreation opportunities to develop physical and mental health while building social competence. Rosenberg[10] discussed the increased willingness and availability of community-based resources for children with disabilities. Although studies of the effectiveness of community options for motor development and impairments is limited, a few community options have been explored that support the development of motor skills and physical well-being. A systematic review of studies measuring the effects of yoga showed preliminary support for benefits for children with disabilities,[8] and aquatic exercise produced positive cardiorespiratory benefits and increased endurance in children with disabilities.[7]

Family Preferences: Liz's mother prefers that Liz concentrate on academics and socialization while at school. The IEP team decided to focus on these areas and not on Liz's motor skills. Liz's mother is concerned with Liz's motor development and is interested in receiving physical therapy at home. She is reluctant to allow Liz to participate in community programs and will need support and

encouragement to consider these options. As a single mother, she has limited financial resources. State insurance financing will pay for physical therapy, but does not pay for most community-based recreation programs. Law and colleagues identified economic status as one of the factors affecting involvement in recreational programs.[12] The physical therapist will work with a social worker and the family to pursue appropriate and affordable community options. It is reasonable to expect that Liz will be capable of participating in recreational activities. Carr[11] found that more than two thirds of adults with Down syndrome in the United Kingdom, followed longitudinally from a young age, participated in at least one recreational sport.

1. Feldman, A., Haley, S. M., & Coryell, J. (1990). Concurrent and construct validity of the Pediatric Evaluation of Disability Inventory. *Physical Therapy, 3*, 177–184.
2. Gemus, M., Palisano, R., Russell, D., et al. (2001). Using the Gross Motor Function Measure to evaluate motor development in children with Down syndrome. *Physical & Occupational Therapy in Pediatrics, 21*, 69–79.
3. Haley, S. M., Coster, W. J., Ludlow, L. H., Haltiwanger, J., & Andrellos, P. (1992). *Pediatric evaluation of disability inventory (PEDI): Development, standardization, and administration manual.* Boston, MA: PEDI Research Group.
4. Nichols, D. S., & Case-Smith, J. (1996). Reliability and validity of the Pediatric Evaluation of Disability Inventory. *Pediatric Physical Therapy, 3*, 177–184.
5. Russell, D., Palisano, R., Walter, S., et al. (1998). Evaluating motor function in children with Down syndrome: Validity of the GMFM. *Developmental Medicine and Child Neurology, 40*, 693–701.
6. Dunst, C. J., Bruder, M. B., Trivette, C. M., et al. (2001). Characteristics and consequences of everyday natural learning opportunities. *Topics in Early Childhood Special Education, 21*, 68–92.
7. Fragala-Pinkham, M., Haley, S. M., O'Neil, M. E. (2008). Group aquatic aerobic exercise for children with disabilities. *Developmental Medicine & Child Neurology, 50*, 822–827.
8. Galantino, M. L., Galhavy, R., & Quinn, L. (2008). Therapeutic effects of yoga for children: A systematic review of the literature. *Pediatric Physical Therapy, 20*, 66–80.
9. Palisano, R. J., Walter, S. D., Russell, D. J., et al. (2001). Gross motor function of children with Down syndrome: Creation of motor growth curves. *Archives of Physical Medicine & Rehabilitation, 82*, 494–500.
10. Rosenberg, A. E. (2000). Conducting an inventory of informal community-based resources for children with physical disabilities: Enhancing access and creating professional linkages. *Physical & Occupational Therapy in Pediatrics, 20*, 59–79.
11. Carr, J. (2007). The everyday life of adults with Down syndrome. *Journal of Applied Research in Intellectual Disability, 21*, 389–397.
12. Law, M., King, G., King, S., et al. (2006). Patterns of participation in recreational and leisure activities among children with complex physical disabilities. *Developmental Medicine and Child Neurology, 48*, 337–342.

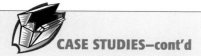

CASE STUDIES—cont'd

The Pediatric Evaluation of Disability Inventory (PEDI)[62] also was administered to provide information on Liz's functional capability and performance in her home and familiar environments, as well as to measure change following intervention. The PEDI is a norm-referenced assessment given in a structured interview format and developed for children with disabilities to provide information on functional capability and performance. The PEDI has shown content and construct validity for children aged 6 months to 7.5 years.[43] The PEDI assesses functional abilities in three content areas (Liz's standard scores are in parentheses; the mean score for typical children her age is 50, with a standard deviation of 10): Self-Care (31.4), Mobility (<10), and Social Function (24.1). Liz's Self-Care scores are within two standard deviations of the mean achieved by typical children, but her Social Function and Mobility skills are significantly delayed compared with those of typically developing children. The PEDI also measures Caregiver Assistance in the same areas and gives standard scores relative to the amount of assistance required by typical peers. Liz's standard scores for Caregiver Assistance were similar to her functional skills: Self-Care Caregiver Assistance 29.3, Mobility Caregiver Assistance <10, and Social Function Caregiver Assistance 24.4.

During the examination, Liz's mother expressed concerns about Liz's endurance, balance, and safety. She identified the stairs and uneven outdoor environments as problematic and requested that therapy focus on these concerns. Liz lives in an apartment complex with steep, open-back stairs. Her younger sister ascends and descends the exterior stairs swiftly and without assistance, whereas Liz requires close supervision, frequent assistance, and extra time to manage the stairs. Her mother would also like to improve Liz's ability to manage community environments. She reports that Liz is unable to keep up with her 3-year-old sister, making it difficult to take both girls out to the store, park, and other public settings.

Physical therapy intervention will focus on improving underlying strength and balance impairments by establishing a home exercise and activity program to help address Liz's mother's identified goals and concerns. Physical therapy will take place in Liz's natural environment of her apartment, the surrounding outside area, and community locations frequented by the family.[40] Strategies will include play, imitation, specific practice on the apartment stairs, and providing multiple opportunities to apply learned skills in different situations. Liz's mother will be encouraged to embed similar activities throughout Liz's day. Liz's younger sister will also join in the physical therapy session to provide both peer modeling and social interaction.

Progress toward goals will be monitored monthly and discharge considered when she meets them. The PEDI and GMFM will be re-administered at that time to measure change and help identify any new areas of concern.

After discussing results of the assessment, the physical therapist and Liz's mother agreed to explore recreational opportunities to help Liz develop her motor skills. The physical therapist will encourage Liz's mother to allow Liz to participate in local recreation activities such as swimming, dance, yoga, soccer, or karate to provide community options to develop both her motor capabilities and social interaction. In addition to her mother's hesitancy to involve Liz with typically developing children because she is afraid they will tease her, economic restraints influence the family's ability to pay for and participate in recreational programs.[84] The therapist will work closely with the family and a social worker to provide suitable and affordable opportunities for Liz's motor development, which should allow direct physical therapy services to be discontinued as recreational activities to address her motor development needs. It is likely that Liz will learn to move safely and efficiently in multiple environments and will develop the ability to participate in social and recreational play and sports.[25]

"Amy"

Amy's case illustrates an application of the Guide to Physical Therapist Practice[4] for a child with intellectual disability in a public school setting. The process for "patient/client management" described in the Guide is not always consistent with the team-oriented process used for making decisions about physical therapy services in schools. The terms patient and client also are inappropriate for school-based practice, where physical therapists usually refer to children as students or children. Notes throughout the case example indicate other variations in the process described in the Guide that are necessary to provide appropriate school-based services.

Based on prior knowledge of Amy, the physical therapist identified the preferred practice pattern as Neuromuscular Pattern 5C: Impaired Motor Function and Sensory Integrity Associated With Nonprogressive Disorders of the Central Nervous System—Congenital Origin or Acquired in Infancy or Childhood. Information about Amy and the process that her school team used to develop her IEP is summarized as follows, according to the Guide's five elements of patient/client (student) management.

Examination History

General demographics: Amy is an 8-year-old girl. English is her family's native language.

Social history: Amy lives with her mother, father, and 12-year-old brother. Her mother is a nurse, and her father owns a heating and air conditioning company. Amy participates in many family activities, such as church, camping, and car trips during the summer.

Employment/work (job/school/play): Amy is in a general third grade class in her neighborhood elementary school, where she, her teacher, and a classroom assistant receive supports and services from a special education teacher, physical therapist, occupational therapist, and speech/language pathologist. For special education eligibility purposes, Amy is classified as having multiple disabilities.

Growth and development: When Amy was about 6 months old, her mother became concerned because she did not seem to look at

Continued

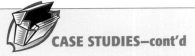

CASE STUDIES—cont'd

people and objects, did not reach for objects, and could not roll over. When she was 8 months old, Amy was diagnosed with spastic quadriplegic cerebral palsy. The most recent norm-referenced developmental test was administered when she was 5 years old. At that time, her age-equivalent scores on the Battelle Developmental Inventory[109] were personal-social, 7 months; adaptive, 5 months; motor, 4 months; communication, 6 months; and intellectual, 5 months. Her severe delay has been established and her school team believes that further norm-referenced testing would not be helpful. Amy weighs 35 pounds and is below the 3rd percentile for weight and height. A report of a nutrition evaluation 6 months ago indicated that Amy was adequately nourished but recommended increasing the amount of calcium and protein in her diet.

Living environment: Amy lives with her parents and brother in a one-story house. The family has a van with a lift for Amy's wheelchair. She also has a bath seat, an upright stander, a four-location communication board, and a Big Mac switch to activate battery-powered toys and devices.

General health status: Amy's health generally is good, although she usually gets pneumonia at least once a year. Her seizure disorder is well controlled with medication. She usually sleeps through the night if someone turns her once.

Social/health habits: Amy moves very little, leading to a low level of physical fitness, which puts her at risk for cardiopulmonary disease as she grows older.

Family history: Not known.

Medical/surgical history: When Amy was 5 years old, she underwent bilateral Achilles tendon and adductor lengthening. Two years later, she had a right varus derotation osteotomy for a subluxed hip.

Current condition(s)/chief complaints: Amy received home-based early intervention services, including physical therapy, from age 9 months to 3 years. From age 3 to 5 years, she was in a half-day neighborhood preschool program, where she received physical therapy, occupational therapy, special education, and speech/language pathology services provided by her school district. When she was 5 years old, she entered her neighborhood kindergarten, and since that time she has been included in general education classes.

Note: The Guide says that the "current condition/chief complaint" should include "patient/client, family, significant other, and caregiver expectation and goals for the therapeutic intervention." Although families may have expectations for physical therapy at this step in the process, a more appropriate process for school-age children is for the child's team, including the family, to identify overall educational goals for the child, then later determine if physical therapy is necessary to achieve those goals.[55]

Amy's parents said that they were concerned because Amy is so passive, does so little, and seems interested in so few things. They have three priorities for her education: (1) that she learn to choose things, people, and activities that she wants; (2) that she become someone that other people like to be with because one of the things she seems to enjoy is being with other children; and (3) that she learn to help more during caregiving activities because she is becoming heavier and more difficult to handle and move.

Functional status and activity level: Amy will look when her name is called, smiles when people she likes talk with her, and enjoys being around other children. She often will close her eyes and drop her head when she does not have the attention of other people. Amy cannot grasp objects, but occasionally will reach toward objects. She eats ground foods fed from a spoon and drinks liquids from a cup. She cannot sit alone or roll over and is dependent on others for all self-care and mobility.

Medications: Amy takes Dilantin twice a day for seizures.

Systems Review

Anatomic and physiologic status: Amy's severe neurologic impairments are likely to influence her cardiopulmonary, integumentary, and musculoskeletal status, which must be kept in mind when identifying goals and interventions. Her anatomic and physiologic status also may require consultation with or referral to a physician.

Communication, affect, cognition, language, and learning style: Amy is a passive child whose communication and intellectual development are far below those of typical 8-year-olds.

Tests and measures: Note: In a school environment, members of students' educational teams other than the physical therapist often administer tests and measures to examine some of the areas listed in the Guide. All team members then share results when developing the IEP. Some information was gathered formally using standardized methods, such as range of motion measurements. Because of Amy's severe limitations, the School Function Measure[35] and other developmental and functional tools were unlikely to be useful, so much of the information was based on observation or prior knowledge. Other students' teams might have different expertise and be responsible for different areas. An occupational therapist on another team, for example, may know more about swallowing than a speech/language pathologist, or a physical therapist may know more about sensory integration than an occupational therapist.

Evaluation: The team met to discuss the information that each contributed to the development of Amy's IEP. Amy has many impairments, activity limitations, and participation restrictions, most of which the team agreed will not improve with intervention. The team also agreed that Amy's parents' concerns should be priorities in determining Amy's IEP goals. The physical therapist expressed concern that range of motion examination indicated that Amy's hip and knee range had decreased since the last measurements, taken 3 months previously.

Diagnosis/classification: The physical therapist used the Gross Motor Function Classification System (expanded and revised)[116] to identify a diagnosis/classification. Amy was functioning at the most limited level, Level V: Self-Mobility Is Severely Limited Even with the Use of Assistive Technology. This diagnosis is not used for special education and related services purposes.

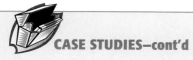

CASE STUDIES—cont'd

EVIDENCE TO PRACTICE 17-2

CASE STUDY "AMY"

CLASSIFICATION DECISION

The decision to use the Gross Motor Function Classification System (GMFCS) to classify Amy's gross motor function is supported by a 1997 study by Palisano and colleagues,[3] which estimated interrater agreement (kappa) to be 0.86 for classification of children over age 2 years at level V.[3] The decision also is supported by 2006 research of Palisano and colleagues, which found that classifications were stable over time, with agreement (kappa) between first and last ratings of 0.89 for children age 6 years and over.[1] The mean time between ratings was 33.5 months, and children classified at levels I and V were the least likely to be reclassified over time. In 2008, Palisano and colleagues published a revised and expanded GMFCS, which clarified the 6- to 12-year age band and distinctions among levels.[2]

Prognosis Decision: The GMFCS indicated that Amy is functioning at Level V, defined as severely limited self-mobility even with the use of assistive technology. In a longitudinal study, Rosenbaum and colleagues administered the Gross Motor Function Measure-66 to children with cerebral palsy every 6 to 12 months for up to 4 years.[4] From the data, they created gross motor development curves that predicted the rate and level of motor development, as measured by the GMFM-66, of children classified at each GMFCS level. Based on these curves, children at level V can be expected to achieve 90% of their maximum GMFM-66 score by an average age of 2.7 years and to achieve an average maximum GMFM-66 score of 22.3. Based on this research, the therapist did not anticipate that Amy's basic gross motor skills would

develop further and focused on functional goals that she could achieve with her current gross motor abilities.

Intervention Decision: A review of research by Chung and colleagues concluded that evidence for the effectiveness of adapted seating in postural control, posture, or function in children with cerebral palsy is limited.[5] Although research evidence does not support the intervention, but does not indicate it is not effective, Amy's team decided to use Amy's adapted wheelchair as her primary positioning device at school. They observed that she is able to maintain a more erect posture when she is seated in her adapted wheelchair than when seated in other types of chairs, and that she seems to engage in more activities when seated in her adapted wheelchair than when in other positioning devices. Regardless of the availability of research evidence, responses of individual children to interventions need to be observed and measured to determine their effectiveness.

1. Palisano, R. J., Cameron, D., Rosenbaum, P. L., et al. (2006). Stability of the gross motor function classification system. *Developmental Medicine & Child Neurology, 48,* 424–428.
2. Palisano, R. J., Rosenbaum, P., Bartlett, D., et al. (2008). Content validity of the expanded and revised Gross Motor Function Classification System. *Developmental Medicine & Child Neurology, 50,* 744–750.
3. Palisano, R., Rosenbaum, P., Walter, S., et al. (1997). Development and reliability of a system to classify gross motor function in children with cerebral palsy. *Developmental Medicine & Child Neurology, 39,* 214–223.
4. Rosenbaum, P. L., Walter, S. D., Hanna, S. E., et al. (2002). Prognosis for gross motor function in cerebral palsy: Creation of motor development curves. *Journal of the American Medical Association, 288,* 1357–1363.
5. Chung, J., Evans, J., Lee, C., Lee J., et al. (2008). Effectiveness of adaptive seating on sitting posture and postural control in children with cerebral palsy. *Pediatric Physical Therapy, 20,* 303–317.

Prognosis: The physical therapist and the rest of the team agreed that the prognosis for improving Amy's primary neuromuscular impairments was poor,[134] but the prognosis for preventing secondary musculoskeletal impairments was more hopeful. The prognosis for improving activities also was poor, but the team agreed that with consistent and appropriate instruction, Amy probably could learn to help herself more, as her parents wished. Because participation does not necessarily require motor performance,[173] Amy's participation in many activities was limited only by the creativity of others who could support her involvement in various life situations.

Plan of Care

Note: The Guide states that as the next step in the prognostic process, the physical therapist should develop the plan of care,

which includes "specific interventions, proposed frequency and duration of the interventions, anticipated goals, expected outcomes, and discharge plans." In the educational environment, physical therapists do not make these decisions unilaterally. With the physical therapist's input, the team, including the student when appropriate, determines all of these elements when developing a student's IEP. In schools, the term plan of care is not used, but the IEP serves a similar purpose.

Amy's team wrote the following goals for her IEP in September:
• Amy will indicate her choice of a person, activity, or object at least 10 times each day at school and 10 times at home for 5 consecutive days by May 20.
• When engaged in an activity with her classmates, Amy will interact with them by such means as looking at them, smiling, reaching, or

Continued

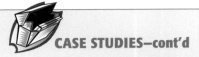

CASE STUDIES—cont'd

vocalizing for at least 3 of 10 minutes during two activities on 5 consecutive school days by May 20.

- Amy will assist in transferring from her wheelchair by leaning forward when touched on the shoulder and asked to stand up, and then will bear her full weight after being assisted to a standing position during 10 consecutive transfers from her wheelchair by May 20.

The team then wrote a sequence of short-term instructional objectives leading to each goal (not mentioned in the Guide or required by IDEA 2004, but helpful for tracking progress in children with severe disabilities). After writing the objectives, the team decided who would be necessary to help Amy achieve each objective and what each would contribute. The team also identified the general supports that Amy needs to attend school and to achieve her goals. Giangreco and associates[55] described five categories of general supports, including supports needed to meet personal, physical, and sensory needs; to teach others about the student; and to provide the student with access and opportunities. The supports identified for Amy were as follows:

- Personal: feeding, diaper changing, and other self-care
- Physical: positioning and mobility
- Sensory: avoiding intense stimuli, which cause Amy to withdraw
- Teaching: teaching other children about Amy, her means of communication, and how to help her participate in activities
- Access: promoting hand use during classroom activities

The team decided that her educational goals could best be met in a general education classroom, with supplemental aids and services. They agreed that not only was a segregated special education setting unnecessarily restrictive, but that a general education classroom was more likely to provide the social and educational environment necessary to help Amy accomplish her goals. Supplemental aids and services in the general education classroom include a half-time assistant assigned to the classroom and ongoing consultation between Amy's classroom teacher and her special education team (a resource teacher, an occupational therapist, a physical therapist, and a speech/language pathologist).

The team decided that Amy's physical therapist was needed to help her achieve the third goal, involving transfers, and with the physical supports of positioning and mobility. The therapist also would help with motor aspects of other goals and would consult with the physical education teacher about how to include Amy in activities that are meaningful for her. The physical therapist proposed and the team agreed that the physical therapist would see Amy and her classroom staff (teachers and classroom assistant) for 1 hour three times a week for the first 2 weeks of school, twice a week for the next 2 weeks, then once a week for 3 months, and then twice a month until the end of the school year. Over the school year, the physical therapist would provide 32 hours of service, or 32 "visits" (a term not used on an IEP).

Intervention

Physical therapists working in schools provide (1) coordination, communication, and documentation; (2) student-related instruction; and (3) procedural interventions, as delineated in the Guide. To provide the necessary positioning and mobility supports, the physical therapist first determined that Amy's wheelchair was adequate for her needs. She also consulted with Amy's classroom teacher to determine which alternatives to wheelchair positioning would be used during which activities and who would be responsible for position changes (procedural intervention). Positions and activities were matched to enable Amy to function as well as possible throughout the day. She uses a supine stander, for example, during a morning science class, which usually involves groups of students standing around tables as they work on a project together. She also stands in the afternoon during art class because her hand use seems to be better when she is standing.

The therapist taught the teacher and assistant how to place Amy in her wheelchair and other positioning devices (student-related instruction), about some of the basic mechanics of the wheelchair, and how to push the chair safely. She also taught Amy's classmates how to push Amy safely and issued wheelchair pushing licenses to those who demonstrated safe pushing techniques (student-related instruction). Other supports provided by the physical therapist were to teach Amy's teacher, the assistant, and her classmates some ways to encourage Amy to raise her head and use her hands during classroom activities, and to teach the assistant methods to use during caregiving activities, especially diaper changing, to help maintain Amy's joint flexibility (student-related instruction). The assistant also used diaper changing, when Amy was supine, as an opportunity to teach basic social interaction skills (facilitating Amy's interaction and then responding contingently).

To help Amy achieve the goal of assisting with transfers, the physical therapist first worked with Amy to identify how best to help her to learn (direct intervention). She found that, although Amy could perform some aspects of a transfer, such as lean forward to prepare to stand, she usually would not, either spontaneously or when asked. She also did not place her feet on the floor as she was moved toward a standing position and did not bear her weight when placed on her feet. To teach Amy to assist with these components of the transfer, the physical therapist consulted with the special education resource teacher to develop a behavioral program. The program included (1) providing verbal and natural cues for a transfer (such as the presence of the supine stander), physical prompts, and reinforcement for leaning forward in her wheelchair, a motor behavior that was already within Amy's repertoire; (2) providing cues, physical prompts, and reinforcement during practice to learn to place her feet on the floor and bear increasing amounts of weight during transfers and other activities, to shape these skills, which were not yet within Amy's

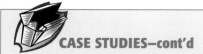

CASE STUDIES—cont'd

repertoire; (3) chaining the various components of the transfer, as Amy began to learn each one; and (4) eventually fading the verbal cues and physical prompts to permit the natural cues surrounding transfers to prompt Amy's participation.

After she was reasonably sure that the program developed to teach Amy to lean forward was effective, the physical therapist taught Amy's teacher, the classroom assistant, and her parents to implement the techniques whenever Amy transferred (student-related instruction). Because Amy had not demonstrated the ability to place her feet on the floor and bear her weight in standing, the physical therapist worked with Amy during transfers and other classroom activities to determine how best to provide physical prompts and other cues and to teach Amy to begin to learn to stand (direct intervention). She then taught Amy's teacher, the assistant, and her parents how to help Amy continue to develop this skill (student-related instruction).

Re-examination

Part B of IDEA requires that each short-term objective have an evaluation procedure and a schedule for evaluation to determine progress toward goals and objectives. This is consistent with the "reexamination" step of the Guide. The physical therapist and the rest of Amy's team continuously observed her performance to evaluate her progress, and they modified or redirected the intervention, as necessary. Her progress toward meeting each of the IEP objectives was evaluated according to the timelines specified on the IEP. By May, she had achieved all of her objectives.

Criteria for termination of physical therapy services: Note: The Guide says that discharge (a term not used in schools) "occurs based on the physical therapist's analysis of the achievement of anticipated goals and expected outcomes." Reasons for discharge or discontinuing services in schools are consistent with the reasons outlined in the Guide, except that the physical therapist does not independently make the decision. The physical therapist may give the rest of the team, including the parents, her rationale, but the team makes the decision, based on the student's need for physical therapy to achieve goals and obtain necessary supports.

"Jeff"

Jeff is a 20-year-old who recently moved from Sunnyvale, a state residential facility for people with developmental disabilities, to a boarding house in the small town where his parents live. Three other young adults with disabilities live at the boarding house, and they invited Jeff to live with them after he visited with them several months ago.

EVIDENCE TO PRACTICE 17-3

CASE STUDY "JEFF"
PROGNOSIS DECISION

Jeff was classified at level IV of the Gross Motor Function Classification System (GMFCS) when he was 12 years old. Level IV indicates that children have self-mobility with limitations; they are transported or use power mobility outdoors and in the community. Based on evidence provided by McCormick and colleagues, this diagnosis is expected to be stable when Jeff is an adult. McCormick and colleagues found that GMFCS levels were stable from around 12 years of age into adulthood, and if a child uses a wheelchair at age 12, the child has a 96% probability of using a wheelchair as an adult.[1]

Intervention decision: Gough[2] and others who have reviewed the research have not found evidence to support the effectiveness of postural management for prevention of deformities. Jeff and his team, however, decided to try bilateral ankle-foot orthoses and improved positioning in an attempt to limit progression of his musculoskeletal impairments. To determine whether the interventions are effective, the impairments are measured regularly and compared with previous measurements. Gough[2] and others promote an emphasis on participation, rather than on body structures, but Jeff's team decided they could address both.

Intervention decision: Jeff wants to have a job when he graduates from high school, and he and his team decided to

pursue supported employment in the community rather than work in a sheltered environment. Stephens and colleagues conducted a longitudinal study of relations between employment status and adaptive skills in people with developmental disabilities.[3] They found that the type of employment was related to adaptive skills, with more competitive employment (such as supported employment) related to a higher level of adaptive skills than sheltered employment. The researchers observed the same pattern with a change in employment. Although the study was correlational and could not determine a cause–effect relationship between type of employment and adaptive skills, the authors concluded that employment, particularly more competitive employment, may enhance adaptive skills and promote successful living in the community.

1. McCormick, A., Brien, M., Plourde, J., Wood, E., Rosenbaum, P., McLean, J. (2007). Stability of the Gross Motor Function Classification System in adults with cerebral palsy. *Developmental Medicine & Child Neurology, 49,* 265–269.
2. Gough, M. (2009). Continuous postural management and the prevention of deformity in children with cerebral palsy: An appraisal. *Developmental Medicine & Child Neurology, 51,* 105–100.
3. Stephens, D. L., Collins, M. D., Dodder, R. A. (2005). A longitudinal study of employment and skill acquisition among individuals with developmental disabilities. *Research in Developmental Disabilities, 26,* 469–486.

Continued

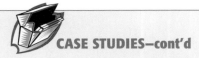

CASE STUDIES—cont'd

Jeff has spastic quadriplegic cerebral palsy and moderate intellectual disability and had lived at Sunnyvale since he was 7 years old. For the first 9 years, he spent most of his time in bed, receiving basic care but little education and few habilitative services other than passive range of motion exercises.

When Jeff was 18, physical therapy and other services were expanded as a result of a court order. Since then, Jeff acquired and learned to use an electronic communication aid and a power wheelchair. The chair has a custom-contoured seat and back to accommodate his moderate scoliosis, pelvic asymmetry with windswept hips, and lower extremity flexion contractures, which developed in spite of the passive range of motion exercises. He also learned to assume a standing position and to bear much of his weight during assisted transfers. Bilateral ankle-foot orthoses, improved positioning in bed and wheelchair, active participation during all transfers, and use of good alternative positioning appear to have helped limit progression of his musculoskeletal deformities.

In preparation for Jeff's transition to the boarding house, his physical therapist, occupational therapist, and mother took him there for an ecologic assessment to determine what skills Jeff needed to live there successfully. He can get help with dressing, bathing, and laundry, if necessary, but he has to be able to use the toilet independently and to transfer to and from his bed without assistance. He also has to be able to use the telephone, make his own breakfast and lunch, and go shopping in a nearby grocery variety store (see ecologic assessment in Table 17-2).

To prepare for his move, Jeff's physical therapist worked with him on the aspects of toilet transfers and shopping identified by

the ecologic assessment, simulating what he will encounter in the community. Before Jeff moved, he, his therapists, and his mother spent several days at the boarding house going through a typical day to help Jeff generalize skills he learned at Sunnyvale to the boarding house and to identify problems and the means to overcome them.

When he moved to the community, Jeff enrolled in the local high school, and a new IEP was written. Two of Jeff's educational goals relate to improving his independence at home and obtaining, learning, and keeping a job. His school physical therapist works with Jeff and his personal care assistant to increase his independence in his home and is working with his supported employment job coach to identify a job that Jeff can learn. Once a job is found, his physical therapist will help Jeff learn to use public transportation and to use the toilet at work and will provide ongoing consultation with the job coach to solve problems as they arise.

The physical therapist's involvement to help Jeff become more independent in his home and work environments is directed toward reducing his disabilities. Positioning and orthoses are used to reduce functional limitations and prevent the development of additional musculoskeletal impairments. For Jeff, it is also important that he maintain or increase his flexibility and endurance. For this reason, the physical therapist helped Jeff find a YMCA in his community that has an accessible swimming pool and a gym in which he can work out. In collaboration with YMCA staff, the therapist and Jeff developed an exercise program that is appropriate for Jeff's needs and that he can carry out with the assistance of YMCA personnel. The physical therapist is available to serve as a consultant as needed.

TABLE 17-2 **Example of an Ecologic Assessment**

Name: Jeff
Activity: Shopping
Environment: Dan's One-Stop

Steps Required	Jeff's Current Performance	Steps Can Acquire	Steps May Not Acquire	Compensatory Strategies	Intervention*
1. Go from home to Dan's and back using electric wheelchair.	Can open front door (outward), go down ramp, and drive to the corner. Cannot go down curb (no curb cut), cross street safely, or go up curb. Once on the sidewalk, can drive to Dan's. Cannot open door from outside. Can maneuver inside store and open door when leaving (outward). Cannot open door of home when returning.	1. Open doors of home and store when the door opens toward him. 2. Go down curb. 3. Ask for assistance and tell someone how to help him up a curb. 4. Cross the street safely.	Go up a curb without assistance.	Curb cuts	1. Teach Jeff to open doors, go down curbs, and cross streets safely (PT, PCA). 2. Talk with city about making curb cuts and with store and house manager about modifying doors (Jeff, CM). 3. Program communication aid to request help with curbs and give instructions (mother, PT).

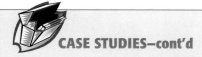

CASE STUDIES—cont'd

TABLE 17-2   **Example of an Ecologic Assessment—cont'd**

Steps Required	Jeff's Current Performance	Steps Can Acquire	Steps May Not Acquire	Compensatory Strategies	Intervention*
2. Select items in the store.	Does not always remember what he needs to get and cannot make or read a shopping list. Can get items that are at hand level, cannot shift weight or extend arm to reach low or high items.	1. Make and use shopping list. 2. Improve ability to reach high and low items. 3. Ask for assistance to get out-of-reach items.	Reach items that are very high or very low.	A reacher?	Teach Jeff 1. To make and use a shopping list (OT, PCA), 2. To use a reacher, if it seems feasible (OT, PCA), and 3. To reach to higher and lower shelves (PT, PCA).
3. Carry items to checkout stand.	Cannot maneuver shopping cart. Items slide off lap, does not want to use tray.	Carry items in a bag or other container on lap or chair.	Push a grocery cart without endangering store and other people.	Bag or other container that is accessible to Jeff	Find container and teach Jeff to use it (OT and PCA).
4. Put items on counter.	Can put items on counter, but is very slow, which annoys people in line behind him.	1. Put container on counter so clerk can remove items, or 2. Ask for assistance.	1. Increase speed sufficiently, or 2. Lift full container to counter.	None	1. Try to improve speed and lifting of container (PT, PCA), and 2. Program communication aid and teach Jeff to ask for assistance (mother and PCA).
5. Pay for purchases.	Cannot get wallet out of pocket, cannot get money out of wallet. Does not recognize denominations of bills or coins, cannot pay correct amount or check change.	1. Get money out of suitable container. 2. Recognize bills and coins. 3. Give sufficient money to cover the purchase.	1. Get wallet out of pocket or money out of wallet. 2. Determine if change is accurate.	1. Use an accessible container for money. 2. Ask personal care assistant to compare bill and change occasionally.	1. Find accessible container for money, and teach Jeff to use it (OT, PCA). 2. Teach Jeff to use money (OT, mother, PCA).
6. Carry purchases home.	Can carry small bag on lap, cannot carry large bag(s).	Carry purchases in container attached to chair.	Carry large or multiple bags on lap.	Alternate container (probably the same as in 3, above)	Find appropriate container for purchases (OT, PCA).

Continued

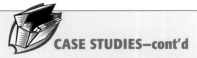

CASE STUDIES—cont'd

TABLE 17-2 **Example of an Ecologic Assessment—cont'd**

Steps Required	Jeff's Current Performance	Steps Can Acquire	Steps May Not Acquire	Compensatory Strategies	Intervention*
7. Put purchases away.	Can open cupboards with flat surfaces or knobs, drawers with knobs, and the refrigerator. Cannot open high or low cupboards or drawers with flat surfaces. Can put purchases away in places he can open and reach.	1. Open all drawers he can reach. 2. Put items away in higher and lower places.	Put items in very high or low places.	1. Make adaptations to allow Jeff to open kitchen drawers he can reach. 2. Rearrange cupboards and drawers so items Jeff uses are accessible.	1. Discuss adaptations and rearrangement with house manager (OT). 2. Improve Jeff's reach (also in 2 above) (PT, PCA).

Note: Those involved with each intervention are determined after the intervention is identified. At this time, Jeff has the assistance of his personal care assistant (PCA), case manager (CM), mother, occupational therapist (OT), and physical therapist (PT).
Format from Baumgart, D., Brown, L., Pumpian, I., et al. (1982). Principle of partial participation and individualized adaptations in educational programs for severely handicapped students. *Journal of the Association for Severely Handicapped, 7,* 17–27.

REFERENCES

1. (2009). *AAIDD Supports Intensity Scale™ information.* Retrieved April 7, 2009, from http://www.siswebsite.org/galleries/default-file/LatestSISpresentation.pdf

2. American Association on Intellectual and Developmental Disabilities. (2009). *AAIDD definition manual on intellectual disabilities.* Retrieved April 6, 2009, from http://www.aaidd.org/content_1196.cfm?navID=187

3. American Association on Mental Retardation. (2002). *Mental retardation: Definition, classification, and systems of supports* (10th ed.). Washington, DC: American Association on Mental Retardation.

4. American Physical Therapy Association. (2001). Guide to physical therapist practice, 2nd ed. *Physical Therapy, 81,* 9–744.

5. Anwar, F. (1986). Intellectual deficit and motor skill. In D. Ellis (Ed.), *Sensory impairments in mentally handicapped people* (pp. 169–183). San Diego: College-Hill Press.

6. Baker, B. J., Cole, K. N., & Harris, S. R. (1998). Intellectual referencing as a method of OT/PT triage for young children. *Pediatric Physical Therapy, 10,* 2–6.

7. Baranek, G. T. (2002). Efficacy of sensory and motor interventions for children with autism. *Journal of Autism and Developmental Disorders, 32,* 397–422.

8. Baranek, G. T., Parham, L. D., & Bodfish, J. W. (2005). Sensory and motor features of autism: Assessment and intervention. In F. R. Volkmar, R. Paul, A. Klin, & D. Cohen (Eds.), *Handbook of autism and pervasive developmental disorders* (pp. 831–857). Hoboken, NJ: John Wiley & Sons

9. Barlow, D. H., & Hersen, M. (1984). *Single case experimental designs: Strategies for studying behavioral change* (2nd ed.). New York: Pergamon Press.

10. Barnhart, R. C., & Connolly, B. (2007). Aging and Down syndrome: Implications for physical therapy. *Physical Therapy, 87,* 1399–1406.

11. Bartlett, D. J., Fanning, J. K., Miller, L., Conti-Becker, A., & Doralp, S. (2008). Development of the Daily Activities of Infants Scale: A measure supporting early motor development. *Developmental Medicine & Child Neurology, 50,* 8:613–617.

12. Benson, J. B., & Uzgiris, I. C. (1985). Effect of self-initiated locomotion on infant search activity. *Developmental Psychology, 21,* 923–931.

13. Bertenthal, B. I., Campos, J. J., & Barrett, K. C. (1984). Self-produced locomotion: An organizer of emotional, intellectual, and social development in infancy. In R. N. Emde & R. J. Harmon (Eds.), *Continuities and discontinuities in development.* New York: Plenum.

14. Bhutta, A. T., Cleves, M. A., Casey, P. H., Cradock, M. M., & Anand, K. J. S. (2002). Intellectual and behavioral outcomes of school-aged children who were born preterm. *JAMA, 288,* 728–737.

15. Bijou, S. W. (1966). A functional analysis of retarded development. In N. R. Ellis (Ed.), *International review of research in mental retardation, Vol 1* (pp. 1–19). New York: Academic Press.

16. Brooks-Gunn, J., Kelbanov, P. K., & Duncan, G. J. (1996). Ethnic differences in children's intelligence test scores: Role of economic deprivation, home environment, and maternal characteristics. *Child Development, 67,* 396–408.

17. Brown, L., Branston, M. B., Hamre-Nietupski, S., Pumpian, I., Certo, N., & Gruenewald, L. (1979). A strategy for developing chronological age appropriate and functional curricular content for severely handicapped adolescents and young adults. *Journal of Special Education, 12,* 81–90.

18. Burgemeister, B. B., Blum, L. H., & Lorge, I. (1972). *Manual: Columbia Mental Maturity Scale* (3rd ed.). New York: Psychological Corporation.

19. Butler, C. (1991). Augmentative mobility: Why do it? *Physical Medicine and Rehabilitation Clinics of North America, 2,* 801–815.

20. Butler, C., Okamoto, G. A., & McKay, T. M. (1983). Powered mobility for very young disabled children. *Developmental Medicine & Child Neurology, 25,* 472–474.

21. Campbell, P. H. (1989). Dysfunction in posture and movement with individuals with profound disabilities. In F. Brown & D. H. Lehr (Eds.), *Persons with profound disabilities: Issues and practices* (pp. 163–189). Baltimore, MD: Paul H. Brookes.

22. Campbell, P. H. (1991). Evaluation and assessment in early intervention for infants and toddlers. *Journal of Early Intervention, 15,* 36–45.

23. Campos, J. J., & Bertenthal, B. I. (1987). Locomotion and psychological development in infancy. In K. M. Jaffe (Ed.), *Childhood powered mobility: Developmental, technical and clinical perspectives: Proceedings of the RESNA First Northwest Regional Conference* (pp. 11–42). Washington, DC: RESNA.

24. Carr, E. G., Dunlap, G., Horner, R. H., et al. (2002). Positive behavior support: Evolution of an applied science. *Journal of Positive Behavior Interventions, 4,* 4–16.

25. Carr, J. (2008). The everyday life of adults with Down syndrome. *Journal of Applied Research in Intellectual Disability, 21,* 389–397.

26. Carr, S. H. (1989). Louisiana's criteria of eligibility for occupational therapy services in the public school system. *American Journal of Occupational Therapy, 43,* 503–506.

27. Chandler, L. S., & Adams, M. A. (1972). Multiply handicapped child motivated for ambulation through behavior modification. *Physical Therapy, 52,* 339–401.

28. Chen, C., Visootsak, J., Dills, S., Graham, J. M., Jr. (2007). Prader-Willi syndrome: An update and review for the primary pediatrician. *Clinical Pediatrics, 46,* 580–591.

29. Chinitz, S. P., & Feder, C. Z. (1992). Psychological assessment. In G. E. Molnar (Ed.), *Pediatric rehabilitation* (2nd ed., pp. 48–87). Baltimore, MD: Williams & Wilkins.

30. Chugani, H. T. (1998). A critical period of brain development: Studies of cerebral glucose utilization with PET. *Preventive Medicine, 27,* 184–188.

31. Cimera, R. E. (1998). Are individuals with severe mental retardation and multiple disabilities cost-efficient to serve via supported employment programs? *Mental Retardation, 36,* 280–292.

32. Cole, C. L., & Levinson, T. R. (2002). Effects of within activity choices on the challenging behavior of children with severe developmental disabilities. *Journal of Positive Behavior Interventions, 4,* 29–37.

33. Connolly, B. H., Morgan, S. B., Russell, F. F., & Fulliton, W. L. (1993). A longitudinal study of children with Down syndrome who experienced early intervention programming. *Physical Therapy, 73,* 170–179.

34. Cornish, K., & Bramble, D. (2002). Cri du chat syndrome: Genotype-phenotype correlations and recommendations for clinical management. *Developmental Medicine & Child Neurology, 44,* 494–497.

35. Coster, W., Deeney, T., Haltiwanger, J., & Haley, S. (1998). *School Function Assessment (SFA).* San Antonio, TX: Pearson.

36. de Vries, B. B., Halley, D. J. J., Oostra, B. A., & Niermeijer, M. F. (1998). The fragile X syndrome. *Journal of Medical Genetics, 35,* 579–589.

37. DiLalla, L. F. (2000). Development of intelligence: Current research and theories. *Journal of School Psychology, 38,* 3–7.

38. Downing, J., Eichinger, J., & Demchak, M. (2002). *Including students with severe disabilities in typical classrooms.* Baltimore, MC: Paul H. Brookes.

39. Dunst, C. (2000). Everyday children's learning opportunities: Characteristics and consequences. *Children's Learning Opportunities Report, 2,* 1–2.

40. Dunst, C. J., Bruder, M. B., Trivette, C. M., Hamby, D., Raab, M., & McLean, M. (2001). Characteristics and consequences of everyday natural learning opportunities. *Topics in Early Childhood Special Education, 21,* 68–92.

41. Eagle, R. S. (1985). Deprivation of early sensorimotor experience and cognition in the severely involved cerebral-palsied child. *Journal of Autism and Developmental Disabilities, 15,* 269–283.

42. Einspieler, C., Kerr, A. M., & Prechtl, H. F. (2005). Is the early development of girls with Rett disorder really normal? *Pediatric Research, 57,* 696–700.

43. Ellis, N. R. (1963). *Handbook of mental deficiency: Psychological theory and research.* London: McGraw-Hill.

44. Fagan, J. F. (2000). A theory of intelligence as processing: Implications for society. *Psychology, Public Policy, and Law, 6,* 168–179.

45. Fagan, J. F., & Shepherd, P. A. (1991). *The Fagan Test of Infant Intelligence training manual.* Cleveland: Infatest Corporation.

46. Falvey, M. A. (1989). Introduction. In M. A. Falvey (Ed.), *Community-based curriculum: Instructional strategies for students with severe handicaps* (pp. 1–13). Baltimore, MD: Paul H. Brookes.

47. Ferguson, D. L., & Baumgart, D. (1991). Partial participation revisited. *Journal of the Association for Persons with Severe Handicaps, 16,* 218–227.

48. Filipek, P. A. (2005). Medical aspects of autism. In F. R. Volkmar, R. Paul, A. Klin, & D. Cohen (Eds.), *Handbook of autism and pervasive developmental disorders* (pp. 534–578). Hoboken, NJ: John Wiley & Sons.

49. Flexer, R. W., Simmons, T. J., Luft, P., & Baer, R. M. (2001). *Transition planning for secondary students with disabilities.* Upper Saddle River, NJ: Merrill Prentice-Hall.

50. Fogel, A., Dedo, J. Y., & McEwen, I. R. (1992). Effect of postural position and reaching on gaze during mother-infant face-to-face interaction. *Infant Behavior and Development, 15,* 231–244.

51. Fombonne, E. (2002). Epidemiological trends in rates of autism. *Molecular Psychiatry, 7*(Suppl. 2), S4–S6.

52. Fragala, M. A., O'Neil, M. E., Russo, K. J., & Dumas, H. M. (2002). Impairment, disability, and satisfaction outcomes after lower-extremity botulinum toxin A injections for children with cerebral palsy. *Pediatric Physical Therapy, 14,* 132–144.

53. Gaytant, M. A., Rours, G. I., Steegers, E. A., Galama, J. M., & Semmekrot, B. A. (2003). Congenital cytomegalovirus infection after recurrent infection: Case reports and review of the literature. *European Journal of Pediatrics, 162,* 248–253.

54. Gemus, M., Palisano, R., Russell, D., Rosenbaum, P., Walter, S. D., Galuppi, B., et al. (2001). Using the gross motor function measure to evaluate motor development in children with Down syndrome. *Physical & Occupational Therapy in Pediatrics, 21,* 69–79.

55. Giangreco, M. F., Cloninger, C. H., & Iverson, V. S. (1998). *Choosing options and accommodations for children: A guide to educational planning for students with disabilities* (2nd ed.). Baltimore, MD: Paul H. Brookes.

56. Gibbs, E. D. (1990). Assessment of infant mental ability: Conventional tests and issues of prediction. In E. D. Gibbs & D. M. Teti (Eds.), *Interdisciplinary assessment of infants: A guide for early intervention professionals* (pp. 77–89). Baltimore, MD: Paul H. Brookes.

57. Green, D., Charman, T., Pickles, A., Chandler, S., Loucas, T., Simonoff, E., et al. (2009). Impairment in movement skills of children with autistic spectrum disorders. *Developmental Medicine & Child Neurology, 51,* 311–316.

58. Guerri, C., Bazinet, A., & Riley, E. P. (2009). Fetal alcohol spectrum disorders and alterations in brain and behaviour. *Alcohol & Alcoholism, 44,* 108–114.

59. Guess, D., Mulligan-Ault, M., Roberts, S., Struth, J., Siegel-Causey, E., Thompson, B., et al. (1988). Implications of biobehavioral states for the education and treatment of students with the most profoundly handicapping conditions. *Journal of the Association for Persons with Severe Handicaps, 13,* 163–174.

60. Gustafson, G. E. (1984). Effects of the ability to locomote on infants' social and exploratory behaviors: An experimental study. *Developmental Psychology, 20,* 397–405.

61. Guzzetta, A., Mazzotti, S., Tinelli, F., et al. (2006). Early assessment of visual information processing and neurological outcome in preterm infants. *Neuropediatrics, 37,* 278–285.

62. Haley, S. M., Coster, W. J., Ludlow, L. H., Haltiwanger, J. T., & Andrellos, P. J. (1992). *Pediatric evaluation of disability inventory.* Boston, MA: Department of Rehabilitation Medicine, New England Medical Center.

63. Haney, M., & Falvey, M. A. (1989). Instructional strategies. In M. A. Falvey (Ed.), *Community-based curriculum: Instructional strategies for students with severe handicaps* (pp. 63–90). Baltimore, MD: Paul H. Brookes.

64. Harris, S. R., & Shea, A. M. (1991). Down syndrome. In S. K. Campbell (Ed.), *Pediatric neurologic physical therapy* (2nd ed., pp. 131–168). New York: Churchill Livingstone.

65. Horn, E. M. (1991). Basic motor skills instruction for children with neuromotor delays: A critical review. *Journal of Special Education, 25,* 168–197.

66. Houghton, J., Bronicki, G. J. B., & Guess, D. (1987). Opportunities to express preferences and make choices among students with severe disabilities in classroom settings. *Journal of the Association for Persons with Severe Handicaps, 12,* 18–27.

67. Hughes, C. (1996). Brief report: Planning problems in autism at the level of motor control. *Journal of Autism & Developmental Disorders, 26,* 99–107.

68. Jelliffe-Pawlowski, L. L., Shaw, G. M., Nelson, V., & Harris, J. A. (2003). Risk of mental retardation among children born with birth defects. *Archives of Pediatrics and Adolescent Medicine, 157,* 545–550.

69. Jobling, A. (1994). Physical education for the person with Down syndrome: More than playing games? *Down Syndrome Research and Practice, 2,* 31–35.

70. Jones, K. L. (1997). *Smith's recognizable patterns of human malformation* (5th ed.). Philadelphia: W. B. Saunders.

71. Jones, M. A., McEwen, I. R., & Hansen, L. (2003). Use of power mobility for a young child with spinal muscular atrophy: A case report. *Physical Therapy, 83,* 253–262.

72. Kaplan, E., Fein, D., Kramer, J., Delis, D., & Morris, R. (2004). *Wechsler Intelligence Scale for Children®—Fourth Edition Integrated.* San Antonio, TX: Pearson Education.

73. Katusic, S. K., Colligan, R. C., Beard, C. M., O'Fallon, W. M., Bergstralh, E. J., Jacobsen, S. J., et al. (1996). Mental retardation in a birth cohort, 1976–1980, Rochester, Minnesota. *American Journal on Mental Retardation, 100,* 335–344.

74. Kermoian, R., & Campos, J. J. (1988). Locomotor experience: A facilitator of spatial intellectual development. *Child Development, 59,* 908–917.

75. King, G., Law, M., King, S., Rosenbaum, P., Kertoy, M. K., & Young, N. L. (2003). A conceptual model of the factors affecting recreation and leisure participation of children with dis-

abilities. *Physical & Occupational Therapy in Pediatrics, 23,* 63–90.

76. King, G. A., Law, M., King, S., et al. (2007). Measuring children's participation in recreation and leisure activities: Construct validation of the CAPE and PAC. *Child: Care, Health & Development, 33,* 28–39.

77. Kolb, B., Forgie, M., Gibb, R., Gorny, G., & Rowntree, S. (1998). Age, experience and the changing brain. *Neuroscience and Biobehavioral Reviews, 22,* 143–159.

78. Kopp, C. B., & McCall, R. B. (1982). Predicting later mental performance for normal, at-risk, and handicapped infants. In P. B. Baltes & O. G. Brim (Eds.), *Life-span development and behavior* (pp. 33–61). New York: Academic Press.

79. Lambert, N., Nihira, K., & Leland, H. (1993). *AAMR Adaptive Behavior Scale-School* (2nd ed.). Austin, TX: Pro-Ed.

80. Landesman-Dwyer, S., & Sackett, G. P. (1978). Behavioral changes in nonambulatory, profoundly mentally retarded individuals. In C. E. Meyers (Ed.), *Quality of life in severely and profoundly mentally retarded people: Research foundations for improvement* (pp. 55–144). Washington, DC: American Association on Mental Deficiency.

81. Larson, J. C. G., Bastian, A. J., Donchin, O., Shadmehr, R., & Mostofsky, S. H. (2008). Acquisition of internal models of motor tasks in children with autism. *Brain, 131,* 2894–2903.

82. Larson, S. A., Lakin, K. C., Anderson, L., Kwak, N., Lee, J. H., & Anderson, D. (2001). Prevalence of mental retardation and developmental disabilities: Estimates from the 1994/1995 national health interview survey disability supplements. *American Journal on Mental Retardation, 106,* 231–252.

83. Law, M., Baptiste, S., Carswell, A., McColl, M. A., Polatajko, H., & Pollock, N. (2005). *Canadian occupational performance measure* (4th ed.). Toronto: Canadian Association of Occupational Therapists.

84. Law, M., King, G., King, S., Kertoy, M., Hurley, P., Rosenbaum, P., et al. (2006). Patterns of participation in recreational and leisure activities among children with complex physical disabilities. *Developmental Medicine & Child Neurology, 48,* 337–342.

85. Leung, A. K. C., Sauve, R. S., & Davies, H. D. (2003). Congenital cytomegalovirus infection. *Journal of the National Medical Association, 95,* 213–218.

86. Lopez, J. M. (2008). Is ZMP the toxic metabolite in Lesch-Nyhan disease? *Medical Hypotheses, 71,* 657–663.

87. Lucyshyn, J. M., Horner, R. H., Dunlap, G., Albin, R. W., & Ben, K. R. (2002). Positive behavior support with families. In J. M. Lucyshyn, G. Dunlap, & R. W. Albin (Eds.), *Families and positive behavior support: Addressing problem behavior in family contexts* (pp. 3–43). Baltimore, MD: Paul H. Brookes.

88. Malian, I., & Nevin, A. (2002). A review of self-determination literature: Implications for practitioners. *RASE: Remedial and Special Education, 23,* 68–74.

89. Maloney, F. P., & Kurtz, P. A. (1982). The use of a mercury switch head control device in profoundly retarded, multiply handicapped children. *Physical & Occupational Therapy in Pediatrics, 2,* 11–17.

90. Mari, M., Castiello, U., Marks, D., Marraffa, C., & Prior, M. (2003). The reach-to-grasp movement in children with autism spectrum disorder. *Philosophical Transactions of the Royal Society of London Series B: Biological Sciences, 358,* 393–403.

91. Martin K. (2004). Effects of supramalleolar orthoses on postural stability in children with Down syndrome. *Developmental Medicine & Child Neurology, 46,* 406–411.

92. McCall, R. B. (1982). Issues in the early development of intelligence and its assessment. In M. Lewis, & L. Taft (Eds.), *Developmental disabilities: Theory, assessment and intervention* (pp. 177–184). New York: SP Medical and Scientific Books.

93. McEwen, I. R. (1992). Assistive positioning as a control parameter of social-communicative interactions between students with profound multiple disabilities and classroom staff. *Physical Therapy, 72,* 634–647.

94. McEwen, I. R. (Ed.). (2001). *Writing case reports: A how-to manual for clinicians.* Alexandria, VA: American Physical Therapy Association.

95. McEwen, I. R., & Shelden, M. L. (1995). Pediatric physical therapy in the 1990s: The demise of the educational versus medical dichotomy. *Physical & Occupational Therapy in Pediatrics, 15,* 33–45.

96. McGonigel, M. J., Woodruff, G., & Roszmann-Millican, M. (1994). The transdisciplinary team: A model for family-centered early intervention. In L. J. Johnson, R. J. Gallagher, M. J. LaMontagne, J. B. Jordan, J. J. Gallagher, P. L. Huntinger, et al. (Eds.), *Meeting early intervention challenges: Issues from birth to three* (2nd ed., pp. 95–131). Baltimore, MD: Paul H. Brookes.

97. Meegan, S., Maraj, B. K., Weeks, D., & Chua, R. (2006). Gross motor skill acquisition in adolescents with Down syndrome. *Down Syndrome: Research & Practice, 9,* 75–80.

98. Meisels, S. J., & Atkins-Burnett, S. (2000). The elements of early childhood assessment. In J. P. Shonkoff, & S. J. Meisels (Eds.), *Handbook of early childhood intervention* (2nd ed., pp. 231–257). Cambridge, MA: Cambridge University Press.

99. Meiser, M. J., & McEwen, I. R. (2007). Lightweight and ultra-light wheelchairs: Propulsion and preferences in two young children with spina bifida. *Pediatric Physical Therapy, 19,* 245–253.

100. Ming, X., Brimacombe, M., & Wagner, G. C. (2007). Prevalence of motor impairment in autism spectrum disorders. *Brain & Development, 29,* 565–570.

101. Missiuna, C., Polluck, N., & Law, M. (2004). Perceived efficacy and goal setting system (PEGS). San Antonio, TX: Psychological Corporation.

102. Morris, C. A., & Mervis, C. B. (2000). Williams syndrome and related disorders. *Annual Review of Genomics & Human Genetics, 1,* 261–284.

103. Mostofsky, S. H., Dubey, P., Jerath, V. K., Jansiewicz, E. M., Goldberg, M. C., & Denckla, M. B. (2006). Developmental

dyspraxia is not limited to imitation in children with autism spectrum disorders. *Journal of the International Neuropsychological Society, 12,* 314–326.

104. Muggli, E. E., Collins, V. R., & Marraffa, C. (2009). Going down a different road: First support and information needs of families with a baby with Down syndrome. *Medical Journal of Australia, 190,* 58–61.

105. National Joint Committee for the Communicative Needs of Persons with Severe Disabilities. (1992). Guidelines for meeting the communication needs of persons with severe disabilities. *ASHA 34*(Suppl. 7), 1–8.

106. National Library of Medicine. (2007). Cornelia de Lange syndrome. Retrieved August 23, 2009, from http://ghr.nlm.nih.gov/condition=corneliadelangesyndrome

107. National Research Council Committee on Educational Interventions for Children with Autism. Division of Behavioral and Social Sciences and Education. (2001). *Educating children with autism.* Washington, DC: National Academy Press.

108. Navajas, D., Farre, R., Mar Rotger, M., Milic-Emili, J., & Sanchis, J. (1988). Effect of body posture on respiratory impedance. *Journal of Applied Physiology, 64,* 194–199.

109. Newborg J. (2005). *Battelle developmental inventory* (2nd ed.). Itasca, IL: Riverside Publishing.

110. Nihira, K. (1999). Adaptive behavior: A historical overview. In R. L. Shalock (Ed.), *Adaptive behavior and its measurement: Implications for the field of mental retardation* (pp. 7–14). Washington, DC: AAMR.

111. Nwaobi, O. M. (1987). Seating orientations and upper extremity function in children with cerebral palsy. *Physical Therapy, 67,* 1209–1212.

112. Nwaobi, O. M., & Smith, P. D. (1986). Effect of adaptive seating on pulmonary function of children with cerebral palsy. *Developmental Medicine & Child Neurology, 28,* 351–354.

113. Orelove, F. P., & Sobsey, D. (1996). Designing transdisciplinary services. In F. P. Orelove & D. Sobsey (Eds.), *Educating children with multiple disabilities: A transdisciplinary approach* (3rd ed., pp. 1–33). Baltimore, MD: Paul H. Brookes.

114. Oswald, D. P., Coutinho, M. J., & Nguyen N. (2001). Impact of sociodemographic characteristics on identification rates of minority students as having mental retardation. *Mental Retardation, 39,* 351–367.

115. Ozonoff, S., Young, G. S., Goldring, S., Greiss-Hess, L., Herrera, A. M., Steele, J., et al. (2008). Gross motor development, movement abnormalities, and early identification of autism. *Journal of Autism & Developmental Disorders, 38,* 644–656.

116. Palisano, R. J., Walter, S. D., Russell, D. J., et al. (2001). Gross motor function of children with Down syndrome: Creation of motor growth curves. *Archives of Physical Medicine & Rehabilitation, 82,* 494–500. 10.1053/apmr.2001.21956

117. Penagarikano, O., Mulle, J. G., & Warren, S. T. (2007). The pathophysiology of fragile X syndrome. *Annual Review of Genomics & Human Genetics, 8,* 109–129.

118. Parette, H. P., Jr., & Hourcade, J. J. (1984). How effective are physiotherapeutic programmes with young mentally retarded children who have cerebral palsy? *Journal of Mental Deficiency Research, 28,* 167–175.

119. Parrish, J. M. (1997). Behavior management. In M. L. Batshaw (Ed.), *Children with disabilities* (4th ed., pp. 657–686). Baltimore, MD: Paul H. Brookes.

120. Pennington, B. F., Moon, J., Edgin, J., Stedron, J., Nadel, L. (2003). The neuropsychology of Down syndrome: Evidence for hippocampal dysfunction. *Child Development, 74,* 75–93.

121. Percy, A. K. (2002). Rett syndrome: Current status and new vistas. *Neurologic Clinics, 20,* 1125–1141.

122. Portney, L. G., & Watkins, M. P. (2009). *Foundations of clinical research: Applications to practice* (3rd ed.). Upper Saddle River, NJ: Prentice Hall Health.

123. Provost, B., Heimerl, S., Lopez, B. R. (2007). Levels of gross and fine motor development in young children with autism spectrum disorder. *Physical & Occupational Therapy in Pediatrics, 27,* 21–36.

124. Rainforth, B. (1991). OSERS clarifies legality of related services eligibility criteria. *TASH Newsletter,* April 1991, p. 8.

125. Rainforth, B. (2002). The primary therapist model: Addressing challenges to practice in special education. *Physical & Occupational Therapy in Pediatrics, 22,* 29–51.

126. Rainforth, B., & York-Barr, J. (1997). *Collaborative teams for students with severe disabilities: Integrating therapy and educational services* (2nd ed.). Baltimore, MD: Paul H. Brookes.

127. Randall, K. E., & McEwen, I. R. (2000). Writing patient-centered functional goals. *Physical Therapy, 80,* 1197–1203.

128. Raven, J. C. (1995). *Raven's progressive matrices.* San Antonio, TX: The Psychological Corporation.

129. Reid, D., Rigby, P., & Ryan S. (1999). Functional impact of a rigid pelvic stabilizer on children with cerebral palsy who use wheelchairs: Users' and caregivers' perceptions. *Pediatric Rehabilitation, 3,* 101–118.

130. Roid, G. H. (2003). *Stanford-Binet intelligence scales* (5th ed.). Chicago, IL: Riverside Publishing.

131. Roizen, N. J. (1997). Down syndrome. In M. L. Batshaw (Ed.), *Children with disabilities* (4th ed., pp. 361–376). Baltimore, MD: Paul H. Brookes.

132. Rozien, N. J., & Patterson, D. (2003). Down's syndrome. *The Lancet, 361,* 1281–1289.

133. Rold, G., & Miller, L. (1998). *Leiter international performance scale—Revised.* Wood Dale, IL: Stoelting.

134. Rosenbaum, P. L., Walter, S. D., Hanna, S. E., et al. (2002). Prognosis for gross motor function in cerebral palsy: Creation of motor development curves. *JAMA, 288,* 1357–1363.

135. Rothstein, J. M., Echternach, J. L., & Riddle, D. L. (2003). The hypothesis-oriented algorithm for clinicians II (HOAC II): A guide for patient management. *Physical Therapy, 83,* 455–470.

136. Russell, D., Palisano, R., Walter, S., et al. (1998). Evaluating motor function in children with Down syndrome: Validity of the GMFM. *Developmental Medicine & Child Neurology, 40,* 693–701.

137. Russell, D J, Rosenbaum, P. L., Avery, L. M., & Lane, M. (2002). *Gross Motor Function Measure (GMFM 66 & GMFM-88): User's manual.* London, England: MacKeith Press.

138. Schalock, R. L., Luckasson, R., Shogren, K. A., et al. (2007). The renaming of *mental retardation*: Understanding the change to the term *intellectual disability. Intellectual and Developmental Disabilities, 45,* 116–124.

139. Shelden, M. L., & Rush, D. D. (2001). The ten myths about providing early intervention services in natural environments. *Infants & Young Children, 14,* 1–13.

140. Shevell, M., Majnemer, A., Platt, R. W., Webster, R., & Birnbaum, R. (2005). Developmental and functional outcomes in children with global developmental delay or developmental language impairment. *Developmental Medicine & Child Neurology, 47,* 678–683.

141. Shumway-Cook, A., & Woollacott, M. H. (1985). Dynamics of postural control in the child with Down syndrome. *Physical Therapy, 65,* 1315–1322.

142. Slater, A. (1997). Can measures of infant habituation predict later intellectual ability? *Archives of Disease in Childhood, 77,* 474–476.

143. Smith-Zuzovsky, N., & Exner, C. E. (2004). The effect of seated positioning quality on typical 6- and 7-year-old children's object manipulation skills. *American Journal of Occupational Therapy, 58,* 380–388.

144. Snell, M. E., & Brown, F. (2006). Designing and implementing instructional programs. In M. E. Snell, & F. Brown (Eds.), *Instruction of students with severe disabilities* (6th ed., pp. 111–169). Upper Saddle River, NJ: Pearson.

145. Sparrow, S. S., Cichetti, C. V., & Balla, D. A. (2005). *Vineland adaptive behavior scales* (2nd ed.). Upper Saddle River, NJ: Pearson Education.

146. Spiker, D., Heebler, K., & Mallik S. (2005). Developing and implementing early intervention programs for children with established disabilities. In M. J. Guralnick (Ed.), *The developmental systems approach to early intervention* (pp. 305–349). Baltimore, MD: Paul H. Brookes.

147. Starr, E. M., Berument, S. K., Tomlins, M., Papanikolaou, K., & Rutter, M. (2005). Brief report: Autism in individuals with Down syndrome. *Journal of Autism & Developmental Disorders, 35,* 665–673.

148. Switzky, H. N., Woolsey-Hill, J., & Quoss, T. (1979). Habituation of visual fixation responses: An assessment tool to measure visual sensory-perceptual intellectual processes in nonverbal profoundly handicapped children in the classroom. *AAESPH Review, 4,* 136–147.

149. TASH force strikes again: Laski and Boyd win Oberti case in New Jersey. *TASH Newsletter,* November 1992, pp. 1–2.

150. Taylor, S. J. (2004). Caught in the continuum: A critical analysis of the principle of the least restrictive environment. *Research and Practice for Persons with Severe Disabilities, 29,* 218–230.

151. Tefft, D., Guerette, P., & Furumasu, J. (1999). Intellectual predictors of young children's readiness for powered mobility. *Developmental Medicine & Child Neurology, 41,* 665–670.

152. Teitelbaum, P., Teitelbaum, O., Nye, J., Fryman, J., & Maurer, R. G. (1998). Movement analysis in infancy may be useful for early diagnosis of autism. *Proceedings of the National Academy of Sciences of the United States of America, 95,* 13982–13987.

153. Telzrow, R. W., Campos, J. J., Shepherd, A., Bertenthal, B. I., & Atwater, S. (1987). Spatial understanding in infants with motor handicaps. In K. M. Jaffe (Ed.), *Childhood powered mobility: Developmental, technical and clinical perspectives: Proceedings of the RESNA first Northwest Regional Conference* (pp. 62–69). Washington, DC: RESNA.

154. Thorndike, R., Hagen, E., & Sattler, J. (1986). *Technical manual for Stanford-Binet intelligence scale* (4th ed.). Chicago, IL: Riverside Publishing.

155. Thorpe, D. E., & Valvano, J. (2002). The effects of knowledge of performance and intellectual strategies on motor skill learning in children with cerebral palsy. *Pediatric Physical Therapy, 14,* 2–15.

156. Turner-Stokes, L. (2009). Goal attainment scaling (GAS) in rehabilitation: A practical guide. *Clinical Rehabilitation, 23,* 362–370.

157. Ulrich, D. A., Lloyd, M. C., Tiernan, C. W., Looper, J. E., & Angulo-Barroso, R. M. (2008). Effects of intensity of treadmill training on developmental outcomes and stepping in infants with Down syndrome: A randomized trial. *Physical Therapy, 88,* 114–122.

158. United Cerebral Palsy National Infant Collaborative Project. (1976). *Staff development handbook: A resource for the transdisciplinary process.* New York: United Cerebral Palsy Association.

159. United States Department of Education. (2000). *Twenty-second annual report to Congress on the implementation of the Individuals with Disabilities Education Act.* Washington, DC: Author.

160. United States Department of Education. (2006). *Twenty-eighth annual report to Congress on the implementation of the Individuals with Disabilities Education Act.* Washington, DC: Author.

161. Vaughn, B. J., Wilson, D., & Dunlap, G. (2002). Family-centered intervention to resolve problem behavior in a fast-food restaurant. *Journal of Positive Behavior Interventions, 4,* 38–45.

162. Verburg, G., Naumann, S., Balfour, L., & Snell, E. (1990). Remote training of mobility skills in persons who are physically and developmentally disabled. In *Proceedings of the RESNA 13th Annual Conference* (pp. 195–196). Washington, DC: RESNA.

163. Vicari, S. (2006). Motor development and neuropsychological patterns in persons with Down syndrome. *Behavior Genetics, 36,* 355–364.

164. Virji-Babul, N., Kerns, K., Zhou, E., Kapur, A., & Shiffrar, M. (2006). Perceptual-motor deficits in children with Down syndrome: Implications for intervention. *Down Syndrome: Research & Practice, 10,* 74–82.

165. Walker, W. O., & Johnson, C. P. (2008). Cognitive and adaptive disabilities. In M. L. Wolraich, D. D. Drotar, P. H. Dworkin, &

E. C. Perrin (Eds.), *Developmental-behavioral pediatrics: Evidence and practice* (pp. 405–443). Philadelphia, PA: Mosby Elsevier.

166. Wang, P. (2008). 10B. Genetics in developmental-behavioral pediatrics. In M. L. Wolraich, D. D. Drotar, P. H. Dworkin, & E. C. Perrin (Eds.), *Developmental-behavioral pediatrics: Evidence and practice* (pp. 317–336). Philadelphia: Mosby Elsevier.

167. Watkins, M. W., Ravert, C. M., & Crosby, E. G. (2002). Normative factor structure of the AAMR Adaptive Behavior Scale-School, 2nd ed. *Journal of Psychoeducational Assessment, 20,* 337–345.

168. Wechsler, D. (1991). *Wechsler intelligence scale for children* (3rd ed.). San Antonio, TX: Harcourt Assessment.

169. Wehmeyer, M. L., & Bolding, N. (1999). Self-determination across living and working environments: A matched samples study of adults with mental retardation. *Mental Retardation, 37,* 353–363, 1999.

170. Wehmeyer, M. L., & Bolding, N. (2001). Enhanced self-determination of adults with intellectual disability as an outcome of moving to community-based work or living environments. *Journal of Intellectual Disability Research, 45,* 371–383.

171. Wehmeyer, M. L., & Schwartz, M. (1997). Self-determination and positive adult outcomes: A follow-up study of youth with mental retardation or learning disabilities. *Exceptional Children, 63,* 245–255.

172. Williams, J. H., Whiten, A., & Singh, T. (2004). A systematic review of action imitation in autistic spectrum disorder. *Journal of Autism & Developmental Disorders, 34,* 285–299.

173. World Health Organization. (2001). *International classification of functioning, disability, and health (ICF).* Geneva, Switzerland: Author.

174. Yan, J. H., Thomas, J. R., & Downing, J. H. (1998). Locomotion improves children's spatial search: A meta-analytic review. *Perceptual & Motor Skills, 87,* 67–82.

175. Ylvisaker, M., & Feeney, T. (2001). Executive functions, self-regulation, and learned optimism in paediatric rehabilitation: A review and implications for intervention. *Pediatric Rehabilitation, 5,* 51–70.

176. Zazula, J. L., & Foulds, R. A. (1983). Mobility device for a child with phocomelia. *Archives of Physical Medicine and Rehabilitation, 64,* 137–139.

177. Zelazo, P. R., & Weiss, M. J. (1990). Infant information processing: An alternative approach. In E. D. Gibbs & D. M. Teti (Eds.), *Interdisciplinary assessment of infants: A guide for early intervention professionals* (pp. 129–143). Baltimore: Paul H. Brookes.

178. Zhang, D., & Katsiyannis, A. (2002). Minority representation in special education: A persistent challenge. *RASE: Remedial & Special Education, 23,* 180–187.

SUGGESTED READINGS

Allen, G., & Courchesne E. (2003). Differential effects of developmental cerebellar abnormality on cognitive and motor functions in the cerebellum: An fMRI study of autism. *American Journal of Psychiatry, 160,* 262–273.

Baumgart, D., Brown, L., Pumpian, I., Nisbet, J., Ford, A., Sweet, M., et al. (1982). Principle of partial participation and individualized adaptations in educational programs for severely handicapped students. *The Journal of the Association for the Severely Handicapped, 7,* 17–27.

Cress, C. J. (2002). Expanding children's early augmented behaviors to support symbolic development. In J. Reichle, D. Beukelman, & J. Light (Eds.), *Exemplary practices for beginning communicators* (pp. 219–272). Baltimore, MD: Paul H. Brookes.

Feldman, A. B., Haley, S. M., Coryell, J. (1990). Concurrent and construct validity of the Pediatric Evaluation of Disability Inventory. *Physical Therapy, 70,* 602–610.

Folio, R. M., & Fewell, R. R. (2000). *Peabody developmental motor scales* (2nd ed.). Austin, TX: Pro-Ed.

Goldman, S., Wang, C., Salgado, M. W., Greene, P. E., Kim, M., Rapin, I. (2009). Motor stereotypes in children with autism and other developmental disorders. *Developmental Medicine & Child Neurology, 5,* 30–38.

Jankovic, J., Caskey, T. C., Stout, J. T., & Butler, I. J. (1988). Lesch-Nyhan syndrome: A study of motor behavior and cerebrospinal fluid neurotransmitters. *Annals of Neurology, 23,* 466–469.

(2000). Prenatal exposure to alcohol. *Alcohol Research & Health, 24,* 32–41.

18 Cerebral Palsy

MARILYN WRIGHT, BScPT, MEd, MSc • LINDA WALLMAN, BScPT

Physical therapists provide an important component of the specialized interdisciplinary services that will help children with cerebral palsy (CP) reach their full potential in their home, educational, and community environments. Their practice encompasses diagnosis of motor deficits and delay, examination of functional performance, evaluation of test results to develop a prognosis and plan of care, consultation, and treatment. Input from physical therapists guides decisions about many interventions such as orthotic prescription, orthopedic surgery, and spasticity management. Physical therapists have great potential to influence the immediate and future lives of children with CP and their families.

NATURE AND CHARACTERISTICS OF CEREBRAL PALSY

"CP describes a group of permanent disorders of the development of movement and posture, causing activity limitations that are attributed to non-progressive disturbances that occurred in the developing fetal or infant brain" (p. 9).[269] Although the brain lesion is static, progressive musculoskeletal impairment is seen in most children.[130,180,269] Secondary musculoskeletal problems such as muscle/tendon contractures, bony torsion, hip displacement, and spinal deformity can contribute to functional deterioration. Many of these problems develop throughout life and are related to physical growth, muscle spasticity and weakness, aging, and other factors.[269]

Motor impairments associated with CP are often accompanied by disturbances of cognition, behavior, communication, sensation, epilepsy, and perception.[269] Cognitive delays (IQ < 70) are present in 23% to 44% of children with CP, and behavioral issues have been recognized in 25%—a rate five times greater than that typically seen in children.[233] Prevalence of impaired speech (42%–81%), hearing (25%), and vision (62%–71%), seizure disorders (22%–40%), urinary incontinence (23%), and constipation (59%) is increased. Tactile sensory impairments, including problems with stereognosis, proprioception, and two-point discrimination, have been reported in 44% to 51% of children with CP. Visual-spatial and visual-perceptual problems are common—90% and 60%, respectively.[253] Rates of coexisting impairments vary with different subtypes. Children with

more significant motor problems experience proportionately higher rates of associated impairments. The degrees of physical and cognitive disability are also related to lifetime costs.[181] Health care, social care, and productivity costs of people with CP contribute to significant societal financial burden.

CLASSIFICATION

CP impairs voluntary motor function and produces a variety of symptoms. Nevertheless, the term *CP* is itself an artificial concept, comprising several causes and clinical syndromes that have been grouped together because of commonalities of management. Classifications based on topography, type of motor disorder, and functional ability describe CP.

Commonly used topographic distributions include diplegia (lower limbs affected more than upper), hemiplegia or hemiparesis (upper and lower limbs on one side of the body), and quadriplegia or tetraplegia (all limbs).[303] Although these designations focus on the limbs, involvement of the head and trunk muscles is typical. A more recent European classification designates spastic CP as bilateral or unilateral.[54] Lack of standardized definitions for topographic designations limits their reliability and validity.[123]

CP is also classified according to movement differences, which to some extent reflect the location of brain damage. Types include spastic, dyskinetic, ataxic, and mixed.[54,284,285] Spastic CP results from involvement of the motor cortex or white matter projections to and from cortical sensorimotor areas of the brain. Spasticity and exaggerated reflexes result in abnormal patterns of posture and movement. Dyskinesia reflects involvement of the basal ganglia. Dyskinetic features include atypical patterns of posture and involuntary, uncontrolled, recurring, and occasionally stereotyped movements of affected body parts. Dyskinetic CP may be classified further into subtypes: dystonic or athetotic. Dystonic movement is dominated by involuntary sustained or intermittent muscle contraction with repetitive movements and abnormal postures. Athetosis is characterized by slow, continuous, writhing movements that prevent maintenance of a stable posture. A cerebellar lesion produces ataxia—an inability to generate normal or expected voluntary movement trajectories that cannot be attributed to weakness or involuntary muscle activity about affected joints.[284] It results in general instability, abnormal patterns of posture, and lack of orderly, coordinated, rhythmic, and accurate movements.[54] In mixed CP, symptoms of spasticity and dyskinesia may be present.[54] The term should be used with an elaboration of the component motor disorders. Proportions of the various subtypes of CP vary with the reporting and sampling sources. Rates also change over time, as causes of CP are altered by advances in prevention and changing rates of prematurity and other medical problems associated with the diagnoses. A population-based study from Sweden based on children born between1990 and 1997 reported that spastic hemiplegia accounted for 30%; spastic diplegia, 38%; spastic quadriplegia, 5.5%; dystonia, 9.5%; athetosis, 5.5%; ataxic forms, 11%, and mixed types 2%.[348]

The functional abilities of people with CP vary greatly. The traditional designations of mild, moderate, and severe have been used widely but are not well defined or used reliably.[268] The Gross Motor Function Classification System (GMFCS) has become the principal system for describing functional gross motor disability in children with CP (Figure 18-1).[53] It is a reliable, five-level, age-categorized system that places children with CP into categories of severity that represent clinically meaningful distinctions in motor function with a particular emphasis on their usual performance in sitting, walking, and wheeled mobility.[242,270]

Examples of young and older children functioning at each of the GFMCS levels are included in the videoclips of GMFCS levels. The GMFCS provides a communication tool on which to base description of research subjects, treatment strategies, and service delivery models. The original system has four age bands, and an expanded and revised version includes an adolescent age band for youth 12 to 18 years of age.[241,268] Children younger than 2 years of age can be classified, but they should be reclassified when they are older. A study of change over time showed that 42% of children classified when younger than 2 years of age were classified at different levels at older ages, most often with a less functional level.[122] The GMFCS has shown strong correlations between classifications in the preschool years and those at 12 years of age and into the adult years.[268] A family questionnaire version has been shown to be reliable in eliciting GMFCS levels from families.[218] Proportions of children falling into the five GMFCS levels vary among studies, and variation sometimes is attributed to the ability to accurately detect all Level I children. A population-based study from Sweden reported the following proportions of children in each GMFCS level: Level I, 48%; II, 18%; III, 12%; IV, 9%; and V, 13%.[348] The Manual Ability Classification System (MACS) is a tool for hand and arm function similar to the GMFCS.[97] It classifies the handling of objects in daily activities by children with CP and reflects typical performance rather than maximal capacity (www.macs.nu). A Communication Function Classification System (CFCS) is being developed.[151]

The Functional Mobility Scale (FMS) classifies mobility in children with CP on a six-point ordinal scale according to the need for assistive mobility devices for moving distances of 5, 50, and 500 meters. These distances reflect home, school, and community settings. Not only is the FMS a reliable and valid classification tool, it also is able to detect change after surgery.[128,144,145]

ORIGIN AND PATHOPHYSIOLOGY

Although the causes of CP are not understood completely, associations have been made with certain prenatal, perinatal, and postnatal events. These include hypoxic, ischemic, infectious, congenital, or traumatic insults affecting the brain. Other contributors include premature birth, atypical uterine growth, multiple births, and genetic factors. Observational research, both controlled population-based studies identifying major causes and prognoses, as well as smaller investigations recognizing less common causes, has added to our understanding of the origin of CP. In particular, advances in magnetic resonance imaging (MRI) have furthered our understanding of the causes and timing of the pathogenesis of CP through visualization of physiologic and pathologic morphologic changes that occur during brain development.[179,180,228]

The pathobiology of CP differs by nature, timing, and location of the brain insult.[180,228,229,277] Recognition of the impact of prenatal factors is increasing. Many perinatal difficulties may occur secondary to preexisting central nervous system pathology. MRI studies estimate that insults contributing to CP occur during the prenatal, perinatal, and postnatal periods in 34%, 43%, and 6% of patients, respectively, and are unable to be estimated in 16%.[179] During the first and second trimesters of gestation, brain pathology is characterized by genetic or acquired impairments. From the late second trimester onward, disturbances are more often a result of infectious or hypoxic-ischemic mechanisms that result in lesions.[180] Most cases of CP diagnosed in infants who were born at term are the result of prenatal influences. Growing awareness that a multiplicity of risk factors contribute to the origin of CP suggests that a causal web is a more realistic model rather than one involving a single event. Single events such as uterine rupture, cord prolapse, or major placental abruption resulting in hypoxic insults to the brain account for a small proportion of cases.[228] Although birth asphyxia can result in CP, it is not a common antecedent. When it is the cause, hypoxic damage is typically bilateral and widespread, including the basal ganglia and gray and white matter, resulting in total body involvement with spastic and dyskinetic features. Additional factors such as inflammation can interact with asphyxia, multiplying the risk of CP.[228]

It has become increasingly clear that cerebral vascular events occurring within the first 28 days after birth are a significant cause of CP. The advent of neuroimaging has contributed significantly to further understanding in this area because neonates with strokes do not present clinically

GMFCS E & R Descriptors and Illustrations for Children between their 6th and 12th birthday

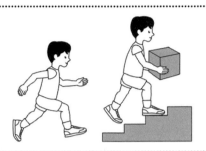

GMFCS Level I

Children walk at home, school, outdoors and in the community. They can climb stairs without the use of a railing. Children perform gross motor skills such as running and jumping, but speed, balance and coordination are limited

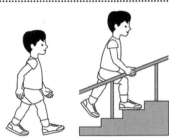

GMFCS Level II

Children walk in most settings and climb stairs holding onto a railing. They may experience difficulty walking long distances and balancing on uneven terrain, inclines, in crowded areas or confined spaces. Children may walk with physical assistance, a hand-held mobility device or use wheeled mobility over long distances. Children have only minimal ability to perform gross motor skills such as running and jumping.

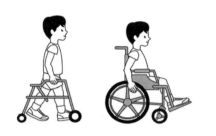

GMFCS Level III

Children walk using a hand-held mobility device in most indoor settings. They may climb stairs holding onto a railing with supervision or assistance. Children use wheeled mobility when traveling long distances and may self-propel for shorter distances.

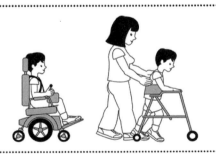

GMFCS Level IV

Children use methods of mobility that require physical assistance or powered mobility in most settings. They may walk for short distances at home with physical assistance or use powered mobility or a body support walker when positioned. At school, outdoors and in the community children are transported in a manual wheelchair or use powered mobility.

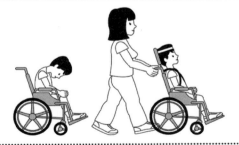

GMFCS Level V

Children are transported in a manual wheelchair in all settings. Children are limited in their ability to maintain antigravity head and trunk postures and control leg and arm movements.

GMFCS descriptors copyright © Palisano et al. (1997) Dev Med Child Neurol 39:214-23
CanChild: www.canchild.ca

Illustrations copyright © Kerr Graham, Bill Reid and Adrienne Harvey,
The Royal Children's Hospital, Melbourne

Figure 18-1   The Gross Motor Function Classification System for children ages 6 to 12 years of age and the Gross Motor Function Classification System – Expanded and Revised for children ages 12 to 18 years of age.

Continued

GMFCS E & R Descriptors and Illustrations for Children between their 12ᵗʰ and 18ᵗʰ birthday

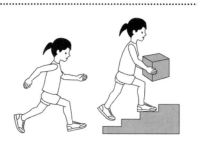

GMFCS Level I

Youth walk at home, school, outdoors and in the community. Youth are able to climb curbs and stairs without physical assistance or a railing. They perform gross motor skills such as running and jumping but speed, balance and coordination are limited.

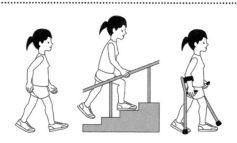

GMFCS Level II

Youth walk in most settings but environmental factors and personal choice influence mobility choices. At school or work they may require a hand-held mobility device for safety and climb stairs holding onto a railing. Outdoors and in the community youth may use wheeled mobility when traveling long distances.

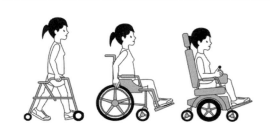

GMFCS Level III

Youth are capable of walking using a hand-held mobility device. Youth may climb stairs holding onto a railing with supervision or assistance. At school they may self-propel a manual wheelchair or use powered mobility. Outdoors and in the community youth are transported in a wheelchair or use powered mobility.

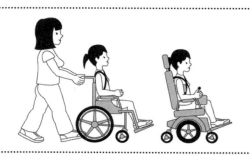

GMFCS Level IV

Youth use wheeled mobility in most settings. Physical assistance of 1-2 people is required for transfers. Indoors, youth may walk short distances with physical assistance, use wheeled mobility or a body support walker when positioned. They may operate a powered chair, otherwise are transported in a manual wheelchair.

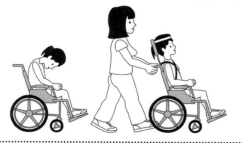

GMFCS Level V

Youth are transported in a manual wheelchair in all settings. Youth are limited in their ability to maintain antigravity head and trunk postures and control leg and arm movements. Self-mobility is severely limited, even with the use of assistive technology.

Figure 18-1, cont'd

with hemiparesis. In contrast to the adult population, approximately one third of perinatal strokes are bilateral. Placental pathology such as thrombotic leisons may be an important factor.[228,229]

Infections such as toxoplasmosis, rubella, cytomegalovirus, herpes virus, hepatitis B, syphilis, human immunodeficiency virus, and streptococcus B can be transmitted from mother to infant, affecting the brain and resulting in CP. Placental inflammation (chorioamnionitis) has also been linked with adverse neurologic outcomes.[228,229] Children with CP have more congenital abnormalities, such as brain malformation, cleft lip or palate, and gut atresia, compared with children who do not have CP. This suggests further the significant contribution of prenatal factors to the origin of CP.[277] Maternal trauma resulting in direct fetal injury, placental abruption, or prenatal vascular insult can also cause CP. Possible mechanisms include reduced placental blood flow and/or placental embolization.[147] Maternal thyroid disease has been linked with cerebral palsy.[154]

Premature birth increases the risk of CP but contributes to one half or fewer of the diagnoses. In such cases, the underlying brain pathology is white matter injury in sensorimotor pathways. Prolonged rupture of the membranes predisposing to intrauterine infection is an important antecedent. Multiple gestation practices, increasingly common as a result of reproductive technology, can contribute to the risk for CP as a result of the tendency for premature birth or the death of a monozygotic fetus, causing malformation in a surviving infant due to vascular collapse.[228,229] The potentially complex medical course, including the use of postnatal steroids, adds to the chain of events that can result in CP.

Infants with atypical intrauterine growth, either small or large for gestational age, are at increased risk for CP. Small birth weight can be associated with infection, preeclampsia, maternal vascular disease, or thrombophilia. Large babies may experience problematic deliveries. Maternal diabetes is a risk factor for macrosomia, but it is not a risk factor for CP. Excessively small or large babies are also at greater risk for perinatal stroke.[228]

Genetic factors can influence the risk of CP at a number of points along the causal pathway. Risk factors with a genetic component include preterm birth, placental abruption, preeclampsia, chorioamnionitis, and thrombophilias or the presence of certain genotypes such as apolipoprotein E.[183] Future research examining gene–gene and gene–environment interactions may provide important information.[228,229] A form of hereditary spastic paresis has also been identified.[84]

Reported rates of various brain pathologies vary. A study of a cohort of 154 children diagnosed with CP for whom MRI was available indicated the following proportions of brain scan findings: 16% normal, 31% periventricular white matter injury, 16% focal ischemic/hemorrhagic lesions, 14% diffuse encephalopathy, 12% brain malformations, 2% infections, and 8% unclassifiable.[259] Sixty-six percent of the children were born at term. Children with brain malformations were more likely to have been born at term and had more severe motor disabilities than other children with a CP diagnosis.

CP is the most common cause of physical disability affecting children in developed countries, with a prevalence of 2.0 to 2.5 per 1000 live births.[303] A review of change in the prevalence of CP shows an increase from below 2.0 per 1000 in the 1970s to above 2.0 per 1000 in the 1990s,[233] with little change over the past few decades despite improvements in neonatal care.[296] Although the overall prevalence of CP has remained relatively steady, changes in the characteristics of CP have occurred. These include an increase in spastic diplegia, possibly reflecting increased survival in preterm and very preterm infants, and a decrease in quadriplegia and an overall reduction in the severity of motor function that is presumed to be indicative of advances in health care.[296]

PROGRESS IN PREVENTION

Perinatal strategies to prevent CP have been both discouraging and encouraging.[229] Bilirubin encephalopathy is now rare in developed countries as a result of the treatment of neonatal jaundice and prevention of rhesus isoimmunization. Continuous electronic fetal monitoring during labor became popular in the 1970s, but studies showed that it does not reduce the frequency of CP. Likewise, no evidence supports the efficacy of treatment of maternal fevers to reduce the risk of CP. Based on outcome assessment at 18 months of age, therapeutic hypothermia has been shown to significantly reduce the combined outcome of infant mortality and major neurodevelopmental disability in term infants with neonatal encephalopathy.[160] Studies are under way to evaluate this intervention for infants with other problems.[229] Trials of administering magnesium sulphate for fetal neuroprotection to women in premature labor have shown potential for decreasing the frequency of moderate or severe CP but not death in very preterm infants.[229,273] Unfortunately, advances in perinatal and neonatal care cannot affect the significant proportion of children who are affected by a variety of prenatal disorders.

A social class gradient has been noted in the prevalence of CP, along with an association between birth weight and socioeconomic status, suggesting that improvements in the education, health, and prenatal care of mothers at risk could improve outcomes.[233] Avoidance of multiple fetus implantation during in vitro fertilization could decrease the incidence of CP due to multiple births.[229]

DIAGNOSIS

Neuroimaging findings and prenatal risk factors can assist in making a diagnosis of CP, but the sensitivity and specificity of single or combined risk factors, such as neonatal seizures, low birth weight, or maternal infection, in predicting CP have been disappointing.[245] As a result, CP remains a clinical diagnosis made when a child does not reach early motor milestones and exhibits abnormal muscle tone or qualitative differences in movement patterns.[265,266] Physical therapists can play an important role in the diagnosis of CP through their involvement in clinics for high-risk infants and early therapy intervention programs.[141] Assessment of asymmetry, involuntary movements, and abnormal primitive reflexes, and the late development of postural responses can contribute to the clinical diagnosis. The use of three-dimensional analysis of spontaneous general movements in infants during the first month of life has shown the potential to objectively differentiate normal from atypical movements in healthy and at risk infants. One study demonstrated 100% sensitivity, 70% specificity, and an overall detection rate of CP of 73%. Such analyses also yield the benefits derived from archiving videos for later comparison and evaluation.[207]

Predictive and discriminative infant neuromotor tests can augment clinical judgment to assist in prediction and identification of CP, respectively. The Alberta Infant Motor Scales (AIMS) demonstrates good psychometric properties, especially between corrected ages 4 and 10 months, and has clinical utility in comparing an infant's development with that of other infants of the same age.[50] The Test of Infant Motor Performance (TIMP) and the NeuroSensory Motor Development Assessment (NSMDA) can be used before as well as after term.[51,63] Prechtl's Assessment of General Movements (GM) has the best combination of sensitivity and specificity for predicting CP in the early months, but the AIMS and the NSMDA are better predictors when the infants are older.[300]

Precise diagnosis can be difficult, especially early in development. No consensus has been reached on how early CP can be identified reliably,[50] although it has been postulated that an experienced physical therapist or pediatrician should be able to identify the signs of CP in all but the mildest cases by 6 months of age.[282] Nevertheless, variation in motor development must be considered and respected and a definitive diagnosis made cautiously in consideration of alternate explanations, while not withholding appropriate services.[54,266] It is important to differentiate between atypical motor trajectories that are indicative of CP and other situations such as recovery from medical conditions, including premature birth. For example, adjusted AIMS norms for infants born prematurely reflect variation in the gross motor trajectories specific to this population.[332] Physical therapists may also play a role in recognizing alternative diagnoses. Transient dystonia presents with similar but resolving neurologic signs of CP.[88,141,266,332]

Diagnosis should be confirmed by a pediatric specialist to rule out other causes of similar clinical signs such as brain tumors or metabolic disorders. Follow-up is necessary to ensure a nonprogressive nature. It is recommended that all children with CP have a brain MRI in cases of unknown origin. Metabolic workups should be considered in children who appear to have CP but have normal brain imaging, because genetic muscle disorders and mitochondrial disease may present similarly to CP.[179,259]

DETERMINANTS OF PROGNOSIS OR OUTCOME

Knowledge of prognosis for gross motor function in children with CP can facilitate communication with families and allow goal setting to be collaborative and realistic.[239] One of the first concerns for parents of children with CP is whether their child will walk. Results from a large database of children with CP indicate that 54% walked independently by 5 years of age, 16% walked with aids, and 30% were unable to walk.[19] Walking ability varied by type of CP. Children with hemiplegic and ataxic CP were more likely to walk, whereas those with dyskinetic and bilateral CP were least likely to do so. Cognitive functioning was the strongest predictor of walking ability for all types of CP. Visual and hearing impairments and the presence of epilepsy also correlated with walking abilities.[19] Independent sitting by 24 months remains the best predictor of ambulation for 15 meters or more with or without assistive devices by age 8 years.[345] If independent sitting is not achieved by age 3, there is very little chance of achieving functional independent walking.[29] Some people with CP experience a decline in their walking abilities in adolescence or adulthood as a result of pain, fatigue, musculoskeletal deterioration, poor surgical outcome, weight and height gains, or fear of falling. Only half of adults with hemiplegia and one third with diplegia have reported maintenance of their walking abilities.[195]

The development of motor growth curves for children with CP has provided clinicians with a practical predictive tool.[139,271] Gross motor curves were based on Gross Motor Function Measure-66 scores of 657 children. The children were stratified by GMFCS level, and data were collected through a prospective longitudinal population-based cohort study of Canadian children with CP. The curves demonstrate that children with CP reach 90% of their motor potential before the age of 3 years for the most severely impaired children (GMFCS Level V) and by the age of 5 years for the least affected children (GMFCS Level I).[271] A continuation of this study following the subjects into adolescence showed that children at GMFCS Levels I and II do not, on average, demonstrate functional decline in GMFM-66 scores, but mean scores for those at Levels III, IV, and V peak at approximately 7 years of age and then decline.[138] It should not be assumed, however, that the average patterns apply to all children with CP because there is large variability within levels. Reference percentile curves have been developed to provide normative interpretation of GMFM-66 scores within GMFCS levels but should be used with caution and only as additional information becomes available to assist with the interpretation of change over time.[137] (Tabulated reference percentiles for the GMFM-66 are available at http://motorgrowth.canchild.ca/en/MotorGrowthCurves/percentiles.asp.) Similar patterns of gross motor development were found in a Swedish study of

319 children between the ages of 1 and 15 years. Variability in GMFM-88 scores was noted among GMFCS levels, and most children reached a plateau at 6 to 7 years.[18] Such studies reflect descriptions of developmental trajectories as influenced by the intervention strategies available in developed countries.

Prognosis for overall functioning as an adult is dependent on many variables, and reports vary greatly. Mean values summarized from six studies showed that 31% of adults with CP lived independently, 12% were married, 24% achieved a tertiary/vocational level of education, and 28% had paid employment.[195] Positive prognostic factors for employment include mild physical involvement, good home support, education, vocational training, and good cognitive skills.[223] Increasing success rates in education and employment over the years have been attributed to advances in and access to technology such as power wheelchairs and computers, environmental access, and supportive legislation.

Life expectancy is associated with severity of motor, cognitive, and visual impairment. A 2-year-old with severe CP has approximately a 40% chance of living to age 20, in contrast to a child with mild CP, for whom the chance is 99%.[157] A decline in mortality of children with severe CP has been noted over the past 20 years, particularly for those with feeding problems, reflecting better management of feeding and swallowing difficulties and overall improvement in the care of medically fragile persons. People with CP have an increased incidence of mortality due to external causes such as drowning and being struck by motor vehicles.[308,309]

ICF-CY AND CEREBRAL PALSY

The International Classification of Functioning, Disability, and Health for Children and Youth (ICF-CY) provides a common language and conceptual framework to explore the complex interactions among a health condition, body structure and function, activity, and participation, in the context of personal and environmental factors of individuals.[355] All domains of this model must be considered when assessing and providing physical therapy and support for children with CP and their families.

BODY FUNCTION/STRUCTURE

Physical therapists address primarily the impairments of neuromusculoskeletal and movement-related body functions and structures in their practice. At the same time, cognitive, behavioral, sensory, cardiovascular, respiratory, digestive, and pain functions and structures are important components of comprehensive care and management. Impairments can be primary or secondary. Primary impairments are an immediate result of the existing pathophysiologic process, whereas secondary impairments develop over time as the result of other impairments, activity limitations, participation restrictions, or environmental and personal factors. Secondary musculoskeletal impairments such as

contractures or skeletal malalignment can have an impact on the capacity for performance of functional activities.[16,130] An understanding of these processes is integral to the prevention of unnecessary disability in children with CP. The following sections discuss the impairments most often addressed directly by physical therapy.

Muscle Tone and Extensibility

Tone is a clinical term used to describe the neural and mechanical properties of muscle. *Muscle tone* is defined as normal resting tension or resistance of muscle to passive movement or muscle lengthening.[54] It excludes resistance as a result of joint, ligament, or skeletal properties. Hypotonia is characterized by diminished resting muscle tone and decreased ability to generate voluntary muscle force. Hypertonia is an abnormal increase in resistance to an external force about a joint resulting from a number of factors, including neurally mediated reflex stiffness, passive muscle stiffness, and active muscle stiffness, all of which contribute to resistance of the muscle to stretch.[107,283] It is difficult to classify abnormal tone as a primary or secondary impairment because (1) it develops over time and with increasing attempts to overcome the force of gravity and gain mobility (except in those with severe impairment), and (2) the early neurally mediated abnormality of tone that is one of the signs leading to the diagnosis of CP is compounded over time by the addition of muscle stiffness and contracture. In children with CP, muscle tone has been found to increase up to 4 years of age and then decrease up to the age of 12.[134]

Spasticity is neural resistance to externally imposed movement, which increases with increasing speed of stretch, and varies with the direction of joint movement. Resistance may rise rapidly above a threshold speed of passive movement or joint angle, resulting in a spastic catch that may represent the threshold for onset of the stretch reflex.[285] Spasticity may be associated with clonus, pathologic reflexes, and particular patterns of posture and movement. Supraspinal and interneuronal mechanisms appear to be responsible for spasticity. Pathophysiologic mechanisms include reduced reciprocal inhibition of antagonist motoneuron pools, decreased presynaptic inhibition, and decreased nonreciprocal inhibition.[285,286] Studies using transcranial magnetic cerebral stimulation have provided evidence of simultaneous activation of antagonistic muscle groups through abnormal alpha motoneuron innervation.[41]

Passive muscle stiffness is the sense of abnormally high tone or hypoextensibility of muscles resulting from abnormal mechanical properties. The muscle offers resistance to passive stretching at a shorter length than that expected in a normal muscle. In addition, if greater than normal amounts of force are required to produce a change in length, the muscle is said to have increased stiffness. This is represented as the passive tension curve for CP (p,CP) in contrast to the normal passive tension curve (p,N) in Figure 18-2, *D*, in

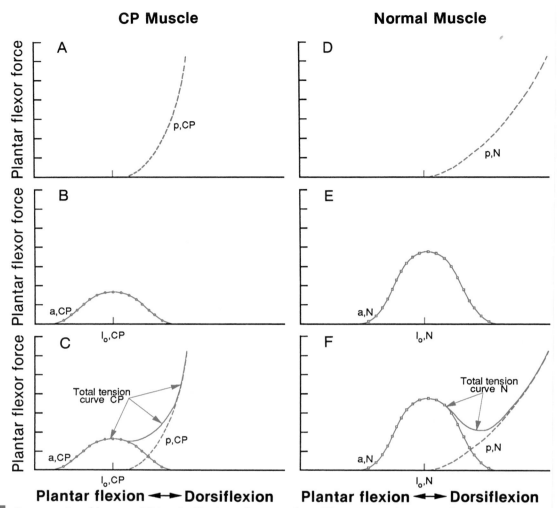

CP Muscle   **Normal Muscle**

Figure 18-2 Representation of force capabilities of ankle plantar flexor muscle at different joint angles in normal muscle (N) and spastic muscle (CP). **A,** Resistance to passive stretch of spastic muscle (p,CP) increasing with more dorsiflexion. **B,** The force of active contraction (a,CP) varying with the joint angle l_0 denoting resting length. **C,** The sum of passive and active effects in spastic muscle. **D,** Resistance to passive stretch in normal muscle (p,N). **E,** Force of active contraction in normal muscle (a,N). **F,** Total tension curve comprising the sum of passive and active effects in normal muscle. Note that (1) the slope (i.e., the stiffness) of p,CP in **A** is greater for the spastic muscle than for normal muscles (p,N) in **D**; (2) the maximal active force achieved by the spastic muscle (a,CP) in **B** is less than the maximal active force of normal muscle (a,N) in **E**; and (3) the maximal active force for spastic muscle (a,CP) shown in **B** occurs at a more plantar-flexed position than that of the normal muscle (a,N) shown in **E**.

response to moving the ankle from a position of plantar flexion to one of dorsiflexion. When a clinician finds that it is not possible to manually stretch the muscle through a normal range using reasonable amounts of manual force, the muscle group is deemed to have a contracture. This is represented as "contracture," the difference between the joint angle at which this extreme resistance is encountered in the CP muscle and that of the normal muscle. Figure 18-2 shows hypothetical active force-length characteristics of spastic plantar flexors (a,CP; see Figure 18-2, *B*) and normal plantar flexors (a,N; see Figure 18-2, *E*), that is, the force generated by the contractile elements of the muscle over the range of muscle lengths from a shortened position (plantar flexed) to a longer position (dorsiflexed). Note that the

maximal force is lower for the CP muscle, and that the peak force occurs at a more plantar flexed position in the CP muscle than in the normal muscle. The sum of the combined effects of active force output and passive stiffness for the CP muscle is shown as total tension curve CP, and the corresponding curve for the normal muscle is shown as total tension curve N (Figure 18-3). The complexity of the representation in Figure 18-3 underscores the difficulty faced by clinicians in correctly determining the cause of increased tone through clinical methods such as passive manipulation of the limb and clinical assessment of muscle strength. The underlying mechanisms of these muscle extensibility alterations in CP are not clearly understood but are important in developing a rationale for interventions.[107] Contractures

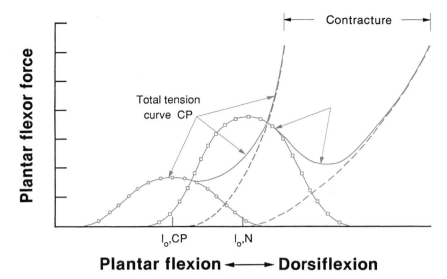

have been characterized by alterations of sarcomere properties; muscle fiber size, type, alignment, and distribution; muscle volume; and muscle cell stiffness.[13,130,190,292] A proliferation of extracellular materials with inferior mechanical properties has been noted in spastic muscle.[107] These abnormal collagen characteristics have been identified in the muscles of children with CP.[28]

Muscles grow and respond to the amount and type of activity they experience during movement. Regular stretching of relaxed muscle under normal physiologic loading occurs in typically developing children. The muscles in children with CP may not relax during activity and may be subject to chronic muscle imbalance, abnormal posturing, and static positioning resulting from spasticity, weakness, and abnormal reflex activity.[130] Muscle growth may not keep up with bone growth during periods of rapid linear growth, thereby contributing to hypoextensibility; conversely, some muscles may become overlengthened as the result of repeated mechanical stretch or orthopedic surgery.[363] Although patterns of tightness vary, the muscles most commonly at risk for contracture are the shoulder adductors; the elbow, wrist, and finger flexors; the hip flexors and adductors; the knee flexors; and the ankle plantar flexors. A population-based study of adolescents with CP demonstrated that although those with lower gross motor function tended to have greater limitations in range of motion (ROM), variation within GMFCS levels could be seen. Some adolescents functioning at GMFCS Level I had contractures; others functioning at Level V did not.[358]

Muscle Strength

Considerable evidence suggests that children with CP are unable to generate normal voluntary force in a muscle or normal torque about a joint.[272,284] This impairment may be expressed as decreased moment of force output, a deficiency in power or, when considered over time, in work.[234] The term

strength may refer to any of these measurable factors, and diminished force production capability is now understood to be a primary impairment in CP. Muscle weakness is consistent with low levels of electromyographic (EMG) activity and has been attributed to decreased neuronal drive, inappropriate co-activation of antagonistic muscle groups, secondary myopathy, and altered muscle tissue properties.[96,99,107,111,272,301] Additionally, muscle shortening and skeletal deformity can lead to changes in lever arm biomechanics, resulting in reduced output of muscle force in terms of torque.[232] Greater weakness has been reported in the distal musculature compared with the proximal musculature, for concentric versus eccentric contractions, and in faster versus slower speeds of movement.[74] Strength has been linked with activity capabilities such as walking speed and gross motor function.[73,232] Strength deficits can also contribute to bone deformity, for example, hip weakness is a postulated cause of hip deformity in ambulatory children and young adults.[209]

Skeletal Structure

Impairments such as weakness, spasticity, abnormal extensibility, and disturbed reflexes can result in excessive and abnormal biomechanical forces. Structures such as joint capsules, joint ligaments, and bones can become compromised. Torsion of long bones, joint instability, and premature degenerative changes in weight-bearing joints can occur.[130] Alignment of the spine and extremities can be affected, particularly during times of physical growth. Reported prevalence of scoliosis in individuals with CP ranges from 15% to 61% and increases with age and GMFCS level.[214,356] Of particular concern is the effect of hip flexion and adduction spasticity on acetabular development and hip joint stability, putting children with CP at risk for hip subluxation and dislocation. A population-based study reported the rate of displacement, defined as a migration percentage of greater than 30%, to be 35.3%. Rates were related to gross motor function based on GMFCS classifications. None of the children with GMFCS Level I had hip displacement or hip surgery compared with 90% of children at Level V.[133,299]

Selective Control

Normal movement is characterized by orderly phasing in and out of muscle activation, co-activation of muscles with similar biomechanical functions, and limited co-activation of antagonists during phasic or free movement. Children with CP have poor selective control of muscle activity. This is defined as the impaired ability to isolate the activation of muscles in a selected pattern in response to demands of a voluntary posture. Individuals with poor selective control exhibit reduced speed of movement, mirror movements, or abnormal reciprocal muscle activation.[110,284,286] They may be unable to move their hip, knee, and ankle joints independently of one another and exhibit coupled flexor and extensor patterns when attempting functional movement.[110] Deficiency in the control of selective movements is a major contributor to impaired motor function.[108] For example, selective control of the lower extremity is related to the ability to extend the knee while flexing the hip during the swing phase of gait.[110] Selective control is an important predictor of improvement after interventions for other impairments such as dorsal rhizotomy to reduce spasticity[98] or orthopedic surgery to lengthen muscle.[110]

Postural Control

Postural control is the ability to control the position of the center of mass over the base of support. (See Chapter 3.) The sensory, motor, and musculoskeletal systems participate in coordinating postural activity. Children with CP have dysfunction in responding to postural challenges and have difficulty in fine-tuning postural activity.[83] Reactive postural adjustments occur in response to unexpected external postural perturbations. Responses in children with CP vary with level of severity. Children with CP functioning at GMFCS Levels I and II have some ability to produce direction-specific adjustments to counteract forces disturbing equilibrium through reactive control, whereas these abilities decrease with higher GMFCS levels and are largely absent in children with GMFCS Level V.[39] Anticipatory postural adjustments are related to expected internal postural perturbations preceding the onset of voluntary movement.[349] In healthy individuals, changes in posture are preceded by preparatory muscle contractions that stabilize the body and allow weight shifts in anticipation of movement, while keeping the center of mass within the stability limits of the body. Children with CP exhibit characteristic disorganization and/or adaptations, including cranial-caudal recruitment of postural muscles, excessive antagonistic co-activation, and reduced or absent capacity to adapt the degree of muscle contraction as appropriate to the specific task or situation.[39,83]

Motor Learning

Motor learning comprises a set of processes associated with practice or experience that leads to relatively permanent changes in the ability to produce skilled action. (See Chapter 4.) Children with CP can be constrained in their ability to learn movement strategies because of impairments such as spasticity, weakness, limitations in sensation, perceptual-motor skills, and cognition, as well as the lack of opportunity to experience motor skills in variable settings. They have difficulty analyzing their own movement and utilizing feedback to improve performance.[322] Motor memory is frequently impaired.[95] These problems might force a child with CP to use additional cognitive resources when planning and performing motor skills. Limited literature exists on the cognitive aspects of motor learning in children with neurologic disability, and more research is needed.[322]

Pain

Pain is a secondary impairment that affects other body functions and structures, levels of participation, and quality of life (QOL) of people with CP.[16,158,319] It can result from primary impairments, overuse syndromes, interventions such as surgery, equipment use, procedures such as injections, and rehabilitation.[204] Chronic pain may contribute to depression, sleep disturbance, fatigue, and reduced overall physical functioning.[16,204,356] Pain was reported by 61% of a group of ambulatory children, and more than half of their parents believed that the pain interfered with activities of daily living.[158] Nonambulatory children also experience pain.

Activity and Participation

In the ICF-CY domains of activity and participation, physical therapists address gross motor skills and mobility and their contributions to involvement in home, school, and community life. Motor skills vary greatly among children with CP, as described by the levels of the GMFCS (see Figure 18-1), and somewhat within GMFCS levels.[271] A number of factors have been identified by pediatric physical therapists as influential in bringing about change in the motor abilities of children with CP.[14] These include muscle tone, movement patterns and selective control, force production, endurance, family factors, and personality characteristics.

Walking is a preoccupation of parents at the time of diagnosis, a frequent goal of families, a predictor of participation, and a skill that can deteriorate over time.[29,236] As a result, ambulating is a major focus of clinical practice and research in children with CP. Walking is not always a realistic or optimal method of mobility. Alternative means of mobility are essential for some children and are chosen by some children and adults for efficiency in certain environments.[323]

Participation in children with disabilities is a complex phenomenon that allows them to pursue the learning of skills, to develop social engagement, and to find satisfaction

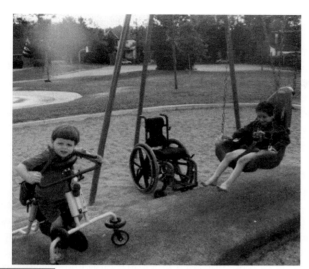

Figure 18-4 Environmental adaptations to playgrounds can facilitate participation in normal childhood activities.

in their lives.[158] Opportunities for children and adolescents with CP to participate in home, school, and community activities are increasing. This can be attributed to advances in technology and a legacy of striving for inclusion that has influenced social attitudes and policies regarding funding and environmental adaptation. Nevertheless, children and adolescents with CP experience restrictions in participation compared with children in the general population.[18,159,211] They may be excluded from playing with peers or bullied; however, many do have positive peer experiences.[159] Adults with CP experience restrictions in participation. They are not fully integrated socially, have less experience with intimate and partner relationships, and have problems securing paid employment.[261]

Many factors are associated with participation. Physical environment (Figure 18-4), GMFCS level, hand function, and cognition are important predictors.[159,219] A European study of participation in children with CP found that walking ability was the most important factor associated with participation.[101] Pain and fine motor, cognitive, and communication abilities were additional predictors, but sociodemographic factors were not. Further analyses revealed that participation varied significantly across countries even when other factors were controlled for. Denmark had higher rates of participation in all areas except relationships. This most likely was reflective of its policies and programs supporting the principle of equal access through public transportation, accessibility, assistive technology, and financial assistance.

Such findings illustrate the impact of the social and legislative environment on the lives of people with disabilities. Other factors that have an impact on participation identified through various studies include the use of aids and adaptations, attitudinal barriers, epilepsy, toileting needs, parental values, parental vigilance, and child motivation.[101,158]

Participation in physical activity is particularly important for children with CP. Child behavior, personality, and family recreational styles predict variation in leisure and recreational participation.[172]

EXAMINATION AND EVALUATION

At all ages, the physical therapy examination and evaluation of children with CP involves the identification of strengths and abilities, as well as participation restrictions, activity limitations, and impairments of body structure and function. Physical therapists integrate this information with prognostic knowledge and information about environmental and personal contextual factors that are potential motivators or barriers. Evaluation involves the synthesis of these pieces of information to determine the difference between current performance and capacity, predict the optimal level of improvement that can be expected, formulate realistic short-term and long-term goals, guide overall clinical decision making, determine specific intervention strategies, and measure outcomes, thereby informing further goals and treatment approaches. Ongoing assessments provide feedback for clinicians, children, and their families that can be motivating or indicative of areas that need more attention. Video and photographic recording of assessments can provide records for ongoing comparison. Information gained from continuously monitoring outcomes, whether in clinical practice or research, enhances overall clinical decision making, promotes best practice, and facilitates the planning of appropriate health services and the allocation of resources.[199,270]

Numerous measurement tools are available. The ICF provides a framework to guide the choice of tests. Selection should be consistent with the purpose of an assessment: discrimination, prognosis, or evaluation. Measurement tools need to be psychometrically strong but also feasible for a particular clinical or research situation. Cost, training, time to administer and score, amount of handling, and child and family acceptance must be considered.

IMPAIRMENT

Muscle Tone and Extensibility

No methods of measuring muscle tone are universally accepted. Choices depend on the purpose of measurement. It is important to consider both neurologic and passive mechanical components of tone and to measure accordingly. The modified Ashworth scale, although commonly used, is really an undifferentiated measure of spasticity and extensibility. It has been shown to have low levels of reliability for children with CP, particularly for the plantar flexor muscles.[64,109] It does not quantify spasticity exclusively as the intrinsic stiffness of the muscles can contribute to hypertonia in addition to a heightened, velocity-dependent stretch reflex response. Measurements evaluating resistance at several speeds may be more useful for planning and evaluating interventions, particularly those that aim to reduce spasticity or manage contracture.[73,237] The modified Tardieu scale measures the point of resistance or "catch" to a rapid velocity stretch, giving an indication of the dynamic neural component of tone or the overactive stretch reflex. Moving the limb slowly into a lengthened position indicates the mechanical component of tone or muscle length at rest, commonly known as ROM.[35] A large difference between the initial catch and the point of mechanical resistance indicates a large reflexive component to motion limitation, and a small difference suggests a more fixed muscle contracture.[35] The Tardieu scale has been found to be more reliable than the modified Ashworth scale, particularly for the plantar flexors, but wide intersessional variations between dynamic and static differences limit use as an outcome measure.[109]

Goniometric errors of 10° to 14° in passive ROM measures occur in same-day goniometric measurements in children with CP and are even greater for those recorded on different days.[203] Some researchers have suggested that a change of more than 15° to 20° between sessions is required to be 95% confident that a true change in ROM has occurred in many joints of children with CP.[171] As a result, caution must be used when relying on goniometric measurements to determine outcomes and make clinical decisions. Regardless of these issues, quantitative measures of joint ROM and skeletal alignment, including rotational and torsional alignment of the pelvis and lower extremities (see Chapter 5), should be documented using consistent procedures. Standardization of testing is necessary, as factors such as testing position and initial length from which the muscle is stretched, and behavioral states such as laughing or fear can affect measures.[286] A major source of error is the difficulty in determining consistent and proper positioning for biarticular muscles such as the hamstrings.[318]

The Spinal Alignment Range of Motion Measure (SAROMM) is a discriminative tool used to estimate limitations of spinal alignment and ROM in children and youth with CP. The SAROMM indicates whether the child has normal alignment and ROM, flexible deviation, or mild, moderate, or severe fixed limitations.[15] It is considered to be sufficiently reliable and valid for use with children with CP in clinical and research settings by rehabilitation therapists.

The Barry-Albright Dystonia Scale provides a tool for rating dystonia.[12] It is a five-point ordinal scale based on severity of posturing and involuntary dystonic movements in eight body regions.

Strength

Testing muscle strength in children with CP may be difficult because of age, cognitive level, spasticity and hyperactive reflexes, abnormal muscle and joint extensibility, or poor selective control. Isokinetic muscle strength testing is available in some settings, allowing for precise stabilization and quantification of strength at different speeds and for

different types of contractions.[7] Clinically, muscle strength is more often measured isometrically by manual muscle testing using an ordinal 6-point scale, or with handheld dynamometry if a child can exert a maximal effort in a consistent manner.[73,111] A make test is more reliable than the break test for lower extremity muscles when handheld dynamometry is used. It has been shown to have high within-session reliability and variable between-session reliability depending on muscle group, positioning, and stabilization.[68,337] As a result, changes in strength should be considered based on measurement error for particular muscle groups.

Strength should also be assessed in a functional context. Observing activities such as moving between sitting and standing positions, or ascending and descending stairs, helps to assess both concentric and eccentric power. Counting the number of repetitions of a functional movement performed over a specific period of time can quantify functional muscle strength. Intertester reliability of 30-second repetitions of lateral step-ups, sit-to-stand, and standing through half kneeling is acceptable, with intraclass correlation coefficient (ICC) values ranging from 0.91 to 0.96 in children with CP 7 to 17 years of age.[337] Muscle strength may differ depending on posture, joint angle, speed of movement, or presence of contracture. Ability to generate force may deteriorate as a result of early fatigue of muscles, reduced endurance, or an inability to generate a sufficiently rapid increase in force, and in some cases, it may be important to measure both the ability to maintain force over time and the ability to generate a brief rapid force.

Endurance and efficiency of movement become increasingly important when children venture into the community on their own or with peers. Endurance can be evaluated by observing the ability to walk age-appropriate distances or propel a wheelchair a comparable span. The 10-meter, 1-minute, 6-minute, and 10-minute walk tests and the 600-yard walk-run test have been found to be reliable in children with CP.[59,321] Ambulation measured over longer distances more closely simulates community ambulation and therefore may more closely represent the ability to participate in the community.[250,321] Reliable and valid shuttle run tests have been developed for children and adolescents with CP at GMFCS Level I or II. These tests are acceptable to children and provide a clinically feasible measure of impairment in aerobic capacity exercise tolerance over time.[338] Sprint running tests can provide information about anaerobic muscle power.[339] Physiologic measures such as the energy expenditure index provide energy cost information in a clinically feasible manner, but these measures have limitations because heart rate may not be an accurate substitute for energy expenditure under all conditions.[104,111] They may be useful when two or more mobility options are compared for the same person.[264] A review of assessments related to physical activity and metabolic issues has been provided by Fernhall and Unnithan.[104]

Selective Control, Postural Control, Motor Learning

Examination of selective control of muscle activity, anticipatory regulation of postural muscle groups, and ability to learn unique movements may be broad, using measures of balance, coordination, and motor control; or specific, for example, using the selective motor control test to quantify active ankle dorsiflexion.[35] The Selective Control Assessment of the Lower Extremity (SCALE) is an objective tool used to quantify lower extremity selective voluntary motor control. It rates the ability to perform specific isolated movement patterns as normal, impaired, or unable.[110,113]

Postural control is measured in many standardized and nonstandardized ways.[143] Sway or response to perturbations can be assessed by disturbing the supporting surface, or by perturbing the subject or environment.[349] Visual observation; kinematic, kinetic, and center of pressure measures; or electromyography (EMG) can be used to assess responses. Analysis of EMG activity during perturbations makes it possible to detect abnormal responses in the timing of muscle activity onset and duration, in the sequencing of agonists, and in the co-contraction of antagonists. Various balance tests such as the Berg Balance Scale can be used for children with CP depending on the abilities of the child and the purpose of measurement.[166]

Pain

Therapists should obtain information about pain routinely, as children with CP may assume chronic pain to be the norm and not offer information spontaneously.[55] Motor, cognitive, and communication problems can complicate but should not preclude the assessment of pain.[131] The Pain Assessment Instrument for Cerebral Palsy is an instrument that allows self-report of pain and may indicate the range of potentially painful activities more accurately than proxy report.[26]

Activity and Participation

When assessing motor abilities in children with CP, a physical therapist must differentiate between capacity ("Can a child perform a task in an ideal environment, representative of the highest probable level of function?"), performance ("Does the child perform the task within the context of his daily life?"), and motivation ("Is the child interested in performing the task?"). Capacity often exceeds performance in children with disabilities.[360] The gap between performance and capacity represents a therapy opportunity to enhance function and participation. When motor skills are assessed, the use of equipment to carry out an activity should be taken into consideration. For example, wearing orthoses in ambulation may substantially affect walking abilities.[275]

The most widely used research and clinical tool for assessment of children with CP is the Gross Motor Function Measure (GMFM).[140] The GMFM is a reliable and valid evaluative instrument designed to detect change in children with CP.[53,276] It has been validated on children 5 months to 16 years of age. The original GMFM has 88 items. A gain of 5 to 7 percentage points is considered a medium positive, clinically important change for an individual child. The GMFM-66 is an interval-level version of the original GMFM developed and validated through Rasch analysis. Relative to the GMFM-88, the GMFM-66 demonstrates improved scoring, interpretation, and overall clinical and research utility; it requires fewer items to be tested and estimates the difficulty of items.[6] A computer program, the Gross Motor Ability Estimator (GMAE), converts scores to an interval scale, plots scores graphically or on an item map, and provides 95% confidence intervals. When GMFM-66 scores are used in conjunction with the gross motor development curves described previously, therapists can determine whether a child's outcomes are consistent with his estimated potential and the extent to which interventions improve gross motor function beyond expectations based on a child's age and GMFCS classification level.[244] Item sets of the GMFM-66 (GMFM-66-IS) have been developed to further improve the efficiency of administration.[274] An algorithm with three decision items indicates which set to use.

The Gross Motor Performance Measure (GMPM) assesses qualitative aspects of motor skills and can help in detecting the fine increments of motor skill gains that are characteristic of children who are severely affected.[34,320] The Quality Function Measure (Quality FM), a further adaptation of the GMPM, is being developed to use video recordings to assess the quality of alignment, selective control (also called dissociated movement), coordination, stability, and weight shift in the stand and walk/run/jump GMFM dimensions. Establishment of the psychometric properties is under way (personal communication, Virginia Wright, 2009).

Walking is an activity that is commonly subject to assessment, because abnormal and compensatory gait patterns are typical in children with CP who are ambulatory. *Gait analysis* is a broad term that refers to many different methods of measuring and studying walking patterns (Figure 18-5). Instrumented gait analysis is promoted as an objective and accurate measurement tool that improves clinical decision making and allows critical evaluation of interventions aimed at better outcomes for children with CP.[114,226]

Findings facilitate a wide range of clinical and research applications, but clinical utility is controversial because of high costs, poorly established reliability of measurement and interpretation, and the questionable validity of laboratory results for representing daily function.[226] Therefore, its value beyond research is controversial. Proponents consider it to be the gold standard measure for clinical practice and research and believe computerized three-dimensional gait analysis is a requirement for the optimal treatment of problems related to ambulation in CP.[231] Others consider it to be an expensive tool that does not contribute sufficiently to warrant its use clinically.[65] A comprehensive gait analysis includes a clinical examination of physical impairments, including spasticity, ROM, bony deformity, strength, and

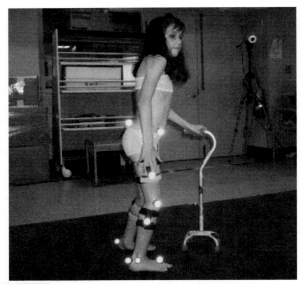

Figure 18-5 Child taking part in gait analysis. Electromyography shows patterns of muscle activities and aids identification of the presence of co-contraction of muscle groups. Markers at joints allow computer calculation of joint movements; force platforms embedded in floor permit measurement of individual muscle group contributions to the work of walking. (Courtesy Human Motion Laboratory at School of Rehabilitation Therapy at Queen's University, Kingston, Ontario, Canada.)

selective control, coupled with a dynamic assessment of the biomechanical and physiologic aspects of walking. Findings from these measures are considered in relation to functional mobility performance outside the gait laboratory and in the context of a child's environment and participation in life activities. Visual observation can be used for subjective descriptions of stability and balance, speed and control, symmetry and movement patterns, weight transfer, foot placement, and the influence of assistive devices. The use of instrumentation to document and quantify temporal, spatial, kinematic, kinetic, and electromyographic information results in objective measures of multiple joints and limb segments simultaneously, providing complex data that could not be detected by visual inspection alone.[58,85] An understanding of power generation and absorption of muscle groups is of particular importance in assessing outcomes.[364]

Visual gait assessment using tools such as the Observational Gait Scale has been found to have moderate interrater reliability and validity based on three-dimensional gait analysis for basic description of key gait parameters.[36,197] The Edinburgh Gait Score was developed for the video gait analysis of people with CP.[152] It includes ratings of gait components in sagittal, coronal, and transverse planes of movement.[255] Accelerometry can be used to quantify physical activity level performance in day-to-day life.[22]

Physical therapists also employ a variety of measures that are not specific to children and adolescents with CP. Infant assessments for diagnosis of delayed motor development include the Test of Infant Motor Performance,[222] (see Chapter 2 for a videoclip illustrating this test), the Alberta Infant Motor Scale,[77] and the Movement Assessment of Infants.[57] The latter includes assessment of primitive reflexes and automatic postural reactions.

The Peabody Developmental Motor Scales can be used to monitor the attainment of motor skills in the preschool and early school years.[342] Tests such as the Timed Up and Go, and Timed Up and Down Stairs, provide measures of functional activities.[5] They may be useful in school or community settings because of their simplicity. The Activity Scale for Kids is a child or parent self-report measure for children with musculoskeletal disorders between the ages of 5 and 15 years and is robust psychometrically for children with CP. It has capacity and performance versions, which assess daily physical activities, including personal care, dressing, eating and drinking, play, locomotion, standing skills, climbing stairs, and transfers.[145,361]

The Pediatric Evaluation of Disability Inventory uses structured interviews to collect parental reports of functional skills in young children with disabilities.[341] The Functional Independence Measure for Children (WeeFIM), a pediatric version of the Functional Independence Measure, measures function as quantified by burden of care for children with developmental disabilities.[8] Chapter 2 provides more information on these tests. The Pediatric Outcomes Data Collection Instrument determines levels of various skills, including transfers and basic mobility, sports, and physical function, and also has a participation component.[11]

Measures of participation in children and adolescents with CP help to ensure that outcomes assessed in clinical situations reflect functional improvements within home, school, and community settings. They can help with goal setting, treatment planning, and overall patient care.[280] The Assessment of Life Habits (LIFE-H) determines the daily life experiences of children.[216,230] It was developed from a theoretical framework aligned with the ICF and rates 11 domains of daily activities and social roles on level of accomplishment, type of assistance, and level of satisfaction. The Children Helping Out: Responsibilities, Expectations, and Supports (CHORES) quantifies the levels of accomplishment and assistance required for self-care and family care, such as feeding pets or performing household chores.[92]

The Children's Assessment of Participation and Enjoyment (CAPE), a child-report instrument, captures diversity, intensity, with whom, location, and enjoyment of participation in formal and informal activities using five scales: recreational, active physical, social, skill-based and self-improvement, and educational. It does not incorporate assistance needed into the scoring system.[174] The Lifestyle Assessment Questionnaire for CP measures physical dependence, restriction of mobility, educational exclusion, clinical burden, economic burden, and restriction of social interaction. The contextual items provide information on the impact of disability on participation of the family unit.[198,216]

The School Function Assessment may be used to assess participation, adaptations, assistance, and activity performance in educational settings, providing information about the environment as well as participation.[81,280] Some measures assess social environments. For example, the Chedoke-McMaster Attitudes Towards Children with Handicaps measures three components of peer attitudes: affective, behavioral, and cognitive.[340]

Although the use of these standardized tools is important for diagnosis and quantification of outcomes, child and caregiver interviews remain the most important clinical tool for collecting useful and meaningful information about participation. A family's recounting of their activities in a typical day and night, including accommodations made for their child with CP, is invaluable.[20,353] Helpful information about the influence of personal and environmental attributes on enabling or creating barriers to function can be gathered through a description of normal daily activities. These range from specific factors internal to a child and his family, to broad factors such as societal attitudes toward children with disabilities. They may include caregiver strain, family or social supports, cultural and family values, economic concerns, physical environments, and many others.[20,346]

Measures of health-related QOL take into account various factors and values believed to be important by health care professionals, parents, and children themselves that contribute toward well-being and ability to fulfill certain life roles.[201,227,344] The Pediatric Quality of Life Inventory (PedsQL), version 3.0, Cerebral Palsy Module, measures health-related QOL dimensions specific to CP. It includes five dimensions: daily activities, movement and balance, pain and hurt, fatigue, and eating.[333] The Caregiver Priorities and Child Health Index of Life with Disabilities (CPCHILD) is a measure of health status and well-being of children with severe CP.[227] The Cerebral Palsy Quality of Life Questionnaire for Children has self-report and parent proxy versions to assess seven domains of QOL, including (1) social well-being and acceptance, (2) feelings about functioning, (3) participation and physical health, (4) emotional well-being, (5) access to services, (6) pain and feeling about disability, and (7) family health.[343] The Child Health Questionnaire is a health-related QOL measure that has been used in children with CP. Various health-related QOL measures such as the Short Form (SF)-36 have been used to study adults with CP.[161]

Evaluation of service delivery can provide valuable information to inform practice. The Measuring Processes of Care tool captures parental satisfaction with services. A 20-question version (MPOC-20) assesses five areas of care: enabling and partnership; providing general information; providing specific information about the child; providing coordinated and comprehensive care; and providing respectful and supportive care.[175] Giving Youth a Voice is an evolution of the MPOC designed to provide youth with disabilities an opportunity to give feedback.[116,294] The perceptions of service providers can be captured with the Measure of Processes of Care for Service Providers.[354]

Tools are available to assist in formulating goals and measuring their attainment. The Canadian Occupational Performance Measure can be used to document and quantify goals that are relevant to a family and to determine whether they are achieved.[188] Goal Attainment Scaling can be used to evaluate whether specific individualized treatment goals or outcomes have been met.[239,304] These forms of assessment complement but are not intended to replace standardized measures. The Rotterdam Transition Profile summarizes goals for the transition of adolescents and young adults with CP to independence in life skills and adult health care through participation in finances, education and employment, housing, intimate relationships, transportation, and leisure activities.[91]

Intervention

The United Nations Convention on the Rights of the Child states that children with disabilities should be able to participate on an equal basis with others in family life, health maintenance, public life, and recreational, leisure, and sporting activities.[327] Children with CP have variable but significant disruptions in these areas, and most are associated with locomotion capabilities.[193] From infancy to adulthood, physical therapy goals for people with CP should focus on the promotion of participation in their specific personal and environmental contexts by maximizing the activity allowed by impairments and compensating for activity limitations when necessary.[237] Specific goals for children in GMFCS Levels I, II, and III include the development of gross motor skills, including standing, walking, running, and jumping. Achievement of these goals requires the promotion and maintenance of musculoskeletal integrity, the prevention of secondary impairment, the enhancement of functional postures and movement, and maintenance of optimal levels of fitness and overall health. Complex relationships between the impairments of spasticity, ROM, selective motor control, and other factors contribute to gross motor function and achievement of tasks in mobility, self-care, and social function.[14] It cannot be assumed that treatment of a specific impairment will lead to improvement in the ability to perform tasks in daily life.[237,357] Skilled physical therapists recognize when tasks and the environment should be adapted rather than impairments remediated to achieve function and participation. Furthermore, the physical therapist must be cognizant of environmental and personal factors that could enhance or create barriers to activity or participation. To help achieve these goals, therapists provide support, guidance, and education for children, families, and communities, in addition to direct treatment.

Relevant and achievable goals are developed for individual children and their families. Goals should be determined in collaboration with families based on their concerns, needs, expectations, priorities, and values.[239,267] Goal setting is an iterative process. Outcome attainment should be regularly reassessed so a therapy plan can be adapted to reflect changes in the child's progress and the family's needs and wishes. Goals should focus on everyday activities in environments typical for the child and should consider elements that enable or constrain their potential achievement.[329]

The concept of family-centered care has been widely accepted as a philosophy for providing services for children with CP and their families. It promotes service delivery that recognizes parents as the experts in their child's needs and promotes supportive partnerships and collaboration between parents and therapists. Families are encouraged to be actively involved in goal setting and decision making regarding services for their child. Therapists are responsive to information needs and share general and specific information in a way that is most useful and meaningful to the family. They recognize the parents' role as advocates for their child and are accepting of a family's choices.[9,176,239] They strive to provide coordinated and comprehensive care in a respectful and supportive manner. Family-centered care improves parents' satisfaction with services and parent–child interaction and reduces associated parental stresses.[189] It can be applied to most treatment approaches.

Families value a therapist's honesty, commitment to their child, and belief that what they are doing is making a difference for their child. This can be promoted by drawing attention to the gains the child is making, listening to parental concerns, and recognizing the personal values and strengths of the child.[247] Therapists need to offer hope but be honest; they may serve as an outlet for a family's anger and fear.[141]

Different approaches to providing physical therapy for children with CP may be used, but many have underlying similarities. Knowledge of a variety of theoretical models, not necessarily pediatric in origin, can help guide a therapist's approach to treating children with CP. Carr and Shepherd's task-related movement science–based approach,[291] the motor control theories of Shumway-Cook and Woollacott,[293] the dynamic systems theory,[76] and neuronal group selection theory[132] can be integrated into physical therapy interventions for children with CP. See Chapter 2 for additional descriptions.

Some physical therapists adhere to specific treatment philosophies. An example is neurodevelopmental treatment (NDT). Traditionally, NDT was based on the theory that inhibiting or modifying the impairments of spasticity and abnormal reflex patterns while facilitating movement patterns could prevent contracture and deformity, promote functional movements, and allow children the greatest degree of independence possible.[25,155] NDT has evolved with advances in rehabilitation, assimilating models of motor control and motor learning, and incorporating different techniques into its approach. Current NDT principles include encouragement of normal movement patterns through therapeutic handling during functional motor activities with gradual withdrawal of therapist facilitation to encourage active participation of the child.[155] Randomized controlled trials (RCTs) on the effectiveness of NDT for children with CP have been inconclusive,[47] but two clinical trials using NDT principles showed improved motor development on the Test of Infant Motor Performance for premature infants at risk for CP.[118,191] Conductive education (CE), an approach originated by Andras Peto in Hungary, integrates education and rehabilitation goals. Children participate in groups that provide motivating, supportive, and challenging atmospheres and allow more time in a therapeutic environment compared with individual treatment. Functional goals are broken down into small steps. Conductors teach children to gain control over their movements and to learn new movements that will result in improved functioning in daily activities through repetition, verbal guidance, and rhythm. As with NDT, research on CE is inconclusive, with reviews of the strongest studies in design and conduct revealing no difference in outcomes between conductive education and comparison groups using conventional approaches.[30,78]

It is difficult to compare the effectiveness of different approaches because discrepancies often are seen in protocol parameters such as frequency, skill level of individual therapists, compliance of families, and age and abilities of individual children. In a study comparing four treatment approaches, Bower and colleagues found that parents were most pleased with therapy when they had requested the services, when they were present during treatment, and when targeted goals were met.[32] They concluded that the most appropriate approach for a child would be one that meets the needs of a particular child.

Parents often consider complementary or alternative therapies for their children. The primary reason is to complement conventional approaches. Other reasons include a desire for more therapy, dissatisfaction with present therapy, the belief that their child could do better, and relief of symptoms.[156,281] For example, some families have had their children participate in hyperbaric oxygen programs, even when studies have shown this treatment not to be effective and to be associated with adverse effects in some children.[202] Alternative therapies are usually expensive, and some professionals may not consider certain choices acceptable. If families choose to take an approach other than the one offered by a therapist, it is necessary to respect their choice. Therapists should not react defensively but rather should provide impartial, objective information about the therapies in question.

INFANCY

Infants grow and develop in response to being loved and nurtured by parents and caregivers in a home environment. Despite being dependent in most aspects of life, infants interact with and develop an understanding of the people in their lives, their surroundings, and themselves. From the time of birth, a child with CP may not experience the usual activities associated with infancy. As a result, some parents of infants with CP may not receive all aspects of positive feedback of a typical nurturing experience and the satisfaction of observing the development of typical motor and social skills. Parents must cope with the impact of the diagnosis and the grieving process that accompanies the awareness that some of their hopes and expectations for their child may not be realized. They may be overwhelmed with the uncertainty that the future holds for them, their child, and their family. Many parents are also concerned with the immediate issues of providing basic infant care and are apprehensive about incorporating the specialized care necessary for their child's optimal development. In addition to coping with these unexpected situations, they find themselves entering into unfamiliar relationships with health care professionals.

Physical Therapy Examination and Evaluation

Infant examination provides information on which to base a prognosis and provides a baseline for the monitoring of improvement or deterioration, growth, maturation, and treatment effects. Therapists must determine the history and environment of an infant and the capabilities and concerns of the family. Normal maturational changes in joint range and alignment must be considered in evaluating the significance of measures.

Various elements of movement and posture combine to produce gross motor skills. These skills include the ability to align one part of the body on another; to bear weight through different parts of the body; to shift weight; to move against gravity; to assume, maintain, and move into and out of different positions; and to perform graded, isolated, and variable movements with an appropriate degree of effort. When functional motor skills are examined, proficiency in incorporating these elements into purposeful and efficient movement must be evaluated. The effects of reflexes and postural reactions on positioning, handling, and movement must be considered. Assessments of seating, feeding, or respiratory problems may be necessary for infants with problems in these areas. Growth is often affected in children with CP; therefore, anthropometric measures, including head circumference, weight, and length in relation to age norms, should be monitored. Growth may influence, or be influenced by, feeding, exercise, and energy efficiency.[52] When assessing infants, it is important to be aware of the influences of temperament, behavioral state regulation, and tolerance of handling on performance.

Physical Therapy Goals, Outcomes, and Intervention

Movement is an important component in the learning and interactions of infants. In babies who have CP, the nature and extent of their impairments affect their potential to develop and learn through movement. This may result in activity limitations related to the development of gross motor skills and may affect their ability to interact with their parents and their environment. Physical therapy in infancy is focused on educating the family, facilitating caregiving and caregiver interaction, and promoting optimal sensorimotor experiences and skills. These allow the infant to reach their potential in interacting with others, developing play skills, and exploring their environment. Intervention and family education must address current and potential problems. Early intervention for children with CP has been advocated to help infants achieve their abilities in the most normal way for them, based on the principles of central nervous system plasticity.[328] Unfortunately, there is no definitive support for its efficacy in changing outcomes.[48,300]

The foremost set of goals at all ages is to educate families about CP to provide support in their acceptance of their child's problems and coping with their child's challenges, and to be of assistance when parents make decisions related to physical therapy management of their child (www.afcp.on.ca/guide.html). Infancy is an important time to introduce the concepts of collaborative goal setting and ongoing communication with families. It may be difficult for families to contemplate specific goals while they are coping with a diagnosis of CP and are uncertain or even unrealistic about prognosis. Parents' goals may be overly optimistic and hopeful during infancy. Therapists must be realistic about the prognosis and the efficacy of physical therapy while remaining hopeful and providing options for intervention.

Abnormal postures and movements resulting from impairments can make an infant difficult to handle and position. These difficulties can affect an infant's interaction with the environment, reaction to caregiving activities, and development of gross motor skills. Therefore, a second physical therapy goal is to promote the parents' skill, ease, and confidence in handling and caring for their infant. These skills alleviate unnecessary stress for parents and child and also help reduce the influence of the impairments, thereby preventing unnecessary secondary impairments and activity limitations. Parents are taught positioning, carrying, feeding, and dressing techniques that promote symmetry, limit abnormal posturing and movement, and facilitate postural stability and functional motor activity. The principles guiding these methods are (1) to use a variety of movements and postures to promote sensory variety, (2) to frequently include positions that promote the full lengthening of spastic or hypoextensible muscles, and (3) to use positions that promote functional voluntary movement of limbs with as little assistance as possible.

A third physical therapy goal in infancy is to facilitate optimal sensorimotor experiences and skills, thereby promoting activity and participation. Therapy should focus on the development of well-aligned postural stability coupled with smooth mobility to allow the emergence of motor skills such as reaching, rolling, sitting, crawling, transitional movements, standing, and prewalking skills. These skills promote the development of symmetry, spatial perception, body awareness, and mobility to facilitate play, social interaction, and exploration of the environment. Movements that include all planes of movement, selective control of body segments, weight shifting, weight bearing, and isolated and bimanual movements should be incorporated into gross motor exercises and activities. These movement components, if experienced with proper alignment, can give the sensory feedback of normal movement patterns and activities. Movements may be facilitated through handling when necessary, but assistance is withdrawn as the child initiates them spontaneously or in response to his environment. Useful examples of activities are noted by Cameron et al.[48] Careful instruction of the family in specific techniques and activities, ongoing reinforcement, encouragement, and support are essential. The therapist should emphasize working therapeutic handling into daily routines to ease the burden of care on the family. Clearly written, illustrated, and updated home programs can be beneficial. Computer-generated programs or videotaping can be used to produce personalized, effective, and efficient information regarding activities, positioning, and exercises.

The normal motor developmental sequence may assist in guiding the progression of motor activities, but a child with CP does not always proceed along the normal developmental sequence, and therapy becomes more functionally oriented. The stage at which this happens depends on the severity of the impairments; in some children, it may occur early in life. The basic goal is to develop the components of posture and movement that underlie many different motor activities.

Equipment may facilitate activities when impairments otherwise prevent their development. For example, the sitting position promotes visual attending, upper extremity use, and social interaction. Infants with CP may be unable to sit independently, may sit statically only with precarious balance, or may not even be able to be seated in commercially available infant equipment. Customized seating or adaptations to regular infant seats may be necessary to allow function in other areas of development to progress. Infants who function at GMFCS Levels IV and V should begin early continuous postural management programs for sleeping, sitting, and standing with postural support for sitting at 6 months of age and standing at 12 months. Infants with limited upper extremity movement may be unable to bring their hands or toys to their mouths to provide normal oral-motor sensory input. In these cases, mouthing activities should be incorporated into therapy. Toys may need to be adapted to facilitate age-appropriate activities.

The care of an infant exhibiting asymmetry, extensor posturing, and shoulder retraction illustrates these approaches. Such an infant should be carried, seated, and fed in a symmetrical position that does not allow axial hyperextension and keeps the hips and knees flexed. Beyond the seated position, however, a variety of postures are necessary to allow elongation of all muscle groups. The therapist should work to ensure that no one position dominates daily activity.

Positioning of or playing with the upper extremities to allow the infant to see his or her hands, practice midline play, reach for his or her feet, or suck on fingers can promote sensorimotor awareness. For infants, handling techniques should encourage active movement, the experience of a variety of normal movement and postural sensations, and the opportunity to organize their own movements.

Active movements that require two hands and that encourage the infant to develop flexor control and symmetry, such as the handling of toys, are incorporated into daily activities. These activities facilitate use of the neck and trunk muscles, promoting anterior and posterior control. The introduction of lateral control is the next step in achieving functional head and trunk control. In some severely affected children, slight gains in head control may be a goal, whereas in minimally affected children, a fairly normal progression of motor development is expected, even without intervention. These therapeutic interventions should not limit infants' spontaneous desires to move and play and explore their environments because even very young children need to be able to assert themselves and manipulate their world.[49] The frequency of treatment should be tailored to meet the needs of a family. Intensive therapy may help parents become comfortable with handling skills but may be challenging for parents to commit to, may be limited by resources, and does not necessarily demonstrate better motor outcomes compared with less frequent interventions.[328] Some settings may provide home-based early intervention programs that emphasize coaching parents in managing daily routines that include therapeutic input.

Role of Other Disciplines

Occupational therapists may be involved in upper extremity function, particularly as it relates to play and eye-hand coordination, as well as in sensory modulation/regulation. In addition, speech and language pathologists may be needed if oral-motor problems are interfering with feeding or early communication development. Community infant development workers may be involved in home-based programs to promote all areas of development. Social workers may help parents through the grieving process, explain programs, and direct them to appropriate resources. Parent support groups or meetings with parents who have been through similar experiences may be helpful. A variety of medical and surgical specialists may be consulted, depending on individual needs.

PRESCHOOL PERIOD

During the preschool years, the development of locomotor, cognitive, communication, fine motor, self-care, and social abilities promotes functional independence in children. The development process is a dynamic one in which all these areas constantly interact with one another. The child's environment remains oriented toward the parents, family, and home during this period, but they begin to interact with the outside world. Child care centers, babysitters, nursery schools, and playmates become part of a preschooler's world.

For children with CP, limitations in motor activities may restrict participation in learning and socialization and may reduce independence. Parents become more aware of the extent and impact of their children's difficulties in all areas of development. These may include their child's ability to participate in and become integrated into normal preschool and community recreational activities, their child's development of cognitive and communication skills, and the long-term effect of their child's disability on future life and independence.

Physical Therapy Examination and Evaluation

Assessment of activity assumes a primary focus, but it is important to determine the interaction of impairment and activity in relation to participation. Tests should be administered at regular intervals to document change resulting from treatment, maturation, or growth and to ensure that goals are appropriate and therapy is being directed appropriately. Assessment should include mobility and transfers, communication, social function, sleep, self-care and a degree of reliance on caregivers, adaptive equipment, and environmental modifications in the performance of activities of daily living (ADLs).

When children in this age group are assessed, environmental and personal factors such as attention, cooperation, the location of the assessment, and the child's reaction to being assessed may affect the evaluation process. Parents or other caregivers should be asked to provide information on whether a child's performance is characteristic of their abilities.

Physical Therapy Goals, Outcomes, and Intervention

During the preschool years, a child's attainable level of motor skills can be predicted with a greater degree of accuracy as the influences of impairments, activity limitations, and personal and environmental factors are more apparent. Families become more skilled at collaborative goal setting and comfortable communicating with service providers. Therapists can work with families to develop goals that are meaningful, realistic, noticeable, and measurable. The continued development of these skills empowers parents to make decisions, solve problems, and set priorities, as well as to become effective advocates for their children and themselves.

Physical therapy goals focus on proactively preventing secondary impairments and optimizing gross motor skills through control and alignment of posture and movements conducive to musculoskeletal development, fitness, and function. Muscles need to be stretched to their limits on a regular basis to maintain extensibility and loaded adequately and frequently to maintain strength; bones need compressive forces to stay strong; and the cardiovascular system needs to be used at moderately intense levels regularly to maintain endurance and fitness.[75,111,351] Functionally, the focus is on

a child's ability to achieve independent mobility. Specific mobility goals will depend on the GMFCS level. Promotion of play, communication, self-care activities, social skills, and problem-solving skills complement motor-based skills to promote participation in the age-appropriate activities of early childhood and family life. Goals for children functioning at GMFCS Levels IV and V may be achieved by using special equipment and adapted toys, rather than progressing through the normal developmental sequence.

In many cases, physical therapy goals may serve as the building blocks for interdisciplinary goals in communication, play, social interaction, and self-care activities. Therapists must be willing to respect the priorities of families and other professionals when determining goals, as it may not be possible to work on all areas at once. They must also be sure that treatment is conducive to achieving the chosen goals and is functional, motivating, and fun for the child.[71,169]

Reducing Primary Impairment and Preventing Secondary Impairment

Physical therapy to improve muscle strength and prevent atrophy involves activities that create increased demand for production of both concentric and eccentric muscle force. Such activities include transitional movements against gravity, ball gymnastics, treadmill use, tricycle riding, and ascending and descending stairs.

Spasticity management may be introduced during the preschool years. Interventions have been directed toward decreasing the impairment of spasticity with the goals of preventing secondary impairment, ensuring comfort and ease of positioning, and improving functional movement. These interventions are used if spasticity is interfering with function or comfort and conversely are not used if a child appears to be dependent on spasticity for function and no other issues need to be addressed. Reducing spasticity will not necessarily improve motor function or participation, as only a single impairment in a multi-impairment condition is addressed.[357] Coexisting impairments such as weakness and selective motor control and contextual child and environment factors influence function.

Spasticity management is considered to be an adjunct to therapy programs, and several options are available. Passive stretching has been shown to cause a short-term decrease in spasticity, but changes are minor.[249] Longer-lasting interventions are operative or pharmaceutical. Selective dorsal rhizotomy (SDR) is a surgical procedure in which the sensory nerve rootlets from the lower extremities are cut selectively to create a balance between elimination of spasticity and preservation of function.[100] Intensive postoperative physical therapy is important to address the resulting weakness (Figure 18-6).

SDR is considered a safe procedure that offers significant and lasting functional gains to properly selected children with spasticity.[100] Abnormalities in patterns of muscle activation may persist after SDR because of continuing problems

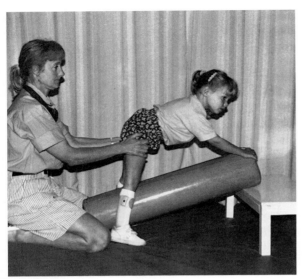

Figure 18-6 Exercises after rhizotomy are frequently directed toward increasing force generation of extensor muscles.

with motor control, which prohibit the proper sequencing of muscle action. A meta-analysis of three RCTs of SDR demonstrated a small but statistically significant improvement for children who had SDR and physical therapy compared with those who received physical therapy only, as measured by the GMFM-66.[205] This meta-analysis suggested that SDR may be most effective for children aged 3 to 8 years with GMFCS Levels III and IV, who have access to and are receptive to physical therapy, but children with GMFCS Levels I and II have also shown improvement.[325] A history of prematurity, good selective control of muscles, lack of contracture or deformity, good cognitive abilities, and motivation, as well as good parental support, are selection criteria and predictors of successful outcomes.[205,325] A prospective 20-year follow-up study, albeit with many confounders and a small sample of 14, showed that improved kinematics and temporal measures measured by gait analysis and gross motor function can last as long as 20 years.[185,186]

A widely used method of spasticity intervention is the injection of small quantities of botulinum toxin A (Botox) into muscles to prevent the release of acetylcholine at the neuromuscular junction. Neuromuscular junctions near the injection site are inactivated for up to 4 months with peak effects observed 2 weeks after injection. The drug is expensive but is often covered by insurance. Targeted muscles are those that have good ROM but exhibit spasticity that interferes with function and those most prone to developing contractures. These muscles include the gastrocnemius, hamstrings, hip flexors, and hip adductors.[126] Evidence is strongest for (1) injections of the calf muscles for equinus varus deformity, (2) the hip adductors for spasticity and pain control in children undergoing adductor-lengthening surgery, and (3) upper extremity spasticity,[17,102,297] but studies of lower limb multilevel injections, including the iliopsoas,

hamstrings, and rectus femoris muscles, have also demonstrated improvements in gross motor functioning measured by the GMFM-66 and gait analysis.[85,286] Phenol injections may be used in conjunction with Botox to allow an increase in the number of injections at the maximal recommended dose.[119] Botox has also been shown to have an analgesic benefit in relieving hip pain in children with CP.[196] Treatment algorithms can provide strategies to treat spasticity with Botox.[67] Studies following children who have received repeated injections of Botox over a period of a few years have had methodologic challenges and report varying results. Continued reduction in spasticity and improved ROM and gross motor function have been noted.[146] Other researchers question whether Botox can prevent contractures and even question whether repeated injections may have a cumulative adverse effect on muscle growth in children with CP.[317]

Longitudinal studies of the effects of Botox on muscle growth and morphology are needed. The severity of adverse effects is low, but concern about respiratory compromise and death has been expressed (www.aacpdm.org.news/fda.php). A systematic review of RCTs concluded that respiratory infection, bronchitis, pharyngitis, asthma, muscle weakness, urinary incontinence, seizures, fever, and unspecified pain have been related to the use of Botox in children with CP.[2] Two deaths have been reported but were believed to be due to seizures rather than to Botox injections.

The use of oral medications has been poorly studied, but these agents may be appropriate for some children.[94,334] A pilot study showed that Artane in children with dystonic CP did not alter their dystonia or upper limb function but was associated with achieving therapeutic goals.[257] Children must be carefully assessed for appropriateness and monitored closely for side effects. Baclofen, a synthetic agonist of gamma aminobutyric acid, has an inhibitory effect on presynaptic excitatory neurotransmitter release, reducing spasticity in individuals with CP.[334] Oral doses high enough to give the proper concentration in the cerebrospinal fluid can, however, cause side effects such as drowsiness. If this is a problem, baclofen can be given intrathecally by a continuous infusion pump implanted in the abdomen that releases the drug at a slow, constant rate into the subarachnoid space once a child weighs 15 kilograms.[334] Intrathecal baclofen reduces spasticity most noticeably in the lower extremities. Improvements in function and ease of care and a reduced need for orthopedic surgery have been documented.[46] It is used most often in children with quadriplegic CP but has also been shown to improve gait in ambulatory children.[38] A high rate of complications has been reported. Some are associated with significant morbidity, but others are common and manageable in most cases.[178] Intrathecal baclofen has also been beneficial in treating patients with generalized dystonia—a difficult problem to manage. In addition to improved dystonia, subjective improvements have been reported in QOL, ease of care, speech, swallowing, posture, and upper and lower extremity functioning.[3,221]

Limitations in ROM can be observed in preschool children, particularly those with more severe involvement. Considerable resources are directed toward maintaining or regaining muscle extensibility and joint mobility.[351] Ideally, muscle length is maintained through active movement, particularly with muscles in a lengthened position. When possible, activities that involve stretching of muscles and movement of joints should be promoted. A classic study by Tardieu found that plantar flexor contractures in children with CP were prevented if the muscles were stretched beyond a minimum threshold length for at least 6 hours during daily activity.[314] Threshold length was the length at which the muscle began to resist a stretch. The data prompting this statement are suggestive rather than conclusive, however. Stretching is unlikely to happen spontaneously in children with spastic CP who have limited active movement, particularly those at GMFCS Levels IV and V. Other options include passive ROM exercises and prolonged muscle stretching. Combinations of these approaches may be used in conjunction with other treatments, making it difficult to assess the usefulness of individual approaches.[23] Passive stretching programs may be useful to maintain muscle length, but evidence of effectiveness and clinical relevance is limited and conflicting.[249,351] Some parents report that ROM exercises cause pain,[131] whereas others believe they relieve muscle cramps.[249] Sustained low load passive stretching of longer duration has been shown to be more effective in increasing ROM and in reducing spasticity.[249] Sustained passive stretching can be achieved through casting, orthoses, or positioning. It is important to not position muscles at their fully lengthened state, as this can cause discomfort. Clinically, a position slightly past the initial catch has been advocated. This can be altered as muscle lengthening occurs. A single cast application or serial casting (the successive application of casts with progressive increases in the amount of stretch) has been used as a method of providing prolonged stretch to the calf muscles.[23,42] After serial casting of the foot and lower leg from 3 to 6 weeks, eight children with CP demonstrated decreased resistance to passive stretch and increased dorsiflexion end range.[42] Peak strength remained unchanged but occurred at longer muscle lengths. Follow-up 6 weeks after cast removal showed substantial reduction in gains, suggesting the need to follow casting with orthotic use. Although it is clear that at least temporary mechanical changes result from casting, the precise nature of the changes and whether they involve an increase in the number of sarcomeres remain unknown.[23] Casting has been shown to be more effective if the hypoextensibility is due to imbalance between the triceps surae and the dorsiflexor muscles, but not if the primary impairment is lack of appropriate muscle growth in response to bone growth.[313,315] Serial casting has also been used for other muscle groups, such as the hamstrings and the upper extremity musculature. Very few researchers have studied casting for its impact on activity or participation.[23] Concern has been expressed that immobilization of growing muscle in a lengthened position can result in sacromere loss and a reduction of the muscle belly girth with adaptation by lengthening of the tendon, exacerbating the altered morphology.[124]

Positioning, serial casting, and Botox injections are often used in combination to achieve optimal improvement.[23] Clinical reasoning suggests that Botox addresses spasticity and casting decreases contracture, but currently, no clear evidence indicates that casting, Botox, or the combination of both is superior to the others in the treatment of equinus. Analyses of research are complex because of differing protocols and other methodologic problems. Ultimately, treatment choices should depend on research evidence combined with considerations such as availability, cost, convenience, family preference, and therapists' expertise and experience with the treatments and follow-up care.[23] Likewise, it is difficult to validate the effectiveness of interventions such as muscle strengthening and functional activities in conjunction with spasticity intervention, but the clinical value of these practices has been observed, and they are strongly advocated.[187]

The integrity of the hip joints is a concern during the preschool years. Early prevention, or identification and intervention, of subluxation can help prevent progression to dislocation, the complete lateral displacement of the femoral head from under the acetabulum.[89,135] Clinical orthopedic assessment at diagnosis and an anteroposterior radiograph at 12 to 24 months of age or at diagnosis if older than 24 months are recommended. Continued surveillance until skeletal maturity is necessary. A program of surveillance based on GMFCS level and radiologic assessment of hip migration percentage, coupled with clinical assessment of changes in ROM, muscle tone, spinal alignment, sitting tolerance, gait, pelvic obliquity, leg length, or hip pain, is recommended. Physical therapists may be the first to recognize warning signs.[117,299,359] An RCT investigating the use of botulinum toxin A and hip abduction orthosis found that the intervention did not alter outcomes for children with hip adductor spasticity and risk of dislocation.[127]

A potential outcome of decreasing spasticity and addressing muscle extensibility during the preschool years is muscle lengthening and growth, which may delay or eliminate the need for extensive orthopedic surgery.[35,213] This impact on surgical intervention has been explored in a prospective study of groups of children receiving differing management.[135] Proactive practices, including early treatment of spasticity through rhizotomy, Botox injections, and intrathecal baclofen, and early detection and surgery to prevent dislocation, were associated with improved ROM in nonambulatory children and a decrease in orthopedic surgery for contracture, rotational deformity, and foot deformity, and salvage operations for dislocated hips, from 40% to 15%.

Early screening of hip positioning may indicate the need for soft tissue lengthening of hypoextensible or spastic hip adductors to allow improved motion and therefore function and prevent the secondary impairment of subluxation or dislocation of the hip joint for preschool-age children.[130,311] Hip adductor surgery with minimal hospitalization or immobilization may be effective if children are followed closely from a young age and surgery is done as soon as a problem arises.[311]

Lower extremity orthoses may be used to reduce primary impairment, prevent secondary impairment, and facilitate efficient and effective walking and other functional activities. Specific goals are to limit inappropriate joint movements and alignment; prevent contracture, hyperextensibility, and deformity; enhance postural control and balance; reduce the energy cost of walking, and provide postoperative protection of tissues.[215] In most studies, the use of ankle-foot orthoses (AFOs) compared with a barefoot condition has shown positive effects on gait kinematics and kinetics, including improvements in ground reaction forces and plantar flexion moments, stride length, foot clearance in swing, heel strike at initial contact, equinus during midstance, related hip and knee movement, temporal-spatial measures, and sometimes function measured by the walking, running, and jumping dimensions of the GMFM.[105,215,217] Research suggests that only orthoses that extend to the knee and have a rigid ankle, leaf spring, or hinged design with plantar flexion stop can prevent equinus deformities.[215,217] Little more than anecdotal observational evidence suggests that using orthoses to control movement into plantar flexion prevents muscle shortening and therefore joint contractures or deformity. Controlled trials are difficult to carry out, as contractures develop over many years. Despite these dynamic benefits, orthoses do not show clinically significant changes in the static bony alignment of the foot and ankle during weight bearing based on radiologic examination.[347] Results are variable depending on the specific gait problems of the child and the type of orthosis, demonstrating the need for individual assessment and prescription.

Many variations of AFOs are available, depending on the biomechanical and functional needs of an individual child. Therapists and orthotists work together closely to decide on the optimal orthosis based on treatment goals. Solid AFOs are used if maximum restriction of ankle movement is desired. Children who would benefit from freedom of movement at the joint can use hinged AFOs, sometimes with stops to prevent movement into plantar flexion. Hinged AFOs permit dorsiflexion, which allows stretching of the plantar flexor muscle group during walking, and have been found to promote a more normal and efficient gait pattern than rigid orthotics without a predisposition to crouch gait. Dynamic or posterior leaf spring orthoses, which are intended to prevent excessive equinus while mechanically augmenting push-off, have been found to reduce equinus in swing, permit ankle dorsiflexion in stance, and absorb more energy during midstance, but actually reduce desirable power generation at push-off.[235] Foot orthoses, or supramalleolar orthoses, may be used for children with pronation who do not require the ankle stabilization of an AFO. Materials from a consensus conference on lower limb orthotic management of CP are available at www.ispoweb.org. The content includes information beyond the scope of orthotics.[217]

Materials such as Lycra, Neoprene, and tape have been used for splints or in garments to assist children biomechanically and facilitate function. Skin tolerance may be an issue, and children and families sometimes find the garments uncomfortable and inconvenient.[106,256]

Daytime and nighttime alignment of the body is important. Children should have a variety of positions in which they can optimally function, travel, and sleep. Children functioning at GMFCS Levels IV and V should have individually tailored postural management programs to prevent the secondary impairments of positional contractures and deformity, prevent skin breakdown, and facilitate function and participation.[117] At all ages, decreased ability to change body position during sleep can cause discomfort, pain, and respiratory problems, which can result in disrupted sleep for children with CP and their families.[356] Physical therapists may be involved in promoting safe, comfortable, and biomechanically optimal sleep positions. Orthoses, splints, and bed positioning systems have been used during sleep, but care must be taken to avoid overstretched muscles, disrupted sleep, or discomfort.[125] Children functioning at GMFCS Levels I, II, and III require programs that emphasize activity from an early age. Comfortable and safe sitting, standing, lying, floor play, and toileting positions are important for the preschooler's fine motor, feeding, communication, and toileting skill development. Children having difficulty with postural control in sitting may need adaptive seating systems. It is necessary to be aware of not only the child's comfort and functional abilities but also the caregivers' concerns and needs and the child's environment. Appropriate adaptive seating can have a positive effect on children by improving the quality and quantity of communication, upper extremity function, level of independence, safety, social interaction, and contentment.[62,133,278] These benefits translate into improvements in the lives of families through valuation of their children's well-being and the added benefits of expending less parental energy in caregiving and supervision.[278] Adaptive seating should be individualized because of the wide variation in postural abilities and alignment.[62] Specific suggestions are included in the assistive technologies section of the Evolve website. Approved car seats and restraints are necessary for safe and comfortable vehicular transportation.[4] Positioning can also contribute to pulmonary health. Children with limited movement are at risk for chest complications because of chest wall biomechanics, feeding difficulties, immobility, and poor coughing abilities. Adaptive seating or orthoses have also been shown to improve pulmonary functioning, but research is very limited.[10]

Weight-bearing programs are thought to reduce or prevent secondary impairments by maintaining lower extremity muscle extensibility, maintaining or increasing bone mineral density, and promoting optimal musculoskeletal integrity, including acetabular development and reduction of fracture. Other assumed benefits include reduced spasticity and improved self-esteem, breathing, circulation, and bowel and urinary function.[248] Optimally, standing involves movement and activity to provide intermittent loading and muscle strain; however, standers are often used, starting at 1 year of age, when children are not able to bear weight effectively on their own. Maintenance of lower extremity weight bearing may allow continued use of standing transfers and reduce the need for older children to be lifted by caregivers. A review of the literature suggests that evidence supports the use of standing programs for increasing bone density in the spine or femur and for reducing spasticity temporarily, but many of the attributes of passive standing remain anecdotal because of a lack of research evidence. Stuberg recommended positioning in standing for 45 minutes two or three times a day to control lower extremity flexor contractures, and for 60 minutes four or five times per week to facilitate bone development, but noted that no definite evidence supports these guidelines.[310] It is important to determine the actual weight being borne through the lower extremities when in a stander, which has been shown to vary from 23% to 102%, with a mean of 68% body weight.[150]

Promotion of Activity

Physical therapy to promote activity is often intensive during the preschool years. Therapists need to recognize when it is realistic to work on a child's impairments to achieve success in an activity, and when it is necessary to adapt a task or the environment to realize success. Treatment often involves components of both; however, children functioning at GMFCS Levels I and II may need very little adaptation, whereas children functioning at Level V may require considerable adaptation. Components of the dynamic systems theory, motor control theory, and motor learning principles and strategies should be integrated into activity-oriented treatment (see Chapters 3 and 4). These elements provide the foundations for organizing a child, tasks, and environments to maximize learning.

Motor learning principles advocate the encouragement of movement exploration and child-initiated solutions to motor tasks, adaptation to changes in the environment, and repetitive practicing of goal-related functional tasks that are meaningful to the child.[169] Ample and variable training in motivating settings is important. Feedback is important in the process of learning skilled movement. Information is received intrinsically through a child's sensory receptors and extrinsically from external sources. Knowledge of results contributes information about movement outcome, and knowledge of performance supplies feedback about the nature of the movement. Trial and error can form the basis for selecting efficient movement patterns.[39] Feed forward mechanisms must also be considered because movement skills have a cognitive component. In some instances,

cognitive strategies may be able to compensate for some of the inherent motor limitations. Children with CP understand concrete instructions much more readily than abstract ones, even if the same tasks are involved. Transfer between tasks may be limited, particularly in children with cognitive limitations, so practice of the target skill is recommended.[329] Integration of skills into functional and cognitively directed tasks may promote carryover.

Therapists should focus on periods most conducive to change, such as alterations or fluctuations in constraining impairments or child engagement in particular goals.[329] Therapy should be challenging and interesting to maintain motivation. For example, kicking a soccer ball is a more functional and fun method of developing balance skills than practicing while standing on one foot. Treatment does not have to focus on normalization of movement patterns. A task can be achieved through many different means based on the child's unique movement capabilities, provided the action is safe and will not cause secondary impairments over time.[329]

Ketelaar and colleagues found that children receiving interventions based on the foregoing principles demonstrated greater improvement in both capability and performance of self-care and mobility activities in daily situations when compared with children receiving intervention designed to normalize movement quality.[169]

Although the body of literature on many aspects of therapy for children with CP is growing, optimal strategies and interventions are not known. Therapists who treat children with CP should modify approaches, as practice expertise and research produce new insights into the areas of motor learning and motor control. For example, constraint-induced therapy, that is, restraining the unaffected limb of children with hemiplegia while intensely training the involved extremity, has shown improved function and evidence of cortical reorganization as measured by functional magnetic resonance imaging (MRI) and magnetoencephalography.[153,312] Intensive training in bimanual upper extremity activities has been shown to increase the frequency and quality of bimanual hand use.[120] Functional relevance, cognitive engagement, and massed practice are aspects of such successful intense programs.[75] See Chapter 4 for more information.

The frequency of intervention varies, depending on the resources available, complementary programming, client goals, parental needs and desires, and the child's response to treatment. Optimal treatment frequency is unknown, but periods of more intensive intervention have resulted in attainment of specific treatment goals at levels that were maintained when frequency was decreased, provided the skills were incorporated into daily functional activities. Bower and colleagues have conducted a number of studies investigating the intensity of treatment.[31-33] An initial study found that bursts of intensive physical therapy directed at achievable specific measurable goals accelerated the acquisition of motor skills compared with conventional physical therapy.[31] In a later study, no difference was noted in gross motor outcomes for children treated five times a week for 6 months compared with those treated twice a week for the same length of time.[33] In addition, families had low compliance and were stressed and tired from the intense therapy.[33] Families and therapists must consider costs, accessibility, time, and the effect of the intervention on family dynamics. A treatment regimen of short periods of intensive therapy separated by periods without therapy may allow for optimal motor gain and may be less demanding for the children and their families.[61,324] The research on intervention intensity provides some guidance for developing service delivery models; however, the treatment frequencies in studies are often much higher than are realistically available in many treatment situations.

Physical therapists may be involved in a variety of roles related to health and well-being. Impairments in oral-motor control and swallowing, drooling, impaired self-feeding, and difficulties in expressing hunger or food preference can result in eating difficulties. Lack of activity can contribute to chronic constipation. Feeding problems can result in inadequate nutritional intake and poor growth, particularly in children with GMFCS Levels III, IV, and V. Growth curves have been developed for children functioning at these levels.[306] Poor growth is associated with poorer health, increased use of health care resources, decreased social participation, missed school days, and limitations in the child's and family's ability to take part in usual activities.[283,306] Gastroesophageal reflux and aspiration can also occur. Oral-motor programs, proper positioning, and parent education and support are important issues to address. In some cases, gastrostomy and antireflux procedures are appropriate. Conversely, increasing rates of obesity in children are a matter of concern. The prevalence of obesity in ambulatory children with CP has increased from 7.7% to 16.5% between 1994 and 2004—an increase similar to that seen in the general pediatric population.[262] Physical therapists can be involved in the promotion of physical activity to address weight gain.

Children with limited mobility or feeding problems may have chronic pulmonary problems, including poor clearance of secretions, aspiration, and susceptibility to pneumonia. Chest physical therapy, suctioning, and other techniques may be necessary to maintain optimal respiratory function.[251]

Failure to develop an appropriate toileting routine during the preschool years can result in participation restrictions and negative reactions from peers. Development of bladder control in children with CP may be delayed in comparison with typically developing children, but most become continent. Cognitive abilities and a diagnosis of quadriplegia can negatively influence the development of control.[263] Therapists may need to recommend appropriate adaptive equipment.

Mobility

Ambulation is a major concern of parents during the preschool years. If the prognosis for walking is good, treatment will include promotion of (1) preparatory ambulation skills,

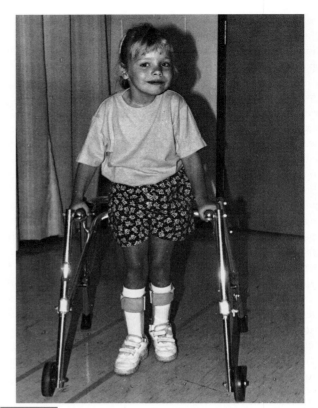

Figure 18-7   Child using a posterior walker, reported to promote upright posture and higher walking speeds than an anterior walker.

such as effective and well-aligned weight bearing, (2) selective control of joint movement and weight shifting needed for gait, and (3) improvement in balance. Body-weight-support harnesses with treadmill training may provide a learning opportunity for the task of walking.[200] Ambulatory aids, such as walkers, crutches, or canes, may be used, either temporarily while a child is progressing to more advanced gait skills, or as long-term aids for independent mobility. The use of posterior walkers has been found to encourage a more upright posture during gait, promote better gait characteristics, and decrease energy expenditure compared with the use of anterior walkers (Figure 18-7).[246]

Body-support walkers may give children at GMFCS Levels IV and V an opportunity for upright positioning and a limited degree of mobility.

Children in this age group are becoming aware of the concept of achievement. Ambulation may be a coveted skill, but it should not become an all-consuming goal, particularly if it may not be attainable or sustainable at older ages. Nonambulatory adults remember walking as the most important goal set for them by their parents and therapists, resulting in feelings of failure from an early age and loss of faith in rehabilitation professionals.[170]

The provision of alternative methods of functional, independent mobility is recommended when ambulation is impossible or inefficient. This need may be met with an

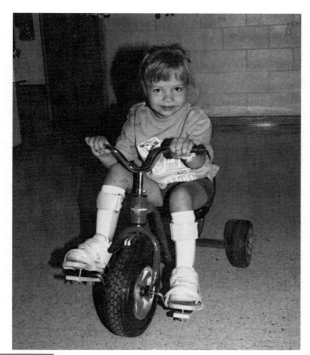

Figure 18-8 An adapted tricycle may meet a child's needs for mobility.

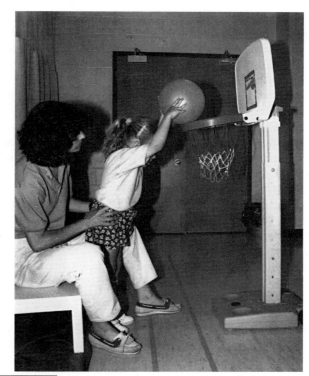

Figure 18-9 Therapeutic exercise programs can include highly motivating play activities. Throwing a basketball may be more motivating than trunk extension exercises.

adapted tricycle (Figure 18-8), a manual wheelchair, or a power mobility device, sometimes with special controls. These devices enable children with CP to explore their environment, achieve a sense of independence and competence, and experience increased social participation. Power mobility may also promote the development of initiative[45] and the acquisition of spatial concepts. The lack of self-propelled locomotion can result in apathy, withdrawal, passivity, and dependent behavior that can persist into later life.[45] If power mobility is being considered, fine motor control, cognitive skills, visual and auditory abilities, behavior, environmental accessibility, transportation, and financial resources must all be taken into account. Children with motor limitations can be safe and effectively mobile in power wheelchairs as young as 17 months of age.[45] Parents initially may be hesitant about introducing power mobility to young children, fearing that it signifies giving up on walking. Power mobility does not preclude ambulation-oriented therapy but provides the child with a method of moving about independently in the meantime and may stimulate self-mobility.[29,350] For children who will continue to be wholly dependent on power mobility for independence, it provides mobility at an appropriate age and gives families an indication of the implications of power mobility for housing, schooling, and transportation needs. For more information, see the Evolve site on assistive technology.

Play

Play, the primary productive activity of children, should be intrinsically motivating and pleasurable. The benefits of play include helping children discover the effects they can have on objects and people in their environment; development of social skills; and enhanced development of perceptual, conceptual, intellectual, and language skills. Children with CP are often constrained in their playfulness even when they have the capacity to be playful. They receive more support in play at home than in community or school environments.[258] Limitations in the play of children with physical disabilities due to physical impairments, time limitations, and social and environmental barriers may affect the experiential learning derived from play and may result in decreased independence, motivation, imagination, creativity, assertiveness, social skills, and self-esteem.[24] Therapy should provide and demonstrate play opportunities and provide input on dealing with social and environmental barriers to play (Figure 18-9).

Appropriate toys and play methods should be suggested to parents and caregivers. If children are physically unable to play with regular toys, a variety of adaptations, such as switch access, can make their toys usable.[184] Environmental control equipment also can be introduced to preschoolers.

It is important to not overprotect children with CP in their attempts to play. Parents should be encouraged to let their children enjoy typical play activities, such as rolling down hills and getting dirty in the mud. Therapists must ensure that therapy and home programs promote, rather than interfere with, normal play experiences. Early integration of children into community recreational activities can introduce a child and family to the benefits of a healthy active lifestyle and social opportunities.

Family Involvement

Planning of interventions should consider the child within the context of their family. Therapists should be sensitive to the family's stresses, dynamics, child-rearing practices, coping mechanisms, privacy, values, and cultural variations. Therapists should be flexible in their approach and programming.

Family involvement is crucial for integrating treatment into everyday life. Home programs are important for optimal therapy results because strengthening, extensibility, and motor learning require more input than can be provided in treatment sessions. Therefore, parents need to gain insight into the rationale behind their child's treatment. Because asking a family to spend 15 minutes on a treatment activity means 15 minutes will be lost from another activity,[20] home therapy activities are ideally integrated into daily life. Therapists need to be sensitive to the well-being of families and must find a balance between providing them with home programs that make them an integral part of their child's therapy and burdening them with activities they cannot realistically be expected to carry out. Obstacles may include constraints on time, energy, skills, or resources, and negative effects on the parent–child relationship. In summary, factors that have a positive influence on the participation of parents in home programs include collaborative decision making regarding the content and intensity of programs, recognition of the needs of individual families, and use of activities that are integrated easily into daily routines and are not stressful for the child or the caregiver.[163]

Siblings can also be included in home programs. Craft and colleagues studied a group of children with CP whose siblings had been educated about the condition and ways in which they could encourage their brother or sister to be more independent.[66] The program resulted in increased ROM and functional independence in the children with CP.

Role of Other Disciplines

Occupational therapists work closely with preschool children to develop independence in activities such as dressing, feeding, toileting, and playing. Speech and language pathologists continue to promote use of efficient methods of communication. Psychologists assess cognitive skills and consult with other professionals on the interaction of intellectual abilities with other areas of development. Social workers and behavior therapists continue to provide ongoing support to families because the stresses involved in parenting a child with a disability persist. Team assessment and intervention are imperative for addressing issues such as feeding problems, augmentative communication, and transition to school. Orthopedic surgeons monitor musculoskeletal development.

SCHOOL-AGE AND ADOLESCENT PERIOD

During the school-age and adolescent years, children typically participate in school and community life while remaining dependent on their families and living in their parental homes. They refine and maintain the basic functional skills they have learned and develop life skills activities that will enable them to cope effectively with the demands of daily living, interaction with peers, and transition to independent adult life. These years, particularly those spent in high school, can be difficult for children with CP.[223] They become increasingly aware of the reality, extent, and impact of their disabilities on themselves, their families, and their relationships with peers. As they strive to contend with the normal stresses of growing up, particularly those of adolescence, they must also cope with being different, acknowledge the potential obstacles to attaining independence, and work to overcome them. Participation in life activities has been shown to be more challenging as children reach adolescence.[158] Problems encountered during these years include lack of independent mobility, poor endurance in performing routine activities, and continued difficulty and slowness with self-care and hygiene skills at a time when privacy is becoming increasingly important. Adolescents may not have normal opportunities to develop socially and sexually or achieve age-appropriate levels of independence from the family. Dating is often delayed and less frequent than for other teenagers.[352] Environmental factors may contribute to reduced access to community and school facilities, limiting opportunities for participation in social, cultural, recreational, and athletic activities.

Parents may be anxious about the effects of their child's disabilities on their participation in age-appropriate endeavors and their future as an adult.[136] They continue to be naturally attentive but have to avoid being overprotective, and must begin to allow their child to take risks and become independent in the outside world.[223] In some cases, financial concerns regarding the need for special equipment, transportation, and home renovations must be addressed. Parents of children who are dependent in ADLs and transfers may suffer from physical stresses, such as back problems.

Physical Therapy Examination and Evaluation

Examination of impairments that could interfere with function or lead to secondary impairment continues to be important. Gross motor assessments may be less frequent as children naturally plateau in this area[138] but are still important for monitoring change resulting from interventions such as spasticity management, surgery, the use of orthoses, or periods of intensive therapy or deterioration. Assessment in a child's natural environment may provide valuable information for differentiating between capacity and performance and determining necessary accommodations to allow participation. For example, the walking speed, endurance, and agility necessary for negotiating school hallways with other children, along with noise and obstacles, may differ from those assessed in a gait laboratory or a structured timed distance test. Studies conducted in school have found that the mean velocity of typical 7-year-old children leading a line of students in a school hallway is 4 feet/second.[80] Information such as this can provide guidelines for the walking abilities necessary for participation in school mobility and for determination of treatment goals.

Privacy of individuals of all ages should be respected, but this is particularly important during these years, when children are becoming more aware of their bodies and their sexuality. They should be appropriately dressed when attending therapy sessions and clinics, particularly if they will be seen by unfamiliar people or will be photographed or videotaped. If it is necessary for children to remove their clothing, a reason should be given for doing so, and their permission should be requested.

Physical Therapy Goals, Outcomes, and Interventions

Goals change to reflect the adolescent's lifestyle and potential for change. Most children with CP achieve their optimal level of gross motor functioning during early school years.[54,138] Some children and adolescents may improve their motor skills, but for most, emphasis is focused on maintaining their achieved level of activity and participating in age-appropriate pursuits. Potential challenges include increasing size, pain, loss of muscle extensibility, puberty, cumulative physical overuse, and a more demanding and competitive lifestyle.[16]

School-age children and adolescents should be active participants in conversations regarding goals and programming if they are cognitively able. They should be encouraged to take increasing responsibility for their own health, nutrition, fitness, personal care, finances, and decision making, so they are prepared to assume these responsibilities in adulthood. It is also important to look ahead and consider appropriate goals for their later life situations and independence. Therapists should strive to foster self-esteem and assertiveness in children and adolescents by emphasizing their abilities, encouraging activities in which they can excel, and helping them to acknowledge their difficulties with a view toward identifying appropriate compensations and use of attendant care. In the case of children with more severe involvement, goals are oriented toward minimizing impairments to facilitate caregiving and comfort.

Secondary impairments must be anticipated and avoided if possible. Maintenance of muscle extensibility, strength, joint integrity, and fitness is important in preventing secondary impairments such as poor endurance, pain, and contracture that can result from the stresses of aging. This age group also needs to develop problem-solving strategies to overcome environmental and societal barriers to become as independent and active as possible in home, school, recreational, social, and community life. Education about their disability is an important but often lacking component of assuming self-management.[261] This may occur because the initial education of families occurs when a child is young, and continued provision of age-appropriate information to the child is often inadequate.

Mobility is important for overall health, well-being, and independence. Adolescents may be capable of using methods of mobility used at younger ages, but environmental and personal factors may influence performance.[268] It is vital to identify underlying causes of excessive energy use, to develop effective strategies to reduce energy-wasteful movements, and to implement physical fitness interventions through community exercise and sport programs. These goals are important for children across the spectrum of GMFCS levels but will be achieved in different ways.[111]

Reducing Primary Impairment and Preventing Secondary Impairment

Progressive resistance training has become a common intervention for children and adolescents with CP. Programs have ranged from 4 to 12 weeks in duration, with a frequency of three times a week, at 80% to 90% of maximal load, with varying levels of repetitions arranged in short sets to allow time for the muscle to rest and recover. Endurance programs use lower intensities with more repetitions. Elastic bands, free weights, isokinetic equipment, and functional movements have been used. Programs have taken place in home, clinic, or community settings. Strengthening should be included in a regular exercise or physical activity regimen to maintain optimal musculoskeletal function throughout the life span.[111] Youth with CP should exercise in positions that are comfortable and allow optimal selective control of targeted muscle groups.

Research has supported the effectiveness of strength training programs for producing significant increases in force production and muscle volume.[90,206] Some studies have reported concurrent improvements in activity as measured by gross motor function, gait parameters such as stride length and kinematics, and perception of body image.[194,326] These improvements have taken place without negative effects such as increased spasticity, increased pain, or decreased ROM. Nevertheless, reviews of strengthening studies in children with CP report different conclusions. Improved strength with inconclusive findings regarding gait, function, and activity level has been reported,[90] as has moderate to large strength and function gains, which were maintained after detraining, and small to moderate gait improvements that partially deteriorated during detraining.[212] Another review with more stringent inclusion criteria—only RCTs—questioned the effectiveness and worth of such programs, as increases in strength were small and nonsignificant, and improvements in activity as measured by the GMFM were statistically but not clinically significant.[288] Strength training is more likely to enhance motor functioning in younger children but may counteract deterioration in youth, thus statistically nonsignificant results may be clinically worthwhile.[212]

Various methods of electrical stimulation have been used as an adjunct to the treatment of CP in attempts to reduce spasticity, increase strength and muscle extensibility, promote the initial learning of selective control, and improve functional activities such as gait.[302] Administration of electrical stimulation over extended periods of time at intensities that do not produce a muscle contraction has not been shown to have a clinical effect.[69] Functional electrical stimulation, that is, stimulation for short durations at high intensities, has been shown to have favorable results on gait parameters when applied to the plantar flexors alone, or in combination with dorsiflexors,[289] although evidence of benefit for proximal muscles is lacking.[331] Placebo effects may be common.[331] Protocols should be individualized for patients after careful analysis of movement, and application should be closely monitored. Although this is a theoretically attractive method because muscle contraction is elicited independent of voluntary control, a review of the literature did not show conclusive evidence of its effectiveness in children with CP.[167]

Spasticity management is still important in this age group. Botulinum toxin continues to be effective and is often complemented with serial casting if contractures are present, to provide more marked and long-lasting effects.[86] Contractures may become more significant in this age group, particularly in more severely affected patients. The interventions described in the preschool section are appropriate, but it is important for therapists to ascertain which structures are causing restriction in movement. Joint hypomobility resulting from capsular or ligamentous tightness can be treated with joint mobilization.[40,142]

Osteopenia with an increased rate of fracture in moderately to severely involved children with CP has been associated with limited ambulation, previous fractures, the use of anticonvulsants, feeding problems, and lower body fat mass.[208] Physical activity that involves weight bearing and bisphosphonate therapy have been shown to have positive effects on bone mineral density in children and adolescents with CP.[56,149]

Although spasticity management and positioning programs may delay or reduce the need for orthopedic surgery, some children may benefit from surgical intervention to address progressive contractures or bone deformity; to improve gait, posture, cosmesis, and hygiene; and to prevent pain.[1,130,311] Possible surgical procedures include muscle/tendon lengthenings and transfers, tenotomies, neurectomies, osteotomies, and fusions. Although some surgeries have been evaluated, few comparative studies or well-controlled studies have focused on the long-term effects of orthopedic surgery in this population.[1,36,311] Single-event multilevel surgery, including procedures for the hip, knee, and ankle, may be performed to prevent progressive deterioration when gross motor function has plateaued. Biomechanical alignment can take place at all joints simultaneously, and the children and families will have to deal with only one hospital admission and one period of rehabilitation.[129,130,311] Children may become progressively flexed in their gait and may develop a crouch gait pattern, which can be worsened by their pubertal growth spurt. This pattern is characterized by excessive ankle dorsiflexion, knee flexion, and hip flexion and may be accompanied by excessive femoral anteversion, hip subluxation, patella alta, excessive external tibial torsion, calcaneal valgus, and knee pain. This problem is also addressed by multilevel orthopedic surgery, which has been shown to relieve stress on the knee extensor mechanism, reduce knee pain, and improve function and independence.[260] More complex surgeries that include procedures such as femoral extension osteotomies and patellar tendon advancements are resulting in promising improvements in knee function and gains in community function.[307]

Physical therapists play important roles in surgical decision making and the management of preoperative and postoperative care. Therapists, surgeons, and families are collaborators in surgical choices based on assessments of gait and other gross motor activities, equipment tolerance, pain, ROM, strength, selective motor control, spasticity, and respiratory function. Child and family goals, resources, motivation, and priorities, as well as surgeon experience, must be considered. As children get older, they should be active participants in making decisions about their care. Their interests, priorities, and concerns about interruptions in their lives as a result of hospitalizations, immobilizations, recovery periods, and commitment to postoperative rehabilitation should be respected. Preoperatively, therapists can educate the family about postoperative needs such as positioning, lifting, transferring, transportation, respiratory care, feeding, sleeping, and pain management, and the potential need for extra help at home. Botox and other forms of spasticity management may be considered to reduce postoperative discomfort.[17] Strengthening and respiratory exercises for preoperative conditioning may be beneficial. Home adaptations and equipment may be put in place in collaboration with occupational therapists, who may provide consultation regarding toileting and bathing needs. Positioning during the immediate postoperative period is important for comfort and muscle extensibility. Caregiver body mechanics are important when dealing with children who are compromised as the result of casts, movement restrictions, and pain. Postoperative rehabilitation contributes to optimal surgical outcomes. Muscle strength, particularly that of the hamstrings, can decrease significantly after surgery.[290] The physical therapist must train control of lengthened and transferred muscle in the context of functional motor tasks such as sit-to-stand, ascent of stairs, and ambulation. Specific exercises will vary according to immobilization and weight-bearing and movement restrictions, but extensibility and strengthening exercises to promote functional motor skills will serve as the basis of training programs.[290] Hydrotherapy may be beneficial. Re-evaluation of orthotic management and walking aids may be necessary to maintain alignment, protect surgical correction, and facilitate functional movement. Surgery may improve posture and gait, but outcomes can be unpredictable, as osteotomies, such as femoral derotations, alter the biomechanics of bones and muscles.

Spasticity, abnormal extensibility of muscles, muscular imbalance, and weakness can result in scoliosis, which, in turn, can affect positioning and respiratory status. Spinal deformity can be a particularly difficult problem in the severely affected patient. Various types of orthoses can be used in the management of scoliosis in individuals with CP without compromising pulmonary function.[192] Evidence does not indicate that they prevent progression of scoliosis in children with CP, but they may provide benefit by stabilizing trunk posture.[217] Surgical correction of spinal deformities may be necessary, usually in those with spastic quadriplegia (see Chapter 8).

Children and youth with CP are less active than their peers.[104,330] They have poorer cardiorespiratory fitness, lower physical work capacity, and higher oxygen costs. Their energy expenditure for walking can be up to three times as great as that of typically developing children, with significant differences across GMFCS levels.[164,336] It is unclear whether their low level of physical activity is related to the physical disability or results from a relatively sedentary lifestyle secondary to their motor problems. Children with CP may have problems exercising caused by inefficiency of breathing, muscle weakness, high muscle tone, increased involuntary movements, abnormal muscle co-activation, poor selective voluntary motor control, contractures, decreased balance, fatigue, and obesity.[111] Various combinations of these impairments can limit a child's ability to play and exercise at intensities necessary to develop cardiorespiratory fitness. Other barriers to physical activity perceived by youth with physical disabilities include pain, lack of time, scarcity of places to exercise with their peers, and people's misconceptions about their abilities and conditions.[165,224]

Physical activity in childhood and adolescence can establish lifestyle habits that continue into adulthood.[336] Exercise programs for children with CP can increase muscle strength and aerobic capacity without causing adverse effects on patterns of movement, flexibility, or spasticity. Cognitive benefits may be derived from physical activity for children with CP.[252] Evidence of the impact on body function, daily activity, participation, self-competence, and QOL is emerging.[112,336] An RCT of task-specific, functional anaerobic and aerobic exercises such as running and changing direction abruptly, step-ups, and stairs in an 8-month, twice per week group training program for children and adolescents with CP classified as GMFCS Levels I and II showed significant effects on aerobic and anaerobic capacity, muscle strength, perceived athletic competence, participation, and QOL.[335] Program specifics can be accessed at www.netchild.nl under fitness. A similar group of children participating in an endurance training program of twice weekly circuit train-

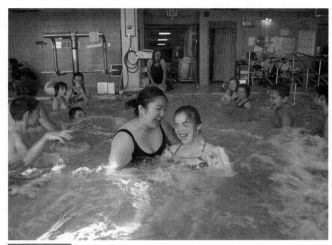

Figure 18-10 Participating in an aquatic class can provide fitness and social opportunities.

ing, including trampoline, running, jumping, treadmill, and cycling activities, demonstrated improved aerobic endurance, walking distance, and stair climbing time. Parents noted that their children could play outside longer and walk for longer periods.[121] Both programs were offered in school settings, possibly contributing to adherence and feasibility. Community fitness programs have been shown to improve muscle strength and perception of physical appearance; participants feel confident and motivated enough to take responsibility for continuing in fitness programs.[79] This can be particularly important if children and adolescents are receiving reduced levels of direct physical therapy intervention. Swimming programs (Figure 18-10) can be enjoyed by those of all ages and GMFCS levels.

Activity and Participation

Although typically, attainment of new gross motor skills levels off, improvements may be possible, even in children with severe physical and cognitive limitations, if goals are realistic, and appropriate behavioral, communication, and motor learning techniques are incorporated into the treatment program.[33,43] Regardless of the lack of potential for large gains in gross motor skills, therapy programs are necessary to maintain optimal levels of functioning and prevent unnecessary deterioration. Treatment principles such as family-centered service remain the same, but goals, tasks, and motivators need to be age appropriate.

Treadmill training with partial-body-weight-support harnesses can provide safe, task-specific gait training, providing multiple repetitions and active participation for children functioning at GMFCS Levels III, IV, and V.[200,225] Studies have small sample sizes but have demonstrated clinically relevant improvements in walking skills, gait velocity, and endurance, as well as improved standing transfers, in nonambulatory children. To date, the quantity and quality of these studies have not been sufficient to conclude that partial-body-weight-support treadmill training results in significant improvements for children with CP. Programs with higher intensities and extended durations have resulted in better outcomes.[72,225] Robotic-assisted treadmill training using a driven gait orthosis requires less personal effort, allowing increased speeds and longer distances during treatment sessions, and possibly enhancing neural reorganization.[210] This intervention shows promise as a therapeutic option to improve walking velocity and gross motor function in children functioning at GMFCS Levels II, III, and IV. Treadmills also are useful for increasing endurance and strength and can be used without harnesses in higher-functioning children.

School-age children have usually developed abstract thinking and sufficient cognitive ability to use biofeedback, which has been found to improve active ROM, strength, and control of movement such as dorsiflexion in children with CP.[93] The use of biofeedback to control posture has also met with some success.[27] Despite positive results, carryover is often limited, generalization to real-life situations is not readily demonstrated, and treatment can be time-consuming.[162] The advent of virtual reality technology may provide an age-appropriate treatment option to enhance exercise motivation, compliance, and effectiveness.[44] The Nintendo Wii (Nintendo Domestic Distributor, College Point, NY) can provide relatively low-cost, commercially available, socially acceptable, and entertaining activities for ambulatory and nonambulatory children and adolescents with CP. It has potential for enhancing visual-perceptual processing, postural control, functional activities, and energy expenditure.[87]

Youth with CP value mobility. The continued use of mobility devices is important for self-sufficiency and participation, particularly as children become larger and need to travel greater distances to participate in their social and educational activities.[243] Youth functioning at GMFCS Levels II to IV often choose to use manual or powered wheeled mobility for safety, practicality, or social appropriateness in school or community settings even if they can walk.[243,323] The use of mobility devices may require environmental modifications, such as entrance ramps or washroom renovations, for accessibility. Driver training offers the freedom to travel independently for those capable of driving a car. When driving is not feasible, instruction in the use of public or special transportation should be provided. Dependence on special transportation programs or parents limits ability to be spontaneous in attending community activities.[243]

Availability of power mobility should not preclude activity to the point of decreased musculoskeletal integrity, motor abilities, or physical fitness. Many adapted or integrated sports activities provide opportunities for exercise and participation.[305] These include horseback riding,[82] swimming, skiing,[305] sailing, canoeing, camping, kayaking, fishing, bungee jumping, yoga, skiing, and tai chi. Adapted games provide exercise, athletic competition, participation in team experiences, and social opportunities (www.medicalhomeinfo.org/health/recreation.html). Therapists need to be aware of and should address factors that may be barriers to participation in recreation and sports pursuits. These include lack of community level support, transportation, and accessibility; family factors such as finances, time, preferences, and involvement; and the adolescent's physical abilities, interests, and self-perceived competence.[173,224]

All athletes are at risk for sports-related injuries, but relatively minor injuries can incapacitate people with CP. They should be encouraged to be responsible for their bodies during sports activities by completing appropriate conditioning, warm-up, and cool-down routines; following comprehensive injury prevention programs, which include strengthening, flexibility, and aerobic and anaerobic training activities and protection of long-term joint integrity; and using appropriate protective and orthotic equipment. Knee injuries commonly involve the patellofemoral joint secondary to spasticity of muscle groups surrounding the joint. Deformities of the ankle and foot, including equinus, equinovarus, and valgus deformities, can lead to increased risk for injury.[177] Injuries should be taken seriously and treated promptly. For more information, see Chapter 15.

School and Community

Tremendous progress has been made in the integration of children with physical disabilities into the educational system and community activities. Although many experiences are very successful, some children experience isolation, marginalization, social or physical exclusion, bullying, or constant adult presence.[159] Physical therapists are involved in school-based therapy programs to support educational integration and participation. Facilities and resources such as support personnel, equipment for accessibility, and computer-based systems may be necessary to meet the physical needs of children in the school system. Therapists work closely with school personnel. They may instruct assistants and teachers in positioning, lifting, and transferring children; carrying out exercise programs; and adapting and developing recess activities and physical education programs. Therapists may also be involved in accessibility, transportation, evacuation, and other safety issues. Therapists working in school settings must be sensitive to the physical and scheduling constraints of the educational environment and must be willing to compromise to meet the educational priorities of students. Therapy may range from consultation and monitoring for students who are thought to have reached their maximal level of functioning, to active therapy for children who have specific treatment goals. When children are seen primarily through the educational system, efforts must be made to keep the family involved in all aspects of care and treatment. See Chapter 30 for further information on this subject based on experiences in the United States.

In addition to educating school staff about the complexities associated with CP, therapists can help educate the other children in the school to reduce teasing and bullying, and to increase acceptance of children with disabilities. In a study by Yude and colleagues, children with hemiplegia who were integrated into regular schools were twice as likely to be rejected and lack friends, and three times more likely to be victimized than their nondisabled peers.[362] Factors associated with more positive attitudes toward peers with disabilities include being female, having a good QOL, being friends with a child with a disability, and acquiring knowledge about people with disabilities through parents or the media.[340] Knowledge about, and positive interactions with, people with disabilities can create positive attitudes, particularly when children are between 7 and 9 years of age because their attitudes about people with disabilities are flexible at this age.[220]

During these years, children learn about their bodies, their sexuality, and appropriate interactions with other people. Children and adults with disabilities can suffer abuse, including sexual abuse, which may result in physical, social, emotional, and behavioral consequences.[298] Some abusers have relationships specifically related to the victim's disability. These people may include personal care attendants, transportation providers, residential care staff, and other disabled individuals. Physical therapists must know how to detect the signs of abuse, be sensitive and receptive to clients who may choose to confide in them, and know the proper procedures to follow if they suspect abuse. They must work with other professionals to promote assertiveness and positive self-esteem in their clients.

All people involved with youth with CP must educate them in being streetwise. Their physical and sometimes cognitive limitations can make them particularly vulnerable to crime. They should be taught to avoid unsafe situations and warned about protecting valuables. Purses or knapsacks slung over a wheelchair handle can be easy to grab. Self-defense courses specifically designed for people with disabilities may be available.

Health care professionals must realize that although parents have been coping with their child's needs for a number of years, parent education is still important because the child and the child's needs are constantly changing. Parents of children with CP are more likely to have a variety of physical and psychological health problems and need to be encouraged to take good care of themselves. Reported health issues include back problems, stomach/intestinal ulcers, migraine headaches, arthritis, emotional problems, pain, and chronic physical conditions.[37] Continued attention to education in lifting and transferring is necessary to prevent injury to caregivers whose children are growing larger and heavier as they, themselves, are aging.

Role of Other Disciplines

Occupational therapists may be involved in promoting independence in ADLs and work closely with physical therapists in managing upper extremity function.[60] Interdisciplinary life skills training can focus on self-care, community living, and interpersonal relationships. Prevocational training and related activities, such as money management and employment searching, may be necessary. Psychologists or social workers may be involved in various aspects of adolescent life such as social and sexuality issues.

TRANSITION TO ADULTHOOD

Adults strive to be independently functioning and self-sufficient individuals who have satisfying social and emotional lives and contribute to society. They typically live independently in the community, alone or with others, with employment to support themselves. They have romantic relationships and sexual experiences, enjoy social outings, often marry, and sometimes have children. Adolescents with CP have the same dreams and aspirations for adult life as all young people.[176] The extent to which these goals can be realized depends on factors such as independence in self-care activities and mobility, level of cognition, communication skills, and available resources and support. Many adults with CP continue to live with their families or in group homes or institutions. Only a small proportion are employed.[195] At a time when most parents are experiencing freedom from caregiving responsibilities, many parents of youth with CP continue to have these obligations.[136] Their concerns focus on how their child can function as an independent adult, how they can continue to care for their child as they themselves age, and who will care for the child when they are unable to do so. They, and their child, may also be coping with a decrease in the number of relatively organized and available programs and equipment resources that were available for the younger child. Continuity of care may be lacking, and they may have difficulty finding medical professionals with experience in managing the health care of people with disabilities.

The transition to adult lifestyle and services is complex. Planning and problem solving should take place throughout adolescence. Successful transition has been characterized by self-determination, enhanced knowledge of self and community, problem-solving and decision-making skills, identification of support systems, and supportive environments, including transition clinics.[21] Areas to be addressed include vocational or postsecondary education, living arrangements, personal management, leisure time, recreational and social activities, and financial planning. The latter involves education about governmental benefits, guardianship, conservatorship, wills, and trusts. Primary and preventive health care services must be organized. These include provision of therapy when needed, medical consultation, primary care, and equipment needs and maintenance. Internet resources from institutions provide guides to assist adolescents and families in navigating the transition to adulthood. These include Bloorview Kids Rehab (www.bloorview. ca/resourcecentre/familyresources/growingupready.php), Ministry of Children and Family Development in British Columbia (www.mcf.gov.bc.ca/spec_needs/pdf/ your_future_now.pdf), and the Alberta Government Planning for Post-Secondary Studies Series (www.alis.gov.ab.ca/ pdf/disabilities/transguidedisabilitystudent.pdf).

Physical Therapy Involvement

Pediatric physical therapists work together with the individual, the family, and the health care team to provide comprehensive planning to facilitate the transition to managing the challenges of adulthood. Major physical therapy goals during this period of transition are aimed at maximizing the capability to maintain function, prevent deterioration, and achieve optimal independent living. Ideally, the medical, therapeutic, and educational outcomes achieved throughout childhood have prepared youth with CP for success in these areas.

Therapists need to encourage problem solving in adolescents who have the potential to live on their own, as they will need to be self-sufficient in managing their health condition. Adults with CP must deal with the normal effects of aging, such as declines in muscle strength and elasticity and bone density, in addition to their preexisting impairments.[238] Strength training can result in improvements in walking ability and may prevent decline in mobility.[5] Community-based strength training programs for adults with CP have been found to increase leg strength by 22% and arm strength by 17%, and to improve performance of sit-to-stand skills during a 10-week intervention.[316]

Poor endurance, pain, fear of falling, and fatigue are factors contributing to ambulatory decline in adults with CP.[29] Fatigue is particularly a problem for those functioning at GMFCS Levels III and IV, suggesting association with overuse. It is associated with pain, lack of physical activity, general health problems, deterioration of physical skills, emotional issues, and low life satisfaction.[161]

Prevention of overuse syndromes, early joint degeneration, progression of contractures, osteoporosis, poor endurance, and pathologic fractures is important. Cervical and back pain, nerve entrapment syndromes, or tendinitis can occur as a result of excessive and repetitive physical stresses.[115] A survey of adults found that 67% reported one or more areas of pain, with lower extremity and back pain most common; 53% had pain of moderate to severe intensity.[287]

Fifty-two percent of ambulatory adults with CP reported deterioration in walking abilities—an increase from 39% seven years earlier in a longitudinal study.[236] Those who reported deterioration had significantly increased pain and physical fatigue with an adverse impact on daily life and participation. They believed that decreased muscle strength and cardiovascular fitness had contributed to their decline. Those who reported improved ambulation attributed the gains to improved balance, strength, and cardiorespiratory fitness. Adults with CP need to find a balance between alleviating unnecessary energy costs in daily living and staying fit to achieve optimal health and functioning.[70] Preventive strategies that may minimize the long-term effects of the neuromuscular dysfunction include choosing exercises that minimize excessive joint stress, using additional mobility aids or devices, such as orthoses, and opting for surgery. Changes to the environment may be necessary to maintain optimal independence.[238] Technological advances provide many options for adults with CP. These include computers for written communication, artificial speech devices, environmental controls, and power mobility. For more information, see the Evolve section on assistive technology.

Adherence to exercise programs of stretching, strengthening, and aerobics may be poor, so encouragement and opportunities should be provided. Poor exercise habits may start during adolescence, if not earlier, and can result in a cycle of poor fitness and endurance.[115] Access to therapy programs may decrease in the adult years, so therapists should encourage the use of community and recreational programs that provide the necessary opportunities to promote fitness and activity.

In many parts of the world, society is becoming more conscious of the rights and needs of individuals with limitations. This recognition has had a positive effect on environmental factors that influence participation. Human rights legislation exists to accommodate people with disabilities and to prevent discrimination in areas such as employment, accessibility, the legal system, and education. Government programs and services are available to people with disabilities. Theaters, restaurants, libraries, museums, government buildings, educational facilities, shopping areas, parks, campground facilities, and parking lots are often accessible through the provision of ramps, appropriate washroom facilities, and other modifications. Air and rail travel is also becoming more available to people with special mobility needs. Some travel organizations cater to people with disabilities. Therapists should be aware of the facilities and resources available to people with physical disabilities. In some situations, funding for assistive devices, living allowances, and housing and tax exemptions help prevent undue hardship. Therapists also should be cognizant of the political policies and issues affecting the lives of those with disabilities and should advocate for advancement of equal access to community and governmental resources.

GLOBAL ISSUES

The treatment of children with CP varies throughout the world. Physical therapists use many different approaches or combinations of approaches, depending on the facilities available, the child's and the family's needs, the therapist's training and background, and the diversity of client values, beliefs, and priorities. Many of the treatments and technologies discussed in this chapter are practiced in developed countries, where services, although variable in their extent, quality, and funding, are generally available and accessible. However, much of the world's population lives in underserved areas, particularly in developing nations or in remote areas of developed nations. In many countries, children with disabilities are not able to realize basic rights and are subject to policies of institutionalization rather than receiving community-based and family-focused care.[254] They may be deprived of opportunities to participate in society, may be denied access to education, and may suffer from stigma. Nevertheless many of the principles and equipment ideas developed elsewhere can be adapted to various situations. Using indigenous materials to fabricate effective and affordable equipment, recycling used equipment, and training local personnel or fostering exchange programs can help to provide resources to underserved areas.

It is important to be sensitive to local customs, cultures, and environmental situations when adapting programs for different settings. Often, the direct application of a certain method is impractical or inappropriate because of economic, geographic, or cultural differences. Throughout the world, increasing emphasis is being placed on community-based rehabilitation, which promotes interventions that are practical and functional for specific settings, lifestyles, and cultures.

PROFESSIONAL ISSUES

Many potential facilitators and barriers to the practice of efficacious, effective, and efficient physical therapy are known. Therapists who care for children with CP must realize that the work can be physically demanding. They must practice appropriate lifting and handling techniques and should maintain a suitable level of fitness if they are treating patients actively. Working with children and their families can be both fulfilling and emotionally stressful. Therapists may be challenged by ethical issues, unrealistic expectations and demands, limited resources, and the pressures of dealing with families during periods of grieving and times of crisis.

Therapists need to concentrate on what is positive and must realize that they cannot control all the variables in their patients' conditions and lives. Professionals must acknowledge their own needs and reactions and feel comfortable in seeking assistance and support from others.

Lifelong physical therapy needs of children with CP and their families are often influenced and constrained by service availability, accessibility, costs, and policy. These parameters can affect wait times for services and may have an impact on service frequency. The psychosocial well-being of families may be affected by long wait periods for therapy.[103] Therapists are often faced with the stressful challenges of providing equitable services within their facility or practice while justifying differences in services among facilities or clients. Intensity of services, including decisions regarding how often, how long, and the duration of an episode, varies considerably among families, therapists, administrators, policy makers, and insurers.[240] Family and fiscal resources challenge therapists to create strategies to provide equitable and appropriate services for all children in their care. Alternatives to continuous therapy include consultation, monitoring, or providing blocks of treatment, while taking into consideration periods of readiness for change. Determining whether children are at a stage of acquiring, improving, maintaining, or generalizing skill, and assessing motivation, supports, and environments, can help indicate optimal times to provide services. Small or large group programs and recreation and sports opportunities can provide alternatives to direct individual therapy.[240] Some families may purchase private services to augment or substitute for publicly funded services if these are deemed insufficient.[103]

CLINICAL RESEARCH AND EVIDENCE-BASED PRACTICE

The number of high-quality studies published on physical therapy for children with CP is increasing, but overall, methodologically robust research is lacking.[182,295] Meta-analyses, systematic reviews, and RCTs provide the highest level of research, but these yield little evidence for many of the traditional therapy approaches used for children with CP. Reviews of physical therapy interventions for children with CP often conclude that evidence is insufficient to support or refute intervention studies; additional studies of more rigorous methodologic quality are recommended.[23,47,78,143,187,248,249] Different reviews of the same intervention may arrive at different conclusions, depending on the particular studies selected for inclusion.[90,212,288] Credibility of pediatric CP research is often affected by lack of the following: randomization, documentation of recruitment procedures, thorough description of subjects, inclusion and exclusion criteria, distribution of GMFCS levels, comparative control groups, blinding of assessors and subjects, analyses to control for attrition, power or sample size calculations, and adequate sample sizes.

Many of these problems result from challenges inherent in conducting research on interventions for children and adolescents with CP. Treatment protocols are often varied and complex. Combinations of treatments may be used intentionally, or concurrent treatments may be provided unintentionally. Measures used may be insensitive to desired outcomes. Recruitment of sufficient numbers of subjects can be affected by the busy schedules of families, "research fatigue," and heterogeneity of subjects. The quality of many studies relies on parent or child compliance with protocols, which is difficult to monitor.[48] Ethical issues surround withholding treatment, using placebos, and defining standards of care. Use of the ICF provides a logical framework for conducting complex research; however, it can be difficult to measure the intricate relationships among the domains of body function/structure, activity, and participation, as well as the impact of contextual factors and their relation to overall health and QOL. Few studies have captured outcomes based on the concept of participation or attitudes.[101]

It is important to use evidence from a variety of designs based on the appropriateness of the design to a particular research question, rather than focusing solely on the hierarchy of levels of evidence, when conducting research on people with CP.[14,138] Alternative designs, when implemented rigorously, provide more realistic and perhaps equally valid results. These include cross-over designs, single-subject designs, longitudinal studies, population-based studies, and methodologically strong qualitative or mixed methods research. Use of the GMFCS provides a common and consistent language for classifying subjects.

It can be challenging for physical therapists to keep current with an ever expanding amount of evidence-based literature and to translate research into clinical practice. Generalizations from research findings to individual children in a clinical setting may be challenging because of the uniqueness of each child. Research evidence may not be transferable into clinical practice, as highly structured and controlled study protocols may not be feasible in clinical settings.[239]

Best practice encompasses the best research evidence available, clinical expertise, and needs and values.[279] These must be considered in the context of a child, the family, and the health care system resources. Physical therapists need to synthesize many factors and decide with the family upon the best approach for each child. They must critically appraise available and appropriate knowledge translation strategies, including accessing recent literature, using the Internet, attending educational sessions, and sharing practice-generated knowledge with colleagues and families to promote optimal decision making. Organizations need to be supportive of these strategies.[13,168]

SUMMARY

Physical therapists play an important role on the team of professionals who work with children with CP and their families. They offer choices and advice and provide interventions to promote development of optimal functional abilities, facilitate independence and participation in all aspects of life, and avoid secondary impairments. The support given during infancy, childhood, and adolescence can have an impact on functioning and quality of life in adulthood. Tools such as the GMFCS and the ICF-CY framework, family-centered values, improved prognostic information, psychometrically strong yet clinically feasible measurement tools, a menu of traditional and innovative treatment approaches, progressive technical advances, and progress in supportive policies combine to make the practice of physical therapy for children and adolescents with CP challenging but exciting.

This chapter concludes with two case studies that illustrate some of the management principles discussed in this chapter.

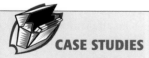

CASE STUDIES

"Noelle"

Noelle was born at 32 weeks of gestation. She weighed 1600 g and had an Apgar score of 8 at 5 minutes. She was admitted to the neonatal intensive care unit and was discharged home to live with her parents and 10 siblings approximately 6 weeks later. She was a healthy, happy baby who was very sociable and interested in play, but her parents felt that she was always behind in her gross motor skills. A developmental pediatrician assessed her at 17 months of age (15 months corrected age). At that time, Noelle could roll in both directions and sit unsupported briefly but was not attempting to crawl. She had increased tone in her lower extremities. A diagnosis was made of asymmetric quadriplegic CP with greater lower extremity than upper extremity involvement. She was referred to the local children's treatment center for physical therapy. She was not seen for a few months because of a waiting list, so her parents enlisted help privately. When she was seen at the children's center at 23 months of age, a physical therapist, an occupational therapist, and a speech and language pathologist assessed her development. Noelle began attending therapy sessions every 2 to 3 weeks and had a home program. She also attended a gross motor group. Physical therapy goals included improving postural control through activities that encouraged righting reactions and weight bearing through the extremities, maintenance of ROM, and accomplishment of gross motor skills such as moving in and out of sitting, and reaching activities that would facilitate play. The GMFM was used to document progress in gross motor skills.

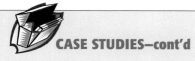

CASE STUDIES—cont'd

EVIDENCE TO PRACTICE 18-1

CASE STUDY "NOELLE"

EXAMINATION DECISION

The GMFM is a reliable and valid evaluative instrument designed to detect change in children with CP. A gain of 5 to 7 percentage points is considered a medium positive clinically important change for an individual child. The GMFM-66, an interval scale-level version of the original GMFM, demonstrates improved scoring, interpretation, and overall clinical and research utility, requires fewer items to be tested, and estimates the difficulty of items.[1] When GMFM-66 scores are used in conjunction with gross motor development curves on the CanChild website, therapists can determine whether a child's outcomes are consistent with their estimated potential,

and the extent to which interventions improve gross motor function beyond expectations based on a child's age and GMFCS classification level. It was possible to see Noelle progress as expected for a child functioning at GMFCS Level III.[2-4]

1. Avery, L. M., Russell, D. J., Raina, P. S., Walter, S. D., & Rosenbaum, P. L. (2003). Rasch analysis of the Gross Motor Function Measure: Validating the assumptions of the Rasch model to create an interval-level measure. *Archives of Physical Medicine and Rehabilitation, 84,* 697–705.
2. CanChild Centre for Childhood Disability Research. Retrieved from http://www.canchild.ca
3. Palisano, R. J., Snider, L. M., & Orlin M. N. (2004). Recent advances in physical and occupational therapy for children with cerebral palsy. *Seminars in Pediatric Neurology, 11,* 66–77.
4. Russell, D., Rosenbaum, P., & Avery, L. M. (2002). *Gross motor function measure (GMFM-66 & GMFM-88) user's manual.* London: MacKeith Press.

AFOs and supportive equipment for standing were prescribed. By 3 years of age, Noelle progressed to walking with a walker using small, adducted steps for short distances and was able to ride an adapted tricycle.

When Noelle was 5 years of age, she had decreased ROM and spasticity in her lower extremities, which had a negative impact on her gross motor skills and other ADLs, such as dressing. She had "scissoring" of her legs and leaned forward when walking. Her parents investigated the possibility of dorsal rhizotomy surgery but decided not to pursue this option. Serial casting to improve ankle ROM resulted in minimal improvement. She proceeded to have orthopedic surgery consisting of bilateral hip flexor (psoas) and adductor releases and medial hamstring and heel cord lengthenings. She had problems with pain management postoperatively and required intensive therapy to maintain ROM and to strengthen muscles after surgery.

Throughout her school years, Noelle received physical therapy services at the children's center, through a school health program, and privately. Communication among therapists was important to provide optimal care. Therapy programs continued to address the impairments of muscle extensibility, strength, and spasticity, and to focus on activities such as self-care and mobility. She rode an adapted bicycle at home and at her family's summer cottage. This activity provided recreational and fitness opportunities. Treatment strategies included treadmill use, exercises such as step-ups, electrical stimulation to tibialis anterior and quadriceps muscles, and functional activities. She received Botox injections and serial casting for her gastrocnemius muscles and also received injections in her hamstrings. She continued to use hinged AFOs and a posterior walker for ambulating but had a manual wheelchair for long distances. Noelle also received occupational and speech and language therapy. A computer was used for written communication.

At 12 years of age, Noelle functions at Level III on the GMFCS. She is in grade 7, and her therapist has addressed issues such as

participation in physical education, safe and functional mobility, and use of adaptive equipment. She continues to ambulate with a posterior walker but uses a wheelchair for long distances. Noelle's goal is to not use her wheelchair too much, so she can maintain her walking abilities. She underwent a gait assessment to document the characteristics of her walking and to gather information that could contribute to treatment decision making. Specific concerns included difficulty with foot clearance during swing phase and the risk of left hip subluxation over time. Step length was reduced compared with normative data, as were single-limb stance time, cadence, and velocity in barefoot trials. She had inappropriate swing phase activity of her rectus femoris muscles bilaterally and delayed and reduced activity of the tibialis anterior muscles (midswing activity only). When her AFOs were worn, gait symmetry, step length, and velocity were improved but were still different from normative values. With the AFOs, a heel strike was observed, her foot remained plantigrade during stance, and heel rise occurred appropriately at terminal swing. Inadequate knee flexion remained a problem with a toe drag in swing bilaterally. Spasticity of the rectus femoris muscle with inappropriate swing phase activity coupled with reduced hip flexor strength could account for the loss of appropriate knee flexion. It was decided that Noelle would receive Botox injections to the rectus femoris muscles and would commence a program of strengthening exercises at a clinic after school, so that therapy would not interfere with educational activities.

A subsequent gait analysis was performed 1 month later to assess changes in gait. She had slight improvement in peak knee flexion bilaterally after Botox injections. A consistent toe drag was noted during initial swing phase on the left, but moderate improvement on the right. To maintain strength and extensibility to allow participation in gross motor activities, an ongoing program of gym exercises and biking was begun. Prolonged low load stretch through positioning at home or through her positioning during sleep was also implemented. Because strengthening of her hip abductors, spinal extensors, and

Continued

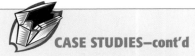

CASE STUDIES—cont'd

knee musculature continues to be important, appropriate exercises have been incorporated into her school gym program.

Noelle participates in many family, school, and community activities such as weddings, horseback riding, and gymnastics. She attends her local school with friends. She was able to ambulate at school with her walker in elementary school but used power mobility once she

entered secondary school. Noelle uses a treadmill at home and is involved in swimming programs.

Noelle has a service dog, Whisper, who can open doors, pick up objects, bark for help, move things out of the way, pull her coat off, and act as a support to help Noelle stand up. See video clips.

EVIDENCE TO PRACTICE 18-2

CASE STUDY "NOELLE"

PLAN OF CARE DECISION AND PATIENT FAMILY PREFERENCES

Youth with CP value mobility, and those functioning at GMFCS Levels II to IV often choose to use manual or powered wheeled mobility for safety, practicality, or social appropriateness in school or community settings even if they can walk. The use of mobility devices was important for Noelle's self-sufficiency and participation, particularly as she

grew and needed to travel greater distances to participate in her social and educational activities. The use of her power chair necessitated environmental modifications such as entrance ramps and washroom renovations at her school.[1,2]

1. Palisano, R. J., Murr, S. (2009). Intensity of therapy services: What are the considerations? *Physical and Occupational Therapy in Pediatrics, 29,* 107–112.
2. Tieman, B. L., Palisano, R. J., Gracely, E. J., et al. (2007). Variability in mobility of children with cerebral palsy in GMFCS levels II-IV. *Pediatric Physical Therapy, 19,* 180–187.

EVIDENCE TO PRACTICE 18-3

CASE STUDY "NOELLE"

PLAN OF CARE DECISION AND PATIENT FAMILY PREFERENCES

Physical activity in childhood and adolescence can establish lifestyle habits that continue into adulthood. Exercise for people with CP can increase muscle strength and aerobic capacity without causing adverse effects on patterns of movement, flexibility, or spasticity. Evidence of the impact on

daily activity, participation, self-competence, and QOL is emerging. Noelle and her family fit physical activity into her busy schedule.[1,2]

1. Fowler, E. G., Kolobe, T. H., Damiano, D., Thorpe, D. E., Morgan, D. W., Brunstrom, A. E., et al. (2007). Promotion of physical fitness and prevention of secondary conditions for children with cerebral palsy: Section on Pediatrics Research Summit Proceedings. *Physical Therapy, 87,* 1495–1510.
2. Verschuren, O., Ketelaar, M., Takken, T., et al. (2007). Exercise programs for children with cerebral palsy: A systematic review of the literature. *American Journal of Physical Medicine and Rehabilitation, 86.*

"Nicole"

Nicole was born at 29.5 weeks of gestation after placental separation. She weighed 1300 g and had an Apgar score of 8 at 5 minutes. She remained in the neonatal intensive care unit for 6 weeks and then went home to live with her parents and 3-year-old sister. Nicole was followed at the screening clinic for high-risk infants, where her parents were given suggestions for handling and positioning because of extensor positioning of her neck and trunk and hypertonicity in her legs. At 5 months of age corrected for prematurity, the diagnosis of CP was made on the basis of hypertonicity in her extremities, affecting lower extremities more than upper; strong, persistent primitive reflex activity; and delayed development of head and trunk control.

Services from a developmental pediatrician, a social worker, an orthopedic surgeon, a physical therapist, and later an occupational therapist were coordinated at the local children's treatment center, a publicly funded facility in Ontario, Canada. Nicole attended physical therapy sessions weekly. Positions that reduced the influence of her

extensor posturing were used to encourage active control of movements and functional skills such as play. Bivalved casts were provided to maintain muscle extensibility and provide optimal alignment of her feet when she was working on standing activities. The casts also reduced some of the extensor posturing in her lower extremities, resulting in improvement in her alignment in sitting and standing and improvement in the quality of functional activities in these positions. These casts were later replaced with solid AFOs when growth slowed down, and Nicole was eager to wear regular shoes. Customized seating and a standing frame gave her a variety of positions in which she could interact with others, use her hands, and experience weight bearing with her body optimally aligned.

At 2 years of age, impairments of hip adductor muscle hypoextensibility and spasticity were treated surgically with bilateral adductor muscle releases and anterior obturator neurectomies. This gave her more functional motion at her hips and put her hip joints in an optimal position for acetabular development to attempt to avoid the potential secondary impairment of hip subluxation or dislocation.

CASE STUDIES—cont'd

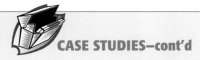

EVIDENCE TO PRACTICE 18-4

CASE STUDY "NICOLE"

PLAN OF CARE DECISION

Young children with mild hip subluxation may benefit from adductor muscle release to prevent further hip subluxation and to provide the potential benefits of easier movement, prevention of pain, ease of perineal hygiene, improved ROM, easier seating, and prevention of pelvic obliquity and scoliosis. Nicole did realize these benefits, but other treatment factors could have contributed to these positive outcomes (http://www.aacpdm.org/publications/outcome/resources/Adductor%20Release%20for%20CP%207-03.pdf).

During her preschool years, Nicole attended an integrated child care program. Her therapists visited the center to discuss Nicole's abilities, programs, handling, and equipment. When Nicole was 5 years old, she was progressing slowly in her gross and fine motor skills. Spasticity in her lower extremities resulted in activity limitations in sitting, standing, transitional movements, fine motor activities, and ADLs, and limited her potential for independence. Ambulation was not functional, but she could move about independently in a power chair and had some limited mobility in a manual wheelchair. The prominence of spasticity, moderate strength, and some degree of selective muscle control of her lower extremity musculature prompted the decision to perform a selective dorsal rhizotomy. After the rhizotomy, her lower extremity spasticity was reduced, and she was weak. Nicole participated in an intensive physical therapy and occupational therapy program for the next year (Figure 18-11).

EVIDENCE TO PRACTICE 18-5

CASE STUDY "NICOLE"

PLAN OF CARE DECISION

SDR has been found to be most effective for children age 3 to 8 years with GMFCS Levels III and IV who have access to and are receptive to physical therapy. A history of prematurity, good selective control of muscles, lack of contracture or deformity, and good cognitive abilities and motivation, as well as good parental support, are selection criteria and predictors of successful outcomes. Nicole had all of these positive indicators.[1,2]

1. McLaughlin, J. F., Bjornson, K. F., Temkin, N., Steinbeck, P., Wright, V., Reiner, A., et al. (2002). Selective dorsal rhizotomy: Meta-analysis of three randomized controlled trials. *Developmental Medicine and Child Neurology, 44,* 17–25.
2. Trost, J. P., Schwartz, M. H., Krach, L. E., Dunn, M. E., Novacheck, T. F. (2008). Comprehensive short-term outcome assessment of selective dorsal rhizotomy. *Developmental Medicine and Child Neurology, 50,* 765–771.

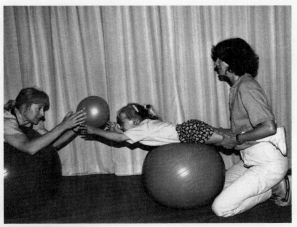

Figure 18-11　Mother and therapist with Nicole, encouraging force generation of trunk and hip extensors.

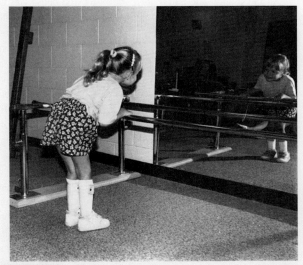

Figure 18-12　Despite many improvements after posterior rhizotomy, Nicole still shows diminished force-generating ability in hip and knee muscles.

A GMFM evaluation was done preoperatively and 1 year after surgery. Her scores improved from 88% to 96% in lying and rolling; from 78% to 87% in sitting; from 19% to 57% in crawling and kneeling; from 13% to 32% in standing (with AFOs); and from 7% to 10% in walking, running, and jumping (with AFOs). She had been able to walk 10 meters at 0.04 meters/second preoperatively but could walk 30 meters at 0.15 meters/second at her 1-year follow-up. Although these findings indicated that her gait had improved, the distance and velocity of her walking were still much below age norms and did not result in functional ambulation. She had improved selective muscle control and active and passive ROM, particularly in motions involving the hamstring muscles. Her strength improved, but she continued to have some weakness, particularly in her hip and knee extensor muscles (Figure 18-12).

Continued

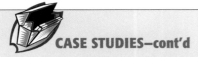

CASE STUDIES—cont'd

Nicole improved in self-care skills such as dressing her lower extremities because she was able to move one leg independently of the other. She was able to function better in activities such as opening jars, printing, and propelling her manual wheelchair. These improvements were believed to be the result of better trunk control and co-contraction in the shoulder musculature rather than of changes in the intrinsic muscles of her hands, motor planning, or visuoperceptual skills—areas that continued to be problems for Nicole.

During her adolescence, Nicole used a power wheelchair in school and community settings but used a manual wheelchair at home. Her inability to support her own weight as she grew taller and heavier was problematic. She was unable to assist any more than minimally with transfers, although the support of her AFOs did assist in her ability to bear weight. Nicole was able to direct her own care with regard to morning showering and dressing routines with help from personal care workers or her mother.

Nicole and her family faced environmental barriers. Their home was in the country and had a gravel driveway. The house was not wheelchair accessible because of stairs into the house, stairs inside, and narrow doorways. Thick carpeting made manual wheelchair pushing and walker maneuvering difficult. As a result of prognostic information from all health care professionals involved in her care, Nicole's family built an addition to their home, which made the downstairs fully accessible. A large deck allowed Nicole to go outdoors on her own and provided a second entrance to the house. The driveway was paved to enable her to reach her taxi or bus. She needed one-person assistance with transfers, toileting, and dressing, but showered and washed her own hair independently using a commode chair in a wheel-in shower.

Nicole attended her neighborhood public grade school and high school. Her parents worked closely with teachers and administrators of the schools. In grade school, a bus with a wheelchair lift provided transportation so she could travel to school with her peers. In high school, she used a taxi adapted for wheelchair use. Renovations were made to washrooms, and equipment was provided, but obstacles such as inaccessible playground equipment limited participation in some activities. Educational assistants were available to help Nicole with self-care and schoolwork. Her above-average knowledge of computer functions allowed her to develop efficient ways of completing her school assignments and communicating with others.

Nicole's therapists provided services at school. Active treatment was provided initially, but during her secondary school years, input consisted of consultation and monitoring of her progress. The responsibility for therapeutic exercises was gradually transferred to Nicole and her family with an emphasis on stretching to maintain ROM. Both found the motivation to continue difficult, although the assistance of her morning personal support worker was helpful. Nicole attended groups focusing on life skills at the children's treatment center. These programs provided opportunities for teens to discuss items of mutual interest.

Nicole was involved with horseback riding, swimming programs, weddings, camps, birthday parties, and sailing. Like many teenagers, she used a chat line on the Internet, and she spoke with her friends on the telephone. Outings with friends, however, were few and far between because of accessibility factors, such as lack of public wheelchair transportation in her township community. Although obstacles have become less common as society becomes more aware of accommodations necessary for people with disabilities, barriers such as buildings without ramps, inadequate parking, and inaccessible washrooms still exist. Impromptu activities, which are so much a part of the teenage lifestyle, are much more difficult when a wheelchair is used for mobility.

Nicole's family has worked with medical, educational, governmental, and community organizations to gain access to services and programs that provide her with normal childhood and adult experiences. They have been active advocates for changes that will provide people with disabilities with a full range of life's opportunities. They believe parents must be prepared to play central, responsible leadership roles within groups and agencies that can assist in these endeavors. They believe that home visits designed to deal with issues of daily routines, integration of treatment goals into home life, and involvement of all family members are important. Nicole's parents believe that it is particularly important for service providers to not withhold any information from the family. They also emphasize the need for feedback and encouragement to the family, especially to the primary caregiver. Nicole's parents found regular conferences to discuss short- and long-term goals invaluable in helping to facilitate effective partnerships among therapists, family, and school staff and in allowing them to become effective advocates for their children. Thorough transition planning beginning in high school facilitated her ability to live independently. Regular meetings identified challenges, focused on immediate and long-term goals, and kept the partners on Nicole's "team" involved and informed.

EVIDENCE TO PRACTICE 18-6

CASE STUDY "NICOLE"

PLAN OF CARE DECISION

The transition to adult lifestyle and services is complex. Planning and problem solving should take place throughout adolescence. Successful transition has been characterized by self-determination, enhanced knowledge of self and community, problem-solving and decision-making skills, identification of support systems, and supportive environments, including transition clinics.[1] Nicole benefited from the efforts of her family and professional staff to plan and organize a successful transition to adult life.

1. Binks, J. A., Barden, W. S., Burke, T. A., Young, N. L. (2007). What do we really know about the transition to adult-centred health care? A focus on cerebral palsy and spina bifida. *Archives of Physical Medicine and Rehabilitation, 88,* 1064–1073.

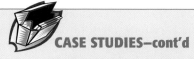

CASE STUDIES—cont'd

After graduation from high school (Figure 18-13), Nicole completed a diploma in travel and tourism and is currently studying public affairs and policy management.

She has a reduced course load because of fatigue. Nicole lived in a residence with 24/7 attendant support but now has her own apartment in an accessible building, where attendant care is available. She travels to university on accessible city transportation. Nicole swims twice a week to maintain her fitness, strength, and extensibility. She takes ½ tablet of Baclofen daily. She functions at a GMFCS Level IV, walking in a complex walker with assistance for exercise. Some programs are available through a rehabilitation center for adults, but therapy services are limited. Her power chair provides independent mobility; however, she uses a manual wheelchair for activities such as shopping and attending concerts. She wears AFOs and can assist in standing transfers. Lower extremity strength continues to be an issue.

Nicole's professional goal is to help people through policy changes. She has already accomplished this by advocating for accessible seating at concerts in her community. This has had the added bonus of her becoming friends with the Backstreet Boys.

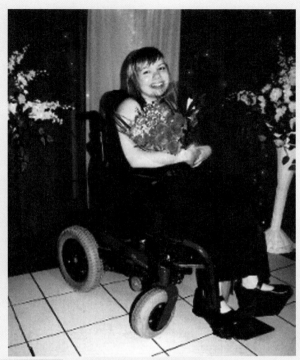

Figure 18-13 Nicole's high school graduation!

ACKNOWLEDGMENTS

Acknowledgments are extended to the children, adolescents, and their families involved in the case studies for their time and valuable perspectives. We also would like to acknowledge the clinical expertise of our colleagues. The literature provides us with research evidence, but best practice would not be possible without our day-to-day learning from each other.

REFERENCES

1. Aiona, M. D., & Sussman, M. D. (2004). Treatment of spastic diplegia in patients with cerebral palsy: Part II. *Journal of Pediatric Orthopaedics B, 13,* S13–S38.
2. Albavera-Hernandez, C., Rodriguez, J. M., & Idrova, A. J. (2009). Safety of botulinum toxin type A among children with spasticity secondary to cerebral palsy: A systematic review of randomized clinical trials. *Clinical Rehabilitation, 23,* 394–407.
3. Albright, A. L., Barry, M. J., Shafron, D. H., & Ferson, S. S. (2001). Intrathecal baclofen for generalized dystonia. *Developmental Medicine and Child Neurology, 43,* 652–657.
4. American Academy of Pediatrics. (1999). Transporting children with special health care needs (RE9852). *Pediatrics, 104,* 988–992.
5. Andersson, C., Grooten, W., Hellsten, M., Kaping, K., & Mattsson, E. (2003). Adults with cerebral palsy: Walking ability after progressive strength training. *Developmental Medicine and Child Neurology, 45,* 220–228.
6. Avery, L. M., Russell, D. J., Raina, P. S., Walter, S. D., & Rosenbaum, P. L. (2003). Rasch analysis of the Gross Motor Function Measure: Validating the assumptions of the Rasch model to create an interval-level measure. *Archives of Physical Medicine and Rehabilitation, 84,* 697–705.
7. Ayalon, M., Ben-Sira, D., Hutzler, Y., et al. (2000). Reliability of isokinetic strength measurements of the knee in children with cerebral palsy. *Developmental Medicine and Child Neurology, 42,* 398–402.
8. Bagley, A.M., Gorton, G., Oeffinger, D., et al. (2007). Outcome assessments in children with cerebral palsy, part II. Discrimatory ability of outcomes tools. *Developmental Medicine and Child Neurology, 49,* 181–186.
9. Bamm, E. L., & Rosenbaum, P. (2008). Family-centred theory: Origins, development, barriers, and supports to implementation in rehabilitation medicine. *Archives of Physical Medicine and Rehabilitation, 89,* 1618–1624.
10. Barks, L. (2004). Therapeutic positioning, wheelchair seating, and pulmonary function of children with cerebral palsy: A research synthesis. *Rehabilitation Nursing, 29,* 146–153.
11. Barnes, D., Linton, J. L., Sullivan, E., et al. (2008). Pediatric outcomes data collection instrument scores in ambulatory

children with cerebral palsy: An analysis by age groups and severity level. *Journal of Pediatric Orthopaedics, 28,* 97–102.

12. Barry, M. J., VanSwearingen, J. M., & Albright, A. L. (1999). Reliability and responsiveness of the Barry-Albright Dystonia Scale. *Developmental Medicine and Child Neurology, 41,* 404–411.

13. Barrett, R. S. & Lichtwark, G. A. (2010). Gross mophology and structure in spastic cerebral palsy: a systematic review. *Developmental Medicine and Child Neurology, 52,*798–804.

14. Bartlett, D. J., & Palisano, R. J. (2002). Physical therapist's perceptions of factors influencing the acquisition of motor abilities of children with cerebral palsy: Implications for clinical reasoning. *Physical Therapy, 82,* 237–248.

15. Bartlett, D., & Purdy, B. (2005). Testing of the spinal alignment and range of motion measure: A discriminative measure of posture and flexibility for children with cerebral palsy. *Developmental Medicine and Child Neurology, 47,* 739–743.

16. Bartlett, D. J., Hanna, S. E., Avery, L., Stevenson R. D., & Galuppi, B. (2010) Correlates of decline in gross motor capacity in adolescents with cerebral palsy in Gross Motor Function Classification System levels III to V: an exploratory study. *Developmental Medicine and Child Neurology, 52,* e155-e160.

17. Barwood, S., Baillieu, C. E., Boyd, R. N., Brereton, K., Nattrass, G. R., & Graham, H. K. (2000). Analgesic effects of botulinum toxin A: A randomised placebo trial. *Developmental Medicine and Child Neurology, 42,* 116–121.

18. Beckung, E., Carlsson, G., Carlsdotter, S., et al. (2002). The natural history of gross motor development in children with cerebral palsy aged 1 to 15 years. *Developmental Medicine and Child Neurology, 49,* 751–756.

19. Beckung, E., Hagberg, G., Uldall, P., & Cans, C. (2008). Probability of walking in children with cerebral palsy in Europe. *Pediatrics, 121,* e187–e192.

20. Bernheimer, L. P., & Weisner, T. S. (2007). "Let me just tell you what I do all day…" The family story at the center of intervention research and practice. *Infants Young Child, 20,* 192–201.

21. Binks, J. A., Barden, W. S., Burke, T. A., et al. (2007). What do we really know about the transition to adult-centred health care? A focus on cerebral palsy and spina bifida. *Archives of Physical Medicine and Rehabilitation, 88,* 1064–1073.

22. Bjornson, K. F., Belza, B., Kartin, D., et al. (2007). Ambulatory physical activity performance in youth with cerebral palsy and youth who are developing typically. *Physical Therapy, 87,* 248–260.

23. Blackmore, A. M., Boettcher-Hunt, E., Jordan, M., & Chan, M. D. Y. (2007). A systematic review of the effects of casting on equinus in children with cerebral palsy: An evidence report of the AACPDM. *Developmental Medicine and Child Neurology, 49,* 781–790.

24. Blanche, E.I. (1997) Doing with - not doing to: Play and the child with cerebral palsy. In Parham, L.D., & Fazio, L.S. (Eds.). *Play in Occupational Therapy for Children.* St. Louis: Mosby, pp 202–218.

25. Bly, L. (1991). A historical and current view of the basis of NDT. *Pediatric Physical Therapy, 3,* 131–135.

26. Boldingh, E. J., van der Bruggen, J., Lankhorst, M. A., et al. (2004). Assessing pain in patients with severe cerebral palsy: Development, reliability, and validity of a pain assessment instrument for cerebral palsy. *Archives of Physical Medicine and Rehabilitation, 85,* 758–766.

27. Bolek, J., Moeller-Mansour, L., & Sabet, A. (2001). Enhancing proper sitting position using a new sEMG protocol, the "minimax" procedure, with Boolean logic. *Applied Psychophysiology and Biofeedback, 26,* 9–16.

28. Booth, C. M., Cortina-Borja, M. J. F., & Theologis, T. N. (2001). Collagen accumulation in muscles of children with cerebral palsy and correlation with severity of spasticity. *Developmental Medicine and Child Neurology, 43,* 314–320.

29. Bottos, M., & Gericke, C. (2003). Ambulatory capacity in cerebral palsy: Prognostic criteria and consequences for intervention. *Developmental Medicine and Child Neurology, 45,* 786–790.

30. Bourke-Taylor, H., O'Shea, R., & Gaebler-Spira, D. (2007). Conductive education: A functional approach for children with cerebral palsy. *Physical and Occupational Therapy in Pediatrics, 27,* 45–62.

31. Bower, E., & McLellan, D. L. (1992). Effect of increased exposure to physiotherapy on skill acquisition of children with cerebral palsy. *Developmental Medicine and Child Neurology, 34,* 25–39.

32. Bower, E., McLellan, D. L., Arney, J., & Campbell, M. J. (1996). A randomised controlled trial of different intensities of physiotherapy and different goal-setting procedures in 44 children with cerebral palsy. *Developmental Medicine and Child Neurology, 38,* 226–237.

33. Bower, E., Mitchell, D., Burnett, M., Campbell, M. J., & McLellan, D. L. (2001). Randomised controlled trial of physiotherapy in 56 children with cerebral palsy followed for 18 months. *Developmental Medicine and Child Neurology, 43,* 4–15.

34. Boyce, W., Gowland, C., Rosenbaum, P., Lane, M., Plews, N., Goldsmith, C., et al. (1995). The Gross Motor Performance Measure: Validity and responsiveness of a measure of quality of movement. *Physical Therapy, 75,* 603–613.

35. Boyd, R., & Graham, H. K. (1999). Objective clinical measures in the use of Botulinum toxin A in the management of cerebral palsy. *European Journal of Neurology, 6*(Suppl. 4), 23–36.

36. Boyd, R., & Hays R. M. (2001). Current evidence for the use of botulinum toxin A in the management of children with cerebral palsy: A systematic review. *European Journal of Neurology, 8*(Suppl. 5), S1–S20.

37. Brehaut, J. C., Kohen, D. E., Raina, P., et al. (2004). The health of primary caregivers of children with cerebral palsy: How does it compare with that of other Canadian caregivers? *Pediatrics, 114,* e182–e191.

38. Brochard, S., Remy-Neris, O., Filipetti, P., et al. (2009). Intrathecal baclofen infusion for ambulant children with cerebral palsy. *Pediatric Neurology, 40,* 265–270.

39. Brogren Carlberg, E., & Hadders-Algra, M. (2005). Postural dysfunction in children with cerebral palsy: Some implications for therapeutic guidance. *Neural Plasticity, 12,* 221–228.

40. Brooks-Scott, S. (1995). *Mobilization for the Neurologically Involved Child.* Tuscon, AZ: Therapy Skill Builders.

41. Brouwer, B., & Ashby, P. (1991). Altered corticospinal projections to lower limb motoneurons in subjects with cerebral palsy. *Brain, 114,* 1395–1407.

42. Brouwer, B., Davidson, L. K., & Olney, S. J. (2000). Serial casting in idiopathic toe-walkers and children with spastic cerebral palsy. *Journal of Pediatric Orthopedics, 20,* 221–225.

43. Brown, D. A., Effgen, S. K., & Palisano, R. J. (1998). Performance following ability-focused physical therapy intervention in individuals with severely limited physical and cognitive abilities. *Physical Therapy, 78,* 934–950.

44. Bryanton, C., Bosse, J., Brien, M., et al. (2006). Feasibility, motivation, and selective motor control: Virtual reality compared to conventional home exercise in children with cerebral palsy. *CyberPsychology and Behavior, 9,* 123–128.

45. Butler, C. (1991). Augmentative mobility: Why do it? *Physical Medicine and Rehabilitation Clinics of North America, 2,* 801–815.

46. Butler, C., & Campbell, S. (2000). Evidence of the effects of intrathecal baclofen for spastic and dystonic cerebral palsy. AACPCM Treatment Outcomes Committee Review Panel. *Developmental Medicine and Child Neurology, 42,* 634–645.

47. Butler, C., & Darrah, J. (2001). Effects of neurodevelopmental treatment (NDT) for cerebral palsy. *Developmental Medicine and Child Neurology, 43,* 772–784.

48. Cameron, E. C., Maehle, V., & Reid, J. (2005). The effects of an early physical therapy intervention for very preterm, very low birth weight infants: A randomized controlled clinical trial. *Pediatric Physical Therapy, 17,* 107–119.

49. Campbell, S. K. (1997). Therapy programs for children that last a lifetime. *Physical and Occupational Therapy in Pediatrics, 17,* 1–15.

50. Campbell, S. K., & Barbosa, V. (2003). The challenge of early diagnosis. *Developmental Medicine and Child Neurology, 45*(Suppl. 94), 5–6.

51. Campbell, S. K., & Hedeker, D. (2001). Validity of the Test of Infant Motor Performance for discriminating among infants with varying risk for poor motor outcome. *Journal of Pediatrics, 139,* 546–551.

52. Campbell, S. K., Wilhelm, I. J., & Slaton, D. S. (1989). Anthropometric characteristics of young children with cerebral palsy. *Pediatric Physical Therapy, 1,* 105–108.

53. CanChild Centre for Childhood Disability Research. Retrieved from http://www.canchild.ca.

54. Cans, C. (2000). Surveillance of cerebral palsy in Europe: A collaboration of cerebral palsy surveys and registers. *Developmental Medicine and Child Neurology, 42,* 816–824.

55. Castle, K., Imms, C., & Howie, L. (2007). Being in pain: A phenomenological study of young people with cerebral palsy. *Developmental Medicine and Child Neurology, 49,* 445–449.

56. Chad, K.E., Bailey, D.A., McKay, H.A., Zello, G.A., & Snyder, R.E. (1999). The effect of a weight-bearing physical activity program on bone mineral content and estimated volumetric density in children with spastic cerebral palsy. *Journal of Pediatrics, 135,* 115–117.

57. Chandler, L.S., Andrew, M.S., & Swanson, M.W. (1980) *Movement Assessment of Infants: A Manual.* Rolling Bay, WA: Infant Movement Research.

58. Chang, F. M., Seidl, A. J., Muthusamy, K., et al. (2006). Effectiveness of instrumented gait analysis in children with cerebral palsy—Comparison of outcomes. *Journal of Pediatric Orthopaedics, 26,* 612–616.

59. Chen, F., DeMuth, S., Knutson, L., & Fowler, E. G. (2006). The use of the 600 yard walk-run test to assess walking endurance and speed in children with CP. *Pediatric Physical Therapy, 18,* 86.

60. Chin, T. Y. P., Duncan, J. A., Johnstone, B. R., & Graham, H. K. (2005). Management of the upper limb in cerebral palsy. *Journal of Pediatric Orthopedics B, 14,* 389–404.

61. Christiansen, A. S., & Lange, C. (2008). Intermittent versus continuous physiotherapy in children with cerebral palsy. *Developmental Medicine and Child Neurology, 50,* 290–293.

62. Chung, J., Evans, J., Lee, C., et al. (2008). Effectiveness of adaptive seating on sitting posture and postural control in children with cerebral palsy. *Pediatric Physical Therapy, 20,* 303–317.

63. Cioni, G., Ferrari, F., Einspieler, C., et al. (1997). Comparison between observation of spontaneous movements and neurological examination in preterm infants. *Journal of Pediatrics, 130,* 704–711.

64. Clopton, N., Dutton, J., Featherston, T., et al. (2005). Interrater and intrarater reliability of the Modified Ashworth Scale in children with hypertonia. *Pediatric Physical Therapy, 17,* 268–274.

65. Cook, R. E., Schneider, I., Hazelwood, M. E., Hillman, S. J., & Robb, J. E. (2003). Gait analysis alters decision-making in cerebral palsy. *Journal of Pediatric Orthopaedics, 23,* 292–295.

66. Craft, M. J., Lakin, J. A., Oppliger, R. A., Clancy, G. M., & Vanderlinden, D. W. (1990). Siblings as change agents for promoting the functional status of children with cerebral palsy. *Developmental Medicine and Child Neurology, 32,* 1049–1057.

67. Criswell, S. R., Crowner, B. E., & Racette, B. A. (2006). The use of botulinum toxin therapy for lower-extremity spasticity in children with cerebral palsy. *Neurosurgical Focus, 21,* e1.

68. Crompton, J., Galea, M. P., & Phillips, B. (2007). Hand-held dynamometry for muscle strength measurement in children with cerebral palsy. *Developmental Medicine and Child Neurology, 49,* 106–111.

69. Dali, C., Hansen, F. J., Pedersen, S. A., Skov, L., Hilden, J., Bjornskov, I., et al. (2002). Threshold electrical stimulation (TES) in ambulant children with CP: A randomized double-blind placebo-controlled clinical trial. *Developmental Medicine and Child Neurology, 44,* 364–369.

70. Damiano, D. L. (2003). Strength, endurance, and fitness in cerebral palsy. *Developmental Medicine and Child Neurology, 45*(Suppl. 94), 8–10.

71. Damiano, D. L. (2006). Activity, activity, activity: Rethinking our physical therapy approach to cerebral palsy. *Physical Therapy, 86,* 1535–1540.

72. Damiano, D. L., & DeJong, S. L. (2009). A systematic review of the effectiveness of treadmill training and body weight support in pediatric rehabilitation. *Journal of Neurologic Physical Therapy, 33*, 27–44.

73. Damiano, D. L., Dodd, K., & Taylor, N. F. (2002). Should we be testing and training muscle strength in cerebral palsy. *Developmental Medicine and Child Neurology, 44*, 68–72.

74. Damiano, D. L., Martellotta, T. L., Quinlivan, J. M., et al. (2001). Deficits in eccentric versus concentric torque in children with spastic cerebral palsy. *Medicine & Science in Sports & Exercise, 33*, 117–122.

75. Damiano, D.L. (2008). Is addressing impairments the shortest path to improving function? *Physical and Occupational Therapy in Pediatrics, 28*, 327–330.

76. Darrah, J., & Bartlett, D. (1995). Dynamic systems theory and management of children with cerebral palsy: Unresolved issues. *Infants and Young Children, 8*, 52–59.

77. Darrah, J., Piper, M., & Watt, M. J. (1998). Assessment of gross motor skills of at-risk infants: Predictive validity of the Alberta Infant Motor Scale. *Developmental Medicine and Child Neurology, 40*, 495–491.

78. Darrah, J., Watkins, B., Chen, L., et al. (2004). Conductive education intervention for children with a diagnosis of cerebral palsy: An AACPDM evidence report. *Developmental Medicine and Child Neurology, 46*, 187–204.

79. Darrah, J., Wessel, J., Nearingburg, P., & O'Connor, M. (1999). Evaluation of a community fitness program for adolescents with cerebral palsy. *Pediatric Physical Therapy, 11*, 18–23.

80. David, K. S., & Sullivan, M. (2005). Expectations for walking speeds: Standards for students in elementary schools. *Pediatric Physical Therapy, 17*, 120–127.

81. Davies, P. L., Soon, P. L., Young, M., et al. (2004). Validity and reliability of the School Function Assessment in elementary school students with disabilities. *Physical and Occupational Therapy in Pediatrics, 24*, 23–43.

82. Davis, E., Davies, B., Wolfe, R., et al. (2009). A randomized controlled trial of the impact of therapeutic horse riding on the quality of life, health, and function of children with cerebral palsy. *Developmental Medicine and Child Neurology, 51*, 111–119.

83. De Graaf-Peters, V. B., Blauw-Hospers, C. H., Dirks, T., et al. (2007). Development of postural control in typically developing children and children with cerebral palsy: Possibilities for intervention? *Neuroscience & Biobehavioral Reviews, 31*, 1191–1200.

84. Depienne, C., Stevanin, G., Durr, A., et al. (2007). Hereditary spastic paraplegia: An update. *Current Opinion in Neurology, 20*, 674–680.

85. Desloovere, K., Molenaers, G., Feys, H., et al. (2006). Do dynamic and static clinical measurements correlate with gait analysis parameters in children with cerebral palsy? *Gait Posture, 24*, 302–313.

86. Desloovere, K., Molenaers, G., Jonkers, I., De Cat, J., De Borre, L., Nijs, J., et al. (2001). A randomized study of combined botulinum toxin type A and casting in the ambulant child with cerebral palsy using objective outcome measures. *European Journal of Neurology, 8*, 75–87.

87. Deutsch, J. E., Borbely, M., Filler, J., et al. (2008). Use of a low-cost, commercially available gaming console (Wii) for rehabilitation of an adolescent with cerebral palsy. *Physical Therapy, 88*, 1196–1207.

88. DeVries, A. M., & deGroot, L. (2002). Transient dystonia revisited: A comparative study of preterm and term children at 2½ years of age. *Developmental Medicine and Child Neurology, 44*, 415–421.

89. Dobson, F., Boyd, R. N., Parrot, J., Nattrass, G. R., Graham, H. K. (2002). Hip surveillance in children with cerebral palsy: impact on the surgical management of spastic hip disease. *Journal of Bone and Joint Surgery, British Volume, 85*, 720–726.

90. Dodd, K., Taylor, N., & Damiano, D. L. (2002). Systemic review of strengthening for individuals with cerebral palsy. *Archives of Physical Medicine and Rehabilitation, 83*, 1157–1164.

91. Donkervoort, M., Wiegerink, D. J. H. G., Van Meeteren, J., et al. (2009). Transition to adulthood: Validation of the Rotterdam Transition Profile for young adults with cerebral palsy and normal intelligence. *Developmental Medicine and Child Neurology, 51*, 53–62.

92. Dunn, L. (2004). Validation of the CHORES: A measure of school-aged children's participation in household tasks. *Scandinavian Journal of Occupational Therapy, 11*, 179–190.

93. Dursun, E., Dursun, N., & Alican, D. (2004). Effects of biofeedback treatment on gait in children with cerebral palsy. *Disability & Rehabilitation, 26*, 116–120.

94. Edgar, T. S. (2003). Oral pharmocotherapy of childhood movement disorders. *Journal of Child Neurology, 18*(Suppl. 1), S40–S49.

95. Ehrsson, H. H., Kuhtz-Buschbeck, J. P., & Forssberg, H. (2002). Brain regions controlling nonsynergistic versus synergistic movement of the digits: A functional magnetic resonance imaging study. *Journal of Neuroscience, 22*, 5074–5080.

96. Elder, G. C., Kirk, J., Stewart, G., et al. (2003). Contributing factors to muscle weakness in children with cerebral palsy. *Developmental Medicine and Child Neurology, 45*, 542–550.

97. Eliasson, A.-C., Krumlinde-Sundholm, L., Rosblad, B., et al. (2006). The Manual Ability Classification System (MACS) for children with cerebral palsy: Scale development and evidence of validity and reliability. *Developmental Medicine and Child Neurology, 48*, 549–554.

98. Engsberg, J. R., Ross, S. A., Collins, D. R., et al. (2007). Predicting functional change from preintervention measures in selective dorsal rhizotomy. *Journal of Neurosurgery, 106*(4 Suppl.), 282–287.

99. Engsberg, J. R., Ross, S. A., Olree, K. S., & Park, T. S. (2000). Ankle spasticity and strength in children with spastic diplegia cerebral palsy. *Developmental Medicine and Child Neurology, 42*, 42–47.

100. Farmer, J., & Sabagh, A. (2007). Selective dorsal rhizotomies in the treatment of spasticity related to cerebral palsy. *Childs Nervous System, 23*, 991–1002.

101. Fauconnier, J., Dickinson, H. O., Beckung, E., et al. (2009). Participation in life situations of 8–12 year old children with cerebral palsy: Cross sectional European study. *British Medical Journal, 338,* b1458.

102. Fehlings, D., Rang, M., Glazier, J., & Steele, C. (2000). An evaluation of Botulinium-A toxin injections to improve upper extremity in children with hemiplegia cerebral palsy. *Journal of Pediatrics, 137,* 331–337.

103. Felman, D. E., Swaine, B., Gosselin, J., et al. (2008). Is waiting for rehabilitation services associated with changes in function and quality of life in children with physical disabilities? *Physical and Occupational Therapy in Children, 28,* 291–304.

104. Fernhall, B., & Unnithan, V. B. (2002). Physical activity, metabolic issues and assessment. *Physical Medicine and Rehabilitation Clinics of North America, 13,* 925–947.

105. Figueiredo, E. M., Ferreira, G. B., Moreira, R. C. M., Kirkwood, R. N., & Fetters, L. (2008). Efficacy of ankle-foot orthoses on gait of children with cerebral palsy: Systematic review of literature. *Pediatric Physical Therapy, 20,* 207–223.

106. Flanagan, A., Krzak, J., Peer, M., et al. (2009). Evaluation of short-term intensive orthotic garment use in children with cerebral palsy. *Pediatric Physical Therapy, 21,* 201–204.

107. Foran, J. R. H., Steinman, S., Barash, I., Chambers, H. G., & Lieber, R. L. (2005). Structural and mechanical alterations in spastic skeletal muscle. *Developmental Medicine and Child Neurology, 47,* 713–717.

108. Forrsberg, H. (1999). Neural control of human motor development. *Current Opinion in Neurobiology, 9,* 676–682.

109. Fosang, A. L., Galea, M., McCoy, A., et al. (2003). Measures of muscle and joint performance in the lower limb of children with cerebral palsy. *Developmental Medicine and Child Neurology, 45,* 664–670.

110. Fowler, E. G., & Goldberg, E. J. (2009). The effect of lower extremity selective voluntary motor control on interjoint coordination during gait in children with spastic diplegic cerebral palsy. *Gait Posture, 29,* 102–107.

111. Fowler, E. G., Kolobe, T. H. A., Damiano, D., et al. (2007). Promotion of physical fitness and prevention of secondary conditions for children with cerebral palsy: Section on Pediatrics Research Summit Proceedings. *Physical Therapy, 87,* 1495–1510.

112. Fowler, E. G., Knutson, L. M., Demuth, S. K., Siebert, K. L., Simms, V. D., Sugi, M. H., et al. (2010). Pediatric endurance and limb strengthening (PEDALS) for children with cerebral palsy using stationary cycling: a randomized control trial. *Physical Therapy, 90,* 367–381.

113. Fowler, E. G., Staudt, L. A., Greenberg, M. B., et al. (2009). Selective control assessment of the lower extremity (SCALE): Development, validation and interrater reliability of a clinical tool for patients with cerebral palsy. *Developmental Medicine and Child Neurology, 51,* 607–614.

114. Gage, J. R., & Novacheck, T. F. (2001). An update on the treatment of gait problems in cerebral palsy. *Journal of Pediatric Orthopaedics B, 10,* 265–274.

115. Gajdosik, C. G., & Cicirello, N. (2001). Secondary conditions of the musculoskeletal system in adolescents and adults with cerebral palsy. *Physical and Occupational Therapy in Pediatrics, 21,* 4967.

116. Gan, D., Campbell, K. A., Snider, A., et al. (2008). Giving youth a voice (GYC): A measure of youth's perceptions of the client-centeredness of rehabilitation services. *Canadian Journal of Occupational Therapy, 75,* 96–109.

117. Gericke, T. (2006). Postural management for children with cerebral palsy: Consensus statement. *Developmental Medicine and Child Neurology, 48,* 244.

118. Girolami, G., & Campbell, S. K. (1994). Efficacy of a neurodevelopmental treatment program to improve motor control in infants born preterm. *Pediatric Physical Therapy, 6,* 175–184.

119. Gooch, J. L., & Patton, C. P. (2004). Combining botulinum toxin and phenol to manage spasticity in children. *Archives of Physical Medicine and Rehabilitation, 85,* 1121–1124.

120. Gordon, A. M., Schneider, J. A., Chinnan, A., et al. (2007). Efficacy of a hand–arm bimanual intensive therapy (HABIT) in children with hemiplegic cerebral palsy: A randomized control trial. *Developmental Medicine and Child Neurology, 49,* 830–838.

121. Gorter, H., Holty, L., Rameckers, E. E. A., et al. (2009). Changes in endurance and walking ability through functional training in children with cerebral palsy. *Physical Therapy, 21,* 31–37.

122. Gorter, J. W., Ketelaar, M., Rosenbaum, P., et al. (2008). Use of the GMFCS in infants with CP: The need for reclassification at age 2 years or older. *Developmental Medicine and Child Neurology, 50,* 46–52.

123. Gorter, J. W., Rosenbaum, P. L., Hanna, S. E., et al. (2004). Limb distribution, motor impairment, and functional classification of cerebral palsy. *Developmental Medicine and Child Neurology, 46,* 461–467.

124. Gough, M. (2007). Serial casting in cerebral palsy: Panacea, placebo, or peril? *Developmental Medicine and Child Neurology, 49,* 725.

125. Gough, M. (2009). Continuous postural management and the prevention of deformity in children with cerebral palsy: An appraisal. *Developmental Medicine and Child Neurology, 51,* 105–110.

126. Graham, H. K., Aoki, K. R., Autti-Ramo, I. A., et al. (2000). Recommendations for the use of botulinum toxin type A in the management of cerebral palsy. *Gait and Posture, 11,* 67–79.

127. Graham, H. K., Boyd, R., Carlin, J. B., et al. (2008). Does botulinum toxin A combined with bracing prevent hip displacement in children with cerebral palsy and 'hips at risk'? A randomized, controlled trial. *American Journal of Bone and Joint Surgery, 90,* 23–33.

128. Graham, H. K., Harvey, A., Rodda, J., et al. (2004). The Functional Mobility Scale (FMS). *Journal of Pediatric Orthopaedics, 24,* 514–520.

129. Graham, H.K., Baker, R., Dobson, F., & Morris, M. E. (2005). Multilevel orthopedic surgery in group IV spastic hemiplegia. *Journal of Bone and Joint Surgery-British Volume, 87,* 548–557.

130. Graham, H. K., & Selber, P. (2003). Musculoskeletal aspects of cerebral palsy. *British Journal of Bone and Joint Surgery, 85,* 157–166.

131. Hadden, K. L., & vonBaeyer, C. L. (2002). Pain in children with cerebral palsy: Common triggers and expressive behaviors. *Pain, 99,* 281–288.

132. Hadders-Algra, M. (2000). The neuronal group selection theory: Promising principles for understanding and treating developmental motor disorders. *Developmental Medicine and Child Neurology, 42,* 707–715.

133. Hadders-Algra, M., van der Heide, J. C., Fock, J. M., et al. (2007). Effect of seat surface inclination on postural control during reaching in preterm children with cerebral palsy. *Physical Therapy, 87,* 861–871.

134. Hagglund, D., & Wagner, P. (2008). Development of spasticity with age in a total population of children with cerebral palsy. *BMC Musculoskeletal Disorders, 9,* 150.

135. Hagglund, G., Andersson, S., Duppe, H., et al. (2005). Prevention of severe contracture might replace multilevel surgery in cerebral palsy: Results of a population-based health care programme and new techniques to reduce spasticity. *Journal of Pediatric Orthopaedics B, 14,* 269–273.

136. Hallum, A. (1995). Disability and the transition to adulthood: Issues for the disabled child, the family, and the pediatrician. *Current Problems in Pediatrics, 25,* 12–50.

137. Hanna, S. E., Bartlett, D. J., Rivard, L. M., & Russell, D. J. (2008). Reference curves for the Gross Motor Function Measure: Percentiles for clinical description and tracking over time among children with cerebral palsy. *Physical Therapy, 88,* 596–607.

138. Hanna, S. E., Rosenbaum, P. L., Bartlett, D. J., et al. (2009). Stability and decline in gross motor function among children and youth with cerebral palsy aged 2 to 21 years. *Developmental Medicine and Child Neurology, 51,* 295–302.

139. Hanna, S. E., Law, M., Rosenbaum, P. R., et al. (2003). Development of hand function among children with cerebral palsy: growth curve analysis for ages 16 to 70 months. Measurement practices in pediatric rehabilitation: A survey of physical therapists, occupational therapists, and speech-language pathologists in Ontario. *Developmental Medicine and Child Neurology, 45,* 448–455.

140. Hanna, S. E., Russell, D. J., Bartlett, D. J., et al. (2007). Measurement practices in pediatric rehabilitation: A survey of physical therapists, occupational therapists, and speech-language pathologists in Ontario. *Physical and Occupational Therapy in Pediatrics, 27,* 25–42.

141. Harris, S. R. (2006). Listening to patients' voices: What can we learn. *Physiotherapy Canada,* 39–47.

142. Harris, S. R., & Lundgren, B. D. (1991). Joint mobilization for children with central nervous system disorders: Indications and precautions. *Physical Therapy, 71,* 890–896.

143. Harris, S. R., & Roxborough, L. (2005). Efficacy and effectiveness of physical therapy in enhancing postural control in children with cerebral palsy. *Neural Plasticity, 12,* 229–243.

144. Harvey, A., Graham, K., Morris, M. E., et al. (2007). The Functional Mobility Scale: Ability to detect change following singe event multilevel surgery. *Developmental Medicine and Child Neurology, 49,* 603–607.

145. Harvey, A., Robin, J., Morris, M. E., et al. (2008). A systematic review of measures of activity limitation for children with cerebral palsy. *Developmental Medicine and Child Neurology, 50,* 190–198.

146. Hawamdeh, Z. M., Ibrahim, A. I., Al-Qudah, A. A. (2007). Long-term effect of botulinum toxin (A) in the management of calf spasticity in children with diplegic cerebral palsy. *Europa Medicophysica, 43,* 311–318.

147. Hayes, B., Ryan, S., Stephenson, J. B. P., et al. (2007). Cerebral palsy after maternal trauma in pregnancy. *Developmental Medicine and Child Neurology, 49,* 700–706.

148. Heinen, F., Desloovere K., Schroeder, A.S., Berweck, S., Borggraefe, I., van Campenhout, A., et al. (2010). The updated European Consensus 2009 on the use of Botulinum toxin for children with cerebral palsy. *European Journal of Paediatric Neurology, 14,* 45–66.

149. Henderson, R. C., Lark, R. K., Kecskemethy, H. H., Miller, F., Harcke, H. T., & Bachrach, S. J. (2002). Bisphosponates to treat osteopenia in children with quadriplegic cerebral palsy: A randomized, placebo-controlled clinical trial. *Journal of Pediatrics, 141,* 644–651.

150. Herman, D., May, R., Vogel, L., et al. (2007). Quantifying weight-bearing by children with cerebral palsy while in passive standers. *Pediatric Physical Therapy, 19,* 283–287.

151. Hidecker, M. J. C., Paneth, N., Rosenbaum, P., et al. Development of the communication function classification system (CFCS) for individuals with cerebral palsy. *Developmental Medicine and Child Neurology, 51*(Suppl. 2), 48, 2009.

152. Hillman, S. T., Hazelwood, M. Z., Schwartz, M. H. (2007). Correlation of the Edinburgh Gait Score with the Gillette Gait Index, the Gilletter Functional Assessment Questionnaire, and dimensionless speed. *Journal of Pediatric Orthopaedics, 27,* 7–11.

153. Hoare, B., Imms, C., Carey, L., et al. (2007). Constraint-induced movement therapy in the treatment of the upper limb in children with hemiplegic cerebral palsy: A Cochrane systematic review. *Clinical Rehabilitation, 21,* 675–685.

154. Hong, T., & Paneth, N. (2008). Maternal and infant thyroid disorders and cerebral palsy. *Seminars in Perinatology, 32,* 438–445.

155. Howle, J. (2003). *Neuro-developmental treatment approach: Theoretical foundations and principles of clinical practice.* Laguna Beach, CA: North American Neuro-developmental Treatment Association.

156. Hurvitz, E. A., Leonard, C., Ayyangar, R., & Simon Nelson, V. (2003). Complementary and alternative medicine use in families of children with cerebral palsy. *Developmental Medicine and Child Neurology, 45,* 364–370.

157. Hutton, J. L., & Pharoah, P. O. D. (2006). Life expectancy in severe cerebral palsy. *Archives of Disease in Childhood, 91,* 254–258.

158. Imms, C., Reilly, S., Carlin, J., et al. (2008). Diversity of participation in children with cerebral palsy. *Developmental Medicine and Child Neurology, 50,* 363–369.

159. Imms, C. (2008). Children with cerebral palsy participate: a review of the literature. *Disability & Rehabilitation, 30,* 1867–1884.

160. Jacobs, S., Hunt, R., Tarnow-Mordi, W., et al. (2007). Cooling for newborns with hypoxic ischaemic encephalopathy. *Cochrane Database System Reviews, 4,* CD003311.

161. Jahnsen, R., Villien, L., Stanghelle, J. K., & Holm, I. (2003). Fatigue in adults with cerebral palsy in Norway compared with the general population. *Developmental Medicine and Child Neurology, 45,* 296–303.

162. James, R. (1993). Biofeedback treatment for cerebral palsy in children and adolescents: A review. *Pediatric Exercise Science, 24,* 198–212.

163. Jansen, L. M. C., Ketalaar, M., & Vermeer, A. (2003). Parental experience of participation in physical therapy for children with physical disabilities. *Developmental Medicine and Child Neurology, 45,* 58–69.

164. Johnston, T. E., Moore, S. E., Quinn, L. T., et al. (2004). Energy cost of walking in children with cerebral palsy: Relation to the Gross Motor Function Classification System. *Developmental Medicine and Child Neurology, 46,* 34–38.

165. Kang, M., Zhu, W., Ragan, B. G., et al. (2007). Exercise barrier severity and perseverance of active youth with physical disabilities. *Rehabilitation Psychology, 52,* 170–176.

166. Kembhavi, G., Darrah, J., Magill-Evans, J., et al. (2002). Using the Berg Balance Scale to distinguish balance abilities in children with cerebral palsy. *Pediatric Physical Therapy, 14,* 92–99.

167. Kerr, C., McDowell, B., McDonough, S., et al. (2004). Electrical stimulation in cerebral palsy: A review of effects on strength and motor function. *Developmental Medicine and Child Neurology, 46,* 205–213.

168. Ketelaar, M., Russell, D. J., Gorter, J. W. (2008). The challenge of moving evidence-based measures into clinical practice: Lessons in knowledge translation. *Physical and Occupational Therapy in Pediatrics, 28,* 191–206.

169. Ketelaar, M., Vermeer, A., Hart, H., van Petegem-van Beek, E., & Helders, P. J. M. (2001). Effects of a functional therapy program on motor abilities of children with cerebral palsy. *Physical Therapy, 81,* 1534–1545.

170. Kibele, A. (1989). Occupational therapy's role in improving the quality of life for persons with cerebral palsy. *American Journal of Occupational Therapy, 43,* 371–377.

171. Kilgour, G., McNair, P., & Stott, S. (2003). Intrarater reliability of lower limb sagittal range-of-motion measures in children with spastic cerebral diplegia. *Developmental Medicine and Child Neurology, 45,* 391–399.

172. King, G., Law, M., Hanna, S., et al. (2006). Predictors of the leisure and recreation participation of children with physical disabilities: A structural equation modeling analysis. *Child Health Care, 35,* 209–234.

173. King, G., Law, M., King, S., Rosenbaum, P., Kertoy, M. K., & Young, N. (2003). A conceptual model of the factors affecting the recreation and leisure participation of children with disabilities. *Physical and Occupational Therapy in Pediatrics, 23,* 63–90.

174. King, G. A., Law, M., King, S., et al. (2007). Measuring children's participation in recreation and leisure activities: Construct validation of the CAPE and PAC. *Child: Care, Health, and Development, 33,* 28–39.

175. King, S., King, G., & Rosenbaum, P. (2004). Evaluating health service delivery to children with chronic conditions and their families: Development of a refined Measure of Processes of Care (MPOC-20). *Children's Health Care, 33,* 35–57.

176. King, S., Teplicky, R., King, G., Rosenbaum, P.(2004). Family-centred service for children with cerebral palsy and their families: a review of the literature. *Seminars in Pediatric Neurology, 11,* 78–86.

177. Klenck, C., & Gebke, K. (2007). Practical management: Common medical problems in disabled athletes. *Clinical Journal of Sport Medicine, 17,* 55–60.

178. Kolaski, K., & Logan, L. R. (2007). A review of the complication of intrathecal baclofen in patients with cerebral palsy. *Neurorehabilitation, 22,* 383–395.

179. Korzeniewski, S. J., Birbeck, G., DeLano, M. C., et al. (2009). A systematic review of neuroimaging for cerebral palsy. *Journal of Child Neurology, 23,* 216–227.

180. Kragloh-Mann, I., & Horber, D. (2007). The role of magnetic resonance imaging in elucidating the pathogenesis of cerebral palsy: A systematic review. *Developmental Medicine and Child Neurology, 49,* 144–151.

181. Kruse, M., Michelsen, S. I., Flachs, E. M., Bronnum-Hansen, H., Madsen, M., & Uldall, P. (2009). Lifetime costs of cerebral palsy. *Developmental Medicine and Child Neurology, 51,* 622–629.

182. Kunz, R., Autti-Ramo, I., Antilla, H., et al. (2002). A systematic review finds that methodological quality is better than its reputation but can be improved in physiotherapy trials in childhood cerebral palsy. *Journal of Clinical Epidemiology, 59,* 1239–1248.

183. Kuroda, M. M., Weck, M. E., Sarwark, J. F., et al. (2007). Association of apolipoprotein E genotype and cerebral palsy in children. *Pediatrics, 119,* 303–313.

184. Lagone, J., Malone, D. M., & Kinsley, T. (1999). Technology solutions for young children with developmental concerns. *Infants & Young Children, 11,* 65–78.

185. Langerak, N. G., Lamberts, R. P., Fieggen, A. G., et al. (2008). A prospective gait analysis study in patients with diplegic cerebral palsy 20 years after selective dorsal rhizotomy. *Journal of Neurosurgery: Pediatrics, 1,* 180–186.

186. Langerak, N. G., Lamberts, R. P., Fieggen, A. G., et al. (2009). Functional status of patients with cerebral palsy according to the International Classification of Functioning, Disability and Health Model: A 20-year follow-up study after selective dorsal rhizotomy. *Archives of Physical Medicine and Rehabilitation, 90,* 994–1003.

187. Lannin, N., Scheinberg, A., & Clark, K. (2006). AACPDM systematic review of the effectiveness of therapy for children

with cerebral palsy after botulinum toxin A injections. *Developmental Medicine and Child Neurology, 48,* 533–539.

188. Law, M., Baptiste, S., McColl, M. A., Opzoomer, A., Polatajko, H., & Pollock, N. (1990). The Canadian Occupational Performance Measure: An outcome measure for occupational therapy. *Canadian Journal of Occupational Therapy, 57,* 82–87.

189. Law, M., Hanna, S., King, G., et al. (2003). Factors affecting family-centred service delivery for children with disabilities. *Child: Care, Health, and Development, 29,* 357–366.

190. Leiber, R. L., Steinman, S., Barash, I. A., et al. (2004). Structural and functional changes in spastic skeletal muscle. *Muscle & Nerve, 29,* 615–627.

191. Lekskulchai, R., & Cole, J. (2001). Effect of a developmental program on motor performance in infants born preterm. *Australian Journal of Physiotherapy, 47,* 169–176.

192. Leopando, M.T., Moussavi, Z., Holbrow, J., Chernick, V., Pasterkamp, H. (1999) Effect of a Soft Boston Orthosis on pulmonary mechanics in severe cerebral palsy. *Pediatric Pulmonology, 28,* 53–58.

193. Lepage, C., Noreau, L., & Bernard, P. (1998). Association between characteristics of locomotion and accomplishment of life habits in children with cerebral palsy. *Physical Therapy, 78,* 458–469.

194. Liao, H.-F., Liu, Y.-C., Liu, W.-Y., et al. (2007). Effectiveness of loaded sit-to-stand resistance exercise for children with mild spastic diplegia: A randomised clinical trial. *Archives of Physical Medicine and Rehabilitation, 88,* 25–31.

195. Liptak, G. S. (2008). Health and well being of adults with cerebral palsy. *Current Opinion in Neurology, 21,* 136–142.

196. Lundy, C. T., Doherty, G. M., & Fairhurst, C. B. (2009). Botulinum toxin type A injections can be an effective treatment for pain in children with hip spasms and cerebral palsy. *Developmental Medicine and Child Neurology, 51,* 705–711.

197. Mackey, A. H., Lobb, G. L., Walt, S. E., & Stott, N. S. (2003). Reliability and validity of the Observational Gait Scale in children with spastic diplegia. *Developmental Medicine and Child Neurology, 45,* 4–11.

198. Mackie, P. C., Jessen, E. C., & Jarvis, S. N. (1998). The lifestyle assessment questionnaire: An instrument to measure the impact of disability on the lives of children with cerebral palsy and their families. *Child: Care, Health, and Development, 24,* 473–486.

199. Majnemer, A., & Mazer, B. (2004). New directions in the outcome evaluation of children with cerebral palsy. *Seminars in Pediatric Neurology, 11,* 11–17.

200. Mattern-Baxter, K. (2009). Effects of partial body weight supported treadmill training on children with cerebral palsy. *Pediatric Physical Therapy, 21,* 12–22.

201. McCarthy, M. L., Silberstein, C. E., Atkins, E. A., Harryman, S. E., Sponseller, P. D., & Hadley-Miller, N. A. (2002). Comparing reliability and validity of pediatric instruments for measuring health and well-being of children with spastic cerebral palsy. *Developmental Medicine and Child Neurology, 44,* 468–476.

202. McDonagh, M. S., Morgan, D., Carson, S., & Russman, B. S. (2007). Systematic review of hyperbaric oygen therapy for cerebral palsy: the state of the evidence. *Developmental Medicine and Child Neurology, 49,* 942–947.

203. McDowell, B. C., Hewitt, V., Nurse, A., Weston, T., & Baker, R. (2000). The variability of goniometric measurements in ambulatory children with spastic cerebral palsy. *Gait and Posture, 12,* 114–121.

204. McKearnan, K. A., Keickhefer, G. M., Engel, J. M., et al. (2004). Pain in children with cerebral palsy: A review. *Journal of Neuroscience Nursing, 36,* 252–259.

205. McLaughlin, J. F., Bjornson, K. F., Temkin, N., Steinbeck, P., Wright, V., Reiner, A., et al. (2002). Selective dorsal rhizotomy: Meta-analysis of three randomized controlled trials. *Developmental Medicine and Child Neurology, 44,* 17–25.

206. McNee, A. E., Gough, M., Morrissey, M., et al. (2009). Increases in muscle volume after plantarflexor strength training in children with spastic cerebral palsy. *Developmental Medicine in Child Neurology, 51,* 429–435.

207. Meinecke, L., Breitbach-Faller, N., Bartz, C., et al. (2006). Movement analysis in the early detection of newborns at risk for developing spasticity due to infantile cerebral palsy. *Human Movement Science, 25,* 125–144.

208. Mergler, S., Evenhuis, H. M., Boot, A. M., et al. (2009). Epidemiology of low bone mineral density and fractures in children with severe cerebral palsy: A systematic review. *Developmental Medicine and Child Neurology, 51,* 773–778.

209. Metaxiotis, D., Accles, W., Siebel, A., & Doederlein, L. (2000). Hip deformities in walking patients with cerebral palsy. *Gait and Posture, 11,* 86–91.

210. Meyer-Heim, A., Ammann-Reiffer, C., Schmartz, A., et al. (2009). Improvement of walking abilities after robotic-assisted locomotion training in children with cerebral palsy. *Archives of Disease in Childhood, 94,* 615–620.

211. Michelsen, S. I., Flachs, E., Uldall, P., et al. (2008). Frequency of participation of 8–12-year-old children with cerebral palsy: A multi-centre cross-sectional European study. *European Journal of Paediatric Neurology, 13,* 165–177.

212. Mockford, M., & Caulton, J. M. (2008). Systematic review of progressive strength training in children and adolescents with cerebral palsy who are ambulatory. *Pediatric Physical Therapy, 20,* 318–333.

213. Molenaers, G., Desloovere, K., Fabray, G., & De Cock, P. (2006) The effects of quantitative gait assessment and botulinum Toxin A on musculoskeletal surgery in children with cerebral palsy. *Journal of Bone and Joint Surgery, 88-A,* 161–169.

214. Morrell, D. S., Pearson, J. M., & Sauser, D. D. (2002). Progressive bone and joint abnormalities of the spine and lower extremities in cerebral palsy. *Radiographics, 22,* 257–268.

215. Morris, C. (2002). A review of the efficacy of lower-limb orthoses used for cerebral palsy. *Developmental Medicine and Child Neurology, 44,* 205–211.

216. Morris, C. (2005). Child or family assessed measures of activity performance and participation for children with cerebral

palsy: A structured review. *Child: Care, Health, and Development*, 31, 397–407.

217. Morris, C. (2009). Aiming to improve the health care of people with cerebral palsy worldwide: A report of an International Society for Prosthetics and Orthotics conference. *Developmental Medicine and Child Neurology*, 51, 689.

218. Morris, C., Galuppi, B. E., & Rosenbaum, P. L. (2004). Reliability of family report for the Gross Motor Function Classification System. *Developmental Medicine and Child Neurology*, 46, 455–460.

219. Morris, C., Kurinczuk, J. J., Fitzpatrick, R., et al. (2006). Do the abilities of children with cerebral palsy explain their activities and participation? *Developmental Medicine and Child Neurology*, 48:954–961.

220. Morrison, J. M., & Ursprung, A. W. (1987). Children's attitudes toward people with disabilities: A review of the literature. *Journal of Rehabilitation*, 53, 45–49.

221. Motta, F., Stignani, C., & Antonello, C. E. (2008). Effect of intrathecal Baclofen on dystonia in children with cerebral palsy and the use of functional scales. *Journal of Pediatric Orthopedics*, 28, 213–217.

222. Murney, M. E., & Campbell, S. K. (1998). The ecological relevance of the Test of Motor Performance elicited scale items. *Physical Therapy*, 78, 479–489.

223. Murphy, K. P., Molnar, G. E., & Lankansky, B. A. (2000). Employment and social issues in adults with cerebral palsy. *Archives of Physical Medicine and Rehabilitation*, 81, 807–811.

224. Murphy, N. A., & Carbone, P. S. (2008). Promoting the participation of children with disabilities in sports, recreation, and physical activities. *Pediatrics*, 121, 1057–1061.

225. Mutlu, A., Krosschell, K., & Gaebler Spira, D. (2009). Treadmill training with partial body-weight support in children with cerebral palsy: A systematic review. *Developmental Medicine and Child Neurology*, 51, 268–275.

226. Narayanan, U. G. (2007). The role of gait analysis in the orthopedic management of ambulatory cerebral palsy. *Current Opinion in Pediatrics*, 19, 38–43.

227. Narayanan, U. G., Fehlings, D., Weir, S., et al. (2006). Initial development and validation of the Caregiver Priorities and Child Health Index of Life with Disabilities (CPCHILD). *Developmental Medicine and Child Neurology*, 48, 804–812.

228. Nelson, K. B. (2008). Causative factors in cerebral palsy. *Clinical Obstetrics and Gynecology*, 51, 749–762.

229. Nelson, K., & Chang, T. (2008). Is cerebral palsy preventable? *Current Opinion in Neurology*, 21, 129–135.

230. Noreau, L., Lepage, C., Boissiere, L., et al. (2007). Measuring participation in children with disabilities using the Assessment of Life Habits. *Developmental Medicine and Child Neurology*, 49, 666–671.

231. Novacheck, T. F., & Gage, J. R. (2007). Orthopedic management of spasticity in cerebral palsy. *Child Nervous System*, 23, 1015–1031.

232. Nystrom, E. M., & Beckung, E. (2008). Walking ability is related to muscle strength in children with cerebral palsy. *Gait & Posture*, 28, 366–371.

233. Odding, E., Roebroeck, M. E., & Stam, H. J. (2006). The epidemiology of cerebral palsy: Incidence, impairments and risk factors. *Disability & Rehabilitation*, 28, 183–191.

234. Olney, S. J., MacPhail, H. E. A., Hedden, D. M., et al. (1990). Work and power in hemiplegic cerebral palsy gait. *Physical Therapy*, 70, 431–438.

235. Oonpuu, S., Bell, K. I., Davis, R. B., & De Luca, P. A. (1996). An evaluation of the posterior leaf spring orthosis using joint kinematics and kinetics. *Journal of Pediatric Orthopedics*, 16, 378–384.

236. Opheim, A., Jahnsen, R., Olsson, E., et al. (2009). Walking function, pain, and fatigue in adults with cerebral palsy: A 7-year follow-up study. *Developmental Medicine and Child Neurology*, 51, 381–388.

237. Ostensjo, S., Brogren Carlberg, E., Vollestad, N. K., et al. (2004). Motor impairment in young children with cerebral palsy: Relationship to gross motor function and everyday activities. *Developmental Medicine and Child Neurology*, 46, 580–589.

238. Overeynder, J. C., & Turk, M. A. (1998). Cerebral palsy and aging: A framework for promoting the health of older persons with cerebral palsy. *Topics in Geriatric Rehabilitation*, 13, 19–24.

239. Palisano, R. J. (2006). A collaborative model of service delivery for children with movement disorders: A framework for evidence-based decision making. *Physical Therapist*, 86, 1295–1305.

240. Palisano, R. J., & Murr, S. (2009). Intensity of therapy services: What are the considerations? *Physical and Occupational Therapy in Pediatrics*, 29, 107–112.

241. Palisano, R. J., Rosenbaum, P., Bartlett, D., & Livingston, M. H. (2008). Content validity of the expanded and revised Gross Motor Function Classification System. *Developmental Medicine and Child Neurology*, 50, 744–750.

242. Palisano, R. J., Rosenbaum, P., Walter, S., et al. (1997). Development and reliability of a system to classify gross motor function in children with cerebral palsy. *Developmental Medicine and Child Neurology*, 39, 214–223.

243. Palisano, R. J., Shimmell, L. J., Stewart, D., et al. (2009). Mobility experiences of adolescents with cerebral palsy. *Physical and Occupational Therapy in Pediatrics*, 29, 133–153.

244. Palisano, R. J., Snider, L. M., & Orlin, M. N. (2004). Recent advances in physical and occupational therapy for children with cerebral palsy. *Seminars in Pediatric Neurology*, 11, 66–77.

245. Palmer, F. B. (2004). Strategies for the early diagnosis of cerebral palsy. *Journal of Pediatrics*, 145, S8–S11.

246. Park, E. S., Park, C. I., & Kim, J. Y. (2001). Comparison of anterior and posterior walkers with respect to gait parameters and energy expenditure in children with spastic diplegic cerebral palsy. *Yonsei Medical Journal*, 42, 180–184.

247. Piggot, J., Paterson, J., & Hocking, C. (2002). Participation in home therapy programs for children with cerebral palsy: A compelling challenge. *Qualitative Health Research*, 12, 1112–1129.

248. Pin, T. W. (2007). Effectiveness of static weight-bearing exercises in children with cerebral palsy. *Pediatric Physical Therapy*, *19*, 62–73.

249. Pin, T., Dyke, P., & Chan, M. (2006). The effectiveness of passive stretching in children with cerebral palsy. *Developmental Medicine and Child Neurology*, *48*, 855–862.

250. Pirpiris, M., Wilkinson, A. J., Rodda, J., Hguyen, T. C., Baker, R. J., Nattrass, G. R., et al. (2003). Walking speed in children and young adults with neuromuscular disease: Comparison between two assessment methods. *Journal of Pediatric Orthopedics*, *23*, 302–307.

251. Plioplys, A. V., Lewis, S., & Kasnicka, I. (2002). Pulmonary vest therapy in pediatric long-term care. *Journal of the American Medical Directors Association*, *3*, 318–321.

252. Ploughman, M. (2008). Exercise is brain food: The effects of physical activity on cognitive function. *Developmental Neurorehabilitation*, *11*, 236–240.

253. Pueyo, R., Junque, C., Vendrell, P., et al. (2009). Neuropsychologic impairment in bilateral cerebral palsy. *Pediatric Neurology*, *40*, 19–26.

254. Puras, D. (2009). Developmental disabilities: Challenged for research practices and policies in the 21st century. *Developmental Medicine and Child Neurology*, *51*, 415.

255. Read, H. S., Hazelwood, M. E., Hillman, S. J., et al. (2003). Edinburgh visual gait score for use in cerebral palsy. *Journal of Pediatric Orthopaedics*, *23*, 296–301.

256. Rennie, D. J., Attfield, S. F., Morton, R. E., et al. (2000). An evaluation of lycra garments in the lower limb using 3-D gait analysis and functional assessment (PEDI). *Gait & Posture*, *12*, 1–6.

257. Rice, J., & Waugh, M. (2009). Pilot study on trihexyphenidyl in the treatment of dystonia in children with cerebral palsy. *Journal of Child Neurology*, *24*, 176–182.

258. Rigby, P., & Gaik, S. (2007). Stability of playfulness across environmental settings: A pilot study. *Physical and Occupational Therapy in Pediatrics*, *27*, 27–43.

259. Robinson, M. N., Peake, L. J., Ditchfield, M. R., et al. (2008). Magnetic resonance imaging findings in a population-based cohort of children with cerebral palsy. *Developmental Medicine and Child Neurology*, *50*, 39–45.

260. Rodda, J. M., Graham, H. K., Nattrass, G. R., et al. (2006). Correction of severe crouch gait in patients with spastic diplegia with use of multilevel orthopedic surgery. *American Journal of Bone and Joint Surgery*, *88*, 2653–2664.

261. Roebroeck, M. E., Jahnsen, R., Carona, C., et al. (2009). Adult outcomes and lifespan issues for people with childhood-onset physical disability. *Developmental Medicine and Child Neurology*, *51*, 670–678.

262. Rogozinski, B. M., Davids, J. R., Davis, R. B., Christopher, L. M., Anderson, J. P., Jameson, G. G., et al. (2007). Prevalence of obesity in ambulatory children with cerebral palsy. *American Journal of Bone and Joint Surgery*, *89*, 2421–2426.

263. Roijen, L. E., Postema, K., & Kuppevelt, V. H. (2001). Development of bladder control in children and adolescents with cerebral palsy. *Child Neurology*, *43*, 103–107.

264. Rose, J., & McGill, K. C. (2005). Neuromuscular activation and motor-unit firing characteristics in cerebral palsy. *Developmental Medicine and Child Neurology*, *47*, 329–336.

265. Rosenbaum, P. L. (2003). Cerebral palsy: What parents and doctors want to know. *British Medical Journal*, *326*, 970–974.

266. Rosenbaum, P. (2006). Variation and abnormality: Recognizing the differences. *Journal of Pediatrics*, *149*, 593–594.

267. Rosenbaum, P., King, S., Law, M., King, G., & Evans, J. (1998). Family-centred service: A conceptual framework and research review. *Physical Therapy and Occupational Therapy in Pediatrics*, *18*, 1–20.

268. Rosenbaum, P. L., Palisano, R. J., Bartlett, D. J., Galuppi, B. E., Russell, D. J. (2008). Development of the Gross Motor Classification System for cerebral palsy. *Developmental Medicine and Child Neurology*, *50*, 249–253.

269. Rosenbaum, P., Paneth, N., Goldstein, M., Bax, M., Damiano, D., et al. (2007). A report: The definition and classification of cerebral palsy. *Developmental Medicine and Child Neurology Suppl*, *109*, 8–14.

270. Rosenbaum, P., & Stewart, D. (2004). The World Health Organization International Classification of Functioning, Disability and Health: a model to guide clinical thinking, practice and research in the field of cerebral palsy. *Seminars in Pediatric Neurology*, *11*, 5–10.

271. Rosenbaum, P. L., Walter, S. D., Hanna, S. E., Palisano, R. J., Russell, D. J., Raina, P., et al. (2002). Development and reliability of a system to classify gross motor function in children with cerebral palsy. *Journal of the American Medical Association*, *288*, 1357–1363.

272. Ross, S. A., & Engsberg, J. R. (2002). Relation between spasticity and strength in individuals with spastic diplegic cerebral palsy. *Developmental Medicine and Child Neurology*, *44*, 148–157.

273. Rouse, D. J., Hirtz, D. G., Thon, E., Varner, M. W., Sprong, C. Y., Mercer, B. M.,et al. (2008). A randomized, controlled trial of magnesium sulfate for the prevention of cerebral palsy. *New England Journal of Medicine*, *359*,895–905.

274. Russell, D. J., Avery, L. M., Walter, S. D., Hanna, S. E., Bartlett, D. J., Rosenbaum, P. L., et al. (2010). Development and validation of item sets to improve efficiency of administration of the Gross Motor Function Measure (GMFM-66) in children with cerebral palsy. *Developmental Medicine and Child Neurology*, *52*, e48–e54.

275. Russell, D. J., Gorter, J. W. (2005). Assessing functional differences in gross motor skills in children with cerebral palsy who use an ambulatory aid or orthoses: Can the GMFM-88 help? *Developmental Medical and Child Neurology*, *47*, 462–467.

276. Russell, D., Rosenbaum, P., & Avery, L. M. (2002). *Gross Motor Function Measure (GMFM-66 & GMFM-88) user's manual.* London: MacKeith Press.

277. Russman, B. S., & Ashwal, S. (2004). Evaluation of the child with cerebral palsy. *Seminars in Pediatric Neurology*, *11*, 47–57.

278. Ryan, S., Campbell, K. A., Rigby, P. J., Fishbein-Germon, B., Hubley, D., & Chan, B. (2009). The impact of adaptive seating

devices on the lives of young children with cerebral palsy. *Archives of Physical Medicine and Rehabilitation, 90,* 27–33.

279. Sackett, D. L., Straus, S. D., Richardson, W. S., Rosenberg, W., & Haynes, R. B. (2000). *Evidence-based medicine: How to practice and teach EBM* (2nd ed.). Edinburgh: Churchill Livingstone.

280. Sakzewski, L., Boyd, R., & Ziviani, J. (2007). Clinimetric properties of participation measure for 5- to 13-year-old children with cerebral palsy: A systematic review. *Developmental Medicine and Child Neurology, 49,* 232–240.

281. Samdup, D. Z., Smith, R. G., & Song, S. II. (2006). The use of complementary and alternative medicine in children with chronic medical conditions. *American Journal of Physical Medicine and Rehabilitation, 85,* 842–846.

282. Samson, J. F., Sie, L. T. L., & de Groot, L. (2002). Muscle power development in preterm infants with periventricular flaring or leukomalacia in relation to outcome at 18 months. *Developmental Medicine and Child Neurology, 44,* 734–740.

283. Samson-Fang, L., Fung, E., Satlings, V. A., Conaway, M., Worley, G., Rosenbaum, P., et al. (2002). Relationship of nutritional status to health and societal participation in children with cerebral palsy. *Journal of Pediatrics, 141,* 637–643.

284. Sanger, T. D., Chen, D., Delgado, M. R., Gaebler-Spira, D., Hallett, M., Mink, J. W.; Taskforce on Childhood Motor Disorders. (2006). Definitions and classification of negative motor signs in childhood. *Pediatrics, 118,* 2159–2167.

285. Sanger, T. D., Delgado, M. R., Gaebler-Spira, D., Hallett, M., Mink, J. W.; Taskforce on Childhood Motor Disorders. (2003). Classification and definition of disorders causing hypertonia in childhood. *Pediatrics, 111,* e89–e97.

286. Scholtes, V. A. B., Beelen, A., & Lankhorst, G. J. (2006). Clinical assessment of spasticity in children with cerebral palsy: A critical review of available literature. *Developmental Medicine and Child Neurology, 48,* 64–73.

287. Schwartz, L., Engel, J. M., & Jensen, M. P. (1999). Pain in persons with cerebral palsy. *Archives of Physical Medicine and Rehabilitation, 80,* 1243–1246.

288. Scianni, A., Butler, J. M., Ada, L., & Teixeira-Salmela, L. F. (2009). Muscle strengthening is not effective in children and adolescents with cerebral palsy: A systematic review. *Austrian Journal of Physics, 55,* 81–87.

289. Seifart, A., Unger, M., & Berger, M. (2009). The effects of lower limb functional electrical stimulation on gait of children with cerebral palsy. *Pediatric Physical Therapy, 21,* 23–30.

290. Seniorou, M., Thompson, N., Harrington, M., et al. (2007). Recovery of muscle strength following multi-level orthopedic surgery in diplegic cerebral palsy. *Gait & Posture, 26,* 475–481.

291. Shepherd, R. B. (1995). Training motor control and optimizing motor learning. In R. B. Shepherd (Ed.), *Physiotherapy in paediatrics* (3rd ed.). Oxford: Butterworth-Heinemann.

292. Shortland, A. P., Harris, C. A., Gough, M., & Robinson, R. O. (2002). Architecture of the medial gastrocnemius in children with spastic diplegia. *Development Medicine and Child Neurology, 44*(3), 158–163.

293. Shumway-Cook, A., & Woollacott, M. (1995). *Motor control: Theory and practical applications* (2nd ed.). Baltimore, MD: Lippincott, Williams & Wilkins.

294. Siebes, R. C., Winjroks, L., Ketelaar, M., van Schie, P. E., Vermeer, A., & Gorter, J. W. (2007). Validation of the Dutch Giving Youth a Voice Questionnaire (GYV-20): A measure of the client-centredness of rehabilitation services from an adolescent perspective. *Disability & Rehabilitation, 29,* 373–380.

295. Siebes, R. C., Wijnroks, L., & Vermeer, A. (2002). Qualitative analysis of therapeutic motor intervention programmes for children with cerebral palsy: An update. *Developmental Medicine and Child Neurology, 44,* 593–603.

296. Sigurdardottir, S., Thorkelsson, T., Halldorsdottir, M., Thorarensen, O., & Vik, T. (2009). Trends in prevalence and characteristics of cerebral palsy among Icelandic children born in 1990 to 2003. *Developmental Medicine and Child Neurology, 51,* 356–363.

297. Simpson, D. M., Gracies, J. M., Graham, H. K., Miyasaki, J. M., Naumann, M., Russman, M. et al. (2008). Assessment: Botulinum neurotoxin for the treatment of spasticity (an evidence-based review): Report of the Therapeutics and Technology Assessment Subcommittee of the American Academy of Neurology. *Neurology, 70,* 1691–1698.

298. Sobsey, D., & Doe, T. (1991). Patterns of sexual abuse and assault. *Sexualtiy and Disability, 9,* 243–259.

299. Soo, B., Howard, J. J., Boyd, R. N., Reid, S. M., Lanigan, A., Wolfe, R., et al. (2006). Hip displacement in cerebral palsy. *American Journal of Bone and Joint Surgery, 88,* 121–129.

300. Spittle, A. J., Doyle, L. W., & Boyd, R. N. (2008). A systematic review of the clinimetric properties of neuromotor assessments for preterm infants during the first year of life. *Developmental Medicine and Child Neurology, 50,* 254–266.

301. Stackhouse, S. K., Binder-MacLeod, S., A., & Lee, S. C. (2005). Voluntary muscle activation, contractile properties, and fatigability in children with and without cerebral palsy. *Muscle and Nerve, 31,* 594–601.

302. Stanger, M., & Bertoti, D. (1997). An overview of electrical stimulation for the pediatric population. *Pediatric Physical Therapy, 9,* 95–143.

303. Stanley, F., Blair, E., & Alberman, E. (2000). *Cerebral palsies: Epidemiology and causal pathways: Clinics in developmental medicine no. 151.* London: MacKeith Press.

304. Steenbeek, D., Ketelaar, M., Galama, K., & Gorter, J. W. (2007). Goal attainment scaling in pediatric rehabilitation: A critical review of the literature. *Developmental Medicine and Child Neurology, 49,* 550–556.

305. Sterba, J. A. (2006). Adaptive downhill skiing in children with cerebral palsy: Effect on gross motor function. *Pediatric Physical Therapy, 18,* 289–296.

306. Stevensen, R. D., Conaway, M., Chumlea, W. C., et al. (2006). Growth and health in children with moderate-to-severe cerebral palsy. *Pediatrics, 118,* 1010–1018.

307. Stout, J., Gage, J. R., Schartz, M. H., et al. (2008). Distal femoral extension osteotomy and patellar tendon advancement to

treat persistent crouch gait in cerebral palsy. *Journal of Bone and Joint Surgery, 90*, 2470–2484.

308. Strauss, D., Brooks, J., Rosenbloom, L., & Shavelle, R. (2008). Life expectancy in cerebral palsy: An update. *Developmental Medicine and Child Neurology, 50*, 487–493.

309. Strauss, D., Shavelle, R., Reynolds, R., Rosenbloom, L., & Day, S. (2007). Survival in cerebral palsy in the last 20 years: Signs of improvement? *Developmental Medicine and Child Neurology, 49*, 86–92.

310. Stuberg, W. A. (1992). Considerations related to weight-bearing programs in children with developmental disabilities. *Physical Therapy, 72*, 35–40.

311. Sussman, M. D., & Aiona, M. D. (2004). Treatment of spastic diplegia in patients with cerebral palsy: Part I. *Journal of Pediatric Orthopaedics B, 13*, S1–S12.

312. Sutcliffe, T. L., Gaetz, W. C., Logan, W. J., Cheyne, D. O., Fehlings, D. L. (2007). Cortical reorganization after modified constraint-induced movement therapy in pediatric hemiplegic cerebral palsy. *Journal of Child Neurology, 22*, 1281–1287.

313. Tardieu, C., Huet de la Tour, E., Bret, M. D., & Tardieu, G. (1982). Muscle hypoextensibility in children with cerebral palsy: I. Clinical and experimental observations. *Archives of Physical Medicine and Rehabilitation, 63*, 97–102.

314. Tardieu, C., Lespargot, A., Tabary, C., & Bret, M. D. (1988). For how long must the soleus muscle be stretched each day to prevent contracture? *Developmental Medicine and Child Neurology, 30*, 3–10.

315. Tardieu, G., Tardieu, C., Colbeau-Justin, P., & Lespargot, A. (1982). Muscle hypoextensibility in children with cerebral palsy: II. Therapeutic implications. *Archives of Physical Medicine and Rehabilitation, 63*, 103–107.

316. Taylor, N. F., Dodd, K. J., & Larkin, H. (2004). Adults with cerebral palsy benefit from participating in a strength training programme at a community gymnasium. *Disability & Rehabilitation, 26*, 1128–1134.

317. Tedroff, K., Granath, F., Forssberg, H., & Haglind-Akerlund, Y. (2009). Long-term effects of botulinum toxin A in children with cerebral palsy. *Developmental Medicine and Child Neurology, 51*, 120–127.

318. ten Berge, S. R., Halbertsma, J. P., Maathuis, P. G., Verheij, N. P., Dijkstra, P. U., Maathuis, P. G. (2007). Reliability of popliteal angle measurement, a study in cerebral palsy patients and healthy controls. *Journal of Pediatric Orthopedics, 27*, 648–652.

319. Tervo, R. C., Symons, R., Stout, J., & Novacheck, T. (2006). Parental report of pain and associated limitations in ambulatory children with cerebral palsy. *Archives of Physical Medicine and Rehabilitation, 87*, 928–934.

320. Thomas, S. S., Buckon, C. E., Phillips, D. S., Aiona, M. D., & Sussman, M. D. (2001). Interobserver reliability for the gross motor performance measure: Preliminary results. *Developmental Medicine and Child Neurology, 43*, 97–102.

321. Thompson, P., Beath, T., Bell, J., Phair, T., Salbach, N. M., & Wright, F. V. (2008). Test-retest reliability of the 10-metre fast walk test and 6-minute walk test in ambulatory school-aged children with cerebral palsy. *Developmental Medicine and Child Neurology, 50*, 370–376.

322. Thorpe, D. E., & Valvano, J. (2002). The effects of knowledge of performance and cognitive strategies on motor skill learning in children with cerebral palsy. *Pediatric Physical Therapy, 14*, 2–15.

323. Tieman, B. L., Palisano, R. J., Gracely, E. J. et al. (2007). Variability in mobility of children with cerebral palsy in GMFCS levels II-IV. *Pediatric Physical Therapy, 19*, 180–187.

324. Trahan, J., & Malouin, F. (2002). Intermittent intensive physiotherapy in children with cerebral palsy: A pilot study. *Developmental Medicine and Child Neurology, 44*, 233–239.

325. Trost, J. P., Schwartz, M. H., Krach, L. E., Dunn, M. E., & Novacheck, T. F. (2008). Comprehensive short-term outcome assessment of selective dorsal rhizotomy. *Developmental Medicine and Child Neurology, 50*, 765–771.

326. Unger, M., Faure, M., & Frieg, A. (2006). Strength training in adolescents learners with cerebral palsy: A randomized controlled trial. *Clinical Rehabilitation, 20*, 469–477.

327. United Nations. (2006). *Convention on the rights of persons with disabilities. Resolution 60/232.* Adopted 13 December 2006. New York: United Nations.

328. Ustad, T., Sorsdahl, A. B., & Ljunggren, A. E. (2009). Effects of intensive physiotherapy in infants newly diagnosed with cerebral palsy. *Pediatric Physical Therapy, 21*, 140–149.

329. Valvano, J. (2004). Activity-focused motor interventions for children with neurological conditions. *Physical and Occupational Therapy in Pediatrics, 24*, 79–107.

330. van den Berg-Emons, R. J., Van Baak, M. A., Speth, L., et al. (1998). Physical training of school children with spastic cerebral palsy: Effects on daily activity, fat mass and fitness. *International Journal of Rehabilitation Research, 21*, 179–194.

331. van der Linden, M. L., Hazlewood, M. E., Aitchison, A. M., Hillman, S. J., & Robb, J. E. (2003). Electrical stimulation of gluteus maximus in children with cerebral palsy: Effects on gait characteristics and muscle strength. *Developmental Medicine and Child Neurology, 45*, 385–390.

332. Van Haastert, I. C., de Vries, L. S., Helders, P. J., & Jongman, M. J. (2006). Early gross motor development of preterm infants according to the Alberta Infant Motor Scale. *Journal of Pediatrics, 149*, 617–622.

333. Varni, J. W., Burwinkle, T. M., Berrin, S. J., Sherman, S. A., Artavia, K., Melcarne, V. L., et al. (2006). The PedsQL in pediatric cerebral palsy: Reliability, validity, and sensitivity of the Generic Core Scales and Cerebral Palsy Module. *Developmental Medicine and Child Neurology, 48*, 442–449.

334. Verrotti, A., Greco, R., Spalice, A., Chiarelli, F., & Iannetti, P. (2006). Pharmacotherapy of spasticity in children with cerebral palsy. *Pediatric Neurology, 34*, 1–6.

335. Verschuren, O., Ketalaar, M., Gorter, J. W., et al. (2007). Exercise training program in children and adolescents with cerebral palsy: A randomized controlled trial. *Archives of Pediatric and Adolescent Medicine, 161*, 1075–1081.

336. Verschuren, O., Ketelaar, M., Takken T., et al. (2007). Exercise programs for children with cerebral palsy: A systematic review of the literature. *Am J Phys Med Rehabil, 86*.

337. Verschuren, O., Ketelaar, M., Takken, T., et al. (2007). Reliability of hand-held dynamometry and functional strength tests for the lower extremity in children with cerebral palsy. *Disability and Rehabilitation* 1–9.

338. Verschuren, O., Takken, T., Ketelaar, M., Gorter, J. W., & Helders, P. J. M. (2006). Reliability and validity of data for 2 newly developed shuttle run tests in children with cerebral palsy. *Physical Therapy, 86,* 1107–1117.

339. Verschuren, O., Takken, T., Ketelaar, M., Gorter, J. W., & Helders, P. J. (2007). Reliability for running tests for measuring agility and anaeobic muscle power in children and adolescents with cerebral palsy. *Pediatric Physical Therapy, 19,* 108–115.

340. Vignes, C., Godeau, E., Sentenac, M., Coley, N., Navarro, F., Grandjean, H., et al. (2009). Determinants of students' attitudes towards peers with disabilities. *Developmental Medicine and Child Neurology, 51,* 473–479.

341. Vos-Vromans, D. C., Ketelaar, M., & Gorter, J. W. (2005). Responsiveness of evaluative measures for children with cerebral palsy: The Gross Motor Function Measure and the Pediatric Evaluation of Disability Inventory. *Disability & Rehabilitation, 27,* 1245–1252.

342. Wang, H. H., Liao, H. F., & Hseich, C. L. (2006). Reliability, sensitivity to change, and responsiveness of the Peabody Developmental Motor Scales second edition for children with cerebral palsy. *Physical Therapy, 86,* 1351–1359.

343. Waters, E., Davis, E., Mackinnon, A., Boyd, R., Graham, H. K., Kai Lo, S., et al. (2007). Psychometric properties of the quality of life questionnaire for children with CP. *Developmental Medicine and Child Neurology, 49,* 49–55.

344. Waters, E., Davis, E., Ronen, G. M., Rosenbaum, P., Livingston, M., & Saigal, S. (2009). Quality of life instruments for children and adolescents with neurodisabilities: How to choose the appropriate instrument. *Developmental Medicine and Child Neurology, 51,* 660–669.

345. Watt, J., Robertson, C. M. T., & Grace, M. G. A. (1989). Early prognosis for ambulation of neonatal intensive care survivors with cerebral palsy. *Developmental Medicine and Child Neurology, 31,* 766–773.

346. Welsh, B., Jarvis, S., Hammal, A., Colver, A.; North of England Collaborative Cerebral Palsy Survey. (2006). How might districts identify local barriers to participation for children with cerebral palsy? *Public Health, 120,* 167–175.

347. Westberry, D. E., Davids, J. R., Shaver, J. C., Tanner, S. L., Blackhurst, D. W., & Davis, R. B. (2007). Impact of ankle-foot orthoses on static foot alignment in children with cerebral palsy. *American Journal of Bone and Joint Surgery, 89,* 806–813.

348. Westbom, L., Hagglund, G., & Nordmark, E. (2007). Cerebral palsy in a total population of 4–11 year olds in southern Sweden: Prevalence and distribution according to different CP classification systems. *BMC Pediatrics, 7,* 41.

349. Westcott, S. L., & Burtner, P. (2004). Postural control in children: Implications for pediatric care. *Physical and Occupational Therapy in Pediatrics, 24,* 5–55.

350. Wiart, L., & Darrah, J. (2002). Changing philosophical perspectives on the management of children with physical disabilities: Their effect on the use of powered mobility. *Disability & Rehabilitation, 24,* 492–498.

351. Wiart, L., Darrah, J., & Kembhavi, G. (2008). Stretching with children with cerebral palsy: What do we know and where are we going? *Pediatric Physical Therapy, 20,* 173–178.

352. Wiegeriak, D. J., Roebroeck, M. E., Donkervoort, M., et al. (2006). Social, intimate and sexual relationships of adolescents with cerebral palsy compared with able-bodies agemates. *Journal of Rehabilitative Medicine, 40,* 112–118.

353. Woods, J. J., & Lindeman, D. P. (2008). Gathering and giving information with families. *Infants & Young Children, 21,* 272–284.

354. Woodside, J. M., Rosenbaum, P. L., King, S. M., et al. (2001). Family-centred service: Developing and validating a self-assessment tool for paediatric service providers. *Journal of Child Health Care, 30,* 237–252.

355. World Health Organization. (2007). *International classification of functioning, disability and health: Children and youth version.* Geneva: Author.

356. Wright, M.J., Yundt, B., Tancredi, A. M., & Larin, H. (2003). Sleep issues in families of children with physical disabilities. *Physical and Occupational Therapy in Pediatrics, 26,* 55–72.

357. Wright, F. V., Rosenbaum, P. L., Goldsmith, C. H., Law, M., Fehlings, D. L. (2008). How do changes in body functions and structures, activity, and participation relate in children with cerebral palsy? *Developmental Medicine and Child Neurology, 50,* 283–289.

358. Wright, M., & Bartlett, D. J. (2010). Distribution of contractures and spinal malalignments in adolescents with cerebral palsy. *Developmental Neuroehabilitation, 13,* 46–52.

359. Wynter, M., Gibson, N., Kentish, M., Love, S. C., Thomason, P., & Graham, H. K. (2008). Consensus statement on hip surveillance for children with cerebral palsy: Australian standards of care. Retrieved from www.cpaustralia.com/au/ausacpdm

360. Young, N. L., Williams, J. I., Yoshida, K. K., et al. (1996). The context of measuring disability: Does it matter whether capability or performance is measured? *Journal of Clinical Epidemiology, 49,* 1097–1101.

361. Young, N. L., Williams, J. I., Yoshida, K. K., & Wright, J. G. (2000). Measurement properties of the Activity Scales for Kids. *Journal of Clinical Epidemiology, 53,* 125–137.

362. Yude, C., Goodman, R., & McConachie, H. (1998). Peer problems of children with hemiplegia in mainstream primary schools. *Journal of Child Psychology and Psychiatry, 39,* 533–541.

363. Ziv, I., Blackburn, N., Rang, M., & Koreska, J. (1984). Muscle growth in normal and spastic mice. *Developmental Medicine and Child Neurology, 26,* 94–99.

364. Zwick, E. B., Saraph, V., Linhart, W. E., & Steinwender, G. (2001). Propulsive function during gait in diplegic children: Evaluation after surgery for gait improvement. *Journal of Pediatric Orthopedics (British), 10,* 226–233.

DARL W. VANDER LINDEN, PT, PhD

Brachial plexus injuries (BPIs) can occur from a wide variety of traumas to the shoulder and spine. This chapter focuses on obstetric brachial plexus injuries (OBPIs), yet the concepts presented apply to resultant impairments, activity limitations, and participation restrictions caused by brachial plexus injury in children at any age. Physical therapists may work with infants and children with OBPI in a variety of settings, including early intervention programs, acute care hospitals, and specialty clinics. Physical therapists may also be involved with these children after neurosurgery to repair damage to nerves in the brachial plexus in infants or after orthopedic surgery to address impairments of muscle strength in toddlers and preschool-aged children. This chapter discusses etiology and pathophysiology, physical therapy examination, physical therapy procedural interventions, family education, and medical management of children with OBPI. A case study of a child with OBPI is presented at the end of the chapter and a video illustrates the outcomes of a late-treated child who underwent surgical intervention.

ETIOLOGY AND INCIDENCE

Injury to the brachial plexus (Figure 19-1) usually occurs during a difficult vaginal delivery. Traction on the newborn's shoulder during delivery of the head in a breech delivery can injure the cervical roots, fracture the clavicle or humerus, or sublux the shoulder. Forceful traction and rotation of the head during a vertex presentation to deliver the shoulder tends to injure the C5 and C6 roots. Associated damage to the phrenic nerve at C4 is less common but will cause ipsilateral hemiparesis of the diaphragm. Congenital anomalies such as cervical rib, abnormal thoracic vertebrae, or shortened scalenus anticus muscle can also cause pressure on the lower plexus.[47]

Factors that may contribute to OBPI include birth weight greater than 3500 g, shoulder dystocia (difficult delivery of the shoulder), prolonged maternal labor, maternal diabetes, a sedated hypotonic infant during delivery, and breech delivery.[4,49,58] Bager reported that the risk of OBPI increased as birth weight increased and those infants with a birth weight of over 4500 g had a risk of OBPI 45 times that of infants born at weights less than 3500 g.[4] Gilbert and colleagues found that infants from vaginal breech deliveries of normal weight (2500–3800 g) had a nine times greater risk of OBPI than those from cephalic vaginal deliveries.[19] The risk associated with breech delivery was even five times greater than for macrosomic infants (>4000 g) with cephalic delivery. For infants delivered vaginally with cephalic presentation, high birth weight was found to be the most important risk factor.[58] In a prospective study of 62 infants with OBPI of whom 17 had permanent impairment, 16 of the 17 infants had birth weights over 3500 g and only 1 of the 17 had a birth weight less than 3500 g. Twelve of 13 infants (92%) diagnosed with OBPI at birth who weighed less than 3500 g had full recovery of function, but only 67% of infants (33 of 49) who weighed more than 3500 g had full recovery.[58]

In prospective studies in a variety of countries, the incidence of OBPI has been reported at 1.6 per 1000,[4] 2.9 per 1000 live births,[10] 4.6 per 1000,[58] and 5.1 per 1000.[28] These rates are generally higher than the incidence reported earlier by Hardy of 0.9 per 1000[24] and by Sjoberg and associates of 1.9 per 1000.[49] The reasons for the increased incidence are not entirely clear but may be due in part to more thorough examination of newborns in the studies, which identified a higher percentage of children with OBPI. The incidence reported in prospective studies may be greater than that reported in retrospective studies because of the number of children who were identified who exhibited complete recovery within the first 3 weeks.[28] Bager, however, did find that the incidence increased in Sweden from 1.3 per 1000 in 1980 to 2.2 per 1000 in 1994, a statistically significant difference.[4]

PATHOPHYSIOLOGY

Damage can occur at the level of the nerve rootlet attached to the spinal cord, at the anterior or posterior rootlets, or distal to where the rootlets coalesce to form the mixed nerve root that exits the vetebral canal.[14] Roots, trunks, divisions, cords, and peripheral nerves can all suffer neurotmesis (complete rupture), axonotmesis (disruption of axons while neural sheath remains intact), or neurapraxia (temporary nerve conduction block with intact axons). Partial or complete rupture may evolve into a neuroma and a mass of fibrous tissue as disorganized neurons on the proximal end attempt to reach their distal end. Hemorrhage into the subarachnoid space leads to presence of blood in the

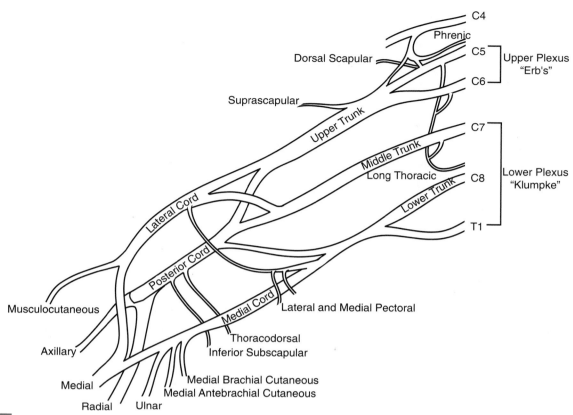

Figure 19-1 The brachial plexus. The variability in the impairments that a brachial plexus injury can cause is easily understood, because the injury can occur at any point along the nerves as they branch off the spinal cord and weave into the brachial plexus.

cerebrospinal fluid, which can be diagnostic of this more serious injury.[47]

Recovery is usually very limited after ruptures. Prognosis after axonotmesis is better as the neurons reconnect more successfully through the intact neural sheath. As axon regrowth proceeds at approximately 1 mm per day, the majority of recovery usually takes 4 to 6 months in the upper arm and 7 to 9 months in the lower arm. Continued recovery can occur for up to 2 years in the upper arm and 4 years in the lower arm.[18] Early recovery after neurapraxia occurs as edema resolves and is usually quick and complete, sometimes within days or weeks.[28] In children with OBPI, a combination of these types of lesions is common, which may explain the variability of return of motor function in individual muscles.

CHANGES IN BODY STRUCTURE AND FUNCTION (IMPAIRMENTS)

Injury can occur at any level of the brachial plexus, but the most common injury is to the upper roots (C5 and C6) resulting in a condition referred to as Erb's palsy. Strombeck and colleagues reported that of 247 children followed for OBPI, 52% had C5-C6 involvement and an additional 34% had C5-C7 involvement.[50] As a result of injury to the fibers

from the upper roots, the child's shoulder is usually held in extension, internal rotation, and adduction; the elbow is extended; the forearm is pronated; and the wrist and fingers are flexed in the textbook "waiter's tip" position (Figure 19-2). Paralysis of the rhomboids, levator scapulae, serratus anterior, subscapularis, deltoid, supraspinatus, infraspinatus, teres minor, biceps, brachialis, brachioradialis, supinator, and long extensors of the wrist, fingers, and thumb can be expected. Grasp is left intact, but sensory loss may be present. Elbow and finger extension is compromised if C7 is also involved.

Erb-Klumpke palsy is a combination of the injury to the upper and lower roots (C5-T1) resulting in total arm paralysis and loss of sensation. Strombeck and colleagues reported that 13% of the children with OBPI in their follow-up study had involvement of the C5-T1 roots.[50] Involvement is usually unilateral but has been reported to be bilateral in 4% of cases.[33] In Erb-Klumpke palsy, the extent of the initial paralysis frequently recedes, with a total paralysis becoming limited to muscles innervated by the upper roots. The pattern of motor loss does not always fit the classic definitions, indicating incomplete or mixed upper and lower types. Horner's syndrome, usually a result of avulsion of T1 roots, can cause deficient sweating, recession of the eyeball, abnormal pupillary contraction, myosis, ptosis, and irises of different colors.

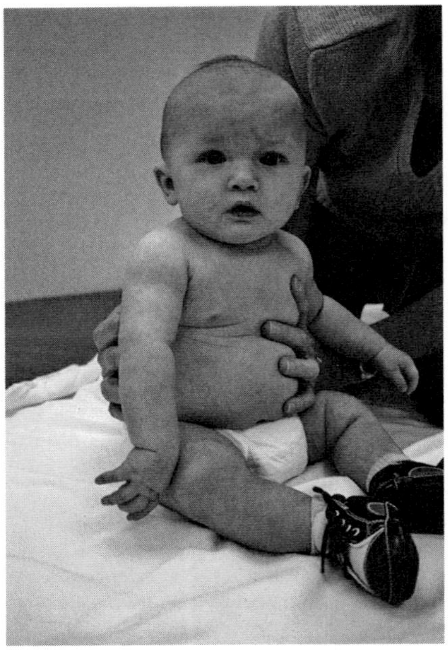

Figure 19-2 Infant with Erb's palsy, a C5-C6 brachial plexus injury, resulting in the "waiter's tip" position of the upper extremity, which is typically observed with this type of injury.

Considered rare, Eng and colleagues reported 8 of 135 infants with BPI had Horner's syndrome.[14]

Klumpke's palsy by definition involves only the lower roots of C7-T1. Some authors have reported the incidence of Klumpke's palsy to be 2% of all OBPI cases,[26] but in a 1995 review Al-Qattan and colleagues found Klumpke's palsy in only 20 of 3508 cases of OBPI reported in papers they reviewed, for an incidence of only 0.6%.[1] When pure Klumpke's palsy is present, the child's shoulder and elbow movements are not impaired, but the resting position of the forearm is typically in supination and there is paralysis of the wrist flexor and extensor muscles and the intrinsic muscles of the wrist and hand.

During the period of neural regeneration following BPI, children use abnormal muscle substitutions that are the most advantageous given the innervated muscles available.[47] For example, they may use a medially rotated shoulder with forearm pronation and wrist flexion when grasping an object. They may also neglect the extremity because of sensory loss or the comparative ease with which the opposite arm and hand accomplishes a task. These patterns of neglect or substitution are reinforced with repetition. The problems that arise from these repetitive patterns include soft tissue contracture and abnormal bone growth. The contractures most likely to develop are scapular protraction; shoulder extension, adduction, and internal rotation; elbow flexion or extension; forearm pronation; and wrist and finger flexion. These will obviously vary depending on the individual pattern of paralysis. Common orthopedic abnormalities include flattening of the humeral head, abnormally short clavicle, hypoplasia of the humeral head, or abnormal glenoid fossa.[27,32]

Positional torticollis can develop as a result of the child's head being habitually positioned away from the involved arm or may be present from the same trauma that caused the OBPI.[7] See Chapter 9 for more information regarding examination of and interventions for torticollis.

NATURAL HISTORY AND PROGNOSIS

The natural history and recovery of OBPI have been difficult to determine because few studies have followed children over a long period of time and authors have primarily used outcome measures of impairment, but not of activity and participation. In addition, many different measures of impairment have been used, but none consistently in a majority of studies, which makes it difficult to determine even the natural history of impairments in children with OBPI. To further complicate matters, neurosurgery as well as secondary orthopedic surgery may be performed on a subset of children studied, and outcomes of these children are often included in data with children who have not had surgical intervention.

A recovery rate of 80% to over 90% was reported in early studies.[7,21,24,37] As a result, the prognosis has been perceived as quite favorable for the majority of infants with OBPI. More recent studies, however, have reported recovery rates of 73%,[29] 66%,[40] 66%,[28] and 69%.[12] In a systematic review designed to improve description of the natural history of OBPI, Pondaag and colleagues reviewed the literature on OBPI outcomes.[45] The inclusion criteria for articles to be used in their systematic review included (1) prospective design, (2) all children with OBPI from a demographic area be followed, (3) minimum of 3-year follow-up with less than 10% lost to follow-up, and (4) outcome well defined with reproducible scoring system and no surgical intervention. Of 103 articles that were identified in the literature, none met all four or even three of the four criteria defined for the systematic review, but 27 of the 103 met two criteria. As a result of their findings, Pondaag and colleagues concluded that the excellent prognosis often cited for OBPI was not based on sound scientific evidence.[45] It should be noted that studies by Hoeksma and colleagues[28] and DiTaranto and colleagues[12] were not published early enough to be included in the systematic review.

Estimates of spontaneous recovery from OBPI are difficult to establish because many children have neurapraxic lesions that resolve within a few days or weeks so these children are not included in many follow-up studies. Hoeksma and colleagues found, in fact, that 34% of infants (19 of 56) diagnosed with OBPI at birth had full recovery by 3 weeks of age.[28] They also found that 32% (18 of 56) had "late" recovery by 1 year of age, but 19 of 56 (34%) did not have full recovery of muscle strength when assessed at a mean age of 3 years. The authors indicated that if the criteria for a "good" outcome as described by Michelow and colleagues of "more than 1/2 of normal range of shoulder and elbow motion"[37] had been used with their cohort of 56 children, 93% would have had a "good" outcome.[28] DiTaranto and colleagues followed 91 infants in Argentina who did not have access to neurosurgical intervention for at least 2 years.[12] They reported that although 69% had full recovery, 18% of infants had minimal recovery and 13% had global OBPI with flaccid and insensate arms.

In an earlier study, Eng and colleagues classified 135 children with incomplete recovery from OBPI into three groups based on residual deformities.[14] The mildly affected group (70%) had minimal scapular winging, shoulder abduction of 90° or more, minimal limitation of shoulder rotation and forearm supination, normal hand function, and normal sweat and sensation. These patients were not considered to have functional problems but some of their involved limbs were shorter and smaller with some shoulder instability. The moderately affected group (22%) had moderate winging of the scapula, shoulder abduction less than 90° with substitution of the trapezius and serratus anterior muscles in shoulder elevation, flexion contracture of the elbow, no forearm supination, weak wrist and finger extensors, good hand intrinsic muscles, and some loss of sweat and sensation. The third group (8%) was considered to have severe impairment with marked winging of the scapula, total loss of scapulohumeral rhythm, shoulder abduction less than 45°, severe elbow flexion contracture, no forearm supination, poor or no hand function, and severe loss of sweat and sensation resulting in a small atrophic extremity or agnosia in the arm.

The differences reported in the natural history and outcomes for children with OBPI make it difficult for parents and professionals to predict with any accuracy to what extent children with OBPI will recover. Unfortunately, the differences reported may be due primarily to the methodology of the studies as most authors operationally define outcome measures for a specific study, report no information on the reliability or validity of their operationally defined outcome measures, and provide no information on whether the raters were blinded to any interventions that may have taken place. In addition, although more recent reports have specifically defined outcomes based on strength of specific muscle groups,[28,29] what is still lacking are studies that report outcomes not only of impairments but also of activity limitations and participation restrictions in children, adolescents, and adults with OBPI. As we shall see later, however, many adults report significant degrees of disability following a BPI in infancy.

ACTIVITY LIMITATIONS

Activity limitations will vary greatly, depending on the extent of the initial pathology, neurologic regeneration, and residual impairments. The primary activity limitations in children with OBPI relate to an inability to reach, grasp, and perform tasks requiring bilateral manual abilities such as catching a large ball or lifting a large object. Activities of daily living (ADLs) that require bilateral upper extremity use will also be compromised. These activities would include donning and removing shirts and pants, tying shoes, and buttoning. Dressing aids may be necessary to achieve maximum independence. Studies have documented range of motion (ROM) limitations of these children's affected arms, but no quantitative studies have reported on the nature and extent of activity limitations such as dressing and eating, or participation restrictions.

Typical developmental activities may be compromised as a result of OBPI. Movement from prone or supine to sit may always be done from one side, thereby asymmetrically strengthening one side of the trunk or delaying development of balance reactions. The developmental milestone of creeping on all fours may not occur because the child may not be able to bear weight on the involved arm, and as a result the child may scoot around in sitting or progress directly to walking at the appropriate age.

Neglect of the involved limb or even self-abusive behavior such as biting can occur because of absent or abnormal sensation. Injuries such as burns, insect bites, and abrasions may go unnoticed if sensation is severely compromised.

Shoulder pain and neuritis in adults is a complication that can interfere not only with the function of the involved arm but also with other aspects of the individual's social or vocational activities.

PHYSICAL THERAPY EXAMINATION

Children may be referred to physical therapy in the days, weeks, months, or years after the initial injury. Physical therapy examination of these children's active and passive ROM and sensory status is key in establishing a baseline of function and abilities. Screening the developmental status of the infant or child will ensure that other pathologic conditions are not missed. In the neonate, frequent reexamination serves to document motor recovery as neural regeneration occurs. These data aid in program planning whether it be therapeutic exercise, splinting, identification of surgical candidates, or discharge from intervention.

Grossman recommended that newborns with OBPI be followed at 2 weeks and at 1, 2, and 3 months of age.[23] Infants not showing evidence of recovery may undergo a magnetic resonance imaging (MRI) scan to define the integrity of the nerve roots. Advances in MRI, electromyography, computed tomography (CT), and CT with metrizamide (CT-myelogram) have aided in preoperative diagnosis and surgical planning, yet they do not replace the careful physical examination of the clinical and functional consequences of neurologic damage and neural regeneration.

Electromyography (EMG), although of little prognostic value, can determine the extent of involvement and is often recommended as a preoperative baseline. Repeated EMG testing can alert the physical therapist to muscles that are undergoing reinnervation before obvious motor changes occur. Findings from diagnostic EMG have been used to attempt to assess the extent and severity of the lesion, but they may not correlate well with findings upon surgical exploration.[25,33] Reinnervation after microsurgery can be identified by EMG immediately following surgery or in the following weeks and months, before clinical signs of motor return are present. This information may change a therapist's goals and intervention, and it may change a patient's prognosis significantly.

RANGE OF MOTION

Physical therapy examination of the neonate with OBPI may be requested before discharge from the hospital. In any age child, ROM measurements of the involved arm and cervical area are performed and compared with the contralateral side. All movements should be performed with great care because the child's joints can be unstable and the limbs may have sensory loss. Baseline ROM data are essential for future identification of secondary contractures that could be avoided with appropriate intervention and to judge the effectiveness of interventions. Newborn infants, however, may have more limited range of motion than adults, especially in the lower extremities. See Gajdosik and Gajdosik[16] or Chapter 5 in the current volume for a more thorough discussion.

MUSCLE STRENGTH AND MOTOR FUNCTION

In the infant, the physical therapist can observe limb movement or palpate muscle contractions when testing a variety of reactions and reflexes such as visual tracking, neck righting, the Moro reflex, the Galant reflex, or the hand-placing reaction. Arm and head movement can be observed during wakeful play periods as a child tries to bring the hand to the mouth or reach for a toy. Care should be taken to document whether movements are with gravity eliminated or against gravity. Asymmetry of abdominal and thoracic movement may indicate phrenic nerve paralysis. A muscle grading system, called the Active Movement Scale, has been developed specifically for children with OBPI to capture subtle but significant changes in active movement of the arm (Table 19-1).[7] This assessment tool has been shown to have adequate interrater reliability and validity to accurately measure motor function of the upper extremity in infants younger than 1 year of age.[9] Curtis and colleagues also provided a review of other measures of impairment that have been used for children with OBPI including the British Medical Research Council (BMRC) system of manual muscle testing and the modified BMRC that uses a 4-point scale (M0–M3) to measure muscle activity.[9]

Older children can be examined using standard manual muscle tests and dynamometers, which can provide objective

TABLE 19-1 Hospital for Sick Children Muscle Grading System: Active Movement Scale*

Observation	Muscle Grade
Gravity eliminated	
No contraction	0
Contraction, no motion	1
Motion $\leq \frac{1}{2}$ range	2
Motion $> \frac{1}{2}$ range	3
Full motion	4
Against Gravity	
Motion $\leq \frac{1}{2}$ range	5
Motion $> \frac{1}{2}$ range	6
Full motion	7

*Full active range of motion with gravity eliminated (muscle grade 4) must be achieved before active range against gravity is scored (muscle grades 5 to 7). From Clarke, H. M., & Curtis, G. C. (1995). An approach to obstetrical brachial plexus injuries. *Hand Clinics, 11*(4), 567.

measures of muscle and grasp strength (see Chapter 5 for more information on strength testing in children). Patterns of movement, abnormal substitutions, and posturing of the arm as a result of muscle imbalance and sensory loss should also be documented. Mallet's classification of upper extremity function (Figure 19-3) as described by Gilbert[17] can be used for older children and has been shown to be reliable when used with children with OBPI.[3]

The impairments present in OBPI do not include spasticity. As a result, any spasticity identified during the examination would suggest an upper motoneuron lesion warranting further diagnostic evaluation by the child's primary physician or neurologist.

SENSATION

Examination of sensory loss in infants is not sensitive or reliable enough to document the clinical progression of neural regeneration. Attempts should be made, however, to identify areas on the involved extremity that may have compromised sensation. Narakas has developed the Sensory Grading System for children with BPI.[38] A grade of S0 is no reaction to painful or other stimuli; S1 is reaction to painful stimuli, none to touch; S2 is reaction to touch, not to light touch; and S3 is apparently normal sensation. Sensory loss does not necessarily correspond to the extent of motor involvement[14]; therefore, care should be taken not to ignore this component of the examination in children with milder involvement.

As neural regeneration proceeds, sensory loss may change to hyperesthesia before achieving normal sensation.[38] Infants or older children may experience pain or discomfort in reaction to sensory stimulation and simple touch. This change should be documented and may indicate progression of

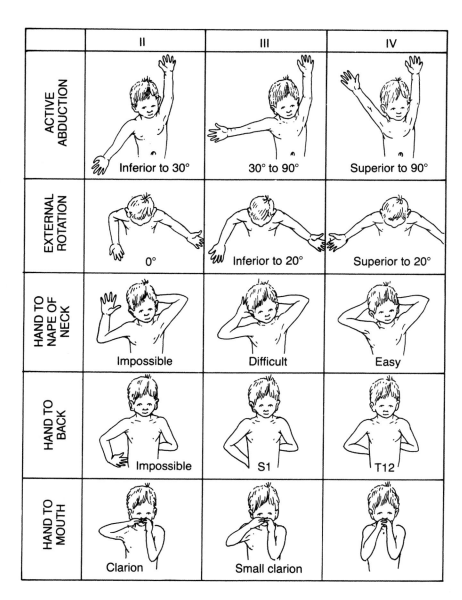

Figure 19-3 Mallet's classification of function in obstetric brachial plexus palsy. Grade 0 (not shown) is no movement in the desired plane, and grade V (not shown) is full movement. (From Gilbert, A. [1993]. Obstetrical brachial plexus palsy. In R. Tubiana (Ed.), *The Hand* [Vol. 4]. Philadelphia: WB Saunders, p. 579.)

regeneration. More definitive sensory testing to a variety of stimuli such as heat, cold, light touch, and two-point discrimination is possible in older children, and specific areas of sensory loss can be mapped. Sensation may take as long as 2 years to recover.[38]

Activity and Participation

Developmental tests of gross and fine motor performance can be used to establish and track any delays caused by the upper extremity impairment in infants and toddlers. Although no research exists on its use in OBPI, the Test of Infant Motor Performance may be useful for infants younger than 5 months of age to document changes in motor function because it has nine activities that are scored independently for each side of the body.[6] Older children who can follow verbal commands or copy body positions can be assessed in their abilities to perform functional activities such as bringing the hand to mouth for eating, bringing the hand to the head for brushing hair, and holding a variety of tools (e.g., toothbrush) sufficiently for their intended use. Videotaping of these activities is helpful.

Although several measures have been developed to assess impairments such as muscle strength and sensation as previously described, no specific measure of activity or participation for use with children who have OBPI could be found in the existing literature. Some authors have reported anecdotal information about activity limitations and participation such as difficulty with ADLs, carrying a tray at school for lunch, or playing a recorder.[49,52]

PHYSICAL THERAPY GOALS

The ideal outcome for the neonate with OBPI is complete return of motor control and sensation with no activity limitations or participation restrictions. The physical therapy goals during the first few months after diagnosis are to support any spontaneous recovery that is occurring and to prevent secondary impairments of muscle contractures and joint injury. If it becomes evident that complete return is not occurring, outcomes and goals must be revised. Depending on the extent of impairment, full ROM and normal strength may remain a goal in the first 2 years of life, because continued neural regeneration or restored motor control through a variety of orthopedic and neurosurgical procedures may still be possible. The majority of spontaneous recovery occurs by 9 months of age, but continued recovery may occur up to 2 years after the injury.[18]

At some point between 9 and 24 months of age, it may be apparent that significant neural regeneration is no longer occurring. Goals would need to be revised for children who lose range or plateau in their recovery over several months. Even with the most diligent implementation of a home program, full ROM is difficult to maintain when muscle imbalance is present. Children with OBPI continue to need monitoring of their ROM and functional status. Every attempt should be made to continue encouraging functional bilateral activities. The desired outcomes at this time (2 years of age) would be that the child develop age-appropriate self-care skills such as dressing and grooming using either extremity and participate in age-appropriate movement activities and preschool programs. Goals would include maintaining or increasing ROM and strength in movements critical to specific activities that the child is currently unable to perform. An example might be increasing elbow flexion motion and strength in order to pick up objects from the ground with both hands and put them on a table.

PHYSICAL THERAPY PROCEDURAL INTERVENTIONS AND FAMILY EDUCATION

The majority of infants with birth-related BPI require only physical therapy and no surgical intervention.[33] A consultation before discharge from the hospital may be performed; however, an initial rest period of 7 to 10 days is required to allow for reduction of hemorrhage and edema around the traumatized nerves. During this time, no ROM or other interventions are initiated as the involved limb is positioned gently across the abdomen. Lying on the involved limb is to be avoided.

After this initial period of immobilization, the physical therapist performs the baseline examinations described earlier in this chapter. A home program is developed for the parents that addresses all ranges of motion at risk for contractures, including precautions about any joints at risk for subluxation or dislocation. The physical therapist explains precautions regarding any areas of sensory loss and teaches the parents how to use positioning and therapeutic play during everyday activities to maintain ROM and strengthen weak muscles. Parents can be referred to the following for additional information about physical therapy interventions: Office of Physical Therapy Affairs, Kuwait Ministry of Health (www.pta-kw.com/pages.aspx?page=12).

ACTIVE MOVEMENT

The objective of the physical therapy program is to facilitate the highest functional outcome possible for the child, particularly in the areas of reach and grasp as they relate to meaningful, developmentally appropriate activities. As previously mentioned, children will use abnormal muscle substitutions that are the most advantageous given the innervated muscles available. The therapist intervenes in several ways, including facilitation of normal movement patterns while inhibiting substitutions during reaching and weight-bearing activities.[47] This intervention should be in the context of performing concrete versus abstract tasks. For example, strengthening of the shoulder flexors could be done by asking the child to lift 10 toy people up and into a dollhouse (a concrete task) instead of performing 10 repetitions of shoulder flexion (an abstract task).[55]

Careful attention to the scapula is critical during reaching activities, because paralysis of the rhomboids and contracture of the muscles that link the humerus to the scapula interfere with the normal 6:1 humeroscapular rhythm in the first 30° of shoulder movement. The scapula can be manually stabilized as the shoulder is assisted in active flexion while the child reaches for a toy. This activity facilitates correct motor training and stretching at the same time.

A variety of opportunities should be provided for weak muscles to participate in normal movement patterns by eliminating gravity for very weak muscles, preventing substitutions, and manually guiding the extremity through movements to accomplish a task. Examples include hand to mouth; transferring objects; weight shifting on propped upper extremities in the prone position, the quadruped position, and in sitting with hands in front or back; creeping; and reaching for toys placed at a variety of angles and heights from the child. Figure 19-4, *A*, illustrates a nonfunctional position that an infant with a classic C5, C6 injury may assume. Figure 19-4, *B*, demonstrates how manually guiding the shoulder into flexion and external rotation allows the infant to experience a more normal, functional movement pattern and obtain more appropriate sensory information through an open palm. The scapula is stabilized at the same time to allow for stretching of the soft tissues connecting the scapula to the humerus. Because active shoulder external rotation and forearm supination is typically lacking in children with C5-C6 injuries, toys should be presented and the upper extremity facilitated such as to encourage these movements during therapy.[47]

Infants should be placed in a side-lying position on their uninvolved arm to avoid stresses on the involved arm and to free the weak arm to reach and play with toys placed in front

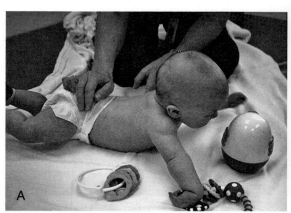
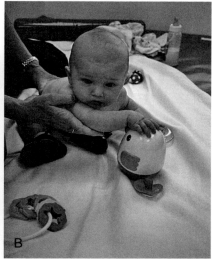

Figure 19-4 **A,** Infant with C5–C6 brachial plexus injury trying to prop and reach. **B,** Infant assisted in reaching and grasping with manual guidance.

of them. Gravity or toys held in the hand can be used as resistance as muscles gain strength. At times, the uninvolved arm may need to be gently restrained when encouraging the child to use the involved arm. Tactile stimulation or facilitation of the weak muscles with gentle joint compression in weight bearing is also helpful.

Normal posture and developmental activities may be compromised as a result of OBPI. Transitional movement into sitting may always be done from one (i.e., the uninvolved) side, and as a result, posture of the trunk may be asymmetrical and balance reactions may be delayed on the involved side. To address reliance on the uninvolved side, movement into sitting and other transitional movements can be practiced from the involved side using manual guidance and facilitation as needed. When sitting is achieved, challenging protective reactions to the involved side can facilitate shoulder abduction. Normal bilateral upper extremity use will likely be delayed. Opportunities for the child to experience and practice two-handed activities such as holding balls or swinging can be provided. In the older child who has not experienced full return of motor function, adaptations and products to assist in ADLs and recreational activities should be made available for the child's consideration. Many products are available for performing a variety of daily tasks using only one hand, and families can be encouraged to design their own adaptations. Not every child or family wants to use these devices, and their opinions should be respected.

RANGE OF MOTION

Passive ROM can be done in the context of normal developmental activities as described previously or during positioning as described later in this chapter. Maintaining ROM is important, as up to 65% of children with incomplete recovery of OBPI have been found to have limited ROM at the shoulder.[29] Passive ROM should never cause pain and should always be gentle. Overstretching can be harmful to joints and joint capsules that are already unstable. For example, forced supination of the elbow may compound the problem of radial head dislocation and ulnar bowing.[14] Picking the child up under the axilla or by pulling on the arms is discouraged because these actions can damage the unprotected shoulder joint.

Prevention of scapulohumeral adhesions is an important goal of physical therapy intervention. Parents should be educated about the anatomy and kinesiology of the glenohumeral joint. During reach, the scapula can be stabilized or restrained to allow for stretching of the muscles that link the scapula to the humerus during the first 30° of abduction. Beyond 30°, the scapula must rotate along with humeral external rotation to avoid harmful impingement of soft tissues on the acromion process. For a visual demonstration of scapulohumeral rhythm, the reader is encouraged to search for appropriate videos on the Internet by using the search term "scapulohumeral rhythm."

The use of botulinum toxin has been shown to improve active motion in muscles antagonist to those injected with the toxin.[11] Basciani and Intiso also reported that botulinum toxin and casting were effective in improving active elbow extension in 22 children with a mean age of 5.6 years.[5] This intervention is relatively benign when compared to surgical intervention and should be studied further as an intervention to maintain ROM in children with OBPI. Whether function is improved along with the reduction in impairment also needs study.

SENSORY AWARENESS

Sensory loss can lead to neglect or even self-mutilation. Parents must be cautioned about the risk of injury to body areas where sensation is compromised and should watch for any signs of self-mutilation such as biting an insensate area. Enlisting the participation of the involved limb in play activities or in holding a bottle allows the child to perceive the extremity as being a purposeful part of the body. Sensory perception can be enhanced by placing objects of different textures and temperatures in the hand, playing games such as finding toys under sudsy water or in rice with the involved hand, or in the case of older children having them name familiar objects placed in their hand while blindfolded. ROM can be incorporated into these activities by guiding the hand to different areas of the child's body to experience tactile stimulation. Parents themselves should be encouraged not to neglect the arm but to caress and play with it as usual while holding or guiding it through patterns that need reinforcement.

POSITIONING AND SPLINTING

Placing the child's arm in optimal positions is a time-efficient way to stretch soft tissue restrictions because this can be done during feeding, carrying, or positioning in a car seat. When the child is sleeping, the arm can be placed toward abduction, external rotation, elbow flexion, and forearm supination on a pillow to the child's side. As the child's arm relaxes during sleep, even more range can be attempted.

Intermittent splinting of the wrist and fingers may sometimes be indicated. Wrist splints may preserve the integrity of the tendons of the fingers and wrist until motor function returns. Resting night splints can help prevent wrist and finger flexion contractures. A wrist cock-up splint maintains a neutral alignment of the wrist yet frees the fingers for play. In an attempt to prevent shoulder adduction and internal rotation contractures, a "statue of liberty" splint or an abduction splint may be used, although some have suggested that these splints may contribute to abduction contractures, hypermobility, and pathology of the glenohumeral and elbow joint.[47]

Restraining splints such as air splints can be used on the uninvolved extremity to encourage use of the involved arm and hand. For example, if elbow flexion is restrained on the uninvolved side, the child would need to use his involved arm to bring a toy to his mouth or self-feed. These restraints should be used for only brief periods during the day with frustration levels monitored carefully. Some children will not tolerate them at all, particularly if it is unrealistic that the involved arm can perform functional activities with some independence.

ELECTRICAL STIMULATION

Although Eng and colleagues promoted the use of electrical stimulation for children with OBPI, and electrical stimulation may be used after neurosurgery, there have been few reports on the efficacy of electrical stimulation for this population.[14] Okafor and colleagues recently reported that electrical stimulation paired with conventional physical therapy resulted in improved active shoulder abduction and elbow flexion when compared with conventional therapy after 6 weeks, but there were only eight children in each group.[42] Further research is needed.

MEDICAL MANAGEMENT

NEUROSURGERY

Neurosurgery to repair the brachial plexus has typically been reserved for the 5% to 10% of children with OBPI who do not exhibit substantial spontaneous recovery. Neurosurgical techniques used in the treatment of OBPI include nerve grafting, neuroma dissection and removal, neurolysis (decompression and removal of scar tissue), and direct end-to-end nerve anastomosis of the nerve ends. These microsurgery techniques have been used to attempt to improve function in those children with OBPI who have significant impairments and activity limitations and who are no longer exhibiting spontaneous improvement.

INDICATIONS FOR AND TIMING OF NEUROSURGERY

A lack of biceps function and elbow flexion has been used in the past to predict which infants would lack complete recovery and therefore be candidates for surgery,[18] but Hoeksma and colleagues found that shoulder external rotation and forearm supination were more accurate predictors of full recovery than elbow flexion.[28] Fisher and colleagues reported that lack of active elbow flexion is also not as useful in determining candidates for surgery as the Active Movement Scale. Hence, lack of active external rotation and forearm supination, as well as scores on the Active Movement Scale may be more useful when determining if an infant should have surgery to repair the brachial plexus lesion.[15]

Neurosurgeons have typically recommended that brachial plexus repair by microsurgery be done between 3 and 8 months of age for optimal results;[7,33] however, Grossman and colleagues found that children who underwent late nerve reconstruction (9 to 21 months of age) demonstrated significant improvement in shoulder function.[22] Because a small number of children (3 of 19) who demonstrated incomplete elbow flexion at 9 months of age went on to have full elbow flexion function at 12 months,[28] it may be prudent to delay neurosurgery until 12 months of age in those children with only upper nerve root involvement. However, Terzis and Kokkalis found in a group of 67 infants that those that had surgery before 3 months had somewhat better outcomes than those who had surgery between 4 and 6 months.[54]

OUTCOMES OF NEUROSURGERY

Although some authors have reported improvement in 75% to 95% of children who have had neurosurgery,[33,34,48] Strombeck and colleagues reported that for children with total arm involvement (C5-T1), those who had surgery had no significant improvements in active motion at the shoulder, elbow, or hand when compared to a group of children who did not have surgery.[50] They did, however, report that children with C5-C6 lesions who had surgery had slightly better shoulder function than children who did not have surgery.[50] In a more recent study, Lin and colleagues reported that neurosurgical repair that included resection and grafting (n = 92) as opposed to neurolysis only (n = 16) had better outcomes as measured by the Active Movement Scale.[35]

In a systematic review of outcomes for children with OBPI who underwent neurosurgery, McNeely and Drake found no randomized controlled trials that reported the effects of neurosurgery compared to conservative treatment for children with OBPI.[36] Although outcomes from case-series studies without control groups (level III evidence) were generally favorable, the authors concluded that there was no conclusive evidence demonstrating a benefit of surgery over conservative management in the treatment of children with OBPI.[36]

Additional caution regarding nerve reconstruction has recently been suggested by Nath and Liu, who reported that of children with C5-6 lesions, the group that had nerve reconstruction (n = 23) did not have improved shoulder function and experienced more severe shoulder glenohumeral deformities than did a group that had only secondary orthopedic surgery (n = 52).[39]

Because most of the studies related to timing of neurosurgery and outcomes of neurosurgery used a case series design, it would seem essential that randomized, controlled trials of the effects of neurosurgery on outcomes in children with OBPI be conducted. These trials should use standardized, reliable, and valid outcome measures in each of the three domains of impairment, activity, and participation. Because some authors have demonstrated that late nerve reconstruction resulted in improvement of shoulder function,[22] whereas others have found only small differences favoring early surgery, it would seem reasonable that a control group for these trials could include a group of children who have late rather than early surgery if the parents so choose after a period of conservative treatment. Only through such randomized controlled trials can it be determined if neurosurgery improves outcomes for children with OBPI.

ORTHOPEDIC CONCERNS AND ORTHOPEDIC SURGERY

Despite therapy and neurosurgery, contractures and secondary deformities are likely to occur in children who do not experience complete return and may even occur in children who have been categorized as having full return of muscle strength and activity.[27] Several authors have reported that glenohumeral deformity is present in up to 67% of children with OBPI.[27,32,53] These osseous deformities were even found to be present in children who had full passive ROM of the shoulder and full functional recovery. Hoeksma and colleagues found that even mild contracture is strongly associated with osseous deformity of the shoulder.[27] Ter Steeg and colleagues suggested that physical therapists may want to consider the use of splints to protect the shoulder during the flaccid period of OBPI before muscle function returns.[53]

The severity and type of contracture will vary depending on the pattern of return and type of intervention the child has undergone. The most common injury, to C5 and C6, will likely result in absence or weakness of shoulder external rotation and abduction, elbow flexion, and forearm supination. Therefore, the most common contractures are shoulder adduction and internal rotation, elbow flexion or extension (depending on the involvement of the triceps), and forearm pronation.

The main goal of orthopedic surgery is to provide the necessary active and passive ROM that will enable the patient's hand to reach the head and mouth for meaningful ADLs. Price and Grossman provided a thorough discussion of historical and current orthopedic surgery for patients with OBPI.[46] Common surgeries include soft tissue releases (at muscle insertions or by Z-plasty), reductions of glenohumeral joint dislocations, transfers of muscles, and osteotomies.[13,25,56] Hoffer and Phipps achieved an increase in abduction of one grade and external rotation of two grades by releasing the pectoralis major, latissimus dorsi, and teres major muscles and then transferring the latissimus dorsi and teres major to the rotator cuff.[30] Functionally, the patients could then reach above their head for a variety of ADLs. Transferring a muscle can be expected to result in the loss of one muscle strength grade; therefore, the muscle chosen for transfer should be as strong as possible before surgery. Grossman reported releasing the subscapularis by 2 years of age in children with persistent internal rotation contractures.[23] He recommended delaying hand and wrist reconstruction until 8 years of age when spontaneous recovery has reached a plateau and the child can fully participate in postoperative hand therapy.

In a more recent study, 23 children with glenohumeral deformity had transfers of the latissimus dorsi and the teres major tendons to the rotator cuff for weakness in external rotation, as well as lengthening of the pectoralis major or the subscapularis muscles.[57] For these children at a mean follow-up of 31 months, active external rotation improved significantly on the Mallet (pre-op score of 2 and post-op score of 4) and on the Active Movement Scale (pre-op score of 3 and post-op score of 6). Any parents pursuing orthopedic surgery for their child should become intimately knowledgeable of the most current research on the technique and outcome of any procedure being considered. For an excellent review of the evaluation and management of shoulder problems in infants and children with OBPI, parents and therapists are referred to Pearl.[44] Clearly identified functional goals should be established before any surgery.

OUTCOMES

The information available on long-term outcomes in adults with a history of OBPI suggests that disability in daily activities can be lifelong and is frequently associated with orthopedic complaints and pain. Gjorup published a long-term follow-up study of adults that included clinical examinations and a lengthy questionnaire on their functional and social status, their vocational and avocational activities, and their feelings about how OBPI had affected their lives.[20] Although this study is descriptive in nature, it is unique in its attempt to document how OBPI affects people as adults. Out of 222 respondents, approximately one third thought they had a usable arm, one third thought they had a useless arm, and the remainder reported transitional stages between these extremes.[20] Slightly more than one third thought they were disabled. Gjorup concluded that patients with OBPI manage well socially, and no correlation was found between the severity of the arm defect and social status achieved by the patient.[20]

Strombeck and colleagues evaluated long-term changes in function in a group of 70 participants aged 7 to 20 years of age.[51] Of this group, 43% had improvements in shoulder function, whereas about 50% had decreased active elbow extension at follow-up. Interestingly, 75% of participants perceived they had no difficulty with ADLs. In a group of 36 adults aged 21 to 72 years with OBPI, however, Partridge and

Edwards found that 60% had painful arthritic joints and 27% had scoliosis.[43] In this group, 80% reported trouble with dressing, 55% with bathing and 66% with cooking. Further, 33 of 36 participants surveyed (91%) reported experiencing pain with 28 of those 33 reporting that their pain was "getting worse." Further outcomes research using health-related quality-of-life measures as described by Jette[31] would be extremely helpful for physical therapists and parents to help in long-term planning for children with OBPI.

PREVENTION

Risk factors for OBPI can be identified before birth. O'Leary identified maternal birth weight, prior shoulder dystocia, abnormal pelvis, maternal obesity, multiparity, and advanced maternal age as risk factors for delivering a child with shoulder dystocia.[41] Cesarean section should be considered when a mother has multiple risk factors for a child being born with shoulder dystocia.

SUMMARY

Shoulder dystocia as a result of macrosomia is the most common cause of OBPI. Children with OBPI present with impairments of flaccidity or reduced muscle activity that are readily apparent at birth. Physical therapists can provide important early intervention for these children by working with parents to ensure that the joints of the flaccid extremity are protected during the first few weeks. If spontaneous recovery does not occur within a few weeks, physical therapists provide interventions to maintain muscle extensibility and joint ROM as well as developmental activities to enhance motor recovery of the involved extremity. Neurosurgery may be considered if substantial spontaneous recovery is not apparent by the age of 6 to 9 months; however, the evidence for the benefits of neurosurgical intervention compared to conservative treatment is not strong. Long-term outcome studies suggest that OBPI affects ADLs and causes disability in adulthood without effects on social participation.

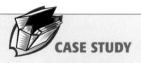

CASE STUDY

"Blair K."

Mrs. K. was at 36 weeks of gestation with her third child. She requested an ultrasound to determine the size of her baby because her second child had been born at 38 weeks postmenstrual age (PMA) weighing 9.7 pounds with the complication of shoulder dystocia. Her obstetrician reluctantly agreed. The fetus was estimated to be 7 pounds at 36 weeks PMA. The physician declined Mrs. K.'s request to be induced or to have a cesarean section at 40 weeks. At 42 weeks PMA, Mrs. K. was induced and delivered an 11-pound baby after a difficult delivery complicated by shoulder dystocia. Blair was in fetal distress with a limp left arm. Radiographs were inconclusive in establishing if there

was a clavicular fracture. The intern told the family that Blair had Erb's palsy and that her hand would be in the waiter's tip position for life. On seeing the pediatric neurologist, the family was told that Blair had a "mild stretching" of the nerves, that the condition was not permanent, and that she would recover fully.

Physical Therapy Diagnosis

The physical therapist saw Blair on her second day of life, before discharge from the hospital. The family was educated about the disorder, including precautions and prognosis. Instruction in ROM

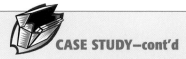

CASE STUDY—cont'd

exercises and positioning was provided, with the parents given the opportunity to practice on a doll. They were told not to begin the exercises until the next week. They were given a packet of information on the diagnosis, exercises, terminology, support groups, and the National Brachial Plexus Association.

Physical Therapy Examination at 2 Days of Age

Blair's left arm demonstrated no movement in the shoulder or arm except for palpable contractions in the pectoralis muscle. Her upper trapezius was active, which she used to splint the shoulder area, causing her left shoulder to be held close to her left ear. ROM was full in all joints. No reaction to pinching of the skin on the left arm was observed. A screening of her motor development was normal for a newborn. Based on the examination, birth history, and previous medical diagnosis of Erb's Palsy, which is a form of obstetrical brachial plexus injury, the preferred practice pattern according to the Guide to Physical Therapist Practice was 5F–Impaired Peripheral Nerve Integrity and Muscle Performance Associated with Peripheral Nerve Injury.[2]

Prognosis and Plan of Care

Because spontaneous recovery can occur, even in infants who have very limited muscle activity at birth, a prognosis was difficult to provide. Because of her obvious movement deficits, however, plans were made to provide Blair with physical therapy procedural interventions on a weekly basis in her home for 3 months. In addition, during these weekly visits her parents would be instructed about positioning and facilitation of muscle function in the involved extremity.

Physical Therapy Interventions

Physical therapy was begun once a week at 3 weeks of age. Direct therapy was provided in the form of guided movements through developmentally appropriate gross and fine movement patterns as the weeks progressed. Tactile stimulation to individual muscles began to elicit muscle contractions in the triceps and pectoralis muscles after 4 weeks. About the same time, a weak grasp was developing when a finger was placed in Blair's hand. ROM in the cervical area and all upper extremity joints remained full. Internet sites such as those for the Brachial Plexus Palsy Foundation (www.brachialplexuspalsyfoundation. org/information.html) and the United Brachial Plexus Network (www.ubpn.org/awareness/A2002newparents.html) as well as a local OBPI support group provided a great deal of information to Blair's family in the ensuing weeks. Additional information is available at the NIH Brachial Plexus Information page (www.ninds.nih.gov/disorders/brachial_plexus/brachial_plexus.htm). The support group informed them about a hospital specializing in the management of OBPI. Their local neurologist was not supportive of their pursuing surgical options for Blair because the neurologist thought the surgery was too experimental, but the family decided to visit this new hospital when Blair was 3 months of age. At the hospital Blair was assessed and the parents were asked to return when Blair was 6 to 7 months of age.

Age 3 Months

ROM was full for all joints. Strength (as measured through observation of spontaneous movement using a manual muscle testing scale of 0 to 5) was returning to some muscle groups as follows: shoulder flexion (2), shoulder abduction (0), shoulder extension (2), elbow flexion (1), elbow extension (2), supination (0), wrist extension (1), and wrist flexion (3). Finger flexion and extension strength appeared normal. It was difficult to determine whether elbow flexion was being performed by the brachioradialis or the biceps brachii muscle. Sensation was returning but was not normal because responses to light touch did not elicit a response in the lower left arm.

Therapy continued once a week, and Blair continued to gain more strength in her shoulder, elbow, and hand. Her home program was modified weekly to add resistance in the form of gravity, handheld toys, or bracelet weights to muscle groups gaining strength in the grade 3 to 4 range. The family members were taught manual guidance techniques to use with emerging gross motor activities. Careful attention was paid to identifying muscles regaining innervation and facilitating them appropriately. Other aspects of the treatment program were implemented as described in the intervention section of this chapter.

Age 6 Months

ROM continued to be full. Blair no longer elevated her shoulder toward her ear. Strength was as follows: shoulder flexion (2+), shoulder abduction (0), shoulder extension (3), elbow flexion (1+), elbow extension (3), supination (0), wrist extension (1), and wrist flexion (3). Finger flexion and extension appeared normal. Wrist flexion was accompanied by a strong pull into ulnar deviation. A wrist cock-up splint to support weak wrist extension and prevent the ulnar deviation was provided for daytime use.

It was still unclear whether elbow flexion was being performed by the biceps, brachialis, or brachioradialis muscle. Developmentally, Blair progressed normally except for assuming quadruped and creeping, which she could not do. Sitting was asymmetrical because she was afraid to shift her weight to the left (there were no functional protective reactions to that side). Weight-shifting activities while seated on balls and the caregiver's lap while Blair was supported at the trunk were done while she was encouraged to reach for toys.

Age 7 Months

Blair returned to the hospital specializing in OBPI. The family was instructed to come on a Monday and be prepared for possible exploratory surgery, if indicated, on the following day. Exploratory surgery was recommended. Decisions on the surgery to be performed were determined at the time of exploration during which EMG was performed. Conduction of neural impulses to the deltoid was confirmed to be present but not to the biceps. Surgery included removal of a neuroma and nerve grafting using the sural nerve as a donor. Blair was discharged on postoperative day 4, and her arm was placed in

Continued

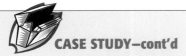

CASE STUDY—cont'd

a sling for 10 days because of the nerve graft. Therapy resumed 10 days after surgery, twice a week. At this time, deltoid muscle activity could be palpated, but biceps strength remained at 1+. Two months after surgery, elbow flexion strength increased from 1+ to 2.

Age 1 Year

Passive ROM continued to be full except for some mild scapulohumeral tightness. The left arm was slightly smaller in girth. Blair continued to prefer to use her right hand for ADLs, yet she would use her left hand if encouraged to do so or if bilateral participation was required. Scapular winging was minimal, and based on Mallet's functional classification (see Figure 19-3), Blair had grade III function. Active ROM was not full yet was functional for activities such as hand to mouth, using some shoulder abduction to substitute for decreased elbow flexion. She also used substitutions for the lack of wrist supination. Therapy continued once a week, and sensation and muscle strength continued to improve. Substitutions were being replaced with more normal movements, and new strategies for gaining and maintaining shoulder range were needed. Therapy activities included picking up objects from the floor and then placing them up on a table while a caregiver facilitated shoulder flexion with external rotation and forearm supination; use of a vibrator on the biceps during activities requiring elbow flexion, such as self-feeding; and practice of fine motor skills (such as stacking rings), which require elbow flexion and supination.

Age 18 Months

Electrical stimulation was prescribed at this time to stimulate the deltoid and biceps muscles. Shoulder abduction strength was at 3–,

elbow flexion 3–. Use of a stimulator that provided alternating current assisted these two active contractions to achieve close to full-range motions against gravity (3+). After 1 month of experimentation and parent instruction with the stimulator, therapy was reduced to once a week, and the parents used the stimulator at home 3 to 5 days a week for 30- to 60-minute sessions. At this age, Blair loved being prone on a platform swing doing push and pull activities that encouraged bilateral shoulder and elbow movements as well as fast movements while prone over bolsters that elicited protective reactions and shoulder flexion.

Age 2 Years

Residual impairments at this time included mild sensory loss, decreased active shoulder and elbow ROM (grade IV on Mallet's scale), and smaller limb girth. Passive ROM was full, and the family had learned that the shoulder would quickly become tight if exercises were neglected. Active ranges, as mentioned, were slightly limited yet functional for toothbrushing and hair brushing, with some substitution of shoulder abduction for lack of full elbow flexion. Some neglect of the involved arm was noticed in situations such as stair climbing because she would only use her uninvolved arm on a railing and in crayon-to-paper activities. No residual disability was apparent at this age; Blair performed all gross and fine motor activities at age-appropriate levels, with some abnormal movement substitutions for weak muscles. Electrical stimulation was discontinued because strength gains were occurring minimally. The frequency of physical therapy was decreased to once a month to monitor progress or regression and continue working on the acquisition of bilateral upper extremity skills without abnormal movement substitutions.

EVIDENCE TO PRACTICE 19-1

CASE STUDY "BLAIR K."

EXAMINATION DECISION

Mallet's scale was used at 1 year of age to determine function.[2] Although this is a widely used functional measure, the Active Movement Scale (see Table 19-1) would provide more detail about the integrity of individual muscle and joint function and should be used in conjunction with Mallet's scale whenever possible to provide a more complete description of muscle strength and function.[1] A decision to have surgery to resect and graft the injured fibers of the brachial plexus was made at 7 months of age. Whenever possible, the physical therapist should consult with the family about the potential risks and benefits of surgery and provide them with appropriate literature about the outcomes of surgical intervention for OBPI. Although some authors have suggested that better outcomes are observed with early surgery (3 to 8 months of age),[3,5] the evidence supporting improved outcomes following surgery this early is not strong.[4]

PLAN OF CARE DECISION

Early intervention to maintain ROM and to develop functional strength and active, functional movement in the involved arm was based on the recommendations by Shepherd[7] and Laurent and Lee.[6] The decision to use electrical stimulation to assist active contraction of the deltoid and biceps muscles was based on the theoretic concept that electrical stimulation would help maintain muscle fiber integrity while waiting for repaired nerve fibers to reestablish functional connections.

PATIENT/FAMILY PREFERENCES

Because the impairments (weakness and lack of arm movement) of Blair's brachial plexus injury were obvious at birth, early physical therapy was offered and accepted by the parents. In cases where the injury to the brachial plexus nerves is less severe and the impairments are less obvious, a decision to monitor the infant's progress may be appropriate

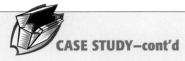

CASE STUDY—cont'd

EVIDENCE TO PRACTICE 19-1—cont'd

as many children with less severe brachial plexus injuries have a good deal of spontaneous recovery.[8] The decision to provide physical therapy should be made in conjunction with the parents and the physician.

1. Clarke, H. M., & Curtis, C. G. (1995). An approach to obstetrical brachial plexus injuries. *Hand Clinics, 11,* 563–580.
2. Gilbert, A. (1995). Obstetrical brachial plexus palsy. In R. Tubiana (Ed.), *The hand* (Vol. 4., p. 79). Philadelphia: WB Saunders.
3. Lin, J. C., Schwentker-Colizza, A., Curtis C. G., & Clarke, H. M. (2009). Final results of grafting versus neurolysis in obstetrical brachial plexus palsy. *Plastic and Reconstructive Surgery, 123*(3), 939–948.
4. McNeely, P. D., & Drake, J. M. (2003). A systematic review of brachial plexus surgery for birth-related brachial plexus injury. *Pediatric Neurosurgery, 38,* 57–62.
5. Strombeck, C., Krumlinde-Sundholm, & Forssberg, H. (2000). Functional outcome at 5 years in children with obstetrical brachial plexus palsy with and without microsurgical reconstruction. *Developmental Medicine and Child Neurology, 42,* 148–157.
6. Laurent, J. P., & Lee, R. T. (1994). Birth related upper brachial plexus injuries in infants: Operative and nonoperative approaches. *Journal of Child Neurology, 9,* 111–117.
7. Shepherd, R. B. (1991). Brachial plexus injury. In S. K. Campbell (Ed.), *Pediatric neurologic physical therapy* (2nd ed., pp. 101–130). New York: Churchill Livingstone.
8. Hoeksma, A. F., ter Steeg, A. M., Nelissen, R. G., van Ouwerkerk, W. J., Lankhorst, G. J., & de Jong, B. A. (2004). Neurological recovery in obstetric brachial plexus injuries: An historical cohort study. *Developmental Medicine and Child Neurology, 46,* 76–83.

ACKNOWLEDGMENTS

We would like to thank Barry Chapman, PT, Developmental Services Center, Champaign, Illinois, for completing the video case for a child with obstetrical brachial plexus injury that accompanies this chapter.

REFERENCES

1. Al-Qattan, N. M., Clarke, H. M., & Curtis, C. G. (1995). Klumpke's birth palsy: Does it really exist? *Journal of Hand Surgery (British), 20B,* 19–23.
2. American Physical Therapy Association. (2001). Guide to physical therapist practice, 2nd ed. *Physical Therapy, 81,* 9–744.
3. Bae, D. S., Waters, P. M., & Zurakowski, D. (2003). Reliability of three classification systems measuring active motion in brachial plexus birth palsy. *Journal of Bone and Joint Surgery, 85A,* 1733–1738.
4. Bager, B. (1997). Perinatally acquired brachial plexus palsy: A persisting challenge. *Acta Paediatrica, 86,* 1214–1219.
5. Basciani, M., & Intiso, D. (2006). Botulinum toxin type-A and plaster cast treatment in children with upper brachial plexus palsy. *Pediatric Rehabilitation, 9,* 165–170.
6. Campbell S. K., Wright B. D., Linacre J. M. (2002). Development of a functional movement scale for infants. *Journal of Applied Measurement, 3*(2), 191–204.
7. Clarke, H. M., & Curtis, C. G. (1995). An approach to obstetrical brachial plexus injuries. *Hand Clinics, 11,* 563–580.
8. Reference deleted in page proofs.
9. Curtis, C., Stephens, D., Clarke, H. M., & Andrews, D. (2002). The active movement scale: An evaluative tool for infants with obstetrical brachial plexus injury. *Journal of Hand Surgery (American), 27A,* 470–478.
10. Dawodu, A., Sankaran-Kutty, M., & Rajan, T. V. (1997). Risk factors and prognosis for brachial plexus injury and clavicular fracture in neonates: A prospective analysis from the United Arab Emirates. *Annals of Tropical Pediatrics, 17,* 195–200.
11. Desiato, M. T., & Risina, B. (2001). The role of botulinum toxin in the neuro-rehabilitation of young patients with brachial plexus palsy. *Pediatric Rehabilitation, 4,* 29–36.
12. DiTaranto, P., Campagna, L., Price, A. E., & Grossman, J. A. (2004). Outcome following nonoperative treatment of brachial plexus birth injuries. *Journal of Child Neurology, 19,* 87–90.
13. Dodds, S. D., & Wolfe, S. W. (2000). Perinatal brachial plexus palsy. (2000). *Current Opinion in Pediatrics, 12,* 40–47.
14. Eng, G.D., Koch, B., & Smokvina, M.D. (1978). Brachial plexus palsy in neonates and children. *Archives of Physical Medicine and Rehabilitation, 59,* 458–464.
15. Fisher D. M., Borschel G. H., Curtis C. G., & Clarke H. M. (2007). Evaluation of elbow flexion as a predictor of outcome in obstetrical brachial plexus palsy. *Plastic and Reconstructive Surgery, 120,* 1585–1590.
16. Gadjosik, C. G., & Gajdosik, R. L. (2006). Musculoskeletal development and adaptation. In Campbell, S., Vanderlinden, D. W., & Palisano, R. J. *Physical Therapy for Children* (3rd ed., pp 191–216).
17. Gilbert, A. (1993). Obstetrical brachial plexus palsy. In R. Tubiana (Ed.), The Hand (*Vol. 4,* p. 579). Philadelphia: WB Saunders.
18. Gilbert, A. (1995). Long-term evaluation of brachial plexus surgery in obstetrical palsy. *Hand Clinics 11,* 583–593.
19. Gilbert, W. M., Hicks, S. M., Boe, N. M., & Danielsen, B. (2003). Vaginal versus cesarean delivery for breech presentation in

California: A population-based study. *Obstetrics & Gynecology*, *102*, 911–917.

20. Gjorup, L. (1965). Obstetrical lesion of the brachial plexus. *Acta Neurologica Scandinavica (Supplementum)*, *18*, 31–58.

21. Gordon, M., Rich, H., Deutschberger, J., & Green, M. (1973). The immediate and long-term outcome of obstetric birth trauma. I. Brachial plexus paralysis. *American Journal of Obstetrics and Gynecology*, *117*, 51–56.

22. Grossman, A. L., Ditaranto, P., Yaylali, I., Alfonso, I., Ramos L. E., & Price, A. E. (2004). Shoulder function following late neurolysis and bypass grafting for upper brachial plexus birth injuries. *Journal of Hand Surgery (British)*, *29B*, 356–358.

23. Grossman, J. A. I. (1996). Multidisciplinary treatment of patients with obstetrical brachial plexus palsy. *Acta Neuropediatrica*, *2*, 151–152.

24. Hardy, A. F. (1981). Birth injuries of the brachial plexus; incidence and prognosis. *Journal of Bone and Joint Surgery (British)*, *63B*, 98–101.

25. Hearle, M., & Gilbert, A. (2004). Management of complete obstetrical brachial plexus lesions. *Journal of Pediatric Orthopedics*, *24*, 194–200.

26. Hernandez, C., & Wendel, G.D. (1990). Shoulder dystocia. *Clinical Obstetrics and Gynecology*, *33*, 526–534.

27. Hoeksma, A. F., ter Steeg, A. M., Dijkstra, P., Nelissen, R. G., Bellen, A., & de Jong, B. A. (2003). Shoulder contracture and osseous deformity in obstetrical brachial plexus injuries. *Journal of Bone and Joint Surgery (American)*, *85A*, 316–322.

28. Hoeksma, A. F., ter Steeg, A. M., Nelissen, R. G., van Ouwerkerk, W. J., Lankhorst, G. J., & de Jong, B. A. (2004). Neurological recovery in obstetric brachial plexus injuries: An historical cohort study. *Developmental Medicine and Child Neurology*, *46*, 76–83.

29. Hoeksma, A. F., Wolf, H., & Oei, S. L. (2000). Obstetrical brachial plexus injuries: Incidence, natural course and shoulder contracture. *Clinical Rehabilitation*, *14*, 523–526.

30. Hoffer, M. M., & Phipps, G. J. (1998). Closed reduction and tendon transfer for treatment of dislocation of the glenohumeral joint secondary to brachial plexus birth palsy. *Journal of Bone and Joint Surgery (American)*, *7*, 997–1001.

31. Jette, A. M. (1993). Using health related quality of life measures in physical therapy outcomes research. *Physical Therapy*, *73*, 528–537.

32. Kon, D. S., Darakjian, A. B., Pearl, M. L., & Kosco, A. E. (2004). Glenohumeral deformity in children with internal rotation contractures secondary to brachial plexus birth palsy: Intraoperative arthorgraphic classification. *Radiology*, *231*, 791–795.

33. Laurent, J. P., & Lee, R. T. (1994). Birth related upper brachial plexus injuries in infants: Operative and nonoperative approaches. *Journal of Child Neurology*, *9*, 111–117.

34. Laurent, J. P., Lee, R., Shenaq, S., Parke, J. T., Solis, I. S., & Kowalik, L. (1993). Neurosurgical correction of upper brachial plexus birth injuries. *Journal of Neurosurgery*, *79*, 197–203.

35. Lin J. C., Schwentker-Colizza A., Curtis C. G., & Clarke H. M. (2009). Final results of grafting versus neurolysis in obstetrical

brachial plexus palsy. *Plastic and Reconstructive Surgery*, *123*, 939–948.

36. McNeely, P. D., & Drake, J. M. (2003). A systematic review of brachial plexus surgery for birth-related brachial plexus injury. *Pediatric Neurosurgery*, *38*, 57–62.

37. Michelow, B. J., Clarke, H. M., Curtis, C. G., Zuker, R. M., Seifu, Y., & Andrews, D. F. (1994). The natural history of brachial plexus palsy. *Plastic and Reconstructive Surgery*, *93*, 675–680.

38. Narakas, A. O. (1987). Obstetrical brachial plexus injuries. In D. W. Lamb (Ed.), *The hand and upper limb* (*Vol. 2*: The Paralyzed Hand, p. 116). Edinburgh: Churchill Livingstone.

39. Nath, R. K., & Liu, X. (2009). Nerve reconstruction in patients with obstetrical brachial plexus injury results in worsening of glenohumeral deformity: A case-control study of 75 patients. *Journal of Bone and Joint Surgery, British Volume*, *91*, 649–654.

40. Noetzel, M. J., Park, T. S., Robinson, S., & Kaufman, B. (2001). Prospective study of recovery following neonatal brachial plexus injury. *Journal of Child Neurology*, *16*, 488–492.

41. O'Leary, J. A. (1992). Shoulder dystocia and birth injury: prevention and treatment. New York: McGraw-Hill, pp 11–24, 106–144.

42. Okafor, U. A., Akinbo, S. R., Sokunbi, O. G., Okanlawon, A. O., Noronha, C. C. (2008). Comparison of electrical stimulation and conventional physiotherapy in functional rehabilitation in Erb's palsy. *Nigerian Quarterly Journal of Hospital Medicine*, *18*, 202–205.

43. Partridge C., & Edwards, S. (2004). Obstetric brachial plexus palsy: Increasing disability and exacerbation of symptoms with age. *Physiotherapy Research International*, *9*, 157–163.

44. Pearl, M. (2009). Shoulder problems in children with brachial plexus birth palsy: Evaluation and management. *Journal of the American Academy of Orthopedic Surgeons*, *17*, 242–254.

45. Pondaag, W., Malessy, M. J., van Dijk, J. G., & Thomeer, R. T. (2004). Natural history of obstetric brachial plexus palsy: A systematic review. *Developmental Medicine and Child Neurology*, *46*, 138–144.

46. Price, A. E., & Grossman, J.A.I. (2004). A management approach for secondary shoulder and forearm deformities following obstetrical brachial plexus surgery. *Hand Clinics*, *11*, 607–614, 1995.

47. Shepherd, R. B. (1991). Brachial plexus injury. In S. K. Campbell (Ed.), *Pediatric Neurologic Physical Therapy* (2nd ed., pp. 101–130). New York: Churchill Livingstone.

48. Sherburn, E. W., Kaplan, S. S., Kaufman, B. A., Noetzel, M. J., & Park, T. S. (1997). Outcome of surgically treated birth-related brachial plexus injuries in twenty cases. *Pediatric Neurosurgery*, *27*, 19–27.

49. Sjoberg, I., Erichs, K., & Bjerre, I. (1998). Cause and effect of obstetric (neonatal) brachial plexus palsy. *Acta Paediatrics Scandinavia*, *77*, 357–564.

50. Strombeck, C., Krumlinde-Sundholm L., & Forssberg H. (2000). Functional outcome at 5 years in children with obstetrical brachial plexus palsy with and without microsurgical reconstruction. *Developmental Medicine & Child Neurology*, *42*, 148–157.

51. Strombeck, C., Krumlinde-Sundholm, L., Remalh, S., & Sejersen, T. (2007). Long-term follow-up of children with obsteric brachial plexus I; functional aspects. *Developmental Medicine and Child Neurology, 49,* 198–203.

52. Sundholm, L. K., Eliasson, A. C., & Forssberg, H. (1998). Obstetric brachial plexus injuries: Assessment protocol and functional outcome at age 5 years. *Developmental Medicine and Child Neurology, 40,* 4–11.

53. Ter Steeg, A. M., Hoeksma, A. F., Kijkstra, P. F., Nelissen, R. G. H. H., & De Jong, B. A. (2004). Orthopedic sequelae in neurologically recovered obstetrical brachial plexus injury. Case study and literature review. *Disability and Rehabilitation, 25,* 1–8.

54. Terzis, J. K., & Kokkalis, Z. T. (2008). Primary and secondary shoulder reconstruction in obstetric brachial plexus palsy. *Injury, 39S,* S5–S14.

55. van der Weel, F. R. R., van der Meer, A. L. H., & Lee, D. N. (1991). Effect of task on movement control in cerebral palsy: Implications for assessment and therapy. *Developmental Medicine and Child Neurology, 33,* 419–426.

56. Waters, P. M. (1999). Comparison of the natural history, the outcome of microsurgical repair, and the outcome of operative reconstruction in brachial plexus birth palsy. *Journal of Bone and Joint Surgery (American), 81,* 649–659.

57. Waters, P. M., & Bae, D. S. (2008). The early effects of tendon transfers and open capsulorrhaphy on glenohumeral deformity in brachial plexus birth palsy. *Journal of Bone and Joint Surgery (American), 90,* 2171–2179.

58. Wolf, H., Hoeksma, A. F., Oei, S. L., & Bleker, O. P. (2000). Obstetric brachial plexus injury: Risk factors related to recovery. *European Journal of Obstetrics & Gynecology and Reproductive Biology, 88,* 133–138.

20 Spinal Cord Injury

CHRISTIN H. KREY, PT, MPT, ATP • THERESE E. JOHNSTON, PT, PhD, MBA • KRISTINE A. SHAKHAZIZIAN, PT • TERESA L. MASSAGLI, MD

Acquired lesions of the spinal cord occur far less commonly in children than in adults, but the unique aspects of growth and development can make treatment of the child with spinal cord injury (SCI) a challenge for pediatric physical therapists. The rehabilitation process may take years because the young child requires time to achieve adequate strength, adult body proportions, and cognitive skills for maximal independence. The child who is not skeletally mature may develop orthopedic problems during growth, which may result in altered function. Direct intervention, monitoring skill acquisition, education, and assessing equipment needs are important roles for the physical therapist.

This chapter describes the pathophysiology, resulting neurologic changes, changes in body functions and structures, and their impact on activity and participation of children with SCI. Examination, prognosis, goals, and outcomes, and physical therapy intervention for the child with SCI are discussed.

EPIDEMIOLOGY

The overall incidence of pediatric SCI in the United States is nearly 20 cases per million children.[129] Motor vehicle crashes (MVCs), sports, falls, and violence are the leading causes of traumatic SCI.[30,129] MVCs are the most prevalent cause in infants, followed by falls in the 2- to 9-year-old age group and sports in the 10- to 14-year-old age group.[13,30] Motor vehicle crashes in children younger than 4 years of age usually result in a high cervical lesion, with continued risk for cervical level injuries through age 8.[37,38] Lap belt injuries tend to occur in children between 5 to 8 years of age. Lap belt injuries frequently occur when a child transitions too early out of a car seat into sitting in a passenger seat, causing the lap portion of a lap/shoulder seat belt to ride high on the abdomen. Spinal injury from a lap belt in an MVC is typically at the thoracolumbar junction, but significant retroperitoneal injury also occurs.[54,111] Teens injured as a result of a MVC typically sustain cervical level injuries.

Child abuse accounts for some cases of SCI, but the frequency of abuse as a cause of SCI is unknown. In one study of child abuse in younger children, all cases resulted in spinal cord injury without radiographic abnormality (SCIWORA defined later).[20]

Boys are almost twice as likely to sustain an SCI as compared to girls.[20,129] African Americans exhibit a significantly higher incidence of pediatric SCI, whereas the Asian population shows a significantly lower incidence than all other races.[129]

Long-term survival rate of a child with an SCI is approximately between 83% of normal life expectancy with an incomplete injury to 50% with a high cervical injury without ventilator dependency,[117] with primary mortality resulting from respiratory complications.[3] Mortality overall seems to follow a different pattern than for individuals with adult-onset SCI as well as the general population of comparable age.[3] A small-scale study suggests that recovery of neurologic function occurs more frequently in pediatric patients than in adults and that recovery can be identified for a longer period of time after injury.[135]

Developmental anomalies of the cervical vertebrae can place the spinal cord at increased risk of injury. These anomalies include instability of the atlantoaxial joint, as seen in Down syndrome, juvenile rheumatoid arthritis, or os odontoideum (a congenital failure of fusion of the odontoid process to the C2 vertebral body) and dysplasia of the base of the skull or upper cervical vertebrae, as seen in achondroplasia.

Nontraumatic myelopathy can be difficult to diagnose because imaging studies may be nonspecific. Nontraumatic causes of SCI in children include tumor (predominantly intramedullary tumors[138]), transverse myelitis, epidural abscess, arteriovenous malformation, multiple sclerosis, and spinal cord infarction due to thromboembolic disorders.

PREVENTION

Proper use of vehicle restraints, water safety instruction, and preparticipation sports physical examinations are important measures in preventing traumatic SCI in children. Lap seat belts must be placed across the pelvis, not across the waist, and shoulder harnesses should cross the clavicle, not the neck, to avoid lumbar or cervical spine injury in the event of a collision. Children should use a booster seat until the lap belt and shoulder harness fit correctly. This typically occurs when the child is about 4 feet 9 inches tall, 8 years old, or 80 pounds. According to the National Highway Transportation and Safety Administration (NHTSA) and federal law, infants should remain in a rear-facing infant car seat to a minimum of 20 pounds and 12 months of age (www.nhtsa.org). Car seat manufacturers have been producing car seats rated to a higher weight rear-facing as it is being suggested the rear-facing position for as long as possible is preferred. Additionally, the current recommendation for a forward-facing 5-point harness is 4 years and 40 pounds; however, the longer a child is restrained in a forward-facing 5-point harness, the better. This again is reflected in the manufacturing of combination car seats with harnesses rated to higher weights. It should also be noted that proper car seat installation as well as proper harness snugness and retainer clip placement are imperative to properly restrain an infant, toddler, or child in an appropriate vehicle safety system.

Organizations, such as Safe Kids Worldwide (www.safekids.org) and the Center for Injury Research and Prevention[27] carry missions to reduce accidental childhood injury. Many health care facilities and schools utilize these organizations to raise awareness and educate the public. Because children with Down syndrome have some risk of atlantoaxial instability, the American Academy of Pediatrics[32] recommends screening radiographs to assess cervical spine stability for this population of children between the ages of 3 and 5 years. This radiographic screening is most helpful for children who may participate in sports or who are symptomatic. The Committee on Genetics[124] also recommends that children with achondroplasia be encouraged to participate in activities such as biking or swimming but to avoid gymnastics and contact sports because of the potential for neck or back injury.

ADVANCES IN RECOVERY

There has been much focus on finding a cure for SCI, with a large thrust occurring after which, in a highly publicized case, a man with C2 ventilator-dependent tetraplegia participated in an intensive 3-year program of electrical stimulation, aqua therapy, and range of motion (ROM) and breathing exercises. Improvements in cardiorespiratory endurance, increased muscle mass, decreased spasticity, less frequent infections, changes in motor strength of some muscles, and improved light touch sensation were reported, but no changes in bladder, bowel, sexual function, or requirement for a ventilator and power wheelchair were noted.[89]

Researchers in spinal cord regeneration are focusing on neuroprotection, neuroplasticity, neuroregeneration, and cellular transplant therapy. Many have tried pharmacologic interventions to halt the chain of secondary events producing neural damage and to protect compromised but viable cells. Antioxidants, free radical scavengers, opiate antagonists, vitamins, thyrotropin-releasing hormone, and calcium channel blockers are a few of the agents that have been tested.[110] The only current practice is the administration of methylprednisolone (corticosteroids) in the acute phase to decrease cord edema and limit cell death. High doses,

administered within the first 8 hours and continued for 24 to 48 hours, have been shown to slightly enhance motor recovery in humans.[16-18,57,76] Data are lacking on the effects of methylprednisolone in the pediatric population. There have been no pediatric-specific studies, and past studies have had a minimal number of subjects in the 13- to 19-years of age category.[18] Currently, the use of the steroid overall is being questioned,[61,62,102,118] and it is even proposed to cause acute myopathy when administered.[110]

More recently, after a professional football player was injured tackling during a game, a treatment of modest hypothermia gained attention.[22] This technique of slowly cooling the body's core temperature to 92°F for a period of time and then slowly rewarming potentially minimizes metabolic demands and edema within an injured spinal cord. This neuroprotective therapy is still being studied in clinical trials.

An international, multicenter, randomized, controlled phase II clinical study was under way to stimulate axonal growth in an acutely injured spinal cord (less than 14 days after injury) through the use of autologous macrophages that were "activated" using proprietary technology of Pro-Neuron Biotechnologies, Inc.,[1] and were then injected directly into the spinal tracts at the injury site.[73] This study lost funding and results are still pending for the data that had been collected. Other studies utilizing various growth factors are under way in animals. Several pharmacologic studies have been conducted with the aim of enhancing axonal transmission in chronic, incomplete SCI, but outcomes have been minimal in published studies, and results of additional studies are still pending.[7]

A major focus in the SCI community most recently has been on stem cell transplants. Various sources have been used, such as olfactory epithelial cells, bone marrow stromal cells, and, most recently, human embryonic stem cells. Several physicians outside the United States[40,113] have injected humans with these cells, but none of these regimens were conducted through rigorous research, and reported results are mixed. In the United States, Geron Corporation (www.geron.com), a biopharmaceutical company, received Food and Drug Administration (FDA) clearance in 2009 to initiate the world's first human clinical trial of embryonic stem cell–based therapy.

It is a slow process to bring new pharmacotherapies into clinical practice, owing to the necessary steps of animal trials, followed by preliminary and then larger-scale trials in humans. Human trials must be placebo controlled and have a sufficient period of follow-up to assess the efficacy of the treatment. Because SCI is not very common, clinical trials usually require collaboration among many medical centers. Approval to move these adult-based studies into the pediatric population is extremely difficult secondary to reluctance to approve studies by human subjects review boards and the FDA in an attempt to protect this vulnerable population. It

---

[1]ProNeuron Biotechnologies, Inc., TelAviv, Israel www.proneuron.com.

is not clear whether the young, immature spinal cord responds exactly the same way to injury as a mature spinal cord. Therefore, additional studies are being conducted in young animals in order to evaluate the sequelae of events after injury.

It is important to realize that patients and their families have been and will continue to be tempted by unproved therapies, often at considerable personal financial expense. Therapists can help them to evaluate the evidence regarding potential therapies. Any purported cure should be subjected to randomized clinical trials before being offered to hopeful but vulnerable patients. It is reasonable for patients and therapists to hold out hope for a cure for SCI. It is often just this hope that motivates patients and caregivers to be meticulous about preventing secondary complications.

MEDICAL DIAGNOSIS, ACUTE MANAGEMENT, AND STABILIZATION

PATHOPHYSIOLOGY

As mentioned earlier, the site or level at which SCI occurs is often related to the cause of injury and the child's age. Many of the nontraumatic causes (tumors, stenosis) of SCI occur in the thoracic spinal cord and result in incomplete injuries.[91] By contrast, vertebral dysplasias place the upper cervical spinal cord or lower brainstem at risk. Birth trauma as a result of traction and angulation of the spine in a breech delivery most commonly causes SCI at the cervicothoracic junction. In the child younger than 8 to 10 years old, the cervical spine has greater mobility than it does in adults because of ligamentous laxity, shallow angulation of the facets, incomplete ossification of vertebrae, and relative underdevelopment of the neck muscles for the size of the head.[137] Young children are therefore more likely to experience injury at the upper cervical spine than are adults,[14] and SCI may occur without any signs of bone damage by radiography, a finding referred to as SCI without radiographic abnormality, or SCIWORA.[15] Studies have reported the incidence of SCIWORA to be anywhere between 6% and 38%.[20,30] In children, 55% of cases of traumatic SCI result in tetraplegia owing to injury between the first cervical and first thoracic root levels, and 45% result in paraplegia from injury below the first thoracic level.[104]

Most cases of traumatic SCI are caused by a blunt, nonpenetrating injury to the spinal cord in which the cord is not lacerated or transected, and in the majority of cases, some white matter tracts remain intact across the lesion. The direct effect of the trauma is immediate disruption of neural transmission in the gray and white matter of the spinal cord at and below the injury site, resulting in spinal shock. Reactive physiologic events evolve over a period of hours and induce secondary injury to the spinal cord.[72] The exact sequence of events between transfer of kinetic energy to the cord and subsequent neuronal death is unknown. Animal models have shown that ischemia, hemorrhage, edema, calcium influx into cells, and generation of free radicals contribute to cell membrane degradation and death of neurons.[57] In gray matter, neurons that die are not replaced. In white matter, axonal segments distal to the injury degenerate and synapses no longer function. Although axonal sprouting does occur to a limited degree in the central nervous system (CNS), it appears to be functionally insignificant, and most of the recovery observed in patients with incomplete lesions is probably due to resolution of neurapraxic injury. Case reports of neurologic improvement years after SCI are rare but provide hope that therapies can be developed to enhance function in the remaining spinal cord tissue.[89]

The zone of injury within the spinal cord is usually large enough to cause a transition in neurologic function from normal to abnormal or from normal to absent over several spinal root levels. Soon after SCI, the level of injury may appear to move cephalad as the secondary or indirect injury processes set in. Later, the level of injury may move caudally as these factors resolve, as sprouting develops (either within the spinal cord or peripherally to denervated muscles), or as hypertrophy of weak muscles occurs. The extent of injury may diminish for as long as 1 year, and it is obvious that until the natural history of SCI and recovery is delineated, experimental treatments may be inappropriately credited with enhancing recovery.

There are several distinct patterns of neuroanatomic incomplete syndromes that have distinct clinical representations. Anterior cord syndrome is usually due to damage of the anterior spinal artery causing infarction to the spinal cord. This injury produces variable motor paralysis, with reduced sensation of pain and temperature but with preserved dorsal column function. Prognosis for return of function is poor. Hemorrhage in the central part of the cervical spinal cord produces flaccid weakness of the arms and strong but spastic legs, with preservation of bladder and bowel function. As a result, ambulation is a potential goal for this population, but hand function may be impaired depending on level of injury. Posterior cord lesions are rare and produce selective loss of proprioception with preserved motor function. Ambulation remains unlikely because of loss of proprioception. A Brown-Sequard lesion results in ipsilateral paralysis and proprioceptive loss and contralateral loss of pain and temperature sensation. Brown-Sequard is primarily seen with penetrating trauma to one side of the spinal cord, such as in a stab wound. Prognosis for ambulation as well as bladder and bowel control is good. Injury to the lumbosacral nerve roots results in cauda equina syndrome, with lower extremity weakness and areflexia of the legs and bladder. Cauda equina lesions are essentially lesions of the peripheral nerve or lower motoneuron and may show recovery over several years owing to resolution of neurapraxia or to regrowth of damaged axons, as well as to peripheral sprouting. The next sections describe the initial management of acute SCI.

EMERGENT STABILIZATION (IN THE FIELD)

Initial management of a child with SCI is focused on stabilization of the spine to prevent further damage to the intact but injured spinal cord. The spine is immobilized during transport and throughout all assessments and procedures. Modified spine boards should be utilized in children younger than years of age to allow for proper neutral alignment of the cervical spine. Because of their larger head-to-torso ratio, their neck will be flexed on a regular spine board, potentially causing further injury. Modifications include either creating an occipital cut-out or elevating the torso on an additional pad (preferred) to allow the cervical spine to be positioned neutrally.[11,12,58] (Figure 20-1).

DIAGNOSTIC STUDIES

At the hospital, a thorough neurologic examination is performed to determine the motor and sensory level of SCI and the completeness of injury. Spinal shock is usually present, although occasionally it has resolved by the time the patient is treated in the emergency department. In spinal shock, the muscles are flaccid below the SCI and all cutaneous and deep tendon reflexes are absent. This state persists for hours to weeks and is said to be over when sacral reflexes, including the bulbocavernous and anal reflexes, are present.

Further evaluation is undertaken with plain radiographs of the whole spine from the first cervical to the

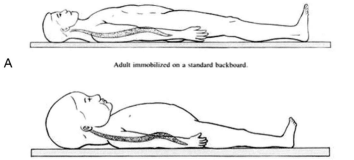

A   Adult immobilized on a standard backboard.

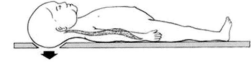

B   Young child on a standard backboard. The relatively large head forces the neck into a kyphotic position.

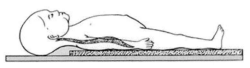

C   Young child on a modified backboard that has a cut-out to recess the occiput, obtaining safe supine cervical positioning.

D   Young child on a modified backboard that has a double-mattress pad to raise the chest, obtaining safe supine cervical positioning.

Figure 20-1   Emergent stabilization: note improved spinal alignment with pediatric spine board modifications cut out (**C**) or elevation of torso (**D**), which is preferred.

sacral vertebrae to identify any fractures, facet subluxations, or dislocations. Full radiographic evaluation is imperative as multiple, noncontiguous fractures occur in 30% of children.[13] Anterioposterior (AP) and lateral radiographs of the entire spine are needed to rule this out.[13] Computed tomography (CT) and magnetic resonance imaging (MRI) are used to diagnose root impingement, presence of bone fragments in the spinal canal, cord compression, and spinal cord hemorrhage. Because of the high incidence of SCIWORA, particularly in children younger than 10 years of age, an MRI is indicated for all children who have sustained an SCI and can show problems that are not seen on plain radiographs.[13]

SURGICAL STABILIZATION

Whether immediate surgical intervention to correct bone injury and decompress the spinal cord is effective in reducing paralysis is unknown because the numerous surgical procedures have never been subjected to randomized clinical trials. The main goal of surgery is to prevent later deformity, pain, or loss of neurologic function. Surgery may not be necessary if spinal alignment can be achieved with traction and maintained with an orthosis. Tonged cervical traction in children under 12 years of age, however, has increased risks as compared with its use in adults. Therefore, halo traction may be safer and preferred,[11] even in axis (C2) fractures.[81] A variant in the use of halo traction is an increase in the number of pins used, while decreasing the amount of torque on each pin. If a halo cannot be applied, a Minerva-type cervicothoracolumbosacral orthosis (CTLSO) would be an option (Figure 20-2). External halo orthoses[81] have also traditionally been used in conjunction with internal posterior wiring in children with atlantoaxial and occipital-cervical instability. However, investigation has identified successful rigid internal fixation for children requiring C1-C2 and occipital-cervical stabilization.[6]

Surgery is indicated if there is a penetrating injury, if traction has failed to reduce a dislocation, if nerve root impingement exists, if the spine is highly unstable and at risk of further damaging the cord, or if bone fragments are

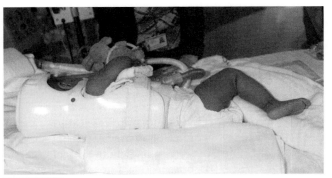

Figure 20-2   Infant wearing CTLSO for acute stabilization secondary to C1-2 injury.

compressing the cauda equina.[45] Regardless of whether surgery is performed, if bone injury has occurred patients usually wear an external orthosis until bone fusion is complete, often for 3 or more months. There is, however, regional variation in practice among orthopedic surgeons in the use of spinal orthoses after spinal fusion. For some lower lumbar (L4 or L5) injuries, the surgeon may have the child wear an orthosis with a thigh piece (see Figure 20-1), which permits only limited hip flexion (e.g., to only 60°). This is done to reduce torque on the immature fusion mass that could occur from pull of the hamstrings on the pelvis in a position of hip flexion.

UNDERLYING INJURIES AND COMORBIDITIES

Traumatic brain injury is one of the most commonly associated comorbidities and has been reported to occur in 38% of the patients with SCI.[20] Traumatic brain injury, which can occur with any type of loss of consciousness, is important to recognize at initial examination as it can significantly affect the rehabilitation process and warrant additional therapies such as speech pathology and neuropsychologic testing (see Chapter 21 on Acquired Brain Injuries for further information).

Another comorbidity that can be easily overlooked, particularly with someone with a cervical level SCI, is injury to the brachial plexus. Brachial plexus injury should be considered if the mechanism of injury included any type of distraction to the shoulder or impingement or fracture of the clavicle in the presence of asymmetrical weakness in the upper extremities.

MEDICAL COMPLICATIONS, LONG-TERM MEDICAL MANAGEMENT, AND PREVENTION OF SECONDARY IMPAIRMENTS

A child's participation in SCI rehabilitation may be affected by a number of medical complications. Each of the following complications must be addressed by the entire rehabilitation team, physicians, nurses, therapists, and caregivers in order to achieve optimum outcomes.

AUTONOMIC DYSREFLEXIA

Autonomic dysreflexia (AD) is a massive reflex sympathetic discharge that occurs after an SCI of T6 or above in response to noxious stimuli below the level of injury, causing a sudden increase in blood pressure (BP > 15 mmHg over baseline systolic).[90] If left untreated, the hypertensive crisis can cause stroke, seizures, or even death. Clinical features include headache, flushing, sweating, pilomotor activity, bradycardia or tachycardia, and hypertension. School-age children and adolescents are capable of reporting headaches, but younger children may have difficulty in verbalizing symptoms and may have more nonspecific symptoms because of their maturing central and peripheral nervous systems. As a result, autonomic dysreflexia is often overlooked in these youngsters. Infants and children who are unusually sleepy, irritable, or crying may be experiencing an AD episode and should have their vital signs checked. Knowledge of baseline BPs are imperative, as infants, toddlers, and children up to 13 years of age have different normals for BP (Table 20-1).[126] Additionally, patients with SCI typically have lower resting BP (i.e., 90/60).[90]

The primary causes of an AD episode/noxious stimulus below the level of injury are overdistended bladder and the need for catheterization or a kinked catheter in the instance of an indwelling system; overdistended bowel and the need to complete a bowel program; and excessive pressure to the skin below the level of injury caused by a wrinkle in clothing, compression hose, or shoes that are too tight/small.

Treatment of AD includes monitoring BP, pulse, and temperature (at least every 5 minutes); elevation of the patient's head (unless contraindicated); removal of compression stockings and abdominal binders; and loosening of tight clothes/shoes. Next perform bladder management steps and, if BP does not decrease, complete bowel regimen. Continuously check vital signs for reduction in BP and return to normal as the various management techniques are completed. If none of the above methods resolve the dysreflexic episode, pharmacologic intervention by a physician or nurse practitioner may be warranted.

RESPIRATORY DYSFUNCTION

Respiratory insufficiency may occur with lesions of the cervical and thoracic spinal cord and is a prominent cause of morbidity and mortality in the population with SCI.[3] Dysfunction ranges anywhere from complete diaphragm paralysis and the requirement of mechanical ventilation (C1-C3 and occasionally C4 depending on age/size of child) to diminished vital capacity or weakened forced expiration during coughing as a result of absent/weakened accessory breathing muscles (lower cervical and thoracic level injuries). Respiratory/breathing exercises are all too often overlooked as part of physical therapy rehabilitation but must be included. Respiratory exercises can occur during any part of treatment sessions, including during mat mobility and sitting balance activities. "Quad coughing" techniques are to be taught to the child and caregivers in order to assist with forced expiration when a cough alone in ineffective in clearing secretions. A quad cough is forced compression of the abdomen with a hand(s) in an inward and upward fashion during expiration.

DEEP VEIN THROMBOSIS

Paralyzed and dependent lower extremities can develop edema and deep vein thromboses (DVTs). Although common in adults with SCI, deep vein thrombosis occurs

TABLE 20-1 90th and 95th Percentiles of Mean Daytime and Nighttime Ambulatory Systolic and Diastolic BP, Stratified According to Gender and Height

| Height, cm | Systolic BP, mm Hg | | | | Diastolic BP, mm Hg | | | |
| | Day | | Night | | Day | | Night | |
	90th pct	95th pct	90th pct	95th pct	90th pct	95th pct	90th pct	95th pct
Boys								
120	120.6	123.5	103.7	106.4	79.1	81.2	61.9	64.1
125	121.0	124.0	104.9	107.8	79.8	81.3	62.2	64.3
130	121.6	124.6	106.3	109.5	79.3	81.4	62.4	64.5
135	122.2	125.2	107.7	111.3	79.3	81.3	62.7	64.8
140	123.0	126.0	109.3	113.1	79.2	81.2	62.9	65.0
145	124.0	127.0	110.7	114.7	79.1	81.1	63.1	65.2
150	125.4	128.5	111.9	115.9	79.1	81.0	63.3	65.4
155	127.2	130.2	113.1	117.0	79.2	81.1	63.4	65.6
160	122.2	132.3	114.3	118.0	79.3	81.3	63.6	65.7
165	131.3	134.5	115.5	119.1	79.7	81.7	63.7	65.8
170	133.5	136.7	116.8	120.2	80.1	82.2	63.8	65.9
175	135.6	138.8	119.1	121.2	80.6	82.8	63.8	65.9
180	137.7	140.9	119.2	122.1	81.1	83.4	63.8	65.8
185	139.8	143.0	120.3	123.0	81.7	84.1	63.8	65.8
Girls								
120	118.5	121.1	105.7	109.0	79.7	81.8	64.0	66.4
125	119.5	122.1	106.4	109.8	79.7	81.8	63.8	66.2
130	120.4	123.1	107.2	110.6	79.7	81.8	63.3	66.0
135	121.4	124.1	107.9	111.3	79.7	81.8	63.4	65.8
140	122.3	125.1	108.4	111.9	79.8	81.8	63.2	65.7
145	123.4	126.3	109.1	112.5	79.8	81.9	63.0	65.6
150	124.6	127.5	109.9	113.1	79.9	81.9	63.0	65.5
155	125.7	128.5	110.6	113.8	79.9	81.9	62.9	65.5
160	126.6	129.3	111.1	114.0	79.9	81.9	92.8	65.4
165	127.2	129.8	111.2	114.0	79.9	81.9	62.7	65.2
170	127.5	130.0	111.2	114.0	79.9	81.8	62.5	65.0
175	127.6	129.9	111.2	114.0	79.8	81.7	62.3	64.7

BP, Blood pressure; pct, percentile.
Adapted from Wühl et al, with permission from Lippincott Williams & Wilkins.

less frequently in children with SCI (5%)[29] but does have a significant occurrence rate in 14- to 19-year-old adolescents.[125] A DVT prophylactic protocol of either insertion of an inferior vena cava filter (typically in older adolescents) or pharmacologic treatment is typically initiated during acute care hospitalization and completed during acute inpatient rehabilitation.

HYPERCALCEMIA/BONE DENSITY/ MUSCLE ATROPHY

Almost unique to children is the problem of immobilization hypercalcemia.[84] During the first 12 to 18 months after SCI, approximately 40% of bone mineral density is lost via calcium excreted in the urine. Children are more likely to

have rapid bone turnover, resulting in a larger load of calcium than the kidneys can excrete. This produces elevated serum calcium level, or hypercalcemia. Nonspecific symptoms include lethargy, nausea, altered mood, and anorexia. Remobilization is an important aspect of treatment in persons without SCI (e.g., the child with a femur fracture), but it is not known if this is effective in reducing hypercalcemia after SCI. The mainstays of treating immobilization hypercalcemia are primarily medical through hydration for improved excretion of the excessive calcium in urine, and administration of Etidronate (Didronel) and Calcitonin (Miacalcin) to avoid excessive calcification in unwanted areas, such as joints (heterotopic ossification) or kidneys (renal stones).

Pathologic fractures, which occur at an increased rate in persons with bone mineral density below 40% of normal, are a potential complication of osteopenia. Deposition of new bone in periarticular soft tissue can also occur in paralyzed extremities. This heterotopic ossification can be asymptomatic, or it may interfere with ROM around a joint or even cause ankylosis. The most commonly affected joints are hips, knees, shoulders, and elbows. Muscle atrophy begins early and occurs at a rapid rate during acute immobilization through 24 weeks postinjury when it begins to plateau at approximately 15% loss of lean muscle mass below the level of injury.[52]

ORTHOSTATIC HYPOTENSION

Orthostatic hypotension, a position-related drop in BP, is a common side effect with SCI. There is a decrease in the venous return of blood from the lower extremities as a result of muscle paralysis, which decreases cardiac output and arterial pressure, causing a quick drop in BP. As a result, the person's BP cannot adjust quickly enough during positional changes such as supine to sit, sit to stand, or coming out of a tilted position in a power wheelchair. Treatment for orthostatic hypotension can include gradient compression stockings, an abdominal binder, utilization of a wheelchair with a reclining back (particularly during acute care mobilization), tilt table, or pharmacologic intervention.

Early physical therapy sessions may address the goal of maintaining a stable BP when transitioning out of bed or while in the wheelchair. The patient's BP should be monitored throughout the treatment session.

THERMOREGULATORY DYSFUNCTION

Persons with SCIs have an impaired ability to regulate body temperature resulting from the loss of hypothalamic thermoregulatory control and interruption of afferent pathways from peripheral temperature receptors below the level of injury. With injuries above T6, there is the complete loss of shivering and sweating and no peripheral circulatory adjustment below the level of injury. Education provided to children and caregivers must include the increased risk of hypothermia and frostbite in cold weather, as well as heat exhaustion and heat stroke in hot weather. Children with SCI should avoid excessive sun exposure and maintain adequate hydration.

SYRINGOMYELIA

Delayed cavitation (syringomyelia) within the damaged spinal cord can occur in patients with complete or incomplete lesions. The occurrence of a cystic cavitation, or syrinx, appears to be common after SCI and may progressively enlarge, resulting in further loss of neurologic function months to years after SCI.[132] Signs and symptoms that may herald presence of a syrinx include loss of motor function, ascending sensory level, increased spasticity or sweating, and new onset of pain or dysesthesia.

SPASTICITY AND PAIN

Spasticity is a frequent occurrence after SCI and usually evolves over a period of 1 to 2 years. Although initially the patient is flaccid, hypertonus gradually appears, and in the first 3 to 6 months after SCI hyperreflexia, clonus and flexor spasms develop. Later, extensor spasms usually predominate. Evolution of spasticity after CNS insult is common and is seen in other conditions such as cerebral palsy and stroke. In SCI, the immediate effects of loss of supraspinal inhibition and the later-developing effects of denervation supersensitivity and sprouting by afferent and collateral neurons probably all contribute to the development of spasticity, but the sequence of events behind the evolution of clinical manifestations of spasticity is not known.

Spasticity can be controlled pharmacologically with oral medications, such as Baclofen, intramuscular injections, such as Botox, or nerve block injections, such as Phenol. Therapeutic interventions to control spasticity include passive ROM, passive and functional electrical stimulation (FES)-assisted cycling, and static standing. Many patients feel a certain amount of spasticity is helpful during transfers, bed mobility or even some activities of daily living so pharmacologic or other therapeutic interventions are usually withheld unless the spasticity is severe enough to limit function.

Neurogenic, or neuropathic, pain can occur after SCI at, above, or below the level of injury. Children and adolescents will describe neurogenic pain as a burning pain, which anecdotally precedes the return of function or sensation at the dermatologic level(s) where pain is experienced. This type of pain can be unbearable but can be pharmacologically controlled with gabapentin (Neurontin) or pregabalin (Lyrica).

SKIN BREAKDOWN AND PRESSURE ULCERS

Pressure ulcers occur as a result of improper positioning, both in bed as well as in a wheelchair, or inadequate pressure relief, which can limit the ability to sit. Pressure ulcers may also occur because of the improper fit of spinal orthoses, upper and lower extremity splints, and braces for ambulation. It is important to remember that skin breakdown is also caused by friction, shear, and moisture. All too often skin breakdown on the buttocks occurs from shearing across the wheel of the wheelchair during transfers and moisture secondary to improper bladder management or continuation of wearing a diaper beyond the age when the child should be dry between catheterizations.

Young children may not exhibit skin breakdown in the typical sense (from poor wheelchair or bed positioning) as seen with adolescents and adults because they are under direct care and guidance of their caregiver; however, young children typically have complete disregard for any body area that is insensate. They often will drag their lower extremities on the ground while crawling, or they may even bite insensate fingertips to the point of self-injury. As children grow older, it is often difficult for them to understand the importance of routine pressure-relief activities, particularly in the adolescent population with their tendency to test boundaries with caregivers. Patients and caregivers must also pay special attention to hot items on insensate skin to avoid burns (e.g., on the thighs from food that has been in the microwave such as popcorn or the heat generated by a laptop computer).

Pressure-relief techniques must also be taught. During acute care hospitalization and rehabilitation, the child/adolescent is turned every 2 hours and frequently is utilizing a specialty low air loss mattress. Children using power mobility can perform pressure-relieving techniques through powered seating, such as tilt and recline. Those using manual wheelchairs can perform wheelchair push-ups or lean laterally and anteriorly. The recommended frequency of pressure-relieving techniques varies between 15 to 30 minutes and should last 1 minute in order to allow return of blood flow to compressed tissue.[34] Children often utilize a watch with a timer to provide an audio reminder to complete weight-shift/pressure-relief measures at designated times.

ORTHOPEDIC MANAGEMENT

Contractures can arise as a result of static positioning, spasticity, or heterotopic bone formation and may interfere with positioning or voluntary movement. As a result, passive ROMs or the prolonged stretches, which an upright stander can provide, are imperative to use as treatments. Tightness is most typically seen in the hip flexor, hamstring, adductor, and ankle plantar flexor muscles. Of note is the fact that children and adolescents with flaccid paralysis may develop "pseudo hip flexion contractures" in which the iliotibial band is actually the tight muscle rather than the iliopsoas and rectus femoris muscles.

Hip subluxation (Figure 20-3) and dislocation are common in children who have onset of SCI before age 10, with an incidence up to 66% in children under 4 years of age.[88] Management to prevent subluxation/dislocation includes stretching of hip adductor and flexor muscles; proper bed positioning in an abducted position with either a wedge or pillow; and wheelchair seating positioning that encourages proper femoral alignment, such as a medial thigh build-up or pommel. Prevention is important, because although typically nonpainful, hip dislocation can lead to pelvic obliquity and other postural changes that will place the child at greater risk of skin breakdown as well as exacerbate a neuromuscular scoliosis. Treatment can include surgical plating and pinning to restore joint alignment.

Pathologic fractures can occur to osteopenic extremities as a result of disregard of lower extremities during transfers, falls, or forceful ROM exercises. The osteopenia has been found to be greatest at the hip and knee as compared to children their age without a disability.[77]

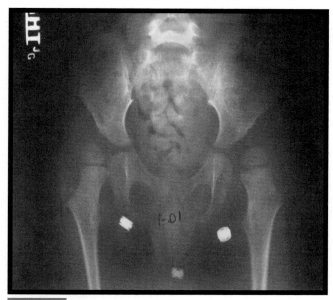

Figure 20-3 Hip instability.

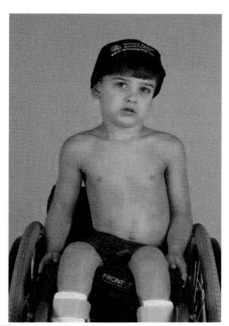

Figure 20-4 Neuromuscular scoliosis.

Neuromuscular scoliosis occurs in virtually all children with SCI (up to 98% has been reported[13]), particularly in patients injured before their adolescent growth spurt, and can affect the comfort of seating and respiratory function. Sixty-seven percent progress to the point of requiring spinal fusion.[13] Although it is important to provide proper pelvic alignment and trunk support in wheelchairs, external support devices in wheelchairs do not seem to ultimately prevent the development of scoliosis (Figure 20-4).

Prophylactic bracing is a controversial topic in therapy because the wear of a thoracolumbosacral orthosis (TLSO) will most likely inhibit independent activities, mobility, and reachable workspace while worn.[28,119] The argument, however, is that wearing the brace prophylactically can prevent (curves <10°) or even delay (curves <20°) spine fusion. If surgery can be delayed until the child has achieved nearly all of her trunk growth, bracing is considered successful. Once a curve nears or surpasses 20°, however, bracing may be futile.[92] Typical brace prescription can range from "while out of bed" for less significant curves to 23 hours a day, for which aggressive brace wear can delay progression when close to the 20° cut-off, particularly during growth spurts. Brace wear compliance is always a question, as many children and teens tend to return for follow-up and leave the brace at home. Surgery for neuromuscular scoliosis becomes indicated once the degree of curve causes respiratory compromise or significant pelvic obliquity that increases the risk of ischial pressure ulcers.

IMPAIRMENTS/OUTCOME MEASURES

THE INTERNATIONAL STANDARDS FOR NEUROLOGIC CLASSIFICATION OF SPINAL CORD INJURY (ISCSCI) OR ASIA EXAMINATION

Professionals should use a common terminology when describing the motor or sensory levels of SCI in children or adults. Most widely used are the International Standards for Neurological Classification of Spinal Cord Injury (ISCSCI), which are published by the American Spinal Injury Association (ASIA).[2] The ISCSCI standards were developed by consensus of a multidisciplinary group of clinical experts and have been revised periodically since their initial publication in 1982. The ISCSCI standards, more commonly referred to as the ASIA Examination, define right and left motor levels, right and left sensory levels, the neurologic level, as well as the severity of injury (i.e., complete versus incomplete). The ISCSCI standards have been used as the primary indicators to predict recovery of neurologic function,[19,82,85] and the exams have been used to determine inclusion for entry into drug and device trials that pertain to SCI,[18,55,89,106,115,122,123] including outcomes of activity-based rehabilitation, a program of intensive cycling, assisted treadmill training, and swimming.[89]

Precise description of the motor and sensory loss after SCI is important for two reasons. First, it helps predict the likelihood of further neurologic recovery in both complete and incomplete syndromes. For instance, in motor complete C5 tetraplegia, most if not all patients gain one full motor level, achieving grade 3 wrist extensor movement (a C6 muscle) during the first 8 months after injury.[39] Researchers have also determined that in SCI above T11, preservation of pinprick sensation has predictive value for return of motor function and independent ambulation, probably because of the proximity of the ascending pain fibers and descending motor fibers in the spinal cord.[106]

The second reason for the importance of precise definition of the level of SCI is that it helps predict the ultimate level of independence a patient can expect to achieve in the areas of mobility, self-care, and even communication. Patients with incomplete SCI may exceed the expectations for any given level of injury. Such expectations for independence must also be tempered by consideration of the child's age, which influences developmental expectations. It can take years for preschoolers to reach the expected level of independence, or they may fall short of expectations if complications, particularly orthopedic problems, arise. Environmental and personal factors also play an important role in determining the child's participation in home life, education, community activities, and social relationships.

Defining the Level of Spinal Cord Injury

The ASIA standards accept the widely used system of muscle grading: 0 = absence, total paralysis; 1 = trace, palpable, or visible contraction; 2 = poor, active movement through full ROM with gravity eliminated; 3 = fair, active movement through full ROM against gravity; 4 = good, active movement through full ROM against moderate resistance; and 5 = normal, active movement through full ROM against full resistance. Motor levels may differ for right and left sides of the body. The key muscles for determination of motor level are listed in Table 20-2. Because all muscles have innervation from more than one root level, the presence of innervation by one root level and the absence by the next lower level results in a weakened muscle. The ASIA-defined motor level is the most caudal root level in which muscle strength is grade 3 or more and the next most rostral muscle a grade 5. By convention, if a muscle has grade 3 strength and the next most rostral muscle is grade 5, the grade 3 muscle is considered to have full innervation by the higher root level, for which it is named. For example, for a patient with a grade 2 C8 key muscle, grade 3 C7 key muscle, grade 4 C6 key muscle, and grade 5 C5 key muscle, the motor level as defined by ASIA is C6. One disadvantage to using only the ASIA key muscles to define a level of function is the omission of examination of hip extensor, hip abductor, and knee flexor muscles. These L5 and S1 muscles play an important role in activities such as transfers, ambulation, and stair climbing. Strength grades of the key muscles can be added together for both sides of the body to create a composite ASIA motor score. This score has been used in research studies assessing efficacy of pharmacologic treatment of SCI.[7,16-18,40,73,76,113] It can also be used to predict function and need for assistance.[112]

The sensory level may not correspond exactly to the motor level. Determining the sensory level is especially helpful in injuries above C5 or to the thoracic spinal cord, where there are no key muscles to define the level of SCI. Rather than relying on dermatome charts, which vary from one text to another, the ASIA standards rely on the presence of normal light touch and pinprick sensation at a key point

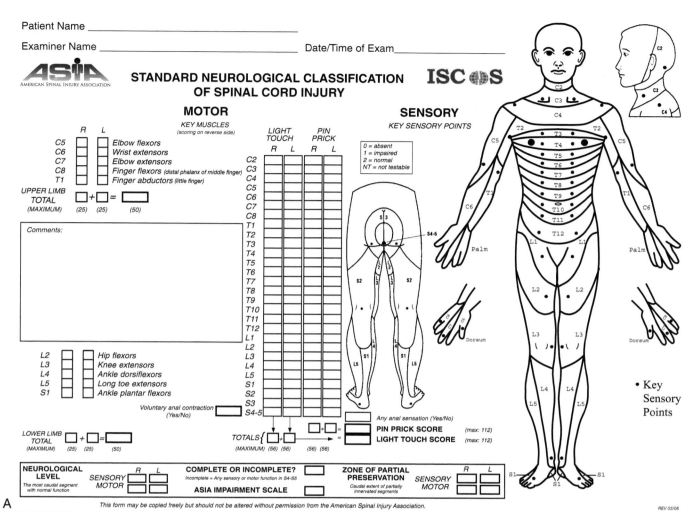

Figure 20-5 **A,** Scoring sheet with key sensory testing areas by dermatome for ASIA Examination. *Note,* Dot in each dermatome indicates exact location within dermatome to complete sensory testing. **B,** Muscle grading, impairment scale, and steps in classification. **C,** Autonomic standards assessment, newly added assessment sheet to complement muscle and sensory testing of ASIA examination. (**A, B,** From American Spinal Injury Association. [2006]. International Standards for Neurological and Functional Classification of Spinal Cord Injury. Chicago, American Spinal Injury Association. **C,** *Spinal Cord, 47,* 36–43, 2009.)

in each of the 28 dermatomes on the right and left sides of the body (see Figure 20-5, A and Table 20-2). Proprioception should also be assessed below the level of injury in patients with incomplete SCI to determine integrity of dorsal column function.

CLASSIFICATION

A complete injury, or ASIA A classification, is defined as the total absence of motor or sensory function in the lowest sacral segments (Figure 20-5, *B*). There may be some preservation of sensation or motor levels below the level of injury. This is defined as a "zone of partial preservation," a term used only with complete injuries.

A patient is said to have an incomplete SCI, ASIA B, C, or D classification, only if motor or sensory function is present in the lowest sacral segment, implying voluntary control of

TABLE 20-2 Key Muscles for Motor Level Classification

C5	Elbow flexors (biceps, brachialis)
C6	Wrist extensors (extensor carpi radialis longus and brevis)
C7	Elbow extensors (triceps)
C8	Finger flexors to the middle finger (flexor digitorum profundus)
T1	Small finger abductors (abductor digiti minimi manus)
L2	Hip flexors (iliopsoas)
L3	Knee extensors (quadriceps)
L4	Ankle dorsiflexors (tibialis anterior)
L5	Long toe extensors (extensor hallucis longus)
S1	Ankle plantar flexors (gastrocnemius, soleus)

From American Spinal Injury Association. (2000, revised 2002). *International Standards for Neurological and Functional Classification of Spinal Cord Injury.* Chicago, American Spinal Injury Association.

MUSCLE GRADING

0   total paralysis

1   palpable or visible contraction

2   active movement, full range of
    motion, gravity eliminated

3   active movement, full range of
    motion, against gravity

4   active movement, full range of
    motion, against gravity and provides
    some resistance

5   active movement, full range of
    motion, against gravity and provides
    normal resistance

5* muscle able to exert, in examiner's
    judgement, sufficient resistance to be
    considered normal if identifiable
    inhibiting factors were not present

NT not testable. Patient unable to reliably
    exert effort or muscle unavailable for test-
    ing due to factors such as immobilization,
    pain on effort or contracture.

B

Figure 20-5, cont'd

ASIA IMPAIRMENT SCALE

☐ **A = Complete**: No motor or sensory
   function is preserved in the sacral
   segments S4-S5.

☐ **B = Incomplete**: Sensory but not motor
   function is preserved below the
   neurological level and includes the
   sacral segments S4-S5.

☐ **C = Incomplete**: Motor function is preserved below the neurological
   level, and more than half of key
   muscles below the neurological
   level have a muscle grade less
   than 3.

☐ **D = Incomplete**: Motor function is preserved below the neurological
   level, and at least half of key muscles below the neurological level
   have a muscle grade of 3
   or more.

☐ **E = Normal**: Motor and sensory function are normal.

CLINICAL SYNDROMES
(OPTIONAL)

☐ Central Cord
☐ Brown-Sequard
☐ Anterior Cord
☐ Conus Medullaris
☐ Cauda Equina

STEPS IN CLASSIFICATION

The following order is recommended in determining the classification
of individuals with SCI.

1. Determine sensory levels for right and left sides.

2. Determine motor levels for right and left sides.
   *Note: in regions where there is no myotome to test, the motor level
   is presumed to be the same as the sensory level.*

3. Determine the single neurological level.
   *This is the lowest segment where motor and sensory function is nor-
   mal on both sides, and is the most cephalad of the sensory and
   motor levels determined in steps 1 and 2.*

4. Determine whether the injury is Complete or Incomplete
   (sacral sparing).
   *If voluntary anal contraction = **No** AND all S4-5 sensory scores = **0**
   AND any anal sensation = **No**, then injury is COMPLETE.
   Otherwise injury is incomplete.*

5. Determine ASIA Impairment Scale (AIS) Grade:

   Is injury Complete?   If **YES**, AIS=A Record ZPP
                              (For ZPP record lowest dermatome or myotome on
       NO ↓   each side with some (non-zero score) preservation)

   **Is injury
   motor incomplete?**   If **NO**, AIS=B
                              (Yes=voluntary anal contraction OR motor
       YES ↓   function more than three levels below the motor
                              level on a given side.)

   **Are at least half of the key muscles below the
   (single) neurological level graded 3 or better?**

       NO ↓   YES ↓

       AIS=C   AIS=D

   If sensation and motor function is normal in all segments, AIS=E
   *Note: AIS E is used in follow up testing when an individual with a
   documented SCI has recovered normal function. If at initial testing
   no deficits are found, the individual is neurologically intact; the
   ASIA Impairment Scale does not apply.*

---

the external anal sphincter or sensation at the mucocutane-
ous junction or both. Further delineation between incomplete classifications occurs based on the extent of preservation
of sensory or motor function below the level of injury.

A recent addition has been the Autonomic Standards
Assessment Form (Figure 20-5, *C*), which highlights autonomic function/dysfunction and can be used to complement
the ISCSCI standards.

APPLICATION TO THE PEDIATRIC POPULATION

Historically, the ISCSCI standards or ASIA examination has
routinely been the clinical tool used for assessing pediatric
patients with SCI. It is considered the gold standard assessment for assessing prognosis and outcomes, yet the actual
utility in the pediatric population has not been assessed until
recently. Recent work suggests that the ISCSCI exams may
have poor utility overall in children under 4 years of age, as
they were unable to complete the exam.[97] Additionally, the
results suggest poor cooperation of children age 10 and
under in terms of anxiety during the pin prick portion of
the discrimination exam. Results also showed low precision
in confidence intervals for total motor scores in children up

to the age of 15, bringing into question the reliability of the
motor examination.[97]

Additional questions revolve around the clinical validity
of the anorectal exam in classification of children with SCI,
particularly children who were injured prior to being potty
trained who have never had to conceptualize holding in a
bowel movement (which is the verbiage typically used during
the anal contraction portion of the exam).[134] Preteens and
teenagers may also have difficulty with the anorectal portion
of the examination because of privacy concerns.

The WeeSTeP, a complement to InSTeP, is an electronic
training module that has been developed to outline
pediatric considerations for the current ISCSCI standards
(www.asialearningcenter.org). Some modifications include
altering the method of approaching child, conducting sensory
testing in a nonthreatening manner, altering vocabulary used
to make it more child friendly, and giving the child sense of
control during test. Alternatives also include an observational
motor assessment or infant motor scale to a certain age. Most
important, however, is explaining to the parents/caregivers
the current standards, how classification may not be able to
be ascertained due to the child's age, and that repeated testing
during various points of follow-up will be used in an attempt

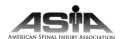

AUTONOMIC STANDARDS ASSESSMENT FORM
Patient Name: _____

ISC◉S

Anatomic Diagnosis: (Supraconal☐, Conal ☐, Cauda Equina☐)

General Autonomic Function

System/Organ	Findings	Abnormal conditions	Check mark
Autonomic control of the heart	Normal		
	Abnormal	Bradycardia	
		Tachycardia	
		Other dysrhythmias	
	Unknown		
	Unable to assess		
Autonomic control of blood pressure	Normal		
	Abnormal	Resting systolic blood pressure below 90 mmHg	
		Orthostatic hypotension	
		Autonomic dysreflexia	
	Unknown		
	Unable to assess		
Autonomic control of sweating	Normal		
	Abnormal	Hyperhydrosis above lesion	
		Hyperhydrosis below lesion	
		Hypohydrosis below lesion	
	Unknown		
	Unable to assess		
Temperature regulation	Normal		
	Abnormal	Hyperthermia	
		Hypothermia	
	Unknown		
	Unable to assess		
Autonomic and Somatic Control of Broncho-pulmonary System	Normal		
	Abnormal	Unable to voluntarily breathe requiring full ventilatory support	
		Impaired voluntary breathing requiring partial vent support	
		Voluntary respiration impaired does not require vent support	
	Unknown		

Lower Urinary Tract, Bowel and Sexual Function

System/Organ		Score
Lower Urinary Tract		
Awareness of the need to empty the bladder		
Ability to prevent leakage (continence)		
Bladder emptying method _____ (specify)		
Bowel		
Sensation of need for a bowel movement		
Ability to Prevent Stool Leakage (Continence)		
Voluntary sphincter contraction		
Sexual Function		
Genital arousal (erection or lubrication)	Psychogenic	
	Reflex	
Orgasm		
Ejaculation (male only)		
Sensation of Menses (female only)		

2 = Normal function, 1=Reduced or Altered Neurological Function
0=Complete loss of control NT=Unable to assess due to preexisting or concomitant problems

Urodynamic Evaluation

System/Organ	Findings	Check mark
Sensation during filling	Normal	
	Increased	
	Reduced	
	Absent	
	Non-specific	
Detrusor Activity	Normal	
	Overactive	
	Underactive	
	Acontractile	
Sphincter	Normal urethral closure mechanism	
	Normal urethral function during voiding	
	Incompetent	
	Detrusor sphincter dyssynergia	
	Non-relaxing sphincter	

Date of Injury_____   Date of Assessment_____   Examiner_____

This form may be freely copied and reproduced but not modified (Sp Cord, 2009, 47, 36-43)
This assessment should use the terminology found in the International SCI Data Set
C (ASIA and ISCoS - http://www.asia-spinalinjury.org/bulletinBoard/dataset.php)

Figure 20-5, cont'd

---

to identify neurologic change until the child is old enough to reliably complete the ISCSCI standards (or until a pediatric version becomes available to use as a clinical tool).

FUNCTIONAL ASSESSMENT

The Functional Independence Measure (FIM) (for adolescents), Functional Independence Measure for Children (WeeFIM),[1,105] Pediatric Evaluation of Disability Inventory (PEDI),[56,103] Pediatric Quality of Life (PedsQL), and Canadian Occupational Performance Measure (COPM) have all been used to describe function and measure outcomes for children with SCI; however, none fully identifies changes with recovery and rehabilitation in children with SCI.

The FIM and WeeFIM are measures used in acute rehabilitation across many diagnoses to determine the "burden

of care." These measures, when used with patients with SCI, may not be sensitive enough to detect change associated with return of function, and some areas tested have ceiling and floor effects. Additionally, a change in FIM or WeeFIM score may be based more on lack of injury severity rather than length of inpatient rehabilitation.[51] For example, in comparing a child with a complete cervical injury to a child with an incomplete thoracic injury, each of whom had a 4-week inpatient rehabilitation stay, the child with the incomplete thoracic injury may show a much larger change in FIM or WeeFIM scores. This change is more related to the fact that, based on level of injury, the amount of functional change is inherently greater as measured by the FIM or WeeFIM, rather than reflecting the amount of rehabilitation received.

Overall, there has not been one measure or test that is the most effective and efficient for children and adolescents with

SCIs. One option may be the Spinal Cord Independence Measure (SCIM), developed in 1994, which measures performance of daily activities in patients with spinal cord lesions. It has been shown to have strong construct validity (.8-1.4, p < .05), inter-rater reliability (SCIM III kappa .64-.84; ICC >.94) and sensitivity to change (SCIM II, 2001),[24-26] even when compared to the FIM.[25] Another option may be Computerized Adaptive Testing (CAT), which employs an algorithm and adapts the number of questions to each specific individual based on previous answers given to achieve the desired precision of scores for all children on a standard metric.[42] Work on development of parent and child-report CAT specifically for children with SCI has been completed,[21,95,96] and preliminary data collection is under way.

Regardless of which assessment tools are used, the physical therapist must establish a thorough baseline report of the child's abilities and activity and determine whether limitations are due to the child's age, primary neurologic changes in body function, secondary changes in body functions such as contractures, the need to wear a spinal orthosis, or other causes. Any standard physical therapy examination includes testing of the child's ability to reach, roll, position in bed, come to sitting, balance in sitting, scoot, crawl, transfer, come to kneel, stand, and ambulate. Some or all of these may not be possible, so the type and amount of assistance needed are recorded, or the therapist may simply record the movement as "unable."

REHABILITATION AND HABILITATION

Research in the adult population has shown that timely referral of patients with SCI to comprehensive, multidisciplinary SCI centers is more cost effective, with improved patient outcomes, reduced hospital and long-term nursing care charges, and an improved prospect for long-term patient earnings, compared with unspecialized care for SCI patients.[23]

The acute rehabilitation and long-term treatment of children with SCI require a comprehensive interdisciplinary approach involving both hospital and school-based personnel. Team members typically include physical therapists, physicians, nurses, a dietician, occupational and speech therapists, therapeutic recreation specialists, a social worker, an orthotist, a clinical psychologist, teachers, the child, and the family.

Physical therapists often work alongside a pediatric physiatrist, who typically provides medical management and serves as a team leader. In some centers, however, an orthopedist, a neurologist, or a pediatrician may fill this role. The lead physician may also request consultation by other physicians such as an orthopedic surgeon or neurosurgeon to monitor spine stability and alignment, a urologist to monitor urinary tract function, and a pulmonologist for ventilator management.

Physical therapists develop age-appropriate ROM, strengthening, and SCI-education programs. They address functional mobility, including bed mobility, transfers, sitting balance, ambulation, and basic and advanced wheelchair skills. The physical therapist makes recommendations on lower extremity orthoses and plays a primary role in the ordering of a wheelchair. Goals must be set according to usual expectations for age. Greater independence with varying degrees of transfers and mobility will be expected the older the child.

PHYSICAL THERAPY EXAMINATION AND INTERVENTION

Physical therapists should include parents as active participants during both the examination and treatment phases. Parents need to receive accurate, understandable information about their child's condition. Because they are trying to adapt to the sudden change in their child's health, they often are unable to generate therapy outcomes for their child beyond wanting the child "to walk again." The therapist and SCI team must assist the family and child in establishing realistic outcomes. One must consider the child's level of injury (see Tables 20-3 and 20-4), the completeness of injury, the age of the child, and the family's expectations for the child. Parents should be included in treatment sessions whenever possible. Although many children work better in therapy sessions in the absence of parents, parents should be regularly included to see the new skills their child can independently accomplish and the emerging skills that require assistance. Parents must become experts in all aspects of their child's mobility and use of adaptive equipment. Parent education and training should be an ongoing process that begins soon after the initial examination and is completed in time for practice on day or overnight outings.

The examination of the infant, young child, or adolescent with SCI is going to encompass many of the same areas of assessment but will require those areas to be tailored based on chronologic as well as developmental age. As previously mentioned, determination of motor and sensory levels in infants and young children is challenging and may require multiple examinations to determine what movement is voluntary and what is reflexively mediated. The therapist can determine activity limitations by comparing the infant's motor skills such as head control, rolling, sitting balance, transitional movements, crawling, and standing with expected developmental milestones. Very young children with SCI require careful follow-up over time to ensure that they meet functional goals and are not infantilized by caregivers.

Quantification of changes in body structure and function in the young child is often unreliable because young children are unable to cooperate consistently with formal testing. Passive ROM measurement is possibly an exception to this, but its rater and test-retest reliability in children with SCI has not been established. In children without SCI and in children with myelodysplasia, manual muscle testing is

TABLE 20-3   **Mobility in Complete Tetraplegia, Expected Function and Necessary Equipment for Level of Injury**

Functional Skill	C1–C4	C5	C6	C7–T1
Bed mobility	D	A, Even with electrical bed	I, May use equipment; electrical bed helpful	I, Electrical bed helpful
Transfers	D, May need mechanical lift	D, May need mechanical lift	Some I with or without sliding board	I, May need sliding board
Wheelchair	I, PWC, head, chin, mouth, or tongue control	I, PWC, hand control with splint	I, MWC, may use adapted rims; likely to use PWC in community	I, MWC
Pressure relief	D, Bed, MWC I, Power tilt PWC	D, Bed, MWC I, Power tilt PWC	I, Leaning to side	I, Push-up on open hands
Transportation	U, Driving; van with lift needed	I, Upper extremity controls; van with lift needed	I, Hand controls A, Load MWC	I, Hand controls I, Load MWC

Adapted from Massagli, T. L., & Jaffe, K. M. (1990). Pediatric spinal cord injury, Treatment and outcome. *Pediatrician, 17,* 244–254. Reprinted with permission of S. Karger, Basel.
A, Assistance required; D, dependent; I, independent; MWC, manual wheelchair; PWC, power wheelchair; U, unable.

TABLE 20-4   **Mobility in Complete Paraplegia, Expected Function and Necessary Equipment for Level of Injury**

Functional Skill	T2–T10	T11–L2	L3–S2
Manual wheelchair	I, Indoors and in community	I, Indoors and in community	May not need MWC except long distances, recreation
Ambulation	SBA, Exercise only; need KAFOs or RGOs and forearm crutches or walker; not practical for T2–T6	I, Indoors with KAFOs or RGOs and forearm crutches; some can do stairs with railing	I, Indoors and community with AFOs; may need forearm crutches or cane
Driving	I, Hand controls I, Load MWC	I, Hand controls I, Load MWC	Can drive automatic transmission; may prefer hand controls

Adapted from Massagli, T. L., & Jaffe, K. M. (1990). Pediatric spinal cord injury, Treatment and outcome. *Pediatrician, 17,* 244–254. Reprinted with permission of S. Karger, Basel.
AFOs, Ankle-foot orthoses; I, independent; KAFOs, knee-ankle-foot orthoses; MWC, manual wheelchair; RGOs, reciprocating gait orthoses; SBA, standby assistance.

generally unreliable if the child is younger than 5 years of age.[88,94] In young children, strength testing is often estimated by encouraging and observing movement. Ideally, the therapist places the child in various positions and encourages him or her to reach for toys with a single extremity. This allows examination of gravity-eliminated and antigravity movements, as well as comparison of left and right extremities. Resistance can be provided with small wrap weights (0.25 lb) or the weight of handheld toys. In reality, the best choice may be for the physical therapist to observe spontaneous play and record descriptions of available movements. The physical therapist also facilitates the child's basic postural responses, such as positive support of the lower extremities or protective extension of the upper extremities. Ruling out substitutions can be challenging. Muscle strength is recorded as 0 through 5, as with adults (rarely with the finer + or − gradations). Scores of 4 and 5 are subjective measures, particularly

in growing children, but with experience the therapist can become an increasingly more accurate evaluator.

Physical therapy intervention sessions will be structured around the child's motivation for play. Within that framework, the therapist designs activities that encourage strengthening, balance, reaching, rolling, sitting, transitions, and mobility in various combinations.

Sitting balance is often one of the major goals of therapy. Balance is impaired by altered strength and sensation and often by the presence of a spinal orthosis. Conversely, a child with tetraplegia or high paraplegia may benefit from a soft orthosis to facilitate sitting, leaving hands free for other activities (Figure 20-6). The seated child is encouraged to progress from therapist support to self-support at a tabletop or on a mat and to independent sitting if this is realistic given the level and completeness of injury. These goals may be achieved by engaging the child in play activities.

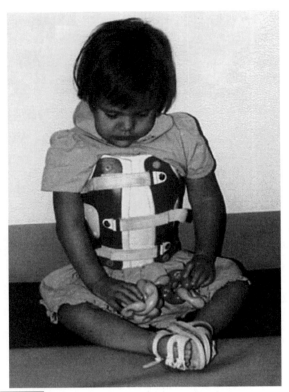

Figure 20-6 A soft orthosis provides external support, improving sitting balance and allowing this child with a high thoracic spinal cord injury to use both hands in play.

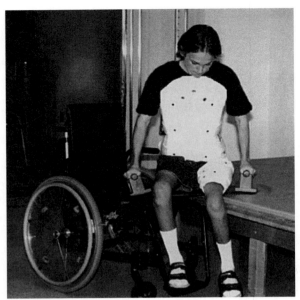

Figure 20-7 Teen wearing a thoracolumbosacral orthosis with a thigh piece that restricts hip flexion uses a sliding board and push-up blocks to begin learning transfers.

All innervated musculature must be strengthened, including muscles that have normal grade 5 strength because they will need to compensate for weakened or paralyzed muscles. Maintaining full ROM, particularly at specific joints, is imperative. For example, full ROM at the shoulders must be maintained for ease of dressing. Historically, patients with tetraplegia who have wrist extension but no hand function were provided with a stretching program that allowed them to develop mild finger flexor tightness to provide for a tenodesis grasp during wrist extension. Current recommendations, however, are to maintain a supple hand and to even splint with metacarpophalangeal flexion and interphalangeal extension ("intrinsic plus" position) to maintain this ROM. The change in practice is due to the evolution of upper extremity reconstructive surgery for the population with tetraplegia, which can augment wrist extension, grasp, lateral pinch, and finger extension. Stretching the hamstrings to allow 100° to 110° of hip flexion, and having adequate hip external rotation is necessary for dressing and self-care. It is important to have excessively flexible hamstrings to prevent overstretching of the low back. Ankle ROM must be maintained at neutral for proper placement on the wheelchair footrest.

A small number of children with tetraplegia have upper cervical injuries (C1-C3) that necessitate mechanical ventilation (see Chapter 23). Physical therapy for these children and for those with C4 tetraplegia has a more narrowed focus because the child is dependent in bed mobility, transfers, and sitting balance (see Table 20-3). Spasticity tends to be more problematic with this population, although daily passive ROM can help reduce tone and facilitate positioning. Physical therapy goals for this population focus on education, as the family must be thoroughly trained in all aspects of the child's mobility and care. Children must also be trained to instruct others in their care, including use and maintenance of the wheelchair, mechanical lift, environmental control unit (ECU), computer access, and any other equipment.

BED MOBILITY AND TRANSFER TECHNIQUES

Bed mobility and transferring techniques for children and adolescents are similar to those used for adults, and extended detail can be found in SCI rehabilitation textbooks.[46,120] Successful mobility focuses on maximizing biomechanics, using momentum, and understanding the head-hips relationship. The head-hips relationship, or concept of moving your head and upper trunk *opposite* to the direction you are moving and looking away from where you are moving in order to unweight the pelvis for transfers or mat mobility, is not intuitive for a child. Mastery of this concept, however, will open up much more opportunity for mobility.

For children with paraplegia and lower level tetraplegia (C6 and below), transfer training may initially include the use of a sliding board. Push-up blocks can also be helpful when first learning transfers (Figure 20-7). As upper extremity strength and balance increases, the child may be able to transfer without a sliding board. Types of transfers learned should include those for level and unlevel surfaces, as well as floor to wheelchair and wheelchair to floor. Older children should also learn how to transfer in and out of a vehicle. Young children can be physically capable in transferring themselves; however, they may require a caregiver's assistance from a safety standpoint as they may totally disregard their legs, putting themselves at risk for a lower extremity fracture. Rather than taking a lateral approach to the surface they wish to transfer to, young children may take more of an anterior approach and scoot forward/backward with their legs in either a long or ring-sit position. Children and adolescents with C5 and above tetraplegia are dependent for transfers and require either a caregiver to lift them or the use of a mechanical lift. In either situation, all caregivers must be educated in proper technique, and the child must be able to verbalize the steps needed to be taken for a safe transfer.

WHEELED MOBILITY

If community ambulation is not an expected outcome, the child needs a wheelchair for mobility. For young children with SCI at or above C6, a power wheelchair is needed for independent mobility. Some young children with lower levels of cervical SCI, or even high thoracic injuries, may be able to propel a manual wheelchair for only limited distances on smooth, level surfaces owing to lack of upper body strength and endurance. For these children to be exposed to a broader range of environments, such as preschool playgrounds or uneven or steep terrain around the family home, prescription of a power wheelchair is justifiable to promote age-appropriate functional mobility. A child as young as 18 to 24 months may be trained to use a power wheelchair but requires adult supervision for safety.[75,93] An ECU and a complex power wheelchair are needed for independent mobility when a joystick is not appropriate due to a higher level of injury. The joystick is replaced with head, tongue, or sip-and-puff controls and the power tilt must allow for ventilator placement. In addition, a manual tilt-in-space wheelchair is necessary to provide these children with a substitute when the power chair needs repairs. The manual wheelchair is also useful for transport in places where the larger, heavier power chair is impractical. Many families do not have a home with hallways or doors large enough to accommodate a power wheelchair, so power mobility may be used primarily in community and school settings and the manual wheelchair is used in the home.

Power-assist wheels are motorized wheels that can be added onto or are already a part of a manual wheelchair. These allow the user to provide some propulsion forces and the motors enhance their propulsion to allow them to be functional. This type of wheel is most applicable for patients with C6-T1 level injuries or where upper body endurance is lacking. Power-assist wheels do add weight to the wheelchair, but the trade-off is that there is still a manual wheelchair that can typically be transported in the trunk of a car, rather than a power chair that requires an adapted van or lift. One case series[31] demonstrates positive outcomes of independent

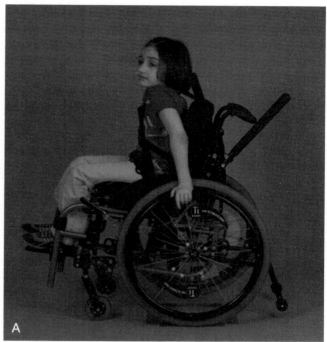

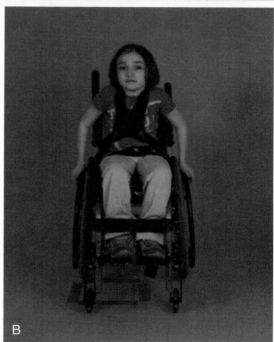

Figure 20-8 Manual wheelchair setup.

propulsion over terrain and ascending ramps in children, ages 7 to 11, with SCI or dysfunction affecting upper extremity strength

For children/adolescents for whom manual wheelchair propulsion is going to be the primary means of independent mobility, extra attention must be paid to the configuration of the wheelchair in addition to the weight of the chair (Figure 20-8). Focus is frequently placed on ultralightweight

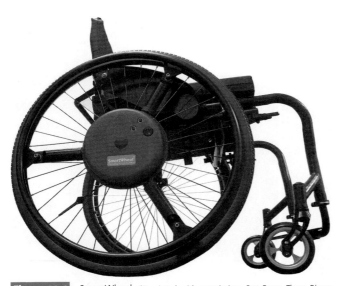

Figure 20-9 SmartWheel. (Reprinted with permission, Out Front, Three Rivers Holdings, LLC.)

materials; however, set-up is just as important, if not more so. Proper set-up details include, overall width and depth of the chair, axle placement, seat-to-floor height, wheel and rim size, caster size, and back type and height. Variances in set-up can now be quantified through the use of the SmartWheel (Figure 20-9), which measures propulsive forces, speed, and cadence.

The Paralyzed Veterans Association (PVA) has also published guidelines on proper wheelchair set-up in the adult population[35,75] to preserve the joints of the upper extremity, and because literature is lacking in the pediatric population,[75] one can only assume best practice is to carry over these same set-up guidelines to the pediatric population. Overuse injuries at the shoulder (rotator cuff impingement, capsular injury) and the wrist (carpal tunnel syndrome) are seen in a large percentage of the adult population. One can only assume that these same injuries occur in pediatrics, as they are pushing wheelchairs for more years, and presumably with more force, because the chair can weigh more than the child. Additionally, the tendency is to add backpacks on the back of the chair, only to increase the overall amount of weight the child needs to propel. Finally, often (Figure times the wheelchairs provided are larger than needed with the anticipation that the child will grow and the chair needs to "grow" with the child, particularly because insurers will only pay for a new chair approximately every 5 years. Manufacturers have designed chairs that can change seat width and depth, but often proper set-up is sacrificed. Other manufacturers have a trade-in program or "growth kit" option to allow for a more appropriately sized and set-up frame to be delivered when needed.

The seating components of either a power or manual wheelchair are prescribed with skin protection and spinal alignment in mind (see the Evolve chapter on assistive technology for additional information). A level pelvis decreases the amount of pressure placed over individual ischial tuberosities of the sacrum, thereby improving overall pressure distribution. A solid seat and back are preferred to sling upholstery in this age group. Many types of wheelchair cushions are available, but none is universally effective for maintaining skin integrity in all persons with SCI, and individual assessment is required to minimize ulcerative forces (pressure, shear, friction and moisture).

Wheelchair positioning and fit can also help to limit development of secondary peripheral neuropathies. Too frequently, peroneal nerve neuropathies are seen as a result of the lateral lower leg, just distal to the head of the fibula, resting against the front end or leg rest of the wheelchair. Additionally, some children and teens use an upper extremity to "hook" around a back cane of a wheelchair for either pressure relief or to assist with balance. Excessive pressure in the antecubital fossa over time may cause median nerve neuropathy.

The wheelchairs must be ordered as soon as possible, but it is likely that they will not arrive before discharge, so rental wheelchairs may be necessary. All wheelchairs and ECUs should be chosen by the rehabilitation team, child, and family in consultation with a knowledgeable vendor (see the Evolve chapter on assistive technology). The therapist should be aware of available funding for wheelchairs and other durable medical equipment. There may be limitations in coverage, and the therapist can assist the family in prioritizing equipment needs.

AMBULATION

Every parent and caregiver wants the child with an SCI to "walk again." Ambulation is feasible and can be tried with certain portions of this population; however, the goals for ambulation must be realistic. In many cases, ambulation does not replace the use of a wheelchair, as braced ambulation is both time and energy consuming. The swing-through gait pattern is, however, much more efficient than other gait patterns. Many adults who have reciprocating gait orthoses (RGOs) or knee-ankle-foot orthoses (KAFOs) prescribed do not use them at all in the long term, and the majority of the remaining patients use them only for standing or exercise. With higher-level injuries, ambulation is more of a therapeutic/exercise goal rather than a true functional goal. The cost of bracing and assistive devices must be balanced against the practicality of ambulation and the willingness of the patient and family to follow through with ambulation after discharge/training sessions. The most common reasons for discontinuing use of the braces are the excessive energy costs and the need for assistance to don and remove them for ambulation. Periodic reexamination of the child's physical abilities and outcomes as an outpatient can be used to determine whether ambulation with braces is a reasonable goal. Many patients become less interested over time in ambulation requiring extensive bracing as the permanence

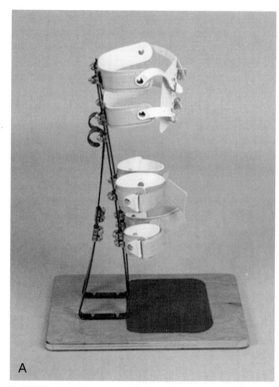

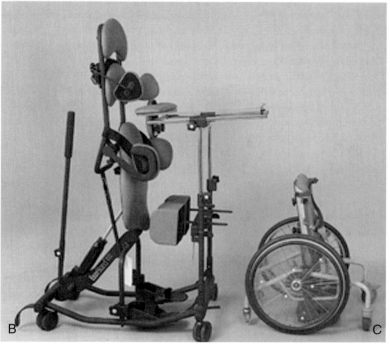

Figure 20-10 A, B, C Options for standing and walking.

of the injury becomes more apparent. Those who remain interested may have specific needs for standing or limited walking that increase the likelihood of long-term use of the orthoses.

The PVA has developed Clinical Practice Guidelines to aid in decision making regarding appropriate clinical goals and suggests using a stander for patients with injuries at T1 and higher, and either a stander or bracing for injuries below T1.[33] These guidelines, however, are based on the adult population; therefore, there may be some outliers in the pediatric population for whom these guidelines are inappropriate.

For those with levels of injury at T1 and below, ambulation is achieved via various types of bracing depending on level of injury and lower extremity muscle strength. For those with absent or limited active hip flexion, a hip-knee-ankle-foot orthosis (HKAFO) is typically prescribed. The hip joint can be locked for a swing-through gait pattern and unlocked to use active hip flexion for a reciprocal gait. Another option is an RGO, which has a cable system that allows for passive reciprocating gait, but the child must be adept at weight shifting and trunk extension. Children who have at least three-fifths strength in the quadriceps muscles or stronger hip flexors can achieve ambulation with KAFOs. Children with lower level injuries and some incomplete injuries may achieve independent ambulation with ankle-foot orthoses (AFOs). Ambulation typically also requires an upper extremity assistive device, particularly for those using H/KAFOs and RGOs. Gait training will typically be initiated in parallel bars and advance to use of an appropriate assistive device (typically front wheeled walkers or Loftstrand crutches) as the child improves in standing balance. Parastance, where the hips and lower trunk are in excessive extension and balance is achieved by resting on the y-ligaments in the hip, must be achieved in order for those ambulating with H/KAFOs to be successful. Donning and doffing, and general orthoses management, must be taught and practiced with both the child and caregivers. Controlled sit-to-stand transitions must also be practiced.

Preschool-age children (5 years and younger) are more likely to pursue ambulation, perform a higher level of ambulation, and ambulate for a longer number of years as compared to older children and adolescents.[133] Once these younger children enter the preteen and adolescent period, however, ambulation is typically abandoned for wheeled mobility beyond an indoor home or school level in order to keep up with peers.

For children who wish to be upright for physiologic and psychologic benefits but do not necessarily wish to ambulate, various devices are available. A standing frame (Figure 20-10, B) can be used for static standing, but there are also parapodiums (Figure 20-10, A) or swivel standers, which have a footplate that, in combination with an assistive device, allows a child to swivel her trunk for very short distance mobility. Mobile standers (Figure 20-10, C) are also available in which a child can assume a standing position while propelling with large, wheelchair-like wheels (see video for chapter 21).

Locomotor training (LT) is an activity-based therapy of assisted ambulation via body-weight-supported (BWS) treadmill training, which is typically followed by overground BWS ambulation or overground gait training with or without an assistive device. The term "activity-based therapy" is used to describe an intervention that results in neuromuscular activation below the level of spinal cord lesion to promote recovery of motor function, thus demonstrating the neuroplasticity of the spinal cord[8,9] A reported goal of LT is to stimulate the locomotor central pattern generators (CPGs) in the spinal cord.[47] It is believed that reflexive movements of ambulation can be restored by stimulating these CPGs through the repetitive motion.[47] This has been shown in a case report of a young child with a documented chronic (>16 months postinjury) incomplete (ASIA C) SCI who regained ambulation even though he had limited ability to isolate his lower extremity muscles.[8] Another case study in which LT was performed as part of a young child's acute inpatient rehabilitation demonstrated the return of isolated volitional contractions of lower extremity muscles and significant gains in functional mobility.[109] Research continues in this area, but early results are promising and suggest the potential value of incorporating LT into physical therapy intervention.

FUNCTIONAL ELECTRICAL STIMULATION CYCLING FOR SCI

Cycling with FES has gained increased popularity as a rehabilitation strategy to encourage neuroplasticity and health gains for people with SCI. FES during cycling can be performed at home, and cycles appropriately sized for children are now available (Figure 20-11). The cycles are FDA approved for children ages 4 years and older; however, the primary limiting factor is the child's size. Typically the bilateral quadriceps, hamstrings, and gluteal muscles are stimulated at the appropriate times during the revolution of the cycle. This intervention has been applied to people with SCI with and without lower extremity sensation. For children

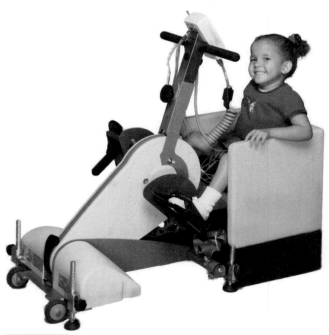

Figure 20-11 Three-year-old child with a T3-T7 SCI using the RT300-P FES cycle (Restorative-Therapies, Inc., Baltimore, Maryland). Photo reprinted with permission.

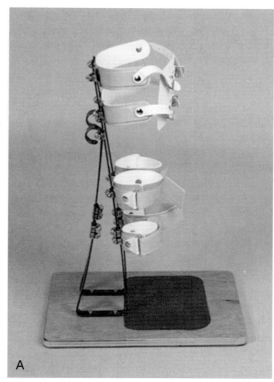

Figure 20-10 A, B, C   Options for standing and walking.

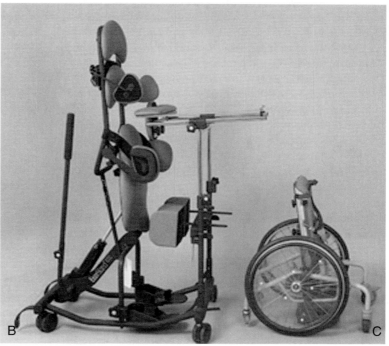

of the injury becomes more apparent. Those who remain interested may have specific needs for standing or limited walking that increase the likelihood of long-term use of the orthoses.

The PVA has developed Clinical Practice Guidelines to aid in decision making regarding appropriate clinical goals and suggests using a stander for patients with injuries at T1 and higher, and either a stander or bracing for injuries below T1.[33] These guidelines, however, are based on the adult population; therefore, there may be some outliers in the pediatric population for whom these guidelines are inappropriate.

For those with levels of injury at T1 and below, ambulation is achieved via various types of bracing depending on level of injury and lower extremity muscle strength. For those with absent or limited active hip flexion, a hip-knee-ankle-foot orthosis (HKAFO) is typically prescribed. The hip joint can be locked for a swing-through gait pattern and unlocked to use active hip flexion for a reciprocal gait. Another option is an RGO, which has a cable system that allows for passive reciprocating gait, but the child must be adept at weight shifting and trunk extension. Children who have at least three-fifths strength in the quadriceps muscles or stronger hip flexors can achieve ambulation with KAFOs. Children with lower level injuries and some incomplete injuries may achieve independent ambulation with ankle-foot orthoses (AFOs). Ambulation typically also requires an upper extremity assistive device, particularly for those using H/KAFOs and RGOs. Gait training will typically be initiated in parallel bars and advance to use of an appropriate assistive device (typically front wheeled walkers or Loftstrand crutches) as the child improves in standing balance. Parastance, where the hips and lower trunk are in excessive extension and balance is achieved by resting on the y-ligaments in the hip, must be achieved in order for those ambulating with H/KAFOs to be successful. Donning and doffing, and general orthoses management, must be taught and practiced with both the child and caregivers. Controlled sit-to-stand transitions must also be practiced.

Preschool-age children (5 years and younger) are more likely to pursue ambulation, perform a higher level of ambulation, and ambulate for a longer number of years as compared to older children and adolescents.[133] Once these younger children enter the preteen and adolescent period, however, ambulation is typically abandoned for wheeled mobility beyond an indoor home or school level in order to keep up with peers.

For children who wish to be upright for physiologic and psychologic benefits but do not necessarily wish to ambulate, various devices are available. A standing frame (Figure 20-10, B) can be used for static standing, but there are also parapodiums (Figure 20-10, A) or swivel standers, which have a footplate that, in combination with an assistive device, allows a child to swivel her trunk for very short distance mobility. Mobile standers (Figure 20-10, C) are also available in which a child can assume a standing position while propelling with large, wheelchair-like wheels (see video for chapter 21).

Locomotor training (LT) is an activity-based therapy of assisted ambulation via body-weight-supported (BWS) treadmill training, which is typically followed by overground BWS ambulation or overground gait training with or without an assistive device. The term "activity-based therapy" is used to describe an intervention that results in neuromuscular activation below the level of spinal cord lesion to promote recovery of motor function, thus demonstrating the neuroplasticity of the spinal cord[8,9] A reported goal of LT is to stimulate the locomotor central pattern generators (CPGs) in the spinal cord.[47] It is believed that reflexive movements of ambulation can be restored by stimulating these CPGs through the repetitive motion.[47] This has been shown in a case report of a young child with a documented chronic (>16 months postinjury) incomplete (ASIA C) SCI who regained ambulation even though he had limited ability to isolate his lower extremity muscles.[8] Another case study in which LT was performed as part of a young child's acute inpatient rehabilitation demonstrated the return of isolated volitional contractions of lower extremity muscles and significant gains in functional mobility.[109] Research continues in this area, but early results are promising and suggest the potential value of incorporating LT into physical therapy intervention.

FUNCTIONAL ELECTRICAL STIMULATION CYCLING FOR SCI

Cycling with FES has gained increased popularity as a rehabilitation strategy to encourage neuroplasticity and health gains for people with SCI. FES during cycling can be performed at home, and cycles appropriately sized for children are now available (Figure 20-11). The cycles are FDA approved for children ages 4 years and older; however, the primary limiting factor is the child's size. Typically the bilateral quadriceps, hamstrings, and gluteal muscles are stimulated at the appropriate times during the revolution of the cycle. This intervention has been applied to people with SCI with and without lower extremity sensation. For children

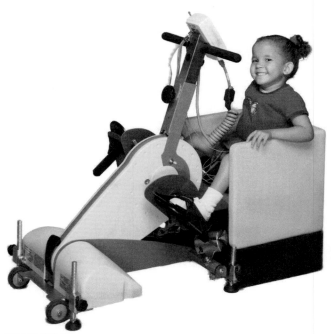

Figure 20-11   Three-year-old child with a T3-T7 SCI using the RT300-P FES cycle (Restorative-Therapies, Inc., Baltimore, Maryland). Photo reprinted with permission.

with sensation, the FES can be gradually applied and limited in intensity in order to not exceed the child's tolerance. Exercise protocols in the literature commonly involve cycling for 30 to 60 minutes three to five times per week at cadences of 40 to 50 revolutions per minute (rpm).[49] The ideal protocol, however, is not known, especially for children. The only published literature with children applied FES cycling for 60 minutes, three times per week, at a cadence of 40 to 50 rpm.[71]

Outcomes reported for FES cycling with adults include improvements in bone mineral density,[10,29,36] strength in stimulated muscles,[71] muscle size,[36,50,59] oxygen uptake,[36,60,71] cardiac output,[44,60] stroke volume,[44] and decreased adiposity.[59,114] There is one report of a man with a high cervical SCI experiencing recovery changing from an ASIA A SCI to an ASIA C.[89] In children, the literature is more limited with changes reported in bone mineral density,[71] oxygen uptake,[69,71] muscle volume,[71] stimulated muscle strength,[71] as well as decreased resting heart rate.[71] In addition, FES cycling has been shown not to increase the degree of hip subluxation after 6 months of cycling.[69]

FES FOR CHILDREN

Most clinically available applications for FES in pediatric SCI use electrodes placed on the skin surface with research applications using surface, percutaneous (inserted into the muscle but exit the skin), or implanted (all beneath the skin) electrodes. Commercially available surface systems are available for specific applications such as foot drop or hand function; however, most of these are not available in pediatric sizes. To provide these applications, a more generic neuromuscular electrical stimulation (NMES) device can be used, and the ability to use a trigger or switch to turn on the stimulation is important for FES applications. Common stimulation parameters for FES include pulse duration sufficient to create a muscle contraction (200 to 400 μsec) and a low frequency, measured in pulses per second (pps) (20 to 30 pps) to minimize fatigue. On and off times will be determined by the activity itself and ramp time can be set for comfort or to minimize spasticity as long as it does not impact the timing of the activity (i.e., during gait when on times are very short).[71]

For all FES applications, a critical portion of the evaluation is the determination of the ability to stimulate the muscle.[98,123] With a lower motor neuron injury, muscle cannot be adequately stimulated and FES is therefore not appropriate.[67] For example, a child with a C5 SCI is likely to have lower motor neuron damage to C6, and thus stimulation for wrist extension may be problematic. A thorough evaluation using electrical stimulation will provide information as to what muscles are appropriate for FES applications.

FES walking options using surface stimulation include the ParaStep[2] system for standing and walking. The ParaStep uses the peroneal withdrawal reflex to mimic a step, allowing the leg to advance.[74] Although the ParaStep is only approved

for use when skeletally mature, the peroneal withdrawal reflex can be obtained using a portable NMES unit and a trigger if desired for children with incomplete SCI who have some ability to maintain stability during stance. For this technique, an electrode is placed near the fibular head and stimulation intensity is set high enough to cause the leg to withdraw into flexion. Another option during gait for a child with an incomplete SCI is to use a portable NMES unit to create dorsiflexion.[108] For both applications during gait, a switch can be placed into the shoe to control the timing of the FES. Commercially available devices specifically designed to aid dorsiflexion for foot clearance can be used, such as the WalkAide[3] and NES L300.[4] Neither of these devices is made in pediatric sizes, but cuff and electrode size modifications with the WalkAide system have made this system successful with some young children.

Implanted devices have been used in pediatric clinical and research applications including facilitation of grasp, standing and walking, bladder and bowel function,[121] and phrenic pacing. The only FDA-approved device for children is the breathing pacemaker.[5] With this device, bilateral phrenic nerve electrodes are placed thoracoscopically and after a period of conditioning can provide full time ventilatory support without a mechanical ventilator.[43] A report of nine children implanted with the breathing pacemaker showed that eight were able to meet their pacing goals.[116]

EXERCISE AND FITNESS

Cardiovascular fitness is a major health concern in the SCI population. Adults with tetraplegia have a 16% increased risk of cardiovascular diseases as compared to the general population, whereas those with paraplegia have a 70% greater risk of coronary artery disease (a subset of the cardiovascular diseases).[99] Greater risk (44%) of cardiovascular diseases is also seen with complete versus incomplete SCI. The prevalence of cardiovascular disease in the SCI population is difficult to estimate because of presence of silent ischemia that goes undetected, but cardiovascular disease has been reported to be the leading cause of death for people with SCI of greater than 30 years duration. These data suggest that interventions are desperately needed to decrease the incidence of cardiovascular disease in the SCI population.[99]

People with SCI tend to lead sedentary lifestyles, which further increases their risk for coronary heart disease (CHD).[63] The level of inactivity seen in the SCI population poses a serious health risk because of the accompanying secondary health complications of CHD, obesity and diabetes.[53,107] Voluntary exercise, however, is difficult for many people with SCI based on the extent of the paralysis, lack of proper exercise equipment, and lack of trained professionals to provide guidance. Although people with paraplegia have more capability to exercise, they are not more fit than people with tetraplegia who have fewer exercise options.[100] In addition, 25% of healthy young people with SCI lack the fitness levels to perform important daily activities.[100] Given the significant impact that SCI has on cardiovascular health, compounded with the lack of availability and need for exercise in this population, there is a dire need for exercise interventions.

Regular exercise can decrease the extent of the metabolic, skeletal, and muscle complications for people with SCI.[97] Some options for exercise include upper extremity ergometry, FES-assisted activity, swimming, and adapted sports.[63,99] Strong level 1 evidence exists for the ability of upper extremity exercise to improve cardiovascular fitness and oxygen uptake.[136] Central effects (heart and lungs) of exercise reported with people with SCI include increases in peak oxygen uptake up to 65%, as well as improvements in stroke volume of approximately 16%.[107] In addition, regular exercise can have a positive impact on lipid profiles[99,136] and glucose homeostasis.[136] The evidence suggests that more intense exercise than currently being performed may be needed to have an impact on lipids post SCI, and that effects are possible with both arm exercise and FES cycling.[136]

Little research has been done on health and fitness in children with SCI, but with the increasing prevalence of obesity among children as a whole, intervening early with children with SCI may help to develop healthy habits that persist into adulthood. The research done indicates that 10- to 21-year-old children with SCI have an increased incidence of metabolic syndrome (present in 11 out of 20 children),[101] decreased lean tissue mass compared to overweight and control subjects,[80] increased fat mass (by 22.9% with paraplegia and 25.9% with tetraplegia),[87] and decreased aerobic capacity compared to controls.[134] In addition, children 5 to 13 years of age have been shown to have decreased aerobic capacity.[68] Exercise interventions targeting some of these deficits have been limited.[79] Liusuwal and colleagues[80] studied the outcomes of a 16-week program targeting nutrition, exercise (aerobic and resistance training), and lifestyle change and reported increases in lean body tissue and in power and efficiency during an upper extremity ergometry test. Johnston and colleagues[70] studied the effects of 6 months of FES cycling and reported increases in peak oxygen uptake during an upper extremity ergometry test. These studies suggest that exercise can have a positive impact on the health of children with SCI; however, more research is needed to determine optimal ways to address the health concerns for people with SCI.

SPORTS AND RECREATION

Therapists should encourage regular aerobic exercise in children and young adults with SCI to help them develop lifelong habits of health promotion, particularly because of their general tendency toward lower-intensity, more sedentary leisure activities.[66] With childhood obesity and type 2 diabetes rates on the rise in the pediatric population, those

with SCIs are at greater risk. A majority of children and teens are not involving themselves in organized activities such as sports, clubs, or those offered by youth centers.[75] Therapeutic recreation specialists facilitate participation in an adaptive physical education program, community-based recreational programs for people with disabilities, or competitive wheelchair sports. Offering specific recreation programs during inpatient rehabilitation or camps after discharge can significantly contribute to overall rehabilitation and quality-of-life outcomes.

MAXIMIZING ACTIVITY AND PARTICIPATION

While hospitalized, the child and adolescent must practice mobility skills outside the structured therapy sessions. For instance, nurses should be updated on progress in mobility skills so that the child can be encouraged to incorporate these abilities into play activities or getting to meals.

Community and school reentry activities are often the combined responsibility of physical therapists, occupational therapists, and therapeutic recreation specialists. Children must become familiar with common architectural barriers such as curbs, heavy doors, and high shelves and learn how to negotiate them or ask for help. Caregivers need to be trained in the type and amount of assistance to provide and cautioned against being overly helpful. Teenagers should be encouraged to problem solve the management of architectural barriers and ask for assistance if safety is jeopardized. Discharge planning and long-term management should address mobility issues in the child's home, school, and community. Whenever possible, a home evaluation should be conducted early in the child's hospital stay. If home modifications are necessary for wheelchair accessibility or safety, the family needs time to gather financial resources and complete modifications. These modifications can be evaluated during weekend passes. Public schools employ physical therapists and occupational therapists who can provide accessibility information while the child is still hospitalized. Upon school entry, the child can be assisted with accommodations under the provisions of Section 504 of the Vocational Rehabilitation Act of 1973.[128] The therapist plays a major role as a consultant to the school administration, faculty, family, and student regarding accessibility issues and needed modifications to architectural barriers or curriculum. For children living great distances from the hospital, physical therapists in the school can provide a local perspective and become a resource to the family.

Another area of concern in community reentry is safe transportation. The physical therapist can assist the family with evaluating safe transportation of their child. If a van will be used, wheelchair tie-downs will be necessary. If the child can sit in a vehicle seat, appropriate car seats, booster seats, or wheelchair tie-down system are needed, depending on the child's age and amount of trunk and neck control. For teenagers, friends may need to be trained in car transfers so that the patient can stay socially active. The teenager returning to driving needs to be independent with transfers and with loading and unloading the wheelchair.

PSYCHOSOCIAL ASPECTS

A team member skilled in mental health should monitor the child's adaptation to disability and be available to help the child verbally process the injury and rehabilitation. This could be a skilled social worker, but if a behavior management program using reinforcers is needed, a clinical psychologist should be consulted. In rare cases, the child may truly be clinically depressed, and a psychiatrist can be consulted if a medication trial is contemplated. As described by Fordyce,[48] acquisition of an SCI accompanied by pain, medical complications, altered cosmesis, and body image, and the new and challenging rehabilitation procedures can be expected to have a significant impact on the patient's affect, self-esteem, and behavior. The child's adjustment to SCI does not necessarily follow predictable stages of crisis response such as shock, denial, depression, and adaptation. Adjustment to SCI probably occurs over several years. The verbal or attitudinal expressions of children with a new SCI are less predictive of outcome than are their behaviors. Physical therapists can facilitate adjustment by actively engaging the child in acquiring the skills needed to maximize independence. Therapists must include parents and caregivers when teaching these skills to children and adolescents, and they must not forget the importance of incorporating peers for adolescents. The psychologist or psychiatrist may also need to confront issues of premorbid risk-taking behavior or even substance abuse. Psychologists, nurses, and pediatric physiatrists collaborate in discussing sexuality and changes in sexual functioning with teenagers who have had SCI. Sexuality is often a difficult topic to approach with teens and their caregivers. If a teen is not ready to verbalize questions or concerns related to sexuality, there are a number of online resources from adult Spinal Cord Injury Model Systems that may provide additional assistance, such as University of Alabama at Birmingham (www.spinalcord.uab.edu).

A concern commonly expressed by teenagers is that of not being able to trust their bodies. The altered motor and sensory processes and potential changes in bowel and bladder function can make their bodies feel foreign to them. In addition, teenagers are accustomed to privacy and independence in their lives. Both their injury and subsequent reliance on a hospital environment, adaptive equipment, and caregivers can disrupt their sense of control. The rehabilitation team should respect their privacy and allow them to participate in scheduling therapy, nursing care, and free time.

QUALITY OF LIFE

Chronic pain has been determined to be one of the most common[63] and limiting factors in terms of quality of life following SCI, resulting in decreased perceived mental and physical health, as well as decreased activity levels[130] (although activity does not seem to decrease as significantly as in the adult population[65]). Musculoskeletal pain is most prevalent in the shoulder, elbow, and wrist. Visceral pain is also frequently identified, particularly originating from the genitourinary tract, as is neuropathic pain.[64]

Depression can hinder quality of life and life satisfaction as it limits community participation and self-inclusion in activities. Adults with pediatric-onset SCI experience depression to varying degrees, which is related to medical complications, perceived mental-health quality of life, occupation, and severity of their injuries (complete versus incomplete).[5]

FOLLOW-UP AND TRANSITION TO ADULTHOOD

The key to ensuring maximal participation in young children with SCI is to provide ongoing examination of impairments and activity and to regularly update expected outcomes that are appropriate. At least two mechanisms are available to accomplish this objective. Children who are discharged from rehabilitation centers are routinely seen in follow-up visits two or more times each year. These reassessments include medical follow-up to reexamine the level and completeness of injury, to evaluate changes in bladder and bowel function and skin integrity, to monitor the spine for development of scoliosis, and to determine the need for medications to treat spasticity or bladder or bowel incontinence.

Reexamination by the physical therapist is an important part of these follow-up visits. Any neurologic changes should be noted, including changes in ROM, strength, sensation, and spasticity. For children, age-appropriate habilitative skills can be taught (i.e., self-catheterization, skin checks, advanced wheelchair skills, and transfers). The wheelchair should be reassessed and adapted as needed to accommodate the child's growth and to ensure that any modifications enhance positioning and propulsion independence.

The physical therapy reexaminations at the rehabilitation facility follow a consultative model. The ongoing progress toward age-appropriate outcomes may occur in a hospital-based outpatient therapy program, but it is more typically accomplished through therapy services offered in early intervention programs or in publicly funded schools. Therapists in these programs ideally are in contact with the rehabilitation centers on a regular basis to update progress and goals and to identify new concerns and equipment needs.

Although the majority of young school-age children with SCI receive direct physical therapy and occupational therapy services in school, few adolescents receive such services. The therapist works from a consultant model, using the faculty and student to carry out programs and recommendations. Issues may include supporting the teen to continue with regular pressure releases, stretching and other home programs, and progressing mobility skills to community distances. The physical therapist and occupational therapist should also consult with the faculty and student regarding an appropriate physical education program; modification of classroom and desk set-up; and accessibility to lockers, bathroom, and lunchroom. In reality, many adolescents with SCI have no physical education program, face problems of accessibility at school, and report that breakdown of wheelchairs (both power and manual) contributes to absences at school.[83] Although completion of education is supported by accommodations and modifications, such supports are more often implemented to enhance the child's participation in classroom activities and are not geared toward competitive performance and productivity. Therapists should assist adolescents in achieving independence with assistive technology for mobility, communication, and environmental control. Skills development in directing and managing human assistants may also be needed.[41] We have also found that few adolescents with SCI receive educational or vocational counseling beyond selection of classes each term.[83] Such students may qualify for transition planning under the Individuals with Disabilities Education Act, Public Law 105-17.[127] School physical therapists might participate in a transition program by assessing functional mobility skills in the community or work-study setting. When teenagers with SCI become 18 years of age, they are eligible in the United States for state vocational counseling services. Such services are often important sources of funding for vocationally related education or even equipment. The importance of facilitating education and employment is underscored by research showing that life satisfaction of adults with pediatric-onset SCI is associated with education, income, satisfaction with employment, and social opportunities, but not with level of, age at, or duration of SCI.[131]

For teenagers, follow-up visits should also include discussions related to sexuality and reproduction.[78] Fertility in women is not impaired by SCI but sexual response and orgasm may be. Pregnant women with SCI should be managed at high-risk medical centers to avoid respiratory and urinary tract complications, detect threatened preterm births, and prevent autonomic dysreflexia during delivery. Although the majority of males with SCI can have erections, these are often fleeting and not adequate for vaginal penetration. Few men with SCI have ejaculations, and sperm quality decreases over time for reasons that are not entirely clear. New techniques for retrieval of sperm and for artificial insemination have helped some men with SCI to father children. In addition to this physiologic information, it is important to include issues of intimacy and relationships in candid discussions of sexuality.

Successful transition to adulthood is a goal of all children/adolescents with SCI. The rehabilitation team plays an important role in fostering success. Transition into a Spinal Cord Injury Model System (www.mscisdisseminationcenter.org) is ideal to continue specialized care; however, travel to such facilities may not be feasible. Continued care from a specialized center will not only provide optimum medical care, but also support services required for seeking education, vocational development, and independent living. Many adults with pediatric-onset SCI do complete an education level equivalent to noninjured peers; however, their employment rate, income, rate of independent living, and marital status do not correlate with noninjured peers.[4] See Chapter 32 for more information.

SUMMARY

Physical therapy for the child with SCI can, at first glance, appear straightforward. Preserving ROM and promoting strength and endurance are the cornerstones for the functional achievement predicted by the level of injury. Yet predicting realistic long-term outcomes and attaining them require respect for the broader and more complex picture. The physical therapist must consider the cause of the injury (progressive versus stable), the completeness of the injury (preserved motor function, sensory function), and the potential for, or presence of, secondary complications (scoliosis, skin breakdown, contractures). The therapist must also be sensitive to the child's age, personal and environmental factors, and the child's ability to meet age-appropriate expectations in the home, school, and community. Unlike adults with SCI, who may be very close to expected levels of independence at discharge from inpatient rehabilitation, children often require years of outpatient therapy to achieve optimal outcomes. Thus, it becomes imperative to provide the child and the family with a team approach incorporating multiple disciplines and settings to maximize the child's potential for functional independence and participation in life roles.

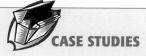

CASE STUDIES

"Stacy"

This case study demonstrates the physical therapy management of a very young child with assumed complete tetraplegia and highlights the importance of parent education and training. The need to monitor the acquisition of skills is also discussed.

Stacy was injured at 9 months of age. She was an unrestrained passenger in an MVC. Although she did not sustain bone injury to the spine, MRI revealed a C6 to T1 intracord hemorrhage. Formal manual muscle testing could not be conducted because of her age, so gross estimates of muscle strength were made, based on observed active movements in play, and documented as such. Shoulder flexion strength was estimated at grade 4, elbow flexion at grade 3, and elbow extension at grade 2. Wrist extension strength was estimated at grade 3, with movements of the fingers graded at trace. Pinprick sensory examination was conducted by looking only for some type of response (facial grimace, withdrawal response), but reactions were difficult to interpret, and she did not appear to have reliable pinprick in the lowest sacral dermatome. Pinprick in the lower extremities induced triple flexion (hip and knee flexion with ankle plantar flexion) involuntary responses. An approximate ISCSCI level/impairment score of C5 ASIA A was determined. Even though the key muscles for C6, the wrist extensors, were grade 3 in strength, the next higher key muscle was not grade 5. Therefore, a level of C5 was assigned.

At her initial physical therapy examination, Stacy had normal passive ROM with the exception of tightness noted at the end range of shoulder flexion and abduction and elbow extension. Functionally, Stacy was unable to roll, and when placed prone on her elbows could sustain the position only very briefly. When placed in sitting with full trunk support, she could raise her head to within about 20° of vertical.

After approximately 2 weeks of acute medical care, Stacy was transferred to an inpatient pediatric rehabilitation facility. Considering her age and level of injury, physical therapy interventions and outcomes were targeted at three major areas (see Table 20-3).

Within approximately 2 weeks, Stacy's caregivers had learned and demonstrated competence in all aspects of her care, and she was discharged to her home. At that time, she continued to show good ROM and some increase in using her upper torso musculature. From an activity standpoint, Stacy was able to reach against gravity when lying supine and to assist minimally in rolling herself to the side. When positioned in prone on her elbows, she was able to maintain her head upright intermittently for 1 to 2 minutes. She was unable to roll out of prone into supine. When in sitting, she was able to prop herself on her arms with some success.

Therapy services were transitioned to a community-based Birth to Three program, and she began to receive physical therapy and occupational therapy two times per week with a focus on trunk control, upper extremity weight bearing, and the facilitation of developmental milestones.

By 1 year after SCI, at 21 months of age, Stacy's elbow extensor strength had improved to an approximate grade 3 and she had a pincer grasp bilaterally but weak finger flexion and no finger extension. She did not show substantial changes in ROM or tone, but she demonstrated continued improvement in her functional skills. She was able to move from prone to supine independently. When placed in a sitting position, she could maintain the position but needed to use her hands for support. Stacy was able to move from sitting to prone by moving onto her forearms over her legs. She was able to "commando crawl" 5 to 10 feet by pulling with her arms.

Stacy's family reported two major concerns. The first was whether Stacy would eventually be able to walk with braces. Her prognosis was discussed, and the concept of the use of a wheelchair was introduced. Benefits of increasing her strength and increasing her independence in mobility were emphasized. It was also emphasized that the use of the wheelchair would in no way hinder her potential ability to walk someday if she were to have neurologic return of function. The other concern was that of headaches and flushing of the face that the family had noted. This raised the question of autonomic dysreflexia. The family was instructed in taking Stacy's BP when these episodes occurred. The visiting home nurse was also contacted to help assess this.

When Stacy was 2.5 years old, her examination revealed continued gains in finger flexion strength but no change in finger extension. Formal manual muscle testing was still not possible because of her age. Her sensory examination revealed no response to pinprick below the C7 dermatome. Her physical therapy examination revealed further improvements in function. Stacy was able to independently commando crawl and transition from a prone position to a sitting position without difficulty. Her sitting balance had improved, and she could reach for and play with toys but needed to keep one hand on the floor for support. She was beginning to scoot backward in sitting and pivot in prone. In addition to notable improvement in hand strength, overall hand function was better. Owing to her growth and improvements in upper extremity function, a trial use of a manual wheelchair was conducted. Stacy was able to sit well with hip guides and a pelvic belt on a solid seat with a solid back. She was able to propel only minimally during the initial trial. A wheelchair prescription was provided, with recommendations for a solid seat and back, hip guides and pelvic belt, and a headrest and chest harness (used for future school-bus transportation). Over the next months, Stacy learned to self-propel short distances with some difficulty.

By age 3.5, Stacy was receiving physical therapy once a week at school and once a week at a local hospital. Stacy was fitted for a pair of HKAFOs because her parents were very interested in a trial of standing and ambulation. It was explained that with Stacy's level of injury, this would probably only be a therapeutic activity and would not result in independent functional ambulation. Her community therapists provided gait training with the orthoses and a posture control walker. The other issue discussed at the SCI clinic was prescription of a car seat. She had outgrown her car seat but had poor trunk control, necessitating an adapted car seat instead of a standard booster seat.

Continued

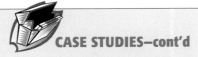

CASE STUDIES—cont'd

Stacy returned to the SCI clinic at age 4. Therapy services were unchanged. She was now able to sit briefly without arm support. With moderate to maximal assistance, she could walk a short distance with a walker and HKAFOs, employing a swing-through gait pattern. Although Stacy exhibited improving upper extremity function, it was discussed with her family that she would probably not attain enough strength in the upper extremities to keep up with her peers at school or in her rural home setting in a manual wheelchair and that a power wheelchair would be necessary. They agreed and tried power wheelchair mobility. Stacy enjoyed the independent movement and demonstrated good control of the chair using a proportional joystick with a small knob. A power wheelchair with head, trunk, and hip supports and belt was ordered for her. A wheelchair cushion was also ordered. Her school therapist supervised a power wheelchair training program. A sliding board was also ordered so she could begin transfer training.

When seen in the SCI clinic at age 6, Stacy was able to scoot in all directions independently. She was able to pull herself up onto furniture. She was able to walk a short distance using HKAFOs and a walker using a swing-through gait pattern, but with great effort and only in therapy. She was lifted for all transfers. She used her power wheelchair at school and used her manual wheelchair at home. She was often pushed in her manual wheelchair, as she had difficulty with directionality and endurance when she self-propelled. It was emphasized to her parents that it was important for Stacy to learn to do transfers and to improve her manual wheelchair skills in order to give her more independence.

Stacy was again seen in the clinic at age 7. At this visit, she was finally able to cooperate for formal manual muscle testing and sensory examination. She had grade 5 shoulder flexion and abduction, elbow flexion, and wrist extension strength and grade 4 elbow extension. Finger flexors were grade 3 and finger abductors grade 2. Grip strength was 1 kg bilaterally. She had intact sensation to C7. Her level of injury was redefined as C7 tetraplegia, ASIA Impairment Scale level A. She was now receiving therapy only at school. She was able to transfer with moderate assistance using the sliding board. She used her HKAFOs infrequently and had become fearful of standing in them. She was able to propel her manual wheelchair only over level indoor surfaces and preferred the power wheelchair for mobility. Adjustments for growth were ordered for her manual wheelchair. It was recommended that therapy continue to focus on transfer training and wheelchair skills. Ambulation training was discussed, and the relative benefits of this for lower extremity ROM and upper extremity exercise were contrasted with the need to develop functional independence in transfers and wheelchair use. It was suggested that Stacy continue to use the orthoses if she was interested and motivated but that the main focus in therapy should be on transfer training and wheelchair skills.

Reflections on Practice

Therapists must be careful, clear, and concise when educating parents and caregivers on ISCSCI Standards/ASIA Impairment scale level, as it is a "label" that tends to follow a patient across the continuum. A better practice may be to utilize an observational motor assessment or infant motor scale early on and use standard testing once the child can participate, as noted by age 7; however, even then sensory testing may not be accurate. Therapists also will frequently encounter families who remain hopeful that their child will ambulate. In fact, even limited ambulation may be more practical at such an early age than using a power wheelchair inside a small home. Note that, by age 7, the child in this case had lost interest in ambulation secondary to fear. At this point, discussions about alternative means of upright positioning should be discussed, such as use of a static or mobile standing frame. Power mobility was not initiated until Stacy was of school age because of space limitations in the home, even though she could have been successful with power mobility much earlier (18 to 24 months). Additionally, the family may not have been psychologically ready to accept the use of a power wheelchair. The family must be on board with equipment prescription; otherwise, there is the risk of technology abandonment. The configuration of the manual wheelchair, as well as strength limitations, may have inhibited Stacy's early success with manual wheelchair mobility. Special attention must be made to the set-up of the manual chair to promote proper biomechanical alignment for propulsion, although because of her young age at initiation of propulsion, Stacy just may not have had the upper extremity strength necessary to propel the chair. Reverse configuration, where the large wheel is in front and small wheel in the back, may have also been an option when she was attempting to propel a manual wheelchair at a young age.

In helping the family and child set realistic goals and outcomes, the therapist must keep an eye to the future, to consider the functional environments a child will face in the home, school, community, and ultimately the workplace. The basic skills of transfers, wheelchair mobility, and being able to direct one's own care must be incorporated at appropriate developmental stages. Stacy would have benefited from the now available soft trunk orthosis (see Figure 20-6) to facilitate sitting and free her hands for play, while helping to limit the development of a neuromuscular scoliosis.

"Alex"

This case study illustrates the acquisition of skills with growth and development in a school-age child with an SCI. Medical complications, both in the acute phase and over time, are discussed because of their impact on function.

Alex was injured in a high-speed MVC at age 5. He was restrained with a lap/shoulder seatbelt but no booster seat. He had an L3-L4 ligamentous tear with right facet dislocation and a right T10 pedicle fracture with cord damage. He was diagnosed with T10 paraplegia, ASIA Impairment Scale level A. He underwent L3-L4 open reduction and internal fixation and fusion, using a right posterior iliac bone graft. He had intestinal injuries and underwent small bowel resection and had a colostomy. A gastrostomy tube was placed several days later to help decompress his stomach. He was fitted with a TLSO with

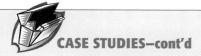

CASE STUDIES—cont'd

a cutout for his gastrostomy tube and colostomy. Two weeks after injury, Alex was transferred to a pediatric inpatient rehabilitation unit.

It took several sessions to complete tests and measures for the physical therapy examination. The therapist initially scheduled short sessions and spent much of the time playing, developing rapport, and employing strategies that helped decrease Alex's anxiety and improve participation. Upper extremity strength was within normal limits, although endurance for activities was decreased. Straight leg raise was to 50° bilaterally. All other passive ROM was within normal limits. Movement was absent, and sensation appeared to be so below the T10 level. There was no lower extremity spasticity. Alex required maximal assistance for all of his mobility, including rolling, getting into and out of sitting, sitting balance, and transfers. He could not self-propel a wheelchair. He frequently complained of stomach pain, and pancreatitis was diagnosed.

Over the next month, Alex adjusted well to the hospital rehabilitation environment. His cooperation and participation improved. Therapy was done in the context of play. Skills were taught starting with small components, and therapy was structured to ensure maximal success. Intervention focused on sitting balance, bed mobility, and transfers. Sliding board, push-up blocks, and leg loops were used to facilitate transfers and bed mobility.

ROM exercise was provided with a focus on hamstring stretching and Alex began learning basic wheelchair skills. Purchase of his own lightweight wheelchair with a pressure-relieving cushion was initiated. Plastic AFOs were fabricated for nightwear to prevent ankle plantar flexion contractures. After 3.5 months, Alex met the discharge outcome expectations, which were set based on his age and level of injury, and went home (Box 20-1).

Integration into school was carefully coordinated with Alex' school district. He began half-day kindergarten and received occupational therapy two times per week at school. Physical therapy was initially provided on a consultative basis through the SCI clinic.

Alex was seen 1 year after injury in the clinic. Lower extremity spasticity had developed, and hip flexor tightness was noted. He was referred for outpatient physical therapy for upper extremity strengthening, lower extremity ROM exercise, and more advanced wheelchair skills (Box 20-2).

In the first years after injury, Alex was introduced to adaptive sports, and he became an enthusiastic and talented skier, swimmer, and track competitor. Mild hip flexion contractures developed during these years, and scoliosis was diagnosed at age 7.

Three years after injury, Alex expressed interest in a walking trial. He did this over the summer with an episode of intense physical therapy at the regional children's hospital. KAFOs were fabricated initially and a pelvic piece was added later. Because of his hip flexion contractures and lower extremity spasticity, he had a difficult time donning the orthotics. He was unable to lock his hips into extension when standing. Thus, while able to walk in the parallel bars, he was unable to independently walk outside of them with a walker. He decided to continue to work on walking with his outpatient physical therapist during the school year. Nine months later, Alex stopped his ambulation attempts because of lack of progress. He asked about the use of FES for ambulation and, after learning that the current state of technology did not result in functional ambulation, decided to not pursue this option. He was discharged from outpatient physical therapy at age 10.

By age 12, wheelchair skills improved to include negotiating steeper inclines and higher curbs. Alex was fully independent in wheelchair mobility with the exception of loading his wheelchair into a vehicle. He competed in sports at the national level. At 12.5 years of age, he developed painful right forearm tendonitis. He used a rental power wheelchair for several months because propelling his manual wheelchair aggravated the tendonitis. Anti-inflammatory drugs were prescribed along with outpatient physical therapy for strengthening. Later that same year at the SCI clinic, he described posterior axillary pain. Examination revealed muscular imbalance with weak external rotators as a likely cause. He was instructed in a home program of strengthening. Hip flexor tightness was worsening despite a program of active stretching and passive stretching using the prone position.

By age 14 Alex's scoliosis had increased to 55° and a posterior spinal fusion was done. Postoperatively, Alex was restricted in his sports activities. At the SCI clinic that year, his hip flexion contractures had increased at −30° on the right and −20° on the left.

BOX **20-1** SKILLS ACQUIRED DURING INPATIENT REHABILITATION AT AGE 5 IN A PATIENT WITH T10 PARAPLEGIA

- Independent bed mobility
- Independent short and long sitting balance
- Independent transfers from wheelchair to bed and back using a sliding board
- Independent push-up pressure releases with reminders
- Self-propel wheelchair over level terrain

BOX **20-2** SKILLS ACQUIRED FROM AGES 6 TO 9 IN A PATIENT WITH T10 PARAPLEGIA

- Independently perform self range-of-motion exercise
- Perform all transfers without a sliding board independently, including from floor to wheelchair
- Independently assume, maintain, and move in a wheelie position
- Ascend and descend low curbs independently
- Self-propel over mild uneven terrain in a wheelie position
- Ascend and descend mild hills

Continued

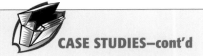

CASE STUDIES—cont'd

Alex was seen again in the SCI clinic at age 15. He was still not very active because of restrictions from his spinal surgery. Hip flexion contractures had increased to −45° on the right and −30° on the left and his right hip was subluxing. The physiatrist discussed hip management options. Alex also complained of upper back pain. He and the physical therapist reviewed posterior shoulder and scapular strengthening and anterior shoulder stretching exercise to avoid impingement syndrome.

Alex was then seen in clinic at age 16 to discuss management of his subluxed hip. Although he was now cleared for sports activities, his lumbar mobility had decreased significantly as a result of the spinal fusion and he could no longer compensate for the limitation in hip extension. Although this did not affect his skiing or track skills, his position in the water during swimming changed because his hips were now in a much greater degree of flexion (Figure 20-12). This caused him to swim more slowly and he sustained a significant loss in his competitive standing.

Reflections on Practice

The need for episodic physical therapy can occur years after initial rehabilitation. The physical therapist must be knowledgeable about typical musculoskeletal problems such as overuse and shoulder impingement syndromes that can occur as a result of an SCI, paralysis, and resulting wheelchair use patterns. Wheelchair athletes propel their chairs with shoulders flexed and internally rotated, placing them at increased risk for impingement. They need to actively exercise humeral depressors, especially external rotators. Compared with adults, children who sustain SCI are at risk for unique orthopedic complications (scoliosis, hip subluxation) that may interfere with achieving maximal function and must be managed throughout childhood and into adolescence.

"Adam"

This case demonstrates the long-term physical therapy management of a teenager with incomplete paraplegia caused by cauda equina

injury. This teenager continued to experience long-term functional improvements owing to a combination of neurologic recovery and active strengthening programs. Four years of treatment and follow-up were needed before he reached a plateau of function.

Adam was injured at age 14 when he fell from a tree. He sustained a burst fracture of the L3 vertebra and a complete anterior dislocation of L3 on the L4 vertebra. On the day after his injury, he underwent surgery to reduce the dislocation, and instrumentation was placed across the two vertebrae for stabilization. Postoperatively, Adam was given a TLSO to wear 24 hours a day for the next 3 to 4 months until fusion was complete. Owing to the instability of the initial injury and the short segment of fusion and instrumentation, a thigh piece was added to the TLSO to prevent hip flexion beyond 80°.

Eight days after his injury, Adam was admitted to a pediatric rehabilitation program. His cauda equina SCI was classified as L2 paraplegia, ASIA Impairment Scale level B. His impairments included deficits in motor and sensory functioning, loss of voluntary bladder and bowel control, and orthostatic hypotension. Motor examination, functional skills, and physical therapy intervention are outlined in Table 20-5. Passive ROM was normal throughout, except straight leg raising was possible to only 30° bilaterally because of posterior thigh pain. His sensory examination to pinprick showed that he had lost normal sensation below the medial femoral condyles and had decreased sensation in the L4 and L5 dermatomes, absent sensation at S1, but preservation of pinprick at S4-S5, perianally. There were no problems with spasticity because cauda equina injuries result in lower motor neuron deficits with flaccid paralysis.

Adam's sitting tolerance was limited by orthostatic hypotension, and he could only sit up with the wheelchair back reclined 45°. From such a position, he could not propel his wheelchair. Support stockings and Ace wraps around his legs were used in conjunction with progressively increasing his angle of inclination during upright sitting. His FIM scores showed complete independence (7) in communication and social cognition. In self-care, he was completely independent (7) for eating and grooming but needed moderate assistance (3) for bathing,

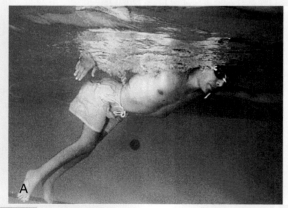
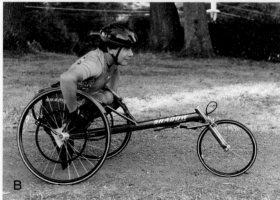

Figure 20-12 Decreased lumbar mobility resulting from back surgery for scoliosis significantly worsens positioning and performance in the water but has no effect on positioning for track events. **A,** Position in water. **B,** No effect for track.

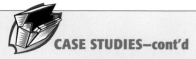

CASE STUDIES—cont'd

TABLE 20-5 **Physical Therapy Intervention during Inpatient Rehabilitation for Teen with Cauda Equina Spinal Cord Injury**

Date	Lower Extremity Strength		Functional Status	Physical Therapy Intervention
Admission to rehabilitation unit	Grade 3 hip flexion and knee extension. Grade 0 for all other lower extremity muscles.		Assist needed for bed mobility and transfers. Unable to self-propel wheelchair, stand, or walk.	Direct intervention for bed mobility, transfers, wheelchair skills, and upper/lower extremity strengthening.
One month after SCI	Grade 3+ hip flexion and knee extension. Grade 0 for all other lower extremity muscles.		Independent bed mobility. Transfers with a sliding board. Independent wheelchair mobility. Beginning to stand in parallel bars.	Direct intervention with focus on upper and lower extremity strengthening and gait training. Referred for solid-ankle AFOs.
Four months after SCI, discharge from inpatient rehabilitation program	Right	Left	Ambulates independently with wheeled walker and AFOs up to 150 ft. Uses wheelchair for long distances.	Direct outpatient intervention for lower extremity strengthening and gait training. School-based consultation for adaptive physical education and mobility in school.
Hip flexion	4–	4–		
Hip abduction	0	2		
Hip extension	1	1		
Knee extension	4+	4+		
Knee flexion	2	2		
Ankle dorsiflexion	0	1		

set-up assistance (5) for upper body dressing, maximal assistance (2) for lower body dressing, and total assistance (1) for toileting and bladder and bowel management. For mobility and locomotion, he needed maximal assistance (2) for all transfers and total assistance (1) for locomotion, using a wheelchair. He was unable to ascend stairs.

Adam's activity limitations on admission included lack of independence in bed mobility, transfers, and indoor and community mobility. With his level of injury, realistic long-term outcomes were independence in bed mobility and transfers and ambulation at home and in the community using AFOs and crutches. Short-term goals included increasing tolerance to the upright position, improved hamstring ROM to allow long-sitting, improved upper extremity strength and endurance to allow independent transfers and wheelchair propulsion, and lower extremity strengthening of the weakened muscle groups.

After 2 weeks, he had only rare episodes of symptomatic orthostatic hypotension. A lighter-weight wheelchair was substituted for the recliner wheelchair.

One month after admission to rehabilitation, there was minimal change in lower extremity strength but significant improvement in Adam's functional skills (see Table 20-5). Hamstring ROM continued to be limited owing to complaints of pain with stretching. Upper body strength improved so that Adam could lift his trunk to do independent pressure relief and could transfer himself without a sliding board to level heights.

Two months after injury, Adam had increased knee extensor strength to grade 4. Solid-ankle AFOs were fabricated, and he began to stand in the parallel bars. Within another month he had adequate

standing balance to begin gait training with a walker. He had also begun to get return of hamstring function. Several weeks later he was independently ambulating with a walker and had met all of his inpatient discharge outcome expectations and so was discharged to his home. Functional skills and lower extremity strength at discharge are shown in Table 20-5. He was reclassified as having L2 paraplegia, ASIA Impairment Scale level C. Passive straight leg raising was to 85° bilaterally, and all other passive ROM was normal. Adam's FIM scores had improved to complete independence (7) in all areas of self-care except bathing; to modified independence (6) for bathing and bladder and bowel management; to complete independence (7) in transfers to bed, chair, wheelchair, and toilet; and to modified independence (6) for transfers to the bathtub chair and for locomotion using a wheelchair or ambulating with the walker and AFOs. He needed moderate assistance (4) to ascend stairs.

At reexamination 1 year after SCI, Adam demonstrated improved strength, particularly in knee flexor, hip extensor, and hip abductor muscles. These strength increases resulted in improved function, but his classification remained L2 paraplegia, ASIA Impairment Scale level C, because he had weakness in the L4, L5, and S1 key muscles used by the ASIA scale. Adam had discontinued his participation in the outpatient physical therapy program the month before but was continuing to work on stretching and strengthening at home. He demonstrated significant improvements in strength and ambulation skills (Table 20-6). His left AFO was changed to one with a hinged ankle to allow free dorsiflexion but no plantar flexion past neutral to allow motion and the possibility of strengthening these muscle groups while

Continued

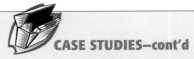

CASE STUDIES—cont'd

TABLE 20-6   Physical Therapy Intervention and Consultation during Outpatient Rehabilitation for Teen with Cauda Equina Spinal Cord Injury

Date	Lower Extremity Strength		Functional Status	Physical Therapy Intervention
One year after SCI,	Right	Left	Ambulates with forearm crutches and AFOs using bilateral reciprocal gait pattern. Starting to walk without crutches. Wheelchair discontinued.	Outpatient physical therapy discontinued; instructed in home exercise program. Consultation through rehab clinic. Home exercise program updated at clinic visit. Hinged AFO on left recommended because of increased plantar-flexion strength.
Hip flexion	4-	4		
Hip abduction	3-	3		
Hip extension	2	3		
Knee extension	5	5		
Knee flexion	3	4		
Ankle dorsiflexion	0	2		
Long toe extensors	0	3		
Ankle plantar flexion	0	2		
Four years after SCI,			Has returned to all preinjury recreational and leisure activities, including hiking, fishing, and hunting.	Consultation through rehab clinic. Recommended hinged AFO on right because of increase in plantar-flexion strength.
Hip flexion	5	5		
Hip abduction	4	4		
Hip extension	3+	4		
Knee extension	5	5		
Knee flexion	4	5		
Ankle dorsiflexion	0	2		
Long toe extensors	0	3		
Ankle plantar flexion	2	3		

walking. Continued home ROM and strengthening exercises were recommended.

Reexamination 2 years after his SCI demonstrated a grade increase in left hip extension and abduction strength and a half-grade increase in right hip extension. This additional strength allowed Adam to ambulate without crutches (see Table 20-6). His level of SCI was now L3 paraplegia, ASIA Impairment Scale level C. He needed new AFOs because of wear and tear. He had developed skin breakdown on the lateral border of his left foot and on his right shin from rubbing against the AFO and the Velcro closure. He no longer used his forearm crutches. ROM was well maintained. He was provided with new AFOs and educated regarding care of insensate skin. Because he was working out in a gym several times a week, specific exercises were recommended for strengthening hip girdle and knee flexor muscles.

At his last examination 4 years after SCI, Adam had shown some improvement in right lower extremity strength of the targeted muscle groups (see Table 20-6). He also demonstrated activity of plantar flexor muscles at the right ankle. Bilateral hinged AFOs with plantar flexion stops were prescribed. Adam was a senior in high school and

worked after school in a gas station. He had returned to an outdoor lifestyle, hiking, fishing, and hunting on a regular basis. He planned to enroll in a community college to study forestry. He was advised of state vocational rehabilitation services available to him and was referred to an adult SCI rehabilitation program for long-term monitoring of renal function and prescription of orthoses.

Reflections on Practice

At various points in his course of recovery, Adam demonstrated functional improvement, sometimes as a result of neurologic improvement and other times as a result of targeted functional skills training, strengthening, and gait training. Comprehensive reexaminations, including precise manual muscle testing, were critical in order to set new goals and implement appropriate interventions to meet these goals.

"JC"

JC is a 4-year-old boy with a history of a T4 ASIA B SCI (previously documented) secondary to a gunshot wound to the chest in August 2008 in Puerto Rico. He was in an acute care facility for 5 weeks,

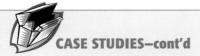

CASE STUDIES—cont'd

including 2 weeks in the Pediatric Intensive Care Unit PICU, before being transferred to a rehab facility where he stayed for a month. There was an approximate 3.5-month lapse between his discharge from rehabilitation in Puerto Rico and his admission to a pediatric SCI rehabilitation facility. Before the injury, JC was potty trained but currently wears a diaper.

On the day of his injury, CT scans showed a right hemopneumothorax, right posterior lung contusion, and comminuted fractures with impacted bullet fragments involving T4-T5 and the fourth and fifth ribs; air was present within the spinal canal. There was no evidence of thoracic vascular injury. CT scan of the neck showed no fractures or dislocations of the cervical spine. CT of the head showed multiple bullet fragments at the left frontotemporal and parietal scalp; there were no intracranial injuries. Repeat CT scan a week later showed

small metallic bullet fragments at the posterior dependent aspect of the right lung, comminuted fracture of the right side lamina of T4 with a bone fragment protruding into the right side aspect of the spinal canal with narrowing of its transverse diameter. There was a comminuted fracture of the costovertebral joints of the fourth and fifth rib as well as the right transverse process of T5. JC remained in the PICU for 2 weeks. He was intubated and ventilated, then placed on O2 via mask with BiPAP at night before weaning to room air. His pain was managed with fentanyl, Versed, morphine, and Ativan. He experienced episodes of dysreflexia with symptoms of increased blood pressure and facial flushing, which were noted and attributed to a urinary tract infection (UTI). He was discharged to inpatient rehabilitation facility 1 month later, where he received inpatient rehabilitation for approximately 1 more month.

REFERENCES

1. Allen, D. D., Mulcahey, M. J., Haley, S. M., et al. (2009, reprinted 2002). Motor scores on the Functional Independence Measure after pediatric spinal cord injury. *Spinal Cord, 47*(3), 213–217.
2. American Spinal Injury Association. (2000). *International Standards for Neurological and Functional Classification of Spinal Cord Injury*. Chicago: American Spinal Injury Association.
3. Anderson, C. J., & DeVivo, M. (2004). Mortality in pediatric spinal cord injury. Paper abstract #10. *Journal of Spinal Cord Medicine, 27*, S113.
4. Anderson, C. J., Vogel, L. C., Betz, R. R., &Willis, K. M. (2004). Overview of adult outcomes in pediatric-onset spinal cord injuries, Implications for transition to adulthood. *Journal of Spinal Cord Medicine, 27*, S98–S106.
5. Anderson, C. J., Vogel, L. C., Chlan, K. M., et al. (2007). Depression in adults who sustained spinal cord injuries as children or adolescents. *Journal of Spinal Cord Medicine, 30*, S76–S82.
6. Anderson, R., Ragel, B., & Brockmeyer, D. (2007). Untitled selection of rigid internal fixation construct for stabilization at the craniovertebral junction in pediatric patients. *Journal of Spinal Cord Medicine, 30*(Suppl), S193–S194 [abstract].
7. Baptiste, D. C., & Fehlings, M. G. (2006). Pharmacological approaches to repair the injured spinal cord. *Journal of Neurotrauma, 23*, 318–334.
8. Behrman, A. L., & Harkema, S. J. (2000). Locomotor training after human spinal cord injury: A series of case studies. *Physical Therapy, 80*, 688–700.
9. Behrman, A. L., & Harkema, S. J. (2007). Physical rehabilitation as an agent for recovery after spinal cord injury. *Physical medicine and rehabilitation clinics of North America, 18*, 183–202.
10. Belanger, M., Stein, R. B., Wheeler, G. D., Gordon, T., & Leduc, B. (2008). Electrical stimulation: Can it increase muscle strength and reverse osteopenia in spinal cord injured individuals? *Archives of Physical Medicine and Rehabilitation, 81*, 1090–1098.
11. Betz, R. R., & Mulcahey, M. J. (2003). Pediatric spinal cord injury. In A. R. Vaccaro, R. R. Betz, & S. M. Zeidman, (Eds.), *Principles and Practice of Spine Surgery*, Philadelphia: Mosby.
12. Betz, R. R., Mulcahey, M. J., Lebby, E., et al. (2004). Sagittal analysis of patients with spinal cord injury, A radiographic analysis and implications for treatment. Poster presentation abstract #36. *Journal of Spinal Cord Medicine, 27*, S135.
13. Bilston, L. E., & Brown, J. (2007). Pediatric spinal injury type and severity are age and mechanism dependent. *Spine, 32*(21), 2339–2347.
14. Bohn, D., Armstrong, D., Becker, L., & Humphreys, R. (1990). Cervical spine injuries in children. *Journal of Trauma, 30*, 463–469.
15. Bosch, P. P., Vogt, M. T., & Ward, W. T. (2002). Pediatric spinal cord injury without radiographic abnormality (SCIWORA): The absence of occult instability and lack of indication for bracing. *Spine, 27*, 2788–2800.
16. Bracken, M. B., Shepard, M. J., Collins, W. F., et al. (1990). A randomized, controlled trial of methylprednisolone or naloxone in the treatment of acute spinal cord injury: Results of the second national acute spinal cord injury study. *New England Journal of Medicine, 332*, 1405–1411.
17. Bracken, M. B., Shepard, M. J., Freeman, D. F., et al. (1984). Efficacy of methylprednisolone in acute spinal cord injury. *Journal of the American Medical Association, 251*(1), 45–52.
18. Bracken, M. B., Shepard, M. J., Holford, T. R., et al. (1997). Methylprednisolone for 24 or 48 hours or tirilazad mesylate for 48 hours in the treatment of acute spinal cord injury: Results of the Third National Acute Spinal Cord Injury Randomized Controlled Trial. National Acute Spinal Cord Injury

Study. *Journal of the American Medical Association, 277*(20), 1597–1604. (*2)

19. Brown, P. J., Marino, R. J., Herbison, G. J., et al. (1991). The 72-h examination as a predictor of recovery in motor complete quadriplegia. *Archives of Physical Medicine and Rehabilitation, 72,* 546–548.

20. Brown, R. L., Brunn, M. A., & Garcia, V. F. (2001). Cervical spine injuries in children: A review of 103 patients treated consecutively at a level 1 pediatric trauma center. *Journal of Pediatric Surgery 36*(8), 1107–1114.

21. Calhoun, C. L., Haley, S. M., Riley, A., et al. (2009). Development of items designed to evaluate activity performance and participation in children and adolescents with spinal cord injury. *International Journal of Pediatrics* Article ID 854904, 7 pages doi:10.1155/2009/854904

22. Cappuccino, A. (2008). Moderate hypothermia as treatment for spinal cord injury. *Orthopedics 31,* 243.

23. Cardenas, D. D., Haselkorn, J. K., McElliot, J. M., & Gnatz, S. M. (2001). A bibliography of cost-effectiveness practices in physical medicine and rehabilitation, American Academy of Physical Medicine & Rehabilitation white paper. *Archives of Physical Medicine and Rehabilitation, 82,* 711–719.

24. Catz, A., & Itzkovich, M. (2007). Spinal Cord Independence Measure: Comprehensive ability rating scale for the spinal cord lesion patient. *Journal of Rehabilitation Research & Development, 44,* 65–68.

25. Catz, A., Itzkovich, M., Agranov, E., et al. (1997). SCIM: Spinal Cord Independence Measure: A new disability scale for patients with spinal cord lesions. *Spinal Cord, 35,* 850–856.

26. Catz, A., Itzkovich, M., Agranov, E., et al. (2001). The Spinal Cord Independence Measure (SCIM), Sensitivity to functional changes in subgroups of spinal cord lesion patient. *Spinal Cord 39,* 97–100.

27. The Center for Injury Prevention and Research at the Children's Hospital Philadelphia, (2006) http://stokes.chop.edu/programs/injury.

28. Chafetz, R. S., Mulcahey, M. J., Betz, R. R., et al. (2007). Impact of prophylactic thoracolumbosacral orthosis bracing on functional activities and activities of daily living in the pediatric spinal cord injury population. *Journal of Spinal Cord Medicine, 30,* S178–S183.

29. Chen, S. C., Lai, C. H., Chan, W. P., Huang, M. H., Tsai, H. W., & Chen, J. J. (2005). Increases in bone mineral density after functional electrical stimulation cycling exercises in spinal cord injured patients. *Disability and Rehabilitation, 27,* 1337–1341.

30. Cirak, B., Ziegfeld, S., Knight, V. M., et al. (2004). Spinal injuries in children. *Journal of Pediatric Surgery, 39*(4), 607–612.

31. Clayton, G. H., Wilson, P. E., & Olezeck, J. (2004). The use of push-rim power-assist wheels in three pediatric patients. Poster presentation abstract #13. *Journal of Spinal Cord Medicine, 27,* S126.

32. Committee on Genetics, American Academy of Pediatrics. (2001). Health supervision for children with Down syndrome. *Pediatrics, 107,* 442–449.

33. Consortium for Spinal Cord Medicine. (1999). *Outcomes following traumatic SCI: Clinical practice guidelines for healthcare professionals.* Washington, DC: Paralyzed Veterans of America.

34. Consortium for Spinal Cord Medicine. (2000). *Clinical practice guideline. Pressure ulcer prevention and treatment following spinal cord injury: A clinical practice guideline for health care professionals.* Washington, DC: Paralyzed Veterans of America.

35. Consortium of Spinal Cord Medicine. (2002). *Clinical practice guideline. Preservation of upper limb function following spinal cord injury: A clinical practice guideline for healthcare professionals.* Washington, DC: Paralyzed Veterans of America.

36. Davis, G. M., Hamzaid, N. A., & Fornusek, C. (2008). Cardiorespiratory, metabolic, and biomechanical responses during functional electrical stimulation leg exercise, Health and fitness benefits. *Artificial Organs, 32,* 625–629.

37. DeVivo, M. J., & Vogel, L. C. (2004). Epidemiology of spinal cord injury in children and adolescents. *Journal of Spinal Cord Medicine, 27,* S4–S10

38. Di Martino, A., Madigan, L., Silber, J. S., & Vaccaro, A. R. (2004). Pediatric spinal cord injury. *Neurosurgery Quarterly, 14*(4), 84–197.

39. Ditunno, J. F., Cohen, M. E., Hauck, W. W., Jackson, A. B., & Sipski, M. L. (2000). Recovery of upper-extremity strength in complete and incomplete tetraplegia: A multicenter study. *Archives of Physical Medicine and Rehabilitation, 81,* 389–393.

40. Dobkin, B. H., Curt, A., & Guest, J. (2006). Cellular transplants in China: Observational study from the largest human experiment in chronic spinal cord injury. *Neurorehabilitation and Neural Repair, 20*(1), 5–13

41. Dudgeon, B. J., Massagli, T. M., & Ross, B. W. (1997). Educational participation of children with spinal cord injury. *American Journal of Occupational Therapy, 51,* 553–561.

42. Dumas, H. M., Haley, S. M., Boyce, M. E., et al. (2009). Self-report measures of physical function for children with spinal cord injury, A review of current tools and an option for the future. *Developmental Neurorehabilitation 12*(2), 113–118.

43. Elefteriades, J. A., Quin, J. A., Hogan, J. F., et al. (2002). Long-term follow-up of pacing of the conditioned diaphragm in quadriplegia. *Pacing and Clinical Electrophysiology, 25,* 897–906.

44. Faghri, P. D., Glaser, R. M., & Figoni, S. F. (1992). Functional electrical stimulation leg cycle ergometer exercise: Training effects on cardiorespiratory responses of spinal cord injured subjects at rest and during submaximal exercise. *Archives of Physical Medicine and Rehabilitation, 73,* 1085–1093.

45. Fehlings, M. G., Sekhon, L. H. S., & Tator, C. (2001). The role and timing of decompression in acute spinal cord injury. *Spine, 26,* S101–S110.

46. Field-Fote, E. C. (2009). *Spinal cord injury rehabilitation.* Philadelphia: F.A. Davis.

47. Field-Fote, E. C., & Behrman, A. (2009). Locomotor training after incomplete spinal cord injury, neural mechanisms and functional outcomes. In E. C. Field-Fote (Ed.), *Spinal cord injury rehabilitation,* Philadelphia: F.A. Davis.

48. Fordyce, W. E. (1981). Behavioral methods in medical rehabilitation. *Neuroscience and Biobehavioral Reviews, 5,* 391–396.

49. Fornusek, C., & Davis, G. M. (2008). Cardiovascular and metabolic responses during functional electric stimulation cycling at different cadences. *Archives of Physical Medicine and Rehabilitation, 89,* 719–725.

50. Frotzler, A., Coupaud, S., Perret, C., et al. (2008). High-volume FES-cycling partially reverses bone loss in people with chronic spinal cord injury. *Bone, 43,* 169–176.

51. Garcia, R. A., Gaebler-Spira, D., Sisung, C., & Heinemann, A. W. (2002). Functional improvement after pediatric spinal cord injury. *American Journal of Physical Medicine and Rehabilitation, 81*(6), 458–463.

52. Giangregorio, L., & McCartney, N. (2006). Bone loss and muscle atrophy in spinal cord injury, Epidemiology, fracture prediction, and rehabilitation strategies. *Journal of Spinal Cord Medicine, 29*(5), 489–500.

53. Ginis, K. A., & Hicks, A. L. (2007). Considerations for the development of a physical activity guide for Canadians with physical disabilities. *Canadian Journal of Public Health, 98* (Suppl 2), S135–S147.

54. Glassman, S. D., Johnson, J. R., & Holt, R. T. (1992). Seatbelt injuries in children. *Journal of Trauma, 33,* 882–886.

55. Glenn, W. W., Phelps, M. L., & Elefteriades, J. A. (1986). Twenty years of experience in phrenic nerve stimulation to pace the diaphragm. *Pacing and Clinical Electrophysiology, 9,* 780–784

56. Haley, S. M., Faas, R. M., Coster, W. J., Webster, H., & Gans, B. M. (1992). *Pediatric evaluation of disability inventory.* Boston: New England Medical Center.

57. Hall, E. D. (2001). Pharmacological treatment of acute spinal cord injury: How do we build on past success? *Journal of Spinal Cord Injury Medicine, 24,* 142–146.

58. Herzenberg, J. E., Hensinger, R.N., Dedrick, D.K. et al. (1989). Emergency transport and positioning of young children who have an injury to the cervical spine. *Journal of Bone and Joint Surgery, 71A,* 15–22.

59. Hjeltnes, N., Aksnes, A. K., Birkeland, K. I., Johansen, J., Lannem, A., & Wallberg-Henriksson, H. (1997). Improved body composition after 8 wk of electrically stimulated leg cycling in tetraplegic patients. *American Journal of Physiology, 273,* R1072–R1079.

60. Hooker, S. P., Figoni, S. F., Rodgers, M. M., et al. (1992). Physiologic effects of electrical stimulation leg cycle exercise training in spinal cord injured persons. *Archives of Physical Medicine and Rehabilitation, 73,* 470–476.

61. Hugenholtz H. (2003). Methylprednisolone for acute spinal cord injury: Not a standard of care. *Canadian Medical Association Journal, 168*(9).

62. Hurlbert, R. J. (2001). The role of steroids in acute spinal cord injury: An evidence-based analysis [review], *Spine, 26* (24 Suppl), S39–S46.

63. Jacobs, P. L., & Nash, M. S. (2001). Modes, benefits, and risks of voluntary and electrically induced exercise in persons with spinal cord injury. *Journal of Spinal Cord Injury Medicine, 24,* 10–18 (and exercise and fitness).

64. Janm F. K., & Wilson, P. E. (2004). A survey of chronic pain in the pediatric spinal cord injury population. *Journal of Spinal Cord Medicine, 27,* S50–S53.

65. Johnson, K. A., & Klaas, S. J. (2007). The changing nature of play, Implications for pediatric spinal cord injury. *Journal of Spinal Cord Medicine, 30,* S71–S75.

66. Johnson, K. A., Klaas, S. J., Vogel, L. C., & McDonald, C. (2004). Leisure characteristics of the pediatric spinal cord injury population. *Journal of Spinal Cord Medicine, 27,* S107–S109.

67. Johnston, T. E., Greco, M. N., Gaughan, J. P., Smith, B. T., & Betz, R. R. (2005). Patterns of lower extremity innervation in pediatric spinal cord injury. *Spinal Cord, 43,* 476–482.

68. Johnston, T. E., Smith, B. T., Betz, R. R., & Lauer, R. T. (2008). Exercise testing using upper extremity ergometry in pediatric spinal cord injury. *Pediatric Physical Therapy, 20,* 146–151.

69. Johnston, T. E., Smith, B. T., Mulcahey, M. J., Betz, R. R., & Lauer, R. T. (2009). A randomized controlled trial on the effects of cycling with and without electrical stimulation on cardiorespiratory and vascular health in children with spinal cord injury. *Archives of Physical Medicine and Rehabilitation, 90,* 1379–1388

70. Johnston, T. E., Smith, B. T., Mulcahey, M. J., Betz, R. R., & Lauer, R. T. (in press). A randomized controlled trial on the effects of cycling with and without electrical stimulation on cardiorespiratory and vascular health in children with spinal cord injury. *Archives of Physical Medicine and Rehabilitation.*

71. Johnston, T. E., Smith, B. T., Oladeji, O., Betz, R. R., & Lauer, R. T. (2008). Outcomes of a home cycling program using functional electrical stimulation or passive motion for children with spinal cord injury: A case series. *Journal of Spinal Cord Medicine, 31,* 215–221.

72. Kakulas, B. A. (1999). A review of the neuropathology of human spinal cord injury with emphasis on special features. *Journal of Spinal Cord Injury Medicine, 22,* 119–124.

73. Kigerl, K., & Popovich, P. (2006). Drug evaluation, ProCord, A potential cell-based therapy for spinal cord injury. *IDrugs 9*(5), 354–360 [abstract].

74. Klose, K. J., Jacobs, P. L., Broton, J. G., et al. (1997). Evaluation of a training program for persons with SCI paraplegia using the Parastep 1 ambulation system, Part 1. Ambulation performance and anthropometric measures. *Archives of Physical Medicine and Rehabilitation, 78,* 789–793.

75. Krey, C. H., & Calhoun, C. L. (2004). Utilizing research in wheelchair and seating selection and configuration for children with injury/dysfunction of the spinal cord. *Journal of Spinal Cord Medicine, 27* (Suppl 1), S29–S37.

76. Lammertse, D. P. (2004). Invited review: Update on pharmaceutical trials in acute spinal cord injury. *Journal of Spinal Cord Medicine, 27,* 319–325.

77. Lauer, R., Johnston, T. E., Smith, B. T., et al. (2007). Bone mineral density of the hip and knee in children with spinal cord injury. *Journal of Spinal Cord Medicine, 30,* S10–S14.

78. Lisenmeyer, T. A. (2000). Sexual function and infertility following spinal cord injury. *Physical Medicine and Rehabilitation Clinics of North America, 11,* 141–156.

79. Liusuwan, R. A., Widman, L. M., Abresch, R. T., et al. (2007). Behavioral intervention, exercise, and nutrition education to improve health and fitness (BENEfit) in adolescents with mobility impairment due to spinal cord dysfunction. *Journal of Spinal Cord Medicine, 30* (Suppl 1), S119–S126.

80. Liusuwan, R. A., Widman, L. M., Abresch, R. T., et al. (2007). Body composition and resting energy expenditure in patients aged 11 to 21 years with spinal cord dysfunction compared to controls, Comparisons and relationships among the groups. *Journal of Spinal Cord Medicine, 30* (Suppl 1), S105–S111.

81. Mandabach, M., Ruge, J. R., Hahn, Y., & McLone, D. G. (1993). Pediatric axis fractures: Early halo immobilization, management and outcome. *Pediatric Neurosurgery, 19,* 225–232; doi: 10. 1159/000120737.

82. Mange, K. C., Ditunno, J. F., Herbison, G. J., et al. (1990). Recovery of strength at the zone of injury in motor complete and motor incomplete cervical spinal cord injured patients. *Archives of Physical Medicine and Rehabilitation, 71,* 562–565.

83. Massagli, T. L., Dudgeon, B. J., & Ross, B. W. (1996). Educational performance and vocational participation after spinal cord injury in childhood. *Archives of Physical Medicine and Rehabilitation, 77,* 995–999.

84. Massagli, T. L., & Reyes, M. R. L. Hypercalemia and Spinal Cord Injury (2008) http://emedicine.medscape.com/article/322109

85. Maynard, F. M., Reynolds, G. G., Fountain, S., et al. (1979). Neurological prognosis after traumatic quadriplegia. *Journal of Neurosurgery, 50,* 611–616.

86. McCarthy, J. J., Chafetz, R. S., Betz, R. R., & Gaughan J. (2004). Incidence and degree of hip subluxation/dislocation in children with spinal cord injury. *Journal of Spinal Cord Medicine, 27,* S80–S83.

87. McDonald, C. M., Abresch-Meyer, A. L., Nelson, M. D., & Widman, L. M. (2007). Body mass index and body composition measures by dual x-ray absorptiometry in patients aged 10 to 21 years with spinal cord injury. *Journal of Spinal Cord Medicine, 30* (Suppl 1), S97–S104.

88. McDonald, C. M., Jaffe, K. M., & Shurtleff, D. B. (1986). Assessment of muscle strength in children with meningomyelocele, Accuracy and stability of measurements over time. *Archives of Physical Medicine and Rehabilitation, 67,* 855–861.

89. McDonald, J. W., Becker, D., Sadowsky, C. L., Jane, J. A., Conturo, T. E., & Schultz, L. M. (2002). Late recovery following spinal cord injury, Case report and review of the literature. *Journal of Neurosurgery (Spine 2), 97,* 252–265.

90. McGinnis, K. B., Vogel, L. C., McDonald, C.M., et al. (2004). Recognition and management of autonomic dysreflexia in pediatric spinal cord injury. *Journal of Spinal Cord Medicine, 27,* S61–S74.

91. McKinley, W. O., Seel, R. T., & Hardman, J. T. (1999). Nontraumatic spinal cord injury, incidence, epidemiology, and functional outcome. *Archives of Physical Medicine and Rehabilitation, 80*(6), 619–623 [abstract].

92. Mehta, S., Betz, R. R., Mulcahey, M. J., et al. (2004). Effect of bracing on paralytic scoliosis secondary to spinal cord injury. *Journal of Spinal Cord Medicine, 27,* S88–S92.

93. Meyer, A. Pediatric mobility issues. (2008). *Rehabilitation Management, 21*(10), 20–23.

94. Molnar, G. E., & Alexander, M. A. (1999). History and examination. In G. E. Molnar (Ed.), *Pediatric rehabilitation* (3rd ed., pp. 1–12). Philadelphia: Hanley & Belfus.

95. Mulcahey, M. J., Calhoun, C. L., Riley, A., & Haley, S. M. (in press). Children's reports of activity and participation after sustaining a spinal cord injury: A cognitive interviewing study. *Developmental Neurorehabilitation.*

96. Mulcahey, M. J., DiGiovanni, N., Calhoun, C. L., et al. Children's and parent's perspectives about activity performance and participation following spinal cord injury, Themes from a cognitive interview study [thematic paper].

97. Mulcahey, M. J., Gaughan, J., Betz, R. R., et al. (2006). The International Standards for Neurological Classification of Spinal Cord Injury, Reliability of data when applied to children and youths. *Spinal Cord, 45,* 1–8.

98. Mulcahey, M. J., Smith, B. T., & Betz, R. R. (1999). Evaluation of the lower motor neuron integrity of upper extremity muscles in high level spinal cord injury. *Spinal Cord, 37,* 585–591.

99. Myers, J., Lee, M., & Kiratli, J. (2007). Cardiovascular disease in spinal cord injury, An overview of prevalence, risk, evaluation, and management. *American Journal of Physical Medicine & Rehabilitation, 86,* 142–152.

100. Nash, M. S. (2005). Exercise as a health-promoting activity following spinal cord injury. *Journal of Neurologic Physical Therapy, 29,* 87–103, 106.

101. Nelson, M. D., Widman, L. M., Abresch, R. T., et al. (2007). Metabolic syndrome in adolescents with spinal cord dysfunction. *Journal of Spinal Cord Medicine, 30* (Suppl 1), S127–S139.

102. Nesathurai, S. (1998). Steroids and spinal cord injury: Revisiting the NASCIS 2 and 3 trials. *Journal of Trauma, 45,* 1088–1093.

103. Nichols, D. S., & Case-Smith, J. (1996). Reliability and validity of the Pediatric Evaluation of Disability Inventory. *Pediatric Physical Therapy, 8,* 15–24.

104. Nobunaga, A. I., Go, B. K., & Karunas, R. B. (1999). Recent demographic and injury trends in people served by the Model Spinal Cord Injury Care Systems. *Archives of Physical Medicine and Rehabilitation, 80,* 1372–1382.

105. Ottenbacher, K. J., Taylor, E. T., Msall, M. E., et al. (1996). The stability and equivalence reliability of the Functional Independence Measure for children (WeeFIM). *Developmental Medicine and Child Neurology, 38,* 907–916.

106. Peckham, P. H., Keith, M.W., Kilgore, K.L. et al. (2001). Efficacy of an implanted neuroprosthesis for resorting hand grasp in tetraplegia: A multicenter study. *Archives of Physical Medicine and Rehabilitation, 82,* 1380–1388.

107. Phillips, W. T., Kiratli, B. J., Sarkarati, M., et al. (1998). Effect of spinal cord injury on the heart and cardiovascular fitness. *Current Problems in Cardiology, 23*, 641–716.

108. Pierce, S. R., Orlin, M. N., Lauer, R. T., Johnston, T. E., Smith, B. T., & McCarthy, J. J. (2004). Comparison of percutaneous and surface functional electrical stimulation during gait in a child with hemiplegic cerebral palsy. *American Journal of Physical Medicine & Rehabilitation, 83*, 798–805.

109. Prosser, L. A. (2007). Locomotor training within an inpatient rehabilitation program after pediatric incomplete spinal cord injury. *Physical Therapy, 87*(9), 1224–1232.

110. Rhoney, D. H., Luer, M. S., Hughes, M., & Hatton, J. (1996). New pharmacological approaches to acute spinal cord injury. *Pharmacotherapy, 16*, 382–392.

111. Rumball, K., Jarvis, J. (1992). Seat-belt injuries of the spine in young children. *Journal of Bone and Joint Surgery (British), 74*, 571–574.

112. Saboe, L. A., Darrah, J. M., Pain, K. S., & Guthrie, J. (1997). Early predictors of functional independence 2 years after spinal cord injury. *Archives of Physical Medicine and Rehabilitation, 78*, 644–650.

113. Samdani, A. F. (2007). Commentary: Spinal cord regeneration, Injury modulation, repair strategies, and clinical trials: The Howard H. Steel Conference Precourse. *Journal of Spinal Cord Medicine, 30*(S1), S3–S4.

114. Scremin, A. M., Kurta, L., Gentili, A., et al. (1999). Increasing muscle mass in spinal cord injured persons with a functional electrical stimulation exercise program. *Archives of Physical Medicine and Rehabilitation, 80*, 1531–1536.

115. Sharkey, P. C., Halter, J. A., & Nakajima, K. (1989). Electrophrenic respiration in patients with high quadriplegia. *Neurosurgery, 24*, 529–535.

116. Shaul, D. B., Danielson, P. D., McComb, J. G., & Keens, T. G. (2002). Thoracoscopic placement of phrenic nerve electrodes for diaphragmatic pacing in children. *Journal of Pediatric Surgery, 37*, 974–978.

117. Shavelle, R. M., DeVivo, M. J., Paculdo, D. R., et al. (2007). Long-term survival after childhood spinal cord injury. *Journal of Spinal Cord Medicine, 30*, S48–S54.

118. Short, D. J., El Masry, W. S., & Jones, F. W. (2000). High dose methylprednisolone in the management of acute spinal cord injury: A systematic review from a clinical perspective, *Spinal Cord, 38*, 278–286.

119. Sison-Williamson, M. Bagley, A., Hongo, A., et al. (2007). Effect of thoracolumbosacral orthoses on reachable workspace volumes in children with spinal cord injury. *Journal of Spinal Cord Medicine, 30*, S184–S191.

120. Sisto, S. A., Druin, E., & Sliwinski, M. M. (2009). *Spinal cord injuries, management and rehabilitation.* St. Louis, MO: Mosby.

121. Spoltore, T., Mulcahey, M. J., Johnston, T., Kelly, K. Morales, V., & Rebuck, C. (2000). Innovative programs for children and adolescents with spinal cord injury. *Orthopedic Nursing, 19*, 55–62.

122. Stein, R. B., Belanger, M., Wheeler, G., et al. (1993). Electrical systems for improving locomotion after spinal cord injury: An assessment. *Archives of Physical Medicine and Rehabilitation, 74*, 954–959.

123. Triolo, R. J., Betz, R. R., Mulcahey, M. J., et al. (1994). Application of functional electrical stimulation to children with spinal cord injuries, Candidate for selection for upper and lower extremity research. *Paraplegia, 32*, 824–843.

124. Trotter, T. L., Hall, J. G., Committee on Genetics, American Academy of Pediatrics. (2005). Health supervision for children with achondroplasia. *Pediatrics, 116*(3), 771–783.

125. Ugalde, V., White, R., Shtutman, N., et al. (2004). Incidence of venous thromboembolism in patients with acute spinal cord injury by age. Paper abstract #6. *Journal of Spinal Cord Medicine, 27*, S112.

126. Urbina, E., Alpert, B., Flynn, F., et al. (2008). Ambulatory blood pressure monitoring in children and adolescents, recommendations for standard assessment: A scientific statement from the American Heart Association Atherosclerosis, Hypertension, and Obesity in Youth Committee of the Council on Cardiovascular Disease in the Young and the Council for High Blood Pressure Research. *Hypertension, 52*, 433–451.

127. U.S. Department of Education. (1997). 105th Congress, *Public Law* 105–117.

128. U.S. Equal Employment Opportunity Commission. (1973). The Rehabilitation Act of 1973, sec. 504.

129. Vitale, M. G., Goss, J. M., Matsumoto, H., et al. (2007). Epidemiology of pediatric spinal cord injury in the United States, 1997 and 2000. *Journal of Spinal Cord Medicine, 30*, S196.

130. Vogel, L. C., Anderson, C. J., Chlan, K. M., et al. (2007). Pain and its impact in adults with pediatric onset spinal cord injury. *Journal of Spinal Cord Medicine, 30*, S193.

131. Vogel, L. C., Klaas, S. J., Lubicky, J. P., & Anderson, C. J. (1998). Long-term outcomes and life satisfaction of adults who had pediatric spinal cord injuries. *Archives of Physical Medicine and Rehabilitation, 79*, 1496–1503.

132. Vogel, L. C., Krajci, K. A., & Anderson, C. J. (2002). Adults with pediatric-onset spinal cord injury, Part 2, musculoskeletal and neurological complications. *Journal of Spinal Cord Medicine, 25*(2), 117–123.

133. Vogel, L. C., Mendoza, M. M., Schottler J.C., et al. (2007). Ambulation in children and youth with spinal cord injuries. *Journal of Spinal Cord Medicine, 30*, S158–S164.

134. Vogel, L. C., Samdani, A., Chafetz, R., et al. (2009). Intra-rater agreement of the anorectal exam and classification of injury severity in children with spinal cord injury. *Spinal Cord*, in print. doi: 10. 1038/sc. 2008. 180.

135. Wang, M. Y., Hoh, D. J., Leary, S. P., et al. (2004). High rates of neurological improvement following severe traumatic pediatric spinal cord injury. *Spine, 29*(13), 1493–1497; doi: 10. 1097/01. BRS. 0000129026. 03194. 0F.

136. Warburton, D. E. R., Sproule, S., Krassioukov, A., & Eng, J. J. (2006). Cardiovascular health and exercise following spinal cord. In J. J. Eng, R. W. Teasell, W. C. Miller, et al. (Eds.), *Spinal cord injury rehabilitation evidence* (Vancouver, British Columbia), 7, 1–7, 28.

137. Wilberger, J. E. (1986). *Spinal cord injuries in children*. New York: Futura.

138. Wilson, P. E., Oleszek, J. L., Clayton, & G. H. (2007). Pediatric spinal cord tumors and masses. *Journal of Spinal Cord Medicine, 30*, S15–S20.

SUGGESTED READINGS

Behrman, A. L., Nair, P. M., Bowden, M. G., et al. (2008). Locomotor training restores walking in a nonambulatory child with chronic, severe, incomplete cervical spinal cord injury. *Physical Therapy, 88*(5), 580–590.

Betz, R. R., Mulcahey, M. J., D'Andrea, L. P., et al. (2004). Acute evaluation and management of pediatric spinal cord injury. *Journal of Spinal Cord Medicine, 27*, S11–S15.

Brown, R., DiMarco, A. F., Hoit, J. D., & Garshick, E. (2006). Respiratory dysfunction and management in spinal cord injury. *Respiratory Care, 51*(8), 853–868.

Chen, D., Apple, D. F., Hudson, L. M., & Bode, R. (1999). Medical complications during acute rehabilitation following spinal cord injury—current experiences of the model systems. *Archives of Physical Medicine and Rehabilitation, 80*, 1397–1401.

Curtis, K. A., Tyner, T. M., Zachary, L., et al. (1999). Effect of a standard exercise protocol on shoulder pain in long-term wheelchair users. *Spinal Cord, 37*, 421–429.

DeVivo, M. J., Richards, J. S., Stover, S. L., & Go, B. K. (1991). Spinal cord injury, rehabilitation adds life to years. *Western Journal of Medicine, 154*, 602–606.

Giovanini, M. A., Reier, P. J., Eskin, T. A., Wirth, E., & Anderson, D. K. (1997). Characteristics of human fetal spinal cord grafts in the adult rat spinal cord: Influences of lesion and grafting conditions. *Experimental Neurology, 148*, 523–543.

Greene, A., Barnett, P., Crossen, J., Sexten, G., Ruzicka, P., & Neuwelt, E. (2002). Evaluation of the THINK FIRST For KIDS injury prevention curriculum for primary students. *Injury Prevention, 8*, 257–258.

Johnston, T. E. (2005). Muscle weakness and loss of motor performance. In S. L. Michlovitz & T. P. Nolan (Eds.), *Modalities for therapeutic intervention* (pp. 247–270). Philadelphia, F.A. Davis.

Johnston, T. E., Betz, R. R., & Lauer, R. T. (2009). Impact of cycling on hip subluxation in children with spinal cord injury. *Journal of Pediatric Orthopedics, 29*, 402–405.

Keith, M. W., Peckham, H. P., Thrope, G. B., et al. (1989). Implantable functional neuromuscular stimulation in the tetraplegic hand. *Journal of Hand Surgery, 14A*, 524–530.

Lenke, L. G., & Betz, R. R. (2003). Neuromuscular scoliosis, Surgical treatment. In A. R. Vaccaro, R. R. Betz, & S. M. Zeidman (Eds.), *Principles and Practice of Spine Surgery*, Philadelphia, Mosby.

Meiser, M. H., & McEwen, I. R. (2007). Lightweight and ultralight wheelchairs: Propulsion and preferences of two young children with spina bifida. *Pediatric Physical Therapy, 19*(3), 245–253.

Mulcahey, M. S., Betz, R. R., Smith, B. T., Weiss, A. A., & Davis, S. E. (1997). Implanted functional electrical stimulation hand system in adolescents with spinal injuries: An evaluation. *Archives of Physical Medicine and Rehabilitation, 78*, 597–607.

Poynton, A. R., O'Farrell, D. A., Shannon, F., Murray, P., McManus, F., & Walsh, M. G. (1997). Sparing of sensation to pin prick predicts recovery of a motor segment after injury to the spinal cord. *Journal of Bone and Joint Surgery, 79*, 952–954.

Qian, T., Guo, X., Levi, A. D., et al. (2005). High-dose methylprednisolone may cause myopathy in acute spinal cord injury patients. *Spinal Cord, 43*(4), 199–203.

Schmid, A., Huonker, M., Barturen, J. M., et al. (1998). Catecholamines, heart rate, and oxygen uptake during exercise in people with spinal cord injury. *Journal of Applied Physiology, 85*, 635–641.

Sipski, M. L., Alexander, C. J., & Harris, M. (1993). Long term use of computerized bicycle ergometry for spinal cord injured subjects. *Archives of Physical Medicine and Rehabilitation, 74*, 238–241.

van Middendorp, J. J., Hosman, A. J., Pouw, M. H., EM-SCI Study Group, & Van de Meent, H. (2009, May 26). Is determination between complete and incomplete traumatic spinal cord injury clinically relevant? Validation of the ASIA sacral sparing criteria in a prospective cohort of 432 patients. *Spinal Cord.* [Epub ahead of print] doi: 10. 1038/sc. 2009.44.

van Middendorp, J. J., Hosman, A. J., Pouw, M. H., EM-SCI Study Group, & Van de Meent, H. (2009). ASIA impairment scale conversion in traumatic SCI: Is it related with the ability to walk? A descriptive comparison with functional ambulation outcome measures in 273 patients. *Spinal Cord, 47*(7), 555–560.

Widman, L. M., Abresch, R. T., Styne, D. M., & McDonald, C. M. (2007). Aerobic fitness and upper extremity strength in patients aged 11 to 21 years with spinal cord dysfunction as compared to ideal weight and overweight controls. *Journal of Spinal Cord Medicine, 30* (Suppl 1), S88–S96.

Wong, A. M. K., Leong, C., Su, T., Yu, S., Tsai, W., & Chen, C. P. C. (2003). Clinical trial of acupuncture for patients with spinal cord injuries. *American Journal of Physical Medicine and Rehabilitation, 82*, 21–27.

21 Acquired Brain Injuries: Trauma, Near-Drowning, and Tumors

MICHAL KATZ-LEURER, LPT, MPH, PhD • HEMDA ROTEM, PT, BPT, MSc(PT)

Acquired brain injury (ABI) in children is a highly stressful event for the child and the family. Damage occurring at a time of development extensively affects the child's abilities to do what children usually do: Play, learn, establish friendships, and gradually develop to be independent young adults. The injury commonly causes a variety of physical, emotional, cognitive, and behavioral impairments. Suddenly, the child's expectations from life and the parents' aspirations for their child may be dramatically changed. These unique emotional, social, and developmental needs of the child and family demand a holistic and inclusive approach by a multidisciplinary team, both as a team and by each member of the team as a specialist in a unique specialty. The following chapter focuses on the physical therapist's role and describes the elements of patient/client management: Examination, assessment procedures, diagnosis, prognosis, and intervention strategies, with emphasis on the child with ABI and his parents and family throughout the rehabilitation process.

ABI is a general categorization that describes any sudden, nonprogressive injury to the brain that occurs after birth and may be the result of trauma (e.g., head injury after traffic accidents, falls) or anoxia (e.g., near-drowning) or a non-traumatic event (e.g., stroke, brain tumor, infection). ABI is the most common cause of morbidity and mortality in children and in young adults.[25] ABI might cause a variety of disorders involving motor dysfunction, cognitive impairment, behavioral disturbance, emotional difficulties, and abnormal function of the autonomic nervous system. Even a mild injury might result in a serious disability that interferes with the child's daily functioning and activities for the rest of his life.

Different theories have been put forth regarding the recovery and adaptation processes of brain function following a brain injury. One suggests that intact areas of the brain that are anatomically linked to the damaged site might be functionally depressed. Because return of activity occurs in these functionally depressed areas, recovery of function might also occur. Another theory suggests that recovery and adaptation of brain function might occur as the original brain area responsible for that function recovers, or through adaptation of noninjured brain regions that normally contribute indirectly to that function. Furthermore, recovery of function occurs as a result of behavioral substitution in which new strategies are learned to compensate for the behavioral deficit.[86]

These theories serve as the foundation for a variety of interventions used by physical therapists for children with ABI, ranging from preventive treatment with the expectation for brain function recovery at one end of the spectrum, to a structured motor training program to facilitate compensation processes of brain function at the other. The latter is the source of many innovative treatment strategies for patients with brain damage. Recent advances in basic science have demonstrated morphologic changes in neural structures within the motor cortex during the process of motor skill acquisition, resulting in behavioral changes in motor performance.[70] The use of functional neuroimaging techniques may assist researchers and clinicians to clarify the effect of treatment on neural reorganization and to identify the sequence and timing of interventions that will optimally and efficiently improve function. Although the outcome of the injury depends largely on the nature and severity of the injury itself, appropriate and timely treatment may play a vital role in determining the level of recovery.[57]

The first part of this chapter describes the epidemiology, pathology, and prognosis of ABI among children and adolescents. Three common examples of causes of brain injury among children—trauma, near-drowning as an example of an anoxic event, and brain tumor—are described in detail. The second part focuses on the physical therapy examination and evaluation techniques and interventions throughout the rehabilitation process. Finally, a detailed case study of a 6-year-old boy with a severe traumatic brain injury is presented and discussed. Two video files illustrate material from this chapter. The first presents and illustrates the above case study. The second (by Ginette A. Kerkering) presents the physical rehabilitation process of a young child with a brain tumor.

TRAUMATIC BRAIN INJURY

EPIDEMIOLOGY

Traumatic brain injury (TBI) is the most common cause of acquired disability in childhood, with an incidence death rate of 4.5, a hospitalization rate for nonfatal TBI of 63, and an emergency department visit rate of 731 cases, all per

100,000 children aged 0 to 14 years per year in the United States.[51] The most frequent causes of injury are motor vehicle accidents and falls, the latter being the primary cause among younger, preschool children; adolescents and young adults are more commonly injured in motor vehicle accidents. The incidence is higher in boys and highest in boys between the ages of 15 and 20 years, followed by children between the ages of 6 and 10 years.[44] Other demographic and socioenvironmental factors associated with an increased risk of TBI include poverty, crowded neighborhoods, family instability, history of alcohol or drug abuse, and learning disability.[48] Preexisting behavioral characteristics such as impulsivity and hyperactivity, as well as attention deficit disorder, have been associated with an increased risk of accidental injury[13]; the "shaken baby syndrome" resulting from vigorous shaking of an infant or small child by the shoulders, arms, or legs can also be a cause of brain injury.[10] Preventive efforts are essential and should include educational programs for children, adolescents, and parents. The effectiveness of preventive activities regarding risky behavior and the use of protective equipment have been described, for example, the notoriety of head injury in children not wearing helmets during bicycle riding arose during the early 1980s, when it was noted that only approximately 15% of riders younger than 15 years of age wore helmets. Societal interest resulted in the implementation of helmet laws that reduced the incidence of pediatric TBI. The results of a case-control study in Seattle in 1989 indicated that the use of bicycle helmets reduced the risk of bicycle-related head injury by 74% to 85%.[82]

PATHOLOGY

Brain damage due to TBI is typically divided into primary and secondary damage. *Primary damage* is related to the forces that occur at the time of initial impact; *secondary damage* occurs as the result of processes evoked in response to the initial trauma.

Primary Brain Damage

Primary brain damage can be classified according to the mechanism of injury, including acceleration-deceleration injury, crush injury, and penetration injury. *Acceleration-deceleration* injuries occur when the force applied is translational (Figure 21-1) or rotational (Figure 21-2) and commonly results from motor vehicle accidents; the head hits an immobile object, or a mobile object hits the immobile head. Such injuries can lead to lesions that might be microscopic or combined with a focal macroscopic lesion with a predilection for the midbrain, pons, corpus callosum, and white matter of the cerebral hemispheres.[63] Acceleration-deceleration injuries, particularly the rotational component, produce differential displacement of adjacent brain tissue layers. This shearing force has its greatest effect in areas where the density differences of the tissues are greatest. Therefore approximately two thirds of lesions of this type,

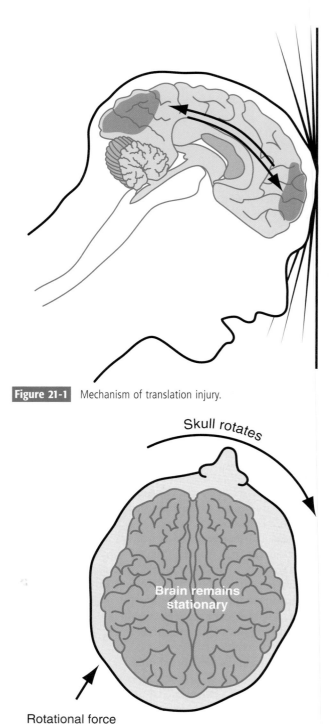

Figure 21-1 Mechanism of translation injury.

Figure 21-2 Mechanism of rotational injury.

that is, diffuse axon injury (DAI), occur at the gray-white matter interface.[71] The child's brain has a higher water content (88%) than the adult brain (77%), meaning that the brain is softer and more prone to acceleration-deceleration injury. *Contusion or crush injuries* are usually frontal or temporal. These injuries result from relatively low-velocity impact such as blows to the head or falls. Skull fractures may be associated, which is significant only when underlying compression of the brain or hemorrhage occurs. Or multiple small intracerebral hemorrhages and occasionally more extensive bleeding may be observed. *Penetration injuries* constitute a minority of pediatric TBI and are classified as non-missile penetrating injuries and missile penetrating injuries. Children are prone to nonmissile penetrating injuries that result from a fall or from a home or playground accident. These injuries often involve nails, pencils, and sharp sticks, which, in most cases, cause focal damage. Missile injuries caused by gunshots or air pellet rifles lead to substantive intracranial damage.

Secondary Brain Damage

Secondary brain damage usually results from hypoxia or ischemia, which can be caused by *intracranial factors* or *extracranial factors* such as hypoxemia or hypotension (systolic blood pressure <90 mm Hg).[12] The main *intracranial causes* of secondary injuries are hemorrhage and brain swelling. Intracranial hemorrhage is due to laceration of blood vessels within the brain or on its surface, resulting in an epidural, subdural, or subarachnoid hematoma, according to the site. Displacement of the brain can occur as the result of a rise in intracranial pressure due to edema, or caused by a mass lesion. Diffuse swelling is more common in infants and children than in adults. It has been suggested that the relatively compliant skull and membranous suture properties of the infant skull allow a significant cranial shape change and a more diffuse pattern of brain distortion than is seen in adults after TBI. Experimental studies have suggested that the edema setting in early after injury might be related to enhanced diffusion of excitotoxic neurotransmitters in the immature brain, or to an enhanced inflammatory response in the developing brain, or to enhanced blood-brain barrier permeability after central nervous system (CNS) injury in the immature versus the adult brain.[47]

Further brain damage may occur as the result of complications such as infection, hydrocephalus, hygroma, or convulsions. Infection of the brain may occur after an open fracture or cerebrospinal fluid (CSF) rhinorrhea, or it may be iatrogenic, caused by intracranial monitoring or surgery.[3] A hygroma develops as the result of localized CSF collection, or resolution of a hematoma. Posttraumatic seizures typically are divided into three types, depending on their time of onset as related to the trauma. Seizures that occur within minutes are referred to as immediate seizures, early seizures occur within 1 week of the trauma, and late seizures occur beyond the first week of injury. A child who suffers two or more late seizures is diagnosed as having posttraumatic epilepsy.

PROGNOSIS

Studies designed to identify prognostic factors for survival and function after TBI have resulted in an overall conclusion

that no single factor adequately predicts outcome from an injury as complex and heterogeneous as TBI. Nevertheless, the severity of the brain injury seems to be directly associated with the outcome.

The most commonly used parameters for determining brain damage severity are the Glasgow Coma Scale, coma duration, and posttraumatic amnesia. The Glasgow Coma Scale (GCS) is a widely accepted method of initially evaluating and characterizing trauma patients with head injuries.[90] The scale has been adapted for infants and young children as the Pediatric Coma Scale.[78] The GCS assesses the level of coma by ranking three aspects of function: Motor response, verbal performance, and eye opening; the best response for each is noted on a scale from 1 to 5. The sum of the scores (3 to 15 points) is used as an indication of the depth of the coma and the severity of injury. A GCS score of 13 to 15 points is considered mild, a GCS score of 9 to 12 points is considered moderate, and a GCS score of 3 to 8 points is considered severe. A limitation of the GCS is that it is a time-dependent assessment tool designed to assess injury severity within the first 48 hours after the trauma.

Coma duration classifies injury severity as mild—coma lasting less than 20 minutes, moderate—coma lasting 20 minutes to 6 hours, severe—coma lasting 6 to 24 hours, and very severe—coma for longer than 24 hours.[4] Depth and duration of impaired consciousness are negatively associated with functional outcome. Coma duration may be a better predictor of motor and cognitive recovery than coma depth measured with the GCS. The longer the duration of the coma, particularly a duration of coma of longer than 4 weeks, the less likely is a good recovery.[38] Nevertheless it has been noted that coma duration as brief as 1 hour may lead to attention deficits, behavioral disturbances, and irritability.[76]

Posttraumatic amnesia (PTA) is defined as a period of variable length after trauma, during which the patient is confused and disoriented; retrograde amnesia is defined as an inability to remember and recall new information. The longer the duration of PTA, the worse is the outcome. It is unlikely that a person will have an outcome of severe disability if the duration of PTA is less than 2 months. Conversely, it is unlikely that a person will have a good recovery if the duration of PTA extends beyond 3 months.[38]

Of all children who sustain TBI, 95% survive.[48] Among those with severe TBI, that percentage drops to 65%. The highest mortality rate is seen in children younger than 2 years of age, with a decline in mortality rate until age 12 years, and then a second peak at age 15 years.[44] Death is seldom due to the primary damage but is more often the result of secondary intracranial or extracranial complications of brain damage or other related injuries.

NEAR-DROWNING

Hypoxic injury refers to any injury caused by tissue oxygen deficiency and includes drowning and near-drowning, inhalation of a foreign body, hanging and strangulation, suffocation and asphyxia, apnea, and others.[32] Although near-drowning is unique in some aspects, it can serve as a model for understanding many of the pathophysiologic, therapeutic, and prognostic aspects of all types of hypoxic injury in the pediatric population.

EPIDEMIOLOGY

Drowning, defined as death within 24 hours of a submersion incident, and near-drowning, defined as survival for at least 24 hours following a submersion incident, represent significant causes of morbidity and mortality in children.[106] In the United States in 1999, 10% of deaths due to accidental injury up to the age of 19 years were due to unintentional drowning. Males were more likely to die of drowning than were females in all age groups; boys 0 to 4 years of age had the highest rate of drowning (3.6 per 100,000), followed by boys 15 to 19 years of age (3.25 per 100,000).[15] Efficient preventive procedures include adult supervision of young children in bathtubs and pools and well-maintained four-sided pool fencing that prevents direct entry to the pool from the house or yard.[87]

PATHOLOGY

Submersion of a child usually leads to panic and a struggle to surface. In attempting to breathe, the child may aspirate water (wet drowning), or laryngospasm may occur without aspiration (dry drowning).[94] The most significant factors causing morbidity and mortality from near-drowning are hypoxemia and a decrease in oxygen delivery to vital tissues. Sustained hypoxemia causes neuronal injury and finally leads to circulatory collapse, myocardial damage, and dysfunction of multiple organ systems, with further ischemic brain damage. During the first few minutes, the brain is deprived of oxygen (hypoxic injury). As the cardiovascular system fails, cerebral blood flow decreases and ischemic injury occurs. The vulnerability of the brain tissue to hypoxic-ischemic injury varies in the white matter and the gray matter. Areas of greatest susceptibility to ischemic injury are usually in vascular end zones, in the hippocampus, insular cortex, and basal ganglia. Even within the hippocampus itself, vulnerability to hypoxic-ischemic damage varies.[49] More severe hypoxia-ischemia leads to more extensive and global cortical damage.

PROGNOSIS

CNS damage and its outcomes determine survival and long-term morbidity. About one third of all children who survive will have significant neurologic damage caused by hypoxic-ischemic encephalopathy.[17] The prognosis for those who are severely injured may be difficult to determine in the first hours after the hypoxic-ischemic event, although prolonged

cardiopulmonary resuscitation, fixed and dilated pupils, and GCS of 3 suggest a poor outcome.[32] Attention to adequacy of oxygenation with optimal ventilator strategies to minimize brain and lung injury, provide cardiovascular support, and avoid iatrogenic complications may help to minimize secondary brain damage.[32]

BRAIN TUMORS

EPIDEMIOLOGY

Brain tumors are the most common form of solid tumors in children and the second most common form of pediatric cancer overall.[26] The annual incidence rate in the United States of brain tumors is about 38 cases per million children. Brain tumors occasionally are congenital, occur most frequently in children ages 1 to 10 years, and are slightly more common in boys than in girls.[26]

PATHOLOGY

Brain tumors may be benign or malignant, primary or metastatic. The term *benign* may imply that a complete cure is possible, but it can be life threatening if it is large, or if it results in increased intracranial pressure, cerebral edema, or brain herniation, especially if it is located in a critical area of the brain for maintaining vital functions, such as the pons or medulla. Malignant brain tumors, which make up 80% of brain tumors among children, are life threatening. Primary brain tumors are those that originate directly from cells in the brain and rarely spread outside of the CNS. Metastatic brain tumors originate from tissues outside the brain.

Tumors can cause symptoms directly, by penetration or compression of an area of the brain, or indirectly, by causing an increase in intracranial pressure. Most common symptoms include headache, nausea, vomiting, irritability, balance disturbances, ataxia, seizures, hemiparesis, and visual problems.[53]

Young children have a relatively high incidence of cerebellum and brainstem tumors.[27] The tumors are classified according to their cellular characteristics and location (Figure 21-3). The most common entities throughout childhood and adolescence are astrocytoma and medulloblastoma, which occur predominantly in the cerebellum. Early signs are those of increased intracranial pressure, as well as cerebellar signs such as ataxia. Metastases may occur throughout the meninges and may involve sites outside the brain. Ependymoma is a primary brain tumor that may occur in the posterior fossa and the cerebral hemispheres. Initial signs and symptoms include those related to increased intracranial pressure in the posterior fossa, seizures, and focal cerebellar deficits.[53] Craniopharyngiomas are histologically benign and occur primarily at the midline of the suprasellar region. Visual disturbances, headaches, and vomiting,

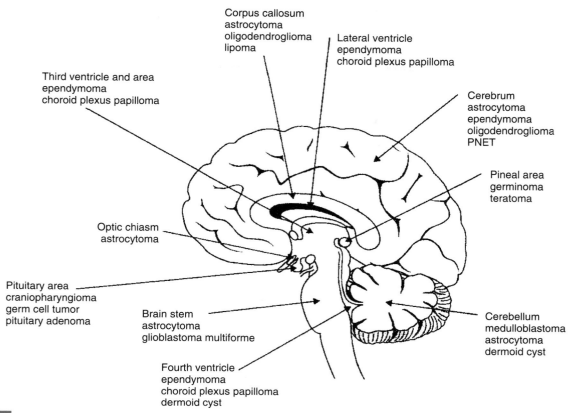

Corpus callosum
astrocytoma
oligodendroglioma
lipoma

Lateral ventricle
ependymoma
choroid plexus papilloma

Third ventricle and area
ependymoma
choroid plexus papilloma

Cerebrum
astrocytoma
ependymoma
oligodendroglioma
PNET

Pineal area
germinoma
teratoma

Optic chiasm
astrocytoma

Pituitary area
craniopharyngioma
germ cell tumor
pituitary adenoma

Brain stem
astrocytoma
glioblastoma multiforme

Cerebellum
medulloblastoma
astrocytoma
dermoid cyst

Fourth ventricle
ependymoma
choroid plexus papilloma
dermoid cyst

Figure 21-3   Common sites of pediatric brain tumors. *PNET,* Primitive neuroectodermal tumor.

as well as endocrine disturbances, are the primary symptoms. Initial signs of brainstem gliomas include progressive cranial nerve dysfunction and gait disorders.

PROGNOSIS

Treatment of brain tumors usually includes surgical resection, radiation therapy, and chemotherapy. Radiation therapy must be used cautiously in young children because of late-onset effects on cognition and learning. Chemotherapy effectiveness is often limited owing to difficulty in crossing the blood-brain barrier. Shunt placement may be necessary to relieve hydrocephalus resulting from blockage of CFS flow by the tumor. The survival rate has been growing continuously in recent years, but in general, it depends on the grade of the malignancy and age. The prognosis is better the older the child is at onset, for example, and the prognosis is better for astrocytomas than for medulloblastomas. A rough estimate of the 5-year survival rate for malignant brain tumors in children is about 70%.[26] In spite of generally encouraging prognostic data, many long-term survivors continue to have major neuropsychological or cognitive deficits.[65]

ACQUIRED BRAIN INJURY— DIAGNOSTIC TECHNIQUES

Imaging techniques can provide specific and accurate information on the structure of the brain, its metabolic activity, and its functional activity. The techniques assist in making a diagnosis and planning treatment strategy and may provide insight as to the prognosis.

Imaging techniques that provide information about brain structure include magnetic resonance imaging (MRI), x-ray (least informative), computed tomography (CT), and angiography.[45] MRI is based on signals produced by tissue protons when placed in a magnetic field. MRI is sensitive in detecting hemorrhage or hypoxic-ischemic damage, and it can often discriminate between benign and malignant masses and other changes in tissue density. CT illustrates thin slices through the brain based on x-rays. This technique can be used to distinguish among many soft tissues and can indicate the location, density, and presence of a tumor or edema. CT is particularly effective in identifying foreign bodies and bone abnormalities. MRI has greater tissue contrast resolution than does CT; it does not use ionizing radiation and has not been shown to produce side effects. On the other hand, CT is less expensive, faster, and safer because an MRI scan requires the child to lie still for an extended period of time, often under sedation. Angiography is used primarily to diagnose and to map vascularization. It is particularly helpful in providing information on blood supply to the brain.[5]

Imaging techniques that provide information about cellular metabolic activity and thereby assist with functional mapping of the brain include functional magnetic resonance imaging (fMRI), positron emission tomography (PET), and magnetic resonance spectroscopy (MRS). The advantages of these techniques are their superior resolution with reference to spatial relationships that define areas of activated brain tissue. fMRI takes a rapid succession of scans that can detect small changes in the level of oxygen consumption and blood flow taking place in areas of the brain that are activated during a test protocol. PET detects the differing levels of glucose uptake that occur in brain tissue. Brain tumors, for example, have a higher level of glucose uptake than normal brain tissue, whereas necrotic tissue has little to no glucose uptake. MRS is another imaging technique that detects metabolic changes; it is noninvasive and does not require contrast agents or labeled tracers.[80]

Techniques that provide information about brain functional activity include electroencephalography (EEG) and evoked potential tests (EPTs)—sensory, motor, or cognitive. Advantages of these techniques are their superior resolution in relation to time. The EEG is a recording of ongoing electrical brain activity, which presents frequency, amplitude, and organization of the waveform at rest and as a response to stimuli. EPT is an electrical potential recorded from the brain after presentation of a stimulus, as opposed to spontaneous potentials as detected by EEG. Sensory EPs are recorded from the brain after stimulation of sense organs, for example, visual—elicited by a flashing light, auditory—by a click or tone stimulus presented through earphones, or tactile or somatosensory evoked potentials—elicited by touch or electrical stimulation of a sensory or mixed nerve in the periphery. In motor evoked potentials, an area of the brain is stimulated electrically, and the response is recorded in the peripheral musculature.[58] The appropriate choice of tests depends on the suspected pathology, and tests are often repeated to monitor the progress of treatment.

PHYSICAL THERAPY MANAGEMENT FOR A CHILD WITH ABI

Physical therapy management for a child with ABI should be targeted to identifying those functions that the child and his family wish to assume or reassume after the injury. The therapist needs to identify the skills needed to successfully achieve these goals, while remaining aware of the physical limitations and cognitive processes that are impaired and that contribute to functional deficits. The therapist

can then design a plan of care that includes the interventions needed to address the physiologic mechanisms of recovery and adaptation at both impairment and activity skill levels.

Numerous therapeutic strategies are employed by physical therapists to address issues of motor control. Traditional approaches that were commonly used to facilitate motor and postural control, such as Neuro-Developmental Treatment (NDT), proprioceptive neuromuscular facilitation (PNF), and the Brunnstrom approach, were derived from the concept that proprioceptive afferent sensory stimulation can be used to modify abnormal tone and facilitate movement patterns, and that recovery from brain damage occurs in a predictable sequence that corresponds to normal development.[56] Another treatment approach may be to target the impairment, as in, for example, muscle strengthening. Current approaches to task-specific training are based on the hypothesis that the most effective form of motor re-education and learning occurs when performance during practice matches performance during retention and transfer (see Chapter 4 on motor learning).

Unfortunately, clinical trials that specifically examine treatment efficacy in children with ABI are sparse. Evidence from work done on children with cerebral palsy (CP) and on adults post stroke might provide a basis for the design of future trials with children with ABI targeted to identify the interventions that optimally and efficiently improve function. A systematic review of physical therapy interventions for patients post stroke reveals a greater benefit from task-oriented specific training than from impairment-focused intervention, and almost no evidence suggests improved functional outcome to support the use of traditional approaches.[95] Nevertheless, traditional approaches continue to influence practice today: Proximal control and midline alignment, isolated joint movement and selective control as a sign of recovery, and the use of developmental postures to enhance outcome for functional tasks are all components of therapy sessions.

The treatment approaches for children with ABI presented in this chapter are based on available evidence from research. As with most research, more mysteries are revealed as we progress.

BEHAVIORAL AND COGNITIVE DISORDERS

Assessing and treating a child with brain injury is a unique and challenging process. The varied clinical presentation and the unpredictable and varied recovery processes obligate the therapist to carry out frequent assessments and, as a consequence, modification of the treatment plan, including its goals and intervention techniques. Additionally, evaluation of assessment results and treatment planning should relate to the age of the child. The child as opposed to the adult with brain injury continues to mature and refine cognitive and functional abilities. Selected examinations and treatment techniques for different age groups are briefly reviewed in this chapter.

Often the clinical situation is complicated in that not only does neuronal injury directly interfere with motor function, but damage to the cognitive processes *associated* with motor performance and learning has been reported. In the period after the injury, children present with a variety of organic, behavioral, and cognitive disorders, as well as with individual emotional reactions to injury and disability, which might influence their ability to participate in assessment and therapy sessions. Common situations include the following:

- Low tolerance to frustration, poor social judgment, aggression, and impulsivity are frequent phenomena among children with ABI.[105] Attention deficits might include inability to concentrate, increased distractibility, or even perseveration. Children tend to experience global attention difficulties, which often persist beyond the acute recovery phase and may affect performance and learning capabilities.

- Memory disorders in children with brain injury are varied. Memory is assessed with respect to the child's ability to learn new material. *Explicit* memory, which is memory for facts and events, is mediated by medial temporal cerebral areas that include the hippocampus and the diencephalic nuclei.[88] *Implicit* memory is the ability to develop skills and habits. Motor skill learning is a form of implicit learning in which changes in motor performance with practice can accrue without conscious awareness of all the movement-related abilities that are being learned. Areas associated with implicit learning include the sensory, motor, and prefrontal cerebral cortices, the basal ganglia, and cerebellar areas, which include the neural network for movement. Explicit and the implicit learning systems are functionally and neuroanatomically distinct. For example, it is possible that children will present with cognitive deficits that interfere with their ability to have explicit recall but may not interfere with their ability to learn new motor skills.

- Language skill impairment, expressive or receptive, might be due to temporal lobe lesions and can obstruct the child's ability to follow instructions.[105] Expressive disorders impair the child's ability to communicate with others, leading to frustration and aggravation.

- Visuospatial and perceptual impairments may affect the child's perception of the environment, for example, the ability to distinguish a given shape from its surroundings.[105] A child may not be able to put on an orthosis and thereby becomes dependent in functional mobility, even though the child is able to ambulate independently once the orthosis is on. Areas associated with these impairments involve the temporal or occipital lobes of the cerebral cortex.

These cognitive and psychological impairments are frequently present to various degrees and often interfere with the child's ability to participate in assessment and treatment procedures. Although the neuropsychologist formally performs specific testing of these areas, the therapist needs to grossly determine the child's level of cognitive ability before engaging in assessment and determining treatment goals. The Rancho Levels of Cognitive Functioning (RLCF) is a simple ordinal scale that uses behavioral observation to categorize the child's cognitive functioning level and classifies the level of pediatric consciousness by three age groups: infants (6 months to 2 years), preschool-aged children (2 to 5 years), and school-aged children (5 years and older). The levels of each scale range from V (no response to stimuli) to I (oriented). Behavioral expectations at each level are variable, depending on the age group (Table 21-1). Cognitive function of children 12 years of age and older can be assessed using the RLCF for adults. This scale is reversed in order compared with pediatric forms and delineates adult cognitive functioning into eight levels (Table 21-2).

Table 21-3 provides the physical therapist with a basic frame for examination and evaluation that would be appropriate at various stages of cognitive functional recovery of a child with ABI. In the next section, we describe assessments of impairment and functional activity appropriate for the child with ABI.

PHYSICAL THERAPY EXAMINATION: ASSESSMENTS AND MEASUREMENTS

Most children with brain injury change their environmental settings during the rehabilitation process from the acute care unit, to the inpatient rehabilitation ward, outpatient therapy departments, community services, and educational settings. A systematic examination and evaluation should be performed upon entry into each new setting. The examination process should include a review of the medical record and a family interview, which provide the therapist with the basic background for the evaluation process and development of a plan of care for implementing a treatment strategy.

Medical data should include medical history before the injury, cause of injury, earliest GCS, imaging reports specifying locations and extent of injury, other injuries, procedures and surgeries performed, medications, complications, and previous therapy progress reports. Consultations with other rehabilitation personnel and education professionals enable every team member to have a greater understanding of the child's needs and abilities.

Data to be collected from the family as part of the examination procedure include information regarding developmental history, including learning ability, behavior, and cognitive level. Talking with the parents and family enables the therapist to more fully understand the family's perception of the extent of the injuries and their impact on the previous level of function, and allows the family to express expectations and desired outcomes, all of which must be taken into account for goal setting and treatment planning.

TABLE 21-1   Rancho Pediatric Levels of Consciousness

Rancho: Pediatric Level	Infants: 6 months to 2 years	Preschool: 2 to 5 years	School Age: 5 years and older
I	Interacts with environment a. Shows active interest in toys; manipulates or examines before mounting or discarding b. Watches other children at play, may move toward them purposefully c. Initiates social contact with adults; enjoys socializing d. Shows active interest in bottle e. Reaches for or moves toward person or object	Oriented to self and surroundings a. Provides accurate information about self b. Knows he or she is away from home c. Knows where toys, clothes, etc., are kept d. Actively participates in treatment program e. Recognizes own room, knows way to bathroom, nursing station, etc. f. Is potty trained g. Initiates social contact with adults, enjoys socializing	Oriented to time and place a. Provides accurate detailed information about self and present situation b. Knows way to and from daily activities c. Knows sequence of daily routine d. Knows way around unit, recognizes own room e. Finds own bed; knows where personal belongings are kept f. Is bowel and bladder trained
II	Demonstrates awareness of environment a. Response to name b. Recognizes mother and other family members c. Enjoys imitative vocal play d. Giggles or smiles when talked to or played with e. Fussing is quieted by soft voice or touch	Is responsive to environment a. Follows simple commands b. Refuses to follow command by shaking head or saying "no" c. Imitates examiner's gestures or facial expressions d. Response to name e. Recognizes mother and other family members f. Enjoys imitative vocal play	Is responsive to environment a. Follows simple verbal or gestured requests b. Initiates purposeful activity c. Actively participates in therapy program d. Refuses to follow request by shaking head or saying "no" e. Imitates examiner's gestures or facial expressions
III	Gives localized response to sensory stimuli a. Blinks when strong light crosses field of vision. b. Follows moving object passed within visual field. c. Turns toward or away from loud sound. d. Gives localized response to painful stimuli.		
IV	Gives generalized response to sensory stimuli. a. Gives generalized startle to loud sound. b. Responds to repeated auditory stimulation with increased or decreased activity. c. Gives generalized reflex response to painful stimuli.		
V	No response to stimuli. Complete absence of observable change in visual, auditory, or painful stimuli.		

Adapted from Professional Staff Association of Rancho Los Amigos Hospital, Inc. (1982). *Rehabilitation of the head injured child and adult: Pediatric levels of consciousness, selected problems* (pp. 5–7). Downey, CA: Rancho Los Amigos Medical Center. Pediatric Brain Injury Service and Los Amigos Research and Education Institute Inc.

TABLE 21-2   Rancho Levels of Cognitive Functioning

RANCHO ADULT LEVEL		
I	No response	Completely unresponsive to any stimuli
II	Generalized response	Inconsistent and nonpurposeful response to stimuli
III	Localized response	Specific yet inconsistent response to stimuli; response is related to type of stimuli (turning head toward sound).
IV	Confused–agitated	Heightened state of activity. Demonstrates bizarre and nonpurposeful behaviors relative to the environment.
V	Confused–inappropriate	Inconsistently follows simple commands. Shows gross attention to environment, but is easily distractible and lacks ability to focus attention on specific task. Memory is severely impaired, new information is very difficult to learn.
VI	Confused–appropriate	Goal direction behavior appropriate, responds to environment. Can consistently follow simple commands and demonstrates carryover of relearned tasks. Dependent on external cues for direction. Shows little carryover to independent performance of newly learned tasks.
VII	Automatic–appropriate	Appears appropriate and oriented to self and environment. Participates in automatic daily routines. Recent memory is impaired, resulting in shallow recall of activities and decreased rate of learning new information.
VIII	Purposeful–appropriate	Recalls and integrates past and recent events. Adapts responses to environment. Demonstrates carryover of new learning and does not require supervision once an activity is learned. Deficits remain in the areas of abstract reasoning, tolerance to stress, and judgment in emergencies.

Adapted from Malkmus, D., Booth, B., & Kodimer, C. (1980). *Rehabilitation of head injured adult: Comprehensive cognitive management* (p. 2). Downey, CA: Los Amigos Research and Education Institute. Inc.

TABLE 21-3   Examination Strategy Based on RLCF Categories

Rancho Adult Level	Rancho Pediatric Level	Global Description	Assessment/Evaluation Strategies
I-III	V-III	None to early response	Assessment should focus on passive manipulation and observation of spontaneous or stimulus-induced movements.
IV-V	II	Agitated, confused	Assessment should focus on observation of spontaneous and simple instructed tasks.
VI-VIII	I	Higher level response	Assessment should focus on more complex, two or more staged, functional and nonfunctional instructed tasks.

During these discussions, the therapist builds up a picture of the child's personality before the injury, his favorite music or television programs, specific heroes for the younger children, special hobbies, leisuretime activities, and information on friends and siblings. This information may enable the therapist to incorporate familiar, attractive, and motivating components into the treatment sessions, and to plan for participation in home and community activities.

In the next stage, the therapist selects appropriate tests and measures to complete the evaluation procedure targeted to diagnosis of impairments and activity limitations, and to define appropriate short- and long-term treatment goals in the design of a plan of care. Tests for functional limitations and activity and participation restrictions, frequently seen in children with brain injuries, are described in the following section. It should be emphasized that many of the described tests have not yet been validated or assessed for reliability in children with ABI. One must consider that children who have experienced trauma or near-drowning might sustain other injuries that impair their ability to perform a test according to its guidelines, and that may affect the test's outcomes. Such problems must be noted as limitations when test results are evaluated.

Range of Motion (ROM)

ROM limitation might be associated with one or more different factors, such as prolonged bed rest, immobilization, pain, peripheral nerve injury, spasticity, side effects of medical treatment, and skeletal injury due to periarticular new bone formation (PNBF), known also as heterotopic ossification (HO).[18] PNBF is a localized and progressive formation of pathologic bone that develops in the soft tissues adjacent to large joints (hips, elbows, shoulders, and knees). The risk of development of PNBF in a child with TBI is about 20%, and this risk increases with severity of the injury, length of immobilization, duration of coma, and presence of spasticity or fracture, especially if the fracture involves an open reduction with internal fixation or joint dislocation.[31] Assessing the ROM in a child who is unable to follow commands might be problematic as the child may resist the movement and cry in response to pain. Observations of spontaneous movements and performance of gentle passive ROM exercises will enlighten the therapist regarding joint limitations.

Spasticity is characterized by muscles that are perceived as "stiff," in which velocity-dependent resistance to passive movement produces increased muscle tone; spasticity is assessed by the Modified Ashworth Scale,[11] which is a simple, quick, but subjective tool with questionable reliability.[19]

Ataxia is primarily a disorder of balance and control in the timing of coordinated movement. Oscillations during movement, along with an increase in oscillations as the task increases in difficulty, can be detected during functional activities and documented by clinical observation. Ataxia might express itself in the limbs and be observed in tasks such as active reaching or in the trunk, and then is evident in upright postures with increasing antigravity demands. Common causes of ataxia are injuries to the cerebellum or to sensory structures. Sensory ataxia worsens when the child's eyes are closed.[6]

Muscle Strength

Muscle atrophy and weakness typically result after prolonged bed rest or sedentary behavior. For example, bed rest for 30 days can result in an 18% to 20% reduction in knee extensor peak torque.[9] Peripheral or spinal nerve damage due to trauma or chemotherapy can cause a reduction in muscle strength. Manual muscle testing (MMT) demands careful attention and the ability of the examinee to follow simple commands—not suitable requirements for the confused child. At this stage, the therapist must evaluate strength simply by observation. Movement should be observed in varied situations with gravity eliminated, as well as against gravity in lying, sitting, and standing, statically and dynamically, and with variable task demands. When a child can follow simple commands such as standing from sitting or lifting weights (e.g., plantar flexor muscle strength might be assessed by asking the child to raise his heels in standing),[61] then this simple procedure might provide information about the functional strength of the muscle groups. Among children with TBI older than 7 years who can fulfill simple instructions, lower extremity muscle strength can be reliably tested using a standardized measurement protocol and a handheld dynamometer[43]; hand strength may be measured objectively in children aged 5 years and older with quantitative analyses of precision-grip forces.[24]

Sensory testing in children with ABI is challenging. Children may have cognitive deficits that impair their ability to accurately respond to sensory input. Their young age may also lead to difficulty in perceiving and expressing sensations. Sensory stimuli should be introduced selectively with careful observation to determine the response. Responses are noted as being generalized, with a full-body response, or localized. Localized responses are more appropriate, with the response being specific to the system that is being stimulated.

Motor Performance

In young children with brain injury, neuromotor developmental assessments are important. Status and change in motor performance in the severely injured child who is confused might be carried out by using a structured observational assessment of motor performance, for example, the Gross Motor Function Measure (GMFM), designed and validated to measure change in gross motor function over time in children with CP.[84] Maximum performance detectable is that of a typical 5-year-old child (see Chapters 2 and 18 for more information on the GMFM). It is important to note that this measure was not developed and has not been validated for children with brain injury, even though it may provide the therapist with objective information for identifying the child's abilities and may assist in planning intervention and assessing the child's progress in motor function.

Several standardized tests are available to assess motor development and postural control. These include the Alberta Infant Motor Scale (AIMS) for children from birth to 18 months,[74] the Bayley Scales of Infant Development III, appropriate for children from birth to 42 months of age,[7] the Peabody Developmental Motor Scales (PDMS),[77] appropriate for children from birth to 83 months of age, and the Bruininks-Oseretsky Test of Motor Proficiency (BOTMP), with age standards for children from 4.5 to 21 years of age (see Chapters 2 and 3 for further psychometric information on these tests).[21]

Upper limb motor performance can be assessed using the PDMS fine motor scale or the BOTMP. Fine motor coordination can be evaluated using the Purdue Pegboard Test, in which the child places pegs into board holes in three 30-second test sessions as fast as possible; the numbers of pegs from these trials are then averaged and compared with age standards.[1] The Developmental Hand Function Test measures the time required to complete seven standardized timed subtests: writing, page turning, small object manipulation, simulated feeding with a spoon, stacking checkers, lifting light objects, and lifting heavy objects.[35]

Postural Control and Balance

Several studies have reported long-lasting deficits in the motor proficiency of children with TBI, leading to significant balance impairment and functional disability.[42,50]

Postural orientation problems may result from sensory impairment such as hemianopsia—impaired proprioception or tactile sensation—or may be due to other CNS deficits, including the inability to coordinate sensory inputs from the vestibular, visual, and somatosensory systems. Postural responses may be affected by neurologic impairment or biomechanical constraint. The effect of perceptual deficits on a child's postural control may vary with age and postural development. Younger children have a greater reliance on visual input; the adult-like patterns might be present at the age of 7 years and older.[99] With an increase in active movement and in the use of anti-gravity positions, impairments in equilibrium and righting reactions may be observed. These reactions can be tested in a variety of positions and activities. Completion, symmetry, and speed of the reactions constitute qualitative information that should be noted when testing. Structured assessment of postural control and balance can be performed only in children who can respond accurately to at least simple instructions. The Pediatric Clinical Test of Sensory Interaction for Balance, for children 4 to 9 years,[79] and the Clinical Test of Sensory Interaction for Balance, for children 8 years and older,[85] require the child to maintain standing balance under six sensory conditions that assist in the identification of impairments in motor responses in variable sensory environments. Tests that assess balance in relation to gross motor skills include the Berg Balance Scale, which contains 14 tasks including sitting and standing unsupported, lifting an object from the floor in standing, and turning 360°.[23] The Functional Reach Test measures the difference between the arm's length and the point of maximal reach forward and sideward in standing.[69] This test has excellent within-session test-retest reliability for children with TBI. The Timed Up and Go test assesses the time required for the child to get up from a sitting position, walk 3 meters, turn, and come back to sit.[101] The test exhibits good within-session test-retest reliability values. Taking the average of two trials showed minimal measurement error for both tests.[41] The balance subtest of the BOTMP is a static and dynamic balance assessment. It focuses primarily on the assessment of the child's anticipatory postural control.[21]

Gait

The walking items of motor assessments can be used as a measure of gait function. For those children who ambulate and achieve the highest scores on these items, it is often useful to include assessment of other gait parameters such as walking speed, distance, and temporal and spatial assessments. Broad-based gait, prolonged time of double limb support, and increased step length variability have been observed in children with TBI.[42] The electronic walkway may provide the therapist with a reliable and valid (i.e., as demonstrated by concurrent assessment with a three-dimensional motion analysis system) measure for assessing walking improvement in those children who showed a ceiling effect in the functional gait measures.[98] The timed walking tests and the shuttle walk-run assessment have good test-retest reliability with normative data available; the last has been designed specifically for the patient after TBI.[97]

Cardiorespiratory Status and Fitness

Autonomic instability is common following severe traumatic, hypoxic, or ischemic brain injury, often presenting with signs and symptoms of hyperstimulation of the sympathetic nervous system (including tachycardia, rhythm disturbances, and decreased heart rate variability). The prevalence of these symptoms decreases with neurologic recovery.[46] Respiratory or pulmonary complications noted after ABI include those directly related to the trauma, such as pneumothorax, hemothorax, and flail chest, and those directly related to the drowning event. A number of pulmonary complications may occur that are related, at least in part, to subsequent neurologic dysfunction, including respiratory failure, aspiration pneumonia, neurogenic pulmonary edema, and tracheal-airway complications.[100] Cardiorespiratory status should be assessed in the physical therapy examination by monitoring heart rate, respiratory rate, blood pressure, and oxygen saturation during activities. These assessments are particularly important at the initial therapy session in a child with impaired consciousness or after prolonged bed rest, as responses to muscle stretch, pain, or position change may be abnormal. Once the child achieves ambulation, endurance limitations and difficulties in performance may become evident. It has been noted that peak exercise capacity and cardiorespiratory fitness of patients with moderate to severe brain injury are significantly lower compared with the capacity of normal healthy adults of a similar age.[67] Heart rate monitoring as an indicator of exercise intensity is important during endurance training. A functional fitness battery for children and adolescents with TBI aged 8 to 17 years has been described by Rossi and Sullivan.[83] The battery includes items assessing flexibility, strength, cardiorespiratory endurance, agility, power, balance, speed, and coordination.[83]

Functional Assessment

The Pediatric Evaluation of Disability Inventory (PEDI) and the WeeFIM[93] are standardized criterion-referenced indicators of status and change in functional skills such as mobility and self-care. The PEDI, which was designed for the functional assessment of children between the ages of 6 months and 7 years,[28] measures the child's capability and functional performance in self-care, mobility, and social function. The PEDI yields normative and scale scores that can be used to compare the child's performance over time. The PEDI focuses on the function of specific tasks and also rates caregiver assistance and modification. It has demonstrated good sensitivity to both global and item-specific changes in children with ABI.[91] About 11 points on a 0 to 100 scaled score

is considered to be a minimal clinically important difference for change on the PEDI Functional Skills and Caregiver Assistance scales.[33] The WeeFIM and the adult Functional Independence Measure (FIM) from which it was derived measure 18 items related to independence in daily functions, including self-care, sphincter control, mobility, locomotion, communication, and social cognition. Each item is scored by indicating the amount of assistance needed to complete the activity. The WeeFIM was designed for use with children 6 months to 7 years of age; the FIM might be used for children 7 years of age and older.[93]

FORMULATING INTERVENTION GOALS AND TREATMENT STRATEGIES

In consideration of the knowledge obtained during discussions and consultations with other therapeutic disciplines, the therapist needs to formulate appropriate treatment goals and to decide which treatment approach is most appropriate for the specific child. The therapist needs to consider all injuries present, the time elapsed since the brain damage event, the rate of recovery, prior interventions, the age of the child, and the child's consciousness and cognitive state. A detailed description of the assessment procedure, the treatment goals formulated, and the treatment approach are presented in the case study with reference to specific guidelines. General concepts related to global treatment goals and treatment strategies can be outlined using the RLCF grade of a child as a framework (Table 21-4). Next we provide information on some of the typical intervention needs of children at each level of cognitive functioning.

TABLE 21-4 Intervention Strategy Related to RLCF Level

Rancho Adult Level	Rancho Pediatric Level	Global Description	Global Treatment Goals and Strategies
I–III	V–III	None to early response	Prevent musculoskeletal complications Sensory stimulation Family education
IV–V	II	Agitated, confused	Directed activity Increase child's motivation for activity Family education
VI–VIII	I	Higher level response	Practice progressively challenging tasks Reduce environmental restrictions Increase physical conditioning

INTERVENTION

Nonresponse to Early Response Stage

A child with severe cognitive impairment functioning at RLCF adult level I-III, pediatric level V-III is unable to follow commands. The physical therapist's primary purpose in treatment is to prevent complications associated with prolonged immobilization while creating an environment conducive to recovery. Procedural interventions and patient-related instruction include the following:
1. Prevention of musculoskeletal complications
2. Sensory stimulation
3. Family education

Prevention of Musculoskeletal Complications

The main treatment strategies to achieve this goal include positioning in bed, passive movement, splints or serial casting, and assisted sitting and standing.

Positioning

Positioning includes prevention of contractures and minimization of asymmetry. The supine position should be avoided if possible because this position stimulates dystonic posturing or reflex hyperactivity. The child is positioned in sidelying or semi-prone. A pillow placed between the slightly flexed legs prevents them from adducting. The upper limb may be positioned on a pillow with the shoulder girdle protracted and the elbow extended.

Passive ROM Exercise

It is unclear whether or not passive ROM exercise has any effect on preventing development of contractures, unless the muscle at risk is stretched for at least 30 minutes every day.[102] In addition, passive ROM exercise may have harmful effects on soft tissue; movements performed too vigorously or in too large a range may cause microtears in muscle, resulting in bleeding into the muscle and subsequent risk for development of PNBF.[62] In paralyzed or very weak muscle, exercises performed at the end of the range might overstretch the periarticular connective tissue, and if performed too quickly, may cause an increase in spasticity.[2] Therefore passive ROM exercises should be performed only if no other way of moving the child's joints is known. It should be done slowly, with care taken to avoid overstretching at the end of the range. While doing the exercise, the therapist (or parent) should verbally describe to the child what is being done. An alternative is continuous passive motion (CPM) by an external motorized device, which enables a joint to be moved passively throughout an arc of motion and assists in attaining and increasing the ROM. When CPM is used, the range and arc of motion should be carefully determined and re-assessed periodically.

Serial Casting or Positional Splints

Serial casting and splints have been found to be effective in the short term in preventing and correcting muscle contractures[66] and increasing ROM in the elbow and ankle joints among adults with brain injury.[52] Few studies among adults with brain injury reported an improvement in spasticity.[16,30] Whereas splints are used early, mainly for prevention, serial casting is used once a developing contracture is evident. When a two-joint muscle is casted, a lengthened position is easily achieved if the cast is applied while the muscle is not lengthened over both joints (i.e., by first addressing one joint with the other flexed, and then extending the cast). Casts should be well padded and particularly well moulded. Casts should be changed regularly for assessment of skin status and for gradual achievement of further correction with each change. A little overcorrection is useful to allow for loss of correction and the need to repeat the casting.[54,55]

Passive Sitting and Standing

As soon as the vital signs are stable, particularly blood pressure and pulse rate, periods of sitting and standing with external constraints are implemented. The standing position on a tilt table loads bones and cartilage, stretches soft tissues, stimulates internal functions such as bowel movement and bladder emptying, and promotes lung expansion, and as a result improves ventilation. The child needs to be stood up slowly while blood pressure changes are monitored. Passive standing for at least 30 minutes, 7 times a week, should be part of the daily routine until the child achieves the ability to stand unsupported.[92]

Multisensory Stimulation

The therapist typically stimulates the five senses directly, and the child's responses are assessed with the intent of advancing the stimulation as the complexity of the response increases. The efficacy of a prolonged sensory stimulation program is controversial. Cochrane's review of sensory stimulation in individuals with TBI in a comatose or vegetative state revealed that most of the literature in this particular area of cognitive-physical rehabilitation is mainly at the level of case studies or case series, and as such does not provide strong evidence of its efficacy in raising the level of consciousness.[60]

Family Education

Family members are encouraged to participate in intervention sessions as much as possible to facilitate carryover of treatment and practice. In the early stages, the child is dependent in all functional mobility and self-care activities. The parent should therefore be instructed on how to safely and effectively perform all caregiving (i.e., dressing, grooming, bathing, and feeding), as well as on how to perform bed mobility activities and transfers into and out of bed to the wheelchair. The caregiver may also contribute to carrying out interventions such as contracture prevention and maintenance of optimal skin integrity.

Vegetative State and Minimal Conscious State

The vegetative state is defined as the absence of an adequate response to the outside world and absence of any evidence of reception or projection of information in the presence of a sleep-wake cycle.[36] Children may have periods of restlessness with open eyes and movement, but responsiveness is limited to primitive postural and reflex movements of the limbs. Children in a minimal conscious state have limited self-awareness, but they do feel pain and have sleep-wake cycles. The vegetative and minimal conscious states are directly due to primary brain pathology and are not an extension of coma. Coma is a transient state, characterized by an inability to obey commands, utter recognizable words, or open the eyes with the absence of sleep-wake cycles.[75] The vegetative state and the minimal conscious state may be masked by the state of coma, thus hindering diagnosis.

Spasticity and muscle contractures are two common features associated with the vegetative and minimal conscious states. For a child in these states, maintaining an ROM is important for hygiene and nursing. Pharmacologic intervention and neurosurgical procedures to reduce muscle spasticity and improve ROM must be followed by physical therapy. Intervention to maintain passive ROM as described above was found to be effective in a few studies among adults with TBI.[104] Botulinum toxin type A combined with a cast or splint and intensive physical therapy resulted in improvement on the Modified Ashworth scale and in ROM.[96]

Agitation/Confused Stage

A child functioning at RLCF adult levels IV-V, pediatric level II, may follow simple commands but would have impaired judgment and problem-solving ability, thereby necessitating constant supervision to prevent injury. The therapist's aim is to encourage successful performance through adaptive task practice.

The main procedural interventions and patient-related instructional strategies to achieve treatments goals include the following:
1. Directed activity
2. Increasing the child's motivation for activity
3. Family education

Directed activity and increasing child motivation may be achieved through the following components of intervention:
- Simple task training
- Modification of tasks to ensure success
- Building a structured environment
- Carrying out many short-interval treatments

Simple Task Training

Functional activities might be learned using procedural memory and implicit learning through repetition of tasks

with appropriate orientation to time, self, and place. At this stage, the child exhibits frequent errors and variable performance. Practice and feedback are two of the more important training variables that can affect motor performance and learning. Children are mainly dependent on visual and verbal cues to organize their movements. At this early stage of learning, therapists serve as important sources of augmented verbal, visual, or tactile feedback that provides information on outcome and error. Some children with TBI simply fail to act without extensive cueing. A highly structured, consistent, and reinforcing environment is required to ensure active participation in training. Adequate session training time is needed to work on each task to improve performance. When errors decrease, other forms of feedback such as kinesthetic information will be used for error detection and correction.

Modification of the Task to Ensure Success

Often, the physical therapist needs to be creative to keep the child focused on treatment and to increase his motivation. The therapist ensures that the activities practiced are relevant to the child's needs on the one hand, but at the same time acts to motivate the child to participate (Figures 21-4 and 21-5). Too much input or a request for difficult or complex movements may result in frustration and agitation at this stage of recovery.

Building a Structured Environment

A calm environment with structured stimuli may enhance the child's ability to follow commands for a short time. The therapist should observe the child's behavior in different settings and with different people and should identify the environmental variables that affect the child's behavior either positively or negatively. Negative factors should be eliminated and should be replaced by those that reinforce desired behavior. This procedure is dynamic, and the

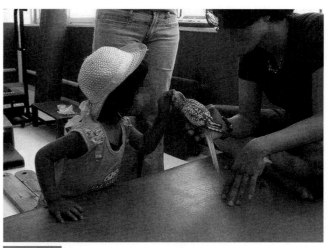

Figure 21-4 Training facilitated by animal-assisted therapy.

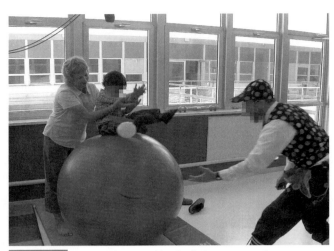

Figure 21-5   Training facilitated by the "Clown Doctors."

therapist needs to re-evaluate the effects of environmental modification on progress and modify intervention to facilitate further improvement.

Carrying Out Many Short-Interval Treatments

At this stage, the child's tolerance of and attention span during treatment is short. Multiple short treatment sessions are preferred to maximize the child's alertness and attention to therapy demands.

Family Education

At this stage, the caregiver is usually with the child all day long. The child has impaired judgment and a short attention span, and as such needs close supervision. A consistent schedule of daily activities and therapy is most effective. Educating the caregiver on how to implement treatment goals as part of the daily routine is extremely important. The expectation is that repetitive task practice during this stage will lead to gradual improvement in motor performance as the child re-acquires motor skills that may be independent of any verbal recollection of the task training.

It is often noted that the child may at times become bored and even frustrated during the rehabilitation period. At such times, innovations such as an outing appropriate to the child's condition might be a good solution. A visit to a park with younger children while practicing intervention-related activities in the playground enables the child to enjoy himself while the therapist achieves treatment goals. Observation of the child in a natural environment might lead to formulation of additional treatment goals. In addition, parents may pick up clues on working toward treatment goals during free-time play activities.

Higher-Level Response Stage

At this level (RLCF pediatric level I or RLCF adult levels VI-VIII), less confusion is noted than in the previous stage, as are an improvement in short-term memory, more

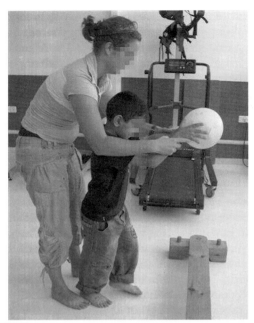

Figure 21-6   Ball exercise.

appropriate and focused behavior, and increased interaction with others and the environment. Limitations of insight, abstract reasoning, and problem solving, however, can still exist. Although the child is relatively independent at this level, complexities in activities of daily living and therapy may require focus on the tasks and skills needed to facilitate community re-integration. Focus is on skill acquisitions that will assist the child in meeting self-care, social, and educational goals. Muscle strengthening and endurance activities are assessed and trained if needed. The main procedural intervention strategies to achieve treatment goals include the following:

1. Practice progressively challenging tasks.
2. Reduce environmental restrictions.
3. Increase physical conditioning.

Practice Progressively Challenging Tasks

The therapist should provide opportunities for the child to actively participate and practice meaningful and motivating activities (Figures 21-6 and 21-7). Functional, relevant, and varied skills should be practiced in an effective manner and in a variety of environmental circumstances. It is common, however, for children to show improvement in the practiced tasks but not be able to transfer the skills to other contexts.[68] Determining the number of repetitions needed to learn a new task, the ability of the child to do the same task the following day, and the ability to do the same task in different contexts provides additional clues to the child's learning capabilities.[68]

More recently introduced therapies include the constraint-induced technique and the use of treadmill training with and without body-weight support (Figure 21-8).

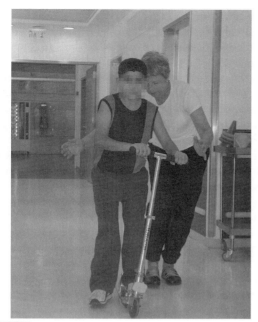

Figure 21-7   Riding on a scooter.

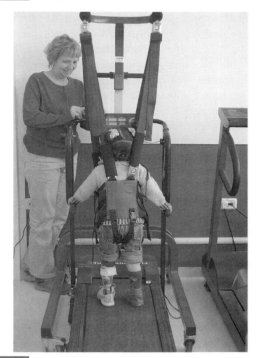

Figure 21-8   Treadmill walking with suspension.

These treatment strategies have come about as the result of basic research in neuroplasticity and neurorecovery. The feasibility of such interventions has been assessed among adults with brain damage and among children with CP. The strength of the evidence that exists in relation to the efficacy of treadmill training with body-weight support among children with CP is generally weak,[20] and this approach has not yet been found to be preferable to regular gait therapy in improving

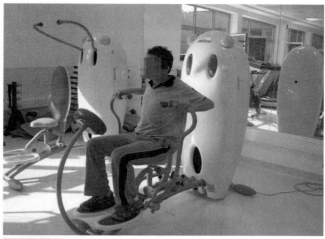

Figure 21-9   Muscle strengthening exercise—Upper extremities.

functional parameters among adults with ABI.[14] Recent evidence suggests that children with hemiplegia due to CP may benefit from constraint-induced movement therapy to improve hand function.[89,103] For children with severe ABI participation in constraint-induced movement therapy may be problematic given the required practice intensity and the frustration that constraint may induce over time. In a multiple case study of children with ABI, it has been noted that constraint-induced movement protocols are possible to implement only if the whole team including parents, totally adhere to the treatment regimen.[37]

Reduce Environmental Restrictions

The therapist may modify the task or the environment to adjust the difficulty of the functional activity. For example, ambulation can be practiced progressively first indoors and then outdoors and then on different surfaces and so on.

Increase Physical Conditioning

Weakness is a common impairment in children with ABI. An adolescent might participate in a standard muscle-strengthening program, with repetitions and duration as needed, or perhaps the adolescent would prefer to participate in gym activities with peers (Figures 21-9 and 21-10). For a younger child, the therapist has to choose appropriate developmental activities that will facilitate muscle strengthening (e.g., play activities combined with stair climbing).

Cardiorespiratory fitness may be reduced by impaired motor abilities, due to prolonged bed rest and inactivity, or due to lesions that affect the autonomic nervous system. Among children with TBI, the mean heart rate at rest was found to be significantly higher and heart rate variability significantly lower as compared with healthy controls.[40a] Only a few studies have investigated the outcome of challenging the cardiovascular system of the child with ABI, making it difficult for clinicians to make an evidence-based decision concerning the applicability of a fitness program for

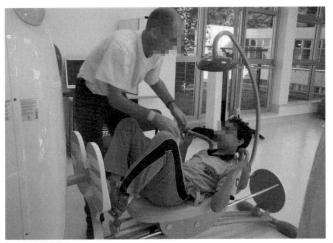

Figure 21-10 Muscle strengthening exercise—Lower extremities.

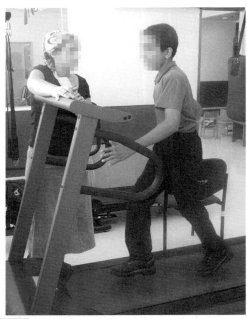

Figure 21-11 Aerobic exercise on the treadmill.

a child. Responsiveness and tolerance of adult patients at the sub-acute stage following moderate to severe brain injury to aerobic training has been demonstrated.[8,34] Evidence suggests that this is a safe, well-accepted, and feasible intervention (Figure 21-11). In the light of insufficient data for children, the therapist must monitor and adhere to acceptable physiologic parameters during endurance therapy sessions.[73]

BACK AT HOME

Once the child is discharged from the rehabilitation setting, outpatient services should continue as necessary to maximize independence at home, at school, and in the

community. High cognitive functions of decision making, judgment, and problem solving usually have not fully recovered, and activities that demand these skills usually require close supervision to ensure safety.

At this time, parents, siblings, and the child all try to adapt to a new family constellation. Many aspects of family life, from emotional to financial, might be influenced directly as a result of the injury or its consequences. Siblings frequently experience adverse effects: About half of the families reported that siblings exhibited behavioral problems such as withdrawal from their injured sibling, or symptoms such as increased fearfulness, or, on the other hand, became over-involved in family issues.[64] Approximately one third of families reported deterioration in their financial status after the child's injury.[72] Parents need help and guidance to re-build the family framework, and they need time to reinforce continued development of the child and his siblings while getting on with their own lives.

An outpatient treatment program in combination with a home-based program might be proposed to the family because the rehabilitation process might need to continue throughout childhood, and intervention provided in the educational system may be inadequate for addressing medical, as opposed to educational, needs. A home-based program was found to be effective among children with ABI[39,40] with the advantage of reducing travel time. In adults with TBI, home-based exercise programs were found to be effective in improving cardiorespiratory fitness.[29] In addition, home-based activity that educates the child to perform exercise as a part of his daily routine might have a long-lasting advantage in preventing secondary impairments such as weight gain, contractures, and pain.[81]

Few studies have examined the effects of repetitive practice of weight-bearing exercises that share similar characteristics to those found in typical functional activities involving the lower limbs (support, balance, and force).[59] For example, sit-to-stand and step-up exercises are mechanically demanding functional activities that children perform many times during their daily routine. Both require muscle strength to raise the body mass, and both require the ability to transfer the center of mass from a larger to a relatively smaller base of support, thereby challenging the muscular system, as well as the equilibrium system. As such, these exercises have the potential to train aspects of motor performance such as balance, strength, and endurance. It was found that a short task-oriented exercise program of sit-to-stand and step-up exercises for children with severe ABI carried out at home resulted in increased functional balance performance[39] and walking performance,[40] which were maintained even after the training had ended.

Because adherence to an exercise program is crucial for its success, simple adjustments to increase compliance were found to be effective. For example, a phone call once a week to the child and parent encouraged them to continue with the program, as did providing each child and family with written information about the program, a detailed explanation and practice run on how to perform each task, and providing a diary in which the child is requested to keep a record of the number of sets he performs each day. All of these tactics have the potential to increase compliance and adherence to the program to well over 50%.[22,39]

For school-aged children, involvement in sports and physical leisuretime activities should be encouraged. These have the potential to increase self-esteem and acceptance by peers. Bicycle riding, horse riding, and other challenging sports activities for children with special needs are recommended, and these days are available in many areas.

ASSISTIVE DEVICES

Nonambulatory children need appropriate assistive technology, and proper use of this technology can be one of the most important aspects of therapeutic intervention. The process of selecting the right equipment requires considerations regarding availability, cost, source of funding, portability, stability, ease of adjustment, ease of modification, construction materials, and aesthetics. Re-evaluation of equipment is needed more frequently than in adults as a result of functional changes and growth.

For preschool children, exploring the environment is crucial for their development. For those children who cannot

ambulate, a device such as a tricycle is a fun alternative to a wheelchair. Many options for adapted equipment are commercially available. When choosing the equipment, one should consider the environment in which the child functions and the needs of caregivers. Another factor that has to be dealt with consists of family lifestyle and typical activities. For teenagers, who are often greatly concerned about their physical appearance and social acceptance by their peers, the prescribed equipment and devices should be as cosmetic and minimal as possible.

SUMMARY

The rehabilitation of children post ABI is a complex and challenging process characterized by varied clinical presentations and unpredictable and varied recovery rates. Although the outcome of the injury depends largely on the nature and severity of the injury itself, appropriate and timely treatment may play a vital role in determining the level of recovery. Physical treatment varies from preventive treatment with the expectation of recovery of brain function, up to a structured motor training program aimed at facilitating compensation processes using existing brain function. Parents are encouraged to take an active role in this lifelong rehabilitation process by enlightening the therapist regarding the child's needs, aspirations, and resources and by carrying over the treatment to the context of daily activities.

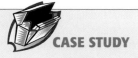

CASE STUDY

"Said"

Said is a 6-year-old boy who lives with his parents, four siblings, his grandmother, and four uncles in a four-bedroom apartment in an underprivileged neighborhood. His father was employed, and his mother was a housewife who cared for the entire extended family. While crossing the street, Said was hit by a car. He was unaccompanied at the time of the accident, and an anonymous passenger in the car called the emergency service. At the accident site, Said's GCS was determined to be 4, and he was immediately intubated and ventilated.

Acute Care

On admission to the acute care unit, a CT scan was performed, which showed bilateral fronto-parietal skull fractures, left parietal subarachnoid hematoma, diffuse cerebral, midbrain, and corpus callosum edema, and bleeding into the third ventricle. CT scan of the chest and abdomen showed fractures of the right inferior ramus of the pubis, ilium fracture with minimal displacement, and bilateral lung contusion. An intracranial pressure (ICP) monitor was inserted; the pelvic fractures did not require intervention. A repeat cranial CT scan a few days later revealed a right fronto-parietal subdural hygroma, and an urgent decompression fronto-parietal craniotomy was performed. A few days later, the ICP monitor was removed. A trial of extubation

failed, and 2 weeks after the accident, a tracheostomy was performed. One week later, Said started to breathe room air without ventilator assistance. A percutaneous endoscopic gastrostomy was placed for nutritional support.

Rehabilitation Center Management

One month after his injury, Said was transferred to our rehabilitation center. His father stayed with him day and night. He described Said as a typically developed young boy, right hand dominant, who loves animals, likes to paint and create with colors and clay, and enjoys playing outside with friends, especially ball games; he is a good pupil at school, has just acquired reading and writing skills, and is a sweet and caring child at home. The father stated repeatedly that the family's greatest wish was to bring Said back home able to ambulate.

General and Neurologic Status on Admission

Said could breathe spontaneously, at a respiratory rate of 24 breaths per minute; he needed supplemental oxygen and assistance in secretion removal. His heart rate at rest was 128 beats per minute. Both pupils responded to light, and he opened his eyes spontaneously but did not follow. Said gave a generalized response to painful stimuli and a generalized startle to loud sounds. The right fourth cranial

Continued

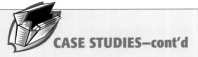

CASE STUDIES—cont'd

(trochlear) nerve and the seventh cranial (facial) nerve appeared to be damaged, and hypotonia was present in all four limbs and trunk.

One Month After Injury

First Physical Therapy Examination and Evaluation

Said's cognitive functioning based on RLCF pediatric level was IV, and examination focused on passive manipulation and observation of spontaneous or stimulus-induced movements. Physical assessment revealed a limited ROM in both ankles (dorsiflexion <90°), hypotonia in all four limbs, no directed movement observed in the head or extremities, and no head control. PEDI admission normative standard scores were zero in all functional skill domains. Scaled scores, which theoretically could provide an individual baseline and thereby give the therapist some idea about progress at outcome assessment, were zero.

Plan of Care and Intervention

The physical therapist's short-term goals were to prevent complications associated with prolonged immobilization and to create an environment most conducive to recovery. The pelvic fractures did not inhibit treatment or weight-bearing activities. The therapist along with the nursing staff carried out bed positioning in sidelying or semi-prone position. His father was trained to do the same. Because Said exhibited hypotonia, and because passive ROM exercises may have harmful effects on soft tissues, only the physical therapist was permitted to do these exercises. Plastic splints were fitted for both lower extremities, and the therapist instructed the father on how to apply them and how to inspect for pressure areas. Suctioning and respiratory therapy were part of the routine management.

Periods of sitting and standing with external constraints were instituted, with gradual increases in duration. Falls in blood pressure were noted at the beginning, and Said's head control was poor. The supported sitting position was in recline with head support, and the standing position on the tilt table was targeted to be less than 90°. After 3 weeks, Said could tolerate both sitting and standing positions for up to 20 minutes each, with a normal blood pressure response. Both the physical therapist and the occupational therapist trained Said's father on how to safely and effectively perform all self-care, as well as on how to perform bed mobility activities and transfers to the wheelchair or to the tilt table. In addition, the father was shown how to do chest therapy and secretion drainage. Although the efficacy of a prolonged sensory stimulation program is still doubtful,[60] the team asked the parents to bring family photographs, which were placed in Said's visual field, and his favorite songs were played to him throughout the day. One month after admission to our rehabilitation department, Said started to respond to the environment.

Two Months After Injury

Second Physical Therapy Examination and Evaluation

At 2 months after the injury, Said's cognitive functioning improved and the RLCF pediatric level was graded as II. Assessment focused on observation of spontaneous and simple instructed tasks. Said's head

control was improved, and some spontaneous movement appeared in his left hand. He squeezed his hand in response to the therapist's request, and he moved his head to the sides when refusing to follow a request. It was noted that Said's muscle tone was still low, both ankles were still limited in dorsiflexion to about 90°, and ataxia was apparent in the limbs, as well as in his trunk. The lying and rolling section of the GMFM revealed initiation of movement in supine but no initiation in any of the prone dimensions. No evident changes in functional ability were noted on any of the domains of the normative scores of the PEDI, but the scaled scores showed improvement (Table 21-5).

Revised Plan of Care and Intervention

Short-term intervention goals included increasing head control and promoting active movement to achieve independence in bed mobility and assisted transfers. At this RLCF level II, simple task training with adjustment of the tasks to achieve success is a useful treatment strategy. Said was provided with graded active facilitation of movement; emphasis was on head control in various positions and on movement from one position to another. The therapist encouraged and facilitated functional activities such as rolling and prone lying with weight bearing through the upper extremities. Sitting up from sidelying and sitting balance were encouraged. The treatment was provided under age-appropriate conditions, incorporating play and motivation that were progressively modified. Because Said demonstrated very short attention and tolerance spans, the team, including the occupational therapist and the speech therapist, decided to split his treatment into multiple short sessions. The physical therapist, who knew that Said loves animals, decided to assess the contribution of animal therapy to treatment. The presence of a guinea pig or parrot during the intervention session motivated and facilitated Said's willingness to participate in treatment, and the duration of each session could then be increased. Changes in tasks and the environment (e.g., practicing moving from sidelying to a sitting position in bed, on the floor, in the treatment hall, or on the playground) were also used to encourage learning. Being in the playground yard was a wonderful

TABLE 21-5   **Said's GMFM Percentage Scores and PEDI Scaled Scores: One, Two, Five, and Eight Months Post Injury**

	Time Post Injury (Month)	1	2	5	8
GMFM	Lying and rolling	0	17	84	100
	Sitting	0	0	78	93
	Crawling and kneeling	0	0	47	71
	Standing	0	0	8	23
	Walking running and jumping	0	0	0	10
PEDI	Self-care	0	30	46	54
	Mobility	0	18	45	56
	Social	0	31	42	49

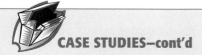

CASE STUDIES—cont'd

opportunity for active practice, providing useful and meaningful functional activities that gave Said the sensation of successful and efficient movement. Said enjoyed sitting in a large swing, which was a great opportunity for multisensory input and a useful means of improving truncal ataxia and trunk stabilization.

Five Months After Injury

Third Physical Therapy Examination and Evaluation
During the fifth month post injury, Said showed remarkable improvement. Although his RLCF level did not change, remaining at grade II, his muscle tone increased, he achieved head control while sitting, and he could perform anti-gravity movement in all four extremities but was still weak. Manual muscle testing performed for knee extensor and hip abductor and extensor muscles resulted in scores of 4/5, with the right side somewhat better than the left side. Outcomes on the PEDI and GMFM 5 months after injury showed that Said had made remarkable improvement (see Table 21-5): He could crawl independently and sit independently, but could not reach forward with either arm to shoulder level while crawling, and could not maintain kneeling without support. Ataxia of the limbs and trunk was increasingly evident in upright postures and increased with anti-gravity demands, making independent transfers, standing, and walking difficult. Bilateral solid ankle-foot orthoses were fitted to contribute to stability in standing and walking.

Continuation of hospitalization in the rehabilitation center was discussed at staff meetings. At about this time, Said went home for a weekend for the first time since the injury. It was very hard for him to come back, as he did not want to leave his mother and siblings, and afterward his motivation in therapy decreased. His mother's visits were few and were brief each time, as she had to take care of Said's four siblings, the youngest of whom was still a baby and the oldest of whom was only 8 years old. Said's father was unemployed since the injury, had been with Said all that time, and was tiring. His little boy was often aggressive and was restless most of the time and needed constant supervision. On the other hand, Said lived in an underprivileged neighborhood, the bathroom and the kitchen were outside of the apartment, and no rehabilitation center was nearby for continuation of therapy. Said's parents expressed their desire that he remain in the rehabilitation center despite their family difficulties, so his achievements could be maximized. In consideration of all these factors, the team together with Said's parents, decided to continue inpatient hospitalization.

Revised Plan of Care and Intervention
Short-term intervention goals now included a focus on reduction of impairments and development of efficient mobility skills to achieve independent transfers and mobility. The therapist's main strategies to achieve treatments goals included the practice of progressively challenging tasks, while reducing environmental restrictions and increasing physical conditioning.

Sessions of treadmill training with body-weight support to facilitate postural control and trunk stabilization compromised by ataxia

and muscle weakness were started. Sit-to-stand activities in various situations were introduced; a strengthening program based on Said's known love for ball games was added (e.g., a basketball game while sitting on a variety of platforms: Floor, comfortable chair, lower chair, moving platform, or a cylinder, or while standing with support). Said played in the treatment room as well as outdoors; he played with his therapist and with other children from the center. In addition, in our rehabilitation department, we have a special gym for children, which Said enjoyed very much.

Because Said could not walk independently, his cardiorespiratory fitness was assessed while riding on a tricycle. A heart rate monitor chest strip and watch were used to assess his heart rate at rest and after 2 and 6 minutes of riding. Few studies have investigated the influence of challenging the cardiovascular system of the child with ABI, making it difficult to make an evidence-based decision about the execution of a fitness program. In light of insufficient data, we adhered to accepted physiologic parameters during endurance therapy sessions.[73] We trained Said by using a tricycle and hand pedaling while in a standing frame. The heart rate monitor was constantly attached to Said's chest, and we gradually increased training time up to 20 minutes, then increased surface difficulties such as riding up a ramp. The "Clown Doctors" incorporated these treatments and improved Said's mood and willingness to tolerate longer exercise sessions.

Eight Months Post Injury—Upcoming Discharge

By the last outcome assessment before his upcoming discharge, 8 months post injury, Said was oriented to time and place, but he still could not provide accurate and detailed information about himself and the present situation. He did know the way to and from daily activities and the sequence of his daily routine. He knew his way around the ward, recognized his own room, could identify his own bed, and knew where his personal belongings were kept. At 8 months after ABI, Said still has not regained his bowel and bladder control and continues to have a tracheostomy as a result of subglottic stenosis; surgery for this is planned for the near future.

The assessment procedure at this stage focused on more complex functional and nonfunctional instructed tasks. It was noted that Said's hypotonic muscle tone had increased to an Ashworth score of 1, his upper extremity and knee strength was 4/5, and pelvic musculature strength was scored at 5/5. His balance performance was assessed by the Pediatric Balance Scale, on which he scored 26/56, with lowest scores on the standing items. Said could stand for 30 seconds but was unable to keep his eyes closed for 3 seconds; he could stand unsupported with feet placed together but was unable to hold the position for 30 seconds and needed assistance to turn 360°. On the GMFM, it was noted that recovery in the lying and sitting dimensions was almost complete (see Table 21-5). Said still cannot remain in high kneeling without support and cannot walk without some support. His PEDI score on all three subscales improved (see Table 21-5). He could walk 100 meters with a posterior walker but

Continued

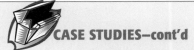

CASE STUDIES—cont'd

needed constant supervision. Recommended treatment goals still focused on reduction of impairments and the development of efficient mobility skills, so Said could achieve independent transfers and mobility.

On discharge, just before the summer holidays, Said was referred to a special education school in his community. In Israel, every child with special needs between the ages of 3 and 21 years may receive rehabilitation services integrated within the education system (see Chapter 30 on services in the United States). Because the interval between discharge from our rehabilitation center and initiation of services in the new education setting was considered too long, we proposed a home-based exercise program for the interim (Evidence Box 21-1). Such a program is designed to increase functional balance performance[40] and walking performance.[39] A wheelchair for community mobility and a walker for in-house mobility were ordered.

EVIDENCE TO PRACTICE 21-1

CASE STUDY "SAID"

EXAMINATION DECISION

Said's father's priorities for intervention after discharge from the rehabilitation department included improvement in Said's safety in transfers from sit to stand and to sit again, in walking, and to improve his ability to climb stairs.

The therapist wanted to assess Said's balance performance in relation to functional abilities. The decision to use the Pediatric Balance Scale[1] was supported by the test structure. It contains 14 tasks, including sit-to-stand, turning in place, and picking up an object from the floor; child performance on each task is scored by a 5-stage ordinal scale. The test has been found to have good test-retest and intraobserver reliability when assessed among children with mild to moderate motor impairment.

PLAN OF CARE DECISIONS

a. The decision to offer Said a home program was based on the lack of easy access to community services and on the available clinical trial results, which provide support for the efficacy of a home program for improving balance and walking performance among children with ABI.[3,4]

b. The therapist prescribed three simple exercises, which had been adapted to the home environment based on publications suggesting that adherence to home exercise programs decreases if more than 4 activities are used.[2]

c. The decision to integrate balance training into functional tasks is based on the "specificity of training" principle. Learning is optimized by practice approximating to the target skill and within the environmental conditions in which the skill will be performed.[5]

d. Based on available evidence, which provides support for the efficacy of sit-to-stand and step-up exercise programs for improving balance and walking performance among children with ABI,[3,4] a modification of these exercises was prescribed: sit-to-stand, step-up exercises with hand support, and in addition, walking with supervision for 20 minutes a day. Said's father took on the responsibility of supervising Said in performing exercises once a day, 4 days a week.

The available restricted exercise protocol consists of limitations, but repetition of the exercise over and over might reduce the child's motivation for practicing. Another limitation relates to the unknown long-term effect of this program among children with ABI.

1. Franjoine, M. R., Gunther, J. S., & Taylor, M. J. (2003). Pediatric Balance Scale: A modified version of the Berg Balance Scale for the school-age child with mild to moderate motor impairment. *Pediatric Physical Therapy*, *15*, 114–128.
2. Henry, K. D., Rosemond, C., & Eckert, L. B. (1998). Effect of number of home exercises on compliance and performance in adults over 65 years of age. *Physical Therapy*, *78*, 270–277.
3. Katz-Leurer, M., Eizenstein, E., & Lieberman, D. G. (2008). Effects of home-based treatment in acquired brain injury children using a task-oriented exercise program. *Physiotherapy*, *94*, 71–77.
4. Katz-Leurer, M., Rotem, H., Keren, O., & Meyer, S. (2009). The effects of a 'home-based' task-oriented exercise programme on motor and balance performance in children with spastic cerebral palsy and severe traumatic brain injury. *Clinical Rehabilitation*, *23*, 714–724.
5. Schmidt R.A., & Wrishberg, C. A. (2004). *Motor learning and performance* (3rd ed.; p. 194). Champaign, IL: Human Kinetics Inc.

REFERENCES

1. Aaron, D. H., & Jansen, C. W. (2003). Development of the Functional Dexterity Test (FDT): Construction, validity, reliability, and normative data. *Journal of Hand Therapy*, *16*, 12.

2. Ada, L., Canning, C., & Paratz, J. (1990). Care of the unconscious head-injury patient. In L. Ada, & C. Canning (Eds.), *Key issues in neurological physiotherapy* (pp. 249–286). Oxford: Butterworth Heinemann.

3. Adamo, M. A., Drazin, D., & Waldman, J. B. (2009). Decompressive craniectomy and postoperative complication

management in infants and toddlers with severe traumatic brain injuries. *Journal of Neurosurgery and Pediatrics, 3,* 334–339.

4. Asikainen, I., Kaste, M., & Sarna, S. (1998). Predicting late outcome for patients with traumatic brain injury referred to a rehabilitation programme: A study of 508 Finnish patients 5 years or more after injury. *Brain Injury, 12,* 95–107.

5. Bariddy, J., Morales, D., Hayman, L., & Diaz-Marchan, P. (2007). Static neuro-imaging in the evaluation of TBI. In N. Zasler, D. I. Katz, & R. D. Zafonte (Eds.), *Brain injury medicine.* New York: Demos Medical Publishing, LLC.

6. Bastian, A. J. (1997). Mechanisms of ataxia. *Physical Therapy, 77,* 672–675.

7. Bayley, N. (1993). *Bayley Scales of Infant Development II.* San Antonio: Psychological Corporation.

8. Bhambhani, Y., Rowland, G., & Farag, M. (2005). Effects of circuit training on body composition and peak cardiorespiratory responses in patients with moderate to severe traumatic brain injury. *Archives of Physical Medicine and Rehabilitation, 86,* 268–276.

9. Bloomfield, S. A. (1997). Changes in musculoskeletal structure and function with prolonged bed rest. *Medicine & Science in Sports and Exercise, 29,* 197–206.

10. Blumenthal, I. (2002). Shaken baby syndrome. *Postgraduate Medicine Journal, 78,* 732–735.

11. Bohannon, R. W., & Smith, M. B. (1987). Interrater reliability of a modified Ashworth scale of muscle spasticity. *Physical Therapy, 67,* 206–207.

12. Bouma, G. J., & Muizelaar, J. P. (1995). Cerebral blood flow in severe clinical head injury. *New Horizons, 3,* 384–394.

13. Brehaut, J. C., Miller, A., Raina, P., & McGrail, K. M. (2003). Childhood behavior disorders and injuries among children and youth: A population-based study. *Pediatrics, 111,* 262–269.

14. Brown, T. H., Mount, J., Rouland, B. L., Kautz, K. A., Barnes, R. M., & Kim, J. (2005). Body weight-supported treadmill training versus conventional gait training for people with chronic traumatic brain injury. *Journal of Head and Trauma Rehabilitation, 20,* 402–415.

15. Centers for Disease Control, National Center for Injury Prevention and Control. (February 2002). WISQARS. Retrieved from: http://www.cdc.gov/ncipc/wisqars.

16. Childers, M. K., Biswas, S. S., Petroski, G., & Merveille, O. (1999). Inhibitory casting decreases a vibratory inhibition index of the H-reflex in the spastic upper limb. *Archives of Physical Medicine and Rehabilitation, 80,* 714–716.

17. Christensen, D. W., Jansen, P., & Perken, R. M. (1997). Outcome and acute care hospital costs after warm water near drowning in children. *Pediatrics, 99,* 715–721.

18. Citta-Pietrolungo, T. J., Alexander, M. A., & Steg, N. L. (1992). Early detection of heterotopic ossification in young patients with traumatic brain injury. *Archives of Physical Medicine and Rehabilitation, 73,* 258–262.

19. Clopton, N., Dutton, J., Featherston, T., Grigsby, A., Mobley, J., & Melvin, J. (2005). Interrater and intrarater reliability of the Modified Ashworth Scale in children with hypertonia. *Pediatric Physical Therapy, 17,* 268–274.

20. Damiano, D. L., DeJong, S. L. (2009). A systematic review of the effectiveness of treadmill training and body weight support in pediatric rehabilitation. *Journal of Neurologic Physical Therapy, 33,* 27–44.

21. Deitz, J. C., Kartin, D., & Kopp, K. (2007). Review of the Bruininks-Oseretsky Test of Motor Proficiency, Second Edition (BOT-2). *Physical and Occupational Therapy in Pediatrics, 27,* 87–102.

22. Fragala-Pinkham, M. A., Haley, S. M., Rabin, J., & Kharasch, V. S. (2005). A fitness program for children with disabilities. *Physical Therapy, 85,* 1182–1200.

23. Franjoine, M. R., Gunther, J. S., & Taylor, M. J. (2003). Pediatric Balance Scale: A modified version of the Berg Balance Scale for the school-age child with mild to moderate motor impairment. *Pediatric Physical Therapy, 15,* 114–128.

24. Gölge, M., Müller, M., Dreesmann, M., Hoppe, B., Wenzelburger, R., & Kuhtz-Buschbeck, J. P. (2004). Recovery of the precision grip in children after traumatic brain injury. *Archives of Physical Medicine and Rehabilitation, 85,* 1435–1444.

25. Greenwald, B. D., Burnett, D. M., & Miller, M. A. (2003). Congenital and acquired brain injury. I. Brain injury: epidemiology and pathophysiology. *Archives of Physical Medicine and Rehabilitation, 84,* S3–S7.

26. Gurney, J. G., Kadan-Lottick, N. (2001). Brain and other central nervous system tumors: Rates, trends, and epidemiology. *Current Opinion in Oncology, 13,* 160–166.

27. Gurney, J. G., Smith, M. A., & Bunin, G. R. (1999). *CNS and miscellaneous intracranial and intraspinal neoplasms. SEER pediatric monograph.* Washington, DC: National Cancer Institute.

28. Haley, S. M., Coster, W. J., & Ludlow, L. H. (1992). *Pediatric Evaluation of Disability Inventory: Development standardization and administration manual.* Boston, MA: Trustees of Boston University.

29. Hassett, L. M., Moseley, A. M., Tate, R. L., Harmer, A. R., Fairbairn, T. J., & Leung, J. (2009). Efficacy of a fitness centre-based exercise programme compared with a home-based exercise programme in traumatic brain injury: A randomized controlled trial. *Journal of Rehabilitation Medicine, 41,* 247–255.

30. Hill, J. (1994). The effects of casting on upper extremity motor disorders after brain injury. *American Journal of Occupational Therapy, 48,* 219–224.

31. Hurvitz, E. A., Mandac, B. R., Davidoff, G., Johnson, J. H., & Nelson, V. S. (1992). Risk factors for heterotopic ossification in children and adolescents with severe traumatic brain injury. *Archives of Physical Medicine and Rehabilitation, 73,* 459–462.

32. Ibsen, L. M., & Koch, I. (2002). Submersion and asphyxial injury. *Critical Care Medicine, 30,* 402–408.

33. Iyer, L. V., Haley, S. M., Watkins, M. P., & Dumas, H. M. (2003). Establishing minimal clinically important differences for

scores on the Pediatric Evaluation of Disability Inventory for inpatient rehabilitation. *Physical Therapy, 83,* 888–898.

34. Jackson, D., Turner-Stokes, L., Culpan, J., Bateman, A., Scott, O., Powell, J., & Greenwood, R. (2001). Can brain-injured patients participate in an aerobic exercise programme during early inpatient rehabilitation? *Clinical Rehabilitation, 15,* 535–544.

35. Jebsen, R. H., Taylor, N., Trieschmann, R. B., Trotter, M. J., & Howard, L. A. (1969). An objective and standardized test of hand function. *Archives of Physical Medicine and Rehabilitation, 50,* 311–319.

36. Jennett, B., & Plum, F. (1972). Persistent vegetative state after brain damage: A syndrome in search of a name. *Lancet, 1,* 734–737.

37. Karman, N., Maryles, J., Baker, R. W., Simpser, E., & Berger-Gross, P. (2003). Constraint-induced movement therapy for hemiplegic children with acquired brain injuries. *Journal of Head Trauma Rehabilitation, 18,* 259–267.

38. Katz, D. I., & Alexander, M. P. (1994). Traumatic brain injury: Predicting course of recovery and outcome for patients admitted to rehabilitation. *Archives of Neurology, 51,* 661–670.

39. Katz-Leurer, M., Eizenstein, E., & Lieberman, D. G. (2008). Effects of home-based treatment in acquired brain injury children using a task-oriented exercise program. *Physiotherapy, 94,* 71–77.

40. Katz-Leurer, M., Rotem, H., Keren, O., & Meyer, S. (2009). The effects of a "home-based" task-oriented exercise programme on motor and balance performance in children with spastic cerebral palsy and severe traumatic brain injury. *Clinical Rehabilitation, 23,* 714–724.

40a. Katz-Leurer, M., Rotem, H., Keren, O., & Meyer, S. (2010). Heart rate and heart rate variability at rest and during exercise in boys who suffered a severe traumatic brain injury and typically-developed controls. *Brain Injury, 24,* 110–114.

41. Katz-Leurer, M., Rotem, H., Lewitus, H., Keren, O., & Meyer, S. (2008). Functional balance tests for children with traumatic brain injury: Within-session reliability. *Pediatric Physical Therapy, 20,* 254–258.

42. Katz-Leurer, M., Rotem, H., Lewitus, H., Keren, O., & Meyer, S. (2008). Relationship between balance abilities and gait characteristics in children with post-traumatic brain injury. *Brain Injury, 22,* 153–159.

43. Katz-Leurer, M., Rotem, H., & Meyer, S. (2008). Hand-held dynamometry in children with traumatic brain injury: Within-session reliability. *Pediatric Physical Therapy, 20,* 259–263.

44. Keenan, H. T., & Bratton, S. L. (2006). Epidemiology and outcomes of pediatric traumatic brain injury. *Developmental Neuroscience, 28,* 256–263.

45. Kemp, A. M., Rajaram, S., Mann, M., Tempest, V., Farewell, D., Gawne-Cain, M. L., Jaspan, T., & Maguire, S.; Welsh Child Protection Systematic Review Group. (2009). What neuroimaging should be performed in children in whom inflicted brain injury (iBI) is suspected? A systematic review. *Clinical Radiology, 64,* 473–483.

46. Keren, O., Yupatov, S., Radai, M. M., Elad-Yarum, R., Faraggi, D., Abboud, S., Ring, H., & Groswasser, Z. (2005). Heart rate variability (HRV) of patients with traumatic brain injury (TBI) during the post-insult sub-acute period. *Brain Injury, 19,* 605–611.

47. Kochanek, P. M. (2006). Pediatric traumatic brain injury: Quo vadis? *Developmental Neuroscience, 28,* 244–255.

48. Kraus, J. F. (1995). Epidemiological features of brain injury in children: Occurrence, children at risk, causes and manner of injury, severity, and outcomes. In S. H. Broman, & M. E. Michel (Eds.), *Traumatic head injury in children* (pp. 22–39). New York: Oxford University Press.

49. Kreisman, N. R., Soliman, S., & Gozal, D. (2000). Regional differences in hypoxic depolarization and swelling in hippo-campal slices. *Journal of Neurophysiology, 83,* 1031–1038.

50. Kuhtz-Buschbeck, J. P., Hoppe, B., Gölge, M., Dreesmann, M., Damm-Stünitz, U., & Ritz, A. (2003). Sensorimotor recovery in children after traumatic brain injury: Analyses of gait, gross motor, and fine motor skills. *Developmental Medicine & Child Neurology, 45,* 821–828.

51. Langlois, J. A., Rutland-Brown, W., & Thomas, K. E. (2005). The incidence of traumatic brain injury among children in the United States: Differences by race. *Journal of Head Trauma Rehabilitation, 20,* 229–238.

52. Lannin, N. A., Cusick, A., McCluskey, A., & Herbert, R. D. (2007). Effects of splinting on wrist contracture after stroke: A randomized controlled trial. *Stroke, 38,* 111–116.

53. Laws, E. R., Thapar, K. (1993). Brain tumors. *CA A Cancer Journal for Clinicians, 43,* 263–271.

54. Leong, B. (2002). Critical review of passive muscle stretch: Implications for the treatment of children in vegetative and minimally conscious states. *Brain Injury, 16,* 169–183.

55. Leong, B. (2002). The vegetative and minimally conscious states in children: Spasticity, muscle contracture and issues for physiotherapy treatment. *Brain Injury, 16,* 217–230.

56. Lettinga, A. T. (2002). Diversity in neurological physiotherapy: A content analysis of the Brunnstrom/Bobath controversy. *Advances in Physiology, 4,* 23–36.

57. Levin, M., Kleim, J., & Wolf, S. (2009). What do motor "recovery" and "compensation" mean in patients following stroke? *Neurorehabilitation and Neural Repair, 23,* 313–319.

58. Lew, H., Lee, E., Pan, S., & Chiang, J. (2007). Electrophysiologic assessment technique: Evoked potentials and electroencephalography. In N. Zasler, D. I. Katz, & R. D. Zafonte (Eds.), *Brain injury medicine* (pp. 150–157). New York: Demos Medical Publishing LLC.

59. Liao, H. F., Liu, Y. C., Liu, W. Y., & Lin, Y. T. (2007). Effectiveness of loaded sit-to-stand resistance exercise for children with mild spastic diplegia: A randomized clinical trial. *Archives of Physical Medicine and Rehabilitation, 88,* 25–31.

60. Lombardi, F., Taricco, M., De Tanti, A., Telaro, E., & Liberati, A. (2002). Sensory stimulation for brain injured individuals in coma or vegetative state. *Cochrane Database of Systematic Reviews, CD001427,* 2002.

61. Lunsford, B. R., & Perry, J. (1995). The standing heel-rise test for ankle plantar flexion: Criterion for normal. *Physical Therapy, 75*, 694–698.

62. Melamed, E., Keren, D., Robinson, D., Halperin, N., & Mrosswasser, Z. (2000). [Periarticular new bone formation following traumatic brain injury]. *Harefuah, 139*, 368–371.

63. Meythaler, J. M., Peduzzi, J. D., Eleftheriou, E., & Novack, T. A. (2001). Current concepts: Diffuse axonal injury-associated traumatic brain injury. *Archives of Physical Medicine and Rehabilitation, 82*, 1461–1471.

64. Montgomery, V., Oliver, R., Reisner, A., & Fallat, M. E. (2002). The effect of severe traumatic brain injury on the family. *Journal of Trauma, 52*, 1121–1124.

65. Moore, B. D., Copeland, D. R., & Ater, J. (1998). Neuropsychological outcome of children diagnosed with brain tumor during infancy. *Child's Nervous System, 14*, 504.

66. Mortenson, P. A., & Eng, J. J. (2003). The use of casts in the management of joint mobility and hypertonia following brain injury in adults: A systematic review. *Physical Therapy, 83*, 648–658.

67. Mossberg, K. A., Ayala, D., Baker, T., Heard, J., & Masel, B. (2007). Aerobic capacity after traumatic brain injury: Comparison with a nondisabled cohort. *Archives of Physical Medicine and Rehabilitation, 88*, 315–320.

68. Neistadt, M. E. (1994). Perceptual retraining for adults with diffuse brain injury. *American Journal of Occupational Therapy, 48*, 225–233.

69. Niznik, T. M., Turner, D., & Worrell, T. W. (1995). Functional reach as a measurement of balance for children with lower extremity spasticity. *Physical and Occupational Therapy in Pediatrics, 15*, 1–15.

70. Nudo, R. J., Milliken, G. W., Jenkins, W. M., & Merzenich, M. M. (1996). Neural substrates for the effects of rehabilitation training on motor recovery after ischemic infarct. *Science, 171*, 1791–1794.

71. Ommaya, A. K., Goldsmith, W., & Thibault, L. (2002). Biomechanics and neuropathology of adult and paediatric head injury. *British Journal of Neurosurgery, 16*, 220–242.

72. Osberg, J. S., Kahn, P., Rowe, K., & Brooke, M. M. (1996). Pediatric trauma: Impact on work and family finances. *Pediatrics, 98*, 890–897.

73. Peel, C. (1996). The cardiopulmonary system and movement dysfunction. *Physical Therapy, 76*, 448–455.

74. Piper, M. C., Pinnell, L. E., Darrah, J., Maguire, T., & Byrne, P. J. (1992). Construction and validation of the Alberta Infant Motor Scale (AIMS). *Canadian Journal of Public Health, 83*, S46–S50.

75. Plum, F. (1991). Coma and related global disturbances of the human conscious state. *Cerebral Cortex, 9*, 25–42.

76. Ponsford, J., Willmott, C., Rothwell, A., Cameron, P., Ayton, G., Nelms, R., Curran, C., & Ng, K. (2001). Impact of early intervention on outcome after mild traumatic brain injury in children. *Pediatrics, 108*, 1297–1303.

77. Provost, B., Heimerl, S., McClain, C., Kim, N. H., Lopez, B. R., & Kodituwakku, P. (2004). Concurrent validity of the Bayley Scales of Infant Development II Motor Scale and the Peabody Developmental Motor Scales-2 in children with developmental delays. *Pediatric Physical Therapy, 16*, 149–156.

78. Reilly, P. L., Simpson, D. A., Sprod, R., & Thomas, L. (1988). Assessing the conscious level in infants and young children: A pediatric version of the Glasgow Coma Scale. *Child's Nervous System, 4*, 30–33.

79. Richardson, P. K., Atwater, S. W., Crowe, T. K., & Deitz, J. C. (1992). Performance of preschoolers on the Pediatric Clinical Test of Sensory Interaction for Balance. *American Journal of Occupational Therapy, 46*, 793–800.

80. Ricker, J., & Arenth, P. (2007). Functional neuro-imaging in TBI. In N. Zasler, D. I. Katz, & R. D. Zafonte (Eds.), *Brain injury medicine* (pp. 130–149). New York: Demos Medical Publishing LLC.

81. Rimmer, J. H., Riley, B., Wang, E., et al. (2004). Physical activity participation among persons with disabilities: Barriers and facilitators. *American Journal of Preventive Medicine, 26*, 419–425.

82. Rodgers, G. B. (1993). *Bicycle and bicycle helmet use patterns in the United States: A description and analysis of national survey data.* Washington, DC: U.S. Consumer Product Safety Commission.

83. Rossi, C., & Sullivan, S. J. (1996). Motor fitness in children and adolescents with traumatic brain injury. *Archives of Physical Medicine and Rehabilitation, 77*, 1062–1065.

84. Russell, D., Rosenbaum, P., Gowland, C., Hardy, S., Lane, M., Plews, N., McGavin, H., Cadman, D., & Jarvis, S. (1993). *Gross motor function manual.* Hamilton, Ontario: McMaster University.

85. Shumway-Cook, A., & Horak, F. B. (1986). Assessing the influence of sensory interaction of balance: Suggestion from the field. *Physical Therapy, 66*, 1548–1550.

86. Stein, D. G. (2007). Concepts of CNS plasticity and their implication for understanding recovery after brain damage. In N. Zasler, D. I. Katz, & R. D. Zafonte (Eds.), *Brain injury medicine.* New York: Demos Medical Publishing LLC.

87. Stevenson, M. R., Rimajova, M., Edgecombe, D., & Vickery, K. (2003). Childhood drowning: Barriers surrounding private swimming pools. *Pediatrics, 111*, e115–e119.

88. Squire, L. R., & Zola, S. M. (1996). Structure and function of declarative and nondeclarative memory systems. *Proceedings of the National Academy of the Sciences U S A, 93*, 13515–13522.

89. Taub, E., Ramey, S. L., DeLuca, S., & Echols, K. (2004). Efficacy of constraint-induced movement therapy for children with cerebral palsy with asymmetric motor impairment. *Pediatrics, 113*, 305–312.

90. Teasdale, G., & Jennett, B. (1974). Assessment of coma and impaired consciousness: A practical scale. *Lancet, 13*, 81–84.

91. Tokcan, G., Haley, S. M., Gill-Body, K. M., & Dumas, H. M. (2003). Item-specific functional recovery in children and youth with acquired brain injury. *Pediatric Physical Therapy, 15*, 16–22.

92. Tremblay, F., Malouin, F., Richards, C.L., & Dumas, F. (1990). Effects of prolonged muscle stretch on reflex and voluntary activations in children with spastic cerebral palsy. *Scandinavian Journal of Rehabilitation Medicine, 22,* 171–180.

93. Uniform Data System for Medical Rehabilitation, 2000

94. van Beeck, E. F., Branche, C. M., Szpilman, D., Modell, J. H., & Bierens, J. J. (2005). A new definition of drowning: Towards documentation and prevention of a global public health problem. *Bulletin of the World Health Organization, 83,* 853–856.

95. Van Peppen, R., Kwakkel, G., Wood-Dauphinee, S., Hendriks, H., Van der Wees, P., & Dekker, J. (2004). The impact of physical therapy on functional outcomes after stroke: What's the evidence? *Clinical Rehabilitation, 18,* 833–862.

96. van Rhijn, J., Molenaers, G., & Ceulemans, B. (2005). Botulinum toxin type A in the treatment of children and adolescents with an acquired brain injury. *Brain Injury, 19,* 331–335.

97. Vitale, A. E., Jankowski, L. W., & Sullivan, S. J. (1997). Reliability for a walk/run test to estimate aerobic capacity in a brain-injured population. *Brain Injury, 11,* 67–76.

98. Webster, K. E., Wittwer, J. E., & Feller, J. A. (2005). Validity of the GAITRite walkway system for the measurement of averaged and individual step parameters of gait. *Gait Posture, 22,* 317–321.

99. Westcott, S. L., Lowes, L. P., & Richardson, P. K. (1997). Evaluation of postural stability in children: Current theories and assessment tools. *Physical Therapy, 77,* 629–645.

100. Wiercisiewski, D. R., & McDeavitt, J. T. (1998). Pulmonary complications in traumatic brain injury. *Head Trauma Rehabilitation, 13,* 28–35.

101. Williams, E. N., Carroll, S. G., Reddihough, D. S., Phillips, B. A., & Galea, M. P. (2005). Investigation of the timed 'up & go' test in children. *Developmental Medicine & Child Neurology, 47,* 518–524.

102. Williams, P. E. (1990). Use of intermittent stretch in the prevention of serial sarcomere loss in immobilised muscle. *Annals of Rheumatic Disease, 49,* 316–317.

103. Willis, J. K., Morello, A., Davie, A., Rice, J. C., & Bennett, J. T. (2002). Forced use treatment of childhood hemiparesis. *Pediatrics, 110,* 94–96.

104. Yablon, S. A., Agana, B. T., Ivanhoe, C. B., & Boake, C. (1996). Botulinum toxin in severe upper extremity spasticity among patients with traumatic brain injury: An open-labeled trial. *Neurology, 47,* 939–944.

105. Ylvisaker, M., & Feeney, T. (2007). Pediatric brain injury: Social, behavioral, and communication disability. *Physical Medicine & Rehabilitation Clinics of North America, 18,* 133–144.

106. Zuckerman, G. B., Gregory, P. M., & Santos-Damiani, S. M. (1998). Predictors of death and neurologic impairment in pediatric submersion injuries: The Pediatric Risk of Mortality Score. *Archives of Pediatric and Adolescent Medicine, 152,* 134–140.

SUGGESTED READING

Flanagan, A., Krzak, J., Peer, M., Johnson, P., & Urban, M. (2009). Evaluation of short-term intensive orthotic garment use in children who have cerebral palsy. *Pediatric Physical Therapy, 21,* 201–204.

Katz-Leurer, M., Rotem, H., Keren, O., & Meyer, S. Heart rate and heart rate variability at rest and during exercise in boys with post severe traumatic brain injury and typically developed controls.

22 Myelodysplasia

KATHLEEN A. HINDERER, PT, PhD • STEVEN R. HINDERER, PT, MD • DAVID B. SHURTLEFF, MD

Children and adolescents with myelodysplasia, perhaps more than most diagnostic groups of children with disabilities, challenge pediatric physical therapists to use and integrate many facets of their knowledge and skills. The multiple body systems affected by this congenital malformation make intervention for these patients more complex than the congenital spinal cord defect alone might imply. Awareness of the many possible manifestations of this condition, knowledge of methods to examine and detect their presence, and the ability to evaluate the relative contribution of each manifestation to current activity limitations are important. This knowledge, combined with the ability to anticipate future needs and potential problems, empowers the physical therapist to select interventions that will optimize function and prevent the development of secondary impairments. Conversely, lack of awareness of these issues is not without consequences, as significant secondary permanent impairments can result when clinicians are not aware of or do not recognize early signs and symptoms of preventable complications related to myelodysplasia.

The objectives of this chapter are to familiarize the physical therapist with the numerous manifestations of myelodysplasia; describe its impact on body systems and functional skills; provide developmental expectations and prognosis based on the level of involvement; outline the roles of the various disciplines involved in team management; discuss methods of examination, evaluation, and diagnosis; and highlight intervention strategies for specific problems.

TYPES OF MYELODYSPLASIA

Dorland's Medical Dictionary defines myelodysplasia as "defective development of any part (especially the lower segments) of the spinal cord." The various types of myelodysplasia are illustrated in Figure 22-1. Spina bifida is a commonly used term referring to various forms of myelodysplasia. Spina bifida is classified into aperta (visible or open) lesions and occulta (hidden or not visible) lesions.[95] The degree of motor and sensory loss from these lesions can range from no loss to severe impairment. Regardless of initial level of neurologic impairment, individuals with any of these lesions are at risk for further loss of function over time. Paralysis may occur later in life as a complication of abnormal tissue growth (dysplasia) causing pressure on

nerves (e.g., lipomatous or dermoid tissue). Lack of proper growth of associated connective tissues around the malformed spinal cord can also cause ischemia and progressive neurologic impairment by tethering of the cord.

Spina bifida aperta is commonly thought of as myelomeningocele, which is an open spinal cord defect that usually protrudes dorsally. Myelomeningoceles are not skin covered and are usually associated with spinal nerve paralysis (see Figure 22-1, A and B). Meninges and nerves can also protrude anteriorly or laterally, making them not visible externally but still associated with nerve paralysis. Some individuals with myelomeningocele do not have associated paralysis.

Meningoceles are also classified as spina bifida aperta. They are skin covered and are initially associated with no paralysis (see Figure 22-1, C). Meningoceles contain only membranes or nonfunctional nerves that end in the sac wall.[95] Other skin-covered lesions, however, can be associated with paralysis.

The next most common form of myelodysplasia is a lipoma of the spinal cord. Lipomas are classified as spina bifida occulta, but most are visible. They may be large or small and manifest as distinct, subcutaneous masses of fat, frequently associated with abnormal pigmentation of the skin, hirsutism, skin appendages, and dimples above the gluteal cleft. A lipomatous or fibrous tract descends ventrally from the subcutaneous lipoma to varying extents into the subdural space adjacent to the spinal cord. Lipomas of the spinal cord are therefore classified based on the location of the tract. They can be (1) lipomyelomeningocele with paralysis, (2) lipomeningoceles with no paralysis, (3) lipomas of the filum terminale usually with no paralysis, and (4) lipomas of the cauda equina or conus medullaris with or without paralysis at birth. If paralysis is absent at birth, it is acquired over time, and if present at birth, it will worsen with time. Some lipomas involving the spinal cord are not associated with an extension to subcutaneous fat. Lipomas of the spinal cord may or may not be associated with bifid vertebrae (true spina bifida occulta).

Diastematomyelia is a fibrous, cartilaginous, or bony band or spicule separating the spinal cord into hemicords, each surrounded by a dural sac. It can occur as an isolated defect along with vertebral anomalies or in conjunction with either myelomeningocele or lipomyelomeningocele.

703

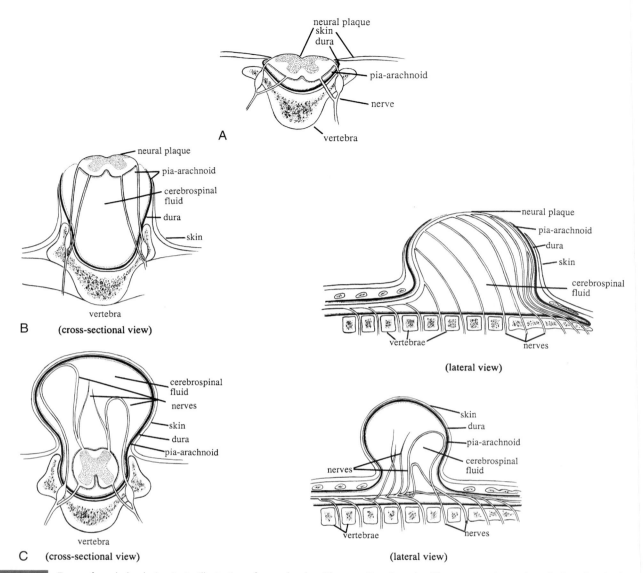

Figure 22-1 Types of myelodysplasia. **A,** An illustration of a myelocele with no cystic subarachnoid space anterior to the spinal cord as is observed with myelomeningocele. **B,** A myelomeningocele may barely protrude from the back or may be a large sessile lesion as pictured here. There is a covering membrane with nerves imbedded in the dome of the sac. These spinal nerves occasionally return to their appropriate neural foramina to exit from the spinal canal. **C,** This type of lesion may be incompletely covered or have a full-thickness skin covering as shown here. When such a lesion is completely skin covered and is associated with no paralysis, it is classified as a meningocele. Meningoceles have only a few or no nerves attached to the dome of the sac. (Adapted from Shurtleff, D. B. [Ed.]. [1986]. *Myelodysplasias and exstrophies: Significance, prevention, and treatment* [pp. 44 and 45]. Orlando, FL: Grune & Stratton.)

Depending on the associated involvement of the spinal cord and meninges, diastematomyelia may be associated with paralysis initially, or progressive weakness can develop later in occulta lesions as a result of cord tethering.

The least common of the myelodysplasias are separate or septated cysts. These myelocystoceles are separate from the central canal of the spinal cord and from the subarachnoid space. They occur in the low lumbar and sacral area and are skin covered. They may or may not be associated with nerve impairment or lipomas of the spinal cord. When a myelocystocele is associated with a primitive gut and an open abdomen, it is classified as an exstrophy of the cloaca. When the bony elements of the sacrum are missing or abnormal, such myelocystic lesions are termed sacral agenesis.

PATHOEMBRYOLOGY

Embryologically, myelodysplastic lesions can be related to two different processes of nervous system formation: abnormal neurulation or canalization. Neurulation is the folding of ectoderm (primitive skin and associated structures) on each side of the notochord (primitive spinal cord) to form a tube that extends from the hindbrain to the second sacral vertebra. Meningoceles can therefore occur both over the skull and along the spinal column. Encephaloceles (containing brain if along the midline of the skull) and myelomeningoceles, which can occur along the spinal canal from the C1 to S2 vertebrae, result from a failure of complete entubulation with associated abnormal mesodermal (primitive connective tissue, muscle, and nervous tissue) development. Abnormal mesodermal development produces epidermal sinus tracts, lipomas, and diastematomyelia, as well as unfused posterior vertebral laminae (i.e., true spina bifida occulta).[95] Neurulation occurs early in development, before day 28 of gestation.

The spinal cord distal to the S2 vertebra develops by canalization. Groups of cells in the dorsal, central midline of the mesoderm, distal to the S2 vertebra, become nerve cells. These cells clump together into masses, which develop cystic structures that join to form many canals. The canals ultimately fuse into one tubular structure that joins with the distal end of the spinal cord, which was developing from the neurulation process described previously. Failure of proper canalization, with subsequent retrogressive development of this region, embryologically explains the occurrence of skin-covered meningoceles, lipomas of the spinal cord, and myelocystoceles, all of which most frequently develop caudal to the L3 vertebra.[95]

The much better formed, essentially normal, central nervous system (CNS) observed in lesions associated with abnormal canalization and the frequency of CNS malformations (e.g., Arnold-Chiari type II, mental impairment, cranial nerve palsies, and hydrocephalus) associated with neurulation can be explained by the way that neurulation takes place. The neural crests first fuse at approximately the C1 vertebra, and closure of the neural tube progresses simultaneously in cephalad and caudal directions. The same embryologic neurulation processes are simultaneously forming the CNS from the tectal plate to the midlumbar area. It is therefore logical that an influence sufficient to interfere with neurulation along the spinal canal would also interfere with development of the cephalad end, producing CNS malformations above the spinal cord level, which are commonly exhibited in this population.[95] Because canalization occurs by different embryologic processes at a different time period than neurulation, any factor interfering with canalization will not necessarily affect neurulation, so the CNS usually forms normally above the midlumbar area (Figure 22-2).

ETIOLOGY

The cause of canalization disorders is unknown. This discussion therefore focuses on disorders of neurulation and, in particular, on myelomeningocele. These causes may also

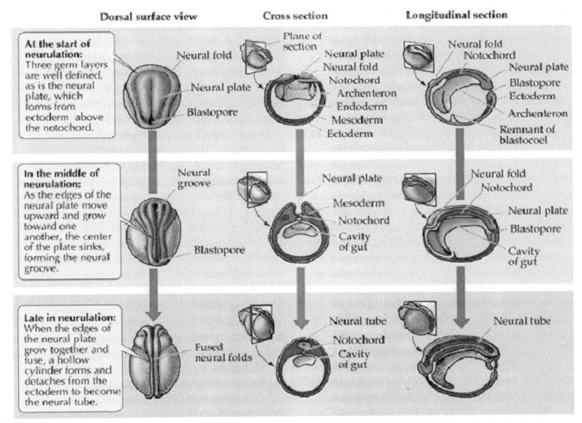

Figure 22-2   Neurulation stages. (From Purves, W.K. [1998]. *Life: the science of biology.* [4th ed]: Sunderland, Pa: WH Freeman.)

apply to other neural tube defects that can result from defective neurulation (anencephaly, encephalocele, meningocele, and lipomyelomeningocele, all with or without diastematomyelia). For brevity, we refer to all these lesions throughout this chapter as MM for myelomeningocele and its associated malformations.[170]

GENETICS

MM is often associated with genetic abnormalities, including chromosomal aberrations and other classic "syndromes." Each child born with MM, therefore, warrants a careful physical examination by a pediatrician because the "syndrome" is usually more important than the spinal lesion for defining prognosis. The recurrence risk for siblings in the United States is 2% to 3%.[170]

The occurrence of MM varies among races and regions of the world. African blacks have the lowest incidence at 1 in 10,000. Celts (Eastern Irish, Western Scots, and all Welsh) have had a birth incidence recorded as high as 1 in 80. The Spanish also have a high birth incidence; however, these patients have unusually good leg function and minimal CNS abnormalities considering their thoracic and high lumbar level lesions. Sikhs living in Vancouver, British Columbia, have another form of MM, with a higher frequency in birth incidence than many other genetically related groups. One can conclude from these data that either there are many genetic causes for MM or that there are many genetically determined responses to one or more teratogens.[170]

TERATOGENS

Teratogens can cause MM. Excess maternal alcohol intake can produce a classic fetal alcohol syndrome with MM. Ingestion of valproic acid (an anticonvulsant medication) during pregnancy is also associated with an increased birth incidence of MM. Many other possible teratogens have been studied, but inadequate descriptions of the pathology of the lesions and the relative infrequency of their occurrence have resulted in inconclusive observations. The rachitic lesion illustrated by Jacobson and Berlin[77] suggests that the MM they observed among progeny of street-drug abusers is a specific entity that is probably due to nutritional deprivation, teratogens, or a combination of these influences. More studies combining detailed family histories, pathologic anatomy, and detailed physical examinations must be conducted to determine the relative contribution of teratogens to MM formation.[170]

NUTRITIONAL DEFICIENCIES

Inadequate levels of dietary folic acid have been identified as a cause of MM and anencephaly in some populations. A significant decrease in the incidence of MM births and abortions was observed for MM diagnosed prenatally in the United Kingdom during a placebo-controlled trial of prenatal folic acid administration for women who had given birth to a previous baby with a neural tube defect.[29,126] With the introduction of more foods containing folic acid in the Celtic regions of the United Kingdom, particularly during winter and early spring when such foods were unavailable in the past, there has been a decrease in the birth incidence of MM predating the research on folic acid supplementation.[45]

The decrease in birth incidence in the United Kingdom reflects a current worldwide trend. Four reports have suggested that the European and United Kingdom studies regarding the benefit of supplementation of folic acid can be applied to the culturally and genetically more diverse populations of Canada, Mexico, and China, where there are different racial and regional differences in the birth incidence of MM.[15,37,56,140] The data from the United States does not include pregnancies terminated because of in utero diagnosis of neural tube defects and, therefore, has led to controversy.[16,121,123,155]

Regardless of the applicability of these studies to the population of the United States, we recommend advising women to take folic acid in an effort to reduce both the recurrence in families[126] and the occurrence in families without a member with MM.[15,33] Women with a first-degree relative with MM or with history of having an open neural tube defect in a previous child or fetus should be advised to take 4 mg per day, and women without a positive history should be advised to take 0.4 mg per day. Both should begin the folic acid at least 3 months before conception. Folic acid is believed to be harmless in this age group because the only possible concern is the masking of pernicious anemia resulting from cobalamin deficiency, allowing progression of the subacute combined degeneration of the spinal cord resulting from cobalamin deficiency. Cobalamin deficiency is rare in this age group, and awareness of the possibility of neurologic loss from spinal cord degeneration should lead to early detection before significant harm occurs. The only other precaution is to warn the women that taking folic acid reduces their risk by 70% but does not eliminate the occurrence of open neural tube defects and has no known effect on the occurrence of closed neural tube defects.

INCIDENCE AND PREVALENCE

Superimposed on a general worldwide decrease in the birth incidence of MM are a number of influences to cause both a reduction in birth incidence and increased prevalence resulting from improved survival. Better nutrition mentioned earlier for the Celtic region of the United Kingdom and Ireland applies to many areas of the industrialized world. Wider availability of maternal serum alpha-fetoprotein screening and more highly refined resolution of diagnostic ultrasonography for fetal examination have given parents an option to terminate pregnancies because their fetus has

MM.[6,106] It is estimated that internationally approximately 23% of pregnancies where a prenatal diagnosis of a neural tube defect is made are voluntarily terminated.[130] Conversely, prenatal diagnosis has allowed other parents to select cesarean section prior to rupture of the amniotic membranes and onset of labor, avoiding trauma to the neural sac from vaginal delivery. Diagnosis now occurs frequently at 18 weeks gestation allowing time for parents to deliberate.[183] The outcome of cesarean delivery compared to vaginal delivery has been children with less paralysis and with minimal risk for CNS infection, both of which were previously a cause for increased morbidity and early death.[98,171] Improved medical care has resulted in increased survival and, secondarily, an increased prevalence of MM. Incidence at birth in the United States has been reported to range from 0.4 to 0.9 per 1000 births, depending on the reporting source.[170] Prevalence per 1000 births in the United States is reported to be 4.18 for Hispanic, 3.37 for non-Hispanic white, and 2.90 for non-Hispanic black mothers.[194]

PERINATAL MANAGEMENT

Since the late 1980s, the intervention of MM has changed from a postnatal crisis of horrendous magnitude to a prenatal option of either pregnancy termination or improved pregnancy outcome by prelabor cesarean section birth. This advance has been made possible by widespread use of maternal serum alpha-fetoprotein screening and improved resolution of ultrasonography.[106] Unfortunately, this type of screening will not detect skin-covered neural defects such as meningoceles, lipomyelomeningoceles, or other rare lesions covered by skin.

Technical improvements are being made rapidly in ultrasonography so that minor variations in the frontal bones of the fetus and encapsulation of the midbrain by the cerebellum can be interpreted as the "lemon" and "banana" signs.[6] Ultrasound in the second trimester can detect spina bifida and other neural tube defects by looking at a cross-section view of the fetal head and visualizing the lateral ventricles, which are part of the fluid collecting system in the brain. The "lemon sign" denotes the scalloping (overlapping) frontal bones, which makes the cross section appear lemon shaped rather than oval and is predictive of spina bifida. The "banana sign" refers to the abnormally shaped midbrain and an elongated cerebellum in the Arnold-Chiari malformation. Among fetuses with neural tube defects, the "lemon sign" can be detected in 80% and the "banana sign" in 93% of cases. These ultrasonographic signs are more accurate in defining the cranial malformations associated with MM than in detecting abnormalities of the spine. As discussed in the section on pathoembryology, these ultrasonographic signs are pertinent to neural tube defects cephalad to the S2 vertebra (i.e., neurulation defects) but not to canalization defects, which are usually not associated with cranial malformations responsible for the Arnold-Chiari type II

malformation,[165] the cause of the "lemon" and "banana" signs. Some spinal dysraphic states and dorsal lumbosacral masses consistent with canalization defects such as myelocystocele or lipomyelomeningocele can be identified with ultrasonography. Other anomalies consistent with syndromes or organ malformations that are incompatible with survival beyond intrauterine life (e.g., anencephaly) can also be detected.

A third modality for prenatal diagnosis, amniotic fluid analysis, is critical in the evaluation of a fetus with a neural tube defect. Up to 10% of fetuses with a neural tube defect, detected in the first half of the second trimester or before, have an associated chromosome error, usually trisomy 13 or 18.[103] Chromosome analysis of amniotic cells is therefore essential to the parental decision-making process regarding abortion of the pregnancy. From the same amniotic fluid specimen obtained for chromosome analysis, the acetylcholinesterase level can be determined. This test is more accurate than determination of the amniotic fluid level of alpha-fetoprotein used previously because the former is positive only in a fetus with an open neural tube defect.[106] The presence of a dorsal spine lesion and a negative result of an acetylcholinesterase test suggest a skin-covered meningocele or other skin-covered MM, which is an indication for normal vaginal delivery. A MM lesion containing nerves protruding dorsal to the plane of the back, in the presence of fetal knee or ankle function observed on ultrasonography, warrants prelabor cesarean section, sterile delivery, and closure of the open-back lesion to preserve nerve function.[103]

Prenatal diagnosis has allowed the introduction of repair of the MM sac in utero. Tulipan and associates[187] reported a decreased need for a cerebrospinal fluid shunt when intrauterine repairs are performed. The authors also claimed improvement in the Chiari II malformation, as evidenced solely by improved appearance on magnetic resonance imaging (MRI). Bannister[8] has cautioned that the MRI appearance is not as important as function. Many believe the Chiari II symptoms are the result of abnormalities in neurulation causing failure of brain stem nuclei to develop properly. Tulipan and associates'[187] claims, however, are not substantiated by the results of cases sent for intrauterine repair by several referral centers to the two surgical treatment centers cited by these authors. Twenty-one of the 26 cases have required cerebrospinal fluid shunts. Additional complications for the 26 infants included the following: 3 had severe Chiari II symptoms, 6 had prolonged neonatal intensive care hospitalizations for apnea because of a combination of prematurity (30 to 31 weeks' gestational age) and Chiari II symptoms, and 4 had dehiscence in utero, with 3 of these 4 developing gram-negative meningitis. To resolve the controversial issues surrounding intrauterine MM repair, the U.S. federal government has funded a prospective study, Management of Myelomeningocele (MOMS), in three centers with prior experience with intrauterine surgery. Patients are referred via a fourth center, the Biostatistics

Center of George Washington University (1-866-ASK-MOMS). This center assigns cases to one of three treating centers and to either the treatment group (cesarean section delivery with intrauterine repair) or a control group (cesarean section delivery without intrauterine repair). The results of this study will determine the value of intrauterine repair of MM. Enrollment of the required 200 participants was 80% complete as of June 2010. Follow-up of participants will occur at 12 and 30 months. Further information is available at www.spinabifidamoms.com.

IMPAIRMENTS

The discussions of pathoembryology and diagnosis describe the potential involvement of the brain and brain stem in addition to the spinal cord in individuals with MM. The multifocal involvement of the CNS results in several possible complex problems, making the care of these individuals more challenging than and substantially different from that of children with traumatic spinal cord injuries. The broad spectrum of problems encountered with MM requires a multidisciplinary team approach in a comprehensive care outpatient clinic setting. This section describes the variety of impairments that can occur with MM. In addition, general examination and intervention issues related to each impairment are discussed. Impairment, for the purpose of this discussion, is defined as a change in body structure and function, whereas activity limitation is the inability to perform tasks as a consequence of impairments. Activity limitations and participation restrictions encountered at specific age levels, along with age-specific examination, evaluation, and intervention issues, are discussed in subsequent sections of this chapter.

MUSCULOSKELETAL DEFORMITIES

Spinal and lower limb deformities and joint contractures occur frequently in children with MM. Orthopedic deformities and joint contractures negatively affect positioning, body image, weight bearing (both in sitting and standing), activities of daily living (ADL), energy expenditure, and mobility from infancy through adulthood. Several factors contribute to abnormal posture, limb deformity, and joint contractures, including muscle imbalance secondary to neurologic dysfunction, progressive neurologic dysfunction, intrauterine positioning, coexisting congenital malformations, arthrogryposis, habitually assumed postures after birth, reduced or absent active joint motion, and deformities after fractures.[108,164] The upper limbs can also be involved as a result of spasticity or poor postural habits. The upper limb region most likely to have restricted motion is the shoulder girdle due to overuse of the arms for weight bearing and poor postural habits.

Postural stability is essential to effectively perform functional tasks. Symmetric alignment is important to minimize joint stress and deforming forces and to permit muscles to function at their optimal length. Uncorrected postural deficits can result in joint contractures and deformities, stretch weakness, and musculoskeletal pain. Deficits that may appear insignificant during childhood often become magnified once an individual has adult body proportions, resulting in activity limitations and discomfort (e.g., low back pain resulting from an increased lumbar lordosis and hip flexion contractures). Consequently, limb, neck, and trunk range of motion (ROM), muscle extensibility, and joint alignment should be monitored throughout the life span so that appropriate interventions can be implemented as indicated.

Typical postural problems include forward head, rounded shoulders, kyphosis, scoliosis, excessive lordosis, anterior pelvic tilt, rotational deformities of the hip or tibia (in-toeing, out-toeing, or windswept positions), flexed hips and knees, and pronated feet. It is important to observe posture and postural control after a given position has been maintained for a period of time to determine the effects of fatigue. Static and dynamic balance should be observed in sitting, four-point positioning, kneeling, half-kneeling, and standing, as well as during transitions between these positions. Symmetry and weight distribution should also be noted. In addition, typical sleeping and sitting positions should be identified to determine if habitual positioning is contributing to postural or joint deformities (e.g., "frog-leg" position in prone or supine, W-sitting, ring sitting, heel sitting, cross-legged sitting, and crouch standing). These habitual positions should be avoided because they may produce deforming forces and altered musculotendon length that result in the development of secondary impairments such as the progression of orthopedic deformities, joint contractures, and strength deficits. Photographs or videotapes of sitting and standing postures are often useful to document current status and to provide a visual baseline for future reference.

Postural deviations and contractures that are typical for individual lesion levels are summarized as follows. Individuals with high-level lesions (thoracic to L2) often have hip flexion, abduction, and external rotation contractures; knee flexion contractures; and ankle plantar flexion contractures. The lumbar spine is typically lordotic. Individuals with mid- to low-lumbar (L3-L5) lesion levels often have hip and knee flexion contractures, an increased lumbar lordosis, genu and calcaneal valgus malalignment, and a pronated position of the foot when bearing weight. They often walk with a pronounced crouched gait and bear weight primarily on their calcaneus. Individuals with sacral level lesions often have mild hip and knee flexion contractures and an increased lumbar lordosis, and the ankle and foot can either be in varus or valgus, combined with a pronated or supinated forefoot. They may walk with a mild crouch gait and may bear weight primarily on their calcaneus unless plantar flexor muscles are at least grade 3/5.

Crouch standing is a typical postural deviation that is observed across lesion levels and is characterized by persistent hip and knee flexion and an increased lumbar lordosis. The crouch posture often occurs because of muscle weakness (e.g., insufficient soleus muscle strength to maintain the tibia vertical) and orthopedic deformities (e.g., calcaneal valgus, which results in obligatory tibial internal rotation and knee flexion). Hip and knee flexion contractures often occur secondarily, in response to adaptive shortening of muscles from prolonged positioning in the crouch-standing posture. Altered postures, such as crouch standing, negatively affect both the task requirements (by increasing the muscle torque required to maintain the position) and the torque-generating capacity of the musculoskeletal system.[62] Such increased demands placed on the musculoskeletal system when standing and walking in a crouched posture may negatively impact function and result in secondary impairments.[4,24,62,102,128,129,168,188,196] It is important that appropriate intervention be implemented to ameliorate crouch standing so that the excessive physical demands and stress placed on the musculoskeletal system are reduced and the development of secondary impairments is prevented.

Scoliosis occurring with MM can be congenital or acquired; the congenital form is usually related to underlying vertebral anomalies and the curve is often inflexible, whereas the acquired type is usually caused by muscle imbalance and the curve is flexible until skeletal maturity is reached,[108] at which point little further progression is usually observed.[164] Scoliosis is more frequently observed in higher lesion level groups and becomes more prevalent and increasingly severe with age in all groups.[108]

Other spinal deformities that can occur in conjunction with or separate from scoliosis are kyphosis and lordosis deformities (Figure 22-3). Congenital kyphosis occurs in 10% to 15% of infants with MM.[124,186] Paralytic kyphosis is acquired in approximately one third by early adolescence,[24]

progressing at a rate of 7% to 8% per year.[10] Kyphosis can occur in the lumbar spine with reversal of the lumbar lordosis, or the kyphosis can be more diffusely distributed over the entire spine. Hyperlordosis of the lumbar spine is another commonly observed deformity. Like scoliosis, both kyphosis and lordosis are more commonly observed in children with higher spinal lesions and the curves tend to progress with age.[108] Severe kyphosis and scoliosis can limit chest wall expansion with consequent restriction of lung ventilation and frequent respiratory infections. The resulting restrictive lung condition can limit exercise tolerance and can be life-threatening in extreme cases.[108] Poor sitting posture, muscle imbalance, and recurrent skin ulcerations are additional problems encountered.[24]

The goal of treatment of spinal deformities is to maintain a balanced trunk and pelvis.[81] Orthotic intervention, usually with a bivalved Silastic thoracolumbosacral orthosis (TLSO), is helpful in maintaining improved trunk position for functional activities but does not prevent progression of acquired spinal deformity.[108] For children with progressive spinal deformities, orthotic intervention is continued until the child reaches a sufficient age to allow surgical fusion of the spine to prevent further progression of these deformities. Long spinal fusions before the skeletal age of 10 result in greater loss of trunk height because of ablation of the growth plates of vertebral bodies included in the fusion mass.[108] In addition, surgery at too young a skeletal age is associated with an increased frequency of instrumentation failure as a result of fragile bones and skin breakdown over the bulky spinal instrumentation.[108] The ideal minimum age for spinal fusion is 10 to 11 years old in girls and 12 to 13 years old in boys.[108] In general, children with spina bifida reach puberty and their growth spurt earlier than their able-bodied peers, so only minimal truncal shortening occurs as a consequence of long spinal fusion when it is performed at the appropriate

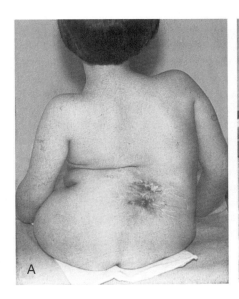
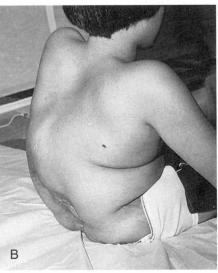

Figure 22-3   Spinal deformities. **A**, Collapsing type of lordoscoliosis. **B**, Kyphotic spinal deformity.

age. It is important to note that a history of recurrent urinary tract infections or poor nutrition increase the risk of perioperative infections with spinal instrumentation procedures for children with MM.[60]

Hip joints also are prone to deformity in children with MM. Fixed flexion deformities often require surgical intervention because they interfere with ambulation and orthotic fit. Correction after surgery should be maintained by encouraging standing and walking.[39,118] Children with high lumbar lesions (L1, L2) have unopposed flexion and adduction forces that gradually push the femoral head superiorly and posteriorly. The resulting contractures and secondary bony deformities of the proximal femur and acetabulum can lead to subluxation or dislocation (Figure 22-4, A and B) in nearly one third to one half of children with MM.[39]

In children with hip subluxation or dislocation, long-term follow-up studies have indicated that reduction of the hips is not a prerequisite for ambulation.[158] Mayfield[108] stated that a level pelvis and good ROM are more important for function than hip reduction. Furthermore, he stated that the presence of the femoral head in the acetabulum does not necessarily improve ROM at the hip or the ability to ambulate. In addition, unlike in children with cerebral palsy, it does not appear to affect the amount of orthotic support

required, hip pain, or gait deviation.[149] The indications for hip surgery in children with MM continue to be controversial; however, a basic principle practiced at many centers is to operate only on children with a lesion level at or below L3, when quadriceps muscle function is present, because these children are more likely to be functional ambulators into adulthood.[108,164] Fixed pelvic obliquity caused by unilateral subluxation or dislocation interferes with sitting or standing posture, contributes to scoliosis, and makes skin care unmanageable. It is another indication for surgical relocation of the hip, regardless of lesion level or ambulatory potential, along with painful hip dysplasia in ambulators.[178]

Shurtleff[164] evaluated the frequency of all types of hip contractures in large numbers of children with various spinal lesion levels. He noted that contractures measured in infancy tended to decrease in severity until approximately age 3 to 4 years, then increased to much higher values by adolescence. The initial decrease in severity of hip contractures can potentially be explained as a normal physiologic phenomenon resulting from intrauterine positioning. The increase in severity of contractures by adolescence, however, is of special concern to physical therapists. Mild contractures of minimal functional significance in young children can increase dramatically during later childhood and adolescence, necessitating persistent intervention and follow-up by the therapist to prevent significant functional loss. Consequently, physical therapists should be proactive in preventing the progression of contractures. Thoracic and high lumbar (L1, L2) groups of children have a higher incidence and greater severity of contractures owing to unopposed iliopsoas muscle function, regardless of whether or not they were participating in a standing program.[97] Shurtleff[164] reported progressively declining frequency and severity of contractures in groups of children with lesions at L3, L4 to L5, and sacral levels, respectively. An unexpected finding from Shurtleff's study was that only a certain percentage of children in each lesion level group had hip contractures, subluxation, or both. These relative percentages were not altered by surgical procedures on the hip and stayed constant across age groups. No clear reasons were discerned why certain individuals were susceptible to contractures, whereas others with similar neurologic function were not.

The knee joints of children with MM frequently have contractures or deformities. These include both flexion and extension contractures; the former more commonly occur in children who primarily use a wheelchair for mobility,[97] and the latter often occur after periods of immobility from fractures, decubitus ulcers, or surgical procedures. Varus and valgus deformities (see Figure 22-4, C and D) are also observed. Flexion deformities may make walking difficult or impossible, and extension deformities may complicate sitting. If either flexion or extension deformities are significant, they may need to be ameliorated via surgical release.[178] Wright and associates[198] reported that 60% of individuals with fixed flexion contractures less than 20° and a lesion level

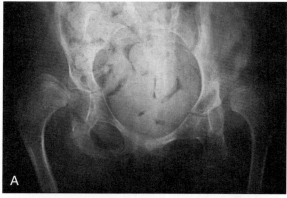
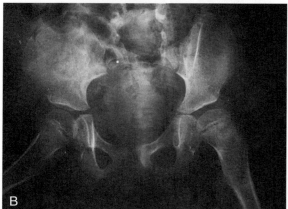

Figure 22-4   Lower limb deformities. **A,** Hip dislocation. **B,** Hip dysplasia and subluxation.

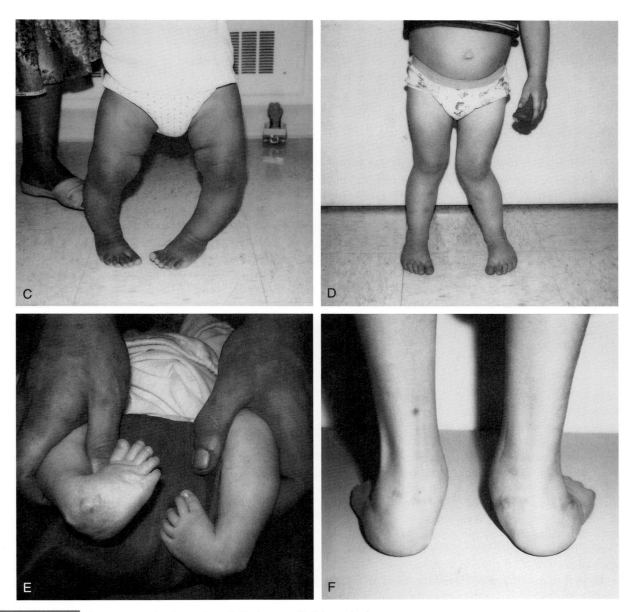

Figure 22-4, cont'd C, Genu varus. D, Genu valgus. E, Equinovarus. F, Calcaneal valgus.

higher than L3 were still biped ambulators in late adolescence, as compared to fewer than 5% of individuals with fixed flexion contractures greater than 20°. They also concluded that muscle imbalance and spasticity do not appear to be major causative factors; rather, the lack of normal joint movement may lead to joint stiffness. As described earlier for the hip joints, Shurtleff[164] studied the frequency of knee contractures and deformities in children with different lesion levels. An initial decrease from the contractures measured in infants was also noted at the knees, with the lowest prevalence occurring at age 4 to 5 years for patients with L3 or higher lesions, and at age 2 to 3 years for children with lesions below L3. The frequency and severity of contractures

increased in all groups from early childhood into adolescence. Knee joint contractures occurred in 65% to 70% of the thoracic and high lumbar groups by age 6 to 8, 20% to 25% of the L4 to L5 group by age 9 to 12, and sporadically among the children with sacral level lesions. Valgus and varus deformities were most frequently observed in the L3 and above groups, with a slight increase during adolescence.

Deformities of the ankles and feet can occur in both ambulatory and nonambulatory children and are most common in children with lesion levels at L5 and above.[164] Partial innervation and consequent muscle imbalance determine the type of deformity that occurs. Even with surgical correction, these deformities will recur unless the deforming forces are removed. Progressive ankle and foot deformities can also be observed in conjunction with the development of spasticity and motor strength loss associated with tethering of the spinal cord. Children with "skip" lesions (see the section on motor paralysis) are particularly prone to progressive foot deformities.[164]

A variety of foot and ankle deformities can occur (see Figure 22-4, *E* and *F*), including ankle equinovarus (clubfeet), forefoot varus or valgus, forefoot supination or pronation, calcaneal varus or valgus, pes cavus and planus, and claw-toe deformities. The most frequent contracture observed is of the ankle plantar flexor muscles. The frequency of foot deformities has been reported to vary from 20% to 50% between lesion level groups[164] and has been reported to be as high as 90% for high level paralysis and 60% to 70% for lower level paralysis.[23,50,178] Although some deformities are more frequently associated with certain neurosegmental levels (e.g., clubfeet in thoracic and high lumbar lesions, claw-toes in sacral lesions), all types of ankle and foot deformities are observed in children at every lesion level. Congenital clubfeet are common, and surgery is indicated once the child is developmentally ready to stand.[24] Other foot deformities may develop over time as a result of muscle imbalance. Dias[38] noted that ankle valgus occurs in the presence of fibular shortening, the latter being highly correlated with paralysis of the soleus muscle. Surgical treatment of a valgus ankle is indicated when the deformity cannot be functionally alleviated with orthotics. The presence of ankle and foot deformities can greatly affect sitting and standing posture, balance, mobility, foot ulcerations, and shoe fit, regardless of lesion level. Weight-bearing forces often result in ankle and foot deformities. Even partial weight bearing on wheelchair footrests in poor alignment over time can result in deformities and foot ulcerations. Consequently, achieving a plantigrade position of the feet is a priority, regardless of ambulatory status. Surgical procedures are often necessary and are effective.[178] Orthoses and assistive devices should be adjusted properly to maintain neutral subtalar alignment and a plantigrade foot position.

Torsional deformities are common. Excessive foot progression angles and windswept positions of the lower limbs are often present (Figure 22-5) as a result of hip anteversion, hip retroversion, or tibial torsion. These torsional deformities negatively affect sitting and standing balance, weight distribution, and walking. See Cusick and Stuberg[32] for factors that contribute to torsional deformities in individuals with developmental disabilities, examination procedures, normative values, and intervention suggestions.

Joint alignment and evidence of abnormal joint stress are often most apparent during dynamic activities, such as walking or wheelchair propulsion. Joint stresses are often magnified when walking on uneven surfaces, stairs, or curbs. Observing wear patterns on shoes and orthoses can provide additional clues to abnormal stress and malalignment. If joint deformities are supple, they may respond to stretching, combined with orthoses or positioning splints to maintain alignment. Fixed deformities may respond to serial casting (e.g., foot deformities) but will often require surgical intervention (e.g., scoliosis, unilateral hip dislocation, or tibial torsion). If muscle imbalance is severe and the deforming forces are not effectively counteracted by stretching, strengthening, or positioning, muscle transfers may be indicated (e.g., partial transfer of the anterior tibialis muscle to the calcaneus to achieve a plantigrade foot position by balancing the unopposed dorsiflexion force in a child with L5 motor function).

There are several reasons for maintaining joint ROM. Limited ROM can interfere with ADL, bed mobility, and transfers. Bed mobility is more efficient and self-care is easier for individuals who have maintained their flexibility.[64] Restricted ROM, combined with muscle weakness, can result in poor postural habits and gait deviations. Adequate ROM must be maintained to perform ADL, such as bathing and toileting. Restricted joint motion can result in overlengthening of weak muscles, not permitting them to function in the optimal range of the length-tension curve. Limited ROM may result in discomfort, especially when lying down (e.g., tight hip flexors pulling on the lumbar spine). Severe contractures also can negatively affect body image. Contractures that may seem insignificant during childhood may become functionally limiting once the individual has adult-sized body proportions (e.g., knee extension contractures can interfere with the ability to maneuver in a wheelchair). In extreme cases, difficulty in managing paralyzed limbs because of joint contractures can put individuals at risk for skin breakdown and possibly amputations because of the increased incidence of injury.[64] The impact of limited ROM on functional performance should be considered before deciding whether intervention is indicated.

ROM and positioning of paralytic limbs should be done carefully, without excessive force, to avoid fractures.[153] Caution should also be exercised when adducting the hips to avoid hip dislocation. The prone hip extension test[179] for measuring hip extension is the method of choice in this population because of interference of spinal and pelvic deformities and lower limb spasticity with the traditional Thomas test method.[12] Ankle ROM should always be measured with the ankle joint in subtalar neutral so that measurements are comparable across time and therapists.

The long-term effects of surgical interventions and weight bearing on insensate joints are becoming evident as individuals with MM reach adulthood.[24] Secondary impairments of knee joint deterioration and arthritis occur with increased frequency in older individuals.[102] Nagankatti and associates[129] reported a prevalence of 1 per 100 cases of Charcot arthroplasty in the MM population.

There are several ways to minimize musculoskeletal stress and reduce the incidence of acquired orthopedic

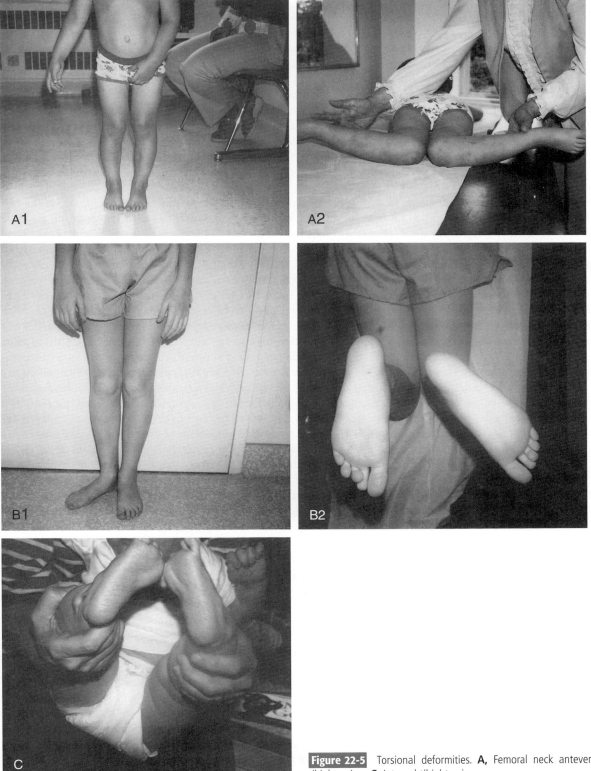

Figure 22-5 Torsional deformities. **A,** Femoral neck anteversion. **B,** External tibial torsion. **C,** Internal tibial torsion.

deformities. Improving traction of the hands by providing biking gloves for community wheelchair mobility reduces the grip forces required for wheelchair propulsion. Wheelchair seat positions influence propulsion effectiveness and the amount of stress on upper limb joints and muscles.[107] For ambulators, shoes with nonskid soles improve foot traction. Symmetric neutral joint alignment should be maintained in both sitting and standing via appropriate orthotics or seating devices. It is important to avoid shifting weight to one leg when standing and to avoid crossing the legs when sitting. Extreme ROM should be avoided, especially when bearing weight. Crutch and walker handgrips should be angled to avoid hyperextension of the wrists, and weight should be distributed across a broad, cushioned area. Orthoses should provide total contact to minimize the risk of development of pressure areas. Excessive pressure on tendons and the palms of the hand should be avoided to reduce the risk of developing carpal tunnel syndrome. Overhead reaching and work activities should be minimized by adapting the home, school, and work environments. In addition, long-distance mobility options should be provided to reduce joint stresses. When sitting, weight bearing should be symmetric, pelvic tilt should be neutral with a slight lumbar lordosis, the hips and knees should be at 90°, and the feet should be flat on the floor. Good lumbar support should be provided. Inclining the seat backward 15° minimizes stress on the lumbar spine and helps keep the pelvis seated back in the chair.[27] Tilting the desk or table top upward improves the position of the upper trunk, head, and shoulders.

OSTEOPOROSIS

Decreased bone mineral density, thought to be secondary to hypotonic or flaccid musculature combined with decreased loading of long bones from altered mobility, is frequently observed in children with MM and often results in osteoporotic fractures. Stuberg[181] suggested that standing programs are beneficial for children with developmental disabilities. He reported that the use of a standing program (60 minutes four or five times per week) appears to increase bone mineral density and enhance acetabular development in children with cerebral palsy. These issues must be studied further in the MM population, however. Bone responses in children with flaccid paralysis may be quite different. Rosenstein and associates[147] examined this issue in the MM population and reported that bone mineral density was 38% to 44% higher in household or community ambulators compared with nonfunctional ambulators (exercise-only ambulators or nonambulators). Salvaggio and associates[150] reported that walking ability was a highly significant determinant of bone density in prepubertal children with MM. Because the effects of lesion level were not controlled in either of these studies, however, the potential contribution of muscle activity versus weight-bearing status to the differences in bone mineral density cannot be determined. In addition, neither study

addressed the issue of reduction of the incidence of osteoporotic fractures.

Studying the frequency of fractures is a more direct and clinically significant method of examining the benefits of standing programs. Shurtleff[164] asked the question, "Are fractures less common among those patients in standing or ambulatory programs than among similarly paralyzed sedentary peers?" Asher and Olson[5] showed no correlation between fractures and the use of wheelchairs. DeSouza and Carroll[36] reported no fractures in 7 nonambulators and 38 fractures in 16 ambulators. Their data implied that exposure to forces that can produce fractures (i.e., upright mobility) is the important risk factor for fractures, rather than the level of flaccid paralysis, as would be expected. Liptak and associates[97] found no difference in the frequency of fractures between a group of children who were wheelchair users and a comparable group of children who ambulated with orthoses. Clinically, the use of standing frames, parapodiums, or hip-knee-ankle-foot orthoses (HKAFOs) in children with high lumbar and thoracic lesions does not appear warranted for the purpose of fracture prevention. For children with lower lumbar and sacral lesion levels, for whom upright positioning and mobility is an important functional skill, undue restriction of physical activity for fear of a fracture is not indicated. The fact that passive weight bearing does not decrease the risk of fractures in these children makes sense if one considers that bone density is more likely maintained by torque generated from volitional muscle activity. Active muscle contraction generates forces through the long bones that are several times greater than the forces from passive weight bearing.

Fractures often present subacutely because of lack of sensation, with swelling and warmth at the fracture site and a low-grade fever often being the only symptoms. Fractures frequently occur after surgery, immobilization in a cast, or as a sequela to foot arthrodesis. Because of the correlation between the duration of casting and the incidence of fracturing, immobilization in a cast is kept to a minimum and fractures are contained in soft immobilization for alignment.[24] Weight bearing is resumed as soon as possible to avoid the risk of additional fractures.[81]

MOTOR PARALYSIS

The inherently obvious manifestation of MM is the paraplegia resulting from the spinal cord malformation. Upper limb weakness can also occur in this population, regardless of lesion level, and is often a sign of progressive neurologic dysfunction. Knowledge of the motor lesion level is useful for predicting associated abnormalities and for prognostication of functional outcome. A detailed discussion regarding developmental and functional expectations for each motor lesion level is provided later in the section on outcomes and their determinants. Strategies for assessing strength and planning intervention programs to enhance motor function are provided in the section on age-specific examination and physical therapy intervention strategies.

The motor level is defined as the lowest intact, functional neuromuscular segment. For example, an L4 level indicates that the fourth lumbar nerve and the myotome it innervates are functioning, whereas segments below L4 are not intact. Table 22-1 provides the International Myelodysplasia Study Group (IMSG) criteria for assigning motor levels from manual muscle strength test results.[76] The IMSG criteria have been shown to best reflect the innervation patterns of individuals with MM as opposed to other spinal segment classification systems. MM spinal lesions can be asymmetric when motor or sensory functions of the right and left sides of the body are compared. Consequently, motor function should be classified individually for the right and left sides.

Neuromuscular involvement of individuals with MM may manifest in one of three ways: (1) lesions resembling complete cord transection, (2) incomplete lesions, and (3) skip lesions.[164] Lesions resembling complete cord transection manifest as normal function down to a particular level, below which there is flaccid paralysis, loss of sensation, and absent reflexes. Incomplete lesions have a mixed manifestation of spasticity and volitional control. Skip lesions are also observed, where more caudal segments are functioning despite the presence of one or more nonfunctional segments interposed between the intact more cephalad spinal segments. Individual skip motor lesions manifest either with isolated function of muscles noted below the last functional level of the lesion or with inadequate strength of muscle groups that have innervation higher than the lowest functioning group.[139] Consequently, it is important to evaluate muscles with lower innervation than the last functional level to determine whether a skip lesion exists. The presence of spasticity and reflexes should also be carefully documented.

McDonald and associates[113] demonstrated that muscle strength grades for the gluteus medius and medial hamstring muscles correlate more highly with strength grades of the hip adductors, hip flexors, and knee extensors than lower limb anterior compartment muscles that have been previously described as being innervated by the L4, L5, and sacral nerve roots. These data potentially explain the clinical observation that individuals with MM often have functional strength in the gluteus medius and medial hamstrings, despite having weak or nonactive lower limb anterior compartment muscles. It was concluded from this study that it is more useful clinically to group individuals with MM by the strength of specific muscle groups, as outlined in Table 22-1, rather than by traditional neurosegmental levels.

SENSORY DEFICITS

Sensory deficits are not clear-cut in this population, because sensory levels often do not correlate with motor levels and there may be skip areas that lack sensation. Because skip areas can occur within a given dermatome, it is important

TABLE 22-1   **International Myelodysplasia Study Group Criteria for Assigning Motor Levels**

Motor Level	Criteria for Assigning Motor Levels
T10 or above T11	Determined by sensory level or palpation of abdominal muscles.
T12	Some pelvic control is present in sitting or supine (this may come from the abdominals or paraspinal muscles). Hip hiking from the quadratus lumborum may also be present.
L1	Weak iliopsoas muscle function is present (grade 2).
L1–L2	Exceeds criteria for L1 but does not meet L2 criteria.*
L2	Iliopsoas, sartorius, and the hip adductors all must be grade 3 or better.
L3	Meets or exceeds the criteria for L2 plus the quadriceps are grade 3 or better.
L3–L4	Exceeds criteria for L3 but does not meet L4 criteria.
L4	Meets or exceeds the criteria for L3 and the medial hamstrings or the tibialis anterior is grade 3 or better. A weak peroneus tertius may also be seen.
L4–L5	Exceeds criteria for L4 but does not meet L5 criteria.
L5	Meets or exceeds the criteria for L4 and has lateral hamstring strength of grade 3 or better plus one of the following: gluteus medius grade 2 or better, peroneus tertius grade 4 or better, or tibialis posterior grade 3 or better.
L5–S1	Exceeds criteria for L5 but does not meet S1 criteria.
S1	Meets or exceeds the criteria for L5 plus at least two of the following: gastrocnemius/soleus grade 2 or better, gluteus medius grade 3 or better, or gluteus maximus grade 2 or better (can pucker the buttocks).
S1–S2	Exceeds criteria for S1 but does not meet S2 criteria.
S2	Meets or exceeds the criteria for S1, the gastrocnemius/soleus must be grade 3 or better, and gluteus medius and maximus are grade 4 or better.
S2–S3	All of the lower limb muscle groups are of normal strength (may be grade 4 in one or two groups). Also includes normal-appearing infants who are too young to be bowel and bladder trained (see "no loss").
"No loss"	Meets all of the criteria for S2–S3 and has no bowel or bladder dysfunction.

Adapted with permission from Patient Data Management System. Myelodysplasia Study Data Collection Criteria and Instructions, 1994. (Available from D. B. Shurtleff, MD, Professor, Department of Pediatrics, University of Washington, Seattle, WA 98195.)
*When description states "meets criteria …," strength of muscles listed for preceding levels should be increasing respectively.

to test all dermatomes and multiple sites within a given dermatome to have an accurate baseline examination. Deficits should be recorded on a dermatome chart with areas of absent and decreased sensation color coded for the various sensory modalities (e.g., light touch, pinprick, vibration, and thermal). Proprioception and kinesthetic sense should also be evaluated in both the upper and lower extremities.

Based on the results of a study conducted on 30 adults with MM, testing with both light touch and pinprick stimuli is not necessary in this population because there is little discriminating value for detecting insensate areas.[66] In contrast, vibratory stimuli could be felt one dermatome below light touch and pinprick sensation. Based on these results, vibration sensation should be evaluated in addition to either light touch or pinprick sensation.

It is important for individuals with MM to be aware of their sensory deficits and to be taught techniques to compensate by substituting other sensory modalities (e.g., vision). The impact of decreased sensation on safety should be emphasized, especially when checking temperature (e.g., bath water or when sitting near a fireplace) and when barefoot. Skin inspection and pressure relief techniques should be taught early so that they are incorporated into the daily routine. The importance of pressure relief cushions and sitting push-ups for pressure relief should be emphasized. Proper intervention of lower limbs and joint protection techniques should be taught when learning how to perform ADL, such as transfers.

The impact of sensory deficits on functional performance should be kept in mind when teaching functional tasks. Individuals with MM may rely heavily on vision to compensate for sensory deficits.[156] They may lack kinesthetic acuity that permits subconscious completion of many repetitive motor tasks. Consequently, visual attention may not be available to be directed at other factors in the environment.[3] Adding small amounts of weight to the ankles or a walker may enhance proprioceptive awareness and facilitate gait training. Use of patellar tendon-bearing orthoses (Figure 22-6) instead of traditional ankle-foot orthoses (AFOs) may also facilitate foot placement for individuals with innervation through L3 because the orthosis contacts the skin in an area of intact sensation.

HYDROCEPHALUS

Hydrocephalus is excessive accumulation of cerebrospinal fluid (CSF) in the ventricles of the brain. Approximately 25% or more of children with MM are born with hydrocephalus. An additional 60% develop it after surgical closure of their back lesion.[143] If left untreated, the continued expansion of the ventricles can cause loss of cerebral cortex with additional cognitive and functional impairment. Cerebellar hypoplasia with caudal displacement of the hindbrain through the foramen magnum, known as the Arnold-

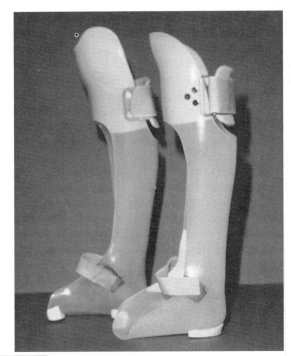

Figure 22-6 Ground-reaction ankle-foot orthosis. Polypropylene patellar tendon-bearing ground-reaction ankle-foot orthoses molded with the foot in a subtalar neutral position. Note the zero heel posts and posts under the first metatarsal heads.

Chiari type II malformation, is usually associated with hydrocephalus.

The hydrocephalus will occasionally arrest spontaneously; however, 80% to 90% of children with hydrocephalus will require a CSF shunt.[170] A ventriculoperitoneal catheter shunts excess CSF from the lateral ventricles of the brain to the peritoneal space, where the CSF is resorbed. Because a shunt is a foreign body, it can be a nidus for infection or can become obstructed, requiring neurosurgical intervention. Repeated or prolonged shunt dysfunction and infections often lead to additional functional and cognitive decline of the child. Shunt dysfunction is often gradual, with subtle symptoms. Therapists should be familiar with these symptoms to facilitate early detection and appropriate referral to a physician for further evaluation. Box 22-1 provides a list of early symptoms and signs of shunt obstruction. Of particular interest are the findings of Kilburn and associates,[84] which suggest that static or declining grip strength measurements are potentially an early indicator of neurologic dysfunction such as shunt malfunction or symptomatic Arnold-Chiari malformation. Hydrocephalus persists throughout life with consequent need of ongoing follow-up by a physician who is familiar with the medical complications associated with MM.

COGNITIVE DYSFUNCTION

Early closure of spinal lesions with antibiotic intervention to prevent meningitis and improved CSF shunt intervention has increased the expected cognitive function of children born with MM. The majority of children without hydrocephalus or with uncomplicated hydrocephalus (no infections or cerebral hemorrhage) will have intellect falling within the normal range on intelligence testing. The distribution of scores tends to be skewed toward the upper and lower ends of normal, however, with fewer children scoring in the middle of the curve and a greater proportion scoring at the lower end of the range.[156] The intellectual performance of children who have had significant CNS infections is lower than those who have not had infection.[162] Intelligence scores tend to be higher in lumbar and sacral lesion level groups than in thoracic lesion level groups.[156] Verbal subtest scores usually exceed performance subtest scores.[156] The poorer scores on performance subtests, however, may not represent true differences in verbal versus nonverbal reasoning skills. Instead, these differences can potentially be explained by upper limb dyscoordination (discussed later) and by memory deficits.[156] Dyscoordination and memory deficits are manifested as distractibility on subtests assessing acquired knowledge (e.g., arithmetic), integrated right-left hemisphere function (e.g., picture arrangement, block design, and coding), speed of motor response (e.g., coding), and memory (e.g., digit span, coding, and arithmetic). Further controlled studies must be conducted to determine the source or sources of discrepant verbal versus performance intelligence scores observed in individuals with MM.

Dise and Lohr[41] demonstrated the need for individual analysis of "higher-order" cognitive functions, including conceptual reasoning, problem solving, mental flexibility, and efficiency of thinking for individuals with MM, regardless of lesion level or general intelligence level. They contend that such neuropsychologic deficits underlie the "motivational" and academic difficulties observed in this population, especially for those with an average IQ.

The "cocktail party personality" is a cognitively associated behavioral disorder that occurs in some individuals with hydrocephalus, regardless of age or intelligence level.[74] These individuals are articulate and verbose, superficially appearing to have high verbal skills. Close examination of the content of their speech, however, shows frequent and inappropriate use of clichés and jargon. Individual words are often misused. Despite the initial appearance of being capable, these individuals are often impaired, their performance in daily life is below what they superficially appear capable of,[74] and they lack social skills.[173] It is important for the physical therapist to directly observe skills that these children report that they can perform and to confirm regular performance of the task at home with parents and care providers to determine if information provided by the patient is accurate.

LANGUAGE DYSFUNCTION

Children with MM and hydrocephalus have been observed to have deficits in discourse, characterized by a high frequency of irrelevant utterances and poorer performance with abstract rather than concrete language. Culatta and Young[31] administered the Preschool Language Assessment Instrument (PLAI) at four levels of abstraction to children with MM and comparable language-age control children. Children with MM performed comparably to control subjects on concrete tasks of the PLAI, but they produced more "no response" and irrelevant responses than control participants on abstract tasks.

LATEX ALLERGY

A range of up to 73% of children with MM have been reported to have latex allergies[157,199] compared to 1% to 5% of control groups. Unfortunately, 2% of latex is major IgE sensitizing proteins that are ubiquitous in our culture, and some children with MM have life-threatening anaphylaxis. Latex-containing materials are most common in operating rooms but are also present in many products used elsewhere in the hospital and in the general community. Furthermore, these proteins are present in wheelchair seats and tires, foam rubber lining on splints and braces, elastic on diapers and clothes, pacifiers, balls, examination gloves used for bladder and bowel programs, and many other everyday objects. Whereas almost all children's hospitals have latex precaution policies, it is important for therapists in schools and clinics in the community to be aware of the need for children with MM to avoid exposure to latex products.

UPPER LIMB DYSCOORDINATION

Children with MM frequently display upper limb dyscoordination, especially those with hydrocephalus.[156] The dyscoordination can potentially be explained by three possible causes: (1) cerebellar ataxia most likely related to the Arnold-Chiari type II malformation; (2) motor cortex or pyramidal tract damage secondary to hydrocephalus; or (3) motor learning deficits resulting from the use of upper limbs for balance and support rather than manipulation and exploration. These children perform poorly on timed fine motor skill tasks.[156] Their movements can be described as halting and deliberate, rather than the expected smooth, continuous motion of able-bodied children. It often appears that there is a heavy reliance on visual feedback instead of kinesthetic sense. Consequently, even with extensive training, these children often have difficulty integrating frequently used fine motor movements at a subconscious level.[156] Practicing fine motor tasks has been found to be beneficial, however, and often carries over into functional tasks.[47] These coordination deficits have been described by some authors as apparent motor apraxias or motor learning deficits.[25,91] Given the frequent occurrence of upper limb dyscoordination in these children, true apraxias are probably less common than these studies indicate.

An additional factor that may contribute to upper limb dyscoordination is delayed development of hand dominance.[156] A large number of children with MM have mixed hand dominance or are left-handed, suggestive of possible left hemisphere damage.[156] Brunt[25] indicated that delayed hand dominance may contribute to deficits in bilateral upper limb function integration, resulting in further difficulty with fine motor tasks.

VISUOPERCEPTUAL DEFICITS

Studies assessing visual perception have not clearly determined whether deficits in children with MM are common, as has been described in the literature.[119,151,185] Tests that require good hand-eye coordination, such as the Frostig Developmental Test of Visual Perception, may artificially lower scores of children with MM as a result of the upper limb dyscoordination described earlier. When upper limb motor function has been removed as a factor in testing by using the Motor Free Visual Perception Test, children with MM have performed at age-appropriate levels.[156] Consequently, results of visuoperceptual tests must be interpreted

carefully, in conjunction with other examinations, before a diagnosis of a visuoperception deficit is made.

CRANIAL NERVE PALSIES

The Arnold-Chiari malformation, along with hydrocephalus or dysplasia of the brain stem, may result in cranial nerve deficits. Ocular muscle palsies can occur,[165] such as involvement of cranial nerve VI (abducens) with consequent lateral rectus eye muscle weakness and esotropia on the involved side. Correction with patching of the eye, prescription lenses, or minor outpatient surgery is necessary to prevent amblyopia and for cosmesis.[143] Gaston[52] studied 322 children with MM for 6 years to monitor them for ophthalmic complications. Forty-two percent of these children had a manifest squint, 29% had an oculomotor nerve palsy or musculoparetic nystagmus, 14% had papilledema, and 17% had optic nerve atrophy. Only 27% of those surveyed had definite normal vision. Seventy percent of proven episodes of raised intracranial pressure (ICP) from CSF shunt malfunction had positive ophthalmologic evidence of the ICP. Shunt surgery is the first priority but may not restore normal ocular motility and visual function, requiring further compensatory interventions.

Cranial nerves IX (glossopharyngeal) and X (vagus) can also be affected with pharyngeal and laryngeal dysfunction (croupy, hoarse cry) and swallowing difficulties.[165] Apneic episodes and bradycardia may occur with a severely symptomatic Arnold-Chiari type II malformation and can potentially be life threatening. These severe symptoms usually appear within the first few weeks of life but can occur at any time.[143] The survival rate is only about 40% in these severe cases.[163] Those infants who do survive, however, have been noted to have gradual improvement in cranial nerve function. Neurosurgical posterior fossa decompression and high cervical laminectomies do not seem to substantially improve the outcome.[54,163] In contrast, surgical decompression of the Arnold-Chiari malformation has been shown to be beneficial for the intervention of progressive upper and lower limb spasticity.[54]

SPASTICITY

The muscle tone of infants and children with MM can range from flaccid to normal to spastic. Stack and Baber[177] found that some upper motoneuron signs were present in approximately two thirds of children with MM whom they examined; however, only about 9% had true spastic paraparesis. The remainder of this group had predominantly a lower motoneuron presentation with scattered upper motoneuron signs (e.g., flexor withdrawal reflex). In the group of children without upper motoneuron signs, most had totally flaccid paralysis below the segmental level of their spinal lesion, but a small percentage had normal tone. In contrast, Mazur and Menelaus[110] stated that approximately 25% of individuals with MM exhibit lower extremity spasticity because of associated CNS abnormalities. As with other CNS conditions, spasticity and abnormal reflexes can affect function, positioning, or comfort in individuals with MM.

PROGRESSIVE NEUROLOGIC DYSFUNCTION

Minor improvements in strength or development of sensation, although rare, can occur even as late as the fourth decade of life. More important, however, is the deterioration from neurologic changes that are due to treatable complications. These changes that can occur in the upper or lower extremities or trunk include loss of sensation, loss of strength, pain at the site of the sac repair, pain radiating along a dermatome, initial onset or worsening of spasticity, development or rapid progression of scoliosis, development of a lower limb deformity not explained by previously documented muscle imbalance, or change in bowel or bladder sphincter control. Such changes can be due to CSF shunt obstruction, hydromyelia (syringohydromyelia, syrinx), growth of a dermoid or lipoma at the site of repair, subarachnoid cysts of the cord, or spinal cord tethering and can be detected via MRI. Cord tethering occurs from scarring of the neural placode or spinal cord to the overlying dura or skin with resultant traction on neural structures.[167] The tethered cord syndrome may also result from other congenital anomalies, including thickening of the filum terminale and diastematomyelia.[144] An acquired cause of progressive spinal cord dysfunction that has been reported is severe herniation of intervertebral disks into the spinal canal, causing compression of the cord.[168] Lais and associates[90] stated that slow deterioration of neurologic function is not uncommon.

Progressive deterioration of spinal cord function resulting from any of these causes can be arrested by neurosurgical interventions. Deterioration of the gait pattern is frequently the first complaint by patients or their parents. Because physical therapists see these patients more frequently than physicians or surgeons, the therapist is often the first to observe these changes and should be alert to the need for immediate referral to a neurosurgeon. Owing to this risk of progressive loss of function, it is essential that individuals with MM be closely monitored throughout their life span.

SEIZURES

Seizures have been reported to occur in 10% to 30% of children and adolescents with MM.[168] The etiologies of seizure activity include associated brain malformation, CSF shunt malfunction or infection, and residual brain damage from shunt infection or malfunction. Anticonvulsant medications, which are necessary for prophylaxis against seizures, unfortunately can also accentuate any cognitive deficits or dyscoordination already present.[51,145] Untreated seizures, however, can lead to permanent cognitive or neurologic functional loss, or even death.

NEUROGENIC BOWEL

Fewer than 5% of children with MM develop voluntary control of their urinary or anal sphincter.[143] Abnormal or absent function of spinal segments S2 through S4, which provide the innervation to these organs, is the primary reason for the incontinence. The anal sphincter can be flaccid, hypotonic, or spastic, causing different manifestations of dysfunction during defecation. Anorectal sensation is also often impaired, preventing the individual from receiving sensory input of an imminent bowel movement so that he or she can take appropriate action. In addition to incontinence, constipation and impaction can also occur. Fortunately, conscientious attention to individually designed bowel programs can have effective results, minimizing problems of incontinence and constipation.[86,143,191,192] The presence of a bulbocavernosus or anal cutaneous reflex (indicating that lower motoneuron innervation of the sphincter is present) is highly predictive of success with a bowel training program.[86] King and associates[86] also reported that instituting bowel training before age 7 years correlates with improved outcomes by means of better compliance. When stool incontinence is interfering with a child's school and social activities, the physical therapist may want to become involved to help address the problem. Incontinence often affects feelings of self-image and competence, which in turn can affect performance in other activities pertinent to the therapist's intervention program.

NEUROGENIC BLADDER

Just as the nerves to control defecation are impaired, so are the nerves that produce bladder control. A variety of different types of dysfunctions can occur, depending on the relative tonicity of the detrusor muscle in the bladder wall and the outlet sphincters of the bladder. Bladder intervention strategies are directed toward the point or points of dysfunction. The goal is infection-free social continence with preservation of renal function. Retrograde flow of urine from the bladder up the ureters to the kidneys, termed "vesicoureteral reflux," can occur without symptoms or signs being evident until the later stages of irreversible renal failure. Inadequate emptying of the bladder with residual urine retention within the bladder provides an optimal culture medium for bacteria, causing recurrent urinary tract infections and possible generalized sepsis. Adequate bladder intervention is therefore an essential component of health maintenance and normal longevity of people with MM, in addition to being an important social issue.

The bladder dysfunction can begin in utero (5% to 10% of newborns with MM show evidence of hydronephrosis and reflux). This is typically due to dyssynergy between the detrusor muscle of the bladder and the external urethral sphincter (i.e., the bladder contracts but the sphincter does not relax to allow the flow of urine out of the urethra). This results in high bladder pressures and vesicoureteral reflux. It is now standard practice for all newborns with MM to undergo an extensive urologic work-up 7 days post partum. Early implementation of intermittent catheterization in infancy helps to prevent later problems with detrusor muscle function from overstretching the bladder wall.[14]

For most individuals, effective bladder intervention is achieved with clean intermittent catheterization on a regularly timed schedule for voiding. A small catheter is inserted into the bladder through the urethra until urine begins to flow. After the bladder is empty or urine stops flowing, the catheter is withdrawn, cleansed with soap and water, and stored for future use. It has been shown that the clean method of catheterization, as opposed to sterile technique, is sufficient for prevention of urinary tract infections.[143] The risk of injury to the urethra or bladder from clean intermittent catheterization is sufficiently low to allow young children to be taught to catheterize themselves. Mastery of the technique is usually achieved by age 6 to 8 years depending on the severity of the involvement.[172] Supplementation of clean intermittent catheterization with oral medication for spastic detrusor muscle function (e.g., oxybutynin [Ditropan], tolterodine [Detrol], glycopyrrolate [Robinul injection], hyoscyamine [Levsin], trospium [Sanctura]), spastic sphincter function (phenoxybenzamine), or hypotonic sphincter function (ephedrine, pseudoephedrine, phenyl-propanolamine) is required in some children to achieve intervention goals. It is recommended that individuals with MM have regular follow-up with a urologist every 6 months until age 2, and yearly thereafter, throughout the life span.[85] The physical therapist must be aware of the method used for urine drainage as it relates to wheelchair positioning, transfer techniques, and orthoses so that assistive devices do not interfere with effective performance of urine drainage techniques. It is important to allow adequate time for patients with MM to attend to bowel and bladder needs before and after examination and therapy sessions so that they are comfortable and continent during physical activities. Discomfort from a distended bladder or rectum may impair performance. Patients are often not assertive in requesting necessary time for personal care, and therapists should encourage them to do so to avoid embarrassing accidents.

Sexual function is also impacted, especially by diminished or absent sensation of the genitalia. For males, a nerve transposition of the ilioinguinal nerve to the dorsal nerve of the penis can provide sensation for sexual activity.[135] The procedure has helped to contribute to the quality of life and overall adjustment to adulthood for adolescents and young men who have undergone the procedure.

SKIN BREAKDOWN

Decubitus ulcers and other types of skin breakdown have previously been shown to occur in 85% to 95% of all children with MM by the time they reach young adulthood.[161] Okamoto and associates[132] performed an extensive study of skin breakdown on 524 patients with MM who were 1 to 20 years old. Perineal decubiti and breakdown over the apex of the spinal kyphotic curve (gibbus) occurred in 82% of children with thoracic level lesions, 62% of those with high lumbar level lesions, and 50% to 53% of those with lower level lesions. Lower limb skin breakdown was approximately equivalent in all lesion level groups (30% to 46%). Although the sites and causes of skin breakdown varied among lesion level groups, the overall frequency was the same. The prevalence of skin breakdown at any one time was 20% to 25% for the population sampled. Several etiologies for skin breakdown were ascertained. In 42% of the children, tissue ischemia from excessive pressure was the cause. In 23% a cast or orthotic device produced the breakdown. In another 23% urine and stool soiling produced skin maceration. Friction and shear accounted for another 10%; burns accounted for 1%; and 1% of causes were not recorded or were unknown. Other authors have described additional causes of skin breakdown.[161] These include excessive weight bearing over bony prominences of the pelvis as a result of spinal deformity, obesity, lower limb autonomic dysfunction with vascular insufficiency or venous stasis, and tenuous tissue postoperatively over bony prominences. One might expect at least modest improvement in the prevalence of skin breakdown for children with MM owing to improved wheelchair cushion technologies and seating options; however, no recent studies have been performed to assess the breadth or severity of this problem.

Age is an important factor in the etiology of skin breakdown. Shurtleff[161] showed that young children who are not toilet trained have the greatest problem with breakdown from skin soiling (ammonia burns). Young active children with MM have the greatest frequency of friction burns on knees and feet from scooting along rugs, hot water scalds, and pressure ulcers from orthoses or casts. Older children, adolescents, and young adults develop skin breakdown over lower limb bony prominences (even if they did not have ulcers when they were younger) from the increased pressure of a larger body habitus, asymmetric weight bearing resulting from deformities, abrasions of the buttocks or lower limbs resulting from poor transfer skills, improperly fitted orthoses, and lower limb vascular problems. Strategies for prevention taught by the physical therapist therefore should be directed to the likely causes of skin breakdown for the age of the individual. Helping the child develop an awareness of his insensate extremities is important during the early years in order to later develop independence with personal care. Mobley and associates[125] found that preschoolers with MM exhibited altered self-perception as evidenced by their drawing fewer trunks, legs, and feet on self-portraits than their able-bodied peers.

Pressure sores can result in a delay or loss of ambulation.[40] Skin breakdown of the insensate foot is often a cause of decreased ability to ambulate. Predictors of skin breakdown resulting from excessive pressure during ambulation or while resting feet on wheelchair footrests are foot rigidity, non-plantigrade position, and surgical arthrodesis.[109] Clawing of the toes may be another contributing factor that also affects shoe wear. To avoid foot ulcerations, physical therapists should examine and document foot deformity, level of sensation, and pressure areas. The insensate foot can be protected with appropriate footwear, orthotics, or surgery. Total contact casting can be useful in healing ulcers.[24]

OBESITY

Obesity is a common and difficult multifactorial problem occurring in children with MM that complicates orthotic and wheelchair fitting and can affect independence and proficiency with transfers, mobility, and self-care activities. For children who are ambulatory, a greater expenditure of energy is required to participate in physical play activities, so it is likely that less time will be spent engaged in physical play and that more sedentary activities (e.g., watching television) will be adopted. Children with mobility limitations, whether they are ambulatory or wheelchair mobile, may not be well accepted by able-bodied peers when they attempt to participate in physically challenging play, or they may feel conspicuous because they have difficulty keeping up. The likelihood of participation under these circumstances is diminished. As obesity develops, this further complicates participation and negatively affects self-image, creating an undesirable cycle perpetuating weight gain. In addition, children with MM probably are at a disadvantage physiologically. Studies evaluating the caloric intake required for children with MM[162] have shown that the intake should be lower than for able-bodied obese peers. This is probably not just a function of the decreased activity level of children with MM. Decreased muscle mass of large lower limb muscle groups diminishes the ability to burn calories (i.e., the basal metabolic rate of children with MM is probably lower than normal). This is consistent with the observation that children with high lumbar and thoracic lesions have greater problems with obesity. Decreased muscle mass coupled with lower extremity inactivity reduces the daily caloric needs such that a young adult who uses a wheelchair as his primary means of mobility will need fewer than 1500 calories a day to maintain his current weight.[104] Liusuwan and associates[99] showed that in a population of children ages 11 to 21, children with spina bifida, when compared to a control group, have significantly less lean body mass measured using dual energy x-ray absorptiometry as well as significantly lower resting energy expenditure measured with an open-circuit indirect calorimeter.

An easy and readily available mechanism to screen for obesity in the general population is height-weight ratios; however, arm span-weight ratios are more appropriate for monitoring individuals with MM. Shurtleff[162] noted that height-weight ratios are not useful in children with MM because of their short stature, decreased linear length secondary to spine or lower limb deformities, and decreased growth of paretic limbs. He recommended monitoring individuals with MM by measuring serial subscapular skinfold thickness, linear length measured along the axis of long bones to take into consideration hip and knee joint contractures, arm span measured with a spanner, and weight measured on a platform scale (subtracting the weight of the wheelchair or adaptive aids). Results should be recorded on National Center for Health Statistics percentile charts.[58] Arm span measurements should be adjusted using correction factors to avoid underestimating body fat content: 0.9 arm span for children with no leg muscle mass (thoracic and high-lumbar levels), 0.95 arm span for those with partial loss of muscle mass (mid- and low-lumbar lesions), and 1.0 arm span for children with minimal or no muscle mass loss. Del Gado and associates[35] reported that in comparison to a control group, 32 children with MM had significantly lower stature, higher weights, and greater subcutaneous fat deposits in their trunks, the latter being associated with cardiovascular disease risk factors.

Weight control is not just a function of decreased caloric intake for children with MM, however, and must involve a regular exercise program. The challenge of the physical therapist is to find age-appropriate physical activities for their clients that are fun and at which they can succeed; in this way, physical activity is positively reinforced and a lifelong pattern of engaging in such activities is developed. Liusuwan and associates[100] piloted a program combining behavioral intervention, exercise, and nutrition education that showed promise as a method for improving health and fitness of adolescents with spinal cord dysfunction.

AGE-SPECIFIC EXAMINATION AND PHYSICAL THERAPY INTERVENTION

There are issues of particular importance for specific age groups with MM. Intervention should be provided to keep pace with the normal timing of development.[17,160] Throughout the life span, it is important to keep in mind the overall picture of the needs of the patient and family. The medical problems and the number of health care professionals involved in the care of individuals with MM can be overwhelming. Many members of other disciplines, in addition to the physical therapist, may also be making requests of the family's time. Each professional should prioritize his or her goals, relative to those of other disciplines and coordinate planning so that the demands placed on the patient and the family are realistic. It is best to work as a team with the family and other disciplines to integrate appropriate intervention programs into the patient's daily routine. In addition, if conflicting information is provided to parents, they often become confused and may lack appropriate information to set realistic goals for their children and adolescents (e.g., goals for mobility, self-care, employment, and independent living). Consequently, multidisciplinary team collaboration with the family is important to establish appropriate goals and expectations.

The following sections focus on special considerations throughout the life span. Four age groups are discussed: infancy, preschool age, school age, and adolescence. Participation restrictions that are typically present, as well as the causes and impact of activity limitations on expected life roles are discussed for each of the four age groups. Examination and evaluation of body structure and function, activity limitations, and participation restrictions, along with recommendations for ongoing monitoring, typical physical therapy goals, intervention, and strategies to prevent secondary impairments and activity limitations, are also discussed. In addition, typical secondary participation restrictions and activity limitations encountered during adolescence and their impact on the transition to adulthood are discussed in the section on adolescence and transition to adulthood. The information presented in this latter section has important implications for preventive intervention during childhood and adolescence to minimize the incidence of acquired impairments and activity limitations that often surface later in life.

It is important to keep in mind that the interaction of a multitude of impairments may affect an individual's functional performance, yet only a few key impairments are discussed for each age group. The reader is referred to the previous section on impairments for a more thorough discussion of other factors. Similarly, only key examination and intervention strategies that are specific to a given age category are discussed in each section. Common goals across the life span are to prevent joint contractures, correct existing deformities, prevent or minimize the effects of sensory and motor deficiency, and optimize mobility within natural environments.[110]

INFANCY

Typical Participation Restrictions: Causes and Implications

The multiple impairments and overwhelming medical needs of a newborn with MM may interfere with parent-infant interaction. Parents are often afraid to handle their infant with MM, and the opportunities for handling and interacting with their child may be further limited by medical complications. Parents and extended family members may be cautious in handling the infant, resulting in decreased stimulation. Naturally occurring opportunities for early environmental stimulation, observation, exploration, and social interaction also may be limited as a result of somatosensory and motor deficits, hypotonia, and visual deficits. Family and infant interaction may be further impeded by the additional parental duties required (e.g., bowel and bladder

intervention), frequent medical visits, and hospitalizations for complications.

The achievement of fine motor and gross motor developmental milestones is usually delayed during infancy because of multiple impairments, including joint contractures and deformities, motor and sensory deficits, hypotonia, upper limb dyscoordination, CNS dysfunction, visual and perceptual disorders, and cognitive deficits. The lack of normal infant movements, combined with impaired sensation, decreases kinesthetic awareness and inhibits perceptuomotor development. Independence with early ADL, such as holding a bottle or finger feeding, is also negatively affected by impairments resulting from MM, especially swallowing disorders, upper limb dyscoordination, and visuoperceptual deficits.

Examination of Impairments

As discussed in Chapter 5, therapists must be aware of normal physiologic flexion of the hips and knees when assessing newborns. Limitations of up to 35° are present in normal newborns. These contractures may be more pronounced at birth in the infant with MM after prolonged intrauterine positioning of the relatively inactive fetus. Physiologic flexion spontaneously reduces in able-bodied infants from the effects of gravity and spontaneous lower limb movements. Physiologic flexion of infants with MM typically does not spontaneously reduce, because of decreased or absent spontaneous lower limb activity secondary to muscle weakness. Consequently, contractures may develop even in children with sacral level function if they lack full strength of the gluteal muscles.

Two primary orthopedic concerns during this period are to identify and manage dislocated hips and foot deformities. Early orthopedic intervention of these deformities results in improved potential for standing balance and more timely achievement of motor milestones such as sitting and walking.[108,117] Achieving a plantigrade foot position is important, regardless of ambulatory prognosis. Plantigrade alignment is optimal for shoe fit, positioning and weight distribution in sitting, and stability when bearing weight for standing pivot transfers or ambulation.

When assessing muscle tone in infants, either the Harris Infant Neuromotor Test[59] (HINT) or the Movement Assessment of Infants[28] are useful tools. Hypotonia is typical in infants with MM, even if sacral level function is present.[197] Poor head control, delayed neck and trunk righting, automatic reactions, and low trunk and lower limb muscle tone are typical. A mixture of hypotonia, hypertonia, and spastic movements may be present in the limbs. It is important to distinguish between voluntary and reflexive movements when assessing muscle function.

One of the key physical therapy considerations in managing the newborn with MM is to establish a reliable baseline of muscle function before and after back closure. This baseline is important for predicting future function and for monitoring status. In addition, it is important to identify muscle imbalance around joints and existing joint contractures that are unlikely to reduce spontaneously.

In the newborn, muscle function is assessed before and after surgical closure of the back to determine the extent of motor paralysis. Side lying is usually the position of choice for testing the newborn, to avoid injury to the exposed neural tissue.[153] The state of alertness must be considered and documented when testing newborns or infants. Repeated examinations may need to be conducted at different times of the day to observe the infant's muscle activity in various behavioral states. Optimal performance cannot be elicited if the infant is in a sleepy state. Muscle activity is best observed when the infant is alert, hungry, or crying. Several techniques can be used to arouse the drowsy infant, including assessing limb ROM, rocking vertically to stimulate the vestibular system, and providing tactile and auditory stimulation.[65,153] Ideally, the infant's spontaneous activity should be observed in supine, prone, and side-lying positions before the examiner starts handling the infant. Handling the infant may suppress spontaneous activity. Movement can often be elicited through sounds, visual tracking, reaching for toys, tickling, placing limbs in antigravity positions to elicit holding responses, and moving limbs to end-range positions to see if the infant will move out of the position.[65] For older infants, muscle activity can be observed, palpated, and resisted in developmental positions. If leg movements in myotomes caudal to the MM occur concurrently with performance of general movements in infants, functional neural conduction through the MM is implicated.[174]

Therapists often do not record specific strength grades for infants and young children. Instead, either a dichotomous scale (present or absent) or a 3-point ordinal scale (apparently normal, weak, or absent) is often advocated.[127,137,153] This 3-point scale, however, lacks sensitivity and predictive validity.[127] In contrast, specific manual muscle test strength scores (grades 0 to 5) have been found to provide useful information for infants and young children with MM and are predictive of later function.[112] Consequently, when strength is assessed manually, we recommend using the full manual muscle testing scale, regardless of age. The estimated quality of the examination should also be recorded, indicating the examiner's degree of confidence in the results, based on the child's level of cooperation. Neck and trunk musculature should be graded as "normal for age" if the child is able to perform developmentally appropriate activities.[82]

Testing sensation in infants and young children presents special challenges. Complete testing of multiple sensory modalities is not possible until the child has acquired sufficient cognitive and language abilities to accurately respond to testing.[153] Parents can often provide useful information to help focus on probable insensate areas. It is best to test the child in a quiet state. Testing with a pin or other sharp object should begin at the lowest level of sacral innervation and progress to more proximally innervated dermatomes until a noxious response is noted (e.g., crying or facial grimace).

Teulier and associates[184] used a motorized treadmill to evaluate stepping responses of infants with MM from 1 to 12 months of age. Treadmill practice elicited steps and increased motor activity. Holding infants with MM on a moving treadmill resulted in 17% more motor activity of their entire body during the year than holding them on a nonmoving treadmill. Infants with MM stepped less than typically developing infants (14.4 versus 40.8 steps/minute), however, and they were less likely to produce alternating steps than typically developing infants at any age level. Responses were affected by lesion level but varied markedly among infants because of other confounding factors such as shunt revisions, medications, joint and ligament structures, and family support resources. Infants with the highest lesion levels (L1-3) exhibited a very low step rate over time, which the authors proposed was due to marked delays in muscle strength and limb control, rather than an innate lack of capacity as three of four infants in this group developed the ability to walk with walkers by 44 months of age. In contrast to interlimb stepping patterns, the within-limb step parameters of infants with MM were quite similar to typically developing infants. The authors plan to study the potential for treadmill practice to produce positive outcomes for infants with MM such as increasing muscle and cardiovascular strength, bone density, and neuromotor control required for upright locomotion.

Ongoing Monitoring

During the first year of life, it is important to monitor joint alignment, muscle imbalance, and the development of contractures. Typical lower limb contractures that develop are hip and knee flexion contractures, combined with external rotation at the hips. Children with weak or absent hip musculature often lie in a "frog-legged" position with the hips flexed and externally rotated and the knees flexed. Consequently, these muscle groups are typically in a shortened position. It is important to closely monitor ROM and muscle extensibility during periods of rapid growth. Soft tissue growth typically lags behind skeletal changes, resulting in decreased extensibility. Stretching exercises should be initiated early on, if indicated, when contractures are relatively flexible and respond well to intervention. If orthoses or night-positioning splints are used to correct orthopedic deformities, the fit of these devices should be monitored to prevent skin breakdown.

Changes in muscle tone and muscle function are observed with progressive neurologic dysfunction. Baseline measurements, therefore, are essential, and these parameters should be closely monitored. Therapists should also watch for behavioral changes, decreases in performance, and other subtle signs of shunt malfunction (see Box 22-1) or seizure disorders. Motor development must also be observed to determine whether an infant is keeping pace with normal developmental expectations. Abnormalities in any of these areas should be reported to the child's primary care physician.

Typical Physical Therapy Goals and Strategies

During the newborn period, physical therapists must be sensitive to the feelings and needs of parents and other extended family members who are learning to cope with the overwhelming problems of a child with MM. Parents go through a period of tremendous adjustment. They are required to meet the demands of a normal infant, plus deal with the extensive medical and surgical needs of their newborn and adjust to the long-term implications of their child's multiple impairments. Not all instructions may be assimilated at any one time given the large amount of information to which parents are asked to attend. Often instructions must be reviewed and reinforced during subsequent visits. Written instructions should be provided to augment verbal explanations.

If ROM is limited, parents should be instructed in positioning techniques. It is optimal to maintain ROM by means of positioning because little additional time is required of the family. If contractures do not resolve with positioning, or if contractures are not supple, parents should also be instructed in stretching exercises and soft tissue mobilization techniques. It is usually most efficient to perform stretching exercises and soft tissue mobilization techniques in conjunction with diaper changes.

For infants who exhibit hypotonia, parents should be instructed in handling techniques to facilitate head and trunk control. Techniques advocated for children with hypotonic cerebral palsy[20] are often beneficial. Parents should be encouraged to provide sitting opportunities for the infant to facilitate the development of head and trunk control. Additional head and trunk support is often required in high chairs, strollers, and car seats. If motor development is significantly delayed and requires therapeutic intervention, a combination of neurodevelopmental intervention and proprioceptive neuromuscular facilitation techniques is beneficial. Therapeutic interventions and adaptive equipment should ideally be planned to keep pace with the normal timing of development so that the child is provided with typical developmental experiences. During the latter half of the first year, preparatory activities for mobility are indicated. Emphasis should be placed on balance, trunk control, and facilitating an upright posture as the child progresses through the developmental sequence.

Prevention of Secondary Impairments and Activity Limitations

Parents should be instructed in proper positioning, ROM, and handling techniques with the lower limbs in neutral alignment to prevent the development of contractures. If the hips are dislocated or subluxed, parents should be instructed in proper positioning, double diapering, and the use of a night-positioning orthosis, if indicated.[148,152] If surgery is indicated to relocate hip dislocations (see previous section on orthopedic deformities), it is generally performed after 6 months of age. Foot deformities are generally treated through serial casting or positioning splints.

Parents should also be instructed to inspect insensate skin areas during diaper changes and dressing for signs of pressure or injury. Parents need to understand the importance of skin inspection and that insensate areas should be inspected on a daily basis throughout the life span.

TODDLER AND PRESCHOOL YEARS

Typical Participation Restrictions: Causes and Implications

The achievement of fine motor and gross motor developmental milestones continues to be delayed. Mobility is typically impaired in this population owing to orthopedic, motor, and sensory deficits. As the child nears the end of the first year of life, it is important to provide opportunities for environmental exploration. If the child does not have an efficient, effective mode of independent mobility by the end of the first year, provision of a mobility device is indicated.

Environmental exploration is essential for the development of initiative and independence. Limited early mobility may result in a lack of curiosity and initiative and may negatively affect other aspects of development.[13,26,164] If a toddler does not have an effective means of independently exploring and interacting with the environment, he or she may learn to be passively dependent. The negative influence of limited early mobility on personality and behavior development can persist throughout life. Passive-dependent behavior is a commonly observed personality trait of adolescents and adults with MM.

Limited mobility also negatively affects socialization, especially interaction with other children. If a stroller is used as the primary mode of community mobility beyond the normal age of weaning a child from a stroller, other children will view the child with MM as a "baby." Play opportunities are also limited if a child does not have an effective means of mobility.

Independence with ADL is often impaired in this population because of fine and gross motor impairments, upper limb dyscoordination, and CNS dysfunction. Children who are not independent with ADL may miss out on normal childhood experiences (e.g., play time) while waiting for others to assist them with basic skills. Their self-esteem may also be negatively affected if other children tease them regarding their dependency.

It is important that parents, child care personnel, and preschool teachers be aware of other motor deficits that are often exhibited in this population, such as poor eye-hand coordination. The potential impact of these deficits on functional performance in handwriting and the acquisition of

ADL skills such as feeding and dressing should be realized so that reasonable goals can be established and the use of appropriate adaptive equipment implemented.

Examination and Evaluation of Impairments and Activity Limitations

By the end of the first year, ROM is expected to be within normal limits. If limited ROM persists, it is important to distinguish between fixed and supple contractures, determine muscle extensibility, and evaluate orthopedic deformities to determine whether they are fixed or flexible.

To assess strength, functional muscle testing techniques are advocated for children 2 to 5 years old because they may not cooperate with traditional test procedures.[65,137] Functional activities that are helpful in determining the strength of key lower limb muscle groups include gait observations, heel- and toe-walking, climbing up and down a step, one-legged stand, toe touching, squat to stand, bridging, bicycling while supine, the Landau position, prone kicking, the wheelbarrow position, sit-ups, pull to sit, and sitting and standing push-ups. It is often possible for young children to cooperate with isolated muscle actions by having them push against a puppet to show how strong they are. To elicit the cooperation of older preschoolers (3- to 4-year-olds), it is often helpful to name the muscle and describe its "job" (the muscle action). The children think that the muscle names are humorous, maintaining their attention. Asking children to have the muscle do its "job" makes strength testing more understandable.[65] We have found it possible to obtain objective, reliable measures of strength from children as young as 4 years of age using handheld myometry techniques.[65] The degree of confidence regarding whether the child's optimal performance was elicited should be recorded.

Once the child is 2 years of age, light touch and position sense can usually be assessed by eliciting tickling responses or having the child respond to the touch of a puppet. Other sensory modalities can ordinarily be accurately tested once the child is 5 to 7 years old. The accuracy of responses often must be double-checked because of short attention span and response perseveration. Two sensory testing techniques minimize perseveration of responses. The first is to randomly alternate between testing light touch and pinprick and have the child identify the type of sensation. The second is to have the child point to the spot that was touched and correctly state when no area was touched.

Fine and gross motor development should be assessed using appropriate standardized tests such as those discussed in Chapter 2. Examination of ADL should focus on what the individual actually does on a daily basis, in addition to what she or he is capable of doing. If independence with ADL is limited, appropriate adaptations and interventions should be implemented to foster independence. The Functional Activities Assessment[133,175,176] is useful for this population (Figure 22-7). Items may be scored by direct observation or by parent report. Assistive devices required to perform a given task are also documented. The "Can" and "Does" scoring format permits the examiner to record what the child can do versus what the child actually does on a regular basis. In addition, if the child is directly observed performing the task, the degree of independence and the time to complete the task are recorded.

Ongoing Monitoring

Joint alignment, muscle imbalance, contractures, posture, and signs of progressive neurologic dysfunction should continue to be monitored. Contractures that seem insignificant during childhood may become functionally limiting once the individual has adult-sized body proportions. For example, knee extension contractures can interfere with the ability to maneuver in a wheelchair.

Typical Physical Therapy Goals and Strategies

Joint alignment, contractures, muscle strength, and postural alignment should continue to be treated, as necessary. Proper positioning in sleeping and sitting should continue. If stretching or strengthening exercises are indicated, it is often helpful to involve other family members in the exercise program so that the child does not feel singled out. For ambulatory candidates with weak hip and knee musculature, strengthening activities may be beneficial if the child is cooperative. In addition to traditional posture exercises,[82] many play activities promote strengthening and the development of good posture.[46] The use of therapy ball techniques to strengthen postural muscles is also beneficial. Muscle re-education techniques, such as functional electrical stimulation and biofeedback, are useful to teach muscles to function in new ROM after stretching exercises. Electrical stimulation has also been found to be beneficial in increasing strength and enhancing functional performance in this population.[80]

During the preschool years, the focus is on improving the independence, efficiency, and effectiveness of ADL and mobility. Development of independence with dressing and feeding should be encouraged. Appropriate guidance should be provided so that parents have age-appropriate expectations. It is important for young children to actively participate in skin inspection, bowel and bladder intervention, donning and removing orthoses, wheelchair intervention, and other ADL tasks. Teaching these skills early on and actively involving the child facilitates independence and incorporation of these activities into the daily routine. As a result, these extra responsibilities required of the child with MM become as natural as other ADL, such as brushing teeth. Waiting to introduce tasks until the child is older often is met with resistance, especially when the child observes that siblings do not have the same requirements.

By kindergarten age, children without disabilities are able to dress and toilet themselves (with the exception of some

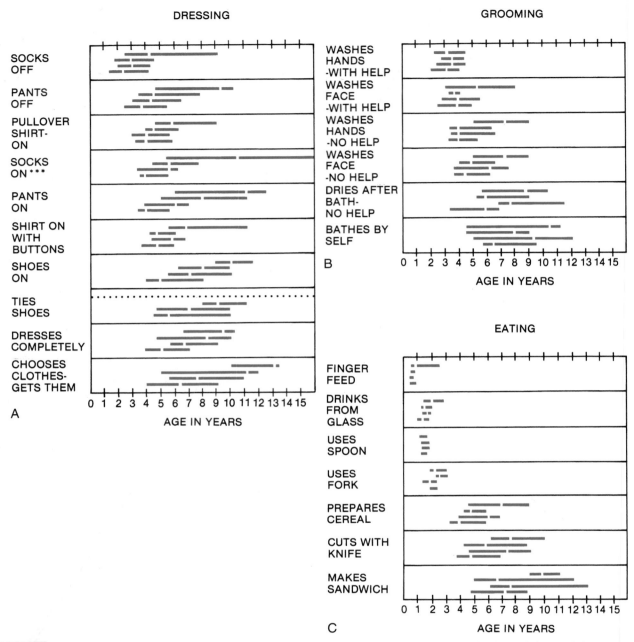

Figure 22-7 Functional activities assessment. The age at which 20%, 50%, and 80% of a group of 173 children learned dressing **(A)**, grooming **(B)**, and eating **(C)** skills is indicated by the beginning of, space between (white space), and end of the black bars, respectively. Triple asterisks indicate that this group never achieved an 80% learning proportion. Dotted line indicates activity was attempted with this group. The bars in each category represent, from top to bottom, (1) thoracic and L1–L2; (2) L3 and mixed lesions, L2–L4; (3) L4–L5; and (4) sacral-level groups. All data were recorded as the child achieved the skill during the 2.5-year period of the study, within 4 months of entering the study, or when the caretaker entered a specific date of achievement in the child's diary. These charts were created from data published by Okamoto and associates[133] and Sousa and associates.[176] (From Shurtleff, D. B. [Ed.]. [1986]. *Myelodysplasias and exstrophies: Significance, prevention, and treatment* [p. 376]. Orlando, FL: Grune & Stratton.)

fasteners), eat independently, and be mobile.[47] These skills must be emphasized at an early age in children with MM so that they achieve independence by the time they begin school. A wide range of age of achievement of independence with ADL is evident in this population when examining the normative data provided on the Functional Activities Assessment (see Figure 22-7). This wide variability in age of achieving skills within a given motor level suggests that a significant percentage of children are delayed in ADL skill acquisition because of attitudes and expectations. Fay and associates[47] suggested that these delays may be partially caused by low parental expectations and protective attitudes, perceptions that it is faster for the parent to perform the task, and parental difficulty accepting the reality of the child's activity limitations. Showing parents the ADL normative data for children with MM and promoting positive parental expectations of independence are beneficial. It is important for parents to positively reinforce the child's attempts to be independent so that she or he is motivated to achieve. It is also important to help the parents understand how incontinence retards their child's normal sexual exploration, learning, and social inhibitions that normal preschool children learn. Alternative opportunities should be offered to children with MM.[21]

Skin inspection and pressure relief techniques should be taught early so that they are incorporated into the daily routine. Proper intervention of lower limbs and joint protection techniques should be taught to avoid injury of insensate areas when learning how to perform ADL, such as transfers. The impact of sensory deficits on functional performance should be kept in mind during gait training and when teaching other functional tasks.

Provision of an effective means of independent mobility is essential for young children. Consequently, if a child does not begin maneuvering effectively within the environment by 1 year of age, alternative means of mobility must be considered to achieve independent home and short-distance community mobility.[26,164] Mobility options should be explored and implemented as frequently as is needed so that the child is able to actively participate in normal childhood activities. Various mobility options are available, from manual devices such as a caster cart to electric wheelchairs. Electric wheelchair use has been found to be feasible and beneficial for children as young as 24 months of age.[26] If a wheelchair is indicated, it is important to present this option to the parents in a positive way. The use of a wheelchair does not preclude walking. In fact, children who use wheelchairs at an early age generally are more interested in mobility, independence, and environmental exploration. Consequently, they tend to be more independent in all forms of mobility later in life. Ryan and associates[149] recommended introducing a wheelchair as early as 18 months to enable children to keep up with their peers, boost self-confidence, facilitate independence, and increase activity levels. A more recent case report[105] suggests that it is potentially feasible to train infants as young as seven months old to safely operate a power mobility device.

Preparatory activities for mobility are indicated for 1- to 2-year-olds. Emphasis should be placed on balance, trunk control, and facilitating an upright posture. For ambulatory candidates, once the child begins to pull to stand, the need for orthoses to improve weight-bearing alignment should be considered. It is important to anticipate future ambulatory needs when recommending orthoses to maximize their utility.

For children with high-level lesions (thoracic to L3), preparatory activities for wheelchair mobility should be emphasized (e.g., sitting balance, arm strengthening, transfer training, wheelchair propulsion, and electrical switch operation if indicated). The focus of wheelchair training for toddlers and preschoolers with high-level lesions should include mobility, environmental exploration, safety, and transfer skills. Household distance ambulation using a parapodium, HKAFO, knee-ankle-foot orthosis (KAFO), or reciprocating gait orthosis (RGO) may be attempted, but energy expenditure is very high. Consequently, wheelchairs are generally used for community mobility of children with thoracic to L3 motor function, particularly once body proportions increase.

Effective biped ambulation is feasible for toddlers and preschoolers with L4 and below motor function. They will require wheelchair skills as older children, however, to participate in sports and prolonged activities. It is essential to maintain adequate ROM and to emphasize an upright posture so that weight-bearing forces are properly distributed and muscles can function at their optimal length. Therapeutic activities that promote trunk control and balance are beneficial. Children with lumbar level lesions will require upper limb support for walking. In general, a reverse-facing walker is best when the child is learning to walk because it allows the child to be upright and minimizes upper limb weight bearing. Reverse-facing walkers have been found to promote better postural alignment than anterior-facing walkers.[101] Once an upright gait is established, the child can be advanced to forearm crutches.

If children with sacral level motor function require upper limb support to begin walking, a reverse-facing walker is also usually best to minimize upper limb weight bearing. Alternatively, forearm crutches can be used if the child is able to walk upright while manipulating the crutches. Children with L5 and S1 level lesions often abandon their upper limb aids when they are young and their center of mass is low to the ground. Upper limb aids may still be indicated for endurance and to decrease trunk sway when walking long distances, for balance when walking on rough terrain, or to minimize the stress on weight-bearing lower limb joints. The need for upper limb aids should be reevaluated when the child is older and body proportions and environmental demands have changed.

The use of positive reinforcement is often recommended for this population to enhance cooperation with examination procedures and intervention programs. In general, food is not an appropriate form of reinforcement because obesity is often a concern. Verbal reinforcement is preferred at this age.

Prevention of Secondary Impairments and Activity Limitations

Individuals are at risk for joint contractures when there is muscle imbalance around joints, when a substantial portion of the day is spent sitting, when there is a prolonged period of immobilization or bed rest, following surgery, and during periods of rapid growth when soft tissue growth may lag behind skeletal changes. It is important to closely monitor individuals with MM during these periods so that intervention can be initiated early on, if needed, when contractures are still flexible and respond well to intervention. Early detection and intervention of contractures can prevent fixed deformities and stretch weakness of overlengthened muscles. Similarly, the importance of skin inspection of insensate areas, use of pressure relief cushions, and sitting push-ups for pressure relief should be emphasized at an early age so that these preventive measures become routine. Daily monitoring of insensate areas can be taught at an early age by jointly inspecting the skin and verbalizing that there are no red areas. Body image can be promoted by playing games that involve touching and finding body parts.

Habitual postural positions that contribute to deforming forces should be discouraged. It is essential to emphasize an upright posture when a child is learning to walk. If children are permitted to stand and walk in a crouched posture, habits become established and it is difficult to teach a more upright posture because of the development of secondary impairments (e.g., joint contractures and stretch weakness of excessively lengthened muscles). Therapists should closely observe joint alignment and posture when a child is standing. Postural deviations that look insignificant when a child is young are often magnified once body proportions increase.

SCHOOL AGE

Typical Participation Restrictions: Causes and Implications

Independence with ADL often continues to be impaired in this age group. Children who are not independent with ADL may miss out on normal childhood experiences (e.g., playtime or recess) while waiting for parents or teachers to assist them with basic skills. Their self-esteem may continue to be negatively affected if other children tease them regarding their dependency.

Mobility limitations are magnified once a child begins school because of the increased community mobility distances and skills required. Advanced mobility skills are needed because of environmental barriers such as curbs, ramps, uneven terrain, and steps. Ineffective or inefficient community mobility can further reinforce dependent behaviors if other children carry his or her schoolbooks and lunch tray or push the wheelchair.

The negative effects of limited mobility and physical limitations on socialization become more apparent at this age. Play and recreational opportunities are restricted if a child does not have an effective method of mobility. Often children with MM are excluded from recess or physical education class. Consequently, they miss out on opportunities for social interaction. Even if they are included in these activities, often their involvement is peripheral (e.g., serving as the score keeper during physical education class). Mobility limitations, dependency with ADL, difficulties with toileting, and the difficulty of managing adaptive equipment often interfere with other aspects of peer interaction, such as going over to friends' houses to play or spending the night with friends.

Finally, it is important that parents and teachers be aware of perceptuomotor, visuoperceptual, and sensory deficits. The potential impact of these deficits on writing speed, legibility, and accuracy; the efficiency and effectiveness of performing ADL skills; problem solving; and cognitive abilities should be realized so that reasonable goals can be established and the use of appropriate adaptive equipment can be implemented. Multiple hospitalizations or medical complications can also negatively affect school performance.

Examination and Evaluation of Impairments and Activity Limitations

As with younger children, joint alignment, strength, muscle imbalance, contractures, muscle extensibility, and posture should continue to be monitored. Other parameters that should be assessed include sensation, coordination, fine motor skills, ADL, mobility, gait, body awareness, and functional skills.

Reliable, sensitive, objective measures of strength can be obtained in school-age children.[65] We recommend that objective methods of strength examination, such as handheld myometry, be used to serially monitor strength of individuals with MM who are old enough to cooperate (typically age 4 or older). Stationary isokinetic or strain gauge devices can also provide objective measures of strength, but these devices are not available in the typical clinic or school setting.

Independence with ADL should be assessed. In addition to the basic ADL skills evaluated in the Functional Activities Assessment, the school-age child's ability to carry items and assist with basic household chores should be evaluated. The physical therapist also assesses the adequacy of clearance, duration, frequency, and reliability of performance of wheelchair push-ups. A nurse usually evaluates bowel and bladder function and the degree of continence. It is important that the physical therapist understand these and degree of independence with bowel and bladder function, however, because positioning, adaptive equipment, and mobility issues can often restrict independence with bowel and bladder intervention programs.

The home, school, and community environments should be accessible so that individuals with MM can participate fully in all activities. The Americans with Disabilities Act of 1990 mandates access to all buildings, programs, and services used by the general public in the United States. Even partial exclusion from a school program can have lasting negative effects on a student's social and emotional development.[7] Providing accessibility to the entirety of school, home, and community activities lets individuals with MM know that they have the same opportunities and rights of access as everyone else. Limited access broadcasts a message of exclusion and estrangement. Both physical and social barriers to participation must be addressed. For a more thorough discussion of evaluating environmental accessibility in the school setting, see Baker and Rogosky-Grassi.[7] Community accessibility should also be evaluated. Ideally, the patient should have access to the community school, church, grocery and drug stores, post office, bank, cleaners, stores and shopping malls, library, restaurants, theaters, sports arenas, hospital, physician's office, work environment, and public transportation. Streets, sidewalks, crosswalks, and parking lots should also be accessible.

Ongoing Monitoring

Joint alignment, muscle imbalance, contractures, posture, and signs of progressive neurologic dysfunction should continue to be monitored. As school-age children mature, they should become more responsible for daily inspection of insensate skin areas when they are bathing and dressing. Appropriate performance of pressure relief strategies should also be monitored. Areas of skin breakdown should be noted so that appropriate adjustments in equipment and preventive behaviors can be implemented or reviewed.

School-age children should be observed closely during periods of rapid growth because they are at risk for loss of function as a result of cord tethering. Parents and teachers should be made aware of signs of progressive CNS complications so that they know when to refer the child to a primary care physician.

Typical Physical Therapy Goals and Strategies

The stretching and strengthening strategies discussed for the two previous age groups also apply to the school-age child. Improving the flexibility of low back extensor, hip flexor, hamstring, and shoulder girdle musculature should be emphasized. When possible, stretching and strengthening exercises should also be incorporated into the physical education program. It is important that children with MM participate in physical education classes and sports activities in a meaningful way. As noted earlier, if children dependent on braces and crutches learn wheelchair skills and use at an early age, they will not be depressed and perceive wheelchair use as a failure when they arrive at adolescence.

Proper positioning while sleeping and sitting should continue. In the classroom, seating should provide stability and symmetric alignment. Feet should be flat on the floor or on wheelchair footrests. The seat and desk height should be adjusted to fit the child's body proportions. The desktop should be tilted up to improve neck and upper trunk alignment. Appropriate cushioning should be provided. The child's chair should be positioned in the room so that the teacher and blackboard can easily be viewed while maintaining neutral alignment, without having to turn in the chair.

If a child has not achieved independence with a given ADL task by the age at which 50% of the normative group achieved independence on the Functional Activities Assessment, the child's performance should be assessed to determine if adaptive equipment is required or if further interventions are indicated. Goals for ADL performance should include efficiency in addition to independence. If the child is not as efficient as the primary caretaker, the caretaker will most likely perform the task. The target goal, therefore, is for the child to be able to perform the task as efficiently as the primary caretaker. Showing parents the ADL normative data for children with MM and promoting positive parental expectations of independence are beneficial (see Figure 22-7). It is important for parents to positively reinforce the child's attempts to be independent so that he or she is motivated to achieve. Pressure relief techniques should be incorporated into the daily routine. Joint protection measures should also be implemented early on to prevent the development of future degenerative changes.

Once children with MM begin school, it is important that they have an independent, efficient, and effective means of mobility for home and long community distances. Alternative means of mobility may need to be considered for long distances to ensure that children with MM are able to keep up with their peers and still have energy left to attend to classroom activities. Various mobility options should be evaluated according to the criteria outlined in Box 22-2 to determine the most effective means of mobility for a given environment. Community-level wheelchair and ambulation skills should be taught, emphasizing efficiency and safety. Community, home, and school environments should be assessed to determine if there are architectural barriers that interfere with daily activities. It is essential for normal social development to permit accessibility to all school, home, and community activities, including recess, physical education, and field trips.[7]

A functional environment should be created at home and school by removing obstacles and adapting the environment to facilitate efficient and independent function. Adaptive equipment and effective mobility devices should be provided to maximize function. Community mobility skills may need to be practiced to facilitate independent function. Endurance training may also be indicated to ensure that the individual has sufficient endurance and efficiency to function effectively in all activities.

Recreation and physical fitness are important for physical, psychologic, and social reasons. Psychosocial benefits of participation in recreational activities include enhancing confidence and self-esteem, increasing socialization, improving group participation skills, provision of a means of exercising in a more normal way, and increasing interest and motivation in maintaining flexibility, strengthening, and endurance. In contrast, perceived physical restrictions result in a sedentary lifestyle, potentially predisposing these individuals to problems with obesity and degenerative diseases. It is

---

BOX **22-2** FEASIBILITY OF WHEELCHAIR AND BIPED AMBULATION: CRITERIA FOR EVALUATION

HOUSEHOLD DISTANCES

Endurance

Adequate to go between rooms in house?
Adequate to get to yard and car?

Efficiency

Record heart rate and calculate energy expenditure.
Record normal and fast household walking speeds.
Is fast pace adequate for emergency situations?
Is normal pace practical for everyday activities?

Effectiveness

Independent with all transfers?
Able to carry, reach, lift, and climb?
Able to perform activities of daily living?
Able to go forward, backward, sideways, and turn?

Safety

Has good stability and balance?
Observes joint and skin protection?
Able to maneuver around obstacles?
Safe on smooth surfaces and rugs?
Safe when turning?

Accessibility

Maneuvers in and out of house independently?
Necessary household rooms accessible?
Emergency exit routes accessible?

COMMUNITY DISTANCES

Endurance

Sufficient at a functional speed for average community distances (e.g., going to school, store, medical appointments, and social activities)?

Adequate for play and recreational activities (e.g., playground, park, beach, theater, sports arenas, sports participation)?
Adequate for long-distance community distances (e.g., shopping mall, zoo, concert, sporting events, hiking)?

Efficiency

Record heart rate and calculate energy expenditure.
Record normal and fast walking paces.
Adequate speed to cross intersections?
Is typical pace practical for community distances?

Effectiveness

Independent with all transfers?
Able to maneuver in all directions?
Able to climb and step over obstacles?
Able to carry packages and groceries?
Able to reach and lift items from shelves?

Safety

Has good stability and balance?
Observes joint and skin protection?
Safe on wet or slippery surfaces?
Able to maneuver around obstacles?
Able to maneuver in congested areas?
Safe on uneven terrain, curbs, inclines, and steps?

Accessibility

Maneuvers in and out of car and bus independently?
Necessary community buildings accessible?

---

important to stimulate a lifelong interest in fitness and recreation. In addition, community resources, feasibility of transportation, and the family's lifestyle must be taken into account.

Recreation activities must be carefully selected to ensure that they are beneficial and feasible yet enjoyable so they will be continued on a regular basis. Ideally, recreation activities should incorporate forms of aerobic exercise, along with socialization. It is important for individuals with MM to be involved in regular aerobic exercise to maintain their physical fitness and effectively control their weight. Recreational and physical fitness goals include maintaining and improving flexibility, strength, endurance, aerobic capacity, cardiovascular fitness, and coordination and controlling

weight. Low-impact aerobics are preferred to minimize stress on joints. Aerobic exercise videotapes have been developed for individuals with disabilities. Swimming is an ideal sport for this population, because they are often able to be competitive with their able-bodied peers and there is minimal stress on joints (www.brighthub.com/education/special/articles/44574.aspx). Other low-impact activities include cycling, rowing, cross-country skiing, roller and ice skating, and aerobic dance (www.cureourchildren.org/sports.htm).

Verbal reinforcement or implementation of a token economy system to earn special privileges is preferred at this age to enhance cooperation with examination procedures and intervention programs. As mentioned above, food is not an appropriate form of reinforcement.

Prevention of Secondary Impairments and Activity Limitations

Deficits that may appear insignificant during childhood often become magnified once an individual has adult body proportions, resulting in activity limitations and discomfort (e.g., low back pain resulting from an increased lumbar lordosis and hip flexion contractures). Joint protection is also important, beginning in early childhood. Joint trauma from excessive stress is cumulative over the life span. Children do not typically complain of pain, and children with MM may not be able to reliably detect pain in insensate areas. Consequently, sources of excess joint stress must be identified by carefully observing children while they perform ADL and transfers, walk, and propel their wheelchair. Permitting school-age children to assume responsibility for daily skin inspection checks with supervision prepares them for independence in adolescence.[141] One method of teaching careful skin inspection involves letting the child locate a small colored adhesive dot that is placed randomly on insensate skin.

Children and their parents should be involved as much as possible in the decision-making process and intervention for their disability. The rationale for assistive devices and therapeutic interventions should be explained so that they agree with intervention plans and become knowledgeable regarding acquisition of medical care and services, rather than being passive recipients.

ADOLESCENCE AND TRANSITION TO ADULTHOOD

Typical Participation Restrictions: Causes and Implications

If normal stages for early childhood development have not been successfully accomplished, adolescence can present a crisis. The preparation of individuals with MM for a successful transition into adult life must be based on developmental concerns and timely issues from infancy through all stages of development to young-adult life.[141] Adolescence brings expanded domains of travel for individuals with MM. School buildings become larger, with more environmental barriers for people with physical disabilities. To keep up with peers, community mobility must include mobility skills to travel long distances quickly and efficiently between classrooms, out to athletic fields as a participant or spectator, around shopping malls, and into crowded movie theaters, dances, and nightclubs. Independent adult living also requires mobility and balance skills that permit completion of advanced ADL tasks such as cooking, cleaning, clothes washing, shopping, yard work, house and equipment maintenance, driving, riding on public transportation, and going to work. Children who have gotten by with slow, inefficient ambulation skills using cumbersome adaptive equipment or

who have had basic wheelchair mobility on level surfaces but suddenly cannot handle ramps, hills, curbs, and uneven ground find themselves lagging behind their peers. Nearly all of the adults in a study of 30 individuals with MM[68] required referral to a physical therapist to address advanced mobility or equipment issues. It has been the observation of the authors that many adolescents and young adults do not have sufficient mobility skills to succeed independently in the community and must play catch-up to achieve their functional potential. The price paid for this delayed development of functional community mobility and lack of independence is social incompetence, dependence for advanced living skills, and unemployability, all of which must subsequently be addressed once mobility skills are improved. It is also important to train for competence and self-reliance. Blum and associates[18] reported that young people with MM who perceived that they were overprotected had less happiness, lower self-esteem, higher anxiety, lower self-perceived popularity, and greater self-consciousness.

Changes in functional mobility skills often occur concurrently with the rapid changes of adolescence. Individuals who have previously been ambulatory often become more reliant on a wheelchair. Dudgeon and associates[42] reported that adolescents with MM often exhibit changes in ambulation that are not explained by progressive complications. They suggested that these changes reflect adaptation of mobility to new environmental and social demands that require different speed, accessibility, and energy demands than those encountered in childhood. If orthotic stabilization of the hip, knee, or both is required, it is unlikely that adolescents with MM will maintain community ambulation; instead, most become nonambulators.[42] Brinker and associates[22] reported a decline in the ability to walk in 11 of 35 adults with sacral level MM (19 to 51 years old). Of the 34 adults who were initially community ambulators, 5 had become household ambulators, 2 were nonfunctional ambulators, and 4 were nonambulators. The one adult who had been a household ambulator became a nonambulator. The most common reasons for their declining ambulatory status were foot ulcerations, infections, and amputations. Wheelchair transfer skills have also been observed to decline during the transition from adolescence to adulthood. In a study of 30 adults with MM who had thoracic through sacral level motor function, the mobility status for 43% had declined since previous examinations performed during adolescence.[68] Several potential factors can play a role in this decreased function.

Changes in body proportions and body composition occur throughout the growing years, but the rate of these changes is accelerated dramatically during adolescence.[65] Increases in limb length affect the torque generated by muscles because of altered muscle length and resistance force moment arms. In addition, increases in height raise the location of the center of mass higher off the ground, making upright balance more difficult and energy expenditure greater to perform mobility tasks. Changes in body composition also alter the biomechanics of movement and affect performance. The relative percentage of force-generating muscle to fat and bone tissue changes the ratio of force-producing tissue to the load of the limbs. The development of obesity often occurs during adolescence and can further accentuate these changes. Banta[9] stated that body mass increases by the cube or volume whereas strength increases only by the square or cross-sectional area. The inevitable result during the adolescent growth spurt is that walking efficiency declines as the energy demands increase. Furthermore, during the adolescent growth spurt, the rate of skeletal growth exceeds the increase in muscle mass; the latter catches up after skeletal growth slows in late adolescence. Decreased flexibility of the trunk and two-joint limb muscles is often observed as part of this process. Normal adolescents frequently become clumsy during this period of adjustment while learning how to coordinate their longer limb lengths and increased muscle mass. Adolescents with MM already have a mechanical disadvantage and are consequently more susceptible to dyscoordination and decreased flexibility. It is likely that these developmental changes contribute to the decline in mobility that often occurs in adolescents with MM.

Progression of the neurologic deficit is another potential cause for decline in mobility function, and adolescents are particularly at risk during rapid periods of growth. Forty percent of the participants in our adult follow-up study[68] had lower limb strength loss compared with previous strength examinations as adolescents. Twenty-seven percent had a reduction in lower limb sensory perception. The greatest motor and sensory losses occurred in the group with lesions at L5 and below—the individuals with the most function to lose. In addition, 10% of study participants demonstrated upper limb strength loss. Progressive neurologic loss, therefore, appears to be an important factor in the changes in mobility status of many individuals during the transition from adolescence to adulthood.

Immobilization for intervention of secondary complications of MM can also contribute to decreased mobility skills. The development of decubiti, fractures, and orthopedic surgeries such as spinal fusions often require extended periods of immobilization with consequent disuse weakness, decreased endurance, and contracture development, all of which can decrease performance of mobility and transfer tasks.

Prolonged periods of bed rest are often necessary to heal decubitus ulcers to avoid bearing weight on pressure areas. Adolescents often have an increased incidence of decubiti compared with younger children. This is due to their increased body mass causing greater pressure over bony prominences around the buttocks and because of the development of adult sweat patterns in these areas. Fifty-six percent of the adults evaluated in our study[68] had a history of skin breakdown since their last examination as

adolescents; nearly 17% had breakdown present at the time of the examination. An alarming number of these people had little insight into the causes or methods for preventing skin breakdown despite their previous care in a large multidisciplinary pediatric clinic. Even more disturbing was the fact that three individuals (10%) had sustained lower limb amputations since adolescence (two bilateral, one unilateral) as a result of nonhealing ulcers that had progressed to osteomyelitis. Clearly, functional mobility is affected by decubitus ulcers and especially by limb loss.

Musculoskeletal problems can also affect the mobility of adolescents. Progression of spinal deformities often occurs during the growth spurt or in conjunction with one of the neurologic complications previously discussed. Sitting and standing balance can be affected by these spinal changes, leading to decreased mobility and transfer skills. Spinal orthoses prescribed to maintain optimal postural alignment also limit trunk ROM and hip flexion, interfering with wheelchair transfers and moving from sitting to standing. Surgical fusion of the spine to correct deformity and prevent its further progression can lead to immobilization with its consequent effects on mobility described earlier. Lower limb fractures secondary to osteoporosis can also necessitate immobilization with increased risk of functional loss.

Adolescents often begin to develop degenerative changes of weight-bearing joints and overuse syndromes as a result of the excessive loading of these joints necessitated by their neurologic deficit. Joint pain, ligamentous instability, or tendinitis can further limit mobility capabilities. Fifty percent of the adult study participants[68] complained of joint pain and 100% had joint or spinal deformities noted at the time of their examination.

Several other issues become important for the physical therapist to be cognizant of during adolescence. Independence with self-care and other daily activities is essential for normal socialization and for preparing individuals to lead normal adult lives. Bowel and bladder continence and independent intervention of bowel and bladder emptying are essential for social acceptance by peers and are even more critical at this stage because of the impact on dating, sexuality, higher education, employment, and independent living. Design and fit of wheelchair equipment, mobility aids, and orthoses affect independence with these tasks. Cosmesis is also a consideration with regard to equipment selection because body image and appearance become increasingly important issues during adolescence. Improper design or fit of equipment can significantly limit normal development in these areas.

Examination and Evaluation of Impairments and Activity Limitations

Based on the discussion of participation restrictions and their causes, the physical therapist should assess several impairments. Emphasis of specific impairments should be based on the known or suspected concurrent medical problems.

Joint ROM and muscle extensibility of two-joint muscles (especially hip and knee flexors) and trunk muscles should be assessed. Neck and low back motions are often restricted, particularly in adolescents and adults, because of muscle imbalance and poor postural habits. Joint swelling, ligamentous instability, crepitus, and pain with or without joint motion should be documented. If these conditions are progressive or severe enough to interfere with function, the patient should be referred to a physician for further evaluation and intervention. The distribution of degenerative joint changes should be noted with regard to performance of mobility tasks and obesity to determine the contribution of abnormal joint stresses to joint pain and dysfunction.

Muscle strength should continue to be monitored for all major upper and lower limb muscle groups. When progressive neurologic dysfunction is suspected, coordination testing and serial grip strength measurements can also be helpful. Posture and trunk balance in sitting and standing (for ambulators) should be assessed. Real or apparent leg length discrepancy may be present in individuals with foot and ankle deformities, lower limb contractures, unilateral or bilateral hip dislocation, or pelvic obliquity related to spinal curves.

Thorough examination of bed mobility, floor mobility, wheelchair mobility and transfers, and appropriateness and fit of wheelchair equipment is essential for wheelchair users. Endurance and effectiveness of mobility should be assessed to determine whether the individual's current mode of mobility is practical for community-level function. Box 22-2 provides further detail regarding important areas to assess. When orthoses are needed to maintain proper alignment or to facilitate efficient ambulation, the physical therapist must assess their appropriateness and fit. Boxes 22-3 and 22-4 provide further information regarding lower limb orthoses used in this population.

Ongoing Monitoring

Given the multitude of potential problems that can occur during adolescence and adulthood, comprehensive examinations should continue on at least a yearly basis, and potentially more frequently when problems are suspected or known to be present. Without regular reexamination, these individuals often fall through the cracks and endure permanent loss of function that was avoidable. An unfortunate example was one of the adult study participants with a diagnosis of lipomeningocele and a neurosegmental classification of "no loss" as an adolescent. His lesion level was reclassified at an L5 level at the time of our study. His loss of neurologic function was caused by a recurrent lipoma on his spine that went undetected and was not surgically removed until permanent neurologic loss had occurred. This individual thought that because his original lesion was removed as an infant with preservation of his spinal cord

function, he had no risk of future problems; therefore, he did not seek medical care until neurologic loss was irreversible. Early detection of progressive muscle strength loss, scoliosis, progression of spasticity, or contractures by the physical therapist with timely referral to a physician familiar with the potential complications associated with MM, along with aggressive physical therapy to reverse lost function (see section on prevention of secondary impairments and activity limitations), can prevent this scenario. This patient's story underscores the need for all individuals with MM to be followed throughout life, even if there are seemingly no current problems or their lesion has been classified as "no loss" after surgical closure.

Typical Physical Therapy Goals and Strategies

Functional goals for adolescents and adults are based on a number of factors that have been discussed in preceding sections of this chapter. The section on outcomes and their determinants provides guidelines for outcome expectations based on neurologic system function. In general, the goal for all but the most severely involved patients is to achieve independent basic and community mobility skills. The physical therapist must, therefore, be aware of all environments, distances, and barriers the individual is required to negotiate to adequately prepare the patient for all eventualities. Instruction in advanced community skills, along with endurance training, is often indicated. Physical and occupational therapists often need to be involved with driver's education programs and with the provision of adaptive equipment required for driving.

Goodwyn[53] expanded the Functional Activities Assessment format to include adolescent skills required for independent living. The items were selected from existing adult-oriented skill achievement tests, and normative data were studied in this population. The Assessment of Motor and Process Skills (AMPS) was also studied in a group of individuals ranging in age from 6 to 73 years old (mean = 21.3 years) and was found to be a valid assessment of ADL performance.[88] The AMPS assesses motor and process skills in terms of efficiency, effort, safety, and level of independence. The Kohlman Evaluation of Living Skills[115] is also a useful screening tool for determining independence with adult living skills such as self-care, safety, health maintenance, money management, transportation, telephone use, and work and leisure activities. For adolescents and adults, the ability to lift and carry items such as a hot dish, grocery bags, a laundry basket, and heavy household items is also important to assess. It is particularly important to observe safety issues and the use of proper body mechanics for advanced living skills. In addition, the maximum carrying distance should be determined and contrasted with functional demands. If independence and effectiveness with ADL are limited, appropriate adaptations and interventions should be made to foster independence. Environmental adaptations or assistive devices required to perform

Box 22-3 INDICATORS FOR LOWER LIMB ORTHOSES

FOOT ORTHOSES AND SUPRAMALLEOLAR ORTHOSES

Advantages

Permits full active dorsiflexion and plantar flexion
Maintains the subtalar joint in neutral alignment
Provides medial and lateral ankle stability

Motor Function

S1 to "no loss"
Must have adequate toe clearance and sufficient gastrocnemius/
    soleus strength to provide adequate push-off and decelerate
    forward movement of tibia

Indications

Unequal weight distribution, resulting in skin breakdown, foot
    deformities, or abnormal shoe wear
Medial and lateral ankle instability, resulting in balance
    problems, especially difficulty traversing uneven terrain
Poor alignment of the subtalar joint, forefoot, or rearfoot

ANKLE-FOOT ORTHOSES (STANDARD AFOS AND GROUND-REACTION FORCE AFOS)

Advantages

In general, the ground-reaction force (see Figure 22-6) is
advantageous for this population. The proximal trim line can be
extended medially to control genu valgus. The ground-reaction
force AFO also facilitates push-off and knee extension during
the stance phase and improves static standing balance. The
ground-reaction force AFO has a patellar tendon-bearing design.
This design distributes pressure across a broad area, preventing
skin breakdown and lower leg deformities, which are common
when traditional AFO anterior straps have been worn for an
extended period of time. If traditional AFOs are used in this
population, the anterior straps must be well padded.

Motor Function

L4 to S1
Weak or absent ankle musculature
Knee extensors at least grade 4

Indications

Medial and lateral instability of knee or ankle
Insufficient knee extension moment (ground-reaction force AFO)
Lack of or ineffective push-off
Inadequate toe clearance
Crouched gait pattern

KNEE-ANKLE-FOOT ORTHOSES

Advantages

If unable to maintain upright posture because of joint
    contractures or muscle weakness, or if the knee joints are
    unstable, KAFOs are indicated.

If the knee joint is primarily required for medial and lateral
    stability so the knee joint is unlocked, or if there is potential
    to progress to ambulation with the knee joints unlocked, it is
    best to incorporate the ground-reaction force AFO
    component into the KAFO design to provide the advantages
    listed earlier in the AFO section.

Motor Function

L3 to L4
Weak knee musculature
Absent ankle musculature

Indications

Medial and lateral instability of knee
Weak quadriceps (grade 4− or less)

RECIPROCATING GAIT ORTHOSES OR HIP-KNEE-ANKLE-FOOT ORTHOSES

Advantages

The reciprocating gait orthosis (RGO) cable system facilitates hip
    extension during stance phase and hip flexion during swing
    phase by coupling flexion of one hip with extension of the
    opposite hip.
Release of both cables permits hip flexion when sitting.
The RGO reduces the energy required for ambulation compared
    with walking with traditional KAFOs.

Motor Function

L1 to L3 (some centers also advocate for thoracic level).
Weak hip flexion is required to effectively operate the cables.

Indications

Unable to maintain an upright posture with the hip joints
    extended.
RGO is indicated to facilitate hip extension and swing phase.

THORACIC-HIP-KNEE-ANKLE-FOOT ORTHOSES, PARAPODIUMS, OR VERLOS

Advantages

Upright positioning for high-level lesions
Generally for exercise walking only

Motor Function

Thoracic to L2. Walking is usually nonfunctional for these
    high-level lesions because of the high energy expenditure
    required and the slow, cumbersome walking pace.

Indications

Limited distance mobility
Upright positioning
"Exercise" walking

BOX 22-4   LOWER LIMB ORTHOTIC SPECIFICATIONS, OBJECTIVES, AND EXAMINATION CRITERIA

ORTHOTIC SPECIFICATIONS

Shoe Heel Height

A low heel ($\frac{1}{4}$ to $\frac{1}{2}$ inch) may improve balance by shifting the center of gravity forward in a person with a calcaneal weight-bearing position.

A low heel ($\frac{1}{4}$ to $\frac{1}{2}$ inch) may decrease knee hyperextension by shifting the center of gravity forward.

A high heel shifts the center of gravity too far forward and causes balance problems in a person with weak plantar flexors.

A high heel may result in increased hip and knee flexion, combined with an increased lordosis or swayback posture.

Ankle Angle

Ideally molded or set in 5° plantar flexion with a rigid anterior and posterior stop to reduce energy requirements and to increase the knee extension moment (Lehmann et al., 1995), as long as toe clearance is adequate and the knee does not hyperextend. If foot clearance is a problem, set angle more acutely, no higher than neutral, at the minimum angle required to clear the foot during swing phase. Plastic orthoses must enclose the malleoli to effectively resist dorsiflexion and provide a rigid anterior stop.[94]

Do not set ankle angle more acutely than a neutral angle unless trying to control a knee hyperextension problem, because the energy expenditure will increase.

Keel

Generally, keel should be rigid to the distal aspect of the metatarsal heads (to decrease energy expenditure by providing a longer lever). The plastic should extend to the end of the toes to maintain proper toe alignment, but it must be pulled thin distal to the metatarsal heads to provide a flexible toe break. If a flexible toe break is not provided, the knee extension moment may be excessive, resulting in knee hyperextension. The alternative is to trim the plastic at the metatarsal heads, but the toes are not adequately supported in this latter case.

Extending a rigid keel out to the end of the toes may be indicated to increase the extension moment at the knee. Do not extend the rigid lever arm to the end of the toes if it results in knee hyperextension or difficulty with balance (especially on stairs).

Plantar Aspect

Posting may be required to accommodate the hindfoot and rearfoot position so that the subtalar joint is maintained in a neutral position, yet a plantigrade position is achieved.[190]

Posting helps distribute the weight across the plantar aspect and prevents varus or valgus.

Straps

All straps should be well padded.

An instep strap angled at 45° helps hold the heel in place and prevents pistoning and friction.

KAFOs should have a three-point pressure distribution.

A combined suprapatellar and infrapatellar strap distributes the pressure best. A spider kneecap pad can also be used but results in greater shear forces through the knee joint.

An infrapatellar strap often deforms the lower leg when worn for a prolonged period of time because the pressure is not well distributed. The patellar tendon-bearing orthotic trim line is preferred in this population because the pressure is better distributed.

ORTHOTIC FABRICATION OBJECTIVES

Increase Medial and Lateral Stability

Mold in subtalar neutral position.[87,190]

Proximal trim line should be sufficiently proximal and anterior to provide adequate leverage to control the ankle and to distribute pressure evenly.

Increase base of support and equalize weight-bearing forces by means of external posting.

Valgus or Pronated Foot

Post medially under first metatarsal head and medial aspect of calcaneus.

Flare posting medially to increase the base of support and to prevent deviation into valgus.

Varus or Supinated Foot

Post medially under first metatarsal head to accommodate supinated position of forefoot and equalize pressure distribution.

Zero posting under calcaneus (with lateral flare if needed) to prevent deviation into supination at heel strike.

Orthoses must sit level in shoes, and the shoes should be fastened securely so they do not slide on orthoses.

Decrease Energy Expenditure

Ankle angle ideally molded or set at 5° plantar flexion with rigid anterior stop (see ankle angle, earlier).

Distal trim line at metatarsal heads to provide a long rigid lever arm.

Provide adequate toe clearance and simulate push-off.

Plantar flexion stop, ideally set at 5° of plantar flexion if able to adequately clear toe without increasing knee flexion during swing phase (see ankle angle, earlier).

Generally a rigid dorsiflexion stop is required, unless the patient has sufficient plantar flexor strength to control forward movement of tibia during stance phase.

Increase Knee Extension Moment

Ground-reaction force, patellar tendon-bearing orthosis.

Solid ankle, cushioned heel, or wedge heel anteriorly to move ground-reaction force forward at heel strike.

Continued

BOX 22-4   LOWER LIMB ORTHOTIC SPECIFICATIONS, OBJECTIVES, AND EXAMINATION CRITERIA—cont'd

Rigid dorsiflexion stop set in 5° plantar flexion (see ankle angle, earlier).

Keel rigid to distal aspect of metatarsal heads to provide a long rigid lever and yet still permit a flexible toe break (see keel, earlier). An even greater extension moment can be provided by extending the rigid lever to the end of the toes. This is usually contraindicated, however, because it results in difficulties with balance (especially on stairs).

Prevent Knee Hyperextension

Prevent knee hyperextension by increasing knee flexion moment.

Flare heel posteriorly to move ground-reaction force behind knee joint axis at heel strike to produce a flexion moment.

Ankle set at neutral angle with rigid dorsiflexion and plantar flexion stop (if this does not adequately prevent knee hyperextension, the angle may need to be set more acutely, into dorsiflexion). The more acute the angle, however, the greater the energy expenditure.[93]

A low heel ($\frac{1}{4}$ to $\frac{1}{2}$ inch) may decrease knee hyperextension by shifting the center of gravity forward.

Keel rigid to the distal aspect of the metatarsal heads to provide a long rigid lever to decrease energy expenditure. Plastic must be pulled thin beyond this point, however, to provide a flexible toe break (do not extend the rigid keel to the end of the toes because this will increase the knee extension moment at push-off).

If knee hyperextension cannot be adequately controlled with previously described modifications, use KAFOs with knee extension stops.

Improve Pressure Distribution

Use total contact orthoses.

All straps should be well padded.

Bony prominences should be padded (e.g., malleoli, prominent naviculi, patellar tendon region).

Posting to equalize pressure distribution on foot and minimize pressure on malleoli and naviculi.

Patellar tendon-bearing orthosis distributes pressure better than a proximal strap.

KAFOs: the combination of a suprapatellar and infrapatellar strap distributes pressure most effectively.

Improve Balance

Adding a low heel ($\frac{1}{4}$ to $\frac{1}{2}$ inch) may improve balance by shifting the center of gravity forward in a person with a calcaneal weight-bearing position.

A high heel shifts the center of gravity too far forward and causes balance problems, particularly in a person with weak or absent plantar flexors.

ORTHOTIC EXAMINATION CRITERIA

Check for pressure areas.

Heel must seat well in orthosis.

Check for rigid keel and flexible toe break.

Check knee alignment and congruency of knee joint axis.

All straps and bony prominences should be well padded.

Check medial and lateral alignment, and make sure the orthosis is posted properly with subtalar joint in neutral.

Check angle at ankle (anterior/posterior and medial/lateral).

Check anterior and posterior stops to make sure they adequately control motion, facilitate push-off, and permit toe clearance during swing phase.

Insert orthosis in shoe to check alignment. If molded properly, the orthosis should be able to balance and stand without support on a flat surface.

---

functional tasks should be determined and specifically selected for application to social, educational, vocational, and work capacity requirements of the adolescent and adult. Vocational counseling and planning should begin early during the high school years. A social worker may need to assist the family with the transition to independent living because a mutually dependent relationship is often fostered by the intense lifelong involvement of parents and siblings in assisting the individual with MM. Recreation therapy may be used to assist with shopping for and purchasing personal items, use of public transportation, and developing appropriate adult leisure activities. Occupational therapy is useful to address advanced living skills such as cooking, cleaning, laundry, money management, and driver's training for appropriate candidates. A social worker can assist with locating accessible housing and obtaining appropriate support services for physical tasks that are too difficult for the patient. Depending on the practice setting, however, it may be necessary for the physical therapist to manage these areas. The expectation for individuals with MM who have intelligence in the normal range and sufficient motor function to care for themselves is the ability to thrive as an independent adult in our society. See Chapter 32 for more information on transition to adulthood.

Prevention of Secondary Impairments and Activity Limitations

The physical therapist plays an important role in anticipating the potential for functional loss when one of the medical complications of MM previously described increases the risk of secondary impairments. For example, when an adolescent undergoes a surgical procedure that requires extended bed rest, maintenance of muscle extensibility, joint ROM, and strength at the bedside followed by resumption of physical mobility tasks as soon as possible postoperatively can prevent long-term or permanent decline in mobility skills. Unfortunately, care providers are often not aware of these issues and intervention is not instituted until it is too late to recover lost function. The physical therapist must serve as an advocate for the patient under these circumstances. Regular skin inspection continues to be important to monitor skin integrity. Another mechanism for preventing secondary impairments is education of patients and their parents regarding the fit, specifications, condition, and maintenance of their adaptive equipment. They should know how to monitor skin tolerance and the fit of adaptive equipment. They should also understand the rationale for equipment and design features that are recommended. Knowledgeable consumers can detect and report potential problems before they result in complications such as decubiti. They need to be aware of the potential consequences of poorly fitted equipment so that they can advocate for quality equipment. The majority of adults in our follow-up study had improperly fitted equipment or lacked equipment that was essential for optimal function. These adults were also unaware of proper equipment maintenance techniques.[68] As a result, many adults were functioning well below their capabilities and had skin breakdown, back pain, or joint pain as a result of poorly fitted orthoses or improper wheelchair design and seating.

OUTCOMES AND THEIR DETERMINANTS

Survival, disability, health, and lifestyles were investigated in a complete cohort of adults with MM in Cambridge, England.[72] Outcomes were investigated at age 35 for 117 individuals who were born between 1963 and 1971. Sixty-three (54%) had died, primarily the most severely affected. The mean age of the survivors was 35 years (range 32 to 38), and 39 of the 54 survivors had an IQ above 80. Sixteen could walk for community distances (50 meters or more) with or without aids. These 16 individuals all had a sensory lesion level at or below L3. Thirty had pressure sores, 30 were overweight, and only 11 were fully continent. In terms of independent living status, 22 survivors lived independently in the community, 12 lived in sheltered accommodations where help was available if required, and 20 needed daily assistance. Twenty of the survivors drove cars and another nine had given up driving. Thirteen were employed, with five of them being in wheelchairs. Seven females and two males had had a total of 13 children (none with visible MM). Hunt and colleagues[73] also reported that shunt revisions, particularly after the age of 2, were associated with poor long-term achievement in this same group of adult survivors with MM. Achievement was operationally defined according to their independent living status, employment,

and use of a car. McDonnell and McCann[114] in a commentary to Hunt and associates' article reported more optimistic outcomes in terms of mobility and employment for shunt-treated survivors of MM in Belfast, Northern Ireland. Hunt[71] reported that only 50% of adults were capable of living independently based on a sample of 69, of whom 68% had normal intelligence. In a sample of 18 patients 16 to 47 years old in Japan, Oi and associates[131] reported that patients with spina bifida occulta (spinal lipoma) have a risk of neurologic deterioration, whether or not they have undergone radical preventive surgery in infancy. This deterioration is primarily related to lower spinal functions, such as ambulation and bowel and bladder control, which likely result from tethered cord, reexpansion of the residual lipoma, or syringomyelia. In contrast, these authors reported psychologic problems in patients with spina bifida aperta. Padua and associates[138] reported that adolescents with MM who have relatively mild activity limitations (i.e., they are able to walk and run) but who have urologic problems need psychologic support to a greater extent than adolescents with severe activity limitations and limited independence. There are many factors that contribute to the observed outcomes.

The motor function present is an important factor for predicting outcomes. Common characteristics of each lesion level are described in this section. The functional motor level does not always correspond to the anatomic lesion level because of individual variations in nerve root innervation of muscles. The information presented here is intended to serve as general guidelines for expectations at a given level of motor function. Many factors besides muscle strength influence an individual's functional potential and result in variations of performance within a given lesion level group. These factors include age, body proportions, weight, sensation, orthopedic deformities, joint contractures, spasticity, upper limb function, and cognition. The relative contribution of these factors is highly individual, and a thorough examination and follow-up of each child is necessary to maximize potential capabilities.

THORACIC LEVEL

Individuals with thoracic level muscle function have innervation of neck, upper limb, shoulder girdle, and trunk musculature, but no volitional lower limb movements are present. Banta[9] stated that at the thoracic level the orthopedic goals are to maintain a straight spine, level pelvis, and symmetric lower limbs. Neck, upper limb, and shoulder girdle muscle groups are innervated by the C1 to T4 spinal nerves; back extensors by the C2 to L4 spinal nerves; intercostals by the thoracic nerves; and abdominals by T5 to L1. Consequently, individuals with motor function at or above T10 have strong upper limbs and upper thoracic and neck motions, but their lower trunk musculature is weak. They have difficulty with unsupported sitting balance and may have decreased respiratory function. Sliding boards may be required to perform wheelchair transfers because of the combination of poor trunk control and upper limb dyscoordination.

Individuals with motor function at T12 have strong trunk musculature and good sitting balance and may have weak hip hiking by means of the quadratus lumborum (innervated by T12 to L3). Ambulation may be attempted for exercise at this level using a parapodium; however, it is generally not an effective means of mobility.[97] A wheelchair is required for functional household and community mobility.

Children with thoracic level lesions also tend to have greater involvement of other areas of the CNS, with corresponding cognitive deficits. Consequently, even though many of these people achieve independence with basic self-care skills and mobility by late childhood, they often require a supervised living situation throughout life. They are rarely competitively employed but often participate in sheltered workshop settings or perform volunteer work.[68]

HIGH LUMBAR (L1-L2) LEVEL

Individuals with high lumbar motor function have weak hip movements. The iliopsoas muscle is supplied by nerve roots L1 through L4, with its primary innervation at L2 and L3. The sartorius muscle is supplied by L2 and L3 and the adductors by L2 through L4. With L1 motor function, weak hip flexion may be present, and with L2 motor function the hip flexors, adductors, and rotators are grade 3 or better. According to Schafer and Dias,[152] unopposed hip flexion and adduction contractures are often present at the L2 motor level, and this muscle imbalance often results in dislocated hips. Short-distance household ambulation is possible with high lumbar innervation (L1 and L2) when body proportions are small, using KAFOs or RGOs and upper limb support. These children generally use a wheelchair for community distances. By the second decade of life, a wheelchair is typically the sole means of mobility commensurate with increased energy requirements and enlarged body proportions.[68,164]

The prognosis of children with high lumbar lesions for function and independent living as adults is similar to that of the thoracic group described earlier.[68] More individuals in this group, however, achieve independent living status (approximately 50%), but they are rarely able to maintain competitive employment as adults.

L3 LEVEL

Individuals with L3 muscle function have strong hip flexion and adduction, weak hip rotation, and at least antigravity knee extension. The quadriceps muscle group is innervated by nerve roots L2 through L4. Children with grade 3 quadriceps strength usually require KAFOs and forearm crutches to ambulate for household and short community distances and a wheelchair for long community distances. By

adulthood, most individuals with L3 level lesions are primarily wheelchair mobile.[68,169,180]

Approximately 60% of individuals with lesions at this level achieve independent living status as adults.[68] Despite their higher level of independence, only a small percentage (about 20%) actively participate in full-time competitive employment.[68]

L4 LEVEL

At the L4 motor level, antigravity knee flexion and grade 4 ankle dorsiflexion with inversion may be present. The medial hamstrings are innervated by nerve roots L4 through S2, and the anterior tibialis is innervated primarily by L4 and L5, with some innervation from S1. An individual is considered to have L4 motor function if the medial hamstrings or anterior tibialis is at least grade 3. Calcaneal foot deformities are common at this motor level as a result of the unopposed action of the tibialis anterior muscle.[152] Knee extension is usually strong, and these individuals are generally functional ambulators with AFOs and forearm crutches. When first learning to walk, however, KAFOs, a walker, or both may be required. A wheelchair is often needed for long distances.

In the adult follow-up study that we conducted, only 20% of individuals with L4 motor function continued to ambulate as adults.[68] Many individuals stopped ambulation after their adolescent growth spurt. Others were unable to maintain ambulation because of ankle and knee valgus joint deformities and elbow and wrist pain resulting from years of weight bearing in poor alignment. To increase the likelihood of maintaining biped ambulation for individuals with L4 motor function throughout adulthood, upright posture should be emphasized when ambulating to minimize the weight-bearing stress on upper limb joints. Orthoses must be aligned properly and posted to support the ankle in a subtalar neutral position. If the ankle joint is malaligned, the knee joint position is adversely affected. It is essential to maintain the knee and ankle in neutral alignment when weight bearing. A flexed and valgus position should not be permitted. Ounpuu and associates[134] demonstrated that 30% of the mechanical work occurs at the ankle during normal gait, underscoring the importance of controlling the ankle in order to provide proper alignment of the body to the ground reaction force. Often a patellar tendon-bearing, ground-reaction force orthotic design is optimal to protect the knee and increase the knee extension moment. The proximal medial trim line can be extended higher to provide additional medial knee support, if needed, to reduce a genu valgus deformity (see Figure 22-5). Knee musculature should be strengthened to help maintain the knee in neutral alignment when weight bearing. Every effort should be made to progress ambulation to using AFOs and forearm crutches to allow short-distance ambulation to easily be combined with long-distance wheelchair mobility. Crutches can be transported on the wheelchair, and AFOs are optimal because, unlike KAFOs, they do not interfere with dressing or toileting and do not cause skin breakdown when sitting. The prognosis for independent living and employment is similar to that for the group with L3 lesions.

L5 LEVEL

According to the IMSG criteria, classification of an L5 motor level is based on the presence of lateral hamstring muscles with at least grade 3 strength, and either grade 2 gluteus minimus and medius muscles (L4-S1), grade 3 posterior tibialis muscles (L5-S1), or grade 4 peroneus tertius muscles (L4-S1). Therefore, an individual with an L5 motor level has at least antigravity knee flexion and weak hip extension using the hamstrings and may have weak hip abduction, as well as weak plantar flexion with inversion, strong dorsiflexion with eversion, or both. Weak toe movements may also be present. Hindfoot valgus deformities or calcaneal foot deformities are common as a result of muscle imbalance. Individuals with motor function through L5 are able to ambulate without orthoses, yet require them to correct foot alignment and substitute for lack of push-off. A gluteal lurch is typically evident unless upper limb support is used. Bilateral upper limb support is usually recommended for community distances to decrease energy expenditure, decrease gluteal lurch and trunk sway, maintain symmetric alignment, protect lower limb joints, and improve safety. The need for upper limb support often becomes more apparent with increased height following growth spurts. Traversing uneven terrain is often difficult. A wheelchair may be required when there is a rapid change in body proportions (e.g., pregnancy) or for long distances on rough terrain. A bike is also useful for long community distances.

Approximately 80% of individuals with lesions at L5 and below achieve independent living status as adults.[68] About 30% are employed full time and an additional 20% part time, well below the average employment rate of the general adult population.

S1 LEVEL

With muscle function present through S1, at least two of the following additional muscle actions are present: gastrocnemius/soleus (grade 2), gluteus medius (grade 3), or gluteus maximus (grade 2). Individuals with S1 motor function have improved hip stability and can walk without orthoses or upper limb support. A weak push-off is evident when running or climbing stairs. A mild to moderate gluteal lurch is often present. Vankoski and associates[189] documented the benefits of crutch use for this lesion level, which resulted in improved pelvis and hip kinematics during gait. Gait deviations and activity limitations are often more pronounced after the adolescent growth spurt. The toe musculature is generally strong. Foot deformities

are less common at this level, but foot orthoses or AFOs may be required to improve lower limb alignment and permit muscle groups to function at a more optimal length. Medial and lateral stability at the ankle is required for adequate function of the plantar flexor muscles during push-off.[92]

S2, S2-S3, AND "NO LOSS" LEVELS

Motor function is classified at the S2 level if the plantar flexor muscles are at least grade 3 and the gluteals grade 4. The only obvious gait abnormality present at this level is generally a decreased push-off and stride length when walking rapidly or running as a result of the decreased strength of the plantar flexor muscles. If all lower limb muscle groups have grade 5 strength except for one or two groups with grade 4 strength, the motor level is classified as S2-S3, according to the IMSG criteria. The term "no loss" is used if the bowel and bladder function normally and lower limb strength is judged to be normal through manual muscle testing. Functional deficits may be present, however, for individuals classified as having no loss. Foot orthoses are often beneficial to maintain the ankle in the subtalar neutral position and optimize ankle muscle function by maintaining optimal muscle length.

EXAMINATION, EVALUATION, AND DIRECT INTERVENTIONS FOR MUSCULOSKELETAL ISSUES, MOBILITY, AND FUNCTIONAL SKILLS

There are three primary reasons for assessing the individual with MM: (1) to define an individual's current status so that appropriate program planning can occur, (2) to identify the potential for developing secondary impairments so that preventive measures can be implemented, and (3) to monitor changes in status that could indicate progressive neurologic dysfunction. Because of the complexity of problems associated with MM, numerous dimensions of disability must be assessed by various disciplines. The physical therapist provides essential information to other team members for program planning and to monitor status. Careful documentation is important for communication among team members and for serial comparisons over time. General examination and intervention strategies will be discussed in this section. Considerations that are specific to certain age categories are discussed in the section on age-specific examination and physical therapy interventions.

EXAMINATION STRATEGIES

The dimensions typically assessed by physical therapists include ROM, muscle extensibility, joint alignment or orthopedic deformities, muscle tone, muscle strength and endurance, sensation, posture, motor development, ADL, mobility skills, equipment needs, and environmental accessibility. It is important to use standardized protocols, when available, that have good reliability and validity to permit comparison within and between individuals.[67] If more than one measurement method exists (e.g., hip extension ROM), the specific method employed should be documented and used consistently. Comprehensive examinations should be conducted at regular intervals throughout the life span on all individuals with MM. In addition, to avoid potential biases it is recommended that therapists remain blind to previous results of the more subjective measures (e.g., manual muscle testing scores or gait deviations) until the examination is complete. Videotapes and photographs are often a useful adjunct to clinical examination of gait, joint deformities, and posture. These visual records provide an excellent baseline for comparison purposes if deterioration in status is suspected. It is beneficial to conduct examination of activities that are influenced by environmental or endurance factors (e.g., wheelchair mobility, gait, or ADL) in more natural settings.

The IMSG recommends a comprehensive, multidisciplinary assessment for all individuals with MM, regardless of functional level, because they all are at risk for progressive neurologic dysfunction, as discussed earlier. The following examination intervals are recommended: newborn preoperatively, newborn postoperatively, 6 months, 12 months, 18 months, 24 months, and annually thereafter, continuing through adulthood.[163] Annual examinations are suggested to occur around an individual's birth date so that they are not forgotten. ROM, muscle extensibility, strength, endurance, coordination, and functional parameters should be monitored more closely during periods of rapid growth, when individuals with MM are at increased risk for loss of function. Preintervention and postintervention measurements should be obtained for individuals undergoing surgery or other therapeutic procedures. More frequent evaluation of specific goal attainment is indicated for individuals receiving ongoing therapeutic intervention. Mobility and independence with ADL should be assessed when body proportions or environmental demands change to determine if the individual has the strength, endurance, coordination, and adaptive equipment required to function effectively.

Shurtleff[163,166] advocated using the Patient Data Management System (PDMS) standardized protocol and recording format to serially monitor individuals with MM. The PDMS is composed of a comprehensive, interdisciplinary recording format, which consists of the dimensions typically assessed by each discipline. In addition, intervention data (e.g., surgery, medications, and therapy) are also documented. Scoring and recording criteria can be obtained by contacting the IMSG.[76] The PDMS computerized recording format is beneficial for monitoring this population because serial test results from birth to present can be efficiently scanned for each parameter to detect improvements or deterioration in status. In addition, an individual patient's status can be directly compared with that of other individuals with similar characteristics by using the interactive database. The

standardized format facilitates communication between and within disciplines and intervention centers and promotes clinical research. Duplication of effort by the various health care professionals involved in the intervention of individuals with MM is minimized because each discipline is assigned specific PDMS areas to assess, yet all disciplines share the information in the combined database. The PDMS format has also been applied to several other pediatric populations, including those with cerebral palsy, cystic fibrosis, hemophilia, and traumatic brain injury.[166]

Individuals with MM should be assessed on at least a yearly basis by multiple disciplines at a comprehensive care center. It is important, however, for comprehensive care centers and local school and intervention settings to coordinate their examinations, goals, and intervention programs to avoid duplication of effort and to ensure appropriate prioritization of intervention goals. The use of the PDMS facilitates communication and coordination of services between team members. The School Needs Identification and Action Forms[148] also provide a useful format for identifying impairments, academic and activity limitations, and the remedial action recommended. The areas assessed by the school needs forms include health-related services required, physical intervention instructions, accessibility, safety and fire drills, preparation for school entry, educational rights and related services, academic difficulties, psychologic evaluation, perceptuomotor deficits, visuoperceptual deficits, self-help skills, social acceptance, social and emotional issues, parent and school relationships, transitional services, and other needs. The School Function Assessment (SFA) measures needs and abilities during school-related functional tasks for kindergarten through sixth-grade students.[30] The SFA consists of three sections: (1) participation in a variety of school activity settings, (2) task supports required (physical and cognitive/behavioral assistance and adaptations), and (3) activity performance in school-related functional activities (e.g., using materials, following rules, and communicating needs). The School Function Assessment Technical Report available at www.pearsonassessments.com/NR/rdonlyres/ D50E4125-86EE-43BE-8001-2A4001B603DF/0/SFA_TR_ Web.pdf describes the standardization sample of 676 students, including 363 students with special needs from 112 sites in 40 U.S. states and Puerto Rico.

INTERVENTION STRATEGIES

Once primary and secondary impairments, activity limitations, and participation restrictions are identified through a comprehensive examination and evaluation, the functional significance must be determined to plan appropriate intervention strategies. Intervention of an impairment is indicated if it currently interferes with function or if the deficit can progress to a point where it may negatively affect future function. Intervention is also indicated if the efficiency, effectiveness, or safety of performance can be improved.

Strength, endurance, and efficiency of performing tasks should be emphasized. Weight-bearing joints must be protected to prevent early onset of osteoarthritis and pain and to prolong mobility. In addition, the most efficient and effective means of mobility for a given environment should be determined. Goal setting for intervention must consider the impact of the multiple impairments discussed earlier on functional performance expectations. The cognitive, social, and behavioral issues discussed in the impairments section should also be considered.

Fay and associates[47] recommended three specific intervention approaches for developmental delays in this population. The first is developmental programming in which children are encouraged by parents, teachers, and therapists with a "high dose" of normal developmental activities in "at-risk" areas. The philosophy behind this approach is that supplemental early emphasis and practice in potential problem areas will minimize later deficits. These early intervention programs are often initiated for children with MM before measurable delays are identified. The second approach, remediation, is implemented once problem areas are clearly identified. This approach consists of repeating a set of graded tasks in the domain of concern. Improved performance through practice theoretically carries over into functional activities. The third approach is teaching compensatory skills. Compensation is often implemented when the other two approaches have not produced sufficient results or when the child is older or more severely impaired. This intervention approach involves identifying and developing strategies to help the child become as independent as possible or providing adaptive equipment to compensate for underlying problems and minimize disability in daily life.

SPECIFIC EXAMINATION AND INTERVENTION STRATEGIES

Specific examination and intervention strategies as they pertain to strength, mobility, gait, and equipment issues are highlighted in this section because of the magnitude of the impact of these factors on function in this population, regardless of age or lesion level. Suggestions for impairment-specific parameters (e.g., ROM, orthopedic deformities, and sensation) were discussed in the section on impairments. Developmental issues were discussed in the section on age-specific examination and physical therapy interventions.

Strength

Upper limb, neck, and trunk musculature should be screened for weakness. If evidence of weakness exists, a more specific examination of strength should be conducted. For individuals with thoracic or high lumbar level involvement, it is important to palpate trunk musculature to determine which portions of muscle groups are functioning. Dynamometer values of grip and pinch strength should also be obtained. Kilburn and associates[84] suggested that grip strength

measurement can be a sensitive gauge of progressive neurologic dysfunction. Level[96] provided a standardized protocol for obtaining grip strength measurements and normative values for children.

Specific testing of isolated motions of lower limb muscles is essential to determine if individual muscles are functioning. Standardized test protocols should be used.[69,78,82] It is essential to detect changes in strength in this population as soon as possible, because loss of strength can be a sign of progressive neurologic dysfunction. As a result, we recommend using quantitative strength measurements in conjunction with traditional manual muscle testing techniques. It is also important to distinguish between reflexive and voluntary movements. Reflexive movements should be documented, but they should not be considered when determining motor lesion levels.

Manual muscle testing is the most common method used to assess strength in this population because of its adaptability in a typical clinic setting. Manual muscle testing is the method of choice for screening muscle strength to determine the presence of volitional activity in specific muscles and to determine whether an individual muscle's function varies throughout the ROM. There are several limitations to relying only on manual muscle testing scores for serially monitoring strength, as discussed in Chapter 5.

Manual muscle testing has limited interrater and test-retest reliability.[65] Manual muscle test scores must change more than one full grade to be confident that a true change in strength has occurred. In addition, manual muscle testing has poor concurrent validity compared with more quantitative measures. Several studies have demonstrated that deficits in strength exceeding 50% are not detected by manual muscle testing.[1,2,19,55,120] Agre and colleagues[1] examined this issue in 33 adolescents with MM. Individuals who had been classified as having "no motor deficits" by means of manual muscle testing actually had strength deficits compared with normative data. These deficits were 40% for the hip extensor and 60% for the knee extensor muscles. The lack of concurrent validity of manual muscle testing compared with quantitative measurements demonstrates that the sensitivity of manual muscle testing in detecting weakness is limited and is inadequate for detecting early strength loss in individuals with MM.

The predictive validity of manual muscle testing has been examined in two studies on children with MM. Murdoch[127] examined the predictive validity of neonatal manual muscle testing examinations using a truncated 3-point scale. The correlation between muscle power of the newborn and subsequent mobility of the child at age 3 to 8 years was "very poor." In contrast, McDonald and associates[113] examined the predictive validity of manual muscle testing for individual muscle groups on 825 children with MM using the complete 0- to 5-point grading scale. Predictive validity of manual muscle testing generally increased from birth to age 5. The probability that a given manual muscle test score precisely predicted future scores varied with age and the particular muscle group tested. These probabilities ranged from 23% to 68% for newborns and from 54% to 87% for older children. The probability that a single test score predicted future strength within ±1 manual muscle test grade, however, was considerably higher, ranging from 70% to 86% for newborns and from 87% to 97% for older children. These results indicate that manual muscle testing is useful for predicting future muscle function within one manual muscle test grade. Strength test results obtained in infancy using the complete manual muscle test scale, therefore, appear to provide useful information for prognosis and for planning the course of intervention.

The limited reliability and concurrent validity of manual muscle testing indicates that it is not the method of choice for monitoring changes in strength over time. In contrast, strength testing using handheld instruments has been found to be a reliable and sensitive method for assessing strength in children and adolescents with MM. Intraclass interrater and test-retest correlation coefficients using this technique ranged from 0.73 to 0.99.[44,61] Other authors report good to high levels of reliability when testing the strength of other populations of children and adolescents with handheld instrumentation.[49,63,65,70,75,116,182] Several portable, handheld instruments are available for use in conjunction with manual muscle testing.[65] The advantages of these tools over nonportable instruments are that they are easily applied in typical clinic settings and can be used with standard manual muscle testing techniques to obtain objective force readings from most muscle groups.

It is best to obtain three myometry trials and report the average score because the mean is more stable over time and between raters.[57,61] Torque values should be reported (force times lever arm length) to permit comparison over time, regardless of changing body proportions, at least until skeletal maturity has been attained. Torque values also permit direct comparison of force production capabilities between individuals with different body proportions. Standardized testing techniques must be implemented when assessing strength with handheld instruments to ensure the consistency of measurements. Many factors influence test results and must be controlled for when testing, including test positions, instructions and commands provided, use of reinforcement and feedback, application of resistance, the type of contraction, and the examiner's body mechanics. For more information regarding techniques used in testing with handheld instruments, see Hinderer and Hinderer.[65]

Several factors should be considered when testing the muscle strength of children with MM, including age, developmental level, cognitive level, ability to follow directions, attention span, motivation, motor planning skills, sensation, and proprioception. The examiner must carefully watch for muscle substitutions. This is particularly challenging in the MM population because of altered angles of pull from orthopedic deformities. It is often difficult for multijoint

muscles such as the hamstrings to initiate motions. Any differences in function between end-range and midrange positions should be noted. Special considerations when testing infants and young children are discussed in the section on age-specific examination and physical therapy interventions.

As discussed in the impairments section, several CNS complications can account for loss of muscle function in this population, necessitating serial strength testing for early detection. There are many factors that can result in normal variations in strength, however, that should also be considered when interpreting test results. These factors include changes in body proportions, hormonal influences, motor learning, illness, injury, surgery, immobilization, physical or psychologic fatigue, the prior state of activity, seasonal variations, temporal factors, motivation, cooperation, and comprehension. Discussion of the specific influences of these factors is beyond the scope of this chapter. For further information regarding the impact of these factors on force production, see Hinderer and Hinderer.[65] Because of the multiple factors that can influence force production, it is important to repeat the testing at more frequent intervals, if strength loss is suspected, to determine whether consistent test results are obtained. Several variables should be considered when interpreting muscle test results, including the reliability and standard error of measurement of the testing method used, the concurrent and predictive validity of test results, and factors that can account for fluctuations in strength.[65]

Static strength measurements should be correlated with functional measures to observe the effects of fatigue and to determine the effect of reduced strength and limited endurance on function. Individuals with neurogenic muscle weakness may have a higher degree of variability in force production as a result of the lower threshold of fatigue and slower rate of recovery of weak musculature. Local muscle endurance appears to be deficient in some neuromuscular diseases.[11,122] Although this issue has not been specifically tested in the MM population, these results suggest that force production may be more variable in weak muscle groups of individuals with MM.

If function is present but weakness exists in muscle groups that are important for postural stability, ADL, mobility, or balance of muscle forces around joints, strengthening exercises are indicated. The specific muscle groups to emphasize vary depending on the lesion level and functional requirements. In general, strong upper limb muscle groups are required for performing transfers, for wheelchair propulsion, and when using assistive devices to walk. Increasing the strength of trunk musculature improves sitting balance and postural stability. Increasing the strength of key lower limb muscle groups that are critical for ambulation can improve gait and can possibly minimize the need for orthoses and assistive devices. For example, increasing the quadriceps and hamstrings strength in an individual with L4 motor function may enable progression of ambulation from using KAFOs to using AFOs (see the case study at the end of this chapter).

Muscle groups should be strengthened within functional ROM. In addition to traditional strengthening exercises, many play activities promote strengthening.[46] Muscle reeducation techniques such as functional electrical stimulation and biofeedback are useful to teach muscles to function in new parts of the ROM. Electrical stimulation has also been found to be beneficial to increase strength and enhance functional performance in this population.[80] Strengthening programs should be implemented during periods when an individual is at risk for loss of muscle strength and endurance (e.g., after recent surgery, immobilization, illness, or bed rest) and during periods of rapid growth when individuals often lose function as a result of changes in body proportions.

Endurance activities are also important for weight control and to enhance aerobic capacity. Individuals with MM must have adequate endurance to meet the challenges of community mobility. Low-impact aerobic activities to minimize joint stress are preferable. In general, jumping activities should be avoided because joint stress is increased as a result of the inadequate deceleration provided by weak lower limb muscles. Indications for endurance training and instruction in energy conservation techniques include decreased aerobic capacity, high energy cost of mobility, and limited endurance.

Mobility

Ineffective mobility is a hallmark of MM. Effective mobility is defined as any efficient and effective means of moving about in space that enables the individual to easily traverse and explore the environment, grow and develop, and independently pursue an education, vocation, or avocation.[164] Mobility options provided should meet these criteria for all environments encountered by the individual so that lifestyle is not limited by endurance and difficulty traversing uneven terrain.

Changes in body proportions can significantly affect mobility. Mobility options, orthoses, and assistive device requirements that are ideal at one time may not be effective once body proportions, environmental demands, or both change. Consequently, the appropriateness of adaptive equipment and mobility options must be reevaluated throughout the life span. Health care providers should emphasize this point to patients to help prevent the feeling of failure if alternative mobility options are required in the future. Too often, individuals with MM grow up being praised for walking instead of using a wheelchair or for walking without assistive devices, depending on their lesion level. This emphasis gives the impression that normal biped ambulation is the only socially acceptable form of mobility. Several of the adults in our follow-up study reported that it was difficult to accept the use of a wheelchair or other assistive devices as they grew up

because they felt that they were a failure or that they would disappoint their parents and health care providers.[68] It is important to emphasize that wheelchairs and other assistive devices are aids for effective mobility and that their use does not represent a failure of biped ambulation.

Bed mobility, floor mobility, wheelchair mobility, ambulation, and transfers should be assessed and compared with the requirements for independent function. Criteria for assessing mobility parameters are endurance, efficiency, effectiveness, safety, degree of independence, and accessibility. Objective information regarding these parameters is often helpful to convince patients and their parents that alternative methods of mobility should be considered. Efficiency can be estimated by measuring the time required to complete a task. Energy expenditure can be estimated by measuring heart rate (HR). Regression equations have been determined for this population to equate heart rate with the energy expenditure required for a given task.[195] The regression equations for energy expenditure and efficiency of this population are as follows:

$$\text{Energy cost (mL O2/kg min)} = 0.073\,(\text{HR}) + 6.119$$

$$\text{Energy efficiency (mL O2/kg meter)} = 0.006\,(\text{HR}) - 0.313$$

Criteria for determining the most practical and effective mode of mobility for household and community distances are provided in Box 22-2. Standardized tests that are useful for assessing mobility in the population with lower level lesions are discussed in Chapter 2. In addition, the Timed Test of Patient Mobility[79] is beneficial for assessing the efficiency of mobility because the time required to perform bed mobility, transfers, wheelchair mobility, and gait mobility tasks is documented. Normative data are available for comparison purposes. We suggest augmenting the efficiency time score of the Timed Test of Patient Mobility with a rating scale for the level of independence, safety, practicality, and assistive devices required for each task.[68] Other tests that are specific to function in wheelchairs include the Functional Task Performance Wheelchair Assessment of positioning, reaching, and driving tasks[34] and the Seated Postural Control Measure for sitting posture and functional movements.[48]

GAIT

Delays in achieving ambulation can be expected for all children with MM, including those with sacral level lesions, and children with high level lesions may cease walking after a period of 3 to 4 years of biped ambulation.[193] Thorough examination and documentation of gait status are essential to monitor functional motor status and to watch for signs of progressive neurologic dysfunction. Patients or their parents typically notice changes in gait patterns and walking endurance before they notice increased muscle weakness. Careful gait observation is also needed to determine the most appropriate orthoses and assistive devices. Examination of orthoses and assistive devices for wear patterns helps determine if they are being used on a regular basis or just to perform in the clinic setting. Gait should be assessed in a natural environment on a variety of walking surfaces. Patients should be observed walking for typical household and community distances to determine the effects of fatigue.

All too often, decisions regarding gait problems and the need for orthoses and assistive devices are made by observing short-distance ambulation on a smooth clinic floor. Performance in the home or community environment may be vastly different than in a clinic situation, especially when walking around a number of obstacles, when in congested areas, when traversing uneven terrain, or with inclement weather. The impact of these factors must be considered when making recommendations.

Requirements for orthoses and ambulatory aids should be documented. Gait deviations should be closely observed and recorded. If possible, gait deviations and efficiency parameters both with and without orthoses and assistive devices should be observed. Typical gait parameters assessed include arm swing, trunk position and sway, pelvic tilt and rotations, compensated or uncompensated Trendelenburg position, excessive hip flexion and rotation, excessive knee flexion or hyperextension, toe clearance, foot position, push-off effectiveness, and foot progression angle.

Observational gait analysis is the technique used most commonly to assess gait in clinical settings.[89] Video analysis augments clinical observations by allowing the evaluator to observe gait multiple times at slow speeds and by providing a permanent record that is invaluable for comparison purposes if deterioration of functional status is suspected. The interrater reliability of observational analysis through videotapes, however, has been reported to be low to moderate.[43,89] Footprint analysis is a low-cost method of obtaining objective information regarding velocity, cadence, foot progression angle, base of support, toe clearance, stride length, and step length.[159] More sophisticated methods of objective gait analysis are described by Stout in the Evolve chapter on Gait.

Criteria for the effectiveness, efficiency, and safety of household and community ambulation are provided in Box 22-2. Efficiency and practicality of ambulation can be estimated by monitoring heart rate, normal and fast walking velocity, and maximum walking distance. Other time-distance variables (e.g., step and stride length, cadence, and cycle time) provide useful information regarding symmetry, stability, and function. These variables can be used for comparison purposes if they are normalized (adjusted) for stature.[146]

Time-distance variables provide information about gait symmetry by comparing right-left differences in step lengths and stance-to-swing phase ratios. Examining cadence and the percentage of time spent in the stance phase versus the swing phase provides information regarding the stability of gait. For instance, a high cadence or an imbalance in the stance versus swing phase duration may indicate instability. Parameters such as walking velocity and cadence provide information regarding the functional practicality of gait. If the velocity is too low or step rate is too high, the individual may not be able to meet environmental demands.

It is essential to normalize time-distance variables for stature to compare these parameters serially over time for a given individual or to compare between individuals of different stature (e.g., comparing with normative data). These parameters are normalized by dividing by leg length. An alternative but less precise method of normalizing time-distance parameters is to divide by height because overall height is closely correlated to individual limb lengths. If these parameters are not normalized for stature, conclusions regarding differences in function may be confounded by changes in body proportions over time.

Indications for lower limb orthoses are provided in Box 22-3. Specifications and their effect on gait are outlined in Box 22-4. Indications for gait training include when a child is first learning to walk; when there is potential for progression to a new type of orthosis or upper limb aid; for progression to a more efficient gait pattern (e.g., from a four-point to a two-point alternative gait); when there is potential for improving gait (e.g., crouched gait pattern, excessive foot progression angle); to improve safety and confidence with advanced walking activities (e.g., walking on inclines, rough terrain, steps; learning to fall safely and stand up independently from floor; carrying and lifting objects); and to improve the efficiency and safety of gait, transfers, and intervention of aids.

Strength of the quadriceps muscles has been suggested by some authors to be the best predictor of ambulatory potential in children with MM;[154,195] others indicate that iliopsoas muscle strength is better.[111] McDonald and associates[111] examined the relationship between the patterns of strength and mobility in 291 children with MM who had received at least three serial standardized strength examinations after age 5 and who were classified for their mobility status as community ambulators, partial (household) ambulators, and nonambulators. Iliopsoas muscle strength was found to be the best predictor of ambulation. The quadriceps, anterior tibialis, and gluteal muscles also were determined to have significant importance for ambulation in these children. Grade 0 to 3 iliopsoas strength was always associated with partial or complete reliance on a wheelchair. Patients with grade 4 to 5 iliopsoas and quadriceps muscle strength were almost all community ambulators, and no members of this group were completely wheelchair dependent. Children with grade 4 to 5 gluteal and anterior tibialis muscle strength were all classified as community ambulators and did not require the use of an assistive device or orthosis.

Key muscle groups for community ambulation, listed in order of importance, are the iliopsoas, gluteus medius and maximus, quadriceps, anterior tibialis, and hamstring muscles.[11] Specific strength of these muscles accounted for 86% of the variance in mobility status. Gluteus medius muscle strength was found to be the best predictor of requirements for aids or orthoses. In individuals with gluteus medius strength grade 2 to 3, 72.2% required aids, orthoses, or both. If activity in this muscle was absent or trace, 95.7% required aids, orthoses, or both. In contrast, if gluteus medius strength was grade 4 to 5, only 11.2% required aids, orthoses, or both. Mazur and Menelaus[110] reported that 98% of all individuals with quadriceps strength of grade 4 to 5 were at least household ambulators, with 82% being community ambulators. In contrast, for individuals with quadriceps strength of grade 3 or less, 88% were exclusive wheelchair users.

Agre and associates[1] reported that maximum walking velocity was correlated with hip and knee extensor muscle strength. They compared the energy expenditure and efficiency of ambulation in children with MM versus able-bodied peers and found that children with MM used almost twice as much energy when walking and had a 41% lower ambulation velocity. They also reported that mobility in a wheelchair was considerably more efficient than walking, approximating normal gait in terms of energy requirements. In addition, individuals classified as having "no loss" by means of manual muscle testing had a decreased walking velocity and increased energy expenditure compared with able-bodied peers.

Equipment

A wide variety of adaptive equipment typically is required for individuals with MM. Equipment needs vary considerably with level of lesion and age. Therapists must be aware of the available options and be able to select the most appropriate type of equipment for a given situation. In addition, it is important to educate parents and patients regarding the fit and appropriateness of adaptive equipment so that they can be knowledgeable consumers. It is beyond the scope of this chapter to discuss specific equipment items. See Baker and Rogosky-Grassi,[7] Knutson and Clark,[87] and Pomatto[142] for further information regarding adaptive equipment and orthoses for this population. Indications for lower limb orthotics are provided in Box 22-3. Design specifications, objectives, and considerations when assessing the components and fit of orthoses are included in Box 22-4.

Examinations of adaptive equipment and orthotics should be conducted on at least a yearly basis. Examinations should occur more often during periods of rapid growth; when environmental demands change (e.g., changing school or work settings); when there are changes in lifestyle, goals, or vocation; or when there is a change in status that may affect motor control or mobility.

SUMMARY

Few populations challenge the skill and knowledge domains of the physical therapist as extensively as individuals with MM. This discussion has highlighted the multitude and complexity of problems encountered by children and adolescents with MM. Each lesion level group has general functional expectations that help direct physical therapy goals from an early age. Although MM is a congenital-onset problem requiring intervention by the physical therapist during infancy and childhood, most of the impairments and functional deficits described in this chapter occur throughout the life span. Individuals with MM should be followed on a regular basis, even as adults, in multidisciplinary specialty clinics by care providers familiar with this population. Because the physical therapist has extended contact with these individuals from infancy through adolescence, the therapist plays an important role in screening and triaging for potential problems, in addition to more traditional physical therapy roles. The challenges and rewards of working with this population are therefore extraordinary. The following case studies illustrate the principles of examination and intervention discussed in this chapter.

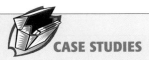

CASE STUDIES

"Sally"

History

Sally is a 6-year-old girl with L4 level paraplegia resulting from a myelomeningocele. She was referred for physical therapy assessment to determine if her ambulation skills could be improved. She had a ventriculoperitoneal CSF shunt placed as an infant with one revision secondary to shunt infection. According to her mother, Sally performs fine motor activities slowly. She is social, happy, and self-confident, however, and makes friends easily.

At 7 months, Sally rolled from prone to supine position but could not sit independently. At 15 months, she commando-crawled and was able to get into quadruped position. She pulled to stand and had a modified quadruped crawl with little lower limb reciprocation at 2 years of age. She did not have an effective method of mobility until 3.5 years of age when she was able to walk with AFOs and a wheeled anterior-facing walker. By 4 years of age, her gait with AFOs and the walker was crouched with little reciprocation and a wheelchair was her primary method of mobility. Her walking improved by switching to use of long leg braces (knees locked) at age 4.5 years, and she began to walk with forearm crutches and KAFOs at age 5 years.

Continued

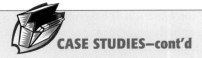

CASE STUDIES—cont'd

Systems Review

Sally has frequent urinary tract infections that often cause her to miss school. Sally's mother performs intermittent catheterization every 4 hours, except when Sally is at school.

Tests and Measures

ROM was within functional limits except for bilateral 15° hip flexion contractures and 20° knee flexion contractures. Her forefeet and hindfeet had a varus inclination when examined in a non-weight-bearing position with her subtalar joint positioned in neutral. This resulted in a valgus, everted position of her feet when bearing weight.

Motor level was L4 with weak quadriceps muscle strength (grade 4−), particularly in the shortened part of the range (from 40° to 20° of active knee extension), and grade 3+ hamstring muscle strength. Weakness in the terminal knee extension range had not been noted previously but was consistent with her history of knee flexion contractures and crouched gait. No volitional activity was present in the gluteal muscles or distal to the knee. Minimal spasticity was present in the hip adductor and hamstring muscles. Sensory level was intact through L3 but absent below this level.

Sally propelled independently in a lightweight wheelchair on level surfaces and on gradual inclines. She was independent for all transfers except to and from the floor because she was unable to independently operate the knee locks on her KAFOs. She walked with locked KAFOs and forearm crutches using a four-point gait pattern and was independent on level surfaces and gradual inclines. She had difficulty traversing uneven terrain and more severe inclines. When she attempted to walk without upper limb support, she had a severe gluteal lurch with lateral trunk sway and lost her balance after a few steps. She was a short-distance community ambulator (primarily walked at home and school and used a wheelchair for long distances). When bearing weight without orthoses or with the knees of her KAFOs unlocked, her hips and knees were severely flexed and her feet were dorsiflexed, everted, and pronated.

Her KAFOs were set in 5° of dorsiflexion and were aligned in valgus at the subtalar joint. The KAFO knee joint axis was not congruent with her anatomic knee joint axis. Only a narrow, infrapatellar anterior knee strap was present, and there was no padding on any of the KAFO straps. She was unable to independently manipulate the knee locks because of her knee flexion contractures. She had pressure marks from the infrapatellar straps and decubiti on her heels.

Evaluation

At the time of her initial assessment, Sally's orthoses did not fit properly and were causing pressure sores. Her parents requested that she progress to AFOs, if possible, so that she could be more independent with transfers. Her hip and knee flexion contractures prevented her from achieving the stable upright stance required for efficient ambulation with AFOs. Her weakness in terminal knee extension, in conjunction with the contractures, presented further difficulties for maintaining upright posture and ambulating with AFOs. Because this weakness had not been noted previously and she exhibited mild lower limb spasticity, it was important to serially monitor her strength and muscle tone over the next several months to determine if she was experiencing progressive neurologic loss. Despite the problems, in Sally's favor were the volitional quadriceps and hamstring muscle function present, a supportive family, and her personality with a willingness to try new and difficult tasks. Hip and knee flexion contracture reduction and healing of the heel decubitus ulcers were initial steps that had to be completed before AFOs could be fabricated. The unavailability of physical therapy at school provided an additional challenge. Her father worked full time and her mother had four other children to care for in addition to Sally, so frequent outpatient physical therapy sessions were not a practical alternative. Discontinuance of the improperly fitting KAFOs and good wound care healed the decubitus ulcers. In the meantime, an aggressive program of stretching and strengthening was implemented.

EVIDENCE TO PRACTICE 22-1

CASE STUDY "SALLY"

EXAMINATION DECISION

The decision to conduct assessments of ROM, joint deformities, muscle strength, sensation, mobility, and assistive devices using the Patient Data Management System in accordance with the International Myelodysplasia Study Protocol was based on the standardized evaluation protocol and the availability of serial data since Sally's birth for monitoring changes over time and comparison data for other individuals from birth to 21 years old who have similar impairments and lesion level classifications.

Sally's L4 motor level was determined based on the strength of specific muscle groups, as outlined in Table 22-1, rather than by traditional neurosegmental levels.

PLAN OF CARE DECISION

Discontinuance of the improperly fitting KAFOs and good wound care was essential for healing the decubitus ulcers. Following 2 weeks of soft tissue mobilization, stretching, and strengthening, a home program of functional electrical stimulation was added to enhance volitional contractions of the quadriceps and hamstring muscles and to assist with muscle reeducation as Sally continued to have difficulty with terminal knee extension and initiation of knee flexion. This resulted in significant increases in strength.

Orthotic recommendations to promote an upright posture and allow versatility during gait training and as Sally made progress were made following consultation with the orthotist. Orthotic specifications included those listed in Box 22-4 for increasing medial and lateral

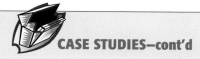

CASE STUDIES—cont'd

EVIDENCE TO PRACTICE 22-1–cont'd

stability, enhancing the knee extension moment, decreasing energy expenditure, providing adequate toe clearance, simulating push-off, distributing pressure evenly, and improving balance. Gait training emphasized an upright posture, initially using a posture-control walker for stability and then progressing to forearm crutches for increased speed and independence. Functional electrical stimulation was used in conjunction with gait training for muscle reeducation.

PATIENT/FAMILY PREFERENCES

The frequency of therapy sessions and Sally's home program took into consideration family constraints. Referral to learn self-catheterization was important for independence and reducing the frequency of recurrent urinary tract infections. Like many individuals with L4 level function, Sally will most likely continue to use the chair for long-distance community mobility as an adolescent and adult. Therefore, it will be important to continue to teach Sally advanced wheelchair skills, including ramps and curbs, so that she is independent with her chair in the community and can participate fully in family and social outings. Educating Sally and her parents on the importance of having a physical therapist assess her ROM, strength, tone, and mobility at least annually across the life span to watch for signs of complications such as orthopedic deformities or tethered cord syndrome is also a priority. Promoting low-impact aerobic exercise and nutrition within the family unit when the patient is still at a young age is important for weight control and fitness across the life span.

IMSG. (1993). International Myelodysplasia Study Group Database Coordination. David B. Shurtleff, MD, Department of Pediatrics, University of Washington. Seattle, WA.

Patient Data Management System. (1994). Myelodysplasia Study Data Collection Criteria and Instructions.

Shurtleff, D. B. (1986). Health care delivery. In D. B. Shurtleff (Ed.), *Myelodysplasias and exstrophies: Significance, prevention, and treatment* (pp. 449–514). Orlando, FL: Grune & Stratton.

Shurtleff, D. B. (1991). Computer data bases for pediatric disability: Clinical and research applications. In K. M. Jaffe (Ed.), *Physical Medicine and Rehabilitation Clinics of North America: Pediatric rehabilitation* (pp. 665–688). Philadelphia: WB Saunders.

McDonald, C. M., Jaffe, K. M., Shurtleff, D. B., & Menelaus, M. B. (1991). Modifications to the traditional description of neurosegmental innervation in myelomeningocele. *Developmental Medicine and Child Neurology, 33,* 473–481.

Karmel-Ross, K., Cooperman, D. R., & Van Doren, C. L. (1992). The effect of electrical stimulation on quadriceps femoris muscle torque in children with spina bifida. *Physical Therapy, 72,* 723–731.

Kieklak, H., & DeVahl, J. (1986). *Respond II: Protocol for pediatric applications.* Minneapolis, MN: Medtronics.

Packman, R. A., & Ewaski, B. (1983). *Respond II: Gait training protocol.* Minneapolis, MN: Medtronics.

Liusuwan, R. A., Widman, L. M., Abresch, R. T., Johnson, A. J., & McDonald, C. M. (2007). Behavioral intervention, exercise, and nutrition education to improve health and fitness (BENEfit) in adolescents with mobility impairment due to spinal cord dysfunction. *Journal of Spinal Cord Medicine 30,* S119–S126.

Direct Interventions

An initial physical therapy session consisting of soft tissue mobilization followed by passive stretching resulted in 10° reductions in the hip and knee contractures. The therapist instructed Sally's mother in techniques for stretching the hip and knee flexors, which Sally performed daily. Strengthening exercises for the quadriceps and hamstring muscles were also implemented, including short arc quads, straight leg raises, knee flexion, and squat-to-stand exercises. The therapist saw Sally biweekly for reexamination and progression of her program. After 2 weeks of therapy, she continued to have difficulty with terminal knee extension and initiation of knee flexion. A home program of functional electrical stimulation was implemented to enhance volitional contractions of the quadriceps and hamstring muscles and to assist with muscle reeducation.[80] Strengthening exercises augmented with functional electrical stimulation resulted in significant increases in strength.

After 2 months of intervention, Sally had only 5° hip flexion contractures and her knees could fully extend. Quadriceps and hamstring muscle strength were grades 4 and 4–, respectively. Her decubiti were fully healed and she was anxious to resume bipedal ambulation. She could stand and walk short distances with her knees and hips extended when she used a reverse-facing walker and concentrated on walking with an upright posture. She fatigued and was distracted easily, however, and still required support at the knees for community distances. The long-term goal remained progression to independent ambulation using AFOs and forearm crutches. Ground-reaction force AFOs (see Figure 22-6) would most likely be the optimal design for advancing her to ambulation with AFOs, for the reasons outlined in Box 22-3. KAFOs were still currently indicated, however, to maintain an upright posture for community distances. If she regressed to a crouch gait pattern, contractures and stretch weakness could recur. After consultation with the orthotist, new KAFOs were fabricated that incorporated a ground-reaction force AFO component, along with removable metal knee joints, uprights, and thigh cuff sections. These orthoses enabled Sally to practice upright walking using a posture-control walker at home, with the knee joints either locked or unlocked. In therapy sessions, and under her mother's supervision, the thigh and knee components could be removed so that she could practice walking with the ground-reaction force AFOs.

Orthotic specifications included those listed in Box 22-4 for increasing medial and lateral stability, enhancing the knee extension moment, decreasing energy expenditure, providing adequate toe clearance, simulating push-off, distributing pressure evenly, and

Continued

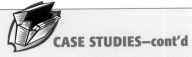

CASE STUDIES—cont'd

improving balance. The orthotist molded the feet in subtalar neutral, and the footplates of the AFOs were posted to accommodate forefoot and hindfoot varus and forefoot supination. The posting provided a wider base of plantigrade support to improve balance and prevented her feet from rolling over into pronation when weight bearing, thus maintaining good biomechanical alignment of the ankles and knees. The ankles were set in 5° of plantar flexion, providing an extensor moment at the knees to encourage more upright stance and gait.

Strengthening exercises and functional electrical stimulation were continued. Gait training began at home and in therapy sessions, initially using a posture-control walker and then progressing to forearm crutches. Gait training emphasized an upright posture and terminal knee extension with the KAFO knee joints unlocked and removed. Functional electrical stimulation was used in conjunction with gait training for muscle reeducation.[83,136] Videotaping of her gait pattern was used throughout the intervention process to provide visual feedback. Sally quickly progressed to ambulation with forearm crutches with the knee joints unlocked. Strength continued to increase; after 3 months of strengthening and gait training, quadriceps and hamstring muscle strength were grades 4+ and 4, respectively, and she was able to walk with ground-reaction force AFOs and forearm crutches for short community distances using a four-point gait pattern. She continued to use a wheelchair for long distances. Progression to a more efficient two-point gait was then emphasized. She mastered the two-point gait pattern following another month of gait training. Strengthening exercises and stretching have continued prophylactically three times a week. Her mother understood that it was essential to avoid regression to a crouched gait pattern and continued to monitor Sally's ROM and posture closely, especially during periods of rapid growth. Sally continues to ambulate independently for short community distances with ground-reaction force AFOs and forearm crutches and uses a wheelchair for longer distances. She also has mastered wheelchair-to-floor transfers.

Sally was referred by the physical therapist for evaluation by a urologist because of her recurrent urinary tract infections. This physician started her on a daily suppressive dose of antibiotic medication and referred her to a nurse to learn self-catheterization. Because of Sally's upper limb dyscoordination, it took her several months to master this skill, but the ability to catheterize herself, especially during school hours so that she no longer went 7 hours between catheterizations from before to after school, resulted in resolution of the recurrent infections.

Prognosis

It will be important to continue to teach Sally advanced wheelchair skills, including ramps and curbs, so that she is independent with the chair in the community; like many individuals with L4 level function, Sally will most likely continue to use the chair for long-distance community mobility as an adolescent and adult. Fortunately, neither Sally's lower limb weakness nor her spasticity progressed to suggest the presence of tethered cord syndrome, but monitoring should continue at least annually throughout her life.

"Megan"

History

Megan is a 6-year-old girl with S1-S2 level paraplegia resulting from a myelomeningocele. She receives physical and occupational therapy through the public schools. She has both ventriculoperitoneal and spinal CSF shunts, which have required multiple revisions. She has also had ophthalmologic surgery for strabismus and three decompressions for Arnold-Chiari malformation. She is very happy, social, self-confident, and makes friends with peers easily, but she prefers to interact with adults.

Megan rolled from prone to supine at 5 months of age and from supine to prone at 7 months. She sat independently at 12 months and crawled on level surfaces and stairs at 18 months. She pulled to stand at 2 years of age and began cruising and walking with a walker using AFOs at 2.5 years of age. Megan's fine motor skills are delayed, which affects her personal care, dressing, and handwriting activities.

Systems Review

Megan has frequent urinary tract infections that are treated with Ditropan. She is catheterized three times a day and is independent with self-catheterization at school. She has no history of skin breakdown or cardiopulmonary complications.

Tests and Measures

Current examination results for Megan at 6 years of age are summarized here. ROM and muscle extensibility were within functional limits. Her forefeet and hindfeet had a varus inclination when examined in a non-weight-bearing position with her subtalar joint positioned in neutral. This resulted in a valgus, everted position of her feet when bearing weight.

Megan's motor level was determined to be S1 on the left and S2 on the right with hip extensors, adductors, and abductors grade 4– on the left and grade 4 on the right; knee extensors were grade 5 bilaterally, and knee flexors, ankle dorsiflexors, invertors, evertors, toe flexors and extensors were grade 4 on the left and grade 5 on the right; and ankle plantar flexors were grade 2 on the left and grade 3 on the right (on a 5-point MMT scale). Sensation was intact through S2.

Megan walked using supramalleolar AFOs with a crouch gait pattern and bilateral gluteal lurch combined with lateral trunk sway. She was independent on level surfaces and gradual inclines. She had difficulty traversing uneven terrain and steeper inclines. She was a short-distance community ambulator with limited endurance. She walked at home and school for distances up to 300 feet and was carried or pushed in a grocery cart for longer distances. The maximum distance she had ever been able to walk with her supramalleolar AFOs was approximately 1 to 4 miles with one hand held, according to her mother. She was beginning to learn to use a tricycle.

Evaluation

Although her supramalleolar AFOs maintained her foot alignment and subtalar joint in neutral in the frontal plane, the strength of her

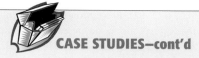

CASE STUDIES—cont'd

plantar flexors was not sufficient to control advancement of the tibia during the stance phase of gait, resulting in a crouch gait posture.

Direct Interventions

The physical therapist determined that ground-reaction force AFOs (see Figure 22-6) would improve her crouch gait pattern for the reasons outlined in Box 22-3. Orthotic specifications included those listed in Box 22-4 for increasing medial and lateral stability, enhancing the knee extension moment, decreasing energy expenditure, providing adequate toe clearance, simulating push-off, distributing pressure evenly, and improving balance. The orthotist molded the feet in subtalar neutral, and the footplates of the AFOs were posted to accommodate forefoot and hindfoot varus and forefoot supination. The posting provided a wider base of plantigrade support to improve balance and prevented her feet from rolling over into pronation when weight bearing, thus maintaining good biomechanical alignment of the ankles and knees. The ankles were set in 5° of plantar flexion, providing an extensor moment at the knees to encourage more upright stance and gait. Gait training began at home and in therapy sessions, using a posture-control walker for balance in combination with walking independently. Gait training emphasized an upright posture, symmetric steps, and reciprocal arm swing. The improvement in Megan's posture and endurance was immediately apparent with the ground reaction AFOs. Her posture was significantly more upright with hip and knee extension. The first weekend that Megan had her new orthoses, she hiked 1.5 miles on uneven terrain with one hand held, only requiring three short rest periods. Megan continues to ambulate independently for short distances in the community with ground-reaction force AFOs.

Prognosis

It will be important to continue lower extremity strengthening exercises and to progress Megan to be independent with community ambulation, including inclines, uneven terrain, and curbs. It will also be important to encourage alternative means of long distance mobility such as bike riding. Her parents understand that it is essential to avoid regression to a crouched gait pattern and continue to monitor her ROM and posture closely, especially during periods of rapid growth. Monitoring her strength should continue at least annually throughout her life, ideally using objective methods of strength assessment.

REFERENCES

1. Agre, J. C., Findley, T. W., McNally, M. C., et al. (1987). Physical activity capacity in children with myelomeningocele. *Archives of Physical Medicine and Rehabilitation, 68*, 372–377.

2. Aitkens, S., Lord, J., Bernauer, E., Fowler, W., Lieberman, J., & Berck, P. (1989). Relationship of manual muscle testing to objective strength measurements. *Muscle and Nerve, 12*, 173–177.

3. Andersen, E. M., & Plewis, I. (1977). Impairment of motor skill in children with spina bifida cystica and hydrocephalus: An exploratory study. *British Journal of Psychology, 68*, 61–70.

4. Andersson, C., & Mattsson, E. (2001). Adults with cerebral palsy: A survey describing problems, needs, and resources, with special emphasis on locomotion. *Developmental Medicine & Child Neurology, 43*, 76–82.

5. Asher, M., & Olson, J. (1983). Factors affecting the ambulatory status of patients with spina bifida cystica. *Journal of Bone and Joint Surgery (American), 65*, 350–356.

6. Babcook, C. J. (1995). Ultrasound evaluation of prenatal and neonatal spina bifida. *Neurosurgery Clinics of North America, 6*, 203–218.

7. Baker, S. B., & Rogosky-Grassi, M. A. (1992). Access to the school. In F. L. Rowley-Kelly & D. H. Reigel (Eds.), *Teaching the student with spina bifida* (pp. 31–70). Baltimore: Paul H. Brookes.

8. Bannister, C. M. (2000). The case for and against intrauterine surgery for myelomeningocele. *European Journal of Obstetrics, Gynecology & Reproductive Biology, 92*, 109–113.

9. Banta, J. V. (1999). Bracing for ambulation: Basic principles, brace alternatives by motor level and predictive long-term goals. In S. Matsumoto & H. Sato (Eds.), *Spina bifida* (pp. 307–311). New York: Springer Verlag.

10. Banta, J., & Hamada, J. (1976). Natural history of the kyphotic deformity in myelomeningocele. *Journal of Bone and Joint Surgery, 58A*, 279.

11. Bar-Or, O. (1986). Pathophysiological factors which limit the exercise capacity of the sick child. *Medicine and Science in Sports and Exercise, 18*, 276–282.

12. Bartlett, M. D., Wolf, L. S., Shurtleff, D. B., & Staheli, L. T. (1985). Hip flexion contractures: A comparison of measurement methods. *Archives of Physical Medicine and Rehabilitation, 66*, 620–625.

13. Becker, R. D. (1975). Recent developments in child psychiatry: I. The restrictive emotional and cognitive environment reconsidered: A redefinition of the concept of therapeutic restraint. *Israeli Journal of Psychiatry and Related Sciences, 12*, 239–258.

14. Bauer, S. B. (2008). Neurogenic bladder: Etiology and assessment. *Pediatric Nephrology, 23*, 541–551.

15. Berry, R. J., Li, Z., Erickson, J. D., et al. (1999). Prevention of neural-tube defects with folic acid in China. *New England Journal of Medicine, 341*, 1485–1491.

16. Birth Defects and Genetic Diseases Branch of Birth Defects and Developmental Disabilities Office, National Center for Environmental Disease and Injury. (1991). Use of folic acid prevention of spina bifida and other neural tube defects, 1983–1991. *Morbidity and Mortality Weekly Report, 40,* 1–4.

17. Bleck, E. E., & Nagel, D. A. (1982). *Physically handicapped children: A medical atlas for teachers.* Orlando, FL: Grune & Stratton.

18. Blum, R. W., Resnick, M. D., Nelson R., & St. Germain, A. (1991). Family and peer issues among adolescents with spina bifida and cerebral palsy. *Pediatrics, 88,* 280–285.

19. Bohannon, R. W. (1986). Manual muscle test scores and dynamometer test scores of knee extension strength. *Archives of Physical Medicine and Rehabilitation, 67,* 390–392.

20. Bower, E. (Ed.). (2009). *Finnie's handling the young child with cerebral palsy at home.* Burlington, MA: Butterworth-Heinemann.

21. Brazelton, T. B. (1992). *Touchpoints: Your child's emotional and behavioral development.* Reading, MA: Perseus Books.

22. Brinker, M., Rosenfeld, S., Feiwell, E., Granger, S., Mitchell, D., & Rice, J. (1994). Myelomeningocele at the sacral level: Long-term outcomes in adults. *Journal of Bone and Joint Surgery, 76A,* 1293–1300.

23. Broughton, N. S., Graham, G., & Menelaus, M. B. (1994). The high incidence of foot deformity in patients with high-level spina bifida. *Journal of Bone and Joint Surgery, 76B,* 548–550.

24. Brown, J. P. (2001). Orthopedic care of children with spina bifida: You've come a long way, baby! *Orthopaedic Nursing, 20,* 51–58.

25. Brunt, D. (1980). Characteristics of upper limb movements in a sample of meningomyelocele children. *Perceptual Motor Skills, 51,* 431–437.

26. Butler, C., Okamoto, G. A., & McKay, T. M. (1984). Motorized wheelchair driving by disabled children. *Archives of Physical Medicine and Rehabilitation, 65,* 95–97.

27. Chaffin, D. B., Andersson, G. B. J., & Martin, B. J. (1999). *Occupational biomechanics* (3rd ed.). New York: John Wiley & Sons.

28. Chandler, L. S., Andrews, M. S., & Swanson, M. W. (1980). *Movement assessment of infants: A manual.* Rolling Bay, WA: Authors.

29. CIBA. (1994). *CIBA Symposium No. 191: Neural tube defects.* London: CIBA Foundation.

30. Coster, W., Deeney, T. A., Haltiwanger, J. T., & Haley, S. M. (1998). *School function assessment.* Boston: Boston University.

31. Culatta, B., & Young, C. (1992). Linguistic performance as a function of abstract task demands in children with spina bifida. *Developmental Medicine and Child Neurology, 34*(5), 434–440.

32. Cusick, B. D., & Stuberg, W. A. (1992). Assessment of lower extremity alignment in the transverse plane: Implications for management of children with neuromotor dysfunction. *Physical Therapy, 72,* 3–15.

33. Czeizel, A. E., & Dudas, I. (1992). Prevention of first occurrence of neural tube defects by periconceptual vitamin supplementation. *New England Journal of Medicine, 327,* 131–137.

34. Deitz, J. C., Jaffe, K. M., Wolf, L. S., Massagli, T. L., & Anson, D. K. (1991). Pediatric power wheelchairs: Evaluation of function in the home and school environments. *Assistive Technology, 3,* 24–31.

35. Del Gado, R., Del Gaizo, D., Brescia, D., Polidori, G., & Tamburro, A. (1999). Obesity and overweight in a group of patients with myelomeningocele. In S. Matsumoto & H. Sato (Eds.). *Spina bifida* (pp. 474–475). New York: Springer Verlag.

36. DeSouza, L., & Carroll, N. (1976). Ambulation of the braced myelomeningocele patient. *Journal of Bone and Joint Surgery (American), 58,* 1112–1118.

37. De Villarreal, L. M., Perez, J. Z., Vasquez, P. A., et al. (2002). Decline of neural tube defects after a folic acid campaign in Neuvo Leon, Mexico. *Teratology, 66,* 249–256.

38. Dias, L. (1999a). Management of ankle and hindfoot valgus in spina bifida. In S. Matsumoto & H. Sato (Eds.), *Spina bifida* (pp. 374–377). New York: Springer Verlag.

39. Dias, L. (1999b). The management of hip pathology in spina bifida. In S. Matsumoto & H. Sato (Eds.), *Spina bifida* (pp. 321–322). New York: Springer Verlag.

40. Diaz Llopis, I., Bea Munoz, M., Martinez Agullo, E., Lopez Martinez, A., Garcia Aymerich, V., & Forner Valero, J. V. (1993). Ambulation in patients with myelomeningocele: A study of 1500 patients. *Paraplegia, 31,* 28–32.

41. Dise, J. E., & Lohr, M. E. (1998). Examination of deficits in conceptual reasoning abilities associated with spina bifida. *American Journal of Physical Medicine and Rehabilitation, 77,* 247–251.

42. Dudgeon, B. J., Jaffe, K. M., & Shurtleff, D. B. (1991). Variations in midlumbar myelomeningocele: Implications for ambulation. *Pediatric Physical Therapy, 3,* 57–62.

43. Eastlack, M. E., Arvidson, J., Snyder-Mackler, L., Danoff, J. V., & McGarvey, C. L. (1991). Interrater reliability of videotaped observational gait-analysis assessments. *Physical Therapy, 71,* 465–472.

44. Effgen, S. K., & Brown, D. A. (1992). Long-term stability of hand-held dynamometric measurements in children who have myelomeningocele. *Physical Therapy, 72,* 458–465.

45. Elwood, J. M., & Elwood, J. H. (1980). *Epidemiology of anencephalus and spina bifida.* Cambridge: Oxford University Press.

46. Embrey, D., Endicott, J., Glenn, T., & Jaeger, D. L. (1983). Developing better postural tone in grade school children. *Clinical Management in Physical Therapy, 3,* 6–10.

47. Fay, G., Shurtleff, D. B., Shurtleff, H., & Wolf, L. (1986). Approaches to facilitate independent self-care and academic success. In D. B. Shurtleff (Ed.), *Myelodysplasias and exstrophies: Significance, prevention, and treatment* (pp. 373–398). Orlando, FL: Grune & Stratton.

48. Fife, S. E., Roxborough, L. A., Armstrong, R. W., Harris, S. R., Gregson, J. L., & Field, D. (1991). Development of a clinical

measure of postural control for assessment of adaptive seating in children with neuromotor disabilities. *Physical Therapy, 71,* 981–993.

49. Florence, J. M., Pandya, S., King, W., Schierbecker, J., et al. (1988). Strength assessment: Comparison of methods in children with Duchenne muscular dystrophy (Abstract). *Physical Therapy, 68,* 866.

50. Frawley, P. A., Broughton, N. S., & Menelaus, M. B. (1998). Incidence and type of hindfoot deformities in patients with low-level spina bifida. *Journal of Pediatric Orthopedics, 18,* 312–313

51. Gadow, K. (1986). *Children on medication.* San Diego, CA: College Hill Press.

52. Gaston, H. (1991). Ophthalmic complications of spina bifida and hydrocephalus. *Eye, 5,* 279–290.

53. Goodwyn, M. A. (1990). *Biomedical psychological factors predicting success with activities of daily living and academic pursuits.* Unpublished doctoral dissertation. Seattle: University of Washington.

54. Griebel, M. L., Oakes, W. J., & Worley, G. (1991). The Chiari malformation associated with myelomeningocele. In H. L. Rekate (Ed.), *Comprehensive management of spina bifida* (pp. 67–92). Boca Raton, FL: CRC Press.

55. Griffin, J. W., McClure, M. H., & Bertorini, T. E. (1986). Sequential isokinetic and manual muscle testing in patients with neuromuscular disease: Pilot study. *Physical Therapy, 66,* 32–35.

56. Gucciardi, E., Pietrusiak, M. A., Reynolds, D. L., & Rouleau, J. (2002). Incidence of neural tube defects in Ontario, 1986–1999. *Canadian Medical Association Journal, 167,* 237–240.

57. Hack, S. N., Norton, B. J., & Zahalak, G. I. (1981). A quantitative muscle tester for clinical use (Abstract). *Physical Therapy, 61,* 673.

58. Hamill, P. V., Drizd, T. A., Johnson, C. L., Reed, R. B., Roche, A. F., & Moore, W. M. (1979). Physical growth: National Center for Health Statistics percentiles. *American Journal of Clinical Nutrition, 32,* 607–629.

59. Harris, S. R., Megans, A. M., & Daniels, L. E. (2010). Harris Infant Neuromotor Test (HINT). *Test User's Manual Version 1.0 Clinical Edition (2009).* Chicago, IL: Infant Motor Performance Scales, L. L. C.

60. Hatlen, T., Song, K., Shurtleff, D., & Duguay, S. (2010). Contributory factors to postoperative spinal fusion complications for children with myelomeningocele. *Spine, 35,* 1294–1299.

61. Hinderer, K. A. (1988). *Reliability of the myometer in muscle testing children and adolescents with myelodysplasia.* Unpublished master's thesis. Seattle: University of Washington.

62. Hinderer, K. A. (2003). *The relationship between musculoskeletal system capacity and task requirements in simulated crouch standing.* Doctoral dissertation. Ann Arbor, MI: University of Michigan.

63. Hinderer, K. A., & Gutierrez, T. (1988). Myometry measurements of children using isometric and eccentric methods of muscle testing (Abstract). *Physical Therapy, 68,* 817.

64. Hinderer, K. A., & Hinderer, S. R. (1988). Mobility and transfer efficiency of adults with myelodysplasia (Abstract). *Archives of Physical Medicine and Rehabilitation, 69,* 712.

65. Hinderer, K. A., & Hinderer, S. R. (1993). Muscle strength development and assessment in children and adolescents. In K. Harms-Ringdahl (Ed.), International perspectives in physical therapy: Muscle strength (*Vol. 8,* pp. 93–140). London: Churchill Livingstone.

66. Hinderer, S. R., & Hinderer, K. A. (1990). Sensory examination of individuals with myelodysplasia (Abstract). *Archives of Physical Medicine and Rehabilitation, 71,* 769–770.

67. Hinderer, S. R., & Hinderer, K. A. (1998). Quantitative methods of evaluation. In J. A. DeLisa & B. M. Gans (Eds.), *Rehabilitation medicine: Principles and practices* (3rd ed., pp. 109–136). Philadelphia: Lippincott-Raven.

68. Hinderer, S. R., Hinderer, K. A., Dunne, K., & Shurtleff, D. B. (1988). Medical and functional status of adults with spina bifida (Abstract). *Developmental Medicine and Child Neurology, 30*(Suppl 57), 28.

69. Hislop, H. J., & Montgomery, J. (2002). *Daniels and Worthingham's muscle testing,* 7th ed. Philadelphia: WB Saunders.

70. Hosking, G. P., Bhat, U. S., Dubowitz, V., & Edwards, R. H. T. (1976). Measurements of muscle strength and performance in children with normal and diseased muscle. *Archives of Disease in Childhood, 51,* 957–963.

71. Hunt, G. M. (1990). Open spina bifida: Outcome for complete cohort treated unselectively and followed into adulthood. *Developmental Medicine and Child Neurology, 32,* 108–118.

72. Hunt, G., & Oakeshott, P. (2003). Outcome in people with open spina bifida at age 35: Prospective community based cohort study. *British Medical Journal, 326,* 1365–1366.

73. Hunt, G. M., Oakeshott, P., & Kerry S. (1999). Link between the CSF shunt and achievement in adults with spina bifida. *Journal of Neurology, Neurosurgery, and Psychiatry, 67,* 591–595.

74. Hurley, A. D. (1992). Conducting psychological assessments. In F. L. Rowley-Kelly & D. H. Reigel, (Eds.). *Teaching the student with spina bifida* (pp. 107–124). Baltimore: Paul H. Brookes.

75. Hyde, S., Goddard, C., & Scott, O. (1983). The myometer: The development of a clinical tool. *Physiotherapy, 69,* 424–427.

76. IMSG. (1993). International Myelodysplasia Study Group Database Coordination. David B. Shurtleff, M. D., Department of Pediatrics, University of Washington, Seattle.

77. Jacobson, C. B., & Berlin, C. M. (1972). Possible reproductive deterrent in LSD users. *Journal of the American Medical Association, 222,* 1367–1373.

78. Janda, V. (1983). *Muscle function testing.* Boston: Butterworths.

79. Jebsen, R. H., Trieschman, R. B., Mikulic, M. A., Hartley, R. B., McMillan, J. A., & Snook, M. E. (1970). Measurement of time in a standardized test of patient mobility. *Archives of Physical Medicine and Rehabilitation, 51,* 170–175.

80. Karmel-Ross, K., Cooperman, D. R., & Van Doren, C. L. (1992). The effect of electrical stimulation on quadriceps femoris muscle torque in children with spina bifida. *Physical Therapy, 72,* 723–731.

81. Karol, L. (1995). Orthopedic management in myelomeningocele. *Neurosurgery Clinics of North America, 6,* 259–268

82. Kendall, F. P., McCreary, E. K., & Provance, P. G. (1999). *Muscles: Testing and function* (4th ed.). Baltimore: Williams & Wilkins.

83. Kieklak, H., & DeVahl, J. (1986). *Respond II: Protocol for pediatric applications.* Minneapolis, MN: Medtronics, Inc.

84. Kilburn, J., Saffer, A., Barnes, L., Kling, T., & Venes, J. (1985). *The Vigorimeter as an early predictor of central neurologic malformation in myelodysplastic children.* Paper presented at the meeting of the American Academy for Cerebral Palsy and Developmental Medicine, Seattle.

85. Kimura, D. K., Mayo, M., & Shurtleff, D. B. (1986). Urinary tract management. In D. B. Shurtleff (Ed.), *Myelodysplasias and exstrophies: Significance, Prevention, and Treatment* (pp. 243–266). Orlando, FL: Grune & Stratton.

86. King, J. C., Currie, D. M., & Wright, E. (1994). Bowel training in spina bifida: Importance of education, patient compliance, age, and anal reflexes. *Archives of Physical Medicine and Rehabilitation, 75,* 243–247.

87. Knutson, L. M., & Clark, D. E. (1991). Orthotic devices for ambulation in children with cerebral palsy and myelomeningocele. *Physical Therapy, 71,* 947–960.

88. Kottorp, A., Bernspang, B., & Fisher, A. G. (2003). Validity of a performance assessment of activities of daily living for people with developmental disabilities. *Journal of Intellectual Disability Research, 47(8),* 597–605.

89. Krebs, D. E., Edelstein, J. E., & Fishman, S. (1985). Reliability of observational kinematic gait analysis. *Physical Therapy, 65,* 1027–1033.

90. Lais, A., Kasabian, N. G., Dryo, F. M., Scott, R. M., Kelly, M. D., & Bauer, S. B. (1993). The neurosurgical implications of continuous neurological surveillance of children with myelodysplasia. *Journal of Urology, 150,* 1879–1883.

91. Land, L. C. (1977). Study of the sensory integration of children with myelomeningocele. In R. L. McLaurin (Ed.), *Myelomeningocele* (pp. 115–140). Orlando, FL: Grune & Stratton.

92. Lehmann, J. F., Condon, S. M., de Lateur, B. J., & Price, R. (1986). Gait abnormalities in peroneal nerve paralysis and their corrections by orthoses: A biomechanical study. *Archives of Physical Medicine and Rehabilitation, 67,* 380–386.

93. Lehmann, J. F., Condon, S. M., de Lateur, B. J., & Smith, C. (1995). Ankle-foot orthoses: Effect on gait abnormalities in tibial nerve paralysis. *Archives of Physical Medicine and Rehabilitation, 66,* 212–218.

94. Lehmann, J. F., Esselman, P. C., Ko, M. J., de Lateur, B. J., & Dralle, A. J. (1983). Plastic ankle-foot orthoses: Evaluation of function. *Archives of Physical Medicine and Rehabilitation, 64,* 402–404.

95. Lemire, R. J., Loeser, J. D., Leech, R. W., & Alvord, E. D. (Eds.). (1975). *Normal and abnormal development of the human nervous system.* Hagerstown, MD: Harper & Row.

96. Level, M. B. (1984). *Spherical grip strength of children.* Unpublished master's thesis. Seattle: University of Washington.

97. Liptak, G. S., Shurtleff, D. B., Bloss, J. W., Baitus-Hebert, E., & Manitta, P. (1992). Mobility aids for children with high-level myelomeningocele: Parapodium versus wheelchair. *Developmental Medicine and Child Neurology, 34,* 787–796.

98. Liu, S. L., Shurtleff, D. B., Ellenbogen, R. G., Loeser, J. D., & Kropp, R. (1999). 19 year follow up of fetal myelomeningocele brought to term. Proceedings of the 43rd Annual Meeting of the Society for Research into Hydrocephalus and Spina Bifida. *European Journal of Pediatric Surgery, 9*(Suppl 1), 12–14.

99. Liusuwan, R. A., Widman, L. M., Abresch, R. T., Styne, D. M., & McDonald, C. M. (2007a). Body composition and resting energy expenditure in patients aged 11 to 21 years with spinal cord dysfunction compared to controls: Comparisons and relationships among the groups. *Journal of Spinal Cord Medicine, 30,* S105–S111.

100. Liusuwan, R. A., Widman, L. M., Abresch, R. T., Johnson, A. J., & McDonald, C. M. (2007b). Behavioral intervention, exercise, and nutrition education to improve health and fitness (BENEfit) in adolescents with mobility impairment due to spinal cord dysfunction. *Journal of Spinal Cord Medicine, 30,* S119–S126.

101. Logan, L., Byers-Hinkley, K., & Ciccone, C. D. (1990). Anterior versus posterior walkers: A gait analysis study. *Developmental Medicine and Child Neurology, 32,* 1044–1048.

102. Lollar, D. (1994). *Preventing secondary conditions associated with spina bifida or cerebral palsy. Proceedings and Recommendations of a Symposium* (pp. 54–64). Washington, DC: Spina Bifida Association of America.

103. Luthy, D. A., Wardinsky, T., Shurtleff, D. B., et al. (1991). Cesarean section before the onset of labor and subsequent motor function in infants with myelomeningocele diagnosed antenatally. *New England Journal of Medicine, 324,* 662–666.

104. Lutkenhoff, M., & Oppenheimer, S. (1997). *Spinabilities: A young person's guide to spina bifida.* Bethesda, MD: Woodbine House.

105. Lynch, A., Ryu, J., Agrawal, S., & Galloway, J. C. (2009). Power mobility training for a 7-month old infant with spina bifida. *Pediatric Physical Therapy, 21,* 362–368.

106. Main, D. M., & Mennuti, M. T. (1986). Neural tube defects: Issues in prenatal diagnosis and counseling. *Journal of the American College of Obstetrics and Gynecology, 67,* 1–16.

107. Masse, L. C., Lamontagne, M., & O'Riain, M. D. (1992). Biomedical analysis of wheelchair propulsion for various seating positions. *Journal of Rehabilitation Research and Development, 29,* 12–28.

108. Mayfield, J. K. (1991). Comprehensive orthopedic management in myelomeningocele. In H. L. Rekate (Ed.) *Comprehensive management of spina bifida* (pp. 113–164). Boca Raton, FL: CRC Press.

109. Maynard, J., Weiner, J., & Burke, S. (1992). Neuropathic foot ulceration in patients with myelodysplasia. *Journal of Pediatric Orthopedics, 12,* 786–788.

110. Mazur, J. M., & Menelaus, M. B. (1991). Neurologic status of spina bifida patients and the orthopedic surgeon. *Clinical Orthopaedics and Related Research, 264,* 54–63.

111. McDonald, C. M., Jaffe, K. M., Mosca, V. S., & Shurtleff, D. B. (1991a). Ambulatory outcome of children with myelomeningocele: Effect of lower-extremity muscle strength. *Developmental Medicine and Child Neurology, 33,* 482–490.

112. McDonald, C. M., Jaffe, K., & Shurtleff, D. B. (1986). Assessment of muscle strength in children with meningomyelocele: Accuracy and stability of measurements over time. *Archives of Physical Medicine and Rehabilitation, 67,* 855–861.

113. McDonald, C. M., Jaffe, K. M., Shurtleff, D. B., & Menelaus, M. B. (1991b). Modifications to the traditional description of neurosegmental innervation in myelomeningocele. *Developmental Medicine and Child Neurology, 33,* 473–481.

114. McDonnell, G. V., & McCann, J. P. (2000). Link between the CSF shunt and achievement in adults with spina bifida. *Journal of Neurology, Neurosurgery, and Psychiatry, 68,* 800.

115. McGourty, L. K. (1988). Kohlman Evaluation of Living Skills (KELS). In B. J. Hemphill (Ed.), *Mental health assessment in occupational therapy* (pp. 131–146). Thorofare, NJ: Black.

116. Mendell, J. R., & Florence, J. (1990). Manual muscle testing. *Muscle and Nerve, 13*(Suppl), 16–20.

117. Menelaus, M. B. (1976). Orthopedic management of children with myelomeningocele: A plea for realistic goals. *Developmental Medicine and Child Neurology, 18*(Suppl 37), 3–11.

118. Menelaus, M. D. (1999). The hip: Current treatment. In S. Matsumoto & H. Sato (Eds.), *Spina bifida* (pp. 338–340). New York: Springer Verlag.

119. Miller, E., & Sethi, L. (1971). The effect of hydrocephalus on perception. *Developmental Medicine and Child Neurology, 13*(Suppl 25), 77–81.

120. Miller, L. C., Michael, A. F., Baxter, T. L., & Kim, Y. (1988). Quantitative muscle testing in childhood dermatomyositis. *Archives of Physical Medicine and Rehabilitation, 69,* 610–613.

121. Mills, J. L., Rhoads, G. G., Simpson, J. L., et al. (1989). The absence of a relation between the periconceptual use of vitamins and neural tube defects. *New England Journal of Medicine, 321,* 430–435.

122. Milner-Brown, H. S., & Miller, R. G. (1989). Increased muscular fatigue in patients with neurogenic muscle weakness: Quantification and pathophysiology. *Archives of Physical Medicine and Rehabilitation, 70,* 361–366.

123. Milunsky, A., Jick, H., Jick, S. S., et al. (1989). Multivitamin/folic acid supplementation in early pregnancy reduces the prevalence of neural tube defects. *Journal of the American Medical Association, 262,* 2847–2852.

124. Mintz, L., Sarwark, J., Dias, L., & Schafer, M. (1991). The natural history of congenital kyphosis in myelomeningocele. *Spine, 16*(Suppl. 5), 348–350.

125. Mobley, C., Harless, L., & Miller, K. (1996). Self perceptions of preschool children with spina bifida. *Journal of Pediatric Nursing, 1,* 217–224.

126. MRC Vitamin Study Research Group. (1991). Prevention of neural tube defects: Results of the Medical Research Council vitamin study. *Lancet, 338,* 131–137.

127. Murdoch, A. (1980). How valuable is muscle charting? A study of the relationship between neonatal assessment of muscle power and later mobility in children with spina bifida defects. *Physiotherapy, 66,* 221–223.

128. Murphy, K. P., Molnar, G. E., & Lankasky, K. (1995). Medical and functional status of adults with cerebral palsy. *Developmental Medicine & Child Neurology, 37,* 1075–1084.

129. Nagankatti, D., Banta, J., & Thomson, J. (2000). Charcot arthropathy in spina bifida. *Journal of Pediatric Orthopedics, 20,* 82–87.

130. Oi, S. (2003). Current status of prenatal management of fetal spina bifida in the world:worldwide cooperative survey on the medico-ethical issue. *Child's Nervous System 19,* 596–599.

131. Oi, S., Sato, O., & Matsumoto, S. (1996). Neurological and medico-social problems of spina bifida patients in adolescence and adulthood. *Child's Nervous System, 12,* 181–187.

132. Okamoto, G. A., Lamers, J. V., & Shurtleff, D. B. (1983). Skin breakdown in patients with myelomeningocele. *Archives of Physical Medicine and Rehabilitation, 64,* 20–23.

133. Okamoto, G. A., Sousa, J., Telzrow, R. W., Holm, R. A., McCartin, R., & Shurtleff, D. B. (1984). Toileting skills in children with myelomeningocele: Rates of learning. *Archives of Physical Medicine and Rehabilitation, 65*(4), 182–185.

134. Ounpuu, S., Davis, R. B., Banta, J. V., & DeLuce, P. A. (1992). The effects of orthotics on gait in children with low-level myelomeningocele. *Proceedings of the North American Congress on Biomechanics,* Chicago, IL, 323–324.

135. Overgoor, M. L. E., Kon, M., Cohen-Kettenis, P. T., Strijbos, S. A. M., de Boer, N., & de Jong, T. P. V. M. (2006). Neurological bypass for sensory innervations of the penis in patients with spina bifida. *Journal of Urology, 176,* 1086–1090.

136. Packman, R. A., & Ewaski, B. (1983). *Respond II: Gait training protocol.* Minneapolis, MN: Medtronics.

137. Pact, V., Sirotkin-Roses, M., & Beatus, J. (1984). *The muscle testing handbook.* Boston: Little, Brown.

138. Padua, L., Rendeli, C., Rabini, A., Girardi, E., Tonali, P., & Salvaggio, E. (2002). Health-related quality of life and disability in young patients with spina bifida. *Archives of Physical Medicine and Rehabilitation, 83,* 1384–1388.

139. Patient Data Management System. (1994). Myelodysplasia Study Data Collection Criteria and Instructions.

140. Persad, V. L., Van den Hof, M. C., Dube, J. M., & Zimmer, P. (2002). Incidence of open neural tube defects in Nova Scotia after folic acid fortification. *Canadian Medical Association Journal, 167,* 241–245.

141. Peterson, P., Rauen, K., Brown, J., & Cole, J. (1994). Spina bifida: The transition into adulthood begins in infancy. *Rehabilitation Nursing, 19,* 229–238.

142. Pomatto, R. C. (1991). The use of orthotics in the treatment of myelomeningocele. In H. L. Rekate (Ed.), *Comprehensive management of spina bifida* (pp. 165–183). Boca Raton, FL: CRC Press.

143. Reigel, D. H. (1992). Spina bifida from infancy through the school years. In F. L. Rowley-Kelly & D. H. Reigel (Eds.), *Teaching the students with spina bifida* (pp. 3–30). Baltimore: Paul H. Brookes.

144. Rekate, H. L. (1991). Neurosurgical management of the newborn with spina bifida. In H. L. Rekate (Ed.), *Comprehensive management of spina bifida* (pp. 1–28). Boca Raton, FL: CRC Press.

145. Reynolds, E. H. (1983). Mental effects of antiepileptic medication: A review. *Epilepsia, 24*(Suppl 2), S85–S95.

146. Rose, S. A., Ounpuu, S., & DeLuca, P. A. (1991). Strategies for the assessment of pediatric gait in the clinical setting. *Physical Therapy, 71,* 961–980.

147. Rosenstein, B. D., Greene, W. B., Herrington, R. T., & Blum, A. S. (1987). Bone density in myelomeningocele: The effects of ambulatory status and other factors. *Developmental Medicine and Child Neurology, 29,* 486–494.

148. Rowley-Kelly, F. L., & Kunkle, P. M. (1992). Developing a school outreach program. In F. L. Rowley-Kelly & D. H. Reigel (Eds.), *Teaching the student with spina bifida* (pp. 395–436). Baltimore: Paul H. Brookes.

149. Ryan, K. D., Pioski, C., & Emans, J. B. (1991). Myelodysplasia— The musculoskeletal problem: Habilation from infancy to adulthood. *Physical Therapy, 71,* 935–946.

150. Salvaggio, E., Mauti, G., Ranieri, P., et al. (1999). Ability in walking is a predictor of bone mineral density and body composition in prepubertal children with myelomeningocele. In S. Matsumoto & H. Sato (Eds.), *Spina bifida* (pp. 298–301). New York: Springer Verlag.

151. Sand, P. L., Taylor, N., Rawlings, M., & Chitnis, S. (1973). Performance of children with spina bifida manifest on the Frostig Developmental Test of Visual Perception. *Perceptual Motor Skills, 37,* 539–546.

152. Schafer, M. F., & Dias, L. S. (1983). *Myelomeningocele: Orthopaedic treatment.* Baltimore: Williams & Wilkins.

153. Schneider, J. W., Krosschell, K., & Gabriel, K. L. (2001). Congenital spinal cord injury. In D. A. Umphred (Ed.), *Neurological rehabilitation* (4th ed., pp. 454–483). St. Louis, MO: Mosby.

154. Schopler, S. A., & Menelaus, M. B. (1987). Significance of strength of the quadriceps muscles in children with myelomeningocele. *Journal of Pediatric Orthopaedics, 7,* 507–512.

155. Seller, M. J., & Nevin, N. C. (1984). Periconceptual vitamin supplementation and the prevention of neural tube defects in south-east England and northern Ireland. *Journal of Medical Genetics, 21,* 325–330.

156. Shaffer, J., Wolfe, L., Friedrich, W., Shurtleff, H., Shurtleff, D., & Fay, G. (1986). Developmental expectations: Intelligence and fine motor skills. In D. B. Shurtleff (Ed.), *Myelodysplasias and exstrophies: Significance, prevention, and treatment* (pp. 359–372). Orlando, FL: Grune & Stratton.

157. Shapiro, E., Kelly, K. J., Setlock, M. A., Suwalski, K. L., & Meyers, P. (1992). Complications of latex allergy. *Dialogues in Pediatric Urology, 15,* 1–5.

158. Sherk, H., Uppal, G., Lane, G., & Melchionni, J. (1991). Treatment versus nontreatment of hip dislocations in ambulatory patients with myelomeningocele. *Development Medicine & Child Neurology, 33,* 491–494.

159. Shores, M. (1980). Footprint analysis in gait documentation. *Physical Therapy, 60,* 1163–1167.

160. Shurtleff, D. B. (1966). Timing of learning in the myelomeningocele patient. *Journal of the American Physical Therapy Association, 46*(2):136–148.

161. Shurtleff, D. B. (1986a). Decubitus formation and skin breakdown. In D. B. Shurtleff (Ed.), *Myelodysplasias and exstrophies: Significance, prevention, and treatment* (pp. 299–312). Orlando, FL: Grune & Stratton.

162. Shurtleff, D. B. (1986b). Dietary management. In D. B. Shurtleff (Ed.), *Myelodysplasias and exstrophies: Significance, prevention, and treatment* (pp. 285–298). Orlando, FL: Grune & Stratton.

163. Shurtleff, D. B. (1986c). Health care delivery. In D. B. Shurtleff (Ed.), *Myelodysplasias and exstrophies: Significance, prevention, and treatment* (pp. 449–514). Orlando, FL: Grune & Stratton.

164. Shurtleff, D. B. (1986d). Mobility. In D. B. Shurtleff (Ed.), *Myelodysplasias and exstrophies: Significance, prevention, and treatment* (pp. 313–356). Orlando, FL: Grune & Stratton.

165. Shurtleff, D. B. (1986e). Selection process for the care of congenitally malformed infants. In D. B. Shurtleff (Ed.), *Myelodysplasias and exstrophies: Significance, prevention, and treatment* (pp. 89–116). Orlando, FL: Grune & Stratton.

166. Shurtleff, D. B. (1991). Computer data bases for pediatric disability: Clinical and research applications. In K. M. Jaffe (Ed.), *Physical Medicine and Rehabilitation Clinics of North America: Pediatric rehabilitation* (pp. 665–688). Philadelphia: WB Saunders.

167. Shurtleff, D. B., Duguay, S., Duguay, G., Moskowitz, D., Weinberger, E., Roberts, T., & Loeser, J. (1997). Epidemiology of tethered cord with meningomyelocele. *European Journal of Paediatric Surgery, 7*(Suppl 1), 7–11.

168. Shurtleff, D. B., & Dunne, K. (1986). Adults and adolescents with myelomeningocele. In D. B. Shurtleff (Ed.), *Myelodysplasias and exstrophies: Significance, prevention, and treatment* (pp. 433–448). Orlando, FL: Grune & Stratton.

169. Shurtleff, D. B., & Lamers, J. (1978). Clinical considerations in the treatment of myelodysplasia. In D. B. Crandal & M. A. B. Brazier (Eds.). *Prevention of neural tube defects: The role of alpha-fetoprotein* (pp. 103–122). New York: Academic Press.

170. Shurtleff, D. B., Lemire, R. J., & Warkany, J. (1986). Embryology, etiology and epidemiology. In D. B. Shurtleff (Ed.), *Myelodysplasias and exstrophies: Significance, prevention, and treatment* (pp. 39–64). Orlando, FL: Grune & Stratton.

171. Shurtleff, D. B., Luthy, D. A., Benededetti, T. J., & Mack, L. A. (1994). Meningomyelocele: Management in utero and post

partum. *Neural tube defects* (pp. 270–286). CIBA Foundation Symposium 181.

172. Shurtleff, D. B., & Mayo, M. (1986). Toilet training: The Seattle experience and conclusions. In D. B. Shurtleff (Ed.), *Myelodysplasias and exstrophies: Significance, prevention, and treatment* (pp. 267–284). Orlando, FL: Grune & Stratton.

173. Simeonsson, R. J., Huntington, G. S., McMillen, J. S., Halperin, D., & Swann, D. (1999). Development factors, health, and psychosocial adjustment of children and youths with spina bifida. In S. Matsumoto & H. Sato (Eds.). *Spina bifida* (pp. 543–551). New York: Springer Verlag.

174. Sival, D. A., Brouwer, O. F., Bruggink, J. L. M., et al. (2006). Movement analysis in neonates with spina bifida aperta. *Early Human Development, 82,* 227–234.

175. Sousa, J. C., Gordon, L. H., & Shurtleff, D. B. (1976). Assessing the development of daily living skills in patients with spina bifida. *Developmental Medicine and Child Neurology, 18*(Suppl 37), 134–142.

176. Sousa, J. C., Telzrow, R. W., Holm, R. A., McCartin, R., & Shurtleff, D. B. (1983). Developmental guidelines for children with myelodysplasia. *Journal of the American Physical Therapy Association, 63,* 21–29.

177. Stack, G. D., & Baber, G. C. (1967). The neurological involvement of the lower limbs in myelomeningocele. *Developmental Medicine and Child Neurology, 9,* 732.

178. Staheli, L. T. (2001). *Practice of pediatric orthopedics.* Philadelphia: Lippincott Williams & Wilkins.

179. Staheli, L. T. (1977). Prone hip extension test: Method of measuring hip flexion deformity. *Clinical Orthopedics, 123,* 12–15.

180. Stillwell, A., & Menelaus, M. B. (1983). Walking ability in mature patients with spina bifida. *Journal of Pediatric Orthopedics, 3,* 184–190.

181. Stuberg, W. A. (1992). Considerations related to weight-bearing program in children with developmental disabilities. *Physical Therapy, 72,* 35–40.

182. Stuberg, W. A., & Metcalf, W. K. (1988). Reliability of quantitative muscle testing in healthy children and in children with Duchenne muscular dystrophy using a hand-held dynamometer. *Physical Therapy, 68,* 977–982.

183. Sutton, L. N. (2008). Fetal surgery for neural tube defects. *Best Practice Research in Clinical Obstetrical Gynaecology 22,* 175–188.

184. Teulier, C., Smith, B. A., Kubo, M., et al. (2009). Stepping responses of infants with myelomeningocele when supported on a motorized treadmill. *Physical Therapy, 89*(1), 60–72.

185. Tew, B., & Laurence, K. M. (1975). The effects of hydrocephalus on intelligence, visual perception, and school attainments. *Developmental Medicine and Child Neurology, 17*(Suppl 35), 129–134.

186. Torode, I., & Godette, G. (1995). Surgical correction of congential kyphosis in myelomeningocele. *Journal of Pediatric Orthopedics, 15,* 202–205.

187. Tulipan, N., Sutton, L. N., & Cohen, B. M. (2003). The effect of intrauterine myelomeningocele repair on the incidence of shunt-dependent hydrocephalus. *Pediatric Neurosurgery, 38,* 27–33.

188. Turk, M. A. & Weber, R. J. (1998). Adults with congenital and childhood onset disability disorders. In J. B. DeLisa & B. M. Gans (Eds.). *Rehabilitation medicine: Principles and practice* (3rd ed., pp. 953–962). Philadelphia: Lippincott-Raven.

189. Vankoski, S., Moore, C., Satler, K., Sarwark, J. F., & Dias, L. (1995). The influence of forearm crutches on pelvic and hip kinematic parameters in childhood community ambulators with low-level myelomeningocele—Don't throw away the crutches. *Developmental Medicine & Child Neurology, 37*(Suppl 75), 5–6.

190. Weber, D., & Agro, M. (1993). *Clinical aspects of lower extremity orthotics.* Winnipeg, Manitoba: Canadian Association of Prosthetists and Orthotists.

191. Wicks, K., & Shurtleff, D. B. (1986a). An introduction to toilet training. In D. B. Shurtleff (Ed.), *Myelodysplasias and exstrophies: Significance, prevention, and treatment* (pp. 203–219). Orlando, FL: Grune & Stratton.

192. Wicks, K., & Shurtleff, D. B. (1986b). Stool management. In D. B. Shurtleff (Ed.), *Myelodysplasias and exstrophies: Significance, prevention, and treatment* (pp. 221–242). Orlando, FL: Grune & Stratton.

193. Williams, E. N., Broughton, N. S., & Menelaus, M. B. (1999). Age-related walking in children with spina bifida. *Developmental Medicine & Child Neurology, 41,* 446–449.

194. Williams, L. J., et al. (2002). Prevalence of spina bifida and anenecephaly during the transition to mandatory folic acid fortification in the United States. *Teratology, 66,* 33–39.

195. Williams, L. V., Anderson, A. D., Campbell, J., Thomas, L., Feiwell, E., & Walker, J. M. (1983). Energy cost of walking and of wheelchair propulsion by children with myelodysplasia: Comparison with normal children. *Developmental Medicine and Child Neurology, 25,* 617–624.

196. Winter, D. A. (1983). Knee flexion during stance as a determinant of inefficient walking. *Physical Therapy, 63,* 331–333.

197. Wolf, L. S., & McLaughlin, J. F. (1992). Early motor development in infants with myelomeningocele. *Pediatric Physical Therapy, 4,* 12–17.

198. Wright, J., Menelaus, M., Broughton, N., & Shurtleff, D. (1991). Natural history of knee contractures in myelomeningocele. *Journal of Pediatric Orthopedics, 11,* 725–730.

199. Zsolt, S., Seidl, R., Bernert, G., Dietrich, W., Spitzauer, S., & Urbanek, R. (1999). Latex sensitization in spina bifida appears disease-associated. *Journal of Pediatrics, 134,* 344–348.

23 Children Requiring Long-Term Mechanical Ventilation

HELENE M. DUMAS, PT, MS • M. KATHLEEN KELLY, PT, PhD

Mechanical ventilation (MV) is a life-sustaining form of medical technology that either substitutes for or assists a child's respiratory efforts. Children require MV as a treatment modality because of underlying disease processes resulting in respiratory insufficiency.

By definition, an individual is considered to be a *long-term* ventilator user if MV is required for longer than 6 hours per day for at least 3 weeks.[74] Although the degree of care and support varies from child to child, each child dependent on long-term MV requires high-cost care that demands sophisticated equipment and round-the-clock vigilance and monitoring.

The child with ventilator dependence represents a unique challenge for all health care professionals, as providers have moved beyond the goal of increasing survival rates and are now in the era of defining best practices that result in optimal quality-of-life outcomes. For the pediatric patient dependent on long-term MV, goals include minimizing impairments, reducing the incidence of activity limitations and disabilities, and ultimately maximizing participation in home, school, and community. The role of the pediatric physical therapist is an important one in addressing these issues.

Children dependent on MV may be seen by physical therapists in a hospital-based setting such as a neonatal or pediatric intensive care unit (NICU or PICU), in a tertiary care hospital, or in a hospital-based inpatient pulmonary rehabilitation program. Children dependent on MV may also be seen by a physical therapist in the community in a public or private school-based program, a medical day care setting, a home- or center-based early intervention program, and/or at home. This chapter suggests a framework for examination, diagnosis, and intervention strategies for children based on their need for long-term ventilatory assistance. The pathophysiologic processes that are commonly seen in pediatric practice are discussed, as are the common modes of ventilatory support. The reader is referred to several sources for a more in-depth discussion of ventilator equipment and medical management.

INCIDENCE

Although children dependent on long-term MV remain a small percentage of the overall group of children with special health care needs, population studies indicate that this group of children is growing. As a result of continuing advances in medical care, use of aggressive respiratory management for critically ill infants and children, and improved technology, the number of children who are dependent on MV continues to increase.[45,47] In the United States, prevalence estimates are available for the states of Utah[42] and Massachusetts.[45] In Massachusetts, the number of children dependent on MV has increased nearly threefold in a recent 15-year span from an estimated 70 children in 1990[94] to 197 in 2005.[45] In Utah, the number of children using MV at home increased by 33% from 1996 to 2004.[42] Outside the United States, studies also identify a steadily growing prevalence.[58,92]

Geographic differences in the prevalence of children with ventilator dependence may exist as a result of differing medical practices, parental expectations of long-term survival, and the expectation of being able to care for a child on a ventilator at home.[8,17,34,42,45,62,69] In addition, the ongoing introduction of new respiratory equipment for home care use and the presumption of an overall reduced cost of care have added to the positive expectations of care for children at home on a ventilator in various geographic regions.[5,33,34,108] Unfortunately, no central tracking system exists for documenting ventilator use, outcomes of care, or care settings for children dependent on long-term MV.[5,43,45]

Recent Massachusetts census data indicates that the highest percentage of children requiring MV is no longer due to the chronic lung disease associated with premature birth but rather is the result of congenital and neurologic disorders and neuromuscular diseases.[45] This shift is of particular importance to physical therapists because children with congenital, neurologic, and neuromuscular diagnoses are common diagnostic groups referred to physical therapists, and it is thus increasingly more likely that physical therapists will encounter a child who is dependent on MV. In a recent study of children requiring MV and admitted to one of six inpatient pulmonary rehabilitation programs in the Northeastern United States, 83% received rehabilitation services during their hospitalization, and 50% of those children discharged using ventilators required rehabilitation services following discharge from the hospital.[90]

CHRONIC RESPIRATORY FAILURE

The need for long-term MV is due to ongoing impaired respiratory function. Adequate respiratory function requires the effective exchange of oxygen and carbon dioxide with an organ for gas exchange (the lungs), a "pump" mechanism (the rib cage and respiratory muscles), and the neural control centers for breathing. Under normal conditions, one's respiratory function adapts to satisfy the changing metabolic needs that may occur during exercise, hyperthermia, or other demands, but when these systems are unable to deliver oxygen and remove carbon dioxide from the pulmonary circulation, respiratory failure ensues and gas exchange is impaired.[6]

Acute respiratory failure may develop in minutes or hours, whereas chronic respiratory failure develops over several days or weeks. Chronic respiratory failure is the result of an uncorrectable imbalance in the respiratory system in which a failure of the exchange of oxygen and carbon dioxide occurs within the alveoli, along with failure of the muscles required to expand the lungs and/or failure of the brain centers controlling respiration. In this situation, ventilatory muscle power and central respiratory drive are inadequate to overcome the respiratory load.[21] A distinctive aspect of children requiring long-term ventilator assistance is that they are united by chronic respiratory failure and dependence on technology and not by a common medical or rehabilitation diagnosis (Box 23-1).

In a wide variety of medical diagnoses, chronic respiratory failure is the result. Causes of chronic respiratory insufficiency in children have been grouped into the following categories: Conditions that affect the lungs, lung parenchyma, and airway (e.g., bronchopulmonary dysplasia [BPD], tracheobronchomalacia); conditions which cause central dysregulation of breathing (e.g., ischemic encephalopathy, traumatic brain injury, spinal cord injury); and diseases/disorders of the chest wall and thorax that affect the "respiratory pump" (e.g. spinal muscular atrophy, scoliosis)[5,6,88] (Table 23-1).

LUNGS, LUNG PARENCHYMA, AND AIRWAY

A common cause of primary lung failure is respiratory distress syndrome (RDS), in which primary lung or airway disease compromises pulmonary gas exchange. Respiratory distress syndrome, associated with preterm birth, pulmonary immaturity, and deficiency of surfactant, is a common cause of ventilator dependence in infants, as well as a major cause of neonatal death. Because of anatomic and physiologic immaturities, infants are predisposed to respiratory dysfunction such as atelectasis, airway obstruction, increased

---

Box **23-1** SIGNS OF CHRONIC RESPIRATORY FAILURE

CLINICAL SIGNS

Decreased inspiratory breath sounds
Use of accessory muscles/chest wall retractions
Altered depth and pattern of respiration (deep, shallow, apnea, irregular)
Weak cough
Nasal flaring
Wheezing/expiratory grunting/prolonged expiration
Retained airway secretions/incompetent swallowing/weak or absent gag reflex (neurologic, neuromuscular, and skeletal conditions)
Cyanosis
Tachycardia
Hypertension
Bradycardia
Hypotension

Cardiac arrest
Fatigue/Decreased level of activity
Poor weight gain
Excessive sweating
Changes in mental status
Retained airway secretions
Restlessness/irritability
Headache
Papilledema
Seizures
Coma

PHYSIOLOGIC/LABORATORY FINDINGS

Hypoxemia (acute or chronic): PaO_2 < 65 mm Hg
Hypercapnia (acute or chronic): $PaCO_2$ > 45 mm Hg
O_2 saturation <95% breathing room air (metabolic or respiratory)

From Laghi, F., & Tobin, M. (2006). Indications for mechanical ventilation. In M. Tobin (Ed.), *Principles and practice of mechanical ventilation* (2nd ed.; pp. 129–162). New York: McGraw-Hill Companies; American College of Chest Physicians.
Mechanical ventilation: Beyond the ICU quick reference guide. (July 2009). Retrieved from: http://www.chestnet.org/education/cs/mech_vent/qrg/p14.php.

TABLE 23-1 **Common Pathophysiologic Mechanisms Leading to Chronic Respiratory Failure**

Lungs, Lung Parenchyma, and Airway	Central Dysregulation of Breathing	Diseases/Disorders of the Chest Wall and Thorax (Pump Failure)
Bronchopulmonary dysplasia	Congenital central hypoventilation syndrome	Congenital myopathies
Respiratory distress syndrome	Infectious disease of the brain/brainstem	Muscular dystrophies
Chronic lung disease of infancy	Brain tumor	Phrenic nerve trauma
Tracheobronchomalacia	Arnold-Chiari malformation	Diaphragmatic dysfunction
Tracheomegaly	Traumatic brain injury	Botulism
Tracheoesophogeal fistula	Spinal cord injury	Dwarfism
Subglottic stenosis	Intracranial hemorrhage	Scoliosis
Laryngeal atresia	Hypoxic encephalopathy	Guillain-Barré syndrome
Bronchial atresia		

Data from O'Brien et al., 2006; Amin & Fitton, 2003; and American Thoracic Society, 2003.

pulmonary vascular resistance, and pulmonary edema. As well, they are predisposed to diaphragmatic fatigue and instability in the neural control of breathing. Recent additions to the armamentarium for treatment of neonatal respiratory distress include antenatal steroids, surfactant replacement therapy, oxygen therapy, and high-frequency ventilators used in the early neonatal period.[12]

As smaller and more immature babies survive requiring prolonged MV, they are at risk for the unfortunate sequelae of ventilator-induced lung injury resulting in bronchopulmonary dysplasia (BPD) and chronic lung disease of infancy (CLDI).[7,97] BPD, first described by Northway et al. in 1967,[85] is diagnosed when an infant is 28 days of chronologic age, continues to require supplemental oxygen, and has an abnormal clinical examination and chest radiograph.[5] CLDI is diagnosed at 36 weeks of postmenstrual age if the clinical examination and chest radiographs continue to be abnormal and the need for oxygen is still present. BPD accounts for the majority of cases of CLDI.[5]

BPD is associated with low birth weight, prematurity, and severe initial lung disease. It is thought that structural changes in the lung parenchyma occur as a result of both increased ventilatory pressures over a period of time and prolonged exposure to high levels of oxygen tension. A newer and milder form of BPD has emerged as a result of surfactant administration and improved critical care practices that are more lung-protective.[25,96] The classification of BPD is based on several factors, first defined by the age at birth being older or younger than 32 weeks. From that point, disease severity is categorized as mild, moderate, or severe based on the need for supplemental oxygen or positive-pressure ventilation at 36 weeks of postmenstrual age for infants born before 32 weeks or 56 days of postnatal age for infants born at 32 weeks or after. This new phenotype is characterized by impaired/disrupted alveolar development, rather than the airway damage and fibrosis seen in the classical form of BPD.[5,57,96]

Although no major breakthroughs have occurred in the prevention of BPD, long-term outcomes have improved and disease severity is reduced as a result of improvements in medical and pharmacologic treatment. For example, the goal of high-frequency ventilation is to adequately ventilate at lower intrapulmonary pressures and smaller tidal volumes, thereby reducing the degree of barotrauma and volutrauma to the immature airways, and to reduce the risks of pulmonary air leaks.[54,59,104] The use of surfactant therapy is now standard practice, and its use has contributed substantially to reduced morbidity rates. A wide variety of surfactant types are available, including both artificial surfactant and surfactant derived from animal sources.[59]

In addition to respiratory support, the treatment of BPD includes nutritional support; pharmacologic interventions such as bronchodilators, anti-inflammatory drugs, sedatives, and diuretics; and developmental care and follow-up. These infants require ongoing monitoring of their physiologic status to ensure physiologic stability. Although many infants "recover" from BPD and eventually function independent of assisted ventilation and supplemental oxygen if conditions for growth are optimized, a small proportion go on to require prolonged ventilation.[5] The reader is referred to Chapter 28 for more detailed information on RDS, BPD, and CLDI.

Congenital and acquired anomalies of the airway may also be primary causes of chronic respiratory failure leading to a dependence on MV. Airway abnormalities of the trachea such as tracheomalacia, tracheomegaly, tracheal atresia; abnormalities of the bronchi such as bronchial atresia, bronchial stenosis, and bronchomalacia; laryngeal atresia; tracheal and esophageal fistulas; and subglottic stenosis can all prevent alveolar ventilation and necessitate positive pressure and MV.[6]

CENTRAL DYSREGULATION OF BREATHING

Central dysregulation of breathing is characterized by disorders affecting the central respiratory centers (i.e., brainstem or cervical spinal cord). An example of this is congenital central hypoventilation syndrome (CCHS) (previously known as Ondine's curse), a rare disorder that presents very shortly after birth or early in infancy. CCHS is characterized by failure of the autonomic control of ventilation in the absence of primary pulmonary or neuromuscular disease or in the absence of a brainstem lesion. CCHS is postulated to be due to a defect in the *PHOX2B* homeobox gene, the product of which is a transcription factor important for regulation of neural crest cell migration (see chapter on Genomics and Genetic Syndromes Affecting Movement) on the Evolve website.[10,68,72] This disorder is generally diagnosed in the neonatal period when the infant experiences apneic episodes during sleep or while awake. CCHS is known to be associated with genetic or oncologic conditions such as Hirschsprung's disease[66,98,101] and neuroblastoma.[98] Although the incidence of CCHS is low, this group of patients faces a lifelong dependence on MV, almost exclusively with positive-pressure ventilators or diaphragmatic pacemakers. Early treatment is essential to minimize the neurologic effects of hypoxia.[68]

Disorders of the brainstem that affect respiration typically result from trauma, infectious disease processes, brainstem tumors, or complications of Arnold-Chiari malformations.[112] In these instances, chronic respiratory failure may be transient or long term and may present as apnea or other sleep-disordered breathing. Traumatic injuries or acquired disorders of the spinal cord can also result in chronic respiratory failure, leading to dependence on MV. The prognosis for dependence on MV depends on the level of the lesion, the extent of nerve damage, and the nature of the lesion.[26,63,93] Typically, with injuries involving the upper cervical or cervicothoracic area, respiration is compromised because of phrenic and intercostal nerve root damage affecting the function of the diaphragmatic and accessory muscles of respiration. Patients with cervical-level injuries usually require MV throughout the entire day and night or, occasionally, only at night.[63] The rate and extent of recovery of respiratory sufficiency and motor function after a spinal cord injury are contributing factors to quality-of-life outcomes.[83]

RESPIRATORY PUMP FAILURE

Failure of the respiratory pump may be caused by impaired neural control of respiration or by inadequate force generation of the respiratory muscles as the result of primary muscle disease, spinal cord injury, chest wall defects, or muscle fatigue. As a result, the respiratory pump is unable to facilitate and sustain adequate alveolar ventilation[6] (Figure 23-1).

For example, spinal muscular atrophy, a hereditary and progressive anterior horn cell disease, results in generalized hypotonia and paralysis of the limb and trunk musculature. If respiratory involvement is present and noted in the early postnatal period, it is usually severe, leading to ventilator dependence very early in the child's life (see Chapter 12).

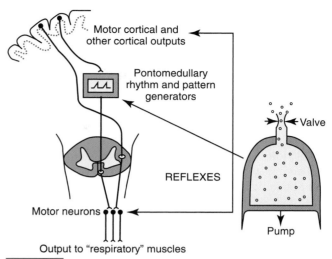

Figure 23-1   Schema illustrating the cortical control of respiration. Corticospinal and bulbospinal pathways with direct input to the respiratory motor neurons and the connection between the motor cortex and pontomedullary centers in the brainstem are shown. The respiratory motoneuron output directs the activity of the respiratory "pump," as well as the upper airway ("valve"). Reflex pathways provide feedback to the motor neurons, medulla, and cortex.

Intrinsic muscle disease is another common cause of chronic respiratory failure in children. Those with congenital myopathies typically manifest symptoms of respiratory failure early in the course of the disease, whereas those with muscular dystrophies typically do not present with respiratory compromise until late childhood or early adolescence. In either case, MV may be warranted to compensate for the significantly reduced respiratory muscle function.[108]

Infants have an increased chest wall compliance that decreases with age as the ribs move in a downward vertical direction with growth and development. Congenital anomalies of the thorax and rib cage may result in pulmonary hypoplasia and significantly decreased lung volumes due to reduced chest wall compliance or structural abnormalities that restrict lung and chest expansion. Thoracic abnormalities are associated with a variety of syndromes such as asphyxiating thoracic dystrophy, arthrogryposis (Chapter 10), osteogenesis imperfecta (Chapter 11), and dwarfism, as well as scoliosis (Chapter 8). Treatment of these various impairments varies; however, in some cases, the child may require MV.

MECHANICAL VENTILATION

Although the underlying disease processes and severity of respiratory failure differ considerably among individuals, MV is the final common treatment approach for individuals with chronic respiratory failure.[6] MV and the artificial airways used to facilitate it are designed to assist or substitute for a person's respiratory efforts (i.e., moving air into and out of the lungs).[70,110]

The decision to institute long-term MV is often made as a lifesaving measure, and MV is increasingly used electively to preserve physiologic function and improve quality of life. In many instances involving infants and children, the clinical decision is made to take advantage of the growth and maturational potential of the lungs,[74] and to maximize the child's overall developmental potential. Thus, the desired outcome for many children is medical stability with adequate growth and healing of the lungs, and eventual withdrawal of assisted ventilation.

Because so many combinations of ventilatory attributes can obtain desirable results, practices are far from uniform, and often scientific research is lacking.[16,74,75] The optimal settings for each patient vary and are determined by the patient's metabolic requirements, respiratory drive, and pulmonary mechanics.[6,100] The type of MV and the various parameters chosen depend on a number of considerations. These include the age of the patient, an understanding of the underlying disease process that precipitated ventilatory failure, available equipment, knowledge of the current literature, previous experience with specific types of machines, and site of care (e.g., pediatric intensive care unit [PICU], home environment)[108] (Table 23-2). In general, ventilators are adjusted to maintain an oxygen saturation >95% and a CO_2 tension within the range of 35 to 45 mm Hg while the child is awake or asleep.[6]

TABLE 23-2 Selection Criteria for Mechanical Ventilation

Parameter	Findings
CLINICAL	
Respiratory*	Apnea; decreased breath sounds; rigorous chest wall movement; weakening ventilatory effort
Cardiac	Asystole; peripheral collapse; severe bradycardia or tachycardia
Cerebral	Coma; lack of response to physical stimuli; uncontrolled restlessness; anxious facial expression
General	Limpness; loss of ability to cry
LABORATORY†	
$PaCO_2$	Newborn: >60–65 mm Hg
	Older child: >55–60 mm Hg
	Rapidly rising >5 mm Hg
PaO_2	Newborn: <40–50 mm Hg
	Older child: <50–60 mm Hg

From Laghi, F., & Tobin, M. (2006). Indications for mechanical ventilation. In M. Tobin (Ed.), *Principles and practice of mechanical ventilation* (2nd ed.; pp. 129–162). New York: McGraw-Hill Companies.
*More than one episode of apnea with bradycardia or an episode of cardiac arrest is an adequate indication for initiating mechanical ventilation (MV), even in the absence of blood gas data.
†Laboratory values less extreme than those indicated must be supplemented by clinical evidence of severity to warrant initiating MV.

Since the beginning of the modern era of MV in the 1950s, ventilators have undergone, and continue to undergo, significant technologic advances.[74] Specifically, pediatric MV has undergone continual changes that reflect increased knowledge, understanding, and appreciation of the developing cardiorespiratory system. Currently, ventilation approaches utilize protective strategies to avoid atelectotrauma and lung overdistention through the use of maximal alveolar pressures, minimal positive end-expiratory pressure, and permissive hypercapnia.[35,40,74] Contemporary knowledge of respiratory physiology and a more detailed understanding of the pathophysiologic mechanisms underlying diseases of the respiratory system continue to drive research and development in this area. Although it is beyond the scope and intent of this chapter to detail available technical information on MV, a brief overview of MV will be provided.

Positive-pressure ventilation (PPV) is the most commonly used assisted ventilation strategy. Most often, PPV is delivered invasively via an endotracheal (for the short term in the tertiary care hospital) or tracheostomy tube (for the long term) with pressurized gas delivered into the airways and ventilator circuit during inspiration until the ventilator breath is terminated. As the airway pressure drops to zero, elastic recoil of the chest accomplishes passive exhalation by pushing the tidal volume out.

Positive-pressure ventilators are classified by their method of cycling from the inspiratory phase to the expiratory phase. Thus, they are named after the parameter that signals the termination of the positive-pressure inspiratory cycle of the machine. The signal to terminate the inspiratory activity of the ventilator may be a preset *volume* (for a volume-cycled ventilator), a preset *pressure* limit (for a pressure-cycled ventilator), a preset *time* factor (for a time-cycled ventilator), or a preset *flow* with a constant tidal volume (Table 23-3). In addition, some modes of ventilation are based on the patterns of ventilation that are being produced (Box 23-2).

Positive-pressure ventilatory support may also be accomplished noninvasively.[23,39,51,102] Positive pressure via face mask can be accomplished using continuous positive airway pressure (CPAP) or bi-level positive airway pressure (BiPAP). CPAP applies continuous distending pressure to the alveoli throughout the entire respiratory cycle, keeping the alveoli partially inflated so that they may expand more easily with each cycle. CPAP may be delivered nasally, thus minimizing discomfort.[30] BiPAP uses cycling variations between two CPAP levels, allowing spontaneous breathing during every ventilatory phase[56] and has been used effectively to wean children from long-term MV.[95]

In addition to the obvious advantage of avoiding a tracheostomy, noninvasive forms of PPV reduce the risk of acquired infection and allow patients to be more mobile.[23,64] Difficulties with noninvasive ventilation in children, however, such as poor mask fit, inadequate ventilation because of leaks, and eye irritation and nasal dryness due to high flow, have been reported. In addition, the use of

TABLE 23-3   **Classification of Positive-Pressure Ventilators**

Control Variables	Phase Variable Categories
Variables that the ventilator manipulates to cause inspiration; only one variable can be controlled at a time	Control variables measured and used by the ventilator to initiate some phase of the breath cycle
Pressure: Ventilator has a set pressure, thus mechanical ventilation terminates when a preselected inspiratory pressure is achieved	Trigger variables: These variables reach some preset peak threshold to begin inspiration
Volume: Ventilator maintains a constant volume irrespective of changes in pulmonary mechanics	Limit variables: These variables reach a preset level before inspiration ends
Flow: Ventilator maintains a constant tidal volume	Cycle variables: These control variables are used to end inspiration
Time: Ventilator maintains a constant time between inspiration and expiration	Baseline: These control variables are controlled during expiratory time

Adapted from Chatburn, R. L., & Primiano, F. P. (2001). A new system for understanding mechanical ventilation. *Respiratory Care, 46,* 604–621.

Box **23-2**   MODES OF INVASIVE POSITIVE-PRESSURE VENTILATION

- Continuous mandatory ventilation (CMV)—All breaths are mandatory; full ventilator support
- Continuous spontaneous ventilation—All breaths are spontaneous
- Intermittent mandatory ventilation (IMV)—Intermittent breaths are at a fixed rate and are not synchronized to the patient
- Assist/control (AC) ventilation—Mandatory breaths are triggered by patient's inspiratory effort (or within a preset time)
- Synchronized intermittent mandatory ventilation (SIMV)—Patient can take unassisted spontaneous breaths, which are synchronized with mandatory breaths at some preset volume and rate
- Proportional assisted ventilation—Every ventilator breath is proportional to the patient's respiratory effort

Note: Portable positive-pressure ventilation may not be designed to operate within certain limits and may not be able to handle dynamic changes in respiratory physiology.
Adapted from numerous sources, listed in the references at the end of the chapter (Chatburn & Primiano, 2001; Donn & Sinha, 2002; Gali & Goyal, 2003; and Make et al., 1998).

---

noninvasive ventilation is limited in patients with congenital facial anomalies, which may preclude a tight-fitting mask, and with conditions that have the potential for infection, such as facial trauma or burns.[64] Rapid technological and medical advances should continue to lead to increased utilization of this mode of assisted ventilation in the future.

Another strategy for noninvasive MV is the use of negative-pressure ventilation (NPV). NPV provides a pressure gradient, which is established by creating a negative pressure around the person's entire body (from the neck down) during inspiration, causing air to enter the lungs. The typical interface used with this type of ventilation is a customized chest shell, a wrap/poncho, or a tank ventilator. A major advantage of NPV is that it avoids or delays the need for a tracheostomy, thereby reducing the risk of infection. Another advantage of NPV is that ventilation is not interrupted when secretions are suctioned.[74,108] NPV has been used most successfully for patients with normal lung mechanics and hypoventilation, as seen in patients with neuromuscular disease and pulmonary disease requiring periodic or nocturnal ventilatory support.[78] The limitations of NPV are that airway occlusion may occur in infants and young children during sleep, and the chest shell or wrap is not effective for children who require high respiratory rates, tidal volumes, or distending pressures; thus NPV is not commonly used in the latter.[75]

To avoid complications related to controlled MV, emphasis on the use of partial ventilatory assistance is increasing. Ideally, the desirable mode of ventilation is one with optimal synchrony and patient-ventilator interface, along with the use of lung-protective strategies.[30,81] With the advent of microprocessor technology, newer models of ventilators are able to offer greater flexibility with respect to their modes of ventilatory delivery.[16,22,30]

Although long-term MV has decreased mortality rates for infants and children, complications that have an impact on overall health, growth and development, and quality of life are frequently reported. Long-term invasive PPV requires a tracheostomy, which increases the complexities of care. Complications due to tracheotomy such as tracheitis, accidental decannulation, tracheal ulceration, or granuloma development are common.[20] Tracheostomy placement and/or complications require routine surgical surveillance or surgical intervention (bronchoscopy),[60] placing the child at further risk. An artificial airway also interferes with speech and nutrition.[75] Secondary illnesses such as ventilator-associated pneumonia[106] and respiratory syncytial virus infection[114] have been reported.

Although MV has had a significant impact on the outcomes of children with respiratory failure, one needs to

---

BOX 23-3 COMPLICATIONS ASSOCIATED WITH MECHANICAL VENTILATION

RESPIRATORY

Tracheal lesions (erosion, edema, stenosis, granuloma, obstruction, perforation)

Accidental endotracheal tube displacement or actual extubation

Air leaks (pneumothorax, pneumomediastinum, interstitial emphysema)

Infection (tracheitis, pneumonitis)

Trapping of gas (hyperinflation)

Excessive secretions (atelectasis)

Oxygen hazards (depression of ventilation, bronchopulmonary dysplasia)

Pulmonary hemorrhage

CIRCULATORY

Impairment of venous return (decreased cardiac output and systemic hypotension)

Oxygen hazard (retrolental fibroplasia, cerebral vasoconstriction)

Septicemia

Intracranial hemorrhage

Hyperventilation (decreased cerebral blood flow)

GASTROINTESTINAL

Gastrointestinal hypomotility

Stress ulcer

METABOLIC

Increased work of breathing ("fighting the ventilator")

Alkalosis (potassium depletion, excessive bicarbonate therapy)

RENAL AND FLUID BALANCE

Antidiuresis

Excess water in inspired gas

EQUIPMENT MALFUNCTION

Power source failure

Improper humidification (overheating of inspired gas, inspiratory line condensation)

Improper tubing connections (kinked line, disconnection)

Ventilation malfunction (leaks, valve dysfunction)

From Epstein, S. K. (2006). Complications associated with mechanical ventilation. In M. Tobin (Ed.), *Principles and practice of mechanical ventilation* (2nd ed.). New York: McGraw-Hill Companies; Mutlu, G. K. M., Mutlu, E. A., & Factor, P. (2001). GI complications in patients receiving mechanical ventilation. *Chest, 119,* 1222–1241; and Attar, M. A., & Donn, S. M. (2002). Mechanisms of ventilator-induced lung injury in premature infants. *Seminars in Neonatology, 7,* 353–360.

---

appreciate the unwanted effects of secondary lung injury that can occur with PPV.[23] Numerous complications can occur with invasive PPV (Box 23-3). It is essential that individuals who work with children who require long-term MV understand normal and pathologic respiratory physiology, the anatomic and physiologic changes of the developing respiratory system, and how the machine interfaces with the patient's physiology.[16,23,65,75]

ENVIRONMENT OF CARE

Infants in a neonatal intensive care unit (NICU) may be placed on MV because of lung or airway anomalies, neurologic disorders affecting respiration, or disorders of the respiratory pump. A study by Vohr et al. indicated that length of time on MV in the NICU ranged from 16 to 40 days across multiple centers for infants who were born prematurely.[113] Children in a PICU may be placed on MV for postsurgical indications; as the result of recent trauma, illness, or organ failure; or because of a history of chronic respiratory failure. Only a small percentage of these children will require long-term MV.[44,111] Once the decision has been made to mechanically ventilate an infant or child for an extended length of time, immediate thoughts should be

toward the long-term impact of a prolonged hospitalization and the alternatives.

In recent years, the locus of inpatient care for children dependent on MV has shifted from acute care hospital neonatal and pediatric ICUs to post-acute inpatient pulmonary rehabilitation programs. ICUs are referring children to rehabilitation units, where they can spend longer periods of time at a lower financial cost. In the post-ICU environment, children may be weaned from their oxygen or ventilators or weaned to a less invasive mode of ventilation.[18,61,89,90] Weaning ventilator support to the least invasive mode possible to optimize safe discharge home while providing a developmentally appropriate environment with necessary rehabilitation services appears to be an appropriate expectation.[2,90] Parent–child interaction, parent education, and growth and development can be promoted along with achievement of medical stability. This is an important consideration for referring children to rehabilitation programs and for setting realistic expectations for referral sources, patient and families, clinical staff, and payers. A limited number of rehabilitation facilities, however, admit children who are ventilator dependent.[89,90]

Whether fully weaned, weaned to fewer hours per day of MV, or weaned to a less invasive mode of ventilation, the ultimate goal is to discharge children home. When medically stable on a ventilator suitable for nonhospital use and with appropriate caregiver support, children dependent on MV can be cared for at home and can participate in community activities.[34,41,87] Technological advances in design, efficiency, and portability have contributed to an increase in the use of MV outside the hospital environment. This option is dependent on many factors, but primarily on a stable airway, an oxygen requirement typically less than 40%, a $PaCO_2$ level not more than 10% above baseline, and an adequate nutritional intake to maintain growth and development.[88] Home ventilation minimizes nosocomial infections and improves children's psychosocial development, social integration, and quality of life.[71,83]

Over the past decade or longer, emphasis on home care and its impact on improving quality of life for children with ventilator dependence has been increasing.[19,47] Barriers to discharge from the hospital exist, however, including the inability to recruit qualified home nursing staff; inadequate or delayed funding of home care resources; unsuitable housing; delays in obtaining the appropriate equipment; and a limited number of capable family caregivers.[34,76,86]

It is imperative that the family or designated caregivers be involved in, and capable of learning, all aspects of the child's care.[34,41,86] This care includes not only managing the ventilator and other monitoring equipment, but also being able to provide emergency medical procedures if the child experiences distress and, most important, the ability to recognize signs of distress. The high degree of medical and technological expertise required by parents or caregivers can be a tremendous drain on a family.[34,62,115,116] The critical nature of this type of family teaching goes beyond our normal expectations of the family unit, so caregivers may need extensive support from various health care team members.

The transition to home carries with it other circumstances that can contribute to increased stress such as financial burden and significant changes in a family's routine, lifestyle, and relationships. The shift in responsibility for medical care from health care professionals to the family has resulted in a myriad of issues that require psychological, social, ethical, financial, and policy solutions.[13,115,116] In many cases, an often overlooked indirect cost is that the primary caregiver has to leave the work force to care for the child.[115] Although these added burdens do not necessarily outweigh the tremendous benefits of children being raised at home and integrated into their communities, they can be overwhelming and can have an impact on the quality of life of the child and family.[47,91] Fortunately, efforts to formulate social and public policies around the unique needs of this population have expanded.[79,115] It has been suggested that a social model of disability more appropriately captures the needs of these individuals and their families and highlights the responsibilities of society to meet the needs of individuals with disabilities.[115]

As the degree and complexity of impairment, activity limitations, and disabilities increase, quality of life usually decreases—especially when financial, psychosocial, and emotional supports dwindle. With this in mind, one of the most important roles of the various health care providers is to work closely with family members as a child is being considered for discharge from the hospital and while at home. Parents should expect health care professionals to give them as much information as needed to make an informed decision about their abilities to care for their child at home, as well as the risks and benefits.[52] A family's coping skills and lifestyle needs should always be at the forefront of any parent–professional relationship and a major consideration of any rehabilitation program that might be recommended.[115] It is essential that the child's therapy program be integrated into the family's daily routine and not be the sole focus of a family's daily schedule.

For children using MV at home, however, hospital re-admissions are common following an acute respiratory illness or surgical procedure.[11,27,34,41,87] Burdens of a hospital re-admission for the child and family may include separation from family, coping with the illness itself, and financial concerns such as loss of income and the cost of the hospital admission.[82] Children and families can also face the possibility of a breakdown in their established network of community service providers caused by the interruption in service. Unplanned re-admissions to the acute care or rehabilitation hospital may cause a strain on inpatient staffing as the medical acuity of these children is high.[62]

ACTIVITY LIMITATIONS ASSOCIATED WITH LONG-TERM MECHANICAL VENTILATION

As was noted previously, a wide range of pathophysiologic mechanisms underlie dependence on MV, hence this "medical" diagnosis represents a diverse and heterogeneous group of children with varying impairments and functional capabilities. Despite differences, these children are similar in that they may be medically fragile and at risk for physical, mental, and psychosocial disabilities. Although the predictive value of any one risk factor is not well established, it appears that long-term outcome depends on the interaction of biologic and environmental factors.

The literature base on long-term developmental, motor, or functional outcomes for infants and children requiring prolonged MV is limited. The group that has been studied most extensively consists of infants and children with BPD. The morbidity associated with BPD includes not only associated chronic respiratory problems but other growth- and development-related factors.[9] For example, linear and anthropometric growth are often adversely affected by BPD.[55]

Singer and colleagues reported poorer performance on developmental indices for infants with BPD than for infants not affected by BPD and followed longitudinally to 3 years of age; 98% of the infants with BPD had required MV.[103] Thomas et al. reported in a study of 417 preterm infants with very low birth weight (VLBW), that a greater proportion of those infants with prolonged and continuous MV as opposed to discontinuous ventilation had a poorer neurodevelopmental outcome at 1 year of age.[109] Gaillard and colleagues reported that at 3 years of age, infants receiving prolonged MV for >49 days were more likely than those ventilated for <49 days to have a severe disability.[38] Similarly, Wocadlo and Rieger reported that 31% of preterm infants (<30 weeks of gestation) assessed at 8 years of age had a developmental coordination disorder (DCD) (see Chapter 16), and that those with DCD had required more MV support during their hospital admission.[118]

The child dependent on long-term MV is at risk for activity limitations related to communication[53] and oral feeding[1] because of tracheostomy placement. Limitations in motor activities may be due to fatigue, cardiorespiratory endurance, or access to environmental surroundings because of tubing length and the ventilator itself. The lack of variable practice opportunities makes motor skill acquisition difficult, and thus the repertoire of skills in a variety of developmental domains is limited (see Chapter 4 for additional details on motor learning concepts). As a point of illustration, the acquisition of independent mobility in typically developing children allows them to acquire information about their world and develop perceptions upon which they can act. Thus, development of cognitive skills such as object permanence is facilitated through motoric competencies. This interweaving of developmental domains and their interdependence is a well-known phenomenon, so the impact of atypical circumstances and lack of environmental affordances can be substantial. Thus, it is apparent why children dependent on long-term MV may present with global developmental delays, despite having no history of neurologic insults.

A recent case study described the achievement of independent ambulation while a child was using CPAP. An 18-month-old child with CLDI and tracheobronchomalacia was provided a new CPAP device that allowed compressed air to be delivered via tracheostomy tube with extended tubing. It was hypothesized that the shorter, heavier tubing of the traditional CPAP device had severely restricted the child's mobility, but the application of the new CPAP device afforded the child the space to move up to 10 meters, and thus, psychomotor development was stimulated.[28] Unfortunately, no studies documenting the relationship of physical therapist interventions and ventilator weaning or motor/mobility outcomes are available for children dependent on MV.

In addition to the aforementioned developmental risks, the additive effects of secondary complications such as recurrent hypoxic episodes,[73] recurrent infections, poor weight gain, and poor physical growth can directly result in any number of impairments and subsequent activity limitations.[14,103] For example, because of the often prolonged periods of immobility or restricted activity early in the course of their disease, children may demonstrate impairments such as sensory defensiveness, generalized weakness, and soft tissue or muscular tightness. Likewise, if the child has had some type of hypoxic or ischemic episode, neurologic damage may additionally limit motor skill acquisition and execution.

Regardless of the reason for dependence on MV, appreciation of the fact that the child is at a disadvantage in terms of developmental risk is a compelling reason to begin early intervention as soon as the infant or child is medically stable. Because of the risks for abnormal neurodevelopmental sequelae, physical therapists should be involved with providing developmental intervention early in the course of an infant's hospitalization. Delays in the initiation of rehabilitation or habilitation may place the child at increased risk for developing secondary impairments and activity limitations and may prevent community participation that could otherwise be facilitated.[46,67]

ELEMENTS OF PHYSICAL THERAPIST PATIENT MANAGEMENT

In addition to an understanding of typical and atypical motor skill development, the physical therapist who works with infants, children, and adolescents dependent on MV should have a thorough understanding of cardiorespiratory physiology and the implications of a compromise to that system in the developing infant or child. Physical therapists should be aware of the pathophysiology of chronic respiratory failure, the physiologic conditions requiring MV, the parameters of ventilator machinery, the varied types of MV, and the use of physiologic monitoring devices (Table 23-4). Types and settings of ventilators used will vary according to the child's age and diagnosis, anticipated results, site of care, availability of equipment, and providers' knowledge and experience with specific types of ventilators. Although the infant or child may be medically stable, the presence of an artificial airway creates a critical situation because it may become dislodged or occluded. In addition, the infant or young child may not communicate well, thus it is up to the therapist to interpret any signs of impending or actual distress. The essence of physical therapy intervention is to ensure that no harm be done in the delivery of services while achievement of the child's functional potential is optimized.

Before any examination or intervention session, the therapist should confer with the child's primary nurse or caregiver to determine the child's current medical status, in addition to his baseline physiologic parameters. Depending on the nature and severity of the predisposing condition, cardiorespiratory parameters may vary from what is considered to be typical for the child's age (Table 23-5). It is always prudent to establish safe physiologic parameters within

TABLE 23-4 Commonly Encountered Noninvasive Monitoring Devices*

Equipment	Physiologic Parameters Monitored
Cardiorespiratory monitors	Heart rate and respiratory rate
Pulse oximeter[†]	Transcutaneous arterial oxygen saturation to monitor hypoxemia
Ventilator alarms	Various modes chosen for the individual case, as well as airway pressures, gas concentrations, and expiratory tidal volumes
Transcutaneous PaO_2 and $PaCO_2$	Partial pressure of oxygen and carbon dioxide in the arterial blood
Oxygen analyzers on the ventilator	Oxygen supply in the ventilator circuit
Sphygmomanometer	Blood pressure

*These are some noninvasive devices that one may use to monitor response to activity and general status. Before any examination or treatment session, the therapist should be familiar with all of the equipment used for the child.
[†]Pulse oximeters are not useful for discriminating hyperoxia because the blood is fully saturated at PaO_2 of 150 mm Hg.

which to work. Typically, heart rate, respiratory rate, and oxygen saturation are monitored while the child is on the ventilator. In the home or outpatient setting, one may choose to monitor these parameters periodically; however, no substitute is known for the keen visual observation of signs of distress.

EXAMINATION

As with any child referred for physical therapy services, the therapist must first complete a comprehensive examination that includes a history, a systems review, and specific tests and measures.[4] Because of varying ages, diagnoses and prognoses, and intervention settings for children dependent on MV, tests and measures must be aimed at quantifying a child's aerobic capacity and endurance, adequacy of respiration, motor function, musculoskeletal performance (flexibility, strength, posture), and general adaptive behaviors that are age-appropriate and most relevant to the child and family goals and the clinical setting.

Physical therapists should understand the type of mechanical ventilator being used by the child. The therapist should understand whether the ventilator is doing all the work of breathing for the child, or whether it is assisting the

TABLE 23-5 Normal Ranges of Physiologic Values*

Parameter	Newborn/Infant (<1 year)	Older Infant and Child
Respiratory rate	24–40 40–70 (preterm infant)	20–30 (1–3 years) 20–24 (4–9 years) 14–20 (≥10 years)
Heart rate	100–160 120–170 (preterm infant)	70–120 (1–10 years) 60–100 (≥10 years)
BLOOD PRESSURE, MM HG		
Systolic	60–90 55–75 (preterm infant)	80–130 (1–3 years) 90–140 (>3 years)
Diastolic	30–60 35–45 (preterm infant)	45–90 (≤3 years) 50–80 (>3 years)
PaO_2 (mm Hg)	60–90	80–100
$PaCO_2$ (mm Hg)	30–35	30–35 (≤2 years) 35–45 (>2 years)
Arterial oxygen saturation (%)	87–89 (low) 94–95 (high) 90–95 (preterm infant)	95–100

Data from Bardella, I. J. (1999). Pediatric advanced life support: A review of the AHA recommendations. *American Family Physician. 60,* 1743–1752; Fang, J. C., & O'Gara, P. T. (2007). The history and physical examination: An evidence-based approach. In P. Libby, R. O. Bonow, D. L. Mann, & D. P. Zipes (Eds.), *Braunwald's heart disease: A textbook of cardiovascular medicine* (8th ed.; Chapter 11). Philadelphia, PA: Saunders Elsevier; Sekaran, D. V., Subramanyam, L., & Balachandran, A. (2001). Arterial blood gas analysis in clinical practice. *Indian Pediatrics, 38,* 1116–1128; Chernick, V., Boat, T. F., Wilmott, R. W., & Bush, A. (2006). *Kendig's disorders of the respiratory tract in children* (7th ed.). St Louis, MO: Elsevier; Dieckmann, R., Brownstein, D., & Gausche-Hill, M. (Eds.) (2000). *Pediatric education for prehospital professionals* (pp. 43–45). Sudbury, MA: Jones & Bartlett, American Academy of Pediatrics; American Heart Association ECC Guidelines, 2000.
*These values represent "normal" physiologic values; in the case of infants and children with varying pathophysiologic processes, the "normal" values may be different.

child with the number and/or depth of breaths. Physical therapists should also be aware of the clinical signs that may indicate that the child needs respiratory assistance and should familiarize themselves with the alarm systems of the ventilator, monitors that record oxygen saturation levels, heart and respiratory rates, and the emergency response procedures of the care setting. Therapists should be comfortable observing the patient for signs of respiratory distress, skin color changes indicative of hypoxia, and changes in respiratory rate, breathing pattern, symmetry of chest expansion, posture, and general comfort.[4] Signs of respiratory distress such as retractions, nasal flaring, expiratory grunting, and stridor may not be evident when a child is on a mechanical ventilator. For more information specific to the assessment of the cardiorespiratory system, the reader is referred elsewhere.[80]

The neuromuscular/musculoskeletal examination should provide information about the child's general neurologic and musculoskeletal status and includes assessment of strength, flexibility, sensation, posture, and general movement competencies. Examination procedures will vary, depending on the age and cognitive level of the child, and areas of emphasis may be different, depending on the diagnosis, the care setting, and child and family goals. Last, an important component is the measurement of neuromotor development and motor control. This is an important aspect of the examination for these children because they are at great risk for global developmental delays that may or may not have a pathophysiologic component.

The child needs to be functional within the context of his environment; therefore, an examination of the child's functional level is as important as the respiratory and neuromotor assessments that the physical therapist performs. The functional examination should include age-appropriate basic and instrumental activities of daily living, general mobility skills, communication skills, and an assessment of the child's role within the family and within the relevant environment. The functional assessment provides an indication of how well the child is integrated into his environment, family, and, if applicable, community.

A standardized developmental assessment or functional assessment tool can be used to quantify achievement of motor milestones and/or changes in functional mobility skills. No specific tool has been recommended for children dependent on ventilators, and only a few of the currently available tools have been reported to be used in populations in which children have been ventilator dependent.[15,24,48] When choosing an assessment, therapists should consider the child's age, as well as the care setting, prognosis, diagnosis, and intended outcomes (e.g., developmental milestones such as rolling, functional skills such as transfers, factors influencing quality of life such as accessing transportation to school), while remembering that standardized developmental assessments seldom take into account factors related to endurance for exercise. See Chapter 2 for test reviews.

The physical therapy examination alone does not begin to represent the wide range of competencies that need to be monitored. Ideally, all aspects of the child's development will be assessed periodically by members of the health care team. A multidisciplinary team approach is essential in the management of children with long-term MV and should be the standard of practice, regardless of the physical therapist's practice setting.

EVALUATION AND DIAGNOSIS

Information gathered during the physical therapy examination should be used for the therapist's evaluation and diagnosis. Results of the examination should be synthesized to determine the child's impairments, activity limitations, and participation restrictions, as well as to identify strengths and resources available to minimize disability. Ideally, a multidimensional approach to the use of tests and measures should be employed and the results correlated to relevant activity limitations and disabilities interfering with the child's quality of life. For example, the child with chronic lung disease and mechanical ventilator dependence secondary to BPD may have coexisting neurologic impairments, gastrointestinal abnormalities, and growth disturbance. The physical therapy diagnosis therefore might include developmental delay, aerobic capacity and endurance limitations, and a decreased repertoire of movement patterns. On the other hand, children with the neurologic diagnosis of CCHS may be otherwise medically stable and at risk for developmental delay only if they are hospitalized for a prolonged time. Thus, at this stage of clinical decision making, diagnostic determinations will vary depending on the age of the child, the severity and chronicity of the lung disease, and the coexisting diagnoses.

PROGNOSIS/PLAN OF CARE

The physical therapy prognosis for a child who is dependent on long-term MV may be difficult to establish. The prognosis is the determination of the predicted maximal level of improvement and the estimate of how long it will take the child to achieve that improvement. As this population of children is diverse in its medical diagnoses and age range, the literature base on which to base a prognosis for the reduction of impairments, improvement of function, and facilitation of participation in home and community life is limited.

Decisions regarding the mode, intensity, and frequency of activity need to be made in conjunction with other members of the child's medical team and modified as the disease process changes. The physical therapist must recognize the potential for physiologic jeopardy when implementing any intervention with these infants and children and its potential impact on the child's prognosis. The amount and type of motor activities must be individualized and graded to the child's level of tolerance so that risks associated with the physiologically immature or unstable systems are not magnified.

One of the ultimate goals for pediatric physical therapists, however, should be to promote the concept of lifelong health and fitness.[4] Barring any medical contraindication, physical activity in children who are dependent on a ventilator should be encouraged and incorporated into the plan of care. The long-term benefits of physical activity and lifelong fitness go even farther than physiologic and health-related ones, including mental health benefits such as improved self-esteem and confidence.[32,117]

PHYSICAL THERAPIST INTERVENTION

Regardless of the reason for requiring long-term MV, once a child is diagnosed with chronic respiratory failure and the decision is made to begin artificial ventilation, prevention and treatment of the associated complications need to be primary goals of medical and rehabilitative management. These children require early and aggressive promotion of growth and development and promotion of daily function and participation. Although the degree and intensity may vary, intervention strategies should maximize a child's developmental and functional potential.

No one intervention strategy or intensity is unanimously embraced by physical therapists for any diagnostic group. Similarly, in the case of children with long-term ventilator dependence, physical therapy varies widely because of differing philosophies of management and the wide range of problem areas that might be identified. Thus, the intent of this section is not to recommend specific interventions, but to present a conceptual framework from which one can organize an appropriate plan of care, and to emphasize considerations unique to this group of children.

Infants and children who are typically developing are capable of using a variable repertoire of motor skills to explore and learn. This normal acquisition of skills presumes a smooth interaction of the cardiopulmonary and musculoskeletal systems, as well as the presence of the necessary cognitive requirements. Inactivity in children is never normal, and children usually require minimal encouragement to be active and spontaneous. In the case of a child with chronic respiratory insufficiency, however, compromised physiologic stability alone may limit the seemingly endless exploration and practice in which children typically engage. In children with a chronic illness, a reduced capacity for activity or exercise can be a direct or indirect result of their underlying pathophysiologic process. For example, Smith et al. reported on a large cohort of school-aged children born very preterm and noted significant impairment in exercise capacity despite evidence of only mild small-airway obstruction and gas trapping.[105] Regardless of the cause, a vicious circle of inactivity may ensue: Inactivity → Reluctance to move and explore → Decreased endurance and "fitness" → Inactivity.

Another consideration is that children with long-term MV may associate movement with negative experiences such as fatigue, hypoxia, and pain, which limit their "motivation" to be as active as their peers. A major goal of the physical therapist in the management of children who are dependent on ventilators should be secondary prevention, that is, to prevent deprivation of sensory and motor experiences because of inactivity and the various sequelae that result from that deprivation. Regardless of the child's medical diagnosis, treatment should be aimed at providing a variety of opportunities for movement challenges and for exploration, as well as increasing their capacity for exercise. Depending on whether the child has a specific motor impairment, these goals may be accomplished with or without the use of assistive devices. For example, in the case of a child with BPD who also had an intraventricular hemorrhage, adaptive equipment may be needed for positioning because of poor anti-gravity trunk control, or for ambulation because of lower extremity weakness and spasticity. Alternatively, the child with CCHS and no neurologic injuries leading to motor impairment may be completely independent in all motor skills but may exhibit exercise intolerance.

Coordination, Communication, and Documentation

The multiple medical, emotional, educational, and rehabilitative needs of the child with ventilator dependence are beyond the expertise of a single provider and thus require the care and coordination of an interdisciplinary team. This team will include a primary care physician and multiple specialty physicians. Therapists working with a child dependent on MV should routinely communicate with the child, family, other daily caregivers (e.g., nurse, home health aide), and the child's primary physician. Therapists should also communicate with other medical specialists such as the pulmonologist, physiatrist, orthopedist, and neurologist about the child's therapy goals and physical response to intervention.

Members of the child's team in the home setting may expand to include a case manager, a respiratory equipment provider, and a durable medical equipment vendor. Additionally, team members in a school setting may include teachers, classroom aides, the school nurse, and transportation personnel (bus driver and monitor[s]). In many states, it is typical for a child with a tracheostomy on a ventilator outside the hospital to have a nurse with him at all times. Sharing of successful strategies for communication and motivation, as well as carryover of all rehabilitation goals among physical, occupational, and speech therapists, can facilitate a successful therapist–client relationship and can enhance a consistent approach to the needs of the child and family. Short-term and long-term goals developed by the team should be formulated in conjunction with the family, while the ultimate goal of maximizing function from a physical, cognitive, social-emotional, and family dynamics perspective is kept in mind.

Child- and Family-Related Instruction

Family-centered intervention is mandated by law in the United States, but for reasons other than legal ones, involvement of the parents and family in the life of the child with a disability is essential for optimal child development and family dynamics. The role of the family in shaping the child's environment to be the most conducive to learning, optimal development, and participation is crucial. More important, from a practical point of view, the child's life depends on parents' knowledge of the intensive care needed to maintain the child's health and safety.

Physical therapists can provide the child, family, and other team members with information about the child's diagnosis, indications for ventilator use, and the functional abilities of the child. Therapists can also provide consultation on positioning, orthotic and equipment use, activity tolerance, vital sign monitoring, clinical signs indicating the need for emergency intervention, mobility strategies within the home and school environments, transportation options, and resources for leisure and recreation activities.

Procedural Interventions: Therapeutic Exercise

Therapeutic exercise includes a broad group of activities intended to improve strength, flexibility, muscular and cardiorespiratory endurance, balance, coordination, posture, and motor function or development. Simply stated, the "normal" response to exercise is an increase in heart rate, followed by a return to baseline. Ventilation also increases linearly with the metabolic rate until approximately 60% of oxygen consumption, at which time it increases more rapidly (see Chapter 6 for a summary of the cardiorespiratory and musculoskeletal components of exercise and fitness). These relationships, as well as the other physiologic processes that support adequate ventilation and perfusion during exercise, are altered in conditions of lung disease. Whereas exercise is normally cardiac-limited, in those with chronic lung disease exercise may be ventilatory-limited as a result of deficient exercise capacity and gas exchange, or poor pulmonary mechanics, but the optimal level of physical activity for children with chronic lung disease is not related to disease severity.[107] Each child's specific pathophysiologic process determines the response to exercise and the capacity for improvement.

The beneficial effects of exercise have been well documented in certain populations with respiratory conditions such as those individuals with cystic fibrosis[77] (see Chapter 24) and asthma (see Chapter 25).[36] No studies, however, are available that examine active exercise and strength training for children with ventilators as a group. It has been documented that strength training is useful for children with neurologic[29,37] and neuromuscular disorders[37] and for children born prematurely.[49] As with any diagnostic group, exercise limitations and restrictions should be determined before the start of an exercise program, and with all exercise, children should be supervised closely to avoid musculoskeletal

injury, excessive heart and respiratory rate, and dislodgement of tubing. Studies are needed to determine the effectiveness of exercise programs in the diverse group of children with MV.

Any physical activity in which infants or children dependent on long-term MV engage can be viewed as "exercise" and can be seen as a means of improving their tolerance for movement and endurance. A paucity of literature also exists on the role that developmental intervention plays in improving cardiopulmonary status and exercise tolerance, in addition to achieving developmental goals. As noted earlier, ventilator dependence often dictates limited movement and mobility if the child must remain close to a nonmobile ventilator. For example, time spent in a prone position is often limited and may occur only during physical therapy. Exercise and activity in a prone position are useful for the strengthening of neck and shoulder girdle musculature, and for development of righting reactions. Rotational movements and crossing the midline of the body may be encouraged, as these movements are often constrained by the child's ventilator tubing, but they are important for many functional activities. For a child of any age, upright positioning in sitting or standing is important for physiologic function and bone density and should be encouraged when developmentally and medically appropriate. Activities such as pulling to stand and cruising may occur only in a crib if a child is in a hospital with limited opportunities for playtime on the floor.[31,99]

Procedural Interventions: Functional Training

For children with ventilator dependence, functional training may include bed mobility, transitional movements such as getting up from the floor, or transfer training, including getting into and out of bed and into and out of a wheelchair. Environmental limitations such as tubing length and the need to secure tubing before movement must be addressed.

Prescription, Application, and Fabrication of Devices and Equipment

Appropriate equipment can minimize caregiver dependence and can assist children to attain functional skills, positioning, and mobility unattainable on their own. Adaptive equipment may also be used to minimize the chance of secondary impairments due to the underlying disease process and/or immobility. Young children may require specialized adapted strollers with ventilator-carrying capability. Older children may require manual or power wheelchairs adequately outfitted to transport a ventilator. The ventilator and other equipment must be safely secured to the seating system. If the child is ambulatory, a portable ventilator may be transported in a backpack carried by the child or the care provider.

All systems of transport should meet the Federal Motor Vehicle Safety Standard for car seats and bus transport.[3] This includes securing the ventilator on the seat next to the child. In addition, when transporting a ventilator, it is typical practice in the authors' experience for the child to have a spare tracheostomy tube, ambu bag, oxygen tank, or portable suction unit with sterile catheters, as well as an external battery for the ventilator.

Orthoses may be needed to manage joint contractures, maintain joint flexibility, or provide proper alignment of the trunk, feet, legs, and hands or arms. Of particular importance for a child who may require a trunk orthosis for weak or paralyzed axial musculature to adequately maintain an upright posture and/or prevent or treat a scoliosis is the ability for the rib cage to expand fully and to allow for the fitting of a gastrostomy tube.

Airway Clearance Techniques

Although therapists often focus on strengthening the muscles of respiration and core trunk muscles, maintaining mobility of the rib cage, spine, and shoulder girdle is important to promote any nonassisted ventilation. Physical therapists may also teach a child and family airway clearance techniques and positioning for pulmonary drainage.

RE-EXAMINATION OF OUTCOMES

Re-examination will include performing selected tests and measures to evaluate progress in response to parent/caregiver questions or concerns, physical therapist intervention, growth and development, and medical recovery. Re-examination is indicated at times of new clinical findings or failure to respond to physical therapist intervention, or as dictated by the care setting.[4] For children dependent on MV, a change in type of ventilator or setting, or a decrease in the number of hours of ventilator support per day, may warrant a re-examination of aerobic capacity and endurance for motor tasks or the appropriateness of adaptive equipment.

Video

The video accompanying this chapter illustrates some of the interventions used with a 22-month-old girl with a diagnosis of Moebius syndrome, central respiratory dysfunction, and ventilator dependence.

Weaning

The transition to unassisted breathing is a complex process. Weaning a child from the support of a mechanical ventilator is highly individualized, is accomplished in response to recovery from respiratory insufficiency, and may or may not be the goal for all children. The primary assessment of weaning capability is done to determine at what point the child is capable of maintaining adequate alveolar ventilation while breathing spontaneously. This requires that the child's neural control centers are actively controlling the process, that the ventilatory pump is able to support the work required for breathing,[50] and that the lungs and airway are not severely compromised by disease. Although weaning from MV may be a goal for many children, no standard protocol exists for the discontinuation of long-term ventilator support.

In critical care, the process of endotracheal tube extubation and ventilator weaning is often done by trial and error, whereby time off the ventilator is variable, dependent on when hypercapnia and hypoxia develop. Three commonly used approaches in acute and intensive care settings may be used to wean children from positive-pressure ventilation: (1) Spontaneous breathing trial with the use of a T-piece (with or without CPAP); (2) pressure-support ventilation (PSV), in which all breaths are patient-triggered and pressure-limited (more patient effort is required as the level of pressure support is decreased); and (3) synchronized intermittent mandatory ventilation (SIMV), in which breaths may be mandatory ventilator-controlled or spontaneous. To date, despite the importance of minimizing time on MV, guidance on weaning and extubation is limited in the pediatric literature.[84]

In addition to the increased length of time for the weaning process, weaning strategies for children in a post-acute setting are inherently different from those used in the neonatal or pediatric ICU because of differences between the use of a short-term endotracheal tube and a more permanent stable airway with a tracheostomy. Proposed criteria for weaning readiness in the post-acute pediatric hospital setting include the following: (1) No escalation in ventilator support within 2 days before weaning; (2) stable chest radiograph; (3) blood $PaCO_2$ level not more than 10% above baseline; (4) blood pH within normal range; (5) supplemental FiO_2 of 0.6 or lower; (6) stable blood pressure over the previous 5 to 7 days; (7) heart rate no greater than 95% maximal normal for age; (8) tolerance of adequate nutrition; (9) absence of active infection, acute pain, or other medical problems that might negatively affect the weaning process; and (10) reported understanding by the family/guardian and all health care providers of the desirability of weaning.[88] In pediatric pulmonary rehabilitation, children may be weaned completely off MV; advanced to portable equipment; progressed to milder levels of ventilation (i.e., reduced pressure support); or weaned to a less invasive mode of support (i.e., CPAP).[2,18,88]

Despite the expected financial, clinical, and psychosocial advantages of weaning children with ventilator dependency in a post-acute inpatient setting, only a few studies have reported outcomes on cohorts of children undergoing active weaning programs. In a 1995 study, 42% of infants with BPD were weaned from MV to CPAP, and 29% were weaned to a tracheostomy with supplemental oxygen. However, only 9% of children with diagnoses other than BPD were weaned to a less restrictive form of support.[18] In a more recent inpatient pulmonary rehabilitation single-site study, successful ventilator weaning was achieved during 30% of admission-discharge episodes, with diagnosis (prematurity with BPD) and age (younger) being the strongest predictors of weaning success.[61] Nearly half of children admitted to a prospective multisite study over a 1-year enrollment period who were dependent on MV 24 hours per day at admission no longer required MV at discharge from inpatient rehabilitation. In addition, four children required only 12 or fewer hours per day of ventilator support at discharge.[90]

Even with the home being a less closely monitored situation, reports have described children's dependence on MV being minimized while they are cared for at home. Programs report that up to 57% of children are weaned from MV while at home.[34,42,82,87]

Weaning can be an arduous task, both physiologically and psychologically, and must be done with caution.[43] The weaning prognosis can be enhanced by improvements in cardiorespiratory strength and endurance, adequate nutrition, and overall health; however, both muscular and respiratory fatigue should be avoided during this time. The timing and prognosis for weaning are important for physical therapists to understand, so that physical therapist management may be directed appropriately. It is imperative that the physical therapist coordinate and communicate with the medical team as to the amount of physical exertion that can be tolerated safely. During a time of weaning, the child's schedule of activities may need to be altered. In addition, the observations and ongoing clinical assessments made by the physical therapist may be influential in ventilator weaning. Ventilator settings are often influenced by the child's physical response in areas such as strength, developmental/functional skills, and endurance. When these findings are communicated to the medical care team, weaning may be progressed, halted, or interrupted. Conversely, unpublished clinical observations by the authors indicate that when children are being actively weaned from the ventilator, physical therapy participation may be limited. Infants may sleep more, and older children often do not tolerate the same level of physical activity, until they accommodate to the increased demands of reduced ventilator settings on their respiratory system.

SUMMARY

Children dependent on long-term MV are medically complex, with diagnoses of prematurity and chronic lung disease, cardiac conditions, congenital anomalies, and neuromuscular and/or neurologic conditions. Because of improved medical and technological management, the prevalence of infants and children dependent on MV continues to increase. It is more than likely that the rate of medical and technological progress will continue to keep pace with advances in rehabilitation and prevention of disabilities, as well as policies that support an uncomplicated transition into the home and community.

Children requiring long-term MV are at high risk for secondary illness, recurring hospitalizations, global developmental delays, and clinical compromise secondary to tracheostomy–related complications and equipment failure. Minimized dependence on MV promotes improved quality of life with a reduction in hospital stays, improved physical and mental health, and increased social participation opportunities for children and their families. However, little empirical evidence describes how often successful weaning is achieved.

Although physical therapists can do little to prevent chronic respiratory failure and ventilator dependence, they have an important role to play in fostering children's development and endurance for physical activity. From early on in the NICU through young adulthood, physical therapists are in a unique position to be involved with children dependent on MV and their families. Some aspects of care may include medically related interventions, such as percussion and postural drainage; however, the majority of time may be spent addressing various aspects of the child's development and daily function. As with any population at risk for disability, one of the major roles of the physical therapist is to integrate intervention goals into everyday activities and help caregivers or parents appreciate the relevance of their involvement. The ecologic validity of the intervention and goals increases if those goals are made a part of functionally relevant tasks.

Physical therapists are encouraged to participate in clinical research to contribute to the evidence base supporting management of this clinically diverse population of children. Research is needed to determine effective program planning, program improvements, and appropriate resource utilization, and to set outcome expectations for infants, toddlers, and children dependent on long-term MV. Additional research questions may involve the impact of rehabilitation interventions on the weaning process and the impact of rehabilitation interventions on quality-of-life outcomes for children and their families.

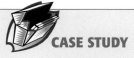

CASE STUDY

"Manny"

This case illustrates the physical therapy management of a child requiring long-term MV and having several co-morbidities. *The Guide to Physical Therapist Practice*[4] and the International Classification of Functioning, Disability and Health (ICF)[19] are used as frameworks.

Manny is a 2-year-old boy with chronic lung disease and history of MV dependence. Manny was born at 28 weeks of gestation to a 29-year-old gravida 3, para 2-3 mother. The pregnancy was remarkable for poor fetal growth for the 2 weeks before delivery. Upon delivery, Manny was intubated in the delivery room. Apgar scores were 4 at 1 minute and 6 at 5 minutes, as Manny demonstrated increased muscle tone, respiratory rate, and heart rate. An echocardiogram revealed a large patent ductus arteriosus (PDA) that was treated successfully. A left grade III intraventricular hemorrhage and mild stage I retinopathy diagnosed at birth have reportedly resolved. A tracheostomy tube was placed at 3 months of age because Manny was unable to be weaned from MV. Before transfer to an inpatient pediatric pulmonary rehabilitation program at 4 months of age (adjusted), Manny spent the first 4 months of his life in a NICU.

The anticipated outcomes of Manny's transfer at 4 months of age to an inpatient pediatric pulmonary rehabilitation program were (1) elimination or reduction of primary body function and structure impairments (chronic lung disease) and of secondary body function and structure impairments (altered muscle tone, decreased force production, diminished aerobic capacity and endurance, decreased tolerance to movement and tactile stimulation), (2) elimination or reduction of activity limitations (mobility, self-care, speech-language, behavior, cognition), and (3) promotion of participation in life situations (readiness for home and family life). Manny's team at the rehabilitation hospital included his family, a pediatrician, a nurse practitioner, a pediatric pulmonologist, a primary nurse, associate nurses, a physical therapist, an occupational therapist, a speech-language pathologist, respiratory therapists, a social worker, a dietitian, a case manager, a pastoral care associate, and a child-life specialist.

Manny was classified into the following physical therapy practice patterns:

Cardiovascular/Pulmonary

Practice Pattern G—Impaired ventilation, respiration/gas exchange, and aerobic capacity/endurance associated with respiratory failure in the neonate

Manny would have been originally placed in this classification of practice patterns because of his chronic lung disease. Because Practice Pattern G includes only infants up to 4 months of age, Manny would need to be re-classified into the following two patterns at his current age of 2 years:

Practice Pattern B—Impaired aerobic capacity/endurance associated with deconditioning

Practice Pattern F— Impaired ventilation, respiration/gas exchange associated with respiratory failure

Neuromuscular

Practice Pattern B—Impaired neuromotor development

Manny's physical therapy problem list and anticipated goals were developed from the projected hospitalization outcomes at admission and the results of his initial physical therapy examination and monthly re-examinations. The initial physical therapy examination at 4 months of age and subsequent re-examinations included a review of his current health status, progress toward projected hospitalization outcomes and physical therapy goals, and application of physical therapy tests and measures. Tests and measures were chosen on the basis of personal contextual factors such as Manny's age, medical diagnosis, medical history/current medical status, and functional capabilities. Tests and measures were also chosen on the basis of environmental factors such as service delivery setting (hospital, hospital crib) and equipment (ventilator or oxygen, physiologic monitoring devices).

The following tests and measures were used:

- Arousal, Attention, and Cognition/Sensory Integrity—Responses to tactile, auditory, and visual stimuli
- Aerobic Capacity and Endurance—Tolerance to physical activity using clinical signs such as shortness of breath, use of accessory muscles, fatigue, and use of pulse oximetry
- Range of Motion/Posture—Passive and active range of motion and postural alignment in age-appropriate developmental positions
- Reflex Integrity—Present or emerging reflexes and reactions
- Muscle Performance—Axial and appendicular muscle tone assessed in gravity-eliminated and anti-gravity positions
- Motor Function/Neuromotor Development and Sensory Integration—Voluntary postures and movement patterns, Bayley Scales of Infant Development II
- Mobility/Functional Performance—The Pediatric Evaluation of Disability Inventory (PEDI) is used to assess functional mobility and caregiver assistance in mobility tasks

Assistive and Adaptive Devices

The child-related/personal factors influencing Manny's recovery include his neuromuscular and cardiopulmonary impairments. In general, the environmental factors influencing Manny's functioning include his dependence on pulmonary support (MV and oxygen) and his extended hospitalization. Manny was given a physical therapy diagnosis of developmental delay (Practice Pattern 5B).

Manny's history of ventilator assistance includes placement on an LP6 continuous PPV at 3 months of age. Manny was slowly weaned from MV by gradually decreasing the pressure and number of assisted breaths per minute, while gas exchange and other clinical indicators (i.e., respiratory rate and oxygen saturation) were carefully

Continued

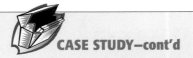

CASE STUDY—cont'd

monitored. Manny was dependent on the ventilator 24 hours per day until 18 months of age, when he progressed to using oxygen mist via a tracheostomy collar, as the length of time off his ventilator was increased each day. Gas exchange and other clinical indicators (i.e., respiratory rate and oxygen saturation) were carefully monitored. Manny progressed to the use of oxygen mist during waking hours and then to using oxygen mist 24 hours per day, with oxygen saturation remaining above 95% as measured by pulse oximetry.

Presently, at 2 years of age, Manny is progressing to using a heat moisture exchanger (HME) over his tracheostomy when not using his oxygen mist. A smaller tracheostomy tube was tried, but Manny was unable to tolerate the downsizing (exhibiting an increased respiratory rate, decreased oxygen saturations) and required that the larger tracheostomy tube continue to be used at the present time.

Using the ICF as a framework, Table 23-6 provides an overview of Manny's cardiopulmonary and physical functioning since his

TABLE 23-6 **Manny's Cardiopulmonary and Physical Functioning**

Adjusted Age	Functioning and Disability	Contextual Factors
4 months	Easily stressed (inaudible cry, distress noted by facial expression, oxygen desaturation) with movement; increased truncal arching at rest; actively moving all extremities; lifts head briefly when held at caregiver's shoulder	Environment—Hospital inpatient with multiple caretakers, excessive noise and lighting, frequent medical interventions, mobility limited by ventilator tubing and cardiac and pulse oximetry wiring, positioning in crib and infant seat
6 months	Easily stressed as described above; actively turning head side to side	Personal—Age, inaudible cry, tracheostomy and gastrostomy tubes in place limiting prone positioning, frequent family visits
9 months	Rolling side to supine; lifts head if propped in prone with support under chest	Environment—As above, now able to be placed in infant swing and highchair outside of crib Personal—As above
1 year	No longer exhibiting stress signals, tolerant of handling and movement, maintains sitting when placed (using arms for propping), able to lift one arm off of the supporting surface; maintains quadruped when placed; assists supine to sit transition	Environment—Continues as hospital inpatient; beginning to participate in physical therapy when on oxygen mist via tracheostomy collar, allowing for increased distance with movement (including provision of physical therapy in unit playroom) Personal—As above, increasing distractibility
15 months	Rolls side to prone; maintains standing with assist when placed (demonstrates lower extremity hypertonia)	
18 months	Transitioning sit to quadruped; creeping with assist; bouncing in standing (decreased lower extremity hypertonia to maintain upright posture); cruises with assist	Environment—Continues as hospital inpatient; on oxygen mist via tracheostomy collar, allowing for movement around unit with caregivers using stroller Personal—As above
21 months	Creeping independently; cruising independently; pulling to stand in crib; beginning to take forward step with hands held	Environment—Continues as hospital inpatient; continuing improved respiratory status—On oxygen mist via tracheostomy collar, allowing for use of body-weight-supported treadmill training off of nursing unit in physical therapy department 2 to 3×/wk, training at 3-min intervals with 5–10 minute rest/play periods ×3–5 trials per session; 40% weight support initially, reduced to 0% over time; manual guidance of foot and lower limb only as needed; initially treadmill at slowest speed and progressed as tolerated
2 years (current status)	Independent ambulation with high guard; wide base of support; creeping up/down stairs (Figure 23-2)	Environment/Personal—Continues as hospital inpatient but able to be out of room off of hospital unit with oxygen mist and trained caregiver

CASE STUDY—cont'd

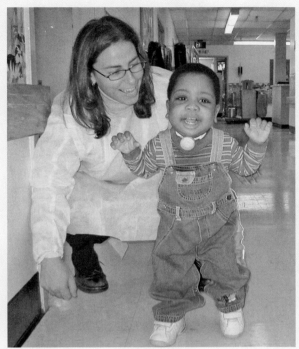

Figure 23-2   At 2 years of age, Manny is beginning to ambulate independently. Manny displays a high guard position of his upper extremities and a wide base of support. Around his neck are his tracheostomy ties with the heat moisture exchanger (HME) in place over his tracheostomy tube.

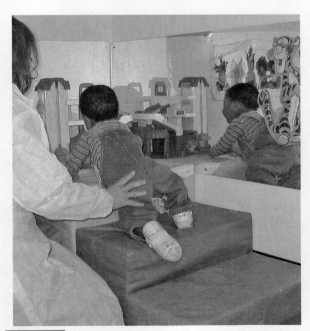

Figure 23-3   Uneven surfaces are a new phenomenon for Manny after spending most of his early life in a hospital crib. In this picture, Manny is learning to creep up the stairs with the help of his physical therapist.

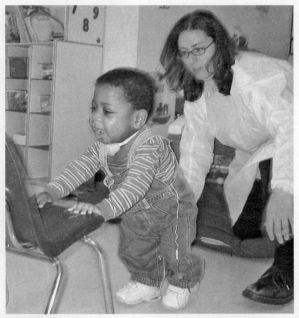

Figure 23-4   At approximately 18 months of age, children typically will climb into a chair without assistance. At 2 years of age, when presented with a child-size chair, Manny did not attempt to climb up onto the chair, but began to push it as if it were a push toy or an assistive device for ambulation. The only chairs Manny has used are a highchair and a stroller, and he has always been lifted by a caregiver from his crib to one of these two seats.

admission to the inpatient pulmonary rehabilitation program at 4 months adjusted age.

Manny has been receiving physical therapy intervention up to three times per week since admission to the inpatient rehabilitation program. Manny's current problem list and goals and objectives are shown in Table 23-7.

The physical therapist interventions utilized as part of Manny's current treatment plan include the following:

a. Coordination, communication, and documentation, with physical therapist participation in patient care rounds; case conferences; family/team meetings; hospital discharge planning; and medical record documentation

b. Patient/client-related instruction: Instruction and education of family and other rehabilitation team members regarding body functions and structures, activity limitations, and participation restrictions; risk factors (i.e., aerobic capacity and endurance); physical therapy plan of care, including positions for play and feeding and activities and equipment for promotion of muscle strength and ambulation; and equipment use

c. Therapeutic exercise: Developmental activities training; task-specific performance training; flexibility exercises; active assistive, active, and resisted exercises; balance and coordination training; body-weight-supported treadmill training; and gait and locomotion training

Continued

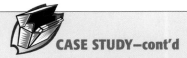

CASE STUDY—cont'd

TABLE 23-7 **Manny's Current Problems and Goals**

Problems	Goals and Objectives
BODY FUNCTIONS AND STRUCTURE: Decreased force production of axial and appendicular musculature in anti-gravity positions with lower extremity extensor muscle hypertonia	Goal: Promote stability and mobility in anti-gravity positions without use of hypertonia for stability in trunk and extremity extensor musculature Short-term objective: Manny will stand unsupported for up to 10 seconds with the supervision of the physical therapist or a caregiver trained to promote safety and assess respiratory response to physical activity.
BODY FUNCTIONS AND STRUCTURE: Diminished aerobic capacity and endurance	Goal: Maximize aerobic capacity and endurance for mobility and self-care tasks Short-term objective: Manny will participate in physical therapy activities as outlined in the plan of care without oxygen saturation declining below preset levels of 95% as measured by pulse oximetry.
ACTIVITY LIMITATION: Delayed motor development and mobility (Figures 23-3 and 23-4)	Goal: Promote age-appropriate motor and mobility skills Short-term objective: Manny will take 1 or 2 unsupported steps with the guarding of the physical therapist or a caregiver trained to promote safety and assess respiratory response to physical activity. Short-term objective: Manny will ambulate up to 50 feet with one hand held once per day with the physical therapist or a caregiver trained to promote safety and assess respiratory response to physical activity.
PARTICIPATION RESTRICTION: Limited mobility for participation in hospital environment secondary to ventilator and oxygen equipment, safety monitoring, and caregiver supervision needs (Figure 23-5)	Goal: Instruct caregivers (family and program staff) to promote safety and assess respiratory response to physical activity with ambulation activities. Goal: Provide appropriate equipment for mobility (walker) and positioning (highchair) to promote participation with family and program staff.

d. Functional training in self-care and home management: Bed mobility and transfer training
e. Prescription, application, and, as appropriate, fabrication of devices and equipment: Seating systems (highchair, stroller, walker)
f. Environmental adaptation: Maximize positioning and mobility options limited by hospital crib, length of ventilator and oxygen tubing, and safety monitoring equipment (pulse oximeter)
g. Airway clearance techniques: Chest percussion, vibration, postural drainage, and suctioning are used by the physical therapist in conjunction with the nursing and respiratory staff to manage Manny's airway.

Manny was admitted to the inpatient pediatric pulmonary rehabilitation program with the anticipation that Manny would wean from his MV. In this case, Manny's decreased dependence on pulmonary support paralleled his gains in physical functioning. The decrease in support from MV to oxygen mist lessened Manny's environmental barriers (short ventilator tubing and being restricted to a hospital crib) and minimized his personal barriers (decreased aerobic capacity and endurance) to promote increased mobility.

Physical therapy is projected to continue throughout Manny's hospitalization to promote Manny's physical functioning. Manny's projected discharge disposition is home to the care of his family, with medical, educational, and social support services provided through a home-based early intervention program. At the time of hospital discharge, Manny will be referred for physical therapy to promote motor function and to address personal and environmental barriers to Manny's current level of physical functioning and health.

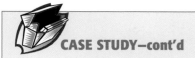

CASE STUDY—cont'd

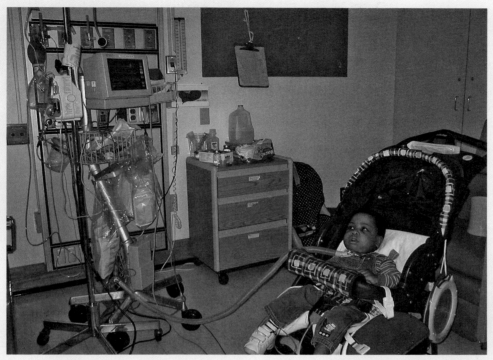

Figure 23-5   Manny in his stroller in his hospital room with his oxygen mist, gastrostomy tube feeding, and cardiac and respiratory monitors connected. The oxygen mist tubing is approximately twice as long as his ventilator tubing used to be, thus significantly increasing his mobility within his crib and within his room.

EVIDENCE TO PRACTICE 23-1

CASE STUDY "MANNY"

EXAMINATION DECISION #1

The decision to use the Bayley Scales of Infant Development II to document Manny's performance in relation to age peers was made because the Bayley measures both mental and motor development of infants from 1 to 42 months of age; it may be used to describe current developmental functioning and to assist in diagnosis and treatment planning for infants and children with developmental delays or disabilities. In addition, the Bayley has been used in evaluating motor outcomes for infants born prematurely and with ventilator dependence and can be used to evaluate changes over time. A third edition is now available.

EXAMINATION DECISION #2

The decision to use the Pediatric Evaluation of Disability Inventory in addition to a motor performance measure was made to assess this child's *functional mobility*. This decision is supported by the availability of normative data reflecting children's capability and level of independence from 6

months to 7.5 years of age. The PEDI has been highlighted as a tool to be used in preschool children at risk for neurodevelopmental disabilities, as it measures functional and adaptive skills, thus providing clinicians with assistance to devise intervention strategies that optimize development, independence, family supports, and community participation.

INTERVENTION FREQUENCY DECISION

Treatment frequency fluctuated throughout Manny's hospitalization. Although no evidence supports a specific intervention frequency, the decision regarding frequency of intervention was based on Manny's medical and physiologic state, period of skill acquisition or potential for regression, and amount of developmental stimulation and interaction while hospitalized; frequency was adjusted throughout his hospitalization on the basis of these factors.

DISCHARGE PLANNING DECISION

The decision to refer Manny for a physical therapy examination through an early intervention program following discharge is supported by the prognosis of ongoing motor

Continued

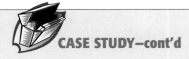

CASE STUDY—cont'd

EVIDENCE TO PRACTICE 23-1—cont'd

deficits due to his premature birth, intraventricular hemorrhage, and prolonged hospitalization. In addition, a study by Graham and colleagues (2008) identified factors contributing to physical and social isolation for children with chronic respiratory needs enrolled in community early intervention programs that may be addressed by a physical therapist.

1. Bayley, N. (2006). *Bayley Scales of Infant and Toddler Development* (3rd ed.). San Antonio, TX: Harcourt Assessment.
2. O'Shea, T. M., Kothadia, J. M., Klinepeter, K. L., et al. (1999). Randomized placebo-controlled trial of a 42-day tapering course of dexamethasone to reduce the duration of ventilator dependency in very low birth weight infants: Outcome of study participants at 1-year adjusted age. *Pediatrics, 104,* 15–21.
3. Koseck, K., & Harris, S. R. (2004). Changes in performance over time on the Bayley Scales of Infant Development II when administered to infants at high risk of developmental disabilities. *Pediatric Physical Therapy, 16,* 199–205.
4. Haley, S. M., Coster, W. J., Ludlow, L. H., et al. (1992). *Pediatric Evaluation of Disability Inventory: Development, standardization and administration manual.* Boston, MA: Trustees of Boston University.

5. Msall, M. E. (2005). Measuring functional skills in preschool children at risk for neurodevelopmental disabilities. *Mental Retardation and Developmental Disability Research Reviews, 11,* 263–273.
6. Bailes, A. F., Reder, R., & Burch, C. (2008). Development of guidelines for determining frequency of therapy services in a pediatric medical setting. *Pediatric Physical Therapy, 20,* 194–198.
7. Schreiber, J. (2004). Increased intensity of physical therapy for a child with gross motor developmental delay: A case report. *Physical and Occupational Therapy in Pediatrics, 24,* 63–78.
8. Gardner, M. R. (2005). Outcomes in children experiencing neurologic insults as preterm neonates. *Pediatric Nursing, 31,* 448,451–456.
9. O'Shea, T. M., Goldstein, D. J., deReginier, R. A., et al. (1996). Outcome at 4 to 5 years of age in children recovered from neonatal chronic lung disease. *Developmental Medicine & Child Neurology, 38,* 830–839.
10. Graham, R. J., Pemstein, D. M., & Palfrey, J. S. (2008). Included but isolated: Early intervention programmes provision for children and families with chronic respiratory support needs. *Child: Care, Health, and Development, 34,* 373–379.

REFERENCES

1. Ambrosino, N., & Clini, E. (2004). Long-term mechanical ventilation and nutrition. *Respiratory Medicine, 98,* 413–420.
2. Ambrosio, I. U., Woo, M. S., Jansen, M. T., & Keens, T. G. (1998). Safety of hospitalized ventilator-dependent children outside of the intensive care unit. *Pediatrics, 101,* 257–259.
3. American Academy of Pediatrics & Committee on Injury and Poison Prevention. (1999). Transporting children with special health care needs (RE9852). *Pediatrics, 104,* 988–992.
4. American Physical Therapy Association. (2001). Guide to physical therapist practice, 2nd edition. *Physical Therapy, 81.*
5. American Thoracic Society. (2003). Statement on the care of the child with chronic lung disease of infancy and childhood. *American Journal of Respiratory Critical Care Medicine, 168,* 356–396.
6. Amin, R., & Fitton, C. (2003). Tracheostomy and home ventilation in children. *Seminars in Neonatology, 8,* 127–135.
7. Attar, M. A., & Donn, S. M. (2002). Mechanisms of ventilator-induced lung injury in premature infants. *Seminars in Neonatology, 7,* 353–360.
8. Bach, J. R., Saltstein, K., Sinquee, D., et al. (2007). Long-term survival in Werdnig-Hoffmann disease. *American Journal of Physical Medicine and Rehabilitation, 86,* 339–345.
9. Barbosa, V., Campbell, S., Sheftel, D., et al. (2003). Longitudinal performance of infants with cerebral palsy on the Test of Infant Motor Performance and on the Alberta Infant Motor Scale. *Physical & Occupational Therapy in Pediatrics, 23,* 7–29.
10. Berry-Kravis, E. M., Zhou, L., Rand, C. M., et al. (2006). Congenital central hypoventilation syndrome: PHOX2B mutations and phenotype. *American Journal of Respiratory Critical Care Medicine, 174,* 1139–1144.
11. Bertrand, P., Fehlmann, E., Lizama, M., et al. (2006). Home ventilatory assistance in Chilean children: 12 years' experience. *Archives of Bronconeumology, 42,* 165–170.
12. Bhandari, V., & Gruen, J. R. (2006). The genetics of bronchopulmonary dysplasia. *Seminars in Perinatology, 30,* 185–191.
13. Boroughs, D., & Dougherty, J. A. (2009). Care of technology-dependent children in the home. *Home Healthcare Nurse, 27,* 37–42.
14. Bos, A. E., Martijn, A., van Asperen, R. M., et al. (1998). Qualitative assessment of general movements in high-risk preterm infants with chronic lung disease requiring dexamethasone therapy. *Journal of Pediatrics, 132,* 300–306.
15. Bourke-Taylor, H. (2003). Melbourne Assessment of Unilateral Upper Limb Function: Construct validity and correlation with the Pediatric Evaluation of Disability Inventory. *Developmental Medicine in Child Neurology, 45,* 92–96.
16. Branson, R. (2004). Understanding and implementing advances in ventilator capabilities. *Current Opinion in Critical Care, 10,* 23–32.
17. Briassoulis, G., Filippou, O., Natsi, L., et al. (2004). Acute and chronic paediatric intensive care patients: Current trends and

perspectives on resource utilization. *Quarterly Journal of Medicine, 97*, 507–518.

18. Buschbacher, R. (1995). Outcomes and problems in pediatric pulmonary rehabilitation. *American Journal of Physical Medicine and Rehabilitation, 74*, 287–293.

19. Carnevale, F. A., Alexander, E., Davis, M., et al. (2006). Daily living with distress and enrichment: The moral experience of families with ventilator-assisted children at home. *Pediatrics, 117*, e48–e60.

20. Carr, M., Poje, C., Kingston, L., Kielma, D., & Heard, C. (2001). Complications in pediatric tracheostomies. *Laryngoscope, 111*, 1925–1928.

21. Carrozzi, L., & Make, B. (2008). Chronic respiratory failure as a global issue. In N. Ambrosino, & R. Goldstein (Eds.), Ventilatory support for chronic respiratory failure. lung biology in health and disease (*Vol. 225*; pp. 27–38). New York: Informa Healthcare.

22. Chatburn, R. L., & Primiano, F. P. (2001). A new system for understanding modes of mechanical ventilation. *Respiratory Care, 46*, 604–621.

23. Cheifetz, I. M. (2003). Invasive and noninvasive pediatric mechanical ventilation. *Respiratory Care, 48*, 442–453.

24. Chung, B., Wong, V., & Ip, P. (2004). Spinal muscular atrophy: Survival pattern and functional status. *Pediatrics, 114*, e548–e553.

25. Coalson, J. J. (2003). Pathology of new bronchopulmonary dysplasia. *Seminars in Neonatology, 8*, 73–81.

26. Como, J. J., Sutton, E. R., McCunn, M., et al. (2005). Characterizing the need for mechanical ventilation following cervical spinal cord injury with neurologic deficit. *Journal of Trauma, 59*, 912–916.

27. Cushman, D. G., O'Brien, J. E., Dumas, H. M., et al. (2002). Re-admissions to inpatient pediatric pulmonary rehabilitation. *Pediatric Rehabilitation, 5*, 133–139.

28. Dieperink, W., Goorhuis, J. F., de Weerd, W., et al. (2006). Walking with continuous positive airway pressure. *European Respiratory Journal, 27*, 853–855.

29. Dodd, K., Taylor, N., & Graham, H. (2003). A randomized clinical trial of strength training in young children with cerebral palsy. *Developmental Medicine & Child Neurology, 45*, 652–657.

30. Donn, S. M., & Sinha, S. K. (2002). Newer techniques of mechanical ventilation: An overview. *Seminars in Neonatology, 7*, 401–407.

31. Dudek-Shriber, L., & Zelazny, S. (2007). The effect of prone positioning on the quality and acquisition of developmental milestones in four-month old infants. *Pediatric Physical Therapy, 19*, 48–55.

32. Dykens, E., Rosner, B., & Butterbaugh, G. (1998). Exercise and sports in children and adolescents with developmental disabilities: Positive physical and psychosocial effects. *Child & Adolescent Psychiatric Clinics of North America, 7*, 757–771.

33. Edwards, E. A., Hsaio, K., & Nixon, G. M. (2005). Paediatric home ventilatory support: The Auckland experience. *Journal of Paediatric Child Health, 41*, 652–658.

34. Edwards, E. A., O'Toole, M., & Wallis, C. (2004). Sending children home on tracheostomy dependent ventilation: Pitfalls and outcomes. *Archives of Disease in Childhood, 89*, 251–255.

35. Elixson, E. M., Myrer, M. L., & Horn, M. H. (1997). Current trends in ventilation of the pediatric patient. *Critical Care Nurses Quarterly, 20*, 1–13.

36. Fanelli, A., Cabral, A. I., Neder, J. A., et al. (2007). Exercise training on disease control and quality of life in asthmatic children. *Medicine & Science in Sports and Exercise, 39*, 1474–1480.

37. Fragala-Pinkham, M. A., Haley, S. M., & Goodgold, S. (2006). Evaluation of a community-based group fitness program for children with disabilities. *Pediatric Physical Therapy, 18*, 159–167.

38. Gaillard, E. A., Cooke, W. I., & Shaw, N. J. (2001). Improved survival and neurodevelopmental outcome after prolonged ventilation in preterm neonates who have received antenatal steroids and surfactant. *Archives of Disease in Childhood, Fetal and Neonatal Edition, 84*, F194–F196.

39. Gali, B., & Goyal, D. (2003). Positive pressure mechanical ventilation. *Emergency Medicine Clinics of North America, 21*, 453–473.

40. Gannon, C. M., Wiswell, T. E., & Spitzer, A. R. (1998). Volutrauma, $PaCO_2$ levels, and neurodevelopmental sequelae following assisted ventilation. *Clinical Perinatology, 25*, 159–175.

41. Gilgoff, R. L., & Gilgoff, I. S. (2003). Long-term follow-up of home mechanical ventilation in young children with spinal cord injury and neuromuscular conditions. *Journal of Pediatrics, 142*, 476–480.

42. Gowans, M., Keenan, H. T., & Bratton, S. L. (2007). The population prevalence of children receiving invasive home ventilation in Utah. *Pediatric Pulmonology, 42*, 231–236.

43. Gracey, D. R., & Hubmayr, R. D. (2001). Weaning from long-term mechanical ventilation. In N. S. Hill (Ed.), *Long-term mechanical ventilation: Lung biology in health and disease* (Vol. 152; pp. 431–448). New York: Marcel Dekker.

44. Graham, R. J., Dumas, H. M., O'Brien, J. E., et al. (2004). Congenital neurodevelopmental diagnoses and an intensive care unit: Defining a population. *Pediatric Critical Care Medicine, 5*, 321–328.

45. Graham, R. J., Fleegler, E. W., & Robinson, W. M. (2007). Chronic ventilator need in the community: A 2005 pediatric census of Massachusetts. *Pediatrics, 119*, e1280–e1287.

46. Graham, R. J., Pemstein, D. M., & Palfrey, J. S. (2008). Included but isolated: Early intervention programmes provision for children and families with chronic respiratory support needs. *Child Care Health Development, 34*, 373–379.

47. Haffner, J., & Schurman, S. (2001). The technology-dependent child. *Pediatric Clinics of North America, 48*, 751–764.

48. Haley, S. M., Fragala, M., & Skrinar, A. M. (2003). Pompe disease and physical disability. *Developmental Medicine & Child Neurology, 45*, 618–623.

49. Hebestreit, H., & Bar-Or, O. (2001). Exercise and the child born prematurely. *Sports Medicine, 31*, 591–599.

50. Hess, D. (2001). Ventilator modes used in weaning. *Chest, 120,* 474S–476S.

51. Hess, D. R. (2002). Mechanical ventilation strategies: What's new and what's worth keeping? *Respiratory Care, 47,* 1007–1017.

52. Hewitt-Taylor, J. (2004). Children who require long-term ventilation: Staff education and training. *Intensive and Critical Care Nursing, 20,* 93–102.

53. Hull, E. M., Dumas, H. M., Crowley, R. A., et al. (2005). Tracheostomy speaking valves for children: Tolerance and clinical benefits. *Pediatric Rehabilitation, 8,* 214–219.

54. Hummler, H., & Schulze, A. (2009). New and alternative modes of mechanical ventilation. *Seminars in Fetal and Neonatal Medicine, 14,* 42–48.

55. Huysman, W. A., Ridder, M., Bruin, N. C., et al. (2003). Growth and body composition in preterm infants with bronchopulmonary dysplasia. *Archives of Disease in Childhood, Fetal and Neonatal Edition, 88,* F46–F51.

56. Jaarsma, A. S., Knoester, H., van Rooyen, F., et al. (2001). Biphasic positive airway pressure ventilation (PeV+) in children. *Critical Care, 5,* 174–177.

57. Jobe, A. H., & Bancalari, E. (2001). Bronchopulmonary dysplasia. *American Journal of Respiratory Critical Care Medicine, 163,* 1723–1729.

58. Kamm, M., Burger, R., Rimensberger, P., et al. (2001). Survey of children supported by long-term mechanical ventilation in Switzerland. *Swiss Medicine Weekly, 131,* 261–266.

59. Keszler, M., & Durand, D. (2001). Neonatal high-frequency ventilation: Past, present, and future. *Clinical Perinatology, 28,* 579–607.

60. Kharasch, V. S., Dumas, H. M., Haley, S. M., et al. (2008). Bronchoscopy findings in children and young adults with tracheostomy due to congenital anomalies and neurological impairment. *Journal of Pediatric Rehabilitation Medicine, 1,* 137–143.

61. Kharasch, V. S., Haley, S. M., Dumas, H. M., et al. (2003). Oxygen and ventilator weaning during inpatient pediatric pulmonary rehabilitation. *Pediatric Pulmonology, 35,* 280–287.

62. Kirk, S., & Glendinning, C. (2004). Developing services to support parents caring for a technology-dependent child at home. *Child Care Health Development, 30,* 209–218.

63. Kirshblum, S. C., & O'Connor, K. C. (2000). Levels of spinal cord injury and predictors of neurologic recovery. *Physical Medicine and Rehabilitation Clinics of North America, 11,* 1–27.

64. Kissoon, N., & Adderley, R. (2008). Noninvasive ventilation in infants and children. *Minerva Pediatrics, 60,* 211–218.

65. Kondili, E., Prinianakis, G., & Georgopoulos, D. (2003). Patient-ventilator interaction. *British Journal of Anaesthesiology, 91,* 106–119.

66. Lai, D., & Schroer, B. (2008). Haddad syndromes: A case of an infant with central congenital hypoventilation syndrome and Hirschsprung disease. *Journal of Child Neurology, 23,* 341–343.

67. Lekskulchai, R., & Cole, J. (2001). Effect of a developmental program on motor performance in infants born preterm. *Australian Journal of Physiotherapy, 47,* 169–176.

68. Lesser, D. J., Ward, S. L., Kun, S. S., et al. (2009). Congenital hypoventilation syndromes. *Seminars in Respiratory and Critical Care Medicine, 30,* 339–347.

69. Lorenz, J. M., Paneth, N., Jetton, J. R., et al. (2001). Comparison of management strategies for extreme prematurity in New Jersey and the Netherlands: Outcomes and resource expenditure. *Pediatrics, 108,* 1269–1274.

70. Luce, J. M. (1996). Reducing the use of mechanical ventilation. *New England Journal of Medicine, 335,* 1916–1917.

71. Lumeng, J. C., Warschausky, S. A., Nelson, V. S., et al. (2001). The quality of life of ventilator-assisted children. *Pediatric Rehabilitation, 4,* 21–27.

72. Macey, P. M., Valderama, C., Kim, A. H., et al. (2005). Temporal trends of cardiac and respiratory responses to ventilatory challenges in congenital central hypoventilation syndrome. *Pediatric Research, 55,* 953–959.

73. Majnemer, A., Riley, P., Shevell, M., et al. (2000). Severe bronchopulmonary dysplasia increases risk for later neurological and motor sequelae in preterm survivors. *Developmental Medicine & Child Neurology, 42,* 53–60.

74. Make, B. J. (2001). Epidemiology of long-term ventilatory assistance. In N. S. Hill (Ed.), Long-term mechanical ventilation: Lung biology in health and disease (*Vol. 152*; pp. 1–18). New York: Marcel Dekker.

75. Make, B., Hill, N., Goldberg, A. I., et al. (1998). Mechanical ventilation beyond the intensive care unit: Report of a consensus conference of the American College of Chest Physicians. *Chest, 113,* 289–344.

76. Margolan, H., Fraser, J., & Lenton, S. (2004). Parental experience of services when their child requires long-term ventilation: Implications for commissioning and providing services. *Child: Care, Health, and Development, 30,* 257–264.

77. McIlwane, M. (2007). Chest physical therapy, breathing techniques and exercise in children with CF. *Paediatric Respiratory Reviews, 8,* 8–16.

78. McPherson, S. (1995). *Respiratory care equipment.* St Louis: Mosby.

79. Mentro, A. (2003). Health care policy for medically fragile children. *Journal of Pediatric Nursing, 18,* 225–232.

80. Moffat, M., & Frownfelter, D. (2007). *Cardiovascular/pulmonary essentials: Applying the preferred physical therapist practice patterns.* Thorofare, NJ: Slack Incorporated.

81. Navalesi, P., & Costa, R. (2003). New modes of mechanical ventilation: Proportional assist ventilation, neurally adjusted ventilatory assist, and fractal ventilation. *Current Opinion in Critical Care, 9,* 51–58.

82. Nelson, V. S., Carroll, J. C., Jurvitz, E. A., & Dean, J. M. (1996). Home mechanical ventilation of children. *Developmental Medicine & Child Neurology, 38,* 704–715.

83. Nelson, V. S., Dixon, P. J., & Warschausky, S. A. (2004). Long-term outcome of children with high tetraplegia and ventilator dependence. *Journal of Spinal Cord Medicine, 27,* S93–S97.

84. Newth, C. J., Venkataraman, S., Willson, D. F., et al. (2009). Weaning and extubation readiness in pediatric patients. *Pediatric Critical Care Medicine, 10*, 126–127.

85. Northway, W. H. Jr., Rosan, R. C., & Porter, D. Y. (1967). Pulmonary disease following respiratory therapy of hyaline-membrane disease: Bronchopulmonary dysplasia. *New England Journal of Medicine, 276*, 357–368.

86. Noyes, J. (2002). Barriers that delay children and young people who are dependent on mechanical ventilators from being discharged from hospital. *Journal of Clinical Nursing, 11*, 2–11.

87. Noyes, J. (2006). Health and quality of life of ventilator-dependent children. *Journal of Advanced Nursing, 56*, 392–403.

88. O'Brien, J. E., Birnkrant, D., Dumas, H. M., et al. (2006). Weaning children from mechanical ventilation in a post-acute setting. *Pediatric Rehabilitation, 9*, 365–372.

89. O'Brien, J. E., Dumas, H. M., Haley, S. M., et al. (2002). Clinical findings and resource use of infants and toddlers dependent on oxygen and ventilators. *Clinical Pediatrics, 41*, 155–162.

90. O'Brien, J. E., Dumas, H. M., Haley, S. M., et al. (2007). Ventilator weaning outcomes in chronic respiratory failure in children. *International Journal of Rehabilitation Research, 30*, 171–174.

91. O'Brien, M. E., & Wegner, C. B. (2002). Rearing the child who is technology dependent: Perceptions of parents and home care nurses. *Journal for Specialists in Pediatric Nursing, 7*, 7–15.

92. Oktem, S., Ersu, R., Uyan, Z. S., et al. (2007). Home ventilation for children with chronic respiratory failure in Istanbul. *Respiration, 76*, 76–81.

93. Padman, R., Alexander, M., Thorogood, C., et al. (2003). Respiratory management of pediatric patients with spinal cord injuries: Retrospective review of the DuPont experience. *Neurorehabilitation and Neural Repair, 17*, 32–36.

94. Palfrey, J.S., Haynie, M., Porter, S., et al. (1994). Prevalence of medical technology assistance among children in Massachusetts in 1987 and 1990. *Public Health Reports, 109*, 226–233.

95. Reddy, V. G., Nair, M. P., & Bataclan, F. (2004). Role of non-invasive ventilation in difficult-to-wean children with acute neuromuscular disease. *Singapore Medical Journal, 45*, 232–234.

96. Robin, B., Kim, Y. J., Huth, J., et al. (2004). Pulmonary function in bronchopulmonary dysplasia. *Pediatric Pulmonology, 37*, 236–242.

97. Rodriguez, R. J. (2003). Management of respiratory distress syndrome: An update. *Respiratory Care, 48*, 279–287.

98. Roher, T., Traschel, D., Engelcke, G., et al. (2002). Congenital central hypoventilation syndrome associated with Hirschsprung's disease and neuroblastoma: Case of multiple neurocristopathies. *Pediatric Pulmonology, 33*, 71–76.

99. Salls, J. S., Silverman, L. N., & Gatty, C. M. (2002). The relationship of infant sleep and play positioning to motor milestone achievement. *American Journal of Occupational Therapy, 56*, 577–580.

100. Shneerson, J. M. (1996). Techniques in mechanical ventilation: Principles and practice. *Thorax, 51*, 756–761.

101. Silvestri, J., Chen, M., Weese-Mayer, D., et al. (2002). Idiopathic congenital central hypoventilation syndrome: The next generation. *American Journal of Medical Genetics, 112*, 46–50.

102. Simonds, A. (2003). Home ventilation. *European Respiratory Journal Supplement, 47*, 38s–46s.

103. Singer, L., Yamashita, T., Lilien, L., et al. (1997). A longitudinal study of development outcome of infants with bronchopulmonary dysplasia and very low birth weight. *Pediatrics, 100*, 987–993.

104. Sinha, S. K., & Donn, S. M. (2008). Newer forms of conventional ventilation for preterm newborns. *Acta Paediatrica, 97*, 1338–1343.

105. Smith, L. J., van Aspereen, P. P., McKay, K. O., et al. (2008). Reduced exercise capacity in children born very preterm. *Pediatrics, 122*, e287–e293.

106. Srinivasan, R., Asselin, J., Gildengorin, G., et al. (2009). A prospective study of ventilator-associated pneumonia in children. *Pediatrics, 123*, 1108–1115.

107. Sritippayawan, S., Harnruthakorn, C., Deerojanawong, J., et al. (2008). Optimal level of physical activity in children with chronic lung disease. *Acta Paediatrica, 97*, 1582–1587.

108. Teague, W. G. (2001). Long term mechanical ventilation in infants and children. In N. S. Hill (Ed.), Long-term mechanical ventilation: Lung biology in health and disease (*Vol. 152*; pp. 177–214). New York: Marcel Dekker.

109. Thomas, M., Greenough, A., & Morton, M. (2004). Prolonged ventilation and intact survival in very low birth weight infants. *European Journal of Pediatrics, 162*, 65–67.

110. Tobin, M. J. (2001). Advances in mechanical ventilation. *New England Journal of Medicine, 344*, 1986–1996.

111. Traiber, C., Piva, J. P., Fritsher, C. C., et al. (2009). Profile and consequences of children requiring prolonged mechanical ventilation in three Brazilian pediatric intensive care units. *Pediatric Critical Care Medicine, 10*, 375–380.

112. Van den Broek, M. J., Arbues, A. S., & Chalard, F. (2008). Chiari type I malformation causing central apnoeas in a 4-month-old boy. *European Journal of Pediatric Neurology, 13*, 463–465.

113. Vohr, B. R., Wright, L. L., Dusick, A. M., et al. (2004). Center differences and outcomes of extremely low birth weight infants. *Pediatrics, 113*, 781–789.

114. von Renesse, A., Schildgen, O., Klinkenberg, D., et al. (2009). Respiratory syncytial virus infection in children admitted to hospital but ventilated mechanically for other reasons. *Journal of Medical Virology, 81*, 160–166.

115. Wang, K. W. K., & Barnard, A. (2004). Technology-dependent children and their families: A review. *Journal of Advanced Nursing, 45*, 36–46.

116. Wang, K. W., & Barnard, A. (2008). Caregivers' experiences at home with a ventilator-dependent child. *Quality Health Research, 18*, 501–508.

117. Weiss, J., Diamond, T., Demark, J., et al. (2003). Involvement in Special Olympics and its relations to self-concept and

actual competency in participants with developmental disabilities. *Research on Developmental Disabilities, 24,* 281–305, 2003.

118. Wocadlo, C., & Rieger, I. (2008). Motor impairment and low achievement in very preterm children at eight years of age. *Early Human Development, 84,* 769–776.

119. World Health Organization. (2001). International classification of functioning, disability and health. impairments, disabilities and health. Geneva: World Health Organization.

SUGGESTED READING

American Thoracic Society. (1999). Idiopathic congenital central hypoventilation syndrome: Diagnosis and management. *American Journal of Respiratory Critical Care Med, 160,* 368–373.

Cutz, E., Ma, T. K. F., Perrin, D. G., et al. (1997). Peripheral chemoreceptors in congenital central hypoventilation syndrome. *American Journal of Respiratory Critical Care Medicine, 155,* 358–363.

Dick, C., & Sassoon, C. (1996). Patient-ventilator interactions. *Clinics in Chest Medicine, 17,* 423–438.

Downes, J. J., & Parra, M. M. (2001). Costs and reimbursement issues in long-term mechanical ventilation of patients at home. In N. S. Hill (Ed.), *Long-term mechanical ventilation: Lung biology in health and disease* (Vol. 152; pp. 353–374). New York: Marcel Dekker.

Gregoire, M. C. L., Lefebvre, F., & Glorieux, J. (1998). Health and developmental outcomes at 18 months in very preterm infants with bronchopulmonary dysplasia. *Pediatrics, 101,* 856–860.

Jardine, E., O'Toole, M., Payton, J. Y., et al. (1999). Current status of long term ventilation of children in the United Kingdom: Questionnaire survey. *British Medical Journal, 318,* 295–299.

Kercsmar, C. M. (2003). Current trends in neonatal and pediatric respiratory care: Conference summary. *Respiratory Care, 48,* 459–464.

Keszler, M. (2009). State of the art in conventional mechanical ventilation. *Journal of Perinatology, 29,* 262–275.

Northway, W. H. Jr. (1979). Observations on bronchopulmonary dysplasia. *Journal of Pediatrics, 95,* 815–817.

Noyes, J., Hartmann, H., Samuels, M., et al. (1999). The experiences and views of parents who care for ventilator-dependent children. *Journal of Clinical Nursing, 8,* 440–450.

O'Shea, T. M., Goldstein, D. J., deReginier, R. A., et al. (1996). Outcome at 4 to 5 years of age in children recovered from neonatal chronic lung disease. *Developmental Medicine & Child Neurology, 38,* 830–839.

Randolph, A. G., & Wypij, D., Venkataraman, S. T., et al. (2002). Effect of mechanical ventilator weaning protocols on respiratory outcomes in infants and children: A randomized controlled trial. *Journal of the American Medical Association, 288,* 2561–2568.

Restrepo, R. D., Fortenberry, J. D., Spainhour, C., et al. (2004). Protocol-driven ventilator management in children: Comparison to nonprotocol care. *Journal of Intensive Care Medicine, 19,* 274–284.

24 Cystic Fibrosis

JENNIFER L. AGNEW, BScPT, BHK • BLYTHE OWEN, MScPT, HBSc

ystic fibrosis (CF) was first defined as a clinical entity over 70 years ago, when Andersen published a paper describing the clinical course of a number of children who had died of pulmonary and digestive problems. She labeled the disorder "cystic fibrosis of the pancreas."[3] This disease thereafter was classified as a disorder of exocrine gland function, influencing the respiratory system, pancreas, reproductive organs, and sweat glands. At times, the first presenting sign has been the subjective report, "My child tastes salty to kiss"; the "sweat test" often confirms the diagnosis. Subsequent study and interest led to a clearer understanding of the disease and a coordinated approach to treating the associated impairments. Over time, the disorder that had so intrigued Andersen has come to be known as cystic fibrosis, and research has continued, yielding a vast knowledge base about this chronic illness.

Classified as a hereditary disease, CF has long been understood to be inherited in an autosomal recessive pattern.[110] Two copies of the gene responsible for CF are inherited by an affected individual. Both parents of a child diagnosed with CF are, therefore, known to be carriers of at least one copy of a mutation at the gene locus responsible for CF. Those persons with one copy of the CF gene are termed heterozygote carriers and are not diagnostically positive for CF. In 1989 a major scientific breakthrough occurred with discovery of the precise locus on chromosome 7 of the gene responsible for CF.[164] Investigations and research have followed to define the pathologic basis of the physical manifestations of CF.

Although at present the time-honored definition of this disease as the most commonly inherited life-shortening illness in the white population remains appropriate, our present growing understanding of CF may prove to temper its impact. More research must be done before treatment may allow people with CF to lead lives free of the complications currently implicit in this diagnosis. Current management of the manifestations of CF has, however, promoted improved quality of life and a better prognosis for life expectancy for people with CF.[51] In the United States, 45% of the approximately 30,000 individuals diagnosed with CF are over the age of 18; therefore CF is no longer thought of as exclusively a childhood disease. The median age of survival for individuals with CF is currently 37.4 years.[190]

CF is diagnosed in 1 in 3000 children born to white American parents, and statistical analysis of this incidence yields a best estimate of the rate of heterozygote carriers as about 5% of the population in areas of the world where significant white populations have settled.[16,143] The incidence of CF in black and Asian peoples is considerably lower than that in whites—approximately 1 in 17,000 births in the black population, and an estimated 1 in 90,000 births in Asian societies.[16] Several reports have documented the incidence of CF in the South Asian population, estimated to be 1 in 10,000 to 1 in 40,750.[121]

Recent research and new possibilities for carrier screening are producing more precise statistical estimates of the actual incidence of individuals who are heterozygote CF carriers, suggesting that previous rates were underestimated.[202] Prenatal diagnosis of CF is now sometimes possible, as is screening for carrier status, which is discussed in detail later in this chapter.

The gene responsible for CF was identified in 1989 by an international team of researchers, led by Drs. Tsui, Collins, and Riordan.[93] This discovery was an extraordinary achievement in molecular genetics and has led to subsequent research advances in the understanding of genetic and pathologic components of CF worldwide. More than 1500 distinct mutations within the CF gene have been identified in many ethnic groups, although fewer than 10 mutations occur with a frequency greater than 1%. A specific trinucleotide deletion, delta-F508, is the most common mutation associated with clinical CF, occurring in 66% of patients worldwide.[161] This mutation results in loss of the amino acid phenylalanine from the product protein, which ultimately affects its production, regulation, and/or function. The specific genetic mutation cannot be used to predict the manifestation of disease severity nor the prognosis in terms of survival.

The nature of the disease, its multisystemic involvement, and the variety of needs of affected individuals and their families dictate that professional intervention in the management of CF is generally concentrated in regional CF clinics. Comprehensive treatment programs for CF were established over 55 years ago[55] and are now the primary mode of delivery of associated health care needs. CF centers changed the practice of focusing on the treatment of ongoing disease to taking a proactive approach of early intervention, maintenance of health, and preservation of lung function.[190] CF centers can offer their clients the services of respirologists, gastroenterologists, physical therapists, respiratory therapists, pharmacists, dietitians, genetic counselors, social workers, psychologists, exercise physiologists, and specialty care nursing personnel. The multidisciplinary team is dedicated to the delivery of the most effective and palatable treatments available in promoting the optimal level of well-being for patients with CF and their families. CF centers worldwide work collaboratively in sharing their clinical expertise and their knowledge base to develop new treatment possibilities and to renew hopes for an ultimate cure for CF.

In this chapter considerations for choosing appropriate intervention for patients with CF are outlined. An increasing number of people with CF are reaching the fifth decade of life,[43] with a few patients living into their 60's and 70's.[16] Surgical advances in lung transplantation offer hope of prolonging life for people with chronic pulmonary disabilities. Physical therapists are serving an expanded role in management programs for people with CF. It is of crucial importance that clinical decisions be directed by careful consideration of available scientific evidence, and that therapists continue to seek out the means to scientifically evaluate empirical experiences. A clear understanding of pathophysiology, etiology, diagnostic indicators, methods of examination, and medical management is essential for the physical therapist working with the CF population to ensure comprehensive incorporation of the issues into the development of management strategies and goals. A discussion of the evolution of self-management through infancy, for preschool and school-age children, and during adolescence and adulthood is included. Improving adherence to a plan of care through the promotion of self-efficacy may prove to enhance the effectiveness of treatment and help prevent or delay the onset of disability characteristic of this disorder. As a result, well-being and improved quality of life will be promoted.

PATHOPHYSIOLOGY

The CF gene defect leads to absent or malfunctioning CFTR protein, which results in abnormal chloride conductance on the epithelial cell. The consequence is obstruction of mucus-secreting exocrine glands by hyperviscous secretions.[108] The main organ systems affected are the respiratory system and the gastrointestinal system, although the reproductive system, sinuses, and sweat glands are also impaired. Blockage of exocrine gland products prevents their delivery to target tissues and organs and creates clinical abnormalities in these body systems.

In the lung, abnormal CFTR protein leads to depletion of the airway surface liquid layer (ASL), which can lead to ciliary collapse and decreased mucociliary transport. The accumulation of hyperviscous secretions leads to progressive

airway obstruction, secondary infection by opportunistic bacteria, inflammation, and subsequent bronchiectasis and irreversible airway damage. This vicious cycle can be complicated by bronchoconstriction of the airways and chronic lung hyperinflation. Deconditioning of the respiratory muscles and malnutrition also affect the functional limitations of the respiratory system.[161]

Obstruction of the small airways in CF and subsequent air trapping and atelectasis result in ventilation and perfusion mismatch, which leads to hypoxemia. Long-standing hypoxemia may result in pulmonary artery hypertension and cor pulmonale or right ventricular failure. Large airway bronchiectasis combined with small airway obstruction reduces vital capacity and tidal volume and results in decreased volumes of airflow at the alveolar level. Consequently, progressively increasing arterial carbon dioxide concentration ($PaCO_2$) occurs, which may lead to hypercapnic respiratory failure.[204] Respiratory failure accounts for 95% of the mortality rate in CF.[140]

In the gastrointestinal tract, viscous secretions begin to obstruct the pancreatic duct in utero, and periductal inflammation and fibrosis cause the loss of pancreatic exocrine function. The resulting maldigestion of fats and proteins leaves the pancreatic-insufficient patient with clinical steatorrhea[57]; the stools are described as bulky, frequent, and "greasy" and as having a strongly offensive odor. In infancy, patients with CF can display evidence of protein-calorie malnutrition with a protruding abdomen, muscle wasting, and initial diagnosis of failure to thrive despite reports from parents of these children's hearty appetites.[110] Compensating for loss of pancreatic function remains a critical feature of management throughout these children's lives.

Another pathologic finding that presents in 10% to 20% of diagnosed cases of CF is meconium ileus, which is demonstrated in neonates.[129] The combination of abnormal pancreatic function and hyperviscous secretions of the intestinal glands creates an altered viscosity of the meconium, which causes an obstruction at the distal ileum, thus preventing passage of meconium in the first neonatal days.[110] Distal intestinal obstruction is seen in some older patients, associated with abnormal intestinal secretions and increased adherence of mucus in the intestines.[56]

Hepatobiliary disease has been reported with greater frequency among patients with pancreatic insufficiency. CF-related liver disease occurs in up to 30% of people with CF, but it is a significant clinical problem only in the minority of individuals (cirrhosis, portal hypertension). Patients with CF and pancreatic sufficiency have an increased risk of developing acute pancreatitis.[60] CF-related diabetes mellitus (CFRD) is an increasingly systemic complication as the patient with CF transitions from childhood to adulthood. CFRD is currently present in 2% of children, 19% of adolescents, and 40% to 50% of adults. Incidence and prevalence are higher in females age 30 to 39, but otherwise, no gender difference is noted.[125]

In the reproductive system, obstruction of the vas deferens causes infertility in 98% of males with CF.[200] Older studies reported that the fertility rate for females with CF was 20% to 30% of normal,[62] but more recent data have suggested that the reproductive tract in females is normal in most women with CF. Therefore, females with CF who have good weight and lung function can expect to have normal hormone levels that contribute to regular ovulation and menstruation. The only mechanical barrier present in females with CF is the cervical mucous plug.[58]

In the upper respiratory tract, sinusitis may cause persistent headache, and nasal polyps occur in 6% to 36% of patients with CF, often necessitating surgical resection. Within 12 months, the recurrence rate of nasal polyps is 60% once polypectomy is performed.[110] Hypertrophic pulmonary osteoarthropathy is often associated with advanced severity of pulmonary disease and is most noticeable in the clinical finding of "clubbing" or rounded hypertrophic changes in the terminal phalanges of the fingers and toes.[109] Osteopenia is present in up to 85% of adult patients, and osteoporosis in 10% to 34%. In children, the reported prevalence is not consistent because of comparisons with different control populations and corrections for bone size in growing children.[174]

ETIOLOGY

The cause of CF is traced to the abnormal gene product, the cystic fibrosis transmembrane conductance regulator (CFTR) protein, which seems to be most abundantly expressed in the apical membrane surface of epithelial cells of the respiratory, gastrointestinal, and reproductive systems, and in the sweat glands.[36] Normal epithelial cells secrete fluid by allowing chloride (a negatively charged ion) to pass through the luminal membrane of the cell. Because this membrane is permeable to sodium (positively charged), it passively follows; increased levels of sodium chloride then stimulate fluid secretion. Fluid levels in the airways must be maintained at a sufficient level to provide for normal mucociliary transport. Structural defects in the CFTR protein lead to abnormalities in cell membrane function, conductance, and regulation. The resulting electrolyte abnormality (chloride impermeability and sodium hyperpermeability) leads to abnormal amounts of fluid being removed from the airway lumen, resulting in reduced airway surface liquid (ASL) volume and underhydrated mucus. These impairments in turn lead to impaired mucociliary clearance and retention of mucus in the lower airways.[19,110] Abnormal expression or regulation of the CFTR protein in airway epithelial cells is the primary cause of the respiratory manifestations of CF.

DIAGNOSIS AND MEDICAL MANAGEMENT

Early diagnosis, including prenatal determination of the presence of the CF gene mutation, has enabled researchers to follow the expression and progression of the disease from birth in many patients. Impairment of the respiratory system may not manifest immediately, and at birth the lungs often appear normal on radiologic examination. In the most distal small airways, however, dilation and hypertrophy of mucus-secreting goblet cells begin early in life, and subsequent impaired mucociliary clearance can cause obstructive mucous plugs and associated air trapping and atelectasis, which can be detected by radiography. The presentation of infants with failure to thrive and nutritional losses through steatorrhea accounts for up to 85% of the cases of CF diagnosed in infancy. A history of respiratory illness such as repeated respiratory tract infections, recurrent bronchiolitis, or even pneumonia is often reported, but in 80% of newly diagnosed cases, no family history of CF is known.[110]

A diagnosis of CF can be made if the patient has one or more characteristic clinical features of the disease, a history of CF in a sibling, or a positive newborn screening test, plus laboratory evidence of an abnormality in the CF transmembrane conductance regulator (CFTR) gene or protein. Acceptable evidence of a CFTR abnormality includes biological evidence of channel dysfunction (i.e., abnormal sweat chloride concentration or nasal potential difference) or identification of a CF disease-causing mutation in each copy of the CFTR gene (i.e., on each chromosome).[61] An elevated level of sodium chloride in the sweat has been the principal diagnostic indicator for CF for more than 50 years.[66] A positive sweat test occurs if the chloride concentration is greater than 60 mmol/L or is within the intermediate range (30–59 mmol/L for infants younger than 6 months of age, and 40–59 mmol/L for older individuals).[143]

In the few centers with the capacity (specialized laboratory and trained personnel), another diagnostic test, nasal potential difference (PD), is possible. This test measures the electrical charge (potential difference) across the epithelial surface (mucous membrane) of the nose. In normal subjects, a small charge of −5 to −30 mV is present, whereas subjects with CF demonstrate values between −40 and −80 mV.[140]

Screening tests for prospective parents who are known carriers (with prior offspring with CF or with CF themselves) are now possible and raise a number of ethical issues when CF is suggested prenatally. Genetic counseling therefore is available at CF centers. Analysis of the blood of known heterozygote parents and of tissue from the fetus obtained through amniocentesis or chorionic villus sampling can determine the presence of the CF gene mutation common to the family history.

Newborn screening is being performed increasingly in many states and provinces within North America and around the world. A sample of blood is taken, and the IRT/DNA test is a two-stage test that is used to screen for CF. The first stage of the test looks for high levels of an enzyme called IRT (immunoreactive trypsinogen) in the blood sample from the baby's foot. If the amount of IRT is above a certain level, a DNA test is performed on the same blood sample. The DNA test looks for the most common genetic mutations associated with CF. A positive screening result indicates that the child is at increased risk of CF and a sweat test must be performed to confirm the diagnosis. Without the onset of newborn screening, children with CF were not diagnosed with the disease until they became symptomatic with respiratory signs or failure to thrive. Several studies have shown that newborn screening for CF leads to improved nutritional outcomes, which in turn lead to improved pulmonary outcomes later in life.[143]

The diagnosis of CF may even be discovered in adulthood because these patients usually present with milder lung disease and pancreatic sufficiency. Their diagnosis is often delayed because of the belief that CF is a pediatric disease and the finding that some adults have normal to borderline sweat test results. The criteria for making a diagnosis are the same for adults and children.[206]

Patients should be followed periodically at CF clinics (usually every 3–4 months although this can vary) by a multidisciplinary team. This center system has contributed to improving national survival considerably.[51] Radiologic assessment, pulmonary function testing (PFT), sputum cultures, nutritional status and patterns of weight loss, blood analysis, exercise testing, and subjective reports of treatment adherence are examined. All of these factors assist the CF clinical team to address the changing therapeutic needs of patients with CF and to initiate treatment regimens with the aim of preventing or slowing development of the functional limitations of CF. Increased frequency of monitoring and increased use of appropriate medications have been associated with an improvement in forced expired volume in 1 second (FEV$_1$—see section on Measuring Pulmonary Function) in CF centers.[89]

Most of the morbidity seen in CF is associated with deteriorating pulmonary status. Past therapeutic management focused on limiting the effects of the pathogenesis of pulmonary impairments. Specifically, treatments would aim to decrease airway obstruction due to chronic bronchorrhea (abnormal mucous secretions) and the progressive inflammation that occurs secondary to chronic bacterial infection.[108]

Irreversible airway damage is caused by bacteria that infect the respiratory tract at an early age (which may be difficult to eradicate) and the associated aggressive host inflammatory response. The development of antibiotic resistance after multiple antibiotic courses leads to chronic persistent infection. In infants and younger children, *Staphylococcus aureus* and *Haemophilus influenzae* predominate, although the most common CF pathogen is *Pseudomonas aeruginosa*. It has been suggested that inhaled *Pseudomonas aeruginosa* has a high affinity for CF airways, which may explain the high prevalence of this organism in patients with CF. Some bacteria such as *Pseudomonas aeruginosa* and *Burkholderia cepacia* complex can also produce biofilms that protect themselves, explaining the persistence of bacterial infection in the majority of CF patients despite attempts at eradication.[49] Chronic *Pseudomonas* infection is associated with a reduction in lung function and a poorer prognosis.

Antibiotic therapy appears to have significantly influenced the effects of the chronic endobronchial infection that typifies CF and has been a mainstay of treatment regimens for over 60 years.[51] Optimally, the choice of antibiotics should be based on the results of sputum culture and sensitivity tests.[16] Sputum cultures show infection by a number of organisms in a common pattern that changes with severity of disease and with the age of the patient. Opportunistic bacteria, such as *Pseudomonas aeruginosa, Staphylococcus aureus, Haemophilus influenzae, Burkholderia cepacia* complex, *Stenotrophomonas maltophilia,* and *Achromobacter xylosoxidans,* are the organisms most frequently seen. Combinations of infectious organisms are common, particularly when disease severity and age of the patient advance. Some evidence suggests that early and vigorous use of antibiotics produces better results than delaying their administration until symptoms are well developed or advanced.[16]

Inhaled antibiotics, such as tobramycin and colistin, are beneficial in suppressing bacterial pulmonary infection because aerosolized medications can be delivered in higher doses directly to the airways while minimizing systemic exposure and toxicity. Ramsey and colleagues showed that inhaled preservative-free tobramycin twice a day resulted in a significant increase in FEV$_1$ and a 36% reduction in the use of intravenous antibiotics for pulmonary exacerbations.[2,159] In the Early Intervention TOBI Eradication (ELITE) trial, a 1-month course of inhaled TOBI (preservative free tobramycin solution) monotherapy achieved an eradication rate >90%. Approximately 70% of patients remained culture-negative for >800 days after the short-course eradication protocol. Delaying the onset of chronic *Pseudomonas aeruginosa* and the development of a mucoid strain may help to preserve lung function over the longer term, but the benefits of this approach need to be assessed in long-term studies.[162] Intravenous antibiotics such as ceftazidime and other aminoglycosides are used to target *Pseudomonas* infections in hospitalized patients when oral or inhaled antibiotics do not improve their respiratory symptoms related to a pulmonary exacerbation.

Burkholderia cepacia complex is an opportunistic pathogen in CF patients and other compromised hosts. Although normally nonpathogenic in healthy immunocompetent individuals, patients with CF are at significant risk of infection.[110] *Burkholderia cepacia* complex is recognized as a particularly virulent pathogen because of its high level of intrinsic antibiotic resistance, its tenacity to persist in the lungs, and its association with more advanced pulmonary disease. Synergy studies combining antibiotics may help identify a more effective antimicrobial therapy for patients with these organisms.[21] This species is highly transmissible from person to person and is highly virulent, which has led to initiation of segregation practices and attempts to control cross-contamination of equipment in many centers. Infection with *Burkholderia cepacia* complex can cause a rapid decline in pulmonary function and can increase mortality in patients with CF. Occasionally, the invasive, fatal bacteremia called "cepacia syndrome" can result.[143]

An organism that can be present in the airways without causing infection is *Aspergillus fumigatus,* but an intense allergic response to this fungus, allergic bronchopulmonary aspergillosis (ABPA), is seen in up to 15% of patients with CF. Clinical manifestations of ABPA include wheezing, pulmonary infiltrates, and central bronchiectasis.[143]

Several of the virulent products of bacterial infection cause airway inflammation and progressive epithelial destruction and therefore contribute significantly to the severity of the pulmonary impairment in CF,[110] but it has also been reported that inflammation can precede infection, as was observed in bronchoalveolar lavage (BAL) studies in infants.[96] Anti-inflammatory corticosteroids may slow progressive pulmonary deterioration[7] but are associated with numerous side effects when used on a long-term basis and require careful consideration before use.[110] They may be used in a small percentage of patients for specific indications such as fungal infection and ABPA.[16]

Influenza, rubella, and pertussis infections are particularly harmful to individuals with CF and can trigger a downward spiral of lung function. Early immunization is highly recommended, and a routine yearly influenza vaccine should be addressed in the regular clinic routine.[16]

The use of inhaled hypertonic saline has been suggested as an inexpensive treatment option to improve mucociliary clearance and pulmonary function in patients with CF. Hypertonic saline is associated with bronchospasm, so patients should be pretreated with bronchodilators. Recent studies have shown that hypertonic saline (7%) may increase the ASL layer and produce a short-term improvement in lung function.[194] Most studies have been performed in patients with moderate to severe lung disease. Sustained improvement in lung function is not yet documented, although ongoing early intervention studies in infants and toddlers may provide further information.

Malnutrition is a key feature of CF, as defective CFTR in the pancreatic epithelium results in obstruction of the pancreatic duct. CF patients become pancreatically insufficient when more than 95% of total pancreatic exocrine function is lost. These patients develop nutrient malabsorption and are at risk for vitamin and mineral deficiencies.[2] Nutrition and lung function are linked such that poor nutritional status and poor somatic growth affect the ability to repair lung disease. Similarly, pulmonary disease affects growth through appetite suppression and increased energy expenditure. Special attention to a properly balanced, high-calorie diet with supplementary pancreatic enzymes and vitamins requires acceptance and compliance in patients. During acute episodes of respiratory exacerbations, the

anorexia that accompanies the frequent racking cough, the increase in mucous production, and the increased work of breathing pose a challenge to provision of adequate nutritional intake. Levels of resting energy expenditure have been shown to be in excess of 150% of normal in patients with CF with more progressive pulmonary disease or malnutrition.[110] Oral nutritional supplements are available, but if patients fail to improve their weight, a gastrostomy feeding tube may be inserted for additional nutritional supplementation.[2]

Cystic fibrosis–related diabetes (CFRD) can develop in CF patients, with the average age of onset between 18 and 21 years. Annual screening for CFRD with an oral glucose tolerance test starts at age 10. Hyperglycemia during times of stress, such as pulmonary exacerbations or while on steroids, can occur.[2] Female patients with CFRD have a poorer survival than male patients.[143] Intermittent CFRD can be treated with insulin, with the goal of normalizing glucose levels.

In patients with CF, the airway lumen is compromised not only by secretions but also by airway edema, smooth muscle hypertrophy, and bronchoconstriction. Inhaled steroids, although never proven effective in CF in controlled clinical trials, may reduce airway edema. Bronchodilators such as β-adrenergic agonists or theophylline, intended to relax airway smooth muscle, are routinely administered, although not all patients respond to them in direct testing. Some patients may have paradoxical decreases in pulmonary function likely due to extensively damaged airways, which normally are held open by muscle tone.[51] When used immediately before exercise or pulmonary physical therapy, bronchodilators may help prevent induced bronchospasm in some patients and therefore are often prescribed as an important adjunct to physical therapy.[110]

Many medications employed in the treatment of CF require nebulization. As a result, the performance characteristics of the nebulizer must be considered when a method of delivery for inhaled medications is selected. Studies comparing the efficiency of different aerosol delivery systems found a significant difference among systems in terms of particle size, total delivery of fluid, and time taken to deliver the medication.[34,104] Less drug wastage, reduced treatment time, and more specific matching of the delivery system to the breathing pattern of the individual are possible.[34]

Effective clearance of mucus-obstructed airways benefits the pulmonary environment by allowing for improved ventilation and gas exchange and by limiting the tissue damage associated with recurrent infection. Physical therapy techniques to promote airway clearance include postural drainage and percussion, positioning, expiratory vibrations, positive expiratory pressure (PEP) therapy, oscillating PEP therapy, high-frequency chest wall oscillations (HFCWO), directed breathing techniques such as the active cycle of breathing technique (ACBT), and autogenic drainage. In addition, huffing and coughing are essential elements of all airway clearance techniques. Exercise, thoracic mobility, and postural realignment exercises are often prescribed to maximize pulmonary fitness.

More research is needed to scientifically support the efficacy of the use of pulmonary physical therapy modalities in CF. Most studies assess only short-term effects on airway clearance by measuring qualities of sputum (i.e., volume, weight, and viscosity) or rates of clearance of radiolabeled aerosol from the lung. Although some modalities yield short-term improvements in these markers, few measure long-term and clinically important end points like health-related quality of life or rates of exacerbation, hospitalization, and mortality. The ethics of performing long-term randomized trials that withhold airway clearance from patients with CF is problematic, as this treatment is considered to be the standard of care and has an established short-term benefit in increasing expectorated sputum volume and enhancing mucous clearance.[116]

A comparative study of the literature and a meta-analysis demonstrated the need for more adequate controls, randomized design and sampling, larger sample sizes, and use of valid outcome measures.[17,187] Studies reviewed by Boyd and colleagues were evaluated and classified according to the level of evidence supported by the research design as proposed by Sackett.[168] The analysis suggested support for exercise, "conventional" physical therapy (postural drainage, percussion, and vibration), and PEP mask therapies in treatment of children with CF in chronic stages of the disease when PFT results were used as an outcome measure. In acute exacerbations of respiratory status, both PEP mask therapy and conventional physical therapy showed some evidence of improving pulmonary function scores. A 2-year study of 66 subjects found that PEP therapy is a valid alternative to conventional physical therapy.[65] In another long-term study, pulmonary function scores improved in subjects using PEP versus conventional physical therapy, which indicated that PEP was preferred by subjects, thereby increasing adherence.[119] A recent study demonstrated the physiologic basis for the efficacy of PEP by confirming that both low PEP and high PEP improve gas mixing in individuals with CF, and that these improvements are associated with increased lung function, sputum expectoration, and arterial blood oxyhemoglobin saturation.[45] Oscillating PEP has gained popularity as an airway clearance technique, and studies indicate its usefulness as an alternative modality to conventional physical therapy.[127] Exercise should be included in the management of CF. In a study at the Hospital for Sick Children in Toronto that evaluated the effects of a 3-year home exercise program, it was found that pulmonary function declined more slowly in the exercise group than in the control group, suggesting a benefit for patients with CF participating in regular aerobic exercise.[169]

Increased understanding of how CFTR dysfunction causes lung disease has resulted in new therapies that target

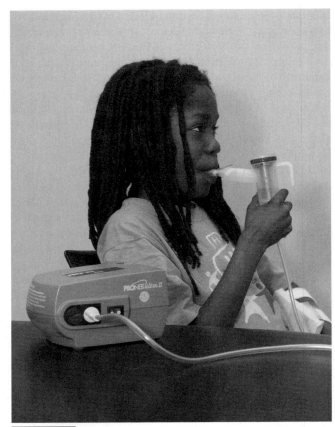

Figure 24-1 Receiving inhalation therapy with reusable breath-enhanced nebulizer with mouthpiece.

the basic defect. Cystic fibrosis transmembrane regulator replacement therapy involves the use of gene transfer therapy. This approach has been limited by the selection of an appropriate vector because of adverse side effects, transfection efficiency, and short-lived gene expression. Another treatment alternative is CFTR pharmacotherapy, which affects the trafficking, expression, or functioning of CFTR, depending on the class mutation. However, chloride secretion in airway epithelial cells is not limited to CFTR; alternative chloride channels can be stimulated to compensate for the lack of CFTR-mediated chloride secretion with specific drugs. Short-term clinical studies look promising and long-term studies are under way. In contrast to stimulating chloride channels, inhibition of sodium absorption through the epithelial sodium channel is being investigated as another novel therapy. Finally, because inadequate ASL is associated with the development of CF lung disease, the inhalation of an osmotic agent may increase the airway fluid layer (Figure 24-1). These exciting therapies are being developed to treat the early and root causes of CF, which will improve outcomes and potentially reduce the burden of care.[161] The unprecedented volume of current research and the emergence of new, successful therapies for CF dictate a need for conscientious practitioners to remain educated and receptive to adjusting their management plans and critical pathways for care of patients with CF.

LUNG TRANSPLANTATION

Organ transplantation is now a treatment option in many different terminal illnesses, including CF. Advances in surgical technique and postoperative care with improved immunosuppressive therapies have given some patients with CF a new lease on life. (See Chapter 26 for a more detailed discussion of the involvement of physical therapy in postsurgical care.)

In North America, both heart-lung and double-lung transplants have been performed on patients with CF with end-stage pulmonary disease. The Toronto Lung Transplant Group included pioneers in this field who performed the world's first successful double-lung transplant in 1987.[152] Cystic fibrosis has steadily increased as an indication leading to lung transplantation and accounts for 67% of adolescent lung recipients and 16% of adults.[15] Survival rates in pediatric lung transplantation are similar to those reported in adults, with a median survival of 4.3 years. Between 2002 and 2006, survival rates improved slightly, with 1-year and 4-year survival rates being 81% and 58%, respectively, compared with 65% and 44% for recipients transplanted between 1988 and 1994.[8]

Living-donor lobar lung transplantation has been performed since 1993, but because it involves recruitment of two donors and the surgical procedure carries inherent risks to the donors, it is not without its problems. The impact of this technique on survival statistics appears comparable with that of other approaches, but long-term analysis is needed.[179] Most complications arise from infections or graft rejection in the early posttransplant period. Development of obliterative bronchiolitis may be evidence of chronic rejection and is a leading cause of death after pediatric lung transplantation.[15] The problem with malabsorption in patients with CF dictates difficulties with the therapeutic regimen for adequate immunosuppression after transplantation. Individual transplant centers should direct and monitor the immunosuppressive regimen because close monitoring of serum levels and adjustment of doses are vital to successful posttransplant management.[205]

Guidelines for listing a patient with CF for lung transplantation include FEV_1 <30% of predicted or rapidly declining lung function (increased frequency and duration of hospitalizations for pulmonary exacerbations, increasing antibiotic resistance of infectious bacteria, and increasing oxygen requirements, hypercapnia, and pulmonary hypertension). Patients should also have a history of compliance with medical treatment, an acceptable psychosocial profile, and functional vital organs.[99,205] A referral for transplant (and acceptance onto the waiting list) must be made early enough to allow for a substantial wait for a suitable donor and creates a need for the development of a preoperative

program of conditioning for these patients, which is a component of the lung transplantation program in many centers. These conditioning programs are designed to optimize the patient's functional ability and exercise tolerance and to help maintain emotional well-being during the long wait for a transplant.[42] Physical therapists play a primary role in the development and implementation of both preoperative and postoperative exercise programs, which are described later in this chapter.

Double-lung transplantation is now most often performed by bilateral anterolateral thoracotomies using bilateral submammary incisions, as first described in 1990.[145] The lungs are transplanted as sequential single-lung grafts. The lung with the worst pulmonary function is replaced first, while oxygenation and ventilation are maintained by the native lung. Replacement of the second lung can then proceed with the newly implanted lung supporting the patient.[201] Use of this technique has reduced to 30% to 35% the number of patients requiring anticoagulation and cardiopulmonary bypass during surgery.[201] This surgical innovation has also reduced the degree of complications from perioperative bleeding, which can be a significant problem for patients with CF because of the presence of inflammatory adhesions within the pleural space.[201]

Single-lung transplants are not performed on patients with CF because the remaining native lung continues to be ventilated after transplantation, and its overexpansion will compress the transplanted lung.[109] Contamination of the native lung could also spread infection to the transplanted lung.[59]

BODY FUNCTIONS AND STRUCTURES

EXAMINATION AND IMPLICATIONS

The primary physiologic abnormalities in CF include (1) a dysfunctional chloride channel in transepithelial electrolyte transport, creating abnormal increases in the concentrations of sodium and chloride in serous gland secretions; (2) blocked exocrine gland function due to obstruction by hyperviscous secretions; and (3) an extraordinary susceptibility to chronic endobronchial infection by specific groups of bacteria, apparently compounded by impaired or deficient mucociliary clearance. Although patients with CF show significant differences in levels of clinical impairment, all patients with CF have these three abnormalities.[109]

The degree of limitations that the abnormal pathology imposes varies greatly among people with CF. Proper measurement of these limitations is crucial to determining the proper interventions. Examination techniques to quantify the abnormal pathology seen in CF measure the functioning of the respiratory and gastrointestinal systems and the limitations in exercise tolerance. Quality-of-life questionnaires and other subjective reports provide information on the patient's perceived level of functioning.

MEASURING PULMONARY FUNCTION

Pulmonary function tests (PFTs) are used to evaluate lung function. PFTs are indicated to determine the presence or absence of lung disease, to quantify the effects of a known lung disease on lung function, and to determine the beneficial or negative effects of various types of therapy.

PFTs consist of a number of different tests, and the type of test ordered depends on the question to be answered. The most common question for patients with CF is "What is the degree of obstruction?" This parameter is easily measured with spirometry, which measures forced vital capacity (FVC), forced expired volume in 1 second (FEV_1), and airflow rates (forced expired flow between 25% and 75% of the vital capacity) during different phases of expiration, yielding an indication of the amount of bronchial obstruction present. The measure of FEV_1 chronicles the early portion of expiration and is often reported as a ratio of FVC. In a healthy individual, FEV_1/FVC is 0.70 to 0.80, indicating that 70% to 80% of the FVC is expired in the first seconds of a forced exhalation.[77] A decrease in this ratio reflects an obstructed expiratory airflow.

Early detection of abnormalities in lung function in CF is critical, as these initial changes involve the small airways.[122] Miller suggests that forced expiratory flow (FEF) 25–75% is more sensitive than FEV_1 or FEV_1/FVC in detecting changes in small airway obstruction.[123] Timed volumes at high lung volumes (e.g., FEV_1) may remain within typical limits because the contribution of the small airways to overall resistance is low.[91] FEV_1 therefore is not a sensitive test in early lung disease but indicates obstruction of the central bronchi and becomes markedly abnormal as disease progresses.[110]

Another form of PFTs is plethysmography, in which the patient breathes through a mouthpiece to measure changes in air pressure within a sealed chamber (body box) while the volume of air remains constant. The volumes that can be measured include functional residual capacity (FRC), total lung capacity (TLC), and residual volume (RV), which can also be assessed by gas dilution methods.[167] Both of these techniques can further evaluate severity of lung disease by determining the degree of gas trapping that occurs in an obstructive disease such as CF.

Although PFTs are informative and invaluable for early detection in advance of lung disease, these tests are not always easily performed. Patients must be cooperative, must be able to follow specific instructions, and must give maximum effort. Children younger than age 6 years usually cannot perform the standard test of forced expiration in 1 second in a reliable manner. Recent reports document that children between 3 and 6 years can successfully undergo spirometry.[134] Another study examining children age 2 to 5 years found that modifying the FEV_1 test to $FEV_{0.75}$ gave a reliable measure of pulmonary function for young children.[8] Various techniques are being developed to measure pulmonary function in infants, such as the raised-volume rapid thoracoabdominal compression (RVRTC) technique and fractional lung volumes. Revised techniques of rapid thoracic compression following increasing lung volumes near TLC and multiple breath washouts have also been investigated. Infant PFTs, however, require special equipment and trained personnel, which currently are available in only a few centers.[197]

In older children and adults, many other factors, such as sputum retention, poor nutrition, and fatigue, can influence the individual's performance during spirometry. Notably, many children with CF show performance scores on repeat tests that have a significantly greater range of variability than scores of typical test subjects.[39] Performing the body plethysmography test can help to more accurately assess lung function by measuring the patient's lung volumes (FRC, TLC, and RV). Some claustrophobia may be experienced by patients undergoing testing in the "body box," and plethysmography may not be appropriate for all young children.

The lung-clearance index is a more sensitive test than spirometry at the early stages of disease. The test consists of multiple-breath washout of a nonabsorbable gas (sulfur hexafluoride) to measure ventilation inhomogeneity caused by airways narrowing from inflammation or partial obstruction by mucus. The technique is easy to perform, requiring only tidal breathing; no additional coordination or forced maneuvers are needed, making it possible to use the technique in infancy and during preschool ages to generate repeatable and reproducible results. One disadvantage is that the inhaled gas does not reach regions of the lung that are completely obstructed, and therefore may underestimate disease severity. Additional longitudinal studies are needed to confirm its practicality and superiority to PFT.[48]

The U.S. National Institutes of Health's comparative review of 307 cases of CF reported that PFT scores showed a common pattern: progressive decline in flow rates and vital capacity (VC) and an increase in the RV/TLC ratio, correlating with clinically gauged worsening of disease.[54] As pulmonary disease becomes progressively more severe, deteriorating PFT scores can be used to help predict life expectancy. In one study, patients with poor arterial gases and an FEV_1 of less than 30% of predicted value had 2-year mortality rates of greater than 50%.[94] Individuals with CF demonstrate a characteristic decline in mid-expiratory flow rate (FEF25–75%); noting the rate of this decline becomes an important prognostic indicator.[75] Steadily worsening PFT scores reliably correlate with declining clinical conditions and are used as an indicator in assessment for lung transplantation.[95] FEV_1 has been shown to be the strongest predictor of mortality in CF and has been the primary outcome measure in many clinical trials.[197]

Signs and Symptoms

Progressive hypoxemia is one of the earliest signs of increasing pulmonary disease and can occur before any other detectable abnormality in lung function.[100] Mucous plugging and bronchiolitis in the patient's airways cause ventilation-perfusion abnormalities, and the subsequent hypoxemia worsens as severity of the obstruction increases.[109] Further declines in arterial oxygenation can occur during sleep, so blood gases may have to be monitored throughout the night to assess the need for nocturnal supplementary oxygen.[128] Increased oxygen demands during exercise can be a contributing factor to hypoxemia in the patient with CF. Although arterial blood gas measures are considered the "gold standard" in blood gas analysis,[209] they are not commonly used in patients with CF because of their invasive nature. Other noninvasive techniques are preferred, such as pulse oximetry, which measures the level of oxygen saturation in the blood. This assessment tool can be used to evaluate the suitability of supplemental oxygen during exercise performance.

Other changes in blood gas readings forewarn of serious advanced pathology. Hypercapnia in CF indicates advanced pulmonary disease and carries a poor prognosis. In a study of survival patterns of patients with CF who demonstrated hypercapnia, it was found that death usually occurred within 1 year of the development of chronic hypercapnia[193] without interventions such as noninvasive ventilation or lung transplantation.

Chest radiographs can provide detailed evidence of the progressive nature of pulmonary disease in CF (Figure 24-2). In the initial stages of pulmonary involvement, the chest radiograph may reveal signs of hyperinflation and peribronchial thickening. As the disease progresses, bronchiectasis can become apparent, particularly in the upper lobes, and pulmonary infiltrates appear as nodular shadows on radiographs. With severe pulmonary disease, the hyperexpanded lungs can precipitate flattening of the diaphragm, thoracic kyphosis, and bowing of the sternum—all detectable on radiography.[109] Confirmation of the development of a pneumothorax can also be provided by examining the chest radiographs. When pulmonary disease is advanced, pulmonary artery hypertrophy may be noticed on radiography as a sign of the pulmonary hypertension associated with cor pulmonale.[109]

Cultures from sputum of a patient with CF identify the variety of bacteria that have infected the lower respiratory tract.[67] Sensitivity studies can then be performed to identify effective antibiotic therapies.[140] CF centers perform regular sputum bacteriologic tests to ensure adequate antibiotic coverage for their patients and to help monitor the state of bacterial infection.[108]

Physical examination of the patient also gathers valuable information. Chest assessment includes inspection, palpation, percussion, and auscultation. Inspection can reveal postural abnormalities (Figure 24-3), modifications of breathing pattern (Figure 24-4), or signs of respiratory distress. Evidence of a chronic productive cough may be apparent. Examination of the comparative dimensions of the chest in the anterior-posterior and transverse planes may reveal the barrel chest deformity common to obstructive lung

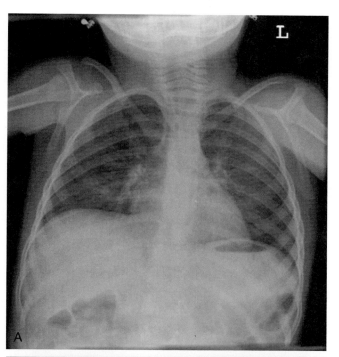

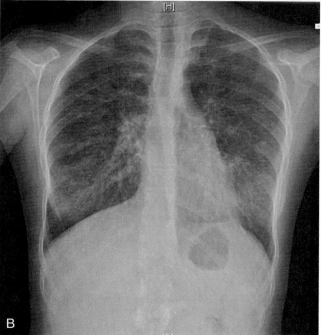

Figure 24-2 Two chest radiographs of the same individual showing marked deterioration over the course of 10 years. **A,** At age 4, there is already evidence of bilateral perihilar peribronchial thickening and patchy infiltrates in the right middle lobe, suggestive of mucous plugging. **B,** Diffuse bilateral bronchiectasis associated with cystic fibrosis with hyperinflation and bilateral areas of consolidation.

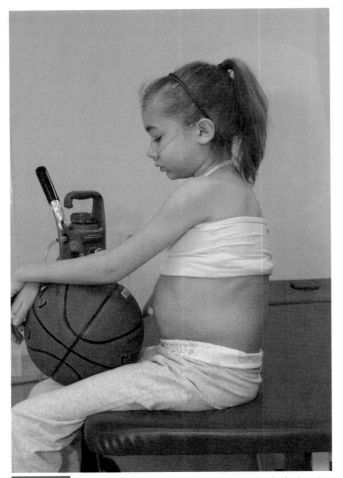

Figure 24-3 An example of postural changes in an individual: elevation of the shoulders and protracted scapulae and increased anterior-posterior diameter of the chest. Note intercostal indrawing.

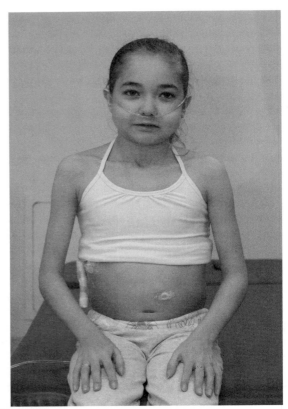

Figure 24-4 Use of accessory muscles of respiration, tracheal tug, and supraclavicular indrawing is apparent on physical inspection. Note the gastrostomy tube and the port-a-catheter line.

diseases.[87] Inspection of the fingers and toes may reveal bluish nail beds and clubbing of the digits, which reflect a change in the amount of soft tissue at the nail bed associated with lung disease. Palpation of the chest wall for chest wall excursion and for tactile fremitus may reveal atelectasis, pneumothorax, or large airway secretions. Examination of the resonance pattern of the chest, as demonstrated by audible changes on percussion, can provide an indication of abnormally dense areas of the lungs.[87] Age of the patient may highly influence the reliability and clinical usefulness of different components of the physical examination. In an infant, measurement of chest wall expansion may be difficult and percussion may not be appropriate.[41]

Careful auscultation of the chest can contribute information on the quality of airflow and evidence of obstruction in different areas of the lungs. Reduced ventilation is suggested by decreased breath sounds or the presence of inspiratory crackles (also called *rales*). If crackles are heard throughout the ventilatory cycle, this suggests impaired secretion clearance. Diffuse airway obstruction may cause polyphonic wheezing. The examiner must be aware that chronically hyperinflated lungs tend to mask or make it difficult to hear adventitious sounds on auscultation.[87] Familiarization with the usual pattern of a patient's lung sounds can be a critical component of evaluation of examination results because an alteration of the typical pattern may signal a pulmonary change that might otherwise have gone undetected.

NUTRITION

In children, studies have indicated that the degree to which a child with CF is underweight was an independent factor that adversely affected survival; more recently short stature has been identified as an independent risk factor for survival. Patients need to work diligently to consume adequate calories to meet increased needs caused by the increased work of breathing and the altered digestive absorption. Patients who are pancreatically insufficient need oral supplementary enzymes to enable them to absorb adequate nutrients from their diet. Pancreatic function may be determined by a number of testing methods, including fecal fat assessment, pancreatic substrate assays, and direct collection of pancreatic secretions by duodenal intubation.[110] Individuals with CF who have significant preservation of pancreatic function and therefore can maintain normal fat absorption have less pulmonary dysfunction and a better prognosis than those individuals who have pancreatic insufficiency.[40] Because pulmonary function is strongly linked with adequate nutrition and weight gain, treatment goals aim to prevent the cascade of wasting precipitated by reduced lung function, increased energy expenditure, decreased intake due to poor appetite, and increased losses due to malabsorption.

Other factors that are associated with a preferred prognosis include single-organ involvement at diagnosis, absent or single-organism sputum colonization, and a normal chest radiograph 1 year after diagnosis. Multiple organ involvement, abnormal chest radiographs at diagnosis, colonization of multiple organisms in the sputum, a falloff from typical growth curves, and recurrent hemoptysis are all factors associated with a poor prognosis. There also appears to be a gender bias in severity of disease expression, with male patients possessing a better prognosis than their female counterparts.[108]

PHYSICAL THERAPY: EXAMINATION AND INTERVENTION

INFANCY

Newborn screening for CF is currently carried out in many countries around the world, including the United States and within some provinces of Canada. The current method of screening suggests that many but not all newborns with CF can be identified. Studies have suggested that through newborn screening, nutritional deficits are detected and that early intervention may be useful to protect against loss of lung function.[16]

A diagnosis of CF for their child can mean many things to parents. At the most basic level, it means they have a child with "special needs," and those needs can be seen to influence the family dynamics.[103] The child's family members are forced to familiarize themselves with CF and with the psychological and practical demands inherent in this diagnosis. Education of the family is a crucial goal, which is best met at regional CF centers that have the expertise and availability of a variety of specialty services. A physical therapist at a CF center is part of a cohesive team of interested investigators and caregivers. Educating patients and their families while measuring and treating the myriad complications that accompany this disease is the ongoing goal of a CF center's staff. The Cystic Fibrosis Foundation (http://www.cff.org) can be a valuable educational and supportive resource at this time.

Promoting Function: Parental Education

Intervention often must be implemented immediately upon diagnosis, and the family needs assistance in making the necessary adjustments and provisions to ensure adherence with any suggested therapeutic regimen. Physical therapists

evaluate which essential elements of the child's care must be addressed by them and then provide instruction for the family on proper administration of the appropriate physical therapy techniques. The therapist should demonstrate sensitivity and equanimity while interacting with these children and their families, remembering that this is a very stressful time for those involved, and that what the family may "hear" can differ from what is actually said to them.[23]

What families seem to need most is information that acknowledges the seriousness of the disease while emphasizing the likelihood of a happy and fulfilling family life. Developing the types of strategies that permit some flexibility in intervention regimens promotes better integration of the child's treatment needs into the family's routines.[113] Parents may have many concerns and a host of questions and can be especially confused by all the uncertainty that typifies the disease. Because the progression of CF is so variable from case to case, ongoing examination of the child's status is the only way to ensure meeting the child's individual requirements. This means that family members must have continued association with the CF center and need to appreciate their role as integral members of the caregiving team.

Children with a chronic condition have been shown to have increased risk of psychosocial dysfunction, particularly when parental anxiety is overwhelming.[28,71] Because excessive parental overprotection is strongly linked to the existence of psychosocial maladjustment in children, the parents of a child with CF must be alerted to the dangers of unnecessarily shielding their child from aspects of normal life. In infancy, this may take the form of overdressing the child to guard against drafts or neglecting to allow the child to participate in normal exploratory play. Physical therapists should reassure parents that infants with CF have the same requirements as other infants with respect to physical and emotional development. Excellent reference materials are available in most CF centers. Teaching manuals, designed to supplement the information imparted by the CF center staff, are often distributed to families and can be made available to other interested caregivers such as child care workers or school teachers. Orenstein's book, *Cystic Fibrosis: A Guide for Patient and Family*,[140] is highly recommended.

Management of Body Functions and Structures

In the neonate, the most frequently seen symptoms of CF are meconium ileus, malabsorption of nutrients, and failure to thrive, all of which are associated with involvement of the gastrointestinal tract.[166] Overt pulmonary involvement is not apparent in the neonatal period because the lungs are morphologically normal at birth.[80,109] Within a few months, however, some infants with CF develop signs of impaired respiratory function, manifesting symptoms suggesting bronchiolitis. Pronounced wheeze, an indication of hyperactive airways, is sometimes apparent, and chest radiographs can reveal evidence of hyperinflation.[149] Obstruction of airflow in these infants may be related to airway inflammation, mucosal edema, copious mucus secretion retention, and increased airway tone.[184] The bronchioles are considered the main site of airflow obstruction in infancy.[182] Studies using bronchoalveolar lavage revealed that every infant with CF—whether symptomatic or not—has evidence of small airway obstruction in the form of bronchial mucous casts.[203]

Measurements to assess possible limitation of pulmonary function cannot be taken in the conventional way (e.g., spirometry) in infants; therefore, researchers have had to modify standard methods by using the raised-volume rapid thoracoabdominal compression technique (RVRTC). $FEV_{0.5}$ was measured and was found to be significantly lower in infants with CF shortly after diagnosis (median age of 28 weeks) and 6 months later on retest.[160]

Infants with CF demonstrate low values of pulmonary compliance,[147] decreased lung compliance, and a less homogeneous distribution of ventilation when compared with typical control subjects.[185] Tepper and colleagues found these changes in both symptomatic and asymptomatic infants.[186] Abnormalities in flow-volume curves[69] and low values of maximal expiratory flow[84] indicate that limitations to airflow in infancy are associated with bronchoconstriction.[80] Infants with CF have indeed displayed altered bronchial tone after the administration of a bronchodilator, as revealed by the fact that airflow rates showed significant increases not seen in a control group.[84] Methacholine challenge testing also revealed heightened airway responsiveness.[1]

These research studies have yielded valuable insight into the early pulmonary manifestations of CF in infancy. The formal PFTs used in these studies, however, are not feasible or practical for the infant population of most clinics or CF centers. Examination of pulmonary involvement in infancy is usually limited to physical findings, history of respiratory symptoms, and chest radiographs. Carefully observing for signs of respiratory distress, such as nasal flaring, expiratory grunting, retractions of the chest wall, tachypnea, pallor, or cyanosis, produces an indication of respiratory status. Interpretation of auscultation of an infant or young child is more challenging because of easily transmitted sounds from close structures underlying the thin chest wall,[41] but careful auscultation is necessary to ascertain if there is any evidence of wheezing. Changes visible on radiography are the most reliable indication of early pulmonary involvement because it has been demonstrated that airflow obstruction may precede the presence of overt respiratory symptoms. Historical accounts of respiratory illness must also be carefully considered.

The rate of deterioration of pulmonary function in individuals with CF may be slowed by early initiation of treatment. Bronchoalveolar lavage findings in infants with CF show the presence of infection and inflammation within the airways as early as 4 weeks postpartum even before clinical manifestations, which can damage the respiratory epithelium resulting in an impairment of mucociliary transport

and secretion retention. The airways of infants with CF have also been shown to be morphologically abnormal with greater diameter and thicker walls.[105] The change in respiratory patterns and mechanics suggests that early therapeutic intervention might actually delay the onset of overt symptoms of respiratory impairment, but the value of initiating pulmonary treatment before development of symptoms remains controversial, although various theoretical arguments for initiating therapy as soon as possible can be presented. The time before onset of structural changes provides an opportunity for intervention and prevention of onset of progressive airway damage.[20] Adherence to a therapy routine may be improved if it is incorporated as a part of one's lifestyle, and prevention of respiratory impairment can be emphasized early in the treatment plan.[203]

A study was conducted to evaluate the combined effects of a bronchodilator and cardiopulmonary physical therapy on infants newly diagnosed with CF, addressing the controversy surrounding treatment for asymptomatic children.[80] Baseline, preintervention measurements of the mechanics and energetics of breathing were obtained for all subjects. Twenty minutes after the inhalation of a bronchodilator, cardiopulmonary physical therapy was given to the subjects, consisting of 20 minutes of chest percussions and vibrations applied in five different postural drainage positions. Immediately after the physical therapy session, repeat pulmonary function measurements were taken. Most of the infants (10 of 13) demonstrated decreases from baseline values in pulmonary resistance, with subsequent decreases in the work of breathing, after administration of the bronchodilator and physical therapy.[80] Researchers postulated that the bronchodilator relieved subclinical bronchospasm and aided the reduction of mucosal edema, and that physical therapy, assisting the immature mucociliary system, was effective in mobilizing secretions, thereby improving the patency of the airways.[80] When serial PFTs are possible, objective measures of the progression of impairment and the effects of specific treatments may provide future evidence of the efficacy of early intervention.[80]

Prevention of obstructive mucous plugging is the initial goal of pulmonary physical therapy in this population. The primary modalities used for promotion of clearance of secretions for infants with CF are modified postural drainage, percussion, and vibrations. The physiologic rationale and precise method of these modalities are well described in most comprehensive texts on physical therapy,[64,88,107,157] but important modifications to the proper use of these modalities for infants will be discussed.

In obstructive airway diseases such as CF, the effectiveness of the antireflux mechanism at the esophagogastric junction is reduced.[141] Increases in intra-abdominal pressure that can be associated with coughing also promote gastroesophageal reflux.[170] Of newly diagnosed infants with CF, 35% had symptomatic gastroesophageal reflux in one study,[189] and 24-hour esophageal monitoring revealed abnormalities in 10 successive infants newly diagnosed with CF in another.[44] There are suggestions that reflux can worsen lung disease in CF[112] and cause upper respiratory symptoms.[207] A 5-year comparative study by Button and colleagues compared the standard tipped position versus the modified position (no tip) in 20 asymptomatic infants.[25] Investigators found that the modified group had significantly fewer days with upper respiratory tract symptoms and shorter courses of antibiotics in the first year of life than those with standard conventional physical therapy. They also had better chest x-ray scores at 2.5 years of age and better pulmonary function at 5 years.

Timing physical therapy around feeding schedules may also be necessary to reduce the risk of gastroesophageal reflux. Postural drainage positions are easily achieved by arranging the infant in the required manner on the caregiver's lap. Holding the small child in this way also seems to offer the child an extra measure of security. Adapting hand position (by "tenting" the middle finger) or using a rubber palm cup suits the application of percussion on a tiny chest wall (Figure 24-5). The applied force of percussion should vary with the size and condition of the infant, and conscientious monitoring of the infant's response to treatment should guide the amount of vigor used in percussion. Timing of manual vibrations to coincide with the expirations of an infant is difficult because of the infant's rapid respiratory rate, and this technique may be very challenging to teach to parents.

Some studies have investigated the use of a positive expiratory pressure mask in infants compared with postural drainage. Constantini and colleagues studied 26 newborns with CF over 12 months using PEP and postural drainage as airway clearance techniques.[37] The use of PEP was associated with less severe gastroesophageal reflux compared with the postural drainage group. No significant difference in the effectiveness of airway clearance was noted between the two groups, and patients and parents preferred PEP. Assisted autogenic drainage is a newer approach that is being investigated in Europe as an alternative airway clearance technique for infants.[188] Another noteworthy factor is the encouragement of achievement of regular developmental milestones to encourage chest mobility, leg strengthening, and endurance training.

Education for the family on the application of prescribed physical therapy modalities should be ongoing. Periodically asking the parent or caregiver to demonstrate treatment positions and manual technique allows the therapist to identify possible problems with proper application. Instructing parents to play breathing games with their infants and toddlers can eventually lead them to perform diaphragmatic breathing and huffing.[47] Breathing exercises can promote use of collateral ventilation and can introduce concepts of techniques that will be used in the future. In some CF centers, the physical therapist is also responsible for ordering, demonstrating, and arranging for the maintenance of the equipment necessary for the aerosol delivery of medications. Instruction on the care and use of these nebulizers is vitally important to ensure correct delivery of prescribed medications.

Adherence with any suggested therapeutic regimen requires commitment on the part of the caregiver. The demands of caring for a child with CF can seem extreme when considering the extra attention to nutritional issues, medications, and physical therapy that this diagnosis entails. Signs of excessive stress or evidence that the family is having difficulty in coping with the caregiving requirements may become obvious. Referral to a social worker or a psychologist might help identify the family in crisis and aid the family in developing strategies to enable adjustment to the various challenges that lie ahead of them as they nurture their child with CF.

PRESCHOOL- AND SCHOOL-AGE PERIOD

Approximately 75% of children with CF are now diagnosed before their third birthday.[103] When there is a positive family history of CF, parents are familiar with the disease, but in many cases, there is no prior knowledge of the disorder and the diagnosis can be startling. Initial shock may be followed by disbelief, anger, or grief.[103] The age of the child when diagnosed affects parental reaction to some extent. The longer the prediagnostic stage (the older the child), the greater the likelihood that the parents may experience extreme shock at the time of diagnosis.[22] Sensitivity for the anguish experienced by the family must be shown.

The clinical status of children with CF is highly variable. Some toddlers may have already experienced pulmonary complications and been hospitalized repeatedly, whereas others exhibit little or no detrimental impact on their

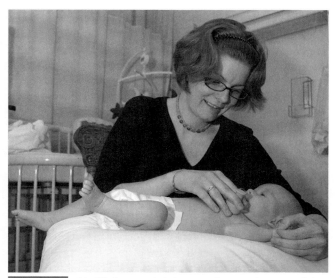

Figure 24-5 Modified postural drainage and percussion on an infant performed by a parent using a palm cup.

respiratory status. The effects of protein-calorie deficits due to malabsorption may be manifest in stunted development such as small stature or a lower than average weight-to-height ratio; therefore, a difference in appearance from their healthy siblings or friends may already be perceptible.

Participation

Young children need to develop the ability to function socially outside the family circle. Demands of school and new friendships dictate a lessening of parental attachments and a capacity for some measure of independence.[103] This type of autonomy may be difficult to achieve for the child with CF. If parents perceive that their child is fragile with exceptionally vulnerable health, they may become overprotective. McCollum and Gibson examined issues of family adaptation to CF and found that 47% of parents in the study admitted granting less independence to their child with CF than to their healthy children.[115] Cappelli and colleagues found a strong correlation between parental overprotection and psychological maladjustment in the child.[28] Behavior problems such as restlessness, excessive daydreaming, and inattentiveness are found more often in children with medical conditions such as CF than in their healthy peers.[115] Encouraging children with CF to participate in a variety of social and physical activities could prove beneficial for their physical and emotional health. The physical therapist should stress the importance of incorporating an active lifestyle into the family dynamic.

Assisting children to gain a sense of self-efficacy is an important goal at this time. A key factor of lifelong adherence to necessary treatment is incorporating a sense of self-efficacy (the confidence that one has the ability to perform a behavior). This results from exposure to a credible role model, encouragement to perform tasks of self-management, and development of competency.[11] Individual care plans are developed with each child, and a self-care manual is provided to the families to act as a guide. By initiating this education when the child is young, it is hoped that it may influence the negative correlation between adherence and aging identified by Passero and colleagues.[146]

The CF Family Education Project at Baylor College of Medicine and Texas Children's Hospital developed an educational program that emphasized self-management by providing individual learning packages for parents and patients in early childhood, middle childhood, and adolescence. Curricula were developed on the basis of social cognitive theory and target behavioral capability, self-efficacy, and outcome expectations. The program was designed to be implemented as an integral component of the health care of these families, facilitating learning through reciprocity between clients and the health care environment.[10]

Measurement of Function and Activity

Measurement of impairment and activity limitations in the young child includes history, physical examination, chest radiographs, blood gases, oximetry, and sputum bacteriology. The pulmonary function of children who are able to execute the necessary voluntary maneuver (usually by age 6) can be assessed by spirometry.

Examination by the physical therapist should include thorough history taking, a physical examination including posture, and, when applicable, some type of exercise tolerance testing. Young children with CF may have chronic cough, hypoxemia, and decreased compliance of the lungs,[185] leading to restrictions in maximal oxygen consumption, an increase in the work of breathing, and an increase in resting energy expenditure.[175] These factors all compromise exercise tolerance.

Exercise testing is an objective method by which the physical therapist can quantify the patient's disease severity and functional ability.[158] Individuals with CF often will not be aware of the extent of their physical limitations owing to the slow progression of their disease.[30] An exercise test can detect mild pulmonary dysfunction, which may go undetected during investigations at rest, and will also help reveal how individuals cope with work despite their disability.[68]

When an exercise test protocol is chosen, the purpose of the test and the age and disease severity of the subject should be carefully considered. Choosing the appropriate exercise test depends on the specific question being asked.[137] For example, to assess activity limitations in aerobic performance, the exercise test should be progressive and should stress the subject's cardiorespiratory system to a symptom-limited maximum. The test should also be reproducible and capable of providing meaningful results.[177]

Cycle ergometers are often used for testing exercise capacity in children with pulmonary disease.[31,133] An accurate prediction of oxygen consumption can be obtained because the mechanical efficiency for pedaling a cycle is independent of body weight and therefore is almost identical for all individuals.[30] Although the treadmill test generally yields higher oxygen consumption values, the cycle ergometer offers the advantages of being relatively inexpensive, portable, and safe. Because cycling is a familiar exercise for many people, it is less likely to cause apprehension. As with the treadmill test, cycle ergometry is reproducible.[63] In addition, the subject is relatively stationary, and therefore vital signs are more easily monitored. Most ergometers have adjustable seat heights suitable for children, and it is important to be able to adjust handlebars and pedal crank length.

Several progressive exercise protocols are used on the cycle ergometer to determine maximum oxygen consumption or individual peak work capacity (Figure 24-6; see Chapter 6). Cerny and colleagues examined subjects with CF matched to a typical control sample to monitor cardiopulmonary response to incrementally increased workloads with cycle ergometry.[31] Workloads were increased every 2 minutes until the subject could not continue. The study demonstrated that control subjects needed an increased workload of 0.32 W/kg on average for an increase in heart rate of 10

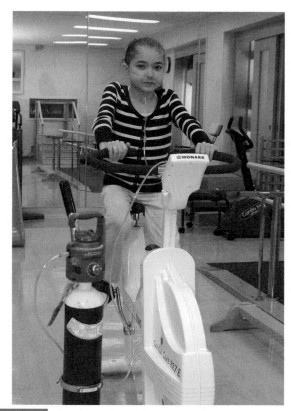

Figure 24-6 Exercise testing with a young patient on oxygen.

beats per minute. Subjects with CF required workload increases ranging from 0.15 to 0.35 W/kg, depending on the severity of their disease, to demonstrate the same change in heart rate. Cerny and colleagues concluded that the limiting factor in exercise tolerance was severity of pulmonary involvement, and not cardiovascular limitation.[31]

If the child is too small to successfully use a cycle ergometer, a treadmill can be used because only the ability to walk is required. The child should be monitored closely to maintain a sense of confidence during the test. Elevation and speed are adjusted according to the size and skill of the subject and should be selected to allow even the subject with severe dysfunction to exercise at two to three levels of difficulty.[30] Two frequently used protocols for children with CF are the Godfrey protocol for cycle tests and the Bruce protocol for treadmill testing.[158]

For individuals with severe lung disease, field walking tests such as 6- or 12-minute walks[24] or the shuttle walking test[171] may be preferred. The reliability and validity of the 6-minute walk test[74] and the shuttle test[172] with children with CF have been demonstrated, and normative values for children who are healthy have been published.[158] Walking tests are simple, are inexpensive, and can be performed by individuals of all ages and abilities with little risk of injury.[153] Because they are highly reproducible, walking tests correspond closely to the demands of everyday activity.[76]

Another quick and portable test that may prove useful in a clinical setting is the 3-minute step test, which illustrated similar results as the 6-minute walk test when outcome measures were arterial oxygen saturation, maximum pulse rate, and the Modified Borg Dyspnea Scale.[9] Narang and colleagues, however, found that when the 3-minute step test was compared with the cycle ergometer, the 3-minute step test provided limited information related to exercise performance in a group with mild lung disease.[130] They suggest that a more suitable test for this group must be given at a higher intensity and must equate better to typical levels of physical activity.

Subjects performing an exercise test must be closely monitored and special attention must be given to signs of increased work of breathing that are disproportionate to what is expected.[30] Subjective measures of the perceived level of respiratory labor with a dyspnea scale such as Borg's Scale of Ratings of Perceived Exertion[14] can be taken before, during, and after the exercise test. Borg's scale is a good indicator of physiologic and psychological strain and allows individuals to interpret the intensity of their exercise according to subjective impressions.[144] For more information on quantifying increased work of breathing, a 15-count breathlessness scale is an objective measure that can be used with the Borg scale or a visual analog scale.[155]

Maximal work capacity is limited by ventilation in individuals with pulmonary disease.[30] Deficiencies in gas exchange and poor pulmonary mechanics compound the effects of decreased exercise capacity.[31,82] The limitation to exercise caused by pulmonary restrictions is further evidenced by failure to reach predicted peak heart rates in exercise test subjects with CF, suggesting that exercise capacity is not limited by cardiovascular factors.[27]

A complete physical examination should assist in revealing the individual's level of fitness, thus aiding the physical therapist in choosing the most appropriate exercise testing protocol. Individual exercise programs can then be designed to improve exercise capacity and fitness level and to encourage patients with CF to be physically active.

Management of Body Functions and Structures

People with CF demonstrate wide variance in the severity of illness because the disease progresses in individuals at different rates, but some amount of chronic airflow obstruction is often already present in childhood. The small peripheral airways are the site of most of these early pulmonary changes, and patchy atelectasis and ventilation-perfusion abnormalities lead to increases in functional dead space and discernible hypoxemia.[109]

The goals of a physical therapy program for the young child should encompass the improvement of exercise tolerance with continued attention to secretion clearance techniques. Correction and maintenance of proper postural alignment are also stressed. Goals of treatment should be designed with the child and her or his family and should account for the developmental stage of the child and the uniqueness of the family's circumstances. The learning environment must accommodate the child's learning style and avoid prescriptive tasks that are beyond the child's capabilities to promote self-efficacy and adherence. Education of the caregivers must incorporate similar strategies because their full cooperation and participation are essential.

Postural drainage, percussion, and vibration (conventional physical therapy) are common modalities for secretion mobilization in this population. Mechanical percussors may be used to ease the work involved with manual percussion and to provide the child with an aid for self-treatment. Children with a chronic illness should be encouraged to assume a degree of responsibility for their own treatment. Feeling some level of control over one's own health fosters self-esteem and helps subdue anxiety.[92] Children with CF may find it difficult to sustain the performance of manual percussion, even on easily accessible lung segments, and mechanical percussors therefore can help alleviate this problem.

Although conventional physical therapy has long been used in the treatment of CF, it has been criticized as being too time-consuming and difficult to perform independently. Adherence with a daily physical therapy regimen is reported as lower than with all other aspects of treatment.[146] Proof of efficacy might promote adherence, but research studies to examine the effectiveness of conventional physical therapy are difficult to evaluate because they use a wide variety of outcome measures, including different PFTs, volume of secretions produced, and participants' subjective impressions.[180] It is also problematic to compare studies done at different stages of the disease or with differences in study populations. Identifying the independent variable is sometimes troublesome because of the diverse combinations of techniques used; for example, percussion is rarely performed independently of postural drainage and coughing, making it difficult to definitively state which aspect of the treatment investigated has proved effective. Recent reviews suggest the usefulness of designing studies comparing treatment versus no treatment, but the ethical considerations of withholding treatment have prevented researchers from conducting this type of study at the present time.[83]

In a study by Lorin and Denning, the short-term effect of conventional physical therapy for patients with CF, compared with cough alone, was production of more sputum.[106] Other studies support the effectiveness of conventional physical therapy in increasing amounts of sputum expectorated by subjects when excess secretion production is already a feature of the patient's condition.[12,114] The amount of sputum produced may be quantified by volume or weight, but caution must be used when interpreting the findings from this type of measurement. Because many individuals may swallow a portion of their sputum, the output can underestimate the true volume produced. The amount of saliva that contaminates the product is difficult to determine, and this has resulted in measurement of the dry weight of sputum in some studies. Measurement of dry weight is not practical in most clinical settings. In addition, the amount of sputum produced does not indicate where it originated.

Alternative methods for mobilizing secretions and stimulating cough have been suggested, usually involving directed breathing techniques. These include huffing, PEP, oscillating PEP (Flutter and Acapella), autogenic drainage, and active cycle of breathing (formerly known as forced expiratory technique, or FET).

The rationale for use of huffing, a type of forced expiration with a similar mechanism to coughing, was suggested by a study that bronchoscopically demonstrated that maintenance of an open glottis throughout the maneuver stabilized the collapsible airway walls of subjects with chronic airflow obstruction.[85] The glottis normally closes in the compression phase of a cough, translating high compressive pressures on the tracheobronchial tree that may cause bronchiolar collapse.[180] Uncontrolled coughing is often nonproductive and exhausting. To perform huffing, the subject is asked to take a deep inspiration and then, without allowing the glottis to close, to render a strong contraction of the abdominal muscles to aid in forceful expiration. Maintaining an open glottis can be compared with vocalizing "ha"[180] or "ho." Huffing is an uncomplicated breathing technique that can be easily taught to young children, and performing huffs can introduce the child to the concept of controlled or directed breathing techniques.

Descriptions of the FET vary in the literature. Generally, it employs forceful expirations combined with an open glottis as in huffing, interspersed with controlled breathing at mid to low lung volumes. A 3-year study was conducted by Reisman and associates to compare the treatment effects of FETs in isolation (without postural drainage) versus conventional physical therapy in subjects with mild to moderate pulmonary involvement.[163] The study assessed the rates of deterioration in PFT scores, exercise challenge tests, and Shwachmann clinical scores for all study subjects. (The Shwachmann score[176] grades the clinical state of patients with CF. Points are allocated for general activity, physical examination, nutrition, and radiographic findings, with a total of 100 points possible. A higher score indicates a better clinical condition.) Subjects who performed only FETs had significantly greater rates of decline in measures of FEV_1, mid-expiratory flow rates (FEF25–75%), and Shwachmann score than the group performing conventional physical therapy.

Clarification of the use of FET that always includes finer breathing control techniques and thoracic expansion exercises required that FET be reclassified as active cycle of breathing techniques by Pryor and associates.[156] The three components are combined in a set cycle: relaxation and breathing control and three to four thoracic expansion

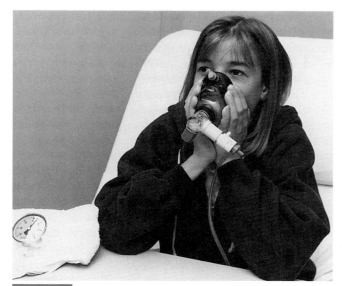

Figure 24-7 Use of a positive expiratory pressure mask.

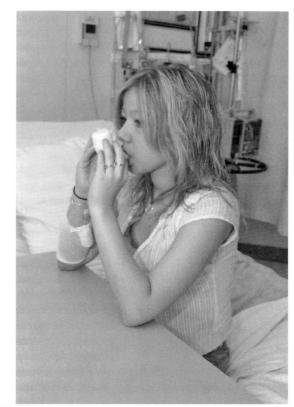

Figure 24-8 Use of Flutter.

exercises repeated twice, then relaxation and breathing control followed by one or two forced expirations. The number of breaths within a cycle can be modified to suit the patient's need. When secretions reach the larger, proximal airways, they may be cleared by a huff or a cough at high lung volume. Postural drainage positions may augment the effect, but the sitting position may be used if a gravity-assisted position is contraindicated.[196]

Use of PEP (Figure 24-7) as a means of secretion mobilization for individuals with CF has been proposed. Introduced for use in this population in the 1980's in Denmark, PEP has been shown to be as effective as traditional cardiopulmonary physical therapy both in chronic (baseline) stages of CF[65,119,135] and during an acute exacerbation of pulmonary complications.[136] The transmural pressure generated by maintaining resistant pressure throughout the expiration phase is thought to allow airflow to reach some obstructed alveoli through use of collateral airway channels. Airways are "splinted open" through the maintenance of PEP, thereby facilitating movement of peripheral secretions toward central airways.[102] The reader is urged to refer to the studies mentioned earlier to gain a better understanding of PEP as an airway clearance modality for CF.

Oscillating PEP (Flutter therapy and the Acapella) was developed to generate a controlled oscillating positive pressure and interruptions to airflow during expiration through a handheld device (Figure 24-8). The Flutter uses the force of gravity, whereas the Acapella uses the force of magnetic attraction.[191] Flutter may be useful as an adjunct to other airway clearance techniques, and short-term studies indicate its usefulness.[98] A long-term comparative study in children found that using Flutter in isolation from other airway clearance techniques did not prove as effective as PEP in maintaining pulmonary function, and that it was more

costly because of the increased number of hospitalizations and antibiotic use.[120] The Flutter technique has been altered since this study. Newbold and colleagues reported no significant difference between PEP and Flutter in terms of pulmonary function and health-related quality of life in adult patients using the now recommended technique.[131] The Acapella is a new device for which little research has been conducted. One study comparing Acapella versus Flutter found that they had similar performance characteristics. Investigators suggested that Acapella may have some advantages over Flutter because it is not position-dependent and can be used at very low expiratory flows.[191] Main and colleagues compared the RC Cornet, a type of oscillatory PEP, versus PEP alone, and showed that neither PEP nor Cornet was associated with significant changes in lung function over 6 or 12 months.[111]

High-frequency chest wall oscillation (HFCWO) consists of an inflatable fitted vest attached to a pump that generates high-frequency oscillations applied to the external chest wall. It is proposed that HFCWO enhances mucociliary transport in three ways: by altering the rheologic properties of mucus, by creating a cough-like expiratory flow bias that shears mucus from the airway walls and encourages its movement upward, and by enhancing ciliary beat frequency.[78] No long-term studies, however, have been performed to validate the benefits or examine the risks of this therapy. Short-term studies have found that HFCWO and conventional physical therapy are comparable for airway clearance,[70,183,195] but caution must be used when comparing these studies because a number of manufacturers producing this device use different protocols.[150] The device is also very costly. The Canadian Cystic Fibrosis Foundation is currently supporting a long-term multicenter randomized controlled trial in Canada that is comparing PEP and HFCWO in patients with CF. For more information on various airway clearance techniques, please visit http://www.cfww.org/ipg-cf/.

Activity

Exercise has been shown to be a useful therapeutic modality for secretion clearance, as evidenced by improved expiratory flow rates in subjects with stable CF with mild pulmonary disease.[208] A 30-month study of the effects of discontinuing other airway clearance modalities in favor of participation in aerobic exercise activities demonstrated no significant declines in clinical status, radiographic results, or PFT outcomes.[4] In an acute exacerbation, exercise proved as effective as conventional physical therapy for the study subjects when pulmonary function was reviewed. The group assigned to "exercise" continued to receive one bronchial hygiene treatment session by a physical therapist daily, whereas the conventional physical therapy group received three of these sessions per day. Cerny concluded that hospitalized patients could substitute exercise for part of the standard in-hospital care.[29]

Benefits of an exercise program extend beyond increases in peak oxygen consumption, increased maximal work capacity, improved mucus expectoration, and improved expiratory flow rates.[81,138,208] Exercise also improves general fitness, self-esteem, and measures of quality of life.[137] Exercise is socially acceptable and helps to normalize the patient's life rather than adding a therapy that accentuates differences from peers. Fitness level also has implications as a prognostic indicator. An improved survival rate is found in individuals with CF who demonstrate higher levels of aerobic fitness. Although this may simply reflect less severe illness, the ability to maintain aerobic fitness appears to have value in improving longevity.[133] In a habitual physical activity study of 187 (n = 99 female) patients age 7 to 25 years, subjects were divided into high and low activity groups and were followed over a 6-year period. Those in the low activity group had a significantly steeper rate of decline in FEV_1 compared with those in the high activity group. The authors conclude that higher activity levels are clearly associated with a slower rate of decline of FEV_1.[199] Selvadurai and colleagues discovered that prepubescent activity levels were similar between genders in patients with CF and between patients with CF and controls.[173] After puberty, girls with similar severity of CF were significantly less active than boys. In another habitual physical activity study, Nixon found that children with CF engage in less vigorous physical activities than their non-CF peers despite having good lung function.

Therefore, it was concluded that individuals with CF should be encouraged to engage in more vigorous activities to promote aerobic fitness that may ultimately have an impact on survival.[132]

Low activity levels are also related to low bone mineral density and vice versa. It is important to encourage patients with CF to optimize nutrition and to participate in regular physical activity to maximize the potential to acquire bone mass in childhood.[198] Prevention and treatment of CF-related bone disease must address the myriad of risk factors. These factors include decreased absorption of fat-soluble vitamins and poor nutritional status due to pancreatic insufficiency, altered sex hormone production, chronic lung infection with increased levels of bone active cytokines, physical inactivity, and glucocorticoid therapy. Chronic pulmonary inflammation leads to increased serum cytokine levels, which are thought to increase bone resorption and decrease bone formation. Decreased quantity and quality of bone mineral density can lead to pathologic fractures and kyphosis in late childhood. Kyphosis contributes to diminished stature, pain and debilitation, rib and vertebral fractures, and chest wall deformities that reduce lung function, inhibit effective cough, hinder airways clearance, and ultimately accelerate the course of CF. The prevalence of bone disease appears to increase with the severity of lung disease and malnutrition. Cross-sectional studies have reported a higher incidence of fractures in individuals with CF.[5]

Young children with CF should be encouraged to use the treatments that best suit their requirements for adequate secretion clearance and prevention of deterioration of clinical status. Attitudes toward adherence with treatment can greatly influence the effectiveness of any therapeutic regimen, and the challenge for the physical therapist is to design an intervention strategy that is useful for both efficacy and practicality. Factors that must be considered in designing a therapy program include disease presentation and severity; patient's age; motivation and ability to concentrate; physician, caregiver, and patient goals; documented effectiveness; training considerations; work required; need for assistance or equipment; and costs.[79] Children who learn to adopt their physical therapy as an aspect of daily living, as opposed to a burden or punishment, will be more likely to comply with treatment plans.

ADOLESCENCE

Adolescence is a time of rapid transformation in many areas of development. Sexual maturation comes about as a result of major changes in circulating hormones occurring around the time of maturity of the skeletal system, typically when the child is about 11 or 12 years old. These hormonal secretions cause a "growth spurt" in the adolescent.[72] "Delay of maturity" occurs when there has been slowed or prolonged skeletal maturation. This is often the cause of delayed puberty in adolescents with CF.[54,124] Arrested sexual development, combined with a smaller than average physical build, can intensify feelings of isolation from healthy peers.[115] Osteopenia (low bone mass) is a possible complication of CF that may be linked to nutritional factors, delayed puberty, reduced exercise or weight-bearing activities, treatment with corticosteroids, and chronic infection.[38] The prevention of osteoporosis and the risk of fracture in patients with signs of osteopenia must be considered when developing a therapy program. The need for increasing independence can conflict with the demands of daily medical care, making adherence with the routine seem arduous. Adolescents with CF who look and feel disparate from the perceived "norm" may rebel against continuation of time-consuming treatments that reinforce their sense of being dissimilar or abnormal.[18]

Management of Body Functions and Structures

Adherence with the "conventional" physical therapy routine of daily postural drainage and percussion sessions is poor in the adolescent population.[115,146] One challenge with this population is to promote self-efficacy with alternative methods of treatment. The use of PEP, an active cycle of breathing technique, or a program of regular exercise may help to promote independence and has already been discussed. Autogenic drainage (AD) is another treatment modality involving self-controlled breathing techniques.

AD requires no equipment or special environment to execute and relies on the user's ability to control both inspiratory and expiratory airflow to generate maximum airflow within the different generations of bronchi.[32] Three separate phases of the technique are believed to "unstick" mucus in the peripheral airways, "collect" the mucus in the middle airways, and "evacuate" it from the central airways according to the volume level of controlled breaths.[116] Mobilization of airway secretions by AD does not rely on the gravity assistance needed for postural drainage and can be performed in a sitting position.

Research studies validating the long-term efficacy of AD are scarce. A study was published comparing AD with conventional physical therapy and PEP in patients with CF,[118] and a 2-year comparison trial of AD and conventional physical therapy has also been reported that showed no significant differences between treatment groups when clinical status and PFT scores were used as outcome measures.[46]

Learning the technique of AD poses difficulties for both the subject and the trainer. It requires concentration and the ability to use proprioceptive and sensory cues to localize secretions in the various levels of bronchi. A hands-on approach is essential, with a minimum of environmental distractions. Frequent training sessions and reviews are necessary. This type of concentrated self-directed activity usually is not achievable by children younger than age 12. The mechanism for collateral ventilation through the channels of Lambert and the pores of Kahn is not fully developed in young children,[52] providing another limitation to the use of AD.

Maintenance of proper posture is important for individuals with CF to provide efficient breathing mechanics. Changes in the length-tension relationships of the respiratory musculature that may occur with increases in FRC create a mechanical disadvantage and contribute to increased work of breathing and muscle fatigue.[30] Several postural changes are found in CF to varying degrees, associated with chronically hyperinflated lungs, including increased anterior-posterior diameter of the chest, shoulder elevation, and forward protraction and abdominal flexion.[165] The incidence of thoracic kyphosis in CF is approximately 15%,[53] which predisposes affected individuals to chronic back pain. Estimates of the rate of back pain among people with CF are as high as 80%.[165]

The physical therapist must examine the patient for postural deviations and signs of osteoporosis and determine which changes may be reversible or amenable to treatment. Exercises to promote improved posture include a strengthening program for the supporting muscles of the back and spine, stretching of contractured musculature, and training the subject to develop a keener sense of his or her postural alignment. Weight-bearing exercises should be included to promote bone formation. An innovative way to keep the adolescent active that can address the above issues is "ball therapy" (Figure 24-9). Ball therapy can also be used to promote aerobic fitness, balance, coordination, and relaxation.[178] Projecting a good appearance is usually very important to adolescents, and informing the teenager with CF of the benefits of a good postural maintenance and weight-bearing program may provide the incentive necessary to ensure adherence to recommendations for exercises.

Secondary effects of strength training with weights may be an improvement in self-confidence in the adolescent because training has been shown to be beneficial in promoting weight gain.[181] As pulmonary impairment worsens, nutritional status is a consideration that requires a great deal of focus. Reduced anaerobic performance in CF is predominantly due to poor nutritional status.[97] The dietitian serving the population with CF contributes considerable expertise in identifying situations in which intervention is necessary and may be a valuable ally in reinforcing the message that exercise can promote weight gain when appropriately managed. A liaison with the dietitian can ensure coordination of dietary and physical therapy recommendations.

TRANSITION TO ADULTHOOD

When CF was first described in 1938, fewer than half of the patients survived their first year,[50] but CF is no longer a purely pediatric disease. The currently reported median age of survival is 37.4 years, although many patients live well into

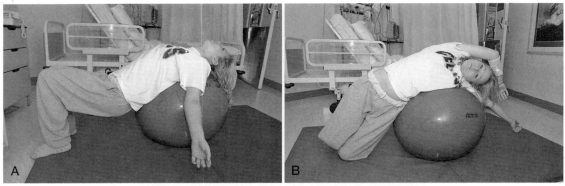

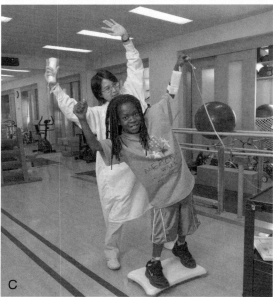

Figure 24-9 **A** and **B,** Therapy ball stretches to promote proper posture and thoracic mobility. **C,** Using new forms of technology: Nintendo Wii Fit System for exercise.

their fifth decade of life.[190] Although many of the issues physical therapists are concerned with in the pediatric patient are similar for adults, some special differences should be considered.

Standard programs of transition from a pediatric to an adult center should include all team members to ensure continuity of the patient's care.[61] Continuity of care enhances the effectiveness of care and minimizes uncertainty and distress for young individuals and their families. Transition from the pediatric to the adult CF team is an important milestone for patients and must be handled sensitively. Transfer is more easily achieved when the pediatric and adult clinics work closely together.[101]

The psychosocial issues in adulthood are distinct because the normal progression of psychological maturation brings new concerns with each developmental stage.[50] Greater clinical awareness, early treatment, and more effective management of CF have all contributed to improvement in prognosis.[151] Choices regarding education, employment

(medical insurance), marriage, and family will have to be made. These choices are more complex than usual for the adult with CF, who not only has to consider present health status but also must attempt to predict and prepare for future health status.

Consideration should be given to medical insurance coverage, flexible work hours, and sick time when choosing employment.[206] Physically demanding occupations may not be appropriate for the adult with CF with pulmonary limitations; therefore, careful consideration of the physical demands of any task must be undertaken. Jobs involving constant exposure to dust, chemical fumes, or smoke should be avoided.[50,140] Adults with CF will face few restrictions on choice of employment; however, infection control issues should be well thought out when choosing a career in health care.[206] Physical therapists should help to accommodate the adult's busy lifestyle and help to incorporate strategies for fitting treatment into work schedules. Methods that are more convenient and promote independence, such as the PEP mask, Flutter, or AD, may be more agreeable to the adult at work or school.

Because many adults with CF witness death among their peers, deterioration of their own health may have heightened significance for them. The adult who as an adolescent chose to be nonadherent with a physical therapy regimen may decide to initiate one again. Generally, individuals with CF have a strong positive outlook and are able to fully enjoy many of the typical pleasures of adulthood despite having to contend with unusual difficulties.[140] Patients' attitudes and outlook on life can have a tremendous influence on the medical progression of CF and are considered in prognostic scores.[50]

Because of the progressive nature of CF, many adults will have more symptoms and activity limitations than they had as children.[140] Minor hemoptysis occurs in up to 60% of adults with CF[54]; in most cases, the cause is an increase in bronchial infection that has irritated a blood vessel.[138,139] Massive hemoptysis, which is also strongly related to advancing age,[50] is defined as rupture of a bronchial blood vessel into the airways, producing greater than 300 ml of blood in 24 hours.[35] It is reported to occur in 5% to 7% of adults with CF[154] and warrants hospitalization and possible blood transfusion.[103]

Pneumothorax, which is one of the most common respiratory complications of adulthood, occurs in approximately 19% of individuals older than 13 years of age.[109] A common cause of pneumothorax is the spontaneous rupture of apical bullae, which develop as the result of increased air trapping and microabscess formation in the diseased lung.[109]

Episodes of hypertrophic pulmonary osteoarthropathy also increase in prevalence with advancing age.[50] Digital clubbing can become more noticeable in people whose pulmonary disease is severe.[140]

In general, cardiac status is related to severity of pulmonary involvement: the more severe the pulmonary adaptation to hypoxemia, the worse the pulmonary hypertension and right-sided heart strain. With comparable degrees of pulmonary disease, adults, especially those with mild lung disease, have more severe echocardiographic abnormalities than children. This may reflect the accumulative effects of episodes of mild hypoxemia and nocturnal oxygen desaturation that occur in even minimally affected individuals.[50]

Many adult females with CF experience urinary incontinence, with reported prevalence ranging from 30% to 68% on anonymous questionnaires. Respondents indicated that this problem was not reported because of embarrassment.[126,142] The repeated physical strain of coughing, physical therapy, and exercise may contribute to its development. Addressing this issue should become part of routine management and follow-up appointments in CF centers.

Management of Body Functions and Structures

Because the incidence of respiratory complications increases with age, physical therapists must work with the individual to adapt the treatment program accordingly. For the individual experiencing hemoptysis, physical therapy may have to be altered, although there are conflicting opinions in the literature as to the extent of modification necessary. Orenstein believes that if the cause of minor hemoptysis is an increase in bronchial infection irritating a blood vessel, treatment should be the same as for other types of increased infection.[140] He believes that bleeding within the lungs can worsen infection by providing a more hospitable environment for bacteria. He does caution that if a particular treatment position aggravates the bleeding, that position should be avoided. Webber and Pryor also believe that physical therapy should be continued with blood streaking; however, with frank hemoptysis, downward chest tilt and chest percussions should be discontinued.[196] The use of postural drainage, percussion, and shaking, along with huffing or FETs, may be less likely to increase the amount of bleeding than the frequent uncontrolled coughing that may occur with abandonment of manual techniques.[180] In summary, it would seem logical that if a particular technique, such as percussion, makes the individual's situation worse, it should be discontinued. Other modalities using breathing techniques may be beneficial at this time.

Cardiopulmonary physical therapy is contraindicated in the presence of an untreated, progressing, or tension pneumothorax[52]; however, treatment can continue with a small, stable pneumothorax[52,107] and with a pneumothorax that has resolved through treatment with a thoracotomy and insertion of a chest tube for vacuum drainage of air.[52] Percussion must not be performed directly over the chest tube site owing to the danger of displacement, but percussion may be safely performed elsewhere on the thorax as tolerated. The PEP mask is a relative contraindication because theoretically it could make the pneumothorax worse as a result of repetitive increased pressure generated in the airways.

Standard anti-inflammatory agents are used to treat the joint pain associated with hypertrophic pulmonary osteoarthropathy.[148] Physical therapists have a role in helping to relieve pain while maintaining joint range of motion (ROM). A home treatment program consisting of stretching, muscle strengthening, and ROM exercises for the specific joints involved can be easily added to the individual's existing exercise program.

Management of urinary incontinence can be addressed by physical therapists prescribing pelvic floor muscle strength training. In the general population, it was reported that pelvic floor muscle training was effective in 53% of patients studied, with this group demonstrating a 66% success rate in the management of urinary incontinence for at least 10 years.[26]

When pulmonary disease becomes so disabling that the individual is having difficulty performing activities of daily living, physical therapy goals should encompass these needs. The patient may have to be instructed on energy

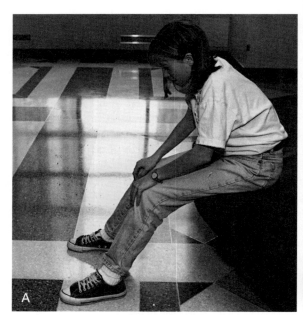
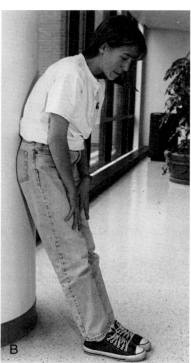

Figure 24-10   **A** and **B,** Positioning for energy conservation, promoting relaxation and ease of breathing.

conservation techniques such as diaphragmatic pursed-lip breathing and assuming positions that relieve breathlessness. These positions should promote comfort and relaxation and should encourage mobility of the thorax and support of the spinal column. They should also include hip flexion to relax the abdominal musculature and aid in increasing intra-abdominal pressure for coughing.[52] Examples of energy conservation positions are shown in Figure 24-10. Retraining of the respiratory pattern using pursed-lip breathing in conjunction with diaphragmatic excursion has shown temporary benefits in increased tidal volume, decreased respiratory rate, reduction in $PaCO_2$ levels, and improved PaO_2 levels, as well as subjective benefits reported by patients.[33] It may be that pursed-lip breathing improves confidence and decreases anxiety by providing some temporary control over oxygenation.[33]

Oxygen needs with exercise may have to be assessed at this time. Continuation of an active lifestyle should be promoted for all individuals with CF to optimize physical condition and maintain an optimistic outlook. If the individual is considering lung transplantation as an option, physical therapists must involve the individual in a formalized exercise program. The Toronto Lung Transplant Program at the Toronto Hospital has a well-established rehabilitation program. Exercise capacity is determined by using a 6-minute walk test and ear oximetry, or the Modified Bruce Protocol on the treadmill.[42] For a 6-minute walk test, the subject is instructed to walk as quickly and comfortably as possible on

a level, measured distance for 6 minutes. If the patient becomes short of breath or too exhausted to continue, he or she is allowed to rest but then must continue the test as soon as symptoms subside. The distance traveled and the rest periods the subject takes are recorded. Subjects' pulse and respiratory rates and oxygen saturation are measured and recorded before, during, and at the conclusion of the test. The purpose of performing a test of exercise capacity is to help determine if severity of disability warrants consideration for transplant. A 6-minute walk test result of less than 400 meters was found to be a significant indicator for a patient to be listed for transplantation.[90]

Individuals can also be monitored at regular intervals with these tests to gauge potential deterioration in their functional status. Once accepted into the lung transplantation program, most centers require attendance at a formal rehabilitation program[73] featuring aerobics, muscle strengthening, stretching, and light calisthenics.

Expected physical therapy outcomes for the adult with CF include optimizing functional ability, physical exercise tolerance, and emotional well-being. For individuals awaiting a lung transplant, improvement in overall function should enable them to handle the actual surgery and immediate postoperative period with less difficulty.[42] Arnold and associates found that 13 patients with end-stage CF showed improvement in their functional exercise capacity by participating in pulmonary rehabilitation while awaiting double-lung transplantation.[6] Pulmonary rehabilitation entailed treadmill walking and lower extremity ergometry three to five times per week, initiated at the time of listing for double-lung transplant. Six-minute walks were performed biweekly to assess changes in functional exercise capacity, and workload on the treadmill and bicycle ergometer was recorded. Six-minute walk distances and treadmill and bicycle workloads all increased significantly. Conclusions from this data confirm the possibility of improving functional exercise capacity in patients with end-stage CF awaiting double-lung transplantation, despite severe limitations in pulmonary function.

Noninvasive ventilation, most commonly biphasic positive airway pressure (BIPAP), may benefit CF patients who are experiencing respiratory failure and awaiting lung transplantation. Although nocturnal oxygen therapy has not been shown to improve long-term prognosis, nighttime BIPAP reduces hypoxia, hypercarbia, and work of breathing and may enhance airway clearance and reduce pulmonary hypertension.[192]

The physical therapist's contact with those individuals in the terminal stages of their disease should not be discontinued. Intervention at this stage must include the provision of comfort measures and must be directed by the patient's wishes. Treatment sessions may have to decrease in duration and be offered with increased frequency throughout the day. Adaptations to postural drainage positions may have to be adopted so treatment can be tolerated. As the work of coughing becomes too tiring or painful, other modalities such as splinting and huffing can be reviewed. Pain control measures and relaxation and anxiety-reducing techniques, such as massage, may be the primary need of the dying patient. Simply listening to the concerns of these patients can be therapeutic. The value of a compassionate ear should not be underestimated. Physical therapists treating terminally ill patients should be careful to incorporate the families' needs, respecting the fact that this is an emotionally volatile time for all involved.

SUMMARY

The management of CF poses many challenges for physical therapists. The multisystemic involvement and chronicity of the disorder compel physical therapists to continually interact with a team of professionals to shape appropriate treatment plans. Collaboration with this type of multidisciplinary health care team is always stimulating and fosters creative and fulfilling practice of physical therapy. New advances suggest exciting possibilities for the future care of people with CF, and physical therapists serving this population are required to continually adapt their management approach in light of new research and increasing longevity. The aspiration to discover a cure seems to be approaching fulfillment. Meanwhile, the challenge for all those involved lies in finding effective means to slow (or prevent) the disabling effects of this disease.

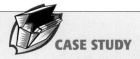

CASE STUDY

"Tristan"

The following case study documents the diagnosis and symptoms of a male with CF, whom we will call Tristan, over the course of a 16-year period.

Tristan's state of health has fluctuated a great deal, especially during times of poor adherence to both the suggested physical therapy regimen and the diet and medications prescribed. Tristan's history of poor adherence does not represent all CF patients but is illustrated in this case history to identify the challenges that multidisciplinary team members struggle with. His parents have often reported having difficulty obtaining cooperation from Tristan, and frequent residential moves have tended to exacerbate the problem of establishing beneficial routines. We can draw inferences from the evidence, which demonstrates correlations between adherence and overall health or frequency of admission to hospital. Perhaps the greatest benefit of examining a case such as this one is to ask ourselves if more could have been done to stimulate or inspire Tristan and his parents to engage in a proactive way with the treatment regimen.

Tristan was diagnosed with CF and pancreatic insufficiency at the age of 2 months with a sweat chloride reading of 124 mEq/L, and his genetics testing showed that he was homozygous for delta 508 deletion. As is common among children diagnosed in infancy, Tristan had been admitted to hospital because of his failure to thrive. Tristan's parents underwent the newly diagnosed CF teaching program to learn how to care for Tristan once he was discharged home. They were instructed by all team members including the doctor, nurse, dietitian, social worker, and physical therapist. Tristan's parents were provided with information and education from the physical therapist regarding anatomy and physiology of the lungs, how CF affects the lungs, the purpose of physical therapy, signs of respiratory distress, and the importance of exercise. His parents obtained a compressor and nebulizer for inhalation treatments and were instructed through a home program consisting of postural drainage (today modified positions would be taught vs. head down positioning) and manual percussion. Goals for physical therapy were established and included maintaining good ventilation and promoting secretion clearance.

Continued

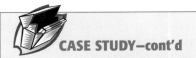

Tristan was seen again for a follow-up appointment 2 weeks later to ensure that the family was on track with the physical therapy program, and that he was gaining weight appropriately. He then was followed on the normal clinic routine of appointments every 3 to 4 months, where breathing exercises such as blowing bubbles and huffing into a tissue or trying to steam up a mirror were introduced when age appropriate. At age 4, Tristan presented to clinic with increased cough, elevated sputum quantity, decreased appetite, and poor exercise capacity. His mother reported that he was having difficulty keeping up with his brothers. His sputum cultures grew *Staphylococcus aureus* and *Streptococcus pyogenes* and his cough was persistently harsh, often culminating in vomiting. This greatly affected his ability to gain weight, and he presented below the third percentile in growth for his age. At this time, Tristan was admitted to the hospital. Fecal fat collection, upper gastrointestinal series, and immunologic workups were initiated upon admission. The dietitian believed that the abnormally high fecal fat percentage in his stool and low vitamin levels were due to poor adherence with enzymes at home. This admission provided an opportunity for the social worker to interview and offer aid to the family. The importance of enzyme therapy was reviewed and assistance with the physical therapy regimen was requested by the family. A referral was initiated to obtain physical therapy services through the home care program. This was welcomed by the parents, who had been feeling overwhelmed with all the time demands of Tristan's treatment and raising three other boys. During the admission, Tristan received ceftazidime and tobramycin intravenously, and a physical therapy program of postural drainage, manual percussions, expiratory vibrations, breathing exercises (three times a day), and an exercise program were performed. Near the end of the admission, he showed marked improvement in his clinical presentation and in his ability to clear secretions comfortably with minimal vomiting after being taught proper huffing technique. He was discharged home on oral cephalexin owing to his acquisition of *Staphylococcus aureus* infection.

At age 4 years 9 months, Tristan's sputum cultures grew *Pseudomonas aeruginosa* and he was started on inhaled tobramycin.

Since the referral to home care, no problems with the physical therapy regimen were identified; however, the importance of regular activity was reviewed. At age 5 years 6 months, Tristan's first PFT revealed an FEV_1 of 69% predicted. His chest x-ray findings demonstrated mild air trapping with increased peribronchial thickening and some small nodular cystic areas. His medications included inhaled tobramycin and albuterol three times daily. Over the next few years, his FEV_1 fluctuated from 54% to 64% to 71%. These changes seemed directly related to his adherence to therapy. At the time of his eighth birthday, Tristan's mother reported that there was some friction between Tristan and herself; there was an ongoing struggle around adherence to the treatment regimen, in particular, physical therapy.

A chest x-ray revealed bronchiectatic changes, particularly in the left lower lobe. It was suggested that Tristan and his family attend the annual teaching day focusing on self-management skills, in the hope that Tristan would take responsibility and have a better understanding of his disease. In an attempt to improve his self-efficacy, a log book (Junior Passport) was provided to Tristan to keep track of his treatments and any questions he may have for the clinic team. (Because of new research on infection control, children with CF are no longer able to attend group workshops together, so education is provided on an individual basis.)

Over the next year, Tristan had no admissions to the hospital. He reported that his spirits improved after meeting other children with CF at the teaching day. Having the chance to discuss how CF affects other kids' lives and how they cope with the heavy treatment regimen gave him new motivation to improve his adherence. The Ability Online Support Network (www.AbilityOnline.org), a Canadian charitable organization, provides an electronic mail forum for children and young adults with disabilities. Using a computer and a modem, persons of all ages can dial into a central computer, where messages can be exchanged with others. There is no charge to participate. This form of interaction is now encouraged over person-to-person contact. Many countries have their own online support groups, which can be accessed by CF patients and their families for support.

Tristan, however, was hesitant to change his physical therapy program from postural drainage and percussion to a more independent treatment (PEP therapy), demonstrating his continued reliance on his parents to assist in his treatment.

Tristan's pulmonary function values continued to decline despite all efforts to improve his adherence. This steady decline was accompanied by noticeable respiratory changes such as tachypnea and indrawing. Tristan also continued to experience frequent emesis with coughing. His chest x-ray showed new markings in the upper lobes and continued deterioration of his lower lobes. His parents resisted having him hospitalized but finally agreed to an admission when his FEV_1 was 57% predicted. He was feverish with cough and vomiting and had significant weight loss. During this admission, physical therapy of manual percussions and expiratory vibrations in modified positions was supplemented by 20 to 30 minutes of stationary bike riding. Tristan was discharged home on inhaled tobramycin and oral cephalexin, as well as a home exercise program designed to accommodate his interests and routine.

A few months later, Tristan required another admission to the hospital with a chest exacerbation. By this time Tristan was 11 years old and was showing evidence of stubbornness and an urgent need for an independent method of chest therapy. In consultation with the physical therapist, Tristan and his parents decided to pursue PEP therapy. During his time in hospital, Tristan was supervised with five to six cycles of PEP therapy, including abdominal breathing and

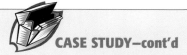

CASE STUDY—cont'd

huffing. Tristan demonstrated good technique and tolerance and was able to produce large amounts of sputum. At the time of discharge, his FEV_1 had improved to 77% predicted. At his next clinic appointment, 5 months later, Tristan admitted to using the PEP mask only sporadically, but reported that he was enjoying learning to play the saxophone at school, which was encouraged by the CF team.

Once again, an attempt was made through counseling to impress on him the importance of adhering to the treatment regimen. Less than a year later, Tristan was again admitted to hospital, with an FEV_1 of 56%. His coughing was extremely harsh and frequently caused vomiting, which had led to weight loss. On auscultation, Tristan had diffuse crackles and decreased air entry to the bilateral bases, with very little airflow audible on the left side. During this stay, consistent exercise and PEP mask treatment three times a day after albuterol inhalation therapy were performed. Tobramycin inhalations in the morning and evening were administered after airway clearance to maximize medication deposition. His FEV_1 climbed back up and was measured a month later as 80% predicted. The dietitian suggested that he eat frequent smaller meals and reviewed high-energy caloric foods.

Over the next few years, admissions to hospital increased in frequency. His adherence to airway clearance was monitored as an inpatient, and Tristan also participated in exercises using ball therapy, bicycling, and stair climbing. He continued to lose weight, however, and at age 15, in April, was admitted for a G-tube insertion. Within a month, he had gained 1.4 kg (3.08 lb) but was readmitted with a chest exacerbation, blood-streaked sputum, and a racking cough. During this admission, the team discovered that his frequent absences from school had resulted in his failing the year, prompting his mother to request summer admissions in the future so as not to jeopardize his schooling. Counseling was offered to both Tristan and his mother, and again, a social work referral was initiated through his local home care agency. Tristan's FEV_1 was at a new low of 41%, and he was complaining of chest tightness. Additional physical therapy techniques such as autogenic drainage and active cycle of breathing were initiated in an attempt to find the most effective airway clearance technique for his current chest status. Tristan demonstrated the technique of AD very effectively and was able to clear secretions even with his feelings of chest tightness and felt that he would be able to keep up this technique at home. He also enjoyed

working on postural chest expansion exercises on a therapy ball, and on discharge had resolved to continue with this combination of treatments.

Three months later, at the end of the summer, Tristan was readmitted to hospital with the by now familiar scenario of falling FEV_1 and vomiting with heavy coughing. A 1-month trial of Pulmozyme was initiated with an initial increase in PFTs. Within 1 month, he was back to the clinic again with an FEV_1 of 36%, daily vomiting and fevers, and significant weight loss. Evidence of his deteriorating respiratory status was apparent in his chest x-rays: nodular densities in the lateral aspects of both right and left upper lobes and worsening lesions that likely represented areas of mucoid impaction. Tristan's ranitidine dosage was adjusted and his gastrointestinal symptoms decreased. He reported continued difficulty sleeping, night sweats, and fevers. He was prescribed a course of azithromycin, an anti-inflammatory agent, and a course of prednisone. Unfortunately, financial difficulties arose, and Tristan was not able to afford the recommended therapy. Fortunately, the social worker investigated external funding for the azithromycin, which resulted in the new therapy, to which Tristan had a good response.

The next few months were quiet ones. Tristan continued to do well, but things deteriorated again when he stopped taking his ranitidine (the excuse for this was that it got misplaced during a residential move). As this situation came to light, Tristan also revealed that he had not been taking azithromycin during the last few weeks because he had also lost this medication. He was complaining of abdominal pain again and was demonstrating low PFT scores with an FEV_1 of 43% predicted. Tristan was skipping school and was lying in front of the television all day. A referral to psychology was made because he was despondent. Tristan was given the opportunity to relate to the psychologist his fears and concerns regarding his future, and life strategies were discussed. The correlation between adhering with the prescribed treatment regimen and his overall health status appeared to be finally accepted by Tristan. Quality of life issues and ideas to boost both his energy levels and his mood were proposed by all members of the team. Once again, Tristan appeared to understand and agreed to try to be more diligent with the treatment program.

As he left the clinic, he was boosted by the support of the team, and we remain hopeful that as he continues to mature, he will be able to apply himself with a new resolve.

Continued

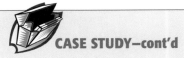

CASE STUDY—cont'd

EVIDENCE TO PRACTICE 24-1

CASE STUDY "TRISTAN"
CHANGE IN PRACTICE

Side effects of postural drainage have been observed and recorded by physical therapists. These include desaturation, discomfort, pain and gastroesophageal reflux (GER). GER is an abnormal tendency to regurgitate gastric contents into the esophagus, which may lead to aspiration of acidic gas, microaspiration, or macroaspiration. Esophageal irritation can also lead to vagal nerve stimulation and reflex bronchospasm. It is well documented that episodes of increased GER occur during postural drainage in children and adolescents with CF. Button and colleagues studied 20 infants with CF in standard postural drainage (PD) positions using head-down tilt positions and modified postural drainage, which avoided head-down tilt.[1,2] Significantly more episodes of GER were

associated with the standard PD group compared with the modified PD group. Moreover, after 5 years, infants randomized to the modified PD group at diagnosis had better FEV$_1$ and forced vital capacity and fewer radiologic changes than those in the standard PD group. Thus, modified PD without head-down tilt is now the recommended therapy for infants and children with CF.

1. Button, B. M., Heine, R., Catto-Smith, A., Olinsky, A., & Phelan, P. D. (1997). Postural drainage and gastro-esophageal reflux in infants with cystic fibrosis. *Archives of Disease in Childhood, 76,* 148–150.
2. Button, B. M., Heine, R., Catto-Smith, A., Olinsky, A., & Phelan, P. D. (2003). Story I. Chest physiotherapy in infants with cystic fibrosis: To tip or not? A five-year study. *Pediatric Pulmonology, 35,* 208–213.
3. Foster, A. C., Voyles, J. B., & Murphy, S. A. (1983). Twenty-four hour pH monitoring in children with cystic fibrosis: Association of chest physiotherapy to gastro-esophageal reflux. *Pediatric Research, 17,* 188A.

EVIDENCE TO PRACTICE 24-2

CASE STUDY "TRISTAN"
PLAN OF CARE DECISION

The decision to treat acquisition of *Pseudomonas aeruginosa* with inhaled tobramycin was aimed at decreasing the bacterial load during pulmonary declines. Ramsey and colleagues showed that inhaled preservative-free tobramycin (300 mg twice a day) for 28 days alternating with 28 days off treatment resulted in significant increases in FEV$_1$ and a 36% reduction in the use of IV antibiotics for pulmonary exacerbations.[1] More recently, therapies are aimed at eradicating *Pseudomonas aeruginosa* to limit the transformation from nonmucoid to mucoid strains, regardless of an associated pulmonary decline. Currently, two large trials are under way for CF patients with early *Pseudomonas aeruginosa* infection: the

EPIC (Early Pseudomonas Infection Control) trial and the ELITE (Early Intervention TOBI Eradication) trial.[3] The CF community worldwide has accepted the decision to treat early infection with antibiotics. As a result, these important studies are not trying to determine if we should treat infection early, but rather how we should treat it.[2]

1. Ramsey, B. W., Pepe, M. S., Quan, J. M., et al. (1999). Intermittent administration of inhaled tobramycin in patients with cystic fibrosis. Cystic Fibrosis Inhaled Tobramycin Study Group. *New England Journal of Medicine, 340,* 23–30.
2. Flume, P., O'Sullivan, B., Robinson, K., et al. (2007). Cystic fibrosis pulmonary guidelines: Chronic medication for maintenance of lung health. *American Journal of Respiratory and Critical Care Medicine, 176,* 957–969.
3. Ratjen, F., Munck, A., & Kho, P. (2008). Short and long-term efficacy of inhaled tobramycin in early *P. aeruginosa* infection: The ELITE study. *Pediatric Pulmonology, 31*(suppl 31):319–320.

EVIDENCE TO PRACTICE 24-3

CASE STUDY "TRISTAN"
CHOICES OF TECHNIQUES

The technique of PEP therapy was introduced to the family when Tristan was able to perform PFTs reliably. The PEP mask was compared with conventional postural drainage and percussion (PD&P) in a 1-year randomized controlled

trial involving 40 children age 6 to 17 years. Clinical status, pulmonary function, and compliance with physical therapy were monitored. A significant improvement in FVC and FEV$_1$ was seen in the PEP group compared with the PD&P group. Participants preferred the PEP technique compared with PD&P, implying that improved adherence may be achievable.[1,2] Reasons for this preference included comfort,

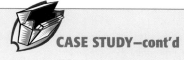

CASE STUDY—cont'd

EVIDENCE TO PRACTICE 24-3—cont'd

convenience, independence, ease of use, greater control and flexibility regarding treatment times, and less interruption of daily living. The individual circumstances for each patient will help dictate the choice of airway clearance regimen. Advantages and disadvantages are associated with each of the therapeutic options, and decisions regarding prescription of airway clearance may include age of the patient, patient preference, severity of disease, availability of a caregiver, and observed efficacy based on patient reporting and objective measures. It should be noted that prescribed therapies may change as the patient's situation changes, thus the efficacy and appropriateness of airway clearance therapy should be periodically reassessed.[3]

1. McIlwaine, P. M., Wong, L. T., Peacock, D., & Davidson, A. G. (2001). Long-term comparative trial of conventional postural drainage and percussion versus positive expiratory pressure physiotherapy in the treatment of cystic fibrosis. *Journal of Pediatrics, 131*, 570–574.
2. Gaskin, L., Corey, M., Shin, J., Reisman, J. J., Thomas, J., & Tullis, D. E. (1998). Long term trial of conventional postural drainage and percussion vs. positive expiratory pressure [abstract]. *Pediatric Pulmonology, 17*(suppl), 345.
3. Flume, P. A., Robinson, K. A., O'Sullivan, B. P., Finder, J. D., Vender, R. L., Willey-Courand, D., White, T. B., & Marshall, B. C. (2009). The Clinical Practice Guidelines for Pulmonary Therapies Committee. Cystic fibrosis pulmonary guidelines: Airway clearance therapies. *Respiratory Care, 54*, 522–537.

REFERENCES

1. Ackerman, V., Montgomery, G., Eigen, H., & Tepper, R. (1991). Assessment of airway responsiveness in infants with cystic fibrosis. *American Review of Respiratory Disease, 144*, 344–346.
2. Amin, R., & Ratjen, F. (2008). Cystic fibrosis: A review of pulmonary and nutritional therapies. *Advances in Pediatrics, 55*, 99–121.
3. Andersen, D. H. (1938). Cystic fibrosis of the pancreas and its relation to celiac disease: A clinical and pathologic study. *American Journal of Diseases of Children, 56*, 344–395.
4. Andreasson, B., Jonson, B., Kornfalt, R., Nordmar, E., & Sandstrom, S. (1987). Long-term effects of physical exercise on working capacity and pulmonary function in cystic fibrosis. *Acta Paediatrica Scandinavica, 76*, 70–75.
5. Aris, R. M., Merkel, P. A., Bachrach, L. K., Borowitz, D. S., Boyle, M. P., Elkin, S. L., Guise, T. A., Hardin, D. S., Haworth, C. S., Holick, M. F., Joseph, P. M., O'Brien, K., Tullis, E., Watts, N. B., & White, T. B. (2005). Consensus statement: Guide to bone health and disease in cystic fibrosis. *Journal of Clinical Endocrinology and Metabolism, 90*, 1888–1896.
6. Arnold, C. D., Westerman, J. H., Downs, A. M., & Egan, T. M. (1991). Benefits of an aerobic exercise program in C.F. patients waiting for double lung transplant. *Pediatric Pulmonology Supplement, 6*, 287.
7. Auerbach, et al. (1985). Auerbach, HS, Williams, M, Kirkpatrick, JA, & Colten, HR. Alternate-day prednisone reduces morbidity and improves pulmonary function in cystic fibrosis. *Lancet, 2*, 686–688.
8. Aurora, P., Stocks, J., Oliver, C., Saunders, C., Castle, R., Chaziparasidis, G., & Bush, A. (2004). Quality control for spirometry in pre-school children with and without lung disease. *American Journal of Respiratory and Critical Care Medicine, 169*, 1152–1159.
9. Balfour-Lynn, I. M., Prasad, S. A., Laverty, A., Whitehead, B. F., & Dinwiddie, R. (1998). A step in the right direction: Assessing exercise tolerance in cystic fibrosis. *Pediatric Pulmonology, 25*, 223–225.
10. Bartholomew, L. K., Czyzewski, D. I., & Swank, P. R. (1996). Short-term outcomes of the CF Family Education Program (CF FEP): What we know and what we don't know. *Pediatric Pulmonology Supplement, 13*, 154–155.
11. Bartholomew, LK, Parcel, GS, Swank, P.R., & Czyzewski, DI. (1993). Measuring self-efficacy expectations for the self-management of cystic fibrosis. *Chest, 103*, 1524–1530.
12. Bateman, J. R. M., Newton, S. P., Daunt, K. M., Pavia, D., & Clarke, S. W. (1979). Regional lung clearance of excessive bronchial secretions during chest physiotherapy in patients with stable chronic airway obstruction. *Lancet, 1*, 294–297.
13. Boas, S. (2008). The evidence for exercise. *Pediatric Pulmonology Supplement, 31*, 161–163.
14. Borg, G. A. V. (1982). Psychophysical bases of perceived exertion. *Medicine and Science in Sports and Exercise, 14*, 377–381.
15. Boucek, M. M., Edwards, L. B., Keck, B. M., Trulock, E. P., Taylor, D. O., Mohacsi, P. J., & Hertz, M. I. (2003). The registry of the International Society for Heart and Lung Transplantation: Sixth official pediatric report—2003. *Journal of Heart and Lung Transplantation, 22*, 636–652.
16. Boucher, R. C., Knowles, M. R., & Yankaskas, J. R. (2000). Cystic fibrosis. In *Textbook of respiratory medicine* (3rd ed., Vol. 2; pp. 1291–1323). Toronto: WB Saunders.

17. Boyd, S., Brooks, D., Agnew-Coughlin, J., & Ashwell, J. (1994). Evaluation of the literature on the effectiveness of physical therapy modalities in the management of children with cystic fibrosis. *Pediatric Physical Therapy, 6,* 70–74.

18. Boyle, I. R., di Sant'Agnese, P. A., & Sack, S. (1976). Emotional adjustment of adolescents and young adults with cystic fibrosis. *Journal of Pediatrics, 88,* 318–326.

19. Brennan, G. (2004). Brennan, AL & Geddes, DM. Bringing new treatments to the bedside in cystic fibrosis. *Pediatric Pulmonology, 37,* 87–98.

20. Brody, A. S. (2004). Early morphological changes in the lungs of asymptomatic infants and young children with cystic fibrosis. *Journal of Pediatrics, 144,* 145–146.

21. Burns, J.L. (1997). Treatment of cepacia: In search of the magic bullet. *Pediatric Pulmonology Supplement, 14,* 90–91.

22. Burton, L. (1975). *The family life of sick children: A study of families coping with chronic childhood disease.* London: Routledge & Kegan Paul.

23. Bush, A. (1997). Giving the bad news—Your child has cystic fibrosis. *Pediatric Pulmonology Supplement, 14,* 206–208.

24. Butland, R. J. A., Pang, J., Gross, E. R., Woodcock, A. A., & Geddes, D. M. (1982). Two, six and 12-minute walking test in respiratory disease. *British Medical Journal, 284,* 1607–1608.

25. Button, B. M., Heine, R., Catto-Smith, A., Olinsky, A., Phelan, P. D., & Story, I. (2003). Chest physiotherapy in infants with cystic fibrosis: To tip or not? A five-year study. *Pediatric Pulmonology, 35,* 208–213.

26. Cammu, H., Van Nylen, M., & Amy, J. J. (2000). A 10-year follow-up after Kegel pelvic floor muscle exercises for genuine stress incontinence. *British Journal of Urology International, 85,* 655–658.

27. Canny, G. J., & Levison, H. (1987). Exercise response and rehabilitation in cystic fibrosis. *Sports Medicine, 4,* 143–152.

28. Cappelli, M., McGrath, P. J., MacDonald, N. E., Katsanis, J., & Lascelles, M. (1989). Parental care and overprotection of children with cystic fibrosis. *British Journal of Medical Psychology, 62,* 281–289.

29. Cerny, F. J. (1989). Relative effects of bronchial drainage and exercise for in-hospital care of patients with cystic fibrosis. *Physical Therapy, 69,* 633–639.

30. Cerny, F. J., & Darbee, J. (1990). Exercise testing and exercise conditioning for children with lung dysfunction. In S. Irwin, & J. S. Tecklin (Eds.), *Cardiopulmonary physical therapy* (pp. 461–475). St Louis: Mosby.

31. Cerny, F. J., Pullano, T. P., & Cropp, G. J. A. (1982). Cardiorespiratory adaptations to exercise in cystic fibrosis. *American Review of Respiratory Disease, 126,* 217–220.

32. Chevaillier, J. (1984). Autogenic drainage. In D. Lawson (Ed.), *Cystic fibrosis: Horizons* (p. 235). New York: Wiley.

33. Ciesla, N. (1989). Postural drainage, positioning and breathing exercises. In C. F. Mackenzie (Ed.), *Chest physiotherapy in the intensive care unit* (pp. 93–133). Baltimore: Williams & Wilkins.

34. Coates, A. L., MacNeish, C. F., Lands, L. C., Meisner, D., Kelemen, S., & Vadas, E. B. (1998). A comparison of the availability of tobramycin for inhalation from vented vs. unvented nebulizers. *Chest, 113,* 951–956.

35. Cohen, A. M. (1992). Hemoptysis: Role of angiography and embolization. *Pediatric Pulmonology Supplement, 8,* 85–86.

36. Collins, F. S. (1992). The C.F. gene: Perceptions, puzzles and promises. *Pediatric Pulmonology Supplement, 8,* 63–64.

37. Constantini, D., Brivio, A., et al. (2001). PEP-mask versus postural drainage in CF infants: A long-term comparative trial. *Pediatric Pulmonology Supplement, 22,* 308, A400.

38. Conway, S. P. (2001). Impact of lung inflammation on bone metabolism in adolescents with cystic fibrosis. *Paediatric Respiratory Review, 2,* 324–331.

39. Cooper, P. J., Robertson, C. F., Hudson, I. L., & Phelan, P. D. (1990). Variability of pulmonary function tests in cystic fibrosis. *Pediatric Pulmonology, 8,* 16–22.

40. Corey, M., Gaskin, K., Durie, P., Levison, H., & Forstner, G. (1984b). Improved prognosis in C.F. patients with normal fat absorption. *Journal of Pediatric Gastroenterology and Nutrition, 3*(suppl 1), 99–105.

41. Crane, L. (1990). Physical therapy for the neonate with respiratory disease. In S. Irwin, & J. S. Tecklin (Eds.), *Cardiopulmonary physical therapy* (pp. 389–416). St Louis: Mosby.

42. Craven, J. L., Bright, J., & Dear, C. L. (1990). Psychiatric, psychosocial, and rehabilitative aspects of lung transplantation. *Clinics in Chest Medicine, 11,* 247–257.

43. Cystic Fibrosis Foundation. (2008). *Patient registry annual data report for 2007.* Bethesda, MD: Cystic Fibrosis Foundation.

44. Dab, I., & Malfroot, A. (1988). Gastroesophageal reflux: A primary defect in cystic fibrosis. *Scandinavian Journal of Gastroenterology Supplement, 143,* 125–131.

45. Darbee, J. C., Ohtake, P. J., Grant, B. J., & Cerny, F. J. (2004). Physiologic evidence for the efficacy of positive expiratory pressure as an airway clearance technique in patients with cystic fibrosis. *Physical Therapy, 84,* 524–537.

46. Davidson, A. G. F., McIlwaine, P. M., Wong, L. T. K., & Pirie, G. E. (1992). Long-term comparative trial of conventional percussion and drainage physiotherapy versus autogenic drainage in cystic fibrosis. *Pediatric Pulmonology Supplement, 8,* 298.

47. Davidson, K. L. (2002). Airway clearance strategies for the pediatric patient. *Respiratory Care, 47,* 823–828.

48. Davies, J. C., & Alton, E. (2009). Monitoring respiratory disease severity in cystic fibrosis. *Respiratory Care, 54,* 606–617.

49. Davies, J. C., & Bilton, D. (2009). Bugs, biofilms, and resistance in cystic fibrosis. *Respiratory Care, 54,* 628–638.

50. Davis, P. B. (1983). Cystic fibrosis in adults. In J. D. Lloyd-Still (Ed.), *Textbook of cystic fibrosis* (pp. 351–370). Stoneham, MA: Wright.

51. Davis, P. B. (2006). Cystic fibrosis since 1938. *American Journal of Respiratory and Critical Care Medicine, 73,* 475–482.

52. DeCesare, J. A., & Graybill, C. A. (1990). Physical therapy for the child with respiratory dysfunction. In S. Irwin, & J. S.

Tecklin (Eds.), *Cardiopulmonary physical therapy* (pp. 417–460). St Louis: Mosby.

53. Denton et al. (1981) Denton, JR, Tietjen, R, & Gaerlan, PF. Thoracic kyphosis in cystic fibrosis. *Clinical Orthopaedics and Related Research, 155,* 71–74.

54. di Sant'Agnese, P. A., & Davis, P. B. (1979). Cystic fibrosis in adults: 75 cases and a review of 232 cases in the literature. *American Journal of Medicine, 66,* 121–132.

55. Doershuk, C. F., Matthews, L. W., & Tucker, A. S. (1964). A five-year clinical evaluation of a therapeutic program for patients with cystic fibrosis. *Journal of Pediatrics, 65,* 1112–1113.

56. Durie, P. R. (1988). Gastrointestinal motility disorders in cystic fibrosis. In J. P. Willa (Ed.), *Disorders of gastrointestinal motility in childhood* (pp. 91–99). New York: Wiley.

57. Durie, P. R., Gaskin, K. J., Corey, M., Kopelman, H., Weizman, Z., & Forstner, G. G. (1984). Pancreatic function testing in cystic fibrosis. *Journal of Pediatric Gastroenterology and Nutrition, 3,* 89–98.

58. Edenborough, F. P. (2001). Women with cystic fibrosis and their potential for reproduction. *Thorax, 56,* 649–655.

59. Egan, T. M. (1992). Overview of lung transplantation for cystic fibrosis. *Pediatric Pulmonology Supplement, 8,* 204–205.

60. Elborn, J. (2007). How can we prevent multi-system complications of cystic fibrosis? *Pediatric Pulmonology, 28,* 303–311.

61. Farrell, P.M., Rosenstein, B.J., White, T.B., Accurso, F.J., Castellani, C., Cutting, G.R., Durie, P.R., LeGrys, V.A., Massie, J., Parad, R.B., Rock, M.J., Campbell III, P.W. (2008). Guidelines for diagnosis of cystic fibrosis in newborns through older adults: cystic fibrosis foundation consensus report. *The Journal of Pediatrics, 153,* s4–s14.

62. Flume, P. A., & Yankaskas, J. R. (1999). Reproductive issues. In J. R. Yankaskas, & M. R. Knowles (Eds.), *Cystic fibrosis in adults* (pp. 449–464). Philadelphia: Lippincott-Raven.

63. Fox, E. L., & Mathews, D. K. (1981). *The physiological basis of physical education and athletics* (3rd ed.). Philadelphia: Saunders College.

64. Frownfelter, D. L. (Ed.), (1996). *Chest physical therapy and pulmonary rehabilitation.* Chicago: Year Book Medical.

65. Gaskin, L., Shin, J., Reisman, J. J., Thomas, J., & Tullis, E. (1998). Long term trial of conventional postural drainage and percussion vs. positive expiratory pressure. *Pediatric Pulmonology Supplement, 15,* 345a.

66. Gibson, L. E., & Cooke, R. E. (1959). A test for concentration of electrolytes in sweat in cystic fibrosis of the pancreas utilizing pilocarpine by iontophoresis. *Pediatrics, 23,* 545–549.

67. Gilljam, H., Malmborg, A., & Strandvik, B. (1986). Conformity of bacterial growth in sputum and contamination free endobronchial samples in patients with cystic fibrosis. *Thorax, 41,* 641–645.

68. Godfrey, S. (1974). *Exercise testing in children.* Philadelphia: WB Saunders.

69. Godfrey, S., Bar-Yishay, E., Arad, I., Landau, L. I., & Taussig, L. M. (1983). Flow-volume curves in infants with lung disease. *Pediatrics, 72,* 517–522.

70. Grece, C. A. (2000). Effectiveness of high frequency chest compression: A 3-year retrospective study. *Pediatric Pulmonology Supplement, 20,* 302.

71. Green, M., & Solnit, A. J. (1964). Reactions to the threatened loss of a child: A vulnerable child syndrome. *Pediatrics, 34,* 58–66.

72. Green, O. C. (1983). Endocrinological complications associated with cystic fibrosis. In J. D. Lloyd-Still (Ed.), *Textbook of cystic fibrosis* (pp. 329–349). Stoneham, MA: Wright.

73. Grossman, R. F. (1988). Lung transplantation. *Medical Clinics of North America, 24,* 4572–4579.

74. Gulmans, V. A. M., van Veldhoven, N. H. M. J., de Meer, K., & Helders, P. J. M. (1996). The six-minute walking test in children with cystic fibrosis: Reliability and validity. *Pediatric Pulmonology, 22,* 85–89.

75. Gurwitz, D., Corey, M., Francis, P. J., Crozier, D., & Levison, H. (1979). Perspectives in cystic fibrosis. *Pediatric Clinics of North America, 26,* 603–615.

76. Guyatt, G. H., Sullivan, M. J., Thompson, P. J., Fallen, E. L., Pugsley, S. O., Taylor, D. W., & Berman, L. B. (1985). The 6-minute walk: A new measure of exercise capacity in patients with chronic heart failure. *Canadian Medical Association Journal, 132,* 919–923.

77. Hancox, B., & Whyte, K. (2006). *Pocket guide to lung function tests* (2nd ed.). New York: McGraw-Hill.

78. Hansen, L. G., Warwick, W. J., & Hansen, K. L. (1994). Mucus transport mechanisms in relation to the effect of high frequency chest compression (HFCC) on mucus clearance. *Pediatric Pulmonology, 17,* 113–118.

79. Hardy, K. A. (1994). A review of airway clearance: New techniques, indications, and recommendations. *Respiratory Care, 39,* 440 –452.

80. Hardy, K. A., Wolfson, M. R., Schidlow, D. V., & Shaffer, T. H. (1989). Mechanics and energetics of breathing in newly diagnosed infants with cystic fibrosis: Effect of combined bronchodilator and chest physical therapy. *Pediatric Pulmonology, 6,* 103–108.

81. Heijerman, H. G. M., Bakker, W., Sterk, P., & Dijkman, J. H. (1991). Oxygen-assisted exercise training in adult cystic fibrosis patients with pulmonary limitation to exercise. *International Journal of Rehabilitation Research, 14,* 101–115.

82. Henke, K. G., & Orenstein, D. M. (1984). Oxygen saturation during exercise in cystic fibrosis. *American Review of Respiratory Disease, 129,* 708–711.

83. Hess, D. R. (2001). The evidence for secretion clearance techniques. *Respiratory Care, 46,* 1276–1293.

84. Hiatt, P., Eigen, H., Yu, P., & Tepper, R. S. (1988). Bronchodilator response in infants and young children with cystic fibrosis. *American Review of Respiratory Disease, 137,* 119–122.

85. Hietpas, B., Roth, R., & Jensen, W. 1979) Huff coughing and airway patency. *Respiratory Care, 24,* 710173.

86. Reference deleted in page proofs.

87. Humberstone, N. (1990). Respiratory assessment and treatment. In S. Irwin, & J. S. Tecklin (Eds.), *Cardiopulmonary physical therapy* (pp. 283–322). St Louis: Mosby.

88. Irwin S., J.S. Tecklin (1990). *Cardiopulmonary physical therapy.* St Louis: Mosby.

89. Johnson, C., Butler, S. M., Konstan, M. W., Morgan, W., & Wohl, M. E. (2003). Factors influencing outcomes in cystic fibrosis. *Chest, 123,* 20–27.

90. Kadikar, A., Maurer, J., & Kesten, S. (1997). The six-minute walk test: A guide to assessment for lung transplantation. *Journal of Heart and Lung Transplantation, 16,* 313–319.

91. Kattan, M. (1987). Pediatric pulmonary function testing. In A. Miller (Ed.), *Pulmonary function tests: A guide for the student and house officer* (pp. 199–212). Philadelphia: WB Saunders.

92. Kellerman, J., Zeltzer, L., & Ellenberg, L. (1980). Psychological effects of illness in adolescence: Anxiety, self-esteem and perception of control. *Journal of Pediatrics, 97,* 126–131.

93. Kerem, B. S., Rommens, J. R., Buchanan, J. A., Markiewicz, D., Cox, T. K., Chakravarti, A., Buchwald, M., & Tsui, L. C. (1989). Identification of the cystic fibrosis gene: Gene analysis. *Science, 245,* 1073–1080.

94. Kerem, E., Reisman, J., Corey, M., Canny, G. J., & Levison, H. (1992). Prediction of mortality in patients with cystic fibrosis. *New England Journal of Medicine, 326,* 1187–1191.

95. Khaghani, A., Madden, B., Hodson, M., & Yacoub, M. (1991). Heart-lung transplantation for cystic fibrosis. *Pediatric Pulmonology Supplement, 6,* 128–129.

96. Khan, T. Z., Wagener, J. S., Bost, T., Martinez, J., Accurso, F. J., & Riches, D. W. (1995). Early pulmonary inflammation in infants with cystic fibrosis. *American Journal of Respiratory and Critical Care Medicine, 151,* 1075–1082.

97. Klijn, P. H., Terherggen-Largo, S. W., van der Ent, C. K., van der Net, J., Kimpen, J. L., & Helders, P. J. (2003). Anaerobic exercise in pediatric cystic fibrosis. *Pediatric Pulmonology, 36,* 223–229.

98. Konstan, M. W., Stern, R. C., & Doershuk, C. F. (1994). Efficacy of the flutter VRPI in airway mucus clearance in cystic fibrosis. *Pediatrics, 124,* 689–693.

99. Kreider, M., & Kotloff, R. M. (2009). Selection of candidates for lung transplantation. *Proceedings of the American Thoracic Society, 6,* 20–27.

100. Lamarre, A., Reilly, B. J., & Bryan, A. C. (1972). Early detection of pulmonary function abnormalities in cystic fibrosis. *Pediatrics, 50,* 291–298.

101. Landau, L. I. (1995). Cystic fibrosis: Transition from paediatric to adult physician's care. *Thorax, 50,* 1031–1032.

102. Lannefors, L. (1992). Different ways of using positive expiratory pressure to loosen and mobilize secretions. *Pediatric Pulmonology Supplement, 8,* 136–137.

103. Lloyd-Still, D. M., & Lloyd-Still, J. D. (1983). The patient, the family and the community. In J. D. Lloyd-Still (Ed.), *Textbook of cystic fibrosis* (pp. 443–446). Stoneham, MA: Wright.

104. Loffert, D. T., Ikle, D., & Nelson, H. S. (1994). A comparison of commercial jet nebulizers. *Chest, 106,* 1788–1792.

105. Long, F. R., Williams, R. S., & Castile, R. G. (2004). Structural airway abnormalities in infants and young children with cystic fibrosis. *Journal of Pediatrics, 144,* 154–161.

106. Lorin, M. I., & Denning, C. R. (1971). Evaluation of postural drainage by measurement of sputum volume and consistency. *American Journal of Physical Medicine and Rehabilitation, 50,* 215–219.

107. Mackenzie, C. F. (1989). Undesirable effects, precautions, and contraindications of chest physiotherapy. In C. F. Mackenzie (Ed.), *Chest physiotherapy in the intensive care unit* (pp. 321–344). Baltimore: Williams & Wilkins.

108. MacLusky, I. B., Canny, G. J., & Levison, H. (1987). Cystic fibrosis: An update. *Paediatric Reviews and Communications, 1,* 343–384.

109. MacLusky, I. B., & Levison, H. (1990). Cystic fibrosis. In V. Chernick, (Ed.), *Kendig's disorders of the respiratory tract in children* (Vol. 5; pp. 692–730). Philadelphia: WB Saunders.

110. MacLusky, I. B., & Levison, H. (1998). Cystic fibrosis. In V. I. Chernick (Ed.), *Kendig's disorders of the respiratory tract in children* (Vol. 6; pp. 838–882). Philadelphia: WB Saunders.

111. Main, E., Tannenbaum, E., Stanojevic, S., Scrase, E., & Prasad, A. (2006). The effects of positive expiratory pressure (PEP) or oscillatory positive pressure (RC Cornet) on FEV1 and lung clearance index over a twelve month period in children with CF. *Pediatric Pulmonology Supplement, 29,* 351.

112. Malfroot, A., & Dab, I. (1991). New insights on gastro-oesophageal reflux in cystic fibrosis by longitudinal follow-up. *Archives of Disease in Childhood, 66,* 1339–1345.

113. Maxwell, B. (1991). Nursing aspects of C.F. care. *Pediatric Pulmonology Supplement, 6,* 85–86.

114. Mazzacco, M. C., Owens, G. R., Kirilloff, L. H., & Rogers, R. M. (1985). Chest percussion and postural drainage in patients with chronic bronchiectasis. *Chest, 88,* 360–363.

115. McCollum, A. T., & Gibson, L. E. (1970). Family adaptation to the child with cystic fibrosis. *Journal of Pediatrics, 77,* 571–578.

116. McCool, F. D., & Rosen, M. J. (2006). Nonpharmacologic airway clearance therapies: ACCP evidence-based clinical practice guidelines. *Chest, 129*(1 suppl), 250S–259S.

117. McIlwaine, P. M., Davidson, A. G. F., Wong, L. T. K., & Pirie, G. E. (1992). Autogenic drainage. *Pediatric Pulmonology Supplement, 8,* 134–135.

118. McIlwaine, P. M., Davidson, A. G. F., Wong, L. T. K., Pirie, G. E., & Nakielna, E. M. (1988). Comparison of positive expiratory pressure and autogenic drainage with conventional percussion and drainage therapy in the treatment of cystic fibrosis. *Pediatric Pulmonology, 4*(suppl 2), 132a.

119. McIlwaine et al. (1997) Long-term comparative trial of conventional postural drainage and percussion versus positive expiratory pressure physiotherapy in the treatment of cystic fibrosis. *Journal of Paediatrics, 131*(4), 570–574.

120. McIlwaine, P. M., Wong, L. T., Peacock, D., Davidson, A. G. (2001). Long-term comparative trial of positive expiratory pressure versus oscillating positive expiratory pressure (flutter) physiotherapy in the treatment of cystic fibrosis. *Journal of Pediatrics, 138,* 845–850.

121. Mei-Zahav, M., Durie, P., Zielenski, J., Solomon, M., Tullis, E., Tsui, L.-C., & Corey, M. (2005). The prevalence and clinical characteristics of cystic fibrosis in South Asian Canadian immigrants. *Archives of Disease in Childhood, 90,* 675–679.

122. Mellins, R., Levine, O. R., Ingram, R. H. Jr., & Fishman, A. P. (1968). Obstructive disease of the airways in cystic fibrosis. *Pediatrics, 41,* 560–573.

123. Miller, A. (1987). Spirometry and maximum expiratory flow-volume curves. In A. Miller (Ed.), *Pulmonary function tests: A guide for the student and house officer* (pp. 15–32). Philadelphia: WB Saunders.

124. Mitchell-Heggs, P., Mearns, M., & Batten, J. C. (1976). Cystic fibrosis in adolescents and adults. *Quarterly Journal of Medicine, 45,* 479–504.

125. Moran, A., Dunitz, J., Nathan, B., Saeed, A., Holme, B., & Thomas, W. (2009). Cystic fibrosis related diabetes: Current trends in prevalence, incidence and mortality. *Diabetes Care, 32,* 1626–1631.

126. Moran, F., Bradley, J. M., Boyle, L., Elborn, J. S. (2003). Incontinence in adult females with cystic fibrosis: A Northern Ireland survey. *International Journal of Clinical Practice, 57,* 182–183.

127. Morrison, L., & Agnew, J. (2009). Oscillating devices for airway clearance in people with cystic fibrosis. *Cochrane Database of Systematic Reviews, 1,* CD006842.

128. Muller, N., Frances, P., Gurwitz, D., Levison, H., & Bryan, A. C. (1980). Mechanisms of hemoglobin desaturation during rapid-eye movement sleep in normal subjects and in patients with cystic fibrosis. *American Review of Respiratory Disease, 119,* 338.

129. Munck, A., Gerardin, M., Alberti, C., Ajzenman, C., Lebourgeois, M., Aigrain, Y., & Navarro, J. (2006). Clinical outcome of cystic fibrosis present with or without meconium ileus: A matched cohort study. *Journal of Pediatric Surgery, 41,* 1556–1560.

130. Narang, I., Pike, S., Rosenthal, M., Balfour-Lynn, I. M., & Bush, A. (2003). Three-minute step test to assess exercise capacity in children with cystic fibrosis with mild lung disease. *Pediatric Pulmonology, 35,* 108–113.

131. Newbold, E., Tullis, E., Corey, M., Ross, B., & Brooks, D. (2005). The Flutter device versus the PEP mask in the treatment of adults with cystic fibrosis. *Physiotherapy Canada, 57,* 199–207.

132. Nixon, P. A., Orenstein, D. M., & Kelsey, S. F. (2001). Habitual physical activity in children and adolescents with cystic fibrosis. *Medicine and Science in Sports and Exercise, 33,* 30–35.

133. Nixon, P. A., Orenstein, D. M., Kelsey, S. F., & Doershuk, C. F. (1992). The prognostic value of exercise testing in patients with cystic fibrosis. *New England Journal of Medicine, 327,* 1785–1788.

134. Nystad, W., Samuelsen, S. O., Nafstad, P., Edvardsen, E., Stensrud, T., & Jaakkola, J. (2002). Feasibility of measuring lung function in preschool children. *Thorax, 57,* 1021–1027.

135. Oberwaldner, B., Evans, J. C., & Zach, M. S. (1986). Forced expirations against a variable resistance: A new chest physiotherapy method in cystic fibrosis. *Pediatric Pulmonology, 2,* 358–367.

136. Oberwaldner, B., Theissl, B., Rucker, A., & Zach, M. S. (1991). Chest physiotherapy in hospitalized patients with cystic fibrosis: A study of lung function effects and sputum production. *European Respiratory Journal, 4,* 152–158.

137. Orenstein, D. M. (1998). Exercise testing in cystic fibrosis. *Pediatric Pulmonology, 25,* 223–225.

138. Orenstein, D. M., Franklin, B. A., Doershuk, C. F., Hellerstein, H. K., Germann, K. J., Horowitz, J. G., & Stern, R. C. (1981). Exercise conditioning and cardiopulmonary fitness in cystic fibrosis. *Chest, 80,* 292–298.

139. Orenstein D. M. (1997) *Cystic fibrosis: A guide for patient and family.* (2nd ed.)., Philadelphia: Lippincott-Raven,

140. Orenstein, D. M. (2003) *Cystic fibrosis: A guide for patient and family,* (3rd ed.)., New York: Lippincott-Raven,

141. Orenstein, S. R., & Orenstein, D. M. (1988). Gastroesophageal reflux and respiratory disease in children. *Journal of Pediatrics, 112,* 847–858.

142. Orr, A., McVean, R. J., Webb, A. K., & Dodd, M. E. (2001). Questionnaire survey of urinary incontinence in women with cystic fibrosis. *British Medical Journal, 322,* 1521

143. O'Sullivan, B., & Friedman, S. (2009). Cystic fibrosis. *Lancet, 373,* 1891–1904.

144. Paley, C. A. (1997). A way forward for determining optimal aerobic exercise intensity? *Physiotherapy, 83,* 620–624.

145. Pasque, M. K., Cooper, J. D., Kaiser, L. R., Haydock, D. A., Triantafilloy, A., & Trulock, E. P. (1990). Improved technique for bilateral lung transplantation: Rationale and initial clinical experience. *Annals of Thoracic Surgery, 49,* 785–791.

146. Passero, M. A., Remor, B., & Solomon, J. (1981). Patient-reported compliance with cystic fibrosis therapy. *Clinical Pediatrics, 20,* 264–268.

147. Phelan, P. D., Gracey, M., Williams, H. E., & Anderson, C. M. (1969). Ventilatory function in infants with cystic fibrosis. *Archives of Disease in Childhood, 44,* 393–400.

148. Phillips, B. M., & David, T. J. (1986). Pathogenesis and management of arthropathy in cystic fibrosis. *Journal of the Royal Society of Medicine, 79*(suppl 12), 44–49.

149. Phillips, B. M., & David, T. J. (1987). Management of the chest in cystic fibrosis. *Journal of the Royal Society of Medicine, 80*(suppl 15), 30–37.

150. Phillips, G. E., Pike, S. E., Jaffe, A., & Bush, A. (2004). Comparison of active cycle of breathing and high-frequency oscillation jacket in children with cystic fibrosis. *Pediatric Pulmonology, 37,* 71–75.

151. Pinkerton, P., Trauer, T., Duncan, F., Hodson, M., & Batten, J. (1985). Cystic fibrosis in adult life: A study of coping patterns. *Lancet, 2,* 761–763.

152. Pizer, H. F. (1991). *Organ transplants: A patient's guide.* Cambridge, MA: Harvard University Press.

153. Porcari, J. P., Ebbeling, C. B., Ward, A., Freedson, P. S., & Rippe, J. M. (1989). Walking for exercise testing and training. *Sports Medicine, 8*, 189–200.

154. Porter, D. K., Van Every, M. J., Anthracite, R. F., & Mack, J. W., Jr. (1983). Massive hemoptysis in cystic fibrosis. *Archives of Internal Medicine, 143*, 287–290.

155. Prasad, S. A., Randall, S. D., Balfour-Lynn, I. M. (2000). Fifteen-count breathlessness score: An objective measure for children. *Pediatric Pulmonology, 30*, 56–62.

156. Pryor, J. A. (1991). The forced expiratory technique. In J. Pryor (Ed.), *Respiratory care* (pp. 79–100). London: Churchill Livingstone.

157. Pryor, J., & Prasad, A. (2002). *Physiotherapy for respiratory and cardiac problems* (3rd ed.). Philadelphia: Churchill Livingstone.

158. Radtke, R., Stevens, D., Benden, C., & Williams, C. (2009). Clinical exercise testing in children and adolescents with cystic fibrosis. *Pediatric Physical Therapy, 21(3)*,275–281.

159. Ramsey, B. W., Pepe, M. S., Quan, J. M., et al. (1999). Intermittent administration of inhaled tobramycin in patients with cystic fibrosis. Cystic Fibrosis Inhaled Tobramycin Study Group. *New England Journal of Medicine, 340*, 23–30.

160. Ranganathan, S. C., Stocks, J., Dezateux, C., Bush, A., Wade, A., Carr, S., Castle, R., Dinwiddie, R., Hoo, A., Price, J., Stroobant, J., Wallis, C., & The London Collaborative Cystic Fibrosis Group. (2004). The evolution of airway function in early childhood following clinical diagnosis of cystic fibrosis. *American Journal of Respiratory and Critical Care Medicine, 169*, 928–933.

161. Ratjen, F. A. (2009). Cystic fibrosis: Pathogenesis and future treatment strategies. *Respiratory Care, 54*, 595–602.

162. Ratjen, F., Munck, A., & Kho, P. (2008). Short and long-term efficacy of inhaled tobramycin in early *P. aeruginosa* infection: The ELITE study. *Pediatric Pulmonology Supplement, 31*, 319–320.

163. Reisman, J. J., Rivington-Law, B., Corey, M., Marcotte, J., Wannamaker, E., Harcourt, D., & Levison, H. (1988). Role of conventional physiotherapy in cystic fibrosis. *Journal of Pediatrics, 113*, 632–636.

164. Riordan, J. R., Rommens, J. M., Kerem, B. S., Alon, N., Rozmahel, R., Grzelczak, Z., Zielensky, J., Lok, S., Plavsic, N., Drumm, M. L., Iannuzzi, M. C., Collins, F. S., & Tsui, L. C. (1989). Identification of the cystic fibrosis gene: Cloning and characterization of complementary DNA. *Science, 245*, 1066–1073.

165. Rose, J., & Jay, S. (1986). A comprehensive exercise program for persons with cystic fibrosis. *Journal of Pediatric Nursing, 1*, 323–334.

166. Rosenstein, B., & Langbaum, T. (1984). Diagnosis. In L. M. Taussig (Ed.), *Cystic fibrosis* (pp. 85–115). New York: Thieme-Stratton.

167. Ruppel, G. (1998). *Manual of pulmonary function testing* (7th ed.). St Louis: Mosby.

168. Sackett, D. L. (1986). Rules of evidence and clinical recommendations on the use of antithrombotic agents. *Chest, 89*(suppl), 25–35.

169. Schneiderman-Walker, J., Pollock, S., Corey, M., Wilkes, D., Canny, G., Pedder, L., & Reisman, J. (2000). A randomized controlled trial of a 3-year home exercise program in cystic fibrosis. *Journal of Pediatrics, 136*, 304–310.

170. Scott, R. B., O'Loughlin, E. V., & Gall, D. G. (1985). Gastroesophageal reflux in patients with cystic fibrosis. *Journal of Pediatrics, 106*, 223–227.

171. Scott, S. M., Walters, D. A., Singh, S. J., Morgan, M. D. L., & Hardman, A. E. (1990). A progressive shuttle walking test of functional capacity in patients with chronic airflow limitation. *Thorax, 45*, 781a.

172. Selvadurai, H. C., Cooper, P. J., Meyers, N., Blimkie, C. J., Smith, L., Mellis, C. M., & Van Asperen, P. P. (2003). Validation of shuttle tests in children with cystic fibrosis. *Pediatric Pulmonology, 35*, 133–138.

173. Selvadurai et al. (2005). Selvadurai HC, Blimkie J, Cooper PJ, Mellis CM, Van Asperen PP. Gender differences in habitual activity in children with cystic fibrosis. *Archives of Disease Childhood, 89*, 928–933.

174. Sermet-Gaudelus, I., Castanet, M., Retsch-Bogart, G., & Aris, R. (2009). Update on cystic fibrosis-related bone disease: A special focus on children. *Pediatric Respiratory Reviews, 10*, 134–142.

175. Shepherd, R., Vasques-Velasquez, L., Prentice, A., Holt, T. L., Coward, W., & Lucas, A. (1988). Increased energy expenditure in young children with cystic fibrosis. *Lancet, 2*, 1300–1303.

176. Shwachman, H., & Kulczycki, L. L. (1958). Long-term study of 105 patients with cystic fibrosis. *American Journal of Diseases of Children, 96*, 6–15.

177. Singh, S. (1992). The use of field walking test for assessment of functional capacity in patients with chronic airways obstruction. *Physiotherapy, 78*, 102–104.

178. Spalding, A., Kelly, L., Santopietro, J., & Posner-Mayor, J. (1999). *Kid on the ball: Swiss balls in a complete fitness program.* Windsor: Human Kinetics.

179. Starnes, V. A., Bowdish, M. E., Woo, M. S., Barbers, R. G., Schenkel, F. A., Horn, M. V., Pessotto, R., Sievers, E. M., Baker, C. J., Cohen, R. G., Bremner, R. M., Wells, W. J., & Barr, M. L. (2004). A decade of living lobar lung transplantation: Recipient outcomes. *Journal of Thoracic and Cardiovascular Surgery, 127*, 114–122.

180. Starr, J. A. (1992). Manual techniques of chest physical therapy and airway clearance techniques. In C. C. Zadai (Ed.), *Pulmonary management in physical therapy* (pp. 99–133). New York: Churchill Livingstone.

181. Strauss, G. D., Osher, A., Wang, C. I., Goodrich, E., Gold, F., Colman, W., Stabile, M., Dobrenchuk, A., & Keens, T. (1987). Variable weight training in cystic fibrosis. *Chest, 92*, 273–276.

182. Taussig, L. M., Landau, L. I., & Marks, M. I. (1984). Respiratory system. In L. M. Taussig (Ed.), *Cystic fibrosis* (pp. 115–174). New York: Thieme-Stratton.

183. Tecklin, J. S., Clayton, R. G., & Scanlin, T. F. (2000). High frequency chest wall oscillation vs. traditional chest physical therapy in CF: A large, 1-year, controlled study. *Pediatric Pulmonology Supplement, 20*, 304.

184. Tepper, R. S. (1992). Assessment of pulmonary function in infants with cystic fibrosis. *Pediatric Pulmonology Supplement, 8*, 165–166.

185. Tepper, R. S., Hiatt, P., Eigen, H., Scott, P., Grosfeld, J., & Cohen, M. (1988). Infants with cystic fibrosis: Pulmonary function at diagnosis. *Pediatric Pulmonology, 5*, 15–18.

186. Tepper, R. S., Hiatt, P. W., Eigen, H., & Smith, J. (1987). Total respiratory compliance in asymptomatic infants with cystic fibrosis. *American Review of Respiratory Disease, 135*, 1075–1079.

187. Thomas, J., Cook, D. J., & Brooks, D. (1995). Chest physical therapy management of patients with cystic fibrosis. A meta-analysis. *American Journal of Respiratory Critical Care Medicine, 151*(3 Pt 1), 846–850.

188. Van Ginderdeuren, F., Malfroot, A., & Dab, I. (2001). Influence of 'assisted autogenic drainage (AAD),' 'bouncing' and 'AAD combined with bouncing' on gastro-oesophageal reflux (GOR) in infants. *Journal of Cystic Fibrosis*, Book of abstracts, p. 112.

189. Vinocur, C. D., Marmon, L., Schidlow, D. V., & Weintraub, W. H. (1985). Gastroesophageal reflux in the infant with cystic fibrosis. *American Journal of Surgery, 149*, 182–186.

190. Volsko, T. A. (2009). Cystic fibrosis and the respiratory therapist: A 50-year perspective. *Respiratory Care, 54*, 587–593.

191. Volsko, T. A., DiFiore, J. M., & Chatburn, R. L. (2003). Performance comparison of two oscillating positive expiratory pressure devices: Acapella versus Flutter. *Respiratory Care, 48*, 124–130.

192. Wagener, J. S., & Headley, A. A. (2003). Cystic fibrosis: Current trends in respiratory care. *Respiratory Care, 48*, 234–244.

193. Wagener, J. S., Taussig, L. M., Burrows, B., Hernried, L., & Boat, T. (1980). Comparison of lung function survival patterns between cystic fibrosis and emphysema or chronic bronchitis patients. In J. M. Sturgess (Ed.), *Perspectives in cystic fibrosis* (pp. 236–245). Mississauga, Canada: Imperial Press.

194. Wark, P., & McDonald, V. M. (2009). Nebulized hypertonic saline for cystic fibrosis. *Cochrane Database of Systematic Reviews, 2*, CD001506.

195. Warwick, W. J., & Hansen, L. G. (1991). The long term effect of high frequency chest compression therapy on pulmonary complications of cystic fibrosis. *Pediatric Pulmonology, 11*, 265–271.

196. Webber, B. A., & Pryor, J. A. (1998). *Physiotherapy for respiratory an cardiac problems* (2nd ed.). New York: Churchill Livingstone.

197. Weiser, G., & Kerem, E. (2007). Early intervention in CF: How to monitor the effect. *Pediatric Pulmonology, 42*, 1002–1007.

198. Wilkes, D. L., Schneiderman-Walker, J., Atenafu, E., Wells, G., Tullis, E., Lands, L., Corey, M., Coates, A. L., & Ratjen, F. (2008). Bone mineral density and habitual physical activity in cystic fibrosis. *Pediatric Pulmonology Supplement, 31*, 436.

199. Wilkes, D. L., Schneiderman-Walker, J., Corey, M., Atenafu, E., Li, Y., Lands, L., Tullis, E., Coates, A. L., & Ratjen, F. (2007). Long-term effect of habitual physical activity on lung function

in patients with cystic fibrosis. *Pediatric Pulmonology Supplement, 30*, 358.

200. Wilschanski, M., Corey, M., Durie, P., Tullis, E., Bain, J., Asch, M., Ginzburg, B., Jarvi, K., Buckspan, B., & Hartwick, W. (1996). Diversity of reproductive tract abnormalities in men with cystic fibrosis. *Journal of the American Medical Association, 276*, 607–608.

201. Winton, T. (1992). Double lung transplantation for cystic fibrosis: Operative technique and early post-operative care. *Pediatric Pulmonology Supplement, 8*, 208–209.

202. Witt, D. R., Blumberg, B., Schaefer, C., Fitzgerald, P., Fishbach, A., Holtzman, J., Kornfeld, S., Lee, R., Nemzer, L., Palmer, R., Sato, M., & Jenkins, L. (1992). Cystic fibrosis carrier screening in a prenatal population. *Pediatric Pulmonology Supplement, 8*, 235.

203. Wood, R. E. (1993). Why commence conventional chest physiotherapy for CF at diagnosis? *Pediatric Pulmonology Supplement, 9*, 89–90.

204. Yankaskas, J. R. (1992). Respiratory failure in CF: Pathophysiology and treatment, including the role of mechanical ventilation. *Pediatric Pulmonology Supplement, 8*, 87–88.

205. Yankaskas et al. (1998). Yankaskas, JR, Mallory, GB, and the Consensus Committee. Lung transplantation in cystic fibrosis: Consensus conference statement. *Chest, 113*(1):217–226, 1998.

206. Yankaskas, J. R., Marshall, B. C., Sufian, B., Simon, R. H., & Rodman, D. (2004). Cystic fibrosis adult care: Consensus conference report. *Chest, 125*, 1S–39S.

207. Yellon, R. F. (1997). The spectrum of reflux-associated otolaryngologic problems in infants and children. *American Journal of Medicine, 103*, 125–129.

208. Zach, M. S., Purrer, B., & Oberwaldner, B. (1981). Effect of swimming on forced expiration and sputum clearance in cystic fibrosis. *Lancet, 2*, 1201–1203.

209. Zadai, C. C. (1992). Comprehensive physical therapy evaluation: Identifying potential pulmonary limitations. In C. C. Zadai (Ed.), *Pulmonary management in physical therapy* (pp. 55–78). New York: Churchill Livingstone.

SUGGESTED READING

Doershuk, C. F., Downs, T. D., Matthews, L. W., & Lough, M. D. (1970). A method for ventilatory measurements in subjects one month to five years of age: Normal results and observations in disease. *Pediatric Research, 4*, 165–174.

Flume, P., O'Sullivan, B., Robinson, K., et al. (2007). Cystic fibrosis pulmonary guidelines: Chronic medication for maintenance of lung health. *American Journal of Respiratory and Critical Care Medicine, 176*, 957–969.

Folkins, C. (1972). The effects of physical training on mood. *Journal of Clinical Psychology, 32*, 583–588.

Goodwin, B. (May 2005). Nutritional issues in gastroenterology. Series #27: Nutrition issues in cystic fibrosis. *Practical Gastroenterology*, 76–94.

Lewiston, N., & Moss, R. (1987). Interobserver variance in clinical scoring for cystic fibrosis. *Chest, 91*, 878–882.

Mellins, R. (1969). The site of airway obstruction in cystic fibrosis. *Pediatrics, 44,* 315–318.

Orenstein, D. M. (2004). *Cystic fibrosis: A guide for patient and family* (3rd ed.). Philadelphia: Lippincott-Raven.

Orenstein, D. M., Henke, K. G., & Cerny, F. J. (1983). Exercise and cystic fibrosis. *Physician and Sports Medicine, 2,* 57–63.

Park, R. W., & Grand, R. J. (1981). Gastrointestinal manifestations of cystic fibrosis: A review. *Gastroenterology, 81,* 1143–1161.

International Physiotherapy Group for Cystic Fibrosis Mucoviscidosis Association. (2002). Physiotherapy in the treatment of cystic fibrosis (CF). Retrieved from the secretary of IPG/CF at: www.ipg-cf.fw.hu.

Schneiderman-Walker, J., Wilkes, D. L., Strug, L., Lands, L. C., Pollock, S. L., Selvadurai, H. C., Hay, J., Coates, A. L., & Corey, M. (2005). Sex differences in habitual physical activity and lung function decline in children with cystic fibrosis. *Journal of Pediatrics, 147,* 321–326.

Selvadurai, H. C., Blimkie, J., Cooper, P. J., Mellis, C. M., & Van Asperen, P. P. (2004). Gender differences in habitual activity in children with cystic fibrosis. *Archives of Disease Childhood, 89,* 928–933.

Solomon, M. P., Wilson, D. C., Corey, M., Kalnins, D., Zielenski, J., Tsui, L. C., Pencharz, P., Durie, P., & Sweezey, N. B. (2003). Glucose intolerance in children with cystic fibrosis. *Journal of Pediatrics, 142,* 128–132.

Wilkes, D., Schneiderman-Walker, J., Strug, L., Selvadurai, H. C., Lands, L. C., Corey, M., & Coates, A. L. (2003). Habitual activity and disease progression in boys and girls with cystic fibrosis. *Pediatric Pulmonology Supplement, 25,* 330.

25 Asthma: Multisystem Implications

MARY MASSERY, PT, DPT

Nearly one in ten children in the United States has a diagnosis of asthma (CDC 2010). This frequency has been increasing for decades both in the United States and abroad for reasons that are not yet clearly understood.[21a,22,23,47,63,110,123] According to the U.S. Centers for Disease Control and Prevention (CDC), from 1979 to 1995 the incidence of asthma increased over 160% for children ages 0 to 4 years and 74% for children ages 5 to 14 years. Similarly, the morbidity rate increased 63% for children ages 0 to 4 years and 20% for children ages 5 to 14 years, whereas the mortality rate increased 12% for children ages 0 to 4 years and 146% for children ages 5 to 14 years.[22] Follow-up data in a CDC report on the state of childhood Asthma in the United States indicated that asthma morbidity and mortality rates may have peaked in the mid/late 1990s.[2]

Pragmatically, the incidence figures mean that nearly 10% of all children seen by pediatric physical therapists may have asthma. Does this disease impact a child's motor performance? If so, what kind of impact does it have and what clinical implications does the presence of asthma have for the physical therapist treating pediatric patients?

The purpose of this chapter is to achieve the following:

1. Define asthma and discuss the medical ramifications of the disease.
2. Demonstrate the process of a differential physical therapy diagnosis for potential physical and activity limitations secondary to asthma through the illustration of a clinical case.
3. Identify the types of cardiopulmonary, neuromuscular, musculoskeletal, integumentary, and gastrointestinal impairments that may be associated with this diagnosis.
4. Present possible treatment strategies and specific PT procedural interventions.
5. Present potential long-term outcomes of physical therapy procedural interventions on the maturation and physical performance of a child with asthma.
6. Through a case study, illustrate participation benefits when a child's health is well supported.

PATHOPHYSIOLOGY

Asthma is a pulmonary disease with three significant characteristics: (1) airway inflammation, (2) airway obstruction that is often reversible either spontaneously or with pharmacologic intervention, and (3) bronchial hyperresponsiveness to stimuli that are classified as either extrinsic or intrinsic.[92,95,131] It is a disease of both the large and the small airways with recurrent episodes of shortness of breath, wheezing, chest tightness, and coughing. Bronchial hyperresponsiveness to a variety of extrinsic and intrinsic stimuli is increased. Extrinsic or allergic stimuli include but are not limited to pollen, mold, animal dander, cigarette smoke, foods, drugs, and dust. Intrinsic or nonallergic stimuli include but are not limited to viral infections, inhalation of irritating substances, exercise, emotional stress, and environmental factors such as the weather or climate changes. An individual may be sensitive to either type of stimuli or to both types.

Researchers have found genetic causes for the development of asthma, but genetics alone does not account for all types and severities of the expression of the disease.[7,15,46] The physical, environmental, neurogenic, chemical, and pharmacologic factors that are associated with asthma are specific to each individual. They stimulate or trigger the immune system to release chemical mediators, which in turn cause constriction of the bronchial muscles, increased mucus production, and swelling of the mucous membranes. Mucus accumulation, which has been shown to be abnormal in asthma, may cause blockage of the airways, resulting in further air trapping and hyperinflation, and is a primary cause of death associated with asthma.[70]

Over the decades, inflammation has been identified as a central component of asthma and may be a primary contributor to airway remodeling leading to chronic inflammation. This structural change may make the airways less responsive to medications.[95]

In addition to the pulmonary manifestation of asthma, numerous studies have shown that a diagnosis of asthma in childhood results in frequent hospitalizations, poorer growth and development than peers, sleep disorders, and a reduction in overall quality of life.[1,13,60,64,86,100,104,132,134] These factors result in an increased number of missed school/work days and limitations on the child's participation in typical childhood activities.[17,29,35]

Asthma and other chronic respiratory diseases have been shown in recent years to be associated with the presence of gastroesophageal reflux disease (GERD).[67,69,89,96,121,135] Children with asthma should be screened for the possibility of underlying reflux. In some cases, chronic cough can be misdiagnosed as asthma, when in fact the primary cause is GERD.[102,124] This has obvious implications for the medical management of cough symptoms.

PRIMARY IMPAIRMENT

DIAGNOSIS

The diagnosis of asthma is made on the basis of history, physical examination, auscultation and palpation, and pulmonary function tests (PFTs), especially in response to a methacholine challenge.[61] Wheezing and rhonchi may be detected by auscultation even when the child does not show difficulty breathing. Breathing is often reported as worse at night or early in the morning. Hyperexpansion of the thorax, increased accessory muscle breathing, postural changes, increased nasal secretions, mucosal swelling, nasal polyps, "allergic shiners" (darkened areas under the eyes), and evidence of an allergic skin condition may be noted on physical examination. During an acute asthma attack, the child may show an increased respiratory rate, expiratory grunting, intercostal muscle retractions and nasal flaring, an alteration in the inspiration-expiration ratio, and coughing. In severe cases, a bluish color of the lips and nails may be noted (oxygen desaturation).

Attempts have been made to produce a national classification system for the severity of the disease based on clinical findings, but follow-up studies found those systems to inconsistently reflect the severity of the disease.[10,16,104] In spite of the shortcomings, one of the most common severity classification systems was published by the U.S. National Institutes of Health (NIH) Heart, Lung and Blood Institute in 1997 and the details are listed in Table 25-1.[94] The NIH classification system lists asthma by clinical symptoms as (1) intermittent, (2) mild persistent, (3) moderate persistent, or (4) severe persistent. A recently updated Expert Panel Report #3 emphasizes initially diagnosing asthma by the severity of the disease, but then emphasizes controlling asthma rather than continuing to classify the severity[95] (www.nhlbi.nih.gov/guidelines/asthma/asthgdln.pdf).

Pulmonary Function Tests (PFT)

PFTs are performed to determine the location and degree of the respiratory impairment as well as the reversibility of bronchoconstriction following administration of a bronchodilator (methacholine challenge). Test values are compared with predicted values based on age, sex, and height.[24] PFT measurements may reveal (1) decreased forced vital capacity (FVC), (2) decreased forced expiration during the first second of FVC (FEV_1) as well as FEV_6 (6th second of exhalation), (3) decreased forced expiratory volume compared with forced vital capacity (FEV/FVC), (4) decreased peak expiratory flow rate (PEFR) because of airway obstruction in large or small airways, (5) forced expiratory flow (FEF) during 25% to 75% of FVC (FEF25% to 75%) because of airway obstruction in the small airways, (6) increased residual volume (RV), and (7) increased functional residual capacity (FRC) because of air trapping.[95] Generally, patients with asthma are instructed to monitor their daily pulmonary fluctuations and adjust their medication levels by testing their PEFR with a peak flow meter. However, recent studies have shown that FEV_1 and midexpiratory FEF25% to 75% are better indicators of disease status than PEFR.[45a] Peak flow meters are cheaper and more readily available in a home environment, so they will probably

TABLE 25-1 Clinical Classification of the Disease Severity of Asthma

Classification	Indications and Behaviors
Step 1 Intermittent	Intermittent symptoms occurring less than once a week
	Brief exacerbations
	Nocturnal symptoms occurring less than twice a month
	Asymptomatic with normal lung function between exacerbations
	FEV_1 or PEFR rate greater than 80%, with less than 20% variability
Step 2 Mild persistent	Symptoms occurring more than once a week but less than once a day
	Exacerbations affect activity and sleep
	Nocturnal symptoms occurring more than twice a month
	FEV_1 or PEFR rate greater than 80% predicted, with variability of 20–30%
Step 3 Moderate persistent	Daily symptoms
	Exacerbations affect activity and sleep
	Nocturnal symptoms occurring more than once a week
	FEV_1 or PEFR rate 60–80% of predicted, with variability greater than 30%
Step 4 Severe persistent	Continuous symptoms
	Frequent exacerbations
	Frequent nocturnal asthma symptoms
	Physical activities limited by asthma symptoms
	FEV_1 or PEFR rate less than 60%, with variability greater than 30%

Practical Guide for the Diagnosis and Management of Asthma Based on Expert Panel Report 2. NIH Publication No. 97-4053. Bethesda, MD: National Institute of Health, National Heart, Lung and Blood Institute, 1997, p. 10; and Morris, M. & Perkins, P. Asthma. e-Medicine, available at http://www.emedicine.com/med/topic177.htm, last updated 5/9/04.

continue as the home equipment of choice until FEV_1 and FEF25% to 75% can be readily tested at home. The child under the age of 5 or 6 years, however, cannot perform pulmonary function tests and needs to be monitored on the basis of clinical signs and symptoms.[19]

IMPAIRMENT IN INFANCY TO ADULTHOOD

A diagnosis of asthma is not typically made until the child is 3 to 6 years of age when numerous episodes of pulmonary problems have been demonstrated and are consistent with asthma.[61] In the meantime, children may be diagnosed with "reactive airway disease." More sophisticated tests such as PFTs are not possible until children are around 6 years of age when they are capable of cooperating and performing the tests.[19] The young child diagnosed with asthma will typically present with a family history of asthma or atopic predispositions, prematurity, lung abnormalities, exposure to second hand smoke, history of episodes of wheezy bronchitis, croup, recurrent upper respiratory tract infections, chronic bronchitis, recurrent pneumonia, respiratory distress syndrome, difficulty sleeping, bronchopulmonary dysplasia, or respiratory syncytial virus (RSV) infection.[127]

Severe RSV infection in infancy is highly associated with a later diagnosis of asthma. Currently, it is not known if children with asthma have a more severe reaction to the virus or if a severe infection with RSV actually causes asthma to develop later in childhood.[40,97,117] In addition to normal childhood illness, complications associated with prematurity and very low birth weight also have a high correlation with a later diagnosis of asthma. Like RSV infection, it is not known if prematurity causes asthma or simply makes infants more predisposed to asthma.[65,66] Respiratory problems following preterm births were also associated with eczema and GERD.[65]

By adolescence, asthmatic symptoms often decrease. Even when free of clinical symptoms, however, the adolescent may have significant impairment revealed by PFT measures. In several long-term studies, children who were preterm babies with respiratory problems, such as bronchopulmonary dysplasia (BPD) or respiratory syncytial virus (RSV) infection, were more likely to have lung and airway restrictions later in childhood, especially noted in reduced expiratory flows.[33,42,88,118] Preterm babies with chronic lung conditions are more likely to have asthma, and it is speculated that they may be more likely to develop emphysema-like conditions in middle age.[11] This remains an hypothesis, however, as survivors of extreme prematurity have not yet reached middle age.

Pediatric physical therapists should pay careful attention to a child's medical history to note evidence of a risk for asthma and consider all the ramifications on that child's health, growth, and development when planning procedural interventions.

MEDICAL MANAGEMENT

Episodes of asthma attacks are usually reversible and can be prevented or modified to some degree when the individual-specific triggers have been identified. The frequency, duration, and severity of attacks are highly variable even for the same individual.[4,101] Acute treatment is aimed at reversing the bronchoconstriction. Bronchodilator medications are administered by inhalation or injection. If the asthma attack is severe and does not respond to bronchodilator medications, the diagnosis of status asthmaticus may be made. This is considered a life-threatening medical emergency.[99] Hospitalization will be required to administer medications intravenously, to monitor blood gases, and to administer oxygen.

The goals of long-term management are to prevent chronic and troublesome symptoms, to maintain pulmonary function and physical activity level, to prevent recurrent exacerbations, to minimize the need for emergency room visits or hospitalizations, to provide optimal pharmacotherapy, and to meet the patient's and family's expectations of and satisfaction with asthma care.[95] This is accomplished through pharmacologic support as well as periodic examination, ongoing monitoring, and education. The patient should be taught to self-monitor asthma symptoms and patterns, response to medications, quality of life, and functional status and to perform and record peak flow readings. A written action plan should be developed and reviewed and revised periodically. This action plan should be shared with school and other personnel who are involved with the child. Some allergens such as cigarette smoke, animal dander, and dust can be handled by environmental control. Desensitization ("allergy shots") may be used for triggers such as pollen or mold. Triggers such as emotional stress may be handled by relaxation exercises and education.[25]

There is no cure for asthma. The pharmacologic management is intended to stop, control or prevent symptoms through short-term relief or long-term management of the condition. Most patients take more than one medication to control their symptoms.

The current National Institutes of Health (NIH) Publication on the Guidelines for Asthma describes a terraced approach to pharmacologic management of asthma[95] (www.nhlbi.nih.gov/guidelines/asthma/asthgdln.pdf). The key recommendations of the NIH publication describe dosing medication according to the severity of the disease in three distinct age groups: 0 to 4 years, 5 to 11 years, and 12 years and older, as recent evidence indicates that children respond differently to asthma medications than their adult counterparts. Inhaled corticosteroids continue to be the drug of choice across all age groups for long-term management of asthmatic symptoms. Inhaled medications deliver a concentrated dose most effectively with fewer systemic side effects and a quicker onset of action than other means of administration, but children with persistent asthma need both long-term and short-acting agents to manage their disease. A press release accompanying the NIH report on August 29, 2007, summarizes the recommendations for persistent asthma as follows:

> Expert Panel Report 3 includes new recommendations on treatment options such as leukotriene receptor antagonists and cromolyn for long term control; long acting beta agonists as adjunct therapy with inhaled corticosteroids; omalizumab for severe asthma; and albuterol, levalbuterol, and corticosteroids for acute exacerbations. http://public.nhlbi.nih.gov/newsroom/home/GetPressRelease.aspx?id=2442

Newer drugs are constantly being researched and brought on the market; thus, any listing of medications is relevant only within a limited time frame.[44,58] The overall goal of medication research is to find drugs that will stop the inflammatory process at an earlier point or prevent the presentation of asthma altogether. As the understanding of the pathophysiology and genetics of asthma increases, new medications with more specific but fewer side effects will probably be developed. Medications to address coexisting conditions such as allergies and GERD will also contribute to the effective management of the child's asthma.[32,41,58,121] Physical therapists should check with the child's physician about current medications. A consumer-friendly website from the Mayo Clinic describes asthma medications for children and adults (www.mayoclinic.com/health/asthma-medications/ap00008).

SECONDARY IMPAIRMENTS

QUALITY OF LIFE

Recurrent asthma attacks or poorly controlled asthma may result in the child or family deciding to restrict normal childhood activities out of fear of asthma exacerbations or social retributions.[128] In fact, it is not only the child who suffers. Adult caregivers are forced to miss days of work just like the child is forced to miss days of school; taken together they reduce the quality of life for the entire family.[114] Growing up with this chronic disease is bound to play a role in the child's choice of an adult vocation and living situation.

MEDICATION SIDE EFFECTS

Although the medications used in the management of asthma are necessary, the side effects of these medications also may have an impact on daily life. For example, oral corticosteroids may cause an increased appetite and weight gain, fluid retention, increased bruising, and mild elevation of blood pressure. Other side effects reported from a variety of asthma medications are nervousness, headache, trembling, heart palpitations, dizziness or light-headedness, dryness or irritation of the mouth and throat, heartburn,

nausea, bad taste in the mouth, restlessness, difficulty concentrating, and insomnia, to mention a few.[92] To determine if motor, cognitive, or emotional behaviors are related to the medication, consult with the child's physician.

GROWTH AND DEVELOPMENT

Another aspect of asthma that is particularly important for self-esteem in adolescence is growth and development. There is conflicting data on whether children with asthma eventually catch up to their peers in terms of skeletal maturation.[3,12,79] For example, Baum[12] found that children with severe asthma have a significantly shorter stature, skeletal retardation, and delayed puberty. Researchers have questioned whether asthma itself or the prolonged use of steroids is responsible for such findings. In 2009, however, Mainz showed that adherence to current inhaled corticosteroid (ICS) dosing recommendations was more beneficial to the growth and development of a child with severe persistent asthma than not taking corticosteroids. In fact, the 9-year-old child who was the subject of the study had an additional skeletal impairment (thoracic deformity) caused by the pulmonary hyperinflation that resulted from his poor asthma management. Thus, proper use of ICS and other asthma medication may actually promote normal growth.

IMPACT ON FINANCIAL COSTS TO THE FAMILY AND SOCIETY

Asthma is associated with the highest related costs of routine pediatric care, reportedly topping $3 billion a year in the United States.[87] A study of 71,818 children ages 1 to 17 years who were enrolled in a health maintenance organization,[78a] was conducted to measure the impact of asthma on the use and cost of health care. The children with asthma incurred 88% more costs than children without asthma. Thus, having a child with asthma not only increases the family's focus on its medical needs but also consumes a family's financial resources. For some families, this cost may be at the expense of other needs, placing a financial burden on the family and the community.

SUMMARY OF THE MEDICAL ASPECT OF ASTHMA

Asthma is a common childhood disease that can result in severe functional limitations and restrictions in childhood activities. There are three primary components of asthma: often reversible airway obstruction, airway inflammation, and airway hyperresponsiveness that can affect the large and the small airways causing shortness of breath. The disease itself is complex with multiple system interactions such that each child's presentation of asthma is unique. The physical therapist needs to know how this disease affects that particular child's ability to participate in physical activities and what role the therapist can play in optimizing the child's potential for normal development, participation, and health.

PHYSICAL THERAPY EXAMINATION, EVALUATION, AND INTERVENTIONS

Physical therapists are traditionally involved in exercise programs for children with asthma, and studies have shown the efficacy of such programs in improving endurance and decreasing asthmatic symptoms.[93,103,129] The specifics of exercise testing and the development of a fitness program are covered in Chapter 6 and will not be covered here. Endurance programs such as treadmill training, which are also common, will not be covered either, as this author prefers to find ways to improve fitness and endurance through participation in typical childhood activities rather than in contrived activities, circumstances permitting. If physical fitness is seen as an "exercise duty," it is this author's experience that the child and family are less likely to follow through, seeing physical exercise as a chore rather than an opportunity for growth. Thus, the intent for the physical therapy section of this chapter is to (1) help the clinician understand the process of a differential diagnosis for the potential physical and activity limitations that may occur secondary to the interaction of asthma with growing and maturing bodies and (2) to present strategies and interventions that endeavor to get these children back among their peers, playing and competing in age-appropriate physical activities, rather than participating in adult-supervised exercise programs.

Nevertheless, the child with asthma may need more than a nudge and emotional support to engage in age-appropriate physical activities. Few studies address possible secondary physical impairments, such as adverse musculoskeletal changes/alignments, and neuromuscular recruitment problems that could limit the child's functional potential.[27,79,125] In the Guide to Physical Therapist Practice, physical therapy is defined as a "profession with ... widespread clinical applications in the restoration, maintenance and promotion of optimal physical function."[6] Thus, if physical and functional limitations were identified as occurring secondary to asthma, then physical therapy would be the appropriate service to restore, maintain, and promote optimal physical functioning. Physical therapy examinations

---

Box **25-1**	MOTOR IMPAIRMENT CATEGORIES

1. Neuromuscular system
2. Musculoskeletal system
3. Integumentary system
4. Cardiovascular/pulmonary system
5. Internal organs, especially gastrointestinal system*

Adapted from American Physical Therapy Association. Guide to Physical Therapist Practice, 2nd ed., *Physical Therapy*, 81(1), 29, 2001.
*The APTA's impairment categories do not have a category for dysfunction of internal organ systems other than the cardiovascular/pulmonary system; thus, "internal organs" was added by this author to correct for this deficit.

---

and evaluation and considerations for physical therapy interventions will be discussed within the context of a single case to illustrate how to perform a differential diagnosis through a multisystem review and how to appropriately plan procedural interventions to address both the medical and physical deficits. Impairment categories listed in the Guide, plus an additional category of "internal organs," will be specifically evaluated for their impact on movement potential for the child with asthma (Box 25-1). Long-term outcomes from these interventions are also presented.

SUMMARY

This chapter presented the pathophysiology and current medical management strategies associated with childhood asthma. In addition, through the use of a single case, ideas for the physical therapy diagnosis and management of physical limitations associated with asthma and its resultant functional limitations were presented through a multisystem and multidiscipline perspective. Impairments in the cardiopulmonary, neuromuscular, musculoskeletal, integumentary, and gastrointestinal systems were assessed for their contribution to the activity and participation limitations that could not be fully explained by asthma alone. An individualized physical therapy program was then presented as a template for other pediatric physical therapy programs. Short-term and long-term results from the physical therapy procedural interventions used with this single case were presented to give the reader an indication of the potential success of such interventions. Obviously, each individual case is unique and must be developed within the context of that particular patient's situation.

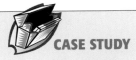

CASE STUDY

"Jonathan"

"Jonathan" was referred to physical therapy by his pediatric pulmonologist at 9 years of age. He was in fourth grade and lived with both parents and two older siblings in a large metropolitan area with access to excellent pediatric care. He had two significant diagnoses: exercise-induced asthma (EIA) and a pectus excavatum. Figure 25-1 shows Jonathan at 10 years old.

A pectus excavatum is an anterior chest wall deformity, particularly of the body of the sternum and the surrounding costal cartilage. The cartilage is collapsed inward giving the visual presentation of a hollowing out of the chest, otherwise called a "cavus," "caving-in," or a "funnel" deformity of the lower sternum[48] (Figure 25-2). Jonathan's mother reported that his chest "always looked that way" from birth (Figure 25-3). The thoracic surgeon recommended surgery to correct the deformity, but the family refused a surgical intervention.

Jonathan's mother reported a history of frequent bouts of recurring bronchitis from 3 to 6 years old before the eventual diagnosis of asthma at age 6 by a pediatric pulmonologist. He had no history of pneumonia or hospitalizations. Jonathan's asthma has been managed with medications since then, including Flovent twice a day (two puffs), and Intal and Ventolin as necessary before participation in soccer. In spite of the medications, the patient and his mother reported frequent episodes of extreme EIA symptoms, including chest tightness, wheezing, and shortness of breath after 5 to 10 minutes of soccer, resulting in a termination of the activity. The pulmonary physician reported that Jonathan's pulmonary function tests (PFTs) indicated that his pulmonary limitations were minor (i.e., minor peripheral airway resistance). No other significant deficits were found on four different testing dates over a year's time. Cardiac testing was negative. Even on an exercise challenge test by the pulmonologist, Jonathan showed no significant change in lung function, nor a positive response to a bronchodilator challenge. The diagnosis of EIA was made primarily on the basis of the child's clinical presentation rather than pulmonary tests.

If his lung function tests did not show significant impairment from his EIA, and his chest deformity was not causing lung or heart impairments, then what could explain his level of functional limitations? The pulmonologist believed that the medical status of his EIA alone could not have caused such a severe activity limitation. She knew that the patient and his family were motivated to follow his asthma management program, especially because Jonathan wanted to qualify for the travel soccer team. As a result, she referred Jonathan to physical therapy to rule out physical impairments that might account for some of the severity of his disease presentation.

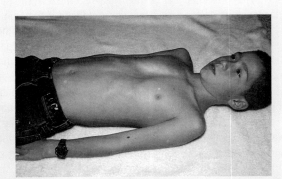

Figure 25-1 Jonathan at age 10 years. Note pectus excavatum (cavus deformity of the lower chest and sternum).

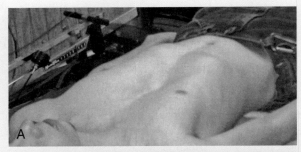

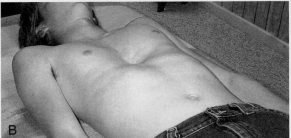

Figure 25-2 **A**, This 16-year-old male has asthma and a more severe congenital pectus excavatum deformity. **B**, Note lower sternal depression (or funnel), bilateral rib flares, and elevated and protracted shoulders.

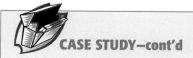

CASE STUDY–cont'd

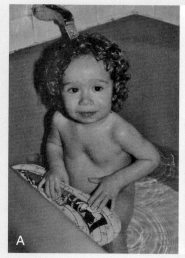 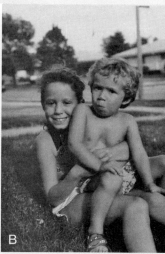

A

B

Figure 25-3 Comparison picture of Jonathan at ages 2 and 3 years old. Note the pectus excavatum is more severe at 3 years of age.

EVIDENCE TO PRACTICE 25-1

CASE STUDY "JONATHAN"

EXAMINATION DECISION

The decision to look at Jonathan's musculoskeletal and neuromotor systems was based on years of clinical experience of the therapist following long-term, complicated pediatric cardiopulmonary cases, and the referring physician's impression that Jonathan's endurance and lifestyle limitations could not be fully accounted for by the asthma alone. At the time of the referral, there was no evidence published on the consequential physical impairments for kids with pulmonary or chest wall deformities, but today we have two case studies that show improved postural alignment (musculoskeletal changes) and other physical improvements for such children following physical therapy interventions (Canavan & Cahalin, 2008; Massery, 2005). A Cochrane systematic review in 2001 by Hondras and colleagues (2001) showed insufficient evidence yet to support manual therapy for asthma. That finding does not mean that manual therapy is not effective. It means more research needs to be done in this area before broader conclusions can be drawn. Holloway and Ram (2004) reported similar findings for neuromotor retraining for breathing.

PLAN OF CARE DECISION

The decision to treat Jonathan's secondary physical problems, primarily musculoskeletal and neuromotor control issues, was based on Jonathan's personal goals and motivation, his mother's motivation, the clinical experience of his physician

and therapist, and limited research on chronic diseases at the time that physical therapy was initiated. Now, however, we have multiple research studies confirming this decision to treat. Asthma negatively impacts the quality of life for children with asthma and other chronic health issues, and these effects carry over into adulthood. Children with asthma are (1) less likely than their peers to participate in ongoing physical activities without additional support by the family or medical community, (2) more likely to report poorer quality of life across the life span, (3) more likely to miss days of school or work, and (4) more likely to be obese in adulthood, to name a few (Fletcher et al., 2010; Philpott et al., 2010; van den Bemt et al., 2010). The good news is that these trends can be reversed when quality of life measures are included in the child's asthma management (Bravata et al., 2009).

PATIENT/FAMILY PREFERENCES

Jonathan's family was motivated to try a nonsurgical (pectus excavatum), minimal medication approach to managing his asthma and chest wall deformity with the long-term goal of maximizing his participation in childhood activities. Jonathan himself had a specific goal: to make the travel soccer team. This goal was made the epicenter of his physical therapy plan. Every intervention was introduced as a way to improve Jonathan's odds of making the team, demonstrating relevance to Jonathan's goals, not just the therapist's desired outcome. Studies, such as that by Robinson and colleagues (2008), have shown patient-centered programs result in better long-term

Continued

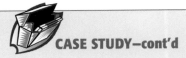

CASE STUDY—cont'd

EVIDENCE TO PRACTICE 25-1—cont'd

adherence to medical management programs and improve health and quality-of-life outcomes.

Canavan, P. K., & Cahalin, L. (2008). Integrated physical therapy intervention for a person with pectus excavatum and bilateral shoulder pain: A single-case study. *Archives of Physical Medicine and Rehabilitation, 89*(11), 2195–2204.

Holloway, E., & Ram, F. S. (2004). Breathing exercises for asthma. [Update of *Cochrane Database Systematic Reviews,* 2000, (3), CD001277; PMID: 10908489.] *Cochrane Database of Systematic Reviews, 1,* CD001277.

Hondras, M. A., Linde, K., et al. (2001). Manual therapy for asthma. [Update of *Cochrane Database Systematic Reviews,* 2000, (2), CD001002; 10796578.] *Cochrane Database of Systematic Reviews, 1,* CD001002.

Massery, M. (2005). Musculoskeletal and neuromuscular interventions: A physical approach to cystic fibrosis. *Journal of the Royal Society of Medicine, 98*(Suppl 45), 55–66.

Bravata, D. M., Gienger, A. L., et al. (2009). Quality improvement strategies for children with asthma: a systematic review. *Archives of Pediatrics & Adolescent Medicine, 163*(6), 572–581.

Fletcher, J. M., Green, J. C., et al. (2010). Long term effects of childhood asthma on adult health. *Journal of Health Economics 29*(3), 377–387.

Philpott, J. F., Houghton, K., et al. (2010). Physical activity recommendations for children with specific chronic health conditions: juvenile idiopathic arthritis, hemophilia, asthma, and cystic fibrosis. *Clinical Journal of Sport Medicine, 20*(3), 167–172.

van den Bemt, L., Kooijman, S., et al. (2010). How does asthma influence the daily life of children? Results of focus group interviews. *Health Quality of Life Outcomes, 8,* 5.

Robinson, J. H., Callister, L. C., et al. (2008). Patient-centered care and adherence: Definitions and applications to improve outcomes. *Journal of the American Academy of Nurse Practitioners 20*(12), 600–607.

Medical History and Multisystem Screening of the Neuromuscular, Musculoskeletal, Integumentary, Cardiovascular/Pulmonary, and Gastrointestinal Systems

A multisystem approach to screening medical and physical deficits was performed starting with an extensive medical history, followed by identifying the child's limitations in activities and participation, and then working "backward" with this information to try to uncover the primary impairment(s) that might explain the presenting signs and symptoms. In this case, the pulmonologist had already done an extensive medical history and pertinent tests to rule out other underlying medical pathologies that could account for his participation limitations. Other medical reasons for an increase in asthmatic symptoms could have included gastroesophageal disease (GERD), sleep disordered breathing, pulmonary ciliary dysfunction, or vocal fold dysfunction to name a few.[34,108,124,130] Jonathan never had any overt clinical symptoms of reflux or nocturnal dysfunction; thus, no tests were done. His mother did not recall any testing for ciliary dysfunction (which results in impaired airway secretion motility because of dysfunction of the beating cilia), and the lack of any recurrent respiratory infection, such as repeat pneumonias, made this diagnosis unlikely.[26] At the time of the physical therapy examination, vocal fold dysfunction and supra-esophageal manifestations of GERD were not commonly understood to be a possible cause of asthmatic symptoms, and this possibility was thus not explored. However, physical therapists currently assessing children with asthma should try to rule out gastric and vocal fold disorders as a routine part of the asthma medical screening.[8,14,59,62,133,135]

Screening Assessment of Functional Limitations Related to Asthma

Following a medical history review, the physical therapy examination and evaluation focused on assessment of Jonathan's breath support throughout everyday activities to determine if there was a specific area of impairment or a pattern of limitation that could explain his endurance limitations (Table 25-2).

Soda-Pop Can Model of Postural Control and Respiration

Before describing Jonathan's examination results, the dual nature of the respiratory and postural muscles needs to be understood. External and internal forces affect respiration and postural control strategies. This concept is illustrated in the following model[80,81] (Figure 25-4).

The aluminum shell of a can of soda pop is thin, flimsy, and inherently weak. Yet when unopened, it is functionally strong. It is almost impossible to compress or deform the unopened can unless the exterior shell is punctured. However, when it is opened, it loses its "strength" and is easily crushed. It is the internal pressure from the carbonation, not the aluminum exterior, that gives the can strength. The trunk of the body embodies a similar concept, using its muscular contractions to prevent its flimsy casing, the skeleton, from being "crushed" by external forces such as gravity. The trunk is composed of two chambers (thoracic and abdominal cavities), which are completely separated by the diaphragm, thus rendering each chamber capable of creating different internal pressures. The diaphragm is the trunk's primary pressure regulator. The chambers are functionally sealed at the top by the vocal folds and at the bottom by the pelvic floor muscles. The entire system is dynamically supported by muscles that generate, regulate, and maintain internal pressures in both chambers. As a result, these muscles must simultaneously meet the respiratory and postural needs of that person. In other words, the trunk muscles act as one continuous functional unit, providing the core support for pressure regulation that allows the individual to multitask, enabling "walking, talking, and chewing gum" to occur simultaneously and effortlessly.[14,38,51,53,57,120]

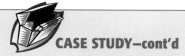

CASE STUDY—cont'd

TABLE 25-2 Assessing Functional Limitations Associated with Asthma or Other Ventilatory Dysfunction*

Functional Activity	Secondary Problems[†]
Breathing	Inadequate breath support and inefficient trunk muscle recruitment at rest or with activities such that breathing or postural control are compromised
	Asthmatic triggers such as rapid airflow caused by sudden increase in physical activity, dry air or extreme air temperatures, or other triggers that trip an asthmatic reaction
Coughing	Ineffective mobilization and expectoration strategies
Sleeping	Breathing difficulties, signs of obstructive or central sleep disorders
	Nocturnal reflux (GERD)
Eating	Swallowing dysfunction
	Reflux (GERD)
	Dehydration
	Poor nutrition
Talking	Inadequate lung volume and/or inadequate motor control for eccentric and concentric expiratory patterns of speech
	Poor coordination between talking (refined breath support) and moving (postural control)
Moving	Inadequate balance between ventilation and postural demands
	Breath holding with more demanding postures: use of the diaphragm as a primary postural muscle for trunk stabilization
	Inadequate lung volume to support movement
	Inadequate and/or inefficient muscle recruitment patterns for trunk/respiratory muscles causing endurance problems or poor motor performance
	Ineffective pairing of breathing with movement, especially with higher level activities

*The following activities require adequate lung volumes and coordination of breathing with movement for optimal performance.
[†]These typical secondary problems associated with asthma should be screened for to determine their possible contribution to the child's motor impairment or motor dysfunction.

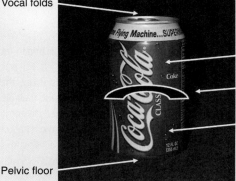

Vocal folds

Thoracic cavity

Diaphragm

Abdominal cavity

Pelvic floor

Figure 25-4 A postural control model using a soda pop can.

The functions of the internal organs are supported by these pressures as well, especially the lungs, heart, vascular structures, gastrointestinal system, and lymphatic systems. For example, following a lower cervical spinal cord injury, the diaphragm is still functioning, but the intercostals and abdominal muscles are paralyzed. As a result, normal pressures cannot be generated. Without the other muscles' support, the diaphragm is mechanically compromised resulting in impaired inspiratory lung volumes, impaired expiratory force (weak cough), low blood pressure, and frequent constipation.[83,113,119] In Jonathan's case, his pectus excavatum became his "weak spot." The postural/respiratory implications will be discussed in the next section.

Breathing

Increased effort was noted with Jonathan's quiet breathing pattern, including (1) occasional paradoxical breathing (i.e., inward

Continued

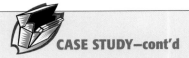

movement of the chest or abdomen during inhalation) and (2) frequent forced exhalations. Paradoxical breathing is thought to be due to the significant negative inspiratory pressures that the child with asthma must exert to overcome inspiratory resistance in the airways.[21,45,81]

The paradoxical movements of his chest wall indicated a muscle imbalance between the respiratory muscles, usually associated with weaker intercostals and abdominal muscles in relation to the diaphragm.[9] This weakness in the chest muscles, combined with the unbalanced descent of the diaphragm, may be the result of the pectus excavatum or it may have contributed to the further development of the pectus (the "chicken and the egg" syndrome). On the other hand, Jonathan's forced exhalations were probably secondary to the obstructive lung component of asthma, which constricts the conducting airways during exhalation. This forces the child to recruit expiratory muscles (primarily the abdominals and internal intercostals) to push the air out of the chest, even during quiet exhalation, causing increased work of breathing even at rest.

These patterns indicated that Jonathan's motor planning for ventilation muscle recruitment did not appear to be optimal for activities that required greater oxygen consumption because he was already overusing his diaphragm and recruiting his upper accessory muscles at rest, all the while underutilizing his intercostal muscles. All these observations led me to believe that his respiratory muscle imbalance may be significantly contributing to his decreased endurance and poor musculoskeletal alignment of his chest and overall postural alignment, and it may account for the endurance limitations not attributed to asthma itself by the pulmonologist.

Coughing

The patient demonstrated an effective cough. The only reports from the family of ineffective coughing or impaired airway clearance strategies during respiratory episodes came from his mother, noting that sometimes when he is sick, his secretions are so thick that they get "stuck" in his chest. Jonathan reported that he rarely drank water at school. This would indicate a need for increased hydration and a possible screening for ciliary dysfunction to rule out the possibility that the cilia themselves were dysfunctional rather than that the mucus was simply thicker because of dehydration.[130] He did not report vomiting associated with forceful coughing as many children with asthma report. Gagging or vomiting is a common occurrence following a hard cough, likely because of the lower esophageal sphincter (LES) succumbing to the high abdominal pressures associated with a series of coughs. When the LES fails, the intraabdominal pressure of cough will force the abdominal contents up into the thoracic esophagus. This is clinically noted as a severe reflux presentation: a dry gag, or a full vomit at the end of the cough.[116]

Sleeping

The patient reported that he sleeps on his back with his arms by his side, and occasionally he sleeps on his side. No breathing difficulties (including apnea, snoring, or irregularities), coughing, or drooling at night were reported that could indicate upper airway obstruction or

GERD.[126] A preference for the supine position at night, however, may indicate a recruitment of upper accessory muscles even while sleeping owing to the optimal length-tension relationship of those muscles in supine along with increased posterior stabilization.[18] Jonathan reports that he does not "curl up" to sleep. It is my clinical observation that children who are primarily upper chest breathers instead of diaphragmatic breathers will often choose to sleep supine with their arms up over their head rather than prone or curled up on their side, probably because of the improved length-tension relationship of all the anterior and superior chest muscles in supine. They may also report that they start out on their side or stomach, but find themselves on their backs in the morning. Depending on the rest of the findings, one may want to recommend a change in sleep postures for Jonathan, but only if that still allows him to sleep through the night as sleep-disordered breathing is a common consequence for children with asthma. Increased negative pressure during inhalation because of asthma's restricted airways, combined with a recumbent position, may predispose patients to nocturnal GERD and disrupted sleep.[100,132]

Eating

Jonathan did not report problems with chewing or swallowing any foods or textures, nor did he report any difficulties with drinking any type of liquid at any speed. In addition, there was no history of aspiration, choking, or gagging episodes. He did not present with any clinical signs of GERD, which is a common association with asthma and should be ruled out as a contributor to the motor or health restrictions.[124] Asthma is typically associated with a higher sensitivity or reactivity to dry air in the airway; thus, adequate hydration to keep the airway moist (humidity) is necessary to decrease external triggers to asthmatic reactions.[90] Hydration is also necessary to keep secretions thin and mobile.[5] Jonathan did not have a "feeding problem," but he did have a hydration problem, which most likely exacerbated his EIA symptoms.

Talking

Jonathan demonstrated a normal number of syllables per breath (at least 8 to 10) as noted during conversational speech.[30,49] He was capable of excellent sustained vocalization: 20 seconds (twice the expected length).[30] He could also talk in all postures at multiple volume levels with good postural control and controlled eccentric breath support. This was clearly the patient's strongest demonstration of breath control within a functional task. I anticipated using this strength to reinforce eccentric trunk control and pacing activities with soccer. Speech breathing is primarily eccentric control of the inspiratory muscles; thus, I could use his excellent eccentric motor planning for the trunk muscles during speech to recruit the same muscles for eccentric control during other eccentric trunk and postural maneuvers.[37]

Moving

Jonathan reported episodes of extreme shortness of breath (dyspnea) and asthmatic episodes within 5 to 10 minutes of participating in strenuous activities such as soccer. He reported that he "warms up for a minute" before starting to run in soccer. This quick change from

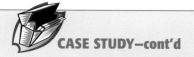

CASE STUDY—cont'd

rest to running would cause a rapid acceleration in inspiratory volume and flow rates and could possibly trigger his EIA response secondary to upper airway hyperresponsiveness or increased airway resistance.[5,91] He also reported that he used his bronchodilator inhaler immediately before team practice, which doesn't allow for maximal benefit of the drug; thus, incorrect use of medications may also be contributing to his EIA. It was interesting that Jonathan did not report breathing problems with quiet activities, in spite of the fact that his breathing demonstrated inconsistent recruitment patterns and an increased work of breathing at rest. No breath holding was noted with any developmental posture or transitional movement. Poor coordination between breathing and movement appeared to be contributing to his limitations in higher-level activities such as sport participation but not during quiet activities.

Summary of Functional Screening

The functional screening indicated impairment at the level of muscle recruitment for breath support at rest and during strenuous exercise, with resultant endurance impairments. Activities that demanded greater oxygen consumption and faster inspiratory flow rates, such as soccer, immediately used up his pulmonary reserves, causing Jonathan to hit an early "ceiling" effect, forcing him to terminate the activity because of dyspnea and asthmatic symptoms. It also caused a rapid influx of dry air, which most likely triggered the EIA response. No significant problems were noted with functional tasks requiring less oxygen demand and slower inspiratory flow rates such as sleeping, coughing, eating, or talking. In fact, breath support for talking was extremely well developed and was noted as his strongest asset on the functional assessment. Inadequate daily hydration, which would decrease his secretion mobility and produce heightened airway hyperresponsiveness (bronchospasm), was also a significant finding. Jonathan's functional screening results are summarized along with his other examination and evaluation findings in Table 25-3.

TABLE 25-3 **Synopsis of Jonathan's Initial Physical Therapy Examination and Evaluation**

Evaluation	Jonathan's Results
Medical diagnoses (pathology)	Asthma, primarily exercise induced (EIA) Pectus excavatum
Impairment (summary of body functions and structure)	**Cardiopulmonary:** Inflammation and hyperresponsiveness of airways particularly after initiation of exercise with PFTs indicating mild peripheral airway resistance Marked endurance limitations (5–10 minute tolerance) especially with higher level activities (particularly soccer) Occasional dehydration and decreased secretion mobility Increased work of breathing even at rest, RR 20 breaths/min (high end of normal) Auscultation clear in all lung fields No cardiac deficits per cardiologist **Musculoskeletal:** Marked pectus excavatum and elevated sternal angle Rib flares, L > R, with weakness noted in oblique abdominal muscles L > R (patient is right-handed) Functional midthoracic kyphosis of the spine particularly at the level opposite the pectus Decreased lateral side bending, indicating chest wall and quadratus lumborum restrictions Rib cage mobility restrictions greatest in mid chest nearest the pectus Mid trunk "fold" in sitting (rib cage collapsing onto the abdomen in sitting) "Slouched" sitting and standing postures: shoulders protracted and internally rotated Shortened neck musculature, hypertrophy No shoulder range-of-motion limitations **Neuromuscular:** Muscle imbalances in trunk muscles with significantly weaker/underutilized intercostal muscles, oblique abdominal muscles, and scapular adductors Inefficient neuromuscular recruitment patterns for inspiratory and expiratory efforts as well as for postural demands **Integumentary:** No restrictions noted **Internal organs, especially gastrointestinal system:** No reflux, constipation, or other gastrointestinal dysfunction

Continued

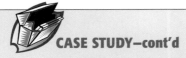

CASE STUDY—cont'd

TABLE 25-3   **Synopsis of Jonathan's Initial Physical Therapy Examination and Evaluation—cont'd**

Evaluation	Jonathan's Results
Functional limitations (breathing, coughing, sleeping, eating, talking, moving)	Breathing pattern was inefficient showing muscle imbalance among the diaphragm, abdominals, intercostals, and upper accessory muscles
	Movement and participation limitations secondary to medical impairments, endurance impairments, postural impairments, and breath support impairments
	In addition to movement limitations due to the medical component of asthma, his movements were limited by the simultaneous postural and respiratory demands presented during higher level activities such as soccer and the ventilatory needs to support such tasks
	No functional breath support limitations noted in sleeping, eating, coughing, or talking activities
Activity and participation limitations	According to mother, Jonathan was beginning to withdraw from participation in physical activities, especially organized athletics, secondary to his "deformed chest" and fear of asthmatic episodes
	EIA caused him to stop playing soccer after typically 5 to 10 minutes
	Patient had already stopped swimming to avoid taking off his shirt among his friends
Diagnosis	9-year-old boy, with history of severe EIA and marked pectus excavatum
	Significant restrictions in chest wall mobility and posture, as well as motor planning deficits, contributed to limitations in adequate breath support, postural control and endurance for desired functional activities and contributed to the continued development of the pectus and other postural deformities
	Dehydration also appeared to play a significant role in triggering a bronchospasm (EIA) during the rapid change in inhalation volume and negative force associated with participation in sports such as soccer
Prognosis	Excellent
	Capable of developing new motor plans
	Musculoskeletal deformities were functional, not fixed; still prepubescent
	Motivated by his desire to "make" the traveling soccer team, and be "normal"
	Supportive family
	Good medical care

Assessing the Impairments Related to Functional Limitations

When limitations are noted during the functional limitation screening assessment, further impairment testing should be done (age appropriately) to assess the extent of the initial limitations and as a baseline for assessing future progress. A baby or young child would not be capable of performing or cooperating with some tests, such as PFTs; thus, the physical therapist must assess the appropriateness of any impairment test for each specific patient.

According to Jonathan's pulmonologist, his lung pathology alone could not have caused his marked functional limitations noted during athletics such as soccer. Results of our functional screening concur with that opinion; thus, further impairment tests and measures were taken. A few key findings from his examination will be interpreted here to explain their relevance to his functional limitations.

Jonathan demonstrated a muscle imbalance between his three primary respiratory muscles (diaphragm, abdominals, and intercostals) and his upper accessory muscles of respiration. As previously described, all play a dual role in simultaneously meeting his breathing needs and his postural needs. Because of his asthma, Jonathan had to overcome increased inspiratory resistance even at rest, which likely led him to over-recruit the upper accessory muscles from a

very young age, setting up a pattern of overuse, which leads to fatigue (endurance factor). When he needed more oxygen during exercise, he recruited those same accessory muscles even more so, reaching a ceiling on his respiratory reserves. There were no muscles left to recruit when he needed more oxygen (again with an impact on endurance). Thus, when his postural demands increased, such as during soccer, his oxygen requirements limited the activity. As Hodges described in 2001, when faced with increasing oxygen demands, the diaphragm will decrease its active role in postural control in order to concentrate on its survival role as a respiratory muscle.[53]

Typical of many patients who have an increased work of breathing, Jonathan used his accessory muscles of respiration at the expense of his diaphragm and external intercostals, seen clinically as occasional paradoxical breathing and forced expiratory maneuvers at rest. I suspect this pattern contributed to the sternal abnormalities (elevated sternal angle and pectus excavatum) that formed early in his life. In my clinical observations, children with an early onset of asthma or other chronic respiratory conditions who overuse their sternocleidomastoid (SCM), scalenes, and trapezius muscles, cause a greater force on the anterior-superior pull on the sternal angle, resulting in an elevated sternal angle. The manubrium (the top portion of

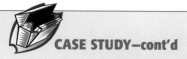

CASE STUDY—cont'd

the sternum) is calcified at birth, whereas the body of the sternum is primarily cartilaginous.[31] Perhaps that is why the solid manubrium tilts superiorly with the pull of the SCM muscles, whereas the less stable sternal body is less likely to be drawn upward. This in turn causes greater superior expansion of the chest at a loss of anterior chest excursion (decreased circumferential chest wall excursion), leading to chest wall restrictions. In addition, children like Jonathan tend to initiate inspiration with a greater effort to overcome the increased airway resistance from asthma, creating a larger negative inspiratory force (NIF) and more collapsing forces on the chest wall.[21,98] Clinically, this is observed as an excessive inferior descent of the diaphragm (low abdominal excursion) with flat or paradoxical intercostal movement (inward movement of the middle or lower chest wall). I believe that, over time, the repeated excessive NIF contributed to a decreased developmental stimulus for the activation of the intercostal muscles, thus setting up a pattern of muscle imbalance along Jonathan's chest wall and contributing to the further development of his pectus excavatum and associated rib cage and thoracic spine restrictions.

This is a pattern that I see repeated in numerous other cases in which asthma limits the child's participation in normal activities from infancy through puberty. I believe that the neuromuscular recruitment patterns developed early in life because of the child's ventilatory needs result in musculoskeletal abnormalities and neuromuscular imbalance of the respiratory/postural trunk muscles for movement. This is unique to childhood asthma because of the maturation and development of their systems versus adult-onset asthma where the motor systems have already completed typical development.

Evaluation of Examination Results: Impairments of the Neuromuscular, Musculoskeletal, Integumentary, Cardiovascular/ Pulmonary, and Gastrointestinal Systems

1. From a medical perspective, Jonathan's asthma was well managed, but it was still limiting participation in typical childhood activities. Thus, his cardiopulmonary system was not the only impaired system. Typical secondary medical impairments such as GERD were not overtly present, but daily underhydration was likely a significant contributor to his EIA response.

2. Jonathan demonstrated muscle imbalance in quiet and strenuous breathing. It appeared that he could benefit from learning new motor strategies to breathe effectively and efficiently (neuromuscular retraining) in order to better support ventilatory needs simultaneously with the postural demands of the task.

3. Jonathan demonstrated numerous chest wall and spine restrictions, but no integumentary restrictions. He needed more musculoskeletal mobility to support adequate internal lung expansion at low energy cost and decrease the triggers that caused his EIA response, such as rapid inspiratory airflows. This mobility was necessary before neuromuscular retraining could be effectively undertaken, and before adaptive cardiopulmonary strategies could be optimized. Thus, with his asthma well managed from a medical perspective, the musculoskeletal system presented the first obstacle to his optimal physical function and endurance.

Therefore, in spite of the fact that his primary diagnosis was cardiopulmonary, this examination pointed to significant musculoskeletal and neuromuscular impairments associated with Jonathan's medical diagnosis. Large-scale literature reviews of breathing retraining such as the Cochrane Reviews have been more plentiful in the past few years, but they generally apply to adult populations. Although authors of these reviews continue to conclude that the evidence for strengthening respiratory muscles or neuromuscular retraining of breathing patterns is inconclusive based on a lack of controlled studies or the small number of available controlled studies, they specifically express the opinion that the current state of the evidence is such that one cannot conclude that breathing retraining doesn't work, just that there is not enough hard evidence to make a decision either way.[39,55,105] The result is similar for manual therapy musculoskeletal interventions.[56]

Diagnosis

Jonathan is a 9-year-old boy with a history of severe EIA and marked pectus excavatum. Significant restrictions in his chest wall mobility and posture, as well as motor planning deficits and underhydration, appear to contribute to limitations in breath support and endurance for his desired functional activities and contribute to the continued development of the pectus excavatum and other postural deformities by perpetuating trunk muscle imbalance and an increased work of breathing.

Prognosis

Jonathan's parents have rejected a surgical option to reduce his pectus, and thus his prognosis was related to the potential success of a noninvasive physical therapy program. I believed that Jonathan had an excellent prognosis for the following reasons: (1) he was closely followed from a medical perspective, (2) he was neurologically intact and capable of developing new motor strategies, (3) his musculoskeletal deformities were functional, not fixed, and he was still prepubescent, and (4) just as important, Jonathan was extremely motivated by his desire to "make" the traveling soccer team and his desire to be able to take his shirt off without embarrassment because of the pectus. His mother was completely committed to helping her son maximize any opportunity to improve his health and well-being, including doing daily exercises at home under her supervision, if necessary. With this high level of support from the patient and his family, I anticipated making maximal progress with about 6 to 12 visits over a 1-year time frame.

Physical Therapy Procedural Interventions and Outcomes

The goals of Jonathan's physical therapy program are listed in detail in Tables 25-4 and 25-5, and the physical therapy interventions are summarized in Tables 25-5 and 25-6. These represent typical goals and intervention strategies for many children with

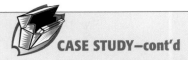

CASE STUDY—cont'd

TABLE 25-4   **Goals of Physical Therapy Program**

Physuical Therapy Goals	Jonathan's Goals
Long-term goal	**Reduce secondary impairments** that limit Jonathan's ability to achieve his desired level of physical activity performance and participation (soccer, baseball, swimming etc.) and health (missed days of school, ER visits, sicknesses).
Short-term goals	**Increase joint mobility** of rib cage and thoracic spine to promote full ROM for optimal breath support, full trunk movements to optimize skilled movements of the trunk musculature, decrease forces promoting developing kyphosis, as well as decrease forces promoting developing pectus excavatum.
	Improve muscle strength and muscle balance between diaphragm, intercostals, abdominals, paraspinals, scapular retractors, and neck muscles to normalize forces on the developing spine (decrease kyphosis), ribs (increase individual rib movement potential), sternum (decrease pectus forces), and shoulder (decrease anterior humeral head positioning and potential shoulder ROM losses).
	Improve motor planning of trunk muscle recruitment for respiration and posture by: Changing the sequence of activation of respiratory muscles to promote sooner activation of intercostal muscles, thus preventing paradoxical chest wall movement, which increases pectus forces (greater negative inspiratory forces reinforce development of a pectus if intercostals are weak, paralyzed, or delayed).
	Refining the respiratory pattern during quiet and stressful breathing to improve endurance by teaching Jonathon to utilize his diaphragm (endurance muscle) for a greater percentage of the ventilatory workload, and to decrease his over-recruitment of accessory muscles (short burst supporters) during quiet breathing.
	Refining recruitment pattern of postural muscle to:
	Increase recruitment of intercostals, oblique abdominal and transverse abdominal muscles, scapular retractors, and paraspinals.
	Decrease over-recruitment of rectus abdominus and sternocleidomastoid (SCM).
	Improve core trunk movements so that the intercostals, oblique abdominals, and transverse abdominal muscles become the primary stabilizers of the mid trunk, thus avoiding the SCM being overutilized as the primary trunk flexor, which can cause rib elevation, forward head, and eventually rib flares from underuse of oblique abdominals.
	Improve coordination of breathing with movement to improve oxygen transport during an activity (improving endurance) and to optimize the coordination between the respiration and postural demands of any physical task in order to improve overall physical performance from simple tasks such as activities of daily living to demanding tasks such as soccer.
	Improve patient and family's understanding of how they can more effectively manage the adverse effects of asthma on Jonathan's posture and movement patterns in order to reduce external triggers that precipitate his asthma attacks. This includes improving his overall hydration levels especially during athletic activities, decreasing activities that result in rapid changes in inspiratory airflow demands (slower warm-ups), and improving the timing of his asthma medications with strenuous activities.

TABLE 25-5   **Physical Therapy Interventions**

Impairment Category	Interventions for Jonathan
Asthma (cardiopulmonary) management strategies	Increased hydration to decrease extrinsic EIA triggers
	Improved timing of medications with activity level to get maximal benefit of medication
	Developed and implemented a new warm-up protocol for soccer practices and games that slowly increased his respiratory work load to avoid dramatic changes in inspiratory lung volumes and speed to avoid EIA trigger such as initiating a walk/run warm-up rather than running only, with gradual increase in running time and speed and stretching all trunk musculature prior to soccer
	Coordinated ventilatory strategies with movement and stretching to decrease respiratory workload and EIA trigger
	Improve efficiency of movement with resultant improved endurance
	Implement breath control techniques to prevent or minimize EIA attacks
	Improve awareness of oncoming EIA symptoms
	Use controlled breathing techniques to ward off EIA attack when possible

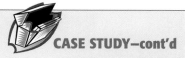

CASE STUDY—cont'd

TABLE 25-5   Physical Therapy Interventions—cont'd

Impairment Category	Interventions for Jonathan
Musculoskeletal interventions	Rib cage mobilization to increase chest wall and thoracic spine mobility in order to reduce respiratory workload and increase likelihood of recruiting intercostal muscles for more efficient respiration and support for developing thorax (reducing pectus excavatum forces)
	Intercostal muscle release to optimize length-tension relationship
	Quadratus lumborum muscle release to promote activation of oblique and transverse abdominis muscles for lower trunk stabilization instead of quadratus
	Active assistive anterior and axial glides to thoracic spine
	Home program to maintain newly gained trunk mobility
Neuromuscular interventions	Specific diaphragmatic training from recumbent to upright positions, and eventually to sporting conditions
	Emphasis on slow, easy effort during initiation of inhalation to prevent overpowering developing intercostal muscles
	Increased recruitment and strength of intercostals for all breathing patterns, postural control, and skeletal development (reducing pectus, paradoxical breathing, and thoracic kyphosis)
	Specific coordination of inhalation/exhalation patterns with all activities (ventilatory strategies)
	Increased recruitment and strength of scapular adductor, shoulder external rotators, and paraspinals for increased posterior stabilization
	Lengthening of neck accessory muscles through active stretching
	Midtrunk stabilization exercises (reducing rib flares and improving midtrunk interfacing between intercostals abdominals)
Integumentary interventions	None needed at this time
Internal organs (gastrointestinal) interventions	Increase hydration, especially during sporting activities

TABLE 25-6   Lateral Trunk Flexion Mobility Test for Rib Cage and Quadratus Lumborum

Test	Initial Date	Discharge Date 11 Months Later	Reevaluation 4 Years After Discharge
Lateral side bend toward L: mobility of right rib cage	2¼"	4½"	3⅝"
Lateral side bend toward L: mobility of right quadratus lumborum	1"	3"	2⅜"
Lateral side bend toward R: mobility of left rib cage	1½"	3¾"	3"
Lateral side bend toward R: mobility of left quadratus lumborum	1¼"	2½"	2⅜"

Note: From initial evaluation to discharge 11 months later, Jonathan's rib cage mobility doubled on the right, and more than doubled on the left. His quadratus lumborum length tripled on the right and doubled on the left. At the 4-year follow-up examination, he had lost some mobility at all levels except the left quadratus lumborum.

asthma and can be adapted for other cases or age ranges. All goals are developed in the context of a patient-centered care plan as research and clinical experience shows better long-term outcomes and carryover.[107,109]

Asthma (Cardiovascular/Pulmonary and Gastrointestinal) Procedural Interventions

Jonathan was instructed in immediate changes that he could implement at school, home, and on the soccer field to decrease the triggers

that set off his EIA response. He was extremely sensitive to a sudden increase in inspiratory volumes and flow rates that occurred secondary to soccer warm-ups, which started with laps around the soccer field. It was likely that the combination of (1) the dryness in his airway caused by the change from nose breathing to mouth breathing because of the sudden need for increased inspired air during the running activity and (2) the large, fast moving volume of air required to perform this high level of exercise played a significant role in

Continued

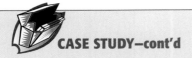

CASE STUDY—cont'd

triggering an acute attack.[5,90] Within 5 to 10 minutes of soccer, he would typically experience such extreme shortness of breath that he was forced to stop playing. Often he did not recover in time to rejoin his teammates.

Jonathan's management program included several steps:

1. He was instructed in ways to increase his hydration overall, and specifically to use hydration before and throughout the games and practices in order to keep his upper airway moist.

2. He began to take his medications sooner, at least 15 to 30 minutes before the start of soccer, to receive the maximum benefit from the drugs.

3. He started a new warm-up that slowly increased his activity level so that the oxygen demand gradually increased, allowing him to breathe through his nose for a longer period of time and allowing the necessary inspired air volume to also increase slowly.

4. He stretched his trunk, spine, rib cage, and shoulders before the game to maximize mobility (compliance) of his chest wall movements, thus decreasing his work of breathing and reducing the negative pressures (NIF) that he needed to generate to inhale adequate volumes of air, which in turn reduced the collapsing forces on his chest wall.

5. He coordinated his breathing specifically with the relationship of the trunk movement and rib cage during each stretching exercise and movement in general to reinforce normal pattern combinations of movement and breathing (ventilatory strategies).[37,72]

6. He was taught two particular breath control techniques to help him regain control of breathing during the early stages of an asthmatic attack: (a) repatterning controlled breathing technique and (b) an enhanced Jacobsen's progressive relaxation technique. These techniques were developed by Frownfelter.[37]

Repatterning controlled breathing technique

6a. The patient is asked to start with exhalation. "Try to blow out easily with your lips pursed. Don't force it just let it come out." Suggesting that the patient visualize a candle with a flame which their exhalation makes flicker but not go out will help to produce a prolonged, easy exhalation. Doing this allows the respiratory rate to decrease automatically. When the patient feels some control of this step, then ask him or her to "hold your breath at the top of inspiration just for a second or two." Make sure the patient does not hold his or her breath and bear down as in a Valsalva maneuver. Last, ask the patient to take a slow breath in, hold it, and let it go out through pursed lips. Patients learn that when they are short of breath, this technique often helps them to gain control, making them feel less panicky.[37] Jacobsen's progressive relaxation technique.

6b. Utilizes ventilatory strategies to help the patient experience the difference between inhaling and contracting the upper trapezius versus exhaling and relaxing the trapezius in order to develop new motor strategies to keep the trapezius from being over recruited.[37]

Using a mirror for feedback, the patient is instructed to lift his shoulders while inhaling and is then asked to hold his breath at the peak of shoulder elevation. The therapist applies maximal downward resistance while telling the patient to "hold." The patient is then instructed to "let go" slowly and to exhale with gentle pursed lip breathing while the therapist slowly applies axial rotation to the spine through the shoulders. The purpose of the activity is to help the patient feel and see the difference between excessive recruitment of the trapezius and relaxation of the trapezius.

Asthma Management Outcomes

Jonathan rigorously followed the regimen including carrying a water bottle with him everywhere, even in the classroom. He noticed an immediate decrease in chest tightness and dyspnea during soccer practice and games. Of particular note, before using the repatterning controlled breathing technique, Jonathan said he had no way to stop the progression of his asthma attack once it started. Now he said that if the attack was mild he was able to "work through it" with the repatterning, and it did not develop into a full-blown attack. He could now play a whole game of soccer without EIA preventing his participation. In fact, he made the travel soccer team and could play four consecutive games of soccer in 1 day without EIA symptoms. As a consequence of decreasing EIA triggers, Jonathan began having fewer and fewer asthmatic attacks, such that all asthma medications were discontinued 2 months after starting physical therapy. This was not an intended consequence of physical therapy, but a welcomed one. Jonathan reported only one incident of bronchitis in the following year and no asthma attacks after 2 months of physical therapy.

Musculoskeletal Interventions

Jonathan needed increased chest wall and spine mobility before attempting neuromuscular training of muscles along that tight rib cage. Jonathan was positioned in side lying with a large towel roll placed under his lower ribs to maximize rib expansion on the uppermost side (Figure 25-5, A). Manual rib mobilization was performed to all 10 ribs bilaterally to increase individual rib movement potentials, to increase rib cage compliance, and to increase the potential for axial rotation of his thoracic spine (a tight rib cage makes lateral or axial movements of the thoracic spine less possible).[80] From the results of my testing, the intervention was focused more on the left side than the right, and more in the midchest than the upper or lower chest (Figure 25-5, B). This was followed by intercostal muscle release techniques to maximize intercostal spacing and optimize their length-tension relationship for neuromuscular retraining (Figure 25-5, C). Finally, his quadratus lumborum was released bilaterally to allow for more separation between the rib cage and the pelvis (Figure 25-5, D). Posteriorly, the thoracic spine was only mildly restricted in anterior glides (extension of spine) and axial rotation, so active assisted mobilizations were incorporated into his home program. Jonathan worked on maintaining his newfound trunk mobility with a home stretching program.

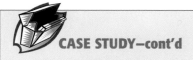

CASE STUDY—cont'd

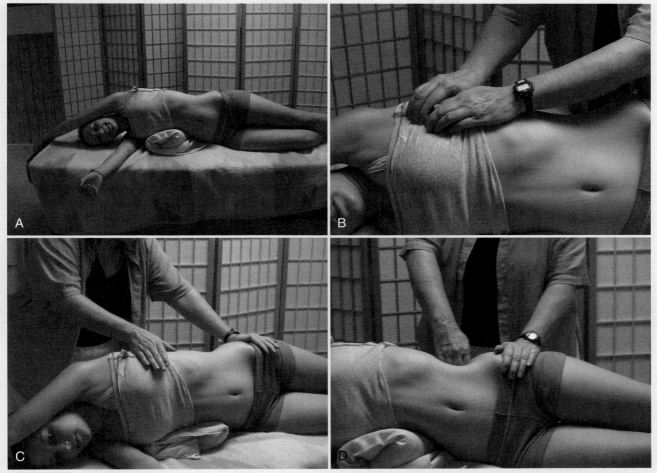

Figure 25-5 PT musculoskeletal interventions to increase chest wall mobility (demonstrated with a female, not with Jonathan). **A,** Start position. Note towel roll under the patient's lower ribs to maximize chest expansion. **B,** Rib mobilization technique for the midribs. Similar positioning would be used for other ribs. **C,** Intercostal muscle release (lengthening technique) on lower ribs. In this picture, the therapist's thumb is between ribs 8 and 9 in the intercostal spacing. The release movement proceeds from posterior to anterior on the chest wall. **D,** Quadratus lumborum (QL) muscle release (lengthening technique). The therapist's right hand is lengthening the QL while the left hand is stabilizing the pelvis.

Musculoskeletal Outcomes

Jonathan made tremendous progress in trunk mobility as measured by range of motion in lateral trunk flexion (Figure 25-6). His rib cage mobility doubled on the right and more than doubled on the left. His quadratus lumborum length tripled on the right and doubled on the left (see Table 25-6). His anterior glides and axial rotation glides of thoracic spine were now normal.

His pectus excavatum volume, which was measured using a water displacement method, was 34 mL H2O when measured 4 months into treatment (Figure 25-7). The volume was reduced by half to 18m L H2O at discharge 7 months later (Table 25-7). (Pectus volume was not measured on initial evaluation.)

Postural assessment showed elimination of functional kyphosis in sitting and standing postures. Jonathan no longer showed a midtrunk

"fold" in a sitting posture. Mother and son reported that his teachers no longer continually reminded him to sit up straight in school. Inferior rib flares were no longer apparent as his abdominal muscles now adequately stabilized the rib cage at the midtrunk and his primary neuromuscular recruitment pattern now utilized his abdominal muscles instead of his sternocleidomastoid muscles as his primary trunk flexor. His sternal angle elevation appeared slightly reduced but was not objectively measured.

Neuromuscular Interventions

The priorities of Jonathan's physical therapy were to address his medical needs first, then his musculoskeletal restrictions, and finally his neuromuscular impairments. Jonathan needed to balance the strength and recruitment patterns of his respiratory and postural muscles to optimize breath control at a low energy cost, while

Continued

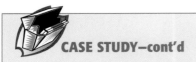

CASE STUDY—cont'd

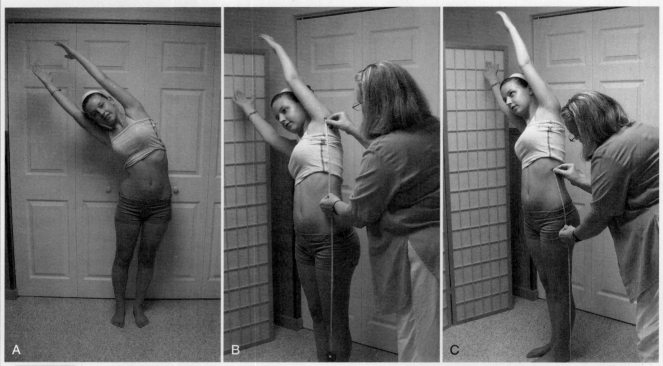

Figure 25-6 Lateral trunk flexion measurement sites. **A,** Lateral trunk flexion movement. Total excursion was measured in two segments. **B,** Rib cage mobility was measured from a full upright position to the end lateral trunk flexion position. The starting points for the tape measure were the midaxillary line (head of the humerus) superiorly to rib 10 (lowest palpable rib) inferiorly. Total movement in inches was recorded. **C,** The mobility of the quadratus lumborum, and to a lesser extent the gluteus medius, was measured likewise from rib 10 superiorly to the greater trochanter inferiorly.

TABLE 25-7 **Other Tests and Measures**

Test	Initial Date	Discharge Date 11 Months Later	Reevaluation 4 Years after Discharge
Pectus volume displacement (typical: zero or minimal volume)	34 mL (taken 4 months after initial evaluation)	18 mL	17 mL
Respiratory rate (typical 10–20)	20	11	–
Auscultation	Clear	Clear	Clear
Phonation (typical 10 seconds)	20 sec	25.5 sec	28.6 sec
PFTs (pulmonary function tests)	Normal lung volumes and flow rates	Not taken	Normal lung volumes and flow rates

Note that Jonathan's pectus excavatum, which was 34 mL H_2O when measured 4 months into treatment, was reduced by half to 18 mL H_2O at discharge and was maintained relatively at the same level when remeasured 4 years later.

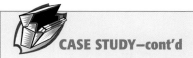

CASE STUDY—cont'd

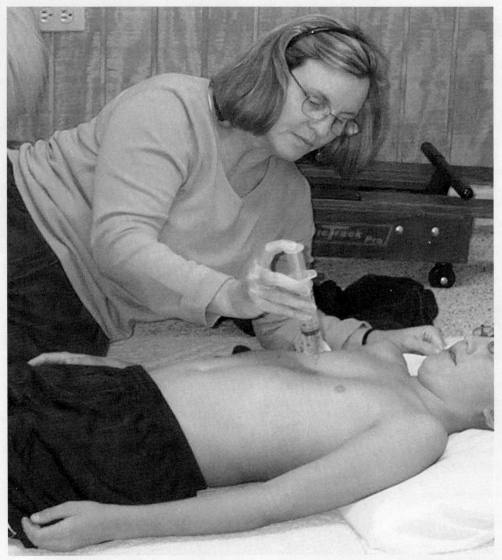

Figure 25-7 Pectus excavatum volume displacement measurement. The patient is positioned supine with the pectus deformity parallel to the floor (in this picture, the patient is slightly tilted superiorly and would need to have his upper trunk raised slightly with pillows to make the pectus parallel to the surface). A volume displacement measurement is used as a crude estimate of the extent of the volume of the pectus. Water from a measured syringe fills the pectus until spilling over the deformity. The test is repeated three times or more until consistent. If a consistent measurement cannot be made, the measurement is discarded.

simultaneously providing appropriate muscle force to his developing spine and rib cage—quite a balancing act.[28,43,52,54,75,76,111,112,115]

The neuromuscular retraining of Jonathan's respiratory muscles started with specific diaphragmatic training in a sidelying posture to facilitate a more optimal length-tension relationship of the diaphragm while simultaneously facilitating a less optimal length-tension relationship of the upper accessory muscles to minimize their

recruitment during quiet breathing. Jonathan did not respond with increased diaphragmatic recruitment and excursion with positioning and verbal cues alone, so manual facilitation techniques were added.

Several techniques were used, but the one that produced the greatest consistency, reproducibility, and appropriate timing of activity in the diaphragm was the "diaphragm scoop" technique, which is an indirect facilitation technique to the diaphragm's central tendon

Continued

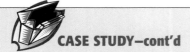

CASE STUDY—cont'd

area.[37] This technique provided specific quick stretch input to the central tendon of the diaphragm via the patient's abdominal viscera at the end of the expiratory cycle in an effort to recruit the central tendon as the initiator of the next inspiratory effort. Continued manual cueing was provided throughout the entire inspiratory phase to facilitate greater inferior excursion of the diaphragm. An emphasis was placed on initiating inspiration with an "easy, slow onset" to avoid recruitment of the upper accessory muscles and an overpowering of his intercostal muscles (paradoxical breathing). Once the patient could consistently succeed in recruiting his diaphragm in sidelying, he was challenged by decreasing manual input and increasing postural demands by using positions such as sitting and standing. At this point Jonathan was instructed to practice this technique using visualization at home just before sleeping to take advantage of a relaxed state. Eventually, he was trained to use the diaphragm breathing technique in sports as well as static postural holds. Auditory cues for the rate, rhythm, and depth of inspiration were included in all breathing retraining techniques. Objective measures of his success were taken with assessment of chest wall excursion (CWE).[73,74,85]

Jonathan demonstrated poor recruitment of his external intercostal muscles, which are needed to stabilize the chest wall during inspiration to prevent paradoxical breathing and the potential development of a pectus excavatum secondary to this inward force.[9,21] Jonathan demonstrated this paradoxical chest wall movement even at rest in his mid–rib cage. Thus, weak intercostals could be, in part, responsible for the development of his pectus. I used manual facilitation techniques with (1) upper extremity flexion, abduction, and external rotation activities (D2) diagonals from proprioceptive neuromuscular facilitation (PNF)[68] combined with (2) thoracic extension and rotation; intentionally paired with (3) large inspiratory efforts, to utilize optimal length-tension relationships and function of the external intercostals; and (4) a maximal inspiratory effort followed by a

peak inspiratory hold to increase positive outward pressure on the anterior chest wall (Figure 25-8). Jonathan was instructed to visually follow his arm motions to maximize the trunk rotation because thoracic rotation produces greater intercostal muscle recruitment than straight plane motions.[57,106] Jonathan was instructed to continue the exercises at home once he could demonstrate the proper recruitment pattern.

Another chest wall exercise was added. Jonathan was positioned supine lying on a vertical thoracic towel roll to maximize his thoracic spine extension and to stabilize the costotransverse junctions (junction of the ribs to the transverse process of the thoracic spine). Jonathan was then instructed to externally rotate his shoulders while pinching his shoulder blades back to the towel roll to maximize anterior chest expansion by recruiting the external intercostals and the pectoralis muscle (using the pectoralis muscles to act as a chest wall expander rather than an upper extremity adductor). The position also stretched his neck flexors. During this activity, he was instructed to take in a deep breath and hold it during a PNF hold-relax technique to maximize the response from his scapular retractors.[122] This provided maximal positive pressure from within his chest cavity, which provided a significant counterforce to the pectus, thus lifting his anterior chest.[9,78] This concept can be achieved independently by substituting a resistive band instead of the therapist's hands (Figure 25-9).

Jonathan's abdominal muscles were often recruited concentrically for exhalation. To retrain the abdominals for quiet breathing, Jonathan was given eccentric trunk exercises to be done during his warm-up for soccer where he had a history of asthma exacerbations. He was instructed to pair eccentric exhalation (quiet speech) with eccentric trunk movements to reinforce the natural coupling of breathing and postural control responses.[71,84] For example, during knee lunge exercises, Jonathan would count out loud while going into a controlled lunge (eccentric task) and then purposely inhale as he

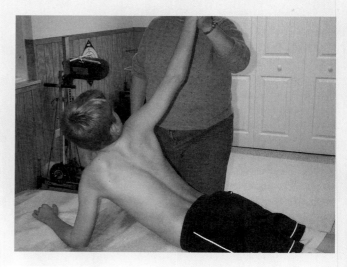

Figure 25-8   Home exercise program. Prone on elbows. This is one activity that Jonathan did at home to promote intercostal muscle activation and strengthening as well as to promote spinal axial rotation and chest wall expansion.

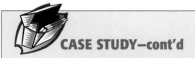

CASE STUDY—cont'd

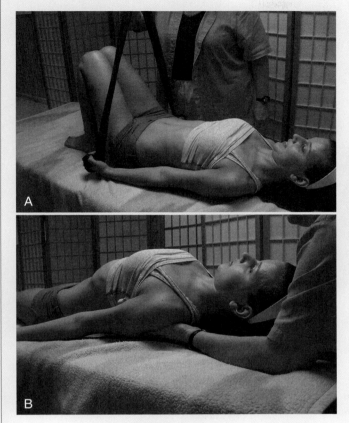

Figure 25-9   Home exercise program. Supine over a vertical towel roll. **A,** This exercise is a variation of the one used for Jonathan in the clinic. It is used to increase thoracic extension and to elevate the anterior rib cage. Resistance is applied to trunk extension, rib cage expansion, and shoulder external rotation via a resistive band such as Thera-Band as the patient pulls the band downward toward the floor. **B,** In Jonathan's case, resistance was applied via the therapist's hands in the clinic (demonstrated here with a female, not with Jonathan).

came back up to stance. Jonathan would adapt this concept to the variety of soccer warm up exercises.

Lastly, Jonathan was instructed in specific recruitment of internal intercostals and oblique abdominal muscles as the primary stabilizers of the inferior rib cage to (1) decrease the rib flare deformity, (2) improve midtrunk stabilization to offer the diaphragm better mechanical support, (3) reduce his overdependence on the rectus muscle for stabilization, which again reinforced the development of the pectus, and (4) provide stability of the rib cage during activation of the SCM muscles to prevent the chest from being lifted toward the head when Jonathan's intended movement was to bring his head to the chest. Once again, a PNF D2 upper extremity pattern was used.[68] This time, the patient was positioned supine with his arm positioned in flexion, abduction, and external rotation while lying over a vertical towel roll. The patient's arm was stabilized distally. The patient was asked to "try to lift his arm up in the diagonal pattern" but was not allowed any movement. The result was a strong isometric contraction of the midtrunk muscles (oblique and transverse abdominis and internal intercostals), which are required for stabilization of the trunk before the distal extremity could be moved off the ground. This allowed him to perform small concentric contractions of his internal intercostals and external obliques without being overpowered by the rectus. When the patient successfully demonstrated consistency in recruiting these muscles, which was observed by a flattening of the rib flares during the active contractions of the intercostals and obliques, he was instructed to carry over the training independently with higher level postures and longer periods of dynamic stabilizations such as holding his trunk while continuing to breathe through longer segments of activities like running.

To improve recruitment of thoracic paraspinal muscles, rather than primarily lumbar extensors (to decrease kyphotic forces), Jonathan was instructed in (1) full upper extremity swings in standing during soccer warm-up routine, (2) coordinating slow inhalation with shoulder abduction and scapular adduction, and (3) coordinating eccentric exhalation (counting out loud) when he returned his arms down to his side. He was instructed to focus on recruiting diaphragm and intercostal muscles during inhalation (which should recruit more thoracic extensors) and to concentrate on controlling the eccentric component of the arm and trunk muscles during exhalation. If Jonathan was my new patient today, I would include more specific

Continued

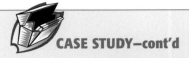

CASE STUDY—cont'd

TABLE 25-8   **Chest Wall Excursion (CWE) in Sitting and Supine Positions**

Tidal Volume Sitting (Quiet Spontaneous Breathing)	Initial Date	Discharge Date 11 Months Later	Reexamination 4 Years after Discharge
Upper chest (level of 3rd rib) upper accessory muscles	½"	½"	–
Mid chest (level of xiphoid) intercostals	¼"	⅜"	–
Lower chest (half the distance from xiphoid process to navel) lower intercostals and diaphragm	⅛"	⅜"	–

Tidal Volume Supine (Quiet Spontaneous Breathing)	Initial Date	Discharge Date 11 Months Later	Reexamination 4 Years after Discharge
Upper chest (level of 3rd rib) upper accessory muscles	⅛"	½"	1/16"
Mid chest (level of xiphoid) intercostals	0"	¼"	0"
Lower chest (half the distance from xiphoid process to navel) lower intercostals and diaphragm	⅜–½"	⅝"	¾"

Note that, in sitting, improvements were noted in mid and lower chest expansion. No 4-year follow-up measurements.
In supine, all levels increased by discharge, but at the 4-year follow-up examination, the gains in the mid and upper chest had disappeared. Only the lower chest expansion continued to show similar levels to the discharge values.

training for the transverse abdominis which has been shown to be associated with diaphragmatic movements.[38,52,50]

Neuromuscular Outcomes

Jonathan now demonstrated an effective balance between the primary respiratory muscles (diaphragm, intercostals, and abdominals) during volitional and spontaneous breathing in both quiet breathing and maximal inspiratory maneuvers in multiple postures and activities. Paradoxical movement of the chest wall was no longer noted (improved functional strength of intercostal muscles). No functional thoracic kyphosis was noted during quiet stance or during active recruitment of trunk extensors. Quiet breathing now demonstrated a normal recruitment pattern: (1) initiation of inhalation with the diaphragm and simultaneous chest wall movement, (2) easy inspiratory onset, no apparent effort (low work of breathing, low negative inspiratory force which reduces pectus forces), and (3) smooth continuous movements throughout the inspiratory cycle. Objectively, this was seen with (1) significant increases in mid–chest wall excursion measurements (intercostal recruitment) during quiet breathing (tidal volume) in both supine and standing (Table 25-8), (2) a respiratory rate that decreased from 20 to 11 breaths/minute, and (3) phonation support in syllables/breath that increased by 28% (see Table 25-7). Midtrunk stabilization showed marked improvement in strength of oblique abdominal muscles, right still stronger than left. Posturally, this was noted by the minimization of his rib flares and appropriate timing recruitment of the abdominals during trunk stabilization activities both in therapy and, as reported by the patient, during sports activities. Functionally, Jonathan reported that he could now run the mile at school without excessive dyspnea or asthmatic symptoms.

Jonathan needed maximal sensory and motor input to change his motor strategies for respiration. Verbal cues alone did not produce satisfactory results. Manual, visual, auditory, and positional input in each activity was specifically applied to assist Jonathan in developing new motor plans to improve breathing efficiency and appropriate skeletal forces that promoted normal development of his rib cage and spine.

Integumentary Interventions: None needed.

Functional Outcomes and Quality of Life Issues

Following his physical therapy program, Jonathan and his mother noted important functional improvements (Table 25-9). He made the travel soccer team and could play four consecutive games without EIA attacks. His last EIA episode occurred 2 months after starting physical therapy. Before physical therapy, he had an EIA episode almost every time he played soccer. At discharge, he could also run the mile in gym class at school without EIA or excessive dyspnea.

He did not miss any days of school for EIA after initiating physical therapy. His mother said that before the physical therapy program, "he would miss 5 to 8 days a year because of sickness related to EIA, but those sick days don't take into account the weekends, holidays, and summer days that Jonathan was incapacitated with asthma-related problems." He had two severe EIA episodes before physical therapy that resulted in emergency room (ER) visits. During his physical therapy interval, he did not have any ER visits.

His mother said that in addition to making it possible for him to rejoin his classmates in regular physical activity such as soccer and baseball, following the year of physical therapy Jonathan began to go

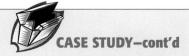

CASE STUDY—cont'd

TABLE 25-9 **Functional Outcomes**

Functional Outcomes	Initial Date	Discharge Date 11 Months Later	Reexamination 4 Years after Discharge
EIA attacks or symptoms during sports activities	Frequent	None	None
Length of participation in a sporting activity	5 to 10 minutes before EIA symptoms forced him to stop	Full participation: up to four soccer games per day	Full participation: plays baseball in high school
Complete the "mile test" in gym class	No	Yes	Yes
Average number of days absent from school due to asthma-related complications	5 to 8	0	0
Emergency room visits	2	0	1
Hospitalizations	0	0	0
Daily asthma medications	Yes	No	No

Note that Jonathan's greatest improvements are in activity and health gains.

swimming again. He had all but given up swimming the year before because of "his deformed chest" and the derogatory comments that were directed at him by other children.

When asked for a general statement about how the physical therapy program affected her son's quality of life, Jonathan's mom said: "It was a miracle. Before we began to see you, Jonathan and I had to focus on his medical condition rather than focusing on being a kid. It completely changed his life." Jonathan and his mother no longer saw him as "disabled" by his pulmonary disease.

Discussion

Jonathan was seen for eight visits over 11 months. The family's motivation to follow through diligently on home programs, and the child's excellent ability to learn new motor strategies, resulted in a minimal number of visits to accomplish the goals of treatment. Under different circumstances, achieving the procedural intervention goals in a similar case may take longer or goals may be less attainable.

The results of this particular case were marked, but not unrepeatable. Jonathan's physical therapy program was developed from a multisystem perspective to develop better "external support" for his "internal" asthma. I believe the keys to his success were threefold:

1. A team approach to his condition: recognition by his pulmonologist that his functional limitations were more severe than his medical condition alone indicated, her belief that physical interventions are an integral part of effective management of pulmonary diseases, and her belief that a surgical intervention for his pectus should be the last, not his first, option.
2. A detailed physical therapy examination that focused on identifying the underlying impairments outside of his "asthma and the pectus diagnoses alone," examining both medical and physical impairments to determine which system(s) could account for the severity of his functional limitations.

3. A specific intervention program targeted to reverse or minimize those impairments with a major emphasis on the patient's responsibility in the program (education), and on applying new strategies directly into his daily life (functional).

Although it is possible that his changes were due to maturation, it is unlikely according to his mother, who noted that all of his improvements came after the initiation of physical therapy compared to the previous school year without physical therapy.

Following physical therapy, Jonathan's pulmonary symptoms went into complete remission, which neither this author nor his pulmonologist had anticipated. Physical therapy does not "cure" asthma. Could it be that the EIA diagnosis was not completely accurate? Jonathan had all the symptoms of EIA, but his PFTs did not confirm the diagnosis. Recently, doctors have begun to explore other possible explanations for EIA symptoms that do not fit the classic picture of asthma, such as vocal fold dysfunction or supraesophageal manifestations of GERD, which present with similar symptoms: high sensitivity to fast inspiratory flow rates, a lack of typical asthmatic responses on PFTs, and a lack of significant improvement with asthma medications. Because of Jonathan's dramatic improvement with physical interventions, his pulmonologist is now reconsidering his original diagnosis.

The tests and measures used in this case have varied levels of reliability and validity. The medical tests, such as PFTs and respiratory rates, have long-established reliability and validity.[24,77] Tests for the physical impairments are not as well established. Tests for phonation length were established in the speech therapy field.[30] Inter- and intratester reliability for chest wall excursion (CWE) measurements have been established, but normative standards were not found to be predictable by age and sex. The patient served as his own control.[73,74,85] Lateral trunk flexion and the pectus volume measurement have not been validated by research.

Continued

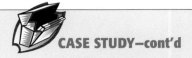

CASE STUDY—cont'd

Four-Year Follow-up at Age 14 Years

Jonathan participated in physical therapy for 1 year. Four years after discharge (5 years after initiating physical therapy), Jonathan was contacted, interviewed, and reexamined to assess the long-term effects of this program on his pathology (asthma), his impairments, activity limitations, and participation. Jonathan was 14 years old and a freshman in high school (Figures 25-10, 25-11, and 25-12).

Medical Update

An examination by his pulmonologist showed no limitations noted in PFT volumes or flow rates. He was also revaluated by his cardiologist who diagnosed an asymptomatic mitral valve prolapse, which is not uncommon with a pectus excavatum.[36] No cardiac intervention was needed. He had had only one respiratory episode in the last 5 years: a croup-type virus that resulted in a severe bronchitis and his only trip to the emergency department. He did not have any EIA episodes during the 4-year interval. He did not use daily asthma medication. He did, however, report use of his bronchodilator prophylactically when he had a cold, "just in case."

Test and Measures

See Tables 25-6, 25-7, and 25-8 for results of the tests.

Functional Outcomes and Quality of Life Update

See Table 25-9 for Jonathan's functional outcomes.

Jonathan received a "perfect attendance award" in eighth grade, which his mother commented was a complete reversal of his school years before physical therapy. Endurance is no longer a limitation according to both Jonathan and his mother.

Jonathan's mother reported that he continues to gain confidence both socially and athletically following the physical therapy intervention. She no longer sees any signs of self-consciousness regarding his

chest wall deformity. This may be a result of maturation, but she thought it was worth noting because it changed so significantly during and following the intervention period.

Even with 4 to 5 years' reflection since the onset of physical therapy, Jonathan's mother still says that the physical, medical, and emotional benefits to her son were incredible. She said that they kept up the home exercises for approximately 4 months after his discharge from physical therapy, but slowly drifted away from them, which may explain some of the minor loss of chest wall mobility upon reexamination. Jonathan did keep using the strategies that he learned in physical therapy such as maintaining adequate hydration levels and proper warm-up before exercise.

Impression

Jonathan has maintained his pulmonary health since discharge 4 years ago with no apparent signs of EIA or its impairments, especially as it affected his endurance and participation in activities and his overall health. At this point, it appears that his asthma or other undiagnosed pulmonary disease is resolved or benign. His spinal alignment is now completely normal, avoiding what appeared to be the likely development of a true thoracic kyphosis. His chest wall deformities are still minimally present and more localized, less noticeable, and do not cause any activity limitations. Recent medical tests also show that his chest wall deformities do not have any measurable impact on his cardiac or pulmonary function. His remarkable gains in individual rib cage mobility from the initial visit to discharge (lateral side bending test) have been nearly retained. Jonathan and his mother stated that they wished they had continued with periodic physical therapy rechecks to maintain all the gains he made during that first year.

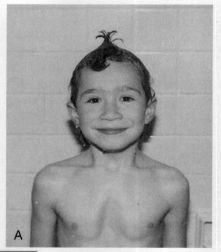
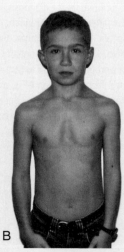
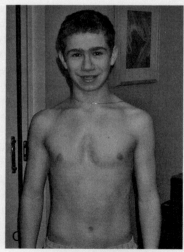

Figure 25-10 Comparison of pectus excavatum and postural alignments. **A**, Jonathan at 6 years old. **B**, Jonathan at 10 years old. **C**, Jonathan at 14 years old. By age 14, Jonathan's pectus has become narrower and more localized. Shoulders are less protracted, resulting in a more neutral resting position. His trapezius is less elevated, and although no rib flare is noted in either standing posture, adequate abdominal stability is more apparent at age 14.

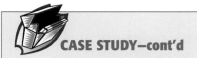

CASE STUDY—cont'd

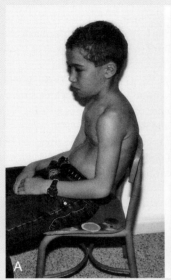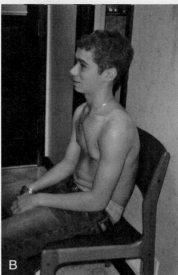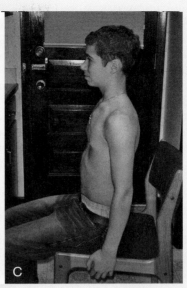

Figure 25-11   Comparison of sitting postures. **A,** Typical sitting posture in school per his mother: age 9 and younger. This is a reenactment picture taken at age 10. Jonathan was too embarrassed to have his picture taken of his "deformed chest" when he was initially evaluated at age 9. Note slouched posture (functional kyphosis) with midtrunk fold, pectus, elevated sternal angle. By age 10, patient no longer regularly postured himself like this in sitting. **B,** Jonathan at 14 years old. When asked to slouch in sitting, the midtrunk fold and kyphosis are barely noticeable. Prominent sternal angle is still noticeable. **C,** Straight sitting posture at age 14 years old. Note normal back posture. Mild pectus and mild rib flare still present at base of sternum.

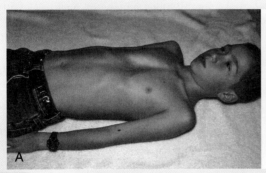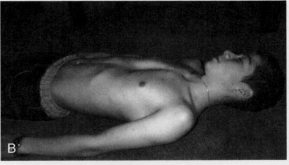

Figure 25-12   Comparison of supine postures. **A,** Discharge picture at age 10. Pectus was reduced almost in half from 34 to 18 mL H_2O displacement measurement during the 11 months of physical therapy. Lower rib flares functionally integrated with abdominal muscles. Neck muscles more elongated. Slight shoulder protraction still noted. **B,** Four years later at age 14. Pectus slightly deeper, but narrower (volume unchanged from discharge at 17 mL). Rib flares more prominent than at discharge. Patient stated that he stopped doing his trunk exercises about 4 months after discharge because he was doing so well. Neck muscles more elongated. Shoulders less protracted.

I believe Jonathan's physical therapy program worked so well because it was tailored to address his specific EIA pattern and chest wall deformities from a multisystem perspective and included educational, medical, psychologic, and physical perspectives. Interventions by physical therapists can have a tremendous positive impact on the impairments, activity limitations, and resultant disabilities that occur as a result of a primary pulmonary pathology, especially in a maturing system. If the patient cannot breathe efficiently and effectively, then that patient cannot function at his or her highest level. The concepts presented here for Jonathan can certainly be adapted to infants and toddlers as well as older children. The key is to develop a program that keeps the patient, his family, and his resources in mind while developing a targeted intervention strategy.[20,82]

Following the reexamination, Jonathan's home program was updated and reinitiated with an emphasis on maintaining his musculoskeletal alignment and trunk control. I recommended quarterly check-ups throughout puberty to modify the program as necessary.

REFERENCES

1. Abrams, S. A. (2001). Chronic pulmonary insufficiency in children and its effects on growth and development. *Journal of Nutrition, 131*(3), 938S–941S.

2. Akinbami, L. (2006). *The state of childhood asthma, United States, 1980–2005.* Washington, DC: U.S. Department of Health and Human Services, Centers for Disease Control and Prevention, 1–24.

3. Allen, D. B. (2002). Safety of inhaled corticosteroids in children. *Pediatric Pulmonology, 33*(3), 208–220.

4. Amdekar, Y. K. (2001). Natural history of asthma in children. *Indian Journal of Pediatrics, 68*(Suppl 4), S3–S6.

5. Anderson, S. D., & Holzer, K. (2000). Exercise-induced asthma: Is it the right diagnosis in elite athletes? *Journal of Allergy & Clinical Immunology, 106*(3), 419–428.

6. APTA (2001). Guide to physical therapist practice, ed. 2. *Physical Therapy, 81*(1).

7. Apter, A. J., & Szefler, S. J. (2004). Advances in adult and pediatric asthma. *Journal of Allergy & Clinical Immunology, 113*(3), 407–414.

8. Arguin, A. L., & Swartz, M. K. (2004). Gastroesophageal reflux in infants: A primary care perspective. *Pediatric Nursing, 30*(1), 45–51.

9. Bach, J. R., & Bianchi, C. (2003). Prevention of pectus excavatum for children with spinal muscular atrophy type 1. *American Journal of Physical Medicine & Rehabilitation, 82*(10), 815–819.

10. Baker, K. M., Brand, D. A., & Hen, J., Jr. (2003). Classifying asthma: Disagreement among specialists. [see comment]. *Chest, 124*(6), 2156–2163.

11. Baraldi, E., Carraro, S., & Filippone, M. (2009). Bronchopulmonary dysplasia: Definitions and long-term respiratory outcome. *Early Human Development, 85*(Suppl 10), S1–S3.

12. Baum, W. F., Schneyer, U., & Kloditz, E. (2002). Delay of growth and development in children with bronchial asthma, atopic dermatitis and allergic rhinitis. *Experimental & Clinical Endocrinology & Diabetes, 110*(2), 53–59.

13. Berhane, K., McConnell, R., Gilliland, F., et al. (2000). Sex-specific effects of asthma on pulmonary function in children. *American Journal of Respiratory & Critical Care Medicine, 162*(5), 1723–1730.

14. Bhatia, J., & Parish, A. (2009). GERD or not GERD: The fussy infant. *Journal of Perinatology, 29*(Suppl 2), S7–S11.

15. Birkisson, I. F., Halapi, E., Bjornsdottir, U. S., et al. (2004). Genetic approaches to assessing evidence for a T helper type 1 cytokine defect in adult asthma. *American Journal of Respiratory & Critical Care Medicine, 169*(9), 1007–1013.

16. Braganza, S., Sharif, I., & Ozuah, P. O. (2003). Documenting asthma severity: Do we get it right? *Journal of Asthma, 40*(6), 661–665.

17. Bravata, D. M., Gienger, A. L., Holty, J. E., et al. (2009). Quality improvement strategies for children with asthma: A systematic review. *Archives of Pediatrics & Adolescent Medicine, 163*(6), 572–581.

18. Butler, J. E., & Gandevia, S. C. (2008). The output from human inspiratory motoneurone pools. *Journal of Physiology, 586*(5), 1257–1264.

19. Callahan, K. A., Panter, T. M., Hall, T. M., et al. (2010). Peak flow monitoring in pediatric asthma management: A clinical practice column submission. *Journal of Pediatric Nursing, 25*(1), 12–17.

20. Canavan, P. K., & Cahalin, L. (2008). Integrated physical therapy intervention for a person with pectus excavatum and bilateral shoulder pain: A single-case study. *Archives of Physical Medicine and Rehabilitation, 89*(11), 2195–2204.

21. Cappello, M., Legrand, A., & De Troyer, A. (1999). Determinants of rib motion in flail chest. *American Journal of Respiratory & Critical Care Medicine, 159*(3), 886–891.

21a. CDC. (2010, May 15, 2009). "Asthma Fast Facts." Retrieved May 8, 2010, 2010, from http://www.cdc.gov/nchs/fastats/asthma.htm.

22. Centers for Disease Control and Prevention. (1998, April 24). Surveillance for Asthma—United States, 1960–1995. Retrieved May 30, 2004, from www.cdc.gov/mmwr/preview/mmwrhtml/00052262.htm.

23. Centers for Disease Control and Prevention. (2009, May 15). Asthma Fast Facts. Retrieved May 8, 2010, from www.cdc.gov/nchs/fastats/asthma.htm.

24. Cherniack, R. M., & Cherniack, L. (1983). *Respiration in health and disease* (3rd ed.). Philadelphia: WB Saunders Co.

25. Chiang, L. C., Ma, W. F., Huang, J. L., et al. (2009). Effect of relaxation-breathing training on anxiety and asthma signs/symptoms of children with moderate-to-severe asthma: A randomized controlled trial. *International Journal of Nursing Studies, 46*(8), 1061–1670.

26. Cole, P. (2001). Pathophysiology and treatment of airway mucociliary clearance: A moving tale. *Minerva Anesthesiology, 67*(4), 206–209.

27. Cserhati, E. F., Gegesi Kiss, A., Poder, G., et al. (1984). Thorax deformity and asthma bronchial. *Allergologia et Immunopathologia, 12*(1), 7–10.

28. De Troyer, A., Kirkwood, P. A., & Wilson, T. A. (2005). Respiratory action of the intercostal muscles. *Physiological Reviews, 85*(2), 717–756.

29. Dean, B. B., Calimlim, B. M., Kindermann, S. L., et al. (2009). The impact of uncontrolled asthma on absenteeism and health-related quality of life. *Journal of Asthma, 46*(9), 861–866.

30. Deem, J. F., & Miller, L. (2000). *Manual of voice therapy* (2nd ed.). Austin, TX: PRO-ED.

31. Doskocil, M. (1993). Contribution to the study of the development and ossification of human sternum. *Functional and Developmental Morphology, 3*(4), 251–257.

32. Dowdee, A., & Ossege, J. (2007). Assessment of childhood allergy for the primary care practitioner. *Journal of the American Academy of Nurse Practitioners, 19*(2), 53–62.

33. Doyle, L. W., Cheung, M. M., Ford, G. W., et al. (2001). Birth weight <1501 g and respiratory health at age 14. *Archives of Diseases in Childhood*, *84*(1), 40–44.

34. Eid, N. S., & Morton, R. L. (2004). Rational approach to the wheezy infant. *Paediatric Respiratory Reviews 5*(Suppl A), S77–S79.

35. Fletcher, J. M., Green, J. C., & Neidell, M. J. (2010). Long term effects of childhood asthma on adult health. *Journal of Health Economics*, *29*(3), 377–387.

36. Fonkalsrud, E. W. (2003). Current management of pectus excavatum. *World Journal of Surgery*, *27*(5), 502–508.

37. Frownfelter, D., & Massery, M. (2006). Facilitating ventilation patterns and breathing strategies. In D. Frownfelter & E. Dean (Eds), *Cardiovascular and pulmonary physical therapy evidence and practice* (4th ed., chap. 23). St. Louis, MO, Elsevier Health Sciences.

38. Gandevia, S. C., Butler, J. E., Hodges, P. W., et al. (2002). Balancing acts: Respiratory sensations, motor control and human posture. *Clinical & Experimental Pharmacology & Physiology*, *29*(1–2), 118–121.

39. Garrod, R., & Lasserson, T. (2007). Role of physiotherapy in the management of chronic lung diseases: An overview of systematic reviews. *Respiratory Medicine*, *101*(12), 2429–2436.

40. Gern, J. E. (2004). Viral respiratory infection and the link to asthma. *Pediatric Infectious Disease Journal*, *23*(Suppl 1), S78–S86.

41. Gerson, L. B., & Fass, R. (2009). A systematic review of the definitions, prevalence, and response to treatment of nocturnal gastroesophageal reflux disease. *Clinical Gastroenterology and Hepatology*, *7*(4), 372–378; quiz, 367.

42. Greenough, A., Alexander, J., Boit, P., et al. (2009). School age outcome of hospitalisation with respiratory syncytial virus infection of prematurely born infants. *Thorax*, *64*(6), 490–495.

43. Grimstone, S. K., & Hodges, P. W. (2003). Impaired postural compensation for respiration in people with recurrent low back pain. *Experimental Brain Research*, *151*(2), 218–224.

44. Hallstrand, T. S., & W. R. Henderson, Jr. (2010). An update on the role of leukotrienes in asthma. *Current Opinion in Allergy and Clinical Immunology*, *10*(1), 60–66.

45. Han, J. N., Gayan-Ramirez, G., Dekhuijzen, R., et al. (1993). Respiratory function of the rib cage muscles. *European Respiratory Journal*, *6*(5), 722–728.

45a. Hansen, E. F., J. Vestbo, et al. (2001). "Peak flow as predictor of overall mortality in asthma and chronic obstructive pulmonary disease." *American Journal of Respiratory & Critical Care Medicine 163*(3 Pt 1): 690–693.

46. Harik-Khan, R. I., Muller, D. C., & Wise, R. A. (2004). Serum vitamin levels and the risk of asthma in children. *American Journal of Epidemiology*, *159*(4), 351–357.

47. Hartert, T. V., & R. S. Peebles, Jr. (2000). Epidemiology of asthma: The year in review. *Current Opinion in Pulmonary Medicine*, *6*(1), 4–9.

48. Hebra, A. (2004, February 25). Pectus Excavatum at e-Medicine. Retrieved June 2, 2004, from www.emedicine.com/ped/topic2558.htm.

49. Hixon, T. J. (1991). *Respiratory function in speech and song*. San Diego, CA: Singular Publishing Group.

50. Hodges, P., Kaigle Holm, A., Holm, S., et al. (2003). Intervertebral stiffness of the spine is increased by evoked contraction of transversus abdominis and the diaphragm: In vivo porcine studies. *Spine*, *28*(23), 2594–2601.

51. Hodges, P. W., & Gandevia, S. C. (2000). Activation of the human diaphragm during a repetitive postural task. *Journal of Physiology*, *522*(Pt 1), 165–175.

52. Hodges, P. W., Gurfinkel, V. S., Brumagne, S., et al. (2002). Coexistence of stability and mobility in postural control: Evidence from postural compensation for respiration. *Experimental Brain Research*, *144*(3), 293–302.

53. Hodges, P. W., Heijnen, I., & Gandevia, S. C. (2001). Postural activity of the diaphragm is reduced in humans when respiratory demand increases. *Journal of Physiology*, *537*(Pt 3), 999–1008.

54. Hodges, P. W., Sapsford, R., & Pengel, L. H. (2007). Postural and respiratory functions of the pelvic floor muscles. *Neurourology & Urodynamics*, *26*(3), 362–371.

55. Holloway, E., & Ram, F. S. (2004). Breathing exercises for asthma. [Update of Cochrane Database Systematic Reviews, 2000;(3),CD001277; PMID: 10908489.] *Cochrane Database of Systematic Reviews, 1,* CD001277.

56. Hondras, M. A., Linde, K., & Jones, A. P. (2001). Manual therapy for asthma. [Update of Cochrane Database Systematic Reviews, 2000;(2), CD001002 ; 10796578.] *Cochrane Database of Systematic Reviews, 1,* CD001002.

57. Hudson, A. L., Butler, J. E., Gandevia, S. C., et al. (2010). Interplay between the inspiratory and postural functions of the human parasternal intercostal muscles. *Journal of Neurophysiology*, *103*(3), 1622–1629.

58. Indinnimeo, L., Bertuola, F., Cutrera, R., et al. (2009). Clinical evaluation and treatment of acute asthma exacerbations in children. *International Journal of Immunopathology and Pharmacology*, *22*(4), 867–878.

59. Jadcherla, S. R., & Shaker, R. (2001). Esophageal and upper esophageal sphincter motor function in babies. *American Journal of Medicine*, *111*(Suppl 8A), 64S–68S.

60. Janse, A. J., Sinnema, G., Uiterwaal, C. S., et al. (2008). Quality of life in chronic illness: Children, parents and paediatricians have different, but stable perceptions. *Acta Paediatrics*, *97*(8), 1118–1124.

61. Joseph-Bowen, J., de Klerk, N. H., Firth, M. J., et al. (2004). Lung function, bronchial responsiveness, and asthma in a community cohort of 6-year-old children. *American Journal of Respiratory & Critical Care Medicine*, *169*(7), 850–854.

62. Kabakus, N., & Kurt, A. (2006). Sandifer Syndrome: A continuing problem of misdiagnosis. *Pediatrics International*, *48*(6), 622–625.

63. Kaiser, H. B. (2004). Risk factors in allergy/asthma. *Allergy & Asthma Proceedings, 25*(1), 7–10.

64. Karkos, P. D., Leong, S. C., Benton, J., et al. (2009). Reflux and sleeping disorders: A systematic review. *Journal of Laryngology and Otology, 123*(4), 372–374.

65. Kase, J. S., Pici, M., & Visintainer, P. (2009). Risks for common medical conditions experienced by former preterm infants during toddler years. *Journal of Perinatal Medicine, 37*(2), 103–108.

66. Kennedy, J. D. (1999). Lung function outcome in children of premature birth. *Journal of Paediatrics & Child Health, 35*(6), 516–521.

67. Khoshoo, V., Haydel, R., & Saturno, E. (2006). Gastroesophageal reflux disease and asthma in children. *Current Gastroenterology Reports, 8*(3), 237–243.

68. Knott, M., & Voss, D. E. (1968). *Proprioceptive neuromuscular facilitation.* New York: Harper & Row.

69. Kobernick, A. (2009). Treating GERD in asthma improved lung function. American College of Allergy, Asthma and Immunology. Seattle, WA. *Chest Physician News, 4,* 15.

70. Kuyper, L. M., Pare, P. D., Hogg, J. C., et al. (2003). Characterization of airway plugging in fatal asthma. [see comment]. *American Journal of Medicine, 115*(1), 6–11.

71. Lamberg, E. M., & Hagins, M. (2009). *Evidence supporting the role of breath control in postural stabilization.* American Physical Therapy Association, Combined Sections Meeting 2009. Las Vegas, NV.

72. Lamberg, E. M., & Hagins, M. (2010). Breath control during manual free-style lifting of a maximally tolerated load. *Ergonomics, 53*(3), 385–392.

73. LaPier, T. K. (2002). Chest wall expansion values in supine and standing across the adult lifespan. *Physical and Occupational Therapy in Geriatrics, 21*(1), 65–81.

74. LaPier, T. K., Cook, A., Droege, K., et al. (2000). Intertester and intratester reliability of chest excursion measurement in subjects without impairment. *Cardiopulmonary Physical Therapy, 11*(3), 94–98.

75. Lee, L. J., Chang, A. T., Coppieters, M. W., et al. (2010). Changes in sitting posture induce multiplanar changes in chest wall shape and motion with breathing. *Respiratory Physiology & Neurobiology, 170*(3), 236–245.

76. Lee, L. J., Coppieters, M. W., & Hodges, P. W. (2009). Anticipatory postural adjustments to arm movement reveal complex control of paraspinal muscles in the thorax. *Journal of Electromyography and Kinesiology, 19*(1), 46–54.

77. Leiner, G. C., Abramowitz, S., Small, M. J., et al. (1963). Expiratory peak flow rate; standard values for normal subjects. *American Review of Respiratory Disease, 88,* 644–651.

78. Lissoni, A., Aliverti, A., Tzeng, A. C., et al. (1998). Kinematic analysis of patients with spinal muscular atrophy during spontaneous breathing and mechanical ventilation. *American Journal of Physical Medicine & Rehabilitation, 77*(3), 188–192.

78a. Lozano, P., P. Fishman, et al. (1997). "Health care utilization and cost among children with asthma who were enrolled in a health maintenance organization." *Pediatrics 99*(6): 757–764.

79. Mainz, J. G., Kaiser, W. A., Beck, J. F., et al. (2009). Substantially reduced calcaneal bone ultrasound parameters in severe untreated asthma. *Respiration, 78*(2), 230–233.

80. Massery, M. (2005). Musculoskeletal and neuromuscular interventions: A physical approach to cystic fibrosis. *Journal of the Royal Society of Medicine, 98*(Suppl 45), 55–66.

81. Massery, M. (2006). Multisystem consequences of impaired breathing mechanics and/or postural control. In D. Frownfelter & E. Dean, *Cardiovascular and pulmonary physical therapy evidence and practice* (4th ed., chap. 39). St. Louis, MO., Elsevier Health Sciences.

82. Massery, M. (2009). The Linda Crane Memorial Lecture: The patient puzzle—piecing it together. *Cardiopulmonary Physical Therapy Journal, 20*(2), 19–27.

83. Massery, M., & Cahalin, L. (2004). Physical therapy associated with ventilatory pump dysfunction and failure. In W. DeTurk & L. Cahalin, *Cardiovascular and pulmonary physical therapy* (chap. 19). New York, McGraw-Hill.

84. Massery, M. P. (1994). What's positioning got to do with it? *Neurology Report, 18*(3), 11–14.

85. Massery, M. P., Dreyer, H. E., Bjornson, A. S., et al. (1997). Chest wall excursion and tidal volume change during passive positioning in cervical spinal cord injury. (Abstract). *Cardiopulmonary Physical Therapy, 8*(4), 27.

86. Mellinger-Birdsong, A. K., Powell, K. E., Iatridis, T., et al. (2003). Prevalence and impact of asthma in children, Georgia, 2000. *American Journal of Preventive Medicine, 24*(3), 242–248.

87. Mellon, M., & Parasuraman, B. (2004). Pediatric asthma: Improving management to reduce cost of care. *Journal of Managed Care Pharmacy, 10*(2), 130–134.

88. Metsala, J., Kilkkinen, A., Kaila, M., et al. (2008). Perinatal factors and the risk of asthma in childhood: A population-based register study in Finland. *American Journal of Epidemiology, 168*(2), 170–178.

89. Molle, L. D., Goldani, H. A., Fagondes, S. C., et al. (2009). Nocturnal reflux in children and adolescents with persistent asthma and gastroesophageal reflux. *Journal of Asthma, 46*(4), 347–350.

90. Moloney, E., O'Sullivan, S., Hogan, T., et al. (2002). Airway dehydration: A therapeutic target in asthma? *Chest, 121*(6), 1806–1811.

91. Moloney, E. D., Griffin, S., Burke, C. M., et al. (2003). Release of inflammatory mediators from eosinophils following a hyperosmolar stimulus. *Respiratory Medicine, 97*(8), 928–932.

92. Morris, M., & P. Perkins. (2004, May 9). Asthma. Retrieved June 1, 2004, from www.emedicine.com/med/topic177.htm.

93. Morris, P. J. (2008). Physical activity recommendations for children and adolescents with chronic disease. *Current Sports Medicine Reports, 7*(6), 353–358.

94. National Institutes of Health. (1997). Practical Guide for the Diagnosis and Management of Asthma Based on Expert Panel Report 2. NIH Publication No. 97-4053, National Institutes of Health: National Heart, Lung and Blood Institute, 60, Bethesda, Md.

95. National Institutes of Health. (2007). Expert panel report 3: Guidelines for the diagnosis and management of asthma. NIH Publication 07-4051, National Institute of Health: National Heart, Lung, and Blood Institute, Bethesda, Md.

96. Nordenstedt, H., Nilsson, M., Johansson, S., et al. (2006). The relation between gastroesophageal reflux and respiratory symptoms in a population-based study: The Nord-Trondelag health survey. *Chest, 129*(4), 1051–1056.

97. Openshaw, P. J., Dean, G. S., & Culley, F. J. (2003). Links between respiratory syncytial virus bronchiolitis and childhood asthma: Clinical and research approaches. *Pediatric Infectious Disease Journal, 22*(Suppl 2), S58–S64; discussion S64–S65.

98. Papastamelos, C., Panitch, H. B., & Allen, J. L. (1996). Chest wall compliance in infants and children with neuromuscular disease. *American Journal of Respiratory and Critical Care Medicine, 154*, 1045–1048.

99. Papiris, S., Kotanidou, A., Malagari, K., et al. (2002). Clinical review: Severe asthma. *Critical Care (London) 6*(1), 30–44.

100. Parish, J. M. (2009). Sleep-related problems in common medical conditions. *Chest, 135*(2), 563–572.

101. Parsons, J. P., & Mastronarde, J. G. (2009). Exercise-induced asthma. *Current Opinion in Pulmonary Medicine, 15*(1), 25–28.

102. Peterson, K. A., Samuelson, W. M., Ryujin, D. T., et al. (2009). The role of gastroesophageal reflux in exercise-triggered asthma: A randomized controlled trial. *Digestive Diseases and Sciences, 54*(3), 564–571.

103. Philpott, J. F., Houghton, K., & Luke, A. (2010). Physical activity recommendations for children with specific chronic health conditions: Juvenile idiopathic arthritis, hemophilia, asthma, and cystic fibrosis. *Clinical Journal of Sports Medicine, 20*(3), 167–172.

104. Powell, C. V., Kelly, A. M., & Kerr, D. (2003). Lack of agreement in classification of the severity of acute asthma between emergency physician assessment and classification using the National Asthma Council Australia guidelines (1998). *Emergency Medicine* (Fremantle, WA), *15*(1), 49–53.

105. Ram, F. S., Wellington, S. R., & Barnes, N. C. (2003). Inspiratory muscle training for asthma. *Cochrane Database of Systematic Reviews* (4), CD003792.

106. Rimmer, K. P., Ford, G. T., & Whitelaw, W. A. (1995). Interaction between postural and respiratory control of human intercostal muscles. *Journal of Applied Physiology, 79*(5), 1556–1561.

107. Robinson, J. H., Callister, L. C., Berry, J. A., et al. (2008). Patient-centered care and adherence: Definitions and applications to improve outcomes. *Journal of the American Academy of Nurse Practitioners, 20*(12), 600–607.

108. Roger, G., Denoyelle, F., & Garabedian, E. N. (2001). Dysfonction laryngee episodique. *Archives de Pediatrie, 8*(Suppl 3), 650–654.

109. Rothman, R. L., Yin, H. S., Mulvaney, S., et al. (2009). Health literacy and quality: Focus on chronic illness care and patient safety. *Pediatrics, 124* (Suppl 3), S315–S326.

110. Rudd, R. A., & Moorman, J. E. (2007). Asthma incidence: Data from the National Health Interview Survey, 1980–1996. *Journal of Asthma, 44*(1), 65–70.

111. Saboisky, J. P., Gorman, R. B., De Troyer, A., et al. (2007). Differential activation among five human inspiratory motoneuron pools during tidal breathing. *Journal of Applied Physiology, 102*(2), 772–780.

112. Saunders, S. W., Rath, D., & Hodges, P. W. (2004). Postural and respiratory activation of the trunk muscles changes with mode and speed of locomotion. *Gait Posture, 20*(3), 280–290.

113. Schilero, G. J., Spungen, A. M., Bauman, W. A., et al. (2009). Pulmonary function and spinal cord injury. *Respiratory Physiology & Neurobiology, 166*(3), 129–141.

114. Schmier, J. K., Manjunath, R., Halpern, M. T., et al. (2007). The impact of inadequately controlled asthma in urban children on quality of life and productivity. *Annals of Allergy, Asthma & Immunology, 98*(3), 245–251.

115. Shirley, D., Hodges, P. W., Eriksson, A. E., et al. (2003). Spinal stiffness changes throughout the respiratory cycle. *Journal of Applied Physiology, 95*(4), 1467–1475.

116. Sidhu, A. S., & Triadafilopoulos, G. (2008). Neuro-regulation of lower esophageal sphincter function as treatment for gastroesophageal reflux disease. *World Journal of Gastroenterology, 14*(7), 985–990.

117. Silvestri, M., Sabatini, F., Defilippi, A. C., et al. (2004). The wheezy infant: Immunological and molecular considerations. *Paediatric Respiratory Reviews, 5*(Suppl A), S81–S87.

118. Simoes, E. A. (2008). RSV disease in the pediatric population: Epidemiology, seasonal variability, and long-term outcomes. *Managed Care, 17*(11 Suppl 12), 3–6; discussion, 18–19.

119. Skjodt, N. M., Farran, R. P., Hawes, H. G., et al. (2001). Simulation of acute spinal cord injury: Effects on respiration. *Respiratory Physiology, 127*(1), 3–11.

120. Smith, M. D., Russell, A., & Hodges, P. W. (2009). Do incontinence, breathing difficulties, and gastrointestinal symptoms increase the risk of future back pain? *Journal of Pain, 10*(8), 876–886.

121. Sopo, S. M., Radzik, D., & Calvani, M. (2009). Does treatment with proton pump inhibitors for gastroesophageal reflux disease (GERD) improve asthma symptoms in children with asthma and GERD? A systematic review. *Journal of Investigational Allergology & Clinical Immunology, 19*(1), 1–5.

122. Sullivan, P. E., Markos, P. D., & Minor, M. A. (1982). *An integrated approach to therapeutic exercise: Theory and clinical application.* Reston, VA: Reston Publishing Co.

123. Sunyer, J., Anto, J. M., & Burney, P. (1999). Generational increase of self-reported first attack of asthma in fifteen industrialized countries. European Community Respiratory Health Study (ECRHS). *European Respiratory Journal, 14*(4), 885–891.

124. Sveen, S. (2009). Symptom check: Is it GERD? *Journal of Continuing Education in Nursing, 40*(3), 103–104.

125. Temprado, J. J., Milliex, L., Grelot, L., et al. (2002). A dynamic pattern analysis of coordination between breathing and rhythmic arm movements in humans. *Neuroscience Letters*, *329*(3), 314–318.

126. Teodorescu, M., Consens, F. B., Bria, W. F., et al. (2009). Predictors of habitual snoring and obstructive sleep apnea risk in patients with asthma. *Chest*, *135*(5), 1125–1132.

127. Van Bever, H. P. (2009). Determinants in early life for asthma development. *Allergy, Asthma, and Clinical Immunology*, *5*(1), 6.

128. van den Bemt, L., Kooijman, S., Linssen, V., et al. (2010). How does asthma influence the daily life of children? Results of focus group interviews. *Health Quality of Life Outcomes*, *8*, 5.

129. van Veldhoven, N. H., Vermeer, A., Bogaard, J. M., et al. (2001). Children with asthma and physical exercise: Effects of an exercise programme. *Clinical Rehabilitation*, *15*(4), 360–370.

130. Voynow, J. A., & Rubin, B. K. (2009). Mucins, mucus, and sputum. *Chest*, *135*(2), 505–512.

131. Wagner, C. W. (2003). Pathophysiology and diagnosis of asthma. *Nursing Clinics of North America*, *38*(4), 561–570.

132. Wasilewska, J., Kaczmarski, M., Protas, P. T., et al. (2009). [Sleep disorders in childhood and adolescence, with special reference to allergic diseases]. *Polski Merkuriusz Lekarski*, *26*(153), 188–193.

133. Wiener, G. J., Tsukashima, R., Kelly, C., et al. (2009). Oropharyngeal pH monitoring for the detection of liquid and aerosolized supraesophageal gastric reflux. *Journal of Voice*, *23*(4), 498–504.

134. Yolton, K., Xu, Y., Khoury, J., et al. (2010). Associations between secondhand smoke exposure and sleep patterns in children. *Pediatrics*, *125*(2), e261–e268.

135. Yuksel, H., Yilmaz, O., Kirmaz, C., et al. (2006). Frequency of gastroesophageal reflux disease in nonatopic children with asthma-like airway disease. *Respiratory Medicine*, *100*(3), 393–398.

26 Thoracic Surgery

BETSY A. HOWELL, PT, MS • CHRIS TAPLEY, PT, MS

Approximately 6 to 10 in 1000 children are born each year with moderate and severe forms of congenital heart defects.[111] Early detection, often prenatal, and improved medical and surgical management combine with the type of defect and the individual child characteristics to determine the impact. For example, two children, each diagnosed with a ventricular septal defect, may have entirely different histories. One child may go undiagnosed for several years, whereas the other child may require surgery in infancy. Many children are now diagnosed in utero—an especially important development for children with hypoplastic left heart syndrome (HLHS). Formerly, most congenital heart defects were repaired when the child was at least 1 year old, often older. More of these surgeries are now being performed during the first days and months of life, which is likely to affect how children with congenital heart defects grow and develop. The likelihood of a physical therapist treating a child who has previously had open-heart surgery is greater, now that more children survive open-heart surgery. A large adult population that has survived surgery in childhood for congenital heart defects also exists.

Physical therapists examining this population should closely monitor and document the nature and extent of developmental differences that may result from earlier surgical repair, as well as potential neurologic deficits related to the cardiac defect itself or to postoperative complications. To prepare therapists for this task, this chapter describes congenital heart defects; surgical repairs, including heart and heart-lung transplantation; acute and chronic physical impairments secondary to heart defects and surgery; profound cyanosis or neurologic implications and complications; and physical therapy management for the population of children with cardiac defects. Internet links to several major institutions that perform hundreds of surgeries each year on children with various congenital heart defects are also provided.

CONGENITAL HEART DEFECTS

Although embryologists can identify at what point during fetal development certain defects occur, and what risk factors may contribute to their development, the cause of congenital heart defects remains largely unknown. The presence of more than one child with congenital heart defect in the same family or in the family history suggests a possible genetic component. Approximately 10% of children with congenital heart defects also have other physical malformations.[181] Heart defects may be associated with Down syndrome, Turner syndrome, Williams syndrome, Marfan syndrome, Costello syndrome, DiGeorge syndrome, and the VATERL association, an acronym for the following characteristics: vertebrae, imperforate anus, cardiac anomalies, tracheo-esophageal fistula, renal anomalies and limb anomalies. The American Heart Association published a lengthy statement on current knowledge of the genetic basis for congenital heart defects[195] that describes in detail many of the above syndromes and their chromosomal disorders and associated cardiac defects. The American Heart Association has also published a lengthy statement on noninherited risk factors linked to congenital heart defects.[126]

Infants of diabetic mothers also have an increased incidence of congenital heart disease (CHD).[53] Other noninherited risk factors found to be associated with congenital heart defects are maternal phenylketonuria, rubella, maternal obesity, and many different medications.[126] It was observed that women who used a multivitamin supplement before or just after conception had a significant reduction in the incidence of cardiac defects in their children.[36]

Diagnosis of cardiac problems may occur during prenatal life or at birth. Some congenital heart defects require immediate attention, and others may be followed by further evaluation. Even with improved diagnostic techniques, some infants with severe cyanotic disease are not diagnosed before they are discharged to home, but several weeks later they may be diagnosed with a heart defect, when they develop symptoms of septic shock. Prenatal diagnosis is essential for some diagnoses, especially HLHS. In a review of mortality rates and the number of cardiac cases performed each year by a surgical program, those with smaller programs had increased mortality rates when outcomes of the more severe defects were compared.[256] Other cardiac defects may not be diagnosed until much later, even as late as adolescence. For example, coarctation of the aorta is occasionally diagnosed during a sports physical examination when a large difference between upper and lower extremity blood pressures or an abnormally high upper extremity blood pressure is observed.

The infant with a congenital heart defect often has abnormal respiratory signs, including a labored breathing pattern and an increased respiratory rate. The infant may be diaphoretic and tachycardic. Edema around the eyes and decreased urine output (evidenced by dry diapers) may also be observed. Eating problems result from difficulty in coordinating sucking and swallowing with breathing at an increased rate. Irritability that is difficult to assuage may be noted. These symptoms of congestive heart failure can lead to the diagnosis of a cardiac defect or can provide evidence of worsening of a known defect.

Congenital heart defects are usually classified as acyanotic or cyanotic. With acyanotic lesions, the child is pink and has normal oxygen saturation. If mixing or shunting of blood occurs within the heart, the blood shunts from the left side of the heart to the right side, so oxygenated blood goes to the lungs as well as to the body. Common acyanotic lesions include atrial septal defects (ASDs), ventricular septal defects (VSDs), patent ductus arteriosus (PDA), coarctation of the aorta, pulmonary stenosis, and aortic stenosis.

In cyanotic defects, blood is typically shunted from the right side of the heart to the left side. Unoxygenated blood is then returned to the body, resulting in arterial oxygen saturation levels 15% to 30% below normal values. Common cyanotic lesions include tetralogy of Fallot, transposition of the great arteries, tricuspid atresia, pulmonary atresia, truncus arteriosus, total anomalous pulmonary venous return, and HLHS.

Type and timing of intervention depend on the defect and the child's age. Some defects are repaired immediately, whereas others require a staged procedure, with the first several surgeries being palliative rather than corrective. Some acyanotic defects are not repaired until the child is several years old. Less impairment of growth and weight gain, however, occurs when surgery is performed in the first 2 years of life.[209,231] Concerns regarding neurologic complications following surgery and their impact on long-term functional and cognitive development continue to be examined as an increasing number of infants survive earlier and more complex surgeries.[67,150] Low-flow cardiopulmonary bypass[265] and neurophysiologic monitoring during and after surgery, including measuring cerebral oxygenation,[194] help to minimize the possibility of neurologic complications.[10] Acyanotic and cyanotic defects are further described in the next two sections and may be compared with normal anatomy of the heart (Figure 26-1).

ACYANOTIC DEFECTS

ATRIAL SEPTAL DEFECT

Atrial septal defect, one of the most common congenital heart defects, is an abnormal communication between left and right atria (Figure 26-2). The defect is classified by its location on the septum. Blood is generally shunted from the left atrium to the right atrium. This defect has traditionally been repaired when a child is between 4 and 6

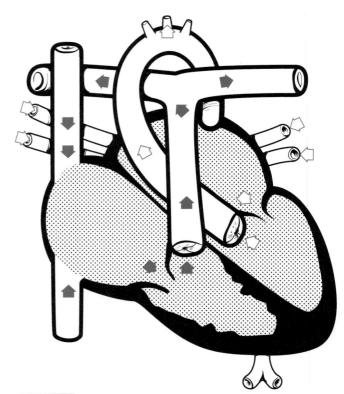

Figure 26-1   Anatomy of the heart.

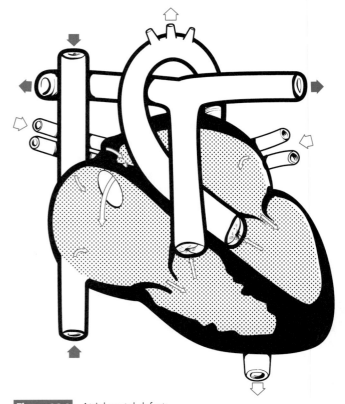

Figure 26-2   Atrial septal defect.

years old because of slow progression of damage to the heart and lungs. If a child has more severe symptoms, the defect is repaired sooner.[172] Some adults with signs of heart failure are found to have a previously undiagnosed ASD. As medical technology advances, late diagnoses should become rare.

Closure is usually done using a device to close the hole. It is inserted via cardiac catheterization. Surgical repair may still occur if the ASD is in an unusual position, making it difficult to close via cardiac catheterization. Surgery was traditionally done through a median sternotomy incision; however, minimal access techniques can be used, which can entail a smaller incision centered over the xiphoid process. These techniques can also result in shortened length of hospitalization.[187] The defect is usually sutured together, or a patch closure is used when surgery is necessary.[137] The timing of surgery depends on the age of the child, when the diagnosis is confirmed, and how symptomatic the child is, but it typically occurs during the first 5 years of life. A longitudinal study of patients undergoing closure of an ASD during childhood showed excellent survival and low morbidity rates.[207]

VENTRICULAR SEPTAL DEFECT

Ventricular septal defect is the most common congenital heart defect (20%–30% of all children with congenital defects).[98] It can be present alone or in association with other defects such as tetralogy of Fallot and transposition of the great arteries. VSD alone is discussed here. A VSD is a communication between the ventricles that allows blood to be shunted between them, generally from left to right (Figure 26-3). The increase in blood flow through the right ventricle to the lungs may lead to pulmonary hypertension. In severe cases, in which pulmonary pressures exceed systemic pressures, shunting switches from right to left, which is often termed Eisenmenger syndrome.[98] A large defect may lead to early left ventricular failure. An infant with a large VSD has signs of severe respiratory distress, diaphoresis, and fatigability, especially during feeding, when the infant's endurance is stressed.[87] The infant's weight is dramatically affected in this situation. A child this severely affected requires a much earlier surgical repair than a child who is asymptomatic.

Small defects may close spontaneously. Defects that compromise the clinical status of the patient must be surgically closed. The timing of surgery varies, depending on the child's tolerance of the defect. A child with a larger defect undergoes surgery earlier to diminish the negative effects on growth and the pulmonary system.

Surgical intervention is provided through a mediastinal approach and usually requires a synthetic patch closure.[6] Transcatheter devices are now being used with regularity and good success to close muscular VSDs but not as successfully as with perimembranous VSDs.[175]

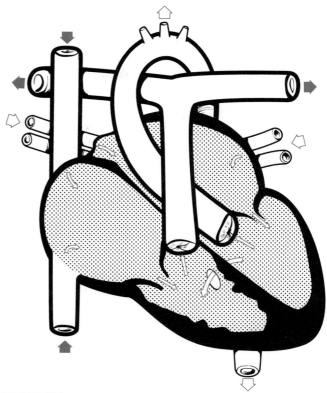

Figure 26-3 Ventricular septal defect.

PATENT DUCTUS ARTERIOSUS

The ductus arteriosus is a large vessel that connects the main pulmonary artery to the descending aorta (Figure 26-4). It usually closes soon after birth but dilates (remains patent) in response to hypoxia or prostaglandins E1 and E2.[147] The ability to maintain patency of the ductus arteriosus becomes important in certain cyanotic heart defects (to be discussed later). Spontaneous closing of the ductus arteriosus can create a critical situation in the infant with an undiagnosed heart defect. A high incidence of patency is found in premature infants because of respiratory distress syndrome and the resulting hypoxia.

Several options are available if the PDA fails to close spontaneously or with medication. One option is video-assisted thoracoscopic surgery, which involves several small thoracostomies and results in no chest wall muscles being cut and no rib retraction.[109] Another option is transcatheter coil occlusion performed by cardiac catheterization, which can be an outpatient procedure. Video-assisted and coil occlusion techniques are less traumatic, can reduce hospital stay,[120] and may decrease the risk of scoliosis, which is associated with thoracotomy. The traditional left thoracotomy incision is the standard operative approach if the above cannot be performed. The ductus is ligated and sutured.

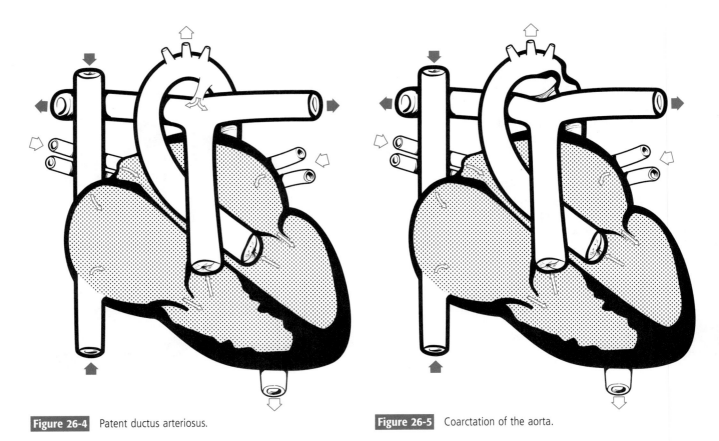

Figure 26-4   Patent ductus arteriosus.

Figure 26-5   Coarctation of the aorta.

COARCTATION OF THE AORTA

Coarctation of the aorta is defined as a narrowing or closing of a section of the aorta (Figure 26-5). PDA was observed in approximately 23% of diagnosed cases of coarctation of the aorta.[249] Infants with a severe narrowing may develop left ventricular failure.[89] Early repair is necessary when a child is severely symptomatic. The child or adult without symptoms may go undiagnosed until a routine physical examination reveals an abnormally high upper extremity blood pressure.

The coarctation can be treated via cardiac catheterization using a balloon that is inflated in the constricted area. Surgical intervention is another method of treating coarctation of the aorta. Access to the aorta is gained through a left thoracotomy, after which the aorta is repaired with an end-to-end anastomosis, a subclavian flap, or a patch aortoplasty.[249]

PULMONARY STENOSIS

Pulmonary stenosis, a narrowing of the right ventricular outflow tract, is classified by the location of the narrowing relative to the pulmonary valve. It often occurs in association with other heart defects. Timing of intervention depends on the severity of the narrowing and the degree of functional compromise, as well as on when pressure in the right ventricle becomes too high. Intervention is generally a valvulotomy that is performed via cardiac catheterization. Surgery when necessary is performed through a median sternotomy; the type of surgical procedure depends on the site of narrowing. A valvotomy may be performed, or, in severe cases, the valve may need to be replaced.[177]

AORTIC STENOSIS

Aortic stenosis, a narrowing of the left ventricular outflow tract, is classified by its relation to the aortic valve (supravalvular, valvular, or subvalvular) (Figure 26-6). The narrowing will cause the left ventricle to work harder to pump blood through the narrowing. An aortic valvotomy is performed via cardiac catheterization in infants and children with symptomatic stenosis. In severe cases, surgery may be required for a valvulotomy, or a valve replacement may be necessary if a valvulotomy cannot be performed.[255]

CYANOTIC DEFECTS

TETRALOGY OF FALLOT

The tetralogy of Fallot is the most common cyanotic cardiac defect, accounting for almost 50% of all cyanotic lesions. The primary abnormalities that occur in the tetralogy of Fallot

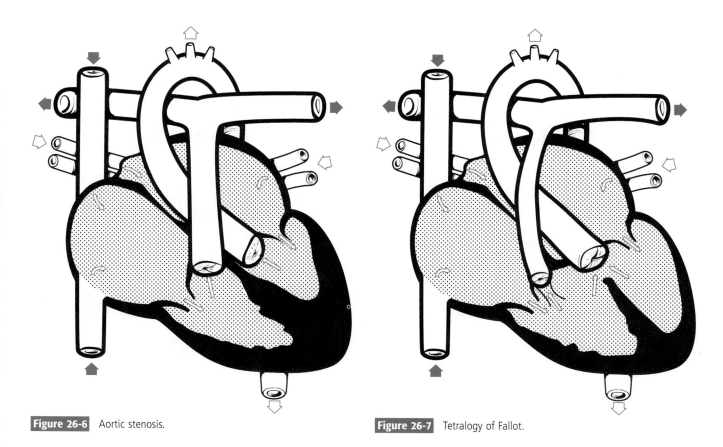

Figure 26-6 Aortic stenosis.

Figure 26-7 Tetralogy of Fallot.

are a VSD, right ventricular outflow tract obstruction, an aorta that overrides the right ventricle, and hypertrophy of the right ventricle (Figure 26-7).[143] Clinical manifestations of the defect depend on the severity of obstruction of the right ventricular outflow tract. With increasing obstruction, an increase in cyanosis is observed that becomes more marked when the child is overexerted or upset. Clubbing of the nail beds occurs and becomes more apparent after the first 6 to 8 months. The child's height and weight are often affected. Cyanotic or blue episodes occur, which are thought to be caused by an abrupt decrease in pulmonary blood flow and are characterized by dyspnea, syncope, and deepening cyanosis.[143,188] Cyanotic episodes are typically relieved by squatting or by bringing the knees to the chest. These maneuvers are believed to increase systemic vascular resistance and ultimately to increase pulmonary blood flow. Oxygen or morphine or both may need to be administered.[143]

Surgical intervention depends on the patient's symptoms and overall clinical picture. If possible, a complete repair is usually done early in life. Early palliation may be necessary if an infant is severely involved and would probably not survive corrective surgery. The palliative procedure used most often is a Blalock-Taussig (BT) shunt performed through a thoracotomy. The BT shunt involves an anastomosis of the subclavian artery to the pulmonary artery, providing increased pulmonary blood flow while the infant

gains more time to grow before undergoing corrective surgery. Mild growth retardation may occur in the upper extremity on the side of the shunt, but it has not been viewed as a major problem.[188] Another important consequence of early palliation is continued cyanosis until complete repair is performed.

Corrective surgery involves closing the VSD and relieving the right outflow tract obstruction. After surgical repair, an exercise stress test is warranted before the initiation of an exercise program because of a 14% incidence of ventricular arrhythmias at rest and a 30% incidence during exercise.[82] Early and late mortality rate was observed to be 4.5%.[47]

TRANSPOSITION OF THE GREAT ARTERIES

In transposition of the great arteries, the pulmonary artery arises from the morphologic left ventricle, and the aorta arises from the right ventricle (Figure 26-8).[42] In the absence of other defects, systemic blood returns to the body unoxygenated and pulmonary blood returns to the lungs fully oxygenated. This situation is obviously not compatible with life unless the ductus arteriosus remains patent. Immediate intervention, usually with infusion of prostaglandin E1, is necessary to keep the ductus arteriosus open. An atrial septostomy is performed by a cardiac catheterization to keep the child alive until surgical intervention occurs.

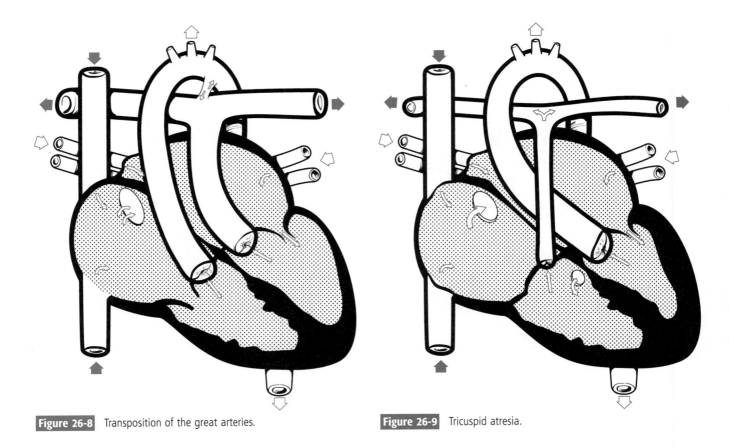

Figure 26-8 Transposition of the great arteries.

Figure 26-9 Tricuspid atresia.

The type of surgical intervention used for correction of transposition of the great arteries depends largely on the surgeon's preference. In most institutions, the arterial switch procedure is performed, correcting the abnormal anatomy. This is the preferred technique, when anatomically possible. Surgery during the first 2 to 4 weeks of life is preferred so that the left ventricle meets the systemic demands. Surgical repair occurs through a median sternotomy and involves transecting the aorta and pulmonary artery. The coronary arteries are excised with a wide button of aortic tissue and are reimplanted in the old pulmonary arterial vessel; the great vessels are then switched and anastomosed, so that the aorta connects to the left ventricle and the pulmonary artery connects to the right ventricle. The arterial switch procedure produces results that are free of the dysrhythmias and right ventricular failure associated with the techniques described previously.[42]

In some institutions, a Mustard or Senning technique is used to redirect the venous return to the atria by baffles or flaps of atrial wall, respectively.[62,240] These techniques leave the right ventricle as the pumping chamber for the systemic system.

The Rastelli procedure is a surgical technique used when a severe left ventricular outflow tract obstruction and a VSD coexist. Repair usually occurs when the child is between 4 and 6 years old. A conduit diverts blood from the left ventricle through the VSD and the right ventricle to the aorta, a right ventricle–to–pulmonary artery conduit is formed, and any previous shunts are eliminated.[259] Therapists may see teenage or young adult patients who have had this repair.

Reoperation for conduit enlargement is not uncommon. Depression of right ventricular function over time has been reported in some patients whose defects were corrected by these procedures.[124,178]

TRICUSPID ATRESIA

Tricuspid atresia is failure of development of the tricuspid valve, resulting in lack of communication between the right atrium and the right ventricle. Usually, an ASD or a VSD or both exist to allow pulmonary blood flow (Figure 26-9). Right-to-left shunt allows mixing of unoxygenated and oxygenated blood, causing the child to be cyanotic. The right ventricle is frequently underdeveloped.

Surgical repair is staged, with the initial operation shunting blood from the body to the lungs with a BT shunt through a thoracotomy. If the VSD is large and too much blood is going to the lungs, however, a band may be placed around the pulmonary artery to decrease blood flow to the lungs. The child remains cyanotic for several years. The next stage of surgical repair is often the Fontan procedure (or a modification thereof), performed through a median sternotomy in which the right atrium is attached to the pulmonary artery or directly to the right ventricle, using a conduit or baffle. The VSD may be surgically closed.[144] It is not uncommon to have significant chest tube drainage for weeks after Fontan surgery, thereby increasing the length of hospital stay.

In some institutions, a bidirectional Glenn procedure performed before the Fontan procedure leads to an improved outcome. In the Glenn procedure, the superior vena cava is anastomosed to the right pulmonary artery. The child remains cyanotic but gains time for growth before undergoing the Fontan operation.

PULMONARY ATRESIA

Pulmonary atresia occurs when the pulmonary valve fails to develop, resulting in obstruction of blood flow from the right side of the heart to the lungs. Blood flow to the lungs is initially maintained by a PDA. An ASD or a VSD may also be present, allowing shunting of blood from the right to the left side of the heart and ultimately back to the body. The size of the right ventricle may vary, affecting later surgical decisions. Early intervention involves maintaining patency of the ductus arteriosus to increase blood flow to the lungs until surgery can be performed. An atrial septostomy is usually performed during the initial cardiac catheterization. A BT shunt is often performed as soon as possible. Later surgery involves ligating the previous shunt, closing the ASD, and opening the pulmonary valve by a valvulotomy, an infundibular graft, or a right ventricle-to-pulmonary artery conduit. If the ventricle is poorly developed, the Fontan procedure may be performed to provide communication through a conduit between the right atrium and pulmonary artery.[198] Children remain cyanotic during their early developmental years until the Fontan operation is performed.

TRUNCUS ARTERIOSUS

Truncus arteriosus occurs when the aorta and the pulmonary artery fail to separate in utero and form a common trunk arising from both ventricles (Figure 26-10). Four grades of the condition are differentiated, depending on the location of the pulmonary arteries. Early surgical intervention is necessary. Surgical repair is provided through a median sternotomy and involves removing the pulmonary arteries from the truncus, closing the VSD, and connecting the pulmonary arteries to the right ventricle by an extracardiac baffle. Mortality rates are lower in patients operated on in the first 6 months of life (9% vs. 18% for later repair).[174,190]

TOTAL ANOMALOUS PULMONARY VENOUS RETURN

Total anomalous pulmonary venous return occurs when the pulmonary veins fail to communicate with the left

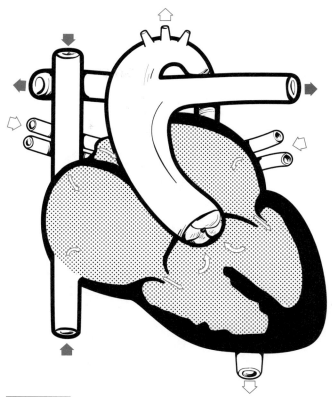

Figure 26-10   Truncus arteriosus.

atrium and instead connect to the coronary sinus of the right atrium or to one of the systemic veins. The ductus arteriosus often remains patent (Figure 26-11). The increase in flow through the right side of the heart and into the lungs may lead to congestive heart failure. Anastomosis of the pulmonary veins to the left atrium through a median sternotomy is usually performed as soon as possible. Postoperative ventilation may be difficult because of stiffness and wetness of the lungs from the previous excessive blood flow.[41,105] Mortality rates continue to improve but remain nearly 30% for infants.[105] There is one reported case of a 48-year-old patient who is 47 years post repair for total anomalous pulmonary venous return.[56]

HYPOPLASTIC LEFT HEART SYNDROME

Hypoplasia (incomplete development or underdevelopment) or absence of the left ventricle and hypoplasia of the ascending aorta make HLHS the most common form of a univentricular heart, often coexisting with severe aortic valve hypoplasia. A PDA provides systemic circulation until surgical intervention. Without surgical intervention, death is certain. Hospital survival rate (the percentage of children who leave the hospital alive after surgery for HLHS) still lags behind the rate for other congenital heart surgeries, but the surgical survival rate is now 90%.[196] Bove reported that

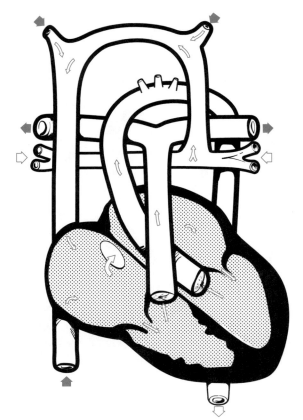

Figure 26-11 Total anomalous pulmonary venous return.

the survival rate after second-stage palliation is now 97%, and the survival rate is 81% after the Fontan operation.[39] Lloyd reported, however, that some of the survivors of the Fontan operation were observed to have neurologic conditions (6%) and respiratory conditions (11%).[152] Five-year survival rates are between 69% and 71%, depending on the patient's anatomy,[39] and 10-year survival rates were observed to be at 55%.[19]

Prenatal diagnosis and care are essential for the parents to prepare for and to be counseled about prognosis and surgical options. They also enable the parents and medical staff to plan for delivery and the immediate postpartum period.[19] Tibballs observed that prenatal diagnosis led to termination of pregnancy at a rate of 44% to 71% in Europe and 18% to 45% in the United States.[236] It was observed by Mahle and colleagues that prenatal diagnosis was found to possibly decrease postoperative neurologic events when compared with those diagnosed postnatally.[157]

Three options are available to parents of infants diagnosed as having HLHS. One option is no surgical intervention. As a second option, the child's name may be placed on a waiting list for a heart transplant; as a third, the child may undergo a series of palliative procedures.[46]

The initial surgical procedure (Norwood I[39]) involves enlarging the ASD, transecting the main pulmonary artery

and anastomosing it to the aorta, and reconstructing the aortic root. A BT or central shunt is placed to allow pulmonary blood flow. Some centers have recently begun using a right ventricle (RV)–to–pulmonary artery (PA) conduit as the first stage.[19,156,196,218] This procedure may require the second stage to be performed sooner, and the potential long-term consequences of cutting into the right ventricle are not known.[39] A third technique just recently offered for the extremely fragile child is a hybrid technique that combines interventional cardiac catheterization with surgery. This involves an atrial septostomy and placing a pulmonary artery band to restrict pulmonary blood flow and a stent in the arterial duct to hold it open. The child does not need to go on cardiopulmonary bypass.[19] Before the second stage, the child's oxygen saturation and activity level may start to decrease. Children may have more difficulty eating, especially with taking a bottle or nursing, which requires more energy. The second stage is a hemi-Fontan or bidirectional Glenn procedure, in which the superior vena cava is anastomosed to the pulmonary arteries and the BT shunt is ligated. The Fontan procedure may be performed several months to a few years later. This procedure provides continuity between the right atrium and the pulmonary artery, and pulmonary venous return is separated from the systemic system. As a result, the right ventricle pumps fully oxygenated blood to the body.[127,183,184] Table 26-1 summarizes the common types of congenital heart defects, their typical surgical repair, and associated impairments and functional limitations.

TRANSPLANTATION

Heart Transplantation

Cardiac transplantation is a viable option for children with end-stage heart failure secondary to congenital malformations or for children with cardiomyopathy. Introduction of immunosuppressive medications to control rejection has increased survival rates to 65% after 5 years, and a 92% survival rate in infants has been reported.[25]

The previous indication for transplantation in children was largely cardiomyopathy (62%). Since 1988, however, the number of transplants for congenital heart defects has surpassed that of cardiomyopathy.[141,191] The increase is related at least in part to the fact that cardiac transplantation is being offered more frequently as an option for children with HLHS. As a result, a greatly increased number of children younger than 1 year of age have received a cardiac transplant.[12,38,191,226] Razzouk and associates have observed 84% 1-year and 72% 7-year survival rates in infants younger than 1 year of age undergoing cardiac transplantation.[200]

Lamour and colleagues conducted a review of age, diagnosis, and previous surgery and their impact on children undergoing heart transplantation, using data from the Pediatric Heart Transplantation Study and the Cardiac Transplant Research Database.[145] They observed that morbidity

TABLE 26-1   **Summary of Congenital Heart Defects, Surgical Repair, and Associated Issues**

Type of Defect	Surgical Repair	Associated Issues	Physical Therapy Issues
Atrial septal defect	Suture or patch closure/device closure		
Ventricular septal defect (VSD)	Dacron patch closure/device closure	Failure to thrive; pulmonary hypertension	Failure to thrive
Atrial ventricular septal defect/ endocardial cushion defect	Pericardial patch	Down syndrome; failure to thrive	Developmental delay
Coarctation of the aorta	Stent or subclavian patch/end-to-end anastomosis	Hypertension	Upper extremity range of motion
Pulmonary stenosis	Valvotomy		
Aortic stenosis	Valvotomy; aortic valve replacement; conduit		
Tetralogy of Fallot	VSD closed; right ventricular outflow tract resected	"Tet" spells	
Transposition of the great arteries (dextro)	Arterial switch operation	Edema; poor left ventricle function	Decreasing exercise tolerance with age
Pulmonary atresia (PA) with a VSD	Blalock-Taussig shunt (BT); VSD closed; right ventricle–to–pulmonary artery conduit	Developmental delay; poor oral intake	Developmental delay; feeding issues
Pulmonary atresia without a VSD	Valvotomy/BT shunt; right ventricular outflow tract patch, ASD closed, Fontan procedure	Very sick postoperatively, low oxygen saturations	Developmental delay
Total anomalous pulmonary venous return	Anomalous veins connected to left atrium; ASD closed	Failure to thrive	Failure to thrive
Tricuspid atresia	1. Atrial septostomy, BT shunt 2. Bidirectional Glenn or hemi-Fontan procedure 3. Fontan procedure	Low oxygen saturations	Failure to thrive
Truncus arteriosus	VSD closure, right ventricle–to–pulmonary artery conduit	Pulmonary hypertensive crisis	Developmental delay; failure to thrive
Hypoplastic left heart syndrome	1. Division of the main pulmonary artery; suture PA to the aorta; BT shunt and patent ductus arteriosus ligation 2. Bidirectional Glenn or hemi-Fontan procedure 3. Fenestrated Fontan procedure	Low oxygen saturations	Poor oral feeders; developmental delay; may not crawl; neurologic and behavioral issues; decreased exercise tolerance, especially with right-to-left shunt

was higher post heart transplant in patients with CHD (86%) than in those with cardiomyopathy (94%). This extensive study revealed a 5-year survival rate of approximately 80% in patients with transplants performed from 1990 to 2002. Other variables related to increased morbidity included long ischemic times, history of Fontan pretransplant, and older recipient age. The mortality rate was less for those undergoing a cardiac transplantation after a Glenn procedure than after a Fontan.[125] Griffiths evaluated patients with failing Fontan physiology and their response to heart transplantation.[100] They found that those patients who were transplanted because of impaired ventricular function had a lower mortality rate than those with preserved ventricular function, but with secondary problems such as protein-losing enteropathy, plastic bronchitis, ascites, and edema. Overall, more than 50% of patients who underwent heart

transplantation as a teenager were still alive 15 years later. This number is even higher for those transplanted as infants.[132] Of those survivors at least 10 years post transplant, 92% had no activity limitations, but 69% had issues with hypertension.

Surgery is performed through a median sternotomy and involves removal of the recipient heart with residual atrial cuffs remaining. The atria are reanastomosed with the donor heart, and then the great arteries are connected.[103] Severing of the vagus nerve and the cervical and thoracic sympathetic cardiac nerves leaves the heart denervated.[54,131] An intrinsic control system exists within the heart, so it is not dependent on innervation for function. Cardiac impulse formation occurs because of spontaneous depolarization of the sinoatrial node.[131] The sinus node firing rate is faster than the usual heart rate in resting humans, so the heart rate of an individual after transplantation is faster than normal.[241]

Several other influences on myocardial contractility remain, including the Frank-Starling effect, the Anrep effect, and the Bowditch effect. The Frank-Starling effect is the increase in cardiac output seen by an increase in stroke volume after increased input or venous return.[131] This is an important effect that helps the body meet its early oxygen needs for exercise after transplantation. With the Anrep effect retained, cardiac muscle increases its contractile force when aortic pressure rises (afterload). The Bowditch effect describes an augmented contractile force of the heart with an increase in heart rate.[54,131] The transplanted heart has an increased sensitivity to circulating catecholamines (epinephrine and norepinephrine). Epinephrine increases the heart rate and the force of myocardial contraction, and norepinephrine increases the peripheral vascular resistance.[54] Hormonal release takes several minutes to have an effect on heart rate and contractility. As a result, it is generally advised that patients perform several minutes of warm-up exercises before vigorous exercise. It also takes several minutes for the body to reduce the hormones to normal levels, so a cooldown period at the end of exercise is also advised. The resting heart rate is higher than usual in transplant recipients, and the peak heart rate is lower; both should be taken into account when transplant patients are exercising.[241]

Antirejection treatment begins with triple therapy of antimetabolites, antiproliferatives, and steroids (www.cumc.columbia.edu/dept/cs/pat/hearttx/medications.html). All serve to combat rejection at different cell lines. The use of steroids is discontinued as soon as possible and is reinstituted only if rejection occurs.[12,191] The use of steroids should be taken into consideration when the weight and height percentiles of transplant recipients are reviewed. Most children increase their weight dramatically without a concomitant increase in height.[78,191] Antirejection medicines can lead to bone loss, photosensitivity, thickening of the gums, muscle and bone weakness, headaches, increased potassium levels, nausea, and increased cholesterol levels.

Rejection is an ongoing issue in all transplant patients. Signs and symptoms of rejection range from fever, malaise, poor appetite, weight gain, tachycardia, tachypnea, and low urine output to poor perfusion, complete heart block, pulmonary edema, and shock.[103] Severe rejection has been observed in several adolescent transplant recipients after just one dose of immunosuppressive medicine is missed.

Several complications are common in the pediatric heart transplant population. Hypertension and seizures have been observed in a number of patients. Seizures are believed to be caused by high immunosuppressive medication levels; however, they generally do not recur once the patient is on a therapeutic dose of anticonvulsants.[78,191] Other central nervous system disturbances have been observed in children, ranging from lethargy and confusion to localized neurologic defects and behavioral disturbances. Central nervous system

dysfunction occurs more commonly in children than in adults; fortunately, the impairment is usually transient.[103] As more children survive successful initial cardiac transplant, the potential need for retransplantation increases. Availability of donors, long-term survival, and functional outcomes are factors that continue to be investigated.

CONDITIONS REQUIRING LUNG AND HEART-LUNG TRANSPLANTATION

More than 200 heart-lung transplantations take place each year, with only 5% of all transplants in children younger than 18 years of age.[115] Primary pulmonary hypertension and Eisenmenger syndrome are the indications for more than 50% of the heart-lung transplants that are being done, with a small percentage performed for CHD, and about 30% performed for cystic fibrosis. Primary pulmonary disease is the usual diagnosis of lung transplant recipients; however, some transplants are necessary secondary to lung failure caused by congenital heart defects. Lung transplants in these cases are usually associated with cardiac repair. Previous thoracotomy is no longer considered a contraindication for heart-lung or lung transplantation; however, it does increase the risk of perioperative bleeding.[258] The 3-month survival rate for children (1990–2002) was 90% after discharge from the hospital, with a 5-year survival rate of 80%.[145] The highest risk of dying is observed to occur within the first 6 months after transplant. The Kaplan-Meier survival rates after lung or heart-lung transplantation (1991–2007) at 1, 3, 5, and 10 years were 69%, 64%, 44%, and 39%, respectively.[97] In his review of pediatric lung transplantation, Sweet observed that the number of lung transplants each year hovers around 50 in the United States and around 70 internationally.[232]

The International Society for Heart and Lung Transplantation (ISHLT) registry reports a median survival of 4.3 years.[9] Survival after lung and heart-lung transplantation remains well below that seen with transplantation of other solid organs.[232]

The surgical procedure for a heart-lung transplantation is performed through a median sternotomy. The recipient heart and then lungs are removed. Donor organs are placed inside the chest cavity, with the trachea anastomosed several rings above the carina. The right atrial anastomosis is performed, followed by anastomosis of the aorta.[34] Because of the risk of tracheal dehiscence, an omentum wrap around the suture line is typically used.[99]

The surgical procedure for single-lung transplantation is performed through a thoracotomy incision. Removal of diseased lung is followed by placement of the donor lung. The bronchial anastomosis is completed with an omentum wrap, followed by anastomosis of the pulmonary artery.[33]

When both lungs are transplanted, pulmonary innervation is lost.[123] An early study observed bronchial hyperresponsiveness to inhaled methacholine, which was thought to be caused by denervation hypersensitivity.[91] Since that time, however, postganglionic cholinergic nerve responses have been observed to be intact, as demonstrated by a normal bronchoconstrictor response to a stimulant. Therefore, airway hypersensitivity is most likely a result of intact postganglionic cholinergic nerve response instead of denervation hypersensitivity.[229] Hypersensitivity was not observed during exercise.[91]

Because secretions below the tracheal anastomosis in the denervated lung do not excite the cough reflex, percussion, postural drainage, and breathing exercises are required to aid expectoration.[34] A certain amount of atelectasis is observed in all patients, especially when the transplanted lungs must be compressed to fit into the thoracic cage.[123] Pulmonary edema is also commonly observed in the early postoperative period. Positive end-expiratory pressure is often used with mechanical ventilation to reduce atelectasis and pulmonary edema.[258]

The diagnosis of rejection is made on the basis of clinical signs and symptoms suggesting a deterioration in function. Chest radiographic findings and pulmonary function test results are noninvasive indicators. If necessary, a transbronchial biopsy is performed when patients are breathless and febrile and have rales and wheezes on auscultation.[117]

Pulmonary infection occurs in most transplant recipients, usually repeatedly. Obliterative bronchiolitis is a common posttransplant complication that has been reported to affect 71% of long-term survivors.[90,225] The acute phase of obliterative bronchiolitis is characterized by varying degrees of bronchiolar obstruction by plugs of granulation tissue; in the chronic phase, the bronchioles are partially to completely occluded.[11] Severe damage may necessitate retransplantation. With improvements in immunosuppression, obliterative bronchiolitis is becoming less common in adults; the same progress is anticipated in children. In spite of all of the progress made in immunosuppression, heart and lung transplant recipients still suffer from many adverse effects including infection, malignancy, organ dysfunction, and toxicity, as well as chronic infection.[201] Bronchiolitis obliterans remains the most common cause of late mortality.[9]

Education of parents and children about the implications and ramifications of a heart, heart-lung, or lung transplantation must be thorough and frank, including discussion of the implications of being on a waiting list and the extent of postoperative care provided after transplantation. Geographic and social dislocation may occur during assessment and during the wait for a transplant.[251] Warner stresses that families must be aware that, although transplantation is a last resort, it still may not be the answer.[251] Many centers require transplant candidates to participate in a formal exercise rehabilitation program before receiving the transplant to minimize postoperative complications, maximize the success of the transplant, and assess compliance. Compliance before transplantation may be an indicator of posttransplant compliance. Noncompliance is a contraindication

for transplantation because rigid adherence to the immunosuppressive regimen is imperative. Missed doses of immunosuppressants can result in death.

INOTROPIC SUPPORT

Intravenous inotropic support is commonly used for end-stage congestive heart failure in the pediatric population.[31] Inotropic agents are drugs that increase stroke work at a given preload and afterload.[228] These drugs include digoxin, dopamine, norepinephrine, epinephrine, isoproterenol, dobutamine, amrinone, and milrinone. Previously, these drugs have often been limited to in-hospital use because of the need for close monitoring and supervision.[31] Recently there has been a trend to complete outpatient inotropic support with medications such as milrinone as a bridge to transplantation. Berg and colleagues reported the use of home inotropic support in 14 children with end-stage congestive heart failure and found minimal complications as well as substantial cost-savings and improved family dynamics.[31] McBride and associates also reported on the safety of a monitored exercise program for pediatric heart transplant candidates on multiple inotropic support.[169] They found that patients were able to engage in an aerobic and musculoskeletal conditioning program three times per week with no adverse episodes of hypotension or significant complex arrhythmias. Physical therapists need to be aware of the increased use of these medications in the home setting. As noted, studies are showing safety with activity while on inotropic support. Patients, however, still need to be carefully monitored when engaging in therapeutic activities while on inotropic support.

TECHNOLOGICAL SUPPORT

Mechanical ventilation is common after open-heart surgery in the pediatric patient but should not deter the physical therapist from beginning treatment. Recent improvements in cardiopulmonary bypass, decreased operating time, and improved postoperative fluid management have allowed early extubation, often within 8 hours of surgery.[197] This has led to decreased costs, early patient mobility, and fewer respiratory complications. Some pediatric patients, however, may require the use of high-frequency jet ventilation in the period after open-heart surgery; this will prevent initiation of early physical therapy. High-frequency jet ventilation introduces a small tidal volume at a very rapid rate. Its use allows delivery of oxygen and removal of carbon dioxide at reduced mean airway and peak inspiratory pressures, and it is often used in unstable patients for whom physical therapy is contraindicated.[182] The three main advantages of high-frequency ventilation over conventional approaches to ventilation are improvement in the ventilation/perfusion ratio, less reduction of cardiac output, and minimized barotrauma.[171]

Nasal intermittent positive pressure ventilation has been used for short periods in the pediatric surgical patient who has had difficulty remaining extubated. This type of ventilation provides respiratory support through a preset tidal volume or inspiratory time, resulting in improved arterial blood gas tensions, improved alveolar ventilation, and decreased work of breathing.[35] Nitric oxide is now being used successfully with patients who have pulmonary hypertension postoperatively.[214]

Extracorporeal membrane oxygenation (ECMO) may be used for cardiovascular support in children after open-heart surgery. Indications for biventricular support by ECMO in the early postoperative period include progressive hypotension, increased ventricular filling pressures, poor peripheral perfusion, decreased urine output, and decreased mixed venous oxygen saturation.[72,135] ECMO is especially effective in treating conditions with right-sided heart failure and has been used as a support while the patient awaits a heart, heart-lung, or lung transplant.[253] The ECMO pump takes over oxygenation and perfusion of the child's body while the heart and lungs are "rested." ECMO is also used as a bridge to surgery in the severely compromised patient who is too ill to undergo repair immediately. ECMO is capable of providing support for several days to at most a few weeks[13] and is associated with severe complications such as cerebral infarction, brain hemorrhage, renal failure, and multiorgan system failure.[118] Patients on ECMO must remain intubated and sedated and therefore are unable to be mobilized while on support.[118] Bautista-Hernandez and associates observed that 62% of their patients survived to discharge from the hospital—patients who probably would not have survived their initial surgery without EMCO first to stabilize them.[26]

VENTRICULAR ASSISTIVE DEVICES

Children in the United States awaiting heart transplantation face the highest waiting list mortality of any solid-organ transplantation procedure.[48] Because of long wait times and limited donor availability, the use of mechanical circulatory support devices for children is increasing. Goldman and associates have suggested that the use of mechanical circulatory support devices as a bridge to transplant has been shown to decrease waiting list mortality and improve the efficiency of organ utilization in children.[96]

As previously noted, young children with the most severe heart failure are most often supported with ECMO.[118] Another approach uses ventricular assistive devices (VADs). VADs, circulatory pumps that supplement or completely replace the pumping function of one or both ventricles, have been used extensively in the adult population as a bridge to a transplant device or to a recovery device for many years. Their use in the pediatric population, however, has been limited because of limited availability of devices that meet pediatric physiology and cardiac flow needs.[13,205,235] Bastardi

and colleagues and others have suggested that despite the lack of pediatric specific devices, VADs are a viable option to be used as a bridge to transplant therapy or in some cases to recovery in the pediatric population.[24,45,108,205]

Currently, a limited number of VADs are available for use in the pediatric population. None at the time of publication have U.S. Food and Drug Administration (FDA) premarket approval for long-term use in children with heart failure.[235] Some devices, including the HeartMate left ventricular assist system (Thoratec Laboratories Corporation, Pleasanton, CA), Thoratec VAD (Thoratec Laboratories Corporation), and Ambiomed BVS 5000 (Ambiomed Inc., Danvers, MA), have been FDA approved to support children and adolescents with body surface greater than 0.7 m^2 for extracorporeal support and 1.4 m^2 for implantable support.[13,234,235,254] The MicroMed-DeBakey VAD (Micromed Technology, Houston, TX), the Jarvik 2000 (Jarvik Heart Inc., New York, NY) and the HeartMate II axial flow pump (Thoratec Laboratories Corporation) can be employed on a case-by-case approval basis for compassionate use in the treatment of pediatric patients with heart failure.[13] The MicroMed-DeBakey VAD Child has received a humanitarian device exemption from the FDA for use in pediatric patients 5 to 16 years of age with class IV end-stage heart failure and for those listed as candidates for transplantation.[13]

In the United States, options are very limited for the infant and young pediatric population. The primary device used in the United States for this population is the Berlin Heart Excor (Berlin Heart AG, Berlin, Germany). This pneumatically driven, pulsatile VAD may be used as a left ventricular assistive device (LVAD) or as a biventricular assistive device (BiVAD). The Berlin Heart Excor supports a variety of blood pumps capable of delivering stroke volumes from 10 to 80 ml, making it suitable for use in children as small as 3 kg through full-size adults.[108,205,235] The Berlin Heart Excor is available for use in infants to adolescents on a case-by-case approval basis through a formal petition of approval from the FDA.

In May 2007, the FDA granted a conditional investigative device exemption approval for the Berlin Heart Excor PVAD.[235] Rockett and associates have reported their experience with use of the Berlin Heart Excor.[205] Between April of 2005 and May of 2008, 17 patients underwent implantation with the Berlin Heart Excor system. Eleven of those patients went on to transplant, 2 patients underwent explantation due to recovery, and 3 died while on support; 1 patient remained on support at the time of publication of the study. Malarisrie and colleagues reported similar findings with 8 patients with the Berlin Heart Excor implanted.[163] Five patients survived until transplant, and 3 died while on support. Of note, in both reports a high incidence of neurologic complications was noted, with 7 of 11 patients reported by Rockett[205] and 5 of 8 patients reported by Malarisrie.[163] Despite the high level of neurologic complications in both studies, many children survived to transplant who would likely have died otherwise without use of a VAD system.

Use of a VAD or other mechanical support system offers other benefits as well. Most notably for physical therapists is the ability to mobilize and engage in aggressive physical therapy soon after implantation of a VAD in children of all ages.[202,205] Experience at multiple centers has shown the benefits and safety of mobilizing patients after VAD implantation.[79,202,205] Early physical therapy should focus on positioning and prevention of contractures during the immediate postoperative period, while patients remain intubated. After extubation, progression will depend on the age and medical status of the patient.

In the infant and toddler population, consideration must be given to early positioning and handling. This stage will include significant family education encouraging holding and positioning and attempting to normalize positioning as much as possible.[202] Many times, families are very hesitant to handle and complete care for the patient soon after implantation. Through education and support, it is essential that parents and other family members gain comfort with handling and transferring the patient as medically appropriate. All care needs to be provided in coordination with the medical and nursing team.

As the infant or toddler becomes more stable, it is essential to provide as much of a normalized routine as possible, incorporating physical therapy, occupational therapy, speech therapy, and school and activity staff as appropriate. Consideration must be given to device limitations, but, as able, patients should be progressed through activities to facilitate achievement of typical developmental milestones. Each different device will present its own unique challenges, and significant collaboration and training among team members of all disciplines are required to provide the most comprehensive and appropriate care.[79,202]

For the older child and adolescent, many of the same considerations as noted for the infant and the toddler apply. An overall team approach should be implemented to normalize the daily schedule as much as possible. Therapy should focus on increasing the patient's independence with activities of daily living (ADLs), transfers, and mobility in early therapy sessions, with progression to higher-level functional activities and strengthening and endurance activities as the patient's condition allows. The goal is to have patients at peak conditioning and level of fitness at the time of transplantation. In this population, it is also important to discuss device safety and limitations with patients as appropriate.[202] If possible, movement and socialization opportunities should be provided off of the medical unit on a regular basis with appropriately trained staff.

Therapists working with the VAD population must be aware of the high neurologic complication rate seen within this population.[24,45] The therapist must be aware of developing symptoms during treatment and the need to aggressively treat deficits after neurologic insult occurs. The pediatric population has demonstrated significant functional recovery after neurologic complications, and the ability of patients to participate in therapy plays a large role in that recovery.[205]

Because of increasing recognition of the integral role that mechanical assistive devices play as a bridge to transplant in the pediatric population, there is a strong push for further development of devices that can be used in the pediatric population.[13,235] In 2004, the National Heart, Lung, and Blood Institute of the U.S. National Institutes of Health issued five contracts to help support the development of five novel pediatric circulatory support devices. These devices remain in various stages of development at this time.[235] If fully developed, these devices stand to greatly increase the routine use of circulatory support devices in the pediatric population.[235] Pediatric therapists are likely to see increased numbers of patients on these devices in a variety of settings. Developing comprehensive programs and management plans will be integral to the functional and developmental progression of these patients.

MANAGEMENT OF ACUTE IMPAIRMENT

EDUCATION

Most acute impairments after thoracic surgical procedures occur in the immediate or early postoperative period. Many institutions are now using a preoperative education approach similar to the one put forth by Rockwell and Campbell, who described a preoperative program to assist in minimizing postoperative complications and to educate the parents of children 3 to 12 years of age.[206] Education today is typically facilitated through a virtual DVD or actual physical tour, role play, and coloring pages or reading a book that shows the child what will happen after surgery. Preoperative programs probably benefit the parents as much as the child in alleviating some anxiety about the surgery. Preoperative education for the child younger than 5 years is also described by Page.[188] The program lists concepts that may be helpful in teaching and preparing the child and family for surgery. A doll is used to educate the child about placement of tubes and incisions; pictures are used for parents. Preparing children before the surgery should assist in obtaining their cooperation after surgery and should minimize their fears. Preoperative education is now generally provided by nursing staff.

PULMONARY MANAGEMENT

The primary area to be addressed after heart repair is the pulmonary status of the patient. Numerous articles describe pulmonary complications and physical therapy in the postoperative pediatric patient.[3,20-23,80,140,233,245,248] Although intervention varies with the age of the child, the primary goals are to mobilize secretions, increase aeration, and increase general mobility (Figure 26-12).

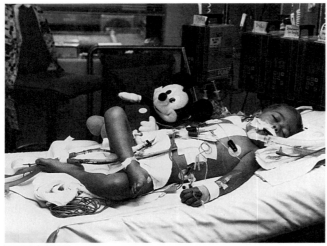

Figure 26-12 Two-year-old boy 24 hours after open-heart surgery.

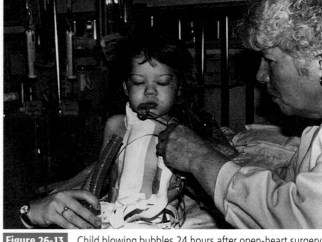

Figure 26-13 Child blowing bubbles 24 hours after open-heart surgery.

Mucous transport is slowed after surgery, which can lead to atelectasis.[80] Atelectasis also occurs secondary to an altered breathing pattern, prolonged positioning in supine, and possible diaphragmatic dysfunction in the early postoperative period.[21] In early studies by Bartlett and coworkers, lack of deep breaths was observed as a causative factor in atelectasis.[20,22] The yawn maneuver or prolonged inspiration with normal or increased inflation prevented atelectasis.[23] Bartlett observed that a collapsed lung expands only after the normal lung is fully inflated.[21] This is achieved with prolonged inspiration. The restriction in ventilation has also been attributed to incoordination and reduction of rib expansion after sternotomy.[153]

Incentive spirometry is an effective tool for reducing the occurrence of atelectasis in the pediatric population.[140] The primary emphasis with incentive spirometry or any other respiratory intervention should be on prolonged inspiration. When the inspiration is held for at least 3 seconds, arterial oxygen tension improves.[250] Huckabay and Daderian observed an increase in compliance with breathing exercises after surgery when children were given a choice and some control regarding breathing exercises.[114] With young children, tools such as bubble blowing or blowing on a windmill can be used (Figure 26-13).[206] Although these are expiratory maneuvers, a child often takes in a large inspiration before exhaling. Other respiratory techniques, such as percussion and postural drainage, vibration, segmental expansion, and assisted cough techniques (Figure 26-14), can be performed to mobilize secretions and increase aeration.[116]

Segmental expansion techniques may be performed to reduce postoperative complications and increase segmental aeration.[248] These techniques are performed by placing a hand over a particular segment and allowing it to move with the ventilator or respiratory cycle. Gentle pressure may be applied to the chest wall during exhalation at the end

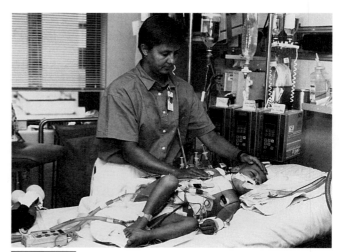

Figure 26-14 Child receiving percussion after open-heart surgery.

of the expiratory phase, just before the inspiratory phase. This facilitates airflow to the specific segment.[165] When a specific lobe or segment has decreased aeration, this technique, used in conjunction with gentle sustained pressure on the opposite upper lobe, may increase aeration to the affected area. When the patient is in a sidelying position, gentle rocking may stimulate segmental expansion and relax the patient.[165] This technique is particularly effective when the child is upset or does not tolerate percussion or other treatment techniques. It may decrease the respiratory rate and is especially useful with infants who cannot respond to verbal relaxation instructions. Segmental expansion techniques are also beneficial when the patient is having excessive bleeding after surgery and use of more vigorous techniques is contraindicated.[128] The authors have used this technique with lung transplant recipients who have been unable to cooperate or follow commands for deep breathing and coughing and found it to work well in decreasing atelectasis and increasing oxygen saturation. Segmental expansion techniques performed before other respiratory techniques may further enhance their benefit. Percussion may need to be performed to assist in removal of excess secretions. Percussion is defined as rhythmic clapping with cupped hands over the involved lung segment performed throughout the respiratory cycle, with the goal of mechanically dislodging pulmonary secretions.[119] Vibration also assists in mobilization of secretions. It is performed by creating a fine oscillating movement of the hand on the chest wall just before expiration and continuing until the beginning of inspiration.[119]

Both percussion and vibration techniques can be performed in conjunction with postural drainage. Optimal positions are described by Crane and are pictured in Frownfelter's text on chest physical therapy.[57] Positioning must be used with caution in the postoperative patient; use of the Trendelenburg position, for example, is often contraindicated after open-heart surgery. It is important to confirm with the nurse or the physician whether it is even suitable for the child to be flat in bed. Despite limitations, percussion and vibration can be performed in the positions available. It has been the authors' experience that children respond well to both percussion and vibration, even on the first postoperative day. Encouraging the child to tell you if the treatment hurts—because it should not be painful—often facilitates cooperation. It may also be helpful to coordinate the treatment with administration of pain medications. Percussion may be contraindicated when platelets are low, pulmonary artery pressures are too high, or the child becomes too agitated with treatment. Vibration can generally be safely used instead. Blood pressure and intracardiac pressures should be closely monitored throughout treatment because they are indicators of intolerance to treatment. The physician usually establishes parameters, set on an individual basis.

Massery described a counterrotation technique for altering respiratory rate in the neurologically impaired patient that has been safely used in children after open-heart surgery through a median sternotomy only.[165] The technique has been used by the authors to slow the respiratory rate and increase expansion of the lateral segment. It generally relaxes patients and increases their tidal volume. When the technique is used in the postoperative cardiac patient, extreme caution must be exercised to avoid disturbing chest tubes and other intravenous lines. This treatment is recommended only after intracardiac lines have been removed. The sternal incision has not been a problem; because it is stable, it does not undergo any mobilization during application of this technique. The counterrotation technique is performed with the therapist standing behind the sidelying patient near the patient's buttocks. One hand is placed on the anterior iliac spine and the other hand is placed on the patient's posterior shoulder. On inspiration the hand on

the buttocks pulls down and posteriorly, while the hand on the shoulder gently pushes up and anteriorly. On expiration, the therapist's hands and the patient's body return to neutral. This is repeated several times in cycle with the patient's breathing. It should be very relaxing and comfortable for the patient.

The techniques just described not only facilitate increased lung expansion but also mobilize secretions. Once mobilized, secretions act as an irritant in the airway when the child takes a deep breath, and a spontaneous cough usually occurs.[21] The child may need some assistance in removing excess secretions, owing to lack of cooperation or to inability to cooperate secondary to age. This may be accomplished by coughing or airway suctioning.

If the child is intubated, suctioning is done to clear secretions and maintain patency of the tube. Children who have cyanotic heart defects, such as HLHS, tend to desaturate during suctioning. It is extremely important to hyperventilate these patients with oxygen and a resuscitation bag before and after suctioning and to monitor their oxygen saturation and other hemodynamic parameters.[37,76,116,208] It is also important to monitor how far the suction catheter is inserted, so it only goes approximately 0.5 to 1 cm past the end of the endotracheal tube and does not touch the patient's carina. During suctioning, normal sterile saline may be instilled through the endotracheal tube to thin the thickened secretions. If the child is not intubated and is unwilling to cough, nasal pharyngeal suctioning may be performed to stimulate a cough and clear secretions. If the child is able to drink, a small sip of water or juice may also stimulate a cough. During coughing, a blanket or a soft stuffed animal may be used to help splint the incision and minimize discomfort.[128]

PAIN

Most major institutions that perform cardiac surgery on children have pain management teams that assist the surgical team in monitoring and managing the child's postoperative pain because uncontrolled pain can be detrimental to the child's recovery. The FLACC scale is now used frequently to determine if the child is in pain (Table 26-2).

Pain medications must be given regularly, not only to reduce anxiety (which further increases pain from splinting) but also to encourage deeper breathing. A child in pain does not take deep breaths, even spontaneously. Morphine, a commonly used postoperative narcotic, depresses spontaneous sighing; patients receiving morphine should be encouraged to voluntarily take deep breaths.[69] Other techniques now being used to manage postoperative pain include epidural morphine administration and patient-controlled analgesia.[7,260] Both have proved effective in management of postoperative pain, especially in thoracotomy patients. Proper pain management is also extremely important in mobilizing the patient.

TABLE 26-2 **FLACC Scale**

Categories	Scoring		
	0	**1**	**2**
Face	No particular expression or smile	Occasional grimace or frown, withdrawn, disinterested	Frequent to constant quivering chin, clenched jaw
Legs	Normal position or relaxed	Uneasy, restless, tense	Kicking, or legs drawn up
Activity	Lying quietly, normal position, moves easily	Squirming, shifting back and forth, tense	Arched, rigid or jerking
Cry	No cry (awake or asleep)	Moans or whimpers; occasional complaint	Crying steadily, screams or sobs, frequent complaints
Consolability	Content, relaxed	Reassured by occasional touching, hugging, or being talked to; distractable	Difficult to console or comfort

Merkel, S. (1997). The FLACC: A behavioral scale for scoring postoperative pain in young children. *Pediatric Nurse, 23,* 293–297. Copyright 1997 by Jannetti Company, University of Michigan Medical Center.

EARLY MOBILIZATION

Early mobilization is generally performed by the nursing staff. For physical therapists who may be involved, the following section reviews the importance of early mobilization and how to begin early mobilization. Postoperative immobility can lead to a variety of problems, including reduced ventilation and perfusion distribution,[193] shallow breathing,[203,219] fever,[50] retention of secretions,[189] fluid shifts,[213] and generalized discomfort from immobility. The child should be mobilized as soon as possible to minimize these deleterious effects.

Range of motion (ROM) exercises should be initiated as soon as possible. It may not be possible to attain normal ROM immediately, because of discomfort or intravenous or arterial lines, but any movement helps to mobilize the patient. ROM exercises are extremely important for the child with a thoracotomy incision because this incision tends to produce more guarding than is produced by a median sternotomy. Passive to active-assisted shoulder ROM to 90 degrees of flexion is usually tolerable. Discomfort often occurs when the arm is returned to a neutral position. The therapist may apply gentle resistance to the arm as the child attempts to return the arm to a neutral position because contraction of the arm muscles tends to minimize discomfort.[128]

The child's position should be changed regularly to avoid retention of secretions in the dependent portion of the lung.[189] Regular turning has been observed to decrease postoperative fevers.[50] It also assists in decreasing postoperative chest wall immobilization, which is thought to decrease ventilation.[193] The supine position alone contributes to airway closure[60,203] and a shift in blood volume to the dependent side.[213]

Arterial oxygen saturation is also affected by body position because of ventilation and perfusion matching.[60] The supine position tends to decrease ventilation, which affects ventilation and perfusion matching and may ultimately decrease oxygen saturation. Positioning the patient effectively can reduce the pulmonary dysfunction that occurs most commonly when perfusion is greater than ventilation.[60] The prone position has been observed to be associated with a significantly higher arterial oxygen tension than the supine position,[75] as well as an increased tidal volume and improved lung compliance.[60] This position can be especially beneficial in preventing respiratory difficulty in a child who is extubated. The sidelying position has been observed to be a better position than the supine position for improving oxygenation.[15,60] In studies, adult patients became better oxygenated when the "good" lung was in the dependent position.[15,237] In children, however, the opposite was observed, namely, gas exchange improved with the good lung uppermost.[59] It has been observed in lung transplant recipients that regional differences in blood flow distribution produced by position changes may lead to significant changes in oxygenation. Positioning the patient in a sidelying position, with the best lung dependent, may improve ventilation and perfusion matching.[237] The best lung may or may not be the transplanted lung in the early postoperative period; thus tolerance to having the transplanted lung dependent should be confirmed with the surgeons before the patient is placed in this position.

Early ambulation after surgery reduces both pulmonary and circulatory complications.[252] It has been observed to be as effective as deep-breathing exercises in minimizing complications in adults.[65] Ambulation was observed to be beneficial in returning respiratory function toward normal by inducing more frequent and deeper sigh respirations.[219] Activity and mobility have been clinically observed to minimize chest tube output. At our center, children ambulate as soon as atrial lines and groin lines are removed and the child is extubated. Children often ambulate for the first time with

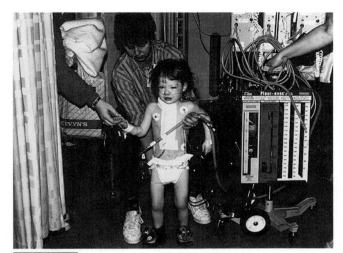

Figure 26-15   A child walking 1 day after open-heart surgery.

any or all of the following: central venous pressure line, peripheral intravenous line, arterial line, chest tubes, temporary pacemakers, and oxygen (Figure 26-15). The first walk is often only for 5 to 10 feet and may be difficult for the patient. Anxiety often plays as great a role in the perceived difficulty as does the discomfort. It may be beneficial for the patient to receive some pain medication before the first walk. Parents are anxious, so the benefits of early ambulation should be explained to them ahead of time, with emphasis on the problems that can occur by remaining in bed. This is also a good time to review with parents the importance of picking their child up under the bottom and back as they did when the child was an infant. They should avoid picking up the child under the child's arms for 4 to 6 weeks after surgery to allow the sternum time to heal.

MEDICAL COMPLICATIONS

Several medical complications can affect postoperative function. Secondary to phrenic nerve palsy, some children may have a paralyzed diaphragm after surgery that affects their early postoperative course, as well as their long-term respiratory status and endurance. The paralyzed diaphragm may persist but is seldom permanent.[164,176] In a recent study by Ross Russell and associates, phrenic nerve palsy was observed in as many as 20% of infants who underwent cardiac surgery, mechanical ventilation was at least an average of 72 hours in this group, and the risk of death before discharge from the hospital was greater than 10%.[212] The incidence was greater for those younger than 18 months of age, but two thirds of those with phrenic nerve palsy had fully recovered by 3 months postoperatively. Infants have horizontal ribs and lack the normal bucket handle movement, relying primarily on use of the diaphragm for respiration. Paralysis of the diaphragm by unilateral or bilateral phrenic nerve palsy can cause further respiratory problems,

including difficulty in weaning from the ventilator.[116] Noninvasive positive pressure ventilation has been successfully used for bilateral diaphragm paralysis until diaphragm function has returned.[138]

Prolonged mechanical ventilation does occur in some children, especially infants, after surgery for congenital heart defects. This has been associated with nosocomial pneumonia, higher surgical risk, increased postoperative fluid, and low cardiac output.[223] Some incidence of children requiring a tracheostomy and/or gastrostomy after congenital heart surgery has been reported. Performing these procedures sooner may allow for earlier discharge from the hospital. The incidence of tracheostomy after surgery is fairly low at 1% or less,[210] but Kelleher and colleagues reported that 28% of their patients undergoing a Norwood operation required nasogastric tubes for feeding or placement of a gastrostomy tube at discharge from the hospital.[130] Guillemaud and associates found that at least 3% of all children with cardiac defects who underwent surgery had some type of airway problem, the most common being vocal cord paralysis.[102] This should be taken into account when an infant is having difficulty coming off the ventilator or when treating an infant with difficulty with oral feedings.

Peroneal nerve palsy, usually caused by improper positioning of the lower extremity during surgery, is another potential complication of surgery. The resultant drastic alteration in the child's gait must be addressed as soon as possible. An ankle-foot orthosis can improve gait and should be necessary for only a short time.

Neurologic Implications and Complications

Postoperative neurologic impairments were long thought to be largely due to prolonged surgical time, usually related to length of hypothermic arrest, low cardiac output, or arrhythmias after surgery.[73,257] Recent research on infants with congenital heart defects, however, has indicated that preoperatively brain maturation is delayed,[148] cerebral blood flow is diminished,[149] and there is some incidence of mild ischemic lesions associated with periventricular leukomalacia.[149,159] Neurodevelopment has been noted to be affected postoperatively in children with repaired congenital heart defects possibly for several reasons, including how a child is rewarmed after surgery,[217] genetic factors,[84,264] seizures,[83] type of circulatory arrest,[28] and length of stay after surgery.[179] Seizures during the initial postoperative period are associated with a significant increase in abnormal neuromuscular findings. Frontal seizures were found to be associated with a lower Mental Developmental Index (MDI) (p = .03) score on the Bayley Scales of Infant Development II than is seen with nonfrontal seizures.[83]

Hemodynamic instability and coagulation disturbances are risk factors for postoperative neurologic problems in infants as well.[67] Thirty-five percent of premature infants weighing less than 2 kg who had open-heart surgery developed neurologic complications.[211] Neurologic consequences may be the result of an air embolus, a prolonged hypotensive period,[244] or complications of long-term cyanosis.[4] Choreoathetosis has been observed in some children after they have been on cardiopulmonary bypass. When a basal ganglia lesion is also seen, the prognosis is poor.[112] It is encouraging to note that of almost 700 children who underwent a Fontan operation, less than 3% suffered a stroke.[68] In an attempt to reduce the risk of neurologic injury during surgery, some centers are using continuous regional cerebral perfusion, especially during aortic arch reconstruction.[39] Many centers are using near-infrared spectroscopy to monitor cerebral oxygenation in the perioperative period, but in a review of the literature on this topic, Hirsch and colleagues found little substantial evidence to support that the use of perioperative near-infrared spectroscopy has an impact on neurologic outcomes.[110] Low regional cerebral oxygen saturation in the first 48 hours after the Norwood procedure was significantly correlated with an adverse outcome.[194]

This is an area of research that physical therapists could be involved in to correlate forms of monitoring and postoperative neurologic outcomes. The child who has suffered a neurologic insult requires both early intervention and long-term physical therapy. A child with severe extensor tone may benefit from inhibitive casts on the lower extremities and hand splints to decrease the effects of increased tone and to maintain ROM. Parent education concerning the impact of a neurologic insult, including information on handling and positioning the child with increased tone, appropriate stimulation, use of adaptive equipment, and long-term follow-up, should begin as soon as the diagnosis is confirmed.

AGE-SPECIFIC DISABILITIES IN THE IMMEDIATE POSTOPERATIVE PERIOD

The infant who undergoes surgery within the first few days after birth experiences immediate disruption of all aspects of typical newborn life. The infant is often sedated, restrained, and intubated, all of which interfere with being held, bundled, and fed. Parents need education about the areas of stimulation that are withdrawn from their child during this time and instruction in ways to compensate for this deprivation. The fact that their child is born with a congenital anomaly may further impede the attachment process.[154] The therapist assists the process by involving the parents in treatment as soon as possible and by educating them about engaging and calming their baby.

Toddlers who have cardiac surgery often recover very quickly with few impairments. Anxiety over being left alone during the hospitalization may be the biggest problem interfering with function in this age group.[154] The child may feel abandoned and may react by becoming passive and apathetic or, conversely, by becoming aggressive. These behaviors are more commonly observed in the child who is in the hospital for the first time, such as the child with an ASD.

Toddlers tend to be limited more by their parents' restrictions than by their own physical limitations.[52,154] Activity guidelines should be reviewed with parents on an ongoing basis; showing them by example may be even more helpful. Although it is beneficial to explain to the parents ahead of time what their child will experience, it may be helpful to wait to tell the toddler what is happening as it is happening. Connolly and colleagues evaluated children who underwent cardiac surgery at 5 to 12 years of age both preoperatively and postoperatively for posttraumatic stress disorder (PTSD) symptoms.[55] They found PTSD symptoms in 23% of the children, and 12% met criteria for PTSD. They also observed an increased number of symptoms correlated with an intensive care unit stay longer than 48 hours.

Adolescents who have cardiac surgery may need to be encouraged to move and may need to be assisted to become active. The parents are often more reluctant than the child about early mobilization, including ambulation. They should be reassured that it is beneficial for their child to move as soon as possible. Adolescents may choose to assert their independence and try to do everything for themselves, or they may choose to become totally dependent on their parents and hospital staff. Whichever situation occurs, young people benefit from early education about how to move and what they should be doing. This helps them to realize what is expected of them. They should be informed of what they need to do and should not be given a choice when the task is not optional.[244]

CHRONIC DISABILITIES AND ACTIVITY LIMITATIONS

Various disabilities and activity limitations occur as a result of primary impairments incurred by children with congenital heart defects (see Table 26-1). The disabling process may start very early secondary to poor attachment between parent and infant.[95] Infants who had cardiac surgery showed less positive affect and engagement than typical babies, making it even more stressful for mothers who are already distressed.[81] Poor attachment can lead to poor social development. The overprotection and excessive activity restrictions imposed by some parents further compound this disability. Parents have stated that they were afraid to permit activity in their child with CHD.[101] If this attitude is allowed to persist, the child's developmental and functional levels will surely suffer. It has been observed that maternal perceptions of the child's disease severity were a stronger predictor of emotional adjustment than was disease severity.[63] Emotional maladjustment may contribute to the poor self-esteem that is often noted in children with congenital heart defects. Limitations resulting from decreased activity, delayed development, poor self-esteem, overprotection by parents, and physical illness may lead to poor peer interactions. This may further limit a child with CHD from interacting with society. These issues should be addressed with parents and the child as early as possible to try to limit their effects on developmental progression and functional capabilities. Subsequent sections elaborate on various aspects of the disabling process across childhood and adolescence.

INFANCY

Recent research has been important in establishing the preoperative status of the brain, its development, and subsequent neurologic impairment in the infant with a congenital heart defect. Licht and associates assessed infants preoperatively with HLHS and transposition of the great arteries.[148] They found these infants to have head circumferences that were smaller by a whole standard deviation, as well as brain development that lagged a full month behind their gestational age, thus indicating that in utero brain development is affected by the cardiac defect. This group of researchers also found that preoperative cerebral blood is diminished, and was sometimes associated with periventricular leukomalacia.[149] Thus, children with congenital heart defects start off at a disadvantage neurologically and developmentally.

Infants with dextro-transposition of the great arteries who underwent a preoperative balloon atrial septostomy had an increased rate of embolic stroke compared with those who did not undergo balloon atrial septostomy.[179] Surveillance for this risk should be conducted when these patients are seen in the immediate postoperative period, or even later.

In children with CHD, several other contributing factors can lead to impairment and activity limitations in infancy. Common problems include poor feeding, poor growth, and developmental lag. Parents must constantly watch for signs and symptoms of congestive heart failure in their infant. These signs include the onset of rapid breathing, changes in behavior, edema, excessive sweating, fatigue, vomiting, and poor feeding.[52,263] Parental frustration and stress can impair early attachment to the infant. It has been observed during the first year of life that securely attached infants showed greater improvements in health than did insecurely attached infants.[94] Gardner and associates observed infants with cardiac defects to be consistently less engaging with their mothers when compared with infants without defects.[81]

When compared with healthy infants and infants with cystic fibrosis, infants with CHD were the least attached to their mothers, and their parents were the most stressed.[95] Normal attachment may be difficult, particularly with the very sick infant who is frequently hospitalized. The health care team should begin working with the parents as early as possible on how they can interact with their infant to facilitate attachment and avoid overstimulating their infant.

It is not uncommon for infants with CHD to be poor feeders, which further increases parental stress. Infants with corrected cyanotic heart defects had a significantly delayed first feed when compared with those infants who had undergone correction for an acyanotic defect. They also had a longer duration from first feed to discharge.[121] The delay in being able to feed their infant followed by possible difficulty with feeding may add stress to the parents.

Many of the major centers that perform surgical repair for some of the more complex cardiac defects treat children from all over the world. It is important to be aware of the nutritional state of the country of origin, the size of the child's parents, and the issues surrounding the surgery when a child's nutritional state is evaluated. Vaidyanathan and colleagues studied the nutritional status of children in South India after surgical repair for congenital heart defects and found that persistent malnutrition was predicted by birth weight and initial nutritional status as well as by parental anthropometry.[243]

Infants expend most of their energy during eating. In normal infants, decreased ventilation is observed during feeding, creating a decrease in the partial pressure of oxygen and an increase in the partial pressure of carbon dioxide.[166,167] This decrease in ventilation may seriously compromise the child with CHD and is compounded by the increase in metabolic rate. Not only does the child not eat well, but he or she also requires more calories to thrive.[88] When studying infants with CHD after surgery, Nydegger and colleagues found that an increased resting energy expenditure before surgery persisted in those repaired after 10 days of life; by 6 months of age, it was comparable to that in infants without CHD.[185] Abnormalities in mesenteric perfusion are documented in several studies, with mesenteric hypoperfusion noted after the Norwood operation.[61,107] This may lead to feeding intolerance in addition to difficulty in getting enough calories into the child's body.

Watching their child failing to thrive can be devastating to parents and can further increase their anxiety about feeding their child and trying to encourage adequate caloric intake.[88] The prolonged feeding time can be frustrating to parents and can make them feel inadequate.[40,154] If alternative feeding methods are used, such as nasogastric or gastrostomy tube feedings, parents should be educated not only on how to administer the feeding but also on how to hold and nurture their child during the feeding.[154] It may be helpful to tell parents that providing time for normal, nonstressful interaction may improve the parent-infant attachment and ultimately may improve the health of their infant. It is helpful to inform parents that the overall time that supplemental feedings are necessary varies with each child. Some parents have stated that they were able to remove supplemental feedings within 1 week of leaving the hospital; others have stated that it took months for their child to take enough by mouth to be able to discontinue supplemental feedings. Many parents have stated to these authors that their infant ate better at home, where it was possible to eat on demand and to have a more routine day.

Physical therapy assessment is sometimes needed to observe the infant feeding and parental interaction. Other problems unrelated to poor endurance may be exhibited by the infant with CHD. If oral-motor dysfunction exists, it should be addressed with parents as soon as possible. Some parents need assistance in how best to handle and support their child during feeding. It can be beneficial for parents to observe that their child does not feed well for anyone.

Poor growth is closely associated with poor feeding. It has been observed that infants with cyanotic heart disease have poor growth in height and weight, whereas infants with acyanotic heart disease, specifically those with a large left-to-right shunt, are severely underweight secondary to the marked increase in metabolism.[88] The child's growth improves after surgery but may not achieve typical parameters. This lack of catch-up growth is especially remarkable in children with cyanotic defects with a right-to-left shunt.[88,209]

Functional and activity limitations, especially delayed achievement of basic motor skills, can be observed in the infant with cardiac disease. Schultz and associates assessed the development of infants with CHD who had undergone repair before 6 months of age, and compared them with their twin siblings without CHD.[220] They found that infants with CHD had a more marked deficit on the Psychomotor Developmental Index (PDI) on the Bayley Scales of Infant Development II than on the MDI, but both indices were worse than those of their siblings without CHD. Decreased nutritional status and cardiac function may leave the infant too weak to expend the energy required for typical motor activity.[154] Some cyanotic children preferentially scoot around on their buttocks and, even after extensive intervention at home, do not crawl. They often go on to walking without ever crawling,[128] probably because of the increased energy expenditure associated with use of both upper and lower extremities in crawling. Cyanotic children also tend to have an internal mechanism that permits them to do only what they are physically capable of doing, given their oxygen saturation.[52] They often rest without cueing and can rarely be pushed beyond what they are willing to do. Intervention may or may not improve the child's functional abilities; however, it may do a great deal to relieve parental anxiety. Education should be focused on what the child is doing normally, such as using typical movement patterns, instead of on developmental lag based solely on age. Intervention should include parental education concerning areas the parent can work on with the child as part of regular family routines throughout the day, rather than in one focused block of time.

The presence of congestive heart failure is significantly associated with mental and motor developmental delay. Infants with congestive heart failure scored less well than expected on the Bayley Scales of Infant Development I as early as 2 months of age.[2] Haneda and associates observed a significant decrease in Gesell's developmental quotient in infants and children who had circulatory arrest time greater than 50 minutes.[106] This information is useful when working with parents to help them understand that their child is demonstrating typical developmental skills for a child with CHD. This does not mean that intervention cannot improve the situation. Parents should be encouraged to work with their child on developmental tasks that are challenging. If functional and activity limitations are minimized early, the effects of reparative surgery may be dramatic.

Neurologic impairment and functional limitations may also occur from external forces related to the surgical repair. Discrepancy exists among research study findings regarding the effects of deep hypothermia and circulatory arrest on the psychomotor and intellectual development of infants.[32,67,104,173,211,222] Messmer and associates observed no delay in psychomotor and intellectual development in infants after deep hypothermia.[173] Kaltman and associates evaluated neurodevelopmental outcome in infants after an early repair for a VSD.[129] The MDI and PDI for this group fell within the normal range unless they had a suspected or confirmed genetic syndrome. In another study, the researchers did not observe neurologic impairment after surgery, but they did observe mild developmental delays, most profoundly in cyanotic infants.[104] Bellinger and associates observed that children who had total circulatory arrest during the arterial switch operation scored lower on the Bayley Scales of Infant Development at 1 year of age than infants who had low-flow bypass.[29] They were also observed to have expressive language difficulties at 2.5 years of age and exhibited more behavior problems.[29] Deep hypothermic circulatory arrest greater than 40 minutes correlated with a greater occurrence of seizures postoperatively.[84] Clancy and associates observed seizures postoperatively in greater than 11% of infants in the immediate postoperative period.[51] All of the infants had undergone cardiopulmonary bypass during surgery.[51] The presence of a genetic syndrome was a strong predictor of a worse developmental outcome as measured by the PDI and MDI.[84] Gessler and associates performed neurologic examinations on infants preoperatively and postoperatively, which revealed mild asymmetries in muscle tone in just a third of the infants preoperatively and in almost two thirds postoperatively.[85] They also found that the inflammatory response to cardiopulmonary bypass has an adverse effect on neuromotor outcome. Recent research by Sahu and associates indicates that weaning the infant off bypass at lower temperatures lowers the risk for postoperative neurophysiologic dysfunction more than weaning at slightly higher temperatures.[217]

There is further need to identify those factors that can be consistently utilized to determine and lower risk for neurologic damage in young children after cardiac surgery.[238] In light of conflicting information in the literature, therapists should realize the potential for problems. Parents should be advised that their child might take longer than usual to accomplish developmental milestones. In a comprehensive review of the literature from the mid 1970's to the late 1990's, the overall long-term development of children after repair or palliation for CHD as infants was within the expected range for most standardized tests.[160]

PRESCHOOL PERIOD

The preschool child with chronic disabilities caused by CHD has grown up in the medical environment. This may help to alleviate some of the child's and the parents' anxieties when surgery is imminent. Parental anxieties can be exacerbated during this period, however, as they begin to realize the impact that their child's cardiac disease has on growth and development. The child's symptoms could be worsening, and another surgery may soon be needed. The parents' response and interaction during this period are important; it should be recognized that parents already have the tendency to be overprotective of their child, and this may increase during the preschool period.

The emotional adjustment of the child has been observed to be affected by the mother's perception of the severity of the child's illness more than by its actual severity.[63] If the mother perceives the child's disease to be more severe than it is and limits the child accordingly, the child's physical development and social participation may suffer. In acyanotic children, it has been observed that the intelligence quotient (IQ) was lower when associated with poorer adjustment, greater dependence, and greater maternal pampering and anxiety.[199] Activity limitations may be out of proportion compared with what the child is actually capable of doing. Intervention may need to be initiated to instruct parents on what activities the child is capable of performing, and on how the child self-limits activity without parental intervention. It should be noted that Visconti and associates observed that parents who were more stressed when their child with repaired CHD as an infant was 1 year old noted more behavior problems when their child was 4 years old.[247]

Atallah and associates looked at mental and psychomotor outcomes after the Norwood procedure and compared the traditional modified Blalock-Taussig shunt era versus the newer right ventricle–to–pulmonary artery shunt era.[8] The MDI was not different between groups; however, the PDI was significantly lower in the RV-to-PA shunt group. The RV-to-PA shunt group also had more frequent sensorineural hearing loss.

Children with CHD have been observed to have some developmental delay—especially those children with cyanotic disease.[29,71,199] Children with cyanosis scored significantly lower than acyanotic and typically developing children on all subscales of the Gesell Developmental Schedules[106] and on Stanford-Binet and Cattell intelligence tests.[199] Cyanotic children were observed to sit and walk later than acyanotic and typically developing children and were slower in speaking phrases than were children without disabilities.[71,199,224] Curtailment of physical activity in the child with

severe cardiac dysfunction interferes with the active manipulation of objects needed for adequate development of early sensorimotor processes.[199,224] This lack of opportunity may affect IQ scores, psychological development, and participation. Despite these challenges, intelligence and behavior are often within typical parameters.[93] In addition to intelligence, other factors to be considered include functional activities and activities of daily living.[150]

Educating parents about what they should be allowing their child to do is as important as teaching them precautions pertaining to their child. Children were observed to have significant gross motor advances during the second year of life when parental warmth was combined with a decrease in parental restrictions. It was also observed that children with CHD performed better on IQ tests when their parents attempted to accelerate their child's development.[199] Parents should be taught that children with cardiac disease, particularly cyanotic disease, limit their own activity and stop and rest when needed.[52] Children with Down syndrome and a cardiac defect were observed to score higher on developmental tests and achieve feeding milestones earlier if parents followed through appropriately with therapy instructions.[58]

SCHOOL-AGE PERIOD

Cognitive function was not found to be affected in children who underwent an ASD repair between ages 3 and 17 years while on cardiopulmonary bypass.[227] This is an important finding as it has long been believed that this was a primary factor in neurologic problems after surgery for congenital heart defects. Children with an ASD, however, do not have the same associated risk factors, such as unstable hemodynamics, chronic hypoxemia, and metabolic acidosis, that children with other congenital heart defects have, particularly those with cyanotic heart defects. When comparing children who had an ASD closed surgically (using cardiac bypass) versus interventional closure by cardiac catheterization, Visconti and associates found that when using the Wechsler Intelligence Scale for Children-III, the Full-Scale IQ and Performance IQ were significantly lower in the surgical closure group.[246] This was largely due to deficits in visual-motor and visual-spatial components. The device closure group, however, performed significantly worse when sustained attention was required and tested.

Bellinger and associates examined the use of hypothermic circulatory arrest versus low-flow cardiopulmonary bypass during surgery for their effects on development and neurologic status of children. Hypothermic circulatory arrest was associated with significantly lower gross and fine motor scores on the Peabody Developmental Motor Scale.[30] These children also scored worse on balance, nonlocomotor ability, and manual dexterity and had more difficulty with speech, particularly with imitating oral movements and speech sounds. The two management groups did not differ from each other in IQ or overall neurologic examination results, but both were significantly lower than the norms, with lower scores occurring in visual-spatial and visual-motor integration skills. Bellinger and associates confirmed visual-perceptual motor deficits in another group of children who had undergone cardiac surgical repair as infants.[27] Their findings were not associated with operative methods, but still the literature supports that all children undergoing surgical repair for a cardiac defect should be considered at risk for neurodevelopmental problems, especially visual-perceptual problems. Mahle and associates performed a similar study but did not find differences in verbal or performance IQ regardless of whether or not the patient underwent cardiac bypass.[158] Along with congenital heart defects and subsequent surgery, children are at risk for lower IQ scores if they have other defects or a lower socioeconomic status.[74] Physical and psychosocial functioning were influenced negatively by lower family income.[170] Special attention should be paid to this at-risk group of children with a congenital heart defect and a lower socioeconomic status.

School adjustment and peer interaction have been observed to be altered in children with CHD. In a study by Youssef, school absenteeism was high in these children and was proportionate to the severity of their disease.[262] It has been observed that a child's adjustment to school is affected more by strain on the family than by the child's physical limitations related to the CHD.[44] Teachers have noted that children with CHD had more school problems; more behavior problems were observed in boys. Children with more behavior problems had lower self-esteem and more depression.[262] Some of the inability to focus and sustain attention on a task may be related to the surgery, the cardiac defect in and of itself, and frustration with the difficulty associated with visual-motor skills and completing fine motor tasks.[27,133] After surgical intervention, some of the behavioral problems may be alleviated; both missing school and diminished activity level should be improved postoperatively.[151] Children may need rehabilitation after surgical repair, however, to teach them how much they are capable of doing, to assist them with visual-perceptual and fine motor tasks, and to help them deal with any functional limitations or inability to perform a task.

Surgical intervention that corrects a cyanotic defect plays an important role in the child's development. Improvement in IQ has been reported after surgery.[151,186] Intellectual development was essentially normal in children after the Fontan operation.[242] Mahle and associates observed, however, that school-age children with HLHS who had a seizure before their initial surgery scored lower on all IQ subsets.[161] Self-confidence, social confidence, and general adjustment have improved after surgery.[151] Significant improvement in self-perception was observed in children after they had their heart defect repaired.[261] If decreased experiences are a factor in developmental performance, a child who is no longer limited by disease should develop more normally.

Parental overprotectiveness can continue to prove more limiting to a child's development than the defect itself. Parents were found to underestimate their child's exercise tolerance in 80% of the cases studied by Casey and associates.[43] Parents were also found to rate their child lower cognitively than the child scored on standardized neurologic testing administered by a professional.[158] Parental restriction generally begins with the advice of the physician and proceeds from there,[52,136] but what the parents perceive to be the physician's advice can be unclear. Longmuir and McCrindle evaluated by questionnaire to the cardiologist and parents the physical activity restrictions for children after the Fontan operation.[155] Twenty percent of children were being unnecessarily restricted by their parents in their physical exertion. Yet only 40% of parents knew that their child should not participate in competitive sports, and 50% of parents did not understand that their child had body contact restrictions caused by anticoagulation medication.

Social and emotional maladjustment in children with cardiac disease can be due to maternal maladjustment and guilt.[136] Parental stress has been found to be correlated with IQ scores and with receptive language abilities, behavior scores, and socialization skills.[162] Psychosocial or therapy intervention by professionals could be beneficial to preserving a more normal parent-child interaction. Some improvement in maternal interaction and attitude has been noted after surgical correction of the child's cardiac defect.[186] In contrast to these reports is a study by Laane and associates, which found that children with congenital heart defects reported a higher quality of life than healthy children.[142] It was also observed that parents of children with HLHS described their child's health, physical ability, and school performance as average or above.[161] When compared with healthy children, children with repaired pulmonary atresia had an overall equal quality of life.[70] It is important as therapists to remember to treat children with congenital heart defects with this in mind.

ADOLESCENCE

Adolescents who have CHD and physical limitations show increased feelings of anxiety and impulsiveness.[139] Early professional intervention to assist the parents and child to cope best with the child's physical limitations may be helpful.

A delay in the onset of puberty in adolescents with CHD may further complicate their social development and participation. The body structure of the adolescent with CHD was found to be noticeably different from that of typical adolescents. Weight and height were significantly less with the presence of cardiac disease. Adolescents with heart disease had head, neck, and shoulder measurements similar to those of healthy adolescents, but the thorax, trunk, pelvis, and lower extremities were significantly smaller. The anterior-posterior diameter of the pelvis was so reduced that it appeared almost flat.[5] Physical differences of this magnitude can only make adolescents with heart disease feel even more different and intensify their low self-esteem.

Intervention that encourages the adolescent to participate in physical activities, including guidelines on how to participate, may improve peer interaction and ultimately self-esteem. Children who participated in an exercise program were observed to have improvement in their self-esteem, as well as in their strength. Parents were found to be less restrictive and had less anxiety about their child after a formal exercise program.[64]

Physical activity is important for all children, including children with CHD. The defect and surgical intervention, as well as possible alterations in response to exercise, must be understood before an exercise program is prescribed for a child with CHD. The American Heart Association has published an extensive review of exercise testing in the pediatric age group, including recommendations for those with various congenital heart defects.[122] Exercise testing performed by children 5 to 18 years after their operation for a Fontan revealed significantly lower maximal workload, maximal oxygen uptake, and maximal heart rate compared with their peers without CHD. Children post Fontan surgery were also observed to have less efficient oxygen uptake during submaximal exercise.[204] Children post Fontan surgery who had a persistent right-to-left shunt were found to have decreased oxygen saturation levels during exercise.[230] This needs to be taken into account when any kind of therapy is provided to patients who have a history of the Fontan procedure.

Cardiac rehabilitation programs for children with cardiac disease have shown significant and beneficial changes in hemodynamics and improvement in exercise endurance and tolerance.[14,18,92,134,168,192,215] Improvement from physical training allowed adolescents to function at near typical activity levels.[92] A recent study testing exercise tolerance in children 10 years after an arterial switch procedure demonstrated an excellent long-term exercise capacity.[113] The psychological improvements were as noticeable and important as the physical improvements.[64,134,163]

Adolescents who have undergone heart transplantation are able to achieve an increase in cardiac output in response to exercise; however, they do not achieve the same peak workloads or maximal oxygen consumption as do typical adolescents.[49] During the early phase of rehabilitation, many children with transplanted hearts, lungs, or heart-lungs are so debilitated that they are unable to perform at an intensity that would raise their heart rate. The dyspnea index used as part of the Stanford heart transplant protocol is helpful in monitoring the child's physical tolerance during activity.[216] The child counts out loud to 15. The goal initially is to attempt to do this on one breath. At first, it may take three breaths to count to 15 while at rest. Exercise should increase the number of breaths to reach the count of 15 by only one or two breaths and should not be resumed until a return to resting baseline. Most children progress quickly, usually reaching 15 on one breath within 1 week of beginning exercise. The dyspnea index is an easily used measure for self-monitoring of exercise tolerance at home.[128] Children who underwent heart transplantation in infancy were found to have exercise capacities that were not different from those of normal subjects.[1] They did have a slightly lower peak heart rate (p, 0.001) and peak oxygen consumption (p, 0.01) and a lower anaerobic threshold (p, 0.05), but the respiratory exchange ratio was equal and the oxygen pulse index did not differ significantly.

The patient who has had a heart-lung transplantation also has an increased ventilatory response to exercise.[16,17,221] The dyspnea index is again useful with these patients. Heart, heart-lung, and lung transplant recipients have experienced marked rehabilitation after transplantation.[33] The authors have found it highly beneficial for adolescents to be enrolled in a formal rehabilitation program after transplant to change their lifestyle, as well as condition them. The quality of life improves, with most children functioning at an age-appropriate level without developmental delays.[66,146,180]

In their systematic review of studies of long-term survival and morbidity in the presence of CHD, Verheught and associates observed that survival is decreased in anyone with CHD when compared with the normal survival rate. Morbidity was increased further with more complex CHD. Their review also revealed that supraventricular arrhythmias were prevalent in patients with atrial septal defect (ASD), transposition of the great arteries (TGA), and tetralogy of Fallot (TOF); ventricular arrhythmias were more prevalent in TOF, and CVAs were more common with TGA, ASD, and coarctation of the aorta. Heart failure, cyanosis, and complexity of lesions are predictors of increased mortality in adults with CHD.[239] Increased ventilatory response or poor exercise capacity in adults 25 years after a Mustard or Senning operation for transposition of the great arteries was found to have a substantially higher risk for cardiac emergency or death.[86] A recent study by Fredriksen and associates revealed that patients who underwent surgical correction for transposition of the great arteries show a gradual decline in exercise performance with age, leading toward a significantly lower exercise capacity then healthy peers.[77] The International Society for Adult Congenital Heart Disease published an extensive report on the guidelines and management of adults with CHD (*Circulation* 118:e714–e833, 2008). The authors refer you to this useful reference on the ongoing treatment of adult survivors with repaired congenital heart defects.

SUMMARY

This review of congenital heart defects, surgical and therapeutic intervention, and developmental consequences provides therapists with a foundation for working with this patient population. As surgical intervention occurs earlier and corrective techniques are performed sooner, it will be increasingly important to examine and monitor developmental progression. Children with congenital heart defects cannot be made to perform a developmental task that they do not have the energy to perform. The physical therapist plays an integral role in the habilitation and rehabilitation of children with CHD. A major part of this role involves parent education concerning typical developmental sequences in children with cardiac conditions and appropriate parent-child interaction to promote socioemotional development. In light of recent research indicating neurologic issues even preoperatively in all patients with cardiac defects and knowledge of visual-perceptual issues and behavior and attention problems, ongoing research and therapy are essential in this challenging population.

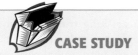

CASE STUDY

The following case study describes a typical course of surgeries, with complications that resolved, in a child with cyanotic heart disease.

"David"

David was born with severe cyanotic CHD. He was diagnosed with total anomalous pulmonary venous return, transposition of the great arteries, hypoplastic left ventricle syndrome, ASD, and pulmonary atresia. He had two surgeries performed within the first month of life. At 10 days of age, he had ligation of the ductus arteriosus and a modified BT shunt. At 4 weeks of age, he required repair of his right pulmonary artery. Then, at 4 months of age, he underwent surgery to repair his total anomalous pulmonary venous return. After this surgery, it took approximately 4 weeks to wean him from the ventilator, owing to a left phrenic nerve palsy. He was discharged to home on nasogastric feedings, which continued until he was 1 year old. He advanced from nasogastric feedings to baby food and liquid from a "tippy" cup.

David experienced some delay in achieving developmental milestones. He sat independently at 9 months of age. At 16 months of age, David had a bidirectional Glenn procedure and his BT shunt was taken down. He did well after this surgery and was discharged to home within 1 week of his surgery date. He developed well over the next 18 months, with marked improvement in his activity level. For instance, David crawled at 17 months of age and then walked at 19 months.

At 3 years of age, David had a Fontan procedure performed, which he tolerated well until seizures occurred on the third postoperative day. Computed tomography scanning revealed a right frontal lobe infarct, and increased tone and briskness of reflexes were noted on his left side. He was irritable and was difficult to console. Initially, David demonstrated left-sided neglect and a decrease in his protective reactions to the left. Within 1 week, his tone was only minimally increased, and he was able to use his left extremities with cueing. Within 2 weeks, his protective reactions were symmetrical, and he was shifting his weight and using either extremity readily. His ambulation was typical of a child after surgery, with slight balance problems and the use of a wide base of support. He did have difficulty coming to a standing position from sitting without support, which resolved within 4 weeks.

David's parents are attentive and recognize tasks that are difficult for him. They have continued home exercises to encourage use of his left extremities and have had better cooperation from him than have the therapists. He continued to be followed for reexamination several times a year to monitor his progress and update his home program.

Four years later at age 7, David goes to school every day and does well. His overall endurance and risk taking are less than his peers, but generally he gets along well.

REFERENCES

1. Abarbanell, G., Mulla, N., Chinnock, R., & Larsen, R. (2004). Exercise assessment in infants after cardiac transplantation. *Journal of Heart & Lung Transplantation, 23,* 1334–1338.

2. Aisenberg, R. B., Rosenthal, A., Nadas, A. S., & Wolff, P. H. (1982). Developmental delay in infants with congenital heart disease. *Pediatric Cardiology, 3,* 133–137.

3. Ali, J., Weisel, R. D., Layug, A. B., Kripke, B. J., & Hechtman, H. B. (1974). Consequences of postoperative alterations in respiratory mechanics. *American Journal of Surgery, 128,* 376–382.

4. Amitia, Y., Blieden, L., Shemtove, A., & Neufeld, H. (1984). Cerebrovascular accidents in infants and children with congenital cyanotic heart disease. *Israel Journal of Medical Sciences, 20,* 1143–1145.

5. Angelov, G., Tomova, S., & Ninova, P. (1980). Physical development and body structure of children with congenital heart disease. *Human Biology, 52,* 413–421.

6. Arciniegas, E. (1991). Ventricular septal defect. In A. E. Baue, A. S. Geha, G. L. Hammond, H. Laks, & K. S. Naunheim (Eds.), *Glenn's thoracic and cardiovascular surgery* (5th ed.; pp. 1007–1016). Norwalk, CT: Appleton & Lange.

7. Asantila, R., Rosenburg, P. H., & Scheinin, B. (1986). Comparison of different methods of postoperative analgesia after thoracotomy. *Acta Anaesthesiologica Scandinavica, 30,* 421–425.

8. Atallah, J., Dinu, I. A., Joffe, A. R., Robertson, C. M. T., Sauve, R. S., Dyck, J. D., Ross, D. B., & Rebeyka, I. M. (2008). Two-year survival and mental and psychomotor outcomes after the Norwood procedure. *Circulation, 118,* 1410–1418.

9. Aurora, P., Boucek, M. M., Dobbels, C. J., Edwards, L. B., Keck, B. M., Rahmel, A. O., Taylor, D. O., Trulock, E. P., & Hertz, M. I. (2007). Registry of the International Society for Heart and Lung Transplantation. Tenth official pediatric lung and heart/lung transplantation report—2007. *Journal of Heart and Lung Transplantation, 26*, 1223–1228.

10. Austin, E. H., III, Edmonds, H. L., Jr., Auden, S. M., Seremet, V., Niznik, G., Sehic, A., Sowell, M. K., Cheppo, C. D., & Corlett, K. M. (1997). Benefit of neurophysiologic monitoring for pediatric cardiac surgery. *Journal of Thoracic and Cardiovascular Surgery, 114*, 707–717.

11. Aziz, S., & Jamieson, S. (1991). Combined heart and lung transplantation. In A. E. Baue, A. S. Geha, G. L. Hammond, H. Laks, & K. S. Naunheim (Eds.), *Glenn's thoracic and cardiovascular surgery* (5th ed.; pp. 1623–1638). Norwalk, CT: Appleton & Lange.

12. Bailey, L. L., Assaad, A. N., Trimm, R. F., Nehlsen-Cannarella, S. L., Kanakriyeh, M. S., Haas, G. S., & Jacobson, J. G. (1988). Orthotopic transplantation during early infancy as therapy for incurable congenital heart disease. *Annals of Surgery, 203*, 279–285.

13. Baldwin, J. T., Borovetz, H. S., Duncan, B. W., et al. (2006). The National Heart, Lung and Blood Institute pediatric circulatory support program. *Circulation, 113*, 147–155.

14. Balfour, I. C., Drimmer, A. M., Nouri, S., Pennington, D. G., Hemkins, C. L., & Harvey, L. L. (1991). Pediatric cardiac rehabilitation. *American Journal of Diseases of Children, 145*, 627–630.

15. Banasik, J. L., Bruya, M. A., Steadman, R. E., & Demand, J. K. (1987). Effect of position on arterial oxygenation in postoperative coronary revascularization patients. *Heart and Lung, 16*, 652–657.

16. Banner, N., Guz, A., Heaton, R., Innes, J. A., Murphy, K., & Yacoub, M. (1988). Ventilatory and circulatory responses at the onset of exercise in man following heart or heart-lung transplantation. *Journal of Physiology, 399*, 437–449.

17. Banner, N. R., Lloyd, M. H., Hamilton, R. D., Innes, J. A., Guz, A., & Yacoub, M. H. (1989). Cardiopulmonary response to dynamic exercise after heart and combined heart-lung transplantation. *British Heart Journal, 61*, 215–223.

18. Bar-Or, O. (1985). Physical conditioning in children with cardiorespiratory disease. In R. L. Terjung (Ed.), *Exercise and sport science review* (pp. 305–334). New York: Macmillan.

19. Barron, D. J., Kilby, M. D., Davies, B., Wright, J. G., Jones, T. J., & Brawn, W. J. (2009). Hypoplastic left heart syndrome. *The Lancet, 374*, 551–564.

20. Bartlett, R. H. (1980). Pulmonary pathophysiology in surgical patients. *Surgical Clinics of North America, 60*, 1323–1338.

21. Bartlett, R. H. (1984). Respiratory therapy to prevent pulmonary complications of surgery. *Respiratory Care, 29*, 667–677.

22. Bartlett, R. H., Brennan, M. L., Gazzaniga, A. B., & Hanson, E. L. (1973a). Studies on the pathogenesis and prevention of postoperative pulmonary complications. *Surgery, Gynecology and Obstetrics, 137*, 925–933.

23. Bartlett, R. H., Gazzaniga, A. B., & Geraghty, T. R. (1973b). Respiratory maneuvers to prevent postoperative pulmonary complications. *Journal of the American Medical Association, 224*, 1017–1021.

24. Bastardi, H. J., Naftel, D. C., Webber, S. A., et al. (2008). Ventricular assist devices as a bridge to heart transplantation in children. *Journal of Cardiovascular Nursing, 23*, 25–29.

25. Bauer, J., Dapper, F., Kroll, J., Hagel, K. J., Thul, J., & Zickmann, B. (1998). Heart transplantation in infants—Experience at the Children's Heart Center in Giessen. *Zeitschrift fur Kardiologie, 87*, 209–217.

26. Bautista-Hernandez, V., Thiagarajan, R. R., Flynn-Thompson, F., Rajagopal, S. K., Nento, D. E., Yarlagadda, V., Teele, S. A., Allan, C. K., Emani, S. M., Laussen, P. C., Pigula, F. A., & Bacha, E. A. (2009). Preoperative extracorporeal membrane oxygenation as a bridge to cardiac surgery in children with congenital heart disease. *Annals of Thoracic Surgery, 88*, 1306–1311.

27. Bellinger, D. C., Bernstein, J. H., Kirkwood, M. W., Rappaport, L. A., & Newburger, J. W. (2003). Visual-spatial skills in children after open-heart surgery. *Developmental and Behavioral Problems, 24*, 169–179.

28. Bellinger, D. C., Jonas, R. A., Rappaport, L. A., Wypij, D., Wernovsky, G., Kuban, K. C. K., Barnes, P. D., Holmes, G. L., Hickey, P. R., Strand, R. D., Walsh, A. Z., Helmers, S. L., Constantinou, J. E., Carrazana, E. J., Mayer, J. E., Hanley, F. L., Castaneda, A. R., Ware, J. H., & Newburger J. W. (1995). Developmental and neurologic status of children after heart surgery with hypothermic circulatory arrest or low-flow cardiopulmonary bypass. *New England Journal of Medicine, 332*, 549–555.

29. Bellinger, D. C., Rappaport, L. A., Wypij, D., Wernovsky, G., & Newburger, J. W. (1997). Patterns of developmental dysfunction after surgery during infancy to correct transposition of the great arteries. *Journal of Developmental and Behavioral Pediatrics, 18*, 75–83.

30. Bellinger, D. C., Wypij, D., duPlessis, A. J., Rappaport, L. A., Jonas, R. A., Wernovsky, G., & Newburger, J. W. (2003). Neurodevelopmental status at eight years in children with dextro-transposition of the great arteries: The Boston circulatory arrest trial. *Journal of Thoracic and Cardiovascular Surgery, 126*, 1385–1396.

31. Berg, A. M., Snell, L., Mahle, W. T. (2007). Home inotropic therapy in children. *Journal of Heart and Lung Transplantation, 26*, 453–457.

32. Blackwood, M. J., Haka-Ikse, K., & Steward, D. J. (1986). Developmental outcome in children undergoing surgery with profound hypothermia. *Anesthesiology, 65*, 437–440.

33. Bolman, R. M., Shumway, S. S., Estrin, J. A., & Hertz, M. I. (1991). Lung and heart-lung transplantation. *Annals of Surgery, 214*, 456–470.

34. Bonser, R. S., & Jamieson, S. W. (1990). Heart-lung transplantation. *Clinics in Chest Medicine, 11*, 235–246.

35. Bott, J., Keilty, S. E., Brown, A., & Ward, E. M. (1992). Nasal intermittent positive pressure ventilation. *Physiotherapy, 78*, 93–96.

36. Botto, L. D., Mulinare, J., Erickson, J. D. (2000). Occurrence of congenital heart defects in relation to maternal multivitamin use. *American Journal of Epidemiology, 151,* 878–884.

37. Boutros, A. R. (1970). Arterial blood oxygenation during and after endotracheal suctioning in the apneic patient. *Anesthesiology, 32,* 114–118.

38. Bove, E. L. (1991). Transplantation after first-stage reconstruction for hypoplastic left heart syndrome. *Annals of Thoracic Surgery, 52,* 701–707.

39. Bove, E. L., Ohye, R. G., & Devaney, E. J. (2004). Hypoplastic left heart syndrome: Conventional surgical management. *Pediatric Cardiac Surgery Annual of the Seminars in Thoracic and Cardiovascular Surgery, 7,* 3–10.

40. Bruning, M. D., & Schneiderman, J. U. (1983). Heart failure in infants and children. In C. R. Michaelson (Ed.), *Congestive heart failure* (pp. 467–484). St Louis: Mosby.

41. Byrum, C. J., Dick, M., Behrendt, D. M., & Rosenthal, A. (1982). Repair of total anomalous pulmonary venous connection in patients younger than 6 months old. *Circulation, 66*(suppl I), 208–214.

42. Callow, L. B. (1989). A new beginning: Nursing care of the infant undergoing the arterial switch operation for transposition of the great arteries. *Heart and Lung, 18,* 248–257.

43. Casey, F. A., Craig, B. G., & Mulholland, H. C. (1994). Quality of life in surgically palliated complex congenital heart disease. *Archives of Disease in Childhood, 70,* 382–386.

44. Casey, F. A., Sykes, D. H., Craig, B. G., Power, R., & Mulholland, H. C. (1996). Behavioral adjustment of children with surgically palliated complex congenital heart disease. *Journal of Pediatric Psychology, 21,* 335–352.

45. Cassidy, J., Haynes, S., Kirk, R., et al. (2009). Changing patterns of bridging to heart transplantation in children. *Journal of Heart and Lung Transplantation, 28,* 249–254.

46. Chang, R. K., Chen, A. Y., & Klitzner, T. S. (2002). Clinical management of infants with hypoplastic left heart syndrome in the United States, 1988–1997. *Pediatrics, 110,* 292–298.

47. Cho, J. M., Puga, F. J., Danielson, G. K., Dearani, J. A., Mair, D. D., Hagler, D. J., Julsrud, P. R., & Ilstrup, D. M. (2002). Early and long-term results of the surgical treatment of tetralogy of Fallot with pulmonary atresia, with or without major aortopulmonary collateral arteries. *Journal of Thoracic Cardiovascular Surgery, 124,* 70–81.

48. Reference deleted in page proofs.

49. Christos, S. C., Katch, V., Crowley, D. C., Eakin, B. L., Lindauer, A. L., & Beekman, R. H. (1992). Hemodynamic responses to upright exercise of adolescent cardiac transplant patients. *Journal of Pediatrics, 121,* 312–316.

50. Chulay, M., Brown, J., & Summer, W. (1982). Effect of postoperative immobilization after coronary artery bypass surgery. *Critical Care Medicine, 10,* 176–179.

51. Clancy, R. R., Sahrif, U., Ichord, R., Spry, T. L., Nicolson, S., Tabbutt, S., Wernovsky, G., & Gaynor, J. W. (2005). Electrographic neonatal seizures after infant heart surgery. *Epilepsia, 46,* 84–90.

52. Clare, M. D. (1985). Home care of infants and children with cardiac disease. *Heart and Lung, 14,* 218–222.

53. Clarke, C. F., Beall, M. H., & Perloff, J. K. (1991). Genetics, epidemiology, counseling, and prevention. In J. K. Perloff, & J. S. Child (Eds.), *Congenital heart disease in adults* (pp. 141–165). Philadelphia: WB Saunders.

54. Clough, P. (1990). The denervated heart. *Clinical Management, 10,* 14–17.

55. Connolly, D., McClowry, S., Hayman, L., Mahony, L., & Artman, M. (2004). Posttraumatic stress disorder in children after cardiac surgery. *Journal of Pediatrics, 144,* 480–484.

56. Cooley, D. A., Cabello, O. V., & Preciado, F. M. (2008). Repair of total anomalous pulmonary venous return. *Texas Heart Institute Journal, 35,* 451–453.

57. Crane, L. D. (1987). The neonate and child. In D. L. Frownfelter (Ed.), *Chest physical therapy and pulmonary rehabilitation* (pp. 666–697). Chicago: Year Book.

58. Cullen, S. M., Cronk, C. E., Pueschel, S. M., Schnell, R. R., & Reed, R. B. (1981). Social development and feeding milestones of young Down syndrome children. *American Journal of Mental Deficiency, 85,* 410–415, 1981.

59. Davies, H., Kitchman, R., Gordon, I., & Helms, P. (1985). Regional ventilation in infancy. *New England Journal of Medicine, 313,* 1626–1628.

60. Dean, E. (1985). Effect of body position on pulmonary function. *Physical Therapy, 65,* 613–618.

61. Del Castillo, S. L., Moromisato, D. Y., Dorey, F., Ludwick, J., Starnes, V. A., Wells, W. J., Jeffries, H. E., & Wong, P. C. (2006). Mesenteric blood flow velocities in the newborn with single-ventricle physiology: Modified Blalock-Taussig shunt versus right ventricle-pulmonary artery conduit. *Pediatric Critical Care Medicine, 7,* 132–137.

62. de Leval, M. R. (1991). Senning operation. In A. E. Baue, A. S. Geha, G. L. Hammond, H. Laks, & K. S. Naunheim (Eds.), *Glenn's thoracic and cardiovascular surgery* (ed 5; pp. 121–126). Norwalk, CT: Appleton & Lange.

63. DeMaso, D. R., Campis, L. K., Wypij, D., Bertram, S., Lipshitz, M., & Freed, M. (1991). The impact of maternal perceptions and medical severity on the adjustment of children with congenital heart disease. *Journal of Pediatric Psychology, 16,* 137–149.

64. Donovan, E. F., Mathews, R. A., Nixon, P. A., Stephenson, R. J., Robertson, R. J., Dean, F., Fricker, F. J., Beerman, L. B., & Fischer, D. R. (1983). An exercise program for pediatric patients with congenital heart disease: Psychological aspects. *Journal of Cardiac Rehabilitation, 3,* 476–480.

65. Dull, J. L., & Dull, W. L. (1983). Are maximal inspiratory breathing exercises or incentive spirometry better than early mobilization after cardiopulmonary bypass? *Physical Therapy, 63,* 655–659.

66. Dunn, J. M., Cavarocchi, N. C., Balsara, R. K., Kolff, J., McClurken, J., Badellino, M. M., Vieweg, C., & Donner, R. M. (1987). Pediatric heart transplantation, at St. Christopher's Hospital for Children. *Journal of Heart Transplantation, 6,* 334–342.

67. duPlessis, A. J. (1997). Neurologic complications of cardiac disease in the newborn. *Clinics in Perinatology, 24,* 807–825.

68. duPlessis, A. J., Chang, A. C., Wessel, D. L., Lock, J. E., Wernovsky, G., Newburger, J. W., & Mayer, J. E., Jr. (1995). Cerebrovascular accidents following the Fontan operation. *Pediatric Neurology, 12,* 230–236.

69. Egbert, L. D., & Bendixon, H. H. (1964). Effect of morphine on breathing pattern. *Journal of the American Medical Association, 188,* 485–488.

70. Ekman-Joelsson, B. M., Berntsson, L., & Sunnegardh, J. (2004). Quality of life in children with pulmonary atresia and intact ventricular septum. *Cardiology in the Young, 14,* 615–621.

71. Feldt, R. H., Ewert, J. C., Stickler, G. B., & Weidman, W. H. (1969). Children with congenital heart disease. *American Journal of Diseases of Children, 117,* 281–287.

72. Fenton, K. N., Webber, S. A., Danford, D. A., Ghandi, S. K., Periera, J., & Pigula, F. A. (2003). Long-term survival after pediatric cardiac transplantation and postoperative ECMO support. *Annals of Thoracic Surgery, 76,* 843–847.

73. Ferry, P. C. (1990). Neurologic sequelae of open-heart surgery in children. *American Journal of Diseases of Children, 144,* 369–373.

74. Forbess, J. M., Visconti, K. J., Hancock-Friesen, C., Howe, R. C., Bellinger, D. C., & Jonas, R. A. (2002). *Circulation, 106*(suppl I), I-95–I-102.

75. Fox, M. D., & Molesky, M. G. (1990). The effects of prone and supine positioning on arterial oxygen pressure. *Neonatal Network, 8,* 25–29.

76. Fox, W. W., Schwartz, J. G., & Shaffer, T. H. (1978). Pulmonary physiotherapy in neonates: Physiologic changes and respiratory management. *Journal of Pediatrics, 92,* 977–981.

77. Fredriksen, P. M., Pettersen, E., & Thaulow, E. (2009). Declining aerobic capacity of patients with arterial and atrial switch procedures. *Pediatric Cardiology, 30,* 166–171.

78. Fricker, F. J., Trento, A., & Griffith, B. P. (1990). Pediatric cardiac transplantation. In A. N. Brest (Ed.), *Cardiovascular clinics* (pp. 223–235). Philadelphia: FA Davis.

79. Furness, S., Hyslop-St. George, C., Pound, B., et al. (2008). Development of an interprofessional pediatric ventricular assist device support team. *ASAIO J, 54,* 483–485.

80. Gamsu, G., Singer, M. M., Vincent, H. H., Berry, S., & Nadel, J. A. (1976). Postoperative impairment of mucous transport in the lung. *American Review of Respiratory Disease, 114,* 673–679.

81. Gardner, F. V., Freeman, N. H., Black, A. M., & Angelini, G. D. (1996). Disturbed mother-infant interaction in association with congenital heart disease. *Heart, 76,* 56–59.

82. Garson, A., Gillette, P. C., Gutgesell, H. P., & McNamara, D. G. (1980). Stress-induced ventricular arrhythmia after repair of tetralogy of Fallot. *American Journal of Cardiology, 46,* 1006–1012.

83. Gaynor, J. W., Jarvik, G. P., Bernbaum, J., Gerdes, M., Wernovsky, G., Burnham, N. B., D'Agostino, J., Zackai, E., McDonald-McGinn, D. M., Nicolson, S. C., Spray, T. L., Clancy, R. R. (2006). The relationship of postoperative electrographic seizures to neurodevelopmental outcome at 1 year of age after neonatal and infant cardiac surgery. *Journal of Thoracic and Cardiovascular Surgery, 131,* 181–189.

84. Gaynor, J. W., Wernovsky, G., Jarvik, G. P., Bernbaum, J., Gerdes, M., Zackai, E., Nord, A. S., Clancy, R. R., Nicolson, S. C., & Spray, T. L. (2007). Patient characteristics are important determinants of neurodevelopmental outcome at one year of age after neonatal and infant cardiac surgery. *Journal of Thoracic and Cardiovascular Surgery, 133,* 1344–1353.

85. Gessler, P., Schmitt, B., Pretre, R., & Latal, B. (2009). Inflammatory response and neurodevelopmental outcome after open-heart surgery. *Pediatric Cardiology, 30,* 301–305.

86. Giardini, A., Hager, A., Lammers, A. E., Derrick, G., Muller, J., Diller, G. P., Dimopoulos, K., Odendaal, D., Gargiulo, G., Piccio, F. M., & Gatzoulis, M. A. (2009). Ventilatory efficiency and aerobic capacity predict event-free survival in adults with atrial repair for complete transposition of the great arteries. *Journal of American College of Cardiology, 53,* 1548–1555.

87. Giboney, G. S. (1983). Ventricular septal defect. *Heart and Lung, 12,* 292–299.

88. Gingell, R. L., & Hornung, M. G. (1989). Growth problems associated with congenital heart disease in infancy. In E. Lebenthal (Ed.), *Textbook of gastroenterology and nutrition in infancy* (2nd ed.; pp. 639–649). New York: Raven Press.

89. Girlando, R. M., Belew, B., & Klara, F. (1988). Coarctation of the aorta. *Critical Care Nurse, 8,* 38–50.

90. Glanville, A. R., Baldwin, J. C., Hunt, S. A., & Theodore, J. (1990). Long-term cardiopulmonary function after human heart-lung transplantation. *Australian and New Zealand Journal of Medicine, 20,* 208–214.

91. Glanville, A. R., Gabb, G. M., Theodore, J., & Robin, E. D. (1989). Bronchial responsiveness to exercise after human cardiopulmonary transplantation. *Chest, 96,* 281–286.

92. Goldberg, B., Fripp, R. R., Lister, G., Loke, J., Nicholas, J. A., & Talner, N. S. (1981). Effect of physical training on exercise performance of children following surgical repair of congenital heart disease. *Pediatrics, 68,* 691–699.

93. Goldberg, C. S., Schwartz, E. M., Brunberg, J. A., Mosca, R. S., Bove, E. L., Schork, M. A., Stetz, S. P., Cheatham, J. P., & Kulik, T. J. (2000). Neurodevelopmental outcome of patients after the Fontan operation: A comparison between children with hypoplastic left heart syndrome and other functional single ventricle lesions. *Journal of Pediatrics, 137,* 646–652.

94. Goldberg, S., Simmons, R. J., Newman, J., Campbell, K., & Fowler, R. S. (1991). Congenital heart disease, parental stress, and infant-mother relationships. *Journal of Pediatrics, 119,* 661–666.

95. Goldberg, S., Washington, J., Morris, P., Fischer-Fay, A., & Simmons, R. J. (1990). Early diagnosed chronic illness and mother-child relationships in the first two years. *Canadian Journal of Psychiatry, 55,* 726–733.

96. Goldman, A. P., Cassidy, J., de Leval, M., et al. (2003). The waiting game: Bridging to paediatric heart transplantation. *Lancet, 362,* 1967–1970.

97. Gorler, H., Struber, M., Ballman, M., Muller, C., Gottleib, J., Warnecke, G., Gohrbandt, B., Haverich, A., & Simon, A. (2009). Lung and heart-lung transplantation in children and adolescents: A long-term single-center experience. *Journal of Heart and Lung Tranplantation, 28,* 243–248.

98. Graham, T. P., Bender, H. W., & Spach, M. S. (1989). Ventricular septal defect. In F. H. Adams, G. C. Emmanouilides, & T. A. Riemen (Eds.), *Moss's heart disease in infants, children, and adolescents* (pp. 189–208). Baltimore: Williams & Wilkins.

99. Griffith, B. P., Hardesy, R. L., Trento, A., Paradis, I. L., Duquesnoy, R. J., Zeevi, A., Dauber, J. H., Dummer, J. S., Thompson, M. E., Gryzan, S., & Bahnson, H. T. (1987). Heart-lung transplantation: Lessons learned and future hopes. *Annals of Thoracic Surgery, 43,* 6–16.

100. Griffiths, E. R., Kaza, A. K., Wyler von Ballmoos, M. C., Loyola, H., Valente, A. M., Blume, E. D., & del Nido, P. (2009). Evaluating failing Fontans for heart transplantation: Predictors of death. *Annals of Thoracic Surgery, 88,* 558–564.

101. Gudermuth, S. (1975). Mothers' reports of early experiences of infants with congenital heart disease. *Maternal-Child Nursing Journal, 4,* 155–164.

102. Guillemaud, J. P., El-Hakim, H., Richards, S., & Chauhan, N. (2007). Airway pathologic abnormalities in symptomatic children with congenital cardiac and vascular disease. *Archives of Otolaryngology Head and Neck Surgery, 133,* 672–676.

103. Haas, G. S., Bailey, L., & Pennington, D. G. (1991). Pediatric cardiac transplantation. In A. E. Baue, A. S. Geha, G. L. Hammond, H. Laks, & K. S. Naunheim (Eds.), *Glenn's thoracic and cardiovascular surgery* (5th ed.; pp. 1297–1317). Norwalk, CT: Appleton & Lange.

104. Haka-Ikse, K., Blackwood, M. A., & Steward, D. J. (1978). Psychomotor development of infants and children after profound hypothermia during surgery for congenital heart disease. *Developmental Medicine and Child Neurology, 20,* 62–70.

105. Hammon, J. W., & Bender, H. W. (1991). Anomalous venous connection: Pulmonary and systemic. In A. E. Baue, A. S. Geha, G. L. Hammond, H. Laks, & K. S. Naunheim (Eds.), *Glenn's thoracic and cardiovascular surgery* (5th ed.; pp. 971–993). Norwalk, CT: Appleton & Lange.

106. Haneda, K., Itoh, T., Togo, T., Ohmi, M., & Mohri, H. (1996). Effects of cardiac surgery on intellectual function in infants and children. *Cardiovascular Surgery, 4,* 303–307.

107. Harrison, A. M., Davis, S., Reid, J. R., Morrison, S. C., Arrigain, S., Connor, J. T., & Temple, M. E. (2005). Neonates with hypoplastic left heart syndrome have ultrasound evidence of abnormal superior mesenteric artery perfusion before and after the modified Norwood procedure. *Pediatric Critical Care Medicine, 6,* 445–447.

108. Hetzer, R., & Stiller, B. (2006). Technology insight: Use of ventricular assist devices in children. *Nature Clinical Practice Cardiovascular Medicine, 3,* 377–387.

109. Hines, M. H., Raines, K. H., Payne, R. M., Covitz, W., Cnota, J. F., Smith, T. E., O'Brian, J. J., & Ririe, D. G. (2003). Video-assisted ductal ligation in premature infants. *Annals of Thoracic Surgery, 76,* 1417–1420.

110. Hirsch, J. C., Charpie, J. R., Ohye, R. G., & Gurney, J. G. (2009). Near infrared spectroscopy: What we know and what we need to know—A systematic review of the congenital heart disease. *Journal of Thoracic and Cardiovascular Surgery, 137,* 154–159.

111. Hoffman, J. I., & Kaplan, S. (2002). The incidence of congenital heart disease. *Journal of the American College of Cardiology, 39,* 1890–1900.

112. Holden, K. R., Sessions, J. C., Cure, J., Whitcom, D. S., & Sade, R. M. (1998). Neurologic outcomes in children with postpump choreoathetosis. *Journal of Pediatrics, 132,* 162–164.

113. Hovels-Gurich, H. H., Kunz, D., Seghaye, M., Miskova, M., Messmer, B. J., & von Bermuth, G. (2003). Results of exercise testing at a mean age of 10 years after neonatal arterial switch operation. *Acta Paediatrica, 92,* 190–196.

114. Huckabay, L., & Daderian, A. D. (1990). Effect of choices on breathing exercises post-open heart surgery. *Dimensions in Critical Care Nursing, 9,* 190–201.

115. Huddleston, C. B., Bloch, J. B., Sweet, S. C., de la Morena, M., Patterson, G. A., & Mendeloff, E. N. (2002). Lung transplantation in children. *Annals of Surgery, 236,* 270–276.

116. Hussey, J. (1992). Effects of chest physiotherapy for children in intensive care after surgery. *Physiotherapy, 78,* 109–113.

117. Hutter, J. A., Despins, P., Higenbottam, T., Stewart, S., & Wallwork, J. (1988). Heart-lung transplantation: Better use of resources. *American Journal of Medicine, 85,* 4–11.

118. Imamura, M., Dossey, A. M., Prodhan, P., et al. (2009). Bridge to cardiac transplantation in children: Berlin heart versus extracorporeal membrane oxygenation. *Annals of Thoracic Surgery, 87,* 1894–1901.

119. Imle, P. C. (1981). Percussion and vibration. In C. F. MacKenzie, N. Ciesla, P. C. Imle, & N. Klemic, N (Eds.), *Chest physiotherapy in the intensive care unit* (pp. 81–91). Baltimore: Williams & Wilkins.

120. Jacobs, J. P., Giroud, J. M., Quintessenza, J. A., Morell, V. O., Botero, L. M., van Gelder, H. M., Badhwar, V., & Burke, R. P. (2003). The modern approach to patent ductus arteriosus treatment: Complementary roles of video-assisted thoracoscopic surgery and interventional cardiology coil occlusion. *Annals of Thoracic Surgery, 76,* 1421–1428.

121. Jadcherla, S. R., Vijayapal, A. S., & Leuthner, S. (2009). Feeding abilities in neonates with congenital heart disease: A retrospective study. *Journal of Perinatology, 29,* 112–118.

122. James, F. W., Blomqvist, C. G., Freed, M. D., Miller, W. W., Moller, J. H., Nugent, E. W., Riopel, D. A., Strong, W. B., & Wessel, H. U. (1982). Standards for exercise testing in the pediatric age group. *Circulation, 66,* 1377A–1397A.

123. Jamieson, S. W., Stinson, E. B., Oyer, P. E., Reitz, B. A., Baldwin, J., Modry, D., Dawkins, K., Theodore, J., Hunt, S., & Shumway, N. E. (1984). Heart-lung transplantation for irreversible pulmonary hypertension. *Annals of Thoracic Surgery, 38,* 554–562.

124. Jarmakani, J. M., & Canent, R. V. (1974). Preoperative and postoperative right ventricular function in children with transposition of the great vessels. *Circulation, 50*(suppl II), 39–45.

125. Jayakumar, K. A., Addonizio, L. J., Kichuk-Chrisant, M. R., Galantowicz, M. E., Lamour, J. M., Quaegebeur, J. M., & Hsu, D. T. (2004). Cardiac transplantation after the Fontan or Glenn procedure. *Journal of American College of Cardiologists, 44*, 2065–2072.

126. Jenkins, K. J., Correa, A., Feinstein, J. A., Botto, L., Britt, A. E., Daniels, S. R., Elixson, M., Warnes, C. A., & Webb, C. L. (2007). Noninherited risk factors and congenital cardiovascular defects: Current knowledge. A scientific statement from the American Heart Association Council on cardiovascular disease in the young. *Circulation, 115*, 2995–3014.

127. Johnson, A. B., & Davis, J. S. (1991). Treatment options for the neonate with hypoplastic left heart syndrome. *Journal of Perinatal and Neonatal Nursing, 5*, 84–92.

128. Johnson, B. A. (1991). Postoperative physical therapy in the pediatric cardiac surgery patient. *Pediatric Physical Therapy, 2*, 14–22.

129. Kaltman, J. R., Jarvik, G. P., Bernbaum, J., Wernovsky, G., Gerdes, M., Zackai, E., Clancy, R. R., Nicolson, S. C., Spray, T. L., & Gaynor, J. W. (2006). Neurodevelopmental outcome after early repair of a ventricular septal defect with or without aortic arch obstruction. *Journal of Thoracic and Cardiovascular Surgery, 131*, 792–798.

130. Kelleher, D. K., Laussen, P., Teizeira-Pinto, A., & Duggan, C. (2006). Growth and correlates of nutritional status among infants with hypoplastic left heart syndrome after stage 1 Norwood procedure. *Nutrition, 22*, 236–244.

131. Kent, K. M., & Cooper, T. (1974). The denervated heart: A model for studying autonomic control of the heart. *New England Journal of Medicine, 291*, 1017–1021.

132. Kirk, R., Edwards, L. B., Aurora, P., Taylor, D. O., Christie, J., Dobbels, F., Kucheryavaya, A. Y., Rahmel, A., & Hertz M. I. (2008). Registry of the International Society for Heart and Lung Transplantation: Eleventh official pediatric heart transplantation report—2008. *Journal of Heart and Lung Transplantation, 27*, 970–977.

133. Kirshbom, P. M., Flynn, T. B., Clancy, R. R., Ittenbach, R. F., Hartman, D. M., Paridon, S. M., Wernovsky, G., Spray, T. L., & Gaynor J. W. (2005). Late neurodevelopmental outcome after repair of total anomalous pulmonary venous connection. *Journal of Thoracic and Cardiovascular Surgery, 129*, 1091–1097.

134. Koch, B. M., Galioto, F. M., Vaccaro, P., Vaccaro, J., & Buckenmeyer, P. J. (1988). Flexibility and strength measures in children participating in a cardiac rehabilitation exercise program. *Physician and Sports Medicine, 116*, 139–147.

135. Kolovos, N. S., Bratton, S. L., Moler, F. W., Bove, E. L., Ohye, R. G., Bartlett, R. H., & Kulik, T. J. (2003). Outcome of pediatric patients treated with extracorporeal life support after cardiac surgery. *Annals of Thoracic Surgery, 76*, 1435–1442.

136. Kong, S. G., Tay, J. S., Yip, W. C., & Chay, S. O. (1986). Emotional and social effects of congenital heart disease in Singapore. *Australian Paediatric Journal, 22*, 101–106.

137. Kopf, G. S., & Laks, H. (1991). Atrial septal defects and cor triatriatum. In A. E. Baue, A. S. Geha, G. L. Hammond, H. Laks, & K. S. Naunheim (Eds.), *Glenn's thoracic and cardiovascular surgery* (5th ed.; pp. 995–1005). Norwalk, CT: Appleton & Lange.

138. Kovacikova, L., Dobos, D., & Zahorec, M. (2009). Non-invasive positive pressure ventilation for bilateral diaphragm after pediatric cardiac surgery. *Interactive Cardiovascular Surgery, 8*, 171–172.

139. Kramer, H. H., Aswiszus, D., Sterzel, U., van Halteren, A., & Clafen, R. (1989). Development of personality and intelligence in children with congenital heart disease. *Journal of Child Psychiatry, 30*, 299–308.

140. Krastins, I. R., Corey, M. L., McLeod, A., Edmonds, J., Levison, H., & Moles, F. (1982). An evaluation of incentive spirometry in the management of pulmonary complications after cardiac surgery in a pediatric population. *Critical Care Medicine, 10*, 525–528.

141. Kriett, J. M., & Kaye, M. P. (1991). The registry of the International Society for Heart and Lung Transplantation: Eighth official report, 1991. *Journal of Heart and Lung Transplantation, 10*, 491–498.

142. Laane, K. M., Meberg, A., Otterstad, J. E., Froland, G., & Sorland, S. (1997). Quality of life in children with congenital heart defects. *Acta Paediatrica, 86*, 975–980.

143. Laks, H., & Breda, M. A. (1991a). Tetralogy of Fallot. In A. E. Baue, A. S. Geha, G. L. Hammond, H. Laks, & K. S. Naunheim (Eds.), *Glenn's thoracic and cardiovascular surgery* (5th ed.; pp. 1179–1201). Norwalk, CT: Appleton & Lange.

144. Laks, H., & Breda, M. A. (1991b). Tricuspid atresia. In A. E. Baue, A. S. Geha, G. L. Hammond, H. Laks, & K. S. Naunheim (Eds.), *Glenn's thoracic and cardiovascular surgery* (5th ed.; pp. 1259–1272). Norwalk, CT: Appleton & Lange.

145. Lamour, J. M., Kanter, K. R., Naftel, D. C., Chrisant, M. R., Morrow, W. R., Clemson, B. S., & Kirklin, J. K. (2009). The effect of age, diagnosis, and previous surgery in children and adults undergoing heart transplantation for congenital heart disease. *Journal of American College of Cardiologists, 54*, 160–165.

146. Lawrence, K. S., & Fricker, F. J. (1987). Pediatric heart transplantation: Quality of life. *Journal of Heart Transplantation, 6*, 329–333.

147. Levitsky, S., & del Nido, P. (1991). Patent ductus arteriosus and aortopulmonary septal defects. In A. E. Baue, A. S. Geha, G. L. Hammond, H. Laks, & K. S. Naunheim (Eds.), *Glenn's thoracic and cardiovascular surgery* (5th ed.; pp. 1017–1025). Norwalk, CT: Appleton & Lange.

148. Licht, D. J., Shera, D. M., Clancy, R. R., Wernovsky, G., Montenegro, L. M., Nicolson, S. C., Zimmerman, R. A., Spray, T. L., Gaynor, J. W., & Vossough, A. (2009). Brain maturation is delayed in infants with complex congenital heart defects. *Journal of Thoracic and Cardiovascular Surgery, 137*, 529–537.

149. Licht, D. J., Wang, J., Silvestre, D. W., Nicolson, S. C., Montenegro, L. M., Wernovsky, G., Tabbutt, S., Durning, S. M., Shera, D. M., Gaynor, J. W., Spray, T. L., Clancy, R. R., Zimmerman, R. A., & Detre, J. A. (2004). Preoperative cerebral

blood flow is diminished in neonates with severe congenital heart defects. *Journal of Thoracic and Cardiovascular Surgery, 128*, 841–850.

150. Limperopoulos, C., Majnemer, A., Shevell, M. I., Rosenblatt, B., Rohlicke, C., Tchervenkov, C., & Darwish, H. Z. (2001). Functional limitations in young children with congenital heart defects after cardiac surgery. *Pediatrics, 108*, 1325–1331.

151. Linde, L. M., Rasof, B., & Dunn, O. J. (1970). Longitudinal studies of intellectual and behavioral development in children with congenital heart disease. *Acta Paediatrica, 59*, 169–176.

152. Lloyd, T. R. (1996). Prognosis of the hypoplastic left heart syndrome. *Progress in Pediatric Cardiology, 5*, 57–64.

153. Locke, T. J., Griffiths, T. C., Mould, H., & Gibson, G. J. (1990). Rib cage mechanics after median sternotomy. *Thorax, 45*, 465–468.

154. Loeffel, M. (1985). Developmental considerations of infants and children with congenital heart disease. *Heart and Lung, 14*, 214–217.

155. Longmuri, P. E., & McCrindle, B. W. (2009). Physical activity restrictions for children after the Fontan operation: Disagreement between parent, cardiologist and medical record reports. *American Heart Journal, 157*, 853–859.

156. Maher, K. O., Pizarro, C., Gidding, S. S., Januszewska, K., Malec, E., Norwood, W. I., & Murphy, J. D. (2003). Hemodynamic profile after the Norwood procedure with right ventricle to pulmonary artery conduit. *Circulation, 108*, 782–784.

157. Mahle, W. T., Clancy, R. R., McGaurn, S. P., Goin, J. E., & Clark, B. J. (2001). Impact of prenatal diagnosis on survival and early neurologic morbidity in neonates with the hypoplastic left heart syndrome. *Pediatrics, 107*, 1277–1282.

158. Mahle, W. T., Lundine, K., Kanter, K. R., Forbess, J. M., Kirshbom, P., Tosone, S. R., & Vincent, R. N. (2004). The short term effects of cardiopulmonary bypass on neurologic function in children and young adults. *European Journal of Cardiothoracic Surgery, 26*, 920–925.

159. Mahle, W. T., Tavani, F., Zimmerman, R. A., Nicolson, S. C., Galli, K. K., Gaynor, J. W., Clancy, R. R., Montenegro, L. M., Spray, T. L., Chiavacci, R. M., Wernovsky, G., & Kurth, C. D. (2002). An MRI study of neurological injury before and after congenital heart surgery. *Circulation, 106*(suppl I), I-109–I-114.

160. Mahle, W. T., & Wernovsky, G. (2001). Long-term developmental outcome of children with complex congenital heart disease. *Clinics in Perinatology, 28*, 235–247.

161. Mahle, W. T., Wernovsky, G., Moss, E. M., Gerdes, M., Jobes, D. A., & Clancy, R. R. (2000). Neurodevelopmental outcome and lifestyle assessment in school age and adolescent children with hypoplastic left heart syndrome. *Pediatrics, 105*, 1082–1089.

162. Majnemer, A., Limperopoulos, C., Shevell, M., Rohlicek, C., Rosenblatt, B., & Tchervenkov, C. (2008). Developmental and functional outcomes at school entry in children with congenital heart defects. *Journal of Pediatrics, 153*, 55–60.

163. Malaisrie, S. C., Pelletier, M. P., Yun, J. J., et al. (2008). Pneumatic paracorporeal ventricular assistive device in infants and children: Initial Stanford experience. *Journal of Heart and Lung Transplantation, 27*, 173–177.

164. Markland, O. N., Moorthy, S. S., Mahomed, Y., King, R. D., & Brown, J. W. (1985). Postoperative phrenic nerve palsy in patients with open-heart surgery. *Annals of Thoracic Surgery, 39*, 68–73.

165. Massery, M. (1987). Respiratory rehabilitation secondary to neurological deficits: Treatment techniques. In D. L. Frownfelter (Ed.), *Chest physical therapy and pulmonary rehabilitation* (pp. 538–544). Chicago: Year Book.

166. Mathew, O. P. (1988). Respiratory control during nipple feeding in pre-term infants. *Pediatric Pulmonology, 5*, 220–224.

167. Mathew, O. P., Clark, M. L., Pronske, M. L., Luna-Solarzano, H. G., & Peterson, M. D. (1985). Breathing pattern and ventilation during oral feeding in term newborn infants. *Journal of Pediatrics, 106*, 810–813.

168. Mathews, R. A., Nixon, P. A., Stephenson, R. J., Robertson, R. J., Donovan, E. F., Dean, F., Fricker, F. J., Beerman, L. B., & Fischer, D. R. (1983). An exercise program for pediatric patients with congenital heart disease: Organizational and physiologic aspects. *Journal of Cardiac Rehabilitation, 3*, 467–475.

169. McBride, M. G., Binder, T. J., & Paridon, S. M. (2007). Safety and feasibility of inpatient exercise training in pediatric heart failure: A preliminary report. *Journal of Cardiopulmonary Rehabilitation and Prevention, 27*, 219–222.

170. McCrindle, B. W., Williams, R. V., Mitchell, P. D., Hsu, D. T., Paridon, S. M., Atz, A. M., Li, J. S., & Newburger, J. W. (2006). Relationship of patient and medical characteristics to health status in children and adolescents after the Fontan procedure. *Circulation, 113*, 1123–1129.

171. McWilliams, B. C. (1987). Mechanical ventilation in pediatric patients. *Clinics in Chest Medicine, 8*, 597–607.

172. Mee, R. B. (1991). Current status of cardiac surgery in childhood. *Progress in Pediatric Surgery, 27*, 148–169.

173. Messmer, B. J., Schallberger, Y., Gattiker, R., & Senning, A. (1976). Psychomotor and intellectual development after deep hypothermia and circulatory arrest in early infancy. *Journal of Thoracic and Cardiovascular Surgery, 72*, 495–501.

174. Milgalter, E., & Laks, H. (1991). Truncus arteriosus. In A. E. Baue, A. S. Geha, G. L. Hammond, H. Laks, & K. S. Naunheim (Eds.), *Glenn's thoracic and cardiovascular surgery* (5th ed.; pp. 1079–1087). Norwalk, CT: Appleton & Lange.

175. Moodie, D. S. (2005). Technology insight: Transcatheter closure of ventricular septal defects. *Nature Clinical Practice Cardiovascular Medicine, 11*, 595.

176. Morriss, J. H., & McNamara, D. G. (1975). Residua, sequelae and complications of surgery for congenital heart disease. *Progress in Cardiovascular Diseases, 18*, 1–25.

177. Moulton, A. L., & Malm, J. R. (1991). Pulmonary stenosis, pulmonary atresia, single pulmonary artery and aneurysm of the pulmonary artery. In A. E. Baue, A. S. Geha, G. L.

Hammond, H. Laks, & K. S. Naunheim (Eds.), *Glenn's thoracic and cardiovascular surgery* (5th ed.; pp. 1131–1163). Norwalk, CT: Appleton & Lange.

178. Nakazawa, M., Okuda, H., Imai, Y., Takanashi, Y., & Takao, A. (1986). Right and left ventricular volume characteristics after external conduit repair (Rastelli procedure) for cyanotic congenital heart disease. *Heart and Vessels, 2,* 106–110.

179. Newberger, J. W., Wypij, D., Bellinger, D. C., Du Plessis, A. J., Kuban, K. C. K., Rappaport, L. A., Almirall, D., Wessel, D. L., Jonas, R. A., & Wernovsky, G. (2003). Length of stay after infant heart surgery is related to cognitive outcome at age 8 years. *Journal of Pediatrics, 143,* 67–73.

180. Niset, G., Coustry-Degre, C., & Degre, S. (1988). Psychosocial and physical rehabilitation after heart transplantation: 1-year follow-up. *Cardiology, 75,* 311–317.

181. Noonan, J. A. (1981). Syndromes associated with cardiac defects. In M. A. Engle (Ed.), *Pediatric cardiovascular disease* (pp. 97–115). Philadelphia: FA Davis.

182. Norwood, S. H., & Civette, J. M. (1991). Ventilatory assistance and support. In A. E. Baue, A. S. Geha, G. L. Hammond, H. Laks, & K. S. Naunheim (Eds.), *Glenn's thoracic and cardiovascular surgery* (5th ed.; pp. 45–66). Norwalk, CT: Appleton & Lange.

183. Norwood, W. I. (1991a). Hypoplastic left heart syndrome. *Annals of Thoracic Surgery, 52,* 688–695.

184. Norwood, W. I. (1991b). Hypoplastic left heart syndrome. In A. E. Baue, A. S. Geha, G. L. Hammond, H. Laks, & K. S. Naunheim (Eds.), *Glenn's thoracic and cardiovascular surgery* (5th ed.; pp. 1123–1130). Norwalk, CT: Appleton & Lange.

185. Nydegger, A., Walsh, A., Penny, D. J., Henning, R., & Bines, J. E. (2009). Changes in resting energy expenditure in children with congenital heart disease. *European Journal of Clinical Nutrition, 63,* 392–397.

186. O'Dougharty, M., Wright, F. S., Loewenson, R. B., & Torres, F. (1985). Cerebral dysfunction after chronic hypoxia in children. *Neurology, 35,* 42–46.

187. Ohye, R. G., & Bove, E. L. (2001). Advances in congenital heart surgery. *Current Opinion in Pediatrics, 13,* 473–481.

188. Page, G. G. (1986). Tetralogy of Fallot. *Heart and Lung, 15,* 390–400.

189. Pairolero, P. C., & Payne, W. S. (1991). Postoperative care and complications in the thoracic surgery patient. In A. E. Baue, A. S. Geha, G. L. Hammond, H. Laks, & K. S. Naunheim (Eds.), *Glenn's thoracic and cardiovascular surgery* (5th ed.; pp. 31–43). Norwalk, CT: Appleton & Lange.

190. Peetz, D. J., Spicer, R. L., Crowley, D. C., Sloan, H., & Behrendt, D. M. (1982). Correction of truncus arteriosus in the neonate using a nonvalved conduit. *Journal of Thoracic and Cardiovascular Surgery, 83,* 743–746.

191. Pennington, D. G., Noedel, N., McBride, L. R., Naunheim, K. S., & Ring, W. S. (1991). Heart transplantation in children: An international survey. *Annals of Thoracic Surgery, 52,* 710–715.

192. Perrault, H., & Drblik, S. P. (1989). Exercise after surgical repair of congenital cardiac lesions. *Sports Medicine, 7,* 18–31.

193. Peters, R. M. (1979). Pulmonary physiologic studies of the perioperative period. *Chest, 76,* 576–585.

194. Phelps, H. M., Mahle, W. T., Kim, D., Simsic, J. M., Kirshbom, P. M., Kanter, K. R., & Maher, K. O. (2009). Postoperative cerebral oxygenation in hypoplastic left heart syndrome after the Norwood procedure. *Annals of Thoracic Surgery, 87,* 1490–1494.

195. Pierpont, M. L., Basson, D. T., Benson, D. W., Gelb, B. D., Giglia, T. M., Goldmuntz, E., McGee, G., Sable, C. A., Srivastava, D., Webb, C. L. (2007). Genetic basis for congenital heart defects: Current knowledge. A scientific statement from the American Heart Association Congenital Cardiac Defects Committee, Council on Cardiovascular Disease in the Young: Endorsed by the American Academy of Pediatrics. *Circulation, 115,* 3015–3038.

196. Pizarro, C., Malec, E., Maher, K. O., Januszewska, K., Gidding, S. S., Murdison, K. A., Baffa, J. M., & Norwood, W. I. (2003). Right ventricle to pulmonary artery conduit improves outcome after stage I Norwood for hypoplastic left heart syndrome. *Circulation, 108*(suppl II), II-155–II-160.

197. Prakanrattana, U., Valairucha, S., Sriyoschati, S., Pornvilawan, S., & Phanchaipetch, T. (1997). Early extubation following open heart surgery in pediatric patients with congenital heart diseases. *Journal of the Medical Association of Thailand, 80,* 87–95.

198. Puga, F. J. (1991). Surgical treatment of pulmonary atresia with ventricular septal defect. In A. E. Baue, A. S. Geha, G. L. Hammond, H. Laks, & K. S. Naunheim (Eds.), *Glenn's thoracic and cardiovascular surgery* (5th ed.; pp. 1165–1177). Norwalk, CT: Appleton & Lange.

199. Rasof, B., Linde, L. M., & Dunn, O. J. (1967). Intellectual development in children with congenital heart disease. *Child Development, 38,* 1043–1053.

200. Razzouk, A. J., Chinnock, R. E., Gundry, S. R., & Bailey, L. L. (1996). Cardiac transplantation for infants with hypoplastic left heart syndrome. *Progress in Pediatric Cardiology, 5,* 37–47.

201. Reddy, S. C., & Webber, S. A. (2003). Pediatric heart and lung transplantation. *Indian Journal of Pediatrics, 70,* 723–729.

202. Rehabilitation of patients on Berlin heart EXCOR pediatric ventricular assist devices at Texas Children's Hospital. Presented at Texas Children's Hospital, May 29, 2009.

203. Risser, N. L. (1980). Preoperative and postoperative care to prevent pulmonary complications. *Heart and Lung, 9,* 57–67.

204. Robbers-Visser, D., Kapusta, L., van Osch-Gevers, L., Strengers, J. L. M., Boersma, E., deRijke, Y. B., Boomsma, F., Bogers, A. J. J. C., & Helbing, W. A. (2009). Clinical outcome 5 to 18 years after the Fontan operation performed on children younger than 5 years. *Journal of Thoracic and Cardiovascular Surgery, 138,* 89–95.

205. Rockett, S. R., Bryant, J. C., Morrow, W. R. (2008). Preliminary single center North American experience with the Berlin heart pediatric EXCOR device. *ASAIO J, 54,* 479–482.

206. Rockwell, G. M., & Campbell, S. K. (1976). Physical therapy program for the pediatric cardiac surgical patient. *Physical Therapy, 56,* 670–675.

207. Roos-Hesselink, J. W., Meijboom, F. J., Spitaels, S. E., van Domburg, R., van Rijen, E. H., Utens, E. M., Bogers, A. J., & Simoons, M. L. (2003). Excellent survival and low incidence of arrhythmias, stroke and heart failure long-term after surgical ASD closure at young age: A prospective follow-up study of 21–33 years. *European Heart Journal, 24,* 190–197.

208. Rosen, M., & Hillard, E. K. (1962). The effects of negative pressure during tracheal suction. *Anesthesia and Analgesia, 41,* 50–57.

209. Rosenthal, A. (1983). Care of the postoperative child and adolescent with congenital heart disease. In L. A. Barness (Ed.), *Advances in pediatrics* (pp. 131–167). Chicago: Year Book.

210. Rossi, A. F., Fishberger, S., Hannan, R. L., Nieves, J., Bolivar, J., Dobrolet, N., & Burke, R. P. (2009). Frequency and indications for tracheostomy and gastrostomy after congenital heart surgery. *Pediatric Cardiology, 30,* 225–231.

211. Rossi, A. F., Seiden, H. S., Sadeghi, A. M., Nguyen, K. H., Quintana, C. S., Gross, R. P., & Griepp, R. B. (1998). The outcome of cardiac operations in infants weighing two kilograms or less. *Journal of Thoracic and Cardiovascular Surgery, 116,* 29–35.

212. Ross Russell, R. I., Helms, P. J., & Elliot, M. J. (2008). A prospective study of phrenic nerve damage after cardiac surgery in children. *Intensive Care Medicine, 34,* 728–734.

213. Rubin, M. (1988). The physiology of bedrest. *American Journal of Nursing, 88,* 50–56.

214. Russell, I. A., Zwass, M. S., Fineman, J. R., Balea, M., Rouine-Rapp, K., Brook, M., Hanley, F. L., Silverman, N. H., & Cahalan, M. K. (1998). The effects of inhaled nitric oxide on postoperative pulmonary hypertension in infants and children undergoing surgical repair of congenital heart disease. *Anesthesia and Analgesia, 87,* 46–51.

215. Ruttenberg, H. D., Adams, T. D., Orsmond, G. S., Conlee, R. K., & Fisher, A. G. (1983). Effects of exercise training on aerobic fitness in children after open heart surgery. *Pediatric Cardiology, 4,* 19–24.

216. Sadowsky, H. S., Rohrkemper, K. F., & Quon, S. Y. M. (1986). *Rehabilitation of cardiac and cardiopulmonary recipients: An introduction for physical and occupational therapists.* Stanford, CA: Stanford University Hospital.

217. Sahu, B., Chauhan, S., Kiran, U., Bisoi, A., Ramakrishnan, L., & Nehra, A. (2009). Neuropsychological function in children with cyanotic heart disease undergoing corrective cardiac surgery: Effect of two different rewarming strategies. *European Journal of Cardio-Thoracic Surgery, 35,* 505–510.

218. Sano, S., Ishino, K., Kado, H., Shiokawa, Y., Sakamoto, K., Yokota, M., & Kawada, M. (2004). Outcome of right ventricle-to-pulmonary artery shunt in first-stage palliation of hypoplastic left heart syndrome: A multi-institutional study. *Annals of Thoracic Surgery, 78,* 1951–1958.

219. Scheidegger, D., Bentz, L., Piolino, G., Pusterla, C., & Gigon, J. P. (1976). Influence of early mobilisation on pulmonary function in surgical patients. *European Journal of Intensive Care Medicine, 2,* 35–40.

220. Schultz, A. H., Jarvik, G. P., Wernovsky, G., Bernbaum, J., Clancy, R. R., D'Agostino, J., Gerdes, M., McDonald-McGinn, D., Nicolson, S. C., Spray, T. L., Zackai, E., & Gaynor, J. W. (2005). Effect of congenital heart disease on neurodevelopmental outcomes within multiple-gestation births. *Journal of Thoracic and Cardiovascular Surgery, 130,* 1511–1516.

221. Sciurba, F. C., Owens, G. R., Sanders, M. H., Bartley, B. P., Hardesty, R. L., Paradis, I. L., & Costantino, J. P. (1988). Evidence of an altered pattern of breathing during exercise in recipients of heart-lung transplants. *New England Journal of Medicine, 319,* 1186–1192.

222. Settergren, G., Ohqvist, G., Lundberg, S., Henze, A., Bjork, V. O., & Persson, B. (1982). Cerebral blood flow and cerebral metabolism in children following cardiac surgery with deep hypothermia and circulatory arrest: Clinical course and follow-up of psychomotor development. *Scandinavian Journal of Thoracic Cardiovascular Surgery, 16,* 209–215.

223. Shi, S. S., Zhao, Z. Y., Liu, X. W., Tan, L. H., Lin, R., Shi, Z., & Fang, X. (2009). Perioperative risk factors for prolonged mechanical ventilation following cardiac surgery in neonates and young infants. *Chest Journal, 134,* 768–774.

224. Silbert, A., Wolff, P. H., Mayer, B., Rosenthal, A., & Nadas, A. S. (1969). Cyanotic heart disease and psychological development. *Pediatrics, 43,* 192–200.

225. Starnes, V. A., Marshall, S. E., Lewiston, N. J., Theodore, J., Stinson, E. B., & Shumway, N. E. (1991). Heart-lung transplantation in infants, children, and adolescents. *Journal of Pediatric Surgery, 26,* 434–438.

226. Starnes, V. A., Oyer, P. E., Bernstein, D., Baum, D., Gamberg, P., Miller, J., & Shumway, N. E. (1992). Heart, heart-lung, and lung transplantation in the first year of life. *Annals of Thoracic Surgery, 53,* 306–310.

227. Stavinoha, P. L., Fixler, D. E., & Mahony, L. (2003). Cardiopulmonary bypass to repair an atrial septal defect does not affect cognitive function in children. *Circulation, 107,* 2722–2725.

228. Stevenson, L. W. (1998). Inotropic therapy for heart failure. *New England Journal of Medicine, 339,* 1848–1850.

229. Stretton, C. D., Mak, J. C. W., Belvisi, M. G., Yacoub, M. H., & Barnes, P. J. (1990). Cholinergic control of human airways in vitro following extrinsic denervation of the human respiratory tract by heart-lung transplantation. *American Review of Respiratory Disease, 142,* 1030–1033.

230. Stromvall-Larsson, E., Eriksson, E., Holgren, D., & Sixt, R. (2004). Pulmonary gas exchange during exercise in Fontan patients at a long-term follow-up. *Clinical Physiology & Functional Imaging, 24,* 327–334.

231. Suoninen, P. (1971). Physical growth of children with congenital heart disease. *Acta Paediatrica Supplement, 225,* 7–50.

232. Sweet, S. C. (2009). Pediatric lung transplantation. *Proceedings of the American Thoracic Society, 6,* 122–127.

233. Thoren, L. (1954). Post-operative pulmonary complications. *Acta Chirurgica Scandinavica, 107,* 193–205.

234. Throckmorton, A. L., Allaire, P. E., Gutgesell, H. P., Matherne, G. P., Olsen, D. B., Wood, H. G., Allaire, J. H., & Patel, S. M.

(2002). Pediatric circulatory support systems. *ASAIO J, 48*(3), 216–221.

235. Throckmorton, A. L., & Chopski, S. G. (2008). Pediatric circulator support: Current strategies and future directions. Biventricular and univentricular mechanical assistance. *ASAIO J, 54,* 491–497.

236. Tibballs, J., & Cantwell-Bartl, A. (2008). Outcomes of management decisions by parents for their infants with hypoplastic left heart syndrome born with and without a prenatal diagnosis. *Journal of Paediatric Child Health, 44,* 321–324.

237. Todd, T. R. (1990). Early postoperative management following lung transplantation. *Clinics in Chest Medicine, 11,* 259–267.

238. Trittenwein, G., Nardi, A., Pansi, H., Golej, J., Burda, G., Hermon, M., Boigner, H., & Wollenek, G. (2003). Early postoperative prediction of cerebral damage after pediatric cardiac surgery. *Annals of Thoracic Surgery, 76,* 576–580.

239. Trojnarska, O., Grajek, S., Katarzynski, S., & Kramer, L. (2009). Predictors of mortality in adult patients with congenital heart disease. *Journal of Cardiology, 16,* 341–347.

240. Trusler, G. A. (1991). The Mustard procedure. In A. E. Baue, A. S. Geha, G. L. Hammond, H. Laks, & K. S. Naunheim (Eds.), *Glenn's thoracic and cardiovascular surgery* (5th ed.; pp. 1203–1209). Norwalk, CT: Appleton & Lange.

241. Uretsky, B. F. (1990). Physiology of the transplanted heart. In A. N. Brest (Ed.), *Cardiovascular clinics* (pp. 23–55). Philadelphia: FA Davis.

242. Uzark, L., Lincoln, A., Lamberti, J. J., Mainwaring, R. D., Spicer, R. L., & Moore, J. W. (1998). Neurodevelopmental outcomes in children with Fontan repair of functional single ventricle. *Pediatrics, 101,* 630–633.

243. Vaidyanathan, B., Radhakrishnn, R., Sarala, D. A., Sundaram, K. R., & Cumar, R. K. (2009). What determines nutritional recovery in malnourished children after correction of congenital heart defects. Retrieved from: www.pediatrics.org/cgi/doi/10.1542/peds.2009-0141.

244. van Breda, A. (1985). Postoperative care of infants and children who require cardiac surgery. *Heart and Lung, 14,* 205–207.

245. Van De Water, J. M., Watring, W. G., Linton, L. A., Murphy, M., & Byron, R. L. (1972). Prevention of postoperative pulmonary complications. *Surgery, Gynecology and Obstetrics, 135,* 229–233.

246. Visconti, K. J., Bichell, D. P., Jonas, R. A., Newburger, J. W., & Bellinger, D. C. (1999). Developmental outcome after surgical versus interventional closure of secundum atrial septal defect in children. *Circulation, 100*(suppl), II145–II150.

247. Visconti, K. J., Saudino, K. J., Rappaport, L. A., Newburger, J. W., & Bellinger, D. C. (2002). Influence of parental stress and social support on the behavioural adjustment of children with transposition of the great arteries. *Journal of Developmental Behavior Pediatrics, 23,* 314–321.

248. Vraciu, J. K., & Vraciu, R. A. (1977). Effectiveness of breathing exercises in preventing pulmonary complications following open heart surgery. *Physical Therapy, 57,* 1367–1371.

249. Waldhausen, J. A., Myers, J. L., & Campbell, D. B. (1991). Coarctation of the aorta and interrupted aortic arch. In A. E. Baue, A. S. Geha, G. L. Hammond, H. Laks, & K. S. Naunheim (Eds.), *Glenn's thoracic and cardiovascular surgery* (5th ed.; pp. 1107–1122). Norwalk, CT: Appleton & Lange.

250. Ward, R. J., Danziger, F., Bonica, J. J., Allen, G. D., & Bowes, J. (1966). An evaluation of postoperative maneuvers. *Surgical Gynecology and Obstetrics, 66,* 51–54.

251. Warner, J. O. (1991). Heart-lung transplantation: All the facts. *Archives of Disease in Childhood, 66,* 1013–1017.

252. Webber, B. A. (1991). Evaluation and inflation in respiratory care. *Physiotherapy, 77,* 801–804.

253. Weinhaus, L., Canter, C., Noetzel, M., McAlister, W., & Spray, T. L. (1989). Extracorporeal membrane oxygenation for circulatory support after repair of congenital heart defects. *Annals of Thoracic Surgery, 48,* 206–212.

254. Reference deleted in page proofs.

255. Weldon, C. S., Behrendt, D. M., & Haas, G. S. (1991). Congenital malformations of the aortic valve and left ventricular outflow tract. In A. E. Baue, A. S. Geha, G. L. Hammond, H. Laks, & K. S. Naunheim (Eds.), *Glenn's thoracic and cardiovascular surgery* (5th ed.; pp. 1089–1106). Norwalk, CT: Appleton & Lange.

256. Welke, K. F., O'Brien, S. M., Peterson, E. D., Ungerleider, R. M., Jacobs, M. L., & Jacobs, J. P. (2009). The complex relationship between pediatric cardiac surgical case volumes and mortality rates in a national clinical database. *Journal of Thoracic Surgery, 137,* 1133–1140.

257. Wells, F. C., Coghill, S., Caplan, H. L., & Lincoln, C. (1983). Duration of circulatory arrest does influence the psychological development of children after cardiac operation in early life. *Journal of Thoracic and Cardiovascular Surgery, 86,* 823–831.

258. Whitehead, B., James, I., Helms, P., Scott, J. P., Smyth, R., Higenbottam, T. W., McGoldrick, J., English, T. A. H., Wallwork, J., Elliott, M., & de Leval, M. (1990). Intensive care management of children following heart and heart-lung transplantation. *Intensive Care Medicine, 16,* 426–430.

259. Williams, W. H. (1991). Rastelli's operation for "anatomic" repair of transposition of the great arteries with ventricular septal defect and left ventricular outflow tract obstruction. In A. E. Baue, A. S. Geha, G. L. Hammond, H. Laks, & K. S. Naunheim (Eds.), *Glenn's thoracic and cardiovascular surgery* (5th ed.; pp. 1217–1226). Norwalk, CT: Appleton & Lange.

260. Wilson, R. S. (1991). Anesthesia for thoracic surgery. In A. E. Baue, A. S. Geha, G. L. Hammond, H. Laks, & K. S. Naunheim (Eds.), *Glenn's thoracic and cardiovascular surgery* (5th ed.; pp. 19–29). Norwalk, CT: Appleton & Lange.

261. Wray, J., & Sensky, T. (1998). How does the intervention of cardiac surgery affect the self-perception of children with congenital heart disease? *Child: Care, Health and Development, 24,* 57–72.

262. Youssef, N. M. (1988). School adjustment of children with congenital heart disease. *Maternal-Child Nursing Journal, 17,* 217–302.

263. Zahr, L. K., & Boisvert, J. (1990). Hypoplastic left heart syndrome repair. *Dimensions in Critical Care Nursing, 9,* 88–96.

264. Zetser, I., Jarvik, G. P., Bernbaum, J., Wernovsky, G., Nord, A. S., Gerdes, M., Zackai, E., Clancy, R., Nicolson, S. C., Spray, T. L., & Gaynor, J. W. (2008). Genetic factors are important determinants of neurodevelopmental outcome after repair of tetralogy of Fallot. *Journal of Thoracic and Cardiovascular Surgery, 135,* 91–97.

265. Zimmerman, A. A., Burrows, F. A., Jonas, R. A., & Hickey, P. R. (1997). The limits of detectable cerebral perfusion by transcranial Doppler sonography in neonates undergoing deep hypothermic low-flow cardiopulmonary bypass. *Journal of Thoracic and Cardiovascular Surgery, 114,* 594–600.

SUGGESTED READING

Almond, C. S., Thiagarajan, R. R., Piercey, G. E., et al. (2009). Waiting list mortality among children listed for heart transplantation in the United States. *Circulation, 119,* 717–727.

Bellinger, D. C., Wypij, D., Kuban, K. C. K., Rappaport, L. A., Hickey, P. R., Wernovsky, G., Jonas, R. A., & Newburger, J. W. (1999). Developmental and neurological status of children at 4 years of age after heart surgery with hypothermic circulatory arrest or low-flow cardiopulmonary bypass. *Circulation, 100,* 526–532.

Neburger, J. W., & Bellinger, D. C. (2006). Brain injury in congenital heart disease. *Circulation, 113,* 183–185.

Verheugt, C. L., Uiterwaal, C., Grobbee, D. E., & Mulder, B. J. M. (2008). Long-term prognosis of congenital heart defects: A systematic review. *International Journal of Cardiology, 131,* 25–32.

Wilkinson, J. L. (1989). Heart and heart/lung transplantation in children. *Australian Paediatric Journal, 25,* 111–118.

27 The Environment of Intervention

THUBI H. A. KOLOBE, PT, PhD, FAPTA • AMANDA AREVALO, PT, MS, PCS • TRICIA ANN CATALINO, PT, MS, PCS

Physical therapy for children relies on parents and other caregivers to positively influence the children's functional outcomes and well-being. Consequently, changes in the profile and aspirations of any contemporary society shapes the demand for specific types of services. Since the 1980s, the role of pediatric physical therapists in the provision of services for children with disabilities has expanded to address the demands for enhancing the *capacity* of the caregiving environment. More recently, the concept of *participation*, proposed in the International Classification of Functioning and Health model (ICF) by the World Health Organization,[159] has challenged professionals to consider how individuals function in their environment as the ultimate outcome of intervention. Participation is defined by the ICF as being involved in life situations and activities.[159] Although planning and providing services that enhance children's participation continues to be a challenge, designing services that enhance both children's participation and the capacity of the caregiving environment is a monumental task.

A better understanding of how physical, social, and attitudinal elements in the environment mediate children's functional skills and participation is critical for effecting change. Simply acknowledging that the caregiving environment is a crucial element in child development is not enough. Neither is accepting the role of the family. Understanding of environmental determinants entails synthesis of information from current research findings on (1) environmental factors that contribute to optimal or nonoptimal functional outcomes in children, (2) how factors interact and directly or indirectly influence outcomes, and (3) the types of intervention programs or approaches that influence the caregiving environment and child outcome directly and indirectly. Also needed are studies, particularly by pediatric physical therapists, on the environment of intervention as it relates to service delivery and motor outcomes in children. Until there are more studies on the impact of physical therapy, literature from psychology, anthropology, and family therapy offers a sizable body of knowledge that can be useful to physical therapists.

This chapter synthesizes the literature with focus on environmental factors as they relate to child development and participation, family functioning, and physical therapy interventions. First, we briefly review theoretic frameworks and findings that support targeting the child's caregiving environment and also may inform intervention strategies. Next, we analyze characteristics of the physical and social environments that have been closely linked to child outcomes and that could form the basis for service delivery models for children with disabilities. In the last section, we offer suggestions for how therapists can plan interventions that are informed by and influence the environment (contextual interventions). Because physical therapists focus their interventions on motor development and its ability to promote participation whereas research on environmental factors has focused on social and cognitive development, the chapter concentrates on environmental factors that we believe (1) may affect or be affected by physical therapy, (2) are important for children's activity and participation in daily life, and (3) are likely to contribute to the differences in the outcomes of children based on family background.

DEFINITIONS

The environment in this chapter is used to describe the *physical and social* settings in which children develop, grow, and function. The *physical* environment may be a home, day care center, school, or neighborhood. It encompasses structural conditions such as space, equipment, and material resources (e.g., toys and books), and relates to safety and access. The *social* environment conveys interactions and relationships that nurture development and shape behavior. It includes relationships, starting with interactions with parents, siblings, extended families, and extending to peers and other adults in the community. The social environment also relates to emotional wellness and the quantity and quality of support. For children and their families, these two environments are inextricably intertwined as they constitute a *caregiving environment*. No one environment can predict child outcome.

The physical environment has always been an important focus of pediatric physical therapy intervention for children with motor delays or disabilities. Concepts of skill acquisition, the principles of motor learning, and the dynamic system theory[54,145,146] emphasize the significance of the environment for motor development and function. Gentile's taxonomy of tasks[54] considers the task and the environment to be interrelated and offers suggestions for using the environment to teach a task or skill. Dynamic system theory considers the interaction of neurologic and psychologic systems and the social environment to be essential for the development of motor function.[145] Studies by Palisano and colleagues[110] and Tieman and colleagues[147] illustrate how environmental setting can affect the methods of mobility used by children with cerebral palsy. For example, children who were capable of walking with support increasingly needed more assistance ambulating at home, school, and in the neighborhood. Because more and more findings seem to point to close associations between social and economic environmental factors and child and caregiver functioning,[88,135] therapists need to also understand and incorporate some of these factors into their interventions to enhance functioning and participation in the physical environment. This is also necessary to cultivate successful partnerships with families and other caregivers.

The question of the *natural environment* often comes up in discussions of the environment of intervention. Initially, therapists and other providers defined the natural environment as a physical setting or space. More recently, however, authors and researchers in early interventionist study have expanded the definition to include both the setting where children actively participate in their everyday lives and naturally occurring routines or rituals.[98,121,129] This definition, which regards the natural environment as contextual, is subsumed in the broader definition of the caregiving environment and incorporated in information that will be discussed in this chapter.

CONCEPTUALIZING THE ENVIRONMENT

GENETICS AND THE ENVIRONMENT

The debate between the genetic versus environmental roles in shaping children's outcomes is long-standing. However, the consensus is that both do (nature-nurture interaction).[90,132] Each child is equipped with biologic and genetic characteristics that are susceptible to environmental factors that in turn influence development and participation.[91] For example, research in the fields of neuroscience, genetics, and developmental psychology report compelling data showing that the quality of early life experiences influences a child's biologic and genetic make-up.[48,74,107,132] The National Scientific Council on the Developing Child[108] explained this relationship and the basic science of early childhood development (ECD) with a set of core developmental concepts that are included in Box 27-1.

Knowledge of the epigenetic response to cumulative exposure to nurturant or suboptimal environmental conditions has implications for understanding the role of the environment in health and well-being.[48,87] Epigenetics is the

---

Box **27-1** CORE CONCEPTS OF CHILD DEVELOPMENT

- Human development is shaped by a dynamic and continuous interaction between biology and experience.
- Culture influences every aspect of development and is reflected in childrearing beliefs and practices designed to promote healthy adaptation.
- The growth of self-regulation is a cornerstone of early childhood development that influences all domains of behavior.
- Children are active participants in their own development, reflecting the intrinsic human drive to explore and master one's environment.
- Human relationships, and the effects of relationships on relationships, are the building blocks of healthy development.
- The broad range of individual differences among young children often makes it difficult to distinguish normal

variations and maturational delays from transient disorders and persistent impairments.
- The development of children unfolds along individual pathways whose trajectories are characterized by continuities and discontinuities, as well as by a series of significant transitions.
- Human development is shaped by the ongoing interplay among sources of vulnerability and sources of resilience.
- The timing of early experiences can matter, but, more often than not, the developing child remains vulnerable to risks and open to protective influences throughout the early years of life and into adulthood.
- The course of development can be altered in early childhood by effective interventions that change the balance between risk and protection, thereby shifting the odds in favor of more adaptive outcomes.

From National Research Council and Institute of Medicine. (2000). *From neurons to neighborhoods: The science of early childhood development.* Committee of Integrating the Science of Early Childhood Development, J. P. Shonkoff & D. A. Phillips (Eds.). Washington, DC: National Academy Press: Executive Summary, pp. 3–4.

study of heritable alterations in gene expression that act independently and do not change the DNA sequence.[27,34] Until recently, scientists believed that genes were the sole carrier of hereditary information from parents. However, children also inherit epigenetic "switches" from their parents that turn genes on or off. These switches can be flipped by exposure to environments and experiences to help or hinder adaptation to challenges, and they can be passed from generation to generation.[21,122,143] Epigenetic research in experimental animals and retrospective research in humans confirm that environmental influences during developmental periods have profound consequences on the phenotypic expression of biologic and behavioral traits during adulthood.[49] These findings suggest that physical therapists have a unique opportunity to influence environmental factors for optimal motor development and function with potential to carry over for generations to come.

DEVELOPMENTAL FRAMEWORKS AND THEORIES

Child development models have also evolved to encompass not only genetic predisposition but also personal characteristics and environmental factors. These include developmental systems theory, ecocultural theory, the ecologic model of human development, developmental "niche," and transactional theory. *Developmental systems theory* considers a range of developmental and evolutionary models to study the interaction of factors that influence development.[59] These factors may include genetics and biology, the physical and social environment, and culture. *Ecocultural theory* is based on the construct that children develop a sense of well-being when they are engaged in ongoing routines and activities with their family and caregivers.[156] These routines and activities are derived from the greater culture and how the family organizes to support the needs of its members and the family as a whole. The *ecologic model of human development* by Bronfenbrenner[15] expanded the transactional model to include concentric layers of influence that begin at the level of the family unit (microsystem) and extend to neighborhoods (mesosystem) and policy (macrosystem). This model emphasizes both the multilevel and multifaceted nature of environmental experiences that influence child development and performance. The *developmental niche* integrates children's development with their unique environments and cultures.[64] Developed by Super and Harkness in 1986, this model stipulates three components that encompass the child's sociocultural environment: (1) the physical and social settings of the child's life, (2) culturally regulated customs and practices of child care, and childrearing, and (3) the psychology of the caretakers.[141] The three components compose the child's microenvironment and interact together to shape the child through daily life routines. The well-known transactional theory, proposed by Sameroff and Chandler,[124] views the child's development as a function of an interaction among the child, family, and the

environment. The relationship is considered dynamic in nature, with all three elements having the power to change the nature of the interaction and the outcome of the child's development. Collectively these models support embedding services within the context of the child's environment and provide a framework for therapists to conceptualize and plan assessments and interventions. Toward the end of this chapter, we will illustrate how developmental frameworks can inform practice.

ENVIRONMENT AS A DETERMINANT OF CHILD HEALTH AND DEVELOPMENT

The World Health Organization (WHO) Commission on the Social Determinants of Health (CSDH) published the *Total Environment Assessment Model for Early Childhood Development: Evidence Report* (TEAM-ECD) supports the mounting evidence that environmental enrichment has positive implications for "sculpting" the developing brain.[135] The TEAM-ECD report explains how the environment, specifically the socioeconomic environment, is an elemental determinant of early childhood development (ECD) and, therefore, the most significant determinant of health and well-being across a life span.[73] As a critical social determinant of health, ECD is therefore viewed as a means to reduce health disparities and promote health and well-being of the population. The commission published *10 Facts About ECD as a Determinant of Health*[160] that expand conceptualizations about child development (www.who.int/child_adolescent_health/topics/development/10facts/en/index.html).

Much of the information from findings that informed the facts described in the TEAM-ECD report is not new. What is new is the emphasis on *nurturance,* attention to social and economic resources and inequities, and focus on the health and well-being as the ultimate goal of ECD—the essence of participation. The following are the Guiding Principles of the TEAM-ECD that, in our opinion, capture this environment-person interplay:
1. Early child development (physical, social/emotional, and language/cognitive development) is the result of interactions between children's biologic factors and the environments in which they are embedded.
2. Successful early child development occurs when the physical, social, and economic environment are nurturant for children.
3. The use of an equity-based approach for providing nurturant environments for children addresses the inequities in socioeconomic resources that result in inequities in early child development. Further, gains in social and economic resources for families of young children result in commensurate gains in children's developmental outcomes.[135]

The WHO Commission together with the National Academy of Sciences reports[134] are the result of an extensive analysis of research on early brain development and the role of early experiences in shaping development. Because children rely on motor function to fulfill expected societal roles (participate), these findings challenge physical therapists to not only concern themselves with the social and economic resources of the children they serve but to continually strive for innovative approaches to intervention. To do so will require current information on the characteristics of the environment that may be closely related to motor function and moderate intervention outcomes of physical therapy. As more and more children with disabilities participate in community events such as team or competitive sports and as technology advances affords such independent endeavors, ignoring socioeconomic barriers is no longer an option. Although research supports the notion of sensitive periods during which environmental experiences appear to greatly influence development such as the early childhood age, motor functioning and memory seem to show remarkable plasticity throughout the life span. Essentially, for as long as therapists rely on caregivers to support their interventions, the caregiving environment will be a major determinant of physical therapy outcomes.

CONTEXTUAL FACTORS

The question that often comes up in discussions of the role of the environment as it pertains to service delivery is that given the multiplicity of potential environmental factors that contribute to child outcome, which factors are more important? There is no simple answer because various factors are closely correlated with different domains of child development, and the relationships vary based on age, diagnosis,

caregiver health status, and family support.[23,88] Also, it is not the number of factors but their relationships and interactions with one another and with caregiving that seem to predict outcomes.[115,132,135] Furthermore, the nature of relationships is complex, suggesting the need for conceptual frameworks or models that can help contextualize these factors. Because no one environmental factor is solely responsible for an outcome, characterization of the environment must reflect interrelationships among factors. In this section we describe environmental factors, and their characteristics, that may be closely linked to physical therapy goals, interventions, and outcomes—in other words, factors that could either influence or be influenced by physical therapy to bring about optimal child and family outcomes. To some extent, some of the factors have distinguished family functioning between families of children with and without disabilities.[88]

We propose a conceptual framework that depicts the factors affecting child and family functioning and participation (Figure 27-1). For example, studies show that factors such as caregiver beliefs about childrearing, culture, stress and depression, resources available to families, and caregiver health are closely linked to optimal or nonoptimal family functioning, particularly in families of children with disabilities.[36,84,90,117,131] These factors manifest themselves in parenting behaviors during parent-child interaction, how caregivers structure the environment, and the extent of social networks. The interplay among the factors and family functioning occurs in both the distal and proximal environments. We will elaborate on each of the factors in the following sections and, as much as possible, highlight the implications for physical therapy.

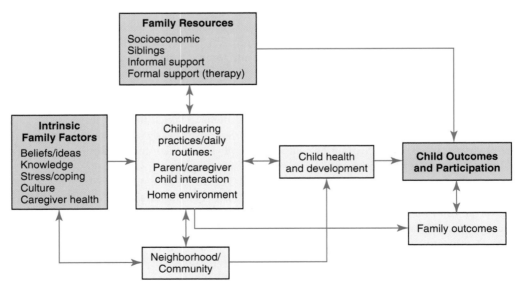

Figure 27-1   Conceptual framework of factors affecting child and family function and participation within home and child care settings (proximal environment).

DISTAL ENVIRONMENT

In this chapter, "neighborhood" and "community" are used interchangeably when referring to the distal environment. Neighborhood refers to a specific geographic area, such as a residential area. Community usually refers to a group of people who share not only a geographic area, but also social goals and institutions.[120] Neighborhoods may contain social institutions such as schools, churches, and hospitals. The extent to which child development is influenced by proximal and distal environments is proportional to the time a child spends in each environment. Younger children are influenced more by proximal environments. At school age, the influence of distal environments increases.[76,135] Research suggests that the impact of distal environments may enhance the effects of the proximal environment. For example, children of families with low incomes who live in neighborhoods with limited resources are doubly susceptible to the deleterious effects of poverty than children of families with low incomes who live in relatively affluent neighborhoods.[76] Darling and Steinberg[29] observed that for older children neighborhood factors explained differences in child outcomes over and above the variance explained by family factors.

The processes by which the factors within the neighborhood and community exert their influence on child development and competence are not clear and are, at best, speculative. Some theorists and researchers propose that frequent contact among parents at common neighborhood places may lead to shared ways of raising children.[82] Parents may use this information to structure family routines and experiences. Others believe that how the family structures and manages resources within their neighborhood determines the types of experiences they will engage in to raise their children.[25] For example, families who live in neighborhoods with high violence and poor employment opportunities may limit their children's exposure or access to social institutional resources such as the YMCA. Yet another view is that because poor employment opportunities are also associated with long working hours, children may spend a significant amount of time in alternative child care settings.[112] Depending on affordability, child care may be of good or questionable quality.

An emerging role of the physical therapist is consultation with families who express interest in their children's participation in community activities, such as sports, and swimming programs offered by park districts, crafts activities offered by most libraries, and children's theater. The extent to which children and families benefit from community activities will depend on what constitutes an optimal environment, access, and the family's level of participation. Because research indicates that availability of an informal social support network of extended family and friends who live nearby may moderate the impact of the neighborhood

on child outcome,[120] therapists should consider intervention plans that incorporate informal support networks. The Family Resources Scale[36] and Network Survey[108] are quick, easy, and family-centered ways of obtaining information on the environment from families. Scales such as the School Function Assessment[26] assess the child's performance in the school setting and can therefore generate information about this environment. The School Function Assessment is described in Chapter 30.

PROXIMAL ENVIRONMENT

The proximal environment represents the microcosm of the child's ecology.[15] Caregiving is embedded in the proximal environment. A significant portion of this chapter focuses on interactions within this environment as they are the vehicle through which nurturance occurs and the family and child shape each other.[16,40,92] Within the proximal environment the family, including the child, develops mutual relationships and a sense of cohesion that allows it to function as a unit and to nurture its members (Figure 27-2). We have developed a framework that conceptualizes how factors within the proximal environment interact to influence child functioning and participation (see Figure 27-1). In families with young children, family functioning centers on parenting behaviors and childrearing routines (e.g., caregiver-child interaction, or amount and variety of stimulation). Parenting behaviors and childrearing routines in turn are shaped by several factors such as beliefs and knowledge parents have about child development and competence, cultural expectations, the caregivers' physical and mental health, availability of resources, physical space and play materials, and the neighborhood environment. The parenting behaviors interact with the child's health and abilities to influence the child's

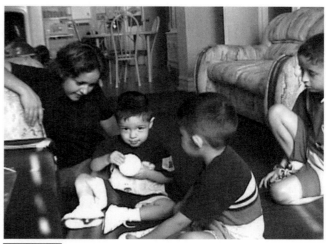

Figure 27-2 Family and its members: Sibling participation in a therapy session.

development, family functioning, and the child's level of participation. Key to this ecology is the family's home which provides the child easily accessible opportunities for social and physical interactions that foster the child's health and development. How the child perceives and responds to these interactions extend beyond the home to other environments such as school and neighborhood.

Family Structure

At the center of the child's proximal environment is the caregiving family and its structure and function.[126] Others refer to structure as household composition.[53] The family as a social system and unit consists of subsystems that represent different levels of interactions. Levels may represent the characteristics of an individual member of the family, a parent-parent, parent-child, and a child-child dyad. Family structure or composition may either be mother-child or father-child households (single parent families), nuclear families (mother, father, and children), extended households (grandparents and aunts and cousins), or foster families. Given the changing demographics in the United States, definitions of what constitutes a family and family functioning are changing, giving way to a more blended or contemporary family and roles. In any given situation, parents or a child are but one subsystem of the family unit; therefore, interventions directed at a child without regard to other subsystems may be limited. The structure of the family also shapes family resources and influences the type of care the child receives. Whether or not families are two-parent versus single-parent families not only affects income, but it also influences the flexibility parents can have in employment arrangements and child care.

A question of the benefits of the ratio of adults to child as they relate to family structure merits special consideration. Research findings on the influence of adult/child ratio on child development suggest that a high caregiver/child ratio is favorable, particularly for social and cognitive development.[71,105] Infants are likely to receive a variety of stimulations when the ratio is high. It is important to point out, however, that the literature on children living in single-family homes suggests that these children have poorer outcomes when compared to those who live in homes with two biologic parents.[18,92,152]

The findings on the adult/child ratio relationship and motor outcome, however, are inconclusive.[53,85,105] Mulligan and associates[105] observed that infants of families with a low caregiver/child ratio had lower motor scores at 9 months but no correlations were found at 6 and 12 months. Garrett and associates[53] and Kolobe[85] found no associations between the caregiver/child ratio and infants' scores on motor tests. The presence of an extended family (versus the number of adults in the family) may play a key role in moderating this relationship. For example, in extended family households, the infant may be indulged by a large number of adults. As a result, the demand on the child to be independent in areas

such as self-help and mobility may not be high. In some instances, other extended family members may influence parents by lowering expectations of the child, particularly a child with a physical disability.

Family structure has several implications for physical therapy. The family structure can have a *protective or stressful* impact on children's development and well-being. For example, a high adult/child ratio that includes extended family members may create more opportunities for caregiver-child interactions that promote the child's well-being and positive social and cognitive developmental outcomes. But, because of the findings on motor outcome, during assessments therapists must not only determine if the child's family is relying on the extended family member as caregivers, but they should also seek to understand the expectations the family members may have for the child's functional independence and participation in family routines. Few studies have examined the benefits of a high adult/child ratio in families of children with physical disabilities. It would appear that situations in which the child requires assistance and multiple services, a high ratio would be beneficial.

Because low socioeconomic status creates the likelihood for overcrowding and limited resources, the appearance of a high adult/child ratio under these conditions may stress the family structure and place more demands on the family. Overcrowding has been associated with poor cognitive development, interpersonal behavior, and mental health.[40,68] Therefore, the appearance of overcrowding must be discussed with the family. Therapists must seek to understand the family's perceptions of the role of the various members of the household as it relates to the child before seeking or consulting social services. Failure to do so may bridge the trust the family may have with the therapist or result in a high cancellation of scheduled appointments.

Family Functioning

Many of the environmental factors that may influence or be influenced by physical therapy exert their influence on the child through family functioning.[115] Family functioning refers to the family's ability to conduct and accomplish everyday activities across various situations.[66] The child, as a subsystem within a family system, influences and is influenced by the interactive nature in which the family performs its functions. A great deal of family functioning centers on parenting behavior and childrearing. Childrearing practices represent goal-directed actions that parents engage in to promote their children's development.[29] A related term used in the literature is *family routines*.[31,33,43] That childrearing is the vehicle through which families shape the behavior and development of children is widely accepted,[29,134,135] although the childrearing practices and behaviors that exert the strongest influence on motor development are unclear. Research on childrearing has focused on cognitive, social, emotional, and language development.[5,77] The few studies that have included the motor domain suggest that how parents interacts with the child and structure the learning and home environment may affect motor development.[2,6,24,53] In turn, parent-child interaction and how the caregiver structures the learning environment are related to parenting beliefs and culture[11,104] with family stress serving as a moderating factor between parenting beliefs and behavior.[131]

Parenting Beliefs

Childrearing practices do not occur in isolation. As depicted in the model presented in Figure 27-1, childrearing practices that families engage in may reflect the beliefs, ideas, perceptions, expectations, and attitudes families have about parenting and child competence.[83,104] Many parents have ideas about how children develop and what they should do to foster specific developmental skills. Parents' beliefs about child development may also influence decisions about why one approach to childrearing is better than the other.[47,136] The belief-behavior link is believed to have contributed to parent education models and programs used by professionals. The underlying assumption is that parents have the power to change the child (change agents) and that educating parents will influence their ideas about parenting and child outcome.

A great deal of information about child development and behavior that shape parents' beliefs about childrearing comes from media that are widely endorsed by society,[84] such as magazines and television. Similar information about children with disabilities, however, is not as readily available, creating information gaps and uncertainty. Indeed, parents of children with disabilities have consistently ranked the need for information high.[148] Parents have also perceived information sharing as one of the most valuable aspects of therapy.[155] These findings have significant implications for therapists. They underscore the importance of therapists sharing information with families about development, assessment findings, various intervention approaches and their evidence, and resources that are available in their communities, including information on the Internet. According to Grosec and associates,[60] "parents who have accurate knowledge of their child's ability are better able to match teaching efforts to their child's developmental level" (p. 266), particularly fathers. Children, as early as infancy (1) initiate actions that may or may not be acceptable to their caregivers, (2) are capable of evaluating the consequences of such actions, (3) express and negotiate their needs, and (4) make decisions to comply with, or resist, the caregivers' actions or instructions.[67]

Parent-Child Interaction

Parent-child interaction is a childrearing component of family functioning that represents an intimate transaction between children and their caregivers; it is considered the basis for subsequent relationships children form.[5] Parent-child interaction refers to any verbal or nonverbal communication between the parent and child that is met with a

verbal or behavioral response.[91] The continual and contingent characteristic of parent-child interaction is what is believed to shape relationships and influences skill acquisition. Parent-child interaction is predicated on the notion that the child and caregiver have a dual responsibility to maintain the interaction.[4] A great deal of parent-child interaction occurs during caregiving and play, which are sensorimotor experiences. When parent-child relationships provide nurture and responsiveness, the result is healthy brain architecture, which can promote positive child outcomes.[131]

Barnard[5] identified four features of successful parent-child interaction:

- Repertoire of behaviors, such as body movements and facial expressions
- Contingent responses to each other
- Rich interactive content in terms of play materials, positive affect, and verbal stimulation
- Adaptive response patterns that accommodate the child's emerging developmental skills

If both the parent and child must have a sufficient repertoire of behaviors, then limitations in either the child's movements or the caregiver's facial expressions may result in interactions that are less then satisfying.[77] Children with motor disabilities often demonstrate slow responses to external stimulation, which may limit the richness of contingent responses between them and their caregiver. Indeed, mothers of children with disabilities were described as initiating play and more directive during play interactions with their children compared to mothers of children with typical development.[100,133] Preliminary findings from a longitudinal study on the influence of parent-child interaction on motor outcome showed a relationship between the dyadic patterns at age 1 and motor performance at age 3 years.[86] Therefore, sharing information with parents about their children's abilities and providing suggestions for encouraging their children's activity and participation may optimize parent-child interactions.

Implications of parent-child interactions to physical therapy are numerous. Of particular relevance are findings that suggest that parent-child interactions are amenable to change and that the quality of interactions can improve with time.[5,79,131,137] Using videotaped recordings of parent-child interactions at 30 months of age, Spiker and associates[137] observed that mothers in the group receiving weekly home visits and center-based program were more supportive and offered more developmentally appropriate stimulation than mothers in the control group. Chiarello and Palisano[24] reported modest gains in the quality of interaction following physical therapy intervention provided in the context of play and parent-child interaction. Given that children with physical disabilities have limitations in their repertoire of motor skills, it would seem that physical therapy interventions should emphasize adaptive responses and synchronous relationships between children and caregivers. Focusing on motor activities that promote parent-child interaction early in the child's life may provide a foundation for later relationships with adults and peers.

Characteristics of positive interactions include flexibility of the caregiver, responsiveness to the child's distress and cues, and contingency in responses by both the child and caregiver. The ability to (1) allow disruption, (2) redirect the child in a supportive manner, and (3) allow the child to initiate an action are reported as distinguishing features of successful and mutually enjoyable interactions.[5,100] This information is particularly relevant for families of children with short attention who need repeated redirecting, and children with cerebral palsy who may need prompts and extra time to initiate actions. Therapists are encouraged to consider these essential ingredients when working with caregivers on new skills for their children.

Therapists can also explore parent-child interactions intervention approaches developed by professionals in other disciplines. For example, the Promoting First Relationships (PFR) curriculum is a training program for providers to help caregivers provide sensitive and responsive care that facilitates positive parent-child relationships. Studies show that when service providers are given PFR training, they learn how to give parents feedback to promote nurturing relationships, improve parent-child interactions, and help mothers learn about their child's feelings and needs.[78,79] The research on PFR shows that when the providers were trained, mothers were more competent in recognizing their child's interactive behaviors and cues. Further, the children were more responsive to their mothers and more contingent in their interactions. When caregivers teach a child a new skill, physical therapists can encourage them to particularly pay attention to the child's cues of engagement and disengagement, such as pleasure and distress. Because children have a wider repertoire of disengagement than engagement cues and because learning a new skill is likely to trigger a cluster of disengagement cues, demonstrating how the caregiver can recognize, prevent, or alleviate the cues may be more effective than simply showing the caregiver how to teach the new skill. Sumner and Spietz[140] provided excellent information on child cues.

Therapists may also share and model the "teaching loop" with parents.[140] The teaching loop has four elements: (1) verbally and nonverbally alerting the child to the task and teaching material, (2) giving clear instructions about how the task it to be performed, (3) allowing the child time to perform the task, and (4) giving the child feedback. Central to the teaching loop is the process of contingency, the immediacy of a response from either the child or the caregiver. An example of instructive feedback is "It's really nice the way you let her figure out how to pull her arm out from underneath while she was lying on her tummy. This opportunity allowed her time to plan and strategize (on how to get her arm out), to engage in trial and error, and to know that you are watching to help if needed." An example of positive feedback is "It is great how you give her eye contact and cheer her on when she tries to eat the cheerios by herself. Praise has been shown to increase the likelihood that the child will repeat the success, and most children like being praised when they are successful." Overall, many of the elements of the teaching loop are consistent with the principles of motor learning described in Chapter 4.

Culture

A family's culture is at the heart of parenting behaviors and transcends beliefs and expectations about child development and societal roles. The notion that many of the childrearing practices that parents engage in are embedded in families' ethnic traditions is also widely accepted.[52] The challenge for professionals continues to be the cultural mismatch that results from development and implementation of culturally inappropriate interventions. Cultural mismatch is also believed to contribute to health disparity, particularly between the majority and minority cultures.[151] The mismatch can also affect the professional-family-child relationships.

A distinction needs to be made between ethnicity and culture as these terms tend to be used interchangeably. Ethnicity is part of one's identity derived from membership through birth in a racial, national, or linguistic subgroup.[93] Individuals can come from the same ethnic group (e.g., Hispanic), but differ in culture. Therefore, defining culture in terms of ethnicity overlooks the variations within groups and often results in stereotyping of families. Culture is considered to be a shared ideology and valued set of beliefs, norms, customs, and meanings evidenced in a way of life.[142] See Box 27-2 for central themes and other terms that are used to describe culture. Culture influences how families understand life processes, define health and illness, and perceive the causes of illness; it also shapes their attitudes toward wellness and influences their beliefs about the cure. This includes physical therapy. Culture is also believed to play a role in the confidence with which childrearing ideas are held by parents, and the flexibility with which parents are amenable to change, particularly in light of new information (e.g., parent education).[52]

Box 27-2   **CENTRAL THEMES PERTAINING TO CULTURE**

- It serves as a blueprint to guide daily behavior.
- It is a system of learned patterns of behavior.
- It is shared by other members of a group.
- It influences peoples' beliefs, values, behaviors, and perceptions.
- It is a way of life.
- It is passed on from one generation to another.
- It is valued by members of the culture and considered to be right.
- Its influences are not always conscious.

Literature on culture is extensive and a detailed discussion on culture and child development is beyond the scope of this chapter. For more information, the following are recommended: Rios Muñoz,[117] Bruns & Corso,[19] Madding,[97] Leavitt,[89] Masten,[101] Rogoff and associates,[119] and Super and Harkeness.[142] A central theme of the literature on culture is that the lack of self-awareness by professionals during family-professional interactions can produce negative emotional responses and hinder collaborations. A therapist's educational background, culture, values, and beliefs may unconsciously influence the goals and hopes they have for children and families. In this section, we will briefly discuss conceptualizations about cultural beliefs and parenting behaviors that we believe enhance collaborations between therapists and families from diverse cultures and promote cultural sensitivity—a step toward cultural competence.

Conceptualizations of the cultural environment and how it is linked to the developing child vary. One such conceptualization, the developmental "niche," has been proposed by Super and Harkness.[142] The developmental "niche" describes three core concepts that we believe could be integrated into frameworks and approaches for interventions with families, particularly team-based interventions. These concepts consider the child's cultural environment as (1) representing culturally shared ideas held by parents that inform childrearing, (2) comprising individuals that have assigned roles and responsibilities within a "given frame of routines of daily life" (p. 4), and (3) consisting of shared childrearing practices that integrate the child into the environment. These concepts are distinctive and yet complementary. Cultural beliefs and parent action have implications for collaborative goal setting. Parents who are concerned about the basic survival of their children will organize their caregiving around protection. Parents may hold their infants more and engage in soothing and tactile type of interactions. On the other hand, parents who believe that the lives of their children are not threatened may engage more in talking with the baby than holding the baby.[116] The implicit nature of cultural beliefs suggests that therapists should listen for information that relates to the hierarchical nature of beliefs (e.g., survival/protection before stimulation) when gathering data during examination and goal development. Skills in interviewing are of utmost importance.

Another conceptualization that provides a good understanding of the link between the cultural beliefs and parenting behaviors comes from the hierarchy of beliefs by Sameroff and Feil:[125] *categorical, compensatory,* and *perspectivistic.* These beliefs influence how parents perceive and respond to their children's behaviors[61] and differ based on acculturation and biculturalism. A categorical belief is associated with attributing a single cause to one outcome. Parents with categorical beliefs are likely to exhibit difficulty in adapting their childrearing practices. A compensatory belief is characterized by a belief that multiple causes lead to multiple outcomes, and parents in this category are likely to pursue several childrearing options. Perspectivistic beliefs are associated with adaptive or flexible parent behaviors. Parents believe that multiple causes may interact with other systems to produce different or alternative outcomes. Take an example of a mother's reaction to her child's inability to crawl at 1 year. A mother who has a categorical belief may suspect heredity and decide to "wait and see." A mother with compensatory beliefs may suspect heredity or illness and consult a professional, whereas a mother with perspective beliefs may acknowledge the possibility that this is something that runs in the family, but may also investigate other potential causes such as illness and the degree of stimulation or expectations in the home, and she may consult both friends and professionals. Guttierez and Sameroff[61] observed that Mexican-American mothers tended to be categorical, but bicultural Mexican-American mothers were more perspectivistic than Anglo-American mothers. These findings highlight the influence of acculturation on cultural beliefs and parent behavior.

How parents perceive their children's development and behavior has significant implications for examination, goal setting, and intervention. The flexibility to accept one or a variety of outcomes is also germane to expectations parents may have about therapists, therapy, and the intervention process as they relate to their children. Perspectivism is associated with ability to accept diversity (of child behavior and outcome). We believe that this would include ideas of outsiders such as health care providers. Although Sameroff and Feil[125] indicated the neither category is good or bad, they suggest that the explanations given by parents for why things occur be put in the context that applies to each category. In a case of a child with a disability, when the cause of the disability is unknown, or there are multiple causes of functional limitations, or multiple interventions, having a perspectivistic view may be helpful. Parents are more likely to change when new information is in agreement with their views and beliefs.[65]

Cultural beliefs that families hold about childrearing and development need to be examined in the context of decisions parents make. One way of understanding families' perspective is to use scenarios or vignettes. Another is to use questions that focus on both the context and content, particularly circumstantial contexts, and to engage in meta-listening in order to hear how parents explain their children's behavior and expectations. For example, therapists may ask questions like, "If one were to understand how and why your child moves the way she/he does, what would one need to know or do?" Or "children with Down syndrome sometimes prefer to sit and not move around, tend to have strong preference for certain foods than others, or to enjoy banging objects. I notice that Kiesha likes to do some of the same things. Why do you think she does these things? Is that what your family thinks? Does this bother you? What about other family members?" What is important is how parents perceive and interpret the child's behavior.[69] Hirsberg suggested listening for anxiety and conflict (in terms of decision making). If shifting parent perspective is considered in the best interest of the child (e.g., from categorical to perspectivism), then the therapist should ask parents how their expectations could be realized, the rationale behind the goals they envisage for their children, and what they perceive as a consequence if a goal is not attained. This is particularly important for parents from minority cultures who may have a harder time participating in decision making and for whom barriers to proactive participation and collaboration may exist.[99] When working with families from culturally diverse populations, therapists also need to be aware of where the decision making power is within each family. In many families, the father is the decision maker; however, in cultures such as Mexican- or African-American families, extended family members may be the decision makers.

Documented negative consequences of cultural mismatch and incompetence on the part of professionals have led to attention directed at training in cultural sensitivity and competence. Knowing about other cultures can be a daunting task. The Think Cultural Health website (www.thinkculturalhealth.org) is a resource for health care professionals to become culturally competent. The website provides materials and tools and helps allocate resources on professional cultural competency. Several cultural awareness self-assessments questionnaires are available (e.g., from the Maternal and Child Health website: www.hrsa.gov/OMH/cultural). Box 27-3 includes a checklist of practical actions. We have compiled the list from information identified by authors cited previouly. Therapists may find the list useful when working with families of diverse backgrounds.

Parenting Stress and Coping

One rationale for intervening with children with disabilities and their families is to reduce levels of stress and burden of care that may be experienced by families. Stress serves as a moderating factor between parenting beliefs and behavior. Shonkoff[131] described the impact of contextual factors on developmental outcomes based on the principle of dynamic stress. Dynamic stress includes positive stress, tolerable stress, and toxic stress. Positive stress is physiologic stress that is short-term and repairable. Tolerable stress can be neutralized by supportive relationships that provide a safe environment and have minimal impact on a child's development. Toxic stress (such as, extreme poverty, physical/emotional abuse, maternal depression, family violence) can disrupt brain architecture, which can lead to developmental delays. The fundamental principle of dynamic stress is important when considering environment and contextual factors in relation to the science of early childhood development—that is, the interconnectedness between genetics neurobiology, developmental psychology, and ecology.

Stress associated with caregiving is not unique to families of children with disabilities, although these families report more stress than their counterparts.[88] All families experience unique stressors. The difference between whether or not stress will disrupt family functioning is in how the family perceives the stressful event. Each family reacts to a stressor according to the family's perception, the number of stressful events they are experiencing simultaneously, the family's resources for managing the stressors, and characteristics of the stressor events themselves.[102] Studies show that the number of child-related stressors and the amount and quality of family resources, such as social support, are the most significant factors in the adjustment of the family. Therapists need to be aware of the real and perceived stressors and the resources or support available to each family unit. Adaptation appears to be a continuous variable that is dependent on the unique combination of stressors and resources.

BOX 27-3   CONCEPTS TO CONSIDER WHEN WORKING WITH FAMILIES OF CULTURALLY DIVERSE BACKGROUNDS

Develop an awareness of one's own values, beliefs, and culture.
Learn about the family culture.
Determine the family's extent of acculturation.
Learn (via observation and interaction with the family) about the family's views on children, childrearing, child development, disability, intervention, medicine and healing, roles of family members, common religious beliefs).
Respect the uniqueness (such as values and beliefs) of each family system:
  • Determine if there is a family member who is the head-of-the household, and address that person when delivering service.
  • Determine which family member is the primary caregiver for the child, and include that person in the therapy session.

• Determine if there is more than one person who is the primary caregiver or who is included in childrearing.
• Communicate in culturally appropriate ways, such as addressing family members in formal or informal tones.
• Use examination procedures, tests and measures, interventions, and activities that are culturally sensitive.
• Recognize that a caregiver might identify with one culture but might not choose to adhere to its beliefs.
• Use translators when needed, and make sure to speak to the caregiver and not the translator.
• At the initial examination, gather only pertinent information about the family's culture in relation to the child, parenting practices, and childrearing beliefs.

Stress seems to also be related to the number of roles a person assumes.[57] Mothers who were the sole responsible provider for their children reported greater stress and poorer psychologic well-being than mothers who were partial providers. Although multiple roles were found to positively influence the mothers' self-esteem, too many roles resulted in depressive symptoms. With more and more single parents working out of the home, the varying and conflicting roles of caregivers should be considered when planning interventions with families. Stress compounds the impact of poverty on children's development. For example, the child outcomes of a parent guidance intervention provided to mothers of low socioeconomic status (SES) were less favorable for mothers experiencing high stress.[14] These findings suggest that therapy interventions, if not well matched with the family's needs, may add to parenting stress.

The findings on stress and coping provide a compelling reason for physical therapists to assess caregiver stress. A therapist with good communication and observations skills should have little trouble identifying stressors in families. However, assessing the level of stress is easier to do when working with a multidisciplinary team. Psychologists or social workers can help guide the interview process or administer evaluations that are related to parental stress, maternal depression, and other toxic stressors. If these professionals are not available, as is sometimes the case in rural areas, tools that assess caregiving within the home environment (e.g., the HOME), maternal stress level and psychosocial level (e.g., the Parenting Stress Index-Short Form (PSI/SF), and socioeconomic status (e.g., Hollingshead scale) may help guide decision making and determination of toxic stressors occurring in the child's life.

Once identified, stressors should be reflected in the type of service delivery, frequency, and duration of intervention. For instance, for a family whose income is far below the poverty line and at risk of being evicted from their home, improving their child's gross motor development and receiving weekly physical therapy services might not be a priority. In such situations, referrals to social services and community resources might be more beneficial than physical therapy.

Caregiver Health

Evidence of the relationship between the health of caregiver and that of children with disabilities continues to grow. Findings from a Canadian population-based study suggest that there may be an increased risk for chronic health conditions among caregivers of children with disabilities such as cerebral palsy, particularly those with behavior problems.[13,88] These caregivers reported more and poorer health conditions such as back problems and ulcers and higher episodes of depression and stress than caregivers of children without disabilities. Although no causal connections are implied, the findings suggest that caring for children with neurodevelopmental disorders, particularly if accompanied by behavior problems, may be an added source of stress for caregivers.[13]

The results also revealed that the majority of families seem to be able to balance caring for a child with a disability with other family demands. These findings suggest that the history component of the physical therapist's examination should include questions about caregiver health. This information exchange is useful for intervention planning but must be voluntary on the part of the family.

Family Resources

Part C of the IDEIA of 2004 mandates determination of family resources as part of child and family assessment and as a basis for the development of the individualized family service plan (IFSP). Family resources, or lack thereof, are a major contributing factor to child outcome and may be part of the proximal or distal environment.[51,103] Within the proximal environment, the family's resources may be internal, such as parents' level of education or knowledge about child development, whereas the distal resource may be external such as income-related resources or support networks. Because family resources are numerous, multifaceted, and need based, not all the resources that are needed to promote optimal family functioning can be provided through the formal service delivery system. Therefore, the approach recommended is to select family resources that may be related to motor development and participation in the home and community and evaluate how they may be impacted by physical therapy interventions. The multifactorial nature of influence suggests that positive childrearing practices can mediate negative factors of a child's physical environment[40,92] but not vice versa. In this section, we will discuss socioeconomic status (SES) and family support. SES is an indicator of parental education, occupation, and family structure.[70]

Socioeconomic Status

Children of families with low SES are overrepresented among children with disabilities and developmental delays[134] and less likely to receive a full complement of services.[103] The influence of poverty on child development is nonlinear. Younger children are more susceptible to the effects of poverty.[35] Children of minority race/ethnicity tend to be the most affected by poverty.[17,51] Two studies reported a positive correlation between SES and motor development of young infants,[53,85] calling attention to the need for physical therapists to examine the relationship more closely.

How SES influences child development and competence is not well understood. Several mechanisms have been proposed. First, SES organizes family life in terms of determining how much money or time parents allocate to raising their children. Second, factors such as poor maternal and infant malnutrition, stress, and pervasiveness of toxic environments that are prevalent in low SES environments affect brain size and growth.[113] Other mechanisms are believed to be the types of neighborhoods that parents choose to raise their children (Figure 27-3), access to community resources that foster

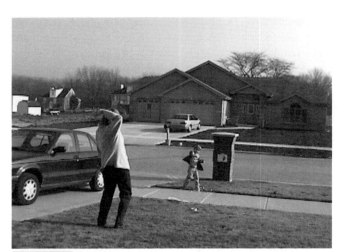

Figure 27-3 Neighborhoods where children grow up influence their development.

child development such as child care, the availability of learning material in the home, and parental stress.[17,53,63]

Research on resilience and protective factors suggests that infants and young children who live in adverse conditions are most vulnerable when protective factors such as maternal competence are stressed.[157] Efforts to ameliorate the negative effects of poverty on children, particularly through parent education, have had mixed results. Halpern[63] performed an extensive review on the outcomes of early intervention for children and families with low SES and concluded that little progress has been made in the early 21st century in improving the lives of families from low SES, including those with children who have special needs.

Of significance to pediatric therapists is the discrepancy that often exists between services provided under research conditions compared with actual practice. Interventions provided under research conditions tend to be more comprehensive and intensive. Depending on program resources, therapists may need to use innovative approaches to service delivery. Frequencies and intensities predetermined by programs may need to be modified to accommodate the families' needs. For example, depending on family needs, therapists may explore with families the feasibility of intensive interventions initially followed by periods of monitoring and consultation. In other words, therapists may need to explore the issue of critical periods for child and family learning. Currently the money allocated to services for children with special needs is far less than the costs associated with providing "best practices" as mandated by IDEA.[16]

Informal and Formal Support

Support represents the relationship between the need perceived by an individual and the appropriateness of the response. Parents of children with disabilities have been reported to have lower perceived social support compared to those without.[88] Two forms of support are described in the literature: social and professional, or informal and formal.[36] Social support refers to mutually rewarding personal interactions from which an individual derives feelings of being valued and esteemed. The need for social support for children with special needs and their families varies throughout the life span. A shift in support occurs as the child matures, from professional support, to family support, to support from friends. The caretakers of younger children rely on spouse interaction[42] and physician information for support, whereas caretakers of older children rely more on friends and community members.[28]

An important source of professional support is information sharing. Positive child and family outcomes have been associated with those interventions that focused on providing parents with information pertaining to child development, caregiving for a child with special needs or a chronic disease, and linking families to community resources.[75,109,128] Therapists are an important source of information for parents in many areas of development, particularly on issues related to mobility and assistive devices.

The impact of social support on parent, child, and family functioning has been studied extensively.[36,139] Overall the findings reveal that social support can buffer the negative effects of stress and impoverished distal and proximal environments. The adequacy of various forms of support enhances positive caregiver interaction styles, positive perception of the child, and family well-being. The authors also have discussed various ways of assessing social support. Not only is support offered in different ways and perceived to have different meanings by families, but also professionals construe the concept of support differentially. Stewart[139] described five social support theories that can be applied to clinical practice and, therefore, are germane to this chapter:

- *Attribution theory* relates to motives for helping, the process of gaining or giving support, and the negative as well as positive aspects of support.
- *Coping theory* refers to the cognitive aspects of support and its costs to those involved.
- *Equity theory* describes the reciprocal nature of support.
- *Loneliness theory* emphasizes the affective aspects of support.
- *Social-comparison theory* addresses the effects of peer support.

Combining these perspectives, Stewart proposed several recommendations for intervention. First is agreement between the health care professionals and persons providing support regarding the intervention approach. Second is the notion that support can foster adaptation to stress and prevent health disorders and that professionals have a role in understanding the sources of stress and proposing ideas for support. For example, therapists can ascertain whether their clients have a social network that mediates potential loneliness. According to Stewart, recognition of the reciprocal role of social support may encourage the professional to share information and offer support to decrease the family's sense of isolation.

Home Environment

For decades the connection between the home environment and children's development and competence has been the subject of research by psychologists, educators, and health professionals.[20] Research during the 1970s and 1980s was largely concerned with understanding the relationship between poverty and child development. As the number of children born prematurely increased, the home environment has again emerged as a topic that merits special attention.[10,12] Traditionally, motor development was believed to be less sensitive to changes in the home environment. This perspective was supported by studies of children younger than 3 years of age that used the Bayley Scales of Infant Development. Later studies of preschool children, however, suggest there is a positive relationship between the quality of the home environment, measured by the Home Observation Measure of the Environment (HOME), and motor development.[10,53,86] These findings suggest that the influence of the home environment on motor development may be gradual. There may not be an immediate impact on function. The HOME assesses the quality of various aspects of child participation in family activities, teaching and learning opportunities, and the appropriateness of toys, which are important for therapists and parents to discuss. The HOME also provides a systematic way of gathering information about the caregiving environment and can be a valuable asset for service delivery in any setting.

Physical therapists have expertise in modification of the physical environment of the home to increase a child's activities and participation. The focus has been on adapting equipment the physical space to accommodate the child with disabilities. This can include architectural changes such as ramps or handrails, and special equipment such as special chairs and standers. The child's home also offers the therapist an opportunity to put interactions in context. Assessment of the caregiving environment is particularly useful for interventions designed to improve a child's participation in family activities and routines. Examination and evaluation of a child's strengths and needs in the home enables informed decisions on whether intervention should focus on changing the child's abilities, the task, the environment, or some combination to improve activity and participation (Figure 27-4). The assessment includes, but is not limited to, type of floor surface, space, curbs and steps, door sizes, table heights, and access to toys. Observations can include how the family organizes tasks, environmental demands placed on the child, and opportunities for play and exploration. Besides the HOME, other assessment tools that consider the child's environment are the Pediatric Evaluation of Disability Inventory (PEDI),[62] and School Function Assessment (SFA),[26] Children's Assessment of Participation and Enjoyment (CAPE).[81] In addition, parent interviews, questionnaires, and surveys are other

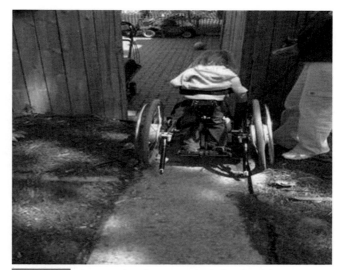

Figure 27-4   Contextual environment: physical and social.

forms of obtaining information about the child's functional abilities in their environment.

IMPLICATIONS FOR INTERVENTION

Despite the overwhelming evidence that supports the importance of the environment in shaping the development and functional independence of children, changing the childrearing environments of children through interventions such as parent education has proved difficult. At the heart of this dilemma is lack of information about the amount of resources or the intensity of interventions that are of sufficient magnitude to bring about change in the child and family. Evidence suggests that families' familiarity with particular teaching strategies, coupled with the importance they place on achievement, plays a major role in the types of activities they will invest in.[55] Yet seldom do professionals take the time to understand these expectations and strategies.

Interventions with children can only be as successful as what the caregiving environment has to offer. The ultimate goal of therapy is to enhance this environment by supporting and promoting positive interactions between the child and the environment and participation in life situations. In the last segment of this chapter, we propose ways for therapists to use the information from the preceding sections when planning assessments and interventions that are contextual. We briefly describe an organizing intervention model that we have developed, which capitalizes on the characteristics of the environment and key features from some of theoretic frameworks previously discussed. We draw attention to how the contextual environment can inform what we consider the "first encounter" between the therapist and the child's family, discuss the skills that the therapist and family must have if they are to form meaningful and successful partnerships necessary to optimize child outcomes, present an example of what we consider a contextual assessment process, and conclude with a brief example of an intervention approach that intended to maximize information exchange between the professional and caregivers.

KNOWLEDGE TRANSLATION FOR CAREGIVERS AND CHILDREN MODEL

Parent (or caregiver) education is the most commonly used intervention approach and is seen as a vehicle through which to bridge professional information and child outcome. A review of programs that focused on parents as teachers of their children and home visitation, however, reported poor correlations between maternal and child outcomes.[58] Overall all program effects have also been short term, suggesting limitations in carry-over or caregiver competency and the need to rethink strategies used in by professionals. We have used information from teaching and learning paradigms and cultural childrearing frameworks to develop and test the Knowledge Translation for Caregivers and Children (KT for CACH), a model of *knowledge translation* from professional to parent to child (Figure 27-5). The model is multifactorial and interactive: First it capitalizes on participation as a form of social learning, communication, and behavior change.[118,119] Second, it carefully titrates *anticipatory forms of guidance* and instruction into the *participatory exchange*.[8] Third, the model maximizes information sharing through vignettes.[9] Fourth, it creates frequent opportunities for self-evaluations as contexts for meta-awareness and behavior change.[3] The model balances professional skill-orientated approaches with social realities of cultural expectations.[8,106] We will apply this information to a case scenario, but first we will explain the concepts included in the model and described in the approach.

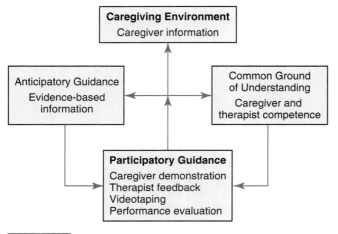

Figure 27-5 The Knowledge Translation for Caregivers and Children model.

Anticipatory Guidance

Anticipatory guidance is a concept and practice that has been used extensively in health care. Telzrow[144] defined it as "the provision of information to parents or children with the expected outcome being a change in parent attitude, knowledge, or behavior" (p. 14). Anticipatory guidance centers on professional opinions, knowledge, and expertise, and often sets the agenda for interventions.[37] Many of the parent education models have used this concept and practice exclusively.

Participatory Guidance

Participatory guidance or guided participation refers to a concept and approach to learning that emphasizes the child as an active and responsible learner in structured and unstructured activities and in forming diverse relationships with caregivers.[119,138] The hallmark of participatory guidance is mutual responsiveness of the individuals involved in that it focuses simultaneously on individual, interpersonal, and cultural processes of learning. Emphasis is placed on how the caregiver structures and guides the child's learning experiences in novel and routine situations by first creating a common ground for understanding. Because the caregiver determines the goal and is guided to discover solutions, there is a greater chance the intervention will carry over and become a habit or routine. This approach relies on understanding the caregiver role within the family system and expectations the family has for the child. Pridham, et al.[114] described the guided participation process to include steps that the guide has in mind from the beginning of the activity to ultimately transfer the responsibility of primary problem-solving from the guide to the caregiver.

APPLICATION TO PRACTICE: AN INTERVENTION ENCOUNTER: SEEKING A COMMON GROUND

Ordinarily, families of children with disabilities begin with little knowledge of the health care and educational systems and lack a sense of their own competence in terms of what may be suitable for their children. Transitions from one setting (e.g., early intervention) to another (preschool) are also accompanied by knowledge gaps and uncertainties. Similarly, therapists start with little information about the child and family other than what may be written on referral forms. The traditional approach has been for physical therapists to begin the encounter with an interview of families to obtain information about the child's birth and developmental history, as well as medical and other interventions. Occasionally the interview may include the family structure and physical home environment. This first step, although appropriate, is limited in that it overlooks that parents of children with developmental delays or disabilities constantly try to bridge the gap between what is known and unknown about their child's condition and prognosis. To begin to bridge the gap, using the Knowledge Translation for Caregivers and Children (KT for CACH) model, the initial encounter should focus on *seeking a common ground for communication and understanding*. In other words, therapists need to reassure the family that the information gaps exist on both sides. Seeking a common ground for communication and understanding involves using information exchange to ensure mutual comprehension.[119] This is particularly important when working with families from diverse cultures or beliefs.

A common ground for understanding is also a central ingredient of collaboration. Collaboration is a shared responsibility whose intent is to capitalize on individual strengths and diversity and to minimize biases. During the initial encounter, families of children with disabilities may rely on physicians, physical and occupational therapists, and case managers for most decisions relating to their child. Yet many families have their own intervention ideas about raising children, including solutions to health-related problems. Some families seek professional help only as a last resort. This puts both the family and the therapist in a learner/expert position. The therapist needs to explain his or her role to the family and at the same time learn about what the family has to offer. Elements of successful collaborations have been proposed.[149] Initially encounters may be stressful, particularly when roles and needs are not well defined. However, the ultimate goal should be to create a *match* between the therapist's understanding of the caregiving environment and the parents' understanding of the diagnosis and intervention process. Collaboration in seeking, gathering, and sharing information happens to also be a hallmark of family-centered intervention. Ultimately, true collaboration occurs when information exchanged has reached a level that enables each partner to guide the planning of the examination and goal setting. True collaboration, however, also hinges on the competencies of the partners.

Caregiver Competence

Most families of children with disabilities are also families of children who are typically developing. As such, most have been successful in caring for and teaching their children without "outside" intervention. Therefore, during the initial encounter, therapists should not only explicitly acknowledge this competence but also use it as a basis for determining information gaps. For example, finding out about the family's daily routines within their proximal and distal environments before or after the diagnosis of the child with disabilities will help determine the extent to which the family has curtailed or enhanced its routines and participation in neighborhood events. Most families may demonstrate the necessary skills to engage in information exchange, but some may need more encouragement. The family-centered approach accepts that power resides within the family, but that the family can elect to share the responsibility with the professional.

Physical Therapist Competencies

Gathering information about children's environments requires advanced competency in skillful interviewing and observation. Skillful interviewing is also characterized by the ability to engage in active listening. A therapist must be able to *hear* expressions of childrearing beliefs, values, isolation, stress, and resilience. A detailed discussion on interview skills is beyond the scope of this chapter. Literature on effective interviewing and observation is extensive.[1,45,46,111,123] Because many of the interactions and relationships discussed previously are nonverbal, therapists must also be skillful observers. Observation of movement, a skill that most therapists are accustomed to, must be extended to include observations of a milieu of social and economic interactions that form the context within which the child functions and participates. A therapist must be able to see dyadic exchanges, responsiveness, parenting styles, stress, engagement, and cues. The long-term benefits that accrue from attempting to understand the milieu of the child and his or her environment can be dramatic, albeit time consuming.

GATHERING INFORMATION ABOUT THE ENVIRONMENT

As pointed out previously, child development and outcome are shaped by so many connected environmental factors that identifying and assessing them all would be difficult if not close to impossible. The assumption made in this chapter is that the intervention encounter should be team based. Woods and Lindeman[153] proposed a framework to gather and share information and described five strategies to engage a family in the intervention process. The five strategies include (1) moving interviews to a conversation, (2) community mapping, (3) having follow-up conversations when using questionnaires and checklists, (4) problem-solving discussions, and (5) environmental scans. The following suggestions are based on problem solving and are aimed at improving reciprocity, encouraging and maximizing information sharing, and building on parent-therapist collaboration:

1. Begin the interview process with open-ended questions, moving on to close-ended questions, and finally to *"why"* questions.
2. Map the caregiving environment. Community mapping is a process in which the family identifies their child's natural learning activities. Ask specific questions about opportunities available in the community that include those activities.
3. Provide families with paper questionnaires and checklists used to gather demographic information and engage them in follow-up conversations and questions about the checklists/questionnaires.

4. Set the stage for problem-solving discussions by engaging in active listening—listen to the caregiver's concerns and problems and follow-up with a discussion in which the therapist is doing most of the probing and facilitating. The goal is to encourage the family to resolve the problem on their own.

5. Together with parents, scan each specific environment where the child and family spend most of their time and discuss how the child can participate in each setting.

How questions are framed holds the key to the quantity, quality, and the flow of information. Methods that have worked well in qualitative research may be valuable to therapists who are inexperienced or having difficulty collaborating with families.[44] The open-ended ethnographic interview method[45] may provide rich qualitative information in areas such as family structure and functioning, family values, cultural childrearing beliefs, daily family routines, stressors and coping strategies, informal and formal support, and level of family participation. However, some families may prefer the questions-and-answers method, self-administered questionnaires or assessment scales, or both.[30]

Several well-known self-report and observational scales can be used to supplement information gathered from interview and to assess other aspects of the caregiving environment. Many address characteristics of the environment and can provide a systematic way of gathering information and most are observational and interview based. Examples include the Home Observation for Measurement of the Environment (HOME), which assesses the quality of caregiving and the home environment that includes aspects of a child's participation in family routines and toys available,[20] the Nursing Child Assessment Teaching Scales (NCATS),[4] which measure parent-child interaction, and the Scale for Assessment of Family Enjoyment within Routines (SAFER),[127] a routines-based interview used to gather information about a family's home and community routines. The Affordances in the Home Environment for Motor Development (AHEMD-SR) is a recently published instrument for parental self-report of the quality and quantity of factor in the home to enhance motor development in children age 18 to 42 months.[50] Other assessment tools address children's participation in leisure and recreation. These include the Children's Assessment of Participation and Enjoyment (CAPE) and Preferences for Activities of Children (PAC).[81] The CAPE examines how children and youth participate in everyday activities outside of their school classes. The PAC supplements the CAPE by examining children's preferences for involvement in each activity.

SUMMARY

The importance of the environment in shaping children's health, development, function, well-being, and participation is widely accepted. A challenge to pediatric therapists is to determine approaches and intervention strategies that are evidence based,

family centered, culturally relevant, and environmentally appropriate. The complex and multifactorial nature of the interactions among environmental determinants that shape child outcomes underscore the need for therapists to continually (1) rethink how they provide services to children and their families, (2) revise family education approaches, (3) reexamine parent-professional collaboration, and (4) reinvest in cultural competence. Four summary considerations are provided. First, conceptual frameworks are necessary to explain the influence of the environment on service provision and vice versa because many of the factors that shape child and family outcomes are intertwined. Second, willingness by both parties to learn from each other is central to effective family-professional collaboration. Therapists must seek to learn from families just as much as they desire to teach them and are encouraged to establish a common ground of understanding and participatory guidance. Third, the process of cultural competence, which begins with the examination of one's own culture and proceeds to learning about families' cultural beliefs and meanings attached to illness or disabilities, is an important aspect of service provision. The caregiving environment can remove or add health inequities seen in children's activity and participation, depending on the therapist's cultural competency. Fourth, the importance of the environment does not take precedence over the role of biologic factors in influencing child development and function. On the contrary, best practice requires therapists, together with the child and family, to address impairments in body functions and structures based on an understanding of the child's condition. Effective intervention plans must simultaneously address both biologic and environmental factors that are important for the child's activity and participation. Therapists are encouraged to consider a child's needs within the larger context of family structure and functioning not only to increase the likelihood of goal attainment but also because recommendations can affect the child and family for years to come (Figure 27-6).

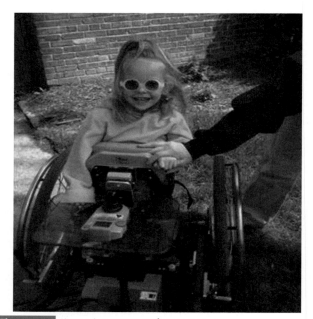

Figure 27-6 Impacting outcomes for years to come.

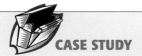

CASE STUDY

The following case scenario examples illustrate how the Knowledge Translation for Caregivers and Children model is applied to organize the physical therapist examination. Rosa is a 5-year-old girl who was diagnosed with medulloblastoma at 8 months with resultant brain stem seizures about six times a day in which her head drops and eyes blink rapidly for about 10 minutes. Rosa walks with a walker because of generalized weakness. She is "home schooled." Rosa has been receiving occupational and speech therapy and recently, at the request of the family, her primary physician has referred her to physical therapy because she still needs help with toileting.

Rosa's father and physician believe that with intensive physical therapy and strength training, she should be able to be independent in toileting. Rosa wears diapers and is placed on the toilet every $1\frac{1}{2}$ hours with rare, if any, success. Her mother believes that Rosa has a general idea of wiping but won't try to do it. Rosa doesn't flush the toilet but will point to the handle. She doesn't help with clothing management; she tells others when she is wet when wearing training pants but "it doesn't seem to bother her" when in diapers.

According to reports from the speech and occupational therapists, Rosa shows little flexibility in dealing with stressful events. Her mother and the therapists disagree on the extent Rosa's behavior is a problem. According to the mother, Rosa is not that difficult to deal with, but "If she wants to do something, she does it, and if you can't do something immediately, she gets upset and cries, and can remain upset for about half an hour. So I just try to be as organized as possible and respond to her needs as best as I can."

Step 1: Establishing a Common Ground of Understanding

There are several key concerns and challenges presented by this scenario that call for the need to first establish a common ground of understanding about the problem and expectations, including (1) disagreements about Rosa's behavior problem, (2) expectations of mother and father, (3) the parents' understanding of Rosa's diagnosis and prognosis, and (4) cultural childrearing expectations regarding self-care.

Interview

To establish a common ground of understanding, the physical therapist needs to find out how the various family members view the problem, why independence in toileting is important for Rosa's father, what the family thinks is preventing Rosa from being independent in this activity, what they have tried, their evaluation of previous efforts, how long they think it will take for Rosa to complete this activity, and what would happen if Rosa cannot be independent in toileting (cultural beliefs and values, understanding of the disability, and consequences). The questions must target the understanding of the parents' and Rosa's perception of her toileting abilities as well as the caregivers' (particularly the mother's) preferred method of teaching and learning. Open-ended questions are well suited not only to allow the family to freely express the information they wish to disclose but to create opportunities for more probing "why" follow-up questions.[46]

Interview techniques such as restating and reframing are believed to be particularly appropriate when trying to understand a sensitive or complex situation.[46]

Observation

Observation of the mother's teaching and Rosa's learning styles is another essential element in establishing a common ground of understanding. If the mother is primarily responsible for Rosa's toileting, asking her to demonstrate how she would ordinarily teach Rosa toileting and self-care is the next step. Before the teaching session, the therapist observes how the mother prepares herself, Rosa, and the environment. During the demonstration, the therapist observes the nonverbal exchanges between the mother and Rosa and listens to instructions and verbal interactions. The therapist pays special attention to the level and timing of assistance.

After the demonstration, the therapist asks the mother and Rosa to explain why they do each step the way they do. In establishing a common ground, and within the framework of participatory guidance, the rationale is as important as the manner in which the mother teaches the activity.[119] Also important is finding out how similar or different the teaching and learning episode would be if performed by other members of the family.

Information Exchange

The process of gathering and exchanging information should be concurrent. Using an anticipatory guidance approach, the therapist provides the family members with information (if they don't already have it) about medulloblastoma and seizures, prognosis, and outcomes of various interventions. Although much of this information is available on the Internet, discussing what parents have found is important. If Rosa's family does not have access to the Internet, the therapist can select and print the information for the family. The therapist is careful to use information that is based on evidence. This requires that the therapist is competent in finding, appraising, and sharing research in a manner that is acceptable to the family.

Based on the Knowledge Translation for Caregivers and Children model, the information exchange precedes and guides the examination process. Only after Rosa's parents have understood the diagnosis and prognosis of her condition will they be in a good position to decide whether or not toileting is still a major or only goal and how they want to proceed with assessment of other areas of function. The information, including findings from the interview and observation, will also allow both parties to further explore goals for participation. The first step of the model, establishing a common ground for understanding, may be a departure from the traditional approach of history taking immediately followed by examination procedures. In essence, we are proposing a two-step process.

Step 2: Exploring Goals and Their Importance to the Family

Based on the information exchange, the family decided to abandon toilet training and instead chose to focus on (1) Rosa's behavior in terms of expressing frustrations more appropriately and reducing her

Continued

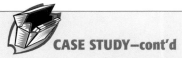

CASE STUDY—cont'd

inflexibility, (2) independence in self-grooming, (3) being able to take a bath with very little help, (4) expressing what she wants so other members of the family can help her, and (5) putting on and taking off her training pants. Although these seem like clearly stated goals, the therapist once again began by developing a common ground of understanding the role of these goals in the context of family functioning, environmental implications, and Rosa's participation. This is where the iterative process of the Knowledge Translation for Caregivers and Children model comes in. The "why" questions need to be answered before the therapist and parents can agree on the assessments and tools needed, such as the Home Observation for Measurement of the Environment[20] and the Pediatric Evaluation of Disability Inventory.[62] The therapist must seek to understand why these goals are important, what the family thinks is preventing Rosa from attaining them, what the family members have tried to help Rosa attain the goals, how long they think it will take for Rosa to achieve the goals, and what would happen if Rosa does not.

This information gets at cultural beliefs and values, understanding of the disability, expectations, and consequences. In return, the therapist can use anticipatory guidance to offer options about tests and measures and explain their strengths and limitations so that the parents understand what each provides. Anticipatory guidance may also provide the information that parents need to refine their understanding of a team approach to examination, Rosa's health condition, and achievement of goals. The therapist must consistently strive to understand the context of the environment that will play a major role in influencing goal attainment. This will take more time, but time well invested. The therapist must also share this information with the speech and occupational therapists and Rosa's primary physician.

Step 3: Goal Setting and Planning

Successful goal setting also hinges on a common understanding of presenting problems and environmental and professional resources. The process of goal setting, therefore, must be a collaborative effort. Family-generated goals are important; however, as illustrated in Rosa's case, families often modify their goals in light of new information. Consequently, the importance of anticipatory guidance cannot be overlooked. The process for goal setting, using the Knowledge Translation for Caregivers and Children model, is similar to that described in step 2.

Given Rosa's limitations in processing information and problem solving, and the different expectations in school and at home, the two environments where she spends most of her time, prioritization of the goals expressed by the family is essential. Although prioritization is also collaborative process, Wolery[158] proposed six considerations that therapists may use to guide the process:

1. What are the family's priorities and judgment regarding goal attainment?
2. Will goal attainment increase ease of caregiving?
3. Will goal attainment allow the child to gain access and participate in an inclusive setting?

4. Will goal attainment allow the child to learn additional skills?
5. Will goal attainment reduce the possibility of the child being stigmatized?
6. Will goal attainment improve the child's function in several environments?

In Rosa's case, the goals were prioritized as follows: (1) expressing what she wants so other members of the family can help her, (2) modifying her behavior in terms of expressing frustrations more appropriately and reducing her inflexibility, (3) putting on and taking off her training pants, (4) obtaining independence in self-grooming, and (5) being able to take a bath with very little help.

Step 4: Intervention Strategies

The approach to implementing intervention strategies using the Knowledge Translation for Caregivers and Children model relies heavily on the participatory guidance approach developed by Rogoff et al.[119] Using a combination of anticipatory and guided participation, therapists must adapt their role as problem solvers to partner with parents to find solutions. During guided participation, the therapist must first observe the caregivers as they teach the various skills stated in the goals and ask the caregivers for explanations of why they use the approaches they do so as to ensure mutual understanding. The therapist may have several ideas to modify the environment (i.e., communication board, chaining events to ensure generalization, physical modifications) to promote independence, but must first ask the parents if they have tried any strategies and what the outcomes were. Based on the principles of participatory guidance, the physical therapist may have the background, experience, and knowledge needed to achieve positive outcomes for the child but must first engage the caregiver to participate in the process.

The following are two examples of intervention strategies for goal 1, expressing what she wants so other members of the family can help her; and goal 5, being able to take a bath with very little help. First, the therapist and family must discuss what has been tried before. The family may be asked to demonstrate the techniques. The caregiver's teaching demonstrations are essential elements of the participatory guidance approach. If none of the techniques are considered helpful, then new options must be developed using a problem-solving approach described by Rogoff et al.[119]

The following options for the goal "expressing what she wants so other members of the family can help her" were discussed and were expanded to address participation:

- Label objects in the house with pictures and their names.
- Verbalize objects and pictures to Rosa every time she looks at them.
- Begin using different picture boards with two choices; upon success, increase the number of picture choices.
- Reward Rosa when she points to a picture cue or gets a question correct (e.g., use points that can be used for a reward).
- Use of the boards at home, during meals, at school, or when visiting relatives.

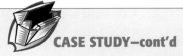

CASE STUDY—cont'd

The strategy for the goal "being able to take a bath with very little help" is as follows.

Establishing a Common Ground

First the therapist describes the activity. Then the therapist asks the mother (or other caregivers) about her preferred method of learning and teaching. The therapist asks about other skills that require similar ability and that are part of Rosa's daily activities, such as getting in and out of bed or the car or getting down to the floor. Participatory guidance is believed to be effective when an activity is taught within the context of daily routines.[119]

Observation

The therapist observes the mother teaching the task and asks the mother and Rosa to demonstrate how they go through the entire routine of taking a bath. Observing the mother's teaching and Rosa's learning styles is another key element in participatory guidance. During the demonstration, the therapist observes the mother's position in relation to Rosa, the level and timing of assistance, and the nonverbal exchanges between the mother and Rosa. The therapist attends to the mother's instructions and verbal interactions. After the demonstration, the therapist asks Rose and her mother why they do each step the way they do.

Sharing Information

The therapist shares her analysis of the bathing activity with Rosa and her mother and relates her analysis to Rosa's functional abilities and constraints. The therapist discusses the various options and guides (verbally or physically) mother and Rosa on how to perform the transfer. The following are three potential methods: (1) Rosa sits on the outside edge of the tub and then moves her legs into the tub, (2) Rosa holds onto a grab bar and puts one leg in the tub at a time, or (3) Rosa uses a bathtub bench to lower herself into the tub. The key is not only to educate Rosa and the mother about potential options but also to allow them to select their preferred method. This is particularly helpful if any of the methods can be generalized to other transfer activities.

Videotaping the Performance

If possible, the therapist might suggest that the family videotape the practice sessions, and then the therapist can review and analyze the tapes with the mother and other caregivers. Research shows that caregivers learn best when they can observe and evaluate their performance. Essentially the therapist's role in participatory guidance is that of a coach.

REFERENCES

1. Adler, P. A., & Adler, P. (1998). Observational techniques. In N. K. Denzin & Y. S. Lincoln (Eds.), *Collecting and interpreting qualitative materials* (pp. 79–109). Thousand Oaks, CA: Sage Publications.

2. Badr (Zahr), K. L. (2001). Quantitative and qualitative predictors of development for low-birth weight infants of Latino background. *Applied Nursing Research, 14*, 125–135.

3. Bandura, A. (1986). *Social foundations of thought and action: A social cognitive theory.* Englewood Cliffs, NJ: Prentice Hall.

4. Barnard, K. E. (1978). *Nursing child assessment teaching scale.* Seattle: University of Washington.

5. Barnard, K. E. (1997). Influencing parent-child interactions for children at risk. In M. J. Guralnick (Ed.), *The effectiveness of early intervention* (pp. 249–267). Baltimore: Paul H. Brookes.

6. Benasich, A. A., & Brooks-Gunn, J. (1996). Maternal attitudes and knowledge of child-rearing: Associations with family and child outcomes. *Child Development, 67*, 1186–1205.

7. Reference deleted in page proofs.

8. Black, M. M., Siegel, E. H., Abel, Y., & Bentley, M. E. (2001). Home and videotape intervention delays early complementary feeding among adolescent mothers. *Pediatrics, 107*, 67–74.

9. Black, M. M., & Teti, L. O. (1997). Promoting mealtime communication between adolescent mothers and their infants through videotape. *Pediatrics, 99*, 432–437.

10. Bradley, R. H. (1993). Children's home environments, health, behavior, and intervention efforts: A review using the HOME inventory as a marker measure. *Genetic, Social, and General Psychology Monographs, 119*(4), 437–490.

11. Bradley, R. H., Caldwell, B. M., & Corwyn, R. F. (2001). The child care HOME inventories: Assessing the quality of family child care homes. *Early Chidhood Research Quarterly, 18*, 294–309.

12. Bradley, R. H., Corwyn, R. F., McAdoo, H. P., & Coll, C. G. (2001). The home environment of children in the United States Part I: Variations by age, ethnicity, and poverty. *Child Development, 72*, 1844–1867.

13. Brehaut, J. C., Kohen, D. E., Garner, R. E., et al. (2009). Rosenbaum PL. Health among caregivers of children with health problems: Findings from a Canadian population-based study. *American Journal of Public Health 99*(7), 1254–1262.

14. Brinker, R. P., Seifer, R., & Sameroff, A. J. (1994). Relations among maternal stress, cognitive development, and early intervention in middle- and low-SES infants with developmental disabilities. *American Journal of Mental Retardation, 98*, 463–480.

15. Broffenbrenner, U. (1986). Ecology of the family as a context for human development research perspectives. *Developmental Psychology, 22*, 723–742.

16. Brooks-Gunn, J., Berlin, L. J., & Fuligni, A. S. (2000). Early childhood intervention programs: What about the family? In

J. P. Shonkoff & S. J. Meisels (Eds.), *Handbook of early childhood intervention* (pp. 549–577). New York: Cambridge University Press.

17. Brooks-Gunn, J., & Duncan, G. J. (1997). The effects of poverty on children and youth. *The Future of Children*, 7(2), 55–71.

18. Brown, S. L. (2004). Family structure and child well-being; The significance of parental cohabitation. *Journal of Marriage*, 66, 351–367.

19. Bruns, D. A., & Corso, R. M. (2001). Working with culturally and linguistically diverse families. *Eric Digest* (EDP-PS-01-4).

20. Caldwell, B. M., & Bradley, R. H. (1984). *Manual for the home observation for measurement of the environment* (rev. ed.). Little Rock, AR: University of Arkansas.

21. Campion, J., Milagro, F. I., & Martinez, J. A. (2009). Individuality and epigenetics in obesity. *Obesity Reviews*, 10, 383–392.

22. Reference deleted in page proofs.

23. Chen, J. Y., & Clark, M. J. (2007). Family function in families of children with Duchenne muscular dystrophy. *Family Community Health*, 30(4), 296–304.

24. Chiarello, L. A., & Palisano, R. J. (1998). Investigation of the effects of a model of physical therapy on mother-child interactions and the motor behaviors of children with motor delay. *Physical Therapy*, 78(2), 180–194.

25. Cook, T. D., Kim, J. R., Chan, W. S., & Setterten, R. (1997). How do neighborhoods matter? In F. F. Furstenburg, T. D. Cook, J. Eccles, G. H. Elder, & A. J. Sameroff (Eds.), *Managing to make it: Urban families in high risk neighborhoods*. Chicago: University of Chicago Press.

26. Coster, W., Deeney, T., Haltiwanger, J., & Haley, S. (1998). School Function Assessment (SFA).

27. Cutfield, W. S., Hofman, P. L., Mitchell, M., & Morison, I. M. (2007). Could epigenetics play a role in the developmental origins of health and disease? *Pediatric Research*, 61, 68R–75R.

28. Darling, R. B. (1979). *Families against society: A study of reactions to children with birth defects*. Beverly Hills, CA: Sage, p. 78.

29. Darling, N., & Steinberg, L. (1993). Parenting style as context: An integrative model. *Psychological Bulletin*, 113, 487–496.

30. Davis, S. K., & Gettinger, M. (1995). Family-focused assessment for identifying family resources and concerns: Parent preferences, assessment information, and evaluation across three methods. *Journal of School Psychology*, 33, 99–121.

31. DeGrace, B. W. (2003). Occupation-based family-centered care: A challenge for current practice. *American Journal of Occupational Therapy*, 57, 347–350.

32. Reference deleted in page proofs.

33. Dickstein S. (2002). Family routines and rituals—the importance of family functioning: Comment on the special section. *Journal of Family Psychology*, 16(4), 441–444.

34. Dupont, C., Armant, D. R., & Brenner, C. A. (2009). Epigenetics: Definition, mechanisms and clinical perspective. *Seminars in Reproductive Medicine*, 27, 351.

35. Duncan, G. J., Brooks-Gunn, J., & Klebanov, P. K. (1994). Economic deprivation and early childhood development. *Child Development*, 65(2), 296–318.

36. Dunst, C. J., Trivette, C. M., & Jodry, W. (1997). Influences of social support on children with disabilities and their families. In M. Guralnick, (Ed.), *The effectiveness of early intervention* (pp. 499–522). Baltimore: Paul H. Brookes.

37. Dworkin, P. H. (2000). Preventive health care and anticipatory guidance. In J. P. Shonkoff & S. J. Meisels (Eds.), *Handbook of early childhood intervention* (2nd ed., pp. 327–338). Cambridge: Cambridge University Press.

38. Reference deleted in page proofs.

39. Reference deleted in page proofs.

40. Evans, G. W. (2006). Child development and the physical environment. *Annual Review Psychology*, 57, 423–451.

41. Reference deleted in page proofs.

42. Flynt, S. W., Wood, T. A., & Scott, R. L. (1992). Social support of mothers of children with mental retardation. *Mental Retardation*, 30, 233–236.

43. Fiese, B. H., Tomcho, T. J., Douglas, M., Josephs, K., Poltrock, S., & Baker, T. (2002). A review of 50 years of research on naturally occurring family routines and rituals: cause for celebration? *Journal of Family Psychology*, 16(4), 381–390.

44. Fontana, A., & Frey, J. H. (2003). The interview from neutral stnce to political involvement. In N. K. Denzin & Y. S. Lincoln (Eds.), *The Sage handbook of qualitative research* (3rd ed., pp. 695–727). Thousand Oaks, CA: Sage.

45. Fontana, A., & Frey, J. H. (2003). The interview: from structured questions to negotiated text. In N. K. Denzin & Y. S. Lincoln (Eds.), *Collecting and interpreting qualitative materials* (pp. 61–106). Thousand Oaks, CA: Sage.

46. Fontana, A., & Frey, J. H. (1998). Interviewing: The art of science. In N. K. Denzin & Y. S. Lincoln (Eds.), *Collecting and interpreting qualitative materials* (pp. 47–78). Thousand Oaks, CA: Sage.

47. Fox, R. A. (1995). Maternal factors related to parenting practices, developmental expectations, and perceptions of child behavior problems. *Journal of Genetic Psychology*, 156, 431–441.

48. Francis, D. D. (2009). Conceptualizing child health disparities: A role for developmental neurogenomics. *Pediatrics*, 124, S196–S202.

49. Frisancho, A. R. (2009). Developmental adaptation: Where we go from here. *American Journal of Human Biology*, 21, 694–703.

50. Gabbard, C., Cacola, P., & Rodrigues, L. (2008). A new inventory for assessing "affordances in the home environment for motor development" (AHEMD-SR). *Early Childhood Education Journal*, 36(1), 5–9.

51. Garcia-Coll, C., & Magnusson, K. (2000). Cultural differences as sources of developmental vulnerabilities and resources. In J. P. Shonkoff & S. J. Meisels (Eds.), *Handbook of early childhood intervention* (2nd ed., pp. 94–114). Cambridge: Cambridge University Press.

52. Garcia-Coll, G., & Magnusson, K. (1999). Cultural influences on child development: Are we ready for a paradigm shift? In A. S. Masten (Ed.), *Cultural processes in child development— The Minnesota Symposia on Child Psychology* (pp. 1–24). Mahwah, NJ: Lawrence Erlbaum.

53. Garrett, P., Ng'andu, N., & Ferron, J. (1994). Poverty experiences of young children and the equality of their home environments. *Child Development, 65*, 331–345.

54. Gentile, A. M. (2000). Skill acquisition: Action, movement, and neuromotor processes. In J. H. Carr & R. B. Shepherd (Eds.), *Movement science: Foundation for physical therapy rehabilitation* (pp. 111–187). Rockville, MD: Aspen.

55. Goodnow, J. J. (1997). Parenting and the transmission and internalization of values: From social-cultural perspectives to within-family analysis. In J. E. Grusec & L. Kuczynski (Eds.), *Parenting strategies and children's internalizations of values: A handbook of contemporary theory* (pp. 331–361). New York: Wiley.

56. Reference deleted in page proofs.

57. Gottlieb, A. S. (2002). Single mothers of children with developmental disabilities: The impact of multiple roles. *Family Relations, 46*(1), 5–13.

58. Gray, R., & McCormick, M. C. (2005). Early childhood intervention programs in the US: Recent advances and future recommendations. *Journal of Primary Prevention, 26*(3), 259–265.

59. Griffiths, P. E., & Gray, R. D. (2005). Discussion: three ways to misunderstand developmental systems theory. *Biology and Philosophy, 20*, 417–425.

60. Grosec, J. E., Rudy, D., & Martini, T. (1997). Parenting cognitions and child outcomes: An overview and implications for children's internalization of values. In J. E. Grusec & L. Kuczynski (Eds.). *Parenting and children's internalization of values: A handbook of contemporary theory* (pp. 259–282). New York: John Wiley & Sons.

61. Gutierrez, J., & Sameroff, A. (1990). Determinant of complexity in Mexican American and Anglo American mothers' conception of child development. *Child Development, 61*, 384–394.

62. Haley, S. M., Coster, W. J., Ludlow, L. H., Haltiwanger, J., & Andrellos, P. (1992). *Pediatric Evaluation of Disability Inventory (PEDI)*, Boston.

63. Halpern, R. (2000). Early intervention for low-income children and families. In J. P. Shonkoff & S. J. Meisels (Eds.), *Handbook of early childhood intervention* (pp. 361–386). New York: Cambridge University Press.

64. Harkness, S., Super, C. M., Sutherland, M. A., et al. (2007). Culture and the construction of habits in daiy life: Implications for the successful development of children with disabilities. *OTJR: Occupation, Participation and Health, 27* (Suppl), 33S–40S.

65. Harwood, R. L., Miller, J. G., & Irizarry, N. L. (1995). *Culture and attachment: Perceptions of the child in context.* New York: Guilford.

66. Hayden, L. C., Schiller, M., Dickstein, S., et al. (1998). Levels of family assessment: I. Family, marital, and parent-child interaction. *Journal of Family Psychology, 12*, 7–22.

67. Hepburn, S. L. (2003). Clinical implications of temperamental characteristics in young children with developmental disabilities. *Infant & Young Children, 16*, 59–76.

68. Hernandez, D. J. (2004). Demographic change and the life circumstances of immigrant families. *The Future of Children: Children of Immigrant Families, 14*(2), 17–47.

69. Hirshberg, L. M. (1996). History-making, not history-taking: Clinical interviews with infants and their families. In S. J. Meisels & E. Fenichel (Eds.), *New visions for the developmental assessment of infants and young children* (85–124). Washington, DC: Zero to Three.

70. Hollingshead, A. B. (1975). *Four factor index of social status.* New Haven: Yale University Press.

71. Howes, C., Guerra, A. W., & Zucker, E. (2007). Cultural communities and parenting in Mexican-heritage families. *Parenting: Science and Practice, 7*(3), 235–270.

72. Reference deleted in page proofs.

73. Irwin, L. G., Siddiqi, A., & Hertzman, C. (2007). *Early child development: A powerful equalizer final report.* Geneva, Switzerland: World Health Organization's Commission on Social Determinants of Health.

74. Jack, G. (2000). Ecological influences on parenting and child development. *British Journal of Social Work, 30*, 703–720.

75. Johnson, C., & Kastner, T. (2005). Helping families raise children with special health care needs at home. *Pediatrics, 115*, 507–511.

76. Kaufman, J., & Rosenbaum, J. (1992). The education and employment of low-income black youth in white suburbs. *Educational Evaluation and Policy Analysis, 14*, 229–240.

77. Kelly, J. F., & Barnard, K. E. (2000). Assessment of parent-child interaction: Implications for early intervention. In J. P. Shonkoff & S. J. Meisels (Eds.), *Handbook of early childhood intervention* (pp. 258–289). New York: Cambridge University Press.

78. Kelly, J. F., Buehlman, K., & Caldwell, K. (2000). Training personnel to promote quality parent-child interaction in families who are homeless. *Topics in Early Childhood Special Education, 20*(3), 174–185.

79. Kelly, J. F., Zuckerman, T., & Rosenblatt, S. (2008). Promoting first relationships. A relationship-focused early intervention approach. *Infants and Young Children, 21*(4), 285–295.

80. Reference deleted in page proofs.

81. King, G., Law, M., King, S., Hurley, P., Rosenbaum, P., & Young, N. (2004). *Children's Assessment of Participation and Enjoyment (CAPE) and Preferences for Activities for Children (PAC).* San Antonio, TX: Harcourt Assessment.

82. Klebanov, P. K., Brooks-Gunn, J., McCarton, C., & McCormick, M. C. (1998). The contribution of neighborhood and family income to developmental test scores over the first three years of life. *Child Development, 69*(5), 1420–1436.

83. Kochanska, G., Kucznski, L., & Radke-Yarrow, M. (1989). Correspondence between mother's self-reported and observed child-rearing practices. *Child Development, 60*, 56–63.

84. Kochanska, G. (1990). Maternal beliefs as long-term predictors of mother-child interaction and report. *Child Development, 61*(6), 1934–1943.

85. Kolobe, T. H. A. (2004). Childrearing practices and developmental expectations for Mexican-American mothers and the developmental status of their infants. *Physical Therapy, 84*, 439–453.

86. Kolobe, T. A., Smith, E., & Ishi, L. (2006). The influence of maternal childrearing beliefs and practices on motor outcome of Mexican American children. *Pediatric Physical Therapy, 18*, 77–78.

87. Kuzawa, C. W., & Sweet, E. (2008). Epigenetics and the embodiment of race: Developmental origins of US racial disparities in cardiovascular health. American. *Journal of Human Biology, 21*, 1–14.

88. Lach, L. M., Kohen, D. E., Garner, R. E., et al. (2009). The health and psychosocial functioning of caregivers of children with neurodevelopmental disorders. *Disability & Rehabilitation, 31*(8), 607–618.

89. Leavitt, R. (1999). *Cross-cultural rehabilitation: an international perspective.* Toronto: WB Saunders.

90. Li, S-C. (2003). Biocultural orchestration of deveopment plasticity across levels: The interplay of biology and culture in shaping the mind and behavior across the life span. *Psychological Bulletin, 129*, 171–194.

91. Leitch, D. (1999). Mother-infant interaction: Achieving synchrony. *Nursing Research, 48*, 55–58.

92. Linver, M. R., Brooks-Gunn, J., & Kohen, D. E. (2002). Family processes as pathways from income to young children's development. *Developmental Psychology, 38*, 719–734.

93. Lynch, E. W. (1992). Developing cross-cultural competence. In E. W. Lynch & M. J. Hanson (Eds.), *Developing cross-cultural competence: A guide for working with young children and their families.* Baltimore: Paul H. Brookes.

94. Reference deleted in page proofs.

95. Lynch, E. W., & Hanson, M. J. (1992). *Developing Cross-Cultural Competence. A guide for working with young children and their families.* Baltimore, MD: Paul H. Brookes.

96. Reference deleted in page proofs.

97. Madding, C. (2000). Maintaining focus on cultural competence in early intervention services to linguistically and culturally diverse families. *Infant-Toddler Intervention, 10*(1), 9–18.

98. Majnemer, A. (2009). Promoting participation in leisure activities: Expanding role for pediatric therapists. *Physical and Occupational Therapy in Pediatrics, 29*(1), 1–5.

99. Marshak, L. E., Seligman, M., & Prezant, F. (1999). *Disability and the family life cycle: Recognizing and treating challenges.* New York: Basic Books.

100. Marfo, K. (1992). Correlates of maternal directiveness with children who are developmentally delayed. *American Journal of Orthopsychiatry, 62*, 219–233.

101. Masten, S. A. (Ed.). (1999). *Cultural processes in child development: The Minnesota Symposia on Child Psychology.* Mahwah, NJ: Lawrence Erlbaum, pp. 123–135.

102. McCubbin, H. I., & Patterson, J. M. (1982). *Systematic assessment of family stress, resources and coping.* St. Paul: University of Minnesota, pp. 7–15.

103. McLoyd, V. C. (1998). Socioeconomic disadvantage and child development. *American Psychologist, 53*, 185–204.

104. Mills, R. S. L., & Rubin, K. H. (1990). Parental beliefs about problematic social behaviors in early childhood. *Child Development, 61*, 138–151.

105. Mulligan, L., Specker, B. L., Buckley, D. D., O'Connor, L. S., & Ho, M. (1998). Physical and environment factors affecting motor development, activity level, and body composition of infants in child care centers. *Pediatric Physical Therapy, 10*, 156–161.

106. Nacion, K. W., Norr, K. F., Barnes-Boyd, C., & Barnet, G. (2000). Validating the safety of nurse-health advocate services. *Journal of Community Health Nursing, 17*(1), 32–42.

107. National Scientific Council on the Developing Child. (2007). The science of early childhood development. Retrieved December 4, 2009, from Center on the Developing Child, www.developingchild.net.

108. NCAST Programs. (1986). *Network survey.* University of Washington. Seattle, WA: NCAST Publications.

109. Nobile, C., & Drotar, D. (2003). Research on the quality of parent-provider communication in pediatric care: Implications and recommendations. *Developmental and Behavioral Pediatrics, 24*, 279–287.

110. Palisano, R. J., Tieman, B. L., Walter, S. D., et al. (2003). Effect of environmental setting on mobility methods of children with cerebral palsy. *Developmental Medicine and Child Neurology, 45*, 113–120.

111. Patton, M. Q. (1990). *Qualitative evaluation and research methods* (2nd ed). Newbury Park, CA: Sage, pp. 277–368.

112. Phillip, M. J., Voran, D., Kisker, E., Howes, C., & Whitebook, M. (1994). Child care for children in poverty: Opportunity or inequity? *Child Development, 65*, 472–492.

113. Pollitt, E., Gorman, K. S., Engle, P. L., Rivera, J. A., & Martorell, R. (1995). Nutrition in early life and the fulfillment of intellectual potential. *Journal of Nutrition, 125*, 1111S–1118S.

114. Pridham, K., Brown, R., Clark, R., et al. (2005). Effect of guided participation on feeding competencies of mothers and their premature infants. *Research in Nursing & Health, 28*, 252–267.

115. Raina, P., O'Donnell, M., Rosenbaum, et al. (2005). The health and well-being of caregivers of children with cerebral palsy. *Pediatrics, 115*:e626–e636.

116. Richman, A., Miller, P., & Levine, R. (1992). Cultural and educational variations in maternal responsiveness. *Developmental Psychology, 28*, 614–621.

117. Rios Muñoz, G. (2005). A seminar to support the supporter: Promotion of provider self-awareness and sociocultural perspective. In K. M. Finello (Ed.), *The handbook of training and*

practice in infant and preschool mental health (pp. 137–161). San Francisco: Jossey-Bass.

118. Rogoff, B., Goodman Turkanis, C., & Bartlett, L. (2001). *Learning together: Children and adults in a school community.* New York: Oxford University Press.

119. Rogoff, B., Mistry, J., Concu, A., & Mosier, C. (1993). Guided participation in cultural activities by toddlers and caregivers. *Monographs of Society for Research in Child Development, 58,* Serial No. 236.

120. Roosa, M. W., Jones, S., Tein, Jenn-Yun, & Cree, W. (2003). Prevention science and neighborhood influences on low-income children's development: Theoretical and methodological issues. *American Journal of Community Psychology, 31,* 55–72.

121. Rosenbaum, P. (2007). The environment and childhood disability: opportunities to expand our horizons. *Developmental Medicine & Child Neurology, 49,* 643.

122. Rothstein, M. A., Cai, Y., & Marchant, G. E. (2009). The ghost in our genes: Legal and ethical implications of epigenetics. *Health Matrix, 19,* 1–62.

123. Rubin, H. J., & Rubin, I. S. (2005). *Qualitative interviewing: The art of hearing data* (2nd ed.). Thousand Oaks, CA: Sage.

124. Sameroff, A. J., & Chandler, M. J. (1975). Reproductive risk and the continuum of caretaking casualty. In F. D. Horowitz, M. Hetherington, S. Scarr-Salapatek & G. Sigel (Eds.), Review of child development research (*Vol. 4,* pp. 187–244). Chicago: University of Chicago Press.

125. Sameroff, A. J., & Feil, L. A. (1985). Parental conception of development. In I. E. Sigel (Ed.). *Parental belief system: The psychological consequences for children* (pp. 83–105). Hillsdale, NJ: Erlbaum.

126. Sameroff, A. J., & Fiese, B. H. (2000). Transactional regulation: The development ecology of early intervention. In J. P. Shonkoff & S. J. Meisels (Eds.), *Handbook of early childhood intervention* (2nd ed., pp. 135–159). New York: Cambridge University Press.

127. Scott, S., & McWilliam, R. A. (2003). *Scale for assessment of family enjoyment within routines.* Chapel Hill, NC: University of North Carolina.

128. Seitz, V., & Provence, S. (1990). Caregiver-focused models of early intervention. In S. J. Meisels & J. P. Shonkoff (Eds.), *Handbook of early childhood intervention* (pp. 400–427). New York: Cambridge University Press.

129. Shikako-Thomas, K., Majnemer, A., Law, M., & Lach, L. (2008). Determinants of participation in leisure activities in children and youth with cerebral palsy: Systemic reviews. *Physical and Occupational Therapy in Pediatrics, 28*(2), 155–169.

130. Reference deleted in page proofs.

131. Shonkoff, J. P. (2006). A promising opportunity for developmental and behavioral pediatrics at the interface of neuroscience, psychology, and the social policy: Remarks on receiving the 2005 C. Anderson Aldrich Award. *Pediatrics, 118*(5), 2187–2191.

132. Shonkoff, J. P., Boyce, W. T., & McEwen, B. S. (2009). Neuroscience, molecular biology, and the childhood roots of health disparities. *Journal of the American Medical Association, 301,* 2252–2259.

133. Shonkoff, J. P., Hauser-Cram, P., Krauss, M. W., & Upshur, C. C. (1992). Development of infants with disabilities and their families. *Monographs of the Society for Research in Child Development, 57*(6, Serial No. 230).

134. Shonkoff, J. P., & Phillips, D. A. (2001). *From neurons to neighborhoods: The science of early childhood development.* Washington, DC: National Academy Press.

135. Siddiqi, A., Irwin, L. G., & Hertzman, C. (2007). *Total environment assessment model for early child development: Evidence report for the Commision on the Social Determinants of Health.* Geneva, Switzerland: World Health Organization, Commision on the Social Determinants of Health.

136. Sigel, I. E. (1992). The belief-behavior connection: A resolvable dilemma? In I. E. Sigel, A. V. McGillicuddy-Delisi, & J. J. Goodnow (Eds.), *Parental belief systems: The psychological consequences for children* (2nd ed., pp. 433–456). Hillsdale, NJ: Lawrence Erlbaum Associates.

137. Spiker, D., Ferguson, J., & Brook-Gunn J. (1993). Enhancing maternal interactive behavior and child social competence in low birth-weight, premature infants. *Child Development, 64,* 754–768.

138. Stern-Bruscheweiler, N., & Stern, D. N. (1989). A model for conceptualizing the role of mothers representational work in various mother-infant therapies. *Infant Mental Health Journal, 10,* 142–156.

139. Stewart, M. J. (1989). Social support: Diverse theoretical perspectives. *Social Science and Medicine, 28,* 1275–1282.

140. Sumner, F., & Spietz, A. (1994). *NCATS/Caregiver/parent-child interaction feeding manual.* Seattle, WA: NCATS Publications.

141. Super, C. M., & Harkness, S. (1986). The developmental niche: A conceptualization at the interface of child and culture. *International Journal of Behavioral Development, 9,* 545–569.

142. Super, C. M., & Harkness, S. (1997). The cultural structuring of child development. In J. W. Berry, P. R. Dasen, & T. S. Saraswathi, (Eds.), *Handbook of cross-cultural psychology* (2nd ed., pp. 1–39). Boston: Allyn & Bacon.

143. Suter, M. A., & Aagaard-Tillery, K. M. (2009). Environmental influences on epigenetic profiles. *Seminars in Reproductive Medicine, 27,* 380–390.

144. Telzrow, R. (1978). Anticipatory guidance in pediatric practice. *Journal of Continuing Education in Pediatrics, 20,* 14–27.

145. Thelen, E. (1995). Motor development. A new synthesis. *American Psychologist, 50,* 79–95.

146. Thelen, E., & Ulrich, B. D. (1991). Hidden skills. *Monographs of the Society for Research in Child Development, Serial No. 223, 56,* 1–97.

147. Tieman, B. L., Palisano, R. J., Gracely, E. J., & Rosenbaum, P. L. (2004). Gross motor capability and performance of mobility in children with cerebral palsy: A comparison across home,

school, and outdoors/community settings. *Physical Therapy*, *84*, 419–429.

148. Turnbull, A., Turbiville, V., & Turnbull, H. R. (2000). Evolution of family-professional relationships: Collective empowerment for the early 21st century. In J. P. Shonkoff & S. J. Meisels (Eds.), *Handbook of early childhood intervention* (pp. 1370–1420). New York: Cambridge University Press.

149. Turnbull, A. P., & Turnbull, H. R. (2001). *Families, professionals, and Exceptionality: A special partnership*, 4th ed. Des Moines, IA: Merrill Prentice-Hall.

150. Reference deleted in page proofs.

151. United States Department of Health and Human Services: Agency for Healthcare Research and Quality. (2008). National healthcare disparities report. Retrieved December 18, 2009, from www.ahrq.gov/qual/nhdr08/Key.htm.

152. Wen, M. (2008). Family structure and children's health and behavior: Data from the 1999 National Survey of America's Families. *Journal of Family Issues*, *29*, 1492–1519.

153. Woods, J. J., & Lindeman, D. P. (2008). Gathering and giving information with families. *Infants and Young Children*, *21*(4), 272–284.

154. Reference deleted in page proofs.

155. Washington, K., & Schwartz, I. (1996). Maternal perception on the effects of physical that occupational therapy services on caregiving competency. *Physical and Occupational Therapy in Pediatrics*, *16*, 33–54.

156. Weisner, T. S. (2002). Ecocultural understanding of children's developmental pathways. *Human Development 45*, 275–281.

157. Werner, E. (2000). Protective factors and resilience. In J. P. Shonkoff & S. J. Meisels (Eds.), *Handbook of early childhood intervention* (pp. 115–132). New York: Cambridge University Press.

158. Wolery, M. (2004). Using assessment information to plan intervention programs. In M. McLean, D. B. Bailey, & M. Wolery (Eds.), *Assessing infants and preschoolers with special needs* (3rd ed., pp. 517–544). Englewood Cliffs, NJ: Prentice Hall.

159. World Health Organization. (2001). *ICIDH2: International Classification of Functioning, Disability and Health*. Geneva: World Health Organization.

160. World Health Organization. (2008). 10 facts about early child development as a social determinant of health. Retrieved December 4, 2009, from www.who.int/child_adolescent_health/topics/development/10facts/en/index.html.

28 The Special Care Nursery

LINDA KAHN-D'ANGELO, PT, ScD • YVETTE BLANCHARD, PT, ScD • BETH MCMANUS, PT, ScD, MPH

Providing services to high-risk infants and their families in the neonatal intensive care unit is a complex subspecialty of pediatric physical therapy requiring knowledge and skills beyond the competencies for entry into practice. The newborns in the neonatal intensive care unit (NICU) are among the most fragile patients that physical therapists will treat, and detrimental effects can occur as the result of routine caregiving procedures. Pediatric physical therapists (PTs) need advanced education in areas such as early fetal and infant development; infant neurobehavior; family responses to having a sick newborn; the environment of the NICU, physiologic assessment and monitoring; newborn pathologies, treatments, and outcomes; optimal discharge planning; and collaboration with the members of the health care team.[256] This chapter describes the neonatal intensive care unit and the role of the physical therapist within this setting. Practice in this setting requires knowledge of neonatal physiology, development, and health complications including prematurity, pulmonary conditions, neurologic conditions, fetal alcohol syndrome, fetal abstinence syndrome, and pain. A framework for physical therapy examination, evaluation, prognosis, and interventions for infants in the special care nursery is presented. The follow-up of infants after discharge from the intensive care nursery is addressed. Two case studies are presented to apply knowledge to practice.

HISTORY OF THE SPECIAL CARE NURSERY

Modern neonatal care was born with the development of the incubator by Couveuse in France in 1880.[130] The first text on the premature infant, *The Nursling*, authored by Budin, a student of Couveuse, was published in 1900. The main principles of neonatal care were support of body temperature, control of nosocomial infection, minimal handling, and provision of special nursing care. Interestingly, nurseries were quiet, and lights were dimmed at night. Dr. Martin Couney, who was one of Budin's students, used these principles of treatment for the premature infant, and in a bizarre entrepreneurial twist, exhibited them in Chicago for a fee.[234] Dr. Julius Hess attended this exhibition and applied these principles in the late 1940s. Dr. Hess achieved a neonatal mortality rate for preterm infants of 20%, which was respectable for the time. In response to the increased survival rate of premature infants reported by Hess, Budin's principles of care were implemented across the United States.

During the 1950s, a number of cities developed centers for the care of premature infants and a number of states developed maternal mortality committees that gathered data to be used as a basis for planning activities directed at preventing maternal death. During the 1960s, Arizona, Massachusetts, and Wisconsin promulgated standards for maternity units and developed regional perinatal care centers. Reports from these three states and several professional organizations, including the American Medical Association, the American College of Obstetricians and Gynecologists, the American Academy of Pediatrics, and the Academy of Family Physicians, stimulated the development of the regional organization of perinatal services.[93]

By the late 1960s, full-term infants with health complications were also being treated in the neonatal nursery. Advances in microlaboratory techniques for biochemical determinations from minute quantities of blood and the development of miniaturized monitoring equipment, ventilatory support systems, and means to conserve body heat improved the care of the neonate with serious illness.[93] Expansion of neonatal pharmacology, widespread use of phototherapy for management of hyperbilirubinemia, and methods of delivery of high-caloric solutions parenterally when oral feeding was not possible also improved the chances for survival of the very sick neonate. In 1975, the emergence of the subspecialties neonatology and perinatology affirmed the need for practitioners skilled in the care of infants in the high-technology nursery.

During the past three decades, the availability of neonatal intensive care has improved outcomes for high-risk infants, including premature infants and those with serious medical or surgical conditions.[15] Improved survival for very low birth weight and extremely low birth weight infants has been reported during the time frame of 1988 to 2002.[94,160,248] This improvement in survival is related to antenatal steroids, more aggressive resuscitation in the delivery room, and advanced treatments given in the special care nursery including surfactant therapy.[153]

ORGANIZATION OF PERINATAL SERVICES

Neonatal intensive care units are designed to meet a wide range of special needs, from the monitoring of apparently well infants at risk of serious illness to the intensive treatment of infants with acute illness. The March of Dimes report *Toward Improving the Outcome of Pregnancy* published in 1976, articulated the concept of regionalized perinatal care with three levels of maternal and neonatal care.[71] A subsequent report restated the importance of regionalization and recommended changes in designations from levels I, II, and III to basic, specialty, and subspecialty with expanded criteria.[199] By the beginning of the 21st century the number of neonatal intensive care units in the United States had increased to 880 (120 level II, 760 level III).[107] The three levels of neonatal care and capabilities within levels recommended by the American Academy of Pediatrics are presented in Box 28-1.[15]

THE NEONATAL INTENSIVE CARE ENVIRONMENT

As depicted in Figure 28-1, the newborn in the intensive care nursery transitions from the buoyant, warm, enclosed, and relatively quiet and dark environment of the womb to a bright, often noisy, technology filled, gravity-influenced environment and is subjected to procedures that often cause pain and discomfort.

The newborn is extremely vulnerable to the environmental effects of the intensive care nursery. Many studies and recommendations have been made to decrease negative effects and actually facilitate development as well as keep the infant alive. Caregivers play an important role in assessing and controlling aspects of the environment such as noise, light, and intensity of medical procedures.

In the 1980s, concern emerged that the typical nursery stay of several weeks may have detrimental effects on later behavior of the infant born at very low birth weight (<1500 grams).[130] At that time, the neonatal intensive care nursery was characterized by bright lights both night and day, high noise levels, and the intrusive medical procedures characteristic of high-technology treatment.[54,108]

Research ensued on the effects of different sensory inputs during the NICU stay and the concept of neonatal care facilitating optimal development. This care included modulation of the environment to facilitate development, recognition of infant distress and discomfort, and family-centered care.[3,8,9,104,111–113,127] More recently, environmental design of the intensive care nursery and the potential impact on neurodevelopmental outcome of the neonate were appraised by representatives from multiple hospitals.[154] Using an evidence-based approach, potentially better practices were identified to support neonatal development. These recommendations included implementation of guidelines for tactile stimulation, providing early exposure to mother's scent, minimizing exposure to noxious odors, developing a system for noise assessment of the NICU, minimizing ambient noise near the isolette, and preservation of sleep. Deep sleep is necessary for development of the neurosensory system and the maturing brain and should be facilitated and protected while the neonate is in the intensive care unit.[183]

BOX 28-1   HOSPITAL PERINATAL CARE LEVELS

LEVEL I: BASIC CARE

Evaluate and provide postnatal care to infants 35 to 37 weeks gestation, stabilize infants <35 weeks' gestation until transfer

LEVEL II - SPECIALTY CARE

IIA: Provides care for moderately ill infants >32 weeks' gestation

IIB: Provides mechanical ventilation for brief periods

LEVEL III: SUBSPECIALTY CARE

IIIA: Provides care for infants >28 weeks, performs minor surgical procedures

IIIB: Provides care for infants <28 weeks' gestation, provides advanced respiratory support (high-frequency ventilation); advanced imaging, pediatric surgical specialists, access to pediatric medical subspecialists

IIIC: Provides extracorporeal membrane oxygenation (ECMO) and complex cardiac surgery with cardiopulmonary bypass

---

NOISE AND LIGHT

The intensive care unit includes many pieces of equipment that contribute to the noise level including respirators and alarms for unacceptable levels of heart rate, respiration, oxygen, temperature, and carbon dioxide exchange. Everyday activities such as conversation, closing drawers, dragging chairs, and tearing tape add to the noise level. Noise is measured on a logarithmic scale and small changes in measured decibels (db) are detectable. As a frame of reference, conversation may be at a 60-db level and dragging a chair may be at an 80-db level. Bremer et al. found that high noise levels from alarms and telephones can cause an increase in autonomic response that puts premature infants at risk for bradycardic and hypoxic episodes.[48] The American Academy of Pediatrics recommends noise levels not exceed 45 db with noise levels above 50 db only 10% of the time and a maximum of 65 db.[275] Darcy, Hancock, and Ware found that noise levels in several NICUs in the mid-Atlantic region of the United States were often louder than the 50-db level and that 60 db levels were exceeded at times.[78] Lasky and Williams followed 22 infants with extremely low birth weight (<1000 grams) throughout their stay in a NICU that was constructed with

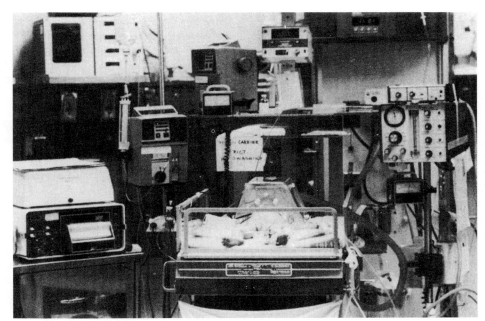

Figure 28-1 Infant surrounded by typical NICU equipment. (Data from American Academy of Pediatrics, Policy Statement, Levels of Neonatal Care, *Pediatrics*, vol 114, No 5, 2004.)

a high priority on noise abatement and found that the neonates were exposed to noise levels averaging 56 db.[152] Noise levels increased with the use of older model ventilators and an open bed rather than an isolette. The authors concluded it is unlikely that newborns in the intensive care nursery consistently experience noise that does not exceed the recommended levels. Hearing loss has not been linked specifically to noise levels, but a synergistic relationship may occur with excessive nose and ototoxic drugs such as gentamicin.[49] Sound levels of the NICU may interfere with frequency discrimination and pattern recognition.[111]

Slevin et al. studied the impact of a designated "quiet period," which included asking staff to keep noise levels at a minimum, switching phones to a flashing light system, and postponing caregiving activities if possible.[236] During the "quiet period," the researchers noted significant reductions in infants' median diastolic blood pressure and mean arterial pressure.[236] Other simple techniques such as covering the isolette with a blanket or placing a sound absorbing panel in the isolette help decrease the sound levels.[12,225] It is interesting to note that approximately half of the neonatal nurses interviewed reported that they never or rarely limit their conversations near the incubators/cribs.[1] Noise can also interfere with the development of sleep patterns in neonates.

Infants younger than 32 weeks gestational age have little ability to limit the amount of light entering the eyes because of thinness of the eyelids.[112] High light levels and decreased light/dark cycles may adversely affect newborn patients.[14] Recommended light levels are less than 646 lux (60 foot-candles) and are reported to be met more often than recommendations for noise levels.[152] Graven

recommended the following strategies to minimize the risk of visual impairments while the infant is in the NICU: protecting REM sleep, dark periods; limiting intense noise and other unnecessary sensory stimulation; and paying careful attention to the sensory environment of each infant.[112]

There is a growing body of evidence on the developmentally appropriate environment for neonates.[64,275] Private rooms are an alternative to the large multi-isolette/crib ward that currently characterizes the NICU. Noise levels decreased and catheter-associated bloodstream infections fell after infants moved from a ward to a single room.[271] An obvious disadvantage of the single room model is staff coverage.

PREMATURITY AND LOW BIRTH WEIGHT

More than 500,000 infants are born prematurely (gestation of less than 37 weeks) in the United States every year.[114] Approximately 1% of live births are very preterm with gestational age younger than 32 weeks.[279] Preterm birth is a leading cause of infant mortality and morbidity, accounting for over 70% of neonatal deaths and half of long-term neurologic disabilities such as cerebral palsy, cognitive impairment, and behavioral problems.[66,178] The preterm birth rate has increased from 9% to 12% since 1981.[114] Infants born prematurely or who are small for gestational age (SGA) are divided into three major categories: low birth weight (LBW), from 1501 to 2500 grams; very low birth weight (VLBW), 1000 to 1500 grams; and extremely low birth weight (ELBW), less than 1000 grams.

The causes of preterm birth are not clear but seem to involve an interaction of multiple factors including genetic, social, and environmental factors.[279] Spontaneous preterm delivery and birth has recently been described as a common complex disorder like heart disease, diabetes, and cancer.[279] Criteria for complex diseases include family history, recurrence, and racial disparities.[114] American black women had 1.5 times the rate of preterm birth and 4 times the rate of infant mortality because of preterm births compared with white women.[146] Approximately 40% of premature births are believed to be caused by intrauterine or systemic infections or both which are not diagnosed until the onset of labor.[32] Pregnancy-specific stress is associated with smoking, caffeine consumption, and unhealthy eating, and it is inversely correlated with healthy eating, vitamin use, exercise, and gestational age at delivery.[167] Maternal hemorrhage and pathologic distention of the uterus are associated with preterm labor.[75] Infants born after assisted reproduction have a lower birth weight and gestational age when compared to matched controls.[172]

There has been a significant increase in survival of infants with VLBW and ELBW[153] as a result of more aggressive delivery room resuscitation, surfactant therapy, and a decreased rate of sepsis.[94,280] Approximately half of children surviving extremely low-birth-weight deliveries have subsequent moderate to severe neurodevelopmental disabilities.[153] Brain injury, retinopathy of prematurity, bronchopulmonary dysplasia, and neonatal infection increase the risk of mortality or neurosensory impairment.[27]

There is a national focus on preventing preterm birth spearheaded by the March of Dimes National Prematurity Campaign of 2003, recently extended to 2020.[176] The Prematurity Research Expansion and Education for Mothers who Deliver Infants Early (PREEMIE) Act (P.L. 109–450) was passed in 2006 with a subsequent Surgeon's General Conference on the Prevention of Preterm Birth in 2008.[191] The conference objectives were to (1) increase awareness of preterm birth in the United States; (2) review key findings on causes, consequences, and prevention of prematurity; and (3) establish an agenda for public and private sectors to address this public health problem. Conference recommendations included (1) increased research in medicine, epidemiology, psychosocial, and behavioral factors relating to prematurity; (2) professional education and training; (3) communication and outreach to the public; (4) addressing racial disparities, and (5) improvement of quality of care and health services.

ASSESSMENT OF GESTATIONAL AGE

The determination of gestational age of infants in the special care nursery is crucial to interpretation of findings from neurologic and behavioral examinations. The New Ballard Score (NBS) is the most widely used assessment of gestational age.[241] The NBS assesses neuromuscular maturity (such as posture), physical maturity (such as presence of lanugo), and external genitalia to determine gestational age from 20 to 44 weeks and is accurate within 1 week.[241]

Gestational age is also determined by ultrasound, measurements such as weight; length; head circumference; wrist, hip, and shoulder ranges of motion; and amniotic fluid analysis.[224] Although gestational age is usually determined by physicians or nurses, the physical therapist should be familiar with how gestational age is determined.

NEONATAL HEALTH CONDITIONS ASSOCIATED WITH IMPAIRMENTS IN BODY FUNCTIONS AND STRUCTURES

Several pulmonary, neurologic, cardiac, and other health conditions in neonates are associated with increased risk for impairments in body functions and structures that affect cognitive, motor, sensory, behavioral, learning, and psychosocial development that may result in long-term activity limitations and participation restrictions.[153] The physical therapist providing services in the NICU should have a working knowledge of physiology of neonates, pathophysiology and associated impairments in body functions and structures, and how impairments affect the infant's behavior. Practice in the NICU is a complex subspecialty of pediatrics and knowledge and skills should be obtained through advanced didactic and practical education. Clinical guidelines and clinical training models for neonatal physical therapy are outlined by Sweeney, Heriza, and Blanchard.[256]

PULMONARY CONDITIONS

RESPIRATORY DISTRESS SYNDROME

Respiratory distress syndrome (RDS), or hyaline membrane disease, is the single most important cause of illness and death in preterm infants and is the most common single cause of respiratory distress in neonates.[247] RDS occurs in 10% of all premature infants in the United States. The percentage increases to 50% to 60% for infants born less than 29 weeks gestational age.[17,68] The principal factors in the pathophysiology of RDS are pulmonary immaturity and low production of surfactant. Low surfactant production results in increased surface tension, alveolar collapse, diffuse atelectasis, and decreased lung compliance. These factors cause an increase in pulmonary artery pressure that leads to extrapulmonary right-to-left shunting of blood and ventilation-perfusion mismatching. Clinical manifestations of RDS include grunting respirations, retractions, nasal flaring, cyanosis, and increased oxygen requirement after birth. Prophylactic use of antenatal steroids to accelerate lung maturation in women with preterm labor of up to 34 weeks significantly reduced the incidence of RDS and decreased mortality.[68]

Treatment goals for RDS include improvement in oxygenation and maintaining optimal lung volume.[144] The type of intervention depends on the severity of the respiratory disorder and includes oxygen supplementation, assisted ventilation, surfactant administration, and extracorporeal membrane oxygenation (ECMO). Continuous positive airway pressure (CPAP) or positive end–expiratory pressure (PEEP) is applied to prevent volume loss during expiration. Nasal and nasopharyngeal prongs are used with positive end-expiratory pressure ventilators. Mechanical ventilation via tracheal tube is used in severe cases of RDS. (See Chapter 23 for a more detailed description of ventilators.) Mechanical ventilation may injure the lungs of premature infants through high airway pressure (barotrauma), large gas volumes (volutrauma), alveolar collapse and refill (atelectotrauma), and increased inflammation (biotrauma).[22]

The new generation of ventilators is equipped with microprocessors enabling effective synchronized (patient-triggered) ventilation.[143] High-frequency oscillatory ventilation (HFOV) was developed with the goal of decreasing complications associated with mechanical ventilation. Conventional intermittent positive pressure ventilation is provided 30 to 80 breaths per minute, whereas HFOV provides "breaths" at 10 to 15 cycles per second or 600 to 900 per minute. At this time, evidence is insufficient to support the routine use of HFOV.[125]

Prophylactic use of surfactant for infants judged to be at risk of developing RDS (infants less than 30 to 32 weeks gestation) has been demonstrated to decrease the risk of pneumothorax, pulmonary interstitial emphysema, and mortality.[247] Early administration of multiple doses of natural or synthetic surfactant extract results in improved clinical outcome and appears to be the most effective method of administration. When a choice of natural or synthetic surfactant is available, natural surfactant shows greater early decrease in requirement for ventilatory support.[240,287] Newer synthetic surfactants include whole surfactant proteins or parts of the proteins (peptides). A recent clinical trial showed that these preparations decreased mortality and rates of necrotizing enterocolitis with other clinical outcomes being similar to those of natural surfactant preparations.[211] A recent pilot study showed that an inhaled steroid, budesonide, delivered intratracheally with surfactant administration to very low birth weight infants with severe RDS reduced mortality and chronic lung disease with no immediate adverse effects.[285]

Extracorporeal membrane oxygenation (ECMO) is a technique of cardiopulmonary bypass modified from techniques developed for open-heart surgery that are used to support heart and lung function (for review of ECMO and implications for pediatric physical therapy, see Pax Lowes & Palisano[207]). In newborns with acute respiratory failure, the immature lungs are allowed to rest and recover to avoid the damaging effects of mechanical ventilation. Because of the need for systemic administration of heparin and the resultant risk of systemic and intracranial hemorrhage, ECMO is reserved for use with infants who are at least 34 weeks of gestational age, weigh more than 2000 g,

have no evidence of intracranial bleeding, require less than 10 days of assisted ventilation, and have reversible lung disease.[250] ECMO is contraindicated for infants younger than 34 weeks of age because of high rates of intracranial hemorrhage, perhaps because of systemic anticoagulation necessary with ECMO or to abnormal cerebrovascular pressures and flows accompanying ECMO. ECMO is used to manage intractable hypoxemia in near-term infants, newborns with meconium aspiration, RDS, pneumonia sepsis, and congenital diaphragmatic hernia.[68]

The prognosis of infants with RDS is correlated with the severity of the original disease, but today few infants die of acute respiratory failure, but rather from complications of extreme prematurity such as infections, necrotizing enterocolitis, and intracranial hemorrhage.[143] Infants who do not require assisted ventilation recover without developmental or medical sequelae, but the clinical course of the very immature infant may be complicated by air leaks in the lungs and BPD. Infants who survive severe RDS often require frequent hospitalization for upper respiratory tract infections and have an increased incidence of neurologic sequelae.[133]

Emerging technologies for management of RDS include inhalation of nitrous oxide, liquid ventilation, or a hybrid of liquid and gas ventilation. The rationale for using liquid ventilation is to decrease alveolar surface tension by eliminating the air-liquid interface by filling the alveolus with liquid.[68] Inhalation of nitrous oxide helps decrease pulmonary artery resistance, cytokine-induced lung inflammation, and increase gas exchange. Findings regarding the use of nitrous oxide (NO) and prevention of chronic lung disease and neurologic injury are inconclusive.[21] Inhaled nitric oxide for severe RDS is an experimental treatment that may decrease chronic lung disease and mortality. However, increase in intracranial hemorrhage caused a termination of a study in 2006.[131]

BRONCHOPULMONARY DYSPLASIA AND CHRONIC LUNG DISEASE OF INFANCY

Bronchopulmonary dysplasia (BPD) and chronic lung disease of infancy (CLD) are two chronic pulmonary conditions that are caused by incomplete or abnormal repair of lung tissue during the neonatal period.[129] The National Institute of Child Health and Human Development defined infants with mild BPD as requiring oxygen supplementation for a total of at least 28 days, whereas infants with moderate or severe BPD require oxygen supplementation or ventilatory support at 36 weeks postmenstrual age and for more than 28 days.[90] CLD is diagnosed at 36 weeks' postmenstrual age, if there is a continued need for supplemental oxygen, abnormal physical examination, and abnormal chest radiograph. Chronic lung disease (CLD) occurs in 57% to 70% of infants born at 23 weeks gestational age; 33% to 89% of infants born at 24 weeks gestational age; and 16% to 71% of infants born at 25 weeks gestational age.

The cause of BPD is multifactorial with pathogenesis being associated with immature lung tissue, barotraumas (high airway pressure), and volutrauma (large gas volumes) resulting from mechanical ventilation. Atelectotrauma (alveolar collapse and reexpansion) occurs with increased inflammation and an imbalance in inflammatory and anti-inflammatory chemical mediators (cytokines) in infants with ELBW.[33] Neonatal sepsis especially because of candidemia, a systemic yeast infection, is associated with CLD.[150] Boys are at greater risk for developing CLDs, perhaps because of a lag of 1 to 2.5 weeks in pulmonary and cerebral maturation compared with girls.

Prevention of premature birth is the most effective preventive measure for BPD.[33] Antenatal steroids are still the most effective intervention in lung maturation. A decreased incidence of BPD was reported after management that included early administration of surfactant, immediately followed by nasal CPAP, lower oxygen saturation targets of 90% to 95%, and early parenteral amino acid supplementation.[103] The use of superoxide dismutase enzymes as an antioxidant has been investigated for treatment of BPD and CLD.[129] Management of BPD includes oxygen supplementation with oxygen saturation less than 95%, avoidance of mechanical ventilation if possible, diuretics after the first week of life, and steroids to help wean from oxygen during later stages of treatment.[33] Chronic lung disease is a major morbidity influencing development and is associated with poor nutrition, growth, feeding, prolonged hospitalization, and episodes of nosocomial infection. Treatment with early corticosteroids is associated with gastrointestinal bleeding and intestinal perforation, and there is a possibility of neurodevelopmental impairment.[120] Up to 50% of infants with BPD are hospitalized in the first year following discharge from the NICU.[137,239] Respiratory symptoms in patients with BPD persist into early adolescence[121,269] although most studies have shown no reduction in exercise capacity in children with BPD.[34] BPD seems to be associated with a global developmental impairment which correlates with BPD disease severity.[90,137] The reader is referred to Chapter 23 for information on children who require long-term ventilator assistance.

MECONIUM ASPIRATION SYNDROME

Meconium aspiration syndrome (MAS) is defined as respiratory distress in an infant born through meconium-stained amniotic fluid whose symptoms cannot be otherwise explained.[92] It can be characterized by early onset respiratory distress in term and near-term infants with symptoms of respiratory distress, poor lung compliance, hypoxemia, and radiographic findings of hyperinflation and patchy opacifications with rales and rhonchi on auscultation.[278] Because of the frequent occurrence of air leaks in these infants, positive pressure ventilation is contraindicated. It is unclear whether the meconium itself causes pneumonitis severe enough to lead to the above symptoms or if the presence of meconium

in the amniotic fluid is a result of other events such as stressed labor, postmaturity, and depressed cord pH that may have predisposed the fetus to severe pulmonary disease.[68] It is recommended that the infant with depressed physiologic function and meconium-stained fluid be suctioned endotracheally as pharyngeal suctioning does not reduce MAS.[263] Antibiotics are often given until bacterial infection is ruled out. The infant is hypersensitive to environmental stimuli and should be treated in the quietest environment possible. According to a Cochrane Review in 2007, surfactant administration may reduce the severity of MAS and decrease the number of infants requiring ECMO.[91,233] Obstetric approaches to the prevention of MAS such as intrapartum surveillance, amnioinfusion, and delivery room management have not demonstrated a decrease in MAS.[284] Approximately 20% of infants with MAS demonstrated neurodevelopmental delays up to 3 years of age even though they responded well to conventional treatment.[30]

NEUROLOGIC CONDITIONS

PERIVENTRICULAR LEUKOMALACIA

Periventricular leukomalacia (PVL) is the predominant form of brain injury and the leading known cause of cerebral palsy (CP) and cognitive impairments in premature infants.[82] PVL is a symmetrical, nonhemorrhagic, usually bilateral lesion caused by ischemia from alterations in arterial circulation.[281] Male gender, premature rupture of membranes, preeclampsia, reduced carbon dioxide in the blood, and intraventricular hemorrhage (IVH) are associated with PVL.[123] PVL is characterized by necrosis of white matter dorsal and lateral to the external angles of the lateral ventricles. The area affected includes the white matter through which long descending motor tracts travel from the motor cortex to the spinal cord. Because the motor tracts involved in the control of leg movements are closest to the ventricles and therefore more likely to be damaged, spastic diplegia is the most common motor impairment (Figure 28-2). If the lesion extends laterally, the arms may be involved, with resulting spastic quadriplegia. Visual impairments may also result from damage to the optic radiations.[281]

PVL is caused by a reduction in cerebral blood flow in the highly vulnerable periventricular region of the brain where the arterial "end zones" of the middle, posterior, and anterior cerebral arteries meet and is often associated with intraventricular hemorrhage (IVH).[268] Decreased cerebral blood flow leads to ischemia and a decrease in antioxidants. This results in generation of free oxygen radicals and glutamate toxicity factors that contribute to periventricular leukomalacia. The incidence of white matter damage in premature infants increases with decreased gestational age because of the immature vascular supply, impairments in cerebral autoregulation, and damage to premyelinating oligodendrites from free radicals.[145,268] PVL also affects subplate neurons

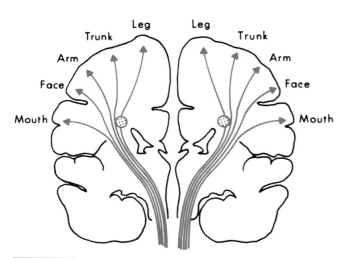

Figure 28-2 Diagram of cortical spinal tracts. Dotted circular areas indicate periventricular leukomalacia that would be expected to affect descending fibers for control of lower extremity. (From Volpe, JJ. *Neurology of the newborn*, 2nd edition, Philadelphia: WB Saunders, 1987, p 314.)

which lie just below the developing cerebral cortex until programmed apoptosis (cell death). Subplate neurons play an essential role in axonal targeting of thalamocortical synapses, and their loss may contribute to motor, visual, and cognitive impairments.[82] Systemic hypotension associated with difficult resuscitation at birth and ECMO are also associated with PVL. Patent ductus arteriosus and severe apneic spells are other contributing factors, particularly after the first week of life.[145]

Serial ultrasonography one week following birth and magnetic resonance imaging are diagnostic tools for periventricular leukomalacia.[82] White matter echodensities and echolucencies on high-resolution cranial ultrasonography are predictive of neurologic sequelae associated with cerebral palsy.[86] Serial ultrasonographic studies are important because the evolution of periventricular echodensity is related to prognosis. Early periventricular echodensity that resolves during the first weeks of life is not correlated with childhood disability. Formation of cysts as a result of dissolution of brain tissue secondary to infarction, however, is correlated with cerebral palsy and cognitive impairments. Cerebral palsy occurs in more than 90% of infants who develop bilateral cysts larger than 3 mm in diameter in the parietal or occipital areas.[86]

Medical management of PVL includes prevention of intrauterine asphyxia, maintenance of adequate ventilation and perfusion, avoidance of systemic hypotension, and control of seizures.[38,268] Prevention of intrauterine asphyxia includes identification of high-risk pregnancies, fetal monitoring, fetal blood sampling, and cesarean section as indicated. Maintenance of adequate ventilation includes avoiding common causes of hypoxemia such as inappropriate feeding, inserting or removing ventilator connections,

painful procedures and examinations, handling, and excessive noise. Adequate perfusion can be maintained with appropriate treatment if the infant exhibits apnea and severe bradycardia. Outcomes of PVL include increased incidence of CP if cysts are visible with ultrasound, whereas cognitive impairment may be the outcome if ultrasound shows increased periventricular echogenicity without cysts.[86]

GERMINAL MATRIX-INTRAVENTRICULAR HEMORRHAGE AND PERIVENTRICULAR HEMORRHAGE

Germinal matrix-intraventricular hemorrhage (GM-IVH) is the most common type of neonatal intracranial hemorrhage. GM-IVH occurs in neonates younger than 32 weeks of gestational age and weighing less than 1500 grams with an inverse relationship between gestational age and incidence of GM-IVH. The incidence of GM-IVH has declined and ranges from 15% to 20%.[173] Most hemorrhages occur within the first 24 hours after birth and progress over 48 hours or more. By the end of the first postnatal week, 90% of hemorrhages have reached their full extent. Papile developed a four-level grading scale based on ultrasound scan to classify hemorrhages.[204] Grade I is an isolated germinal matrix hemorrhage. Grade II is an IVH with normal-sized ventricles that occurs when hemorrhage in the subependymal germinal matrix ruptures through the ependyma into the lateral ventricles. Grade III is an IVH with acute ventricular dilation, and grade IV is a hemorrhage into the periventricular white matter. Perinatal events that can lead to increased cerebral blood flow and GM-IVH include respiratory distress, apnea, hypotension, rapid volume expansion, routine caregiving interventions, and environmental stress such as noise and light.[38]

GM-IVH pathogenesis involves complex interaction of intravascular, vascular, and extravascular factors. This lesion involves bleeding into the subependymal germinal matrix, which is a gelatinous area that contains a rich vascular network supplied mainly by Heubner's artery, a branch of the anterior cerebral artery; branches of the middle cerebral artery; and the internal carotid. This matrix is prominent from 26 to 34 weeks of gestation and is usually gone by term. The vessels that traverse the matrix are primitive in appearance and structure, with a single layer of endothelium without smooth muscle, elastin, or collagen, and the area is devoid of supportive stroma. Hemorrhage occurs from these primitive capillaries. In a small number of preterm infants, hemorrhage may occur from the choroid plexus or the roof of the fourth ventricle (Figure 28-3). Cerebral autoregulation of the blood vessels normally protects the brain from significant alterations in cerebral blood flow. Hypoxia and hypoxemia in the neonate interfere with cerebral autoregulation[85] and increase the risk of vessel rupture.[247] Positive-pressure ventilation can be transmitted to capillaries of the germinal matrix, which can

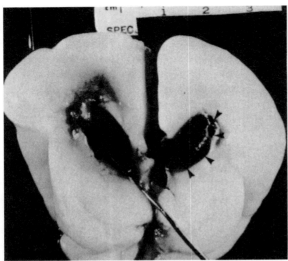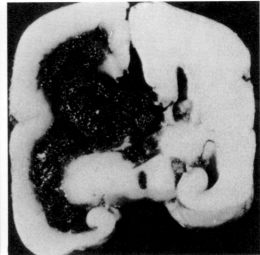

Figure 28-3 Coronal section of cerebrum showing germinal matrix - intraventricular hemorrhage. (From Volpe, JJ. *Neurology of the newborn*, 5ᵗʰ edition, Philadelphia, WB Saunders, 2008, p 519.)

impede venous return, leading to increased pressure and rupture. The most vulnerable area of the venous drainage system is at the level of the foramen of Monro and the caudate nucleus, the most common site of GMH-IVH.[38]

Extravascular factors also contribute to GMH-IVH. The germinal matrix is highly vascularized and the capillary bed is embedded in gelatinous material that provides poor support for the fragile blood vessels. This along with excessive fibrinolytic activity in the periventricular area may result in the extension of a small bleed, which may then rupture into the ventricles.[268] Environmental and genetic factors also may affect the risk for IVH as well as maternal infection such as chorioamnionitis.[182] Neuropathology associated with IVH includes hydrocephalus, germinal matrix destruction, cyst formation, and accompanying hypoxic-ischemic lesions.

The signs and symptoms of GMH-IVH may range from subtle and nonspecific to catastrophic. Clinical signs include a decreasing hematocrit, a full anterior fontanelle, changes in activity level, impaired visual tracking, increased muscle tone of lower limbs, neck flexor hypotonia, and brisk tendon reflexes.[268] Catastrophic deterioration involves major acute hemorrhages with clinical signs of stupor progressing to coma, respiratory distress progressing to apnea, generalized tonic seizures, decerebrate posturing, fixation of pupils to light, and flaccid quadriparesis.

The diagnosis of GMH-IVH is usually made by cranial ultrasonography. The American Academy of Neurology recommends that cranial ultrasonography be done on all preterm neonates less than 30 weeks gestation age between 7 and 14 days of chronologic age and at 36 to 40 weeks gestational age to screen for GMH-IVH.[187] MRI is more accurate than ultrasound and may be used at term as a

predictor of outcome at 2 to 3 years for VLBW preterm infants.[82]

Efforts to prevent IVH have met with varying degrees of success. Lower rates of IVH have been reported in NICUs with higher patient volume and higher neonatologist-to-house staff ratio.[258] Prevention of neonatal hypoxic events as such as respiratory distress, apnea, hypotension and rapid volume expansion, hypercarbia, excessive caregiving interventions, and environmental stress such as excessive noise or light may decrease incidence of IVH.[38] A review of the use of phenobarbital did not reveal a significant decrease in occurrence or severity of IVH, but there was an increased risk for ventilation need.[276] Infants treated with indomethacin have been shown to have a decrease in incidence and severity of IVH.[228] Outcomes for infants treated with indomethacin are better for boys than girls.[188]

Interventions for IVH include acute treatment, pharmacologic therapy, and management of ventricular dilation.[38] Acute treatment includes physiologic support to maintain oxygenation, perfusion, body temperature, and blood glucose level. Physical handling is minimized. The infant should be positioned in prone or side lying with the head in midline or to the side without neck flexion. Management of ventricular dilation includes ventriculoperitoneal shunting or temporary ventricular draining.[38,288]

Outcomes of IVH depend on severity and extent of the hemorrhages and the presence of associated problems. Infants with a small or mild hemorrhage survive and have a low incidence of neurologic complications. Infants with moderate hemorrhage have a mortality rate of 5% to 20%, and ventricular dilation develops in 15% to 20% of survivors. When bleeding is severe, mortality is 50%. The incidence of neurologic conditions such as cerebral palsy, hydrocephalus, cognitive impairment, sensory and attention problems, and learning disorders varies from 15% in infants with moderate hemorrhage to 35% to 90% in infants with severe hemorrhage.[85]

HYPOXIC ISCHEMIC ENCEPHALOPATHY

Hypoxic ischemic encephalopathy (HIE) is a spectrum of neurologic impairment associated with high neonatal mortality and neurologic morbidity.[221] HIE is a lack of oxygen and substrate delivery to the brain as a result of decreased blood flow which may occur from maternal, uteroplacental, or fetal complications.[163] Examples of potential causes include maternal cardiac arrest, placental abruption, and fetomaternal hemorrhage. The incidence of term gestation perinatal HIE ranges from 0.5 to 2 infants per 1000 live births.[105] MRI is the preferred imaging tool in the neonatal period and long-term follow-up.[164] Clinical signs of moderate encephalopathy include lethargy, decreased activity level, hypotonia, weak suck, incomplete Moro reflex, constricted pupils, bradycardia, and periodic breathing. Clinical signs of severe HIE include stupor or coma, no spontaneous activity, decerebrate posturing, flaccid tone, absent Moro and suck reflexes, dilated or nonreactive pupils, variable heart rate, and apnea.[232] The pattern of HIE occurs in two phases. The first phase is a primary energy failure related to the specific insult, which causes the lack of oxygen and glucose. The secondary or delayed brain injury phase energy failure occurs some hours later with symptoms evolving over approximately 72 hours and is postulated to be due to delayed cell death.[266] Delayed cell death is caused by cellular energy failure, acidosis, and neurotoxicity resulting from neurotransmitter (glutamate), calcium, and nitric oxide release and accumulation from the earlier injury phase.[266]

Historically the treatment of neonatal HIE has been limited to supportive care, but hypothermia either of the head or whole body is an emerging treatment to interrupt several critical steps during the process of hypoxic-ischemic injury.[289] Other neuroprotective interventions being studied include oxygen free radical scavengers and excitatory amino acid antagonists such as allopurinol and glutamate receptor antagonists.[118,264] There is a 10% risk of death with moderate HIE and up to 30% of infants manifest spastic quadriparesis and cognitive impairment resulting from cortical and subcortical injury in a parasagittal distribution.[268] In severe HIE mortality is 60% and the majority of all survivors will have long-term morbidity associated with damage to the thalami, basal ganglia, hippocampi, and mesencephalic structures.[232,268] Long-term sequelae include cognitive impairment, spastic quadriparesis, seizure disorder, ataxia, bulbar and pseudobulbar palsy, atonic quadriparesis, hyperactivity, and impaired attention.[268]

NEONATAL SEIZURES

Seizures are the most frequent and distinct neurologic signs that occur in the neonatal period.[268] A seizure is clinically defined as a paroxysmal alteration in autonomic, behavioral, and motor function. The incidence of neonatal seizures has been reported as ranging from 1.5 to 3.5 per 1000 live births in North America, varying with risk factors such as low birth-weight, prematurity, maternal medical conditions, and perinatal obstetrical complications.[186] Causes of neonatal seizures include hypoxia-ischemia, stroke, metabolic disease, and drug intoxication or withdrawal or idiopathic. Seizures are classified by Volpe as subtle, such as tonic horizontal deviation of eyes in term infants and chewing movements in premature infants, tonic involving sustained posturing of a limb, and clonic involving rhythmic and slow movement.[268] The most frequent overt sign of neonatal neurologic disorders is the convulsive seizure. Electroencephalography (EEG) does not record some of the behaviors/signs previously described as seizures by observation. Neonatal seizures documented by EEG with or without clinical manifestations represent the most accurate diagnosis, although there is controversy regarding the possibility of seizures occurring without EEG activity because they are subcortical.[259,268] Although some experts argue that the diagnosis of neonatal seizures should not be based on clinical observation alone, EEGs are not available in most NICUs.[235]

It is imperative to recognize neonatal seizures, determine their origin, and provide specific treatment for the illness/condition causing them. It is also important to decrease their interference with feeding and respiration.[259,268] Management of neonatal seizures includes maintenance of the infant's airway and monitoring of vital signs and blood gases. There is not a consensus of when to treat with anticonvulsant drugs and for how long.[109] The most common anticonvulsant used is phenobarbital with others including phenytoin, and benzodiazepams. These anticonvulsant drugs have many side effects including respiratory, myocardial, and central nervous system depression, and jaundice, and may have toxic effects on the developing brain.[38]

A 2004 Cochrane Review concluded that "there is little evidence to support the use of any of the anticonvulsants currently used in the neonatal period," although it is generally agreed that recurrent or prolonged seizures require treatment to reduce the risk of brain injury.[109,235] Trials of new pharmacologic agents such at bumetanide are currently ongoing.[101] The mortality rate for neonates with seizures has declined from 40% before 1969 to less than 15%. In a recent study, neonatal mortality was 7%, and 28% of infants had poor long-term neurologic outcome such as cerebral palsy, cognitive impairment, and epilepsy.[180] A normal neurologic and behavioral examination and normal to mildly abnormal EEG are associated with a favorable outcome with little or no disability.[180]

CARDIAC CONDITIONS

Cardiac conditions common to neonates in the NICU include congenital heart defects such as patent ductus arteriosis (PDA), pulmonary atresia, tetralogy of Fallot (TOF), coarctation of the aorta (COA), and pulmonary atresia. Cardiac conditions are presented in Chapter 26.

OTHER MEDICAL CONDITIONS

NECROTIZING ENTEROCOLITIS

Necrotizing enterocolitis (NEC) is an acute inflammatory disease of the bowel that occurs most frequently in premature infants weighing less than 2000 grams during the first 6 weeks of life.[110,170] Although the cause is not known, several factors appear to play a role in the pathogenesis of NEC. Many of these factors involve impaired blood flow to the intestine and include asphyxia, congenital heart disease, abdominal wall defects, neural tube defects, intrauterine growth restriction, exchange transfusion, and presence of umbilical catheter.[260] Diminished blood supply results in death of mucosal cells lining the bowel wall, decreasing secretion of lubricating mucus. The thin bowel wall becomes susceptible to proteolytic enzymes, swells, breaks down, and is permeable to exotoxins. Gas-forming bacteria invade the damaged area to produce pneumatosis intestinalis, air in the submucosal, or subserosal surfaces of the bowel. Decreased immunologic factors hamper the ability of the intestinal tract to fight organisms that are not absorbed,[44] and intestinal motility is not mature until the third trimester.[165] The digestive system of premature infants, especially those who are VLBW and ELBW, often is intolerant to enteral (tube) feedings. Enteral feedings contribute to bacterial colonization by directly introducing organisms into the intestine as well as providing substrate for organism growth. Bradshaw reported that nearly all infants who had NEC had enteral feedings.[44] Breast milk may have protective effects against the development of NEC.

Signs of obstruction of the bowels include vomiting, distention of the abdomen, increased gastric aspirates, passing of bloody stools, retention of stools, lethargy, decreased urine output, and alterations in respiratory status. Diagnosis of NEC is made by physical examination, laboratory tests, and radiography. Radiographic or abdominal ultrasonography is used to follow the course of the disease, with lucent bubbles appearing as the gas-forming bacteria enter the intestinal wall.[134] Medical treatment of NEC includes discontinuation of all oral feedings, abdominal decompression via nasogastric suction, administration of intravenous antibiotics, and correction of fluid and electrolyte imbalances.[44] Surgical intervention is indicated when there is radiographic evidence of fixed, dilated intestinal loops accompanied by intestinal distention, perforation, intestinal gangrene, and abdominal wall edema.

Factors that are predictive of poor outcome include prior enteral feeding, patent ductus arteriosus, indomethacin use, and perforation. Improved medical-surgical care and the use of total parenteral nutrition has reduced the mortality rate from 24% to 65% in the 1960s and 1970s to 9% to 28% in the 1990s, with even lower rates for neonates who did not require surgical intervention.[260] Among survivors, 10% to 30% have strictures, especially of the colon, which require surgery. A Cochrane Review recommended further large clinical trials to determine how the timing of introduction of parenteral feeding affects clinical outcomes in infants with VLBW.[43]

GASTROESOPHAGEAL REFLUX DISEASE

Gastroesophageal reflux disease (GERD) is the retrograde movement of acidic stomach contents into the esophagus.[260] GERD occurs frequently in preterm infants because of the horizontal position and immature lower esophageal sphincter function.[37] Signs of GERD include frequent vomiting, regurgitation of feeds, irritability, and pulmonary aspiration. The premature infant may present with more subtle signs such as apnea and bradycardia.[73,87] GERD is associated with failure to thrive, recurrent apnea, recurrent respiratory infections, and ventilator dependence.[260]

Tests for GERD include esophageal pH monitoring, with a tube placed in through a nostril and left in place for 24 hours, and impedance monitoring, which detects the flow of fluids and gas through hollow viscera, or a combination of both techniques.[73] A GERD behavioral scale questionnaire called the Infant Gastroesophageal Reflux Questionnaire (I-GERQ), which has been shown to be valid and specific,[200] has been modified by Birch and Newell for premature infants.[37]

Management of GERD includes positioning the infant in prone or on the left side if cardiorespiratory monitoring is applied, using a feed thickener such as carob, pharmacologic agents; monitoring for apnea, parenteral support, and surgery if the previous treatment strategies are not successful and if there are respiratory symptoms associated with GERD.[37,260] Pharmacologic agents include antireflux drugs such as ranitidine, lansoprazole, and metoclopramide.[26] The most commonly used surgical procedure for the neonate is a fundal plication in which the proximal stomach is wrapped around the distal esophagus, creating a junction that prevents reflux.[201]

RETINOPATHY OF PREMATURITY

Retinopathy of prematurity (ROP) is caused by proliferation of abnormal blood vessels in the newborn retina, which occurs in two phases. Phase I is delayed growth of retinal blood vessels after premature birth. Phase II occurs when the hypoxia created during phase I stimulates growth of new blood vessels. Growth of retinal blood vessels is stimulated by vascular endothelial growth factor (VEGF) and insulin-like growth factor-1 (IGF-1).[175] Use of oxygen supplementation causes hyperoxia and suppresses VEGF and IGF-1 causing apoptosis (death) of vascular endothelial cells, which causes hyperoxia-induced blood vessel damage and scarring of the retinal vessels.[237] As the preterm infant matures, the metabolically active retina triggers release of VEGF and IGF-1, which leads to new vascular proliferation which causes the progression of retinopathy.

The outcome of ROP varies from normal vision to total loss of vision if there is advanced scarring from the retina to the lens resulting in retinal detachment.[252] ROP was called retrolental fibroplasia in the early 1940s and was virtually eliminated with the severe restriction of oxygen use between 1950 and 1970. The condition has recurred as one of the major causes of disability in preterm infants as a result of the increased survival of infants with VLBW. The incidence of ROP increases with lower gestational age, lower birth weight, and BPD.[175]

The classification system for ROP uses a standard description of the location of the retinopathy using zones and clock hours, the severity of the disease or stage, and presence of special risk factors.[135] The classification system was revised in 2005 to include a rapid progressive form of ROP.[136] Classification of ROP includes five stages.[251] Stage 1 is characterized by a visible line of demarcation between the posterior vascularized retina and the anterior avascular retina. Stage 2 is characterized by pathologic neovascularization that is confined to the retina and appears as a ridge at the vascular/avascular junction. Stage 3 includes new vascularization and migration into the vitreous gel. Stage 4 is characterized by a subtotal retinal detachment. Stage 5 is complete retinal detachment.

Prematurity and low birth weight are the most important factors associated with ROP. IVH, use of supplemental oxygen, sepsis, and blood transfusion are other risk factors.[252] Risk factors for infants with ELBW include birth weight less than 1000 grams, steroid use, maternal preeclampsia, number of days on ventilation, continuous positive pressure ventilation, male gender, and fluctuating PaO_2.[286] Prevention and treatment include oxygen administration at PaO_2 between 50 and 70 mm Hg and administration of vitamin A, which is still under investigation.[79] Light reduction was not shown to be effective in altering the incidence of ROP.[220]

All premature infants given supplemental oxygen are at risk for ROP and should be screened. Guidelines approved by the American Academy of Pediatrics include screening 4 to 6 weeks after birth or within 31 to 33 weeks postconceptual age, whichever is later. Subsequent intervals for examination are based on initial findings.[251] A study conducted in Sweden recommended that the screening criterion be lowered to 31 weeks or less to identify infants with severe ROP.[151]

Surgical intervention can be divided into two overlapping objectives: treatment of neovascular process with retinal cryotherapy and surgical intervention for retinal detachment

(laser photocoagulation, cryotherapy, vitrectomy, and scleral buckling).[251] Implementation of an oxygen management policy that included strict guidelines for increasing and weaning of FiO_2 (fraction of inspired oxygen), monitoring oxygen saturation in the delivery room, in-house transport, and hospitalization for infants with birth weights of 500 to 1500 grams decreased the incidence of stages 3 and 4 ROP and decreased the need for laser treatment.[67] The oxygen level that maintains brain perfusion while minimizing the risk of ROP has not been determined.[20] Surgical outcome varies from complete recovery or mild myopia to blindness, depending on the extent of the disease. Emerging treatment modalities include administration of VEGF, IGF-1, and dietary supplementation with omega-3-polyunsaturated fatty acids.[175]

HYPERBILIRUBINEMIA

Hyperbilirubinemia, or physiologic jaundice, is the accumulation of excessive amounts of bilirubin in the blood. Bilirubin is one of the breakdown products of hemoglobin from red blood cells. This condition is seen commonly in premature infants who have immature hepatic function, an increased hemolysis of red blood cells as a result of high concentrations of circulating red blood cells, a shorter life span of red blood cells, and possible polycythemia from birth injuries. The pathogenesis of hyperbilirubinemia may be multifactorial and associated with late preterm gestational age, exclusive breast-feeding, and ABO hemolytic disease (blood incompatibility between mother and fetus), East Asian ethnicity, and jaundice in first 24 hours of life.[273] The primary goal in treatment of hyperbilirubinemia is the prevention of kernicterus, which is the deposition of unconjugated bilirubin in the brain, especially in the basal ganglia, cranial nerve nuclei, anterior horn cells, and hippocampus. Kernicterus can occur in infants with ELBW at low levels of bilirubin; consequently phototherapy is often initiated at low serum bilirubin levels.[13] Phototherapy is administered via a bank of lights or fiberoptic blankets. For phototherapy by lights, the infant is positioned in an open radiant warmer or incubator and the eyes are shielded to avoid retinal damage. Studies show that on/off cycles of more than 1 hour are as effective as continuous treatment. Fiberoptic phototherapy uses light from a halogen lamp transmitted through a fiberoptic bundle to a blanket that is wrapped around the infant. Infants who received continuous phototherapy for 23 hours with a fiberoptic panel held against their back and kangaroo care (skin-to-skin contact with parent) showed comparable declines in bilirubin levels compared with infants who received phototherapy from a bank of lights in an isolette for 24 hours a day.[171] Using a lower bilirubin level threshold for phototherapy treatment (5 mg per deciliter rather than 8 mg) for infants with ELBW significantly reduced bilirubin levels and rate of neurodevelopmental impairment, but not the death rate.[189]

If phototherapy is not effective in reducing the total serum bilirubin concentrations to acceptable levels, or if there is a rapidly rising bilirubin level, exchange transfusion is done.[84] In this technique, approximately 85% of the infant's red blood cells are replaced. Care must be taken so as not to disrupt cerebral blood flow and intracranial pressure. Recent case studies and clinical trials from the 1980s and 1990s demonstrated the beneficial effects of metalloporphyrins such as tin (Sn) mesoporphyrin and tin protoporphyrin for both prophylaxis and treatment to reduce hyperbilirubinemia.[83] These substances are inhibitors of heme oxygenase, the enzyme in the synthesis of bilirubin that limits the rate of degradation of heme to bile. Infants with severe hyperbilirubinemia who are not responsive to phototherapy and whose parents are Jehovah's Witnesses and rejected exchange transfusion have been successfully treated with Sn-mesoporphyrin.[140]

FETAL ALCOHOL SYNDROME

Chronic alcohol exposure in utero may result in a multitude of symptoms at birth, including withdrawal symptoms of irritability, tremors, apnea, hypertonia, hypersensitivity to sensory stimuli, and seizures.[268] Alcohol rapidly crosses the placenta and the blood-brain barrier of the fetus, and there is a dose-dependent relationship between maternal alcohol intake in the first trimester of pregnancy and the occurrence of fetal alcohol syndrome (FAS). FAS is the most recognized outcome of prenatal alcohol exposure and is characterized by pre- and postnatal growth retardation, craniofacial anomalies, as well as CNS dysfunction such as intellectual disabilities and behavior problems.[117] It is now recognized that the effects of prenatal exposure to alcohol make up a continuum of physical anomalies and cognitive and behavioral deficits. The term "fetal alcohol spectrum disorder" (FASD) has been described as a nondiagnostic umbrella term that describes the range of effects including FAS.[117]

Alcohol exposure in utero is associated with a broad range of adverse effects on placental development and function.[51] Symptoms of withdrawal manifest within the first 24 hours after birth. The clinical withdrawal syndrome dissipates within a week, and the treatment includes avoidance of sensory overload and administration of phenobarbital for seizures.

FAS is one of the most common causes of intellectual disability in the world, and it is characterized by a triad of symptoms composed of growth deficiency, cardiac defects, and CNS disturbances, such as microcephaly and dysmorphology (including facial, genital, and joint abnormalities).[268] Neuroimaging studies have demonstrated overall and regional volumetric and surface area reductions; abnormalities of particular areas of the brain including the basal ganglia, corpus callosum, cerebellum, and hippocampus; and reduced and increased densities for white and gray matter with disproportionate reduction in the size of the frontal lobes.[193,268]

Neurobehavioral effects of FASD include a continuum of long-lasting impairments in cognition and behavior, including problems in learning, memory, executive functions, hyperactivity, impulsivity, and poor communication and social skills.[117] Prenatal exposure to alcohol also had adverse effects on neuroendocrine functions including increased activity of the hypothalamic-pituitary-adrenal (HPA) axis, which is the putative regulatory mechanism for response to stressful sensory stimuli.[274] A number of ocular and neuro-ophthalmic impairments occur in FASD such as refractive errors, strabismus, and amblyopia, which can lead to lifelong visual impairment if not treated.[51]

Maternal and family education and support programs play important roles in prevention of FASD.[149] Once FASD is suspected or diagnosed, evidence-based treatment programs that support the family environment through enhancing parenting skills, facilitating parent-child attachment, and early intervention services may improve children's health and cognitive outcomes.[149] Interventions with the child include psychostimulant pharmacologic agents and cognitive control therapy.[216]

NEONATAL ABSTINENCE SYNDROME

Maternal use of narcotics during pregnancy leads to the fetus developing dependency on that drug. The most commonly used drugs that lead to fetal dependence and withdrawal are heroin, cocaine, methadone, and pain medication. There is often maternal use of several drugs during pregnancy, including alcohol and tobacco, which accompanies socioeconomic factors, poor nutrition, stress, infections, and poor perinatal care.[227] The fetus experiences withdrawal or neonatal abstinence syndrome (NAS) when the mother is withdrawn from her drug or drugs or when the fetus is delivered.[77] The onset of withdrawal symptoms usually occurs within 72 hours after birth.[230] Symptoms of withdrawal include irritability, tremors, seizures, apnea, increased muscle tone, inability to sleep, hyperactive deep tendon reflexes, incoordination, inefficient sucking and swallowing, and high-pitched, shrill cry.[267] The diagnosis of NAS is made based on maternal history, maternal and infant toxicology lab tests, and clinical examination of the infant. Measures for evaluation and treatment of neonatal abstinence include the Neonatal Intensive Care Unit Network Neurobehavioral Scale (NNNS), which was designed to provide a comprehensive assessment of both neurologic integrity and behavioral functions,[161] and the Neonatal Drug Withdrawal Scoring System, also known as the Lipsitz tool, which scores tremors, irritability, reflexes, stools, muscle tone, skin abrasions, tachypnea, repetitive sneezing, yawning, vomiting, and fever.[28] Infants with withdrawal symptoms should receive supportive care including swaddling, non-nutritive sucking, and decreased sensory stimulation. Small frequent feedings and additional calories may be needed. If necessary, medications such as tincture of opium, morphine, methadone, and buprenorphine are used.[139,267]

PAIN

Pain is defined as an unpleasant sensory and emotional experience associated with actual or potential tissue damage and is best described by self-report.[119] Obviously the neonate cannot report on pain but may express pain through specific pain behaviors, physiologic changes, changes in cerebral blood flow, and cellular and molecular changes in pain processing pathways. Adverse sequelae may "include death, poor neurologic outcomes, abnormal somatization and response to pain later in life."[119] The peripheral nervous system is capable of responding to stimuli by 20 weeks postconception. Both the number and types of peripheral receptors are similar to those of adults by 20 to 24 weeks of gestation with a resulting increased density of receptors in the newborn as compared with adult. Spinal cord and brain stem tracts are not fully myelinated, therefore, central nerve conduction is slow. There is evidence that pain pathways, cortical and subcortical centers of pain perception, and neurochemical systems associated with pain transmission are functional in premature neonates of 20 to 24 weeks gestational age.[98] Most nociceptive impulses are transmitted by nonmyelinated C fibers but also by A delta and A beta fibers, which transmit light touch and proprioception in adults.[119] However, the pain modulatory tracts, which can inhibit pain through release of inhibitory neurotransmitters such as serotonin, dopamine, and norepinephrine, are not developed until 36 to 40 weeks of gestation. As a consequence, the preterm infant is more sensitive to pain than term or older infants.[119,246] Painful stimuli resulting from medical conditions and medical procedures (such as heel sticks, intubation, ventilation, ocular exam, and IV placement) can lead to prolonged structural and functional alterations in pain pathways that may persist into adult life.[36,99] The infant also may associate touch with painful input, which can interfere with bonding and attachment.

Although it is difficult to assess pain in the neonate, the physical therapist working in the NICU should be aware of methods of examination and nonpharmacologic intervention to alleviate pain. Both physiologic and behavioral responses of the neonate to nociceptive or painful stimuli have been identified. Physiologic manifestations of pain include increased heart rate, heart rate variability, blood pressure, and respirations, with evidence of decreased oxygenation. Skin color and character include pallor or flushing, diaphoresis, and palmar sweating. Other indicators of pain are increased muscle tone, dilated pupils, and laboratory evidence of metabolic or endocrine changes.[217] Neonatal behavioral responses to nociceptive input include sustained and intense crying; facial expression of grimaces, furrowed brow, quivering chin, or eyes tightly closed; motor behavior

such as limb withdrawal, thrashing, rigidity, flaccidity, fist clenching, finger splaying, and limb extension; and changes in behavioral state.[115] Pain may lead to poor nutritional intake, delayed wound healing, impaired mobility, sleep disturbances, withdrawal, irritability, and other developmental regression.[270]

There are 40 methods to assess pain in infants.[217] Recommended pain measures include the Neonatal Facial Coding System,[116] the Neonatal Infant Pain Scale,[157] the CRIES,[148] and the Premature Infant Pain Profile.[246] These measures include biologic items, behavioral items, or both. The Bernese Pain Scale for Neonates was specifically developed for preterm neonates who require ventilation.[69] Recent studies indicate that extremity movements such as extremity flexion, extension, finger splay, hand on face, fisting, and frown are associated with pain, especially at early gestational age and may increase the accuracy of examination of pain.[132] New avenues for assessment of neonatal pain include the use of noninvasive EEG, neuroimaging, and near infrared spectroscopy to attempt to measure perception of pain.[217]

Nonpharmacologic methods to alleviate pain include decreasing the number of noxious stimuli, decreasing stimulation, swaddling, non-nutritive sucking, tactile comfort measures, rocking, containment, and music.[270] Preterm neonates demonstrated a lower mean heart rate, shorter crying time, and shorter mean sleep disruption after heel stick with facilitated tucking (containing the infant with hands softly holding the infant's extremities in soft flexion) than without.[72,272] Administration of breast milk, sucrose solution, and non-nutritive sucking may help decrease the pain response in newborn infants.[159,231] Sensorial saturation, which includes subtle tactile, vestibular, gustative, olfactory, auditory, and visual stimuli, was found to be effective in decreasing pain responses of premature infants receiving heel sticks.[31]

Morphine, fentanyl, and topical mixture of a local anesthetic cream such as a eutectic mixture of lidocaine and prilocaine (EMLA) are the most common analgesics administered to neonates.[19,246] Other pharmacologic agents under investigation include methadone and ketamine.[19,35]

FAMILY RESPONSE TO THE NEONATAL SPECIAL CARE NURSERY

Premature birth, followed by the intensity of the experience of the NICU, is highly stressful and sometimes traumatic not only for the baby but also for the parents and the whole family. The NICU experience for parents may vary depending on the severity of the infant's illness and the level of preparedness parents have prior to the infant's admission to the NICU.[196,265] Although prior knowledge of a possible premature or complicated birth may soften the intensity of the experience at first, all parents of premature infants are particularly vulnerable throughout their infant's neonatal period. The foremost concern is for survival. Once survival is certain, concern shifts to the quality of the infant's developmental outcome. The parents themselves can be considered to be "premature parents" and may be mourning the loss of the "imagined" or "wished for baby" as they struggle to develop a bond with their "real baby."[50,147] Parents report that the NICU experience often leaves them with a temporary loss of their parental role and identity and at time of discharge may feel overwhelmed, worried, and even panicked, especially if their infant had required ventilation while in the NICU.[219] The phase immediately after discharge from the hospital is often one of anxious adjustment during which mothers express their lack of confidence and insecurity in caring for their preterm infant.[184]

The length of stay for infants admitted to the NICU varies widely according to the severity of the condition leading to the admission. Some infants may spend as little as one day in the NICU (respiratory distress); others may spend months (e.g., extreme prematurity, short gut). Research on parental response to having their newborn admitted to the NICU has been fairly consistent in reporting a high level of parental stress and anxiety, which may lead to a posttraumatic stress reaction (PTSR). PTSR is a predictor of infant sleep and eating problems at 18 months.[214] The prevalence of postpartum depression (PPD) in mothers of newborns admitted to the NICU (45%) is higher compared to PPD in first-time mothers of healthy infants (8% to 15%).[29] On a more positive note, a recent study reported that the implementation of the "parent-friendly" changes as seen in most hospitals across the United States contributed to helping parents make a more successful adaptation to having an infant in the NICU.[65]

Admission of the newborn to the NICU happens at a critical time in the development of the family unit. For the infant, biobehavioral transition from intrauterine to extrauterine life occurs in the first months of life.[196] For the parents, the first months are a time when they search for "the goodness of fit" between themselves and their new baby.[261] The core challenge for parents is to engage with their baby in a way that is unique to them and fosters the baby's development.[245] Many factors may render the relationship between parents and their premature infant vulnerable. Premature infants have poor abilities to self-regulate physiologic rhythms and attention is limited, which can disrupt the parent-infant synchrony so critical during interactive episodes.[95] Preterm infants are more irritable, smile less, and have facial signals that are less clear than full-term infants,[242] which affect the parents' ability to read and respond to their infant's cues.[95] Steinberg contended that posttraumatic stress reaction and depression interfere with the parents' ability to read their baby's cues and respond sensitively to the baby's needs.[244] Nevertheless, a number of studies have demonstrated that during this difficult hospital time, helping parents understand their baby's behavior appears to be critical in helping them maintain their role as parents and mitigate levels of stress.[155,169,219] Physical thera-

pists, with their unique skills in infant behavioral observation and developmental intervention, play an important role in the support offered parents during this difficult time. The physical therapist can help the parents read their baby's cues and provide feedback on their baby's responses. Several studies have reported long-term effects ranging from 9 months to 2 years of behaviorally based interventions on infant development, parent-infant interaction, maternal confidence and self-esteem, and paternal attitudes toward and involvement in caregiving.[80,106,206,218] Primarily derived from the Neonatal Behavioral Assessment Scale (NBAS), behaviorally based intervention tools that have been developed to promote parent and child outcomes are summarized in Table 28-1.

FRAMEWORK FOR PHYSICAL THERAPY

The primary role of the physical therapist in the NICU is to promote the neonate's movement; postural control; and adaptation to extrauterine life through collaboration with caregivers of infants identified with, or at risk for, a developmental delay or disability and provision of developmental interventions. Another important role is to support parental adaptation to the experience of having a sick child in the NICU and facilitate their participation in the infant's care. Updated clinical practice guidelines for physical therapists working in the NICU have recently been published in a two-part article series.[256,257] Part 1 articulates the path to professional competence and describes the clinical competencies for physical therapists, NICU clinical training models, and a clinical decision-making algorithm.[256] Part 2 presents the evidence-based practice guidelines and recommendations and theoretic frameworks that support neonatal physical therapy practice.[257] Three theoretic frameworks for serving infants in the NICU are the enablement model, family-centered care, and infant neurobehavioral functioning. Those theoretic frameworks address the three main components of physical therapy intervention: communication and coordination, information sharing with parents, and procedural interventions (for more details, refer to Chapters 1 and 29).

INTERNATIONAL CLASSIFICATION OF FUNCTIONING, DISABILITY, AND HEALTH

The International Classification of Functioning, Disability and Health, commonly referred to as the ICF, is a framework for understanding relationships between health and disability at both individual and population levels (see Figure 1-4).[283] The ICF was developed to create a common language to improve communication among health care providers, researchers, policy makers, and people with disabilities and to provide a scientific basis for understanding and studying health and health-related states, outcomes, and determinants.[202] The health-related domains are classified from body,

TABLE 28-1   **Behaviorally Based Assessments Used to Promote Parent and Child Outcomes**

Assessment	Description
Newborn Behavioral Observation system (NBO)[196]	The NBO is an individualized, infant-focused, family-centered observational system that is designed for use by practitioners to elicit and describe the infant's competencies and individuality. Its explicit goals are to strengthen the relationship between the parent and the child and promote the development of a supportive relationship between the clinician and the family.
Mother's Assessment of the Behavior of the Infant (MABI; Field et al., 1978)	The MABI is an abbreviated version of the Neonatal Behavioral Assessment Scale (NBAS) designed to be administered by parents to their own infant. The 15 items are based on the NBAS items, omitting all reflex testing. The items are grouped into four dimensions (social, motor, state organization, and state regulation) and are scored on a 4-point scale.
Combined Physical and Behavioral Neonatal Examination (CPBNE; Keefer, 1995)	The CPBNE incorporates behavioral items from the NBAS into the routine neonatal physical examination. It allows the practitioner to assess the infant's behaviors and to generate an individual behavioral profile.
Family-Administered Neonatal Activities (FANA; Cardone & Gilkerson, 1990; 1995 NBAS manual)	The FANA is designed to elicit from parents their initial perceptions of their newborn and then to use the behavior of the baby as the vehicle through which parents can affirm or challenge their initial perceptions. The FANA integrates the practices of short-term, focused, psychodynamic interviewing with a family-empowerment approach.

individual, and societal perspectives by means of two lists: a list of body functions and structures and a list of domains of activity and participation. Because an individual's functioning and disability occurs in a context, the ICF also includes a list of environmental and personal factors (for more information, see www.who.int/classifications/icf/en).

High-risk neonates frequently demonstrate impairments in muscle tone, range of motion, sensory organization, and postural reactions. These *impairments in body functions and structures* may contribute to limitations in *activity* such as difficulty in breathing, feeding, visual and auditory responsiveness, and motor activities such as head control and movement of hands to mouth. The interaction between impairments and activity limitations may contribute to restrictions in parent-infant interaction (*participation*). The ICF model also considers personal and environmental factors as relevant influences on body functions and structures, activity, and participation. *Personal factors* include an infant's health complications and temperament. *Environmental factors* range from levels of lighting and noise in the special care nursery to family and community support such as maternity leave that will directly influence the infant's outcome and well-being (see Table 28-2 for an example of the ICF model adapted for the infant in the neonatal intensive care unit).

INFANT NEUROBEHAVIORAL FUNCTIONING

Since the late 1980s, advances in perinatal and newborn intensive care have dramatically decreased the mortality rates of preterm and sick newborns at high risk for developmental problems. As premature infants have become younger in gestational age at birth (as young as 23 weeks

of gestation) and smaller in birth weight (as little as 450 grams), there has been a growing concern among health care professionals not only to assure their survival but to optimize their developmental course and outcome. Better known as developmental care, the intervention model designed to address these issues focuses on the detailed observation of infant neurobehavioral functioning to design highly individualized plans of care and provide developmentally appropriate experiential opportunities for the newborn in the hospital setting and the provision of supportive care for the infant's family.[9] Recent research suggests that individualized developmental care may improve some medical complications and short-term outcomes such as length of stay, level of alertness, and feeding progression.[179,210]

Als's synactive theory provides a theoretic framework for the neurobehavioral functioning of the young infant.[2] Infant neurobehavioral functioning is understood as the unfolding of sequential achievements in four interdependent behavioral dimensions organized as subsystems.[2] The infant (1) stabilizes her autonomic or physiologic behavior, (2) regulates or controls her motor behavior, (3) organizes her behavioral states and her responsiveness through interaction with her social and physical environment, and (4) orients to animate and inanimate objects. Through maturation and experience, the infant is able to organize her behavior subsystems and actively participate in her social world including interactions with caregivers to meet her needs.[2,46] Competency in behavioral organization can be determined through the careful observation of the behaviors displayed by the infant within each of the behavioral dimensions. Als has categorized behaviors within each of the behavioral dimensions as either "*approach/regulatory*" or "*avoidance/stress.*"[2] Regulatory behaviors indicate a state of

TABLE 28-2   **Application of the International Classification of Functioning, Disability, and Health for Infants in the Neonatal Intensive Care Unit**

Health Condition (Includes Disease or injury)

Examples: prematurity, respiratory distress, intraventricular hemorrhage, periventricular leukomalacia, arthrogryposis, spina bifida, failure to thrive, short gut, Down syndrome

Body Functions and Structures	**Activities**	**Participation**
Physiologic and Psychologic Functions of Body Systems	Execution of a Task or Action by an Individual	Individual's Involvement in NICU Life Situations
Examples: muscle tone, postural reactions, range of motion, sensory organization, behavioral state control, neurobehavioral functioning, physiologic stability↓	Examples: breathing, sucking, crying, head control, hand to mouth, kicking, grasping, visual and auditory responsiveness↓	Examples: parent-infant interaction, communication, being held by parents, feeding, sleeping, growing↓
Impairments	Activity Limitations	Participation Restrictions
Examples: skeletal deformity, fluctuating tone, startles, deafness, decreased range of motion, behavioral disorganization	Examples: cannot breathe on own, tube fed, cannot locate sound	Examples: cannot be held by parents because of the inability to maintain physiologic stability and neurobehavioral organization

Environmental Factors	**Personal Factors**
Physical, Social, and Attitudinal Features of the Family and NICU Setting	Personal Characteristics of the Individual
Examples: lighting and noise levels, maternity leave, family support, family's distance to travel to hospital, siblings	Examples: medical complications, temperament, sensitivity, preferences

well-being and are observed when an infant's self-regulatory abilities are able to support the social and environmental demands placed on her; she is then described as *organized*.[76] Stress behaviors indicate a state of exhaustion and are observed when the infant's threshold for self-regulation is exceeded by the demands placed on her; she is then described as *disorganized*.[76]

The application of neurobehavioral observations to clinical practice has been formalized with the Newborn Individualized Developmental Care and Assessment Program (NIDCAP).[3,4] The NIDCAP proposes a structured method of weekly observation and assessment of infant behavior by a developmental specialist or NIDCAP certified physical therapist. Based on these observations and following consultations with the infant's family and medical team, an individualized care plan is developed and implemented. Within this perspective, intervention is aimed at facilitating prolonged periods of organization by reinforcing the infant's individual self-regulatory style while supporting families to nurture and care for their infant.[7,9,42]

FAMILY-CENTERED CARE

Family-centered care (FCC) was first defined in 1987 as part of former surgeon general Everett Koop's initiative for family-centered, community-based, coordinated care for children with special health care needs and their families. The American Academy of Pediatrics (AAP) recognizes the importance of FCC as an approach to health care[192] and stresses the importance of the role that families play in patient outcomes.[174] At the heart of family-centered care is the recognition that the family is the constant in a child's life. For this reason, family-centered care is built on partnerships between families and professionals. The Institute for Family-Centered Care has identified eight core concepts of FCC that guide the delivery of services to families with children with health care needs: (1) respect, (2) choice, (3) information, (4) collaboration, (5) strengths, (6) support, (7) empowerment, and (8) flexibility (www.familycenteredcare.org). Many medical institutions and NICUs across the country have instituted their own FCC guidelines and practices, but for the most part they all share the pursuit of being responsive to the priorities and choices of families. Cleveland published a systematic review of the literature to identify the needs of parents in the NICU and the type of nursing support most helpful during their stay in the NICU (Table 28-3).[70] Parents need accurate information, to have contact with their infant, and to be fully included in their infant's care. Individualized care and knowing that the NICU staff is watching over and protecting their infant is also important to parents. The types of behaviors that best support parents in the NICU are those where they feel welcome at all times,

TABLE 28-3 **Needs of Parents Who Have Infants in the NICU and the Types of Support That Are Most Helpful[70]**

Needs of Parents	Behaviors That Support Parents
1. Accurate information 2. Contact with the infant 3. Inclusion in the infant's care 4. Vigilant watching-over and protecting the infant 5. Being positively perceived by the nursery staff 6. Individualized care 7. A therapeutic relationship with the nursing staff	• Emotional support • Parent empowerment • A welcoming environment with supportive unit policies • Parent education with an opportunity to practice new skills through guided participation

are encouraged to participate in their child's care, and are engaged in a therapeutic relationship with the nursing staff. Parent-to-parent groups provide families with additional emotional support.[70] The physical therapist in the NICU can consider those recommendations in the implementation of family-centered physical therapy interventions in the neonatal intensive care unit.

DEVELOPMENTAL EXAMINATION AND EVALUATION

The purposes of the neonatal physical therapy examination and evaluation are to identify (1) impairments in body function and structure that contribute to activity limitations and participation restrictions, (2) the developmental status of the child, (3) individualized responses to stress and self-regulation, (4) needs for skilled positioning and handling, and (5) environmental adaptations to optimize growth and development. The examination and evaluation of infants in the NICU must support the goals of physical therapy intervention aimed at facilitating the infant's participation in age-appropriate developmental activities (e.g., feeding, tucking, self-soothing, social interaction with caregivers) and interactions with the family (e.g., relationship-building, attachment).

The examination and evaluation of high-risk infants are best conducted using a combination of observation and handling techniques that ideally occur over the course of several sessions. Infants hospitalized in the NICU will often not tolerate a full standardized developmental examination. Rather, the physical therapist often formulates a neurobehavioral profile based on observation of the infant's behaviors. That is, the physical therapist describes the infant's successes and difficulties in achieving and maintaining self-regulation and identifies the strategies that best support the needs and developmental level of the infant (Box 28-2).[42]

As handling of medically fragile infants can impose physiologic stress, physical therapy procedures must be appropriately timed and modulated to match the neurobehavioral competencies of the infant. Under the guidance of family-centered practice, any examination or intervention with an infant should be in partnership with families to assist

> **Box 28-2 RECOMMENDATIONS FOR PHYSICAL THERAPIST EXAMINATION AND EVALUATION OF INFANTS IN THE NICU**
>
> 1. Protect the infant's fragile neurobehavioral system, particularly for infants who may not tolerate handling or a standardized evaluation.
> 2. Repeat observations over time.
> 3. Partner with parents and members of the NICU team.
> 4. Observe, interpret, and communicate infant behaviors to parents and members of the NICU team.

with bonding, facilitate developmentally supportive positioning and handling, and allow for continuous carry-over of therapeutic strategies. Lastly, the physical therapist is part of an interdisciplinary team of health care providers. Consistent with the Guide to Physical Therapist Practice,[18] effective communication and collaboration with professionals from all disciplines and accurate documentation are critical. The next section utilizes a neurobehavioral framework to describe the examination of the high-risk infant with examples of considerations for specific diagnoses.

BEHAVIORAL STATE

States of consciousness were originally proposed by Wolff and have been expanded to include six behavioral states: (1) deep sleep, (2) light sleep, (3) drowsy, (4) quiet awake, (5) active awake, and (6) crying.[282] Als has expanded this paradigm to include 12 states to distinguish between the adaptive and maladaptive self-regulation strategies of fragile infants compared to full-term infants.[3] Increasing gestational age is associated with demonstration of more robust state organization. That is, as infants mature, they are able to transition smoothly and predictably between states. For example, an infant who is 25 weeks corrected gestational age (CGA) will likely spend most of the day in a light sleep state and will have brief periods of quiet awake. Comparatively, an infant who is 40 weeks CGA should have longer periods of quiet awake time, particularly before and following feedings. An infant's ability to achieve and maintain sleep and awake states will be compromised by her medical and neurodevelopmental status. The physical therapist plays a key role in educating parents and staff to identify state transitions and optimize the environment (e.g., modifications to light, sound, and interaction) to facilitate smooth transitions to and from sleep.

Infants with neonatal abstinence syndrome (NAS) demonstrate difficulty with state organization.[226] Examination of the infant with NAS requires careful observation of state transitions. The therapist should observe how readily the infant moves from one state to the next, the duration of each state, and her self-soothing strategies. Before the examination, the infant's care team should be consulted to determine how NAS symptoms are being assessed (e.g., a standardized scoring method) and managed medically.

AUTONOMIC NERVOUS SYSTEM

During the examination of the autonomic system, the physical therapist obtains the infant's heart and respiratory rate from the cardiorespiratory monitor. In the neonate, heart rates range from 120 to 180 beats per minute, and respiratory rate ranges from 40 to 60 breaths per minute.[168] In addition, respiratory effort and digestive function during rest, routine care, handling, and social interaction should be noted. Irregular respirations or paling around the mouth, eyes, and nose; spitting up; straining; bowel movements; and hiccoughs indicate instability or difficulty in achieving self-regulation. Smooth respirations; even color; and minimal startles, tremors, and digestive instability indicate that the demands of the situation have not exceeded the infant's capacity for self-regulation.

Infants with chronic lung disease (CLD) have limited endurance for functional activities. Changes in respiratory effort during the examination should be carefully observed. Costal retractions, head bobbing, and nasal flaring are evidence of increased work of breathing, and their presence, timing, and resolution should be carefully noted.[205] Collaboration with nursing and respiratory therapy staff to facilitate the developmental examination is necessary in order to coincide with optimal timing of diuretic therapy, how modification to oxygen therapy will be managed including the upper and lower parameters of oxygen, and whether the mode of oxygen therapy can be modified for the examination to allow for greater bedside mobility. The examination of the infant with CLD requires frequent breaks, appropriate pacing of activity, and modification of the environment (e.g., lighting, sound, and social interaction) to allow the infant to utilize strategies for self-regulation.

MOTOR SYSTEM

Physical therapists are perhaps the most highly qualified members of the health care team to examine and interpret the motor system of a fragile infant. Examination should include observation of the infant's posture at rest and active flexion movements during quiet awake periods, routine care, social interaction, and feeding. Functional movements should be interpreted according to the progression of active flexion patterns that emerge with increasing gestational age. Typically these occur at 32 weeks for lower extremities, 35 weeks for upper extremities, and 37 to 39 weeks for head and trunk.[265] Thus, the immature neuromotor system of the preterm infant often precludes independent antigravity flexion movements and predisposes the infant to compensations, including retracted scapulae, externally rotated and abducted lower extremities, and extension and rotation postures of the cervical spine and trunk.[255] As contemporary frameworks such as those described in the previous section guide practice, less emphasis is placed on testing a battery of infant reflexes. Rather, the physical therapist examination evaluates reflexes deemed more "functional" (e.g., suck, swallow, palmar and plantar grasp, and early righting responses).[56]

Infants with intraventricular hemorrhage (IVH) are at risk for neuromotor impairments that range from mild to severe.[128,177] When examining an infant with IVH, the therapist should note asymmetries in postural muscles and active movements of the extremities, including absence of isolated distal or rotational movements. Clonus should be tested in both ankles. Changes in muscle tone at rest and during active movement should be observed and noted. The emergence of flexor tone and antigravity movements should be evaluated when the infant is awake and alert, as behavioral state influences motor system activity and hence infant motor control.

SOCIAL INTERACTION

Infants enter this world predisposed to socialize. Many healthy, full-term infants can visually track faces or brightly colored objects and alert to familiar voices.[196] Many preterm or medically fragile infants can complete these tasks with some modifications.[3,40] A developmental examination may include presenting visual and auditory stimulation to an infant. Physical therapists should judiciously offer opportunities for the infant to socially interact, as these complex tasks can be distressful and overwhelm the infant's capacity for self-regulation. The physical therapist plays a critical role in facilitating social interaction between infants and caregivers by modeling developmentally supportive interactions, modifying the environment as needed, and providing parents with anticipatory guidance about the progression of their infant's social interaction skills.

TESTS AND MEASURES

Tests and measures provide (1) objective documentation of infant functioning over time, (2) justification for developmental interventions in the NICU, (3) documentation of

TABLE 28-4 **Tests and Measures Used to Assess Infants in the Neonatal Intensive Care Unit**

Name	Description
Neurological Assessment of the Preterm and Full-Term Newborn Infant (Dubowitz & Dubowitz, 1981)	Purpose: To determine gestational age Divided into six sections examining posture and tone, tone patterns, reflexes, movements, abnormal signs/patterns, orientation and behavior.
Neonatal Behavioral Assessment Scale (NBAS; Brazelton & Nugent, 1995)	Purpose: To assess neurobehavioral functioning Composed of 28 behavioral items, each scored on a 9-point scale, and 18 reflex items, each scored on a 4-point scale. Also includes a set of seven supplementary items designed to summarize the quality of the infant's responsiveness and the amount of examination facilitation needed to support the infant during the assessment.
Newborn Behavioral Observation System (NBO; Nugent et al., 2007)	Purpose: relationship-building tool with parents. Composed of 18 neurobehavioral items designed to help practitioners sensitize parents to their child's competencies and uniqueness, support the development of a positive and nurturing parent-infant relationship, and foster the development of the practitioner-parent relationship.
Newborn Individualized Developmental Care and Assessment Program (NIDCAP; Als, 1986)	Purpose: To identify individualized developmental care strategies Composed of a neurobehavior checklist marked every 2 minutes before, during, and after a caregiving event. A narrative is written that describes the caregiving event from the infant's perspective and offers suggestions for caregiving modification that best support the infant's current level of self-regulatory abilities.
Assessment of Preterm Infant Behavior (APIB; Als et al., 1982a)	Purpose: To assess neurobehavioral functioning of the high-risk infant Composed of behavioral items and reflex items, the APIB provides a valuable resource in support of developmental care (NIDCAP). It is also used as a neurodevelopmental diagnostic instrument for clinicians and developmental consultants in the nursery setting.
NICU Network Neurobehavioral Scale (NNNS; Lester & Tronick, 2004)	Purpose: To assess neurobehavioral functioning of drug-exposed and high-risk infants Composed of 115 items, 45 of which require manipulation of the infant, whereas 70 are observed. Divided into three parts: Examination Scale, Examiner Ratings Scale, and Stress/Abstinence Scale.
Test of Infant Motor Performance (TIMP; Campbell et al., 2001)	Purpose: To assess infant functional motor behavior Composed of 13 items on the Observed Scale, each scored on a dichotomous scale, and 29 items on the Elicited Scale, each scored on a 5-, 6-, or 7- point hierarchic scale.
Neonatal Oral-Motor Assessment Scale (NOMAS; Braun & Palmer, 1985)	Purpose: To measure components of nutritive and non-nutritive sucking Composed of variables such as rate, rhythmicity, jaw excursion, tongue configuration, and movement.
Nursing Child Assessment Feeding Scale (NCAFS; Barnard & Eyres, 1979)	Purpose: To assess parent-infant feeding interaction Observational tool assessing parental responsiveness to infant's cues and signs of distress and social interaction during feeding.
Early Feeding Skills Assessment (EFS; Thoyre, Shaker & Pridham, 2005)	Purpose: To assess infant readiness and tolerance for feeding. Used to create a profile of an infant's feeding skills in relation to predetermined oral feeding competencies.

the effectiveness of those interventions, and (4) identification of infants in need of developmental follow-up and intervention after discharge from the NICU. Most useful to the physical therapist are tests and measures of neurologic function, neurobehavioral functioning, motor behavior, and oral-motor function. Table 28-4 provides a list of tests and measures commonly used by physical therapists in the NICU. Certification on many of these tools requires extensive training (e.g., NBAS, APIB, NIDCAP, and TIMP) and will greatly enhance the clinical skills of physical therapists working with this medically complex population. The use of these tools

varies widely between NICU physical therapists but the TIMP, designed by and for physical therapists working with infants as young as 32 weeks of gestation, has become the most widely used assessment of infant functional motor behavior.[57] The Dubowitz, used to establish the gestational age of the infant at birth, provides physical therapists with an excellent opportunity to learn about neurologic maturity of infants in the weeks before term age.[89] The Newborn Behavioral Observation (NBO) is a relationship-building tool that supports the efforts of the physical therapist to establish a rapport with families and share with them developmental information about their infant in a positive context.[196] Some of these tests require significant time in administration, scoring, and interpretation (NIDCAP, NBAS, APIB); whereas the time required to complete these tests decreases with practice, the physical therapist needs to evaluate the importance of the information gathered and the category of infants most likely to benefit from those tests. A team approach and sharing of information between professionals (e.g., NIDCAP) may help in addressing some of the time and cost issues associated with those tests.

The administration of tests to fragile and medically complex infants in the NICU requires clinical judgment and constant monitoring of physiologic stability to determine whether the administration of the test is well tolerated by the infant. Many infants will not have the physiologic stability required to withstand the stress caused by the handling imposed during the administration of the test (e.g., APIB, TIMP). For infants without sufficient physiologic stability, testing will have to be either postponed or done in multiple brief testing periods in order to gather the necessary information. The following includes a detailed description of tests and measures commonly used by physical therapists in the NICU.

NEUROLOGICAL ASSESSMENT OF THE PRETERM AND FULL-TERM NEWBORN INFANT

The Neurological Assessment of the Preterm and Full-Term Newborn Infant, commonly known as the Dubowitz, is a systematic, quickly administered, neurologic and neurobehavioral assessment developed to document changes in neonatal behavior in the preterm infant after birth, to compare preterm infants with newborn infants of corresponding postmenstrual age, and to detect deviations in neurologic signs and their subsequent evolution.[88,89] The assessment takes 15 minutes or less to administer and is divided into six sections: (1) posture and tone, (2) tone patterns, (3) reflexes, (4) movements, (5) abnormal signs/patterns, and (6) orientation and behavior. Scoring is based on patterns of response rather than a summary or total score. Although the Dubowitz has a long tradition in the NICU, it is mostly used by physicians and medical residents to establish gestational age at birth by observation. For physical therapists working in the NICU, learning to administer the Dubowitz will contribute to the knowledge and expertise in evaluating the tone and posture of very young infants.

NEONATAL BEHAVIORAL ASSESSMENT SCALE

The Neonatal Behavioral Assessment Scale (NBAS) is the most commonly used assessment of infant neurobehavioral functioning in the world today.[47] Used extensively in research, the NBAS includes 28 behavioral items scored on a 9-point scale and 18 reflex items scored on a 4-point

scale. The reflex items can be used to identify gross neurologic abnormalities but are not intended to provide a neurologic diagnosis. The NBAS also includes a set of seven supplementary items designed to summarize the quality of the infant's responsiveness and the amount of examination facilitation needed to support the infant during the assessment. These supplementary items were originally included to better capture the quality of behaviors seen in high-risk infants. Therefore, the NBAS is well suited for use with the high-risk population. The NBAS is appropriate for use with term infants and stable high-risk infants near term age until the end of the second month of life postterm.

The NBAS has been used extensively in research to study and document the effects of prematurity; intrauterine growth retardation; and prenatal exposure to cocaine, alcohol, caffeine and tobacco on newborn behavior.[197] The NBAS has also inspired others to develop scales for use with diverse populations. Examples include the Assessment of Preterm Infant Behavior for use with premature infants[5] and the NICU Network Neurobehavioral Scale for use with drug-exposed infants,[162] both described in this section. The NBAS's central focus on the facilitation of infant competence by a trained and sensitive examiner has also brought to light its powerful qualities as an intervention tool for use with a wide range of families. This subsequently led to the development of a number of NBAS-based relationship-building tools such as the Mother's Assessment of the Behavior of the Infant (MABI),[277] the Combined Physical Exam and Behavioral Exam (PEBE),[141] the Family Administered Neonatal Activities (FANA),[63] and most recently the Newborn Behavioral Observation system described in this section (NBO).[196] More information on the NBAS is available at www.brazelton-institute.com.

NEWBORN BEHAVIORAL OBSERVATION SYSTEM

The Newborn Behavioral Observation system (NBO) is a relationship-building tool designed to help practitioners sensitize parents to their child's competencies and uniqueness, support the development of a positive and nurturing parent-infant relationship, and foster the development of the practitioner-parent relationship.[196] The NBO consists of 18 neurobehavioral items used to elicit infant competencies and make observations of newborn behavior, such as sleep behavior, the baby's interactive capacities and threshold for stimulation, motor capacities, crying and consolability, and state regulation.[195] As it is conceptualized as an interactive behavioral observation, the NBO is always administered in the presence of the family so that it can provide a forum for parents and the practitioner to observe and interpret the newborn's behavior. The NBO takes about 45 minutes or longer to administer and can be completed from the first day of life up to the end of the second month of life postterm. The NBO is designed to be flexible and has been used in diverse settings such as routine pediatric postpartum exams, either in hospital, clinic, or home setting, in a way that is compatible with the demands of clinical practice. Recent research suggests that the NBO may be an effective tool in helping professionals support parents in their efforts to get to know and understand their infants' development and can promote a positive relationship between parents and clinicians.[194,223] More information on the NBO is available at www.brazelton-institute.com.

NEWBORN INDIVIDUALIZED DEVELOPMENTAL CARE AND ASSESSMENT PROGRAM

The Newborn Individualized Developmental Care and Assessment Program (NIDCAP) is a comprehensive approach to care for infants in the NICU that is developmentally supportive and individualized to the infant's goals and level of stability.[3,4] The NIDCAP is inclusive of families and professionals. Completion initially involves direct and systematic observation—without the observer manipulating or interacting—of the preterm or full-term infant in the nursery before, during, and after a caregiving event. Observation is guided by a behavioral checklist to record the caregiving event; positioning; environmental characteristics such as light, sound, and activity; and the infant's behaviors. The observation begins 10 minutes before care, to observe the infant's stability and behavioral reactions when undisturbed; observation continues until care is completed and for another 10 minutes thereafter or until the infant reaches preobservation stability levels. The behavior observation checklist is marked every 2 minutes for heart and respiratory rates, oxygen saturation levels, position of the infant, and the caregiving event taking place. The observation time can be minutes or hours long depending on the caregiving event and the stability of the infant. Following this observation, a narrative is written that describes the caregiving event from the infant's perspective, highlighting in great detail the neurobehaviors of the infant in relationship with the caregiving and environmental events taking place simultaneously. Suggestions for caregiving modifications to support the infant's physiologic maturation and strategies at self-regulation are developed from the narrative. The physical therapist who is NIDCAP trained and certified can share this information with the NICU team and provide suggestions for modifying the environment and caregiving activities. These suggestions may pertain to lighting, noise level, activity level, bedding, aids to self-regulation, interaction, timing of manipulations, and facilitation of transitions from one activity to another. The NIDCAP has been found to be most effective in influencing medical outcome,[7,9] and it is suggested to be a causative agent in altering brain function and structure.[6] More information and a list of NIDCAP training centers may be obtained at www.nidcap.org.

ASSESSMENT OF PRETERM INFANT BEHAVIOR

The Assessment of Preterm Infant Behavior (APIB) is a comprehensive and systematic neurobehavioral assessment of preterm and high-risk infants[5,10,11] that is based on the Neonatal Behavioral Assessment Scale.[47] Also viewed as a neuropsychologic assessment, the APIB provides a detailed assessment of infants' self-regulatory efforts and thresholds to disorganization as viewed through the infant's behaviors. The exam proceeds through a series of maneuvers that increase in vigor as well as tactile and vestibular demands to determine the infant's self-regulatory abilities. The APIB may take up to an hour, depending on the level of stability of the infant, whereas scoring may take between 30 and 45 minutes. Writing the clinical assessment report from the APIB may take up to 3 hours, depending on the complexity of the medical history, developmental issues, and recommendations.[5] To be safely handled for the duration of the assessment, the infant must be physiologically stable and 32 weeks postconceptional age or older. The APIB is appropriate for use with high-risk infants until approximately 44 to 48 weeks of postconceptional age. Training is extensive and available for clinicians and developmental professionals in the NICU and follow-up clinical settings. More information is available at www.nidcap.org.

NICU NETWORK NEUROBEHAVIORAL SCALE

The NICU Network Neurobehavioral Scale (NNNS) is designed for the neurobehavioral assessment of medically stable drug-exposed and other high-risk infants, especially preterm infants between the ages of 30 and 46 to 48 weeks postconceptional age.[162] The NNNS is used to document and describe developmental and behavioral maturation, central nervous system integrity, and infant stress responses. Although similar to the NBAS in its content, the NNNS differs from it in the order of item administration. For example, items are skipped if the infant is not in the appropriate behavioral state, and deviations in administration are recorded. Additionally, the time required to administer the NNNS is shorter than the NBAS, because the NNNS is less focused on infant best performance and the infant-examiner interaction. The NNNS comprises 115 items, 45 of which require specific manipulation of the infant, whereas the other 70 items are observed over the course of the examination. It is divided in three parts: (1) an Examination Scale that includes neurologic items that assess passive and active tone and primitive reflexes and items that reflect central nervous system integrity; (2) an Examiner Ratings Scale that includes behavioral items including state, sensory, and interactive responses; and (3) a Stress/Abstinence Scale that includes seven categories of items designed to capture behavioral signs of stress typical of high-risk infants and signs of neonatal abstinence or withdrawal commonly seen in drug-exposed infants.[162] The

NNNS has been used to describe the neurobehavioral profile of infants exposed to methamphetamine,[208,238] cocaine,[222] and marijuana.[81]

TEST OF INFANT MOTOR PERFORMANCE

The Test of Infant Motor Performance (TIMP) is a test of functional motor behavior in infants for use by physical and occupational therapists and other professionals in the NICU and early intervention or diagnostic follow-up settings.[57] The TIMP can be used to assess the infants between the ages of 34 weeks postconceptional age and 4 months postterm. The test examines postural and selective control of movement needed for functional motor performance in early infancy. The TIMP requires approximately 25 to 45 minutes for administration and scoring.[57] Spontaneous and elicited movements constitute separate subscales. The Observed Scale consists of 13 dichotomously scored items that assess the infant's spontaneous attempts to orient the body, to selectively move individual body segments, and to perform qualitative movements such as ballistic or oscillating movements.[60] Examples of observed behaviors include individual finger and ankle movements, reaching, and aligning the head in midline while supine. The Elicited Scale consists of 29 items scored on a 5-, 6-, or 7-point hierarchic scale.[55] Elicited behaviors reflect the infant's response to positioning and handling in a variety of spatial orientations and to visual and auditory stimuli. Examples include rolling prone with head righting when the leg is rotated across the body and turning the head to follow a visual stimulus or to search for a sound in prone.

The TIMP has been shown to have excellent test-retest and rater reliability,[55] good construct validity,[60,190] concurrent validity,[59] and predictive validity.[57,61,100,243] The TIMP can be used for the early identification of very young infants at risk for poor motor performance[61,100] and cerebral palsy as early as 2 months of adjusted age.[23,24] A shorter version used for screening purposes, the Test of Infant Motor Performance Screening Items (TIMPSI), is now available.[62] The TIMPSI takes half the time to administer when compared to the TIMP and is considered useful for fragile babies or for rapid screening that reduces the need for full TIMP testing in infants who do well on the TIMPSI. Users of the TIMPSI must have previous knowledge and training of the full TIMP in order to use it effectively. More information about the TIMP and TIMPSI can be found at www.timp.com.

ORAL-MOTOR EXAMINATION

Oral-motor examination is an advanced competency. Two useful measures are the Neonatal Oral-Motor Assessment Scale (NOMAS)[45,102] and the Nursing Child Assessment Feeding Scale (NCAFS).[25,254] The NOMAS measures components of nutritive and nonnutritive sucking. Variables assessed during sucking include rate, rhythmicity, jaw excursion, tongue configuration, and tongue movement. A pilot study determined cutoff scores for oral-motor disorganization and dysfunction. The NCAFS assesses parent-infant feeding interaction and evaluates the responsiveness of parents to their infant's cues, signs of distress, and social interaction during feeding. Both of those assessment tools require highly specialized training but provide an excellent diagnostic framework for fragile feeders. Neonatal physical therapists may also find useful the Early Feeding Skills Assessment (EFS) as a tool to assess infant readiness and tolerance for feeding and to identify a profile of an infant's specific skills relative to a developmental progression of oral feeding competencies.[262] There are also instruments to study the pressure generated by each suck and the length of sucking bursts such as the Kron Nutritive Sucking Apparatus and the Actifier,[97] which can also be used as a method for stimulation of intraoral tissue in neonates.

DEVELOPMENTAL INTERVENTIONS

Since the 1980s, state-of-the art medical care has progressed substantially, leading to the increased survival rate of high-risk infants. But surviving premature birth and severe illness in the neonatal period is not sufficient. Attention also has to be given to the developmental outcome of these infants. Because a high proportion of prematurely born children show some degrees of learning disabilities that cannot be linked to a known cerebral insult, it has been suggested that some of the medical and developmental problems resulting from premature birth arise from the immature organism's difficulty in adapting to the caregiving environment outside the womb.[39] Therefore, continual evaluation and modification of care is necessary to ensure that the quality, quantity, and type of care provided to infants and their families promotes optimal developmental outcomes. Because of physiologic, sensory, and neurologic immaturity, neonates admitted to the NICU are vulnerable to environmental conditions, making quality care critical. The pioneering work of Heidi Als and her colleagues on developmental care made us keenly aware that the NICU environment was poorly matched to the needs of preterm infants.[2,9] The goal of developmental interventions, therefore, is to provide sensory experiences that are appropriate in type and intensity and are closely matched to the infant's needs and level of sensory integration capacity, which can be monitored through the infant's behaviors and responses.[39] It is also stressed that interventions of all forms, including physical therapy-based interventions, need to carefully examine the cost-benefit to the infant on an individual basis and should be framed within a 24-hour care perspective. The Annual Graven Conference on the Physical and Developmental Environment of the High Risk Infant held at the University of Florida every year has made the environment in which these infants grow its mission (for more information, visit www.cme.hsc.usf.edu/hri). Spearheaded by Graven, study groups have been formed and have established guidelines for the regulation of sensory stimuli in the NICU.[112,113,154,166,213]

Physical therapists should carefully assess and reflect on the relevance of all interventions provided in the NICU. Intervention of any kind, even though theoretically believed to be helpful or even scientifically shown to be effective, may in fact be harmful unless individualized attention is given to an infant's physiologic, sensory, and neurologic responses to the event. An infant whose sleep is already interrupted numerous times during the day and night may benefit more from sleep protection than from additional handling. Developmental interventions that are integrated into the needs of the infant and her day/night routine are most promising. Therefore, the success of an intervention program such as kangaroo care, along with its effect on the development of infants and their families, is not surprising.[96,138,198] The experience of kangaroo care has been shown to foster maternal attachment, improve maternal confidence in caring for her premature infant,[138] and improve the odds of breastfeeding at discharge from the NICU and into the first year of life.[198] Feldman has shown that preterm infants receiving kangaroo care in the NICU had more mature neurobehavioral profiles on the NBAS when compared to control infants.[95] The approach is now widely accepted and is part of the care of the infant rather than being an intervention approach specific to a particular discipline. Physical therapists should strive toward identifying developmental approaches that could easily be integrated into the routine care of the infant rather than be seen as separate interventions. Taking sound as an example, the Graven group's most recent recommendations on sound exposure to the in utero and ex utero fetus states that sound exposure "should provide an environment that will protect sleep, support stable vital signs, improve speech intelligibility, and reduce potential adverse effects on auditory development."[113]

Infants in the NICU present with a wide range of conditions that have an impact on their later developmental outcome, including prematurity, neonatal seizures, intraventricular hemorrhage, stroke, hydrocephalus, respiratory distress syndrome, bronchopulmonary dysplasia, cystic fibrosis, spina bifida, arthrogryposis, and osteogenesis imperfecta. These conditions lead to impairments that affect the infant's activity levels and participation in interactions with parents and caregivers. A review of the literature on interventions in the NICU indicates that various interventions are provided. Interventions include hammock positioning,[142] handling,[53] nursing staff education on positioning,[209] tucking,[126] and physical therapy.[52] The research is vast and consensus is difficult to reach because of the wide range of intervention protocols and study limitations. But some consensus is available on a range of intervention modalities through the Cochrane Collaboration, an international not-for-profit organization that provides up-to-date systematic reviews

about the effects of health care. Table 28-5 presents statements on Cochrane reviews relevant to the developmental interventions of the high-risk infant in the NICU. For the most part, the Cochrane reviews on kinesthetic stimulation, massage, non-nutritive sucking, and developmental care show modest short-term benefits with no negative effects reported. A review of the literature on the effects of bright lights in the NICU, long believed to play a role in retinopathy of prematurity (ROP), suggests that bright lights are not the cause of ROP.[212] More recently, a Cochrane review concluded that physical activity for hospitalized preterm infants may have small short-term but no long-term effects on bone mineralization and growth; the reviewers do not recommend these programs based on the limited research at this time.[229]

Additional protocols currently being implemented include cycled light; supine versus nonsupine sleep position for preventing short-term morbidity and mortality in hospitalized spontaneously breathing preterm infants, push versus gravity for intermittent bolus gavage tube feeding of premature and low-birth-weight infants, home-based postdischarge parental support to prevent morbidity in preterm infants, body position for spontaneously breathing preterm infants with apnea, instruments for assessing readiness to commence suck feeds in preterm infants, and effects on time to establish full oral feeding and duration of hospitalization.

DEVELOPMENTAL FOLLOW-UP

For many high-risk infants and their families, life after discharge from the NICU may involve referrals to a number of medical specialists (e.g., pulmonary, neurology, neurosurgery, ear nose and throat, gastroenterology, craniofacial, orthopedics), a local early intervention program, and developmental follow-up to a hospital-based multidisciplinary clinic. Public law 108–446, known as the Individuals with Disabilities Education Improvement Act of 2004, or IDEA, ensures access to a free and appropriate public education to all children with disabilities. Part C of that law guarantees access to physical therapy services in the home or other natural settings through local early intervention programs for children from birth up to age 3. Once a child is determined eligible to receive early intervention services, an Individualized Family Service Plan (IFSP) is developed and reviewed every 6 months or as necessary. The IFSP includes statements of developmentally appropriate, measurable annual goals and a description of how the child's progress toward meeting the goals will be measured.[253] More can be found on the role of the physical therapist in Chapter 29.

The physical therapist plays an important role in the transition of infants and families to early intervention services. The physical therapist needs to communicate with the therapist or agency providing services to the infant and

TABLE 28-5 **Cochrane Reviews on Topics Relevant to Developmental Interventions of the High-Risk Infant in the NICU (Full Reviews and Plain Language Summaries Are Available at www.cochrane.org)**

Topic of Review	Conclusive Statement
Developmental care Symington, A. J., & Pinelli, J. (2006). *Cochrane Database Systematic Reviews, 2,* CD001814.	The evidence suggests that these interventions may have some benefit to the outcomes of preterm infants; however, there continues to be conflicting evidence among the multiple studies. Therefore, there is so far no clear evidence demonstrating consistent effects of developmental care interventions on important short- and long-term outcomes.
Light reduction in the prevention of ROP Phelps, D. L., & Watts, J. L. (2001). *Cochrane Database Systematic Reviews, 1,* CD000122.	Considerable research has been done on this, and the evidence suggests that bright light is not the cause of this problem and it does not add to the problem.
Infant position during mechanical ventilation Balaguer, A., Escribano, J., & Roqué, M. (2006). *Cochrane Database Systematic Reviews, 4,* CD003668.	There is no clear evidence that body position during mechanical ventilation in newborn babies is effective in producing relevant and sustained improvement. However, putting infants on assisted ventilation in the face-down position for a short time slightly improves their oxygenation and infants in the prone position undergo fewer episodes of poor oxygenation.
Non-nutritive sucking Pinelli, J., & Symington, A. (2005). *Cochrane Database Systematic Reviews, 4,* CD0010701.	The review of literature suggests that weight gain was similar with and without use of a pacifier. In two studies, preterm infants with pacifiers had shorter hospital stays (lower hospital costs), showed less defensive behaviors during tube feedings, spent less time in fussy and active states during and after tube feedings, and settled more quickly into sleep than those without pacifiers. Their transition to full enteral (by tube or mouth) or bottle feeds (three studies) and bottle-feeding performance, in general (one study), was easier. No negative outcomes were reported.
Cot-nursing versus incubator care Gray, P. H., & Flenady, V. (2003). *Cochrane Database Systematic Reviews, 4,* CD003062.	Four studies (two in developed countries) randomly assigned 173 preterm infants to being cared for in cots or incubators. In one study, the cot-nursed infants had a higher mean body temperature in the first week of life. Another study showed less weight gain for infants in cots when in a heated room for the first week of life. Higher numbers of infants cared for in cots were breast-fed when leaving the health care facilities in a study from Ethiopia, but the authors argued that it is not necessarily comparable to feeding practices elsewhere. Lack of information on infections from cot nursing, lack of comparable data, as well as the small number of babies involved restrict the findings of this review.
Predischarge "car seat challenge" Pilley, E., & McGuire, W. (2006). *Cochrane Database Systematic Reviews, 1,* CD005386.	There is no evidence that undertaking a predischarge "car seat challenge" benefits preterm infants, and it is not clear whether the level of oxygen desaturation, apnea, or bradycardia detected in the car seat challenge is actually harmful for preterm infants. The use of the car seat challenge may cause undue parental anxiety about the safety of transporting the infant in a car seat.
Physical activity programs for promoting bone mineralization and growth Schulzke, S. M., Trachsel, D., & Patole, S. K. (2007). *Cochrane Database Systematic Reviews, 2,* CD005387.	This review found that physical activity might have a small benefit on bone development and growth over a short term. There were inadequate data to assess long-term benefits and harms. Based on current knowledge, physical activity programs cannot be recommended as a standard procedure for premature babies.
Early discharge home with gavage feeding for stable preterm infants Collins, C. T., Makrides, M., & McPhee, A. J. (2003). *Cochrane Database Systematic Reviews, 4,* CD003743.	There is not enough strong evidence regarding the effects of early home discharge for preterm babies who are stable but still need gavage (tube) feeds. Although early discharge of babies who are stable but still need gavage (tube) feeds could unite families sooner and might reduce costs; this could also be a burden for the family and might increase complications in the transition from tube feeding.

TABLE 28-5 **Cochrane Reviews on Topics Relevant to Developmental Interventions of the High-Risk Infant in the NICU (Full Reviews and Plain Language Summaries Are Available at www.cochrane.org)—cont'd**

Topic of Review	Conclusive Statement
Massage Vickers, A., Ohlsson, A, Lacy, J., & Horsley, A. (2004). *Cochrane Database Systematic Reviews, 2,* CD000390.	The review only included randomized controlled trials, studies in which a group of babies received massage or "still, gentle touch," in which nurses put their hands on babies but did not rub or stroke them. In most of these studies, babies were rubbed or stroked for about 15 minutes, three or four times a day, usually for 5 or 10 days. On average, the studies found that babies receiving massage, but not "still, gentle touch," gained more weight each day (about 5 grams). They spent less time in the hospital, had slightly better scores on developmental tests, and had slightly fewer postnatal complications, although there were problems with how reliable these findings are. The studies did not show any negative effects of massage.
Early developmental intervention programs after hospital discharge Spittle, A. J., Orton, J., Doyle, L. W., & Boyd, R. (2007). *Cochrane Database Systematic Reviews, 2,* CD005495.	The early developmental intervention programs in this review had to commence within the first 12 months of life, focus on the parent-infant relationship or infant development, and, although they could commence while the baby was still in hospital, they had to have a component that was delivered postdischarge from hospital. A review of trials suggests those programs for preterm infants are effective at improving cognitive development in the short to medium term (up to preschool age). There is limited evidence that early developmental interventions improve motor outcome or long-term cognitive outcome (up to school age). The variability in the intervention programs limits the conclusions that can be made about the effectiveness of early developmental interventions.
Kinesthetic stimulation for preventing or treating apnea Henderson-Smart, D. J., & Osborn, D. A. (2002). *Cochrane Database Systematic Reviews, 2,* CD000373. Osborn, D. A., & Henderson-Smart, D. J. (2000). *Cochrane Database Systematic Reviews, 2,* CD000499.	Laying preterm babies on oscillating mattresses has not been shown to help prevent apnea. Three controlled studies have used different gentle rocking motions (irregularly oscillating water beds, regularly rocking bed trays, or a vertical pulsating stimulus) to reduce the occurrence of apnea in a total of 49 babies. However, there was no clinically useful reduction of periods of apnea, although only a small number of infants were studied. Shorter breathing pauses were reported to be reduced by one study, but it is not thought to be clinically important. No harm has been reported to have been done to the preterm infants with these interventions.
Positioning for acute respiratory distress Wells, D. A., Gillies, D., & Fitzgerald, D. A. (2005). *Cochrane Database Systematic Reviews, 2,* CD003645.	A total of 21 studies were assessed altogether. Three quarters of the 436 children were preterm babies and were mostly (71%) ventilated by machine. The prone position was better than supine for oxygenating the blood, but the difference was small. The increase in oxygen saturation on average increased by 2%. This finding was based on eight studies (183 children, 153 preterm and 95 ventilated) measuring this outcome. The rapid rate of breathing with respiratory distress was slightly lower in the prone position (on average four breaths/min lower) based on five studies (100 infants aged up to 1 month, 59 ventilated). There were no obvious differences with other positions. Note: It is important to remember that these children were hospitalized. Therefore, given the association of the prone position with sudden infant death syndrome (SIDS), the prone position should not be used for children unless they are in hospital and where their breathing is constantly monitored.
Kangaroo mother care to reduce morbidity and mortality in low birthweight infants Conde-Agudelo, A., & Belizán, J. M. Kangaroo mother care to reduce morbidity and mortality in low birthweight infants. (2003). *Cochrane Database Systematic Reviews, 2,* CD002771.	Kangaroo mother care (KMC) involves skin-to-skin contact between mother and her newborn, frequent and exclusive or nearly exclusive breast-feeding, and early discharge from hospital. Compared with conventional care, KMC was found to reduce severe illness, infection, breast-feeding problems, and maternal dissatisfaction with method of care and improve some outcomes of mother-baby bonding. There was no difference in infant mortality. However, serious concerns about the methodological quality of the included trials weaken credibility in these findings. More research is needed.

family. Ideally, providers from the local early intervention agency would meet the family before the infant is discharged from the NICU and thus ensure a smooth and less stressful transition into the family's community. When this situation is not possible, the physical therapist can make contact with the community therapist and provide as much information as possible on the infant's current development and interventions while in the NICU.

Many level III nurseries have a developmental follow-up clinic for high-risk infants. Clinics vary in staffing and criteria for follow-up care. Factors such as birth weight, gestational age, Apgar scores, time on a ventilator, IVH, seizures, and environmental factors such as maternal drug or alcohol use are commonly used criteria. These follow-up programs monitor the health outcomes of graduates of the NICU and provide feedback to the developmental follow-up clinic.[249]

Results of developmental assessments administered at the follow-up clinic are useful in determining whether specialized therapy services are necessary beyond the provision of general recommendations for development and parent education. Referrals for nutrition, audiology, and ophthalmology are also made when necessary. As a team member in the follow-up clinic or early intervention, the physical therapist plays an important role in the examination and monitoring of neuromotor development, provides parent education and anticipatory guidance, and assists the family with coordination of care and referrals to other professionals and community agencies when appropriate.

On average, infants remain hospitalized in the NICU until 38 to 40 weeks of corrected gestational age.[181] For a subpopulation of infants, although intensive medical care is no longer required, discharge home is not yet appropriate because nutritional needs are not being met through oral feeding.[122] These infants typically present with severe chronic lung disease and concomitant feeding issues, neonatal abstinence syndrome requiring continued medical management, severe neurologic impairments, and in some cases are postsurgical. They typically require more intensive physical therapy than can be provided by admission to a pediatric rehabilitation hospital or a community early intervention program. In both settings, the physical therapist examines and evaluates infants and, in consultation with the physical therapist from the NICU, develops an individualized plan to facilitate progression of developmental milestones, age-appropriate feeding skills, and social interaction.

PRACTICE IN THE NICU: REWARDS AND CHALLENGES

Newborn medicine changes rapidly with the advent of new drugs and technology. The NICU work environment is cutting edge, fast paced, and high stress, but it affords the physical therapist incomparable learning opportunities because of the exceptional range of medical conditions

and level of acuity of the infants, numerous exchanges with health care professionals working together in the NICU, and the opportunity to positively shape this new family unit. This highly technical subspecialty area offers the opportunity for physical therapists to provide developmental services within a framework that is family centered and that views the infant as fully participating in the development process, principles that are central to pediatric physical therapy practice. Although each physical therapist's experience is unique and will differ based on practice setting (e.g., children's hospital, birthing hospital), we highlight three challenges to physical therapist practice in the NICU.

PREPARATION

According to the practice guidelines endorsed by the American Physical Therapy Association (APTA),[256] physical therapists in the NICU should meet a series of competencies across multiple domains of neonatal clinical practice ranging from theoretic frameworks to social policy governing practice involving high-risk infants. In addition, physical therapists should participate in a minimum of 6 months of precepting in the NICU. Many NICUs lack an established training program where experienced clinical specialists provide precepting and ongoing mentoring to physical therapists new to neonatal care. Physical therapists may need to advocate for education and training resources. One resource is the NICU Special Interest Group within the Section on Pediatrics of the APTA (see www.pediatricapta.org/special-interest-groups/neonatology/index.cfm for more information).

METHOD OF SERVICE DELIVERY

Traditional models of service delivery for inpatient pediatric rehabilitation may not match the needs of infants and families in the NICU. Although therapists in other subspecialties within the hospital typically see 8 to 10 patients per 8-hour day (from 9 a.m. to 5 p.m.), physical therapists in the NICU are constrained by frequent medical procedures, strict feeding schedules, evening parental visiting schedules, and infection considerations for patients seen outside of the NICU. As such, the model of service delivery needs to be flexible with regard to productivity demands, work hours, and managing schedules of patients other than those in the NICU. The needs and realities of the rehabilitation department and assuring equity of responsibility among all therapists are additional considerations.

PROFESSIONAL ROLE DELINEATION

Depending on NICU staff resources, physical therapists may work closely with occupational therapists, speech language pathologists, and developmental specialists. As such, professional role delineations related to oral feeding, positioning, infant massage, and facilitation and handling may become blurred. According to the APTA, physical therapists are experts in examination and intervention of impairments in body functions and structures and motor activity limitations of the musculoskeletal and neuromuscular system.[256] To this end, this expertise may cross traditional professional boundaries and physical therapists should work collaboratively with colleagues from other disciplines while advocating for the growth of our profession.

SUMMARY

The special care nursery is a specialized setting for providing high technological medical interventions to newborn infants who are unable to sustain basic physiological processes secondary to premature birth or other neonatal complications. Provision of services to infants and families in the special care nursery is a subspecialty area of pediatric physical therapist practice. Knowledge of fetal and infant development, medical complications, and competency in monitoring vital signs and behaviors are essential for providing therapy services in the special care nursery. The examination and evaluation process includes issues identified by families and members of the team and observation of how the infant is positioned and responds to caregiving procedures. Standardized tests and measures are useful in evaluation of infant development and identification of areas of need.

Depending on an infant's needs and ability to tolerate sensory stimulation and movement, interventions may include positioning, strategies to minimize physiological stress, and sensory-motor development. Prevention of musculoskeletal impairments is an important outcome of intervention. Communication and coordination of care with team members, families, and external agencies such as early intervention providers are important components of intervention. Perhaps the most important role of the physical therapist is education and instruction of family members in the infant's behavioral cues and responses and handling and caring for the infant in anticipation of the transition to home. After discharge, an important role of the physical therapist in high-risk follow-up clinics is to monitor infant motor development, address family information needs and concerns, and coordinate care with community service providers.

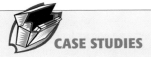

CASE STUDIES

Two case studies are presented to illustrate how the contents of the chapter apply to practice in the NICU. The first case is about a little boy, born extremely preterm, who spent over 4 months in the NICU. He presents with significant respiratory difficulties, which affect his oral feeding development. As a result, the family faces a decision about surgical intervention versus further hospitalization in a rehabilitation setting. The second case is about a little girl, born full-term, with Down syndrome. There is concern from the medical team that the infant's mother has not bonded with her daughter. Following a particularly powerful session with the physical therapist, the parents gain a new appreciation for their daughter's strengths and competencies.

Both patients were hospitalized in the same level III NICU. The NICU rehabilitation team consists of a physical therapist who is an APTA board-certified pediatric clinical specialist employed full time and two therapists (one physical therapist and one occupational therapist) employed half time. Rehabilitation team members are part of a larger interdisciplinary team that includes medicine, social work, nutrition, and nursing. Physical therapists generally spend approximately 30 to 60 minutes with each patient and family, depending on the context of the session (e.g., oral feeding, developmental evaluation, discharge teaching). In addition to patient care, physical therapists participate in daily medical rounds and weekly developmental and feeding rounds.

"Travis"
Examination

History

Travis was born precipitously at 24 2/7 weeks weighing 590 grams. His ApGARS were 4, 7, and 8 at 1, 5, and 10 minutes, respectively. He was intubated in the delivery room, received mechanical ventilation, and was transferred to the NICU. Upon admission, he received one dose of artificial surfactant. During the first 2 weeks of life, he required dopamine, received two blood transfusions, and was treated with hydrocortisone to maintain a stable blood pressure and adequate perfusion. Travis's cardiovascular system was compromised by a patent ductus arteriosus, which was treated with ibuprofen. He required phototherapy treatment for 12 days for hyperbilirubinemia, and he was treated with antibiotics for presumed early-onset infection.

Travis remained on mechanical ventilation until 33 weeks CGA when he transitioned to continuous positive airway pressure (CPAP). Travis remained on CPAP until 36 weeks when he was able to be weaned to 50 ml of oxygen that he received through a low-flow nasal cannula. At 33 weeks, Travis received a 14-day course of antibiotics for medical necrotizing enterocolitis. At 36 weeks, he was diagnosed with gastroesophageal reflux (GER) and was started on antireflux medications. All Travis's head ultrasounds revealed no intraventricular

Continued

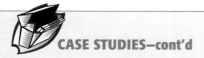

hemorrhage. His eye exams revealed state II retinopathy of prematurity in both eyes.

Travis's mother visits the NICU daily and is very involved in Travis's care. His 13-year-old sister and father visit on weekends. The majority of Travis's extended family resides in Korea, and the family has few social supports.

Travis was referred to physical therapy at 4 weeks of age (28 weeks PCA). His primary nurse reported that Travis was "stiff," "arched a lot," and "seemed irritable" during his routine care.

Observation

Travis was seen at 28 weeks PCA for an initial physical therapy examination. Travis's mother was present. The physical therapist introduced herself and described her role in the NICU. She explained that Travis was referred to physical therapy because he is at risk for developmental difficulties. Moreover, once home, babies like Travis are likely eligible and would benefit from physical therapy as part of early intervention services. There are many interventions, however, that can start even earlier—while Travis is still in the hospital—to promote his development and help family members to care for his needs when he goes home. The physical therapist described for Travis's mother what the examination would consist of—observing Travis's likes and dislikes during his routine care, his ability to self-soothe, and his movements with his arms and legs. The therapist acknowledged that Travis's mother knows him best and asked her to participate in the evaluation.

Travis was supine with his head turned to right side, swaddled, and he had a positioning roll around his lower body. Medical fragility precluded administering a formal, standardized evaluation. The physical therapist completed a neurobehavioral observation during Travis's routine care in order to identify factors with deficits.[257] The developmental evaluation consisted of taking Travis's temperature, changing his diaper, and repositioning him, which took approximately 25 minutes.

Body Functions and Structures

Autonomic. Upon arrival, Travis's heart rate was in the 160s, respiratory rate was in the 60s, and oxygen saturation (SaO_2) was 95% to 98%. His color was pink and his respirations appeared rhythmical. He demonstrated decreased autonomic stability at several points during the evaluation. He paled and startled when his blanket was unwrapped; his movements became tremulous while his temperature was being taken; and he had several oxygen desaturations during his diaper change ($SaO_2 < 85$), especially when his legs were lifted. Travis's autonomic instability resolved with gentle containment to his head and feet during all aspects of his care, offering Travis breaks and opportunities to self-regulate (e.g., tucking, grasping, bracing his feet) and minimizing the environmental stimuli (e.g., shielding the light and speaking softly during his care). Motor. While supine, Travis was observed to retract his scapulae and externally rotate his arms; his legs were externally rotated and abducted, and his trunk and head were not in midline. His grasp was moderately strong on both sides, and his suck was weak and nonrhythmical when tested with

his pacifier in supine. Overall, Travis's tone was low, and he made infrequent attempts at active flexion movements. When repositioned in left side lying, Travis demonstrated more active flexion movements (hands to mouth and midline, tucking of his lower extremities) and the quality of his suck improved.

State and Social Interaction

Travis was in a drowsy state during most of the examination. During his diaper change, he became irritable, demonstrating a weak cry. With containment and environmental modifications (e.g., shielding the light), he was able to open his eyes briefly and make attempts to focus on the therapist's face. At this point, the therapist encouraged Travis's mother to engage in eye contact with him. Travis maintained social interaction for a few brief seconds, and Travis's mother shared that she had never seen him open his eyes for that long.

Throughout the examination, the physical therapist described Travis's thresholds for overstimulation and, more important, his attempts and successes at self-regulation. Travis's mother had already noticed that he was "sensitive" to the bright lights in the room, and she attempted to reduce the light while changing his diaper. During the examination, she learned that Travis benefits immensely from containment during and after diaper changes. She shared with the therapist that she was excited to use this new technique because she often feels "helpless" at the bedside.

Activity and Participation

Travis's immature autonomic, motor, and state systems limit his ability to fully participate in the developmental tasks of a newborn. Travis requires increased supports to achieve and maintain self-regulation during routine care. He has limited ability to achieve a calm awake state to interact with his caregivers. Travis's immature feeding and oral motor skills coupled with his gastroesophageal reflux often prevent feeding from being a positive experience for Travis.

Based on Travis's participation limitations and his mother's concerns (e.g., his sensitivity to light and limited ability to keep his eyes open to look at her), the goals of physical therapy were to (1) minimize signs of autonomic instability during routine care; (2) increase active flexion movements, first in side lying, and then progressing to supine; (3) increase postural control, first in side lying, and then progressing to supported sit; (4) increase strength and coordination of his non-nutritive suck and then his nutritive suck when developmentally appropriate; (5) increase time in calm alert state; and (6) increase visual fixation and auditory processing skills with decreasing environmental modifications.

Outcomes for Travis were to (1) demonstrate age-appropriate neuromotor skills, such as full active flexion patterns in side lying and supine to allow for self-soothing skills (e.g., hands to mouth and midline), maintaining head in midline for brief periods to allow for visual fixation on caregiver's face, and emerging postural reactions to allow for tolerance of a variety of upright positions for caregiving and social interaction; (2) take all nutrition by bottle, demonstrating age-appropriate suck-swallow-breathe coordination, with each feeding lasting no more than 30 minutes; (3) demonstrate organized sleep/

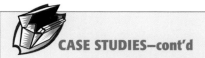

CASE STUDIES—cont'd

wake cycles; (4) have parents be independent in all of Travis's care, handling, and developmental activities; and (5) initiate referrals for family and community supports before discharge.

Intervention

The physical therapist saw Travis two to three times per week. Therapy sessions took place at a care time when Travis's mom was present in order to facilitate parent-infant bonding and shared observations of Travis and to partner with Travis's mother in his physical therapy plan of care (*patient/client instruction*). An individualized developmental care plan was created for Travis, reviewed with his parents, and

incorporated into his medical chart. The plan included a physical therapy clinical pathway, developed by the therapist, that delineated his goals, plan of care (e.g., progression of developmental interventions), and recommendations for caregivers.

Interventions (*procedural interventions*) to promote autonomic stability during care included implementing side-lying diaper change, whereby the diaper change is completed with the infant in side-lying to prevent excessive lifting of the legs, which contributes to autonomic instability (Duplesis, 2008). In addition, gentle containment to Travis's head and feet were provided during routine care to promote self-regulation and autonomic stability.

EVIDENCE TO PRACTICE 28-1

CASE STUDY "TRAVIS"

PLAN OF CARE DECISION

The decision to provide gentle containment during care was based on a review of the literature examining the effect of gentle touch on medically fragile infants. In this review, Harrison included six studies that examined the effect of gentle touch provided daily (ranging from 20 minutes total per day to 10 to 15 minutes, three times per day) to infants in the NICU who were medically fragile. The results suggest that gentle touch is associated with immediate neurobehavioral benefits (e.g., decreased motor activity, fewer stress signals), but the long-term benefit (e.g., decreased length of stay, improved weight gain, fewer days on supplemental oxygen) has not been established.

FAMILY PREFERENCES

In a meta-analysis of literature examining parent preferences, Cleveland examined 60 studies of the needs and preferences of parents of infants in the NICU.[2] A common theme, germane to the intervention of containment, emerged. Parents often reported feeling excluded from the care of their infant and wished to have more contact with their infant (i.e., holding, touching). The authors suggested that NICU practitioners provide opportunities for "guided participation" for parents.

1. Harrison, L. L. (2001). The use of comforting touch and massage to reduce stress in preterm infants in the neonatal intensive care unit. *Newborn and Infant Nursing Reviews, 1*(4), 235–241.
2. Cleveland, L. M. (2008). Parenting in the neonatal intensive care unit. *Journal of Obstetric, Gynecologic, and Neonatal Nursing, 37*, 666–691.

Interventions to increase active flexion movements included side lying positioning with gentle facilitation to decrease scapular retraction, shoulder elevation, hip external rotation, and abduction. Positioning strategies included use of a length-wise towel roll under the abdomen during prone positioning and a long posterio-lateral blanket roll placed at the infant's back and between the legs and in front of the abdomen while side lying. In addition, a large "U"-shaped blanket roll supported the infant's lower body and trunk to provide additional boundaries and containment. Pictures of the infant in optimal positions were taken and hung at the bedside to promote continuity of care (*coordination, communication, and documentation*). When Travis transitioned to a low-flow nasal cannula, the physical therapist treated him at the bedside and encouraged supported upright activities and adapted prone positioning with a small towel roll under Travis's chest. These activities encouraged age-appropriate activation of postural muscles to reduce the likelihood of atypical head molding.[185]

Interventions to promote quiet awake state and age-appropriate social interaction included environmental modifications and parent and staff education. Travis's incubator was covered with a dark blanket to reduce environmental light exposure,[158] his eyes were

shielded during procedures and physical examinations, the ambient lights were kept low as often as possible,[9] and strategies were implemented to reduce noise[138] proximate to Travis's incubator (e.g., not placing items on top of the incubator, opening and closing incubator doors slowly, and speaking quietly during social interaction).

Bottle-feeding was introduced at 39 weeks when Travis's respiratory system was more stable and he began to demonstrate feeding readiness cues (e.g., waking for his feedings, rooting, and bringing his hands to his mouth). To promote age-appropriate feeding skills and feeding as a positive experience, Travis was offered non-nutritive sucking before feeding[215]; the physical therapist externally paced Travis during feeding[156] and utilized a slow-flow nipple.[74]

During each session, the therapist and mother partnered to complete Travis's routine care (i.e., diaper change and temperature), and then the therapist demonstrated increasingly more complex developmental tasks and caregiving activities (e.g., sessions began in the incubator in side lying and progressed to activities on the therapist's lap, first in side lying, then supine, prone, and upright). Typically, when the therapist introduced a new developmental task or caregiving activity, she demonstrated it to Travis's mother, discussed how it could promote Travis's development, and described Travis's response—including his

Continued

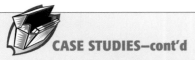

CASE STUDIES—cont'd

strengths and difficulties with the task. Then the therapist encouraged Travis's mother to engage in the development task with Travis and provided support and guidance (oral and hands on) as needed.

Reexamination

Test of Infant Motor Performance (TIMP)

At 36, 38, and 40 weeks, the physical therapist evaluated Travis's development using the TIMP. The TIMP was chosen because (1) the test is appropriate for use from 32 weeks' PCA until 4 months post term; (2) it is a valid and reliable test; (3) the TIMP discriminates infants with various risks for delays; and (4) the TIMP can identify very young infants at risk for poor motor performance.[57,61,100,243] Moreover, the PT chose a time when Travis was awake and alert and would likely tolerate the 45- to 60-minute TIMP session. At 36 weeks, Travis's TIMP raw score was 41, which indicates that Travis is at increased risk for developmental difficulties.[58] He has limited selective motor control, poor postural control, and immature visual and auditory tracking skills.

Neonatal Oral Motor Assessment Scale (NOMAS)

Because of slow progression with bottle-feeding skills (i.e., poor endurance and decreased oral motor coordination) and a hoarse cry, Travis underwent further evaluation of his oral motor skills. The physical therapist completed a feeding evaluation at 40 weeks with Travis using the NOMAS. The NOMAS was chosen because the scale is (1)

appropriate for use with fragile feeders and can be completed in one feeding session, (2) reliable and valid, (3) identifies infants with feeding delays and dysfunction, and (4) identifies very young infants at risk for long-term feeding difficulties.[124,203]

Based on Travis's atypical jaw excursion, tongue movement, and suck-swallow-breathe pattern, his feeding was categorized as dysfunctional. The attending neonatologist ordered a modified barium swallow (videofluoroscopic examination), which revealed that Travis was aspirating thin, but not thick, liquids.

A family meeting with Travis's care team was held when Travis was 40 weeks CGA. The physical therapist reported on Travis's progress with the plan of care. Travis had achieved several of his outcomes. He demonstrated organized sleep/wake cycles, and his parents were independent in all Travis's care and his developmental program. However, Travis's motor skills continued to be delayed and he was not fully bottle-feeding. At the team meeting, discharge plans presented to the parents included transfer to a pediatric short-term rehabilitation hospital or the placement of a gastrostomy tube and transfer home with community supports. Travis's parents were apprehensive about the surgery associated with the gastrostomy tube and opted to transfer Travis to the short-term rehabilitation facility. At this point, the physical therapist completed a full discharge report describing Travis's progress as well as his current physical therapy needs.

EVIDENCE TO PRACTICE 28-2

CASE STUDY "TRAVIS"

PLAN OF CARE DECISION

There is growing evidence to suggest that preterm infants have long-term feeding difficulties.[1] These include coughing and choking with feedings, not tolerating food textures, and developmental of oral aversions. Furthermore, oral feeding difficulties are particularly stressful for parents.

There is a paucity of literature investigating the effect of short-term rehabilitation on improved feeding development of preterm infants. The purpose of a short-term rehabilitation program is to achieve optimal feeding outcomes—that is, take all nutrition by bottle demonstrating age-appropriate suck-swallow-breathe coordination, with each feeding lasting no more than 30 minutes. This is often achieved through interdisciplinary interventions to increase oral motor coordination, promote endurance and self-regulation during feeding, and foster parental independence in positioning, handling, and feeding-specific interventions. This intensity and specificity of therapeutic intervention is not available in the NICU setting. Furthermore, in Travis's NICU, an experienced interdisciplinary feeding team conducts feeding evaluations, creates feeding plans, and facilitates discharge planning for infants who reach 42 weeks

CGA and are not fully bottle or breast-feeding. Based on Travis's presentation, the team drew from its practice knowledge in feeding-related discharge planning to suggest that Julia may be a good candidate for short-term rehabilitation and that her prognosis for safe, efficient bottle-feeding in 8 to 10 weeks was good.

FAMILY PREFERENCES

In a meta-analysis of literature examining parent preferences, Cleveland examined 60 studies of the needs and preferences of parents of NICU hospitalized infants.[2] A common theme, germane to the clinical decision making of discharge planning for infants with feeding difficulty, emerged. Parents often reported feeling excluded from the care of their infant and wished to be more involved in the clinical decision making related to their infant's care. The author suggested that NICU practitioners provide opportunities for parent empowerment and inclusion in decision making.

1. Hawdon, J. M., Beauregard, N., Slattery, J., & Kennedy, G. (2000). Identification of neonates at risk of developing feeding problems in infancy. *Developmental Medicine and Child Neurology, 42,* 235–239.
2. Cleveland, L. M. (2008). Parenting in the neonatal intensive care unit, *Journal of Obstetric, Gynecologic, and Neonatal Nursing, 37,* 666–691.

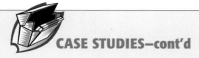

CASE STUDIES—cont'd

"Julia"

Julia is a full-term (38 2/7 weeks) little girl born via cesarean section weighing 3025 grams. She was diagnosed prenatally with Down syndrome and tetralogy of Fallot. Her Apgar scores were 5, 7, and 8 at 1, 5, and 10 minutes, respectively. She received supplemental oxygen via mask initially but then transitioned to room air. She presented with hyperbilirubinemia and received phototherapy treatment. Initially, Julia received intravenous fluids and then began to bottle-feed small amounts. She tolerated increasing amounts of formula but then developed bloody stools. Julia remained on IV fluids for 4 days until a repeat abdominal x-ray revealed normal bowel. She tolerated increasing volumes of formula well.

Julia's parents live 2 hours away and visit every third day. Julia has three older sisters at home, ages 2, 5, and 7. Julia's nurse shared with the physical therapist that Julia's mother had a lot of questions and concerns about Julia's development, and the nurse was concerned that Julia's mom had not yet bonded with Julia.

Observation

Julia was referred to physical therapy at 5 days of life. The physical therapist conducted a neurobehavioral observation, using the Neurobehavioral Observation system (NBO), with Julia's parents.

EVIDENCE TO PRACTICE 28-3

CASE STUDY "JULIA"

PLAN OF CARE DECISION

The decision to use the NBO to guide the initial observation and subsequent interventions is supported by the tool's purpose as a relationship-building instrument to highlight, for parents, the infant's unique strengths and competencies.[3,4] Furthermore, the NBO can be readily implemented in a busy NICU setting, and it is easy and quick to administer, making it ideal for medically fragile infants with limited endurance and low threshold for loss of self-regulation. Evidence suggests that the NBO is effective in helping in promoting the clinician-family relationship and the parent-infant relationship, and it helps parents to better understand their infant's unique strengths.[2] Furthermore, the NBO has been adapted to offer a clinical framework for providing interventions for the medically fragile or developmentally vulnerable infant.[1]

1. Blanchard, Y., & McManus, B. M. (under review). *Clinical framework for physical therapist intervention with families of high-risk infants.* Pediatric Physical Therapy.
2. Nugent, J. K., & Blanchard, Y. (2005). Newborn behavior and development: Implications for health care professionals. In K. M. Thies, & J. F. Travers (Eds.), *The handbook of human development for health care professionals.* Sudbury, MA: Jones & Bartlett.
3. Nugent, J. K., Keefer, C. H., Minear, S., Johnson, L., & Blanchard, Y. (2007). Understanding newborn behavior & early relationships: The newborn behavioral observations (NBO) system handbook. Baltimore: Brookes.
4. Nugent, J. K., Blanchard, Y., & Stewart, J. S. (2008). Supporting parents of premature infants: An infant-focused family-centered approach. In D. Brodsky & M. A. Ouellette (Eds.), *Primary care of the premature infant.* Elsevier.

The physical therapist selected the NBO because it is a relationship-building tool rather than an assessment. That is, although the therapist could develop her clinical impressions of Julia based on the NBO, the main purpose is to partner with parents to observe their baby. Moreover, the NBO utilizes a strength-based approach (i.e., rather than highlighting the infant's impairments), which the therapist employed to empower Julia's parents and encourage them to participate in the social interaction.

During the NBO, the physical therapist engaged the parents by asking questions about Julia's likes and dislikes and the parents' observations of Julia's developmental competencies. For example, when asked what Julia liked, the mother reported, "I don't really know. … She's so different from my other kids." When asked if he noticed if Julia was starting to look and listen to things in her environment, Julia's father responded, "She can't really do any of that. … She has Down syndrome. She failed her hearing exam. … We think she might be deaf." As the physical therapist administered the NBO, the parents moved closer and became more engaged in the observation. At one point when Julia brought her hands to her face and began to suck on her thumb, Mom became teary and stated, "She might be a thumb-sucker; all of her sisters sucked their thumb!" The physical therapist asked the father to call Julia's name. Almost immediately she turned her eyes toward her father. The dad became quite excited and said, "She can hear. She knows my voice!"

Body Functions and Structures

<u>Autonomic.</u> Upon arrival, Julia's heart rate was in the 140s, respiratory rate was in the 40s and oxygen saturation was between 90% to 94%. Julia's color was generally pink with slight paling around her mouth and forehead. Julia demonstrated difficulty regulating her autonomic system (i.e., mottled skin on her chest and increased paling around her mouth, eyes, and nose) when she was unswaddled, was required to hold her head up in supported sit, and while prone. She

Continued

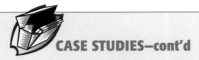

CASE STUDIES—cont'd

demonstrated pink coloring and rhythmical respirations when she was tucked with positional supports with her hands near her face and mouth. Motor. Julia was observed to have generalized hypotonia. She demonstrated difficulty with active flexion movements, hand grasp, and coordinated suck when positional supports were removed. Because she had an initial moderate head lag, the physical therapist opted not to perform pull-to-sit. When supported at the trunk and assistance was provided to maintain flexed and midline position of her extremities, Julia made attempts at righting her head in supported sit. Julia was able to bring her hands to midline and was observed to have a stronger, more coordinated suck while in side lying. State. Julia was able to maintain a quiet awake state when tasks were modulated and appropriately paced to reduce her fatigue. Julia became fussy and then appeared in a diffuse state between sleep and awake while prone and when asked to look and listen simultaneously. Social Interaction/Responsivity. Julia was able to visually fixate to face and the red ball when swaddled and with limited auditory environmental stimuli. She had difficulty coordinating looking and listening.

Activity and Participation

Julia is limited by her ability to fully participate in the developmental tasks of a newborn. She requires increased supports to achieve and maintain self-regulation during routine care. She has limited endurance to maintain a calm awake state to interact with caregivers. Julia's immature feeding and oral motor skills often prevent feeding from being a positive experience for Julia.

Goals and Outcomes

Based on Julia's participation limitations and concerns voiced by Julia's parents, the goals of physical therapy were to (1) tolerate handling and care with less fatigue and autonomic instability, (2) increase active flexion patterns, (3) increase postural control of head and neck muscles, (4) increase time in quiet awake state, and (5) increase visual tracking and auditory processing skills.

Outcomes for Julia were to (1) demonstrate age-appropriate neuromotor skills, such as full active flexion patterns in side lying and supine to allow for self-soothing skills (e.g., hands to mouth and midline) maintaining head in midline for brief periods to allow for visual fixation on caregiver's face and emerging postural reactions to allow for tolerance of a variety of upright positions for caregiving and social interaction; (2) take all nutrition by bottle demonstrating

age-appropriate suck-swallow-breathe coordination with each feeding lasting no more than 30 minutes; (3) demonstrate organized sleep/wake cycles; (4) have parents be independent in all care, handling, and developmental activities for Julia; and (5) initiate referral for family and community supports before discharge.

Intervention

Julia remained in the hospital for an additional week and was seen every other day by the physical therapist. Interventions to increase endurance and promote autonomic stability during motor activities included modulating Julia's activity (e.g., adapting timing, pacing, and activity requirements to match Julia's capacity for self-regulation) and offering frequent rest breaks at regular intervals rather than waiting until she could not maintain self-regulation (Blanchard & McManus, under review). Interventions (*procedural interventions*) to promote active flexion patterns included the use of posterior shoulder and pelvic positional rolls during therapy sessions. Parents were educated (*patient/client instruction*) about the benefits of positional supports (i.e., to promote forward shoulders and flexed hips) while Julia is awake and alert. In addition, the physical therapist reviewed the American Academy of Pediatrics guidelines for safe sleep, including supine sleeping without use of positional rolls or supports.[16] Interventions to increase social interaction skills included presenting one form of stimulation (i.e., visual or auditory) at a time.[41] In addition, social interaction activities were completed when Julia was in a position that supported her motor system (e.g., supine with towel rolls posterior to her shoulders and hips or semiupright and swaddled). The physical therapist wrote a developmental plan of care for Julia. The physical therapist shared the plan of care with Julia's parents and care team and elicited feedback before including the plan in Julia's medical chart (*coordination, communication, and documentation*).

Reexamination

A discharge meeting was held with Julia's family and team. The physical therapist shared updates on Julia's progress from a rehabilitation perspective. Julia made excellent progress with her plan of care and had achieved her developmental outcomes. The physical therapist completed a referral for early intervention and the Down syndrome follow-up clinic at a children's hospital about an hour away from Julia's home.

REFERENCES

1. Aita, M., & Goulet, C. (2003). Assessment of neonatal nurses' behaviors that prevent overstimulation in preterm infants. *Intensive Crit Care Nurs, 19*(2), 109–118.
2. Als, H. (1982). Toward a synactive theory of development: Promise for the assessment and support of infant individuality. *Infant Mental Health Journal, 3*(4), 229–243.
3. Als, H. (1986). A synactive model of neonatal behavioral organization: Framework for the assessment of neurobehavioral development in the premature infant and for support of infants and parents in the neonatal intensive care environment. *Physical and Occupational Therapy in Pediatrics, 6*(3/4), 3–54.
4. Als, H., & Butler, S. (2008). Newborn individualized developmental care and assessment program (NIDCAP), Changing

the future for infants and families in intensive and special care nurseries. *Early Childhood Services, 2,* 1–19.

5. Als, H., Butler, S., Kosta, S., & McAnulty, G. B. (2005). The Assessment of Preterm Infants' Behavior (APIB), Furthering the understanding and measurement of neurodevelopmental competence in preterm and full-term infants. *Mental Retardation and Developmental Disabilities, 11,* 94–102.

6. Als, H., Duffy, F. H., McAnulty, G. B., et al. (2004). Early experience alters brain function and structure. *Pediatrics, 113*(4), 846–857.

7. Als, H., Gilkerson, L., Duffy, F. H., et al. (2003). A three-center randomized controlled trial of individualized developmental care for very low-birth weight infants: Medical, neurodevelopmental, parenting and caregiving effects. *Journal of Developmental and Behavioral Pediatrics, 24*(6), 399–408.

8. Als, H., Lawhon, G., Brown, E., et al. (1986). Individualized behavioral and environmental care for the very low birth weight preterm infant at high risk for bronchopulmonary dysplasia: Neonatal intensive care unit and developmental outcome. *Pediatrics, 78,* 1123–1132.

9. Als, H., Lawhon, G., Duffy, F. H., McAnulty, G. B., Gibes-Grossman, R., & Blickman, J. G. (1994). Individualized developmental care for the very low birthweight preterm infant. *Journal of the American Medical Association, 272*(111), 853–858.

10. Als, H., Lester, B. M., Tronick, E. Z., & Brazelton, T. B. (1982a). Manual for the assessment of preterm infants' behavior (APIB). In H. E. Fitzgerald, B. M. Lester, & M. W. Yogman (Eds.). *Theory and research in behavioral pediatrics* (pp. 65–132). New York: Plenum Press.

11. Als, H., Lester, B. M., Tronick, E. Z., & Brazelton, T. B. (1982b). Toward a research instrument for the assessment of preterm infants' behavior. In H. E. Fitzgerald, B. M. Lester, & M. W. Yogman (Eds.). *Theory and research in behavioral pediatrics* (pp. 35–63). New York: Plenum Press.

12. Altuncu, E., Akman, I., Kulekci, S., Akdas, F., Bilgen, H., & Ozek, E. (2009). Noise levels in neonatal intensive care unit and use of sound absorbing panel in the isolette. *International Journal of Pediatric Otorhinolaryngology, 73*(7), 951–953.

13. Ambalavanan, N., & Whyte, R. K. (2003). The mismatch between evidence and practice. Common therapies in search of evidence. *Clinics in Perinatology, 30,* 305–331.

14. American Academy of Pediatrics. (1974). Committee on Environmental Hazards. Noise pollution: Neonatal aspects. *Pediatrics, 54,* 76–479.

15. American Academy of Pediatrics. (2004). Policy Statement Levels of Neonatal Care. *Pediatrics, 114,* 1341–1347.

16. American Academy of Pediatrics Task Force on Sudden Infant Death Syndrome. (2005). The Changing Concept of Sudden Infant Death Syndrome: Diagnostic Coding Shift, Controversies Regarding the Sleeping Environment, and New Variables to Consider in Reducing Risk. *Pediatrics, 116,* 1245–1255.

17. American Lung Association (ALA). (2006). Lung disease data at a glance: Respiratory distress syndrome (RDS). Available at www.lungusa.org/site/pp.asp?c=dvLUK900E&b=327819.

18. American Physical Therapist Association: Guide to Physical Therapist Practice, 2001.

19. Reference deleted in page proofs.

20. Anderson, C. G., Benitz, W. E., & Madan, A. (2004). Retinopathy of prematurity and pulse oximetry: A national survey of recent practices. *Journal of Perinatology, 24,* 164–168.

21. Arul, N., & Konduri, G. G. (2009). Inhaled nitric oxide for preterm neonates. *Clinics in Perinatology 36,* 43–61.

22. Attar, M. A., & Donn, S. M. (2002). Mechanisms of ventilator-induced injury in premature infants. *Seminars in Neonatology, 7,* 353–360.

23. Barbosa, V. M., Campbell, S. K., & Berbaum, M. (2007). Discriminating infants from different developmental outcome groups using the Test of Infant Motor Performance (TIMP) item responses. *Pediatric Physical Therapy, 19,* 28–39.

24. Barbosa, V. M., Campbell, S. K., Smith, E., & Berbaum, M. (2005). Comparison of Test of Infant Motor Performance (TIMP) item responses among children with cerebral palsy, developmental delay, and typical development. *American Journal of Occupational Therapy, 59,* 446–456.

25. Barnard, K. E., & Eyres, S. J. (1979). *Child health assessment.* Part 2: The first year of life. (DHEW Publication No HRA79-25), Bethesda, MD. US Government Printing Office, Washington D.C.

26. Barney, C. K., Baer, V. L., Schoffield, S. H., et al. (2009). Lansoprazole, ranitidine, and metoclopramide: comparison of practice patterns at 4 level III NICUs within one healthcare system. *Advances in Neonatal Care, 9*(3), 129–131.

27. Bassler, D., Stoll, B. J., Schmidt, B., et al. (2009). Using a count of neonatal morbidities to predict poor outcome in extremely low birth weight infants: Added role of neonatal infection. *Pediatrics, 123,* 313–318.

28. Beauman, S. S. (2005). Identification and management of neonatal abstinence syndrome. *Journal of Infusion Nursing, 28,* 159–167.

29. Beck, C. (1999). Postpartum depression: Stopping the thief that steals motherhood. *AWHONN Lifelines, 3,* 41–44.

30. Beligere, N., & Rao, R. (2008). Neurodevelopmental outcome of infants with meconium aspiration syndrome: Report of a study and literature review. *Journal of Perinatology, 28,* S93–S101.

31. Bellieni, C. V., Buonocore, G., Nenci, A., Franci, N., Cordelli, D. M., & Bagnoli, F. (2001). Sensorial saturation: An effective analgesic tool for heel-prick in preterm infants. *Biology of the Neonate, 80,* 15–18.

32. Berghella, V. (Ed.). (2007). Obstetric and maternal-fetal evidence-based guidelines (2 volumes). UK: Informa Healthcare. Thompson.

33. Bhandari, A., & Bhandari V. (2009). Pitfalls, problems, and progress in bronchopulmonary dysplasia. *Pediatrics, 123,* 1562–1573.

34. Bhandari, A., & Panitch HB. (2006). Pulmonary outcomes in bronchopulmonary dysplasis. *Seminar in Perinatology, 30,* 219–226.

35. Bhutta, A. T. (2007). Ketamine: A controversial drug for neonates. *Seminars in perinatology, 31*, 303–308.

36. Bhutta, A. T., & Anand, K. J. (2002). Vulnerability of the developing brain: neuronal mechanisms. *Clin Perinatol, 29*(3), 357–372.

37. Birch, J. L., & Newell, S. J. (2009). Managing gastro-oesophageal reflux in infants. *Arch Dis Child Fetal Neonatal, 47*, 134–137.

38. Blackburn, S. T., & Ditzenberger, G. R. (2007). Neurologic system. In Kenner C. & Lott J. (Eds.), *Comprehensive neonatal care* (Chap. 12). Philadelphia: Saunders/Elsevier.

39. Blanchard, Y. (1991). Early intervention and stimulation of the hospitalized preterm infant. *Infants and Young Children, 4*(1), 76–84.

40. Blanchard, Y. (2009). Using the Newborn Behavioral Observations (NBO) system with at-risk infants and families: United States. In J. K. Nugent, T. B. Brazelton, & B. Patrauskas (Eds.), *The newborn as a person: Enabling healthy infant development worldwide* (pp. 120–128). Hoboken, NJ: John Wiley & Sons.

41. Reference deleted in page proofs.

42. Blanchard, Y., & Mouradian, L. (2000). Integrating neurobehavioral concepts into early intervention eligibility evaluation. *Infants and Young Children, 13*(2), 41–50.

43. Bombell, S., & McGuire, W. (2008). Delayed introduction of progressive enteral feeds to prevent necrotizing enterocolitis in the very low birth weight infants. *Cochrane Database of Systematic Review, 16*, CD001970.

44. Bradshaw, W. T. (2009). Necrotizing enterocolitis: Etiology, presentation, management, and outcomes. *Journal of Perinatal and Neonatal Nursing, 23*, 87–94.

45. Braun, M. A., & Palmer, M. M. (1985). A pilot study of oral-motor dysfunction in "at-risk" infant. *Physical & Occupational Therapy in Pediatrics, 5*(4), 13–26.

46. Brazelton, T. B. (1962). Crying in infancy. *Pediatrics, 29*, 579–588.

47. Brazelton, T. B., & Nugent, J. K. (1995). *The Newborn Behavioral Assessment Scale*. London: McKeith.

48. Bremer, P., Byers, J. F., & Kiehl, E. (2003). Noise and the premature infant: Physiological effects and practice implication. *Journal of Obstetric, Gynecologic, and Neonatal Nursing, 32*, 447–453.

49. Brown, G. (2009). NICU noise and the preterm infant. *Neonatal Network, 28*(3), 165–173.

50. 50. Bruschweiler-Stern, N. (1997). Mère à terme et mère prématurée (The full-term and preterm mother). In M. Dugnat (Ed.), *Le Monde Relationnel du bébé (The Relational World of the Newborn)* (pp. 19–24). Ramonville Saint-Agne, France: ERES.

51. Burd, L., & Hofer, R. (2008). Biomarkers for detection of prenatal alcohol exposure: A critical review of fatty acid ethyl asters in meconium. *Birth Defects Research, 82*, 487–493.

52. Cameron, E. C., Maehle, V., & Reid J. (2005). The effects of an early physical therapy intervention for very preterm, very low birth weight infants: A randomized controlled clinical trial. *Pediatric Physical Therapy, 17*, 107–119.

53. Cameron, E. C., Raingangar, V., & Khoori, N. (2007). Effects of handling procedures on pain responses of very low birth weight infants. *Pediatric Physical Therapy, 19*, 40–47.

54. Campbell, S. K. (1986). Organizational and educational considerations in creating an environment to promote optimal development of high-risk neonates. *Physical and Occupational Therapy in Pediatrics, 6*(3/4), 191–204.

55. Campbell, S. K. (1999). Test-retest reliability of the Test of Infant Motor Performance. *Pediatric Physical Therapy, 11*, 60–66.

56. Campbell, S. K., & Murney, M. E. (1998). The ecological relevance of the Test of Infant Motor Performance Elicited Scale items. *Phys Ther, 78*, 479–489.

57. Campbell, S. K., & Hedeker, D. (2001). Validity of the Test of Infant Motor Performance for discriminating among infants with varying risk for poor motor outcome. *Journal of Pediatrics, 139*, 546–551.

58. Campbell, S. K., Levy, P., Zawacki, L., & Liao, P. J. (2006). Population-based age standards for interpreting results on the Test of Infant Motor Performance. *Pediatric Physical Therapy, 18*, 119–125.

59. Campbell, S. K., & Kolobe, T. H. A. (2000). Concurrent validity of the Test of Infant Motor Performance with the Alberta Infant Motor Scale. *Pediatric Physical Therapy, 12*, 1–8.

60. Campbell, S. K., Kolobe, T. H. A., Osten, E. T., Lenke, M., & Girolami, G. L. (1995). Construct validity of the Test of Infant Motor Performance. *Physical Therapy, 75*(7), 585–596.

61. Campbell, S. K., Kolobe, T. H. A., Wright, B., & Linacre, J. M. (2002). Validity of the Test of Infant Motor Performance for prediction of 6-, 9-, and 12-month scores on the Alberta Infant Motor Scale. *Developmental Medicine and Child Neurology, 44*, 263–272.

62. Campbell, S. K., Swanlund, A., Smith, E., Liao, P., & Zawacki L. (2008). Validity of the TIMPSI for estimating concurrent performance on the Test of Infant Motor Performance. *Pediatric Physical Therapy, 20*, 3–210.

63. Cardone, I. A., & Gilkerson, L. (1990). Family Administered Neonatal Activities: A first step in the integration of parental perceptions and newborn behavior. *Infant Mental Health Journal, 11*, 127–131.

64. Carlson, B., Walsh, S., Wergin, T., Schwarzkopt, K., & Ecklund, S. (2006). Challenges in design and transition to a private room model in the neonatal intensive care unit. *Advances Neonatal Care, 6*, 271–280.

65. Carter, J. D., Mulder, R. T., Bartram, A. F., & Darlow, B. A. (2005). Infants in a neonatal intensive care unit: Parental response. *Archives of Disease in Childhood. Fetal and Neonatal Edition, 90*, F109–F113.

66. Challis, J. R., Lye, S. J., Gibb, W., Whittle, W., Patel, F., & Alfaidy, N. (2001). Understanding preterm labor. *Annals of New York Academy of Science, 943*, 225–234.

67. Chow, L. C., Wright, K. W., & Sola, A. (2003). Can changes in clinical practice decrease the incidence of severe retinopathy or prematurity in very low birth weight infants? *Pediatrics, 111*, 339–349.

68. Cifuentes, J., & Carlo, W. (2007). Respiratory system. In C. Kenner & J. W. Lott (Eds.), *Comprehensive neonatal care: An interdisciplinary approach* (4th ed.), Philadelphia: Elsevier.

69. Cignacco, E., Mueller, R., Hamers, J., & Gessler, P. (2004). Pain assessment in the neonate using the Bernese Pain Scale for Neonates, *Early Human Development, 78*, 125–131.

70. Cleveland, L. M. (2008). Parenting in the neonatal intensive care unit. *Journal of Obstetrics, Gynecological and Neonatal Nursing, 37*, 666–691.

71. Committee on Perinatal Health. (1976). *Toward improving the outcome of pregnancy: Recommendations for the regional development of maternal and perinatal health services.* White Plains, NY: March of Dimes National Foundation.

72. Corff, K. E., Seideman, R., Venkataraman, P. S., Lutes, L., & Yates, B. (1995). Facilitated tucking: A nonpharmacologic comfort measure for pain in preterm neonates. *Journal of Obstetric, Gynecologic, & Neonatal Nursing, 24*, 143–148.

73. Corvaglia, L., Mariani, E., Aceti, A., Capretti, G., et al. (2009). Combined oesophgeal impedance-pH monitorying in preterm newborn: comparison of two options for layout analysis. *Neurogastroenterology Motil, 21*, 1027–e81.

74. Daley, H., & Kennedy, C. (2000). Meta analysis: Effects of interventions on premature infants feeding. *Journal of Perinatal and Neonatal Nursing, 4*(3), 62–77.

75. Damus, K. (2008). Prevention of preterm birth: A renewed national priority. *Current Opinion Obstetric Gynecology, 20*, 590–596.

76. D'Apolito, K. (1991). What is an organized infant? *Neonatal Network, 10*(1), 23–29.

77. D'Apolito, K., & Hepworth, J. T. (2001). Prominence of withdrawal symptoms in polydrug-exposed infants. *Journal of Perinatal and Neonatal Nursing, 14*(4), 46–60.

78. Darcy, A. E., Hancock, L. E., & Ware E. J. (2008). A descriptive study of noise in the neonatal intensive care unit: Ambient levels and perceptions of contributing factors. *Advanced Neonatal Care, 8*(5 Supplement), S16–S26.

79. Darlow, B. A., &Graham, P. J. (2002). Vitamin A supplementation for preventing morbidity and mortality in very low birthweight infants. *Cochrane Database Systematic Reviews, 4*, CD000501.

80. Das Eiden, R., & Reifman, A. (1996). Effects of Brazelton demonstrations on later parenting. *Journal of Pediatric Psychology, 21*(6), 857–868.

81. De Moraes Barros, M. C., Guinsburg, R., de Araujo Peres, C., Mitsuhiro, S., Chalem, E., & Laranjeira, R. R. (2006). Neurobehavior of full-term small for gestational age newborn infants of adolescent mothers. *Journal of Pediatrics, 149*(6), 781–787.

82. Deng, W., Pleasure, J., & Pleasure, D. (2008). Progress in periventricular leukomalacia. *Archives of Neurology, 65*, 1291–1295.

83. Dennery, P. A. (2005). Metalloporphyrins for the treatment of neonatal jaundice. *Current Opinions in Pediatrics, 17*, 167–169.

84. Dennery, P. A., Seidman, D. S., & Stevenson, D. K. (2001). Neonatal hyperbilirubinemia. *New England Journal of Medicine, 344*(8), 581–590.

85. deVries, L. S., & Rennie, J. M. (2005). Neurological problems of the neonate: Preterm cerebral hemorrhage. In J. M. Rennie (Ed.), *Roberton's textbook of neonatology* (4th ed., pp. 1148–1169). Edinburgh: Churchill Livingstone.

86. De Vries, L. S., Van Haastert, I. L., Rademaker, K. J., Koopman, C., & Groenendaal, F. (2004). Ultrasound abnormalities preceding cerebral palsy in high-risk infants. *Journal of Pediatrics, 144*, 815–820.

87. Dhillion, A. S., & Ewer, A. K. (2004). Diagnosis and management of gastroesophageal reflux in preterm infants in neonatal intensive care units. *Acta Paediatica, 93*, 88–93.

88. Dubowitz, L., & Dubowitz, V. (1981). *The neurological assessment of the preterm and full-term newborn infant.* London: Heinemann.

89. Dubowitz, L., Dubowitz, V., & Mercuri, E. (1999). *The neurological assessment of the preterm and full-term newborn infant* (2nd ed.). London: McKeith.

90. Ehrenkranz, R. A., Walsh, M. C., Vohr, B. R., et al. (2005). Validation of National Institute of Health consensus definition of bronchopulmonary dysplasia. *Pediatrics, 116*, 1353–1360.

91. El Shahed, A. I., Dargaville, P., Ohisson, A., & Soll, R. F. (2007). Surfactant for meconium aspiration syndrome in full term/near term infants. *Cochrane Database Systematic Reviews, 2*, CD002054.

92. Fanaroff, A. A. (2008). Meconium aspiration syndrome: Historical aspects. *Journal of Perinatalogy, 28*, s3–s7.

93. Fanaroff, A. A., & Graven, S. N. (1992). Perinatal services and resources. In A. A. Fanaroff & R. J. Martin, (Eds.), *Neonatal-Perinatal Medicine: Diseases of the Fetus and Infant* (pp. 12–21). St. Louis, MO: Mosby.

94. Fanaroff, A. A., Stoll, B. J., Wright, L. L., et al. (2007). Trends in neonatal morbidity and mortality for very low birthweight infants. *American Journal of Obstetrics and Gynecology, 196*, 147.e1–e8.

95. Feldman, R. (2007). Parent-infant synchrony and the construction of shared timing: Physiological precursors, developmental outcomes and risk conditions. *Journal of Child Psychology and Psychiatry, 48*(3/4), 329–354.

96. Feldman, R., & Eidelman, A. I. (2003). Skin to skin contact (kangaroo care) accelerates autonomic and neurobehavioral maturation in preterm infants. *Developmental Medicine and Child Neurology, 45*, 274–281.

97. Finan, D. S., & Barlow, S. (1996). The actifier: A device for neurophysiological studies of orofacial control in human infants. *Journal of Speech and Hearing Research, 39*, 833–838.

98. Fitzgerald, M., & Anand, K. J. S. (1993). Developmental neuranatomy and neurophysiology of pain. In N. L. Schechter, C. B. Berde, & M. Yaster (Eds.), *Pain in infants, children and adolescents* (pp. 11–32). Baltimore: Williams and Wilkins.

99. Fitzgerald, M., & Beggs, S. (2001). The neurobiology of pain: Developmental aspects. *Neuroscientist, 7*(3), 246–257.

100. Flegel, J., & Kolobe, T. H. A. (2002). Predictive validity of the Test of Infant Motor Performance as measured by the Bruininks-Oseretsky Test of Motor Proficiency at school age. *Physical Therapy, 82,* 762–771.

101. Fukuda, A. (2005). Diuretic soothes seizures in newborns. *Nature Medicine, 11,* 1153–1154.

102. Gaebler, C., & Hanzlik, R. (1996). The effects of prefeeding stimulation program on preterm infants. *American Journal of Occupational Therapy, 50,* 184–192.

103. Geary, C., Caskey, M., Fonseca, R., & Malloy, M. (2008). Decreased incidence of bronchopulmonary dysplasia after early management changes, including surfactant and nasal continuous positive airway pressure treatment at delivery, lowered oxygen saturation goals, and early amino acid administration: A historical cohort study. *Pediatrics, 121,* 89–96.

104. Glass, P., Avery, G. B., Siva Subramanian, K. N., Keys, M. P., Sostek, A. M., & Friendly, D. S. (1985). Effect of bright light in the hospital nursery on the incidence of retinopathy of prematurity. *New England Journal of Medicine, 313,* 401–404.

105. Gluckman, P. D., Wyatt, J. S., Azzopardi, D., et al. (2005). Selective head cooling with mild systemic hypothermia after neonatal encephalopathy: Multicenter randomized trial. *Lancet, 365,* 663–670.

106. Gomes-Pedro, J., de Almeida, J. B., & Costa Barbosa, A. (1984). Influence of early mother-infant contact on dyadic behavior during the first month of life. *Developmental Medicine and Child Neurology, 26,* 657–664.

107. Goodman, D. G., Fisher, E. S., Little, G. A., Stukel, T. A., Chang, C. H., & Schoendorf, K. S. (2002). The relation between the availability of neonatal intensive care and neonatal mortality. *New England Journal of Medicine, 346,* 1538–1544.

108. Gottfried, A. W. (1985). Environment of newborn infants in special care units. In A. W. Gottfried & J. L. Gaiter, (Eds.), *Infant stress under intensive care* (pp. 23–54). Baltimore: University Park Press.

109. Granelli, S. L. P., & McGrath, J. (2004). Neonatal seizures: Diagnosis, pharmacologic interventions and outcomes. *Journal of Perinatal and Neonatal Nursing, 18,* 275–287.

110. Grave, G. D., Nelson, S. A., Walker, W. A., et al. (2007). New therapies and preventive approached for necrotizing enterocolitis: Report of a research planning workshop. *Pediatric Research, 62,* 510–514.

111. Graven, S. N. (1997). Clinical research data illuminating the relationship between the physical environment and patient medical outcomes. *Journal Healthcare Design, 9,* 15–19.

112. Graven, S. N. (2004). Early neurosensory visual development of the fetus and newborn. *Clinics in Perinatology, 31*(2), 199–216.

113. Graven, S. N. (2000). Sound and the developing infant in the NICU: Conclusions and recommendations for care. *Journal of Perinatology, 20*(8), S88–S93.

114. Green, N. S., Damus, K., Simpson, J. L., et al. (2005). Research agenda for preterm birth: Recommendations from the March of Dimes. *American Journal of Obstetrics and Gynecology, 193,* 626–635.

115. Grunau, E., Holsti, L., Whitfield, M., & Ling, E. (2000). Are twitches, startles, and body movements pain indicators in extremely low birth weight infants? *Clinical Journal of Pain, 16,* 37–45.

116. Grunau, R. V. E., Johnston, C. C., & Craig, K. D. (1990). Neonatal facial and cry responses to invasive and non-invasive procedures. *Pain, 42,* 295–305.

117. Guerri, C., Bazinet, A., & Riley, E. (2009). Fetal alcohol disorders and alterations in brain and behavior. *Alcohol & Alcoholism, 44,* 108–144.

118. Gunes, T., Ozturk, M. A., Koklu, E., Kose, K., & Gunes, I. (2007). Effect of allopurinol supplementation on nitric oxide levels in asphyxiated newborns. *Pediatric Neurology, 36,* 17–24.

119. Hall, R. & Anand, K. J. S. (2005). Physiology of pain and stress in the newborn. *NeoReviews, 6,* e61–e68.

120. Halliday, H. L., Ehrenkranz, R. A., & Coyle, L. W. (2003). Delayed postnatal corticosteroids for chronic lung disease in preterm infants. *Cochrane Database Systematic Reviews 1,* CD001145.

121. Halvorsen, T., Skadberg, B. T., Eide, G. E., Røksund, O. D., Carlsen, K. H., & Bakke, P. (2004). Pulmonary outcome in adolescents of extreme preterm birth: A regional cohort study. *Acta Paediatrica, 93,* 1294–1300.

122. Harmon, S. L., & McManus, B. M. (2007). Developmentally Supportive Care. In J. P. Cloherty, E. C. Eichenwald, & A. R. Stark (Eds.), *Manual of Neonatal Care* (pp. 154–158). Baltimore, MD: Lippincott Williams and Wilkins.

123. Hatzidaki, E., Giahnakis, E., Maraka, S., et al. (2009). Risk factors for periventricular leukomalacia. *Acta Obstetricia et Gynecologica Scandinavica, 88,* 110–115.

124. Hawdon, J. M., Beauregard, N., Slattery, J., & Kennedy, G. (2000). Identification of neonates at risk of developing feeding problems in infancy. *Dev Med Child Neurol, 42,* 235–239.

125. Henderson-Smart, D. J., Cools, F., Bhuta, T., & Offringa, M. (2007). Elective high frequency oscillatory ventilation versus conventional ventilation for acute pulmonary dysfunction in preterm infants. *Cochrane Database of Systematic Reviews, 18*(3), CD000104.

126. Hill, S., Engle, S., Jorgensen, J., Kralik, A., & Whitman, K. (2005). Effects of facilitated tucking during routine care of infants born preterm. *Pediatric Physical Therapy, 17,* 158–163.

127. Hilton, A. (1987). The hospital racket: How noisy is your unit? *American Journal of Nursing, 87,* 59–61.

128. Hintz, S. R., Kendrick, D. E., Vohr, B. R., Poole, W. K., & Higgins, R. D. (2005). Changes in neurodevelopmental outcomes at 18 to 22 months' corrected age among infants of less than 25 weeks' gestational age born in 1993–1999. *Pediatrics, 115,* 1645.

129. Ho, L. (2002). Bronchopulmonary dysplasia and chronic lung disease of infancy: Strategies for preventions and management. *Annals of the Academy of Medicine, Singapore, 31,* 119–130.

130. Hodgman, J. E. (1985). Introduction. In A. W. Gottfried & J. L. Gaiter (Eds.), *Infant stress under intensive care* (pp. 1–6). Baltimore: University Park Press.

131. Hoehn, T., Krause, M. F., & Buhrer, C. (2006). Metal-analysis of inhaled nitric oxide in premature infants: An update. *Klinische Pädiatrie, 218,* 57–61.

132. Holsti, L., & Grunau, R. E. (2007). Extremity movements help occupational therapists identify stress responses in preterm infants in the neonatal intensive care unit: A systematic review. *Canadian Journal of Occupational Therapy, 74,* 183–194.

133. Honrubia, D., & Stark, A. R. (2004). Respiratory distress syndrome. In J. P. Cloherty, E. C. Eichenwald, & A. R. Stark (Eds.), *Manual of neonatal care* (5th ed.). Philadelphia: Lippincott Williams & Wilkins.

134. Horton, K. K. (2005). Pathophysiology and current management of necrotizing enterocolitis. *Neonatal Network, 24,* 37–46.

135. International Committee on Retinopathy of Prematurity (ICROP). (1984). An international classification of retinopathy of prematurity. *Pediatrics, 74,* 127–133.

136. International Committee on Retinopathy of Prematurity. (2005). The international classification of retinopathy of prematurity revisited. *Archives of Ophthalmology, 123,* 991–999.

137. Jeng, S. F., Hsu, C. H., Tsao, P. N., et al. (2008). Bronchopulmonary dysplasia predicts adverse and clinical outcomes in very-low-birth-weight infants. *Developmental Medicine and Child Neurology, 50,* 51–57.

138. Johnson, N. N. (2007). The maternal experience of kangaroo holding. *Journal of Obstetrics, Gynecological and Neonatal Nursing, 36*(6), 568–573.

139. Kakko, J., Heilig, M., & Sarman, I. (2008). Buprenorphine and methadone treatment of opiate dependence during pregnancy: Comparison of fetal growth and neonatal outcomes in two consecutive case series. *Drug Alcohol Dependence, 97,* 69–78.

140. Kappas, A., Drummond, G. S., Munson, D. P., & Marshall, J. R. (2001). Sn-Mesoporphyrin interdiction of severe hyperbilirubinemia in Jehovah's Witness newborns as an alternative to exchange transfusion. *Pediatrics, 108*(6), 1374–1377.

141. Keefer, C. H. (1995). The combined physical and behavioral neonatal examination: A parent-centered approach to pediatric care. In T. B. Brazelton & J. K. Nugent, (Eds.), *Neonatal Behavioral Assessment Scale* (pp. 92–101). London: Mac Keith Press.

142. Keller, A., Arbel, N., Merlob, P., & Davidson, S. (2003). Neurobehavioral and autonomic effects of hammock positioning in infants with very low birth weight. *Pediatric Physical Therapy, 15,* 3–7.

143. Keszler, M. (2009). State of the art in conventional mechanical ventilation. *Journal of Perinatology, 29,* 262–275.

144. Kenner, C., & Lott, J. W. (Eds.) (2003). Respiratory system. In *Comprehensive neonatal care* (pp. 1–17). St. Louis: Saunders/Elsevier.

145. Kinney, H. C. (2005). Human myelinization and perinatal white matter disorders. *Journal of Neurological Sciences, 228,* 190–192.

146. Kinney, H. C. (2006). The near-term (late preterm) human brain and risk for periventricular leukomalacia: A review. *Seminars in Perinatology, 33,* 793–801.

147. Klaus, H. H., Kennell, J. H., & Klaus, P. H. (1995). *Bonding.* Reading, MA: Addison Wesley Longman.

148. Krechel, S. W., & Bildner, J. (1995). CRIES: A new neonatal postoperative pain measurement score. Initial testing of validity and reliability. *Pediatric Anaesthesia, 5,* 53–61.

149. Kumpfer, K. L., & Fowler, M. A. (2007). Parenting skills and family support programs for drug-abusing mothers. *Seminars Fetal Neonatal Medicine, 12,* 134–142.

150. Lahra, M., Beeby, P., & Jeffrey, H. (2009). Intrauterine inflammation, neonatal sepsis, and chronic lung disease: A 13-year hospital cohort study. *Pediatrics, 123,* 1314–1319.

151. Larsson, E., & Holmstrom, G. (2002). Screening for retinopathy of prematurity: evaluation and modification of guidelines. *British Journal of Ophthalmology, 86*(12), 1399–1402.

152. Lasky, R. E., & Williams, A. L. (2009). Noise and light exposures for extremely low birth weight newborns during their stay in the neonatal intensive care unit. *Pediatrics, 123,* 540–546.

153. Latal, B. (2009). Prediction of neurodevelopmental outcome after preterm birth. *Pediatric Neurology, 40,* 413–419.

154. Lauderet, S., Liu, W. F., Blackington, S., et al. (2007). Implementing potentially better practices to support the neurodevelopment of infants in the NICU. *Journal of Perinatology, 27,* S75–.

155. Lawhon, G. (2002). Facilitation of parenting the premature infant within the newborn intensive care unit. *Journal of Perinatal and Neonatal Nursing, 16*(1), 71–83.

156. Law-Morstatt, L., Judd, D. M., Snyder, P., Baier, R. J., & Dhanireddy, R. (2003). Pacing as a treatment techniques for transitional sucking patterns. *Journal of Perinatology, 23,* 483–488.

157. Lawrence, J., Alcock, D., McGrath, P., Kay, J., MacMurray, S. B., & Dulberg, C. (1993). The development of a tool to assess neonatal pain. *Neonatal Network, 12,* 59–66.

158. Lee, Y., Malakooti, N., & Lotas, M. (2005). A comparison of the light-reduction capacity of commonly used incubator covers. *Neonatal Network, 24,* 37–42.

159. Leef, K. H. (2006). Evidence-based review of oral sucrose administration to decrease the pain response in newborn infants. *Neonatal Network, 25,* 275–284.

160. Lemmons, J. A., Bauer, C. R., Oh, W., et al. (2001). Very low birth weight outcomes of the National Institute of Child Health and Human Development Neonatal Research Network, January 1995 through December 1996. NICHD Neonatal Research Network. *Pediatrics, 107,* E1.

161. Lester, B. M., & Tronick, E. Z. (2004). History and description of the neonatal intensive care unit network neurobehavioral scale. *Pediatrics, 113,* 634–640.

162. Lester, B. M., & Tronick, E. Z. (2005). *NICU Network Neurobehavioral Scale.* Baltimore: Brookes.

163. Levene, M. I., & de Vries, L. (2006). Hypoxic-ischemic encephalopathy. In *Neonatal-perinatal medicine* (pp. 938–944). Philadelphia: Mosby.

164. Liauw, I., Palm-Meinders, I. H., Van der Grond, J., et al. (2007). Differentiating normal myelination from hypoxic-ischemic encephalopathy on T1 weighted MR images: A new approach. *American Journal of Neuroradiology, 28,* 660–665.

165. Lin, P. W., Nasr, T. R., & Stoll, B. J. (2008). Necrotizing enterocolitis: Recent scientific advances in pathophysiology and prevention. *Seminars in Perinatology, 32,* 70–82.

166. Liu, W. F., Laudert, S., Perkins, B., Macmillan-York, E., Martin, S., & Graven, S. (2007). The development of potentially better practices to support the neurodevelopment of infants in the NICU. *Journal of Perinatology, 27,* S48–S74.

167. Lobel, M. (2008). Pregnancy-specific stress, prenatal health behaviors, and birth outcomes. *Health Psychology, 27,* 604–615.

168. Long, T. (2001). *Handbook of pediatric physical therapy.* Baltimore: Lippincott, Williams, & Wilkins.

169. Loo, K. K., Espoinosa, M., Tyler, R., & Howard, J. (2003). Using knowledge to cope with stress in the NICU: How parents integrate learning to read the physiologic and behavioral cues of the infant. *Neonatal Network, 22*(1), 31–37.

170. Louie, J. P. (2007). Essential diagnosis of abdominal emergencies in the first year of life. *Emergency Medical Clinics of North America, 25,* 1009–1040.

171. Ludington-Hoe, S. M., & Swinth, J. Y. (2001). Kangaroo care during phototherapy: Effect on bilirubin profile. *Neonatal Network, 20,* 41–48.

172. Ludwig, A. K., Sutcliff, A. G., Diedrich, K., & Ludwig, M. (2006). Post-neonatal health and development of children born after assisted reproduction: A systematic review of controlled studies. *European Journal Obstetric Gynecology Reproductive Biology, 127,* 3–25.

173. Madan, A., Hamrick, S., & Ferriero, D. (2005). Central nervous system injury and neuroprotection. In H. W. Taeusch, R. Ballard, C. Gleason, & M. E. Avery, (Eds.), *Avery's diseases of the newborn* (8th ed., pp. 965–992). Philadelphia: Saunders.

174. Malusky, S. K. (2005). A concept analysis of family-centered care in the NICU. *Neonatal Network, 24*(6), 25–32.

175. Mantagos, I. S., Vanderveen, D. K., & Smith, L. (2009). Emerging treatments for retinopathy of prematurity. *Seminars in Ophthalmology, 24,* 82–86.

176. March of Dimes. Premature birth, www.marchofdimes.com/prematurity.

177. Marlow, N., Wolke, D., Bracewell, M. A., & Samara, M. (2005). Neurologic and developmental disability at six years of age after extremely preterm birth. *New England Journal of Medicine, 352*(1), 9–19.

178. Matthews, T. J., Menacker F, & MacDorman, M. F. (2004). Infant mortality statistics from the 2002 period. Linked birth-death data set. *National Vital Statistics Report, 53,* 1–29.

179. McAnulty, G. B., Duffy, F. H., Butler, S., Parad, R., Singer, S., Zurakowski, D., & Als, H. (2009). Individualized developmental care for a large sample of very preterm infants: health, neurobehaviour and neurophysiology.

180. McBride, M. C., Laroia, N, & Guillet, R. (2000). Electrographic seizures in neonates correlate with poor neurodevelopmental outcome. *Neurology, 55,* 506–513.

181. McCormick, M. C., & Richardson, D. K. (1995). Access to neonatal intensive care. *Future Child, 5*(1), 162–175.

182. McCrea, H. J., & Ment, L. R. (2008). The diagnosis, management, and postnatal prevention of intraventricular hemorrhage in the preterm neonate. *Clinics in Perinatology, 35,* 777–792.

183. McGrath, J. M. (2007). Implementation of interventions that support sleep in the NICU. *Journal of Perinatal and Neonatal Nursing, 21,* 83–85.

184. McHaffie, H. E. (1990). Mothers of very low birthweight babies: How do they adjust? *Journal of Advanced Nursing, 15,* 6–11.

185. McManus, B. M., & Capistran, P. S. (2008). A Case Study of Early Intervention of Dolichocephaly in the Newborn Intensive Care Unit: Collaboration Between the Developmental Care Specialist and Primary Nursing Team. *Neonatal Network, 27*(5), 307–315.

186. Memon, S., & Memon, M. M. (2006). Spectrum and immediate outcome of seizures in neonates. *Journal of College of Physicians and Surgeons Pakistan, 16,* 717–720.

187. Ment, L. R., Bada, H. S., Barnes, et al. (2002). Practice parameter: Neuroimaging of the neonate. *Neurology, 58,* 1726–1738.

188. Ment, L. R., Vohr, B. R., Makuch, R. W., et al. (2004). Prevention of intraventricular hemorrhage by indomethacin in male preterm infants. *Journal of Pediatrics, 145,* 832–834.

189. Morris, B. H., Oh, W., Tyson, J. E., et al. (2008). Aggressive vs. conservative phototherapy for infants with extremely low birth weight. *New England Journal of Medicine, 359,* 1885–1896.

190. Murney, M. E., & Campbell, S. K. (1998). The ecological relevance of the Test of Infant Motor Performance Elicited Scale items. *Physical Therapy, 78,* 479–489.

191. National Institute of Child Health and Development. (2008). Surgeon General's Conference on the Prevention of Preterm Birth. Washington, DC. June 16–17, www.nichd.nih.gov/about/meetings/2008/SG_preterm-birth/agenda.clm; presentations can be accessed at http://videocast.nih.gov/PastEvents.asp?c=1.

192. Neff, J. M., Eichner, J. M., Hardy, D. R., Klein, M., Percelay, J. M. et al. (2003). Family-centered care and the pediatrician's role. *Pediatrics, 112*(3), 691–696.

193. Niccols, A. (2007). Fetal alcohol syndrome and the developing socio-emotional brain. *Brain Cognition, 65*(1), 135–142.

194. Nugent, J. K., & Blanchard, Y. (2005). Newborn behavior and development: Implications for health care professionals. In J. F. Travers & K. M. Thies (Eds.), *The handbook of human development for health care professionals* (pp. 79–94). Sudbury, MA: Jones & Bartlett.

195. Nugent, J. K., Blanchard, Y., & Stewart, J. S. (2008). Supporting parents of premature infants: An infant-focused family-centered approach. In D. Brodsky & M. A. Ouellette (Eds.). *Primary Care of the Premature Infant.* New York: Elsevier.

196. Nugent, J. K., Keefer, C. H., Minear, S., Johnson, L. C., & Blanchard, Y. (2007). *Understanding newborn behavior & early relationships: The Newborn Behavioral Observations (NBO) system handbook.* Baltimore: Brookes.

197. Nugent, J. K., Petrauskas, B. J., & Brazelton, T. B. (2009). *The newborn as a person.* Hoboken, NJ: Wiley & Sons.

198. Nye, C. (2008). Transitioning premature infants from gavage to breast. *Neonatal Network, 27*(1), 7–13.

199. Oh, W., & Gilstrap, I. (2002). *Guidelines for Perinatal Care* (5th ed.). Old Grove Village, IL: American Academy of Pediatrics, American College of Obstetrician and Gynecologists.

200. Orenstein, S. R., Cohn, J. F., Shalaby, T. M., et al. (1996). Reflux symptoms in 100 normal infants: Diagnostic validity of the infant gastroesophageal reflux questionnaire. *Clinical Pediatrics, 35,* 607–614.

201. Pacilli, M., Chowdhury, M., & Pierro, A. (2005). The surgical treatment of gastro-esophageal reflux in neonates and infants. *Seminars in Pediatric Surgery, 14,* 34–41.

202. Palisano, R. J. (2006). A collaborative model of service delivery for children with movement disorders: A framework for evidence-based decision making. *Physical Therapy, 86*(9), 1295–1305.

203. Palmer, M. M., Crawley, K., & Blanco, I. A. (1993). Neonatal Oral-Motor Assessment Scale: a reliability study. *J Perinatol, 13*(1), 28–35.

204. Papile, L., Munsick-Bruno, G., & Schaefer, A. (1983). Relationship of cerebral intraventricular hemorrhage and early childhood neurological handicaps. *Journal of Pediatrics, 193,* 273–277.

205. Parad, R. B. (2008). Bronchopulmonary dysplasia/chronic lung disease. In J.P. Cloherty, E. C. Eichenwald, & A. R. Stark (Eds.), *Manual of neonatal care* (6th ed.). Philadelphia: Lippincott Williams & Wilkins.

206. Parker, S., Zahr, L. K., Cole, J. C. D., & Braced, M. L. (1992). Outcomes after developmental intervention in the neonatal intensive care unit for mothers of preterm infants with low socioeconomic status. *Journal of Pediatrics, 120,* 780–785.

207. Pax Lowes, L., & Palisano, R. J. (1995). Review of medical and developmental outcome of neonates who received extracorporeal membrane oxygenation. *Pediatric Physical Therapy, 7,* 215–221.

208. Paz, M. S., Smith, L. M., LaGasse, L. L., et al. (2009). Maternal depression and neurobehavior in newborns prenatally exposed to methamphetamine. *Neurotoxicology & Teratology, 31*(3), 177–182.

209. Perkins, E., Ginn, L., Fanning, J. K., & Bartlett, D. J. (2004). Effect of nursing education on positioning of infants in the neonatal intensive care unit. *Pediatric Physical Therapy, 16,* 2–12.

210. Peters, K. L., Rosychuk, R. J., Hendson, L., Cote, J. J., McPherson, C., & Tyebkhan, J. M. (2009). Improvement of short- and long-term outcomes for very low birth weight infants: Edmonton NIDCAP trial. *Pediatrics, 124*(4), 1009–1020.

211. Pfister, R. H., Soll, R. F., & Wiswell, T. (2007). Protein containing synthetic surfactant versus animal derived surfactant extract for the prevention and treatment of respiratory distress syndrome. *Cochrane Database of Systematic Reviews,* Issue 4, CD006069.

212. Phelps, D., & Watts, J. (2001). Early light reduction for preventing retinopathy of prematurity in very low birth weight infants. *Cochrane Database of Systematic Reviews,* Issue 1, CD000122.

213. Philbin, M. K., Lickliter, R., & Graven, S. N. (2000). Sensory experience and the developing organism: A history of ideas and view to the future. *Journal of Perinatology, 20*(8 Pt 2), S2–S5.

214. Pierrehumbert, B., Nicole, A., Muller-Nix, C., Forcada-Guex, M., & Ansermet, F. (2003). Parental post-traumatic reactions after premature birth: Implications for sleeping and eating problems in the infant. *Archives of Disease in Childhood. Fetal and Neonatal Edition, 88,* 400–404.

215. Pinelli, J., & Symington, (2005). A. Non-nutritive sucking for promoting physiologic stability and nutrition in preterm infants. *Cochrane Database of Systematic Reviews,* Issue 4, CD001071.

216. Premji, S., Benzies, K., Serret, K., & Hayden, K. A. (2007). Research-based interventions for children and youth with fetal alcohol spectrum disorder: revealing the gap. *Child Care Health and Development, 33*(4), 389–397.

217. Ranger, M. (2007). Current controversies regarding pain assessment in neonates. *Seminars in Perinatology, 31,* 283–288.

218. Rauh, V., Achenbach, T., Nurcombe, B., Howell, C., & Teti, D. (1998). Minimizing adverse effects of low birthweight: Four-year results of an early intervention program. *Child Development, 59,* S44–553.

219. Redshaw, M. E. (1997). Mothers of babies requiring special care: Attitudes and experiences. *Journal of Reproductive & Infant Psychology, 15*(2), 109–121.

220. Reynolds, J. D., Hardy, R. J., Kennedy, K. A., Spencer, R., van Heuven, W. A., & Fielder, A. R. (1998). Lack of efficacy of light reduction in preventing retinopathy of prematurity. Light Reduction in Retinopathy of Prematurity Cooperative Group. *New England Journal of Medicine, 28,* 1572–1576.

221. Robinson, T. (2007). Hypothermia and the treatment of the term gestation infant with perinatal hypoxic-ischemic encephalopathy. *Journal of Kentucky Medical Association, 105,* 253–259.

222. Salisbury, A. L., Lester, B. M., Seifer, R., et al. (2007). Prenatal cocaine use and maternal depression: Effects on infant neurobehavior. *Neurotoxicology & Teratology, 29*(3), 331–340.

223. Sanders, L. W., & Buckner, E. B. (2009). The NBO as a nursing intervention. *Ab Initio,* Spring, www.brazelton-institute.com/abinitio2009spring.

224. Sansoucie, D., & Cavaliere, T. (2007). Assessment of the Newborn and Infant. In C. Kenner & J. W. Lott (Eds.). *Comprehensive neonatal care: An interdisciplinary approach* (4th ed.). Philadelphia: Elsevier.

225. Saunders, A. N. (1995). Incubator noise: A method to decrease decibels. *Pediatric Nursing, 21,* 265–268.

226. Schechner, S. (2008). Drug abuse and withdrawal. In J. P. Cloherty, E. C. Eichenwald, & A. R. Stark (Eds.), *Manual of*

neonatal care (6th ed.). Philadelphia: Lippincott Williams & Wilkins.

227. Schempf, A. H. (2007). Illicit drug use and neonatal outcomes: A critical review. *Obstetrical and Gynecological Survey, 62,* 749–757.

228. Schmidt, B., & David, P. (2001). Long-term effects of indomethacin prophylaxis in extremely-low-birth-weight infants. *New England Journal of Medicine, 344,* 1966–1972.

229. Schulzke, S., Trachsel, D., & Patole, S. (2007). Physical activity programs for promoting bone mineralization and growth in preterm infants. *Cochrane Database of Systematic Reviews,* Issue 2, CD005387.

230. Serane, V. T., & Kurian, O. (2008). Neonatal abstinence syndrome. *Indian Journal of Pediatrics, 75,* 911–914.

231. Shah, P. S., Aliwalas, L & Shah, V. (2007). Breastfeeding or breastmilk to alleviate procedural pain in neonates: A systematic review. *Breastfeeding Medicine, 2,* 74–82.

232. Shankaran, S., Laptook, A. R., Ehrenkranz, R. A., et al. (2005). Whole-body hypothermia for neonates with hypoxic-ischemic encephalopathy. *New England Journal of Medicine, 353,* 1574–1584.

233. Short, B. L. (2008). Extracorporeal membrane oxygenation: Use in meconium aspiration syndrome. *Journal of Perinatology, 28,* S279–S283.

234. Silverman, W. A. (1979). Incubator-baby side shows. *Pediatrics, 64,* 127–141.

235. Silverstein, F. S., & Jensen, F. E. (2007). Neonatal seizures. *Annals of Neurology, 62,* 112–120.

236. Slevin, M., Farrington, N., Duffy, G., Daly, L., & Murphy, J. F. (2000). Altering the NICU and measuring infants' responses. *Acta Paediatrics, 89,* 577–581.

237. Smith, L. E. (2004). Pathogenesis of retinopathy of prematurity. *Growth, Hormone, and IGF Research, 14,* S140–S144.

238. Smith, L. M., Lagasse, L. L., Derauf, C., et al. (2008). Prenatal methamphetamine and neonatal neurobehavioral outcome. *Neurotoxicology & Teratology, 30*(1), 20–28.

239. Smith, V. C., Zuponcic, J. A., McCormick, M. C., et al. (2004). Rehospitalization in the first year of life among infants with bronchopulmonary dysplasia. *Journal of Pediatrics, 144,* 799–803.

240. Soll, R., & Morley, C. J. (2001). Prophylactic versus selective use of surfactant in preventing morbidity and mortality in preterm infants. *Cochrane Database of Systematic Reviews,* Issue 2, CD00510.

241. Southgate, W. M., & Pittard, W. B. (2001). Classification and physical examination of the newborn infant. In M. H. Klaus & A. A, Fanaroff (Eds.), *Care of the high risk neonate* (5th ed.). Philadelphia: Saunders.

242. Spiker, D., Ferguson, J., & Brooks-Gunn, J. (1993). Enhancing maternal interactive behavior and child social competence in low birthweight, premature infants. *Child Development, 64,* 754–768.

243. Spittle, A. J., Doyle, L. W., & Boyd, R. N. (2008). A systematic review of the clinometric properties of neuromotor assessments for preterm infants during the first year of

life. *Developmental Medicine & Child Neurology, 50,* 254–266.

244. Steinberg, Z. (2006). Pandora meets the NICU parent or whither hope? *Psychoanalytic Dialogues, 16*(2), 133–147.

245. Stern, D. N. (1995). *The motherhood constellation.* New York: Basic Books.

246. Stevens, B., & Franck, L. (1995). Special needs of preterm infants in the management of pain and discomfort. *Journal of Gynecologic and Neonatal Nursing, 24,* 856–861.

247. Stevens, T. P., Blennow, M., Myers, E. H., & Soll, R. (2007). Early surfactant administration with brief ventilation vs. selective surfactant and continued mechanical ventilation for preterm infants with or at risk for respiratory distress syndrome. *Cochrane Database of Systematic Review,* Issue 4, CD003063.

248. Stevenson, D. K., Wright, L. L., Lemons, J. A., et al. (1998). Very low birth weight outcomes of the National Institute of Child Health and Human Development Neonatal Research Network, January 1993 through December 1994. *American Journal of Obstetrics and Gynecology, 179,* 1632–1639.

249. Stewart, J. (2008). Early intervention and follow-up programs for the premature infant. In D. Brodsky & M. A. Ouellette (Eds.), *Primary care of the premature infant* (pp. 285–288). Philadelphia: Saunders.

250. Stork, E. K. (1992). Extracorporeal membrane oxygenation. In A. A. Fanaroff & R. J. Martin (Eds.), *Neonatal-perinatal medicine: diseases of the fetus and infant* (pp. 876–882). St. Louis: Mosby.

251. Stout, A. U., & Stout, J. T. (2003). Retinopathy of prematurity. *Pediatric Clinics of North America, 50,* 77–87.

252. Strodtbeck, F. (2007). Opthalmic System. In C. Kenner & J. W. Lott (Eds). *Comprehensive neonatal care* (4th ed., pp. 313–332). Philadelphia: Saunders/Elsevier.

253. Stuberg, W., & DeJong, S. (2007). Program evaluation of physical therapy as an early intervention and related service in special education. *Pediatric Physical Therapy, 9,* 121–127.

254. Sumner, G., & Spietz, A. (1994). *NCAST Caregiver/Parent-Infant Interaction feeding manual.* Seattle, WA: NCAST Publications, University of Washington, School of Nursing.

255. Sweeney, J., & Gutierrez, T. (2002). Musculoskeletal implications of preterm infant positioning in the NICU. *Journal of Perinatal and Neonatal Nursing, 16*(1), 58–70.

256. Sweeney, J. K., Heriza, C. B., & Blanchard, Y. (2009). Neonatal physical therapy. Part I: Clinical competencies and NICU clinical training models. *Pediatric Physical Therapy, 21*(4), 296–307.

257. Sweeney, J. K., Heriza, C. B., Blanchard, Y., & Dusing, S. C. (2010). Neonatal physical therapy. Part II: Practice frameworks and evidence-based practice guidelines. *Pediatric Physical Therapy, 22*(1), 2–16.

258. Synnes, A. R., Macnab, Y. C., Qui, Z., et al. (2006). Neonatal intensive care unit characteristics affect the incidence of severe intraventricular hemorrhage. *Medical Care, 44,* 754–759.

259. Thibeault-Eybalin, M. P., Lortie, A., & Carmant, L. (2009). Neonatal seizures: Do they damage the brain? *Pediatric Neurology, 40,* 175–180.

260. Thigpen, J. (2007). Gastrointestinal system. In C. Kenner & J. W. Lott (Eds.), *Comprehensive neonatal care* (pp. 92–131). Philadelphia: Saunders/Elsevier.

261. Thomas, A., & Chess, S. (1977). *Temperament and development.* New York: Brunner-Maze.

262. Thoyre, S. M., Shaker, C. S., & Pridham, K. F. (2005). The early feeding skill assessment for preterm infants. *Neonatal Network, 24*(3), 7–16.

263. Vain, N. E., Szyld, E. G., Prudent, L. M., Wiswell TE, Aguilar, A. M., & Vivas, N. I. (2004). Oropharyngeal and nasopharyngeal suctioning of meconium-stained neonates before delivery of their shoulders: Multicenter, randomized, controlled trial. *Lancet, 364,* 597–602.

264. VanBel, F., Shadid, M., Moison, R. M. W., et al. (1998). Effect of allopurinol on postasphyxial free radiat formation, cerebral hemodynamics and electrical brain activity. *Pediatrics, 101,* 184–193.

265. Vergara, E R., & Bigsby, R. (2004). *Developmental and therapeutic interventions in the NICIU.* Towson, MD: Brookes.

266. Verklan, M. T. (2009). The chilling details: Hypoxic-ischemic encephalopathy. *Journal of Perinatal and Neonatal Nursing, 23,* 59–68.

267. Versaw-Barnes, D., & Wood, A. (2008). The infant at high risk for developmental delay. In J. Tecklin (Ed.), *Pediatric physical therapy* (4th ed., pp. 101–175). Philadelphia: Lippincott, William & Wilkin.

268. Volpe, J. R. (2008). *Neurology of the newborn* (5th ed.). Philadelphia: Saunders/Elsevier.

269. Vrijlandt, E. J., Gerritswen, J., Boezen, H. M., & Duiverman, E. J. (2005). Gender differences in respiratory symptoms in 19-year-old adults born preterm. *Respiratory Research, 6,* 117–121.

270. Walden, M. (2007). Pain in the newborn and infant. In C. Kenner & J. W. Lott (Eds.), *Comprehensive neonatal care.* Philadelphia: Saunders/Elsevier.

271. Walsh, W. F., McCullough, K. L., & White, R. D. (2006). Room for improvement: Nurses' perceptions of providing care in a single room newborn intensive care setting. *Advances Neonatal Car, 6,* 261–270.

272. Ward-Larson, C., Horn, R. A., & Gosnell, F. (2004). The efficacy of facilitated tucking for relieving procedural pain of endotracheal suctioning in very low birthweight infants. *MCN: The American Journal of Maternal Child Nursing, 29,* 151–156.

273. Watchko, J. F. (2009). Identification of neonates at risk for hazardous hyperbilirubinemia: Emerging clinical insights. *Pediatric Clinics of North America, 56,* 671–687.

274. Weinberg, J., Sliwowka, J. H., Lan, N., & Hellemans, KGC. (2008). Prenatal alcohol exposure: Foetal programming, the hypothalamic-pituitary-adrenal axis and sex differences in outcome. *Journal of Neuroendocrinology, 20,* 470–488.

275. White, R. D. (2007). Committee to establish recommended standards for newborn ICU design. Recommended standards for newborn ICU design: Report of Seventh Census Conference on Newborn ICU Design. Retrieved June 19, 2009, from www.nd.edu/~nicudes/index.html.

276. Whitelaw, A., & Odd, D. (2007). Postnatal Phenobarbital for the prevention intraventricular hemorrhage in preterm infants. *Cochrane Database Systematic Reviews, 17,* CD001691.

277. Widmayer, S., & Field, T. (1980). Effects of Brazelton demonstration on early interaction of preterm infants and their teenage mothers. *Infant Behavior and Development, 3,* 79–89.

278. Wiedemann, J. R., Saugstad, A. M., Barnes-Powell, L., & Duran, K. (2008). Meconium aspiration syndrome. *Neonatal Network, 27,* 81–87.

279. Williamson, D., Abe, K, Bean, C., Ferré, C., Henderson, Z., & Lackritz, E. (2008). Current Research in Preterm Birth. *Journal of Women's Health, 17,* 1545–1549.

280. Wilson-Costello, D., Friedman, H., Minich, N., et al. (2007). Improved neurodevelopmental outcomes for extremely low birth weight infants in 2000–2002. *Pediatrics, 119,* 37–45.

281. Wiswell, T. E., & Graziani, L. J. (2005). Intracranial hemorrhage and white matter injury in preterm infants. In A. R. Spitzer (Ed.), *Intensive care of the fetus and neonate* (2nd ed.). St Louis, MO: Mosby.

282. Wolff, P. H. (1959). Observations on human infants. *Psychoanalytic Medicine, 221,* 110–118.

283. World Health Organization. (2001). *International classification of functioning, disability, and health.* Geneva: World Health Organization.

284. Xu, H., Wei, S., & Fraser, W. D. (2008). Obstetric approaches to the prevention of meconium aspiration syndrome. *Journal of Perinatology, 28,* S14–S18.

285. Yeh, T. F., Lin, H. C., Chang, C. H., et al. (2008). Early intratracheal instillation of budesonide using surfactant as a vehicle to prevent chronic lung disease in preterm infants: A pilot study. *Pediatrics, 121,* e1310–e1318.

286. York, J. R., Landers, S., Kirby, R. S., & Arbogast, P. G. (2004). Arterial oxygen fluctuation and retinopathy of prematurity in very-low-birth-weight infants. *Journal of Perinatology, 24,* 82–87.

287. Yost, C. C., & Soll, R. F. (2000). Early versus delayed selective surfactant treatment for neonatal respiratory distress syndrome. *Cochrane Database of Systematic Reviews, 2,* CD001456.

288. Yu, B., Li, S., Lin, Z., & Zhang, N. (2009). Treatment of posthemorrhagic hydrocephalus in premature infants with subcutaneous reservoir drainage. *Pediatrics, 45,* 119–125.

289. Zanelli, S., & Fairchild, K. (2009). Physiologic and pharmacologic effects of hypothermia for neonatal hypoxic ischemic encephalopathy. *Newborn & Infant Nursing Reviews, 9,* 10–17.

29

Serving Infants, Toddlers, and Their Families: Early Intervention Services under IDEA

LISA A. CHIARELLO, PT, PhD, PCS

This chapter focuses on early intervention services in home and community settings under the U.S. Individuals with Disabilities Education Improvement Act (IDEA) of 2004.[97] Part C of the IDEA authorizes federal assistance to states to implement a system of early intervention services for eligible infants and toddlers, birth to 3 years of age, and their families. The law mandates family-centered services in natural environments to promote the child's development and participation in daily activities and routines. Providing services in early intervention can be complex and challenging, but very rewarding. Therapists practicing in early intervention truly have the opportunity to integrate the science and art of physical therapy. This chapter critiques theory, policy, and methods of service delivery and analyzes research. The role of the physical therapist in this unique approach to practice is discussed. The chapter concludes with the presentation of a collaborative model for early intervention service delivery and application, using a case vignette.

Early intervention is a multifaceted process to support infants and toddlers with developmental delay and disability and their families. Early intervention is predicated on the notion that infancy is a sensitive period in development and families assume the primary role of nurturing and providing early learning experiences for their children. The concept of sensitive periods assumes that children are more responsive to experiential learning during the first 3 years of life when there is rapid brain maturation and plasticity.[118] Shonkoff and Meisels[116] defined early intervention as consisting of

> multidisciplinary services … to promote child health and well-being, enhance emerging competencies, minimize developmental delays, remediate existing or emerging disabilities, prevent functional deterioration, and promote adaptive parenting and overall family functioning. These goals are accomplished by providing individualized developmental, educational, and therapeutic services for children in conjunction with mutually planned support for their families (pp. xvii–xviii)

This definition embraces the concepts of prevention, remediation, experiential learning, individuality, and family-centeredness and is consistent with the definition of early intervention in IDEA.

IDEA defines early intervention as

> developmental services that are provided under public supervision, are provided at no cost except where federal or state law provides for a system of payments by families, including a schedule of sliding fees, and are designed to meet the developmental needs of an infant or toddler with disability in any one or more of the following areas: physical development; cognitive development; communication development; social or emotional development; or adaptive development

In addition, IDEA stipulates that services are selected in collaboration with the parent. This definition emphasizes the service delivery aspect of early intervention; the primary premises are that services must be developmental and involve parent collaboration. Hebbeler and colleagues[58] have discussed that the Part C early intervention program is diverse in that it serves as both an intervention program to ameliorate the effects of disability for children with moderate to severe involvement and as a prevention and intervention program for children at-risk for delay or with mild involvement who will attain skills comparable with their peers.

To be effective in early intervention, physical therapists must embrace responsibilities that go beyond technical knowledge and skill. Early intervention providers are required to partner with families and other providers, deliver services in multiple environments, comply with federal and state policy, and provide interventions informed by current evidence and principles of best practice. In addition to expertise in motor development, adaptive function and self-care, physical therapists must have practical knowledge of family ecology and children's social, emotional, cognitive, communication, and language development.[117]

IDEA PART C: INFANTS AND TODDLERS

The Education of the Handicapped Act Amendments of 1986[95] provided for family-centered services for infants and toddlers from birth to 3 years of age. This law was subsequently reauthorized and amended as Part C of the

Individuals with Disabilities Education Act Amendment (IDEA) of 1997[96] and Individuals with Disabilities Education Improvement Act (IDEIA) of 2004[97] commonly referred to as IDEA. Part C mandates early intervention services based on the following declaration:

> [that] Congress finds that there is an urgent and substantial need (1) to enhance the development of infants and toddlers with disabilities and to minimize their potential for developmental delay, and to recognize the significant brain development that occurs during a child's first 3 years of life; (2) to reduce the educational costs to our society, including our Nation's schools, by minimizing the need for special education and related services after infants and toddlers with disabilities reach school age; (3) to maximize the potential for their independently living in society; (4) to enhance the capacity of families to meet the special needs of their infants and toddlers with disabilities; and (5) to enhance the capacity of state and local agencies and service providers to identify, evaluate, and meet the needs of all children, particularly minority, low-income, inner-city, and rural children and infants and toddlers in foster care" (IDEIA, Part C, Sec. 631).

The legislation details the conditions that a state must meet in order to receive federal funding. In addition, Part C clearly articulates particular philosophies of care related to individualized family care, coordination of services, and services in natural environments.

Part C stipulates that early intervention services are designed to meet the developmental needs of an infant or toddler with a developmental delay or disability (or diagnosed physical or mental condition with high probability of resulting in developmental delay) in any one or more of the following areas: physical development, cognitive development, communication development, social or emotional development, and adaptive development. Each state has its own definition of developmental delay, and thus eligibility for early intervention varies from state to state.[58] In Pennsylvania, children have to demonstrate a developmental delay of 25% in one of five areas; in New Jersey, children have to demonstrate a delay of 33% in one area or 25% in two or more areas; and in Oklahoma, children have to demonstrate a delay of 50% in one area or 25% in two or more areas. The list of early intervention services identified in the legislation is provided in Box 29-1. Services are to be provided by qualified personnel based on state licensing or certification requirements. Physical therapists are included under qualified personnel.

The components of service delivery identified in Part C are included in Box 29-2. The five major components are as follows:

- A public awareness program
- A central directory of information
- A comprehensive child find system
- Comprehensive evaluations and assessments
- An individualized family service plan (IFSP)

> **Box 29-1**   EARLY INTERVENTION SERVICES INCLUDED IN THE INDIVIDUALS WITH DISABILITIES EDUCATION IMPROVEMENT ACT
>
> - Family training, counseling, home visits
> - Special instruction
> - Speech-language pathology and audiology services, and sign language and cued language services
> - Occupational therapy
> - Physical therapy
> - Psychologic services
> - Service coordination
> - Medical services only for diagnostic or evaluation purposes
> - Early identification, screening, and assessment services
> - Health services necessary to enable the infant or toddler to benefit from the other early intervention services
> - Social work services
> - Vision services
> - Assistive technology devices and services
> - Transportation and related costs necessary to receive early intervention services

---

> **Box 29-2**   COMPONENTS OF PART C INFANT AND TODDLER PROGRAM OF THE INDIVIDUALS WITH DISABILITIES EDUCATION IMPROVEMENT ACT
>
> - Early intervention services for all infants and toddlers with disabilities (from birth to age 3) and their families
> - Child Find: a system to identify, locate, and evaluate children with disabilities
> - Comprehensive, multidisciplinary evaluation (MDE)
> - Individualized family service plan (IFSP)
> - Procedural safeguards
> - Public awareness program
> - Central directory
> - Comprehensive system of personnel development
> - Administration by a lead agency
> - State interagency coordinating council

To receive funding under Part C, the states must comply with all provisions as detailed in IDEA. The law also states general guidelines on when, how, and where assessments, IFSPs, and interventions must be planned, conducted, and implemented. For detailed information, therapists are advised to read the legislation and regulations, which can be accessed through several websites listed in this chapter's Evolve resource supplement. The document *Providing Physical Therapy Services Under Parts B & C of the Individuals with Disabilities Education Act* (2nd edition) published by the American Physical Therapy Association[83] elaborates on the federal law and the role of the physical therapist.

FAMILY-CENTERED CARE

Although family-centered care is considered best practice in providing health care to all children, in early intervention this philosophy of care is essential because families are considered a direct recipient of services. Family-centered care is based on the premise that the family plays the central role in the life of a child. Research has found that family-arranged experiences have the most direct impact on child outcomes.[53] The underlying tenet is that optimal family functioning promotes optimal child development.[117] Family-centered care is a process that respects the rights and roles of family members while providing intervention to achieve child and family outcomes that promote well being and quality of life. Family-centered care is a comprehensive approach to service that when individualized may include aspects of both child- and parent-centered approaches as therapists support the child's development and function and endeavor to meet the needs of the family.

Several definitions of family-centered intervention have been presented.[45,74,81,113] The common threads are that it is a philosophy and approach to service delivery based on core beliefs of (1) respect for children and families, (2) appreciation of the family's impact on the child's well-being, and (3) family—professional collaboration. The definition by Law et al.[74] is widely used:

> Family-centered service is made up of a set of values, attitudes, and approaches to services for children with special needs and their families. Family-centered service recognizes that each family is unique; that the family is the constant in the child's life; and that they are the experts on the child's abilities and needs. The family works with service providers to make informed decisions about the services and supports the child and family receive. In family-centered service, the strengths and needs of all family members are considered (p. 2).

Perhaps the most important differences between family-centered and professional-driven approaches are that the professional's role is partly defined by the resources and priorities of each child and family, not only by the severity of the child's developmental delay or disability, and that service decisions are not based solely on the professional's knowledge and expertise. Initially, the less-defined role may be unsettling to professionals, whose education and expertise is biased toward addressing a child's impairments and activity limitations.

The key elements of family-centered care, proposed by the National Center for Family-Centered Care, influence provision of services to families and children.[113] The elements are as follows:
- Recognition of the family as the constant in a child's life
- Facilitation of family-to-family networking
- Promotion of parent-professional collaboration at all levels of health care
- Incorporating developmental needs of children into health care systems
- Implementation of programs and policies that provide emotional and financial support to meet the needs of the family
- Honoring diversity (racial, cultural, socioeconomic, ethnic)
- Designing health care services that are accessible, flexible, and responsive to families' needs

These elements appear to be common sense, and these simple statements often conceal the complexity of application to practice. Within professions with a history of working with children with disability, service providers may be inclined to regard family-centered care as not being different from what they have always practiced. Implicit in the family-centered approach is that the role of the family extends beyond involvement in the care of the child, to being beneficiaries of interventions.[10,72] The informational, educational, and health needs of the family are addressed in concert with those of the child, for it is through supporting quality of life for the family that we can promote the child's development.

Family-centered care is founded on a parent-professional partnership. Dunst, Trivette, and Snyder (2000) defined parent-professional partnership as follows[39]:

> Parents and other family members working together with professionals in pursuit of a common goal where the relationship between the family and the professional is based on shared decision-making and responsibility and mutual trust and respect (p. 32).

Service providers recognize and accept the family as the primary decision maker and provide information and support to enable the family to make decisions and to enhance family competency in caring for and nurturing their child.[38] Information sharing is reciprocal and acknowledges that families know their children the best.[125] Families share valuable information about the child and family, needs and concerns, and expectations of early intervention. Service providers inquire about the child's health, development, daily activities and routines, and family resources and supports. Service providers are responsive to the family's need for information about their child, community resources, and preparation for the future. As an example, therapists provide family information regarding their child's diagnosis and prognosis with honesty while embracing hope for the child to participate in life to the fullest potential. Dunst and Dempsey (2007) have found that a positive parent-professional partnership is related to parent's self-efficacy and sense of control.[43]

Themes that emerged from a qualitative study in which families described providers that embraced family-centered care were positiveness, responsiveness, orientation to the whole family, friendliness, sensitivity, and demonstration of skills related to child needs and community resources.[87] Parents value providers who are caring individuals with positive interpersonal and communication skills with families and children.[78] The relationship between the therapist and the family is the foundation for family-centered care[78] and an avenue for promoting caregiver competency.[131] To provide family-centered care, physical therapists are encouraged to expand their knowledge to include understanding of the multidimensional aspects of family functioning including cultural values, child-rearing practices, and the importance of resources and supports. It is important for the early intervention team to address the basic needs of the family.[112] Knowledge of family functioning is critical to avoid the concerns that with family-centered care professionals may be expecting too much from families, thus becoming a source of stress, as opposed to support.[75,78] Family functioning is discussed in Chapter 27.

EFFECTIVENESS OF FAMILY-CENTERED CARE

Several reviews support the effectiveness of family-centered care.[24,45,71,103] Similar to other areas of research in early intervention, a thorough synthesis of findings is challenging because studies vary in how family-centered care is defined, the settings and patient populations investigated, and the outcomes measured. For children with developmental disabilities, family-centered care has been related to improvement in children's developmental skills and functioning, maternal knowledge of child development, maternal participation in intervention programs, developmental appropriateness of the home environment, parenting behaviors, family functioning, and psychosocial well-being of children and mothers. Aspects of family-centered care associated with these outcomes include communication, information sharing, collaboration, fostering family involvement and choice, building on strengths, and providing support.

The complex and multidimensional nature of family-centered care as well as the limitations in research methodology and quality make it difficult to translate findings into practice. Key program characteristics related to more positive outcomes for children and family are emerging: (1) programs that focus on parent-child interaction appear to be more effective than programs that are solely child focused,[11,53,68,79] (2) programs provided within children's everyday experiences are more effective in promoting skill acquisition than those that provide only general support, (3) the impact of parent education programs on development is greatest for children from families who are impoverished,[48] (4) programs that focus on parenting skills and family support may decrease parenting stress,[24] and (5) programs that foster parent involvement and choice are more strongly associated with child and family outcomes than programs that foster the parent-professional relationship.[45]

FAMILY PARTICIPATION

The family-centered approach, in addition to expanding the role of service providers, expands the role of the family,

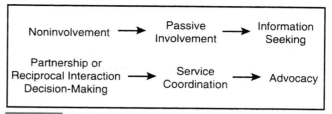

Figure 29-1 Continuum of caregiver involvement.

particularly parents. On one hand, parents are expected to use their skills and resources to meet the needs of their family. On the other hand, they must learn new skills that are related to taking care of a child with special needs, such as advocacy, negotiation, collaboration, and intervention strategies. Because of the fragmented child health system, parents have to coordinate not only developmental services but also services for primary health care, public health programs, specialized medical care, and behavioral health services. Some families may not be receiving the services they need and require assistance in accessing and utilizing services and resources.[80] Families experiencing difficulty in adapting to caring for a child with special needs may need more formal support from the early intervention team.[12]

Family participation in early intervention is encouraged. The extent and type of participation will vary depending on factors unique to each family. The premise is that families have a right and responsibility to select the way in which they will be involved in early intervention services. Family involvement is viewed as a continuum rather than a hierarchy. Figure 29-1 illustrates the continuum of family involvement. Some parents may elect not to be involved at all, either because of unfamiliarity with the service delivery system or because of the difficulty balancing work and family commitments. A family with a demanding work schedule may give permission for professionals to provide early intervention at a child's childcare center but not at home (passive involvement). Another family may actively seek information from the professional team regarding the child's diagnosis, prognosis, and ideas for how the family can enhance the child's development (information seeking). Collaboration and partnership are achieved when a family not only seeks information from professionals but also offers information and actively participates in the development and implementation of service plans. Service coordination and advocacy represent levels of family participation that involve management of services provided and educating others about children with special needs. Ongoing communication between the family and providers and revisiting family needs and participation are integral to family-centered services. It is important for physical therapists to invite parents to participate, identify, and discuss barriers, and provide supports to enable their participation. The Knowledge Translation for Caregivers and Children Model and the accompanying case scenario presented in Chapter 27 illustrate how physical therapists

| Box 29-3 | FAMILIES' PERSPECTIVE OF DESIRED COMPETENCIES OF EARLY INTERVENTION THERAPISTS |

Early intervention knowledge. Therapists have previously acquired or have access to general and disability-specific information relevant to family needs or requests related to their child.

Team coordination. Therapists actively support the coordination and planning among team members, including the family.

Family as part of therapy visits. Therapists are able to actively engage and include family members in therapy sessions.

Information sharing between the therapist and the family. Therapists share and support the use of therapy techniques throughout child and family daily routines and activities.

Commitment of the therapist. Therapists view their role as potentially impacting families and children, not simply as a job.

Flexibility of scheduling. Therapists are willing to juggle their schedules in order to work with families and children.

Respect for individual families. Therapists have respect for families in that they are sensitive to the family context and changes over time, use parent-friendly language, use active listening, and provide families with positive feedback.

Appreciation for the child. Therapists demonstrate appreciation for the child by using a strength-based intervention approach and have the ability to be "in tune" with the child.

Therapist as a person. Therapists possess a personality reflective of them as honest, patient, personable, creative, and humorous.

---

can engage families in identifying priorities, setting goals, and planning intervention and how families often modify their goals in light of new information shared by the therapist, exemplifying collaboration and partnership.

PROVIDING EARLY INTERVENTION SERVICES

THE ROLE OF THE PHYSICAL THERAPIST

Part C of IDEA and the American Physical Therapy Association[4] support the role of physical therapists in early intervention. Acquisition of motor skills is a major part of early development, and young children are sensorimotor learners. Physical therapists, as members of the early intervention team, provide interventions to promote children's activity and participation, including motor learning, environmental adaptations, assistive technology, family support, and education. As health care professionals, we bring expertise to the team related to the neuromuscular, musculoskeletal, cardiopulmonary, and integumentary systems. Physical therapists also have a role in health promotion and prevention. Even though physical therapists have a unique role in early intervention, it is recognized that there is overlap of expertise among professional disciplines. Therefore, in early intervention practice, more so than other areas, communication and skills in teamwork are crucial. It is important for providers to openly discuss the overlap in their areas of expertise and respect the contributions of all service providers. Physical therapists may experience overlap in roles and responsibilities with occupational therapy colleagues in the areas of motor and adaptive development as well as assistive technology. Decisions on how each discipline will contribute to the plan of care for a child and family are made based on who can support the identified outcomes.

It is particularly valuable to consider the role of the physical therapist from the consumer perspective. Thirty-six parents of children with disabilities participated in focus groups to explore their perceptions of competent physical,

occupational, and speech therapists in early intervention.[29,88] Parents discussed the skills and attributes of therapists that were important to them. The discussions were audiotaped, transcribed, and analyzed for themes. The nine themes that emerged are described in Box 29-3. The themes reflect interactions among administration issues, expectations for "best practice," and the importance of the family-therapist relationship.

ELEMENTS OF EARLY INTERVENTION

This section presents five major elements of intervention included in Part C of IDEA. The five elements are team collaboration, evaluation and assessment, the IFSP, providing services in natural environments, and transition. These elements are consistent with the recommendations for children from birth to 8 years of age with special needs developed by the Division for Early Childhood (DEC) of the Council for Exceptional Children.[108] It is through these elements of service provision that therapists implement family-centered care.

Team Collaboration

Team collaboration is the process of forming partnerships among family members, service providers, and the community with the common goal of enhancing the child's development and supporting the family. Communication and coordination are essential skills for effective collaboration. Communication is the process of passing on knowledge and information to other team members to facilitate coordination of services. Each member must be committed to keeping the team informed of important issues. Communication begins with listening. To avoid miscommunication, it is important to restate what was heard and ask for clarification or an example. Prompt follow-through communicates investment in the team. At the same time, being patient reflects understanding of group process. When discussing issues, it is essential to provide suggestions and options, a

> **BOX 29-4** CHARACTERISTICS OF EFFECTIVE TEAMS AND COLLABORATIVE RELATIONSHIPS
>
> - In the developmental phase, team members take time to learn about each other.
> - Members demonstrate honesty, trust, responsiveness, and mutual respect for each other.
> - Membership is stable.
> - All share a common philosophy and goal.
> - The group has a structure for interaction and organization.
> - All members demonstrate commitment.
> - Exchange of information, meaningful discussion, and open communication are practiced.
> - Equal participation is encouraged.
> - Partners contribute specific skills and strengths.
> - Plans, priorities, and decisions are made together.
> - Action plans are used for implementing team recommendations.

solution-focused versus problem-focused approach. A sense of humor helps to bring humanism to day-to-day team struggles.

At the systems level, federal legislation mandates interagency coordination to provide families with efficient and effective mechanisms to access and utilize services from multiple agencies. Service coordination is based on the assumption that integrated and coordinated services will result in improved outcomes for children and families. Within early intervention, the law specifically delineates that service coordinators are responsible for the implementation of the IFSP, coordination with other agencies, and assisting families with access to services. Team collaboration among all service providers and the family, within early intervention as well as with the child's other medical and community teams, is necessary to address child and family needs. Teams that do not effectively communicate and coordinate care may increase family stress rather than serve as a formal support system.

Characteristics of team collaboration described by Briggs[23] and supported by the recommendations for early intervention by the Division for Early Childhood[100] and qualitative research[19] are summarized in Box 29-4. Team members demonstrate respect for each other by valuing cultural differences and acknowledging the expertise and competence each person brings to the team. Positive interpersonal relationships and clear behavioral expectations are important for effective collaboration.[19] Parents and service coordinators have reported that a family-centered program philosophy enhances collaboration.[36] Opportunities for team members to share information and willingness to release traditional roles were viewed as important for collaboration. The following practices have been reported to enhance collaboration:

- Home visits
- Co-visits by team members
- A teacher/therapist as service coordinator
- Regular communication with the service coordinator
- Appropriate use of individual and group intervention
- Center-based programs for parents
- Service options shared with parents
- Flexibility in scheduling and staffing

Barriers to collaboration have also been identified. Lack of consistency of staff and problems with contracted employees were cited as interfering with collaboration.[36] Issues related to funding, interagency coordination, paperwork requirements, and external policies were reported to negatively influence collaboration.[36] Although struggles may exist for "turf," power, or authority, more commonly problems appear to arise from a workplace structure that isolates service providers or one that does not have dedicated time or procedures in place for collaboration.[60] Providing services in natural environments requires time for travel and reduces direct contact among team members. It is important for administration to support procedures and mechanisms for communication such as team meetings at a community-based center, electronic sharing of information, and time in the workload for phone calls and consultation.

Various approaches to team interaction exist in early intervention. In an interdisciplinary approach, team collaboration is necessary because multiple team members with various areas of expertise work together with the family to support one set of outcomes. However, a framework for team collaboration, specifically intensive team interactions, is an essential feature of the *transdisciplinary* approach to service delivery.[70] The transdisciplinary approach involves one primary service provider who implements the IFSP with the family with consultation from other team members. An advantage of the transdisciplinary approach is that the family and child interact with a primary service provider. The transdisciplinary approach is dependent on role release and crossing of disciplinary boundaries. If services are implemented without opportunities for consultation and supervision and do not include the option for additional team members to provide direct service when needed, then a child may not be receiving the services and strategies necessary to support the IFSP. For a resource on the transdisciplinary approach in early intervention, the reader is referred to McGonigel et al.[84]

A specific approach to team interaction associated with the transdisciplinary care termed "coaching" has also been promoted in early intervention.[106] This approach advocates for family involvement in the intervention process and respects the family's strengths and expertise. After collaborative observations and discussions, the therapist models and practices with the family intervention strategies the family can implement throughout the child's daily routines. The therapist follows up with the family to review the strategies and whether they are having the intended effect. Collaboratively the therapist and family determine whether modifications or changes are needed and if the goal has been achieved how to progress to the next step. This collaborative interactive process is also utilized during interactions with other team members.

Communication and coordination of services among health care professionals, early intervention providers, and families has long been recognized.[21] Families of young children with complex medical conditions expend considerable time and resources to meet their children's health, education, and development needs. Collaboration is particularly critical to meet the needs of infants and toddlers who are medically fragile. Even though all team members agree that collaboration is needed, problems in communication and coordination among families, service coordinators, early intervention service providers, physicians, and hospital-based therapists have been reported.[63] Fifty family members and professionals participated in focus groups to discuss their perceptions on communication and coordination between medical and early intervention providers. Overall, concerns were expressed about the ability and time to communicate effectively and the challenges in resolving differences in practice philosophies. The focus groups identified strategies to improve coordination and communication. Strategies included providing funding and resources for comprehensive care coordination services; developing interagency communication systems; conducting communication, teamwork, and advocacy training for families and providers; and providing education on the early intervention system for health and medical providers.

Assessment and Evaluation

IDEA legislation discusses assessment of the child, family, and service needs. IDEA specifies that assessment of the child is performed by qualified and trained personnel and includes review of the child's relevant medical records, observation of the child, informed opinion, and determination of the child's unique strengths and needs and functioning in five areas of development (physical, cognitive, communication, social or emotional, and adaptive). Comprehensive developmental tests and measures may be used for determining eligibility and documenting developmental progress; however, routines-based ecologic assessment of the child's functioning is also indicated to guide the intervention process.[6] The physical therapist synthesizes findings for motor development and adaptive function within the context of findings for all areas of development, social interactions, activities, and daily routines of the child and family. The assessment of the family includes a voluntary interview with the family to identify (1) their resources, priorities, and concerns and (2) the supports and services they need to strengthen their ability to meet their child's developmental needs.

Several key points on the assessment and evaluation process merit emphasis. The legislation dictates that assessment and evaluation must be comprehensive and nondiscriminatory. A team approach supports a holistic view of the child. Information from multiple sources across various situations, including reports from families, is valued.

Professional judgment of therapists and consensus decision making among parents and professionals are important aspects of the assessment and evaluation process.[7] The team uses findings from child and family assessments to determine the child's initial and continued eligibility for early intervention. This determination cannot be made based on a single assessment procedure; however, medical records can be used to determine eligibility without additional assessment if they report information on the child's level of functioning in the five developmental areas. If a child is eligible for early intervention, the team also evaluates the assessment information to determine the child's service needs.

Assessment and evaluation are to be provided in a respectful and collaborative manner with families and children.[34] The purpose and process of the assessment and evaluation should be discussed in advance. Family input is requested in deciding *who* should attend, *what* activities and routines will be observed, *where* the evaluation or assessment should take place, and *when* the session will occur (date and time). Family members can take on many different roles during the assessment and evaluation. Some family members may elect to guide the process, interacting with their child in a variety of activities. Others may prefer to assist the therapist with activities. Another option for a family member is to be a narrator, reflecting on the child's behaviors and providing commentary and elaboration to the other team members. Some families are comfortable with spontaneous exchange of ideas, and other families prefer to answer specific questions. At times, a family member may just want to observe and listen. At the end of the assessment and evaluation, it is important to discuss with the family their perspective on the process.[102]

To maximize the value of assessment and evaluation, consideration should be given to the information needed to make decisions on outcomes, the intervention plan, and how progress will be documented. This process begins with the identification of child and family competencies that serve as a foundation for determining the child's readiness for learning new skills. In addition, an understanding of the family's culture and interests provides the framework for deciding on meaningful intervention strategies. This information is best gathered and discussed through a family interview and systematic naturalistic observation.

Family Interview

An initial step in the process of assessment and evaluation is a family interview. The family interview is considered the first opportunity to establish a trusting relationship and partnership with the family and child as well as a time to promote the relationship between the family and their child.[61] The purpose of the interview is to learn from the family about the child's health, development, and personality; the child and family's daily routines and interests; what resources and strategies are available to enhance the child's development; their perceptions about therapy; and their expectations of early intervention. For some families, the interview process may be a new experience; therefore, therapists encourage, support, and respect the various levels of involvement and value the information that families provide.[15] It is important for therapists to recognize and respect that families are being asked to share personal information.

An effective interview requires sufficient time and is characterized by the ability to have a conversation with the family, listen, acknowledge the child and family's strengths, expand the conversation with appropriate guiding questions, use friendly nonverbal communication, and demonstrate empathy.[61,86] A personable approach facilitates a comfortable environment, welcoming the family to share their thoughts. The manner in which questions are asked also determines the response. Although often unintentional, judgmental questions and comments by service providers not only are a source of parent dissatisfaction, especially with families who represent minority populations, but may contribute to reluctance on the part of these families to offer information.[50] For some families who have difficulty expressing themselves, it is important for therapists to provide guidance while being careful not to misrepresent the family's perspective. Winton and Bailey[134] described three major types of questions that are used to obtain different information. One type is the linear question that is used to obtain specific information or a yes or no response. A second type is an open-ended question that is used to facilitate elaboration on an issue. A third type is circular, in which every response facilitates or dictates an additional response. Table 29-1 provides an example of each type of question. A combination of question types is needed to gather necessary and meaningful information.

Active listening is another key to effective interviewing and to establishing partnerships with families and collaboration on the IFSP. Active listening and acknowledging the family's concerns demonstrates respect and value for the family's priorities and helps the therapist develop a deeper appreciation for the family's daily routines, opportunities for collaboration, how the family frames its resources, and the extent of the family's support network. Another effective interview strategy is the use of silence. There are times when silence is more helpful than questioning. Silence, with some nonverbal gesture of acceptance, may enable a family time to reflect and consider their response.

To support therapy in natural environments, a major component of the interview is gathering information on child and family daily routines in order to identify the context for intervention to promote children's participation in family and community life. Several resources and tools are available to guide this specific process.[16,86,133,135] Through conversations and open-ended questions, such as "tell me about your child" and "describe for me a typical day in your family," therapists gather information on family members' roles, interests, strengths, interactions, and daily experiences. Therapists may need to inquire about specific routines related to play, self-care, and community outings; however, these activities are thoughtfully discussed and not solely presented as a simple checklist. McWilliam and colleagues[86] emphasized the importance of identifying the needs of all family members and considering what the family would like to be able to do. Woods and Lindeman[135] discussed the importance of the interview being a reciprocal process where providers share information on the value of natural learning opportunities and families discuss the activities and routines in their daily life. The interview around daily routines is also an opportunity to begin collaborative problem solving with the family to discover the strategies and resources the family have to address challenges in caring for and promoting their child's development.[135]

Observation

The second step entails observations of the child within his or her natural environment. Natural environment is a broad construct referring to the everyday experiences that are part of the child's home and community settings. Observations in the natural environment may focus on family household routines, parent-child interaction, play, and other daily activities such as feeding, bathing, and dressing. Within the construct of the International Classification of Functioning, Disability and Health,[137] ecologic assessment encompasses the relationships among participation, activity, body function and structures, and environmental and personal factors.

The physical therapist's unique role as part of the team is to focus on postural control and mobility during play, exploration of the physical environment, self-care, and social interactions. The family and therapist select the settings and activities that are most important for the therapist to observe. While observing, the therapist notes the following:
- What the child enjoys doing
- How the child interacts with others
- Opportunities for movement and sensorimotor exploration
- How often and under what circumstances the child moves
- Toys and materials that are available
- Areas of the home accessible to the child
- How much adult assistance or guidance is provided
- Skills or resources the child needs to become more successful
- Musculoskeletal, neuromuscular, cardiopulmonary, integumentary and personal characteristics of the child that may facilitate or be a barrier to the child's participation

TABLE 29-1   **Sample Questions for a Family Interview**

Question Type	Example
Linear	"Is your child taking any medications?"
Open ended	"What does your family like to do for recreation?"
Circular	"Tell me about your child's personality."

During the observation, the physical therapist engages in a conversation with the family members to learn about their perspective of the child's typical performance, abilities, and needs. The therapist also shares information on the child's and family strengths and may begin to discuss or try simple strategies to optimize the child's abilities. Information about the child's activity and participation in settings that are not observed can be gathered during the interview, or the therapist may elect to engage the child in an activity that is not the exact context of the daily routine.

The most meaningful observation occurs when watching a child do something enjoyable with someone who is trusted. "The child's relationship and interaction with his or her most trusted caregiver should form the cornerstone of the assessment."[51] Parent-child interactions are sensorimotor experiences. Motor control, sensory integration, and muscle performance are part of parent-child interactions. In addition to looking at the motor components of the interaction, consideration is also given to social patterns of interaction between the child and caregiver. Kelly and Barnard[67] provided a comprehensive overview of assessment of parent-child interactions. Although not a physical therapist's area of expertise, an appreciation of social interaction helps to focus motor interventions in ways that are holistic and promote a child's self-esteem.

Play is the primary occupational behavior of childhood and is a naturally occurring situation during which children learn and develop new skills. In reference to observing play activities, it is important to look at both independent play as well as play with caregivers, siblings, and peers. Therapists gather information on what toys and play activities the child engages in (sensory/exploratory play, manipulative play, imaginative/dramatic play, or motor/physical play) and the child's likes and dislikes. Therapists consider the interplay between motor abilities and play skills. Is the child able to initiate play experiences? What positions can the child play in? Can the child freely move around to reach toys or play activities that interest him? Further analysis considers if the child's movements are goal directed, the variability of movement to meet environmental demands, and the child's reaction to movement (i.e., level of enjoyment, safety, and body awareness). Lastly, a focus on the process of play provides valuable insights into the child's playfulness. Playfulness is concerned with a child's approach to an activity and includes observations related to the child's enjoyment, engagement, responsiveness, motivation, and locus of control.[26]

In addition to the family interview and ecologic observations, therapists use various tests and measures to evaluate motor development, function, and body functions and structures. These assessment tools are described in Chapter 2 and elsewhere.[77,123] A caution is noted that measures of child development normed on children without delay are valid for determining present level of development and eligibility but often are not valid for planning intervention and measuring change over time. Based on the top-down

approach to evaluation and assessment,[28] measures of body functions and structures are conducted after the team has a clear understanding of the family and child's goals and current abilities and relate to the team's hypothesis for impairments that may be a cause of limitations in activities and restrictions in participation.

Finally, therapists collaborate with the team to document the child's functioning related to three outcome areas of the national accountability system for Part C of IDEA.[59] These areas are: "positive socio-emotional skills (including social relationships), acquisition and use of knowledge and skills (including early language/communication), and use of appropriate behaviors to meet their needs" (p. 8). When children exit early intervention, data in aggregate form is collected to report the percentage of children who made improvements in these areas in relation to their same age peers. This information is for progress monitoring of the early intervention system as a whole and is not meant to capture the individualized experience of a child. The outcome areas do reflect integration of skills in meaningful contexts.

Individualized Family Service Plan

The culmination of the assessment and evaluation process is the development of the individualized family service plan (IFSP). The principle underlying an IFSP is that families have diverse needs based on their individual values and life situations. For intervention to be meaningful for the child, the individuality of each family must be recognized. The team members involved in the development of the IFSP include parents, caregivers, other family members, the family advocate, the service coordinator, persons involved with the assessment and evaluation, and as appropriate, persons who will be providing service.

An initial IFSP must be developed in a timely manner at a meeting time and place convenient for the family. Even though family-centered efforts are made, logistics often make it difficult to arrange the meetings at nights or weekends, thus it is important to recognize that not all key family members may be able to be involved. If a service provider cannot attend, a representative or written information can be sent. These situations have been an area of concern, for without all team members present it is difficult to truly have a collaborative process.

Although the federal law specifies the content of the IFSP (Box 29-5), it does not specify the format of the document or the process for its development. Typically the service coordinator leads the discussion and records the information. Family members can elect, however, to take the role of team leader. During the meeting, the team discusses the assessment and evaluation findings, shares information on the philosophy of early intervention to ascertain if this matches the family's expectations and priorities, and collaborates to develop the IFSP. The team promotes family participation and decisions are made collaboratively. Transferring federal law into practice has been challenging, but more recent

---

Box **29-5**   CONTENT OF THE INDIVIDUALIZED FAMILY SERVICE PLAN

- Statement of present levels of development based on objective criteria: cognitive, communication, physical (motor, vision, hearing, health), social or emotional, adaptive
- Statement of the family's resources, priorities, and concerns related to enhancing the development of the child
- Statement of measurable outcomes expected with criteria, procedures, and timelines to determine progress
- Specific early intervention services based on peer-reviewed research needed to meet the needs of the child and family, including frequency, intensity, and method of delivery
- Statement of the natural environments in which services to be provided (if services are not going to be provided in natural environments, a justification must be included)
- Determination of other services to enhance the child's development and a plan to secure such services through other public or private resources, such as medical resources
- Projected dates for initiation of services and duration of services
- Identification of the service coordinator
- Transition plan: steps to be taken to assure smooth transition to preschool services or other suitable services if appropriate (at age 3)

---

reports indicate that families are participating in the development of the IFSP.[1,58] Aaron,[1] however, reported that family involvement regarding decisions on the types and intensity of services was limited. The findings from a study on quality indicators of IFSP documents were also mixed.[66] A high rating was noted for a focus on child strengths, and 86% of the outcomes were related to family concerns and priorities. However, the documents contained technical jargon and a low rating was noted for evidence of the family's role in the intervention process.

The family should be provided with information that will enable them to make informed decisions and choices *before* the IFSP meeting in order to negotiate for the types of support they need and to ensure equal partnership and ownership in this process. This information may be shared with the family during the information-gathering stages, in the form of a postevaluation interpretive conference, or in writing in the form of an evaluation report. When feasible, questions the family may have pertaining to the evaluation results should also be addressed before the IFSP meeting so that questions related to the logistics of service provision can be fully discussed during the meeting. This will also help reduce the prolonged process that sometimes characterizes

IFSP meetings. Another benefit to sharing the information before the IFSP meeting is that the family members can decide on whom they want to invite to the meeting, something that families consider to be a valuable form of support.

In some regions, administrative efforts to comply with policies on nonbiased evaluations and timely initiation of services have resulted in long meetings where the evaluation and the development of the IFSP occur during the same visit by an independent team who will not be the providers of the service.[1] Although this practice meets the letter of the law it may not support the spirit of the IFSP process. Parents often need to tend to their children during the meeting and have not had an opportunity to assimilate the evaluation findings. It has also been noted that professionals are occupied with completing paperwork for the IFSP; thus, limiting engagement with the family and the required documentation process may be a greater focus than meaningful discussion.[1,135] Therapists working in states where evaluations are conducted by independent teams need to be sensitive to the potential issues that may arise. Therapists on the evaluation team recognize that although their relationship with the family is of short duration, it is still important for them to engage with the family in meaningful ways to support their start with the early intervention system. Therapists who are providers of service recognize that families now have to begin a relationship with another professional and that it may be challenging to have to tell their story again.

Identification of child and family outcomes is often challenging. These outcomes must be based on what is important to the family and determined by the family in collaboration with providers, *not* disciplinary goals. It is important for outcomes to focus on activity and participation within the child's daily routines. Historically, therapists have emphasized child outcomes, and research indicates that the majority of IFSP outcome statements are child focused.[20] The Early Childhood Outcomes Center, funded in 2003 by the U.S. Department of Education, Office of Special Education Programs, has developed a family outcome measure for early intervention.[46] The global outcomes on this measure may assist providers in discussions with families to identify specific individualized family outcomes to guide the supports and services they need. The global family outcomes[9] state that the family does the following:

- Understands their child's strengths, ability, and special needs
- Knows their rights and advocates effectively for their child
- Helps their child develop and learn
- Has support systems
- Can access desired services and activities in their community

Four issues frequently arise regarding the identification of meaningful outcomes. First, some families may look to the professionals for guidance. Therapists can review and discuss with families the information gathered during the family interview regarding the child's daily routines to assist families in identifying outcomes that are important to them. Second, families may express outcomes that the child does not have the readiness or potential to achieve.[3,62] It is important not to dismiss the family's priorities but rather to discuss with the family insights on what the child may be ready to learn related to the outcome area they have identified. Further exploration of why specific outcomes are important to the family and detailed explanations and information about the child's condition may be helpful for informed decision making. Third, outcomes need to be written in measurable terms and family identified outcomes may not meet this requirement. Professionals can add this component, discussing options to phrase the behavior, condition and criterion for the outcome while retaining family-friendly language. Lastly, the team may be overwhelmed with how to address all of the child and family needs identified during the evaluation. Framing outcomes in functional clusters based on participation in daily activities and an open discussion to prioritize outcomes may assist the team in arriving at a consensus.

In recent years, the early childhood education and intervention literature has discussed early learning guidelines[110] as well as advocated for a focus on promoting self-determination of young children.[47,114] Dimensions of self-determination such as self-awareness, self-regulation, engagement, self-initiation, making choices, problem-solving, persistence, and self-efficacy can be nurtured in early childhood. Early intervention provides an avenue to begin to influence children's self-esteem, their belief that they have an impact on their world, and ultimately their quality of life. An understanding of early learning guidelines and the development of self-determination provide a foundation for selecting meaningful outcomes; however, it is important for outcomes to be individualized to the child's unique family context.

Identification of the types and intensity of services to support the child's and family's outcomes requires an open discussion, an understanding of the expertise of various service providers, an appreciation of family preferences, and team collaboration. This discussion also includes options for methods of service delivery, interagency collaboration, financial responsibilities, and transition planning for when the child turns 3 years old. Little is known about the types of supports and services that may be appropriate to address family outcomes.[126] Family-directed service involves providing families with a range of supports including information, access to resources, care coordination, counseling, social work services, and respite care. Although the early intervention team is not expected to be able to provide all of the supports that a family may need, plans are made to assist families in accessing and coordinating appropriate community social services.

Limited knowledge and evidence is available to guide decisions on intensity of services.[54] These decisions are complex and reflect the dynamic interrelationships among numerous child, family, and service system factors. The discussion of the methods of service delivery is essential to promote coordinated and complementary care. Recommendations for strategies to address the child's and family's outcomes and to facilitate mobility, communication, adaptive behavior, self-care, and play enable all team members to contribute their knowledge and provide supports in a comprehensive manner. Physical therapists have a role in sharing their knowledge and skills related to assistive technology. When selecting strategies, the team considers evidence-based practice and the provision of services in natural environments. The methods that will be used to address the outcomes, as well as the individuals who will work together to implement the methods, are agreed upon.

The IFSP is not just a legal document; it is a process of collaboration between the family and providers to design a service plan that is acceptable to the family and addresses the child's needs. The IFSP serves as a means for coordination of services, a guide for intervention, and a standard for evaluating outcomes. The IFSP is reviewed every 6 months, and a formal meeting is held annually. The IFSP can be reviewed at another time at the request of a team member. Periodic IFSP reviews allow for renegotiations or revisions of the service plan, as well as monitoring of goal attainment. During an IFSP review, family satisfaction, effectiveness of the IFSP process, and status of the outcomes are discussed. If outcomes were not achieved, reflection of the appropriateness of the outcomes, service, and strategies is needed to effectively revise the IFSP.

Therapists practicing in early intervention require effective interpersonal and communication skills to be able to invite and support the family to contribute their insights, recommendations, and priorities. Anecdotal stories indicate that the IFSP process can be overwhelming and intimidating for families, especially when families do not believe that their opinions are valued. It is appropriate for therapists to make recommendations, but they should be consistent with information that was gathered from the family during the interview. Recommendations are framed as questions, thus providing the family the opportunity to agree or disagree. Additional recommendations to make these experiences more positive include a focus on child and family strengths, use of lay language, and flexibility to allow informal conversation and sharing of ideas instead of rigidly following a predetermined format. Lastly, it is important to acknowledge that variability exists in how states have implemented the IFSP process. Therapists are encouraged to serve as an advocate to ensure that the spirit of family-centered care and individualization are honored.

Providing Services in Natural Environments

IDEA defines natural environments as "settings that are natural or normal for the child's age peers who have no disabilities." More meaningful is that natural environments are "a variety of settings where children live, learn, and play."[111] The natural environment is not limited to the home but rather is defined as any place where children participate in activities and routines that provide learning opportunities that promote a child's behavior, function, and development. This includes childcare settings, parks, grocery stores, YMCAs, and libraries.

Providing services in natural environments is a general intervention approach, a process, and a conceptualization. Although natural environment implies a physical location, such as a playground, it goes beyond the physical place. It includes the people and relationships, the activities and routines the child and family typically engage in at that location, and the learning opportunities afforded by those activities. Dunst and colleagues[42] have identified with families in a variety of family and community settings and present an approach for discussing with families activities and learning opportunities. These settings include family routines (household chores and errands), caregiving routines (bathing, dressing, eating, grooming, bedtime), family rituals and celebrations (holidays, birthdays, religious events), outdoor activities (gardening, visits to the park/zoo), social activities (visiting friends, play groups), play activities (physical play and play with toys), and learning activities (listening to stories, looking at books/pictures). Physical therapists are encouraged to gain knowledge about activities families and children do, places families and children go, the community they serve, and supports and resources for families.

Natural environments match the purpose of early intervention: "support families in promoting their children's development, learning, and participation in family and community life."[111] This approach embraces family-centered care by recognizing that the family has a primary role in nurturing the child and fostering growth, development, and learning. Campbell and Sawyer found that when service is focused on natural learning environments, caregivers are actively participating in the session and interactions revolve around the caregiver-child dyad.[32] When providing interventions in natural environments, therapists can easily focus on the children's function, promote socialization with their family and friends, and "strengthen and develop lifelong natural supports for children and families" (Section on Pediatrics, APTA, 2008)[111] (Figure 29-2). "The emphasis in early intervention must not be on creating nearly normal children but on enabling children and their families to have normal life opportunities" (p. 3).[101]

For infants and young children, self-determined behavior, parent-child relationship,[68] and play form the foundation to support the child's role in the family and to prepare the child for interactions with peers and school (Figure 29-3). Brotherson and colleagues[25] observed the families and home environments of 30 young children with disabilities and found that families provide a variety of opportunities in the home to promote the development of their children's self-determination. The themes to describe these strategies included choice and decision making, support of self-esteem, engagement with home environment and others, and control

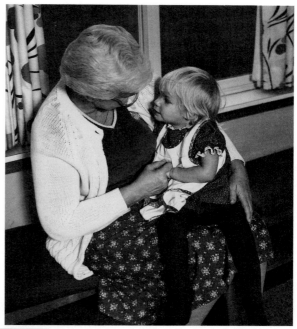

Figure 29-2 When providing therapy in the home, the family and therapist may consider inviting grandmother to participate in the visit to support her role as a resource for the family in nurturing her grandchild. (From Wong, D. L., Hockenberry-Eaton, M., Winkelstein, M. L., Wilson, D., Ahmann, A., & DiVito-Thomas, P. A. [1999]. *Whaley & Wong's nursing care of infants and children* [6th ed.]. St. Louis, MO: Mosby, Figure 4-23, p. 155.)

and regulation of the home environment. Therapists can build on these strategies and reflect with parents on ways to support what the child does, what the family does, and what the environment affords to foster development of self-determination.[47] Chai and colleagues[33] identified socially and culturally based interactions as the common theme across various conceptual frameworks on natural environments. Therapists build a relationship with the family and provide support, feedback, and guidance to promote parent-child interactions that foster trust and competence.[68] Supporting children's play enables the therapist to capture the essence of children in their daily lives. Therapists not only should address the physical components of play, but they should also involve parents, siblings, and friends to promote socialization.

Interventions for caregiving and self-care activities such as sleeping, feeding, bathing, dressing, and moving throughout the environment are essential (Figure 29-4). Families of young children with cerebral palsy have identified self-care as their highest priority.[35] It is important for physical therapists to support feeding and nutrition needs, as this is a primary concern of families and critical for children's energy to move, growth and well-being.[35a] As health care professionals, physical therapists have knowledge and skills in differential diagnosis, feeding disorders, pharmacology, oral-motor functioning, assistive technology, and community resources.

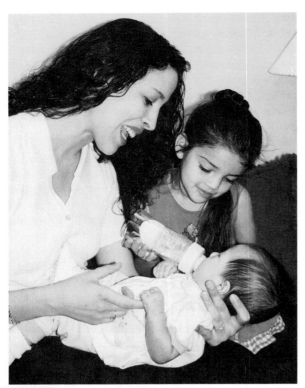

Figure 29-3 Involvement of siblings in caregiving activities during therapy visits promotes family bonds and supports family routines. (From Wong, D. L., Hockenberg-Eaton, M., Winkelstein, M. L., Wilson, D., Ahmann, A., & DiVito-Thomas, P. A. [1999]. *Whaley & Wong's nursing care of infants and children* [6th ed.]. St. Louis, MO: Mosby, Figure 14-6, p. 677.)

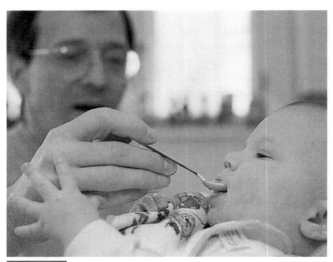

Figure 29-4 It is important for therapists to partner with fathers and support their role in caregiving activities. (From Wong, D. L., Hockenberg-Eaton, M., Winkelstein, M. L., Wilson, D., Ahmann, A., & DiVito-Thomas, P. A. [1999]. *Whaley & Wong's nursing care of infants and children* [6th ed.]. St. Louis, MO: Mosby, Figure 3-7, p. 92.)

Providing services in natural environments is supported by principles of motor learning.[129] Practice and repetition of activities in natural contexts and settings are more effective for learning and generalization. These places and activities are interesting and engaging and thus naturally motivating to children. This includes the opportunity to learn through modeling by peers and family members. Based on the family's daily life, therapists guide families on how to structure practice to promote learning of contextualized motor skills. Therapists help families to provide prompts and cues and, when necessary, physical assistance to enable the child to learn skills in self-care and mobility. Scales, McEwen, and Murray[109] found that parents recognized the benefits that providing instruction to families can have; however, parents noted that this approach may be more stressful to families. Therapists are encouraged to collaborate with families to prioritize the activities and strategies and to support families in this process.

Therapists also provide recommendations to adapt the physical environment, activities, and materials to enhance the child's access and functional participation. Examples include minor changes to the layout of a room or use of adapted toys or positioning and mobility devices. Assistive technology is an important component of intervention for children with severe physical disabilities.[122] Assistive technology, such as switches to activate toys, needs to become more widespread for children under age 3.[37,76] Young children with physical disabilities can successfully learn to operate switches to produce meaningful outcomes.[30] Similarly, power wheelchair mobility may afford children as young as 2 years of age the opportunity for independence.[27] Planning forms and charts are available to guide the team in the decision-making process for designing and implementing adaptations.[31]

On one hand, consumers and professionals value services in natural environments. Research suggests that family routines provide the mechanism through which parents influence child outcomes.[119] Bernheimer and Weisner[17] gathered information on the daily lives of 102 families of children with disabilities and reported, "If there is one message for practitioners from our parents and from our longitudinal studies, it is that no intervention, no matter how well designed or implemented, will have an impact if it cannot find a slot in the daily routines of an organization, family, or individual" (p. 199). In a national survey, families and providers identified critical outcomes of services in natural environments: child mastery, parent-child interactions, inclusion, and child learning opportunities.[40] Furthermore, learning opportunities characterized as being interesting, engaging, competence-producing, and mastery-oriented predicted positive child outcomes.[41]

On the other hand, challenges exist in providing services in natural environments, and therapists are encouraged to seek creative solutions.[55] Challenges include logistic concerns, such as the costs, safety, and time to travel to the child's natural environments as well as philosophical concerns that

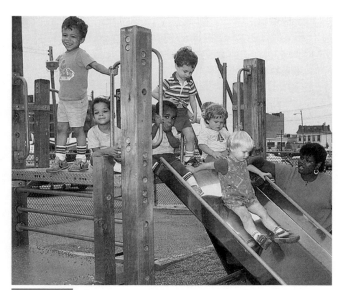

Figure 29-5 Therapy at a childcare setting can focus on promoting social interactions with peers and functional mobility to participate in activities on the playground. (From Wong, D. L., Hockenberg-Eaton, M., Winkelstein, M. L., Wilson, D., Ahmann, A., & DiVito-Thomas, P. A. [1999]. *Whaley & Wong's nursing care of infants and children* [6th ed.]. St. Louis, MO: Mosby, Figure 2-3.)

<table>
<tr><td>Box 29-6</td><td>QUESTIONS TO DISCUSS WITH FAMILIES WHEN ESTABLISHING ACTIVITIES FOR SERVICES IN NATURAL ENVIRONMENTS</td></tr>
</table>

- What activities make up your weekdays and weekends?
- What activities are going well, and which not going well?
- What activities would you like support for?
- What activities does the child prefer to participate in?
- What activities provide natural learning opportunities?
- What activities provide opportunities for child initiation?
- What activities provide opportunities for peer interaction?
- Are there new activities that you would like to try?

---

by mandating a particular approach to service delivery, the system may not be providing options to meet families' individualized needs and circumstances. It is important for agencies to develop and implement policies to ensure staff safety such as the use of cell phones, co-visits, and soliciting advocacy efforts from neighborhood child watch organizations. Visits can occur in a variety of community locations such as the library, town centers, and recreational facilities. When service is provided in a community childcare setting, it is important to schedule periodic visits with the family as well as to collaborate with the childcare providers. Information on childcare regulations, philosophy, and early childhood curriculum will assist the therapist in partnering with childcare providers (Figure 29-5).

Therapists use their expertise to guide families and teach children through meaningful natural learning opportunities. It is important for therapists to advocate for the support and training they need to be able to provide services in natural environments. An annotated bibliography of literature and educational materials provides a useful resource on this topic.[94]

Implementation of intervention in natural environments requires insights and planning. The first step is to consider family-identified outcomes. It is essential for there to be a match between the information from families regarding their concerns, priorities, and resources and the services provided. The next step is to discuss with the family the activities, routines, and people that are part of their daily life. Box 29-6 provides questions to consider when collaborating with families to identify activities. Therapists are encouraged to identify the functional learning opportunities that occur during each activity. If a family outcome is for the child to be able to play at the park, riding a swing may be an activity to consider. The therapist may identify a variety of learning opportunities for the child, such as grasping with two hands, pumping with his or her legs, holding the head and trunk up, understanding high and low, and making sounds. Therapists integrate their therapeutic intervention strategies within the context of family activities and learning opportunities. Therapists are encouraged to balance adult-directed learning opportunities with child-directed activities to promote self-determination.[44] Therapeutic techniques are used to improve the body functions and structures necessary to achieve a functional ability and to prevent secondary complications related to the cardiopulmonary, musculoskeletal, and neuromuscular systems. When possible, therapists are encouraged to integrate impairment-focused interventions into practice of activities.[129] Therapist may struggle with providing interventions in natural environments. A workgroup through the Office of Special Education Programs provides concrete guidelines on intervention practices that support natural environments.[136]

The Transition Plan

The transition plan is part of the IFSP process that deserves special attention because of its essential role in assuring the child's progression in the educational system and participation in the community. The transition process is complex and can be a challenging experience for families. Child, family, program, and community characteristics influence the transition process,[104] and effective practices are comprehensive in order to address all dimensions.[105] Therapists, as early intervention team members, can take an active role in the transition process.

The first step is to become knowledgeable about how Part B Preschool Services (IDEA, 2004)[97] are implemented and about resources and service options in the community. IDEA provides for increased coordination between Part C and Part B programs. With the permission of the parent, a representative from the Part C program is invited to the initial Individualized Education Program (IEP) meeting when the child

---

BOX 29-7 STRATEGIES FOR COLLABORATING WITH FAMILIES TO SUPPORT TRANSITION FROM EARLY INTERVENTION

- Listen to the family.
- Provide positive, but realistic, support for the preschool program.
  - Guide the family in gathering information without introducing your bias.
  - Provide the family with survey and interview guidelines for preschool programs.
  - Visit a program with the family and help orient the family and child to the new agency.
- Discuss separation from the child as a natural process.
- Celebrate graduation from early intervention with the family and child.
- Consider a follow-up communication with the family after transition.

BOX 29-8 STRATEGIES TO PREPARE A CHILD FOR PRESCHOOL

- Provide the child with opportunities to play with other children (i.e., siblings, neighbors, play groups).
- Promote independent playtime.
- Encourage the child to participate in a variety of play experiences.
- Encourage self-care skills.
- Give the child an opportunity to practice following simple directions.
- Make the child responsible for small tasks, like putting away toys.
- Have the child make choices, and encourage the child to express wants and needs.
- Read stories about school.

---

is transitioning to preschool services. In addition, IDEA provides states the flexibility to make Part C services available to children until they enter kindergarten or elementary school.

Second, it is important to make the commitment to collaborate with the early intervention and preschool teams. Focus groups have identified interagency relationships and communication as essential factors in the transition process.[105] This step includes an open discussion regarding the environmental characteristics that will support the child's learning and development including attention to the safety of the child in the new environment and during transportation. Therapists can offer, with the family's permission, to share information that will help the staff of the preschool program to meet the child's needs.

Third, therapists collaborate with families and provide them with resources, information, and support as they prepare for their child's transition. This support enables families to take an active role in the transition process. Most important, therapists serve as advocates, keeping in mind the family's dreams and vision for the child. Box 29-7 outlines strategies for collaborating with families. Finally, therapists can focus on preparing children for the preschool environment and promote the development of school readiness skills. Box 29-8 presents examples of strategies that physical therapists can incorporate during early intervention.

EFFECTIVENESS OF EARLY INTERVENTION

Early intervention services are based primarily on philosophy and knowledge of early childhood development and family function as well as the provisions of federally mandated public laws. Research on the benefits of early intervention are equivocal and vary across children and families.[24,48,52,98]

This reflects the complex and multifaceted nature of early intervention services. Results from the National Early Intervention Longitudinal Study[59] also support that early intervention has positive outcomes for both children and families. However, methodological challenges have contributed to limited research and ability to generalize findings across children and settings. Research has focused on interventions for infants and toddlers experiencing delays who are at environmental or biologic risk. Interventions tend to be broad in scope with little detail on specific strategies and procedures, and the potential range of child and family outcomes has not been explored. Research is recommended to help therapists understand the complex influences, both direct and indirect, of child, family, environment, and service factors on meaningful outcomes for children and families.[14] Consequently, the knowledge of what interventions are most effective based on child and family characteristics remains unclear.

Physical therapists will find it particularly challenging to integrate and apply research findings on early intervention for three reasons: (1) a large proportion of the literature and research comes from the fields of medicine, psychology, sociology, and early childhood education and concentrates on health, cognition, and behavior; (2) the role of physical therapy as part of an early intervention team has seldom been addressed; and (3) well-designed studies with large samples, such as the Infant Health and Development Program[99] have targeted "at-risk populations" of infants at risk for global developmental delay, speech and language disorders, or social-emotional maladjustment.[24,48,82,99]

A systematic review of the effects of early intervention on motor development included studies with children both at high risk for or with developmental motor disorder.[18] This review did consider separate effects of interventions provided in the Neonatal Intensive Care Unit from interventions conducted later in infancy and early childhood. Among studies conducted following discharge from the Neonatal

Intensive Care Unit, positive effects on motor development were found for what was categorized as specific or general developmental programs, whereas no support was found for interventions categorized as neurodevelopmental treatment or Vojta. It is challenging to translate this evidence to practice because of the variety of interventions considered as specific or general developmental programs, ranging from treadmill training to enhancing parent-infant interaction, and differences in method of service delivery including who provided the intervention.

Empirical support for early intervention for children with physical disabilities and their families is inconclusive. Children with motor impairment have shown fewer functional gains compared to children with delays in other areas.[56,57,92] Findings for children with disabilities indicate that severity, not the type of physical disability, is a strong predictor of change; children with mild disabilities showed greater gains than children with severe disabilities, regardless of the intensity of services.[57,115] Collectively, research indicates that norm-referenced developmental assessments are not responsive to changes that children with severe physical disabilities are capable of achieving. Outcomes for adaptive function, participation in family and community life, ease of caregiving, and family functioning have not been adequately studied.

Physical therapists providing services within the early intervention system also need to keep abreast of current research related to therapy approaches and specific procedural interventions that may be appropriate for infants and young children. For children with cerebral palsy, a functional approach to therapy has been shown to improve the ability to participate in daily activities[2,69] and constraint-induced movement therapy has resulted in improved upper extremity motor function.[124] Children with cerebral palsy have demonstrated improvements in self-care activities after receiving adaptive equipment and environmental adaptations[120] and parents have reported that use of assistive devices and environmental modifications has a positive impact on their child's ability to participate in self-care and social activities.[91] For children with Down syndrome, treadmill training has been shown to be effective in helping children to walk earlier.[127] For children with motor delays, those who received aquatic therapy in addition to home-based physical or occupational therapy had greater gains in functional mobility.[85]

Regarding procedural interventions, therapists need to consider how these interventions match the family's desired participation outcomes for the child within the context of early intervention services. New York State's clinical practice guideline for young children with motor disorders[90] provides a synthesis of evidence on various intervention approaches and techniques that physical and occupational therapists typically use to promote motor development. The report emphasizes the collaborative team decision-making process that is needed when selecting and evaluating intervention strategies. Landsman[73] has advised therapists to translate the evidence to practice cautiously, as it only represents quantitative research for one child outcome—motor development.

Evidence on the effects of the intensity of physical therapy services is also hard to interpret and apply to early intervention. In early intervention, the team makes decisions regarding types and intensity of services based on child and family needs. Studies on intensity of services do not account for the confounding effects of practice and learning supported by family and other caregivers throughout a child's daily life. The findings from a recent single subject study on intensive physical therapy for infants with cerebral palsy were inconclusive.[128] Research is needed to examine various intensity schedules in early intervention based on a child's readiness to learn new skills.

PROGRAM EVALUATION

Program evaluation determines the extent to which services are provided in an efficient and effective manner. The primary purpose of a program evaluation is to provide service providers with feedback on family satisfaction with how services are provided and the extent child and family outcomes are achieved. A four-tiered approach to program evaluation has been described.[65,130] Through the first tier, a needs assessment, the needs of the population being served are determined, policy or programs to meet the needs are proposed, and a monitoring system is developed to document progress. Through the second tier, monitoring and accountability, services are systematically documented to assist in program planning and decision making. Through the third tier, quality process, the quality of the services is judged to provide information for program improvement. Through the fourth tier, achieving outcomes, the extent to which IFSP outcomes are met and attributed to early intervention services are determined to provide information for program improvement and contribute to the knowledge base.

Program evaluation in early intervention is advocated to document how early intervention is actually implemented and to determine the impact on families and children. As previously discussed, a national accountability system is now in place to monitor the impact of early intervention on global child and family outcomes. However, individual programs are encouraged to not merely gather the data but to engage in the program evaluation process to guide decisions on service delivery. Stuberg and DeJong[121] provided a useful example of how to implement a program evaluation for physical therapy service within early intervention and school settings. They reported that 91% of the children's individualized objectives were either achieved or progress was made. Children in early intervention and preschool had higher achievements than older children, and children with more severe disability had fewer achievements than children with less severe disability. These findings may guide program developers in how best to establish appropriate and meaningful individualized outcomes. Bailey[8] proposed a framework for program evaluation in early intervention to assess family involvement and support. He discussed three levels of accountability: (1) providing what the legislation requires, (2) providing services that reflect current best practices, and (3) achieving family outcomes. Program evaluation is challenging secondary to the multiple dimensions of early intervention, the variability in the characteristics of children and families served, and the individualized needs of families and children. However, through this process facilitators and barriers to providing quality and effective services are identified and recommendations are provided for program improvements.

IMPLICATIONS FOR PHYSICAL THERAPIST PRACTICE

Research findings underscore the need to consider the interaction among child factors and family characteristics when planning physical therapy interventions. Therapists are encouraged to advocate for services that are comprehensive in nature, family centered, and support multiple outcomes. Consequently, interventions should target all three components of health (body functions and structures, activities, and participation) and contextual factors (environmental and personal) of the International Classification of Functioning, Disability, and Health.[137]

Knowledge and research continue to shape the formulation, refinement, and reexamination of themes for family-centered services such as providing families the opportunity to identify their concerns and needs, sharing information with families, conducting family-friendly culturally sensitive assessments, identifying meaningful outcomes, individualizing services, supporting family efforts, and providing services in natural environments. Because no one discipline can provide services that incorporate all child and family needs, effective interventions will require multiple levels of collaboration.[49,53,64] Equally important, will be the availability of professionals who are adequately prepared to engage in this expanded scope of practice.[132]

A MODEL FOR INTERVENTION

A collaborative team model for early intervention service delivery for children with physical disabilities and their families was developed by Palisano, Chiarello, and O'Neil[93] with input from colleagues and community partners as part of the research activities in the Pediatric Post-Professional Program in Rehabilitation Sciences at Drexel University. The development of the model was supported in part from a leadership training grant of the Maternal and Child Health Bureau. The model provides a framework for implementing the components of early intervention services previously described. Therapists may find intervention strategies from this model useful for their practice as we strive to promote quality service delivery and to support children and family outcomes.

The collaborative model for early intervention service delivery, illustrated in Figure 29-6, integrates the policy embodied in federal law (IDEA, 2004);[97] the processes of enablement outlined by the World Health Organization;[137] theories on family and child development;[107,117] and practice guidelines from physical therapy, occupational therapy, and

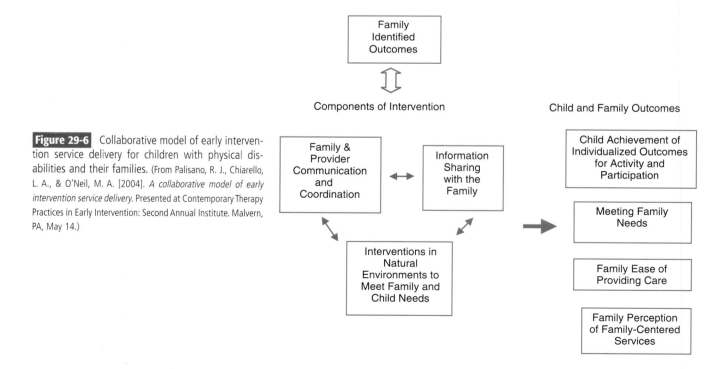

Figure 29-6 Collaborative model of early intervention service delivery for children with physical disabilities and their families. (From Palisano, R. J., Chiarello, L. A., & O'Neil, M. A. [2004]. *A collaborative model of early intervention service delivery.* Presented at Contemporary Therapy Practices in Early Intervention: Second Annual Institute. Malvern, PA, May 14.)

early childhood education.[4,5,83,108] Four broad categories are proposed as outcomes that are meaningful for children with physical disabilities and their families. These outcomes are (1) child achievement of individualized outcomes for activity and participation, (2) meeting family needs, (3) family ease of providing care, and (4) family perception of family-centered behaviors of the service provider team.

The model identifies three components of intervention: *communication and coordination* among the family, service providers, and community; *information sharing* with the family; and *interventions in natural environments* to meet child and family needs. The double-headed and interconnected arrows shown in Figure 29-6 indicate that the three components interact in an iterative fashion. Box 29-9 outlines intervention strategies for implementation of the model. A case scenario is presented to exemplify how strategies are implemented through a collaborative, family-centered team approach in natural environments.

Box **29-9**   STRATEGIES FOR PHYSICAL THERAPIST INTERVENTIONS

COMMUNICATION AND COORDINATION OF SERVICES

- Early intervention team meetings every 3 months
- Co-visits of early intervention team providers every 3 months
- Identification and access of community resources through community mapping
- Visit or phone conference with other health care professionals

INFORMATION SHARING WITH THE FAMILY

Use the Therapeutic Intervention Strategies in Natural Environments Method

- Provide information on family-identified needs.
- Embed intervention strategies into child's and family's daily life (Family Routine and Outcome Matrix).[22]

- Conduct visits when family members who are important in the child's life can participate.
- Conduct visits at a community location identified by the family.
- Provide intervention in different rooms in the home to support a variety of daily activities and routines.
- Implement adaptations, functional training, and restorative/preventive techniques to support self-regulation, parent-child interactions, play, self-care, and mobility.

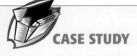

CASE STUDY

"Andrew"

Andrew is a 26-month-old boy with right hemiplegia. His mother, a homemaker, is very involved in his care, and Andrew has two older siblings. The family lives in a two-story row house in an urban environment. Over the past year, Andrew has received early intervention services, including physical, occupational, and speech therapy. Kate, the physical therapist, has been an integral member of the early intervention team and has established a positive relationship with the family. A video clip on the Evolve website accompanies the case scenario.

The county administrator and provider agency support the need for routine coordination and communication among the early intervention team members. In collaboration with the mother, Kate guides early intervention team meetings every 3 months at the family's home. At a recent team meeting, Kate asked the mother to share with the team information about their family and daily routines as well as people and places in the community that are important to them. The mother indicated that she is planning on returning to work in the coming year and would like information on preschool programs in the neighborhood. The mother explained that the immediate neighborhood, including the playground, her older children's schools, and

grandmother's house are visited frequently. She also identified key outcomes for Andrew that were important to her for the next year: (1) interacting with children on the playground including riding a tricycle, (2) walking at home and in the neighborhood without falling, and (3) using his right arm more to help with dressing and feeding.

To foster communication and coordination with community programs, the team discusses possible community resources in the neighborhood such as the community recreation center. The team is committed to identifying and forming relationships with family- and child-oriented community programs located in the neighborhoods served by the early intervention program. As one means of sharing information with the family, the team develops daily routines and outcomes matrix,[23] shown in Table 29-2. The family-identified outcomes are listed across the top row, and the family routines are listed down the first column. The team problem-solves together to decide on strategies that can be used during the family's day to promote the outcomes, and these are listed in the body of the matrix.

To respond to the family's identified need for information on preschools, Kate compiles a list of neighborhood programs and shares it with Andrew's mother at their next visit. To coordinate care

Continued

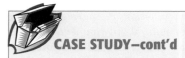

CASE STUDY–cont'd

TABLE 29-2   Sample Activity Matrix for Andrew

	Interacting with Children	Walking at Home and in the Neighborhood without Falling	Using Right Arm to Assist with Dressing and Feeding
FEEDING TIME	Andrew can have a play date over for lunch and build cracker sandwiches together.	Andrew can carry the napkins to the kitchen table at mealtimes.	Andrew can support the bowl with his right hand while scooping food with his left.
OUTSIDE PLAYTIME	With supervision, Andrew can sit on the glider with another child as you sing "Row, row, row your boat."	Support Andrew to walk the block to the playground by having him hold onto your index finger.	Prompt Andrew to push his right arm through his jacket sleeve when getting ready to go outside to play.
BEDTIME	Discuss your visit to the playground, and ask Andrew to tell you what he liked doing with his friend.	Andrew can walk up the flight of stairs for bath time before bed using the railing.	With Andrew sitting in your lap, have him support a cardboard book with his right hand and turn the pages with his left.

with medical services, Kate accompanies the mother and Andrew to their clinic appointment at the children's hospital to see the orthopedic surgeon and orthotist. The group discusses what medical interventions might be needed to support Andrew's goal for safe walking. A plan is established to obtain an orthotic at this time and to keep lines of communication open for the possible need for botulinum toxin injections for management of spasticity of the gastrocnemius muscles.

To support the ability of other family members to interact with and care for Andrew, Kate visits Andrew's grandmother's house and asks the grandmother what is going well and what is not going well when she cares for Andrew. Kate demonstrates strategies to show the grandmother how to provide guidance for Andrew when he goes for walks outside with her. For ongoing communication and coordination among the early intervention team, Kate and the occupational therapist visit Andrew and his mother together to focus on strategies to promote the use of Andrew's right arm during dressing and feeding.

During the summer, Kate and the family have several early intervention visits at the neighborhood playground. Kate adapts Andrew's tricycle with foot pedals, hand rest, and a push handle for the mother. At the playground, Kate and the mother guide Andrew on the climbing gym with the neighborhood children and siblings. Andrew's mother asks Kate to visit their home during lunchtime so a session in their kitchen can focus on feeding. During other visits, Kate provides functional training for independent walking as Andrew goes on a scavenger hunt inside his home and outside in his backyard. She discusses with his mother when it may be appropriate to use verbal and tactile prompts. When the new brace arrives, Kate and Andrew's mother discuss a wearing schedule and the importance of preventing ankle contractures from developing.

At the next team meeting, the therapists and the family discuss Andrew's progress, review the outcomes of the intervention strategies during the past 3 months, and set the stage for working together for the next 3 months to support Andrew and his family.

SUMMARY

Physical therapists in early intervention support the implementation of IDEA by establishing collaborative partnerships with children, families, and professionals from multiple disciplines to provide coordinated and comprehensive care. Therapists integrate knowledge and skill from their professional education with knowledge of early childhood development to promote the child's development and participation in family life, as well as support the family. This unique practice setting enables therapists to embrace the art of caring, prepare children for their roles in school, and foster health and well-being.

REFERENCES

1. Aaron, C. (2009). *Family participation at initial individualized family service planning meeting and decision making on intensity of early intervention services. Doctoral dissertation.* Philadelphia: Drexel University.

2. Ahl, L. E., Johansson, E., Granat, T., & Carlberg, E. B. (2005). Functional therapy for children with cerebral palsy: An ecological approach. *Dev Med Child Neurol, 47*(09), 613–619.

3. American Academy of Pediatrics (Committee on Children with Disabilities). (1998). Managed care and children with special needs: A subject review. *Pediatrics, 102*(3), 657–660.

4. American Physical Therapy Association. (2001). Guide to physical therapist practice. *Physical Therapy, 81*(1), 27–50.

5. American Occupational Therapy Association. (1999). *Occupational therapy services for children and youth under the Individuals with Disabilities Education Act* (2nd ed.). Bethesda, MD: American Occupational Therapy Association.

6. Bagnato, S. J. (2005). The authentic alternative for assessment in early intervention: An emerging evidence-based practice. *Journal of Early Intervention, 28*(1): 17–22.

7. Bagnato, S. J., McKeating-Esterle, E., Fevola, A., Bortolamasi, P., & Neisworth, J. T. (2008). Valid use of clinical judgment

(informed opinion) for early intervention eligibility: Evidence base and practice characteristics. *Infants and Young Children*, 21(4): 334–339.

8. Bailey, D. B. (2001). Evaluating parent involvement and family support in early intervention and preschool programs. *Journal of Early Intervention*, 24(1), 1–14.

9. Bailey, D.B., Bruder, M.B., Hebbeler, K., et al. (2008). Recommended outcomes for families of young children with disabilities. *Journal of Early Intervention*, 28(4):227–251.

10. Bailey, D. B., McWilliam, R. A., Darkes. L. A., et al. (1998). Family outcomes in early intervention: A framework for program evaluation and efficacy research. *Exceptional Children*, 64(3), 313–329.

11. Barnard, K. E. (1997). Influencing parent-child interactions for children at risk. In M. J. Guralnick (Ed.), *The effectiveness of early intervention* (pp. 249–267). Baltimore: Brookes.

12. Barnett, D., Clements, M., Kaplan-Estrin, M., & Fialka, J. (2003). Building new dreams: Supporting parents' adaptation to their child with special needs. *Infants and Young Children*, 16(3), 184–200.

13. Baroni, M., & Sondel, S. (1995). A collaborative model for identifying feeding and nutrition needs in early intervention. *Infants and Young Children*, 8(2), 15–25.

14. Bartlett, D. J., & Lucy, S. D. (2004). A comprehensive approach to outcomes research in rehabilitation. *Physiotherapy Canada*, 56, 237–247.

15. Berman, C., & Shaw, E. (1996). Family-directed child evaluation and assessment under the Individuals with Disabilities Education Act (IDEA). In S. J. Meisels & E. Fenichel (Eds.), *New visions for the developmental assessment of infants and young children* (pp. 361–391). Washington, DC: Zero to Three.

16. Bernheimer, L., & Keogh, B. (1995). Weaving interventions into the fabric of everyday life: An approach to family assessment. *Topics in Early Childhood Special Education*, 15, 415–433.

17. Bernheimer, L. P., & Weisner, T. S. (2007). "Let me just tell you what I do all day …" The family story at the center of intervention research and practice. *Infants and Young Children*, 20(3), 192–201.

18. Blauw-Hospers, C. H., & Hadders-Algra, M. (2005). A systematic review of the effects of early intervention on motor development. *Developmental Medicine and Child Neurology*, 47(6), 421–432.

19. Blue-Banning, M., Summers, J. A., Frankland, H. C., Nelson, L., & Beegle, G. (2004). Dimensions of Family and Professional Partnerships: Constructive Guidelines for Collaboration. *Exceptional Children*, 70(2), 167–184.

20. Boone, H. A., McBride, S. L., Swann, D., Moore, S., & Drew, B. S. (1998). IFSP practices in two states: Implications for practice. *Infants and Young Children*, 10(4), 36–45.

21. Brewer, E. J., McPherson, M., Magrub, P. R., & Hutchins, V. L. (1989). Family-centered, community-based, coordinated care for children with special health care needs. *Pediatrics*, 83, 1055–1060.

22. Bricker, D. (1998). *An activity-based approach to early intervention* (2nd ed.). Baltimore: Paul H. Brookes.

23. Briggs, M. H. (1997). *Building early intervention teams: Working together for children and families*. Gaithersburg, MD: Aspen.

24. Brooks-Gunn, J., Berlin, L. J., & Fuligni, A. S. (2000). Early childhood intervention programs: What about the family? In J. P. Shonkoff & S. J. Meisels (Eds.), *Handbook of early childhood intervention* (pp. 549–577). New York: Cambridge University Press.

25. Brotherson, M. J., Cook, C. C., Erwin, E. J., & Weigel, C. J. (2008). Understanding self-determination and families of young children with disabilities in home environments. *J Early Intervention*, 31(1), 22–43.

26. Bundy, A. (1997). Play and playfulness: What to look for. In L. D. Parham & L. S. Fazio (Eds.), *Play and occupational therapy for children* (pp. 52–66). Philadelphia: Mosby.

27. Butler, C. (1986). Effects of powered mobility on self-initiated behaviors of very young children with motor disability. *Developmental Medicine and Child Neurology*, 28, 325–332.

28. Campbell, P. (1991). Evaluation and assessment in early intervention for infants and toddlers. *Journal of Early Intervention*, 15, 36–45.

29. Campbell, P., Chiarello, L., Wilcoux, M. J., & Milbourne, S. (2009). Preparing therapists as effective practitioners in early intervention. *Infants and Young Children*, 22(1), 21–31.

30. Campbell, P., Milbourne, S., Dugan, L. M., & Wilcox, M. J. (2006). A review of evidence on practices for teaching young children to use assistive technology devices. *Topics Early Child Spec Edu*, 26(1), 3–13.

31. Campbell, P., Milbourne, S., & Wilcox, M. J. (2008). Adaptation interventions to promote participation in natural settings. *Infants Young Children*, 21(2), 94–106.

32. Campbell, P., & Sawyer, L. B. (2007). Supporting learning opportunities in natural settings through participation-based services. *J Early Intervention*, 29(4), 287–305.

33. Chai, A. Y., Zhang, C., & Bisberg, M. (2006). Rethinking natural environment practice: Implications from examining various interpretations and approaches. *Early Child Edu J*, 34(3), 203–208.

34. Chiarello, L. A., Effgen, S., & Levinson, M. (1992). Parent-professional partnership in evaluation and development of individualized family service plans. *Pediatric Physical Therapy*, 4(2), 64–69.

35. Chiarello, L., Palisano, R., Maggs, J., et al. (2010). Family priorities for activity and participation of children and youth with cerebral palsy. *Phys Ther*, 90(9), 1254–1264.

35a. Cloud, H. H. (1997). Update on nutrition for children with special needs. *Topics Clin Nutr*, 13(1), 21–32.

36. Dinnebeil, L. A., Hale, L., & Rule, S. (1999). Early intervention program practices that support collaboration. *Topics in Early Childhood Special Education*, 19(4), 225–235.

37. Dugan, L. M., Campbell, P., & Wilcox, M. J. (2006). Making decisions about assistive technology with infants and toddlers. *Topics Early Child Spec Edu*, 26(1), 25–32.

38. Dunst, C., Johanson, C., Trivetter, C., & Hamby, D. (1991). Family oriented early intervention policies: Family centered or not? *Exceptional Child*, 21(11), 115–118.

39. Dunst, C. J., Trivette, C. M., & Snyder, D. M. (2000). Family-professional partnerships: A behavioral science perspective. In M. J. Fine & R. L. Simpson (Eds.), *Collaboration with parents and families of children and youth with exceptionalities* (2nd ed., pp. 27–48). Austin, TX: PRO-ED.

40. Dunst, C. J., & Bruder, M. B. (2002). Valued outcomes of service coordination, early intervention, and natural environments. *Exceptional Children, 68*(3), 361–375.

41. Dunst, C. J., Bruder, M. B., Trivette, C. M., Hamby, D., Raab, M., & McLean, M. (2001). Characteristics and consequences of everyday natural learning opportunities. *Topics in Early Childhood Special Education, 21*(2), 68–92.

42. Dunst, C. J., Bruder, M. B., Trivette, C. M., Raab, M., & McLean, M. (2001). Natural learning opportunities for infants, toddlers, and preschoolers. *Young Exceptional Children, 4*(3), 18–25.

43. Dunst, C. J., & Dempsey, I. (2007). Family-professional partnerships and parenting competence, confidence, and enjoyment. *Int J Disabil Dev Edu, 54,* 305–318.

44. Dunst, C., Trivette, C., Humphries, T., Raab, M., & Roper, N. (2001). Contrasting approaches to natural learning environment interventions. *Infants and Young Children, 14*(2)48–63.

45. Dunst, C. J., Trivette, C. M., & Hamby, D. W. (2008). *Research synthesis and meta-analysis of studies of family-centered practices.* Ashville, NC: Winterberry Press.

46. Early Childhood Outcomes Center. (2004). *Considerations related to developing a system for measuring outcomes for young children with disabilities and their families.* Department of Education: U.S. Office of Special Education Programs.

47. Erwin, E. J., & Brown, F. (2003). From theory to practice: A contextual framework for understanding self-determination in early childhood environments. *Infants and Young Children, 16*(1): 77–87.

48. Farran, D. C. (2000). Another decade of intervention for children who are low income or disabled: What do we know now? In J. P. Shonkoff & S. J. Meisels (Eds.), *Handbook of early childhood intervention* (2nd ed., pp. 510–548). New York: Cambridge University Press.

49. Filer, J. D., & Mahoney, G. J. (1996). Collaboration between families and early intervention service providers. *Infants and Young Children, 9,* 22–30.

50. Garcia-Coll, G., & Magnusson, K. (1999). Cultural influences on child development: Are we ready for a paradigm shift? In A. S. Masten (Ed.), *Cultural processes in child development—the Minnesota symposia on child psychology* (pp. 1–24). Mahwah, NJ: Lawrence Erlbaum.

51. Greenspan, S. I., & Meisels, S. J. (1996). Toward a new vision for the developmental assessment of infants and young children. In S. J. Meisels & E. Fenichel (Eds.), *New visions for the developmental assessment of infants and young children* (pp. 11–26). Washington, DC: Zero to Three.

52. Guralnick, M. J. (1997). *The effectiveness of early intervention.* Baltimore: Paul H. Brookes.

53. Guralnick, M. J. (1998). Effectiveness of early intervention for vulnerable children: A developmental perspective. *American Journal on Mental Retardation, 102*(4), 319–345.

54. Hallam, R., Rous, B., Grove, J., & LoBianco, T. (2009). Level and intensity of early intervention services for infants and toddlers with disabilities. *Journal of Early Intervention, 31*(2), 179–196.

55. Hanft, E. H., & Pilkington, K. O. (2000). Therapy in natural environments: The means or end goal for early intervention? *Infants and Young Children, 12*(4), 1–13.

56. Harris, S. R. (1997). The effectiveness of early intervention for children with cerebral palsy and related motor disabilities. In M. J. Guralnick (Ed.), *The effectiveness of early intervention* (pp. 327–347). Baltimore: Paul H. Brookes.

57. Hauser-Cram, P., Warfield, M. E., Shonkoff, J. P., & Krauss, M. W. (2001). Children with disabilities: A longitudinal study of child development and parent well-being. *Monographs of the Society for Research in Child Development, 66*(3, Serial No. 266).

58. Hebbeler, K., Spiker, D., Bailey, D., et al. (2007). *Early intervention for infants and toddlers with disabilities and their families: Participants, services and outcomes.* Menlo Park, CA: SRI International.

59. Hebbeler, K., & Barton, L. (2007). The need for data on child and family outcomes at the Federal and State levels. *Young Exceptional Children Monograph Series, 9,* 1–15.

60. Hinojosa, J., Bedell, G., Buchholz, E. S., Charles, J., Shigaki, I. S., & Bicchieri, S. M. (2001). Team collaboration: A case study. *Qualitative Health Research, 11*(2), 206–220.

61. Hirshberg, L. M. (1996). History-making, not history-taking: Clinical interviews with infants and their families. In S. J. Meisels & E. Fenichel (Eds.), *New visions for the developmental assessment of infants and young children* (pp. 85–124). Washington, DC: Zero to Three.

62. Hughes, D. C., & Luft, H. S. (1998). Managed care and children: An overview. *The Future of Children, 8*(2), 25–38.

63. Ideishi, R., O'Neil, M., & Chiarello, L. (2010). Therapist's role in care coordination between early intervention and medical health services for young children with special health care needs. *Physical and Occupational Therapy in Pediatrics, 30*(1), 28–42.

64. Jackson, L. L. (1998). Who's paying for therapy in early intervention? *Infants and Young Children, 11*(2), 65–72.

65. Jacobs, F. H., & Kapuscik, J. L. (2000). *Making it count: Evaluating family preservation services.* Medford, MA: Tufts University.

66. Jung, L. A., & Baird, S. M. (2003). Effects of service coordinator variables on Individualized Family Service Plans. *Journal of Early Intervention, 25*(3), 206–218.

67. Kelly, J. F., & Barnard, K. E. (2000). Assessment of parent-child interaction: Implications for Early Intervention. In J. P. Shonkoff & S. J. Meisels (Eds.). *Handbook of early childhood intervention* (pp. 258–289). New York: Cambridge University Press.

68. Kelly, J. F., Zuckerman, T., & Rosenblatt, S. (2008). Promoting first relationships: A relationship-focused early intervention approach. *Infants and Young Children, 21*(4), 285–295.

69. Ketelaar, M., Vermeer, A., Hart, H., van Petegem-van Beek, E., & Helders, P. J. (2001). Effects of a functional therapy program

on motor abilities of children with cerebral palsy. *Phys Ther*, *81*(9), 1534–1545.

70. King, G., Strachan, D., Tucker, M., Duwyn, B., Desserud, S., & Shillington, M. (2009). The application of a transdisciplinary model for early intervention services. *Infants & Young Children*, *22*(3), 211–223.

71. King, S., Teplicky, R., King, G., & Rosenbaum, P. (2004). Family-centered service for children with cerebral palsy and their families: A review of the literature. *Seminars Pediatr Neuro*, *11*(1), 78–86.

72. Kolobe, T. H. A., Sparling, J., & Daniels, L. E. (2000). Family-centered intervention. In S. K. Campbell, D. W. Vander Linden, & R. J. Palisano (Eds.), *Physical therapy for children* (2nd ed., pp. 881–907). Philadelphia: WB Saunders.

73. Landsman, G. H. (2006). What evidence, whose evidence?: Physical therapy in New York State's clinical practice guideline and in the lives of mothers of disabled children. *Soc Sci Med*, *62*, 2670–2680.

74. Law, M., Rosenbaum, P., King, G., et al. (2003). *What is family-centered services?* FCS Sheet #1. Can Child Centre for Childhood Disability Research, Hamilton, Ontario: McMaster University. http://www.canchild.ca/en/childrenfamilies/resources/FCSSheet1.pdf

75. Leiter, V. (2004). Dilemmas in sharing care: maternal provision of professionally driven therapy for children with disabilities. *Soc Sci Med*, *58*, 837–849.

76. Long, T., Huang, L., Woodbridge, M., Woolverton, M., & Minkel, J. (2003). Integrating assistive technology into an outcome-driven model of service delivery. *Infants and Young Children*, *16*(4), 272–283.

77. Long, T., & Toscano, K. (2002). *Handbook of pediatric physical therapy* (2nd ed.). Philadelphia: Lippincott Willliams & Wilkins.

78. MacKean, G. L., Thurston, W. E., & Scott, C. M. (2005). Bridging the divide between families and health professionals' perspectives on family-centred care. *Health Expect*, *8*, 74–85.

79. Mahoney, G., Boyce, G., Fewell, R. R., Spiker, D., & Weeden, C. A. (1998). The relationship of parent-child interaction to the effectiveness of early intervention services for at-risk children and children with disabilities. *Topics Early Child Spec Edu*, *18*(1), 5–17.

80. Mahoney, G., & Filer, J. (1996). How responsive is early intervention to the priorities and needs of families? *Topics in Early Childhood Special Education*, *16*(4), 437–457.

81. Maternal and Child Health Bureau. (2005). *Definition and principles of family-centered care*. Rockville, MD: Department of Health and Human Services.

82. McCormick, M. C., McCarton, C., Brooks-Gunn, J., & Gross, R. T. (1998). The infant health and development program—Interim summary. *Journal of Developmental and Behavioral Pediatrics*, *19*, 359–370.

83. McEwen, I. (2000). *Proving physical therapy Services under parts B & C of the Individuals with Disabilities Education Act (IDEA), Section on Pediatrics*, Alexandria, VA: American Physical Therapy Association.

84. McGonigel, M. J., Woodruff, G., & Roszmann-Milican, M. (1994). The transdisciplinary team: A model for family-centered early intervention. In L. J. Johnson, R. J. Gallagher, M. J. La Montagne, et al. (Eds.), *Meeting early intervention challenges: Issues from birth to three* (2nd ed., pp. 95–131). Baltimore: Paul H. Brookes.

85. McManus, B. M., & Kotelchuck, M. (2007). Effect of aquatic therapy on functional mobility of infants and toddlers in early intervention. *Pediatr Phys Ther*, *19*(4), 275–282.

86. McWilliam, R. A., Casey, A. M., & Sims, J. (2009). The routines-based interview: A method for gathering information and assessing needs. *Infants and Young Children*, *22*(3), 224–233.

87. McWilliam, R. A., Tocci, L., & Harbin, G. L. (1998). Family-centered services: service providers "discourse & behavior." *Topics in Early Childhood Special Education*, *18*(4), 206–221.

88. Milbourne, S., Campbell, P., & Chiarello, L. A. (2003). *Competent therapist–reflective families: The crossroads of quality early intervention services*. Division for Early Childhood Conference, Washington, DC, October.

89. Reference deleted in page proofs.

90. New York State Department of Health, Division of Family Health, Bureau of Early Intervention. Clinical practice guideline: Report of the recommendations—Motor disorders—Assessment and intervention for young children, 2006.

91. Ostensjo, S., Carlberg, E. B., & Vollestad, N. K. (2005). The use and impact of assistive devices and other environmental modifications on everyday activities and care in young children with cerebral palsy. *Disabil Rehabil*, *27*(14), 849–861.

92. Pakula, A. L., & Palmer, F. B. (1997). Early intervention for children at risk for neuromotor problems. In M. J. Guralnick (Ed.), *The effectiveness of early intervention* (pp. 98–108). Baltimore: Paul H. Brookes.

93. Palisano, R. J., Chiarello, L. A., & O'Neil, M. A. (2004). *A collaborative model of early intervention service delivery*. Presented at Contemporary Therapy Practices in Early Intervention: Second Annual Institute. Malvern, PA, May 14.

94. Pretti-Frontczak, K. L., Barr, D. M., Macy, M., & Carter, A. (2003). Research and resources related to activity-based intervention, embedded learning opportunities, and routines-based instruction; An annotated bibliography. *Topics in Early Childhood Special Education*, *23*(1), 29–40.

95. Public Law 99-457, Education of the Handicapped Amendments Act of 1986, 100 Stat. 1145–1177.

96. Public Law 105-17, Individuals with Disabilities Education Act Amendments of 1997, 111 Stat. 37–157.

97. Public Law 108-446, Individuals with Disabilities Education Improvement Act of 2004, 118 Stat. 2647–2808.

98. Ramey, C. T., & Ramey, S. L. (1998). Early intervention and early experience. *American Psychologist*, *53*(2), 109–120.

99. Ramey, C. T., Bryant, D. M., Wasik, B. H., Sparling, J. J., Fendt, K. H., & LaVange, L. M. (1992). Infant health and development program for low birth weight, premature infants: Program elements, family participation, and child intelligence. *Pediatrics*, *89*(3), 454–465.

100. Rapport, M. J. K., McWilliam, R. A., & Smith, B. J. (2004). Practices across disciplines in early intervention: The research base. *Infants and Young Children, 17*(1), 32–44.

101. Rocco, S. (1994). *New visions for the developmental assessment of infants and young children: A parent's perspective* (pp. 13–15). Washington, DC: Zero to Three.

102. Rocco, S. (1996). Toward shared commitment and shared responsibility: A parent's vision of developmental assessment. In S. J. Meisels & E. Fenichel (Eds.), *New visions for the developmental assessment of infants and young children* (pp. 55–57). Washington, DC: Zero to Three.

103. Rosenbaum, P., King, S., Law, M., King, G., & Evans, J. (1998). Family-centered service: A conceptual framework and research review. *Physical & Occupational Therapy in Pediatrics, 18*, 1–20.

104. Rous, B., Hallam, R., Harbin, G., McCormick, K., & Jung, L. A. (2007). The transition process for young children with disabilities: A conceptual framework. *Infants & Young Children, 20*(2), 135–148.

105. Rous, B., Myers, C. H., & Stricklin, S. B. (2007). Strategies for supporting transitions of young children with special needs and their families. *Journal of Early Intervention, 30*(1), 1–18.

106. Rush, D. D., Shelden, M. L., & Hanft, B. E. (2003). Coaching families and colleagues: a process for collaboration in natural settings. *Infants & Young Children: An Interdisciplinary Journal of Special Care Practices, 16* (1): 33–47.

107. Sameroff, A. J., & Fiese, B. H. (2000). Transactional regulation: The development of ecology in early intervention. In J. P. Shonkoff & S. J. Meisels (Eds.) *Handbook of early intervention* (2nd ed., pp. 135–159). New York: Cambridge University Press.

108. Sandall, S., McLean, M. E., & Smith, B. J. (2000). *DEC recommended practices in early intervention/early childhood special education.* Longmong, CO: Sopris West.

109. Scales, L. H., McEwen, I., & Murray, C. (2007). Parents' perceived benefits of physical therapists' direct intervention compared with parental instruction in early intervention. *Pediatr Phys Ther, 19*, 196–202.

110. Scott-Little, C., Kagan, S. L., Frelow, V. S., & Reid, J. (2009). Infant-toddler early learning guidelines: The content that states have addressed and implications for programs serving children with disabilities. *Infants & Young Children, 22*(2), 87–99.

111. Section on Pediatrics, APTA. Natural Learning Environments Fact Sheet, 2008.

112. Shannon, P. (2004). Barriers to family-centered services for infants and toddlers with developmental delays. *Soc Work, 49*(2), 301–308.

113. Shelton, T. L., & Stepanek, J. S. (1994). *Family-centered care for children needing specialized health and developmental services* (3rd ed.). Bethesda, MD: Association for the Care of Children's Health.

114. Shogren, K. A., & Turnbull, A. P. (2006). Promoting self-determination in young children with disabilities: The critical role of families. *Infants & Young Children, 19*(4): 338–352.

115. Shonkoff, J. P., Hauser-Cram, P., Krauss, M. W., & Upshur, C. C. (1992). Development of infants with disabilities and their families. *Monographs of the society for research in child development, 57*(6, Serial No. 230).

116. Shonkoff, J. P., & Meisels, S. J. (2000). *Handbook of early childhood intervention* (2nd ed.). New York: Cambridge University Press.

117. Shonkoff, J. P., & Phillips, D. A. (2000). *From neurons to neighborhoods: The science of early childhood development.* Washington, DC: National Academy Press.

118. Shore, R. (1997). *Rethinking the brain: New insights into early development.* New York: Families and Work Institute.

119. Spagnola, M., & Fiese, B. H. (2007). Family routines and rituals: A context for development in the lives of young children. *Infants Young Children, 20*(4), 284–299.

120. Stewart, S., & Neyerlin-Beale, J. (1999). Enhancing independence in children with cerebral palsy. *British J Ther Rehabil, 6*(12), 574–579.

121. Stuberg, W., & DeJong, S. L. (2007). Program evaluation of physical therapy as an early intervention and related service in special education. *Pediatr Phys Ther, 19*(2), 121–127.

122. Sullivan, M., & Lewis, M. (2000). Assistive technology for the very young: Creating responsive environments. *Infants and Young Children, 12*(4), 34–52.

123. Tatarka, M. E., Swanson, M. W., & Washington, K. A. (2000). The role of pediatric physical therapy in the interdisciplinary assessment process. In M. J. Guralnick (Ed.), *Interdisciplinary clinical assessment of young children with developmental disabilities* (pp. 151–182). Baltimore: Paul H. Brookes.

124. Taub, E., Ramey, S. L., DeLuca, S., & Echols, K. (2004). Efficacy of constraint-induced movement therapy for children with cerebral palsy with asymmetric motor impairment. *Pediatr, 113*(2), 305–312.

125. Turnbull, A. P., Blue-Banning, M., Turbiville, V., & Park, J. (1999). From parent education to partnership education: A call for a transformed focus. *Topics in Early Childhood Special Education, 19*(3), 164.

126. Turnbull, A. P., Summers, J. A., Turnbull, R., et al. (2007). Family supports and services in early intervention: A bold vision. *Journal of Early Intervention, 29*(3): 187–206.

127. Ulrich, D. A., Ulrich, B. D., Angulo-Kinzler, R. M., & Joonkoo Yun, J. (2001). Treadmill training of infants with Down syndrome: Evidence-based developmental outcomes. *Pediatrics, 108*(5).

128. Ustad, T., Sorsdahl, A. B., & Ljunggren, A. E. (2009). Effects of intensive physiotherapy in infants newly diagnosed with cerebral palsy. *Pediatr Phys Ther, 21*(2), 140–149.

129. Valvano, J., & Rapport, M. J. (2006). Activity-focused motor interventions for infants and young children with neurological conditions. *Infants and Young Children, 19*(4), 292–307.

130. Warfield, M. E. (2002). *Early intervention program evaluation workshop.* Philadelphia: MCP Hahnemann University, May 14.

131. Washington, K., & Schwartz, I. S. (1996). Maternal perceptions of the effects of physical and occupational therapy services on

caregiving competency. *Physical and Occupational Therapy in Pediatrics, 16*(3), 33–54.

132. Widerstrom, A., & Ableman, D. (1996). Team training issues. In D. Bricker & A. Widerstrom (Eds.), *Preparing personnel to work with infants and young children and their families: A team approach* (pp. 23–42). Baltimore: Paul H. Brookes.
133. Wilson, L. L., Mott, D. W., & Bateman, D. (2004). The asset-based context matrix: A tool for assessing children's learning opportunities and participation in natural environments. *Topics in Early Childhood Special Education, 24*(2), 110–120.
134. Winton, P. J., & Bailey, D. B. (1988). The family-focused interview: A collaborative mechanism for family assessment and goal-setting. *Journal of the Division of Early Childhood, 12,* 195–207.
135. Woods, J. J., & Lindeman, D. P. (2008). Gathering and giving information with families. *Infants and Young Children, 21*(4), 272–284.
136. Workgroup on Principles and Practices in Natural Environments (February, 2008) Seven key principles: Looks like / doesn't look like. OSEP TA Community of Practice- Part C Settings. http://www.nectac.org/topics/families/families.asp
137. World Health Organization. (2001). *ICIDH2: International Classification of Functioning, Disability and Health.* Geneva: World Health Organization.

30 The Educational Environment

SUSAN K. EFFGEN PT, PhD, FAPTA • MARCIA K. KAMINKER PT, DPT, MS, PCS

lmost from the start of physical therapy in the United States, physical therapists have worked in educational environments. The civil rights movement of the 1960's and federal legislation of the 1970's, however, marked the beginning of major changes in services for all children with special needs in school settings. As a consequence of continued federal and state mandates for the education of students with disabilities, the school system has become the practice setting that employs the greatest number of pediatric physical therapists. Since 1975, a generation of physical therapists has been instrumental in advocating for school-based practice and the development of standards for practice.[36] The educational setting is unique in emphasizing individualized outcomes for student participation in the education program and continues to present opportunities and challenges for pediatric therapists. This chapter reviews the history of the delivery of physical therapy in educational environments, in addition to discussing federal legislation and court cases that have changed how children with disabilities are educated and receive physical therapy. Key topics related to physical therapy in educational environments are presented, including inclusive education, models of team interaction, service-delivery models, the individualized educational program (IEP), and intervention strategies. Critical issues facing school-based physical therapists are also highlighted.

BACKGROUND

Although the history of physical therapy in the United States is traced to "reconstruction aides" serving the injured of World War I, it can also be traced to the service of "crippled children," especially those with poliomyelitis. In major cities early in the 20th century, children with physical disabilities were served in hospitals and special schools. The children had a variety of diagnoses, including poliomyelitis and spastic paralysis,[16,50] cardiac disorders, "obstetric arms" (brachial plexus injuries), bone and joint tuberculosis, clubfeet, and osteomyelitis.[11,16,89] By the 1930's, numerous articles had been published describing the delivery of physical therapy in these special schools.[11,89,112,125] Epidemics of poliomyelitis increased the need for special schools and physical therapists. After the vaccine for poliomyelitis was developed in the 1950's, the need for special schools was temporarily reduced, until public awareness increased regarding the needs of children with other disabilities.

Historically, most children in special schools had normal or near-normal intelligence. Many schools required children to be toilet trained, and some required children to walk independently. This trend to serve only those with physical disabilities and normal intelligence continued in many areas of the United States until schools were federally mandated in 1975 to serve all children with disabilities by the enactment of Public Law (PL) 94-142, the Education for All Handicapped Children Act.

FEDERAL LEGISLATION AND LITIGATION

A number of social and political events paved the way for the enactment of the Education for All Handicapped Children Act. In 1954, the historic U.S. Supreme Court decision regarding segregated schools was handed down: Brown v. Board of Education of Topeka. Separate-but-equal schools were found inherently unequal. This Supreme Court decision was to end the segregated education of African-American children, but the principles and foundation of this case could also apply to segregated schools for those with disabilities. The call for social equality had begun and would eventually include those with disabilities. President Kennedy's personal experience with his sister who had a disability expedited his establishment in 1961 of the President's Panel on Mental Retardation. Television documentaries exposed institutions in New York, and Blatt and Kaplan's book, *Christmas in Purgatory: A Photographic Essay on Mental Retardation*,[13] raised national concern for the care and treatment of individuals with disabilities. Leaders such as Wolfensberger[130] were influential proponents of deinstitutionalization and normalization. Cruickshank noted that "as is usually the case with major changes in social policy, the normalization trend is not based on empirical data showing greater effectiveness or efficiency of the changes proposed by its advocates" (p. 65).[24] Instead, the normalization trend focused on the civil rights of individuals, a prevailing anti-institutional attitude—especially governmental institutions—and a commitment "to the democratic, the individualistic, and the humanitarian" (pp. 65–66).[24] The federal Developmental Disabilities Assistance and Bill of Rights Act of 1975 (PL 94-103) included a provision that states had to develop and incorporate a "deinstitutionalization and institutional reform plan" (p. 71).[14] Advocacy groups had gained power, and they used the judicial system to win their rights.

The Pennsylvania Association for Retarded Citizens (PARC) *v.* Commonwealth of Pennsylvania (1971) was the historic, decisive court case establishing the uncompromising right to an education for all children with disabilities. This was a class-action suit on behalf of 14 specific children and all other children who were in a similar "class" to those with trainable mental retardation. In Pennsylvania, a child was excluded from public school if a psychologist or other mental health professional certified that attendance at school was no longer beneficial for that child. The local school board could refuse to accept or retain a child who had not reached the mental age of 5 years. Children classified as trainable mentally retarded, therefore, were unable to receive a public education in Pennsylvania. The court sided with the children.

In PARC *v.* Commonwealth of Pennsylvania, the court found that all children between 6 and 21 years of age, regardless of degree of disability, were to be given a "free and appropriate public education (FAPE)." Children with disabilities were to be educated with children without disabilities in the least restrictive environment (LRE). The educational system was ordered to stop applying exclusionary laws, parents were to become involved in the child's program, and re-evaluations were to be conducted. This landmark court case established many important principles that were later incorporated into the Education for All Handicapped Children Act. Simultaneous with the PARC case, other important court cases were being decided. Mills *v.* Board of Education of the District of Columbia (1972) was filed on behalf of all children excluded by public schools for a disability of any kind, including behavioral problems. The major result of this case was that all children, no matter how severe their mental retardation, behavioral problem, or disability, were educable and must be provided for suitably by the public school system. Related services, including physical therapy, were to be part of their educational program.

In *Maryland Association for Retarded Citizens v. Maryland* (1972), it was ruled that children have the right to tuition subsidies, the right to transportation, and the right to be educated with children who are not disabled. These cases and others across the nation began to establish the right of all children to a "free and appropriate public education." It was in this climate that PL 94-142 was enacted.

PL 94-142: EDUCATION FOR ALL HANDICAPPED CHILDREN ACT

PROVISIONS

On November 29, 1975, the U.S. Congress passed PL 94-142, the Education for All Handicapped Children Act. The law included the elements won in individual court cases across the nation and provided for a "free and appropriate public education" for all children with disabilities from ages 6 to 21 years (age 5 years if a state provided public education to children without disabilities at age 5 years). The major provisions of PL 94-142, still in place today, concern the concepts of zero reject, education in the least restrictive environment, right to due process, nondiscriminatory evaluation, individualized educational program, parent participation, and the right to related services, which include physical therapy.

ZERO REJECT

All children, including children with severe or profound disabilities, are to receive an education. These children initially were to receive priority for service because they probably were not receiving appropriate service at that time.

LEAST RESTRICTIVE ENVIRONMENT

Public agencies are to ensure the following:

> To the maximum extent appropriate, children with disabilities, including children in public or private institutions or other care facilities, are educated with children who are not disabled, and special classes, separate schooling, or other removal of children with disabilities from the regular educational environment occurs only when the nature or severity of the disability of a child is such that education in regular classes with the use of supplementary aids and services cannot be achieved satisfactorily. [PL 108-446, 118 Stat. 2677, § 612 (a)(5)(A).]

RIGHT TO DUE PROCESS

The law provides parents with numerous rights. Parents have the right to an impartial hearing, the right to be represented by counsel, and the right to a verbatim transcript of a hearing and written findings. They can appeal and obtain an independent evaluation. Later, under PL 99-372, the Handicapped Children's Protection Act [1986, 20 USC § 1415(e) (4), (f)], parents would be able to get reimbursed for legal fees if they prevailed in a court case.

NONDISCRIMINATORY EVALUATION

Several court cases had noted the discriminatory nature of the testing and placement procedures used in many school systems. Nondiscriminatory tests were to be administered, and no one test could be the sole criterion on which placement was based. Nondiscriminatory testing is critical in the cognitive and language domain; however, physical therapists, too, should be careful to determine that their tests are not biased. When possible, standardized tests that have norms for different racial and cultural groups should be used.

INDIVIDUALIZED EDUCATIONAL PROGRAM

Every child receiving special education must have an individualized educational program (IEP). This is the comprehensive program outlining the specific special education, related services, and supports the child is to receive. It includes measurable annual goals. The IEP is developed annually at an IEP meeting.

PARENT PARTICIPATION

Active participation of parents is encouraged under PL 94-142. Parents are the individuals responsible for continuity of services for their child and should be the child's best advocates. Parents are major decision makers in the development of the IEP: They must give permission for an evaluation, they can restrict the release of information, they have access to their child's records, and they can request due process hearings.

RELATED SERVICES

Related services, such as transportation, speech pathology, audiology, psychologic services, physical therapy, occupational therapy, recreation, and medical and counseling services, are to be provided "as may be required to assist a child with a disability to benefit from special education" [PL 108-446, 118 Stat. 2657, § 602 (26); PL 94-142, 89 Stat. 775]. This quotation from the law has been interpreted in many different ways. Physical therapy "to assist a child with a disability to benefit from special education" in some school systems is limited to only those activities that help the child write or sit properly in class. Other school systems more appropriately interpret the law to mean physical therapy that can help the child explore the environment, perform activities of daily living, improve function in school, prepare for vocational training, and improve physical fitness to be better prepared to learn and participate in a full life after school.

PL 99-457: EDUCATION OF THE HANDICAPPED ACT AMENDMENTS OF 1986; PL 102-119: INDIVIDUALS WITH DISABILITIES EDUCATION ACT AMENDMENTS OF 1991; PL 105-17: INDIVIDUALS WITH DISABILITIES EDUCATION ACT AMENDMENTS OF 1997; PL 108-446: INDIVIDUALS WITH DISABILITIES EDUCATION IMPROVEMENT ACT OF 2004

Congress must reauthorize the law at set intervals. At each reauthorization, the number of the public law changes to indicate which Congress is reauthorizing the law (the first number after PL) and which bill it is for that Congress

(second number). In 1986, the reauthorization, PL 99-457, the Education of the Handicapped Act Amendments of 1986, was particularly critical because this act extended services to infants, toddlers, and preschoolers with disabilities and their families. Services to infants and toddlers, now covered under Part C of the law, are discussed in Chapter 29. On October 7, 1991, PL 94-142 and PL 99-457 were reauthorized and amended as PL 102-119, the Individuals with Disabilities Education Act Amendments of 1991 (IDEA). PL 105-17 was signed into law in June 1997, and PL 108-446, the Individuals with Disabilities Education Improvement Act of 2004, was signed on December 3, 2004. PL 108-446 was to be reauthorized in 2010, but this has been delayed. The reader is urged to check for information on the reauthorization and any new rules and regulations. The key elements of these reauthorizations, really a refinement and reorganization of the previous amendments, are described in this section.

PART A: GENERAL PROVISIONS

Congress found that "disability is a natural part of the human experience and in no way diminishes the right of individuals to participate in or contribute to society. Improving educational results for children with disabilities is an essential element of our national policy of ensuring equality of opportunity, full participation, independent living, and economic self-sufficiency for individuals with disabilities" [PL 108-446, 118 Stat. 2649, § 601(c)]. The recognition that education is not merely the three "R's," but that it is intended to prepare children for independent living and self-sufficiency, is critical for therapists. This expands what goals could be considered "educationally relevant." Also, principles of universal design, which are part of the Assistive Technology Act of 1998, have been added to IDEA 2004. These include the design of products that will be usable by all people, to the greatest extent possible, with minimal need for additional adaptations and accommodations. These elements strengthen the physical therapist's role in providing access to the educational environment and learning materials.[28]

PART B: ASSISTANCE FOR EDUCATION OF ALL CHILDREN WITH DISABILITIES

Part B outlines the right to a free appropriate public education (FAPE) for all children ages 3 to 21 years. Children 3 to 5 and 18 to 21 years of age might not be served if inconsistent with state law. States are mandated to identify, locate, and evaluate all children with disabilities. Children eligible for special education and related services are those having one or more of the disabilities listed in Box 30-1.

Children 3 to 5 years of age are to have IEPs, as are school-age children; however, the 1991 reauthorization, PL 102-119, allowed states the option of using individualized family service plans (IFSPs), required for infants and toddlers, for

Box 30-1   FEDERAL DEFINITIONS OF CHILDREN WITH DISABILITIES

"(1) (i) *Autism* means a developmental disability significantly affecting verbal and nonverbal communication and social interaction, generally evident before age three, that adversely affects a child's educational performance. Other characteristics often associated with autism are engagement in repetitive activities and stereotyped movements, resistance to environmental change or change in daily routines, and unusual responses to sensory experiences.

(ii) Autism does not apply if a child's educational performance is adversely affected primarily because the child has an emotional disturbance, …

(2) *Deaf-blindness* means concomitant hearing and visual impairments, the combination of which causes such severe communication and other developmental and educational needs that they cannot be accommodated in special education programs solely for children with deafness or children with blindness.

(3) *Deafness* means a hearing impairment that is so severe that the child is impaired in processing linguistic information through hearing, with or without amplification, that adversely affects a child's educational performance.

(4) (i) *Emotional disturbance* means a condition exhibiting one or more of the following characteristics over a long period of time and to a marked degree that adversely affects a child's educational performance:

(A) An inability to learn that cannot be explained by intellectual, sensory, or health factors.

(B) An inability to build or maintain satisfactory interpersonal relationships with peers and teachers.

(C) Inappropriate types of behavior or feelings under normal circumstances.

(D) A general pervasive mood of unhappiness or depression.

(E) A tendency to develop physical symptoms or fears associated with personal or school problems.

(ii) Emotional disturbance includes schizophrenia. The term does not apply to children who are socially maladjusted,…

(5) *Hearing impairment* means an impairment in hearing, whether permanent or fluctuating, that adversely affects a child's educational performance but that is not included under the definition of deafness in this section.

(6) *Mental retardation* means significantly subaverage general intellectual functioning, existing concurrently with deficits in adaptive behavior and manifested during the developmental period, that adversely affects a child's educational performance.

(7) *Multiple disabilities* means concomitant impairments (such as mental retardation-blindness or mental retardation-orthopedic impairment), the combination of which causes such severe educational needs that they cannot be accommodated in special education programs solely for one of the impairments. Multiple disabilities does not include deaf-blindness.

(8) *Orthopedic impairment* means a severe orthopedic impairment that adversely affects a child's educational performance. The term includes impairments caused by a congenital anomaly, impairments caused by disease (e.g., poliomyelitis, bone tuberculosis), and impairments from other causes (e.g., cerebral palsy, amputations, and fractures or burns that cause contractures).

(9) *Other health impairment* means having limited strength, vitality, or alertness, including a heightened alertness to environmental stimuli, that results in limited alertness with respect to the educational environment, that—

(i) Is due to chronic or acute health problems such as asthma, attention deficit disorder or attention deficit hyperactivity disorder, diabetes, epilepsy, a heart condition, hemophilia, lead poisoning, leukemia, nephritis, rheumatic fever, sickle cell anemia, and Tourette syndrome; and

(ii) Adversely affects a child's educational performance.

(10) *Specific learning disability*—(i) *General.* Specific learning disability means a disorder in one or more of the basic psychological processes involved in understanding or in using language, spoken or written, that may manifest itself in the imperfect ability to listen, think, speak, read, write, spell, or to do mathematical calculations, including conditions such as perceptual disabilities, brain injury, minimal brain dysfunction, dyslexia, and developmental aphasia.

(ii) *Disorders not included.* Specific learning disability does not include learning problems that are primarily the result of visual, hearing, or motor disabilities, of mental retardation, of emotional disturbance, or of environmental, cultural, or economic disadvantage.

(11) *Speech or language impairment* means a communication disorder, such as stuttering, impaired articulation, a language impairment, or a voice impairment, that adversely affects a child's educational performance.

(12) *Traumatic brain injury* means an acquired injury to the brain caused by an external physical force, resulting in total or partial functional disability or psychosocial impairment, or both, that adversely affects a child's educational performance. Traumatic brain injury applies to open or closed head injuries resulting in impairments in one or more areas, such as cognition; language; memory; attention; reasoning; abstract thinking; judgment; problem-solving; sensory, perceptual, and motor abilities; psychosocial behavior; physical functions; information processing; and speech. Traumatic brain injury does not apply to brain injuries that are congenital or degenerative, or to brain injuries induced by birth trauma.

Continued

Box **30-1** FEDERAL DEFINITIONS OF CHILDREN WITH DISABILITIES—cont'd

(13) *Visual impairment including blindness* means an impairment in vision that, even with correction, adversely affects a child's educational performance. The term includes both partial sight and blindness." (Authority: 20 U.S.C. 1401(3); 1401(30))

Developmental delay: "The term *child with a disability* for a child aged 3 through 9 may, at the discretion of the State and local educational agency, include a

child......experiencing developmental delays, as defined by the State and as measured by appropriate diagnostic instruments and procedures, in one or more of the following areas: physical development, cognitive development, communication development, social or emotional development, or adaptive development, and who, for that reason, needs special education and related services" [PL 105-17, 111 Stat. 43, Sec. 602 (3) (B)].

---

preschool-age children. The 2004 reauthorization also allows states the option to continue to provide early intervention services to children with disabilities until the child enters kindergarten or elementary school [PL 108-446, 118 Stat. 2746, § 632(5)(B)(ii)]. Many professionals believe the problems of preschoolers and their families are better served by the family-centered approach embodied in early intervention.

LEAST RESTRICTIVE ENVIRONMENT

An ongoing area of national effort is the education of children with disabilities in the least restrictive environment (LRE). Children should be educated in their local schools to the maximum extent appropriate. The degree of inclusion in the local school and the general education classroom will vary based on what is appropriate for their needs and age. Children are not merely to be "placed" in general education, but they are to fully participate and have goals related to their academic and social advancement. Since 1990, a significant reduction has occurred in the placement of children with disabilities in separate facilities and segregated classrooms, along with substantial increases in the amount of time they spend in regular classrooms.[123]

TRANSITION

Transition planning was specifically addressed in IDEA 1997 because this important service was often neglected. Transition planning and required services must be included in the IFSP and IEP. Consideration must be given to transition from early intervention to preschool, from preschool to school, at critical points during school, and especially from age 16 years to exit from school. Physical therapists and other related service personnel are to be involved in transition planning for post-school activities, as appropriate. Transition to adulthood is presented in Chapter 32.

ASSISTIVE TECHNOLOGY

Assistive technology devices and assistive technology services allow the child to fully benefit from the educational environment. "The term '*assistive technology device*' means any item, piece of equipment, or product system, whether acquired commercially off the shelf, modified, or customized, that is used to increase, maintain, or improve the functional capabilities of a child with a disability ... '*assistive technology service*' means any service that directly assists a child with a disability in the selection, acquisition, or use of an assistive technology device" [PL 108-446, 118 Stat. 2652, § 602(1)].

Assistive technology services include evaluation, selection, purchasing, and coordination with education and rehabilitation plans and programs. This is an important area, as physical therapists frequently provide assistive devices to improve a child's function and participation at school. Therapists adapt seating so children can function better and safely in the classroom. They assist other team members in devising the most functional communication systems, along with providing access to switching devices and computers. Physical therapists are generally the key related service providers involved in the choice and maintenance of mobility devices, including walkers, crutches, canes, and manual and power wheelchairs. These mobility devices allow children with disabilities to access the school building and grounds and thereby participate in all aspects of their education program. The extent of assistive technology services and the purchasing of devices vary among school systems. For additional information, see Chapter on Assistive Technology (Evolve site).

EARLY INTERVENING SERVICES AND RESPONSE TO INTERVENTION

Early intervening services (EIS) and response to intervention (RTI) are both new to IDEA 2004. EIS focuses on children from kindergarten to grade 3 who would benefit from additional academic services and behavioral support to succeed in the general education environment [34 cfr 300.226(a)][20 u.s.c. 1431(f)(1)]. RTI involves high-quality instruction/intervention, using the student's learning rate and level of performance for decision making. Important educational decisions are based on the student's response to instruction/intervention across multiple tiers.[10] RTI is an evaluation and intervention process used to monitor student progress and make data-based decisions about the need for and provision of instructional modification, research-based intervention, and increasingly intensified services for students having problems in school. The goal of RTI is to prevent the overidentification of children for special education, especially those with potential learning disabilities. RTI is a departure from deficit-based assessments and focuses on possible successful interventions rather than "what is wrong" with the student. It is a multi-tiered service-delivery model with differentiated instruction to meet the individual needs of all students, not just those with specific disabilities.[107]

Response to intervention (RTI) holds many promises in that collaboration and teaming are required to support implementation. RTI is defined by high-quality instruction and provides a curriculum structure that can be implemented in an inclusive setting.[64] RTI allows therapists to participate with the team to meet a student's needs *prior* to establishing eligibility for special education. Therapists may provide expertise in many areas such as in modifying classrooms, suggesting learning strategies, and providing adaptive equipment or any necessary intervention. The goals are to do what is required for the student to succeed in the curriculum with the fewest restrictions.

Questions often arise regarding RTI and the need for written parental approval to perform an evaluation, parental approval to provide services, and the extent of documentation necessary for evaluation and intervention. Answers to those questions will depend on individual state physical therapy practice acts; however, it usually is best to receive written permission from parents for any form of evaluation and intervention. Documentation of interaction with a child is always an important element of ethical practice.

SECTION 504 OF THE REHABILITATION ACT

Section 504 of the Rehabilitation Act of 1973 (PL 93-112) is a broad antidiscrimination statute designed to ensure that federal funding recipients—including schools—provide equal opportunity to people with disabilities (Discipline Under Section 504, 1996). It has been used to broaden a student's eligibility for related services in school. Educational agencies that receive federal funds are not allowed to exclude qualified individuals with disabilities from participation in any program offered by the agency. The definition of qualified *handicapped person* under Section 504 is broader than it is in IDEA. Under Section 504, qualified "*handicapped person* means any person who (i) has a physical or mental impairment which substantially limits one or more major life activities, (ii) has a record of such an impairment, or (iii) is regarded as having such an impairment" [34CFR104.3(j)(1)]. "*Major life activities* means functions such as caring for one's self, performing manual tasks, walking, seeing, hearing,

speaking, breathing, learning, and working" [34CFR104.3(j)(2)(ii)]. The recent Americans With Disabilities Amendments Act of 2008 (ADAAA) includes a "conforming amendment" to Section 504, which means that the expanded coverage of ADAAA also applies to Section 504. The ADAAA retains the definition of disability under Section 504 but emphasizes that the definition should be interpreted broadly.[124] The ADAAA "directs that the ameliorating effects of mitigating measures (other than ordinary eyeglasses or contact lenses) not be considered in determining whether an individual has a disability; expands the scope of 'major life activities' by providing a non-exhaustive list of general activities and a non-exhaustive list of major bodily functions; clarifies that an impairment that is episodic or in remission is a disability if it would substantially limit a major life activity when active."[124]

Thus, it is possible that a child who does not require special education according to the accepted definitions of disabilities under IDEA, but who is a qualified handicapped person, might be able to receive all the aids, services, and accommodations necessary to receive a free and appropriate public education through Section 504. Nationally, only 1.2% of public school students are Section 504 students, with the greatest numbers in middle and high school having attention deficit hyperactivity disorder.[59] The ADAAA now means that more students will qualify for support under Section 504.[67] Interpretation of Section 504 varies among states and even among individual school districts; in some districts, students with 504 plans may receive direct physical therapy services or consultation, but in other districts they may not.

PL 101-336: AMERICANS WITH DISABILITIES ACT

The Americans With Disabilities Act (ADA) (PL 101-336) was signed into law on July 26, 1990. It "extends to individuals with disabilities comprehensive civil rights protection similar to those provided to persons on the basis of race, sex, national origin, and religion under the Civil Rights Act of 1964" (*Federal Register,* July 26, 1991, p. 3540). The regulations cover employment; public service, including public transportation, public accommodations, and telecommunications; and miscellaneous provisions. Although the law is not specific in reference to issues related to children in school, the provisions of ADA assist students with disabilities. The law is especially applicable to day care centers and transition to employment.[97] Public buildings, including schools, must be accessible, and children should be able to use public transportation to get to school, work, and social activities. Children with disabilities should expect to use the skills learned at school in an accessible workplace. The ADA is also discussed in Chapter 32, "Transition to Adulthood for Youth With Disabilities."

ELEMENTARY AND SECONDARY EDUCATION ACT

The Elementary and Secondary Education Act of 1965 (ESEA) was passed as part of the "War on Poverty." ESEA emphasizes equal access to education of all children and encourages high standards and accountability. The law provides federal funding for education programs that are administered by the states.

Congress amended and reauthorized ESEA as the No Child Left Behind Act of 2001 (NCLB) (PL 107-110). This federal legislation was to ensure that all children, including those with disabilities, receive a quality education. To achieve this goal, all children were to be tested and make "adequate yearly progress." There has been considerable criticism of this legislation and more than 151 national organizations have formally expressed concerns regarding NCLB. "Among these concerns are: over-emphasizing standardized testing, narrowing curriculum and instruction to focus on test preparation rather than richer academic learning; over-identifying schools in need of improvement; using sanctions that do not help improve schools; inappropriately excluding low-scoring children in order to boost test results; and inadequate funding."[91] In December 2003, new federal provisions were announced, in recognition of the failure of NCLB to properly address the testing of children with disabilities and to meet annual yearly progress for closing the achievement gap. Under these new provisions, local school systems have greater flexibility in meeting the requirements of NCLB.[44] Each state is now responsible for determining the definition of *significant cognitive disabilities.* To assist with the demands of NCLB, physical therapists working in school systems should make certain that children are properly positioned and have appropriate writing implements or computer access for testing situations. ESEA is being reviewed for reauthorization and the reader should seek information on how the reauthorized law might impact physical therapy service delivery.

CASE LAW

A law as comprehensive and complex as IDEA was bound to lead to some controversy. All possible situations could not be anticipated, and some issues were expected to be resolved by the courts. Disagreements that have led to due process hearings involving physical therapy have generally focused on (1) adequacy of physical therapy services; (2) qualifications and training of personnel; (3) need for services over the summer or during school breaks; (4) compensatory physical therapy; and (5) types of intervention provided.[66] As a result of due process disagreements, a number of significant state and federal court cases have helped define the scope of the law. Those of interest to physical therapists include cases involving related services, best possible education, extended school year (ESY), and LRE.

RELATED SERVICES

Tatro v. Texas (1980) was one of the early major cases involving PL 94-142. Amber Tatro had spina bifida and required clean intermittent catheterization several times during the school day. Her parents wanted assistance with catheterization at school. School officials refused, claiming that catheterization is a medical procedure, and Amber could not attend school unless her parents handled the procedure. The parents then initiated what turned out to be a 10-year legal battle. During the legal process, they were told that although catheterization was necessary to sustain Amber's life, it was not necessary to benefit from education; the school system, therefore, was not obligated to provide the service. After a complicated course through the court system, the case was heard by the U.S. Supreme Court. Amber attempted to attend the proceedings, only to discover that the building was not wheelchair accessible. The Supreme Court ruled that clean intermittent catheterization was a related service that enabled the child to benefit from special education:

> "A service that enables a handicapped child to remain at school during the day is an important means of providing students with the meaningful access to education that Congress envisioned. The Act makes specific provision for services, like transportation, for example, that do no more than enable a child to be physically present in class" (Tatro v. Texas, 1980, p. 891).[79]

This case led to the "bright-line" physician-nonphysician rule that a school district is not required to provide services of a physician (other than for diagnostic and evaluation purposes) but must offer those of a nurse or qualified layperson. This case is important to physical therapists because the realm of related services was expanded, as was the meaning of "required to benefit from special education."

Court cases have also involved related services and children who are medically fragile and require extensive services of a nurse and others. Some states advocate the use of an extent/nature test, in which decision making focuses on the individual case and considers the complexity of and need for services. The U.S. Supreme Court in Cedar Rapids Community School District v. Garret F. (Supreme Court of the United States, No. 96-1793, March 3, 1999) reaffirmed that related services, in this case nursing services, were not excluded medical services under IDEA and must be provided in schools, irrespective of the intensity or complexity of the services. This decision supported the right to an education for children with complex health care needs.

BEST POSSIBLE EDUCATION

Rowley v. Board of Education of Hendrick Hudson Central School District (1982) involved Amy Rowley, who was deaf.

She had a special tutor, her teachers were trained in basic sign language, and she was provided with a sound amplifier. After experimenting with a sign language interpreter in a general education class, the school system decided she did not need the service. Her parents believed she needed the interpreter and went through due process to continue interpreter services. A district court held that Amy was not receiving a free and appropriate public education because she did not have "an opportunity to achieve her full potential commensurate with the opportunity provided to other children." The school district appealed, and the case eventually went to the U.S. Supreme Court. The 1982 Supreme Court decision held that Congress did not intend to give children with disabilities the right to the best possible education (i.e., education that would "maximize their potential"). It rejected the standard used by the lower courts that children with disabilities are entitled to an educational opportunity "commensurate with the education available to nonhandicapped children." The decision set two standards: (1) A state is required to provide meaningful access to education for each child with a disability, and (2) sufficient supportive and related services must be provided to permit the child to benefit educationally from special education instruction.

When the Supreme Court applied these standards in Rowley, it found that Amy did not need interpreter services because she was making "exemplary progress in the regular education system" with the help of the extensive special services. The Supreme Court was careful to point out that merely passing from grade to grade does not mean a child's education is appropriate.

The Rowley decision has had a major impact on the provision of related services, including physical therapy. Unfortunately, in some school systems it has been used to limit the amount of physical therapy provided on the premise that schools are not obligated to provide the "best services." Therapists should recognize that "exemplary progress" may be a reason to terminate services unless an educational need for physical therapy can be substantiated.

EXTENDED SCHOOL YEAR

As children with special needs began to benefit from 9-month educational programs, some parents realized that their children's skills were regressing during the summer and that it took several months to regain those skills when the children returned to school in the fall. Because the U.S. Congress had realized that more than the traditional 12 years of schooling might be necessary for children with disabilities to reach their potential, perhaps it could be inferred that if a child regressed during the summer, extended school year services might be necessary.[79]

Several court cases addressed this issue. In both Battle v. Commonwealth of Pennsylvania (1981) and Georgia Association of Retarded Citizens v. McDaniel (1981), parents sought to extend the school year. In Pennsylvania, it was found that the state's policy of defining a school year as 180 days could not be used to prevent the provision of an extended school year. In Georgia, the court ruled that an extended school year must be based on individual cases. The child must show significant regression following school breaks, the extended year must be part of the IEP, and an extended year does not mean 5 days a week for 52 weeks but must be based on a program to attain goals.

Eligibility for extended school year (ESY) services is now based on several criteria. These include "individual need, nature and severity of the disability, educational benefit, regression and recoupment, self-sufficiency and independence, and failing to meet short-term goals and objectives" (p.16).[106] The possibility of receiving services for the entire year has many implications for physical therapy. The children most likely to require ESY services are usually those with the most severe disabilities, often requiring physical therapy. Some children may be deemed eligible for ESY academic services and may not need ESY physical therapy services. One criterion used to qualify for ESY services is documentation of regression during vacations and the length of time it takes to recoup or relearn skills. It is therefore vital for physical therapists to do an examination and evaluation before and after school breaks. Documentation of regression, especially during short breaks, might enable a child to receive physical therapy over the summer. Using the child's status at the end of the summer as the basis for ESY physical therapy services might be confounded, however, if parents obtain private physical therapy during the summer and regression is prevented.

An ethical dilemma can arise for some physical therapists over the ESY issue. Some school therapists provide private physical therapy during the summer and might prefer that the school system not provide the service. Others might not want the obligation of having to provide services during the summer, either through the school or privately. Therapists must be careful to recognize these potential conflicts of interest.

LEAST RESTRICTIVE ENVIRONMENT

The issue of LRE, also referred to as *inclusion,* has generated much discussion over the years; it has also generated many due process hearings and lawsuits. Outcomes have been mixed. During the early 1990's, the party seeking inclusion, usually the parent, prevailed in a series of court cases, the most noted being Oberti (3d Cir. 1993) and Daniel R.R. (5th Cir. 1989).[133] Later cases ruled against inclusive, general education placements as the LRE for students who were past elementary school age and had severe disabilities.[117] A rational approach must prevail in issues regarding inclusion. As discussed later in the chapter, options must exist for locations and types of services available to the child that can and should change over time.

EDUCATIONAL MILIEU

Although for many years physical therapists have served children with disabilities in the general education setting, educational administrators and teachers vary in their perceptions of the role of physical therapy. Similarly, physical therapists have different perspectives of their role in the educational milieu. Hence, open communication and collaboration are essential. Physical therapists must take the time to develop relationships with administrators, teachers, and staff, and they need to understand the written and unwritten rules of the educational environment, to create an effective working environment.

LEAST RESTRICTIVE ENVIRONMENT

Education of all children in the LRE, no matter how severe their disabilities, is the intent of the federal laws and is considered "best practice" (PL 105-17; PL 108-446).[87,120] The conceptual framework for education in the LRE started in the 1960's. Reynolds[108] advocated a continuum of placement options from most restrictive to least restrictive. Deno[30] named this the *cascade of educational placements.* The cascade of environments, from most to least restrictive, includes the residential setting, homebound services, special schools, special classes in neighborhood schools, general classes with resource assistance in neighborhood schools, and general classes in the neighborhood school without resource assistance. Taylor,[120] a long-time advocate for total integration of people with severe disabilities, proposed that the focus must change from expecting individuals to fit into existing programs to providing services and supports necessary for full participation in community life. Terminology used to describe LRE has evolved from *mainstreaming,* to *integrated,* to *inclusive.* The differences in terms are more than merely a change in language.

Inclusive education at its best involves the whole school where children with disabilities are served in the general education environment with the required "supplementary aids and services."[77] Models for meeting a student's needs in an inclusive setting include (a) general education and special education teachers co-teaching during all or part of the curriculum; (b) indirect, consultative support from the special education teacher; (c) material adaptation by the special education teacher; (d) including the special education teacher as a member of the team serving the child, usually in middle and high school; and (e) a school-wide approach whereby the entire staff takes responsibility for all students.[77] Physical therapists who work in systems using any of these models need to develop collaborative working relationships with all appropriate personnel for maximum communication and team effectiveness, and optimal child outcomes.

Compliance with LRE requirements is occurring to varying degrees across the nation. Therapists must be prepared to work with administrators, teachers, and staff who may know little about children with disabilities and the role of the physical therapist in educational settings. This presents a challenging and potentially rewarding opportunity for therapists to share their knowledge about the disabilities of their students, and their associated activity limitations, participation restrictions, and environmental factors, along with their impairments in body functions and structures. Interaction with other physical therapists is often limited when only a few children receive physical therapy services at each school. Therapists might also need to travel long distances to see a single child, and scheduling services and times to meet with teachers can be difficult. The reader is encouraged to examine other references for a more in-depth discussion of positive outcomes and aspects of inclusion.[19,21,52,81,103,110]

MODELS OF TEAM INTERACTION

There has been an evolution in the models of team interaction over the past several decades. The hierarchy of team interaction is presented in Box 30-2. A unidisciplinary model

---

Box 30-2 Models of Team Interaction

Unidisciplinary: Professional works independently of all others.

Intradisciplinary: Members of the same profession work together without significant communication with members of other professions.

Multidisciplinary: Discipline-specific roles are well-defined and professionals work independently but recognize and value the contributions of other disciplines. "Little or no interaction or ongoing communication occurs among professionals" (p. 225).[122] However, the Rules and Regulations (*Federal Register,* June 22, 1989, p. 26313) for PL 99-457 redefine *multidisciplinary* to mean "the involvement of two or more disciplines or professions in the provision of integrated and coordinated services, including evaluation and assessment."

Interdisciplinary: Discipline-specific roles are well-defined; however, individuals from different disciplines work together cooperatively on planning, implementation, and evaluation of services. Emphasis is on teamwork. Role definitions are relaxed.

Transdisciplinary: Professionals are committed "to teaching, learning and working with others across traditional disciplinary boundaries" (p. 13).[102] Role release occurs when a team member assumes the responsibilities of other disciplines for service delivery.

Collaborative: The team interaction of the transdisciplinary model is combined with the integrated service-delivery model. Services are provided by professionals across disciplinary boundaries as part of the natural routine of the school and community.

is not a team model and should rarely, if ever, be used in school settings. The multidisciplinary model involves several professionals conducting independent evaluations and then meeting to discuss their evaluations and determine goals, objectives, and a plan of action. The meaning of *multidisciplinary* has changed since 1986 because of its usage in PL 99-457. In the law, the term *multidisciplinary* is used to describe an interdisciplinary model, causing frequent confusion.

The definition and application of the transdisciplinary model are also ambiguous. For some, the continuous sharing of information across disciplines is sufficient for a transdisciplinary model. For others, there must be complete role release, which involves not just the sharing of information but also the sharing of performance competencies. Team members teach each other interventions so that all can provide greater consistency and frequency in meeting the child's needs. Occasionally in a transdisciplinary model, only one individual provides the intervention, thereby increasing consistency and allowing rapport to be established with the child and family.

As the team process has developed, several authors have advocated use of the terms that describe the dynamics of team interaction and may include a combination of models based on the specific needs of educators, therapists, children, and families.[57,61,104,115] The defining characteristics of collaborative teamwork, as conceptualized by Rainforth and York-Barr,[104] are summarized in Box 30-3. Advantages of the collaborative model are derived from the diverse perspectives, skills, and knowledge available among individuals on the educational team. This combined talent is an enormous resource for problem solving and support. Collaborative

---

| Box **30-3** | CHARACTERISTICS OF COLLABORATIVE TEAMWORK |

- Equal participation in the team process by family members and service providers
- Consensus decision making in determining priorities for goals and objectives
- Consensus decision making about the type and amount of intervention
- All skills, including motor and communication skills, are embedded throughout the intervention program.
- Infusion of knowledge and skills from different disciplines into the design and application of intervention
- Role release to enable team members to develop the confidence and competence necessary to facilitate the child's learning

Adapted from Rainforth, B., & York-Barr, J. (1997). *Collaborative teams for students with severe disabilities* (2nd ed.). Baltimore: Paul H. Brookes.

---

teams are of vital importance when working with children with multiple disabilities or with those who are severely or profoundly disabled.

When joining a team, physical therapists should ask for clarification regarding models or expectations of team interaction. All individuals should have the same understanding to avoid miscommunication and conflict.

MODELS OF SERVICE DELIVERY

Service-delivery models are frameworks that describe the format in which intervention is provided.[72] Common models include direct, integrated, consultative, monitoring, collaborative, and relational goal-oriented models. In their nationwide survey of school-based physical therapists, Kaminker and colleagues[68] found that therapists reported providing services most often through a combination of these models (Table 30-1).

Direct Model

In the direct model, the therapist is the primary service provider for the child. This is the most common model of physical therapy service delivery across practice settings. Direct intervention is provided when there is emphasis on acquisition of motor skills and when therapeutic techniques cannot be safely delegated. It may take place in the context of the student's natural environment or, if necessary, in an isolated "pull-out" setting; in either case, ongoing consultation with parents, teachers, and other team members is essential.[55] A child may receive direct intervention for one goal, while other models of service delivery are used to achieve other goals. A combination of several models of service delivery is consistent with the integrated and collaborative service-delivery models.

Integrated Model

The Iowa State Department of Education[63] defines the integrated model as one in which (1) the therapist interacts not only with the child but also with the teacher, aide, and family; (2) services are provided in the learning environment; and (3) several people are involved in implementation of the therapy program. Team collaboration is a key feature of the model. The integrated model frequently includes direct and consultative physical therapy services. Goals and objectives should be developed collaboratively, and all individuals serving the child should be instructed on how to incorporate objectives into the child's education program. Direct services, if appropriate, are provided in the least restrictive environment. Only when it is in the best interests of the child should the intervention be provided in a restrictive environment, such as a special room, because skills learned in one setting do not necessarily generalize to other settings.[15] Common examples of when therapy might be acceptable in a more restrictive environment are when the child is participating in academic courses, when extensive equipment is

TABLE 30-1 Physical Therapy Service-Delivery Models in Educational Settings

	Direct	Integrated	Consultative	Monitoring	Collaborative	Relational Goal-Oriented[72]
Therapist's primary contact	Student	Student, teacher, parent, aide	Teacher, parent, aide, student	Student	Entire team, student	Entire team, student
Environment for service delivery	Distraction-free environment (may need to be separate from learning environment) Specialized equipment needed	Learning environment and other natural settings Therapy area if necessary for a specific child	Learning environment and other natural settings	Learning environment Therapy area if necessary for a specific child	Learning environment and other natural settings	Learning environment and other natural settings
Methods of intervention	Educationally related functional activities Specific therapeutic techniques that cannot safely be delegated Emphasis on acquisition of new motor skills	Educationally related functional activities Positioning Emphasis on practice of newly acquired motor skills in the daily routine	Educationally related activities Positioning Adaptive materials Emphasis on adapting to learning environment and generalization of acquired skills	Emphasis on ensuring that child maintains status to benefit from special education	Educationally related activities	Emphasis on overarching goals and desired outcomes that require relationship skills
Amount of actual service times	Regularly scheduled sessions, generally at least weekly	Routinely scheduled Flexible amount of time depending on needs of staff or pupil	Intermittent or as needed, depending on needs of staff or pupil	Intermittent, depending on needs of pupil, may be as infrequent as once in 6 months	Ongoing intervention Discipline-referenced knowledge shared among team members, so relevant activities occur throughout the day	Customized
Implementer of activities	PT, PTA	PT, PTA, teacher, parent, aide, OT, OTA	Teacher, parent, aide	PT	Team	Team
Individualized education plan objectives	Specific to therapy programs as related to educational needs	Specific to educational program	Specific to educational program	Specific to being able to maintain educational program	Organized around life domains in an ecologic curriculum	Short-term to have positive child experience; mid-term to reduce impairment, optimize function, and enhance participation; long-term to optimize adaptation and adjustment

Adapted from *Iowa guidelines for educationally related physical services.* (1996). Des Moines, IA: Department of Education.
OTA, Occupational therapist assistant; *OT,* occupational therapist; *PT,* physical therapist; and *PTA,* physical therapist assistant.

required, when the child is highly distractible, or when it is necessary for the child's safety.

Consultative Model

In the consultative model, the therapist interacts in the learning environment with appropriate members of the educational team, including the parents, who then implement the recommended activities. The physical therapist provides instruction and demonstration without direct intervention. Responsibility for the outcome lies with the individuals receiving the consultation.[34]

Hanft and Place[55] noted that consultation in the school may be included in several service-delivery models. Consultation may be provided for a specific child, as outlined in Table 30-1, but it might also include programmatic consultation with the education staff involving issues related to safety, transportation, architectural barriers, equipment, documentation, continuing education, and improvement of program quality.[76] Programmatic consultation should be the major activity of the therapist at the beginning of each academic year and may often be more important than child-specific goals and objectives. Once the environment is safe, the child is properly positioned throughout the day, and a safe means of mobility is determined, goals pertaining to skill development can be addressed.

Monitoring Model

In the monitoring model, the physical therapist shares information and provides instruction to team members, maintains regular contact with the child to check on status, and assumes responsibility for the outcome of the intervention. Similar to the consultative model, the therapist does not provide direct intervention. Monitoring is important for follow-up of children who have impairments, activity limitations, or participation restrictions that might become more pronounced over time. It allows the therapist to check adaptive equipment and assistive devices. Monitoring may be an important way to determine whether a child is progressing as necessary for transition to the next level of educational or vocational services. It is useful for transition from direct or integrated services to no services, and it provides the family, child, and therapist a sense of security that the child is being observed. If the need for direct services is identified, initiation of services is facilitated because physical therapy is already listed on the IEP.

Collaborative Model

"School-based collaboration is an interactive team process that focuses student, family, education and related service partners on enhancing the academic achievement and functional performance of *all* students in school" (p. 3).[57] It focuses on team operations and management and how to seamlessly interact with team members to select and blend services. Collaboration should be part of all service-delivery models, although not everyone would consider it a model of service delivery.[57] However, because collaboration is frequently defined as a combination of transdisciplinary team interaction and an integrated service-delivery model, it is discussed here as part of service delivery.[104] As noted in Box 30-3 and Table 30-1, services in a collaborative model are provided by all team members, as in an integrated model, but the degree of role release and crossing of disciplinary boundaries is greater. The team assumes responsibility for developing a consensus on the goals and objectives, as well as on implementation of program activities, which are educationally relevant and are conducted in the natural routine of the school and community. In the collaborative model, theoretically, the amount of time the child practices an activity should be greater than in other models because the entire team participates in the program. In reality, this might not be the case because of the varied ability levels of team members, insufficient natural opportunities to practice skills, competing priorities in the student's schedule, and the student's difficulty in performing some activities. Research by Hunt and associates[61] suggests that for students with severe disabilities, collaborative teaming results in increased academic skills, engagement in classroom activities, interactions with peers, and student-initiated interactions. The researchers indicated that parents played a critical role in the development and implementation of the programs, and flexibility was key to the practicality and applicability of suggestions.

In the past, many believed that state physical therapy practice acts prohibited other school personnel from performing procedures that are within the scope of physical therapy practice. Generally, this is not the case as long as the individual does not represent himself or herself as a physical therapist, does not bill for physical therapy, and does not perform a physical therapy evaluation.[101] In fact, a study by Rainforth[101] indicates few limitations on the delegation of procedures by others, especially of the nature likely to occur in an educational environment. Team members do not really perform physical therapy, but rather carry out activities that are recommended to assist the child to learn and practice motor skills in multiple environments.[84]

Relational Goal-Oriented Model

The Relational Goal-Oriented Model (RGM) of service delivery to children was developed by King[72] and builds on the framework of the Life Needs Model of Pediatric Service Delivery.[74] The Life Needs Model addresses the "why" and "what" of service delivery, while the RGM focuses on the "how" of service delivery and incorporates relationship-based practice with goal orientation. The model consists of six elements: (1) overarching goals; (2) desired outcomes; (3) fundamental needs; (4) relational processes; (5) approaches, world-views, and priorities; and (6) strategies. These elements are applied to client-practitioner and practitioner-organization relationships.

PROGRAM DEVELOPMENT

ELIGIBILITY FOR PHYSICAL THERAPY

As was noted previously, for school-age children, a motor delay or disability does not necessarily qualify a student for special education and related services. The child must have an educational need for special education in one of the categories listed in Box 30-1. Once a child meets the criteria for special education in one of these categories, the related service needs are determined as "required to assist a child with a disability to benefit from special education" [PL 108-446, 118 Stat. 2657, § 602 (26)]. Within the requirements of federal law, state and local regulations may include additional elements related to eligibility.

Many states have developed lengthy guidelines for school practice that can assist therapists in their decisions regarding both a student's need for physical therapy and service delivery. These guidelines generally can be found on the website of the state's Department of Education, the state's Physical Therapy Association, or both. For example, the document developed in Maryland (*Occupational and Physical Therapy Early Intervention and School-Based Services in Maryland: A Guide to Practice*), published in December 2008, describes the process for determining the need for school-based occupational and physical therapy services as follows:

> "Once the IEP team agrees on the present levels of the student's performance and IEP goals/objectives, the team then determines whether the unique expertise of an OT or PT is required for the student to be able to access, participate, and progress in the learning environment in preparation for success in his/her postsecondary life. Based on the individual needs of the student, the PLs [present levels], goals and objectives, the IEP team with recommendations from the OT or PT team member(s) determines necessary related services" (p. 28).[80]

The 2006 Kentucky guidelines (*Resource Manual for Educationally Related Occupational Therapy and Physical Therapy in Kentucky Public Schools*) remind therapists to ask a fundamental question: "Is an occupational therapist's or a physical therapist's knowledge and expertise a necessary component of the student's educational program in order for him/her to achieve identified outcomes?" (p. 2).[70] Further key questions regarding service determination listed in the Kentucky guidelines include the following:

- Does the challenge significantly interfere with the student's ability to access the general education curriculum and prepare for employment and independent living?
- Does the challenge in an identified area appear to be caused by limitations in a motor or sensory area?
- Will the student receive appropriate modifications and accommodations and make progress on the IEP goals with

assistance from staff other than the occupational therapist and/or physical therapist?
- Have previous attempts to alleviate the concerns been successful and documented?
- What is the potential for positive or negative change with/without occupational therapy and/or physical therapy services?
- Will the student's educational environment become more restrictive if occupational therapy and/or physical therapy services are not provided? (p. 34)[70]

If a child is not eligible for special education, he or she may be eligible for related services under Section 504 of the Rehabilitation Act. The need for related services must be based on the individual needs of the child. Some school districts have attempted to develop generalized exclusionary criteria such as *performance discrepancy criteria*, also called *cognitive referencing*. Performance discrepancy criteria limit services to children whose cognitive development is below their motor development (p. 506).[18] This assumes a positive correlation between the development of cognition and motor skills. Under this interpretation, the child most appropriate for physical therapy has normal intellectual skills but a delay in motor skills. Children whose cognitive and motor skills are similar would not be eligible for services. Aside from the legal[100] and ethical questions, research does not support cognitive referencing.[9,22]

EVALUATION

Results of the evaluation are used to make decisions about the need for school-based physical therapy services, IEP goals, frequency and duration of services, and ESY services. The elements of patient/client management in the *Guide to Physical Therapist Practice*[2] differ somewhat from those of federal education laws. In the school setting, evaluations are conducted to "assist in determining whether the child is a child with a disability" [PL 108-446, 118 Stat. 27045, § 614(b) (2)]; they are also used to determine the educational needs of the child. The process of evaluation, therefore, is comparable with examination and evaluation in the *Guide*.

A comprehensive team evaluation should be conducted "at least every 3 years, unless the parent and the local educational agency agree that a re-evaluation is unnecessary" [PL 108-446, 118 Stat. 2704, § 614 (a)(2)]. It may be performed no more often than once a year, unless both parent and educational agency agree to more frequent evaluations. Physical therapy evaluation may need to be done more frequently according to the requirements of individual state practice acts and best practice guidelines. All therapists should be familiar with their state's requirements.

Physical therapy evaluation in the educational environment should be consistent with the framework of the World Health Organization's International Classification of Functioning, Disability and Health (ICF), which focuses on both enablement and disablement.[111,131] Although the 2001 edition of the *Guide* incorporates the Nagi disablement model (pathophysiology, impairment, functional limitations, disabilities),[2] the edition that is under revision at the time of this writing will be based on the ICF model.[4] Evaluation should describe the student's participation (engagement in life situations), activities (tasks), and body functions (physiology) and structures (anatomy), with consideration of personal and environmental factors. These elements are reported from the perspective of access, participation, and progress in the educational program. Although the emphasis is on enablement, rather than disablement, the evaluation should incorporate participation restrictions (with required adaptations and assistance), activity limitations, and impairments in body functions and structures.[84] Evaluation should also make the distinction between capacity (what the student *can* do in controlled conditions) and performance (what the student actually *does* in the natural settings of daily life). Intervention strategies to reduce impairments of body functions and structures may be necessary to meet the student's educational needs. Examination should also include a review of body systems from the perspective of school function: musculoskeletal, neuromuscular, cardiopulmonary, and integumentary.

IDEA 2004 mandates that goals and interventions be based on academic demands and functional performance within the educational setting. However, many of the assessments currently used by occupational and physical therapists in school-based settings to create these goals and objectives focus on developmental skills as compared with those of same-age and/or same-grade peers.[29] These developmental assessments provide little information about the student's ability to participate in school-related tasks and reflect a conflict with the principles of IDEA 2004.[29] In addition, these measures do not provide information about performance in context and therefore are not appropriate outcome measures. Based on a model of inclusion for students with disabilities, assessments used in the educational setting should instead focus on participation and functional performance. They should identify to what extent the student requires assistance from an individual, accommodations, and/or modification of the environment to participate in the educational process.

Tests and measures should be technically sound and should be administered by trained and knowledgeable personnel, in accordance with instructions and in the child's native language without racial or cultural bias [PL 108-446, 118 Stat. 2705, § 614(b)(3)]. Selection of standardized tests should be based on professional judgment and dictated by the characteristics of the individual child. Therapists should collaborate with school personnel to identify appropriate tests and measures that gather relevant functional and developmental information. The child's abilities should be assessed in the natural environment when possible: in the classroom, hallway, playground, stairs, and other school settings. The *School Function Assessment* (SFA), developed by

Coster and co-workers,[23] is a standardized measure of participation in all aspects of the educational program for students in kindergarten through sixth grade. Findings may be used to identify IEP goals and develop the intervention plan, including frequency and duration of services. The SFA measures skills that promote participation in the natural environmental settings of regular or special education, addressing both individual and contextual factors. It is a judgment-based, criterion-referenced measure that is both discriminative (identifies functional limitations) and evaluative (measures change over time). It assesses the student's levels of activity, required support, and performance in daily school routines; by contrast, other standardized assessments measure the student's capacity (optimal abilities under controlled conditions). Function is defined by the outcome of performance, not by the methods used. The SFA comprises three major categories of student performance— Participation, Task Supports, and Activity Performance—and includes 21 domains (12 physical tasks and 9 cognitive/behavioral tasks), including the required level of assistance and adaptations. Criterion cut-off scores are provided for children in grades K through 3 and grades 4 through 6, as are item maps that provide a visual (graphic) representation of scores. The SFA can be completed by all members of the school team who are familiar with the student's levels of activity and performance in school-related tasks and environments. It has high internal consistency (ranging from .92 to .98), high test-retest reliability (Pearson *r* ranging from .80 to .99, and intraclass coefficients[ICC] ranging from .80 to .99); it is a valid instrument for use in school settings.[62]

For the student presented in the accompanying case study, the five mobility domains of the SFA were completed collaboratively by the school physical therapist and the classroom teacher, both of whom are well acquainted with the student and her levels of performance. That process took about 30 minutes. Although the test is intended to be conducted in its entirety by staff members representing several disciplines, other staff members chose not to do so; it is not uncommon for some to be reluctant to participate in the full assessment, claiming that it is too time-consuming. Perhaps, in time, the school physical therapist may be successful in persuading other members of the team to appreciate the value of information derived through the SFA.

Another assessment developed specifically for the education setting is the *School Outcomes Measure* (SOM).[6] The SOM is a minimal data set designed to measure outcomes of students who receive school-based occupational therapy and physical therapy.[6] The SOM includes 30 functional status items that cover five general student ability areas traditionally addressed in school-based practice: self-care, mobility, assuming a student's role, expressing learning, and behavior. Data are recorded on student and therapist demographics, as are details on information from the student's IEP, therapy services provided, and therapeutic procedures used.[6] The SOM focuses on the measure of student functional status to enhance participation in the natural environments of school, home, and community. It allows teachers, parents, and others with knowledge of the student to provide information for any areas for which the therapist is not certain of the student's abilities.

Research supports content validity, interrater reliability,[85] and test-retest reliability of the SOM for students who receive occupational and physical therapy.[6] The minimal data set was more responsive to children with mild/moderate functional limitations but less responsive to changes in children with severe disabilities. Arnold and McEwen[6] reported that use of the SOM is suitable on an annual basis in conjunction with IEP goals to evaluate outcomes for students, and that it is an appropriate tool for use in research to address outcomes.

The SOM provides several advantages to the school-based therapist. The tool takes about 10 to 15 minutes to administer once a therapist is familiar with the student; this is clearly an asset for therapists attempting to balance caseload and essential evaluation/outcome data. Another asset is that the SOM requires no manipulatives or supplies—only the test form.

The *Pediatric Evaluation of Disability Inventory* (PEDI)[54] is a judgment-based, criterion-referenced measure that preceded the SFA, is sometimes used in schools, and provides a more global assessment of self-care, mobility, social function, and the need for caregiver assistance. Other standardized tests and measures, as discussed throughout this text, may assist in determining the level of a child's physical functioning.

INDIVIDUALIZED EDUCATIONAL PROGRAM

The IEP is the document that guides the program of special education and related services for the school-age child, 5 to 21 years of age. It is also the document used in most states for the educational program of children ages 3 to 5 years attending preschool. The IEP is developed at a meeting involving the child's parents; at least one regular educator (if the child is or will be participating in the regular education environment); not less than one special education teacher; a representative of the local educational agency who is qualified to provide or supervise specially designed instruction and is knowledgeable about the general education curriculum and resources; an individual who can interpret the instructional implications of the evaluation; and "at the discretion of the parent or the agency, other individuals who have knowledge or special expertise regarding the child, including related services personnel as appropriate; and whenever appropriate, the child" [PL 108-446, 118 Stat. 2709, § 614(d)(1)(B)]. The physical therapist has a professional obligation to participate when decisions regarding physical therapy are being made. The physical therapy contribution to the IEP must relate to the educational needs of the child. Individualized measurable annual academic and functional goals are developed at the IEP meeting. Short-term objectives are no longer required under IDEA 2004, except for those children who take alternate assessments; however, they are essential under "best practice" guidelines, and many school districts continue to expect them. Even if the educational system does not require them, therapists should still develop short-term objectives to monitor and report intervention outcomes as required for the plan of care. Physical therapists must adhere to their state physical therapy practice acts, which may demand more documentation than the educational system requires, including a detailed plan of care. Table 30-2 describes the different elements of outcomes measures.

Attendance at IEP meetings may not be mandatory for all members of the team "if the parent of a child with a disability and the local educational agency agree that the attendance of such a member is not necessary because the member's area of curriculum or related services is not being modified or discussed.... ... A member of the IEP team may be excused... ... if the parent and the local educational agency consent to the excusal; and the member submits, in writing

TABLE 30-2   **Elements of Outcome Measures**

Measure	Part of IEP	Measurable	Time Frame	Dimension	Discipline Specific
Annual goal	Yes	Yes	School year	Activity/participation	No
Long-term objective	Yes	Yes	School year	Activity/participation	No
Short-term	Not required by federal law except for students who take alternate assessments*	Yes	Months, a grading period	Body functions and structures Activity/participation	Varies, some objectives might be within the domain of one discipline
Benchmark	Yes, but not always	Yes	School year or months	Activity/participation	No, although objectives might be within the domain of one discipline

*Might be required by local school system or state physical therapist practice act as part of plan of care.

to the parent and the IEP team, input into the development of the IEP prior to the meeting" [PL 108-460, 118 Stat. 2710, § 614(d)(1)(C)]. Therapists who are providing services for a child are now required to either attend the IEP meeting or receive approval not to attend and then submit their recommendations in writing. This new requirement of written input might encourage greater participation by therapists at IEP meetings.

Under IDEA 2004, the IEP document must include the following:

"(I) a statement of the child's present levels of academic achievement and functional performance, including—
(aa) how the child's disability affects the child's involvement and progress in the general curriculum;
(bb) for preschool children, as appropriate, how the disability affects the child's participation in appropriate activities; and
(cc) for children with disabilities who take alternate assessments aligned to alternate achievement standards, a description of benchmarks or short-term objectives;
(II) a statement of measurable annual goals, including academic and functional goals, designed to—
(aa) meet the child's needs that result from the child's disability to enable the child to be involved in and make progress in the general curriculum; and
(bb) meet each of the child's other educational needs that result from the child's disability;
(III) description of how the child's progress toward meeting the annual goals... ... will be measured and when periodic reports on the progress the child is making toward meeting the annual goals (such as through the use of quarterly or other periodic reports, concurrent with the issuance of report cards) will be provided;
(IV) a statement of the special education and related services and supplementary aids and services, based on peer-reviewed research to the extent practicable, to be provided to the child, or on behalf of the child, and a statement of the program modifications or supports for school personnel that will be provided for the child—
(aa) to advance appropriately toward attaining the annual goals;
(bb) to be involved and progress in the general curriculum...... and to participate in extracurricular and other nonacademic activities; and
(cc) to be educated and participate with other children with disabilities and nondisabled children;
(V) an explanation of the extent, if any, to which the child will not participate with nondisabled children in the regular class;......

(VI) (aa) a statement of any individual accommodations that are necessary to measure the academic achievement and functional performance of the child on State and district wide assessments;......
(bb) if the IEP Team determines that the child shall take an alternate assessment... ...a statement of why the child cannot participate in the regular assessment......
(VII) the projected date for the beginning of services and modifications......and the anticipated frequency, location, and duration of those services and modifications; and
(VIII) beginning not later than the first IEP to be in effect when the child is 16, and updated annually thereafter—
(aa) appropriate measurable postsecondary goals based upon age appropriate transition assessments related to training, education, employment, and, where appropriate, independent living skills;
(bb) transition services (including courses of study) needed to assist the child in reaching these goals; and
(cc) beginning not later than 1 year before the age of majority under State law, a statement that the child has been informed of the child's rights under this title" [PL 108-446, 118 Stat. 2707-2709, § 614(d)(1)(A)].

The IEP is a written commitment by the educational agency of the resources that will be provided to enable a child with a disability to receive necessary special education and related services. The IEP also serves as a management, compliance, and monitoring tool and is used to evaluate a child's progress toward achievement of goals and objectives. IDEA does not require that teachers or other school personnel be held accountable if a child with a disability does not achieve the goals set forth in the IEP; however, calls for greater accountability are increasing.

In the past, the IEP could not be changed without initiating another IEP meeting; however, in IDEA 2004 there are provisions for making changes. The parent "and the local educational agency may agree not to convene an IEP meeting for the purposes of making such changes, and instead may develop a written document to amend or modify the child's current IEP" [PL 108-446, 118 Stat. 2712, § 614(d)(3)(D)]. This change could result in problems for both the child and service providers. For example, therapy services might be added or deleted without input from the therapist. Ongoing team communication and collaboration are essential to ensure that flexibility in modifying the IEP results in positive outcomes.

DEVELOPING GOALS AND OBJECTIVES

The physical therapist, as part of the collaborative team, assists in developing appropriate measurable annual goals, including academic and functional goals. For children requiring alternate assessment, short-term objectives must also be developed. Short-term objectives serve to break down more global, comprehensive goals into manageable elements. They assist in determining whether the child is progressing in reasonable periods of time and help define criteria for the required progress reports. Short-term objectives also assist in clearly identifying when related services might be indicated. For example, instruction by a general or special education teacher might be considered sufficient for an annual goal regarding independently using the cafeteria or the library. A child who is just learning to use a walker around the school, however, may need the services of a physical therapist. General and special education teachers may not have the expertise to teach the child to use a walker and perform the task of opening the library and cafeteria doors, then entering and picking up a book or tray. Achievement of the annual goal might require a physical therapist to teach mobility activities and transfers, an occupational therapist to instruct in feeding activities, and a speech-language pathologist to work on communication in the food line or library.

For establishment of goals and objectives, the desired outcomes must first be identified. Determining desired outcomes might be as simple as merely asking the child, or it might require several team meetings. Outcome statements do not need to be measurable, but they should be functional. Once the desired outcomes are selected, the IEP team must define the goals that are necessary for the student to achieve them. Goals should be context specific, defined by relevant life skills or academic tasks in a school setting.[83] Educational goals should also be discipline-free; that is, they are goals for the student, rather than goals for physical therapy or occupational therapy.[84] They must be measurable, reflecting best practice[2,75,83,105] and the requirements of IDEA 2004 (Public Law 108-446). In an educational setting, goals are written to be achieved within the school year.

For students requiring alternate assessment and others, depending on state law, measurable short-term objectives are developed after desired outcomes and annual goals are identified. "Objectives are developed based on a logical breakdown of the major components of the annual goals, and can serve as milestones for measuring progress towards meeting the goals" (p. 44838).[43] Objectives must relate to the educational program of the child, are based on a task analysis of the annual goal, and are not discipline specific (see Table 30-2). They should be functional and educationally relevant and might be written into the IEP. In some situations, a short-term objective for reduction of impairment is relevant because that step is limiting the child's achievement of the annual goal. Short-term objectives for reducing impairments may be important to document progress toward achievement of the annual goal, but because they are not directly relevant to the educational program, they should not be part of the IEP.

To explain the relationships among impairment, activity limitation, and participation restriction, a therapist might use reading as an analogy. Reading is a very important goal of education, and few teachers would negate the importance of the child's first learning the prerequisite alphabet. The alphabet in itself has little value, just as complete knee range of motion has little value as an objective by itself. But knowing the alphabet is critical for reading and writing, and knee range of motion is critical for walking and stair climbing. The ability to walk or climb stairs expands the child's ability to explore his environment, learn, and, most important, achieve the goal of IDEA of "independent living, and economic self-sufficiency for individuals with disabilities" [PL 108-446, 118 Stat. 2649, Part A, § 601(c)(1)]. Eliminating short-term objectives in the IEP is unfortunate, because they offer an excellent way of monitoring outcomes for progress reports, and they are often better indicators of the services required than are annual goals. Therapists still might have to include short-term goals or objectives in their plans of care, depending on their state practice act requirements.

The physical therapist should participate in the IEP meeting to assist in determining the child's measurable annual goals for the next year. Consensus among experts in pediatric occupational and physical therapy indicate that outcomes should (1) relate to functional skills and activities, (2) enhance the child's performance in school, (3) be easily understood, (4) be free of professional jargon, and (5) be realistic and achievable within the time frame of the IEP.[32] These experts suggested that if a skill or activity cannot be observed or measured during the student's typical school day, then it might not be relevant to the student's educational needs and, therefore, may not be appropriate to include as an IEP goal. The therapists surveyed did not reach consensus on whether generalization of skills across settings is important.

An example of a desired outcome and the objectives involving independent stair climbing is illustrated in Box 30-4. To climb stairs at school independently, a child should have 90 degrees of knee flexion and good strength in the quadriceps muscles. Educationally relevant objectives are included in the child's IEP, and the other short-term objectives, which may or may not be considered educationally relevant, are included in the therapist's plan of care. Documentation of progress toward achievement of each objective is important to share with the child and family. Attainment of short-term objectives should be recognized and rewarded in lieu of waiting, perhaps a long time, for achievement of the long-term goal.

Measurable annual goals and objectives should contain a statement of the behavior to be achieved, under what conditions, and the criteria to be used to determine achievement.[37,75] When performing a task analysis and developing the short-term objectives, several variables should be considered: (1) changes in the behavior itself, (2) changes in the conditions under which the behavior is performed, and (3)

BOX 30-4   EXAMPLE OF DESIRED OUTCOME, ANNUAL GOAL, AND SHORT-TERM OBJECTIVES

DESIRED OUTCOME

Jonathan says: "I want to be able to climb the steps to get into school."

ANNUAL GOAL (LONG-TERM OBJECTIVE) THAT IS MEASURABLE AND EDUCATIONALLY RELEVANT

Jonathan will walk up and down the school stairs independently without using the railing.

SHORT-TERM OBJECTIVES THAT ARE MEASURABLE AND EDUCATIONALLY RELEVANT

1. Jonathan will climb up eight stairs at school with standby supervision using a railing.
2. Jonathan will climb up eight stairs at school with standby supervision without using a railing.
3. Jonathan will climb down eight stairs at school with standby supervision using a railing.
4. Jonathan will climb down eight stairs at school with standby supervision without using a railing.
5. Jonathan will climb up eight stairs at school without supervision or using a railing.
6. Jonathan will climb down eight stairs at school without supervision or using a railing.

SHORT-TERM OBJECTIVES THAT ARE MEASURABLE BUT NOT DIRECTLY EDUCATIONALLY RELEVANT

These objectives, which relate to impairments in body structures and functions, are necessary to achieve the educationally relevant short-term and annual goals and would be part of the therapist's plan of care, but not in the IEP.

1. Jonathan will progress from 30° to 50° of active right-knee flexion.
2. Jonathan will progress from a poor (1/5) to a fair (3/5) muscle-strength grade in his left quadriceps.
3. Jonathan will achieve 90° of active right-knee flexion.
4. Jonathan will achieve a good (4/5) muscle-strength grade in his left quadriceps.

---

or 80% of the time, should be considered carefully for their practicability. Successfully crossing the street only 80% of the time can be fatal! Selection of the behavior, conditions, and criteria for judging attainment of each objective for each individual child must be based on sound professional judgment. Books, computer programs, and other materials that provide lists of potential objectives should not replace professional judgment. In addition to the task variables, consideration should be given to the hierarchy of response competence.[1] A behavior is acquired and then refined as fluency or proficiency develops. The skill must then be maintained and finally generalized or transferred to multiple environments, individuals, and equipment. Acquisition, fluency, maintenance, and generalization of behaviors are the terms used by educators that can be applied to motor learning. The concepts of efficiency, flexibility, and consistency have also been used to define skill components of goals.[99] Use of this terminology is important when there is a need to convey the rationale for providing services past the acquisition phase.

Therapists are encouraged to consider using a prompting system as a strategy to achieve an objective and as a variable in writing the criteria for judging attainment of the objective (Figure 30-1). Systematic delivery of levels of prompting assistance may be implemented in two ways. One is the "system of maximum prompts," and the other is the "system of least prompts."[1,37] The prompts are usually verbal or visual cues, demonstration or modeling, partial assistance or physical guidance, and maximum assistance. In the system of maximum prompts, the therapist initially provides maximum assistance and then gradually, over successive sessions, reduces the amount of assistance as the child achieves more independence. This is also referred to as *fading*. This is a common technique used by therapists, and it allows for maximal success during learning. This system is best suited for acquisition, when it is important to avoid unsafe movement, and for a complex series of tasks such as some activities of daily living.

In the system of least prompts, the child is initially provided the least amount of assistance, usually a verbal or visual cue, and then progresses as necessary to model, guide, or maximal assistance. This approach allows the child to display his or her best effort before the therapist prematurely provides unnecessary assistance. The system of least prompts is best for tasks in which the child has some ability or is developing fluency or generalization to new settings, individuals, or equipment.

Therapists should incorporate other principles of motor learning into the development of short-term objectives and intervention sessions. Increasing muscle strength can contribute to improved motor control and function, particularly improved walking.[88] Practice of motor skills should be structured in ways to promote learning through consideration of part versus whole practice, use of contextual interference, blocked versus random practice, massed versus distributed

changes in the criteria expected for ultimate performance.[1] Changes in behavior may reflect a progression from basic skills to more complex skills or to increasing levels of functional ability. Changes in conditions may range from simple to complex, such as walking in an empty hallway to walking in a hallway with other students. Criteria for progression may be qualitative or quantitative and might include the qualitative measure of perceived exertion during stair climbing or the quantitative measure of walking speed. Use of quantitative criteria, such as judgment by three of four trials,

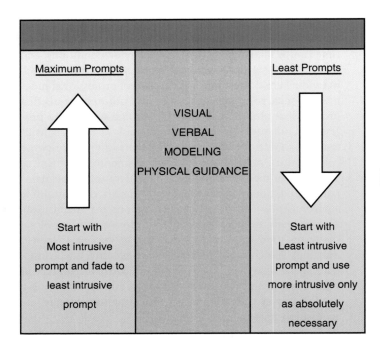

Figure 30-1 Hierarchy of prompting assistance.

practice, schedules of feedback, knowledge of performance, and knowledge of results.[113] Breaking down any of these elements into a progression of simpler to more complex skills can lead to effective objectives. In the education literature, this is referred to as *scaffolding* (see Chapter 4).

FREQUENCY AND INTENSITY OF INTERVENTION

At the IEP meeting, the frequency and intensity of all services should be determined by the entire team. The physical therapist must collaborate with other team members to determine the appropriate amount of physical therapy intervention, combined with the child's other interventions, educational program, and recreation activities. Competing priorities need to be considered so that other areas of importance are not neglected for the child to receive therapy. Appropriate balance among education, therapy, and leisure (play) is an important issue for discussion with parents, particularly with parents who believe that "more is better." The availability of physical therapists should not be a factor in determining the frequency and intensity of the intervention. However, Kaminker and colleagues[69] found regional differences in frequencies of intervention provided by school-based physical therapists, corresponding to ratios of available therapists to students.

The frequency and duration of the physical therapy services required to achieve a specific goal are neither well understood nor well documented.[8,63] Until sufficient peer-reviewed evidence is obtained, decisions on how much intervention is required to achieve a goal largely depend on professional judgment and consideration of the needs of the individual child. Numerous factors enter into decision

making and include potential for improvement; critical period for skill development; amount of training required to carry out an intervention (if anyone can assist with the intervention, then less therapist time is required); and significance of the problem for the child's education.[63] Table 30-3 depicts a matrix of factors to consider when deciding on the extent of physical therapy services required. On this scale, students with several ratings of 4 would probably require more intervention than those with predominant ratings of 1. Physical and occupational therapists from the Cincinnati Children's Hospital used the Iowa guidelines to develop guidelines for frequency of therapy services in a medical setting. They provided guidance on frequency using four modes of service delivery: (1) intensive (3 to 11 times a week), (2) weekly or bimonthly (1 to 2 times a week to every other week), (3) periodic (monthly or less often but at regularly scheduled intervals), and (4) consultative (episodic or as needed).[8]

Without the use of an accepted clinical reasoning tool or objective measure for establishing educational need, school-based physical therapists have difficulties making decisions that support the intent of the IDEA while withstanding outside pressures. The Considerations for Educationally Relevant Therapy for Occupational Therapy and Physical Therapy (CERT) and the Determination of Relevant Therapy Tool (DRTT) are two examples of clinical reasoning models that provide objective data for school-based therapy decision making. Over the past 25 years, therapists in Florida have been developing the CERT, a system intended to assist in determining school-based therapy services. The CERT is not an assessment, but rather "a summary of educational considerations based on a review of student records, evaluations,

TABLE 30-3 **Factors to Consider When Determining the Intensity and Frequency of Physical Therapy**

Factors	1*	2	3	4
Potential to benefit from intervention	Student demonstrates minimal potential for change	Student appears to have potential for change but at a slow rate	Student appears to have a significant potential for change	Student appears to have a very high potential to improve skills
Critical period of skill acquisition or regression related to development or disability	Not a critical period	Minimally critical period	Critical period	Extremely critical period
Amount of motor program that can be safely performed by others	Motor program can be carried out safely by others with periodic intervention by therapist	Many activities from the motor program can be safely performed by others in addition to intervention by therapist	Some activities from the motor program can be safely performed by others in addition to intervention by therapist	A few activities can be safely performed by others but most of the motor program requires the expertise of the therapist
Amount of training provided by therapist to others carrying out the program	Teachers, staff, and parents able to meet student's needs with no additional training required	Teacher, staff, and parents require some training and follow-up	Teacher, staff, and parents could be trained to carry out activities	Teacher, staff, and parents might carry out some activities with extensive training and follow-up
Impact of motor problems and environment on educational program	Environment is accommodating and motor difficulties are minimal	Environment is accommodating and motor difficulties moderately interfere with educational program	Environment is accommodating but motor difficulties are significant and interfere with educational program	Environment is not accommodating; or environment is accommodating but problems are severe

*Numbers are ordered from lowest (1) to highest (4) need for direct services.
Adapted from *Iowa guidelines for educationally related physical therapy services.* (2001). Des Moines, IA: Iowa Department of Education. Reprinted with permission.

observations, progress notes, parent/teacher information and other data" (p. 2).[46] The CERT includes a Summary Sheet, a Student Profile, and a Therapy Profile completed by the therapist. The Student Profile rates the student's abilities in personal care, mobility, gross motor skills, fine motor/visual motor skills, and sensory processing. The Therapy Profile indicates the number of years the student has received educationally relevant therapy, potential response to educationally relevant therapy, students' learning environment, therapy services provided to the student, and support services provided to school staff and/or parents. Contrary to the Iowa guidelines, a rating of 1 suggests that the student has relatively adequate abilities, and a rating of 4 indicates that the student requires intensive training or assistance. Detailed information on the CERT is available at http://www.fldoe.org/ESE/cert.asp.

In Maryland, the DRTT[20] has been developed to assist in occupational therapy and physical therapy service recommendations to the IEP team. For newer therapists, this method encompasses the range of roles and responsibilities of therapists and requires the user to consider all aspects of therapeutic and educational programming prior to decision making. For those therapists who have experience in school

practice, use of the DRTT provides a means to validate decisions related to models and delivery of services, beyond the use of clinical judgment alone. Consistent service delivery among therapists in any jurisdiction helps to alleviate the disputes between families and teams that may arise regarding service recommendations, as well as to support administration with appropriate staffing ratios to meet IEP needs, while managing therapist costs (S. Cecere, personal communication, December 14, 2009).

INTERVENTION

Intervention must be based on the needs of the child, not of the system or professionals. The content, goals, frequency, location, and intensity of intervention are decided collaboratively by the IEP team at the IEP meeting. Effective communication among team members is crucial for the planning, provision, and coordination of services, to avoid overlap of services, missed services, and conflict.[84] The *Guide to Physical Therapist Practice*[2] describes three components of intervention, all of which are essential in the educational environment: coordination, communication, and documentation; patient/client-related instruction; and procedural interventions. The amount of time and effort devoted to each will depend on the needs of the child and may vary at different times of the school year.

COORDINATION, COMMUNICATION, AND DOCUMENTATION

Coordination, communication, and documentation are particularly important in schools where the therapist is in the building only occasionally, and direct interaction with other team members is limited. Frequent communication with parents, teachers, and other related service personnel must be established and maintained. This may be accomplished through regularly scheduled meetings, informal conversation, and written progress reports, as well as by telephone and electronic communication.

Documentation must follow local, state, and national requirements for both education and physical therapy. This means that, although the education agencies might dictate that progress reports are provided to the family only at the same frequency as for children who do not have a disability, the state physical therapy practice act might require documentation after each intervention session. The APTA Defensible Documentation Resource[3] suggests the following: (1) documentation is required for every visit/encounter; (2) documentation should indicate cancellations; (3) documentation must comply with regulatory requirements; (4) entries must be made in ink and properly authenticated; (5) electronic entries should be secure; and (6) documentation in pediatrics should be aligned with family-centered care and should emphasize the functional abilities of the child. Specific to school settings, the physical therapist should "document all strategies, interventions, staff/student training and education, and communication with the student's parents/guardians or community based services" (p. 43).[3] In addition, although the IEP team might decide that physical therapy services are no longer required, discontinuation of physical therapy must be documented by the physical therapist in a final summary to close that episode of care. Services billed through Medicaid and other insurance providers usually require additional documentation. There is great variation across the country with regard to documentation of school-based physical therapy services; therapists must consult their state practice acts to ensure that they are in full compliance.

CHILD-AND FAMILY-RELATED INSTRUCTION

Child- and family-related instruction, along with instruction to other team members, is a critical area of practice in school settings. Practice is essential for acquisition, fluency, and generalization of skills[25,127]; consequently, the family and the IEP team may be largely responsible for assisting the child in carrying out or practicing motor skills. Instruction of parents and appropriate staff members should be a major component of all intervention plans. Instruction should begin and continue as needed: at the start of every school year, at the initiation of physical therapy services, when a child enters a new school, and when a new staff member becomes involved in the care of the child.

In the integrated and collaborative service-delivery models, teachers, staff, and parents participate in the delivery of some aspects of the intervention. Their involvement may be as simple as using proper positioning techniques, or as complicated as handling procedures for transfers and mobility. These individuals must be instructed on proper positioning of the student, safe body mechanics of the caregiver, use of adaptive equipment, and ways to encourage selected motor activities. It is generally prudent for the physical therapist to provide the primary instruction at the initial acquisition stage of motor learning, relinquishing care to the classroom staff at fluency and generalization stages.

Selection of which activities to teach other caregivers is a professional decision that must be based on characteristics of the individual child, the specific activity, and the capabilities and interest of the other individuals. In a series of single-subject design studies, Prieto[98] found that teachers are more likely to encourage children to perform gross motor activities when they have been properly instructed. Soccio[116] compared the frequency of opportunities to practice specific gross motor skills during individual physical therapy sessions and group early intervention classes. There was no difference in the number of opportunities to practice head control when direct physical therapy was compared with integrated group sessions for a child with severe disabilities. Two children with cerebral palsy, however, had more opportunities to practice standing and ambulation activities during direct, individual physical therapy sessions than during integrated group sessions in the classroom. Results suggest that the opportunity to practice motor activities in the classroom varies, based on the type of movement and the class routines. Therapists must carefully select those activities they delegate to others because opportunities for active gross motor movement in classrooms may be limited.[95]

PROCEDURAL INTERVENTIONS

Procedural interventions in school settings are frequently not as important as the other two components of intervention. However, as noted in Table 30-3, some situations would suggest a need for direct intervention, such as (1) when a child is at a critical period of skill acquisition or regression; (2) when the interventions require the expertise of a physical therapist; and (3) when integrating therapy interferes with the educational program. Best practice, research, and federal law indicate that most, if not all, intervention should occur in the natural environment, with an emphasis on providing multiple opportunities to practice specific skills.[5,40,52,56,103,118] When gross motor skills are learned in isolated settings, such as a physical therapy department, there is little generalization to the more natural environment of the home or recreational settings.[15]

Assessment of the school environment and safety considerations take precedence initially over direct interventions. The physical therapist should participate in the development of written plans for emergency evacuation from the school building and the school bus, in addition to instructing appropriate personnel on the implementation of these plans. The physical therapist should be present during evacuation drills and might assist in the practice of safe techniques using weighted dummies and different models of wheelchairs.

The physical therapist's assessment of the student's environment should begin with proper positioning on the bus and in classrooms. Safety of the aisles for walking or wheelchair mobility should be considered. Architectural barriers must be evaluated and appropriate actions taken to eliminate or lessen them. Teachers and family should be consulted regarding their concerns, and they should be instructed in proper handling, positioning, and use of body mechanics.

Direct intervention, if indicated, should start in the natural environment of the classroom. This is accomplished easily with preschoolers.[52] It is more difficult for children whose educational programs consist primarily of academic subjects that occur in the general education classroom. Physical therapy in the algebra class or school library, after the initial consultation, is generally inappropriate. Common sense must prevail. Perhaps therapy can be delivered during gross motor time in a preschool or during physical education. This is not always appropriate, however, because this might be the only time the child has to engage in free play and physical activity with peers. Taking this opportunity away from the child might affect motivation, cooperation, and the development of important social skills that occurs during these activities.

Merely moving traditional intervention from a special room to a more natural environment is also not in the spirit of best practice. The therapist must adjust intervention to the unique opportunities afforded in the natural environment. Available furniture or classroom items should be used, as opposed to bringing in special equipment. Use of these common objects increases the likelihood that the child might use them to practice and develop motor skills when the therapist is not present and allows the therapist to model their use for the parent or teacher. The specific type of intervention provided depends on the needs of the individual child and the education, training, and experience of the therapist. IDEA 2004 requires that interventions be provided "based on peer-reviewed research to the extent practicable" [PL 108-446, 118 Stat. 2707-2709, § 614(d)(1)(A)(IV)]. Although physical therapy intervention has been advancing toward evidence-based practice, many interventions do not have sufficient peer-reviewed research. Throughout this text, peer-reviewed research and evidence-based practice are presented when available. Effgen and McEwen[41,42] published

systematic reviews of common interventions used in educational settings. Therapists must learn to search the literature for recent developments in research to support the interventions they use. If the appropriate intervention cannot be provided for a school-age child because it is not educationally relevant and is not related to the objectives in the IEP, the therapist has a professional obligation to inform the parents. Once the parents are aware of the focus of school-based physical therapy, they might obtain additional therapy elsewhere.

Careful monitoring of progress is critical in determining the effectiveness of and the need for continued intervention. David[27] outlined a measurement process that has been developed for use by collaborative educational teams. The system involves (1) defining the performance problem; (2) identifying the performance expected and outcome criteria; (3) developing a systematic, simple, and time-efficient measurement strategy; (4) having a data-graphing system; (5) providing intervention; (6) monitoring progress; and (7) participating in systematic decision making and intervention changes. David stated that "monitoring without decision making is a waste of valuable time and effort" (p. 56).[27] A simple but comprehensive system of data collection using self-graphing data-collection sheets is recommended.[37] The availability of laptop computers has also made data collection and its graphic presentation much easier for many therapists. Extensive documentation is necessary to support the need to increase, decrease, or discontinue intervention. Documentation of the child's status before and after short and long school breaks is important in determining the need for ESY services.

Physical therapy intervention is not a lifelong activity such as learning and fitness. Both therapists and parents must recognize that, after a period of service delivery with no measurable progress, intervention should be discontinued, or the model should be changed to monitoring. A continued desire for walking, for example, is not justification for continued therapy after due diligence in trying to achieve a goal. Therapists report that the most important factor in successful discontinuation of services is the child's achievement of functional goals.[38] Choosing to discontinue direct intervention when goals have not been met continues to be a challenging area of decision making, although tools like the CERT and DRTT should help in the process.

TRANSITION PLANNING

Change can be difficult for anyone, and the transition from one environment to another can be stressful for both children and their parents, especially for those students with a limited repertoire of response competence. Because all transitions are important, two critical times were identified in IDEA when attention must be paid to transition and the provision of transition services. These times include: (1) when the child is preparing to move from family-centered early intervention services under Part C to preschool services under Part B,[58] and (2) when the student is preparing to transition out of secondary school into the community.[47]

Although the transition from family-centered early intervention services to preschool services is supposed to be "seamless," the transition process is often difficult for both the child and the family. It is usually accompanied by a change in the state agency providing the services, which typically includes a change in the method of service delivery and in personnel. Family-centered services of early intervention are replaced by school system services with reduced family involvement and with service providers focused on educational goals. Communication between parents and providers also becomes more challenging. Physical therapists have not been as engaged as they should be in the transition process for children from early intervention to preschool. They rarely attend transition team meetings and have not received specialized training in transition, but they do report that they work with families during the transition process.[121]

Under IDEA 2004, transition services for post-secondary education comprise "a coordinated set of activities for a child with a disability that... ... is designed within a results-oriented process that is focused on improving academic and functional achievement of the child with a disability to facilitate the child's movement from school to post-school activities, including post-secondary education, vocational education, integrated employment (including supported employment), continuing and adult education, adult services, independent living, or community participation; is based on the individual child's needs, taking into account the child's strengths, preferences, and interests; and includes instruction, related services, community experiences, the development of employment and other post-school adult living objectives, and, when appropriate, acquisition of daily living skills and functional vocational evaluation" [PL 108-446, 118 Stat. 2658, § 602(34)].

Transition assessments and services must begin no later than the first IEP to be in effect when the child is 16 years of age [PL 108-446, 118 Stat. 2709, § 614(d)(1)(A)(VIII)] or younger if determined appropriate by the IEP team.[45] Physical therapists should serve on transition teams for children with physical disabilities who are currently receiving services, as well as for those for whom services have been discontinued. A young adult may no longer have a school-related need for physical therapy, but the therapist can assist in evaluating and intervening to facilitate post-school planning and services.

All transition planning should be determined collaboratively by the school team along with both the student and the family. Emphasis should be placed on self-determination, person-centeredness, and career orientation.[7] The role of the physical therapist in transition planning and in services for students with physical disabilities might include the following:

- Communication with the family and other transition team members regarding daily routines, physical expectations, and demands of the anticipated new environment
- Communication with the student's vocational rehabilitation counselor, occupational therapist, and teachers regarding preparation for mobility and functional activities in the new setting
- Onsite evaluation of the new physical environment and intervention to ensure the student's ability to physically maneuver throughout the setting
- Evaluation of the accessibility of required transportation systems and intervention as required
- Onsite consultation and education of the student, family, and staff related to the student's physical functioning in that environment
- Onsite assessment and identification of assistive technology needs of the student for the new environment
- Assistance in securing assistive technology and instruction in its use
- Attendance at IEP and other meetings as appropriate
- Consultation throughout the transition process to ensure that recommendations are appropriate and that the student is successful[114]

Effective transition services can be impeded by issues related to collaboration and communication among team members. These include lack of shared information across agencies; follow-up data that could improve services; attention to health insurance and transportation; systematic transition planning with the agencies that will have responsibility for post-school services; anticipating the needs of the student post school; and effective management practices.[65] Although the physical therapist is usually not in a leadership role to make major changes in the transition service system, the therapist can provide assistance in several of the problem areas noted. The therapist has the ability to provide information on health insurance; evaluation of transportation needs; equipment for mobility, positioning, and self-care; and anticipation of the physical demands required of the student post school. A therapist's knowledge of the physical demands of post-school settings, such as college or work environments, would help the team to assist the student in effective transitioning to those environments. In Chapter 32, Transition to Adulthood for Youth with Disabilities, preparation of youth with disabilities for adult roles is addressed, including transition services provided within the education and health care systems.

MANAGEMENT OF PHYSICAL THERAPY SERVICES

Successful management and service delivery in educational environments depend on an understanding of the importance of the team process. The physical therapist, as a member of the educational team, must collaborate effectively with the child, the family, and professionals of other disciplines to promote the child's total well-being through each phase of the educational process. Just as team leaders or case managers are needed on intervention teams, so too a manager or director of physical therapy is needed in school settings. A majority of directors of physical therapy services in school systems across the nation are not physical therapists or, indeed, any type of related-service personnel.[40] This has serious implications. To understand professional roles and responsibilities and how to nurture a professional, one must understand the profession. Many of the problems encountered in school systems could probably be prevented if an experienced therapist provided supervision. Therapist managers understand the profession and are able to appropriately address management issues. States such as Iowa and North Carolina, which have therapists working in the state department of education, have become national leaders in setting policy for related-service providers. These therapists help to coordinate services throughout the state and educate both therapists and educators regarding the role of physical therapists in educational environments.

Therapists, unlike teachers, are educated to work in a wide variety of settings, but very few have the opportunity to learn about school-based practice. Those who are new to practice in educational environments in general and those who are new to a particular school system should receive orientation, mentoring, and in-service education. The roles and responsibilities of the therapist and all support staff should be clearly identified in a detailed job description that complies with federal and state laws. As part of a planned orientation program, therapists should be introduced to the entire team of professionals with whom they will be working at all sites. They need to know whom to ask for equipment, space, and other items necessary for successful intervention. Therapists need to know how referrals are received and handled; how workloads and caseloads are determined; how team meetings are planned and when they are scheduled; the written policies and procedures; how peer review or quality improvement is done; emergency procedures; and the policy for continuing education, to name but a few issues. These are not unusual requests, and they can be addressed easily and cost-effectively in any system.

After the therapist is properly introduced and oriented to the system, administrators and therapists must continue to communicate regularly before problems arise. Frequent areas of discontent include too much travel among school buildings and lack of appropriate continuing education opportunities, peer contact, a place to work, and time allotted for administrative tasks and meetings.[40] More time and effort should be spent on retention of physical therapists to reduce the need for recruitment.

Most physical therapy state practice acts in the United States allow a therapist to examine and evaluate without a physician's referral, and 42 states also allow therapists to provide intervention without a referral. In states where physician authorization is required, a system should be developed for obtaining referrals. The referral allows the therapist to examine and evaluate the student, and then to determine and provide appropriate intervention. Depending on the complexity of the child's medical problems and the need for pertinent information, it might be prudent for the therapist to obtain a referral even when not legally required. Collaboration with physicians and all other members of the child's medical and educational team promotes optimal service delivery.

School districts need to develop guidelines to determine therapy workloads and caseloads, as well as for decision making with regard to who should receive intervention and how much intervention should be provided. This can be a difficult task. The CERT, DRTT, and Iowa Guidelines for Educationally Related Physical Therapy Services (see Table 30-3),[63] as discussed, should help with the decision-making process. Children with critical needs for therapy require more intense intervention than do those with lesser needs. A therapist whose caseload primarily includes children with extensive needs for therapy is able to serve fewer children than a therapist whose caseload mostly comprises children with minimal needs. A clear system of documentation is needed to support the complex, sensitive decisions regarding allocation of physical therapy services.

ISSUES IN SCHOOL-BASED PRACTICE

SHORTAGE OF PEDIATRIC PHYSICAL THERAPISTS

A shortage of pediatric physical therapists with the skill set for serving children in the educational setting has been an ongoing problem. It may be attributed to relatively low pay, professional isolation, benefits of other areas of practice, and difficulty in working with children. Solutions are numerous and sometimes complex, but one of the easiest is often neglected. An effective way to train and then recruit new physical therapists is to offer student clinical affiliations in educational settings.

Physical therapy is not the only school-based profession where shortages exist. In 2005, an organization was established to address these issues: the National Coalition on Personnel Shortages in Special Education and Related Services (NCPSSERS). The Coalition represents 30 national, state, and local professional organizations from eight different disciplines. Its stated mission is "to sustain a discussion among all stakeholders on the need for and value of special education, related services, and early intervention; and to identify, disseminate, and support implementation of national, state, and local strategies to remedy personnel shortages and persistent vacancies for the benefit of all children and youth."[92]

SERVICE-DELIVERY SYSTEM

A shortage of qualified physical therapists has affected the type of service-delivery system used and the roles assumed by school personnel. The literature supports integrated or collaborative service-delivery models.[34,57,104] There are obvious advantages to more frequent practice in natural settings with the support of all those who interact with the student. An appropriately administered therapy program in the natural environment might require more, and certainly not fewer, personnel. Training all staff members in a truly integrated or collaborative model requires a great deal of time for instruction and meetings.[49] There are those, however, who incorrectly think that these models can be used to decrease the time required for physical therapy. It should be noted that "Teams Take Time" (the three T's). Instead of direct intervention by a therapist, unqualified staff might perform activities without adequate supervised instruction, or a teacher might be forced to provide an intervention for which he or she is not properly trained. Instead of providing the intervention in a room with necessary equipment, a classroom or hallway is used in the name of natural environment. Rarely are empirical data sufficient to support any service-delivery system. Educators and therapists alike must continually ask themselves if they are truly meeting the needs of each individual child.

PROFESSIONAL ROLES

In school systems with a full staff, professionals can collaborate to decide on the role of each team member. Overlap of professional roles is acknowledged, and divisions of responsibility are made that are best suited to the needs of the child, system, and professional staff.[128] In general, the overlap in physical therapy, occupational therapy, and education is greatest when professionals from these disciplines are serving young children. For older children, less overlap in professional roles exists. Areas of frequent overlap between occupational therapy and physical therapy include programs for strength and endurance, body awareness, classroom positioning and adaptations, enhancement of motor experience, and sensory integration. Areas of overlap between physical therapists and educators might include advanced gross motor skills, endurance training, and transfers. In systems with a critical shortage of physical therapists, the breadth of roles assumed by other staff members increases, based on need and not necessarily on professional skill.

EDUCATIONALLY RELEVANT PHYSICAL THERAPY

McEwen and Shelden[86] summarized a topic of frequent debate: physical therapy that is educationally relevant as compared with that which is not. In school systems that are committed to the comprehensive provision of services to children with disabilities with adequate therapy staff, the definition of educationally relevant physical therapy is comprehensive; it depends on the individual needs of the child, as addressed at the IEP meeting. IDEA clearly indicates that education is intended to prepare students for independent living and economic self-sufficiency, which have broad implications for the provision of physical therapy.

Physical therapy is perceived as more educationally relevant when goals and objectives are mutually agreed upon by the entire educational team. The educational system was never meant to provide for all the child's therapy needs. Physical therapy may be provided outside of the educational system as appropriate; all therapists serving the child should collaborate and coordinate services. Therapists and parents must remember that therapy takes time away from other educational and social opportunities that are vital to the total well-being of the child. These competing priorities must be considered when making decisions regarding service delivery.

LEAST RESTRICTIVE ENVIRONMENT

As more children are educated in the least restrictive environment, therapists must be willing to travel to meet the needs of those students. Unfortunately, travel among many schools is not the most time- and cost-effective method of service delivery. Therapists and administrators must be creative in their approach to serving children in their local schools. Materials have been developed that have successfully encouraged inclusive education, such as *Choosing Options and Accommodations for Children: A Guide to Planning Inclusive Education* (COACH).[48]

REIMBURSEMENT FOR SERVICES

The cost of providing related services in educational environments is a serious concern of program administrators. IDEA provides some federal funding to states, but it has never been enough to cover the full spectrum of services needed by children in special education. To cover the costs of physical therapy, some school systems are charging third-party payers. This can be problematic because of the lifetime cap on many insurance policies, limited therapy coverage, and the possibility of losing insurance if bills are too high. Parents are not required to have their insurance company pay for these services, and they should not be intimidated into thinking that their child will not receive services without insurance payment. School systems may bill Medicaid directly for physical therapy. A concern regarding using Medicaid is that reimbursement is usually based on direct services, and consultation, team intervention, and group treatments are discouraged. Medicaid rules and regulations are determined by each individual state, and therapists should be active at the state level to make certain that these rules and regulations facilitate and do not hinder appropriate school-based intervention.

TRANSPORTATION

Transportation of children receiving special education is a required related service. Ensuring that children are transported safely and efficiently is the responsibility of the school system. Many individuals assist in the transportation process, and the National Highway Traffic Safety Administration[93] has numerous resources to assist in understanding the safe transportation of children. A physical therapist might be asked to assess the safe seating of a student with a disability in a school bus seat or wheelchair; safe embarking and debarking from the bus; and emergency evacuation procedures. Therapists must understand what makes a wheelchair safe for transportation and how to tie down the wheelchair and use occupant-restraint systems. The therapist and the team must discuss and plan for evacuation and must discuss issues related to the student's size, weight, and height; implications of different medical diagnoses (e.g., osteogenesis imperfecta); orthopedic concerns; physical limitations; ability of the student to assist; whether a student stays in the wheelchair; and who gets off the bus first and last.[132] Competence in transportation issues is important for every therapist.

THERAPISTS NEW TO THE EDUCATIONAL ENVIRONMENT

Many school-based physical therapists begin their careers by working in adult or other pediatric settings. Upon entering the educational environment, those who are parents enjoy the benefit of having the same school hours and vacation schedules as their children. Therefore, it is not uncommon for experienced therapists to seek employment in school settings with little or no background in pediatrics, and lacking an understanding of the unique requirements of working under IDEA. Therapists who are new to school practice must immediately learn the rules and regulations of IDEA as outlined in this chapter and as available from the suggested websites and references. In addition, they must be aware of individual state education laws, special education laws, and their state physical therapy practice act. It is the therapists' responsibility to be knowledgeable of the laws that govern practice in schools, just as they should know the rules for reimbursement and practice in hospital settings. In this era of limited resources, administrators have been known to say that services are not appropriate for a child with a disability because they do not want to pay for such a service. They might also say that because a therapist is not available, therapy cannot be recommended in the IEP. Of course, this is incorrect, but most parents and many

therapists will not know that unless they are very familiar with the laws.

School-based therapists need to become effective members of a team, using the various models described in this chapter. Those who have worked in other pediatric settings, such as early intervention and pediatric hospitals, may be accustomed to working with a team, as may therapists who have worked in rehabilitation settings. Therapists who have practiced in outpatient physical therapy settings, however, may not be adequately familiar with team functioning and the degree of role release and collaboration required in the school setting.

Intervention in educational environments is also somewhat different from other settings. As already discussed, goals and objectives must be educationally relevant. Intervention is based on the *Guide*,[2] including coordination, communication, and documentation, as well as patient/client-related instruction. For children who demonstrate high ratings of the factors outlined in Table 30-3, procedural interventions might be provided. However, many students do not require direct intervention, and this change in focus can be difficult for some therapists who are accustomed to providing direct services.

Therapists new to school practice would be wise to seek an experienced mentor, either within or outside the school system. Many school therapists work in isolation, and they do not have access to the guidance and support provided in other clinical settings. They work frequently with teachers, but not necessarily with other therapists who can evaluate their knowledge and skills and with whom they can discuss cases. School administrators need to recognize the effect of this professional isolation for both experienced therapists and those new to the school environment, and they should support the therapist in finding a mentor.

Therapists, especially new graduates and those new to educational environments, should strive to achieve the competencies for school-based physical therapists as outlined in Box 30-5.[39] These competencies may also be shared with administrators to help define the role of school-based physical therapy and to identify the resources necessary for effective service delivery. Therapists should continually read, participate in continuing education, take post-professional courses, and engage in dialogue with colleagues. The Section on Pediatrics of the American Physical Therapy Association offers a wide variety of excellent resources for school-based therapists. Employers need to support therapists' efforts at ongoing professional development.

Box **30-5** COMPETENCIES FOR SCHOOL-BASED PHYSICAL THERAPISTS

CONTENT AREA 1: THE CONTEXT OF THERAPY PRACTICE IN SCHOOLS

1. Describe competencies for school-based physical therapists.
   a. Diagram the functional and supervisory organization of the education system served by the therapist.
   b. Identify the goals and outcomes of the educational curriculum from preschool through high school.
   c. Demonstrate an understanding of the eventual goals of independent living and working.
   d. Apply knowledge of the outcomes-based education curriculum.
2. Demonstrate knowledge of federal (for example, IDEA, Rehabilitation Act of 1973, ADA), state, and local laws and regulations that affect the delivery of services to students with disabilities
   a. Discuss the implications of the laws (national, state and local).
   b. Apply the guidelines of federal, state, and local regulations.
   c. Identify and use information sources for federal, state, and local legislation and regulation changes.
   d. Discuss and demonstrate professional behavior regarding ethical and legal responsibilities.
   e. Discuss professional competencies as defined by professional organizations and state regulations.
   f. Advocate to support services related to educational entitlements.
3. Apply knowledge of the theoretical and functional orientation of a variety of professionals serving students within the educational system
   a. Initiate dialogue with colleagues to exchange professional perspectives.
   b. Disseminate information about the availability of therapy services, criteria for eligibility, and methods of referral.
   c. Describe evaluations and interventions commonly used by psychologists, diagnostic educators, classroom teachers, speech and language pathologists, adaptive physical educators, nurses, physical therapists, occupational therapists, and professionals in other education and health-related disciplines.
4. Assist students in accessing community organizations, resources and activities.
   a. Demonstrate awareness of cultural and social differences that relate to family and student participation in the education program.
   b. In collaboration with the educational team, develop a plan for transition into community activities or adult services.
   c. Identify the need to make appropriate student referrals to community therapy and recreational. services when school services are not able to meet all of the child's needs.

   d. Include the family in the educational process.
   e. Serve as a resource to family and other team members for information and appropriate community resources (medical, educational, financial, social, recreational, and legal).

CONTENT AREA 2: WELLNESS AND PREVENTION IN SCHOOLS

1. Implement school-wide screening program with school nurse, physical education teacher, and teachers.
   a. Apply knowledge of risk factors affecting growth, development, and learning.
   b. Identify the etiology, signs, symptoms, and classifications of common pediatric disabilities.
   c. Identify established biological and environmental factors that affect children's development and learning.
   d. Select, administer, and interpret a variety of screening instruments and standardized measurement tools.
2. Promote child safety and wellness using knowledge of environmental safety measures.
   a. Maintain CPR certification.
   b. Institute an environmental hazards and accident prevention plan.
   c. Recognize child neglect and abuse.

CONTENT AREA 3: TEAM COLLABORATION

1. Form partnerships and work collaboratively with other team members, especially the teacher to promote an effective plan of care.
   a. Demonstrate effective communication and interpersonal skills.
   b. Refer and coordinate services among family, school professionals, medical service providers, and community agencies.
   c. Implement strategies for team development and management.
   d. Develop mechanism for ongoing team coordination.
2. Function as a consultant.
   a. Identify the administrative and interpersonal factors that influence the effectiveness of a consultant.
   b. Implement effective consultative strategies.
   c. Provide technical assistance to other school team members, community agencies, and medical providers.
3. Educate school personnel and family to promote inclusion of the student within the educational experience.
   a. Assist school administrators with development of policy and procedures.
   b. Provide orientation to teachers and classroom aides.
   c. Conduct in-service sessions.
   d. Develop informational resources.

Box 30-5   COMPETENCIES FOR SCHOOL-BASED PHYSICAL THERAPISTS—cont'd

4. Supervise personnel and professional students.
   a. Apply effective strategies of supervision.
   b. Monitor the implementation of therapy recommendations by other team members.
   c. Establish a student clinical affiliation.
   d. Formally and informally teach or train therapy staff.
5. Serve as an advocate for students, families, and school.
   a. Attend public hearings.
   b. Serve on task force or decision-making committees.
   c. Provide necessary information to support student rights.
   d. Actively participate in IEP process.

CONTENT AREA 4: EXAMINATION AND EVALUATION IN SCHOOLS

1. Identify strengths and needs of student.
   a. Interview student, family, teachers, and other relevant school personnel.
   b. Gather information from medical personnel and records.
   c. Observe student in a variety of educational settings.
2. Collaboratively determine examination and evaluation process.
   a. Designate appropriate professional disciplines.
   b. Identify environments and student activities and routines.
   c. Select instruments.
   d. Establish format for conducting examination.
   e. Inform and prepare the student.
3. Determine student's ability to participate in meaningful school activities by examining and evaluating:
   a. Conduct of formal naturalistic observations to determine level of participation and necessary assistance and adaptations;
   b. Functional abilities, including gross motor, fine motor, perceptual motor, cognitive, social and emotional, and ADL;
   c. Impairments related to functional ability, including musculoskeletal status, neuromotor organization, sensory function, and cardiopulmonary status.
4. Utilize valid, reliable, cost-effective, and nondiscriminatory instruments for:
   a. Identification and eligibility;
   b. Diagnostic purposes;
   c. Individual program planning;
   d. Documentation of progress.

CONTENT AREA 5: PLANNING

1. Actively participate in the development of the Individualized Education Plan.
   a. Determine eligibility related to a student's educational program.
   b. Accurately interpret and communicate examination findings collaboratively with family, student, and other team members.

   c. Discuss prognosis of student performance related to curricular expectations.
   d. Discuss and prioritize outcomes related to student's educational needs based on current and future environmental demands and student and family preferences and goals.
   e. Offer appropriate recommendations for student placement and personnel needs in the least restrictive educational setting with intent to serve children in inclusive environments.
   f. In collaboration with the team, determine how therapy can contribute to the development of an individualized educational program (IEP), including:
      i. Meaningful student outcomes;
      ii. Functional and measurable goals and objectives;
      iii. Therapy service recommendations;
      iv. Specific intervention methods and strategies;
      v. Determination of frequency, intensity, and duration.
   g. Develop mechanism for ongoing coordination and collaboration regarding:
      i. Implementation of the IEP;
      ii. Updates or modifications of IEP;
      iii. Transition planning and implementation of the transition plan;
      iv. Interagency activities.

CONTENT AREA 6: INTERVENTION

1. Adapt environments to facilitate student access to and participation in student activities.
   a. Recommend adaptive equipment, assistive technology, and environmental adaptations.
   b. Monitor adaptive equipment, assistive technology, and environmental adaptations.
   c. Be able to instruct student and other team members in the appropriate use of adaptive equipment and assistive technology.
   d. Identify sources for obtaining, maintaining, repairing, and financing adaptive equipment, assistive technology, and environmental adaptations.
2. Use various types and methods of service provision for individualized student interventions.
   a. Employ direct, individual, group, integrated, consultative, monitoring, and collaborative approaches;
   b. Develop generic instruction plans and intervention plans that select and sequence strategies to meet the objectives listed on the student's IEP.
3. Promote skill acquisition, fluency, and generalization to enhance overall development, learning, and student participation.
   a. Use creative problem-solving strategies to meet the student's needs.

Continued

| Box **30-5** COMPETENCIES FOR SCHOOL-BASED PHYSICAL THERAPISTS—cont'd |

b. Explain the basic motor learning theories, and relate them to therapy education programs.

c. Address neuromuscular, musculoskeletal, sensory processing, and cardiopulmonary functions that support motor, social, emotional, cognitive, and language skills.

4. Embed therapy interventions into the context of student activities and routines.

   a. Implement appropriate positioning, mobility, environmental, and ADL strategies into curriculum, classroom schedule, and routines.

   b. Develop a matrix integrating objectives, routines and activities, and strategies.

CONTENT AREA 7: DOCUMENTATION

1. Produce useful written documentation by:

   a. Writing reports in commonly understood and meaningful terms;

   b. Maintaining timely and consistent records;

   c. Concisely summarizing relevant information;

   d. Sharing records with family and other team members.

2. Collaboratively monitor and modify student's IEP.

   a. Establish a mechanism for and record ongoing communication with family and other team members.

   b. Establish a plan of action for re-evaluation.

   c. Schedule pre-established team meetings to review student progress over the course of the school year.

3. Evaluate and document the effectiveness of therapy education programs.

   a. Establish baseline of student's level of participation and functional status.

   b. Collect ongoing data on the student's progress toward stated IEP outcomes.

   c. Summarize data to determine student's progress.

CONTENT AREA 8: ADMINISTRATIVE ISSUES IN SCHOOLS

1. Demonstrate flexibility, priority setting, and effective time management strategies.

2. Obtain resources and data necessary to justify establishing a new therapy program or altering an existing program.

3. Serve as a leader.

   a. Integrate knowledge of education, health, and social trends that affect therapy services.

   b. Identify and educate others on the overall roles, responsibilities, and functions of therapy services.

   c. Identify and differentiate characteristics of alternative approaches for resolving needs of therapy services.

d. Identify the administrative needs of the therapy service within the school setting.

e. Serve as a role model for other therapists regarding professional responsibilities.

4. Serve as a manager.

   a. Develop and analyze job descriptions for therapists.

   b. Implement a recruitment, orientation, mentorship, and professional development program for therapists and staff.

   c. Develop and implement policies and procedures to guide therapy services.

   d. Establish therapy caseloads and staffing needs.

   e. Evaluate the performance of therapy personnel.

   f. Plan and implement a therapy quality assurance plan and program evaluation.

   g. Participate in the assessment of school facilities and educational activities.

   h. Make recommendations, especially related to ensuring accessibility and reasonable accommodations to school environments.

   i. Identify and use appropriate school, home, community, state, and national resources, especially funding sources.

   j. Demonstrate the ability to plan and manage a budget for the therapy component of services.

CONTENT AREA 9: RESEARCH

1. Demonstrate knowledge of current research related to child development, medical care, educational practices, and implications for therapy.

   a. Conduct a literature review.

   b. Seek assistance of experienced researchers in interpreting published research.

   c. Critically evaluate published research.

2. Apply knowledge of research to the selection of therapy intervention strategies, service delivery systems, and therapeutic procedures.

   a. Use objective criteria for evaluation.

   b. Justify rationale for clinical decision-making.

   c. Expand clinical treatment case reports into single-subject studies.

3. Partake in program evaluation and clinical research activities with appropriate supervision

   a. Identify research topics.

   b. Secure resources to support clinical research.

   c. Implement clinical research projects.

   d. Disseminate research findings.

From Effgen, S. K., Chiarello, L., & Milbourne, S. (2007). Updated competencies for physical therapists working in schools. *Pediatric Physical Therapy, 19,* 266–274.

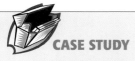

CASE STUDY

"Adrianna"

This case study highlights some of the issues and challenges that are frequently encountered by physical therapists in school-based practice: (1) promotion of the student's participation in the educational program in the least restrictive environment; (2) collaboration with other team members and physicians; and (3) flexibility in selecting models of service delivery based on the student's goals. Adrianna, a child with cerebral palsy (CP), is presented. The format integrates principles outlined in the *Guide to Physical Therapist Practice* ("The *Guide*")[2] and the World Health Organization's International Classification of Functioning, Disability and Health (ICF).[131] The *Guide* provides a framework for physical therapist practice, while the ICF focuses on participation and activities, which are the focus of school-based therapy services, incorporating environmental and personal factors along with body structures and functions. Evaluation includes the elements outlined in the 2001 edition of the *Guide*, but the order of presentation follows the ICF model, first focusing on participation in the educational program and school activities, before identifying associated impairments in body structures and functions. As noted previously, the revision of the *Guide* that is currently under way will be based on the ICF model.[4]

This case study takes place in a suburban school district with more than 9000 students: seven elementary schools (preschool to grade 5, housed in nine buildings), two middle schools (grades 6 to 8), and one high school (grades 9 to 12). The district employs one full-time physical therapist, two occupational therapists (each works 4 days per week), and four certified occupational therapist assistants (three full time and one who works 2 days per week). The physical and occupational therapists report to a supervisor who is a special educator; therefore, the therapists have often needed to inform him about issues related to their disciplines. The physical and occupational therapists have an excellent collaborative relationship.

Adrianna is a young girl with spastic diplegic and ataxic cerebral palsy (CP). She is classified at Level I on the Gross Motor Function Classification System[96]; she walks independently at home, at school, outdoors, and in the community, and she performs gross motor skills with limitations. Adrianna lives in a two-story house with her biological parents and her 4-year-old brother, who is developing typically. Her father is the fitness manager at a large gym, and her mother works part-time. The product of an uneventful 41-week pregnancy and long labor that included the presence of meconium in the amniotic fluid, she was delivered by emergency cesarean section for fetal distress. During the birth process, the umbilical cord was wrapped around her neck and arm. Her birth weight was 8 pounds 2 ounces. Apgar scores were 2, 7, and 5 at 1, 5, and 10 minutes after birth. Adrianna was discharged home at 5 days of age.

Motor development was delayed. Her parents reported that Adrianna began to sit unsupported at about 12 months, crawl at about 15 months, and walk independently at about 28 months. Beginning at 22 months of age, she received home-based physical therapy twice a week for 60-minute sessions through an early intervention program. At 25 months, Adrianna was diagnosed with cerebral palsy.

On her third birthday, Adrianna entered the district's preschool program for children with disabilities, where she received physical, occupational, and speech-language therapy, each in two 30-minute sessions per week. She also participated in the preschool physical education class with her classmates, in one 30-minute session per week. Physical therapy services were delivered primarily in the context of her preschool program: in her classroom, in the physical education class, on the playground, and in her mobility around the school. Occasionally, the therapist removed her from the usual distractions to work on targeted skills. Adrianna had an extraordinarily difficult adjustment to preschool because she was unwilling to separate from her mother. She cried vigorously on a daily basis for the first 3 months of school and thereafter each time her mother departed. Gradually, Adrianna became a joyful student, except when encountering unfamiliar situations, such as assembly programs with the entire school community and the preschool graduation ceremony.

At 5 years and 6 months of age, Adrianna underwent a comprehensive team re-evaluation in preparation for entering kindergarten. Contributing to the process were the school psychologist (who served as case manager), learning consultant, social worker, physical therapist, occupational therapist, speech-language pathologist, and her parents.

Physical Therapist Re-evaluation for IEP: Transition to Kindergarten

In preparation for the re-evaluation, the physical therapist reviewed existing records and discussed Adrianna's functional strengths and challenges with her mother, her classroom teacher, her physical education teacher, and her school occupational therapist. Incorporating the elements outlined in the *Guide*[2] and the ICF model,[131] the evaluation included observation in a variety of school settings, clinical examination, and administration of the School Function Assessment (SFA)[23] and the Gross Motor Function Measure (GMFM).[109]

Seating, Mobility, and Gross Motor Play at Preschool

During circle time in preschool, Adrianna and her classmates sit on preschool-size chairs. When sitting on the floor for play, Adrianna assumes a crossed-legged ("tailor-sit") position. She transfers from the floor to standing by rising from half-kneeling onto her right leg without using her hands for support; she needs to push with one hand on her knee when rising onto her left leg.

Adrianna walks independently and without assistive devices for all preschool activities, for distances of several hundred feet, on level indoor surfaces, uneven outdoor terrain, and ramps without a railing. She falls an average of once or twice per school day. Falls are variably attributable to loss of balance, insufficient ankle dorsiflexion for toe clearance, or inattention to obstacles in her way. Adrianna runs for distances of at least 50 feet. She falls occasionally when running,

Continued

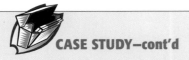

especially on uneven outdoor terrain, and she does not keep pace with her peers when walking around the school, on the playground, or during fire drills. However, her friends wait patiently for her and are eager to help her when she falls.

Two months ago, Adrianna received new supramalleolar orthoses (SMOs) to replace her previous hinged ones. She wears them at school but rarely at home. The new design is fixed, with trimlines that are lower than her previous SMOs; the footplate extends only to the base of the metatarsal heads to allow for push-off during gait. With verbal cues, Adrianna can produce a heel-toe gait for distances of about 20 feet, rarely sustaining it for longer distances. She expresses displeasure at having to wear orthoses, stating that she wants to wear shoes like those of her classmates.

This past year, Adrianna required very close supervision and occasional minimal assistance to negotiate stairs and bus steps; now she does so with greater safety and confidence, requiring continued supervision but without physical assistance. Although Adrianna does not need to access stairs during a typical preschool day, the school physical therapist incorporated stair climbing into intervention sessions during her final preschool year, in anticipation of her transition to kindergarten, where she will need to use stairs. With one hand on a railing, Adrianna walks both up and down stairs using a reciprocal pattern. She no longer needs reminders to advance her hand on the railing before moving her feet to keep her center of gravity over her feet. Without holding a railing and with close supervision to minimal assistance for balance, Adrianna can walk up four or five steps reciprocally and the remaining steps nonreciprocally, leading with either foot; she walks down stairs nonreciprocally, usually leading with the left foot. Adrianna progressed this year to walking up and down bus steps reciprocally, with supervision and holding both railings. She is able to negotiate curbs, sometimes holding one railing but often without holding a railing.

Adrianna has learned to jump up independently to a height of about an inch, generally landing on both feet without losing her balance. She can independently jump forward a distance of about 8 inches but cannot jump backward. With supervision, Adrianna can jump off a 6-inch-high step, usually reaching for the railing and needing to take several steps to recover her balance. Adrianna is now able to perform three consecutive jumping jacks slowly, stopping between them to recover her balance and to maintain appropriate sequencing. She has learned this year to hop once on her right foot with both hands held for minimal assistance, but she is unable to hop on her left foot. Standing at about 8 feet from the therapist, Adrianna can accurately throw or kick an 8.5-inch gym ball in about three of five trials. She can catch a ball with both hands and by trapping it with her body, only when focusing on the task and positioning her hands just right, about once in five trials.

Home and Community Recreational Activities

Adrianna enjoys riding her tricycle at home; she independently climbs on and off and pedals it around her neighborhood, steering accurately. For the past year, she participated in a class for children with disabilities at a climbing gym. Previously, she took part in hippotherapy and aquatic therapy.

Systems Review

Although the focus of a school-based evaluation is on mobility in the educational environment, a systems review can help to identify impairment-level issues that may affect school function.

Cardiovascular and Pulmonary. No problems are evident in Adrianna's cardiopulmonary endurance during functional activities.

Integumentary. Skin integrity is intact, although it should be monitored closely during the first few days of wearing new orthoses.

Musculoskeletal. Adrianna demonstrates mild weakness in her trunk and extremities, with isolated motion at all joints. Range of motion is within functional limits throughout.

Neuromuscular. A moderate degree of spasticity is present in the left biceps and triceps and in the gastrocnemius/soleus of both lower extremities, with minimal spasticity in the right biceps and triceps, as well as in the hamstrings and quadriceps. Hypotonicity is noted in the neck and trunk. Isolated motion is present at all joints, although coordination is impaired. Gross estimation of Adrianna's strength is 4/5 in the upper extremities, 3/5 in the trunk musculature, and 4/5 in the lower extremities.

Body Functions and Structures

Qualitative observations of Adrianna's motor performance during the preschool program indicate problems with motor control, including initiation, timing, sequencing, coordination, modulation, reciprocal inhibition, and force generation of movement, as well as difficulties with anticipatory and reactive postural control.[94,129] The systems review is consistent with these observations regarding range of motion, muscle tone and performance, and orthotic devices. Although Adrianna can accomplish many of the tasks required of her during the school day and can complete many of the test items on some motor assessments, her quality of movement is not refined and she tires more easily than her peers.

Gross Motor Function Measure

The Gross Motor Function Measure (GMFM)[109] was administered by the physical therapist to assess components of motor activities that were described more globally by the SFA. It was designed for children with cerebral palsy and comprises skills that are considered achievable by children at 5 years of age who are developing typically. The measure was completed in about 45 minutes. Adrianna earned maximum scores in these dimensions: (A) Lying and Rolling; (B) Sitting; and (C) Crawling and Kneeling. Her difficulties are in the dimensions of (D) Standing; and (E) Walking, Running, and Jumping. Adrianna's Goal Total Score (dimensions D and E) was 82%, and her Total Score was 93%. Areas of difficulty included unilateral stance, rising from the floor through half-kneeling, hopping, jumping forward, jumping off a step, stepping over a stick at knee level, and negotiating stairs with alternating feet.

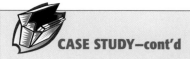

CASE STUDY—cont'd

EVIDENCE TO PRACTICE 30-1

CASE STUDY "ADRIANNA"

EXAMINATION DECISIONS

Gross Motor Function Measure

The decision to use the Gross Motor Function Measure (GMFM)[109] was supported by a study by Bjornson, Graubert, Buford, and McLaughlin[12] of 37 children with spastic diplegia. The GMFM administered at baseline, 12, and 24 months showed high correlations ($P < .001$) with video evaluations for all dimensions except Lying/Rolling. Trahan and Malouin[119] studied 50 children with quadriplegia, hemiplegia, and diplegia at baseline, 4, and 8 months. For the three groups combined, they found changes in GMFM scores ($P < .05$) in each dimension and in total scores at both 4 and 8 months, although the magnitude of changes varied among the groups. Both studies concluded that the GMFM is an effective tool for measuring change over time in the gross motor performance of children with CP.

School Function Assessment

The choice of the School Function Assessment (SFA)[23] was based on research by King et al.[73] that found it to be an appropriate tool for measuring important functional skills in school settings. In a validity study of 64 children, 17 of whom had CP, Hwang, Davies, Taylor, and Gavin[62] measured convergent validity scores that ranged from .56 to .72, when comparing SFA scores with those of the Vineland Adaptive Behavior Scales. Construct validity scores demonstrated significant differences between children with CP and their peers without disabilities.

PLAN OF CARE DECISION

The decision to recommend a rigorous functional physical training program was supported by a study by Gorter et al.[51] of 13 children with CP (age 8 to 13 years) at Gross Motor Function Classification System GMFCS[96] Levels I and II. The authors found improvements in aerobic endurance, walking distance, and walking velocity after a program of rigorous activity in two 30-minute sessions per week for 9 weeks. Valvano[126,127] promoted activity-focused interventions for children with CP, consisting of structured practice and repetition of functional motor tasks. Damiano[25] advocated comprehensive physical activity programs, citing these

important reasons: "(1) preventing secondary musculoskeletal impairments and maximizing physical functioning, (2) fostering the cognitive, social, and emotional development of the child, and (3) developing, maintaining, and perhaps restoring neural structures and pathways" (p. 1535).

Increasing muscle strength can contribute to improved motor control and function, particularly improved gait.[35] Practice of motor skills should be structured to promote learning through consideration of part versus whole practice, blocked versus random practice, massed versus distributed practice, schedules of feedback, knowledge of performance, and knowledge of results.[113] Intervention that is embedded in natural contexts is associated with a higher degree of motivation than activities performed in isolation, resulting in more effective acquisition, retention, and transfer of targeted motor skills.[17] The problem solving of novel skills in natural settings promotes generalization to a variety of real-life situations.[113]

PATIENT/FAMILY PREFERENCES

Orthoses, particularly ankle-foot orthoses (AFOs), are commonly accepted as a component of intervention for individuals with CP.[60,94] However, many children and adolescents reject them in their desire to conform to their peers. Sometimes parents express more dissatisfaction with the orthoses than their children do. Intervention that is not acceptable to the child or the parents will not be used and, therefore, will be of no benefit.[33] Evidence-based practice emphasizes the context of the individual client, including values and personal circumstances.[53] Hence, acceptability of the proposed intervention by the child and caregivers is an essential consideration. Some parents and children opt for less-obtrusive supramalleolar orthoses (SMOs), although their minimal ability to assist in dorsiflexion can result in frequent falls.

Adrianna's parents have an interest in exercise and are motivated to assist her in improving her motor skills. In a systematic review of the evidence, Mattern-Baxter[82] found that body weight–supported treadmill training (BWSTT) may contribute to improvements in gait velocity, gait endurance, and gross motor function among children with CP. However, two other systematic reviews were inconclusive.[26,90] Dieruf and colleagues[31] demonstrated improvements in health-related quality of life indicators following a brief program of intensive BWSTT.

Diagnosis

Although not typically included in documentation in the school setting, according to the *Guide*,[2] Adrianna's physical therapy intervention is addressed through Preferred Practice Pattern 5C: Impaired Motor Function and Sensory Integrity Associated With Nonprogressive

Disorders of the Central Nervous System—Congenital Origin or Acquired in Infancy or Childhood. Adrianna exhibits impaired muscle performance (strength, endurance, and tone) and impaired motor control (balance and coordination), resulting in limitations in her ambulation on all surfaces and in her performance of gross motor skills in her physical education class and on the playground.

Continued

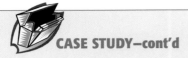

CASE STUDY—cont'd

Prognosis

Adrianna should continue to demonstrate improvement in her mobility and gross motor skills; however, she will remain challenged by activities that require balance and coordination. Although she works hard to keep pace with her classmates in her physical education class, she may become frustrated as the discrepancy widens between her skill level and that of her peers.

IEP Meeting: Transition to Kindergarten

The IEP meeting was conducted during Adrianna's final month of preschool. In attendance were her parents, her classroom teacher, a regular education teacher, the school psychologist (her case manager), learning consultant, school social worker, physical therapist, occupational therapist, and speech-language pathologist. At her age, it was not considered appropriate for Adrianna to attend the meeting, although older students would be invited.

Adrianna has a specific learning disability, and her high level of distractibility impedes her academic achievement. Her speech, like her motor skills, is ataxic; it is slow, dysarthric, and of low volume, with the potential to hinder her social relationships. However, she interacts well with her classmates and has many friends.

Adrianna demonstrates fair coordination in both hands. She is right-hand dominant. To pick up small objects, she often uses a lateral grasp or raking of her fingers instead of a pincer grasp. She is able to hold a crayon with a tripod grasp but requires an adaptive grip when using a pencil. Handwriting is slow and laborious, so it takes her much longer than her classmates to complete assignments. In future years, she is likely to rely on computer skills. Adrianna can generally remove her own clothing, orthoses, shoes, and socks but has difficulty with some areas of dressing, such as opening and closing small buttons and tying shoes. She is working on these skills with her school occupational therapist.

At the IEP meeting, several team members expressed concern about Adrianna's safety on stairs. Her neighborhood school houses kindergarten and some first-grade classes in a two-story building with neither ramps nor elevator. Students generally access both floors during the school day. The adjacent "sister building" houses grades 1 through 5; it is a modern one-story building with barrier-free design. The case manager suggested assigning Adrianna to one of the district's five accessible elementary schools for kindergarten and returning her to her neighborhood school (the accessible building) for first grade.

The physical therapist advocated for Adrianna to be placed in her neighborhood school for kindergarten, the least restrictive environment, with the accommodation of adult supervision on stairs. This would also provide Adrianna with multiple daily opportunities to negotiate stairs. The therapist's rationale was based on evidence of the importance of a large number of practice trials when learning a motor skill.[71,78,113,126,127]

The team agreed to assign Adrianna to a regular-education kindergarten class in her neighborhood school with in-class support for reading and mathematics. Related services specified on the IEP included physical, occupational, and speech-language therapy, each through a combination of integrated and pull-out models of service delivery. She will also participate with her class in two 30-minute sessions per week of physical education, as part of the regular education program. The IEP team discussed Adrianna's social and emotional adjustment to kindergarten, in view of her initial fear of new people and environments. The school physical therapist, who serves students throughout the district, would be the only familiar adult on the first day of kindergarten. For this reason, the physical therapist assured Adrianna, her parents, and the rest of the team that she would be there to greet Adrianna on the first day of school and to assist her in adapting to her new environment.

Goals Contributed by School Physical Therapist

Goals were developed collaboratively by the IEP team. The physical therapist reported that Adrianna stated, "I want to walk like everybody else and I don't want to fall anymore." The following mobility-related goals were identified by the team; the school physical therapist will be among those responsible for assisting Adrianna in achieving them, in one school year. Direct physical therapy services will be provided in two 30-minute sessions per week. (Please note that there is wide variation across the nation regarding the quantity of services provided. Adrianna lives in the northeastern United States, where higher frequencies of service delivery have been reported.)[69]

- Adrianna will keep pace with her classmates when walking independently without falling for distances of at least 300 feet, on level indoor surfaces and uneven outdoor terrain, either with or without her SMOs, in four of five trials.
- Adrianna will walk independently up and down five steps with one hand on a railing and using a reciprocal pattern, in four of five trials. (In the school she will attend for first grade, there are five steps between the two levels of the building, with an adjacent ramp. When walking independently around the building, she can use the ramp; when supervised, she can practice negotiation of stairs.)
- Adrianna will independently walk through the lunch line, place each food and drink item on her tray, and walk with it to her table—a distance of at least 50 feet—in four of five trials.
- Adrianna will independently perform locomotor skills in her physical education class, including jumping, galloping, hopping, skipping, and jumping jacks, in four of five trials.

Kindergarten

At the beginning of Adrianna's kindergarten year, the school physical therapist performed an ecologic assessment through observation in the classroom, on the playground, in the lunchroom, and during physical education class, along with discussions with the classroom teacher and physical education teacher. To promote motor learning,

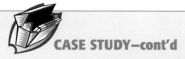

CASE STUDY—cont'd

the therapist asked the staff to closely supervise her walking up and down stairs, while providing physical guidance only when necessary.[113] Adrianna adjusted well to the physical demands of attending a two-story school. After crying frequently during her first several weeks of kindergarten, she has become an enthusiastic participant in the program. Adrianna enjoys climbing on the outdoor playground equipment, where she is remarkably undaunted by her difficulties with some of the activities, described below. She tries to participate fully in her physical education class, although she is unable to perform the higher-level motor skills.

School Function Assessment

During her first few weeks of kindergarten, the five mobility-related domains of the School Function Assessment (SFA) were again administered by the school physical therapist in consultation with her classroom teacher. The SFA measures skills that promote participation in the natural settings of the student's educational program. Mobility domains are in the categories of Activity Performance, Physical Tasks: Travel (19 items), Maintaining and Changing Positions (12 items), Recreational Movement (11 items), Manipulation With Movement (16 items), and Up/Down Stairs (6 items). In the Travel domain, Adrianna shows inconsistent performance in the following tasks: moving on uneven surfaces (e.g., lawns, gravel, doorsills); maneuvering around ruts, holes, and other dangerous surfaces; and moving on slippery surfaces. In Recreational Movement, she demonstrates inconsistent performance in catching a playground ball; running without falling, making changes in direction and speed; throwing and catching a small ball; and playing games involving hitting a target. In Manipulation With Movement, Adrianna is inconsistent in carrying a tray containing more than one item without spilling or dropping things and in safely carrying fragile objects or liquids in open containers. In Up/Down Stairs, she is inconsistent in walking up and down a flight of stairs at regular speed, with or without carrying an object. In all other areas, her performance is fairly consistent.

Plan of Care

Coordination, Communication, and Documentation

The school physical therapist communicates frequently (in person, by telephone, and by email) with Adrianna's parents, classroom teacher, physical education teacher, occupational therapist, speech-language therapist, and case manager. They discuss her functional strengths, participation restrictions, and activity limitations. Physical therapy progress reports are sent home with each academic report card, twice per school year. Formal parent-therapist conferences occur twice during the school year, during designated conference weeks. Through these modes of communication, the therapist suggests exercises, activities, and accommodations, describes Adrianna's progress toward her goals, refers the family to community recreation programs and other resources, and recommends return visits to the orthotist for modification or fabrication of new orthoses. The physical therapist also sends letters to Adrianna's physiatrist as needed.

Student-Related Instruction

During the initial evaluation prior to entry into the district's preschool program, the physical therapist met with Adrianna's parents to discuss her medical history and to check their understanding about CP in general, and Adrianna's condition in particular. Then and subsequently, issues related to her function at school are discussed and recommendations provided for home and community physical and recreational activities.

At the annual review, the school physical therapist discussed with Adrianna's parents current evidence for the benefits of body weight–supported treadmill training (BWSTT) and provided written materials about this intervention.[31,82] There are no treadmills in any of the district's elementary schools, but Adrianna has one available to her, because her father works as fitness manager for a local gym. The family decided to explore the possibility of Adrianna's engaging in a short, intensive treadmill program at her father's gym, supervised by one of her parents and with consultation by the physical therapist. The goal of this intervention would be to promote an increase in the speed of Adrianna's gait over longer distances, to enable her to keep pace with her classmates in her mobility around the school.[82]

At the beginning of each school year and thereafter as appropriate, the physical therapist meets with Adrianna's classroom teacher, physical education teacher, and any other school staff member involved in her educational program, to discuss her functional strengths and challenges and to recommend appropriate accommodations.

Procedural Interventions

School-based direct physical therapy services comprise functional activities, with an emphasis on the particular skills that will enhance Adrianna's participation in her educational program. Muscle strengthening, balance, and coordination exercises are key components. Some intervention sessions are devoted to reinforcing the skills incorporated in her physical education class, such as jumping, galloping, hopping, skipping, and ball skills. Others focus on walking and running throughout the school environment with goals of reducing the frequency of falls and improving her negotiation of stairs. Although on rare occasions the therapist works with Adrianna individually, services are usually conducted with her classmates, in a small group or in the context of her physical education class, outdoor recess, or lunch, or during her mobility around the school. In these natural settings with her peers, she is highly motivated to participate, and they are eager to be chosen, contributing to her positive view of the intervention.

Physical Education Class

Early in the school year, Adrianna had difficulty with some of the gross motor activities in her physical education class. The physical therapist met with the physical education teacher periodically, both formally and informally, to discuss accommodations and strategies to promote Adrianna's participation. Physical therapy intervention sessions often focus on the areas identified, such as locomotor (jumping, galloping,

Continued

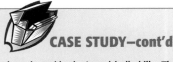

CASE STUDY—cont'd

hopping, skipping) and ball skills. The physical therapist works with Adrianna on these skills in the context of her physical education class, as well as in smaller groups with one or two of her classmates who are developing typically. She now participates in her physical education class to a greater extent, with accommodations as needed.

Playground Activities

Adrianna has made excellent progress in her ability to negotiate the outdoor playground equipment. She is extremely motivated to master increasingly difficult skills and then she seeks new challenges. As soon as Adrianna learned to climb independently to the top of the climbing frame and slowly lower herself, she decided that she wanted to learn to climb up and down the mobile rope ladder and slide down the fire pole, both of which she is now able to do. Adrianna can independently climb on and off a swing and pump her legs to propel it, although she does not swing as high as her peers. She is actively involved in outdoor play with her classmates, although she falls occasionally when running on the wood chips. Classmates include her in their games and are eager to assist her, sometimes even when she is not actually in need of assistance. Rarely do teachers need to intervene.

Transition to First Grade

In preparation for her transition to first grade, the team met to develop Adrianna's IEP. In her neighborhood school, first grade is offered both in the older, two-story building and in the newer one; the team decided to assign her to the barrier-free building. Although she will have fewer opportunities to practice negotiating stairs, she will be able to navigate around the building without adult supervision, promoting her independence. When adult supervision is available, she will work on her stair-climbing goal.

Changes in Episodes of Care and Models of Service Delivery

Adrianna will continue to receive direct school-based physical therapy services for as long as is required to enable her to participate in the educational program. When the team decides that physical education alone is sufficient, the model of service delivery will be changed to consultation or monitoring. For grades 6 through 12, Adrianna will attend much larger, multistory schools that will present new physical challenges for her, with their stairs, long corridors, outdoor tracks, and multiple playing fields. As she prepares to move to the middle school, whether or not she is still receiving direct school-based physical therapy services, it may be appropriate to reassess her mobility within the context of the middle school environment. If endurance and negotiation of stairs remain problematic, the team may decide to resume direct physical therapy. As Adrianna experiences growth spurts, she may present with impairment-level issues, such as reduced range of motion at her knees and ankles, which may adversely affect her mobility and, therefore, may be an indication to resume direct service. At each annual review, or more often if necessary, the IEP team will determine the appropriate level of school-based physical therapy.

The video of Adrianna that accompanies this chapter was filmed at the end of her kindergarten year. It shows her engaging with her classmates in physical education, outdoor play, and lunch, as well as negotiating stairs and bus steps. Physical therapy intervention has been provided in each of these settings to promote Adrianna's ability to access, participate, and progress in her educational program.

SUMMARY

In the United States, physical therapy is mandated as part of federally sponsored programs to serve infants, toddlers, children, and youth with disabilities. For preschool- and school-age children, physical therapy is a related service of the IDEA educational program for those children who require special education, or under Section 504 of the Rehabilitation Act. The school setting is not the high-tech, health-focused environment of the modern hospital setting or the therapy-focused environment of the rehabilitation setting. Rather, the educational needs of students are the highest priority. To provide effective services and attain personal satisfaction, therapists must become knowledgeable of the educational milieu, including federal, state, and local laws, and regulations that govern physical therapy in the educational environment.

Physical therapists working in the educational environment witness first-hand the successes and struggles that students with special needs experience in their everyday lives. As a member of a team of professionals, physical therapists are asked to solve complex problems to enhance the ability of children to participate in education programs. The educational environment is rewarding for physical therapists who are willing and able to meet the unique demands of this practice setting.

REFERENCES

1. Alberto, P. A., & Troutman, A. C. (2008). *Applied behavior analysis for teachers* (8th ed.). Upper Saddle River, NJ: Prentice Hall.
2. American Physical Therapy Association. (2001). Guide to physical therapist practice (2nd ed.). *Physical Therapy, 81,* 1–768.
3. American Physical Therapy Association. (2009). Defensible documentation resource—An introduction. Retrieved from: http://www.apta.org.
4. American Physical Therapy Association. (2010). APTA endorses World Health Organization, ICF model. Retrieved

from: http://www.apta.org/AM/Template.cfm?Section=Home&TEMPLATE=/CM/ContentDisplay.cfm&CONTENTID=50081.

5. American Physical Therapy Association, Section on Pediatrics. (1987). *TASH position statement: On the provision of related services to persons with severe handicaps.* Alexandria, VA: American Physical Therapy Association.

6. Arnold, S. H., & McEwen, I. R. (2008). Item test-retest reliability and responsiveness of the school outcomes measure (SOM). *Physical and Occupational Therapy in Pediatrics, 28,* 59–77.

7. Baer, R. (2001). Transition planning. In R. W. Flexer, T. J. Simmons, P. Luft, & R. M. Baer (Eds.), *Transition planning for secondary students with disabilities* (pp. 333–363). Upper Saddle River, NJ: Prentice-Hall.

8. Bailes, A. F., Reder, R., & Burch, C. (2008). Development of guidelines for determining frequency of therapy services in a pediatric medical setting. *Pediatric Physical Therapy, 20,* 194–198.

9. Baker, B. J., Cole, K. N., & Harris, S. (1998). Cognitive referencing as a method of OT/PT triage for young children. *Pediatric Physical Therapy, 10,* 2–6.

10. Batsche, G., Elliott, J., Graden, J., Grimes, J., Kovaleski, J., Prasse, D., Reschly, D., Schrag, J., & Tilly, D. (2005). *Response to intervention: Policy considerations and implementation.* Alexandria, VA: National Association of State Directors of Special Education.

11. Batten, H. E. (1933). The industrial school for crippled and deformed children. *Physical Therapy Review, 13,* 112–113.

12. Bjornson, K. F., Graubert, C. S., Buford, V. L., & McLaughlin, J. (1998). Validity of the Gross Motor Function Measure. *Pediatric Physical Therapy, 10,* 43–47.

13. Blatt, B., & Kaplan, F. (1966). *Christmas in purgatory: A photographic essay on mental retardation.* Boston: Allyn & Bacon.

14. Braddock, D. (1987). *Federal policy toward mental retardation and developmental disabilities* (p. 71). Baltimore: Paul H. Brookes.

15. Brown, D. A., Effgen, S. K., & Palisano, R. J. (1998). Performance following ability-focused physical therapy intervention in individuals with severely limited physical and cognitive abilities. *Physical Therapy, 78,* 934–949.

16. Cable, O. E., Fowler, A. F., & Foss, H. S. (1938). The crippled children's guide of Buffalo, New York. *Physical Therapy Review, 16,* 85–88.

17. Campbell, P. H., McInerney, W. F., & Cooper, M. A. (1984). Therapeutic programming for students with severe handicaps. *American Journal of Occupational Therapy, 38,* 594–602.

18. Carr, S. H. (1989). Louisiana's criteria of eligibility for occupational therapy services in the public school system. *American Journal of Occupational Therapy, 43,* 503–506.

19. Carter, E., Sisco, L., Brown, L., Brickham, D., & Al-Kahbbaz, Z. (2008). Peer interactions and academic engagement of youth with developmental disabilities in inclusive middle and high school classrooms. *American Journal on Mental Retardation, 113,* 479–494.

20. Cecere, S., Effgen, S. K. & Rechlin, L. (2009, June). *Complex issues: The concept of workload and the determination of frequency and intensity of services.* Baltimore, MD: American Physical Therapy Association Annual Conference.

21. Cole, C., Waldron, N, & Majd, M. (2004). Academic progress of students across inclusive and traditional settings. *Mental Retardation, 42,* 136–144.

22. Cole, K. N., Mills, P. E., & Harris, S. R. (1991). Retrospective analysis of physical and occupational therapy progress in young children: An examination of cognitive referencing. *Pediatric Physical Therapy, 3,* 185–189.

23. Coster, W., Deeney, T., Haltiwanger, J., & Haley, H. (1998). *School function assessment.* San Antonio: The Psychological Corporation.

24. Cruickshank, W. M. (1980). *Psychology of exceptional children and youth* (4th ed.; pp. 65–66). Englewood Cliffs, NJ: Prentice-Hall.

25. Damiano, D. L. (2006). Activity, activity, activity: Rethinking our physical therapy approach to cerebral palsy. *Physical Therapy, 86,* 1534–1540.

26. Damiano, D. L., & Dejong, S. L. (2009). A systematic review of the effectiveness of treadmill training and body weight support in pediatric rehabilitation. *Journal of Neurologic Physical Therapy, 33,* 27–44.

27. David, K. S. (1996). Monitoring process for improved outcomes. *Physical & Occupational Therapy in Pediatrics, 16,* 47–76.

28. David, K. (February 2005). IDEA 2004: PL 108-446, Impact on physical therapy related services. Retrieved from: http://www.pediatricapta.org/csm05/9752.pdf.

29. Davies, P. L., Soon, P. L., Young, M., & Clausen-Yamaki, A. (2004). Validity and reliability of the School Function Assessment in elementary school students with disabilities. *Physical and Occupational Therapy in Pediatrics, 24,* 23–43.

30. Deno, E. (1970). Special education as developmental capital. *Exceptional Children, 37,* 229–237.

31. Dieruf, K., Burtner, P. A., Provost, B., Phillips, J., Bernitsky-Beddingfield, A., & Sullivan, K. (2009). A pilot study of quality of life in children with cerebral palsy after intensive body weight-supported treadmill training. *Pediatric Physical Therapy, 21,* 45–52.

32. Dole, R. L., Arvidson, K., Byrne, E., Robbins, J., & Schasberger, B. (2003). Consensus among experts in pediatric occupational and physical therapy on elements of Individualized Education Programs. *Pediatric Physical Therapy, 15,* 159–166.

33. Domjan, M. (1998). *The principles of learning and behavior* (4th ed.). Pacific Grove, CA: Brooks/Cole.

34. Dunn, W. (1991). Integrated related services. In L. H. Meyer, C. A. Peck, & L. Brown (Eds.), *Critical issues in the lives of people with severe disabilities* (pp. 353–378). Baltimore: Paul H. Brookes.

35. Eagleton, M., Iams, A., McDowell, J., Morrison, R., & Evans, C. L. (2004). The effects of strength training on gait in adolescents with cerebral palsy. *Pediatric Physical Therapy, 16,* 22–30.

36. Effgen, S. K. (1987). *Competencies for school physical therapists.* Philadelphia, PA: Program in Pediatric Physical Therapy, Hahnemann University.

37. Effgen, S. K. (1991). Systematic delivery and recording of intervention assistance. *Pediatric Physical Therapy, 3,* 63–68.

38. Effgen, S. K. (2000). Factors affecting the termination of physical therapy services for children in school settings. *Pediatric Physical Therapy, 12,* 121–126.

39. Effgen, S. K., Chiarello, L., & Milbourne, S. (2007). Updated competencies for physical therapists working in schools. *Pediatric Physical Therapy, 19,* 266–274.

40. Effgen, S. K., & Klepper, S. (1994). Survey of physical therapy practice in educational settings. *Pediatric Physical Therapy, 6,* 15–21.

41. Effgen, S. K., & McEwen, I. (2007). *Review of selected physical therapy interventions for school-age children with disabilities (COPSSE document Number OP-4).* Gainesville, FL: University of Florida, Center on Personnel Studies in Special Education. Retrieved from: http://www.coe.ufl.edu/copsse/docs/PT_CP_090707_5/1/PT_CP_090707_5.pdf.

42. Effgen, S. K., & McEwen, I. (2008). Review of selected physical therapy interventions for school-age children with disabilities. *Physical Therapy Reviews, 13,* 297–312.

43. Federal Register, Part II, Department of Education. (September 29, 1992). 34 CFR Parts 300 and 301: Assistance to states for the education of children with disabilities program and preschool grants for children with disabilities, Final Rule, Vol. 57, No. 189.

44. Federal Register, Part II, Department of Education. (December 9, 2003). 34 CFR Part 200, Title I—Improving the academic achievement of the disadvantaged, Final Rule, Vol. 68, No. 236, pp. 68697–68708. Retrieved from: http://www.ed.gov/legislation/FedRegister/finrule/2003-4/120903a.html.

45. Federal Register, Part II, Department of Education. (June 21, 2005). 34 CFR Parts 300, 301, and 304: Assistance to states for the education of children with disabilities; preschool grants for children with disabilities; and service obligations under special education. Personnel development to improve services and results for children with disabilities: Proposed rule. In print, and retrieved from: http://a257.g.akamaitech.net/7/257/2422/01jan20051800/edocket.access.gpo.gov/2005/05-11804.htm.

46. Florida Department of Education, Exceptional Education & Student Services. (2009). Considerations for educationally relevant therapy (CERT). Retrieved from: http://www.fldoe.org/ESE/cert.asp.

47. Flexer, R. W., Simmons, T. J., Luft, P., & Baer, R. M. (Eds.). (2008). *Transition planning for secondary students with disabilities* (3rd ed.; pp. 3–28). Upper Saddle River, NJ: Pearson Prentice Hall.

48. Giangreco, M. F., Cloninger, C. J., & Iverson, V. (1993). *Choosing options and accommodations for children: A guide to planning inclusive education.* Baltimore: Paul H. Brookes.

49. Giangreco, M. F., York, J., & Rainforth, B. (1989). Providing related services to learners with severe handicaps in educational settings: Pursuing the least restrictive option. *Pediatric Physical Therapy, 1,* 55–63.

50. Givins, E. V. (1938). The spastic child in the classroom. *Physical Therapy Review, 18,* 136–137.

51. Gorter, H., Holty, L., Rameckers, E. E. A., Elvers, H. J. W. H., & Oostendorp, R. A. B. (2009). Changes in endurance and walking ability through functional physical training in children with cerebral palsy. *Pediatric Physical Therapy, 21,* 31–37.

52. Guralnick, M. J. (2001). *Early childhood inclusion.* Baltimore: Paul H. Brookes.

53. Guyatt, G. H., Haynes, R. B., Jaeschke, R. Z., Cook, D. J., Green, L., Naylor, C. D., et al. (2000). Users' guides to the medical literature: XXV. Evidence-based medicine: principles for applying the users' guides to patient care. *Journal of the American Medical Association, 284,* 1290–1296.

54. Haley, S. M., Coster, W. J., Ludlow, L. H., Haltiwarger, J. T., & Andrellas, P. J. (1992). *Pediatric evaluation of disability inventory (PEDI).* San Antonio, TX: The Psychological Corporation.

55. Hanft, B. E., & Place, P. A. (1996). *The consulting therapist: A guide for OTs and PTs in schools.* San Antonio, TX: Therapy Skill Builders.

56. Hanft, B. E., Rush, D. D., & Shelden, M. L. (2004). *Coaching families and colleagues in early childhood.* Baltimore: Paul H. Brookes.

57. Hanft, B., & Shepherd, J. (Eds.). (2008). *Collaborating for student success: A guide for school-based occupational therapy.* Bethesda, MD: American Occupational Therapy Association.

58. Hanson, M. J., Beckman, P. J., Horn, E., Marquart, J., Sandall, S. R., Greig, D., & Brennan, E. (2000). Entering preschool: Family and professional experiences in this transition process. *Journal of Early Intervention, 23,* 279–293.

59. Holler, R. A. & Zirkel, P. A. (2008). Section 504 and public schools: A national survey concerning "Section 504-only" students. *National Association of Secondary School Principals Bulletin, 92,* 19. Retrieved from: http://bul.sagepub.com/cgi/content/abstract/92/1/19.

60. Howle, J. M. W. (1999). Cerebral palsy. In S. K. Campbell (Ed.), *Decision making in pediatric neurologic physical therapy* (pp. 23–83). Philadelphia: Churchill Livingstone.

61. Hunt, P., Soto, G., Maier, J., & Dering, K. (2003). Collaborative teaming to support students at risk and students with severe disabilities in general education classrooms. *Exceptional Children, 69,* 315–332.

62. Hwang, J., Davies, P. L., Taylor, M. P., & Gavin, W. J. (2002). Validation of school function assessment with elementary school children. *Occupation, Participation & Health, 22,* 48–58.

63. Iowa Guidelines for Educationally Related Physical Therapy Services. (2001). Des Moines, IA: Iowa Department of Education.

64. Jackson, S., Pretti-Frontczak, K., Harjusola-Webb, S., Grisham-Brown, J., & Romani, J. M. (2009). Response to intervention: Implications for early childhood professionals. *Language,*

Speech, and Hearing Services in Schools, 40, 424–434. Retrieved from: http://dx.doi.org/10.1044/0161-1461(2009/08-0027).

65. Johnson, D. R., Stodden, R. A., Emanuel, E. J., Luecking, R., & Mack, M. (2002). Current challenges facing secondary education and transition services: What research tells us. *Exceptional Children, 68*, 519–531.

66. Jones, M. & Rapport, M. J. (2009). Court decisions, state education agency hearings, letters of inquiry, policy interpretation, and investigations by federal agencies realted to school-based physical therapy (pp. 147–159). In I. R. McEwen (Ed.), *Providing physical therapy services under Parts B & C of the Individuals With Disabilities Education Act (IDEA).* Alexandria, VA: Section on Pediatrics, American Physical Therapy Association.

67. Kaloi, L., & Stanberry, K. (2009). Section 504 in 2009: Boarder eligibility, more accommodations. National Center for Learning Disabilities. Retrieved from: http://www.ncld.org/on-capitol-hill/federal-laws-aamp-ld/adaaa-a-section-504/section-504-in-2009.

68. Kaminker, M. K., Chiarello, L. A., O'Neil, M. E., & Dichter, C. G. (2004). Decision making for service delivery in schools: A nationwide survey of pediatric physical therapists. *Physical Therapy, 84*, 919–933.

69. Kaminker, M. K., Chiarello, L. A., & Smith, J. A. C. (2006). Decision making for service delivery in schools: A nationwide analysis by geographic region. *Pediatric Physical Therapy, 18*, 204–213.

70. Kentucky Department of Education, Resource manual for educationally related occupational therapy and physical therapy in Kentucky public schools. Retrieved February 26, 2010, from http://www.education.ky.gov/NR/rdonlyres/44B0CBE4-C282-44B6-8DAE-F66E48C2ED7A/0/OTPTFinalResourceOct20065.pdf

71. Ketelaar, M., Vermeer, A., Hart, H., van Petegem-van Beek, E., & Helders, P. J. M. (2001). Effects of a functional therapy program on motor abilities of children with cerebral palsy. *Physical Therapy, 81*, 1534–1545.

72. King, G. (2009). A relational goal-oriented model of optimal service delivery to children and families. *Physical & Occupational Therapy In Pediatrics, 29*(4), 384–408.

73. King, G., Tucker, M. A., Alambets, P., Gritzan, J., McDougall, J., Ogilvie, A., Husted, K., O'Grady, S., Brine, M., & Malloy-Miller, T. (1998). The evaluation of functional, school-based therapy services for children with special needs: A feasibility study. *Physical & Occupational Therapy in Pediatrics, 18*, 1–27.

74. King, G., Tucker, M., Baldwin, P., Lowry, K., LaPorta, J., & Martens, L. (2002). A life needs model of pediatric service delivery: services to support community participation and quality of life for children and youth with disabilities. *Physical & Occupational Therapy in Pediatrics, 22*, 53–77.

75. Lignugaris-Kraft, B., Marchand-Martella, N., & Martella, R. C. (2001). Writing better goals and short-term objectives or benchmarks. *Teaching Exceptional Children, 34*, 52–58.

76. Lindsey, D., O'Neal, J., Haas, K., & Tewey, S. M. (1980). Physical therapy services in North Carolina's schools. *Clinical Management in Physical Therapy, 4*, 40–43.

77. Lipsky, D. K. (2003). The coexistence of high standards and inclusion. *School Administrator, 60*, 32–35.

78. Magill, R. A. (2004). *Motor learning and control: Concepts and applications* (7th ed.). New York: McGraw-Hill.

79. Martin, R. (1991). *Extraordinary children, ordinary lives: Stories behind special education case law* (pp. 45–63). Champaign, IL: Research Press.

80. Maryland State Steering Committee for Occupational and Physical Therapy School-Based Programs. (2010). Occupational and physical therapy early intervention and school-based services in Maryland: A guide to practice. Retrieved from: http://www.marylandpublicschools.org/nr/rdonlyres/954dfc2e-16d9-45fa-b5c4-e713b0134fea/19473/ot_pt_fulldocument_december11_final.pdf.

81. Mastropieri, M., & Scruggs, T. (2010). *The inclusive classroom: Strategies for effective differentiated instruction* (4th ed.). Columbus, OH: Merrill.

82. Mattern-Baxter, K. (2009). Effects of partial body weight supported treadmill training on children with cerebral palsy. *Pediatric Physical Therapy, 21*, 12–22.

83. McConlogue, A., & Quinn, L. (2009). Analysis of physical therapy goals in a school-based setting: a pilot study. *Physical & Occupational Therapy in Pediatrics, 29*, 154–169.

84. McEwen, I. (Ed.). (2009). *Providing physical therapy services under Parts B & C of the Individuals with Disabilities Education Act (IDEA).* Alexandria, VA: Section on Pediatrics, American Physical Therapy Association.

85. McEwen, I. R., Arnold, S. H., Hansen, L. H., & Johnson, D. (2003). Interrater reliability and content validity of a minimal data set to measure outcomes of students receiving school-based occupational therapy and physical therapy. *Physical and Occupational Therapy in Pediatrics, 23*, 77–95.

86. McEwen, I. R., & Shelden, M. L. (1995). Pediatric therapy in the 1990s: The demise of the educational versus medical dichotomy. *Occupational and Physical Therapy in Pediatrics, 15*, 33–45.

87. Meyer, L. H., Peck, C. A., & Brown, L. (Eds.). (1991). *Critical issues in the lives of people with severe disabilities.* Baltimore: Paul H. Brookes.

88. Mockford, M., & Caulton, J. M. (2008). Systematic review of progressive strength training in children and adolescents with cerebral palsy who are ambulatory. *Pediatric Physical Therapy, 20*, 318–333.

89. Mulcahey, A. L. (1936). Detroit schools for crippled children. *Physical Therapy Review, 16*, 63–64.

90. Mutlu, A., Krosschell, K., & Spira, D. G. (2009). Treadmill training with partial body-weight support in children with cerebral palsy: a systematic review. *Developmental Medicine and Child Neurology, 51*(4), 268–275.

91. National Center for Fair and Open Testing. (2009). Joint organizational statement on No Child Left Behind (NCLB) Act.

Retrieved from: http://www.fairtest.org/joint%20statement%20civil%20rights%20grps%2010-21-04.html.

92. National Coalition on Personnel Shortages in Special Education and Related Services (NCPSSERS). (2009). About NCPSSERS. Retrieved from: http://www.specialedshortages.org/aboutus.cfm.

93. National Highway Traffic Safety Administration. (2010). Proper use of child safety restraint systems in school buses. Retrieved from: http://www.nhtsa.dot.gov/people/injury/buses/busseatbelt/.

94. Olney, S. J., & Wright, M. J. (2006). Cerebral palsy. In S. K. Campbell, D. W. Vander Linden, & R. J. Palisano, (Eds.), *Physical therapy for children* (3rd ed., pp. 625–664). St Louis, MO: Saunders Elsevier.

95. Ott, D. A. D., & Effgen, S. K. (2000). Occurrence of gross motor behaviors in integrated and segregated preschool classrooms. *Pediatric Physical Therapy, 12,* 164–172.

96. Palisano, R. J., Rosenbaum, P., Bartlett, D., & Livingston, M. H. (2008). Content validity of the expanded and revised gross motor function classification system. *Developmental Medicine & Child Neurology, 50,* 744–750.

97. Pax Lowes, L., & Effgen, S. K. (1996). The Americans with Disabilities Act of 1990: Implications for pediatric physical therapist. *Pediatric Physical Therapy, 8,* 111–116.

98. Prieto, G. M. (1992). *Effects of physical therapist instruction on the frequency and performance of teacher assisted gross motor activities for students with motor disabilities.* Unpublished master's thesis. Philadelphia: Hahnemann University.

99. Quinn, L., & Gordon, J. (2003). *Functional outcomes documentation in rehabilitation.* St Louis, MO: WB Saunders.

100. Rainforth, B. (1991). OSERS clarifies legality of related services eligibility criteria. *TASH Newsletter, 17,* 8.

101. Rainforth, B. (1997). Analysis of physical therapy practice acts: Implications for role release in educational environments. *Pediatric Physical Therapy, 9,* 54–61.

102. Rainforth, B., MacDonald, C., & York-Barr, J. (1992) *Collaborative teams for students with severe disabilities.* Baltimore, MD: Paul H. Brookes.

103. Rainforth, B., & Kugelmass, J. W. (2003). *Curriculum instruction for all learners: Blending systematic and constructivist approaches in inclusive elementary schools.* Baltimore, MD: Paul H. Brookes.

104. Rainforth, B., & York-Barr, J. (1997). *Collaborative teams for students with severe disabilities* (2nd ed.). Baltimore: Paul H. Brookes.

105. Randall, K. E., & McEwen, I. R. (2000). Writing patient-centered functional goals. *Physical Therapy, 80,* 1197–1203.

106. Rapport, M. J., & Thomas, S. B. (1993). Extended school year: Legal issues and implications. *Journal of the Association for Persons with Severe Handicaps, 18,* 16–27.

107. Ray, L. (2007). Response to intervention. *Section on Pediatrics Newsletter, 12,* 21.

108. Reynolds, M. (1962). A framework for considering some issues in special education. *Exceptional Children, 28,* 367–370.

109. Russell, D., Rosenbaum, P., Gowland, C., Hardy, S., Lane, M., Plews, N., et al. (1993). *Gross motor function measure manual (GMFM)* (2nd ed.). Hamilton, Ontario: Gross Motor Measures Group.

110. Ryndak, D. L., & Fisher, D. (2003). *The foundations of inclusive education: A compendium of articles on effective strategies to achieve inclusive education* (2nd ed.). Baltimore, MD: TASH.

111. Schenkman, M., Deutsch, J. E., & Gill-Body, K. M. (2006). An integrated framework for decision making in neurologic physical therapist practice. *Physical Therapy, 86,* 1681–1702.

112. Sever, J. W. (1938). Physical therapy in schools for crippled children. *Physical Therapy Review, 18,* 298–303.

113. Shumway-Cook, A., & Woollacott, M. H. (2007). *Motor control: Translating research into clinical practice* (3rd ed., pp. 37–38). Philadelphia: Lippincott Williams & Wilkins.

114. Smith, J., & Sylvester, L. (2009). Transition. In I. McEwen (Ed.), *Providing physical therapy services under Parts B & C of the Individuals with Disabilities Education Act (IDEA).* Alexandria, VA: Section on Pediatrics, American Physical Therapy Association.

115. Snell, M. E., & Janney, R. (2000). *Collaborative teaming.* Baltimore, MD: Paul H. Brookes.

116. Soccio, C. A. (1991). *Direct-individual versus integrated-group models of physical therapy service delivery.* Unpublished master's thesis. Philadelphia: Hahnemann University.

117. (1996). Court: Regular class not always LRE. *Special Educator, 11,* 8.

118. TASH. (2000). *TASH resolution on inclusive quality education.* Baltimore, MD: Author.

119. Trahan, J., & Malouin, F. (1999). Changes in the gross motor function measure in children with different types of cerebral palsy: An eight-month follow-up study. *Pediatric Physical Therapy, 11,* 12–17.

120. Taylor, S. J. (1988). Caught in the continuum: A critical analysis of the least restrictive environment. *Journal of the Association for Persons with Severe Handicaps, 13,* 41–53.

121. Teeters Myers, C., & Effgen, S. K. (2006). Physical therapists' participation in early childhood transitions. *Pediatric Physical Therapy, 18,* 182–189.

122. Thurman, S. K., & Widerstrom, A. H. (1990). *Infants and young children with special needs* (2nd ed.). Baltimore, MD: Paul H. Brookes.

123. U.S. Department of Education (2005). *Twenty-seventh annual report to Congress on the implementation of the Individuals with Disabilities Education Act, 2005.* Washington, DC: Author.

124. U.S. Department of Education. (2009). Civil rights discrimination. Retrieved from: http://ed.gov/policy/rights/guid/ocr/disability.html.

125. Vacha, V. B. (1933). History of the development of special schools and classes for crippled children in Chicago. *Physical Therapy Review, 13,* 21–26.

126. Valvano, J. (2004). Activity-focused motor interventions for children with neurological conditions. *Physical and Occupational Therapy in Pediatrics, 24,* 79–107.

127. Valvano, J. (2005). Neuromuscular system: the plan of care. In S. K. Effgen (Ed.), *Meeting the physical therapy needs of children* (pp. 244–245). Philadelphia: FA Davis.

128. Virginia Department of Education. (2004). *Handbook for occupational & physical therapy services in the public schools of Virginia*. Richmond, VA: Author.

129. Westcott, S. L., & Goulet, C. (2005). Neuromuscular system: Structures, functions, diagnoses, and evaluation. In S. K. Effgen (Ed.), *Meeting the physical therapy needs of children* (pp. 185–244). Philadelphia: FA Davis.

130. Wolfensberger, W. (1971). Will there always be an institution? The impact of new service models. *Mental Retardation, 9,* 31–38.

131. World Health Organization (WHO). (2009). International classification of functioning, disability and health (ICF). Retrieved from: http://www.who.int/classifications/icf/en/.

132. Zimmerman, J. M. (2009, June). *School bus transportation: what pediatric physical therapists need to know*. Baltimore, MD: American Physical Therapy Association Annual Conference.

133. Zirkel, P. (1996). Inclusion: Return of the pendulum? *Special Educator, 12*(9), 1, 5.

31

The Burn Unit

MERILYN L. MOORE, PT • LESLEY A. PALMGREN, PT, MPT • CARRIE J. YENNE-LAKER, PT, DPT, CWS

Recovery from severe burn injury is a long and difficult process. Children and their families are confronted by pain, deformity, and in some cases death. Physical therapists have an important role in the management of integumentary and musculoskeletal impairments and optimizing outcomes for physical activity and participation. This chapter describes the role of the physical therapist in the burn unit. An overview of the pathophysiology of burn injury, wound healing, medical and surgical management, and family perspectives is presented as foundation knowledge for the physical therapist to serve as a member of the burn team. Physical therapist management is described based on research, expert opinion, and practice knowledge of the authors. Despite the emotional challenges of the burn unit, therapists oftentimes form rewarding relationships with children and families that are maintained through follow-up over many years.

INCIDENCE AND ETIOLOGY

Recent data from the National Burn Repository of the American Burn Association (www.ameriburn.org/2009NBR AnnualReport.pdf), which represents a reasonable cross section of U.S. hospitals, indicate that children under the age of 5 accounted for 17% of all reported burn injury in 2009, and in this group scald injuries were the most prevalent cause. Other sources have reported that of children age 4 and under who are hospitalized for burn-related injuries, 65% have scald burns, 20% contact burns, and the remainder flame burns.[62]

The majority of scald burns in children are from hot food and liquids spilled in the kitchen or other places where food is prepared and served. Hot tap water burns, which typically occur in the bathroom, tend to be more severe and cover a larger portion of the body surface than other scald burns. Among children (14 years and younger), curling irons, room heaters, ovens and ranges, irons, gasoline, and fireworks are the most common causes of product-related burn injuries. Nearly two thirds of electric injuries in children ages 12 and under are caused by household electric cords and extension cords. Contact with the current in wall outlets causes an additional 14% of such injuries. Boys are at higher risk of burn-related death and injury than girls.

CLASSIFICATION AND SIZE ESTIMATION OF BURNS

Burn injuries occur when energy is transferred from a heat source to the body. If heat absorption exceeds heat dissipation, cellular temperature rises above the point at which cell survival is possible. Tissue damage begins at temperatures of 40°C and increases logarithmically as the temperature rises. At 45°C, denaturation of tissue proteins ensues and leads to cellular necrosis.[15] The extent of injury is related to (1) heat intensity, (2) duration of the exposure, and (3) tissue conductance. Burns are categorized into types according to the primary mechanism of injury including fire/flame, scald, contact, electrical, chemical, and radiation.

The American Burn Association has established guidelines for hospital admission criteria based on size, location, and severity of burn (www.ameriburn.org/BurnCenterReferral Criteria.pdf). People with minor burns may be treated as outpatients. Admission to a burn unit is indicated for partial-thickness burns of greater than 10% of the total body surface area; third degree burns; burns of the hands, face, eyes, ears, feet, and perineum; burns with associated injuries, including electrical, chemical, or inhalation injuries, fractures, or other trauma; burn injury in patients with preexisting medical disorders that could complicate management; prolong recovery; or affect mortality. Other considerations include burn injury in patients who will require special social, emotional, or rehabilitative intervention.

The extent of burn injury, or total body surface area (TBSA), can be estimated in several ways. One approach is referred to as the "rule of nines," which divides the body surface into areas, each representing 9% or a multiple of 9% of body surface area. This method is unreliable in children younger than 15 years of age because it underestimates burned areas of the head and neck and overestimates burned areas of the legs. Another method, the Berkow formula, recognizes that proportions of body surface area change with age. For example, the head and neck of an infant constitute 20% of the body surface compared with 9% of the adult. Some major burn centers now utilize electronic charting tools that can accurately calculate body surface area. The burned areas are "drawn" on a computer image of the body. Based on the drawing, the computer calculates the area of partial-thickness and deep burns.

In children, certain patterns of burn are indicative of abuse. A circumferential burn to an extremity with a clear line of demarcation may indicate abuse when an extremity is immersed in hot water. When a child is dipped in a hot tub of water, burns to the buttocks, feet, and perineum occur sparing backs of knees and anterior hip because the child protectively withdraws into a flexed position.

Burn Depth and Physiology of Wound Healing

Burn injuries are classified as superficial, partial, or full thickness according to the depth of tissue damage. Burn classification characteristics are depicted in Figure 31-1 and listed in Table 31-1. Skin thickness varies in different parts of the body and application of the same intensity of heat for a given period of time results in different burn depth. The skin is thickest on the back, palms of hands, and soles of feet.

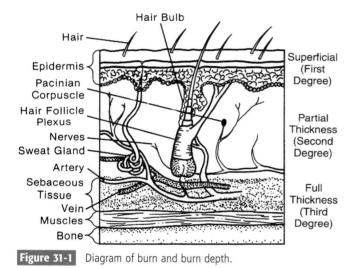

Figure 31-1   Diagram of burn and burn depth.

It is thinnest on the inner thigh and inner arm. In the young child in whom dermal papillae and appendages have yet to develop fully, deeper burns result from heat of the same intensity that produces a partial-thickness burn in the adult.

SUPERFICIAL

Superficial burns affect only the epidermal layer of skin. Because the dermis is not injured, fluid loss does not occur and the superficial area is not included in total body surface area calculations. Superficial burns heal without sequelae.

PARTIAL THICKNESS

Partial-thickness burns affect both the epidermis and dermis and heal by reepithelialization. Basal cells from the basal layer of the epidermis and the lining of dermal appendages (hair follicles, sebaceous, and sweat glands) proliferate and migrate across the burn to heal the wound. The extent of dermal involvement has important consequences for healing and scar formation, especially if the area crosses a joint or involves the face and neck. Partial-thickness burns are divided into two categories, superficial and deep.

Superficial Partial Thickness

Superficial partial-thickness burns involve primarily the papillary dermis, located just below the dermoepidermal junction, which is made mostly of loosely arranged, type III collagen fibers, or reticulin. A burn to the papillary dermis is likely to heal without scar tissue formation, as dermal appendages provide sufficient basal cells to reepithelialize the burned area within 10 to 14 days. As epithelium grows, normal pigmentation gradually returns. As the regenerated epithelium differentiates into layers, the function of the skin in maintaining and conserving core body temperature is restored.

TABLE 31-1   **Classification of Burns**

| | Superficial (First Degree) | Partial Thickness (Second Degree) | | Full Thickness (Third Degree) |
		Superficial	Deep	
Histologic depth	Epidermis only	Epidermis, papillary dermis	Epidermis, papillary, and reticular dermis	Total destruction of the epidermis and dermis; may involve deeper structures (muscle or subcutaneous fat)
Sensation	Painful	Increased sensitivity to pain and temperature	Increased sensitivity to pain and temperature	No pain or temperature sensation present
Color	Bright red	Red, pink	Mottled white to pink	White, khaki/tan, brown-black charred appearance
Surface appearance	Dry, no blisters	Blistered, weeping	Marbled pseudoeschar	Dry, waxy, or leathery
Healing	3 to 7 days, with peeling	7 to 21 days, by reepithelialization; minimal to no scarring with some pigment changes possible	21 to 35 days if no infection; may develop severe hypertrophic scarring with increased healing time	Requires skin grafting

Deep Partial Thickness

A burn extending deeper into the dermis or reticular dermis may take up to 21 days for complete healing. The reticular dermis is made mostly of broad bands of type I collagen, lying in a more structured pattern parallel to the epidermis. Burns to this depth, and beyond the base of the dermal appendages, are likely to result in replacement of normal integument with a mass of metabolically highly active scar tissue lacking the normal architecture of the dermis. Burns that do not heal within 21 days should be considered for skin grafting to minimize the potential for hypertrophic scar formation, scar contracture, and physical impairment.

FULL THICKNESS

Full-thickness burns extend beyond the dermis to the subcutaneous adipose tissue below and usually require skin grafts. Full-thickness burns may extend into fascia, muscle, or bone and are most common on digits, hands, feet, and over bony prominences, such as the iliac crest, patella, anterior tibia, and cranium, because these areas have only a thin covering of subcutaneous tissue.

THE BURN UNIT AND TEAM APPROACH TO CARE

The burn unit is much like any other intensive care unit, but it also has unique characteristics. The sights and smells characteristic of burn injury make for obvious differences from other emergency care settings. Patients in burn centers often have long hospital stays, resulting in intense and prolonged patient-staff interactions. The need for compassion, empathy, guidance, and support is essential.

A multidisciplinary team approach to burn care is fundamental in achieving successful outcomes. The team typically consists of a burn center director, staff physicians, nurse manager, nurses, physical therapists, occupational therapists, speech pathologists, pharmacists, nutritionists, social workers, psychiatrists or psychologists, respiratory therapists, and child life specialists or recreation therapists. Other team members may include residents, fellows, physician extenders, research assistants and when available, schoolteachers, chaplains, orthotists, and prosthetists. Discussions at burn team rounds not only lead to improved patient care but also provide an opportunity for members to gain insight from the experiences of other team members caring for the same child. Daily pressures the team must face include disfigurement, pain, dealing with emergency situations, and confronting death.

MEDICAL MANAGEMENT OF BURNS

When a child is admitted to a burn care facility, an estimate of the burn depth, percentage of total body surface area involvement,[43] and the child's overall condition is made. These decisions determine the need for immediate lifesaving measures, such as endotracheal intubation, ventilatory support, and fluid resuscitation. Thermal destruction of the skin initiates a chain of physiologic changes in the wound, as well as severe multiple systemic responses in almost all organ systems. Damage to the integument places the body at risk for infection, impairs body temperature regulation, and allows body fluid loss resulting in hypovolemia.

Shock as a result of hypovolemia is a critical component of the emergent phase of burn care. The goal is to promptly restore vascular volume to preserve tissue perfusion and minimize tissue ischemia.[43] Intravenous access is achieved, a urinary catheter is placed, and fluid resuscitation is begun. Until capillary leak decreases, intravenous fluid resuscitation is necessary to maintain circulation and perfusion of vital organs.

Loss of capillary integrity is a pathophysiologic feature of burn injury that leads to edema formation. This results in the outpouring of protein-rich intravascular fluid into the interstitium. This process occurs in areas of partial-thickness burns and areas adjacent to full-thickness burns. As the patient voluntarily limits movement because of pain and as a result of direct damage to the lymphatic system, edema accumulates and persists in tissue spaces around tendons, joints, and ligaments. If motion is not restored and edema reduced, new collagen fibers form in this protein-rich fluid and may organize into adhesions.

Escharotomy, incision through full-thickness burned skin, may be necessary to relieve the pressure caused by fluid resuscitation and progressive edema in the extremities and trunk following circumferential burns. Escharotomy is usually performed when tissue pressure exceeds 40 mm Hg. As the burned tissue opens along the incision, tissue tension is relieved, and effective circulation is restored. In patients with deep burns or high-voltage electrical injury involving muscle, fasciotomy may be necessary to relieve elevated pressure in fascial compartments unrelieved by simple escharotomy.

As the child's condition is stabilized, burn wounds are assessed for the purpose of developing a wound closure plan. Evaluation of burn wound depth in children is often difficult; dermal papillae and appendages may not be fully developed, thus the extent of damage may not be determined for several days. Partial-thickness burns will heal with moist dressings. Healing of full-thickness burns must be accomplished with autogenous split-thickness skin grafts.

Aggressive and thorough wound care is important to allow reepithelialization in partial-thickness burns and to define burned areas that may require surgical intervention. Three basic cleansing techniques include (1) local care of a specific area, using water and cleansing agents at bedside or any convenient location; (2) spray hydrotherapy or nonsubmersion, using a shower head to allow the water to run over burn wounds in a tub or shower; and (3) submersion of the child or burned extremity in a tub or tank of water. The choice depends on the extent and location of the burn and the medical condition of the child.

Most burn wound protocols call for daily dressing changes. Various topical antimicrobial creams and solutions are used to promote healing and prevent infection. Different agents may be used concurrently, on different burned areas, or sequentially as the wound and its bacterial flora change. Primary antimicrobial dressings are held in place with secondary gauze dressings (type used is need specific). Gauze should be wrapped so burned surfaces do not touch (e.g., fingers and toes should be wrapped separately, burned ears should not touch the burned head). Such attention to detail helps prevent webbing caused by open surfaces healing together. Wrapping digits individually facilitates active and functional movements.

SURGICAL MANAGEMENT OF BURNS

Excision of full-thickness burned tissue may be initiated a few days after the burn or as soon as the child's circulatory system is stable. Early surgical excision is advantageous in reducing complications, such as burn wound sepsis, and decreasing hospital length of stay. Depending on the depth, location, and total body surface area involvement, excised areas may be immediately autografted or allowed delayed autografting.

AUTOGRAFTING

Autografting or harvesting of one's own skin is required to achieve wound closure for full-thickness burns. Skin grafts may be harvested from virtually any area of the body except the face and hands. Basal cells from the edges of the donor site as well as dermal appendages will reepithelialize the donor site. The scalp is a superior donor site. It has excellent blood supply with deep, closely spaced hair follicles that allow reepithelialization in 4 to 5 days. Regrowth of scalp hair hides the donor site. Donor sites of the torso and extremities reepithelialize in approximately 10 to 14 days.

Split-thickness skin grafts (STSG) are used almost exclusively for full-thickness burn wound coverage. The skin is harvested at a partial thickness of depth, leaving sufficient dermal appendages for reepithelialization. In the majority of instances, burns of the hands, face, and neck take precedence for skin grafting. To produce the best cosmetic outcome for these areas, the donor skin is placed intact as a sheet graft. However, in patients with burns covering a high percentage of total body surface area and limited donor skin, consideration must be given to covering large areas. Donor skin in these situations is often meshed, cutting small holes in the donor skin to allow for expansion over greater body surface area.

Full-thickness skin grafts (FTSG) and flaps are occasionally used in repair of deep burn wounds (e.g., with tendon,

bone, muscle involvement) but are primarily used later in reconstructive procedures. The full thickness of the skin including subcutaneous tissue is excised and used for wound coverage. The full-thickness donor site is typically closed primarily or occasionally with a partial-thickness graft.

Skin grafts must be undisturbed in order to adhere to the excised wound bed. Immobilization is usually accomplished by a splint or bulky dressing secured in place through a variety of methods. Serum fibrin allows for initial adherence of a skin graft. Revascularization of blood vessels between the wound bed and the graft establishes a nutritive blood flow in about 48 hours. Fibroblasts migrate into the wound and begin collagen deposition. In most cases, sufficient collagen deposition occurs between the wound bed and the graft to permit active range of motion (ROM) after the fifth day post operatively.

Early excision of the burn wound has enabled survival of patients with burns up to 98% of total body surface area but presents the problem of wound closure.[35] Temporary methods of wound closure include use of cadaveric skin and biologic dressings, which buy time between autograft procedures. Autograft substitutes such as engineered tissue equivalents and cultured epithelial cells are often necessary for permanent wound closure in a large TBSA burn.

Biologic dressings (Table 31-2) consist of viable or once-viable tissues that are used to temporarily cover wounds in place of either conventional dressings or leaving the wound exposed. Biologic dressings are intended to reduce the risk of wound infection, provide temporary wound closure, and decrease fluid loss through the open wound. They are also effectively used to protect excised burns covered by widely meshed skin graft.

Growth factor technology and innovative combination wound dressings have been introduced, offering improved wound healing, function, and cosmetic result. Engineered tissue equivalents have changed the approach to wound coverage,[37] allowing thinner donor harvesting and multiple reharvesting of the same donor site. Alternative wound closure options are summarized in Table 31-2. Clinical staff must have a substantial base of knowledge and a familiarity with products that are unique to burn care.

IMPAIRMENTS OF BODY FUNCTIONS AND STRUCTURES

BURN SCAR

Scar formation is a natural sequela in the healing process of deep partial-thickness burns and skin grafts. Healing of deep dermal wounds results in the replacement of normal dermis with a mass of metabolically highly active tissues lacking the normal architecture of the skin.[34] Although it cannot be prevented, it can be treated to minimize deleterious effects on function and cosmesis. Children are more susceptible to hypertrophic scarring than adults.[81] It has been long accepted

TABLE 31-2   **Alternative Wound Closure Options and Topical Agents**

Type	Description	Advantages/Indications
TEMPORARY SKIN SUBSTITUTE	Biologic or biosynthetic products provide temporary wound coverage	Used for delayed wound closure
Allograft	Human cadaveric skin	Tests wound bed for autograft preparedness; covers and protects healing of interstices over widely meshed autograft
Xenograft	Pig skin	Limited use as biologic dressing over partial-thickness burns, autoimmune skin disorders; reduces pain, removed as epithelialization occurs
INTEGRA Dermal Regeneration Template (Integra LifeSciences Corporation, Plainsboro, NJ)	Dermal matrix processed from cadaver allograft	Collagen and glycosaminoglycans (GAGs) provide matrix for development of neodermis; provides wound coverage after excision of burn; silicone layer is removed and replaced with thin autograft
AlloDerm (LifeCell Corp, Branchburg, NJ)	Dermal matrix processed from cadaver allograft	Serves as a scaffold for normal tissue regeneration; requires concomitant placement of autograft or secondary healing
Biobrane (Smith & Nephew, London, UK)	Nylon fabric partially imbedded into silicone film	Forms a protective barrier for partial-thickness burns and autoimmune skin disorders; removed as epithelialization occurs; reduces pain and trauma of regular dressing change
ANTIMICROBIAL DRESSINGS	Prevent infection in burn wounds	
Acticoat (Smith & Nephew, London, UK)	Two sheets of polyethylene mesh coated with ionic silver and a rayon/polyester core	Controls bioburden of healing donor sites and partial-thickness burns; removed as epithelialization occurs
Mepilex Ag (Molnlycke Health Care World Wide)	Silver foam dressing with soft silicone backing	Absorbs wound exudate, controls bioburden of moist wound environment; silicone backing reduces pain and trauma of regular dressing change
Aquacel Ag (Convatec, Skillman, NJ)	Silver hydrofiber dressing	Controls bioburden of healing donor sites and partial-thickness burns; removed as epithelialization occurs
Xeroform (Kendall Co., Mansfield, MA)	3% bismuth tribromophenate in petrolatum blend on fine-mesh gauze	Nonadherent, nonabsorbent dressing for partial-thickness burns, healing meshed autograft
ANTIMICROBIAL TOPICALS	Prevent or treat infection in burn wounds	Provide moist wound healing environment
Silver sulfadiazine (Silvadene; Thermazene, Kendall, Mansfield, MA)	Sulfa-based topical antibacterial cream	Common antibacterial used for partial and full-thickness burn; provides moist wound environment for autolytic debridement of necrotic burned tissue
Mafenide Acetate (Sulfamylon, UDL Laboratories, Rockford, IL)	Broad spectrum antibacterial; solution and cream form	Commonly used prophylactically in solution form as a "wet" dressing for meshed autograft
Bacitracin zinc	Petroleum-based antibacterial ointment	Commonly used with xeroform or petroleum gauze to provide increased antimicrobial coverage to healing wounds
Double antibiotic	Bacitracin zinc and polymyxin B in petroleum-based ointment	Effective against gram-positive and negative bacteria
Triple antibiotic (Neosporin)	With neomycin and polymyxin B in petroleum-based ointment	Effective against gram-positive and negative bacteria
Mupirocin (Bactroban, GlaxoSmithKline, Brentford, UK)	Ointment effective against gram-positive bacteria	Effective against staphylococcus aureus
NONADHERENT DRESSINGS		
Petroleum gauze Adaptic (Johnson & Johnson, Arlington, TX), Aquaphor gauze (Smith & Nephew Healthcare Limited, UK)	Petroleum-impregnated gauze	Protects healing burns, grafts, and donor sites from desiccation and mechanical trauma; maintains moist wound environment
Polyurethane dressings OpSite, Tegaderm	Thin polyurethane membrane coated with acrylic adhesive	Permeable to water vapor and oxygen, impermeable to microorganisms; used in minimally exudative superficial wounds; often used as dressing for small donor sites

that the darker a patient's skin, the more predisposed that patient is to hypertrophic scarring.

Several different processes appear to be at work in the healing skin graft. These processes include the following: mass production of large amounts of highly disorganized collagen, replacement of the normal dermal elastic ground substance with inelastic chondroitin sulfate A, involuntary contraction of myofibroblasts, and inflammatory response with increased vascularity and localized lymphedema.

The bonds between collagen and firm inelastic ground substance, coupled with the simultaneous contraction of the myofibroblasts, contribute to the raised appearance of the hypertrophic scar. In addition, voluntary contraction of underlying skeletal muscle reinforces the compaction of the collagen. The position of comfort for most patients is that of flexion of the affected joint. As wound contraction occurs, collagen deposition occurs with the joint in a flexed position. If a flexed joint position is maintained, contracture will occur.

The intensity and duration of the vascular response provides a visible clue to the likelihood of hypertrophic scarring and contracture formation.[79] Hyperemia of scar is indicative of ongoing change within the closed wound. As long as increased blood flow persists, patients are at risk for hypertrophic scarring and contracture. The active phase of scar maturation gradually subsides and is usually complete in 1.5 to 2 years after the burn. The result is a scar that is pale, soft, and pliable.

Use of pressure in the form of tubular stockings or custom pressure garments has been shown to mechanically flatten scar tissue during the scar maturation phase of wound healing. Linares et al. reviewed research on pressure therapy and concluded that 15 mm Hg pressure is necessary for efficacy.[45] Van den Kerckhove demonstrated that more pressure results in a greater flattening effect.[84] Custom therapeutic garments average 24 to 28 mm Hg pressure.[76]

Additional changes in body structure occur as a result of skin grafting. When the split-thickness skin graft is transplanted to the area of full-thickness burn, no hair follicles, sebaceous glands, or sweat glands are included. Dermal appendages will not redevelop. Without oil glands, grafted areas do not produce oil resulting in excessively dry skin. The absence of sweat glands inhibits the ability to dissipate the core body temperature when it is too high. Children who require extensive skin grafting and their families must be cautioned about this problem and warned to avoid environments with high heat and humidity.

Regeneration of nerve endings into the burned areas likely accounts for patients' frequent reports of itching and abnormal or odd sensations in their burn wounds. As the nerve endings grow through the areas of scar tissue, they frequently meet an obstruction that may cause an area of hypersensitivity. Hypersensitivity may also be the result of small neuromas occurring in scattered areas throughout the burned area.

MUSCULOSKELETAL IMPAIRMENTS

Musculoskeletal impairments, including peripheral nerve injury, exposed tendons and joints, heterotopic bone formation, and amputation, are associated with the burn injury, impacting the acute phase of burn rehabilitation. Peripheral nerve damage, occurring in as many as 30% of patients,[26] results from (1) electrical injury by passage of current through the nerve, (2) edema with elevated tissue pressure, (3) metabolic abnormalities and nutritional deficiencies, and (4) localized nerve compression or stretch injury from improper dressings or positioning. The superficial location of the extensor tendons, intrinsic muscles, and joints, as well as the hand's specialized sensory receptors, make management of burns of the hand particularly challenging. Knowing the location and depth of the burn injury to the hand is important. For example, at 4 weeks after burn, the wounds may be closed, but the fact that the terminal extensor tendon was damaged and weakened will not be apparent. If a therapist were to initiate a vigorous splinting or exercise program to regain full distal interphalangeal (DIP) flexion without regard to the status of the tendon, a rupture or attenuation of the terminal extensor tendon might occur.

Heterotopic ossification (HO), abnormal formation of true bone within extraskeletal soft tissues, is a disabling complication that limits ROM in affected joints. The most common site associated with burn injury is the elbow.[30] Physical therapy intervention can be performed in the presence of HO in a pain-free range of motion. In severe cases when excision is indicated, heterotopic ossification usually does not re-form after removal, allowing restoration of functional and even full ROM.[30] The physical therapy goal is remobilization of the joint.

Burn to depth of bone is possible in severe thermal injuries. Necrosis of the periosteum and cortex can occur, especially in superficially located bone such as the skull, fingers, tibia, and olecranon process. Exposed bone presents a challenge for wound closure, as a bed of healthy tissue is needed for successful grafting. Patients with full-thickness burns requiring limb amputation present a number of unique problems,[90] including intolerance of the stump to pressure because of remaining open wounds and fragility of newly healed skin grafts. Following amputation, patients are at risk for developing a joint contracture, especially when there are adjacent burns and skin grafts because of the contractile process of wound healing and scar maturation. Despite the potential for complications, it appears that most patients with burns who require limb amputation can achieve successful prosthetic use.[91]

PRESSURE GARMENTS AND INSERTS

Hypertrophic scarring remains a major problem for the recovering patient. Thin elastic self-adherent wraps, elastic bandages, or custom-fit elastic garments are the mainstay of controlled pressure. See Figure 31-2, *A* and *B*. Inserts of rubber, foam, or gel have been used to improve the response to pressure, particularly over concave surfaces. In the early 1970s, the use of pressure for the treatment of hypertrophic scars, keloids, and severe contractures became a standard of burn care. As previously stated, Linares et al. concluded that 15-mmHg pressure is necessary for efficacy.[45] Although the exact mechanism of action is unknown, pressure appears clinically to enhance scar resolution. A recent meta-analysis demonstrated that pressure garment therapy improved scar height but not global scar score, pliability, vascularity, or pigmentation.[3]

Based on the guidelines on the characteristics of burn treatment, the following features can help the therapist select methods of pressure: (1) healing time of the burn, (2) size of the unhealed areas, (3) fragility or condition of the healed skin, (4) location of the burn, and (5) treatment cost. All patients whose burns require 14 to 21 days to heal or who have skin grafts should have prophylactic pressure therapy. Pressure should be applied as early as possible. The type of pressure, however, depends on the fragility of the newly healed skin and remaining open areas. Pressure therapy can be initiated during the acute phase of recovery using elastic bandages over bulky dressings, and progressing to Tubi-Grip when only thin dressings are required. Custom garments can be applied once the burn is 90% healed. This progression is necessary because new epithelium and grafts are susceptible to shearing. Lower extremity burns may require pressure not only to minimize scarring but also to minimize persistent edema and discoloration. Custom pressure garments are expensive, so anticipated patient compliance should be carefully considered.

Signs that the pressure program has been successful can be seen as early as 24 to 48 hours after the initial application. Immediately after the removal of the garment, indicators of effectiveness include blanching of scar tissue, flattening of the scar, increased softness, and decreased edema. If any of these desirable effects are not observed, the therapist should evaluate garment (1) fit (if the patient has gained or lost more than 10 pounds, this may be enough to decrease the pressure garment's effectiveness) and (2) condition (the average life of custom pressure garments is 3 months). If the garment loses its stretch and does not cause blanching of the scar, it has lost its effectiveness; a new garment must be made. The amount of pressure being provided by the garment can be measured easily and accurately.[49] Trouble spots receiving too much or too little pressure should be located and altered.

Correct application of pressure garments or devices is crucial for effective scar control. External pressure support is prescribed to be worn 23 hours a day until the remodeling phase of healing is complete. Spurr and Shakespeare list the difficulties that arise with a pressure garment program.[78] Pressure garments may need to be

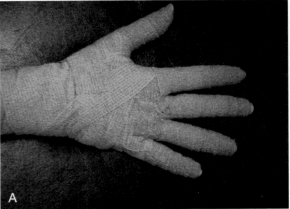

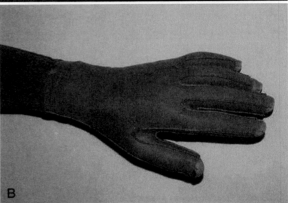

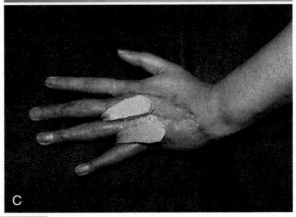

Figure 31-2 Compression can facilitate edema reduction and scar alignment. **A,** Self-adherent elastic wraps can be applied over dressings, providing early compression to reduce edema. **B,** Custom-fit gloves provide long-term protection, support, and scar alignment. Note the slanted web-space design in this glove, included for specific compression of the dorsal web scars. **C,** Further shaping and scar control is obtained with foam or inserts of other materials placed under the glove, in this case the third and fourth web spaces. (From Moore, M. L., Dewey, W. S., & Richard, R. L. [2009]. Rehabilitation of the burned hand. *Hand Clinics, 25,* 529–541.)

worn for up to 2 years. They are inconvenient for patients, may be uncomfortable, and are relatively expensive. There is no guarantee that the child and parents will adhere to recommendations.

As scar tissue approaches maturity, hyperemia fades and the scar flattens and becomes more pliable and soft. When these qualities persist for several weeks after removal of the pressure garments, the scar tissue is mature, and the garments and inserts may then be discontinued.

HAND GARMENTS

Small hands are a challenge to measure and fit properly with pressure garments. For infants, better pressure on the hand may be achieved through the use of self-adherent elastic wrap. Narrow strips of foam padding, worn between the fingers under compression gloves, work well to preserve web spaces and do not macerate the skin or interfere with hand function. If a child's hand is burned only in the palm and does not involve the web spaces, a compression glove alone is contraindicated—gloves tend to pull the thumb into adduction and fold the palm. Instead, a custom molded insert of silicone putty attached to a palmar extension splint is recommended.[54]

FACE GARMENTS

The face is particularly difficult to fit with pressure garments and facemasks. Garments and face masks require frequent monitoring and modification. Caution and close monitoring of face masks is essential, particularly when used in the young growing child. Two studies suggest serious complications in children with head and neck burns. Fricke and colleagues demonstrated changes in growth direction of the mandible and maxilla after consistent application of the total face mask.[29] In addition, Chester and associates claim that the most common cause of obstructive sleep apnea is excessive pressure on the mandible by compression garments, particularly chin straps.[18]

INSERTS

When isolated areas of hypertrophy remain, additional pressure may be required. Areas where this commonly occurs include the sternum, face, volar aspect of the hand, angle of the mandible, web spaces, and across the flexor surface of the joint. To exert sufficient pressure on these areas, custom garments can be supplemented by inserts (see Figure 31-2, C). Characteristics to be considered in choosing the composition of the insert include its texture, flexibility, compressibility, and ability to conform. When used for pressure, the insert must be worn for the same amount of time as the pressure garment (23 hours per day) to be effective.

SILICONE GEL SHEETING

Silicone gel sheeting has been used for treatment of immature burn scars since it was introduced by Perkins and colleagues in 1982.[44] Various silicone sheets, gels, tapes, foam, and adhesive contact products have been introduced to burn scar management, with therapists and other clinicians establishing their personal preferences for products.[1,14,23,47,59,63] Although the mechanism of silicon-based products in the treatment of hypertrophic scar management has not been completely determined, some of the mechanisms of action suggested include an increase in skin temperature, development of a static electric field, increased stratum corneum hydration, and several cellular changes.[4] Silicone gel needs to be in place for at least 12 hours a day for 3 to 6 months.[56]

SCAR ASSESSMENT

The subjective assessment of scar appearance is a widely used method to assess efficacy of pressure devices and scar management treatments. A numeric scar-rating scale has been developed and has proved to be a useful tool for the evaluation of scar surface, thickness, border height, and color differences between a scar and the adjacent normal skin.[92]

PHYSICAL THERAPIST EXAMINATION

The physical therapist's initial examination and evaluation are intended to determine the child's status, identify rehabilitation needs, and anticipate potential problems. Recommendations for examination are presented in Tables 31-3 and 31-4. The expected clinical course and approximate length of hospital stay should be estimated to anticipate potential emotional, physiologic, and rehabilitation difficulties. Identifying the rehabilitation needs of the child requires thorough evaluation of examination findings, as well as an understanding of the implications of different types of burns and their locations. For children with burns that will heal in less than 21 days and don't need grafting, the therapist can anticipate meeting goals for acute care and following up in clinic as needed. For deeper burns, whether or not the area is skin grafted, the child is likely to require outpatient physical therapy to ensure skin healing with minimal scarring and deformity. The child with a deep burn will require periodic team follow-up at the burn center in addition to outpatient physical therapy.

The American Burn Association[2] has published patient outcomes for the different phases of recovery.[80] As part of this document, clinical indicators were established to assist service providers in evaluating patient progress in meeting desired outcomes.

TABLE 31-3 Physical Therapy Examination for Acute Burn Rehabilitation

HISTORY

Demographic Information

Prior level of function (e.g., meeting developmental milestones, physical and scholastic achievement in school-aged children)

Preexisting relevant medical conditions

Caregivers and resources available to assist in recovery

Circumstances of Injury[12a]

Date of injury

Type of burn (e.g., flame, scald, inhalation)

Concomitant injury

Documentation of Burn Wound

Location

Depth of burn (e.g., partial thickness, full thickness)

Extent of burn, percentage TBSA

Exposed anatomic structures (e.g., extensor tendons of dorsal hand)

Wound characteristics (e.g., blisters, moist, pink, dry, leathery)

Dressings

Documentation of Background and Procedural Pain

Oucher[6]

Faces scale[17]

Face, legs, activity, cry, and consolability (FLACC)[51,87]

Physical Examination

Edema and limb circumference[23a]

Joint range of motion: Active and passive (caution with passive range when exposed tendons)

Strength

Mobility and ambulation

Positioning and splinting needs

Respiratory status

Neurologic and psychologic status, including muscle tone, sensation, orientation, behavior, adjustment to injury

TABLE 31-4 Physical Therapy Examination for Intermediate and Long-Term Burn Rehabilitation

HISTORY

Demographic Information

Current level of function (e.g., return to school, age-appropriate play)

Prior level of function (e.g., developmental level, physical and scholastic achievement in school aged children)

Preexisting relevant medical conditions

Caregivers and resources available to assist in recovery

Circumstances of Injury

Date of injury

Date of grafting

Type of graft (split versus full thickness; sheet versus mesh)

Observation of Burn Injury

Scar quality (e.g., evidence of hypertrophic scar, Vancouver Scar Scale)

Signs of infection

DOCUMENTATION OF BACKGROUND AND PROCEDURAL PAIN

Oucher[6]

Faces scale[17]

Face, legs, activity, cry, and consolability (FLACC)[51,87]

Physical Examination

Active and passive range of motion

Strength

Mobility and ambulation

Splinting and positioning device use

Pressure garment use

PHYSICAL THERAPIST INTERVENTION

Once the examination and evaluation are complete, an individualized plan of care is established in collaboration with the child, family, and other members of the burn care team. The plan of care includes the goals, outcomes, and procedural interventions, with the primary focus on prevention of deformities and maximizing cosmesis. There has not been an evidence-based standard of care established for many therapeutic interventions. Positioning, splinting, and ROM exercises are the most frequently used therapeutic interventions with which to combat contractile scar forces. According to the Burn Rehabilitation Summit, there is wide variety among institutions regarding the evaluation and treatment of children with burns.[66] Interventions vary with the stages of wound recovery. Some examples of intervention options by body part are listed in Table 31-5. Recent evidence when available is cited for the listed interventions. Other treatment options are offered anecdotally, based on the combined experience of the authors.

The deforming effects of burn scar contractures can be decreased by use of the following procedural interventions: proper patient positioning and use of splints, ROM and graded resistive exercises, early walking, and scar management techniques. Additionally the plan of care should include play activities and training in functional tasks with a goal of normal and age-appropriate movement and ultimately resuming physical activities and social participation.

PAIN MANAGEMENT

Pain management is an important part of burn care and input by team members, parents, and caregivers as well as by

TABLE 31-5 **Options for Physical Therapy Intervention**

Involved Area	Exercise	Positioning	Splinting	Pressure
Face, head	Massage, facial exercises, eye blinking, mouth opening, chewing, Therabite	No pillow, elevate head of bed	Nasal splints	Custom elastomer mask, custom fabric hood, chin strap, clear mask with silicone, silicone patches or tape
Neck[76a]	Neck ROM, shoulder wedge	No pillow, split mattress	Neck conformer, soft collar, Watusi[38a]	Neck conformer, elastomer insert, silicone wrap
Axilla	Shoulder ROM, abduction/forward flexion exercises, overhead pulleys, finger ladder, wand exercises, prone with upper extremities overhead, shoulder continuous passive motion	Arm trough, papoose, sheepskin slings, bedside table with pillows	Axillary conformer	Padded figure-of-eight wrap, clavicle strap, custom vest, inserts
Elbow	Wall weights, barbells, pronation exerciser	Extension, supination	Anterior conformer, cast	Tubigrip, custom sleeve, silicone sleeve
Wrist, hand[74b]	Hand exercises, gripping devices, hand continuous passive motion (CPM) device	Elevation above heart, flexion wrap	Wrist cock-up splint, burn hand splint, flexion splint, pan extension splint[74a]	Coban, Isotoner gloves, custom gloves, web spacers, silicone inserts
Trunk, buttock, hip	Ambulation, trunk stretches, prone lying	Proning, no pillow under knees, specialty beds	T-shirt splint, hip spica splint, bivalved cast	Custom pantyhose, bicycle shorts, breastplate, silicone patches
Knee	Ambulation, exercise bike, prone lying with feet over end of mat, knee CPM, stairs	No pillow under knees, prevent frog-lying	Knee conformer, knee immobilizer	Tubigrip, custom socks, leggings
Ankle, foot	Ambulation, ankle circles, toe stretches, stairs, tilt table, NuStep, incline treadmill walking	Foam heel protectors	Posterior foot splint, derotational splint, Unna boot, toe flexion splint, burn shoe, cast	Tubigrip, custom socks, toe web spacers, dorsal silicone inserts

the child can help to relieve the pain and distress associated with burn injury. Each child has a particular pain response and how pain is managed early can have lasting effects for future care. The use of self-report tools such as Oucher[6] or Faces Scale[17] and behavioral tools such as Face, Legs, Activity, Cry & Consolability (FLACC)[50,87] or C (COMFORT) score[85] can aid in pain management. Background pain and procedural pain are the two types of pain associated with burn injury. Background pain is described as dull, throbbing, and of a relatively low intensity, and it is managed with long-acting narcotics. Procedural pain occurs when something is done to the child such as wound cleansing, dressing changes, or range of motion. It is described as stabbing and severe. Pharmacologic interventions include scheduled and preprocedural medications such as opioids, nonsteroidal anti-inflammatory drugs (NSAIDS), benzodiazepines, and other facility specific drugs. Virtual reality is also a promising adjunct to pharmacologic management.[55]

Various nonpharmacologic techniques have been developed and tested to promote the compliance of children during wound care.[82] These include educating the child

about the procedure, enhancing child predictability and control, distraction, promotion of self-cleansing and debridement, parent participation, and hypnosis. Anecdotally, these techniques have been modestly effective in the reduction of pain behavior and in increasing cooperation of children. Complete reduction of distress is often not possible; therefore, escape behavior and avoidance conditioning are expected. Escape behavior includes yelling, whining, thrashing, questioning, swearing, and pleading behaviors that are associated with pain. Avoidant behaviors that take place before wound care or therapy can also take many forms, usually some type of procrastination, such as distracting staff, suddenly becoming involved in unrelated activities, or spontaneous complaints of new ailments. The importance of pain management cannot be overemphasized. Any safe and effective method should be used.

POSITIONING

Objectives of positioning include reducing edema, protecting weakened or exposed structures, and maintaining or increasing ROM. Proper positioning can help to reduce general edema incurred during the resuscitation phase by utilizing gravity when elevating and placing the extremities in extension. This is particularly important for the hands and feet, which are especially susceptible to dependent edema and loss of ROM. Contractures associated with dorsal hand burns are metacarpophalangeal (MCP) extension and proximal interphalangeal (PIP) and distal interphalangeal (DIP) flexion, known as the claw hand deformity. Propping and other positioning can aid in ROM and counteract contracture by placing the burned area in a lengthened position, thus maintaining proper flexibility of connective tissue and skin. Positioning is generally achieved with easily available hospital materials such as pillows, bath blankets, towels, and foam wedges (Figure 31-3, A and B). Specialty beds and mattresses can also facilitate optimal positioning. Table 31-6 lists optimal positioning by body part.

SPLINTING

The aims of splinting include graft immobilization, joint protection, contractures prevention, scar elongation and compression, and soft tissue lengthening. Type of splint will vary based on location and depth of burn, stage of recovery, and individual needs of the child. Types of splinting include static splints, dynamic splints, serial casting, or fixators. Factors to consider in a splint include construction, fit, application, and adjustability. A pliable, lightweight, low-heat thermoplastic material is desirable. Bulky dressings should be minimized because they interfere with the fit of the splint and compromise alignment. Splints should be checked at least once daily and necessary adjustments made. Pain, numbness, tingling, inflammation, or maceration of tissue indicate a poor-fitting or improperly applied splint, which can cause pressure necrosis of burned and unburned areas. Immediate adjustment is mandatory to prevent further damage. Examples of splints used for burns are illustrated in Figure 31-3, C through E.

Although the basic principles of splinting and scar contracture alignment must be adhered to for splints to be effective, therapists can be creative with splint design. Recent publications illustrate modified and unusual designs for the neck,[28,75] axilla,[48] and hand.[86]

Acute Phase

Splinting is used in the acute phase to protect joints, tendons, or ligaments. Protective splints put exposed tendons or ligaments on slack until wound closure or integrity of the structure is restored. During the wound-healing phase, splints may be used to prevent contracture and when grafted splints act to immobilize the area to prevent graft interruption. New grafts or biologic dressings are protected by immobilizing adjacent joints and applying gentle, direct pressure to the graft. Splints are typically kept in place at all times until the graft is deemed stable and movement or stretching will be

tolerated, usually 5 to 7 days postoperatively. Most young children are able to continue moving and playing while the splint immobilizes the specific joint involved, as seen in the video clip on the Evolve website.

Intermediate Phase

Children are typically unable to maintain optimal positioning independently after the graft is healed. A splint is the most effective method for optimal positioning during unsupervised periods and during sleep, when positions that contribute to deformity are assumed. If the child achieves full ROM during play activities, the child may only need to wear the splint during naps and at night. If the therapist observes the child has limitations in range of motion during play activities or the child uses compensatory strategies, duration of splint wear should be increased. When voluntary movement is impaired, as in the presence of peripheral neuropathies, a splint must be worn continuously (except during physical therapy and wound care) to avoid joint contracture.

Long-Term Use

Children may continue with a splint-wearing schedule long after wound closure to counteract the detrimental effects of skin contracture and scar formation. Young children are often not strong enough to overcome the resistance of contracting scar. Splints are also used to realign scar tissue or to stretch contracted skin. In these instances, they may be applied at all times to provide a constant stretch or apply pressure. Silicone may be added to splints to attempt to remodel scar as well.

SERIAL CASTING

Serial casting may be an effective alternative to splinting when proper splint alignment cannot be maintained or when the child's adherence to the wearing schedule is unreliable.[76] The goal in serial casting is gradual realignment of the collagen in a parallel and lengthened state by constant circumferential pressure from the cast. When casts are applied well and padded appropriately, there is little risk of pressure areas, because the casts are conforming and do not migrate position. Case studies reported good success with biweekly cast changes until normal ROM is achieved.[40] Procedural interventions may then be continued such as weight-bearing activity in walking for plantar flexion contractures, ROM exercises, and splinting.[40,72] Serial casting has also been shown to be effective in increasing ROM of the burned hand.[33] The fabrication and use of removable digit casts to improve ROM at the proximal interphalangeal joint have also been described.[83]

FIXATORS

External fixators have been introduced in burn management, especially in the case of severe ankle and foot deformities.[39]

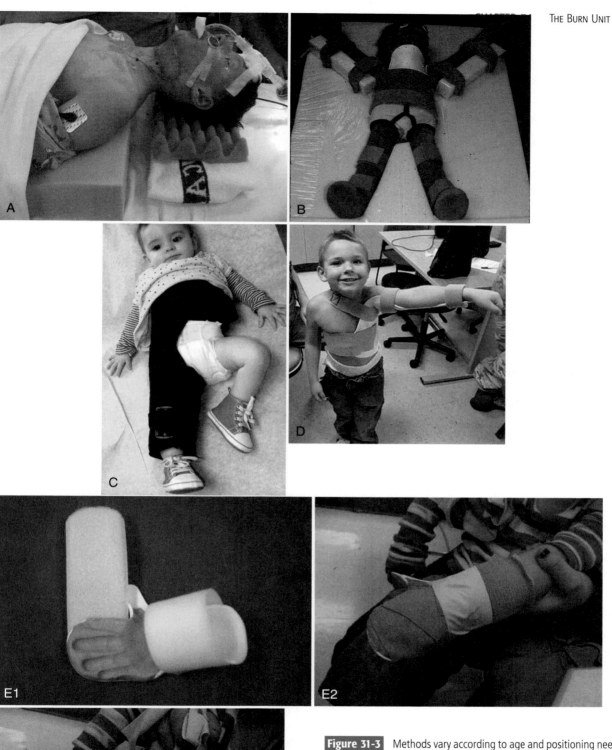

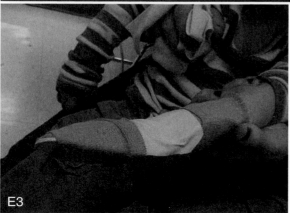

Figure 31-3 Methods vary according to age and positioning needs of the patient. **A,** Teenager positioned in neck extension with foam wedge and egg crate foam pillow. **B,** Bernie the burn puppet demonstrates positioning in a foam papoose, which is used for a very young or heavily sedated child. **C,** Hip extension splint on a baby was fabricated from an adult prefabricated knee immobilizer. **D,** Custom-molded axillary conformer provides supportive positioning of the shoulder and upper extremity, while enabling the child to be ambulatory and to participate in play activities. **E1-E3,** Pan extension splint; elastomer putty insert can be custom molded and attached to the splint to apply pressure and full elongation within it. Optimal position in the splint places the wrist and digits in extension and the thumb in radial abduction. Note the need for overwrapping to keep the splint in place in a young child. (**E,** From Moore, M. L., Dewey, W. S., & Richard, R. L. [2009]. Rehabilitation of the burned hand. *Hand Clinics, 25,* 529–541.)

TABLE 31-6 **Recommendations for Positioning of Burned Areas**

Body Area	Contracture Predisposition	Preventive Positioning
Neck	Flexion	Extension Hyperextension
Anterior axilla	Shoulder adduction	Shoulder abduction
Posterior axilla	Shoulder extension	Shoulder flexion
Antecubital space	Elbow flexion	Elbow extension
Forearm	Pronation	Supination
Wrist	Flexion	Extension
Dorsal hand/ fingers	MCP hyperextension	MCP flexion
	IP flexion	IP extension
	Thumb adduction	Thumb or palmar abduction or opposition
Palmar hand/ fingers	Finger flexion	Finger extension
	Thumb opposition	Thumb radial abduction
Hip	Flexion	Extension
	Adduction	Abduction
	External rotation	Neutral rotation
Knee	Flexion	Extension
Ankle	Plantar flexion	Dorsiflexion
Dorsal toes	Hyperextension	Flexion
Plantar toes	Flexion	Extension

Data from Reginald, R. J., & Marlys, S. J. (1994). *Burn care and rehabilitation principles and practice.* Philadelphia: F.A. Davis Company, 223.

Ilizarov fixators allow a multidimensional application of force to achieve anatomically correct positioning. The use of fixators, and the Ilizarov fixator in particular, is superior to splinting because of the propensity for formation of decubitus ulcers when rigid splints are used.

RANGE OF MOTION AND THERAPEUTIC EXERCISE

Children with burn injuries tend to avoid movement or, at best, move rigidly and slowly. Structured exercise programs are needed to prevent secondary musculoskeletal complications. Although physical therapists have primary responsibility for implementation of these programs, optimal physical restoration will largely depend on the combined and concentrated efforts of the child, family, and all team members.

Many factors influence the therapist's ability to provide adequate exercise for children with burn injuries. Pain, edema, surgical procedures, wound complications, and the child's and the family's adjustment to the injury all affect therapy. The therapist's skill in determining when to initiate exercise, choosing the type of exercise, and then appropriately transferring the care to the child and family are important determinants of functional outcomes and the duration of the rehabilitation program.

Although children recovering from burns share common problems, the exercise program must be customized to each child's unique needs, incorporating age-appropriate functional activities, as illustrated in Figure 31-4, *A–C*. Exercises for specific problems encountered by burn patients have been published.[69]

Emergent Phase

During the emergent or resuscitative period, emphasis is placed on passive range of motion (PROM), positioning, and splinting. However, if the child is alert, he or she may be able to engage in some movement activities such as bed mobility and positioning of extremities for dressing applications. ROM exercise is initiated as soon as the patient is medically stable. Escharotomies do not preclude exercise. Exercises that would compromise or dislodge lines and airways are withheld, and emphasis is placed on positioning of the affected joints.

Acute Phase

The acute phase generally refers to the time period after emergent care through skin grafting, when scarring is beginning to form. Exercises are performed with each joint separately, then with all joints combined in a sustained stretch that elongates the burned area. This is especially important when the burn crosses more than one joint. For example, Richard and colleagues reported that a measurable amount of forearm skin movement occurs to permit wrist extension.[67,68,70] In addition, the position of the elbow influences the amount of elongation of skin tissue necessary for wrist extension.

Multiple vigorous repetitions of movement should be avoided. Repetitions should be performed slowly with prolonged end-range hold. For the therapist or caregiver to gain full ROM, it is best to use nonpainful or less painful exercises and gradually progress to those exercises known to be more painful. Active and active-assistive ROM with terminal stretch assists in maintaining joint mobility and tissue pliability, as well as minimizing loss of strength. Compensatory movements used by children require intervention by a therapist to provide the amount of stretch needed to gain full ROM limited by burn pain or developing scar tissue. Parents can be instructed to assist their child with ROM exercises frequently throughout the day, but they may not be able to deal with the pain or sensation of stretching that it causes their child to experience.

Play and group activities are fun and allow children increased control. Play is perhaps the best method to elicit desired active movement in young children.[51] A report by Mahaney describes a child with a severe burn loss of ability to play and emphasizes the critical importance of play in the development of cognition, affectivity, and social learning (areas related to coping behavior).[46]

Anesthesia Assisted Range of Motion

ROM exercise performed while the patient is under anesthesia is sometimes recommended to determine the extent of

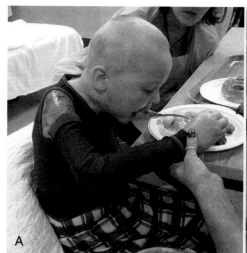

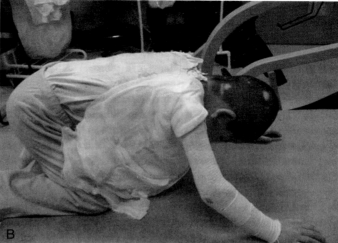

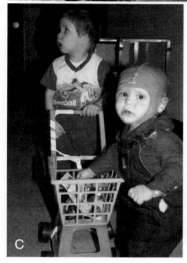

Figure 31-4 Functional activities elicit combined joint motion and stretch of tight scar bands. **A,** Self-care functional activities involve extremity, neck, and torso movement. **B,** Functional weight-bearing stretching and strengthening activities are difficult but essential following prolonged bedrest. **C,** Ambulation; children with burns are more easily motivated to ambulate by incorporating play activities.

joint restriction and as an adjunct to routine exercise sessions.[11] ROM performed while the child is under anesthesia may help the therapist to differentiate the underlying cause of restrictions. In particular, it allows the therapist to determine if the child's pain, fear, apprehension, or behavior is interfering with achieving the goals of exercise sessions.

Range of Motion Post Grafting

After grafting, exercise to the grafted area is discontinued for approximately 3 to 5 days to allow graft adherence. Grafted areas are immobilized at this time. Exercise to joints proximal and distal to the grafted area might influence graft stability and therefore is contraindicated. Active and active-assistive ROM to all other nongrafted areas is continued. If the graft appears stable after 3 to 5 days, gentle active and active-assistive ROM exercise to the grafted area is resumed with approval from the attending physician. It is typical that ROM decreases during the immobilization period after grafting. It is recommended that the physical

therapist observe dressing changes to identify areas of graft slough and possible tendon exposure. Patients who maintain essentially normal ROM during the regrafting phase are expected to have full joint motion in 7 to 10 days.

As healing progresses, with or without grafting, functional strengthening is introduced into the exercise program. Even if the child has open wounds and bandages, the therapist can apply minimal manual resistance. Resistance can be gently applied during isometric or isotonic muscle contraction. The postacute rehabilitative phase begins when the catabolic state reverses and there are few unhealed burn areas. This is the difficult and lengthy phase of wound contracture and hypertrophic scarring in which physical function and appearance can be altered significantly. A child who heals initially with full ROM still has the potential to develop deformities during the postacute period as the healed skin matures and hypertrophic scarring develops. Low load, prolonged stretching is one of the most effective exercise techniques for lengthening bands of scar tissue and increasing

ROM (Figure 31-5, *A–D*). Active-assistive ROM with the therapist applying mild manual stretching at end range of motion is well tolerated. Skin should be stretched to the point of blanching. Whenever possible, multijoint stretching is emphasized because scar tissue may cause profound limitations of motion when multiple joints are involved.

Careful integration of physical conditioning as part of the postacute rehabilitation exercise program enhances the patient's activity and participation. When possible, conditioning exercise incorporates activities enjoyable to the child, such as bicycling, dancing, or swimming, and provides the child not only with a sense of physical well-being but also with an opportunity for social interaction. In some cases, the addition of moderate-intensity progressive resistance and aerobic exercise to standard burn therapy resulted in significant improvements in muscle mass, strength, and cardiovascular endurance.[20] Exercise sessions lasted 1 hour and occurred three times a week for 12 weeks. A clinical trial found that following severe burns children who exercised had a fewer number of surgeries for scar releases up to 2 years after the injury when compared with a control group.[16] Children in the experimental group participated in a supervised exercise program of 60 to 90 minutes three times per week for 12 weeks. The exercise program included resistance and aerobic exercises performed at 70% to 85% maximal effort.

WALKING

Children should begin to walk as soon as their physical and medical condition warrants. For nongrafted lower extremity

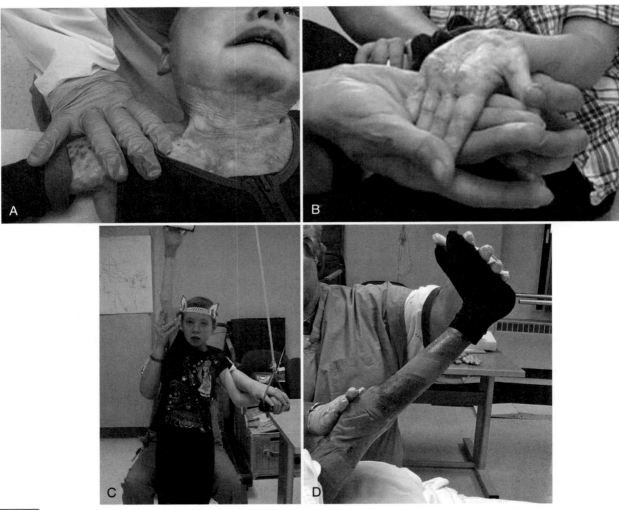

Figure 31-5   Sustained stretch at end of range is key to elongating scar bands. **A,** Prolonged neck stretch places a tethered scar band on maximum stretch by stabilizing the shoulder and trunk and moving the head. **B,** Prolonged palmar stretch is achieved by simultaneously hyperextending all digits with the wrist in extension until blanching is evident throughout the scar. **C,** Prolonged axillary stretch with assistance of an overhead pulley and controlled by the contralateral downward push. **D,** Combined knee extension and ankle dorsiflexion stretch demonstrating skin shortness, which might otherwise not be evident with isolated movement of the joints individually.

burns, walking is initiated once the child is medically stable and cleared by the physician. Mild to moderate burns of the feet do not preclude early ambulation. Children in the burn unit are assisted in ambulation to the limits of their physical endurance and are encouraged to weight bear fully through the lower extremities. If the lower extremities are burned, vascular support should be provided to reduce venous congestion and aid in pain management. Elastic bandages are applied from toe to groin in a figure-8 pattern to provide even distribution of pressure.

Hollowed and associates have developed technical maneuvers and precautions for patients who are intubated to ensure safety during ambulation.[36] Beginning walking while the patient was still intubated was effective in reducing pulmonary complications and increased the survival rate in patients with acute burns from 88% to 95%. In difficult cases, use of a tilt table may be the only way to progress the child to weight bearing. Compared with walking there is less active muscle pumping during static standing, which may have a negative effect on edema and pain.

Early walking after grafting is supported in the literature for adults.[13,32] A prospective study by Schmitt and associates reported a significant reduction (mean of 4.1 days) in length of hospital stay for patients who ambulated on postoperative day 7 compared with patients who ambulated on postoperative day 11.[74] Kowalske and colleagues reported no difference in graft take or time to complete wound closure following lower extremity skin grafting between patients who walked early (postoperative day 3 or 4) and those who walked late (postoperative day 7, 8, or 9).[42] Increased skin graft loss was seen in patients whose physical conditions prohibited ambulation on the randomly assigned day. Ricks and Meagher noted that in children, walking with plaster casting was associated with good lower extremity graft take.[71]

Assistive devices such as walkers, crutches, and canes are not encouraged. A normal gait pattern is encouraged. Young children often show regression in walking, particularly if they had begun to walk before burn injury. Preschool age children may be unwilling to weight bear through burned extremities, and initial attempts to walk are often unsuccessful. Involving the family or child life specialist in intervention may provide the motivation for the child to walk (see Figure 31-4, C).

Dr. Paul Unna's "boot" has been used with lower extremity wounds after grafting to allow patients to ambulate.[19] The Unna boot is a zinc oxide-calamine-gelatin impregnated bandage whose adherent properties secure the graft and provide additional vascular support. The Unna dressing has also proved effective in management of skin grafts to the hands of patients receiving outpatient services.[73]

DESENSITIZATION OF SCARRED AREAS

Desensitization treatment is recommended when healed or scarred areas of the hand are hypersensitive as evidenced by extreme discomfort or irritability in response to normally non-noxious tactile stimulation. Desensitization techniques may include (1) dowel textures, with different textures of material glued onto dowel sticks; (2) contact, with use of particles such as rice or beans; and (3) vibration, with use of battery-operated vibrators.[54]

ADJUNCTIVE THERAPIES

SCAR MASSAGE

Scar massage is used in burn care and appears to be most effective on small areas or linear scar bands. Despite its use, there is limited evidence to support or refute the effect of massage on burn scar. A research study, with a small sample size, specifically addressed manual scar massage for hypertrophic burn scar and found no lasting change in scar resulting from massage.[58] Other articles in the burn literature refer to general systemic effects of massage therapy.[27] Additional effects of scar massage may include reducing hypersensitivity, itch, and pain. Massage may moisturize and soften the scar, allowing easier and greater extensibility with ROM exercises and functional skills training immediately afterward.[66]

THERAPEUTIC HEAT

The use of heat through modalities in patients with burn injury is intended to increase local blood flow and pliability of scar tissue. Warm paraffin has been used in conjunction with stretching for improved tissue extensibility.[41] The superficial heat and lubrication are thought to reduce scar pain and improve scar extensibility. Paraffin is particularly helpful when a painful and contracting scar limits joint ROM. The paraffin mixture is used when it reaches a temperature of 46°C to 48°C or when a light skim covers the top of the mixture. Caution is suggested for newly healed scar tissue, which will blister easily if the standard paraffin bath temperature is used. Pouring or patting of the paraffin is done after the patient is positioned with the affected part in a sustained maximum stretch.

Ultrasound is a likely modality for tissue extensibility given the heating properties, but evidence of effectiveness for burns is limited and has not been studied in children.[89] Ultrasound overgrowth plates is a contraindication for children.

OUTPATIENT THERAPY

After discharge from the burn unit, settings for postacute rehabilitation are highly variable. In acute hospitals, the patient may continue to be seen in outpatient therapy. Burn centers sometimes transfer therapy care of children who travel great distances to a community hospital or local outpatient clinic and follow the child periodically in the burn clinic. Some burn centers have rehabilitation beds or step-down units that provide care until the child and family are ready for discharge to home. Other centers have transitional units, in which children and their families assume responsibility for care in a protective environment.[22] Children with complex injuries, amputations, large body surface area burns, or neurologic involvement may need services for several months in a rehabilitation center.

In our opinion, most children with severe burn injuries would benefit from daily postacute therapy provided by a skilled therapist, although this is usually not feasible. As a consequence, caregivers are responsible for skin care, garment care, therapeutic exercises, and splinting. Housinger and coworkers demonstrated that the success of pediatric outpatient rehabilitation is dependent on the dedicated effort of parents.[3,38] Duration of sessions varies according to parent involvement and the child's tolerance. Although therapy is demanding and crucial during this time, children should also be allowed time for other activities to make the transition to home, school, and community. Reybons stressed that leisure and recreation activities provide an opportunity to reestablish control over leisure time.[65]

Oftentimes the community-based outpatient therapist is responsible to carry out the plan of care. These therapists should not hesitate to contact the burn center with questions, concerns, and information needs. Given the contractile forces of scar tissue, it is imperative that the outpatient therapist prioritize intervention aimed at increasing range of motion and preventing contracture.

RECONSTRUCTION AND LONG-TERM FOLLOW-UP

In most cases it is desirable for the child to return to the burn facility for follow-up outpatient clinic visits. Frequent check-ups will allow the burn team to monitor the child's progress and adherence to the therapy program, and to progress the plan of care when appropriate. The check-ups enable the staff to detect any problems that may develop and to recommend changes to the therapy program as necessary. The burn team can answer questions for the child and family, such as those regarding skin care as healing occurs. Common problems addressed in follow-up clinics include skin breakdown, maceration, dryness, itch, sun intolerance, and impaired thermoregulation. Other issues that are addressed include physical activity level, continued use and fit of pressure garments and splints, maturation of scars, the application of cosmetics, and plans for further surgical procedures. If the family does not live near the primary care facility, local follow-up care can be arranged. In all cases, however, family members should be encouraged to contact the burn unit staff when they have concerns or questions. Open communication minimizes the development of secondary complications.

Persistent cutaneous inflexibility may result in tightening of underlying muscles, tendons, ligaments, joint capsules, and fascia. Chronic limitation of motion, therefore, may continue to affect the physical ability of a child and become more noticeable with growth. Functional outcomes that are also aesthetically pleasing may be more difficult to achieve in children compared with adults. Reconstructive procedures are often required after growth spurts and until bony growth is complete.[21] The child will require further intervention by the physical therapist after each reconstructive procedure for management of the new grafts.

The incidence of surgical release of contractures is higher in children than in adults, even though burn wound size may be similar. The hand and the central body regions (head, neck, and axilla) are likely to have the highest incidence of contracture formation. Central body region contractures, plus contractures at sites that had been previously fascially excised, have the poorest outcome after surgical reconstruction. It has been common practice to delay reconstructive surgery, when possible, until the burn scars have matured. However, early contracture release can be successfully performed in children with severe contractures that limit function.

Surgical and rehabilitative goals for correction of chronic impairments vary according to the age and stated needs of each child. Consideration of length, sensation, mobility, stability, strength, and, to a lesser extent, appearance dictates the reconstructive needs. The emphasis on function versus appearance is different for children of each age group. One of the more challenging areas requiring reconstruction after burn injury is the neck. Perineal contractures are also a frequent problem in the pediatric population. Pisarski and coworkers listed several procedures for correction but reported a high recurrence rate (46%), even with postoperative pressure garments, splints, and exercise.[61]

Scar variables, such as color, texture, dryness, lack of hair, lack of stretch, wrinkles, height, and mesh appearance, are assessed. Older children appear to have a more difficult time accepting the residual scar. When faced with the burden of coping with disfigurement resulting from a burn injury, the adolescent's sense of self-esteem may be diminished. Providing adolescents the opportunity to learn make-up techniques that lessen the impact of their scars is an effective intervention for enhancing self-perception and their perception of how others view them. This was demonstrated in a study of 115 patients attending reconstructive make-up clinics.[5]

FAMILY AND CAREGIVERS

Family or caregivers are an essential environmental factor in the outcome of a child with burn injury. The plan of care developed by the multidisciplinary team should include play activities and training in functional activities to facilitate the development of coping behavior. The child should be allowed to perform as much self-care as is possible, depending on the stage of recovery. Participation in dressing changes, decision making when confronted with choices that are equally acceptable, and personal hygiene must be encouraged to give the child a sense of control.

As the child is getting ready to transition to home, it is crucial that the child's family understand the daily care that will be required. It is best if the family begins early in the child's hospitalization to be instructed in all aspects of care and to ask questions, discuss treatments, and watch demonstrations. Some centers have found it helpful to create manuals to be reviewed with family members before discharge.[12,64] Parents have a chance to absorb written material and to practice the child's care under the supervision of the health care providers before discharge. Thus, when they arrive home with the child, they will feel more confident about their ability to carry out the required therapy. Special patient and family problems such as illiteracy, low learning levels, fluency in English, and deafness have also been addressed with customized guides, including pictorial guides, laminated flip charts, card file systems, audiotapes, videotapes, and photographic guides.[88]

Perhaps the most challenging aspect of transition to home care is adherence to the prescribed home program, which may involve rigorous stretching. This is particularly true if the parents feel guilty about the burn accident. Some children take advantage of feelings of guilt or sympathy and resist therapy at home, even if they were cooperative while in the hospital. In conjunction, some parents also perceive their child to have more problems than the child or his or her teacher reports. Results of a study by Meyer and associates suggest that troubled parents may overestimate the difficulties of their child.[52] Shelby and associates have identified additional family factors.[77] Parents of children who sustained burns reported more depression and anxiety than spouses of adults who were burned. Higher somatic symptom reporting was associated with fewer social resources, higher anxiety, and depression. Lower somatic symptoms were seen in parents reporting high hardiness, esteem, and perceived family social support.

ACTIVITY AND PARTICIPATION

The ultimate goal of a comprehensive program is to assure that children with severe burns heal sufficiently to regain their potential for productive and satisfying lives. The road to recovery is long and complex, requiring meticulous medical and social management after discharge from acute care. The "wellness" of a child and success of intervention should be measured from multiple perspectives, including physical, emotional, and social outcomes. Assessment of these outcomes should take into account factors related to the burn itself, such as severity, as well as adaptations to the consequences of the burn. Successful return to school is an essential part of the "return-to-wellness" process and should be regarded as an important outcome.

Successful recovery of a child with a severe burn can be considered using the International Classification of Functioning, Disability, and Health (ICF).[60] In regard to body function and structures, minimizing the extent and severity of contractures is a primary goal. The length of initial hospitalization, the number of skin graft procedures, the number of joint surface areas requiring skin grafting, the percentage of hospitalization spent in intensive care, septic or bacteremic bouts, and ventilator dependence are factors that may affect the extent and severity of burn-related contractures including the number and complexity of reconstructive surgeries undertaken to improve joint mobility.

Suboptimal management of contractures results in activity limitations and participation restrictions. Poor problem solving, inadequate compensatory strategies, and increased anxiety with physical demands are personal factors that contribute to activity limitations and participation restrictions. Limitations in self-care, mobility, and fine motor skills can restrict social interaction, learning, and leisure pursuits at school and in the community. The child's preinjury status and the need for long-term and periodic treatment are other factors that may influence the child's return to school and potential for future employment.

Physical therapists, as part of the burn team, are often involved in the return-to-school process. The physical therapist may provide school personnel with information regarding the child's current abilities and provide recommendations to school therapists and physical educators. Therapists may also participate in preparing the teachers and students for the child's abilities and needs (by means of individualized videotapes and, when necessary, onsite school visits). School reintegration programs have been developed to enhance a positive sense of self-worth in a child who has been burned. The premise of these programs is that cognitive and affective education about children with burns will diminish the anxiety of the child with a burn, the child's family, faculty and staff of the school, and the students. Five principles guide school reentry programs: (1) preparation begins as soon as possible, (2) planning includes the child and family, (3) each program is individualized, (4) the child is encouraged to return to school quickly after hospital discharge, and (5) burn team professionals remain available for consultation to the school.[8] The student who has sustained a burn injury, the school's personnel, and the student's peer groups benefit from a school reentry program. Concrete, factual information about the burn injury helps open lines of communication between the returning student and his or her peers. The concerns and expectations of school personnel are addressed.[7]

PSYCHOLOGIC ADJUSTMENT

Research on the psychologic adjustment of children following severe burns is encouraging. Blakeney and associates concluded that following severe burns (affecting >80% of total body surface area), children develop positive feelings about themselves and appear no more troubled than a comparable group of children without burns.[9] The impact on the families, however, was significant and must be considered in the rehabilitation process. A follow-up study of 101 young adults with major burn injury during childhood indicates that most are progressing satisfactorily in the domains of education, occupation, and social relationships.[53] Although most children do not have significant psychologic problems despite visible sequelae of their burn injuries, the burn team should carefully observe and inquire about child and family distress and provide support and guidance.

Many patients hospitalized for care of burn injuries show transient psychologic distress independent of such factors as burn size and premorbid function. Patients with severe burns, resulting in extended hospitalization, are particularly vulnerable to development of psychologic distress. The repeated, intrusive, and aggressive nature of burn care, although necessary for survival, may contribute to feelings of loss of control. The symptoms seen in children include regression, anxiety, decreased physical activity, withdrawal, behavior problems, decreased social interaction and play, and other depressive symptoms. The child's psychologic status must be considered when developing the plan of care. The quota system has been shown to be an effective new approach to helplessness behaviors and depressive symptoms that develop in some patients with burn injuries.[25] The quota system as described by Ehde and associates utilizes 80% of a patient's baseline behavior measures as an initial quota value.[25] The behavioral quotas are increased systematically and gradually every day until goals are achieved.

For many children following severe burn injury, recovery is a long and difficult process that challenges the physical and psychologic resilience of the individual. Most burn survivors do eventually adapt well and resume lives of productive activity with satisfactory self-esteem and social interactions.[10] Treatment of children with burns is concerned not only with skin coverage and prevention of infection but also with psychologic and social outcomes. Pediatric burn survivors often live with permanent disfigurement and physical disabilities. A study by Doctor, et al. suggests that people who survive a severe burn injury experience a stable and relatively good health status after their injury.[24] Their health status, however, remains worse than that of the general population. Furthermore, people who survive a major burn indicate that vocation and psychosocial function are often troublesome.

SUMMARY

Physical therapy for children with burns should begin at the time of injury and may extend for years beyond the initial hospitalization. There is no single best physical therapy intervention for children with burns. Each child has unique problems, and specific procedures and techniques are incorporated into an individualized rehabilitation program developed by the team, the child, and the family. The recovery process is long and often complicated, but successful rehabilitation, based on a comprehensive psychologic, social, and physical view of the child, is extremely gratifying.

REFERENCES

1. Ahn, S. T., Monafo, W. W., & Mustoe, T. A. (1989). Topical silicone gel: A new treatment for hypertrophic scars. *Surgery, 106,* 781–786.

2. American Burn Association, Committee on the Organization and Delivery of Burn Care. (1996). Burn care outcomes and clinical indicators. *Journal of Burn Care and Rehabilitation, 17*(2), 17A–39A.

3. Anzarut, A., Olson, J., Singh, P., Rowe, B. H., & Tredget, E. E. (2009). The effectiveness of pressure garment therapy for the prevention of abnormal scarring after burn injury: A meta-analysis. *Journal of Plastic, Reconstructive & Aesthetic Surgery, 62,* 77–84.

4. Armour, A., Scott, P. G., & Tredget, E. E. (2007). Cellular and molecular pathology of HTS: Basis for treatment. *Wound Repair and Regeneration, 15* (Suppl 1), S6–S17.

5. Beattie, D. M., Chedekel, D. S., & Krawczyk, T. (1993). *Utilization of a reconstructive makeup clinic for self-image enhancement in burned adolescents.* Paper presented at the meeting of the American Burn Association, Cincinnati, March.

6. Beyer, J. E., Denyes, M. J., & Villarruel, A. M. (1992). The creation, validation, and continuing development of the Oucher: A measure of pain intensity in children. *Journal of Pediatric Nursing, 7,* 335–346.

7. Bishop, B., & Gilinsky, V. (1995). School reentry for the patient with burn injuries: Video and/or on-site intervention. *Journal of Burn Care and Rehabilitation, 16*(4), 455–457.

8. Blakeney, P. (1995). School reintegration. *Journal of Burn Care and Rehabilitation, 16*(2), 180–187.

9. Blakeney, P., Meyer, W., Moore, P., Murphy, L., Robson, M., & Herndon, D. (1993). Psychosocial sequelae of pediatric burns involving 80% or greater total body surface area. *Journal of Burn Care and Rehabilitation, 14*(6), 684–689.

10. Blakeney, P. E., Rosenberg, L., Rosenberg, M., & Fauerbach, J. A. (2007). Psychological recovery and reintegration of patients with burn injuries. In D. N. Herndon (Ed.), *Total burn care* (pp. 829–843). Philadelphia: Elsevier.

11. Blassingame, W., Bennet, G., Helm, P., Purdue, G., & Hunt, J. (1989). Range of motion of the shoulder performed while patient is anesthetized. *Journal of Burn Care & Rehabilitation, 10*(6), 539–542.

12. Bochke, I., Frauenfeld, A., Hartlieb, D., Zwicker, M., & Inkson, T. (1993). *Patient and family education in burn care: Development of a series of teaching books by a multidisciplinary team.* Poster presented at the meeting of the American Burn Association, Cincinnati, March.

12a. Bombaro, K. M., Engrav, L. H., & Carrougher, G. J., et al. (2003). What is the prevalence of hypertrophic scarring following burns? *Burns, 29,* 299–302.

13. Burnsworth, B., Krob, M. J., & Langer-Schnepp, M. (1992). Immediate ambulation of patients with lower-extremity grafts. *Journal of Burn Care & Rehabilitation, 13*, 89–92.

14. Carney, S. A., Cason, C. G., Gowar, J. P., et al. (1994). Cica-care gel sheeting in the management of hyptrophic scarring. *Burns, 20*, 163–167.

15. Carvajal, H. F. (1990). Burns in children and adolescents: Initial management as the first step in successful rehabilitation. *Pediatrician, 17*, 237–243.

16. Celis, M. M., Suman, O. E., Huang, T. T., Yen, P., & Herndon, D. N. (2003). Effect of a supervised exercise and physiotherapy program on surgical intervention in children with thermal injury. *Journal of Burn Care and Rehabilitation, 24*(1), 57–61.

17. Chambers, C. T., Giesbrecht, K., Craig, K. D., et al. (1999). A comparison of faces scales for the measurement of pediatric pain: Children's and parents' ratings. *Pain, 83*, 25–35.

18. Chester, C. H., Candlish, S., & Zuker, R. M. (1993). *Prevention of obstructive sleep apnea in children with burns of the head and neck.* Paper presented at the meeting of the American Burn Association, Cincinnati, March.

19. Cox, G. W., & Griswold, J. A. (1993). Outpatient skin grafting of extremity burn wounds with the use of Unna Boot compression dressings. *Journal of Burn Care & Rehabilitation, 14*, 455–457.

20. Cucuzzo, N. A., Ferrando, A., & Herndon, D. N. (2001). The effects of exercise programming vs. traditional outpatient therapy in the rehabilitation of severely burned children. *Journal of Burn Care and Rehabilitation, 22*(3), 214–220.

21. Dado, D. V., & Angelats, J. (1990). Management of burns of the hands in children. *Hand Clinics, 6*, 711–721.

22. Daugherty, M. B., DeSerna, C., Barthel, P., & Warden, G. D. (1993). *Moving patients and families toward independence: Establishing a transitional unit.* Poster presented at the meeting of the American Burn Association, Cincinnati, March.

23. Davey, R. B., Wallis, K. S., & Bowering, K. (1991). Adhesive contact media: An update on graft fixation and burn scar management. *Burns, 17*, 313–319.

23a. Dewey, W. S., Hedman, T. L., & Chapman, T. T., et al. (2007). The reliability and concurrent validity of the figure-of-eight method of measuring hand edema in patients with burns. *J Burn Care Res, 28*, 157–162, 2007.

24. Doctor, J. N., Patterson, D. R., & Mann, R. (1997). Health outcome for burn survivors. *Journal of Burn Care and Rehabilitation, 18*(6), 490–495.

25. Ehde, D. M., Patterson, D. R., & Fordyce, W. E. (1998). The quota system in burn rehabilitation. *Journal of Burn Care and Rehabilitation, 19*(5), 436–440.

26. Esselman, P. C., & Moore, M. L. (2007). Issues in burn rehabilitation. In R. L. Braddom (Ed.), *Physical medicine and rehabilitation* (3rd ed., pp. 1399–1413). Philadelphia: Saunders Elsevier.

27. Field, T., Peck, M., Krugman, S., et al. (1998). Burn injuries benefit from massage therapy. *Journal of Burn Care & Rehabilitation, 19*, 241–244.

28. Foley, K. H., Doyle, B., Paradise, P., Parry, I., Palmieri, T., & Greenhalgh, D. G. (2002). Use of an improved Watusi collar to manage pediatric neck burn contractures. *Journal of Burn Care and Rehabilitation, 23*(3), 221–226.

29. Fricke, N. B., Omnell, M. L., Dutcher, K. A., Hollender, L. G., & Engrav, L. H. (1999). Skeletal and dental disturbances in children after facial burns and pressure garment use: A 4-year follow-up. *Journal of Burn Care and Rehabilitation, 20*(3), 239–249.

30. Gaur, A., Sinclair, M., Caruso, E., Peretti, G., & Zaleske, D. (2003). Heterotopic ossification around the elbow following burns in children: Results after excision. *Journal of Bone and Joint Surgery, 85-A*(8), 1538–1543.

31. Ghahary, A., Shen, Y. J., Scott, P. G., Gong, Y., & Tredget, E. E. (1993). Enhanced expression of mRNA for transforming growth factor-beta, type I and type III procollagen in human post-burn hypertrophic scar tissues. *Journal of Laboratory Clinical Medicine, 122*(4), 465–473.

32. Harnar, T., Engrav, L. H., Marvin, J., Heimbach, D., Cain, V., & Johnson, C. (1982). Dr. Paul Unna's boot and early ambulation after skin grafting the leg: A survey of burn centers and a report of 20 cases. *Plastic Reconstructive Surgery, 69*, 359–360.

33. Harris, L. D., Hatler, B., Adams, S., Gilliam, K. S., & Helm, P. (1993). *Serial casting and its efficacy in the treatment of the burned hand.* Paper presented at the meeting of the American Burn Association, Cincinnati, March.

34. Hawkins, H. K., & Pereira, C. T. (2007). Pathophysiology of the burn scar. In D. N. Herndon (Ed.), *Total burn care* (pp. 608–619). Philadelphia: Elsevier.

35. Herndon, D. N., & Rutan, R. L. (1992). Use of dermal templates and cultured cells for permanent skin replacement. *Wounds, 4*(2), 50–53.

36. Hollowed, K. A., Gunde, M. A., Lewis, M. S., & Jordon, M. H. (1993). *Ambulation of intubated burn patients.* Poster presented at the meeting of the American Burn Association, Cincinnati, March.

37. Honari, S. H. (2004). Topical therapies and antimicrobials in the management of burn wounds. *Critical Care Nursing Clinics of North America, 16*, 1–11.

38. Housinger, T., Mortess, C., Dinkler, T., & Warden, G. D. (1992). *Outpatient therapy: Its efficacy in pediatric burns.* Paper presented at the meeting of the American Burn Association, Salt Lake City, UT, April.

38a. Hurlin, F. K., Doyle, B., & Paradise, P., et al. (2002). Use of an improved Watusi collar to manage pediatric neck burn contractures. *J Burn Care Rehab, 23*(3), 221–226.

39. Ilhami, K., Safak, O., & Orhan, G. (2003). Specifically designed external fixators in treatment of complex postburn hand contractures. *Burns, 29*(6), 609–612.

40. Johnson, J., & Silverberg, R. (1995). Serial casting of the lower extremity to correct contractures during the acute phase of burn care. *Physical Therapy, 75*(8), 767–768.

41. Kowalske, K., Holavanahalli, R., & Hynan, L. (2003). A randomized-controlled study of the effectiveness of paraffin and sustained stretch in treatment of burn contractures. *Journal of Burn Care & Rehabilitation, 24*, S67.

42. Kowalske, K., Purdue, G., Hunt, J., & Helm, P. (1993). *Early ambulation following skin grafting of lower extremity burns: A randomized controlled trial.* Paper presented at the meeting of the American Burn Association, Cincinnati, March.

43. Kramer, G., Lund, T., & Beckum, O. (2007). Pathophysiology of burn shock and burn edema. In Herndon, D. N. (Ed.), *Total burn care* (p. 94). Philadelphia: Elsevier.

44. Kwan, P., Keijiro, H., Ding, J., & Tredget, E. E. (2009). Scar and contracture: Biological principles. *Hand Clinic, 25,* 511–528.

45. Linares, H. A., Larson, D. L., & Willis-Galstaum, B. A. (1993). Historical notes on the use of pressure in the treatment of hypertrophic scars or keloids. *Burns, 19,* 17–21.

46. Mahaney, N. B. (1990). Restoration of play in a severely burned three-year-old child. *Journal of Burn Care and Rehabilitation, 11,* 57–63.

47. Malick, M. H., & Carr, J. A. (1980). Flexible elastomer molds in burn scar control. *American Journal of Occupational Therapy, 34,* 603–608.

48. Manigandan, C., Gupta, A. K., Venugopal, K., Ninan, S., & Cherian, R. E. (2003). A multi-purpose, self-adjustable aeroplane splint for the splinting of axillary burns. *Burns, 29*(3), 276–279.

49. Mann, R., Yeong, E. K., Moore, M. L., & Engrav, L. H. (1997). A new tool to measure pressure under burn garments. *Journal of Burn Care and Rehabilitation, 18*(2), 160–163.

50. Manworren, R. C., & Hynan, L. S. (2003). Clinical validation of FLACC: Preverbal patient pain scale. *Pediatric Nursing, 29,* 140–146.

51. Melchert-McKearnan, K., Deitz, J., Engel, J. M., & White, O. (2000). Children with burn injuries: Purposeful activity versus rote exercise. *American Journal of Occupational Therapy, 54*(4), 381–390.

52. Meyer, W., Blakeney, P., Moore, P., Murphy, L., Robson, M., & Herndon, D. (1994). Parental well-being and behavioral adjustment of pediatric survivors of burns. *Journal of Burn Care and Rehabilitation, 15*(1), 62–68.

53. Meyer, W. J., Blakeney, P., Russell, W., et al. (2004). Psychological problems reported by young adults who were burned as children. *Journal of Burn Care and Rehabilitation, 25*(1), 98–106.

54. Moore, M. L., Dewey, W. S., & Richard, R. L. (2009). Rehabilitation of the burned hand. *Hand Clinic, 25,* 529–541.

55. Morris, L. D., Louw, Q. A., & Grimmer-Somers, K. (2009). The effectiveness of virtual reality on reducing pain and anxiety in burn injury patients: A systematic review. *Clinical Journal of Pain, 25*(9), 815–826.

56. Mutalik, S. (2005). Treatment of keloids and hypertrophic scars. *Indian Journal of Dermatology, Venereology and Leprology, 71*(1), 3–8.

57. Nedelec, B., Shen, Y. J., Ghahary, A., Scott, P. G., & Tredget, E. E. (1995). The effect of interferon alpha 2b on the expression of cytoskeletal proteins in an in vitro model of wound contraction. *Journal of Laboratory Clinical Medicine, 126*(5), 474–484.

58. Patino, O., Novick, C., Merlo, A., & Benaim, F. (1999). Massage in hypertrophic scar. *Journal of Burn Care and Rehabilitation, 20,* 268–271.

59. Perkins, K., Davey, R. B., & Wallis, K. A. (1983). Silicone gel: A new treatment for burn scars and contractures. *Burns, Including Thermal Injury, 9,* 201–204.

60. Pidcock, F. S., Fauerbach, J. A., Ober, M., & Carney, J. (2003). The rehabilitation/school matrix: A model for accommodating the non-compliant child with severe burns. *Journal of Burn Care and Rehabilitation, 24*(5), 342–346.

61. Pisarski, G. P., Greenhalgh, D. G., & Warden, G. D. (1994). The management of perineal contractures in children with burns. *Journal of Burn Care and Rehabilitation, 15*(3), 256–259.

62. Pruitt, B. A., Wolf, S. E., & Mason, A. D. Jr. (2007) Epidemiological, demographic, and outcome characteristics of burn injury. In D. N. Herndon (Ed.), *Total burn care* (pp. 14–32). Philadelphia: Elsevier.

63. Quinn, K. J., Evans, J. H., Courtney, J. M., Gaylor, J. D., & Reid, W. H. (1985). Non-pressure treatment of hypertrophic scars. *Burns, Including Thermal Injury, 12,* 102–108.

64. Reed, L., & Heinle, J. (1993). *Meeting the challenge of education for a diversified patient population in a burn treatment center: Design of 2 patient handbooks.* Poster presented at the meeting of the American Burn Association, Cincinnati, March.

65. Reybons, M. D. (1992). Community re-entry and leisure: Reuniting a lifestyle with a burn survivor. *Progress Report, 4*(3), 20–22.

66. Richard, R., Baryza, M. J., Carr, J. A., et al. (2009). Burn rehabilitation and research: Proceedings of a consensus summit. *Journal of Burn Care & Research, 30*(4), 543–573.

67. Richard, R., DerSarkisian, D., Miller, S. F., Johnson, R. M., & Staley, M. (1999). Directional variance in skin movement. *Journal of Burn Care and Rehabilitation, 20*(3), 259–264.

68. Richard, R., Ford, J., Miller, S. F., & Staley, M. (1994). Photographic measurement of volar forearm skin movement with wrist extension: The influence of elbow position. *Journal of Burn Care and Rehabilitation, 15*(1), 58–61.

69. Richard, R. L., Staley, M. J., Miller, S. F., Warden, G. D., & Finley, R. K., Jr. (1993). *Biomechanical basis for physical management of burn patients.* Poster presented at the meeting of the American Burn Association, Cincinnati, March.

70. Richard, R. L., & Staley, M. J. (1994). *Burn care and rehabilitation: Principles and practice* (p. 223). Philadelphia: F.A. Davis Company.

71. Ricks, N. R., & Meagher, D. P., Jr. (1992). The benefits of plaster casting for lower-extremity burns after grafting in children. *Journal of Burn Care & Rehabilitation, 13,* 465–468.

72. Ridgway, C. L., Daugherty, M. B., & Warden, G. D. (1991). Serial casting as a technique to correct burn scar contractures. *Journal of Burn Care and Rehabilitation, 12,* 67–72.

73. Sanford, S., & Gore, D. (1996). Unna's boot dressings facilitate outpatient skin grafting of hands. *Journal of Burn Care and Rehabilitation, 17*(4), 323–326.

74. Schmitt, M. A., French, L., & Kalil, E. T. (1991). How soon is safe? Ambulation of the patient with burns after

lower-extremity skin grafting. *Journal of Burn Care and Rehabilitation, 12,* 33–37.

74a. Schwanholt, C., Daugherty, M. B., & Gaboury, T., et al. (1992). Splinting the pediatric palmar burn. *J Burn Care Rehabil, 13(4),* 460–464.

74b. Scott, J. R., Costa, B. A., & Gibran, N. S., et al. (2008). Pediatric palm contact burns: a ten-year review. *J Burn Care Res, 29(4),* 614–618.

75. Serghiou, M. A., McLaughlin, A., & Herndon, D. N. (2003). Alternative splinting methods for the prevention and correction of burn scar torticollis. *Journal of Burn Care and Rehabilitation, 24(5),* 336–340.

76. Serghiou, M. A., Ott, S., Farmer, D., Morgan, D., Gibson, P., & Sunman, O. E. (2007). Comprehensive rehabilitation of the burn patient. In D. N. Herndon (Ed.), *Total burn care* (pp. 628–629). Philadelphia: Elsevier.

76a. Sharp, P. A., Dougherty, M. E., & Kagan, R. J. (2007). The effect of positioning devices and pressure therapy on outcome after full-thickness burns of the neck. *J Burn Care Res, 28(3),* 451–459.

77. Shelby, J., Groussman, M., Addison, C., Burgess, Y., Sullivan, J., & Saffie, J. (1993). *Stress resiliency in close relatives of thermally injured patients.* Paper presented at the meeting of the American Burn Association, Cincinnati, March.

78. Spurr, E. D., & Shakespeare, P. G. (1990). Incidence of hypertrophic scarring in burn-injured children. *Burns, 16,* 179–181.

79. Staley, M. J., & Richard, R. L. (1994). Scar management. In R. L. Richard & M. J. Staley (Eds.), *Burn care and rehabilitation* (pp. 380–418). Philadelphia: FA Davis.

80. Staley, M., & Richard, R. (1996). Critical pathways to enhance the rehabilitation of patients with burns. *Journal of Burn Care and Rehabilitation, 17(6),* S12–S14.

81. Sullivan, T. (1990). Rating the burn scar. *Journal of Burn Care and Rehabilitation, 11,* 256–260.

82. Thurber, C. A., Martin-Herz, S. P., & Patterson, D. R. (2000). Psychological principles of burn wound pain in children I: Theoretical framework. *Journal of Burn Care and Rehabilitation, 21(4),* 376–387.

83. Torres-Gray, D., Johnson, J., Greenspan, B., Goodwin, C. W., & Naglet, W. (1993). *The fabrication and use of removable digit casts to improve range of motion at the proximal interphalangeal joint.* Poster presented at the meeting of the American Burn Association, Cincinnati, March.

84. Van den Kerckhove, E., Stappaerts, K., Fieuws, S., et al. (2005). The assessment of erythema and thickness on burn related scars during pressure garment therapy as a preventive measure for hypertrophic scarring. *Burns, 31(6),* 696–702.

85. van Dijk, M., de Boer, J. B., Koot, H. M., et al. (2000). The reliability and validity of the COMFORT scale as a postoperative pain instrument in 0- to 3-year-old infants. *Pain, 84,* 367–377.

86. Van Straten, O., & Sagi, A. (2000). "Supersplint": A new dynamic combination splint for the burned hand. *Journal of Burn Care and Rehabilitation, 21(1),* 71–73.

87. Voepel-Lewis, T., Zanotti, J., Dammeyer, J. A., & Merkel, S. (2010). Reliability of the face, legs, activity, cry, consolability behavioral tool in assessing acute pain in critically ill patients. *American Journal of Critical Care, 19:*55–61.

88. Walling, S., Walling, R., & Warden, G. D. (1993). *The development of home program instructional guides to accommodate the special needs of patients and families.* Poster presented at the meeting of the American Burn Association, Cincinnati, March.

89. Ward, R., Hayes-Lundy, C., Reddy, R., Brockway, C., Mills, P., & Saffle, J. (1994). Evaluation of topical therapeutic ultrasound to improve response to physical therapy and lessen scar contracture after burn injury. *Journal of Burn Care & Rehabilitation, 15(1),* 74–79.

90. Ward, R. S., Hayes-Lundy, C., Schnebly, W. A., Reddy, R., & Saffle, J. R. (1990). Rehabilitation of burn patients with concomitant limb amputation: Case reports. *Burns, 16(5),* 390–392.

91. Ward, R. S., Hayes-Lundy, C., Schnebly, W. A., & Saffle, J. R. (1990). Prosthetic use in patients with burns and associated limb amputations. *Journal of Burn Care and Rehabilitation, 11,* 361–364.

92. Yeong, E. K., Mann, R., Engrav, L. H., Goldberg, M., Cain, V., Costa, B., Moore, M., Nakamura, D., & Lee, J. (1997). Improved burn scar assessment with use of a new scar-rating scale. *Journal of Burn Care and Rehabilitation, 18(4),* 353–355.

32 Transition to Adulthood for Youth with Disabilities

NANCY A. CICIRELLO, PT, MPH, EdD • ANTONETTE K. DOTY, PT, MPH • ROBERT J. PALISANO, PT, ScD

Transition to adulthood is a future-oriented process in which youth express their desires and goals and begin planning for adult roles and responsibilities.[20] Tasks associated with the transition to adulthood for youth with disabilities include finding an adult medical home, living outside the family home, obtaining postsecondary education, and participating in work, social, and community activities. The transition process is multifaceted and encompasses the health, psychosocial, and educational-vocational needs of adolescents as they move from child-oriented to adult-oriented lifestyles and systems.[116] Carr et al. defined successful transition as active participation in desired adult roles.[25] Outcomes associated with successful transition of youth with disabilities include (1) enhanced knowledge of self and community; (2) enhanced skills, including physical, communication, problem solving, decision making, social, employment, and leisure; (3) support systems including friends and mentors; (4) assistive technology; and (5) supportive environments.[25] The U.S. Individuals with Disabilities Education Improvement Act of 2004 (PL 108-446) recognized the importance of transition planning. A consensus statement by the American Academy of Pediatrics (AAP), American Academy of Family Physicians, American College of Physicians, and American Society of Internal Medicine advocates for a written health care transition plan for all youth with disabilities by age 14.[2]

Transition to adulthood presents particular challenges for youth with disabilities, their families, health care professionals, and the broader health care system.[2,18,34,102] Adolescents with disabilities demonstrate low rates of high school graduation and are less likely to pursue college education.[96] Blomquist et al. identified low expectations by parents and professionals, lack of knowledge of existing career and vocational education services, and lack of self-advocacy skills as particular challenges for youth with disabilities.[20] Similarly, Stewart identified lack of preparation, limited information, limited supports, lack of skills for adult roles, and disjointed adult services as potential barriers to successful transition.[100] In a national survey conducted by the PACER center, youth with disabilities identified job training, independent living skills, and college or vocational guidance as the transition services they wanted the most.[120] Only 45% reported that someone had discussed with them how to make medical decisions, and less than 50% had been asked about their

work plans.[120] Blomquist surveyed young adults who previously received services from Kentucky's program for children with special health care needs and Shriners Hospitals for Children.[19] Eighty percent of the respondents reported having a usual source of health care, although 29% had no health insurance. Only 44% of the respondents were working; 67% of those did not want to work, whereas 26% were neither working nor in school. In a national survey, only 6% of families reported that their young adult child with special health care needs had achieved core outcomes for successful transition to adulthood.[86] These findings underscore the need for innovative programs to prepare youth with disabilities for adult roles.

Preparing youth with disabilities for adult roles and meeting the needs of adults with childhood onset conditions are emerging areas of physical therapy practice. Youth with disabilities often have needs for (1) personal assistance, (2) assistive technology, (3) instruction in self-advocacy, and (4) development of skills needed for postsecondary education and employment.[46,58,101,109] The International Classification of Functioning, Disability, and Health (ICF),[119] described in Chapter 1, is a *biopsychosocial model* in which the interaction between the person and environment is critical for understanding health, health-related states, and participation outcomes. The ICF provides a useful framework for transition of youth with disabilities to postsecondary education, work, and the adult health system.

The objectives of this chapter are to (1) describe the transition process and challenges for youth with physical disabilities and their families; (2) appraise transition approaches and outcomes; and (3) provide recommendations for the role of the physical therapist in educational, community, and hospital settings. Transition services and supports within education, health care, vocational, and social service systems are addressed, and the roles of physical therapists working in educational, community, and hospital settings are discussed. Two cases, presented at the end of the chapter, illustrate the application of knowledge to practice. One case focuses on the varied roles of the physical therapist as a member of the transition team during a student's last two years in secondary education. The second case describes the experiences and reflections of a pediatric physical therapist as she expands her practice knowledge to include transition of youth with physical disabilities.

PREPARATION OF YOUTH WITH DISABILITIES FOR ADULT ROLES

Transition to adulthood encompasses new roles, responsibilities, and expectations and is influenced by a myriad of personal, familial, community, and societal factors. Havighurst identified tasks of adolescence including (1) forming new and more mature relations with age-mates of both sexes, (2) accepting one's physique and using one's body effectively, (3) achieving emotional independence from parents and other adults, (4) preparing for marriage and family life, (5) gaining economic independence, and (6) desiring and achieving socially responsible behavior.[49]

In 1980, Gliedman and Roth coauthored *The Unexpected Minority*, a report on children with disabilities sponsored by the Carnegie Council on Children.[47] A tenet of the report was that children with disabilities are not going to be "cured," nor are they "sick." This "unexpected minority" is part of the "new age wave" of people with long-term disabilities having increased life expectancies. Factors attributed to increased life expectancy of people with disabilities include advances in medical technologies, decreased institutionalization, and federal legislation. Although adolescents and young adults with childhood onset health conditions are no longer "unexpected," transition services and supports are just emerging and often not well formalized. As such, physical therapists must be prudent in embracing a theoretic shift from solely a medical paradigm to a more inclusive biopsychosocial paradigm that recognizes the importance of personal and environmental contexts for activity, participation, wellness, and prevention. Gliedman and Roth stated that "medical explanation alone negates that which is vital to living with a disability."[47] Merely addressing and viewing problems as individually owned is a "flawed lens," and further obscures "societal forces and responsibilities." These statements are consistent with the perspectives that people with disabilities are consumers with special needs in finding meaningful work, accessing multiple physical environments, and living independently or with self-chosen supports and that successful transition is enabled by the community.[33]

FAMILY INVOLVEMENT

Collaboration among youth with disabilities, their families, and professionals is essential for successful transition.[8] A general expectation is that as adolescents mature they will become more autonomous and assume adult roles and responsibilities. Families of youth with disabilities have expressed needs for future planning[84] and have expressed concerns about what will happen when they no longer are able to care for their adult child.[22,43,76] Parents of students with disabilities are not always involved in transition planning, even though they are often the primary support for their children after high school. McNair and Rush found that parents wanted more information regarding their child's

skill level, work options, adult services, community living, and types of family support, and they desired more involvement in transition planning.[77] Parents who participated in the National Longitudinal Transition Studies expressed the desire for their children with disabilities to graduate from high school with a regular diploma, and their expectations for independent living have increased.[113]

SELF-DETERMINATION

Self-determination is a desirable attribute of youth with disabilities transitioning to adult roles.[38,75,101] Self-determination is defined as the "combination of skills, knowledge, and beliefs that enable a person to engage in goal directed, self-regulated, autonomous behavior."[39] Self-determination is both person centered and person directed and acknowledges the rights of people with disabilities to take charge of and responsibility for their lives.[62] Youth possessing self-determination are thought to have greater ability to take control of their lives and successfully assume adult roles. Youth with cerebral palsy identified being believed in, believing in yourself, and being accepted by others as important for success in life.[66] Social self-efficacy was associated with independence and persistence in a study of adolescents with physical disabilities.[67] Gall et al. have recommended that the transition process involve a gradual shift in responsibilities from the service provider to the parent/family and finally to the young person.[44]

Algozzine et al. conducted a systematic review on interventions to promote self-determination and concluded that approaches using multiple strategies, longer time frames, and involving parents were most effective.[1] Intervention strategies utilized in the studies reviewed included learning and practicing skills, planning, decision making, goal setting, problem solving, and self-advocacy. Evans et al. evaluated a multifaceted transition program that combines self-discovery, skill development, and community experiences.[38] Following participation in the program for 12 months, youth and young adults with multiple disabilities demonstrated statistically and clinically important improvement in self-determination and their sense of personal control, and they spent significantly more time engaged in volunteer/work activities and community leisure activities.

WELLNESS AND SECONDARY PREVENTION

Healthy People 2020 and its predecessor Healthy People 2010[111] are initiatives by the U.S. Department of Health and Human Services to promote health and disease prevention. At the time of publication, the document Healthy People 2020 was available for public comment (www.healthypeople.gov). Goals for people with disabilities include greater access to health, wellness, assistive technology, and treatment programs and a reduction in the proportion of people with disabilities who report encountering environmental barriers to participating in home, school, work, or community activities. Comprehensive and coordinated heath care and self-management of one's health condition, and physical activity are important for wellness and secondary prevention. In Healthy People 2020, in the Disability and Secondary Conditions section, two new objectives are to reduce the proportion of people with disabilities reporting delays in receiving primary and periodic preventive care because of specific barriers and to increase the proportion of parents or other caregivers of youth with disabilities aged 12 to 17 years who report engaging in transition planning from pediatric to adult health care. The objectives reinforce the importance of introducing aging with disabilities and youth in transition into physical therapy education programs and service delivery.

Finding an Adult Medical Home

With medical advances over the past decades, many children with disabilities are now living into adulthood and facing new challenges in the areas of health and wellness.[15] Newacheck et al. reported that in the United States, 18% (12.6 million) of children and adolescents under 18 years of age have a chronic medical condition requiring health and related services of a type or amount beyond that required by children in general.[81] Ninety percent of youth with special health care needs reach their 21st birthday. An estimated 200,000 to 500,000 individuals with lifelong disabilities are over the age of 60, and this number is expected to double by 2030.[10]

An important outcome for youth with disabilities is continuous, comprehensive, and coordinated services in the adult health care system.[2,32,117] Presently, the health care system in the United States is not designed to facilitate the transition between pediatric and adult services, which results in a patchwork approach that is not likely to change in the near future.[15] Typically, people with a lifelong disability have less access to medical providers in the community than the general population. In addition, they have less preventive care, more emergency medical visits, less insurance coverage, and little to no experience managing their own health care. Forty-five percent of youth with special health care needs do not have a physician who is familiar with their health condition. Further, 30% of 18- to 24-year-olds lack a payment source for health care and youth lack access to primary and specialty providers.[15]

In the United States, the medical home model is an effort to improve coordination of services and reduce costs by identifying a primary care provider and coordination of health care and community services. The adult health care system, however, is lacking in primary care providers and the specialized health care and rehabilitation services needed by adults with childhood onset chronic conditions such as cerebral palsy.[16,32,74,82,99] Lack of transition preparation of young people with disabilities and their families is thought to contribute to problems in transition to adult care.[90] The

American Academy of Pediatrics, American Academy of Family Physicians, American College of Physicians, and American Society of Internal Medicine have published a consensus statement recommending that all youth with special health care needs have a written health care transition plan by age 14 years to identify appropriate health care professionals, provide guidelines for primary as well as preventive care, and ensure developmentally appropriate transition services.[2] The Evolve website contains the URL for the American Academy of Pediatrics National Center for Medical Home Initiatives for Children with Special Needs. The website includes resources for families, youth, and providers on finding a medical home and health care transition. Resources for youth include transition notebooks, a portable medical record form, and videos on topics such as talking with your doctor and other health care professionals and planning for the future.

Tonniges and Roberts have investigated health care and transition and found that youth with special health care needs spend more time on crisis management and less on typical life, fun, and activities.[110] Youth with special health care needs are said to live more as a patient and less as a young person, leading to missed school, interruptions in learning, functional declines, social isolation, and low expectations by adults about their abilities and future prospects. Youth express that they would like to live and work independently but often feel they are "treated like a child" and have a loss of control. Many feel they are not seen as unique individuals, separate from their condition, and health care providers often defer to the youths' parents. Families of youth with special health care needs would like more information about resources, referrals to services, a written health transition plan, an advocate to assist and explain, and assistance from their medical home.[15]

Self-Management of Health Condition

To the fullest extent possible, youth with disabilities are encouraged to actively participate in the transition from a pediatric to an adult medical home. The ability to communicate with health care providers, including primary care physicians, specialty physicians, nurses, therapists, and dentists, is an important skill. For youth who require physical assistance for self-care, this includes the ability to instruct care providers. Skills for health promotion, injury prevention, and prevention of secondary impairments also are important. Youth may benefit from experience in coordination of services among their multiple health care providers. Learning to identify their medical home provider and develop strategies for communicating and coordinating their specialty care such as maintaining a record of their health status and care are examples of outcomes for self-management. This may include a transition plan that is shared with each provider. The electronic medical record has potential to improve communication and coordination of care.

Physical Activity

The importance of physical activity is an area of education for youth with disabilities.[42] Promoting lifetime physical fitness is critical for prevention of secondary complications resulting from childhood onset health conditions. The health benefits of regular exercise include decreased risk of heart disease, cancer, age-related physiologic changes, obesity, and increased social well-being. The Surgeon General stated that for people with chronic disabling conditions, regular physical activity can improve stamina, muscular strength, improve quality of life, and prevent disease.[105] The report identifies a lack of available and accessible wellness and fitness programs and recommends implementing community-based programs with safe, accessible environments and including people with disabilities and their families in program planning.

Creating a habit of regular exercise is challenging for individuals with lifelong disabilities. Erson stated that fitness activities should be fun, goal oriented, and contribute to health and well being in order for fitness to become a habit.[37] Exercise can improve academics, reduce maladaptive behaviors, and improve self-esteem and psychosocial functioning of adolescents with disabilities,[36,104] yet as youth advance through the education system, the amount of physical education often decreases. The percentage of school districts providing daily physical education for students in high school decreased from 42% to 27% between 1991 and 1997.[26,79] A survey of recreation preferences found that among adults with childhood onset disabilities, the number one choice for recreation was to watch television followed by listening to music, going to the movies, and playing videogames.[79]

Exposure to diverse recreation and leisure activities enables youth with disabilities to make informed choices. Making choices enhances self-determination and can decrease problem behavior.[103] Furthermore, preferred recreation and leisure activities are more likely to be enjoyable and sustained over time. Exposure to diverse activities enables youth to select alternative activities if initial choices do not work out.

To access community fitness programs, adults with disabilities may require specially designed physical activity education and training programs. The Americans with Disabilities Act (ADA) legislates equitable access of community recreation programs for persons with disabilities. Participation of persons with disabilities in age-appropriate, community-based programs should enhance public awareness that disability does not equate to ill health.

COMMUNITY LIVING

The reauthorization of Individuals with Disabilities Education Act in 1997 included mandates to improve transition of youth from high school to other opportunities such as postsecondary education, employment, and community living. Johnson et al. suggested that transition challenges to community living and employment include (1) access to full spectrum of general education offerings and learning experiences; (2) education placement, curricular decisions, and diploma options that are based on meaningful indicators of learning and skills; (3) options for postsecondary education, community living, and employment; (4) participation of the student and family; and (5) interagency communication and collaboration.[60]

Young adults with disabilities desire options for community living other than the family home. These options may range in descending order of support from residential group homes (agency owned or operated), residential supported living (private housing with flexible supports such as attendant care), and independent living. Howe, Horner, and Newton evaluated supported community living versus residential group homes among 40 adults with cognitive impairments.[55] The authors defined supported living as not facility based but rather as developing supports needed to best match the individual's preferences and needs over time. The number of housemates for adults in supported independent living varied from 0 to 2, whereas the number of housemates for adults in residential living varied from 1 to 19. Housing provision costs were similar for both living arrangements. Young adults in supported living were either the owner of the residence or listed on the rental agreement, and housemates were identified as the preferred choice of each young adult with developmental disabilities. Young adults in supported living experienced significantly more variety in community activities and did preferred activities more frequently compared with young adults living in group homes.

The National Center for the Study of Postsecondary Educational Supports (NCSPES) has identified competencies for successful transition from secondary education.[80] Two competencies are knowledge of self, including one's health condition, and the ability to access services and supports for community living. Life skill curricular content in secondary education such as identifying specific supports needed for living, postsecondary education, or work is recommended for students with special health care needs, regardless of cognitive ability. Curricular content could include accessibility, transportation, and skills for community living and work. For community living, skills may include meal preparation, acquisition of food staples, paying bills, laundry, hiring, managing, or firing personal attendants. Skill sets for work might include the ability to interact with people providing attendant care and to describe and request necessary job accommodations including augmentative communication when needed. Physical therapists working in educational settings are encouraged to anticipate opportunities to be included in life skill programs for students with physical disabilities. Likewise, pediatric physical therapists in clinic and hospital practice settings are encouraged to communicate and coordinate with educators and professionals providing related services (transition coordinator, school-based therapists) and to interact with community organizations and agencies to address transition needs.

POSTSECONDARY EDUCATION

Today, more than ever, students with disabilities are participating in postsecondary education. Postsecondary options include vocational/technical schools, community colleges, liberal arts colleges, and state or private universities. The number of students with disabilities applying and being admitted to institutions of higher education is increasing. In 1996, 9% of college freshmen reported having a disability compared to only 2.6% of freshmen in 1978.[108] Paul, citing the 1996 National Council for Education, stated that 1.4 million students (10.3%) in higher education reported having at least one disability.[85] Forty percent of these students with disabilities had orthopedic and neurology-related disabilities.

Planning for postsecondary education begins early in high school with selection of coursework and academic requirements.[40] Hitchings, Retisch, and Horvath reported that students with disabilities are often not prepared for postsecondary education.[53] Transition plans of 110 students in grades 10 through 12 who attended two Illinois high schools were reviewed. Student interest in postsecondary education declined over a 3-year period from 77% to 47%. Only four students had 4-year transition plans preparing them for postsecondary education. Based on their findings, the authors stated the following recommendations for successful transition to postsecondary education: (1) students must be successful in general education classes to determine if they can learn academic content and meet teacher and workload requirements with or without accommodations, (2) transition planning should begin in the late elementary years and be sustained throughout high school, (3) students must be their own advocates, (4) students must actively engage in the career development process, and (5) educators and professionals providing related services must have knowledge of current policy for transition planning.

Two significant pieces of legislation support students with disabilities admitted to colleges or universities. Section 504 of the Rehabilitation Act of 1973 and the Americans with Disabilities Act (ADA, P.L. 101-336) ensure nondiscriminatory protection for students with disabilities on campuses of higher education. Section 504 stipulates that any institution that receives federal funding must ensure access for all persons with disabilities and specifically stipulates equal opportunity for "otherwise qualified handicapped individuals."[85] The law also requires an "affirmative action obligation" on the part of institutions of higher education. Two purposes of the ADA are to provide "a national mandate for the elimination of discrimination against individuals with disabilities" and to provide strong "enforceable standards addressing discrimination against this population" (p. 201).[85] The ADA

mandates that all public and private businesses and institutions provide reasonable accommodations for persons with disabilities.[52] Federal legislation pertaining to youth with disabilities including the Individuals with Disabilities Education Improvement Act and the Americans with Disabilities Act are presented in Chapter 30.

College Admissions and Enrollment

Whereas education is a given opportunity for all children in the United States through high school, college is a self-chosen endeavor. The guarantees of a free and appropriate public education (FAPE), established under the auspices of IDEA for students with disabilities, do not extend to postsecondary institutions of learning. Instead, colleges and universities use the definition of disability in the ADA. The ADA defines a person with a disability as anyone who has a physical or mental impairment that substantially limits one or more major life activities, has a record of such impairment, or is regarded as having such impairment. Therefore, a qualified student with a disability applying to postsecondary education is one who is able to meet a program's admission, academic, and technical standards either with or without accommodation.[108] Section 504 utilizes the term "otherwise qualified" in extending the same recognition to potential students. Rothstein raised the issues of what can be asked at preadmission and when students should disclose a disability.[92] For example, a student may not want to disclose a physical disability before a campus visit; however, by not disclosing this information, the campus personnel may be put at a disadvantage by not having lead time to make adjustments that could facilitate the visit.

Reasonable accommodations in higher education can include barrier-free design, academic modifications (waiver of certain courses, lighter course loads, and alternative methods of testing) and specific disability services such as translators, tutors, and readers. Important considerations are whether accommodations can be provided without altering the nature of the academic program, without jeopardizing the safety of the student of record or others, and without creating an undue burden of a financial or administrative nature.[92]

The ADA underscores the importance of preparing students with disabilities to articulate their specific needs. For high school students with disabilities, an annual goal could be to plan their individualized education plan (IEP) meeting, which would generalize to skills in articulating requests once enrolled in college. More specifically, students with disabilities could be encouraged to generate the accommodations needed to complete the IEP document as well as list the criteria that would indicate goal attainment. An IEP goal in a high school speech and communication class may be that a student develop a plan of action for requesting accommodations and participate in a mock student service meeting to articulate requests. Zadra suggested preregistration interviews between students with disabilities and college counselors as an excellent strategy for students to communicate their needs and counselors to gather accurate and meaningful information.[85]

Campus Accessibility

Misquez, McCarthy, Powell, and Chu reported that the most significant impetus for making accessibility changes was having students with disabilities on college campuses.[78] Encouraging and supporting high school students with physical disabilities to take advantage of college campus visits will serve a double purpose. First, the students can request to sit in on a college class, they can travel across the campus grounds, and they can visit university resource centers, libraries, and dormitories. This can provide them with a better understanding of the spatial and temporal perimeters of attending a college as compared to a typically enclosed high school campus. Second, as more students with physical disabilities visit and attend colleges and universities, staff, faculty, and administrators will become more cognizant of barriers to campus accessibility. A specific IEP goal for the high school junior or senior may be to evaluate the accessibility of two college campuses using multiple resources such as web page searches, telephone interviews, and onsite visitations. In the state of Oregon, several high schools are converting to portfolios and certificates of initial mastery (CIM) and certificates of advanced mastery (CAM) of projects of interest to students. Researching college campus accessibility could potentially meet the requirements of completing a portfolio while simultaneously discovering important factors that would allow the student to make an informed decision on college applications. A student activity accessibility checklist developed by Roger Smith, Jill Warnke, and Dave Edyburn of the University of Wisconsin, Milwaukee, and Daryl Mellard, Noelle Kurth, and Gwen Berry of the University of Kansas is on the Evolve website. The form provides a comprehensive list of questions for students with disabilities visiting, applying to, and attending a college or university.

Attending college means living away from home for many students. Typically, freshman and sophomore students experience their first extended period away from home living arrangements in college dormitories. Beds, desks, and dressers are standard features, with students bringing the various amenities such as computers, mini-refrigerators, and stereo systems. Students often share living quarters with another student or a group depending on the configurations of the dorm rooms. For the student with a physical disability, room accessibility can be a major challenge. Physical therapists need to think long term when making decisions about interventions with students in primary and secondary education that could generalize to independence in a college dormitory room. If physical independence is not a feasible goal, then the student's ability to direct an attendant in physical management would be a more appropriate goal. In a high school health or physical education class, a student's IEP goals may include competency in directing others for identified tasks where or when physical assistance is needed. Skills for advertising, interviewing, and hiring and firing of attendants would also be critical. These could be experienced through role-play scenarios in a sociology or communication class.

Issues of Confidentiality

Unlike students with "hidden" disabilities such as a learning disability, students with physical disabilities are readily visible. Despite this, issues of confidentiality need to be respected and adhered to. High school students with disabilities need to know that institutions of higher education have policies regarding confidentiality. These policies should include (1) who can be informed, (2) who should be informed, (3) who must be informed, (4) who should not be informed, and (5) when and how any related waivers should be obtained.[92] High school educators and related services staff can assist students to be proactive in determining how they will disclose information. By being proactive, students with disabilities are demonstrating confidence, maturity, and self-esteem to the college personnel. Dukes reported that in higher education, 80% of people who administer disability services have 10 or fewer years of experience.[108] Students who have experienced disability since birth, therefore, may have more experience in disability and education than many college service providers.

Interaction with Instructors

Instructors in postsecondary education programs with different expectations than high-school teachers understandably may exceed a student's comfort zone and create anxiety on the part of both the student and faculty. Amsel and Fichten compared interactions between college students with and without disabilities and their professors.[4] Students with disabilities were less likely to request or accept assistance. Paradoxically, students without disabilities and professors believed it is quite appropriate for students with disabilities to ask for accommodations. The authors concluded that it is imperative that students with disabilities not misperceive the appropriateness of requests for assistance.

A theme that emerged from a qualitative study of faculty-student relationship was to personalize disability through students with disabilities sharing their personal story with their instructors.[11] When faculty members allowed students to share their stories, student empowerment was fostered in the classroom and was accompanied by persistence in higher education. Recommendations based on study findings included providing faculty members the students autobiography and for faculty members to (1) provide student's the opportunity to share information privately with them early in the semester, (2) ensure that all students in the class engage in respectful listening, and (3) use cooperative learning activities, where possible, which will allow for interaction and discussion among small groups of students.

WORK

One of the major life roles of youth transitioning to adulthood is gaining economic independence.[49] Ninety percent of youth with special health care needs reach their 21st birthday, an age when most young adults are either employed are seeking employment.[21] In the National Longitudinal Transition study, 40% of individuals with childhood onset health conditions were employed 2 years after high school as compared to a 63% employment rate for same-age peers at large.[114] Nationally, 23,000 individuals with severe disabilities participated in supported employment in 1988; by 2002, 118,000 individuals participated.[59] Though progress is slow, many youth with special health care needs continue wanting to work.

Employment options for people with disabilities can be viewed on a continuum from least restrictive without supports (community based) to most restrictive (segregated programs with supports) (Figure 32-1). In the 1960s through the 1980s, the primary employment options for people with severe disabilities were adult day programs and sheltered work programs. Supported employment is competitive work in integrated settings for individuals with disabilities for whom competitive employment has not traditionally occurred or for whom employment has been interrupted or intermittent because of a severe disability. These employees need ongoing support services to perform such work.[63] Supported employment includes the following: (1) provision of personalized job development, (2) on-the-job training, (3) ongoing support services, (4) individualized assessment (which is the opposite of norm-referenced assessment and placement), (5) person-centered job selection which relies on the person's personal network, and (6) use assessment and activities that are meaningful and relevant.

Supported employment uses the services of job coaches and on-the-job training and long-term follow-along by an employment specialist following along if needed. Supports provided by friends, family, and coworkers are encouraged. Rusch and Braddock reported a stalled pattern of supported employment since 2000, with work settings limited to people with disabilities outnumbering work settings in the community at large.[93] Competitive employment with supports is a form of customized employment, although not a traditional category of employment. This type of service assists the students who have the ability to work independently but lack the job-seeking skills, interview skills, and organizational skills to obtain employment. With this type of career guidance, students can move on to more challenging careers and postsecondary training.[40]

Recommendations to improve employment of youth with disabilities include development of a national Web-based system to coordinate entry into competitive employment, financial support availability through interagency partnerships, expanded guidance counseling services, and access to long-term support services.[93] Commentaries by Johnson[59] and Test[107] concur with Rusch and Braddock. Johnson concluded that improving graduation from postsecondary education or employment for students with disabilities outside sheltered workshops will depend on collaborative commitment from a wide base of constituents. Test suggested five strategies for achieving successful and meaningful economic independence: "(a) teach all students self-determination skills, (b) expand the mission of programs for 18- to 21-year-olds, (c) focus on interagency collaboration, (d) improve preparation of personnel, and (e) focus on the positive outcomes of supported employment" (p. 248).[107]

Successful work transition is dependent on competencies in essential job functions and provision of appropriate supports or job modifications. Transition services that enable youth to learn essential job functions that are compatible with their abilities should advance individuals toward successful employment. Opportunities for development of work life skills should be incorporated in activities and routines. Examples of work life skills include getting ready for work, transportation, keeping a schedule, appropriate work behavior and dress, communication with supervisors and work mates, eating and toileting, and directing attendants if and when necessary (Figure 32-2).

Learning skills for work transition can be incorporated into physical therapy interventions. For example, a young person receiving physical therapy at an outpatient clinic could be encouraged to schedule or cancel his or her own therapy appointments. Learning how to direct others in physical management is fostered through having youth role play with the therapist in activities such as transfers in and out of a wheelchair, dressing, and donning and doffing orthotics. Youth can be supported to initiate communication with local employment agencies such as Vocational Rehabilitation. Consultation to employers is an unfamiliar area for pediatric physical therapists; however, many colleagues in adult practice have been involved with workplace reentry. Pediatric physical therapists are encouraged to expand their

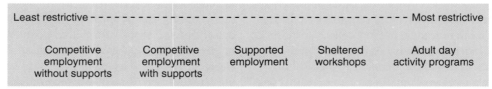

Figure 32-1   Continuum of employment settings for people with disabilities.

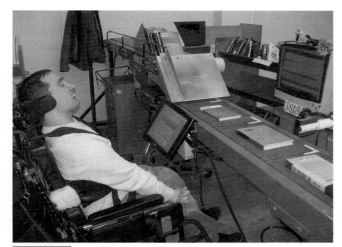

Figure 32-2   Using a Dynavox communication device, Andy enters books into inventory and prices them for sale at Powell's Books. He hits his right head switch, sending a book onto the conveyor belt to be scanned. His right head switch controls the Dynavox, which acts as a keyboard, sending infrared signals to the store's computer, which causes a price label to be printed.

scope of practice to include consultation with community organizations and agencies, such as a job site where specific job-related activities can be observed, analyzed, and solutions with or without accommodations developed.

One of the biggest challenges to work is the potential loss of Supplemental Security Income (SSI) and Social Security Disability Income (SSDI) if an individual makes "too much" income. Requirements of limited income will keep individuals at or below the poverty line as well as sustaining a dependency rather than building on self-determination, which has been emphasized throughout the chapter as an important element of transition to adulthood. Transition to work must include a review of potential income sources to include supplemental security and work-related income. Youth must understand the delicate balance between benefits such as Medicaid or Medicare and work and optimize the benefits of both at appropriate times during the transition process. For some youth and families, exploring trusts for long-term security and support is a component of future planning. Therapists could consider developing their role and skills in advocacy for local, state, and federal policy development that facilitates continued SSI benefits for physical management support regardless of income earnings.

TRANSPORTATION

Transportation is critical for all adult roles: education, work, adult living, and community participation. Youth with disabilities often lack reliable, cost-effective transportation options, which can limit social participation, friendships, and opportunities for work.[115] Learning mobility transportation skills should be addressed as part of a student's IEP and

transition plan. Skills such as using mobility devices independently and safely, accessing public transportation, identifying landmarks, and asking for directions can be developed as part of a community-based training program with assistance from the physical therapist, program staff, and family.[40]

Although the Americans with Disabilities Act mandates include public transportation accessibility, barriers still exist because of limited routes and may necessitate relocation to urban areas to increase transportation options. Students who use assistive walking devices or wheeled mobility may not be able to drive; therefore, they need to access alternative modes of transportation such as rides from coworkers or relatives, accessible public transportation, taxis, or program vans.[98] In 2004, President Bush released an executive order on Human Service Transportation Coordination to improve services for individuals with disabilities, older adults, and people with lower incomes. This was an effort to coordinate the 62 programs funding transportation, thereby reducing service duplication, consumer confusion, and service gaps. Partnership between the Coordinating Council on Access and Mobility (CCAM) and United We Ride was established to provide coordination and common-sense solutions for everyone who needs transportation.[51] In some areas, transportation funding may be offered as part of state Medicaid waiver programs and as part of Impairment Related Work Expenses under the Social Security Administration.

TRANSITION MODELS AND APPROACHES

Contemporary approaches to transition services reflect an ecologic orientation that emphasizes the importance of real-world experiences, supports, and community accommodations.[64,65] King and colleagues appraised the literature to determine the main types of transition approaches and strategies for youth with disabilities, including those with chronic health conditions, and identified four approaches: skills training, prevocational and vocational guidance, youth- and family-centered approaches, and ecologic and experiential options. Transition programs were often guided by more than one approach and utilized multiple strategies.

The focus of *skills training* is to prepare youth for independence and success in chosen adult roles. Kingsnorth, Healy, and Macarthur performed a systematic review and identified six studies that included a comparison group.[69] Five reported short-term improvements in targeted skills such as social skills, assertiveness, and self-efficacy. The programs used a variety of strategies including goal setting, coaching, and experiential learning.

Prevocational and vocational guidance aims to enhance self-awareness strategies including planning and goal setting.[45] Emphasis is on support and guidance, job-seeking skills, and on-the-job skills training.[94] Research findings support the importance of involving youth in decisions about their transition-related goals[95] and teaching skills in real-world contexts.[28,29]

The focus of a *youth- and family-centered* approach is empowerment of youth and families through emotional support and knowledge of community resources and supports. There is evidence of the effectiveness of social support in facilitating positive outcomes and increasing self-esteem.[50] Although family-centered services are considered best practice in pediatric rehabilitation, research is needed on the effectiveness of youth- and family-centered transition approaches.

An *ecologic and experiential* approach is based on the principle that real-world opportunities and experiences optimize skill development.[9,23] The focus is on development of life skills, interpersonal relationships, environmental modifications, and task accommodations. Strategies include linking youth and family to community supports, enhancing knowledge of community opportunities, coaching and mentoring, creating individualized opportunities and experiences, and community education and advocacy. The results of the National Longitudinal Transition study indicate that community-based work experience is more useful than school-based programs.[112] Students with and without disabilities who participated in work experiences in high school were twice as likely to have competitive employment 1 year after graduation from high school than students without work experience.[13]

Service coordination and interagency collaboration are keys to all transition approaches. An interagency transition team should consist of the student, parents, educators, adult service professionals, employers, and community service agencies. Sharing information, expertise, and problem solving are encouraged among team members in order to meet a student's postsecondary goals. Collaborative practices are facilitated through interagency agreements that clearly define roles, responsibilities, and strategies of each community member. Potential barriers to collaboration include ineffective transition planning meetings, intimidating language, and the complexity of agency procedures.[71,72]

Access and accommodation technologies also referred to as assistive technology and assistive technology services are integral to transition services for youth with severe disabilities.[73,89] Assistive technology is defined as technology applied to people with disabilities to enable productivity, communication, self-care, and mobility; to reduce the need for personal assistance; and to promote self-advocacy.[83] The application of assistive technology requires a team approach that begins with a thorough examination that includes assessment of the individual's needs, abilities, preferences, and features of the environment.[27,54]

RESEARCH ON TRANSITION OUTCOMES

In 1983, Congress mandated and funded the first National Longitudinal Transition Study (NLTS). The NLTS was designed to gather data on experiences of students with disabilities during the first 3 to 5 years after high school.

Interviews encompassing many facets of transition were completed with 1990 students and families. Although youth with disabilities made substantial progress, their employment rates, wages, postsecondary education, and residential independence were lower than peers without disabilities. Based on the findings, individualized transition planning that reflects the student's goals, strengths, needs, characteristics, and disability was recommended.[17]

A second National Longitudinal Transition Study (NLTS2) was conducted from 2000 to 2005. The sample included 11,272 students from 501 local education agencies (LEA). Students 13 to 16 years old when the study began were receiving special education across 12 special education categories. Methods were similar to those of the NLTS. In the NLTS2, fewer students were classified with mental retardation, whereas the number of students categorized as having other health impairment increased.[113] More youth with disabilities were living with at least one biologic parent and the heads of households were less likely to be unemployed or high school dropouts. The number of students with mental retardation or emotional disturbances living in poverty with an unemployed head of household increased between 1987 and 2001.

Parents in both National Longitudinal Transition Studies expected their children with disabilities to graduate from high school with a regular diploma. In the NLTS2, parents of youth with speech or hearing impairments had greater expectations for postsecondary education. Overall, 2-year colleges were considered more of an option in 2001 than in 1987 and employment expectations were higher. Parental expectations for employment of youth with mental retardation, hearing impairment, other health impairments, and multiple disabilities increased.[113]

In the NLTS2, participation of students with disabilities in extracurricular activity remained lower than it did for their peers without disability. In 2001, significantly more youth with disabilities had paid jobs 1 year after graduation. The 1-year employment rate was 60%, which is similar to youth in the general population (63%). Youth had an increase in work-study jobs and pay but a decline in the average number of hours worked per week. In social adjustment, more youth with disabilities were suspended or expelled, fired from a job, or arrested in 2001 than in 1987.[113]

Several factors have been identified as predictors of postsecondary education and employment among students who receive transition services. Vocational education, attending a rural school, work-study participation, and having a learning disability (versus another condition) were predictors of full-time employment after graduation in a random sample of 140 graduates from special education programs interviewed 1 and 3 years following graduation.[6] Attending a suburban school and participating in general education curriculum were predictors of postsecondary education. Benz, Lindstrom, and Yovanoff reported that career-related work experience and completion of student identified transition goals were associated with improved graduation and employment outcomes.[12] Students valued individualization of services and personalized attention. Halpern et al. identified the following predictors of success in postsecondary education: (1) high scores on a functional achievement inventory, (2) completing instruction successfully in relevant curricular areas, (3) participating in transition planning, (4) parent satisfaction with secondary education, (5) student satisfaction with secondary education, and (6) parent perception that the student no longer needed help in certain critical skill areas.[48] Critical skills that might pertain to physical therapy include community mobility, use of public transportation, use of restroom, positioning and mobility instruction for personal care attendants, positioning for work or postsecondary education activities, and proficiency with assistive technology.

Betz reviewed 12 studies that examined transition programs for youth with special health care needs and concluded that research is in the exploratory stage of inquiry.[14] None of the studies reviewed identified the program's conceptual or theoretic frameworks. Studies were characterized by a lack of information on the youth receiving transition services and the services that were provided. None of the studies had a control group. Few measures had been examined for reliability and validity. The primary focus of the studies reviewed was on medical aspects of transition.

Stewart et al. performed a comprehensive literature search to identify factors that help or hinder the transition process and the effectiveness of transition services for youth with disabilities.[102] Five review articles were appraised. Skill development, environmental supports, and an individualized approach were identified as important components of transition services. Stewart and associates stated that the reviews focused more on specific strategies rather than the overall approach or service model. Authors of all five reviews stated that there is a need for more research.

Binks et al. performed a systematic review of outcomes specific to the transition from child-centered to adult-centered health care for youth with cerebral palsy or spina bifida.[16] Elements associated with successful transition to adult-centered health care were (1) preparation, (2) flexible timing of transition programs with a suggested age of 14 to 16 years, (3) care coordination that includes an up to date transition plan, (4) transition clinic visits including a consult with both the child and adult health care providers, and (5) interested adult-centered health care providers. A limitation of many of the studies reviewed is that strategies had not been implemented consistently or formally evaluated.

TRANSITION PLANNING IN THE EDUCATION SYSTEM

In 1983, Madeline Will, assistant secretary of the U.S. Office of Special Education and Rehabilitation Services, proposed a *bridges model* for transition of youth from school to work that emphasizes linkages between school and postschool environments.[118] The model identifies three possible bridges: (1) transition without special services, (2) transition with time-limited services, and (3) transition with ongoing services.[41] Subsequently, Halpern proposed *community adjustment* and *work preparation* models.[41] The community adjustment model is based on three pillars of community inclusion: employment, residential environments, and social networks. The work preparation model includes the four elements of transition services described in the Individuals with Disabilities Education Improvement Act (IDEA): (1) based on student needs, preferences, and interests, (2) a coordinated set of activities, (3) an outcome-oriented process, and (4) a progression from school to postschool activities.[41,61] Several promising practices for successful transition have been proposed by advocates, researchers, and policymakers.[70,87] These practices include (1) development of student self-efficacy and social skills, (2) community and paid work experiences, (3) technology to improve accessibility and accommodation, (4) secondary curricular reform, (5) vocational career education, (6) supports for postsecondary education, (7) service coordination and interagency collaboration, and (8) individualized backward planning in which the outcome is first identified and then a transition plan is developed.

The Individuals with Disability Act (IDEA) of 1990 mandated an outcome-oriented process that included transition services, beginning at age 16. The statement of transition services, also known as the individualized transition plan (ITP), ensures that IEP activities help prepare the student for roles following secondary education. In most states, the ITP is included as a page or section of a student's IEP. The plan is reviewed annually and includes coordinated activities that are based on a student's needs and preferences.[41] These might include instruction, community experiences, career development, daily living skills training, functional vocational evaluation, and linkages with adult services.[41] Reauthorization of IDEA in 1997 lowered the age to begin transition services to 14 years. District and state testing was mandated in order to hold schools accountable for the student's progress in the general curriculum. Related services, including physical therapy, were added in the definition of transition services. The Perkins Technical and Vocational Act of 1998 (Public Law 105-332) emphasized the quality of vocational education and the need for supplemental services for individuals with special needs.

The Individuals with Disabilities Education Improvement Act of 2004 redefined the age of transition to 16 years and moved to a "results-oriented" process focusing on improving students' academic and functional achievement to promote postschool outcomes. Accountability was emphasized by requiring the transition plan to include appropriate measurable postsecondary goals. Transition services are defined as follows:

A coordinated set of activities for a student, with a disability, that: (A) is designed within a results oriented process, that is focused on improving the academic and functional achievement of the child with a disability to facilitate the child's movement from school to post-school activities, including postsecondary education, vocational education, integrated employment (including supported employment), continuing and adult education, adult services, independent living, or community participation; (B) is based on the student's needs, taking into account the student's strengths, preferences and interests; (C) includes instruction, related services, community experiences, the development of employment and other post-school objectives, and, when appropriate, acquisition of daily living skills and functional vocational evaluation. (Section 602, IDEA, 2004)

Preparation of students with disabilities for postsecondary education, employment (including supported employment), independent living, and community participation must begin no later than 16 years of age under IDEA but can begin earlier. Goals must be measurable and progress tracked and reported. Local education agencies are required to provide students with a summary of their academic and functional performance along with recommendations for postsecondary environments upon exiting from school. Mandates for databased, coordinated transition planning and reporting of outcomes are ambitious and require considerable personnel development for implementation.[88]

Transition planning begins with determining the student's interests, abilities, strengths, and needs. The family and professionals should discuss future options with the student. The transition plan is completed at the IEP/ITP meeting. Postschool outcomes are identified and activities are coordinated within the school team and with external agencies and organizations. Students should be invited to the IEP/ITP meeting, actively participate, and lead the meeting when able. Representatives from adult service agencies often are present to assist the school team in planning services for students who are eligible for their services. The team, which includes the student, determines the types of transition services (instruction, related services, community experiences, daily living skills, and functional vocational evaluation) necessary to promote movement to postschool environments. Finally, the transition plan includes measurable goals developed by the team. A transition plan for a student with severe disabilities who uses powered mobility and a communication device in vocational environments is included on the Evolve website.

Although in the past, physical therapists have not fully participated in the transition process, they have important roles. Physical therapists are encouraged to (1) prepare youth to be active participants and ideally leaders in developing their IEP; (2) participate in the transition planning process when invited by the student; (3) provide consultation and direct services, as needed, for seating, transfers, mobility, self-care, wellness and fitness, instruction for personal care attendants, assistive technology, and environmental modifications; and (4) work collaboratively with school personnel to ensure that health and physical function are adequately addressed in the school-based ITP. The transition plan on the Evolve website illustrates services and activities that may be supported by a physical therapist.

COMMUNITY- AND HOSPITAL-BASED TRANSITION PROGRAMS

Community- and hospital-based transition programs are emerging and vary considerably in focus and scope. In this section, we summarize four programs. Many of the ideas presented are included in the Life Needs Model.[68] The Life Needs Model (Figure 32-3) is a collaborative approach to service delivery designed to meet the long-term goals of community participation and quality of life for children and youth with disabilities. Core values of community- and hospital-based transition programs for youth with physical disabilities that we propose are listed in Box 32-1.

An early effort was the Children's Healthcare Options Improved through Collaborative Efforts and Services (CHOICES) transition project, one of nine projects in the Maternal and Child Health Bureau's Healthy and Ready to Work Network. As a joint effort of the U.S. Bureau of Maternal and Child Health and Shriners Hospitals for Children, CHOICES was designed to create a continuum of health and social services for young people with disabilities.[20] The recommendation was for a transition plan that included specific goals for independence and self-management and a flexible time frame to support the increasing capacity of youth for choice and self-advocacy. Low expectations, lack of knowledge, and lack of skills were identified as common barriers to successful transition. The Healthy & Ready to Work website (www.hrtw.org/tools/index.html) includes information, resources, assessment tools, and strategies for youth and their families, health care providers, and state and local agencies to achieve successful transition from pediatric to adult health care.

Gall, Kingsnorth, and Healy described a shared management approach to transition services for youth with disabilities implemented at Bloorview Kids Rehab in Toronto, Ontario, Canada.[44] The shared management approach is based on the philosophy that development of a therapeutic alliance between youth, families, and health care providers is essential to allow young people with disabilities to develop into independent and healthy adults. As illustrated in Figure 32-4, the therapeutic alliance is conceptualized as a dynamic relationship in which the roles change over time as the child grows and develops. A gradual shift in responsibilities occurs over time, and leadership is transitioned from the health care provider and parents to the young person, to

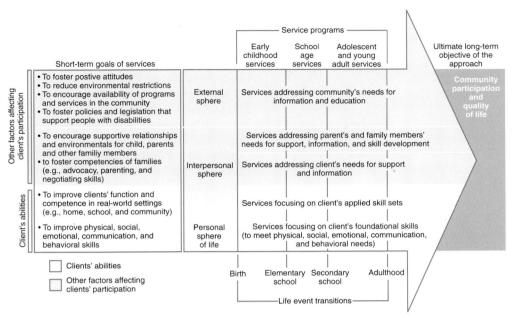

Figure 32-3   Life needs model of service delivery.

<table>
<tr><td>Box 32-1</td><td>PROPOSED CORE VALUES OF COMMUNITY- AND HOSPITAL-BASED TRANSITION PROGRAMS FOR YOUTH WITH PHYSICAL DISABILITIES</td></tr>
</table>

- Youth and family centered
- Partnerships
- Strength-based
- Self-determination
- Experiential learning

---

the maximum extent possible. Youth are encouraged to use experiential learning to gain exposure to opportunities and develop life skills. The program website (www.bloorview. ca/resourcecentre/familyresources/growingupready.php) includes timetables, checklists, and guidelines for service providers.

The Youth En Route Program in London, Ontario, Canada, is distinguished for being one of the first transition programs for youth and young adults with multiple disabilities to systematically evaluate processes and outcomes.[38] Jan Evans, a physical therapist, and Patricia Baldwin, an occupational therapist, were instrumental in development of the program. Youth and young adults 16 to 29 years with multiple disabilities who have completed secondary education are eligible for the program. The program was implemented through a partnership between Thames Valley Children's Centre and Hutton House, a community agency for

adults with disabilities. The service model is based on self-determination and community participation (Figure 32-5). A multifaceted approach is utilized that includes (1) self-discovery, (2) skill development, and (3) community experience. Self-determination is promoted through coaching and supporting youth to define, lead, and guide the services and supports they want as they learn more about themselves and their communities. Efforts are made to support youth goals for employment, education, voluntarism, and leisure with experiential opportunities within the community. The program evaluation consisted of a 1-year pre/posttest of 34 participants in the program. Statistical and clinically significant improvements were found in self-determination and sense of personal control. At posttest, youth reported spending more time on volunteer/work and community leisure activities. The authors emphasize the importance of a flexible, client-centered approach that offers youth opportunities for self-discovery, skill development, and community experiences.

The Center of Innovation in Transition (CITE) and Employment at Kent State University in Ohio provides leadership in graduate education and transition practices for youth 18 to 21 years with disabilities. The center includes several research and demonstration projects for graduate education that serve students with disabilities in the community. The Kent State Transition Collaborative (KSTC) is a joint program between the Transition Center and local public schools. Local high school students with disabilities participate in a continuum of job training and career experiences on the Kent State campus. Graduate students from

Provider →	Parent/family →	Young person
☐ Major responsibility	☐ Provide care	☐ Receives care
☐ Support to parent/family and child/youth	☐ Manages	☐ Participates
☐ Consultant	☐ Supervisor	☐ Manager
☐ Resource	☐ Consultant	☐ Supervisor

Figure 32-4 Shared management model. (Data from Kieckhefer, G. M. [2002]. *Foundations for successful transitions: shared management as one critical component.* Keynote presentation at the Hospital for Sick Children, Toronto, Canada.)

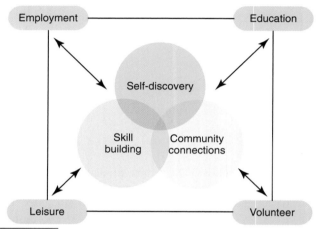

Figure 32-5 Model for Youth En Route Program. (From Evans, J., McDougall, J., & Baldwin, P. [2006]. Printed with permission of authors.)

several disciplines obtain practical experience in providing transition services. The objective of the collaborative is to prepare students with disabilities for competitive employment by providing them opportunities for future planning, skill development, and self-advocacy and to prepare transition coordinators of the future. Since 1985, 20 to 40 high school students with severe disabilities have been provided career exploration and job training each year. In most cases, these students transition to supported employment and community living. More than 100 graduates of the transition coordinator training programs have become transition leaders throughout the state and country.

The Campus Transition Project (CTP), funded by the National Institute on Disability and Rehabilitation Research, is a new program to develop sustainable community-based programs for students with severe disabilities, aged 18 to 21. The project uses the college environment to enable students to experience transitional activities and receive individual instruction to improve skills. Serving 10 students yearly, activities are directed at increasing independence, improving

social skills, self-determination, mobility, and age-appropriate leisure and recreation interests.

The Career and Self Advocacy Program (CASAP) was developed to support educators preparing students with mild to moderate disabilities for adult life. Funded by the U.S. Department of Education, the program focuses around three themes: self-advocacy, goal setting and IEPs, and postsecondary options. A course using content enhancement materials, self-advocacy strategies, life-centered career education, and transition planning is offered for high school students ages 14 through 21. This project served more than 100 middle and high school students over the 4 years of the project. Student participants develop a PowerPoint presentation for leading their IEP meetings, with renewal students presenting at a regional professional meeting. Information on all programs offered by the Center for Innovation in Transition can be accessed at www.ehhs.kent.edu/cite.

Physical therapists may find information on the website useful for implementation of job exploration and self-advocacy programs for high school students with physical disabilities. Of particular interest may be the opportunities for professional development in the area of transition to adulthood that is available to all professionals who work with high school students with disabilities. The center's hands-on programs are unique as they bring together community resources and local high schools in a collaborative model to better serve high school students by giving them opportunities to experience the college environment and training them in self-advocacy and job skills, while giving professionals opportunities for education in the transition field.

ROLE OF THE PHYSICAL THERAPIST IN THE TRANSITION PROCESS

Preparing youth with physical disabilities for transition to the adult care system and postsecondary education, work, and community living is an emerging role of the physical therapist. In 1997, Campbell proposed that preparing individuals with physical disabilities to take personal responsibility for their health and physical fitness should begin at a young age.[24] Although physical therapists have worked in public schools for more than 30 years, the IDEA of 1997 was the first educational law to include related services as mandated services in transition. Several authors have suggested roles for physical therapists in the transition process including the following:[3,24,35,57,97,109]

1. Assessing present or future environments utilizing an ecologic approach
2. Assessing assistive technology needs and instruction of others in use of assistive technology
3. Intervening for positioning, seating, transfers, mobility, and transportation

4. Assisting with job development, coaching, and placement options
5. Anticipating student needs for community living and work
6. Promoting community leisure and health related fitness activities
7. Facilitating transition to adult health care services
8. Collaborating with other professionals, staff, and community-based agencies to coordinate services

Physical therapists working in educational settings may provide consultative services during individualized education program (IEP/ITP) meetings. Therapists may provide direct services during times of the day when the student is on the job, at a postsecondary school, or participating in community recreation. Therapists also provide information and instruction of others including care providers, educators, and family members.[3,97] Though likely more challenging because of the nature of third-party payer systems and no federally mandated school environment practice legislation, therapists working in noneducational practice settings are encouraged to consider these universally shared roles to facilitate youth-to-adult transitions.

The *Guide to Physical Therapy Practice* provides support for the role of the physical therapist, regardless of practice environment, in transition planning and services in all three sections: patient management, preferred practice patterns, and special test and measures.[3,106] The guide states that physical therapists should provide procedural interventions across the life span in the following areas: (1) environmental barriers, (2) self-care and home management (including activities of daily living), (3) work (job/school/play), (4) community and leisure integration, and (5) orthotic, protective, and supportive devices. Box 32-2 lists areas for physical therapist examination for transition services adapted from the guide.

Physical therapist examination, evaluation, and intervention are driven by youth needs and preferences and should occur in specific and relevant environments, present and future. Three environments that physical therapists are encouraged to consider during the transition years are (1) work or postsecondary education settings, (2) adult living environments, and (3) community settings for leisure or social participation. In addition, examination and intervention must be approached from a perspective of future inclusive community living and work rather than segregated living and work. The three components of physical therapist intervention apply to all practice settings and include (1) coordination, communication, and documentation; (2) patient/client-related instruction; and (3) procedural interventions.[3] Box 32-3 lists the types of interventions provided by physical therapists during the transition process. For component 2, the phrase "student- or youth-related instruction" is preferred in the context of transition services.

BOX 32-2 EXAMINATION FOR TRANSITION SERVICES BASED ON THE GUIDE TO PHYSICAL THERAPIST PRACTICE

What should physical therapists examine for transition planning?
• Seating
• Transfers
• Mobility
• Self-care
• Leisure interests and activities
• Device and equipment use

How should therapists examine students for transition planning?
• Measures that describe and quantify
• Checklists/scales
• Logs, interviews (student interest/preferences survey)
• Observations (ecologic assessment/task analysis)
• Transportation assessments
• Questionnaires
• Video/pictures

Where should therapists evaluate students for transition planning?
• Home
• Community sites including recreation facilities
• Postsecondary education environments including university and community
• Job site

What data are generated from a physical therapy examination for transition planning?
• Descriptions of environment and barriers
• Student functioning in the environment
• Ability to participate in environments
• Need for equipment

EXAMINATION AND EVALUATION

The examination begins with identification of the youth's participation goals, reinforcing a person-centered approach. In the *Guide to Physical Therapist Practice*, this is part of the interview phase of the examination. We believe it is important for youth to express interest in self-discovery, experiential learning, and skill development and a need for families to express a willingness to support and engage in activities to prepare their children for adult roles.

Next a task analysis is performed to identify what is necessary to accomplish the goals. The task analysis will guide the examination and evaluation of what the youth can do (strengths) and what problems, challenges, and barriers need to change for achievement of goals. The examination should be interactive with full participation of the youth and her or his family. Areas of examination by physical therapists are

| Box 32-3 | PHYSICAL THERAPY INTERVENTIONS FOR TRANSITION PLANNING BASED ON THE GUIDE TO PHYSICAL THERAPIST PRACTICE |

COORDINATION, COMMUNICATION, AND DOCUMENTATION

- Participation in the IEP process
- Collaboration with agencies: equipment suppliers, transportation agencies
- Data collection/document changes
- Interdisciplinary teamwork
- Referrals to other professional sources

STUDENT/YOUTH-RELATED INSTRUCTION

Instruction, education, and training of student and caregiver regarding:
- Current condition
- Enhancement of performance
- Health wellness, fitness programs
- Transitions across settings
- Transitions to new roles

PROCEDURAL INTERVENTIONS

- Interventions for impairments in body functions and structures
- Functional training in self-care and home management
  Task adaptation
  Travel training
  Eating, dressing, grooming, toileting
  Shopping
- Functional training in work (job/play/school)
  Job program
  Device use
  Task training
  Travel training
  Job coaching
  Safety
  Leisure training
- Prescription, application, fabrication of devices and equipment
  Environmental controls
  Mobility devices, both ambulatory and powered mobility

often directed toward optimization of health status, functional ability, and self-management. Evaluation involves interpretation of examination findings to identify participation restrictions, activity limitations, and contributing impairments in body functions and structures. The physical therapist's examination and evaluation contributes to the assessments performed by other members of the interprofessional team, including future planning, knowledge, skills, supports, and current participation in school and community activities related to transition.

GOALS AND PLAN OF CARE

The collaboration of youth, parent(s), and professionals leads to development of a transition plan (plan of care). This plan will include person-centered, objective, and measurable long-term goals and short-term objectives. Therapists are encouraged to consider long-term goals for activity and participation and short-term objectives for body functions and structures, and personal, and environmental factors hypothesized to contribute to activity limitations and participation restrictions. The plan of care should include collaboration with community providers, organizations, and agencies. Combining the evaluations of all members of the transition team is essential for identifying youth-centered goals for activity and participation that are meaningful in daily life. It is unlikely that a participation goal would be solely single system domain (motor, cognitive, behavioral, self-help, etc.). Key actions, time frames, and individuals responsible for implementation should be noted. Who are the community collaborators you would identify in your practice area to accomplish the goals of the transition plan you created earlier?

Members for the interprofessional team will vary based on each youth's strengths, needs, program staff, and community resources. A transition coordinator ensures communication and coordination among team and external agencies and organizations. Have you ever considered positioning the youth or parent as coordinator to facilitate empowerment and diminish provider dependency? What value does such an approach render? What fears or apprehensions might you have about transferring this responsibility? Although any team member may serve as the transition coordinator, knowledge of community resources and services is important. This knowledge enriches the services and supports phase of the transition process. How well do you know your local, regional, and state resources? Youth and family learning styles and preferred methods of communication are important in determining formats for providing information, self-determination strategies, educational materials, and instruction.

Early communication and correspondence with adult health care providers is a key to transition. Physical therapists can educate youth about maintaining optimal physical function by adopting a lifestyle that promotes health and wellness through activities and sports. Physical therapists in community and hospital settings can develop and utilize linkages with the school-based team and other local resources to ensure effective communication and coordination of services.

The physical therapist may consult and provide procedural interventions for positioning, transfers, mobility, self-care, transportation, recreation, and leisure activities. Environmental modifications, assistive technology, and task

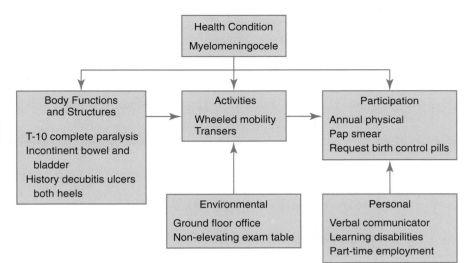

Figure 32-6 ICF framework applied to an 18-year-old female accessing the adult health care system.

accommodations are important for household management, postsecondary education, and vocational training. Services are designed to optimize safety, efficiency, and independence in performance of functional tasks in real-life settings. Before youth leave the pediatric health care system, physical therapists can help them to identify therapy needs and services and to communicate with the adult health care providers they chose.

Progress is monitored and documented at each physical therapist encounter. Services and supports are modified as necessary for achievement of short-term objectives and long-term goals. When objectives are met, services are progressed or altered accordingly. When goals are achieved, the transition plan is updated and new goals written.

The ICF framework is used to present three scenarios for transition services that are presented in Figure 32-6 through Figure 32-8. The first case involves a young woman accessing the adult health care system, the second involves a young man attending a university, and the third involves a young man who has applied for a job. As suggested in Chapter 1, the arrows between the three components of health and environmental and personal factors are specific to each case. Cover up all but the components of activity and participation. What are the environmental contexts for each example? Are the activity and participation entities adult or youth transition oriented? How often have you been future oriented enough to consider such examples? Now think about and list all the steps (task analysis) necessary to fully accomplish each activity. Do not look at the health condition of each youth, to avoid preconceived notions. What physical therapy decisions would you make for each case? What additional information is needed to formulate a plan of care? What tests and measures would you consider administering for each case? What information is specific to physical therapy and what can be acquired through interprofessional collaboration?

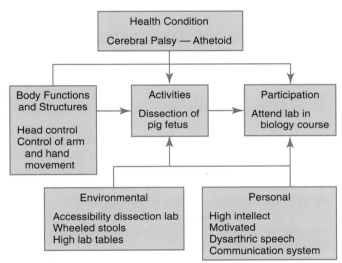

Figure 32-7 ICF framework applied to a 21-year-old male enrolled in a university biology course.

Write a long-term goal and short-term objective for each case. Is your goal person/patient/client centered? Is your goal measurable? Is your goal for activity or participation? Is your objective measurable? Are the measurement criteria appropriate? Based on the goal and objective you wrote for each example, what are indicators that outcomes have been achieved?

What are the current barriers to your embracing this process? Were you able to proceed through this process using the chapter examples without focused attention to the individual health conditions? As an exercise, interchange the health conditions for each example. How does the process change, if at all?

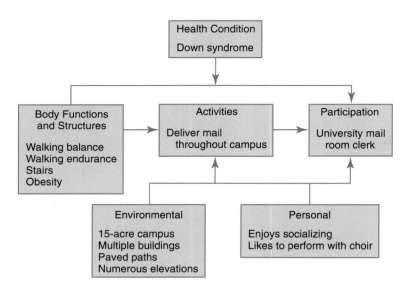

Figure 32-8 ICF framework applied to work considerations for a young adult applying for a job.

PHYSICAL THERAPIST PARTICIPATION IN TRANSITION PLANNING

The extent to which and how physical therapists employed in educational settings participate in transition planning and services are not well understood and even less so in other practice environments. A study conducted in Virginia found that occupational therapists and physical therapists did not participate fully in the transition process for students with severe physical disabilities.[46] In reviewing the attendance at IEP meetings, Getzel and DeFur reported that occupational and physical therapists rarely participated in the meetings, although students received services such as material adaptations and assistive technology from these disciplines.[46] In related studies of occupational therapists' involvement in transition, Inge[56] and Anderson[5] found that therapists were minimally involved in transition planning and transition services. Inge[56] reported that 61% of the respondents did not provide transition services to students 14 to 22 years old. Therapists who were providing services to students in secondary education indicated that the majority of their caseloads consisted of students under age 13. Occupational therapists reported that they did not attend transition planning meetings and did not have time to work with other team members to integrate their interventions into the students' transition plan.

Although it appears that physical therapists are minimally involved with transition planning and services, they have the expertise to intervene in areas that are often barriers to employment, independent living, and recreation for young adults with disabilities.[24,97] In James's qualitative study of five students with multiple disabilities transitioning to adulthood, students, families, and teachers stated that needs for assistive technology, use of transportation, and difficulties with toileting were insurmountable obstacles.[58] In a survey of pediatric physical therapists and occupational therapists, therapists identified themselves as practicing below an optimal level in promoting community recreation and leisure for children and adolescents with disabilities and their families.[109] For example, many therapists stated they were not discussing transportation options, barriers to accessing community facilities, or gathering information on social barriers.

Reasons why physical therapists are not routinely involved with transition services for students with physical disabilities in secondary education and the effects of physical therapist intervention on transition outcomes have not been investigated. Factors associated with professional preparation and cost of services may well impact on physical therapist involvement in transition planning and services in all practice settings (school, hospital, community). Professional education in pediatrics usually focuses on young children, with limited content on young and aging adults with developmental disabilities; physical therapists working with adults in hospitals or outpatient clinics are often not aware of issues common to adults with developmental disabilities.[30]

Practice settings often dictate the parameters for intervention. In contrast to hospitals and clinics, school-based practice is guided by federal and state legislation. Emphasis is on enhancing student participation in the education program. Transition is a natural part of the education process as the student advances through primary, middle, and secondary grades and schools. Interventions by physical therapists working in the hospital setting often emphasize impairments in body functions and structures because of the acute nature of hospital admissions. Outpatient clinics, be they based in a hospital or private practice, generally do not have the typical real-world environment that is the context for activity and participation. Though professional organizations have embraced the ICF model, it is unknown how embedded this model is in any of the practice environments. Hospital and clinic practice settings are more likely to view the youth as a "patient" and are thus more likely to focus on interventions for body functions and structures rather than participation. Communication between practitioners in any or all of these practice environments is especially critical at times of transitions.

ADULTS WITH CHILDHOOD ONSET DISABILITIES

Demographics on adults with childhood-onset conditions underscore the importance of quality services to prepare youth with disabilities to transition to adulthood. Advances in health care since the late 1980s have increased the life span of individuals with childhood onset conditions; 50% to 90% of adolescents with cerebral palsy, spina bifida, and acquired brain injury live into adulthood.[121] Approximately 200,000 individuals with developmental disabilities are over the age of 60, a number that is expected to double by 2030.[30] Further, more students with disabilities are pursuing postsecondary, higher education than ever before.[53]

As pediatric physical therapists strive to assist youth and young adults with physical disabilities in their transition to the adult health care system, a number of issues warrant consideration. Depending on the physical therapy education program attended and years since graduation, physical therapists whose practice is limited to adults may have limited knowledge of childhood onset conditions. As a consequence, they may be uncomfortable providing interventions for secondary impairments such as pain, fatigue, and musculoskeletal contractures in adults with childhood onset conditions. When referring youth who have aged out of the pediatric health care system, pediatric physical therapists are encouraged to enthusiastically offer consultation or shared intervention with their colleagues in adult practice settings. Proactively preparing youth to interact with adult providers is encouraged. For some youth, this might entail creating therapeutic/medical vocabulary for their augmentative communication systems in order to independently express concerns and respond to questions during the examination. We must continually ask ourselves how best to prepare young people with disabilities for transition to adulthood.

PROFESSIONAL RESOURCES FOR PHYSICAL THERAPISTS

The Evolve website includes a list of recommended websites with resources on transition for youth, family, and professionals. The websites include transition manuals, forms for screening and assessment, checklists, and transition activities. For the most part, the psychometric properties of measures and the utility of planning and activity resources have not been evaluated.

ADOLESCENTS AND ADULTS WITH DEVELOPMENTAL DISABILITIES SPECIAL INTEREST GROUP

The Adolescents and Adults with Developmental Disabilities Special Interest Group (AADD SIG) was established by the Section on Pediatrics of the American Physical Therapy Association (APTA) in 2001 to meet the professional development needs of therapists providing services to adolescents and adults with developmental disabilities. The goals are to provide a forum for therapists to meet, network, and promote quality care through education, research, and practice. The focus of the SIG includes (1) examination and prevention of impairments in adults with developmental disabilities to ensure maximum participation in society, (2) development of intervention guidelines for the adult with developmental disabilities, and (3) promotion of advocacy for adults with developmental disabilities through research and education.[31] The membership of the SIG and educational opportunities continue to grow and can be accessed through www.pediatricapta.org.

TASK FORCE ON CONTINUUM OF CARE

In 2005, the House of Delegates of the American Physical Therapy Association passed legislation (RC 34-05) to address issues in transitioning persons with lifelong disabilities to adult-oriented health care by doing the following:

- Identifying core knowledge and skills for delivering care and addressing the transition needs of adolescents and adults with lifelong disabilities
- Incorporating the core knowledge and skills into appropriate association documents
- Developing a plan for communicating and educating physical therapists regarding the importance of these issues in practice

A six-member consultant group was convened to address this initiative. A document that addressed each of these areas was completed in 2006. The following is the summary statement:

> APTA, the Section on Pediatrics, and stakeholders within other APTA Components will share responsibility for developing tools and initiatives to enhance the quality of physical therapist care for individuals with lifelong disabilities and promote the role of the physical therapists in increasing access to and coordination of care for these individuals.

APTA-invited members and consumer representatives subsequently met to discuss the continuum of care for individuals with lifelong disabilities (LLDs).

A task force was formed to address the issues in transition of people with lifelong disabilities to adult-oriented health care and to further the physical therapists' role in the prevention, diagnosis, and treatment of movement dysfunctions of people with developmental disabilities. Four goal areas were identified:

1. Improve the content of entry-level physical therapist education within the context of a doctoring profession.
2. Educate members and stakeholders to create an environment of autonomous practice for physical therapists working with people with LLDs.
3. Explore and promote the role of physical therapists in a variety of practice settings to the membership and public.

4. Explore the magnitude of the issues in providing care to people with lifelong disabilities.

The task force divided responsibilities into the following areas: white paper writing committee, fact sheet development, and education committee. At the time of publication, an APTA-endorsed white paper was under review. Fact sheets and a website on the continuum of care for individuals with lifelong health conditions were in the process of development.

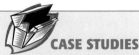

CASE STUDIES

Transition—passage from one state/stage to another—must also transpire for the physical therapist in terms of best practices for youth transitioning to adulthood. It is imperative that physical therapists address the future-oriented participation roles of children and youth through person-centered goals and age-appropriate interventions. This requires consideration of personal and environmental factors pertinent to the youth's goals. Therapists are encouraged to collaborate with adult-oriented colleagues as well as community agencies. The first case study describes a youth transitioning to an employment environment. As you read this case, ask yourself what elements you are implementing in your practice that parallel the case. In the second case, a physical therapist in a school-based setting describes her personal transformation as she serves students who are transitioning from high school to adulthood. Her story illustrates a future-oriented process for expanding the scope of therapy services for youth with disabilities. Choose a young person currently on your caseload and identify changes you will make in your practice based on the second case.

"John"

John is a 22-year-old who recently transitioned from high school to part-time community employment. He has athetoid cerebral palsy. John has no family support and lives in foster care.

He uses a communication device that allows him to select picture/word symbols for communication in a variety of environments and drives a power chair. Limited information is available regarding his cognitive abilities such as reading and computational skills. John's postsecondary school goals include employment and supported living with peers. He attended a public high school and received special education and related services. During high school, John participated in job training programs in the community. The case describes transition services during John's last 3 years of high school to illustrate (1) John's development of employment skills, (2) collaborative activities by education system and adult service providers, and (3) the services provided by the physical therapist. The evidence to practice box summarizes issues pertaining to the case study.

EVIDENCE TO PRACTICE 32-1

CASE STUDY "JOHN"

The extent of how physical therapists are involved with transition-age students is not well understood. There is a paucity of evidence, as only two studies have investigated this role and one is unpublished. Getzel and deFur discovered that physical therapists and occupational therapists rarely participated in transition meetings, even though students received their services.[1] Sylvester found that physical therapists were not addressing postsecondary needs for the students they served.[3]

Often students did not know why they received physical therapy services, and services seemed irrelevant. The goals of the services were impairment focused (e.g., "hold his head up") and irrelevant to future employment, education, and adult living. Further, therapists tended to use the same phrases on multiple IEPs, which did not reflect students'

individualized needs and preferences. The therapists who appeared to be focusing on traditional impairment-focused models of intervention stated that therapy services should decrease as a student ages and that cost was a barrier to providing transition services. Therapists also stated that transition teams did not expect them to be out in the community with students.[3]

1. Getzel, E., & deFur, S. (1997). Transition planning for students with significant disabilities: Implications for student centered planning. *Focus on Autism and Other Developmental Disabilities, 12*(1), 39–48.
2. James, S. (2001). *I was prepared to do nothing; I will do nothing: Why students with multiple disabilities do not have jobs after leaving high school.* Unpublished master's thesis, University of Oklahoma, Oklahoma City.
3. Sylvester, L. (2007, October). *Physical therapy: Achieving postsecondary outcomes.* Presentation at the Division on Career Development and Transition Conference.

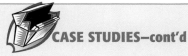

CASE STUDIES—cont'd

EVIDENCE TO PRACTICE 32-1—cont'd

COMMUNITY-BASED VOCATIONAL TRAINING

John's participation in community-based vocational training was an important factor in his ability to obtain community employment at graduation. According to findings from the National Longitudinal Transition Study,[2] community-based work experience is more useful than school-based programs. Students with and without disabilities who participate in work experiences in high school are twice as likely to have competitive employment after graduation than as a student without work experience.[1]

1. Benz, M. R., Lindstrom, L., & Yovanoff, P. (2000). Improving graduation and employment outcomes of students with disabilities: Predictive factors and student perspectives. *Exceptional Children, 66*(4), 509–529.
2. Wagner, M., Cameto, R., & Newman, L. (2003). *Youth with disabilities: A changing population. A report of findings from the National Longitudinal Transition Study (NLTS) and the National Longitudinal Transition Study–2 (NLTS02).* Menlo Park, CA: SRI International.

IMPORTANCE OF ASSISTIVE TECHNOLOGY

John's motor impairments warranted the ongoing process of assistive technology (AT) evaluation and services. AT is a critical service for students with intensive support needs, like John, who cannot express their interests or control their environments resulting from their inability to move and communicate. If AT needs are adequately addressed, reducing the need for personal assistance and increasing self-advocacy should facilitate independence and access to transition services. Assistive technology enables students with severe disabilities to achieve mobility, communicate more effectively, and control their environment. Research demonstrates that the use of AT improves an individual's level of functioning and independence.[4]

The application of AT must be a team approach which may encounter many barriers.[3] Chambers suggested that the AT process starts with a thorough assessment that includes an individual's needs, abilities, preferences, and the physical, social, and attitudinal environment.[2] The following are potential barriers for AT: (1) lack of knowledge of professionals, (2) AT services may not be school based, (3) need for follow-up services, (4) inability to evaluate AT devices prior to purchase, and (5) lack of parental knowledge of AT.[1] For John's team these factors were considered and although the AT process was time intensive, his outcome was successful.

1. Bauder, B. L. (2001). The role of technology in transition planning. In R. Flexer, T. Simmons, P. Luft, & R. Baer (Eds.), *Transition planning for secondary students with disabilities* (2nd ed., pp. 272–301). Upper Saddle River, NJ: Prentice-Hall.
2. Chambers, A. C. (1997). *Has technology been considered? A guide for IEP teams.* Albuquerque, NM: Councils of Administrators in Special Education.
3. Holder-Brown, L., & Parette, H. (1992). Children with disabilities who use assistive technology: Ethical considerations. *Young Children, 47*(6), 73–77.
4. Raskind, M. H. (1997). A guide to assistive technology. *Their World,* 73–74.

Background Information

John began receiving physical therapy in early childhood, and services continued throughout his high school years. Growing up, John did not receive hospital-based physical therapy services; his foster family/guardian felt school-based physical therapy was meeting John's gross motor needs. At a younger age, John walked short distances with a walker with stand-by assistance.

When preparing John for community employment, providing services in a variety of environments was critical. To allow some flexibility within the IEP/ITP, physical therapy services were listed in blocks of time—for example, "4 hours per month for the first month at a new job training followed by 2 hours per month for the remainder of the IEP." This was necessary to meet John's needs while still being in compliance with state special education procedures for the IEP/ITP. A combination of direct and consultative time was needed to implement the transition objectives and was listed as "direct and consultation" on the IEP. Direct services included instruction in skills needed at the job site (powered mobility and restroom transfer). Consultation included working with the office manager or job coaches to explain cerebral palsy and identifying appropriate job tasks. In addition, if a student receives physical therapy in other health care settings, time for collaboration is essential to ensure coordination of services. Finally, travel time to a variety of job sites needed to be calculated and scheduled by the physical therapist as John moved from the high school building to job training sites in the community.

Job Club Program

At age 19, as part of his transition planning and education, John participated in a 6-week summer job club career exploration program at a local university in collaboration with his public school district and as part of his extended school year education program (ESY). To facilitate his participation in the program, a classroom assistant familiar with John accompanied him to the job club program and collaborated with the staff. In addition, the district provided bus transportation. Related service providers (physical therapist, occupational therapist, speech and language pathologist) provided weekly consultation with the staff and direct services as part of John's ESY education program. John had minimal use of his hands and used assistive technology for mobility and communication. He had minimal exposure to vocational options and needed ongoing support for toileting and feeding.

A needs and preferences survey indicated that John had a strong desire to work, was very motivated, was interested in learning computer skills, but had minimal exposure. His preferences included working to make money, learning to dress himself, eating out, and going to dances. John was not interested in postsecondary education, but he wanted to live independently or with friends in accessible housing. Activities and lectures in the job club program were designed for people who could write and talk. Adaptations for John included using eye gaze or head nod to respond to questions on worksheets and allowing extra time to respond with his communication devices.

Continued

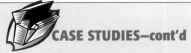

CASE STUDIES—cont'd

The staff stated that it was critical for John to be accompanied by professionals (liaisons) who knew him. They stated that if the student with intensive needs were not provided with technological and physical supports, then the staff would not be able to assess the student's abilities or make adaptations and accommodations.

Role of the Physical Therapist

The physical therapist attended the job club program as part of John's school-based physical therapy extended school year services, which lasted 30 minutes per week. Consultation was provided to work transition coordinators to assist with activity modifications and share information on powered mobility, restroom use, and how to adapt activities for John's motor needs.

Ask yourself these questions if you would like to be more involved in transition services:
- Do I know of any community or job training programs in my area?
- Have I visited programs to observe activities and offer information to the staff about youth with motor disabilities?
- Do I know how education, vocational rehabilitation, and developmental disabilities are coordinated in my community and how to contact key people?
- Do I know that adult services are not mandated and that the IEP/ITP does not carry over into postsecondary education and employment?

Transition Job Training Project

The next year, John participated in a transition job training project at a local university to learn work skills. He used an adapted keyboard with a variety of key sizes and mouse functions in an office environment. He learned office skills including typing, e-mail skills, and Internet access, word processing, document manipulation, and shredding documents. John continued to drive a power scooter, although his athetoid movements were increasing. He experienced difficulty with computer tasks because of poor postural control. The team, with input from John, decided that a power wheelchair with an adapted seating system would provide more support for John's trunk, especially when working at his computer.

Role of the Physical Therapist

John's IEP/ITP included 120 minutes of physical therapy per month. His therapist in collaboration with a local wheelchair vendor examined and evaluated John during computer tasks to determine the need for a new wheelchair and an adapted seating system. The therapist provided consultation by investigating two local transportation systems to check system requirements for wheelchair tie downs to inform the decision-making process for mobility (scooter versus wheelchair). The therapist provided indirect services by completing the Medicaid packet to obtain funding for a new chair. The state Medicaid program required a six-page evaluation/letter of medical necessity. The focus of direct services was on independence in powered mobility and restroom tasks.

Ask yourself these questions if you would like to be more involved in transition services:

- Do I know the process in my state for obtaining powered mobility for students on my caseload, and do I have the information needed to complete the paperwork?
- Do I know the transportation options in the community that are available to students on my caseload? Upon graduation, what is the potential impact of options for wheeled mobility?
- Realizing that students with significant motor impairments need extensive assistive technology (AT) support, am I able to assist with the process of recommending and providing instruction for AT devices? If not, am I aware of educational opportunities in my area?

Last Year of High School

John continued job training at a variety of campus sites during his last year of high school while his school team submitted Medicaid paperwork for a new communication system. The speech language pathologist at the high school completed the evaluation and paperwork for this device. Receipt of a power wheelchair through Medicaid funding provided improved postural positioning. John continued with intensive computer skill and power mobility training at the high school. He was able to drive his chair with a joystick and with intermittent verbal cues for steering when he became distracted.

Role of the Physical Therapist

The physical therapist attended transition planning meetings as a part of the IEP/ITP team. She provided direct intervention for independence with powered mobility skills in multiple environments both in and out of doors. The therapist collaborated with the speech therapist as part of the assistive technology team to determine the best positioning for access to a communication device. John's skills using a variety of school and public transportation modes were evaluated and instruction was provided.

Ask yourself these questions if you would like to be more involved in transition services:
- Do I collaborate with other team members by providing input on positioning to optimize a student's activity and participation in the education program?
- Do I assist with decision making for assistive technology?
- Do I have dedicated schedule times to attend transition planning meetings or to collaborate with families and other professionals?

Six Months before Leaving High School

John mastered powered mobility and was waiting on the new communication device. His school team began to explore the possibility of collaborating with an employer in the community who might be interested in hiring John. In October, the IEP/ITP team (which included an occupational therapist, a physical therapist, and a speech and language pathologist) met with the employer to discuss options and brainstorm about how to make community employment a reality for John. The employer agreed to proceed, and team members began job development and collaboration with the office manager at the job site. An employment proposal was developed and a meeting with the

CASE STUDIES—cont'd

employer and professionals from education, vocational rehabilitation, and developmental disability services was scheduled for November. Figure 32-9 presents an overview of work issues using the ICF framework.

During the interagency team meeting, the employment proposal including skills needed by the student and job tasks were discussed (shredding, computer tasks, possibility of using postage meter, and scanning documents). The proposal included part-time community work (15 hours per week) and a part-time workshop, a collaborative effort between Vocational Rehabilitation and Developmental Disabilities. The transition team decided to start a situational assessment through Vocation Rehabilitation with the school providing transportation and classroom assistance at the job site. The student demonstrated some behaviors (loud vocalizations and choosing not to complete certain tasks) that could become barriers to employment if not addressed early.

In December, the transition team met to update interagency team members. At this time the educational classroom assistant was helping John at the job site. Weekly internal meetings with the office manager were held at the job site. The goal was to brainstorm job tasks and alleviate her concerns about the ability of a worker with cerebral palsy to perform the tasks at hand. There was a 3-week delay for initiation of the situational assessment and rehabilitation engineering input for an adapted keyboard and obtaining a shredder. The interagency team was reminded that educational services for the student ended the first week in January (John's 22nd birthday).

In January, the rehabilitation engineer suggested obtaining and modifying a shredder with a tray to facilitate John's ability to feed paper into the shredder. A suggestion was made to use an adapted keyboard and John's communication device to interface with a computer. Scanning documents as a job task was put on hold because of the multiple tasks at hand. The situational assessment meeting for results was scheduled for February. The evaluators from Vocational Rehabilitation focused on hygiene (drooling) as a main concern of job coaches, although the employer did not see this as a barrier because John was working in his own area.

In March, a job interview was conducted. John communicated yes/no responses using his device. Following the interview, John was hired! The job would initially focus on shredding tasks. John began work the next week; however, the shredder was delayed and when it arrived the chute did not work. John demonstrated increased vocalizations and dependence on the job coach, and a short while later he was hospitalized because of the intestinal issues that his caregivers attributed to stress. Upon his return to work, a specific schedule with breaks was reviewed with John and posted in his work space to give him the sense of control of his environment at work.

Role of the Physical Therapist

During John's last 6 months of high school, the physical therapist provided consultation by assisting with certain case manager tasks delegated by the team such as investigating building code regulations. The therapist communicated by phone with contractors about obtaining ADA-specific railings at the entrance to the work site. She assisted the team with job carving and development, which involved brainstorming possible job tasks required by the employer and matching tasks to John's abilities through consultation and direct services. The therapist also completed ecologic assessments of (1) restroom accessibility and John's use of the restroom to determine supports needed at the job site and (2) John's mobility throughout the work site (from public transportation into the building and around the office).

Ask yourself these questions if you would like to be more involved in transition services:

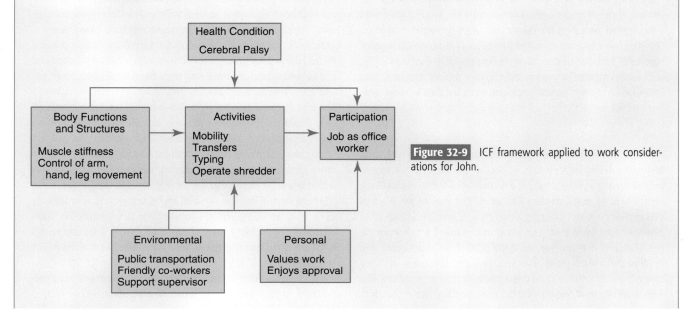

Figure 32-9 ICF framework applied to work considerations for John.

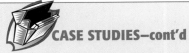

CASE STUDIES—cont'd

- Am I familiar with ADA requirements for employment situations?
- How does my expertise as a physical therapist assist the team in carving out job tasks?
- Am I able to apply what I know about biomechanics and the student's functioning to job tasks in specific employment environments?
- Do I have time in my schedule to brainstorm and problem-solve in the job development process?

Appraisal: What Went Well and What Did Not Go Well?

Team members stated that this was a new experience, never having been involved with this process in the past. They were often unaware of their role in placing a student with intensive support needs into community employment and agreed that communication between educational and adult services was imperative. They went on to state that having an employer in place before John left school facilitated this case. In addition the following were emphasized: needs and preferences and person-centered planning should be a priority, persistence by the case manager is critical, and a team with a similar philosophy and positive view of supported employment was helpful. Finally, they discussed the realization that this process will continue to evolve for John and that team members must be invested for the long term.

This case highlighted the physical therapist in nontraditional roles, at times including certain case manager tasks delegated by the team. Examples include investigating building code regulations and obtaining ADA-specific railings at the entrance to the work site, job carving and development, matching job tasks to the student's abilities, assessing restroom accessibility, and assessing mobility throughout a work site.

Finally, in retrospect, team members valued the importance of community employment with supports and also believed that the challenges proved more difficult compared with placing a student in a segregated workshop for people with developmental disabilities. Qualities that the team members perceived as important to support successful transition of students were persistence and accountability, continuous communication and collaboration among members, data collection on student performance, and using the data to make decisions as necessary.

"Jill"

This case study shares the professional development of a physical therapist working in the public schools as she expands her role to include serving youth with physical disabilities as they transition from high school to postsecondary education. The role of the physical therapist in transition planning, regardless of practice setting, is an emerging area of practice. Our intent in presenting a case from the perspective of the physical therapist is to share experiences and insights that might prove useful to pediatric therapists who are expanding their practice to include adolescents and young adults. The case illustrates how one physical therapist modified her approach to

serving youth in transition within the educational system based on the framework of the International Classification of Functioning, Disability and Health (ICF).

Jill is a physical therapist employed by an educational school district in rural Oregon. She has 21 years of experience in an educational setting. After attending a continuing education course, "College-Bound Students with Physical Disabilities: Do IEPs Reflect the Transition Process to Higher Education?" Jill reflected on new perspectives she gained and how they applied to students on her caseload. Goals of the course were to generate future thinking regarding the next environments and necessary supports and skill sets for activity and role participation in a college environment. These included considering the skills required for living in a dormitory, purchasing items from a college bookstore, self-informing college faculty of needed accommodations for learning, and arranging for one's own visits to the university/college student health services.

Recalling the session of the course that introduced the ICF framework in the context of high school to postsecondary transition, Jill commented that it sounded like the presenter was suggesting that for those college-bound students, physical therapists should also be addressing "life skills." Yes, there was and is more a physical therapist can offer in the youth transition process. This was in sharp contrast to her focus on scheduling physical therapy at times that did not interfere with academic courses. In her own words, Jill stated she was not "looking ahead." Rather she had only been addressing immediate goals to enable students to optimize school performance. Jill left the course armed with ideas and questions to share with the multidisciplinary teams she was part of back at school.

Three years later, Jill shared the following thoughts of how she and her colleagues had altered and expanded their roles in preparing students for transition to postsecondary education. The multidisciplinary team had become more future oriented, asking with increasing regularity what each student will need for new environments upon high school graduation. Previously, "despite many years of experience, I viewed high school as the end of the line ... physical therapy consultation with them [students who are college bound and in academic classes] and with staff must be squeezed into lunchtime, and there was *such* a focus on getting the high school diploma." Knowing that students with disabilities in college settings will not have their "team" of professional supports, decisions regarding assistive technology became anticipatory rather than reactive. She and her teammates recognized how important it was for students to have a more formalized means for requesting assistance in using various technologies. Jill shared that the IEP team became a transition team. "It is unfortunate that it is not until age 16 that we consider students to be in a 'transition' phase, because there is too much 'life skills' work to do in the last 2 years of high school when a student carries a full academic load and has no time for it" (life skills necessary for college life).

Team discussions became more proactive in terms of student-centered issues, especially in terms of supporting and building a student's skill in taking an active role in the IEP meeting. Jill shared how this could empower/prepare students for eventual hiring, directing, or firing of personal attendants while attending college. A specific student-centered goal was crafted collaboratively (with input from the physical therapist, educators, and the specialist in assistive technology), and as a result the student developed a typed explanation of herself to inform future college instructors of her accommodations needs. For example, the student included the statement "my voice/speech isn't clear, but don't underestimate me."

Jill stated that the most challenging part of making the transformation was "in tactfully asking questions and/or pinpointing need areas that were outside the scope of physical therapy, but not outside the scope of the IEP/transition team. That is, as a result of dialogue on the skills a student needed for college success, the workload of some of the IEP team members increased. With parent and student enthusiasm, and all of us wanting college to be a reality, it was easy for team members to 'buy in,' and soon they were formulating ideas on how to prepare the student for college. For example, the teacher removed the educational assistant from the classroom after the assistive technology had been appropriately set up at the start of each class; this required that the student ask his own questions to the teacher and track his own assignments, both vital skills in college. We wanted any problems to be identified in high school, so that we had time to turn them into successes before college."

Jill, as the "medical" professional on the school team, now strives to build the student's "medical ownership" of his or her health condition. Skills sets and accomplishments (objectives) in this area have included having students (1) create a list of routine medical appointments and when they should occur, (2) create a list that includes the name, phone number, and address of each health provider, (3) identify and list specific health impairments (e.g., specifying which hip was most troublesome), (4) learn how to e-mail health providers when oral communication would be challenging, and (5) discuss health concerns (e.g., the potential consequences of insufficient fluid intake in an effort to avert voiding because of an inability to transfer independently). As a physical therapist, Jill had always been involved in optimizing students' mobility. However, she now finds herself asking questions: How will the student carry school materials from building/classroom to building/classroom across a college campus? How will the student access a phone or computer? What self-advocacy skills can be included in therapy so the student will gain confidence to request assistance from other college students who are "natural" supports? How can privacy and dignity for toileting be established when a student requires physical assistance to transfer from the chair to the commode?

As Jill looks ahead for students on her caseload, she has learned the value of initiating transition planning sooner than later. Though an experienced therapist, Jill has been energized to see beyond the final year of high school. She advocates collaboration with the student, family, and professionals from other disciplines to enhance

the participation of youth with disabilities in their post high school roles. Her current thoughts and directions are how best to facilitate/assist a student who will be transitioning out of high school. Jill no longer views the last year of high school as the "end of the story" for students with physical disabilities; instead she sees this time as the beginning of the next chapter of their lives, one that she has a role in helping write.

When asked what advice she would provide to physical therapists interested in building their skills in transition services for youth with physical disabilities, Jill, in her own words, offered the following: "I would advise other physical therapists to look beyond high school mobility, positioning equipment, and transfers and think about if you were the student, how would *you* feel heading off to college? Scared? Helpless? Anxious? Dependent upon others? Do you even believe you can do it? What preparation would help you? Do you need to be more social, to learn to ask for help? Do you feel your toileting assistance is a loss of dignity, and could there be a more dignified way to achieve it, so that you don't impair your urinary system by not voiding? Is your verbal communication difficult for others to understand, so that you need a back-up means of getting your point across? Do you get tired of explaining your ability/disability, and would it be helpful to have a self-prepared handout to handle inquiries? Are you aware of your physical needs for college housing? You can't manage the keys of a mobile phone to text or call, and you can't use speech clearly enough to talk; what are your options to get help, to communicate with your family? Place your body in their shoes, and see what insights it gives you. *Start early.* We might commonly prepare birth to 3 for preschool, or preschool for elementary school. We need to think about the future—prepare in elementary school for college, just as we really do for children without disabilities. With our own children we work on sleepovers to experience other environments and build friendships, phone skills, social skills, advocacy skills, sports that enable living with successes and failures and build confidence, and making healthy "good" choices. It can take many conversations for students to reconcile feelings about their physical disability, understand health issues, and make intelligent decisions."

Jill concluded by saying, "I believe that every IEP team is a transition team readying the student for the future, the question is how far ahead to look. The present has to be addressed, but we need that long-term view to guide us."

As a member of the transition team, Jill expressed the importance of her providing a supporting role in helping each transitioning student to make the ultimate decisions. Selected queries she posed at the transition planning meeting included asking the team the following questions:

- Is the student prepared to hire, instruct, and fire an attendant/assistant in regard to physical needs?
- Has the student identified the technology he or she will need for successful college participation?

Continued

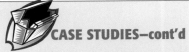

CASE STUDIES—cont'd

• Has the student prepared "his or her story" and described his or her needs for school applications and for the disability coordinator at the higher education institution?

The team, including the student, his family, and the county disability social worker, shared in the responsibility of developing a plan to respond to the preceding questions. One outcome was that 1 hour a day was carved out of the student's academic schedule to address these important issues for activities of daily living, which will be extremely significant in helping the student to transition to a postsecondary academic environment. More specifically, the occupational therapist would address specific concerns regarding voiding, dental hygiene, and issues of drooling. Jill would review the student's ability to demonstrate a self-range of motion program for his upper extremities and to direct an attendant caregiver in lower extremity management.

Jill concluded that she is enthusiastically approaching her role with students so differently now. Jill embraced the challenge posed in the continuing education session, and she now asks, "What are we doing for *that* transition (post high school)?"

SUMMARY

Transition to adulthood is a future-oriented process in which youth begin planning for adult roles and responsibilities including finding an adult medical home, living outside the family home, obtaining postsecondary education, and participating in work, social, and community activities. The transition process encompasses the health, psychosocial, and educational-vocational needs of adolescents as they move to adult-oriented lifestyles and systems. The importance of transition planning is recognized by the Individuals with Disabilities Education Improvement Act of 2004 (PL 108-446) and a consensus statement by the American Academy of Pediatrics (AAP), American Academy of Family Physicians, American College of Physicians, and American Society of Internal Medicine that advocates for a written health care transition plan for all youth with disabilities by age 14.

Contemporary approaches to transition services are youth and family centered, involve youth as active participants, and emphasize real-world experiences, development of life skills, environmental supports, and community accommodations. Although transition planning and services are mandated as part of the education program for students with disabilities, physical therapists working in an educational setting have not fully participated in the transition process. Increasingly, community agencies and children's hospitals are providing transition services, although outcomes are challenged by the lack of coordinated and comprehensive services for adults with childhood onset disabilities.

Pediatric physical therapists are encouraged to embrace a future-oriented process and to help prepare youth with physical disabilities for adult roles. This includes instruction of youth in self-management of their health conditions and instruction of others who provide care. Consultation and direct services are recommended, as needed, for seating, transfers, mobility, self-care, wellness and fitness, assistive technology, and environmental modifications. Potential niche areas of practice include consultation to institutions of higher education, work environments employing persons with disabilities, health clubs interested in being more inclusive in membership recruitment, and adult-oriented physical therapists interested in serving adults with childhood-onset disabilities.

REFERENCES

1. Algozzine, B., Browder, D., Karvonen, M., Test, D., & Wood, W. (2001). Effects of interventions to promote self-determination for individuals with disabilities. *Review of Educational Research, 71*, 219–277.
2. American Academy of Pediatrics, American Academy of Family Physicians, & American College of Physicians-American Society of Internal Medicine. (2002). A consensus statement on health care transitions for young adults with special health care needs. *Pediatrics, 110*(6), 1304–1306.
3. American Physical Therapy Association. *Guide to physical therapy practice.* (2001). Alexandria: VA, American Physical Therapy Association.
4. Amsel, R., & Fichten, C. (1990). Interaction between disabled and nondisabled college students and their professors: A comparison. *Journal of Postsecondary Education and Disability, 8*, 125–140.
5. Anderson, M. A. (2000). *Survey of pediatric occupational therapists in the state of Oklahoma: Is occupational therapy important for secondary level students to assist in successful transition into the community following graduation?* Unpublished master's thesis. University of Oklahoma, Oklahoma City.
6. Baer, R., Goebel, G., Flexer, R. et al. (2003). A collaborative followup study on transition. *Career Development for Exceptional Individuals, 26*(1), 7–25.
7. Reference deleted in page proofs.
8. Baer, R., McMahan, R., & Flexer, R. (2004). *Standards-based transition planning: A guide for parents and professionals.* Kent, OH: Kent State University.
9. Bandura, A. (1986). *Social foundations of thought and action: A social cognitive theory.* Englewood Cliffs, NJ: Prentice Hall.
10. Barnhardt, R. C., & Connolly, B. (2007). Aging and Down syndrome: Implications for physical therapy. *Physical Therapy. 87*(10), 1399–1406.
11. Beilke, J., & Yssel, N. (1998). Personalizing disability. *Journal for a Just & Caring Education, 4*(2), 212–224.

12. Benz, M. R., Lindstrom, L., & Yovanoff, P. (2000). Improving graduation and employment outcomes of students with disabilities: Predictive factors and student perspectives. *Exceptional Children, 66*(4), 509–529.

13. Benz, M. R., Yovanoff, P., & Doren, B. (1997). School-to-work components that predict postschool success for students with and without disabilities. *Exceptional Children, 63*(2), 151–166.

14. Betz, C. L. (2004). Transition of adolescents with special health care needs: Review and analysis of the literature. *Issues in Comprehensive Pediatric Nursing, 27*(3), 179–241.

15. Betz, C., & Nehring, W. (2007). *Promoting health care transitions for adolescents with special health care needs and disabilities.* Baltimore, MD: Paul H. Brooks.

16. Binks, J. A., Barden, W. S., Burke, T. A., & Young, N. L. (2007). What do we really know about the transition to adult-centered health care? A focus on cerebral palsy and spina bifida. *Archives of Physical Medicine and Rehabilitation, 88*(8), 1064–1073.

17. Blackorby, J., & Wagner, M. (1996). Longitudinal postschool outcomes of youth with disabilities: Findings from the national longitudinal transition study. *Exceptional Children, 62*, 399–413.

18. Blomquist, K. B. (2006a). Healthy and ready to work-Kentucky: Incorporating transition into a state program for children with special health care needs. *Pediatric Nursing, 32*(6), 515–528.

19. Blomquist, K. B. (2006b). Health, education, work, and independence of young adults with disabilities. *Orthopaedic Nursing/National Association of Orthopaedic Nurses, 25*(3), 168–187.

20. Blomquist, K. B., Brown, G., Peersen, A., & Presler, E. P. (1998). Transitioning to independence: Challenges for young people with disabilities and their caregivers. *Orthopaedic Nursing/National Association of Orthopaedic Nurses, 17*(3), 27–35.

21. Blum, R. W. (1995). Transition to adult health care: Setting the stage. *Journal of Adolescent Health, 17*(1), 3–5.

22. Breslau, N., Staruch, K. S., & Mortimer, E. A., Jr. (1982). Psychological distress in mothers of disabled children. *American Journal of Diseases of Children (1960), 136*(8), 682–686.

23. Brollier, C., Shepherd, J., & Markley, K. F. (1994). Transition from school to community living. *American Journal of Occupational Therapy: Official Publication of the American Occupational Therapy Association, 48*(4), 346–353.

24. Campbell, S. K. (1997). Therapy programs for children that last a lifetime. *Physical & Occupational Therapy in Pediatrics, 17*(1), 1–15.

25. Carr, E. G., Horner, R. H., Turnbull, A. P., et al. (1999). *Positive behavior support for people with developmental disabilities: A research synthesis.* Washington, DC: American Association on Mental Retardation.

26. Center for Disease Control. (1997). www.cdc.org.

27. Chambers, A. C. (1997). *Has technology been considered? A guide for IEP teams.* Albuquerque, NM: Councils of Administrators in Special Education.

28. Clark, H. B., & Foster-Johnson, L. (1996). Serving youth in transition into adulthood. In B. A. Stroul (Ed.), *Children's mental health: Creating systems of care in a changing society* (pp. 533–551). New York: Brookes.

29. Clement-Heist, K., Siegel, S., & Gaylord-Ross, R. (1992). Simulated and in situ vocational social skill training for youth with learning disabilities. *Exceptional Children, 58*, 336–345.

30. Connolly, B. (2001). Aging in individuals with lifelong disabilities. *Physical and Occupational Therapy in Pediatrics, 21*(4), 23–47.

31. Connolly, B. H. (2005). Issues in aging in individuals with lifelong disabilities. In B. H. Connolly & P. C. Montgomery (Eds.), *Therapeutic exercise in developmental disabilities* (3rd ed., pp. 505–529). Thorofare, NJ: Slack.

32. Cooley, W. C., & American Academy of Pediatrics Committee on Children with Disabilities. (2004). Providing a primary care medical home for children and youth with cerebral palsy. *Pediatrics, 114*(4), 1106–1113.

33. Darrah, J., Magil-Evans J, & Adkins R. (2002). How well are we doing? Families of adolescents or young adults with cerebral palsy share their perceptions of service delivery. *Disability & Rehabilitation, 24*(10), 542–549.

34. Dornbush, S. M. (2000). Transitions from adolescence: A discussion of seven articles. *Journal of Adolescent Research, 15*, 173–177.

35. Doty, A., Hamilton, E., & O'Shea, R. (2008). *The continuum of care for Individuals with lifelong disabilities: Exploring the issues and roles for physical therapists.* Presentation at the Annual Conference of the American Physical Therapy Association, June.

36. Dykens, E. M., Rosner, B. A., & Butterbaugh, G. (1998). Exercise and sports in children and adolescents with developmental disabilities: Positive physical and psychosocial effects. *Child & Adolescent Psychiatry Clinics of North America, 7*(4), 757–771.

37. Erson, T. (2003). *Gross motor activities for inclusive and special needs classrooms: The Courageous Pacers Program.* Framingham, MA: Therapro.

38. Evans, J., McDougall, J., & Baldwin, P. (2006). An evaluation of the "youth en route" program. *Physical & Occupational Therapy in Pediatrics, 26*(4), 63–87.

39. Field, S., Martin, J., Miller, R., Ward, M., & Wehmeyer, M. (1998). Self-determination for persons with disabilities: A position statement of the division on career development and transition. *Career Development for Exceptional Individuals, 21*(2), 113–128.

40. Flexer, R. W., & Baer, R. M. (2008a). Transition planning and promising practices. In R. W. Flexer, R. M. Baer, P. Luft, & T. J. Simmons (Eds.), *Transition planning for secondary students with disabilities* (3rd ed., pp. 3–28). Upper Saddle River, NJ: Prentice-Hall.

41. Flexer, R. W., & Baer, R. M. (2008b). Transition legislation and models. In R. W. Flexer, R. M. Baer, P. Luft, & T. J. Simmons (Eds.). *Transition planning for secondary students with disabilities* (3rd ed., pp. 29–53). Upper Saddle River, NJ: Prentice-Hall.

42. Frey, G. C., Buchanan, A. M., & Rosser Sandt, D. D. (2005). I'd rather watch TV: An examination of physical activity in adults with mental retardation. *Mental Retardation*, *43*(4), 241–254.

43. Friedrich, W. N., Greenberg, M. T., & Crnic, K. (1983). A short-form of the questionnaire on resources and stress. *American Journal of Mental Deficiency*, *88*(1), 41–48.

44. Gall, C., Kingsnorth, S., & Healy, H. (2006). Growing up ready: A shared management approach. *Physical & Occupational Therapy in Pediatrics*, *26*(4), 47–62.

45. Gaylord-Ross, R. (1989). Vocational integration for persons with handicaps. In R. Gaylord-Ross (Ed.), *Integration strategies for students with handicaps* (pp. 195–211). Baltimore: Brookes.

46. Getzel, E., & deFur, S. (1997). Transition planning for students with significant disabilities: Implications for student centered planning. *Focus on Autism and Other Developmental Disabilities*, *12*(1), 39–48.

47. Gliedman, J., & Roth, W. (1980). *The unexpected minority*. New York: Harcourt Brace Jovanovich.

48. Halpern, A. S. (1993). Quality of life as a framework for evaluating transition outcomes. *Exceptional Children*, *59*(6), 486–498.

49. Havighurst R. (1972). *Developmental tasks and education* (3rd ed.). New York: D. McKay.

50. Heal, L. W., Khoju, M., & Rusch, F. R. (1997). Predicting quality of life of youths after they leave special education high school programs. *Journal of Special Education, 31*(3), 279–299.

51. Helfer, B. (2006). *United we ride and safe-T-Lu: New freedom transportation opportunities*. Presentation at Annual TASH Conference, November, Baltimore.

52. Helms, L., & Weiler, K. (1993). Disability discrimination in nursing education: An evaluation of legislation and litigation. *Journal of Professional Nursing*, *9*(6), 358–366.

53. Hitchings, W. E., Retisch, P., & Horvath, M. (2005). Academic preparation of adolescents with disabilities for postsecondary education. *Career Development for Exceptional Individuals*, *28*(2), 26–35.

54. Holder-Brown, L., & Parette, H. (1992). Children with disabilities who use assistive technology: Ethical considerations. *Young Children*, *47*(6), 73–77.

55. Howe, J., Horner, R., & Newton, J. (1998). Comparison of supported living and traditional residential services in the state of Oregon. *Mental Retardation 36*(1), 1–11.

56. Inge, K. (1995). *A national study of occupational therapists in the public schools: an assessment of current practice, attitudes and training needs regarding the transition process for students with severe disabilities*. Unpublished dissertation, Virginia Commonwealth University, Richmond.

57. Inge, K., & Shepherd J. (1999). Occupational and physical therapy. In S. H. De Fur & J. R. Patton (Eds.), *Transition and school based services: Interdisciplinary perspectives enhancing the transition process* (pp. 117–165). Austin, TX: Pro-ed.

58. James, S. (2001). *I was prepared to do nothing; I will do nothing: Why students with multiple disabilities do not have jobs after leaving high school*. Unpublished master's thesis, University of Oklahoma, Oklahoma City.

59. Johnson, D. (2004). Supported employment trends: Implications for transition-age youth. *Research & Practice for Person with Severe Disabilities. 29*(4), 243–247.

60. Johnson, D., Stodden, R., Emanuel, E., Luecking, R., & Mack, M. (2002). Current challenges facing secondary education and transition services: What research tells us. *Exceptional Children, 68*(4), 519–531.

61. Johnson, J., & Rusch, F. (1993). Secondary special education and transition services: Identification and recommendations for future research and demonstration. *Career Development for Exceptional Individuals, 16*(1), 1–18.

62. Kennedy, M., & Lewin, L. (2008). Fact sheet: Summary of self-determination. Retrieved September 1, 2008, from http://thechp.syr.edu/fs_selfdetermination.doc.

63. Kiernan, W., & Schalock, R. (1997). *Integrated employment: Current status and future directions*. Washington, DC: American Association of Mental Retardation.

64. King, G., Baldwin, P., Currie, M., & Evans, J. (2005). Planning successful transitions from school to adult roles for youth with disabilities. *Children's Health Care, 34*(3), 193–216.

65. King, G. A., Baldwin, P. J., Currie, M., & Evans, J. (2006a). The effectiveness of transition strategies for youth with disabilities. *Children's Health Care, 35*(2), 155–178.

66. King, G. A., Cathers, T., Polgar, J. M., MacKinnon, E., & Havens, L. (2006). Success in life for older adolescents with cerebral palsy. *Qualitative Health Research, 10*(6), 734–749.

67. King, G. A., Shultz, I. Z., Steel, K., Gilpin, M., & Cathers, T. (1993). Self-evaluation and self-concept of adolescents with physical disabilities. *American Journal of Occupational Therapy: Official Publication of the American Occupational Therapy Association, 47*(2), 132–140.

68. King, G. A., Tucker, M. A., Baldwin, P. J., & LaPorta, J. A. (2006). Bringing the life needs model to life: Implementing a service delivery model for pediatric rehabilitation. *Physical & Occupational Therapy in Pediatrics, 26*(1/2), 43–70.

69. Kingsnorth, S., Healy, H., & Macarthur, C. (2007). Preparing for adulthood: A systematic review of life skill programs for youth with physical disabilities. *Journal of Adolescent Health: Official Publication of the Society for Adolescent Medicine, 41*(4), 323–332.

70. Kohler, P. D. (1993). Best practices in transition: Substantiated or implied? *Career Development for Exceptional Individuals, 16*, 107–121.

71. Kohler, P. D. (1998). Implementing a transition perspective of education: A comprehensive approach to planning and

delivering secondary education and transition services. In F. R. Rusch & J. Chadsey (Eds.), *Beyond high school: Transition from school to work* (pp. 179–205). New York: Wadsworth.

72. Kohler, P. D., & Field, S. (2003). Transition focused education: Foundation for the future. *Journal of Special Education, 37*(3), 157–163.

73. Lindsey, J. D. (2000). *Technology and Exceptional Individuals* (3rd ed.). Austin, TX: Pro-Ed.

74. Lotstein, D. S., McPherson, M., Strickland, B., & Newacheck, P. W. (2005). Transition planning for youth with special health care needs: Results from the national survey of children with special health care needs. *Pediatrics, 115*(6), 1562–1568.

75. Luther, B. (2001). Age-specific activities that support successful transition to adulthood for children with disabilities. *Orthopaedic Nursing/National Association of Orthopaedic Nurses, 20*(1), 23–29.

76. McGavin, H. (1998). Planning rehabilitation: A comparison of issues for parents and adolescents. *Physical & Occupational Therapy in Pediatrics 18*, 69–82.

77. McNair, J., & Rusch, F. R. (1991). Parental involvement in transition programs. *Mental Retardation. 29*(2), 93–101.

78. Misquez, E., McCarthy, B., Powell, B., & Chu, L. (1997). *University students with disabilities are the chief on-campus accommodation ingredient.* Paper presented at the Annual California State University, Northridge, Conference.

79. Morse, E. (1997). *Recreational Preferences of Children with Special Needs Survey.* Lexington: University of Kentucky.

80. National Center for the Study of Postsecondary Educational Supports (NCSPES). (2000). *Technical report: Postsecondary education and employment for students with disabilities: Focus group discussions on supports and barriers to lifelong learning.* Honolulu: University of Hawaii at Manoa.

81. Newacheck, P., Strickland, B., Shonkoff, J., et al. (1998). An epidemiologic profile of children with special health care needs. *Pediatrics, 102*, 107–123.

82. N.O.D./Harris Survey. (2004). Retrieved March 26, 2010, from www.nod.org/index.cfm?fuseaction=Feature.showFeature&FeatureID=1422.

83. Nosek, M. A. (1991). Personal assistance services: A review of the literature and analysis of policy implications. *Journal of Disability Policy Studies, 2*(2), 1–17.

84. Palisano, R. J., Almasri, N., Chiarello, L., Orlin M., Begley, A., & Maggs J. (2009). Family needs of parents of children and youth with cerebral palsy. *Child Care, Health & Development, 36*(1), 85–92.

85. Paul, S. (2000). Students with disabilities in higher education: A review of the literature. *College Student Journal, 34*(2), 200–211.

86. Pearson, McPherson, M., Weissman, G., Strickland, B. B., van Dyck, P. C., Blumberg, S. J., & Newacheck, P. W. (2004). Implementing community-based systems of services for children and youths with special health care needs: How well are we doing? *Pediatrics, 113*(5):1538–1544.

87. Phelps, L. A., & Hanley-Maxwell, C. (1997). School-to-Work transitions for youth with disabilities: A review of outcomes and practices. *Review of Educational Research, 67*(2), 176–226.

88. Powers, K. M., Gil-Kashiwabara, E., Geenen, S. J., Powers, L. E., Balandran, J., & Palmer, C. (2005). Mandates and effective transition planning practices reflected in IEPs. *Career Development for Exceptional Individuals, 28*(1), 47–59.

89. Raskind, M. H. (1997). A guide to assistive technology. *Their World, 73–74.*

90. Reiss, J. G., Gibson, R. W., & Walker, L. R. (2005). Health care transition: Youth, family, and provider perspectives. *Pediatrics, 115*(1), 112–120.

91. Reference deleted in page proofs.

92. Rothstein, L. (1991). Students, staff, and faculty with disabilities: Current issues for colleges and universities. *Journal of College and University Law, 17*, 471–482.

93. Rusch, F., & Braddock, D. (2004). Adult day programs versus supported employment (1988–2002): Spending and Service practices of mental retardation and developmental disabilities state agencies. *Research & Practice for Person with Severe Disabilities. 29*(4), 237–242.

94. Ryder, B. E., & Kawalec, E. S. (1995). A job–seeking skills program for persons who are blind or visually impaired. *Journal of Visual Impairment & Blindness, 89*, 107–111.

95. Sands, D. J., Spencer, K. C., Gliner, J., & Swaim, R. (1999). Structural equation modeling of student involvement in transition-related actions: The path of least resistance. *Focus on Autism and Other Developmental Disabilities, 14*(1), 17–27.

96. Schultz, A. W., & Liptak, G. S. (1998). Helping adolescents who have disabilities negotiate transitions to adulthood. *Issues in Comprehensive Pediatric Nursing, 21*(4), 187–201.

97. Simmons, T., Flexer, R. W., & Bauder, D. (2008). Collaborative transition services. In R. W. Flexer, R. M. Baer, P. Luft, & T. J. Simmons (Eds.), *Transition planning for secondary students with disabilities* (3rd ed., pp. 203–229). Upper Saddle River, NJ: Prentice-Hall.

98. Sowers, J., & Powers, L. (1991). *Vocational preparation and employment of students with physical and multiple disabilities.* Baltimore: Paul H. Brookes.

99. Stein, R. E. K. (2001). Challenges in long-term health care for children. *Ambulatory Pediatrics, 1*(5), 280–288.

100. Stewart, D. (2006). Evidence to support a positive transition into adulthood for youth with disabilities. *Physical & Occupational Therapy in Pediatrics, 26*(4), 1–4.

101. Stewart, D. A., Law, M. C., Rosenbaum, P., & Willms, D. G. (2001). A qualitative study of the transition to adulthood for youth with physical disabilities. *Physical & Occupational Therapy in Pediatrics, 21*(4), 3–21.

102. Stewart, D., Stavness, C., King, G., Antle, B., & Law, M. (2006). A critical appraisal of literature reviews about the transition to adulthood for youth with disabilities. *Physical & Occupational Therapy in Pediatrics, 26*(4), 5–24.

103. Strand, J., & Kreiner, J. (2004). Recreation and leisure in the community. In R. W. Flexer, T. J. Simmons, P. Luft, & R. M. Baer (Eds.) *Transition planning for secondary students with disabilities* (2nd ed, pp. 460–482). Upper Saddle River, NJ: Prentice-Hall.

104. Strong, W. B., & Wiklmore, J. H. (1998). Unfit kids: An office-based approach to physical fitness. *Contemporary Pediatrics,* April.

105. Surgeon General's Report on Physical Activity and Health. (1996). Washington, DC: U.S. Department of Health and Human Services.

106. Sylvester, L. (2007). *Physical therapy: Achieving postsecondary outcomes.* Presentation at the Division on Career Development and Transition Conference.

107. Test, D. (2004). Invited commentary on Rusch and Braddock (2004): One person at a time. *Research & Practice for Person with Severe Disabilities.* 29(4), 248–252.

108. Thomas, S. (2000). College students and disability law. *Journal of Special Education,* 33(4), 248–258.

109. Thomas, A. D., & Rosenberg, A. (2003). Promoting community recreation and leisure. *Pediatric Physical Therapy,* 15(4), 232–246.

110. Tonniges, T., & Roberts, C. (2007, March 8). *Transitions: A lifelong process and everyone's responsibility.* Presentation for Oklahoma Health Sciences Center Grand Rounds, Oklahoma City, OK, Department of Pediatrics.

111. U. S. Department of Health and Human Services. (2008). *Healthy people 2010.* Retrieved September 1, 2008, from www.healthypeople.gov/Publications/Cornerstone.pdf.

112. Wagner, M., Blackorby, J., Cameto, R., Hebbeler, K., & Newman, L. (1993). *The transition experiences of young people with disabilities: A summary of findings from the national longitudinal transition study of special education students.* Menlo Park, CA: SRI International.

113. Wagner, M., Cameto, R., & Newman, L. (2003). *Youth with disabilities: A changing population.* A report of findings from the National Longitudinal Transition Study (NLTS) and the National Longitudinal Transition Study-2 (NLTS02). Menlo Park, CA: SRI International.

114. Wagner, M., Newman, L., Cameto, R., Levine, P., & Garza, N. (2006). An overview of findings from Wave 2 of the National Longitudinal Transition Study-2 (NLTS2). National Center for Special Education Research. Menlo Park, CA: SRI International.

115. Wehman, P. (2006). *Life beyond the classroom: Transition strategies for young people with disabilities* (4th ed.). Baltimore: Paul H. Brookes.

116. White, P. H. (1997). Success on the road to adulthood; issues and hurdles for adolescents with disabilities. *Rheumatic Diseases Clinics of North America,* 23(3), 697–707.

117. White, P. H. (2002). Transition: A future promise for children and adolescents with special health care needs and disabilities. *Rheumatic Diseases Clinics of North America,* 28(3), 687–703.

118. Will, M. (1983). *OSERS programming for the transition of youth with disabilities: Bridges from school to working life.* Washington, DC: U.S. Department of Education, Office of Special Education and Rehabilitative Services. (ERIC Document Reproduction Service No. ED 256 132).

119. World Health Organization. (2001). *International classification of functioning, disability and health (ICF).* Geneva, Switzerland: World Health Organization. Retrieved March 26, 2010, from www.who.int/classifications/icf/en.

120. Wright, B. (2001). Teens say job training their top need. *Point of Departure,* 2(2), 8.

121. Young, N. L., McCormick, A., Mills, W., et al. (2006). The transition study: A look at youth and adults with cerebral palsy, spina bifida, and acquired brain injury. *Physical & Occupational Therapy in Pediatrics,* 26(4), 25–46.

Index